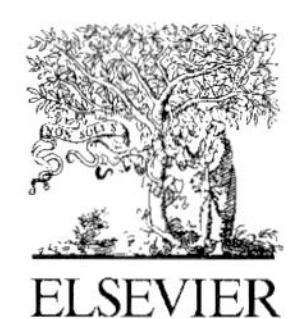

超声心动图临床实践

The Practice of Clinical Echocardiography

第 6 版 6th Edition

中文精要·英文影印版

◎ 主编

[美] 凯瑟琳·M. 奥托（Catherine M. Otto）

◎ 编译

朱振辉 编译委员会主任委员

科学技术文献出版社
SCIENTIFIC AND TECHNICAL DOCUMENTATION PRESS
·北京·

图书在版编目（CIP）数据

超声心动图临床实践：第6版 /（美）凯瑟琳 · M. 奥托（Catherine M. Otto）主编；朱振辉编译. —北京：科学技术文献出版社，2023.5

书名原文：The Practice of Clinical Echocardiography 6th Edition

ISBN 978-7-5189-9609-4

Ⅰ.①超… Ⅱ.①凯… ②朱… Ⅲ.①超声心动图 Ⅳ.① R540.4

中国版本图书馆 CIP 数据核字（2022）第 177298 号

著作权合同登记号 图字：01-2022-5274

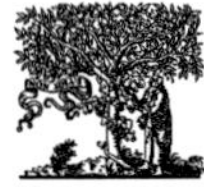

Elsevier (Singapore) Pte Ltd.
3 Killiney Road,
#08-01 Winsland House I,
Singapore 239519
Tel: (65) 6349-0200; Fax: (65) 6733-1817

超声心动图临床实践（第6版）

策划编辑：张　蓉　　责任编辑：张　蓉　段思帆　　责任校对：张永霞　　责任出版：张志平

出 版 者　科学技术文献出版社
地　　址　北京市复兴路15号　邮编　100038
编 务 部　（010）58882938，58882087（传真）
发 行 部　（010）58882868，58882870（传真）
邮 购 部　（010）58882873
官方网址　www.stdp.com.cn
发 行 者　科学技术文献出版社发行　全国各地新华书店经销
印 刷 者　北京地大彩印有限公司
版　　次　2023年5月第1版　2023年5月第1次印刷
开　　本　889 × 1194　1/16
字　　数　1826千
印　　张　71.25
书　　号　ISBN 978-7-5189-9609-4
定　　价　698.00元

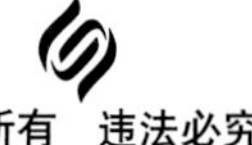

编译主任委员简介

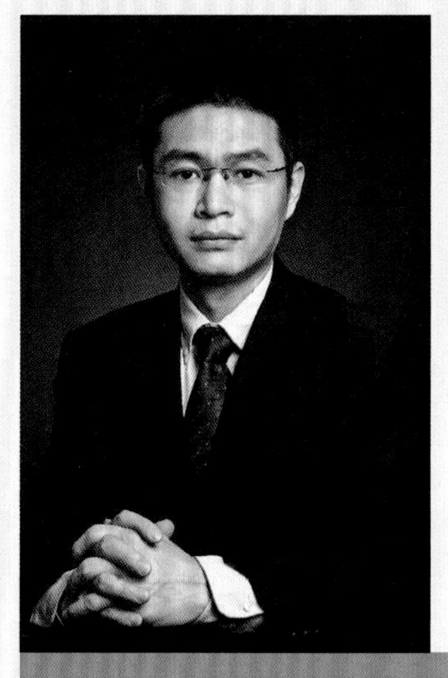

朱振辉

主任医师
中国医学科学院阜外医院超声影像中心超声一科主任

【社会任职】

现任亚太基层卫生协会超声医学分会心脏超声专业委员会副主任委员、中国心胸血管麻醉学会超声分会副主任委员、中国医疗保健国际交流促进会超声医学分会委员、海峡两岸医药卫生交流协会超声医学专家委员会委员、北京慢性病防治与健康教育研究会超声医学专业委员会常务委员、北京医学会超声医学分会第九届委员会心脏超声学组委员；担任《中国分子心脏病学杂志》编委等。

【专业特长】

主要从事心血管病超声诊断的临床和科研工作，对临床各种心血管疾病，包括各种疑难复杂重症疾病的诊断有丰富的经验；擅长开展超声心动图在外科手术和介入手术中的应用，以及经食管超声心动图、三维超声心动图应用等。

【工作经历】

1996年本科毕业于上海医科大学；2005年博士毕业于中国医学科学院北京协和医学院。在中国医学科学院阜外医院超声科工作20余年。

【学术成果】

已发表论文40余篇；参加撰写专著10部；获中华医学科学技术奖三等奖1项，中国医学科学院及中国医学科学院阜外医院医疗成就奖4项。

原书章节编辑

Rosario V. Freeman, MD, MS
Professor of Medicine
Division of Cardiology
Director, Cardiology Fellowship Programs
University of Washington School of Medicine
University of Washington Medical Center
Seattle, Washington
Part II: Echocardiography Best Practices
Part IV: Ischemic Heart Disease

James N. Kirkpatrick, MD
Professor of Medicine, Cardiology, and Bioethics and Humanities
Section Chief, Cardiovascular Imaging
University of Washington School of Medicine
Director, Echocardiography
UW Medicine Heart Institute
Chair, Ethics Committee, UW Medicine
University of Washington Medical Center
Seattle, Washington
Part III: Cardiomyopathies, Tumors, and Pericardial Disease

Eric V. Krieger, MD
Associate Professor of Medicine
Division of Cardiology
Program Director, Adult Congenital Heart Disease Fellowship
University of Washington School of Medicine
Section Chief, Adult Congenital Heart Disease
University of Washington Medical Center and
Seattle Children's Hospital
Seattle, Washington
Part VII: Adult Congenital Heart Disease and the Pregnant Patient

Jason P. Linefsky, MD, MS
Associate Professor of Medicine
Division of Cardiology
Emory University School of Medicine
Assistant Section Chief of Cardiology
Atlanta VA Medical Center
Decatur, Georgia
Part VI: Vascular and Systemic Diseases

原书编者名单

Jamil A. Aboulhosn, MD
Director, Ahmanson/UCLA Adult Congenital Heart Disease Center
Ronald Reagan UCLA Medical Center
Los Angeles, California

Nazem Akoum, MD, MS
Associate Professor of Medicine
Cardiology/Cardiac Electrophysiology
University of Washington School of Medicine
Seattle, Washington

Jose Banchs, MD
Associate Professor
Cardiology
The University of Texas MD Anderson Cancer Center
Houston, Texas

Jeroen J. Bax, MD, PhD
Head, Cardiac Imaging Department
Department of Cardiology
Heart and Lung Center
Leiden University Medical Center
Leiden, the Netherlands

Carmen C. Beladan, MD, PhD
Senior Lecturer in Cardiology
Carol Davila University of Medicine and Pharmacy
Euroecolab
Emergency Institute for Cardiovascular Diseases
Bucharest, Romania

Claire Bouleti, MD, PhD
Professor of Cardiology
Cardiology Department
Miletrie Hospital
University of Poitiers
Poitiers, France

Maria Brosnan, MBBS, PhD
Cardiologist
Department of Cardiology
St Vincent's Hospital Melbourne
Fitzroy, Victoria, Australia

Jonathan Buber, MD
Associate Professor of Cardiology
Division of Cardiology
Department of Internal Medicine
University of Washington Medical Center
Seattle, Washington

Luke J. Burchill, MBBS, PhD
Associate Professor of Medicine
Department of Medicine
Adult Congenital Heart Program
Royal Melbourne Hospital
Melbourne, Victoria, Australia

John D. Carroll, MD
Professor of Medicine
Division of Cardiology
University of Colorado School of Medicine
Director of Interventional Cardiology
University of Colorado Hospital
Anschutz Medical Campus
Aurora, Colorado

David S. Celermajer, MD
Professor of Cardiology
Sydney Medical School
University of Sydney
Director of Echocardiography
Royal Prince Alfred Hospital
Sydney, New South Wales, Australia

Andrew Cheng, MD
Clinical Assistant Professor
Division of Cardiology
Department of Medicine
Veteran Affairs Puget Sound Health Care Center
University of Washington
Seattle, Washington

Richard K. Cheng, MD
Associate Professor
Division of Cardiology
University of Washington School of Medicine
Seattle, Washington

Marie-Annick Clavel, DVM, PhD
Associate Professor at Faculté de Médecine
Institut Universitaire de Cardiologie et de Pneumologie de Québec/Quebec Heart and Lung Institute (IUCPQ)
Université Laval
Québec, Québec, Canada

Jennifer Cohen, MD
Assistant Professor of Pediatrics
Division of Pediatric Cardiology
Mount Sinai Medical Center
New York, New York

Jacqueline Danik, MD, DrPH
Assistant Professor of Medicine
Harvard Medical School
Clinical Director of Echocardiography
Division of Cardiology
Massachusetts General Hospital
Boston, Massachusetts

Jason F. Deen, MD
Associate Professor of Pediatrics
Division of Cardiology
Seattle Children's Hospital
Seattle, Washington

Victoria Delgado, MD, PhD
Cardiologist
Department of Cardiology
Heart and Lung Center
Leiden University Medical Center
Leiden, the Netherlands

Marco R. Di Tullio, MD
Professor of Medicine
Columbia University Irving Medical Center
Department of Medicine
Columbia University
New York, New York

Daniel H. Drake, MD
Surgeon
Department of Surgery
Munson Medical Center
Director, Cardiothoracic Research
Webber Heart Center
Munson Healthcare
Traverse City, Michigan

Arturo Evangelista, MD, PhD
Coordinator of Research
Cardiac Imaging Department
Servei de Cardiologia
Hospital Vall d´Hebron
Barcelona, Spain

Thor Edvardsen, MD, PhD
Head, Department of Cardiology
Oslo University Hospital
Professor
Institute of Clinical Medicine
University of Oslo
Oslo, Norway

Erin A. Fender, MD
Department of Cardiology
Christiana Care
Newark, Delaware

Rosario V. Freeman, MD, MS
Professor of Medicine
Division of Cardiology
Director, Cardiology Fellowship Programs
University of Washington School of Medicine
University of Washington Medical Center
Seattle, Washington

Laura Galian Gay, MD, PhD
Cardiology
Hospital Vall d'Hebron
Barcelona, Spain

Ivor L. Gerber, MD, MBChB
Cardiologist
Department of Cardiology
Green Lane Cardiovascular Service
Auckland City Hospital
Auckland, New Zealand

Holly Gonzales, MD
Assistant Professor
Division of Medicine
Vanderbilt University Medical Center
Nashville, Tennessee

Sally Caroline Greaves, MMedSci, MBChB
Cardiologist
Department of Cardiology
Green Lane Cardiovascular Service
Auckland City Hospital
Auckland, New Zealand

Deepak K. Gupta, MD
Assistant Professor
Division of Cardiovascular Medicine
Vanderbilt University Medical Center
Nashville, Tennessee

Michael L. Hall, MD
Assistant Professor
Department of Anesthesiology
University of Washington School of Medicine
Seattle, Washington

Stephen B. Heitner, MD
Associate Professor of Medicine
Director, OHSU Hypertrophic Cardiomyopathy Center
Knight Cardiovascular Institute
Oregon Health & Science University
Portland, Oregon

Gary Huang, MD
Assistant Professor
Division of Cardiology
University of Washington School of Medicine
Seattle, Washington

Judy Hung, MD
Professor of Medicine
Harvard Medical School
Director of Echocardiography
Division of Cardiology
Massachusetts General Hospital
Boston, Massachusetts

Bernard Iung, MD
Professor
Cardiology Department
Bichat Hospital, APHP
Professor
University of Paris
Paris, France

Nikolaus Jander, MD
Department of Cardiology and Angiology II
University Heart Center Freiburg—Bad Krozingen
Bad Krozingen, Germany

Yuli Y. Kim, MD
Medical Director, Philadelphia Adult Congenital Heart Center
Hospital of the University of Pennsylvania and Children's Hospital of Philadelphia
Philadelphia, Pennsylvania

James N. Kirkpatrick, MD
Professor of Medicine, Cardiology, and Bioethics and Humanities
Section Chief, Cardiovascular Imaging
University of Washington School of Medicine
Director, Echocardiography
UW Medicine Heart Institute
Chair, Ethics Committee, UW Medicine
University of Washington Medical Center
Seattle, Washington

Eric V. Krieger, MD
Associate Professor of Medicine
Division of Cardiology
Program Director, Adult Congenital Heart Disease Fellowship
University of Washington School of Medicine
Section Chief, Adult Congenital Heart Disease
University of Washington Medical Center and
Seattle Children's Hospital
Seattle, Washington

Roberto M. Lang, MD
Professor of Medicine and Radiology
Director Noninvasive Cardiac Imaging Laboratories
Section of Cardiology
Heart & Vascular Center
University of Chicago Medicine
Chicago, Illinois

James Lee, MD
Associate Director of Echocardiography
Division of Cardiology
Henry Ford Heart and Vascular Institute
Detroit, Michigan

Jeannette Lin, MD
Associate Clinical Professor
Ahmanson/UCLA Adult Congenital Heart Disease Center
Ronald Reagan UCLA Medical Center
Los Angeles, California

Jonathan R. Lindner, MD
M. Lowell Edwards Professor of Cardiology
Knight Cardiovascular Institute
Oregon Health & Science University
Portland, Oregon

Jason P. Linefsky, MD, MS
Associate Professor of Medicine
Division of Cardiology
Emory University School of Medicine
Assistant Section Chief of Cardiology
Atlanta VA Medical Center
Decatur, Georgia

G. Burkhard Mackensen, MD, PhD
UW Medicine Research & Education Endowed Professor
Director, Interventional Echocardiography
University of Washington Medical Center
Seattle, Washington

Ahmad Masri, MD
Assistant Professor of Medicine
Oregon Health and Science University
Portland, Oregon

Sofia Carolina Masri, MD
Assistant Professor
Division of Cardiology
University of Wisconsin
Madison, Wisconsin

Shannon McConnaughey, MD
Fellow, Cardiovascular Disease
Division of Cardiology
University of Washington School of Medicine
Seattle, Washington

Jan Minners, MD, PhD
Professor
Department of Cardiology and Angiology II
University Heart Center Freiburg—Bad Krozingen
Bad Krozingen, Germany

William R. Miranda, MD
Department of Cardiology
Mayo Clinic
Rochester, Minnesota

Petros Nihoyannopoulos, MD
Professor
Cardiology, NHLI
Imperial College London
Hammersmith Hospital
London, United Kingdom

Catherine M. Otto, MD
Professor of Medicine
J. Ward Kennedy-Hamilton Endowed Chair in Cardiology
Division of Cardiology
University of Washington School of Medicine
Director, Heart Valve Clinic
Associate Director, Echocardiography
University of Washington Medical Center
Seattle, Washington

David S. Owens, MD
Associate Professor
Division of Cardiology
University of Washington School of Medicine
Seattle, Washington

Donald C. Oxorn, MD
Professor of Anesthesiology
Adjunct Professor of Medicine
University of Washington School of Medicine
Seattle, Washington

Philippe Pibarot, DVM, PhD
Professor at Faculté de Médecine
Institut Universitaire de Cardiologie et de Pneumologie de Québec/Quebec Heart and Lung Institute (IUCPQ)
Université Laval
Québec, Québec, Canada

David Playford, MBBS, PhD
Professor of Cardiology
Faculty of Medicine
University of Notre Dame
Fremantle, Western Australia, Australia

Bogdan A. Popescu, MD, PhD
Professor of Cardiology
Carol Davila University of Medicine and Pharmacy
Head, Department of Cardiology
Institute of Cardiovascular Diseases
Director, Euroecolab
Institute of Cardiovascular Diseases
Bucharest, Romania

David Prior, MBBS, PhD
Deputy Director, Cardiology
Department of Cardiology
St Vincent's Hospital Melbourne;
Associate Professor
St Vincent's Department of Medicine
University of Melbourne
Fitzroy, Victoria, Australia

Jordan M. Prutkin, MD, MHS
Associate Professor of Medicine
Cardiology/Cardiac Electrophysiology
University of Washington School of Medicine
Seattle, Washington

Robert A. Quaife, MD
Professor of Medicine
Division of Cardiology
University of Colorado School of Medicine
Director of Advanced Cardiac Imaging
University of Colorado Hospital
Anschutz Medical Campus
Aurora, Colorado

Florian Rader, MD
Associate Director
Cardiac Non-Invasive Laboratory
Smidt Heart Institute
Cedars-Sinai Medical Center
Los Angeles, California

Vrishank Raghav, PhD
Assistant Professor
Aerospace Engineering
Auburn University
Auburn, Alabama

Carlos A. Roldan, MD
Professor of Medicine
University of New Mexico School of Medicine
New Mexico VA Health Care System
Albuquerque, New Mexico

Ernesto E. Salcedo, MD
Professor of Medicine
Division of Cardiology
University of Colorado School of Medicine
Director of Echocardiography
University of Colorado Hospital
Anschutz Medical Campus
Aurora, Colorado

Zainab Samad, MD
Chair, Department of Medicine
Aga Khan University
Karachi, Pakistan

Stephen P. Sanders, MD
Professor of Pediatrics
Harvard Medical School
Director, Cardiac Registry
Departments of Cardiology, Pathology, and Cardiac Surgery
Boston Children's Hospital
Boston, Massachusetts

Kelly H. Schlendorf, MD
Associate Professor
Medical Director, Heart Transplant
Division of Cardiovascular Medicine
Vanderbilt University Medical Center
Nashville, Tennessee

Richard Sheu, MD
Assistant Professor
Director, Perioperative Echocardiography
Department of Anesthesiology and Pain Medicine
University of Washington Medical Center
Seattle, Washington

David A. Sidebotham, MBChB
Anesthesiologist and Intensivist
Department of Cardiothoracic Anaesthesia and Cardiovascular Intensive Care Unit
Auckland City Hospital
Auckland, New Zealand

Robert J. Siegel, MD
Director, Cardiac Non-Invasive Laboratory
Smidt Heart Institute
Cedars-Sinai Medical Center
Los Angeles, California

Candice K. Silversides, MD
Cardiologist
Department of Medicine
University of Toronto
Toronto, Ontario, Canada

Samuel C. Siu, MD
Cardiologist
Department of Medicine
Western University
London, Ontario, Canada

Otto A. Smiseth, MD, PhD
Professor
Division of Cardiovascular and Pulmonary Diseases
Oslo University Hospital
Oslo, Norway

Raymond F. Stainback, MD
Chief, Non-Invasive Cardiology
Texas Heart Institute at Baylor St. Luke's Medical Center
Associate Professor
Section of Cardiology
Department of Medicine
Baylor College of Medicine
Houston, Texas

Kenan W.D. Stern, MD
Assistant Professor of Pediatrics and Radiology
Department of Pediatrics - Division of Cardiology
Icahn School of Medicine at Mount Sinai
New York, New York

Felix C. Tanner, MD
Professor and Vice Chairman
Department of Cardiology
University Heart Center
Zürich, Switzerland

Hans Torp, DrTech
Professor
Department of Circulation and Medical Imaging
Norwegian University of Science and Technology
Trondheim, Norway

Wendy Tsang, MD
Assistant Professor of Medicine
Division of Cardiology
University of Toronto
Toronto General Hospital
University Health Network
Toronto, Ontario, Canada

Alec Vahanian, MD
Professor of Cardiology
University of Paris
Paris, France

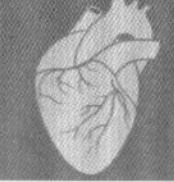

Anne Marie Valente, MD
Director, Boston Adult Congenital Heart Program
Boston Children's Hospital
Brigham and Women's Hospital
Harvard Medical School
Boston, Massachusetts

Pieter van der Bijl, MD, PhD
Research and Imaging Fellow
Department of Cardiology
Heart and Lung Center
Leiden University Medical Center
Leiden, the Netherlands

Rachel M. Wald, MD
Professor of Medicine
University Health Network and Mount Sinai Hospital
University of Toronto
Toronto, Ontario, Canada

Andrew Wang, MD
Professor of Medicine
Vice Chief for Clinical Services
Department of Cardiology
Duke University Medical Center
Durham, North Carolina

Dee Dee Wang, MD
Director, Structural Heart Imaging
Center for Structural Heart Disease
Division of Cardiology
Henry Ford Heart and Vascular Institute
Detroit, Michigan

Terrence D. Welch, MD
Associate Professor of Medicine and Medical Education
Geisel School of Medicine at Dartmouth
Hanover, New Hampshire
Program Director, Cardiovascular Medicine Fellowship
Dartmouth-Hitchcock Medical Center
Lebanon, New Hampshire

Ajit P. Yoganathan, PhD
Emeritus Regents' Professor
Wallace H. Coulter Distinguished Faculty Chair
Wallace H. Coulter School of Biomedical Engineering
Georgia Institute of Technology
Atlanta, Georgia

Ali N. Zaidi, MD
Director, Mount Sinai Adult Congenital Heart Disease Center
Associate Professor
Medicine and Pediatrics
Icahn School of Medicine at Mount Sinai
New York, New York

Karen G. Zimmerman, BS, ACS, RVT
Editor-in-Chief
CASE: Cardiovascular Imaging Case Reports
American Society of Echocardiography
Durham, North Carolina
Facilitator of Clinical Quality
Department of Cardiology
Henry Ford Health System
Detroit, Michigan

编译委员会名单

丛书编译委员会顾问专家

高润霖　（中国医学科学院阜外医院）

汪忠镐　（首都医科大学宣武医院）

丛书编译委员会组长

吴永健　（中国医学科学院阜外医院）

张　健　（中国医学科学院阜外医院）

主任委员

朱振辉　（中国医学科学院阜外医院）

副主任委员（按姓氏笔画排序）

权　欣　（中国医学科学院阜外医院）

吴伟春　（中国医学科学院阜外医院）

委　员（按姓氏笔画排序）

卫　青　（中国医学科学院阜外医院）

王　燕　（中国医学科学院阜外医院）

王剑鹏　（中国医学科学院阜外医院）

牛丽莉　（中国医学科学院阜外医院）

卢宏泉　（中国医学科学院阜外医院）

田莉莉　（中国医学科学院阜外医院）

刘　偈　（中国医学科学院阜外医院）

刘思岐　（中国医学科学院阜外医院）

孙　欣　（中国医学科学院阜外医院）

李　慧　（中国医学科学院阜外医院）

李羽加　（中国医学科学院阜外医院）

李鸣瑶　（中国医学科学院阜外医院）

李晓妮　（中国医学科学院阜外医院）

肖明虎　（中国医学科学院阜外医院）

张　冰　（中国医学科学院阜外医院）

陈慧婷　（福建省三明市第一医院）

赵　莹　（中国医学科学院阜外医院）

施怡声　（中国医学科学院阜外医院）

陶　瑾　（中国医学科学院阜外医院）

戴　莹　（福建省立医院）

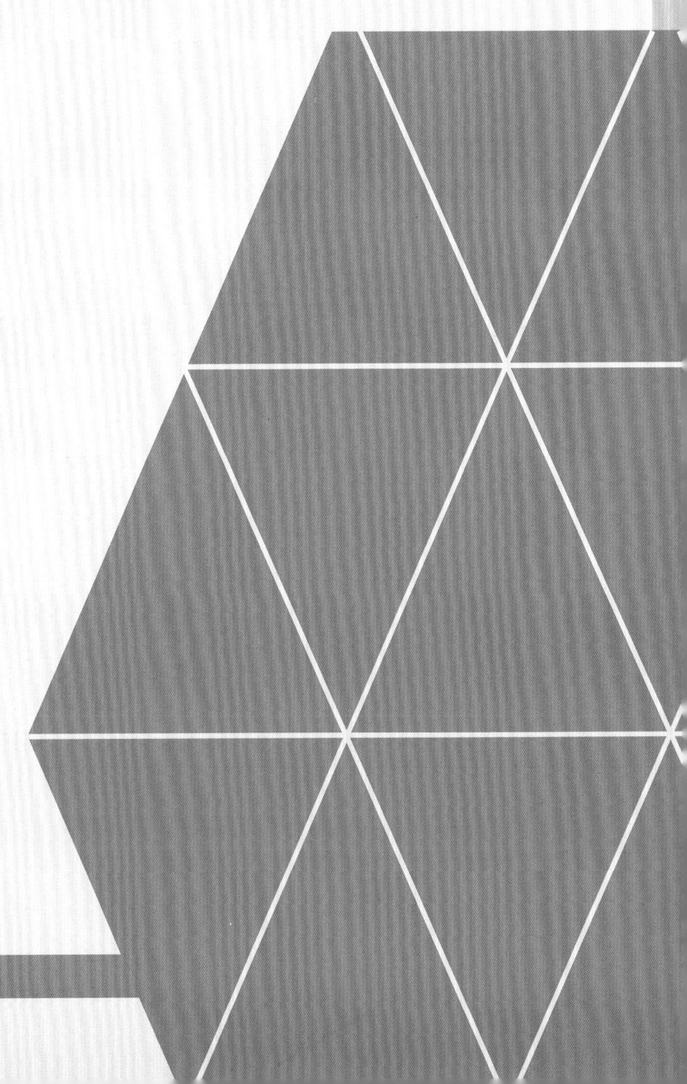

原书前言

The Practice of Clinical Echocardiography 聚焦于超声心动图成像的临床应用，在数据获取和解释、诊断准确性及超声心动图在临床决策中的作用方面提供了先进的参考文本。简而言之，本书反映了我们作为治疗心血管疾病患者的临床医师的角色。第 6 版更新了新的临床知识、新的治疗方法和新的指南，以及高级超声心动图成像的创新。

除了具有超声心动图专业知识的心脏科医师和心脏科培训生，本书也适用于所有临床心脏科医师，包括那些普通心脏科、介入心脏科、电生理学、晚期心力衰竭、成人先天性心脏病、遗传性心血管疾病和瓣膜心脏病的亚专科医师。本书可作为在临床环境中使用超声心动图方法的其他内科医师的参考文献，包括心脏麻醉师、心脏外科医师、放射科医师、急诊内科医师和对心血管疾病有积极兴趣的内科医师。希望想超越超声心动图成像入门阶段的心脏超声医师、心血管技术专家、医师助理、护士从业人员和护理专业人员，会在本书发现有价值的信息。对于临床研究工作者，高级超声心动图方法的细节包含在每一章中。

超声心动图是评估疑似或已知心血管疾病患者的关键组成部分。随着超声心动图技术的发展和成熟，超声心动图医师的作用已从单纯的图像描述转变为将超声心动图结果与其他临床数据相结合，从而提供鉴别诊断或治疗建议。通常，超声心动图可提供临床决策所需的所有数据。当需要其他信息时，超声心动图结果有助于确定需要其他哪种影像学检查方法。实际上，超声心动图已经成为心脏病会诊不可或缺的一项操作。

现在申请医师要求的信息不仅包括对超声心动图图像和多普勒血流数据的定性和定量解释，而且还包括这些信息如何影响临床决策的讨论。具体例子包括介入治疗（如是否适合经导管主动脉瓣置入术）、药物或外科治疗（如治疗心内膜炎、主动脉夹层手术）、慢性心脏病患者（如瓣膜反流、二尖瓣狭窄）的最佳干预时机、预后影响（如妊娠期心脏病、心力衰竭患者），以及定期随访评估（如先天性心脏病，术后患者）的可能需求和频率。此外，超声心动图

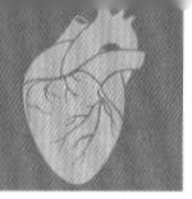

在为每例患者选择最佳治疗方案（如选择植入心脏内除颤器的患者）方面至关重要，并且在监测经皮介入治疗及药物或手术治疗的效果方面也至关重要。

超声心动图的临床实践不再局限于在影像实验室进行的全面诊断性检查。相反，超声心动图已经成为心血管护理的重要组成部分，以至于现在在重症监护病房、急诊科、介入实验室、电生理操作和手术室中都使用了专门的仪器。随着超声仪器变得更容易使用、更小、更便宜，这种成像方式的临床应用可能会继续扩大。

本书每一章都提供了由该领域的专家以本书姊妹篇——*Textbook of Clinical Echocardiography*（*sixth edition*）中的基本材料为基础编写的高阶论述。教科书侧重于影像学的基本原理；相比之下，*The Practice of Clinical Echocardiography* 则侧重于超声心动图在临床决策中的作用，重点还放在最佳数据获取的原则、数据分析的定量方法、潜在的技术限制和研究热点领域。此外，本书还回顾了其他诊断方法的优势和局限性，以对照超声心动图在临床实践中的作用。详细的表格、彩色插图、超声心动图图像、多普勒描记和包含已发表结局研究的关键数据的数字使本书更清晰易懂并具备深度。

第 6 版进行了重组分类，首先第一部分是关于超声心动图医师的高级原则，第二部分是关于影像实验室的超声心动图最佳实践及经胸和经食管超声心动图、术中和介入性超声心动图和床旁心脏超声临床实践。本书的核心是按疾病诊断分类编排：心肌疾病、肿瘤和心包疾病由 James Kirkpatrick 编辑，缺血性心脏病由 Rosario Freeman 编辑，心脏瓣膜病由笔者编辑，血管和系统性疾病由 Jason Linefsky 编辑。其中 Eric Krieger 编辑的最后一部分“成人先天性心脏病和妊娠患者”为该亚专科的培训人员提供了一份简明的“教材中的教材”。

第 6 版的其他主要特点包括以下内容。

（1）表格总结了数据采集和测量的技术细节，并提供了临床疾病和超声心动图结果之间的相关性。

（2）证据表总结了验证和结局研究。

（3）现行指南以表格或图表形式总结。

每一章以一个汇总表结束，其提供了超声心动图数据获取、测量和解读的实用方法。

希望这本书能为读者提供必要的背景来支持和补充临床经验、专业知识。

当然，获取和解读超声心动图和多普勒数据的能力取决于适当的临床教育和培训，这在医师和技师的认证要求中有详细说明，也如专业学会［包括美国超声心动图学会（American Society of Echocardiography，ASE）、美国心脏病学会（American College of Cardiology，ACC）和美国心脏协会（American Heart Association，AHA）］所推荐的那样。我们强烈支持这些教育要求和培训建议；这本书的读者应阅读相关文件。

此外，在图像和血流数据采集的技术方面，以及我们对特定超声心动图结果的临床意义的理解方面，都在不断进步。这本书代表了我们在一个时间点上的知识基础，读者还应查阅当前的文献以获得最新的信息。虽然每一章都提供了大量精心选择的参考文献列表，但超声心动图文献是如此海量，因此纳入所有相关参考文献是不切实际的。如果需要所有相关文献，读者可以使用在线医学文献检索。

对于有兴趣掌握超声心动图的读者，其他资源包括 *Textbook of Clinical Echocardiography*（*sixth edition*），可以在阅读本书之前阅读和研究，由 Rosario Freeman、Becky Schwaegler、Jason Linefsky 和笔者共同撰写的 *Echocardiography Review Guide*（*fourth edition*）提供了一个快速的总结和自我评价问题；以及笔者和 Donald Oxorn 合著的 *Intraoperative and Interventional Echocardiography: Atlas of Transesophageal Echocardiography*（*second edition*）包含 1500 多幅图像和视频，以病例展示的形式呈现，并附有简明的评论。

读者只需要少量的时间就可以获得超声心动图图像获取和解读的基本技能；挑战在于如何将这些技能从“基础”转变为“专家”。随着超声心动图完全融入每个临床机构的医学实践，我们每个人都应该意识到自己的局限性、实践范围和临床实践需求。Otto 系列教材所包含的集中的教学内容和积累的临床经验，不仅为学习超声心动图提供了坚实的基础，而且可以为那些希望挑战自我成为超声心动图大师的人加速学习曲线。

Catherine M.Otto

2021 年 4 月

原书致谢

我要对促成本书出版的每一位致以最深切的感谢。首先我要向章节编辑——Rosario Freeman、James Kirkpatrick、Jason Linefsky和Eric Krieger表示敬意和衷心的感谢，他们花费了大量的时间、精力和编辑技巧来精心设计本书，并帮助章节作者清晰、简洁和完整地呈现信息。其次非常感谢章节作者贡献了学术的、有思想的、深刻的文本和杰出的插图来帮助读者更好地理解超声心动图实践。我们每个机构的支持人员在文稿准备和提供有效沟通方面都值得赞赏。

许多研究对象为我们当前的知识提供了数据，这些研究对象当然也值得感谢。我们所有机构的心脏超声医师对我们在超声心动图临床实践中的合作伙伴，以及本书显示的大多数图像的提供者，一并表示感谢。我真诚地感谢Joe Chovan的杰出插图。此外，感谢Robin Carter、Jennifer Ehlers、Doug Turner，以及Elsevier的整个编辑和制作团队。最后，我衷心感谢华盛顿大学（University of Washington）心脏病学的同事和我的家人，感谢他们一直以来的鼓励和支持。

编译荣誉主任委员序言

中国医学科学院阜外医院作为国家心血管病中心一直致力于提高心血管疾病的医疗水平，超声影像中心作为疾病检出的第一道影像学关卡，一直力求通过精炼的超声报告满足临床医师对于疾病诊疗的诉求。但是实际工作中，临床医师与超声医师之间缺乏有效沟通，难以体现临床所需的关键数据和心脏信息，导致疾病诊疗难度增加。

出于提升超声医师临床思维的考量，中国医学科学院阜外医院超声一科朱振辉主任带领其他超声医师，推进 *The Practice of Clinical Echocardiography*（*6th Edition*）一书在国内的出版。本书由世界著名专家 Catherine M. Otto 博士团队完成，聚焦于超声心动图成像的临床应用，在数据获取和解释、诊断准确性及超声心动图在临床决策中的作用上提供了先进的参考文本，从临床医师的角度出发考虑诊断所需。除此之外，本书回顾了其他诊断方法的优势和局限性，以对照超声心动图在临床实践的作用，适合所有在临床环境中使用和涉及超声心动图检查的医护人员，包括但不限于心脏麻醉师、心脏外科医师、放射科医师、内科医师和护理人员等。

随着超声心动图检查的发展与成熟，超声医师的角色已从单纯的图像描述转变为将超声心动图结果与其他临床数据相结合，从而提供鉴别诊断及治疗建议。由衷希望每一位超声医师能从临床出发，把自己视为真正的临床医师而非简单的检查人员，共同进步。

王　浩

2022 年 10 月

编译主任委员前言

世界知名专家 Catherine M.Otto 博士及其团队撰写的 *The Practice of Clinical Echocardiography* 是一部较为经典的心脏超声专业著作，由世界著名的出版社——Elsevier 出版引进，2021 年已再版到第 6 版。此次改版首先更新了超声心动图的通用技术方法和高级应用技术，包括左、右心功能定量测量方法、床旁超声、术中超声、介入超声及三维超声、心肌力学和应变、声学造影等，详述了高质量超声科室的质控。然后按成人常见的心脏疾病病种如冠心病、心肌病、瓣膜病、先天性心脏病、心力衰竭、结缔组织病、系统性疾病和血栓栓塞等疾病的临床基础和超声表现、诊断要点乃至临床治疗相关超声应用等展开详细的论述。

正如原书作者所言，超声医师的工作已从单纯的图像描述转变为要将超声心动图结果与其他临床资料相结合，从而提供鉴别诊断或治疗建议，以及治疗过程中的评价监测和引导等全治疗周期的应用，发挥全新的更高层次的核心作用，所以从临床应用环境的角度来学习和理解变得必要和迫切。本书可适用于超声心动图专业医师的实践指导，同时也可以作为心内科、心外科、急重症科、结构性心脏病介入科、麻醉科及其他影像科等医师临床实践中超声应用的很好的学习文献和教材。同时辅以大量典型病例超声影像、高度凝练的总结性图表及相关临床研究文献的数据，相信对各相关学科医师都会裨益良多。

经编译委员会、相关专家及出版社商议，编译委员会只为读者作本书每章节的中文导读，正文则按英文版原文，以利于读者原汁原味地高水平理解原意，学习超声心动图专业知识的同时还可以学习相关专业英文表达，提高专业英语水平。

朱振辉

2022 年 10 月

英文目录

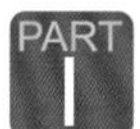

Advanced Principles for the Echocardiographer

Section Editor: Catherine M. Otto

Echocardiography Best Practices

Section Editor: Rosario V. Freeman

Cardiomyopathies, Tumors, and Pericardial Disease

Section Editor: James N. Kirkpatrick

Ischemic Heart Disease

Section Editor: Rosario V. Freeman

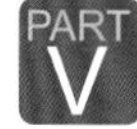

Valvular Heart Disease

Section Editor: Catherine M. Otto

Vascular and Systemic Diseases

Section Editor: Jason P. Linefsky

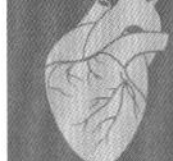

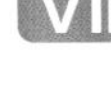

PART VII Adult Congenital Heart Disease and the Pregnant Patient

Section Editor: Eric V. Krieger

中文目录

第五部分　瓣膜性心脏病

第六部分　血管和全身疾病

第七部分　成人先天性心脏病和妊娠患者

词汇表

2D	two-dimensional
3D	three-dimensional
A-long	apical long-axis
A-mode	amplitude mode (amplitude versus depth)
A	atrial transmitral diastolic velocity
A′	diastolic tissue Doppler velocity with atrial contraction
A2C	apical 2-chamber
A4C	apical 4-chamber
ACHD	adult congenital heart disease
ACS	acute coronary syndrome
AcT	acceleration time
AF	atrial fibrillation
AMVL	anterior mitral valve leaflet
ant	anterior
Ao	aortic or aorta
AoV	aortic valve
Ar	pulmonary vein atrial reversal velocity
AR	aortic regurgitation
ARVD	arrhythmogenic right ventricular dysplasia
AS	aortic stenosis
ASD	atrial septal defect
ASE	American Society of Echocardiography
ATVL	anterior tricuspid valve leaflet
AV	atrioventricular
AVA	aortic valve area
AVC	aortic valve closure
AVR	aortic valve replacement
AVSD	atrioventricular septal defect
BAV	bicuspid aortic valve
BMV	balloon mitral valvotomy
BNP	B-type natriuretic peptide
BP	blood pressure
BSA	body surface area
CABG	coronary artery bypass graft
CAD	coronary artery disease
CCTGA	congenitally corrected transposition of the great arteries (*see* L-TGA)
CCU	coronary care unit
CO	cardiac output
COPD	chronic obstructive pulmonary disease
CPB	cardiopulmonary bypass
CRT	cardiac resynchronization therapy
CS	coronary sinus
CSA	cross-sectional area
CT	computed tomography
CTEPH	chronic thromboembolic pulmonary hypertension
CW	continuous wave
Cx	circumflex coronary artery
D	diameter
DAo	descending aorta
DCM	dilated cardiomyopathy
DICOM	Digital Imaging and Communications in Medicine
DORV	double-outlet right ventricle
dP/dt	rate of change in pressure over time
DSE	dobutamine stress echocardiography
DT	deceleration time
D-TGA	complete (D or dextro) transposition of the great arteries

E	early transmitral diastolic velocity
E′	early diastolic tissue Doppler veloctiy
ECG	electrocardiogram
ED	end-diastole
EDD	end-diastolic dimension
EDP	end-diastolic pressure
EDV	end-diastolic volume
EF	ejection fraction
endo	endocardium
EOA	effective orifice area
epi	epicardium
EPSS	E-point septal separation
EROA	effective regurgitant orifice area
ES	end-systole
ESD	end-systolic dimension
ESPVR	end-systolic pressure-volume relationship
ESV	end-systolic volume
ETT	exercise treadmill test
FDA	Food and Drug Administration (USA)
FL	false lumen
FPV	flow propagation velocity
FS	fractional shortening
FSV	forward stroke volume
HCM	hypertrophic cardiomyopathy
HFpEF	heart failure with preserved ejection fraction
HOCM	hypertrophic obstructive cardiomyopathy
HPRF	high pulse repetition frequency
HR	heart rate
HRrEF	heart failure with reduced ejection fraction
HV	hepatic vein
IABP	intraaortic balloon pump
IAS	interatrial septum
ICD	implanted cardiac defibrillator
ICE	intracardiac echocardiography
ICU	intensive care unit
IE	infective endocarditis
inf	inferior
INR	international normalized ratio
IV	intravenous
IVC	inferior vena cava
IVCT	isovolumic contraction time
IVRT	isovolumic relaxation time
IVUS	intravascular ultrasound
L	length
LA	left atrium
LAA	left atrial appendage
LAD	left anterior descending coronary artery
LAE	left atrial enlargement
lat	lateral
LBBB	left bundle branch block
LCC	left coronary cusp
LCx	left circumflex coronary artery
LIPV	left inferior pulmonary vein
LMCA	left main coronary artery
LPA	left pulmonary artery
LSPV	left superior pulmonary vein

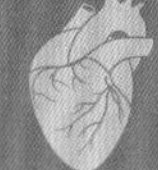

L-TGA L-transposition of the great arteries (*see* CCTGA)
LV left ventricle
LVAD left ventricular assist device
LVEDP left ventricular end-diastolic pressure
LVH left ventricular hypertrophy
LVID left ventricular internal dimension
LVOT left ventricular outflow tract

M-mode motion display (depth versus time)
MAC mitral annular calcification
MAIVF mitral-aortic intervalvular fibrosa
MCE myocardial contrast echocardiography
MFS Marfan syndrome
MI myocardial infarction
MPA main pulmonary artery
mPAP mean pulmonary artery pressure
MPI myocardial performance index
MR mitral regurgitation
MRI magnetic resonance imaging
MS mitral stenosis
MV mitral valve
MVA mitral valve area
MVL mitral valve leaflet
MVP mitral valve prolapse
MVR mitral valve replacement

NBTE nonbacterial thrombotic endocarditis
NCC noncoronary cusp
NYHA New York Heart Association (classification for heart failure symptoms)

OM1 first obtuse marginal branch
OM2 second obtuse marginal branch

ΔP pressure gradient
PA pulmonary artery
PACS Picture Archiving and Communications Systems
PAH pulmonary arterial hypertension
pAn pseudoaneurysm
PAP pulmonary artery pressure
PAPVR partial anomalous pulmonary venous return
PASP pulmonary artery systolic pressure
PCI percutaneous coronary intervention
PCWP pulmonary capillary wedge pressure
PDA patent ductus arteriosus or posterior descending artery (depends on context)
PE pericardial effusion
PEP preejection period
PET positron-emission tomography
PFO patent foramen ovale
PH pulmonary hypertension
PHT pressure half time
PISA proximal isovelocity surface area
PLAX parasternal long-axis
PM papillary muscle
PMVL posterior mitral valve leaflet
post posterior (or inferior-lateral) ventricular wall, or after
PPM patient prosthesis mismatch
PR pulmonic regurgitation
PRF pulse repetition frequency
PRFR peak rapid filling rate
PS pulmonic stenosis
PSAX parasternal short-axis
PV pulmonary vein
PVC premature ventricular contraction
PVOD pulmonary venoocclusive disease
PVR pulmonary vascular resistance
PW pulsed wave
PWT posterior wall thickness

RA right atrium
RAE right atrial enlargement
RAO right anterior oblique
RAP right atrial pressure
RCA right coronary artery
RCC right coronary cusp
RF regurgitant fraction
RIPV right inferior pulmonary vein
RJ regurgitant jet
ROA regurgitant orifice area
RPA right pulmonary artery
RSPV right superior pulmonary vein
RSV regurgitant stroke volume
RT3DE real-time three-dimensional echocardiography
RV right ventricle
RVAD right ventricular assist device
RVE right ventricular enlargement
RVH right ventricular hypertrophy
RVOT right ventricular outflow tract
RWT relative wall thickness

SAM systolic anterior motion
SAS subaortic stenosis
SC subcostal
SD standard deviation
SEE standard error of the estimate
SPECT single photon emission computed tomography
SPPA spatial peak pulse average
SPTA spatial peak temporal average
SR strain rate
SSN suprasternal notch
STE speckle tracking echocardiography
STJ sinotubular junction
STVL septal tricuspid valve leaflet
SV stroke volume or sample volume (depends on context)
SVC superior vena cava
SVR systemic vascular resistance

TAPSE tricuspid annular plane systolic excursion
TAPVR total anomalous pulmonary venous return
TAVI transcatheter aortic valve implantation
TDI tissue-Doppler imaging
TEE transesophageal echocardiography
TGA transposition of the great arteries
TGC time gain compensation
TIA transient ischemic attack
TL true lumen
TOF tetralogy of Fallot
TPV time to peak velocity
TR tricuspid regurgitation
TS tricuspid stenosis
TSV total stroke volume
TTE transthoracic echocardiography
TV tricuspid valve

V volume or velocity (depends on context)
VAD ventricular assist device
VAS ventriculo-atrial septum
V_{cf} velocity of circumferential shortening
V_{max} maximum velocity
VSD ventricular septal defect
VTI velocity-time integral

WPW Wolff-Parkinson-White syndrome

Z acoustic impedance

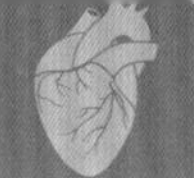

Greek Symbols and Their Meaning

Symbol	*Greek Name*	*Used For*
α	alpha	frequency
γ	gamma	viscosity
Δ	delta	difference
θ	theta	angle
λ	lambda	wavelength
μ	mu	micro-
π	pi	mathematic constant (approximately 3.14)
ρ	rho	tissue density
σ	sigma	wall stress
τ	tau	time constant of ventricular relaxation

Units of Measure

Variable	*Unit*	*Definition*
Amplitude	dB	Decibels = a logarithmic scale describing the amplitude ("loudness") of the sound wave
Angle	degrees	Degree = (π/180)rad. Example: intercept angle
Area	cm^2	Square centimeters. A two-dimensional measurement (e.g., end-systolic area) or a calculated value (e.g., continuity equation valve area)
Frequency (f)	Hz kHz MHz	Hertz (cycles per second) Kilohertz = 1000 Hz Megahertz = 1,000,000 Hz
Length	cm mm	Centimeter (1/100 m) Millimeter (1/1000 m or 1/10 cm)
Mass	g	Grams. Example: LV mass
Pressure	mmHg	Millimeters of mercury, 1 mmHg = 1333.2 dyne/cm^2, where dyne measures force in g · cm/s^2
Resistance	dyne · s · cm^{-5}	Measure of vascular resistance
Time	s ms μs	Second Millisecond (1/1000 s) Microsecond
Ultrasound intensity	W/cm^2 mW/cm^2	Where watt (W) = joule per second and joule = $m^2 \cdot kg \cdot s^{-2}$ (unit of energy)
Velocity (v)	m/s cm/s	Meters per second Centimeters per second
Velocity-time integral (VTI)	cm	Integral of the Doppler velocity curve (cm/s) over time (s), in units of cm
Volume	cm^3 mL L	Cubic centimeters Milliliter, 1 mL = 1 cm^3 Liter = 1000 mL
Volume flow rate (Q)	L/min mL/s	Rate of volume flow across a valve or in cardiac output L/min = liters per minute mL/s = milliliters per second
Wall stress	dyne/cm^2 kdyn/cm^2 kPa	Units of meridional or circumferential wall stress Kilodynes per cm^2 Kilopascals where 1 kPa = 10 kdyn/cm^2

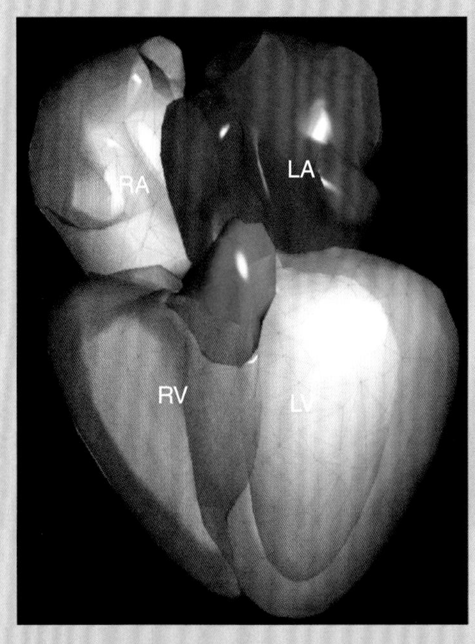

PART I
第一部分

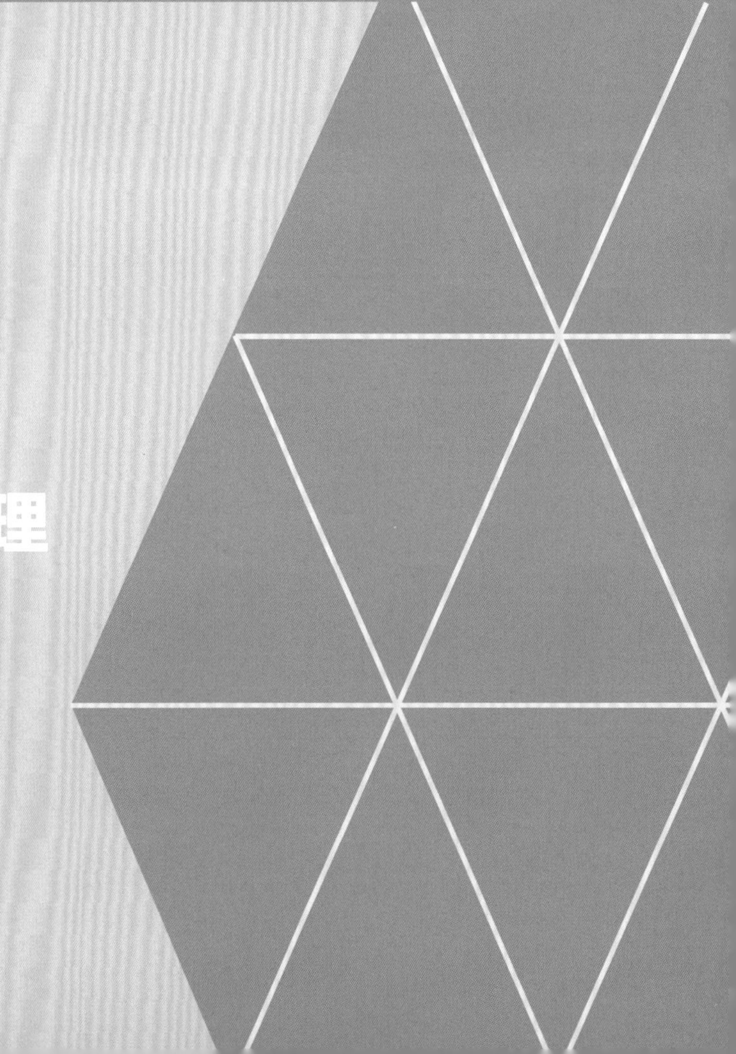

Advanced Principles for the Echocardiographer
超声心动图高级应用原理

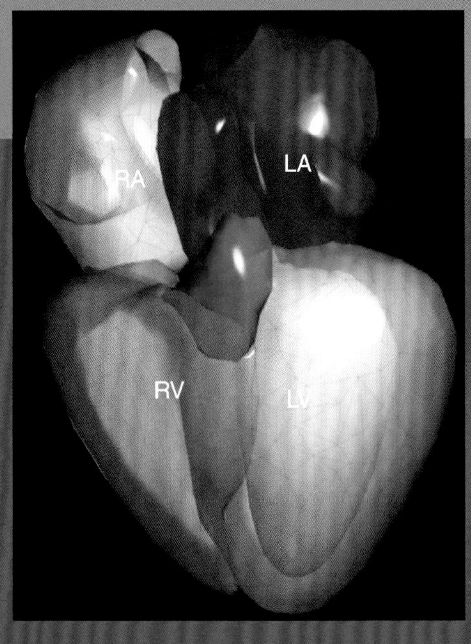

中文导读

第1章
三维超声心动图：图像获取、展示和分析

三维超声心动图是近年来的一项重要创新技术。本章从核心原理上着重讲解了三维超声心动图的图像获取、展示，以及分析。

1.阐述了三维超声心动图的图像获取的物理原理基础、空间分辨率和时间分辨率的关系，以及如何优化，不同三维超声心动图模式的获取及相应的特点：多平面同步显示，三种金字塔容积模式［局部放大三维超声心动图（ZOOM）、窄扇角（实时模式）和宽扇角（全容积）］的获取，该模式的选择取决于想要展示的部位。技术操作的细节方面、心电门控，以及减少探头和患者的移动（呼吸抑制）可以减少拼接伪像，增益、亮度和平滑度的适当调节和伪彩色的应用可以优化三维超声心动图的图像。

2.如何展示三维超声心动图的图像：对获取的容积图像进行切割剪裁可以展示感兴趣区的立体结构，通常有自动切割、方格切割、平面切割和双平面快速切割等方法。获取后的三维超声心动图的图像展示包括容积呈现、表面呈现方式和超声断层切片方式。

3.三维超声心动图的图像分析：可作病理形态分析和定量分析，分析方法则有多平面重建、建模和多普勒血流分析。除在显示器中展示三维超声心动图外，三维结构真实呈现的新技术也涌现出来，包括3D打印、虚拟现实技术和增强现实技术。

最后，本章介绍了特定心脏结构包括左心室、右心室、左心房、二尖瓣、三尖瓣、主动脉瓣，以及彩色多普勒血流的三维超声心动图的图像获取、展示和分析方案，并分别列举三维超声心动图的局限性。

朱振辉

1 3D Echocardiographic Image Acquisition, Display, and Analysis

WENDY TSANG, MD, SM | ROBERTO M. LANG, MD

Three-dimensional (3D) echocardiography (3DE) is one of the most important innovations in the field of cardiovascular ultrasonography.[1–3] To maximize the information obtained from a 3DE data set, image acquisition and analysis should be performed with a deep understanding of the underlying technical principles and using a systematic approach. Although there are differences among cardiovascular ultrasound equipment manufacturers with respect to terminology and technical performance, the underlying fundamental principles among vendors remain the same. The goal of this chapter is to provide a practical guide that focuses on the core principles required to acquire, display, and analyze cardiac structures using 3DE and describes the limitations of this imaging modality. The first part of this chapter describes the physics, technical factors, and terminology related to 3DE. The second part provides a practical description of the clinical use of 3DE with respect to acquisition, display, and analysis of specific cardiac structures.

ULTRASOUND IMAGING SYSTEM FUNCTION

The basis for ultrasound image formation is as follows. To acquire an image, the transducer transmits a high-frequency sound beam. When this beam hits an acoustic interface, such as an intertissue boundary, some of the sound waves are reflected and "echoed" back to the transducer.[4] An image is then created by incorporating information regarding the distances and intensities of the echoes transmitted to the probe from the tissue boundaries based on calculations that incorporate the speed of sound in the tissue and the time required for each echo to return. In the transducer, the piezoelectric element is the component that transmits and receives ultrasound information and transforms it into electric signals, which are then sent to the ultrasound machine. A single-element transducer can acquire and form images only in a single spatial and one temporal dimension. In practice, this is M-mode imaging in that only structures in the beam line are visualized.

Two-dimensional (2D or B-mode) images are acquired using linear phased array transducers in which 48 to 128 piezo elements are arranged in a single row (one-dimensional linear array) with each element functioning separately (Fig. 1.1).[5] (2D images can also be acquired with mechanical transducers, which consist of a rapidly moving single crystal.) Each element is activated according to a specific sequence with a delay in phase with respect to the transmit initiation time (Fig. 1.2). The individual waves generated from each element interact constructively and destructively to form an overall wave that has a direction and is known as a *radially propagating scan line.* Because the elements are arranged in a single row in a 2D linear phased array transducer, the transducer can steer and focus in only two directions (Fig. 1.3), axial and azimuthal (lateral). When the 2D image is formed, the resolution in the elevation plane is fixed by the vertical dimension of the elements, which restricts the slice thickness.

In an ultrasound machine, the transmitting and receiving functions create scan lines through beamforming and summing (Fig. 1.4). Beamforming or spatial filtering is a signal processing technique that uses the array of elements to create directional or spatial selectivity of signal transmission and reception. The time delay before the activation of each element and the strength of the sent signal allow focusing and steering of the transmission beam. Summing is the act of combining signals by summing the pulses from each transducer element to create a scan line. For the ultrasound machine to perform beamforming, the following components are required: high-voltage transmitters, low-noise receivers, analog-to-digital converters, digital delay lines, and delay controllers. In 2D imaging, beamforming does not occur in the transducer but in the ultrasound machine, consuming approximately 100 W of energy and 1500 cm^2 of a personal computer electronic board area.

With 3DE, the transducer elements are organized in a matrix formation (2D array). Early 3D transducers were called *sparse arrays* because not all the elements in the matrix were simultaneously electrically active.[6] These were the first transducers to enable acquisition of 3D images that could be immediately visualized, but because of the sparse array activation pattern, control of the ultrasound beam was not precise, and diffraction effects such as grating lobes were commonly encountered. The 3D transducers used today are fully sampled matrix array transducers in which each element is simultaneously electrically active.[7,8] 3D matrix array transducers are composed of 2000 to 3000 piezoelectric elements with operating frequencies ranging from 1 to 5 MHz for transthoracic and 2 to 8 MHz for

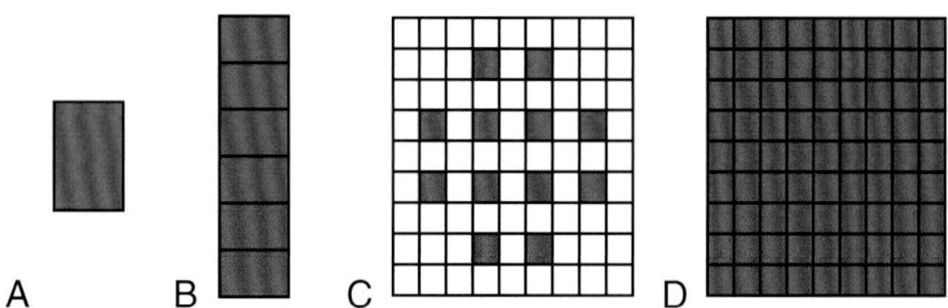

Fig. 1.1 Transducer elements. (A) Single-element transducers have a single active piezoelectric crystal for transmitting and receiving ultrasound beams. (B) Phased array transducers are composed of 48 to 128 electrically active elements in a single row; with a coordinated sequence of firing, they can form a focused wave front that has a direction. (C) A sparse array transducer has approximately 2000 to 3000 elements, but not all of them are electrically active. (D) In a fully sampled matrix array transducer, all elements are electrically active. Active elements are depicted in *red*.

transesophageal transducers.[9,10] Phasic activation of the elements in the matrix array allows 3D transducers to generate a scan line that propagates radially (axial direction) and can be steered in two directions (azimuth/lateral and elevational), creating a pyramidal coordinate system (see Fig. 1.3).

As mentioned previously, in a 2D probe, all components required for beamforming are contained in the ultrasound machine. To maintain this configuration with a fully sampled 3D matrix array probe containing 3000 elements would require a 3000-channel system and cable, 4 kW of power consumption, and a large personal computer electronics board area to contain all the circuitry, which would not be practical.[11] A major hurdle in the development of fully sampled matrix array probes was the need to reduce power consumption and the size of the connecting cable while maintaining the electric interconnections for every element, to ensure that each element remains independent with respect to transmitting and receiving. This was achieved through placement of specifically engineered miniaturized application-specific integrated circuit (ASIC) boards within the transducer.[12–14] The first commercial, fully sampled matrix array transducer had 24 to 26 ASICs, which were connected to the approximately 3000 elements. This allowed the 3000 elements to be independently active while simultaneously keeping the size of the transducer cable reasonably small. With further miniaturization advancements, current transthoracic and transesophageal probes have a single ASIC.

As a result of the placement of the transducer ASICs, beamforming was split into two components (see Fig. 1.4): a microbeamforming stage that uses the beamforming circuitry in the transducer and requires less than 1 W of power and a coarse stage of beamforming that occurs through conventional cables in the ultrasound machine.[15,16] When microbeamforming occurs in the transducer, it is no longer required that each piezoelectric element be connected to the ultrasound machine. The 3000-channel circuit boards within the transducer control the fine steering by delaying (through fine circuitry integrated

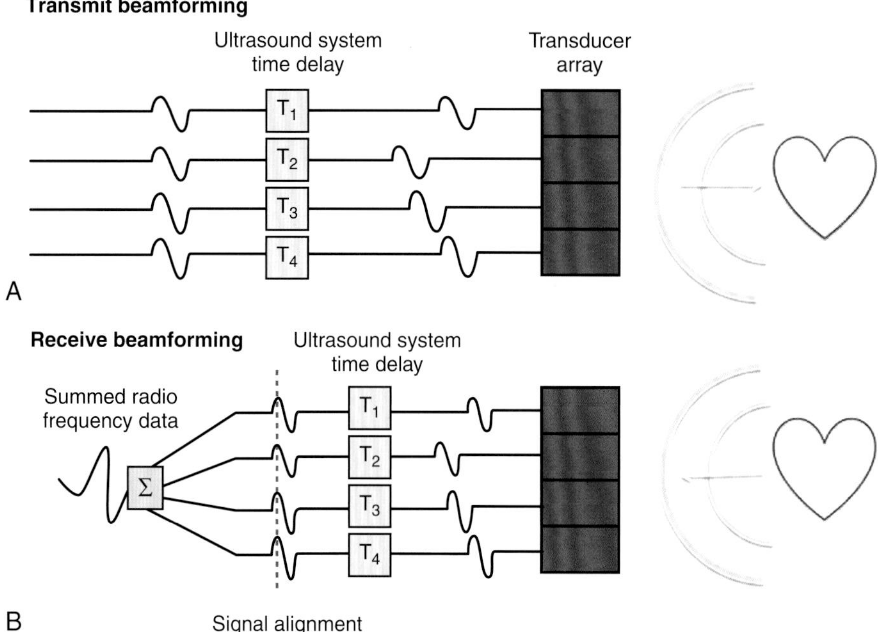

Fig. 1.2 Beamforming. (A) During ultrasound transmission, each piezoelectric element in the transducer array (T_1 through T_4) is activated at different times (phasing), which allows formation of a focused ultrasound beam. (B) During ultrasound receiving, selective delays of the echo signals received by the different piezoelectric elements allow focusing (alignment) of the signals, which can then be summed coherently (Σ).

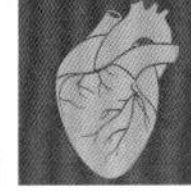

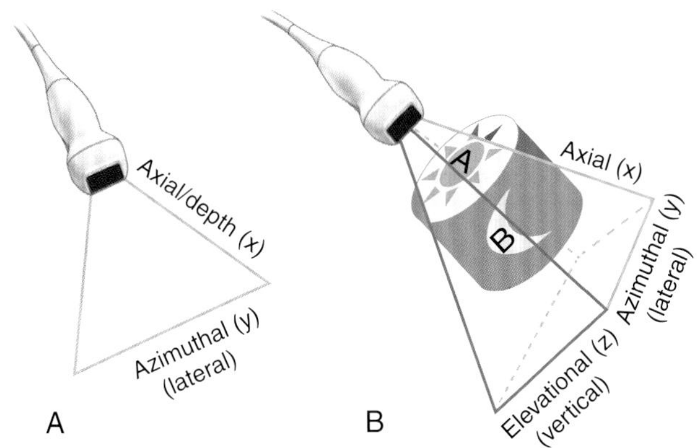

Fig. 1.3 2D and 3D transducers. (A) A 2D transducer can steer and focus in only two directions, axial (x-axis) and azimuthal or lateral (y-axis). (B) 3D transducers generate scan lines that propagate radially (axial) and can be steered in two directions (azimuth or lateral, and elevational), creating a pyramidal coordinate system. In 3DE, image spatial resolution is determined by the direction of the ultrasound beam in relation to the object of interest. If the object is perpendicular to the ultrasound beam, as in object *A*, then the best spatial resolution will be in the axial resolution. In contrast, if the object is parallel to the beam, as in object *B*, then the best resolution will be in the lateral plane.

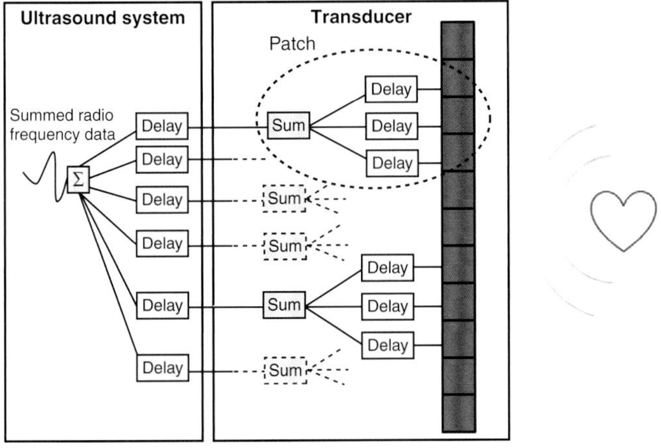

Fig. 1.4 Beamforming in a fully sampled matrix array probe using the cascaded approach. In 3D imaging, the beamforming and steering processes are divided the transducer and the ultrasound system. In the transducer, the 3000 piezoelectric elements, interconnection technology, and fine analog delay circuitry in the single application-specific integrated circuit (ASIC) control transmission and reception of signals by using subsections of the matrix array called patches *(stippled oval)* to control analog microbeamforming and fine steering. Signals from each patch are summed, which reduces the number of control lines required in the transducer coaxial cable that links the transducer to the ultrasound system from 3000 to 128 or 256 channels. Coarse steering is digitally performed within the system, where the analog-to-digital conversion takes place with the use of digital delay lines.

into the ASIC) and summing signals within subsections of the matrix, known as *patches*. This allows the number of cables connecting the transducer to the ultrasound machine to be reduced from 3000 to between 128 and 256. Coarse steering occurs in the ultrasound machine, where digital delay lines convert the analog signals to digital signals.

However, placing the circuitry for microbeamforming in the transducer head generated significant heat proportional to the mechanical index used during imaging. Two different strategies have been taken to address this issue: (1) active cooling, in which the heat is actively transported through the transducer cable, and (2) passive cooling, in which heat production is reduced through improved crystal manufacturing processes that create single-crystal materials with homogenous solid-state domains and piezoelectric properties. These new crystal materials improved the conversion of transmitted power into ultrasound energy and that of received ultrasound into electrical energy. This increase in efficiency during transduction resulted not only in reduced heat production but also in wider bandwidths, increased echo penetration and resolution, improved image quality, reduced artifacts, reduced power consumption, and increased Doppler sensitivity.

More recent developments have resulted in improved sidelobe suppression, increased sensitivity and penetration, and the implementation of harmonic capabilities that can be used for both grayscale and contrast imaging. This has led to significantly smaller matrix transducers with improved image quality and has created the capability for a single transducer to acquire both 2D and 3D images.

RESOLUTION IN 3D ECHOCARDIOGRAPHY

In 3DE, spatial and temporal resolution are inversely linked. Optimizing image quality for either spatial or temporal resolution will adversely affect the quality of the other.

SPATIAL RESOLUTION

The spatial resolution of an imaging system is characterized by its point-spread function. The point-spread function is the image obtained of an infinitesimal point object. A single pixel in an idealized image (point input) will be reproduced as something other than a single pixel in the obtained image. This degree of blurring (spreading) of any point object varies according to the dimensions employed.

Each point in a 3DE pyramidal data set is located using three coordinates (see Fig. 1.3): (1) depth within the 3D volume, which is the distance from the transducer (x-axis); (2) the azimuth plane (y-axis); and (3) the elevation plane (z-axis). Spatial resolution is different along each of these axes and is related to the spacing between scan lines. 3D matrix array transducers generate scan lines that propagate radially (axial direction) and can be steered in two directions: azimuth (lateral) and elevational. Samples within a scan line are more finely spaced, whereas scan lines in the other directions (i.e., elevational or lateral) are farther apart. Overall, the elevational plane has poorer image resolution because the scan lines are farthest apart in this plane.

Generally, spatial resolution along the x-axis is similar to that of 2D scanning, which is one-half wavelength. In the other two planes, it is twofold to threefold worse. The spread in current 3D imaging systems is 0.5 mm in the axial (x) dimension, 2.5 mm in the lateral (y) dimension, and 3 mm in the elevation (z) dimension. Therefore, the best images with minimal blurring are obtained in the axial dimension and the worst ones in the elevation dimension. The portion of an object or region that is perpendicular to the ultrasound beam will be best displayed in the axial resolution, and it will have higher resolution than the region that is parallel (see Fig. 1.3).

In practice, for transthoracic imaging this means that the poorest 3D images are obtained from the apical approach, in which cardiac structures are predominantly imaged using the lateral and elevation dimensions. Conversely, the best 3D images are obtained from the parasternal approach, which uses

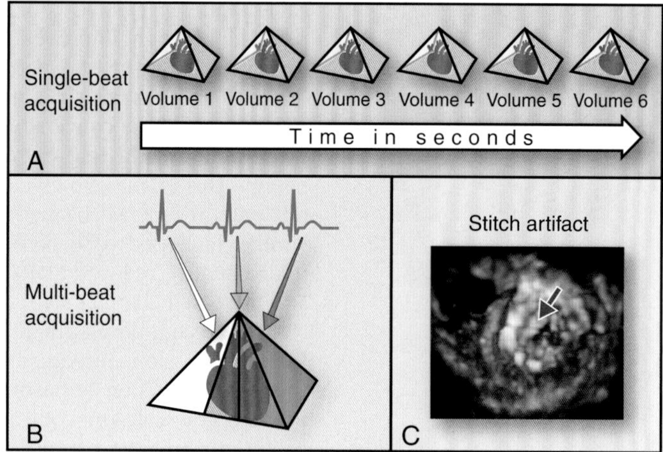

Fig. 1.5 Single-beat versus multibeat acquisition. (A) Single-beat acquisition is the acquisition of multiple 3D volume data sets per second. (B) Multibeat acquisition requires the acquisition of multiple subvolumes, which are then stitched together to form one full volume. (C) Example of a stitch artifact *(red arrow)* in a 3D data set.

the axial and lateral dimensions. For this reason, when using transesophageal echocardiography (TEE), the mitral valve (MV) is visualized with better resolution than the aortic valve (AV).

TEMPORAL RESOLUTION

A major limitation to 3D imaging, and echocardiography in general, is the constant speed of sound in myocardial tissue and blood (1540 m/s). Because of this limitation, the maximum number of pulses that can be transmitted per second without creating interference is obtained by dividing the speed of sound in myocardial tissue and blood by the imaging depth or distance that the pulse has to travel back and forth. The maximum number of pulses limits the number of 3D pyramidal volumes per second that can be imaged given a desired pyramidal size and spatial resolution. Therefore, in 3D imaging, an inverse relationship exists between volume rate (temporal resolution), volume size, and spatial resolution (number of scan lines). However, manufacturers have developed solutions to circumvent the limitation of fixed sound speed. These methods include electrocardiogram (ECG)–gated stitching of subvolumes (multibeat), a real-time zoom feature that reduces the field of view, parallel receive beamforming that allows true real-time large pyramidal (full-volume) acquisition, interpolation of images or image sectors, frame (volume) reordering, virtual array, multiline transmission, and high-pulse repetition frequency. Of these methods, ECG-gating and real-time zoom are options that can be adjusted by the operator. The other methods are either built into the ultrasound system or require post-acquisition software. Each of these methods is discussed in this section except for real-time zoom, which is a pyramidal size option that is discussed in the section on 3D acquisition modes.

Single-Beat or Multibeat Acquisition

Single-beat 3D imaging refers to the acquisition of multiple pyramidal data sets per second during a single heartbeat (Fig. 1.5). This methodology overcomes the limitations imposed by rhythm disturbances or respiratory motion. Historically, its use was limited by poor temporal and spatial resolution; however, technological advances allow current ultrasound machines to acquire 3D data sets of large structures with high temporal resolution using single-beat imaging (Table 1.1).

TABLE 1.1 Strengths and Weaknesses of Single-Beat Versus Multibeat 3D Image Acquisition.

	Single-Beat	*Multibeat*
Artifacts	None	Stitch artifacts from motion or cardiac arrhythmias
Temporal resolution	Lower	Higher

Despite temporal and spatial resolution improvements with single-beat acquisition, multibeat 3D acquisition is still important in patients with structures that require large pyramidal volumes and high temporal resolution. Multibeat acquisitions are pyramidal acquisitions of multiple narrow volumes of data over several heartbeats (ranging from two to six cardiac cycles) that are subsequently stitched together to create a single volumetric data set. In this way, pyramidal volume size can be maintained while the volume rate is increased by obtaining and stitching these subvolumes together. However, multibeat imaging is inherently susceptible to stitch artifacts, which appear as subvolume misalignment and are created by patient or transducer motion, cardiac translation during respiratory or cardiac motion, or changes in cardiac cycle length.

Parallel Beamforming

Parallel beamforming is a method wherein the system transmits one wide beam and receives multiple narrow beams in parallel; this increases the volume rate by a factor equal to the number of receive beams (Fig. 1.6). This parallel processing of the received data allows multiple scan lines to be sampled in the same amount of time that a conventional scanner would take to create a single line. It is achieved by having each beamformer focus along a slightly different direction that was insonified by the broad transmit pulse. However, as the receive beams are steered farther and farther away from the center of the transmit beam, lower energy signals are received, resulting in a reduction of signal strength and resolution. Increasing temporal resolution by increasing the number of parallel beams requires an increase in the size, cost, and power consumption of the beamforming electronics, thereby decreasing the signal-to-noise ratio and the contrast resolution.

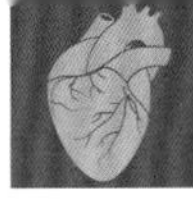

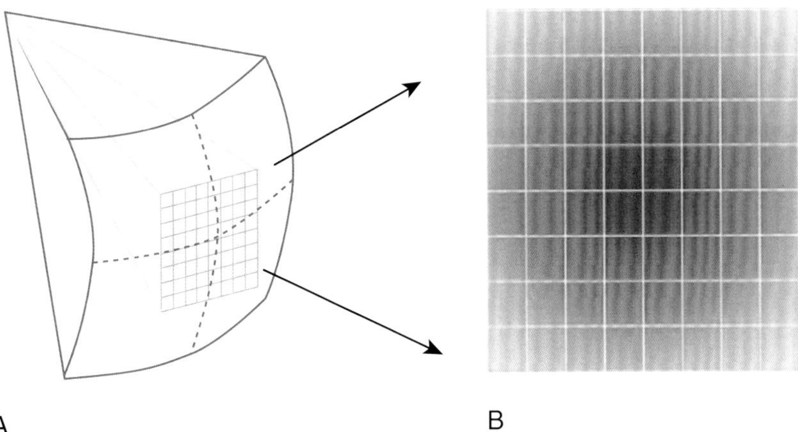

Fig. 1.6 Parallel beamforming. (A) For each transmitted ultrasound pulse, 64 beams are received in parallel. Increasing the number of parallel beams improves the frame rate but leads to an increase in size, cost, and power consumption of the beamforming electronics and broadens the transmit beam. It also results in deterioration in the signal-to-noise ratio and the contrast resolution due to the broader transmit beam. (B) The amplitude of the broader transmit beam is highest *(red)* in the center and lowest *(blue)* in the periphery, which results in lower energy signals from the parallel receiving beams steered farther away from the center of the beam.

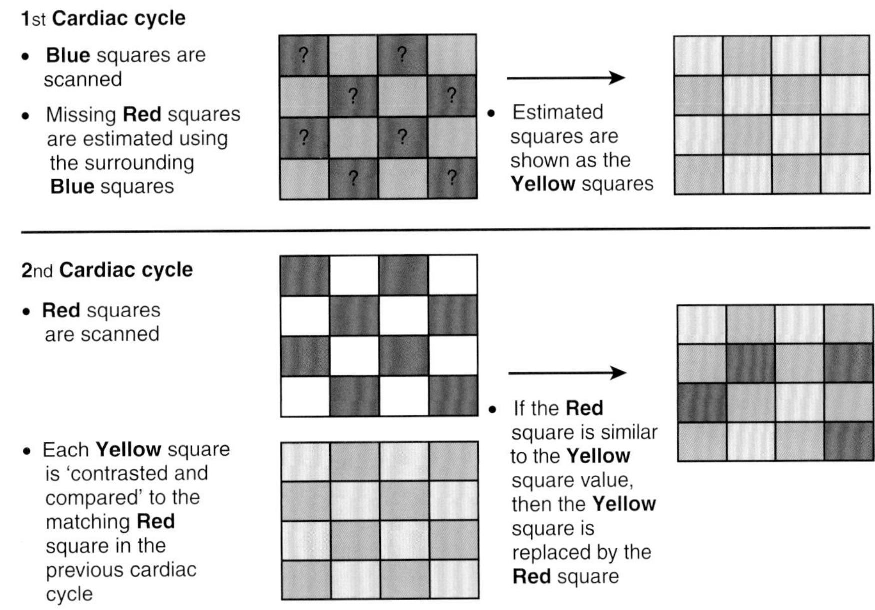

Fig. 1.7 Interpolation of image sectors. Schematic diagram shows how interpolation of image sectors occurs.

Interpolation of Images or Image Sectors

Interpolation is a function in which unknown points are estimated by using known data. In 3DE, this occurs by interpolating results for either image subsections or frames between those acquired. When interpolation occurs within a matrix array, the array functions like a checkerboard (Fig. 1.7). During the first cardiac cycle, some elements are active, and the nonactive elements are interpolated. During the next cardiac cycle, the initially nonactive elements become active, and their results are compared with the interpolated image. If the data acquired by the initially nonactive elements improves the 3D image, those data are used. Otherwise the interpolated data remains in use. Limiting the number of active elements results in faster processing, allowing more volumes to be acquired over a given period of time, thereby increasing the temporal resolution. Similarly, interpolation can be used to construct intermediate volumes from adjacent volumes.

Frame Reordering

In frame reordering, a high frame (volume) rate algorithm is used. It reorders 3D volumes of a periodically moving cardiac structure taken at a number of instants over several cardiac cycles.[17] All of the volumes used are acquired ad hoc, without ECG-gating at different time periods. This results in faster acquisition times (tenths of a second) and volume rates that are higher than those typically achieved by the ultrasound system during a single cardiac cycle. The algorithm functions by identifying the temporal sequence of volumes on either side of the ECG R wave and interleaving these volumes into a coherent ordering with respect to the R-wave peak. By reordering only those frames close to the QRS, the beat-to-beat time interval variability is removed. This results in an increase in 3D volume rate from 10 to 540 frames per second (fps). Weaknesses inherent to this method include the 20-minute processing time per sequence, low beat-to-beat variability of the heart or cardiac

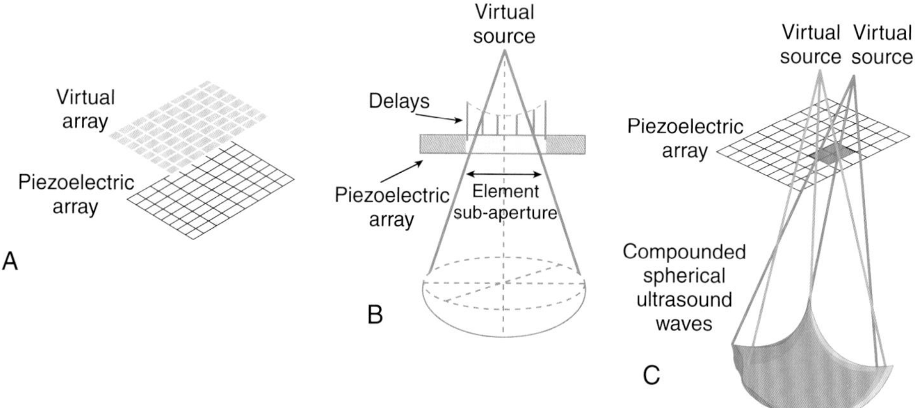

Fig. 1.8 Virtual array. (A) A virtual array is located behind the probe and is used to artificially form an entire imaging volume. (B) For each individual virtual source, delays are computed and a sub-aperture is defined. (C) When the distance between the virtual source and the physical probe is small, the sub-aperture is smaller and the curvature of the emitted waveform is larger, resulting in a wider field of view at the cost of low propagation energy.

structure of interest within the QRS complex, and other factors that affect temporal coherence. An advantage of this methodology is that it can be performed with a standard 3DE ultrasound system and a standard computer.

Additionally, the same algorithm can be used to reorder subcomponents of the 3D volume to improve image quality. In 3DE, different parts of the volume are acquired at different times because of the manner in which scan lines are sent, read, and composed into a Cartesian volume format. Because the frames are not simultaneously acquired, it is possible for individual voxels in a frame to be slightly out of sequence. Reordering these voxels or a subcomponent instead of whole frames can be a solution to this problem.

Virtual Array

Current commercial 3DE ultrasound systems typically rely on hardware-based focused ultrasound beams, limiting the volume rate to a few tens of volumes per second. In contrast, high-volume-rate (ultrafast) 3DE images are those in which thousands of volumes are acquired per second. This is achieved through the transmission of a small number of defocused ultrasound waves that insonify the entire volume of interest.[18] With this method, dynamic focusing is performed in the receive mode. During transmit mode, the coherent synthetic summation of the ultrasonic volume acquired for each transmission occurs, allowing for the restoration of a dynamic focus without compromising the ultrafast volume rate. This is achieved through the use of a virtual array located behind the probe.[18,19]

The virtual array is used to synthetically form the entire imaging volume (Fig. 1.8). For each individual virtual source, delays are computed and a sub-aperture is defined. When the virtual sources are located far behind the probe, a larger sub-aperture is present; this results in greater emitted energy and a smaller field of view. When virtual sources are located near the physical probe, the sub-aperture used is smaller, and the curvature of the emitted waveform is increased. This results in the insonification of a large field of view at the cost of a lower propagated energy. In the extreme case of sources located at infinity behind the probe, tilted plane waves are obtained.

Although this method allows for a high volume rate, limitations still exist with respect to the balance among contrast, resolution, volume rate, and field of view. Additionally, the use of defocused waves may result in poor image quality because of the wide lateral spreading of the transmitted energy, possible high side lobes and motion artifacts, and inability to generate second harmonics. However, this method holds promise because it allows mapping of blood flow and tissue motion in the entire 3D field of view.

Multiline Transmission

Multiline transmission is a technique in which multiple ultrasound pulses focused along different steering directions are transmitted simultaneously.[20–22] The gain in volume (frame) rate is equal to the number of beams. Traditional multiline transmission is susceptible to crosstalk artifacts, which result from the interactions among the ultrasound fields on transmit and receive waveforms. This can be eliminated by simultaneously transmitting beams along the transverse diagonal of the transducer.

High Pulse Repetition Frequency

This method increases color Doppler volume rates by combining multiple narrow beams with high pulse repetition frequency (PRF).[23,24] With high PRF, pulses are transmitted with three times the frequency that is needed to allow the echo from the farthest depth to return. For example, if two pulses are emitted, the echo from the first pulse will return from the farthest depth at the same time the echo from the second pulse returns from an intermediate depth. When this occurs, there is no way to determine whether the signal originates from the deepest level or the intermediate level. The high PRF increases the Nyquist limit, thereby shortening the acquisition time. This method has been demonstrated to have high accuracy compared with cardiac magnetic resonance in quantifying aortic regurgitation.[25]

RELATIONSHIP BETWEEN SPATIAL AND TEMPORAL RESOLUTION

Overall, the relationships among volume rate, number of parallel receive beams, sector width, depth, and line density are described by the following equation:

$$\text{Volume rate} = (1540 \times \text{Number of parallel receive beams}) / [2(\text{Volume width}/\text{Lateral resolution})^2 \times \text{Volume depth}]$$

Thus, on an ultrasound machine, volume rates can be increased by decreasing volume depth or width or by reducing the number of parallel receive beams (Fig. 1.9). However, adjusting the parallel receive beams affects the signal-to-noise ratio, altering image quality. Similarly, changing the scan-line density in the pyramid can alter lateral resolution and affect image contrast.

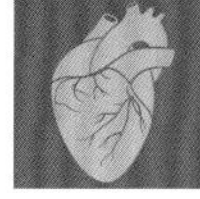

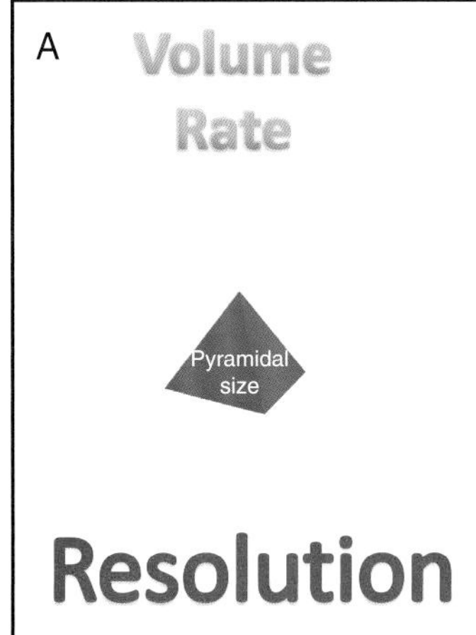

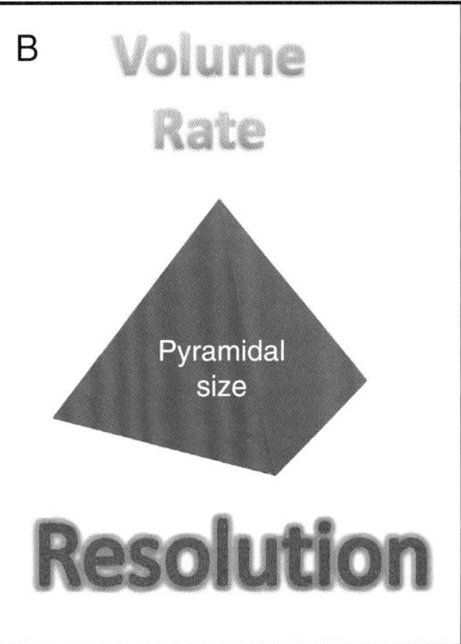

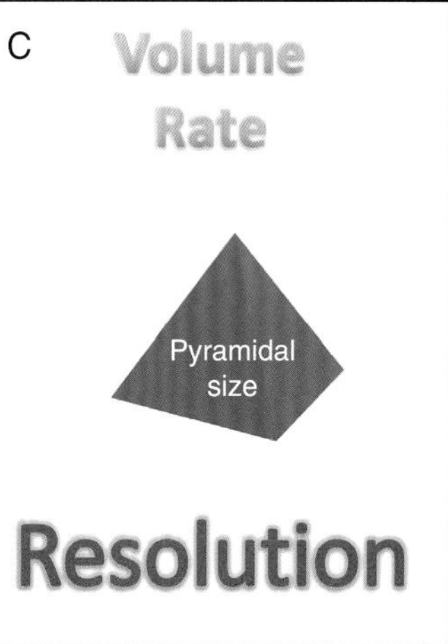

Fig. 1.9 **Relationship between temporal and spatial resolution.** (A) Volume rate (temporal resolution), pyramidal or volume size, and lateral and spatial resolution (scan-line density) are all interrelated, and changes in one affect the others. (B) Volume rate can be maintained when increasing pyramidal size by decreasing lateral resolution through lower scan-line density. (C) Alternatively, volume rate can be maintained with less lateral resolution loss by not increasing pyramid size as large as that in panel B.

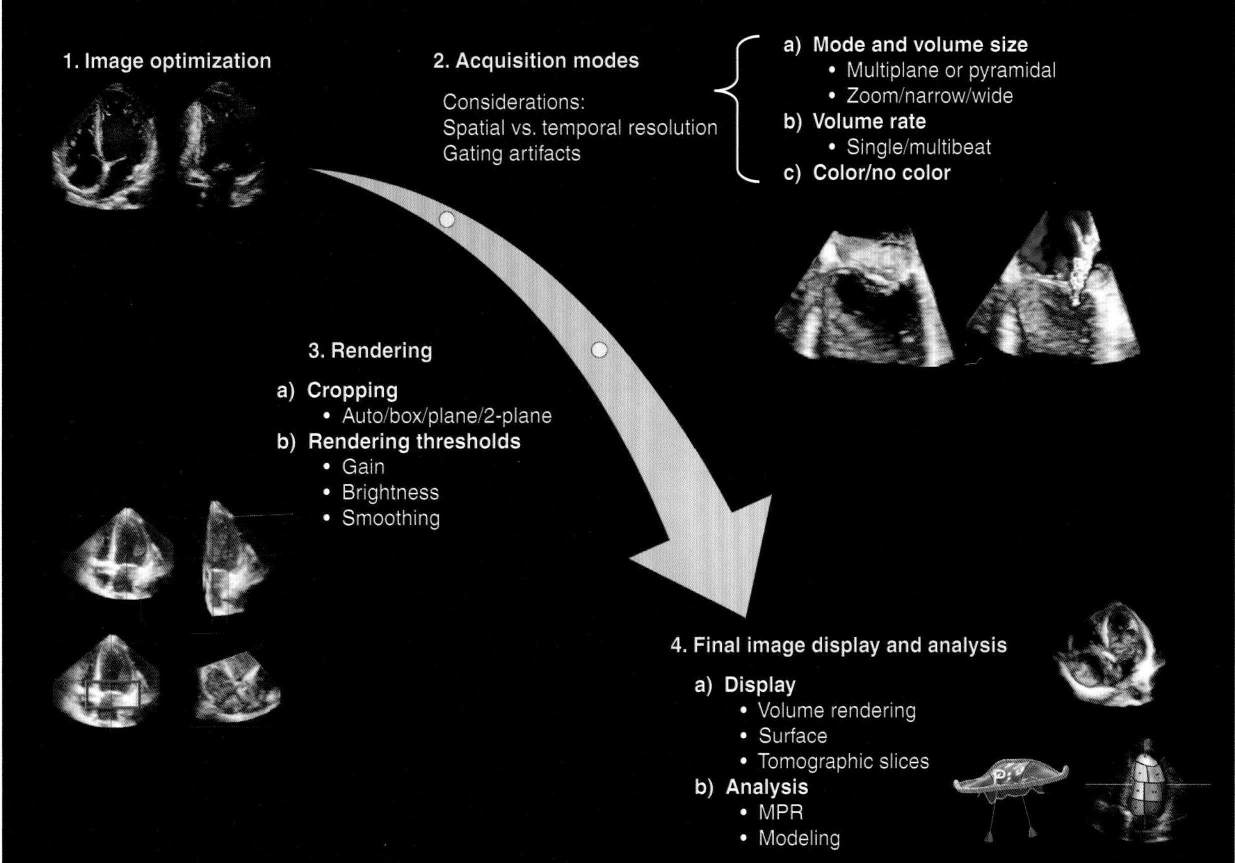

Fig. 1.10 **Steps for 3DE data acquisition.** The steps for 3DE data acquisition are (1) 2D image optimization; (2) decision making regarding volume size and volume rate, which also depend on whether color Doppler images will be obtained; (3) optimization of the 3D image through cropping and adjustment of rendering thresholds; and (4) display and analysis of the 3D data set. *MPR*, Multiplanar reconstruction.

MULTIVIEW 3D ECHOCARDIOGRAPHY IMAGE FUSION

Whereas the discussions here involve 3DE images that are obtained using pyramidal volumes, 3D images can also be generated by fusing multiple 2D images.[26] Typically, these image fusion systems require post-acquisition reconstruction of 2D images acquired with the use of a 2D transducer that is tracked in three dimensions by a spatial tracking system.[27,28] This was the methodology used initially to create 3DE images, but it is now used to improve image quality of structures that are challenging to image, such as the right ventricle.[29–31]

3D ECHOCARDIOGRAPHY DATA ACQUISITION

Overall, 3DE data acquisition can be divided into four main steps (Fig. 1.10). First, the 2D image should be optimized.

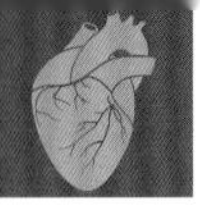

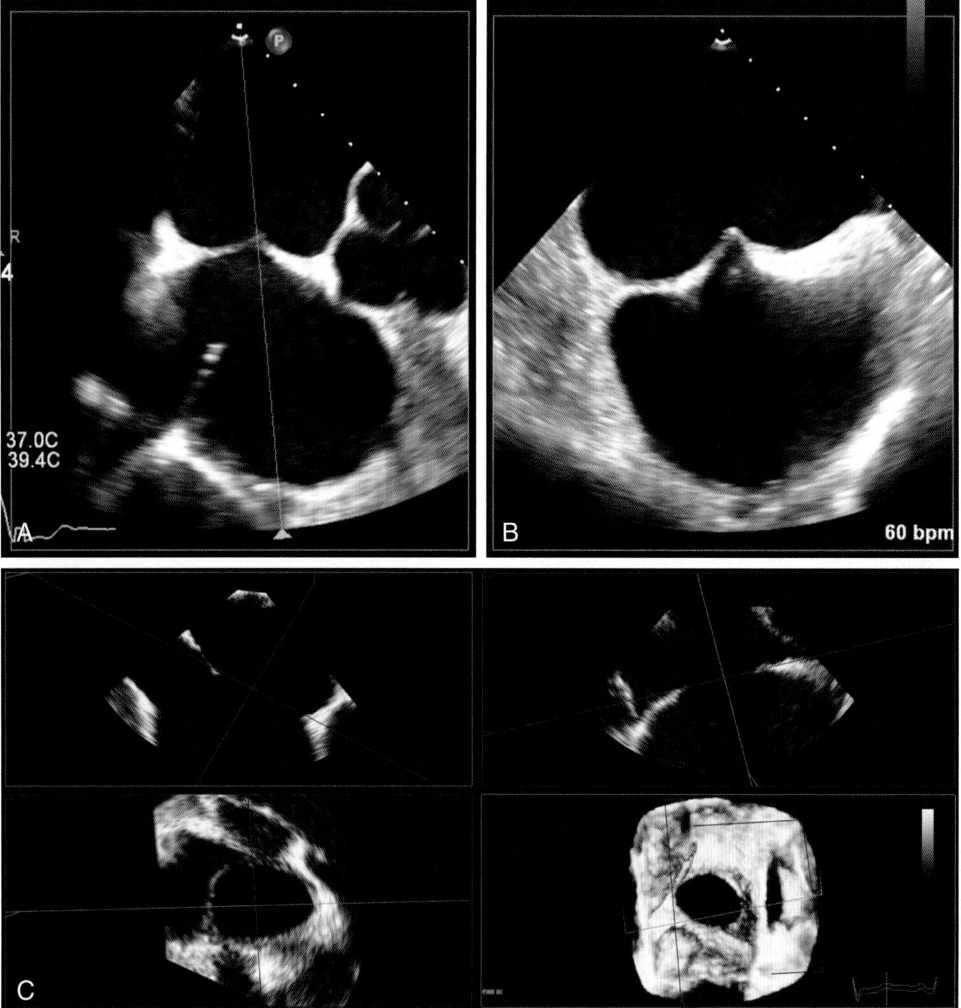

Fig. 1.11 Simultaneous multiplane imaging allows visualization of two to three planes in B-mode. One image is typically the reference view, whereas the other images represent planes rotated at any angle from the reference plane. In this example, an interatrial septal puncture is being performed. In the reference view (A), the catheter appears to be centered in the middle of the septum and away from the aortic root. The cross-sectional view (B), which includes the superior vena cava, demonstrates that the puncture is not too superior. Multiplane images can also be used to optimize placement of the planes to acquire measurements from 3DE data sets. (C) In this example, the planes are aligned to measure the dimensions of an interatrial septal defect. The measurements should be taken from the two cross-sectional planes rather than the en face view of the entire defect because those planes have higher resolution.

Second, based on the structure evaluated, a choice should be made with respect to acquisition viewing mode (multiplane or pyramidal volume) and volume size. These choices will be affected by whether 3D color Doppler images will be obtained. Subsequently, decisions should be made to optimize volume rate (e.g., single vs. multibeat, scan-line density adjustment). Third, depending on the structure of interest, the 3D data set may be cropped and the image optimized. Fourth, the optimal method for displaying the 3D data is determined, and, if needed, the 3D data should be analyzed.

2D IMAGE OPTIMIZATION

2D image quality should be optimized before acquisition of the 3DE data set. Acoustic shadowing and other noise on the 2D image will also appear within the 3D data set.[32] Image optimization can be achieved by using breathing maneuvers to minimize transducer motion and through adjustments to regional and global gain. Most importantly, when setting up the 3D acquisition, multiplane visualization should be used to ensure that the planes perpendicular to the original reference imaging plane are also optimized. This ensures that the entire structure of interest will be included in the 3D pyramid.

3D ACQUISITION MODES

Simultaneous Multiplane Mode

Simultaneous multiplane imaging permits visualization of two to three planes in B-mode or color flow Doppler echocardiography. The first image is typically a reference view of a particular structure, whereas the other images represent planes rotated at any angle from the reference plane (Fig. 1.11 and Table 1.2). Multiplane imaging in the elevation plane is also available.

Pyramidal Size

As described previously, pyramidal size affects spatial and temporal resolution.[33] Ideally, the smallest pyramid that captures the information required should be used. Although original 3DE acquisition was limited to three relatively fixed pyramidal sizes, these and other options are now available on ultrasound equipment as starting points for further adjustment of the pyramidal size. All of these sizes can be acquired using single-beat or multibeat approaches to increase spatial and temporal resolution. Three basic pyramidal sizes are briefly described here (Fig. 1.12 and Table 1.3).

TABLE 1.2 Uses of Multiplane Mode.

Pre-acquisition	• Ensure that the cardiac structure of interest is contained within the 3D pyramid.
Post-acquisition	• Ensure that the structure of interest is contained within the 3D pyramid. • Assess for stitch artifacts when using multibeat acquisition.
Analysis	• Obtain true 2D cross-sectional measurements (e.g., biplane LV ejection fraction) from the 3D data sets. • Display the structure of interest in two cross-sectional 2D planes. • Accurately localize mitral/aortic valve pathology with cross-sectional 2D planes. • Obtain en face measurements of stenotic orifice area, regurgitant orifice area, and vena contracta area.
Interventional procedures	• Assist with identifying the puncture site of the interatrial septum. • Assess placement of atrial septal defect/patent foramen ovale closure devices. • Assess placement of devices such as mitral clips or percutaneous mitral valves. • Assess paravalvular regurgitation after transcatheter aortic valve placement.

Zoom

Zoom is typically the smallest pyramidal size available for acquisition (~30 by 30 degrees) and is used for small cardiac structures. It increases temporal and spatial resolution by decreasing the region of interest in both the azimuth and elevation planes. However, there can be a loss of spatial resolution if the sector is magnified greatly.

Narrow Sector

Depending on the vendor, the narrow sector is also called *bird's eye* or *live mode*. Historically, this size permitted real-time display of a pyramidal volume of 30-to-50 degrees by 60-to-90 degrees. This mode allows imaging of a narrow region of the structure of interest plus the surrounding areas, so is ideal for use during percutaneous procedures.

Wide Sector

Depending on the vendor, the wide sector is also called *full volume* or *large mode*. This pyramidal size is the largest acquisition sector possible and is best used for structures such as the left or right ventricle. The wide sector data set can be cropped or multiplane transected to remove tissue planes; this allows one to identify or extract components of valvular structures within the volume or to visualize 2D cross-sectional x, y, and orthogonal planes using off-line analysis software.

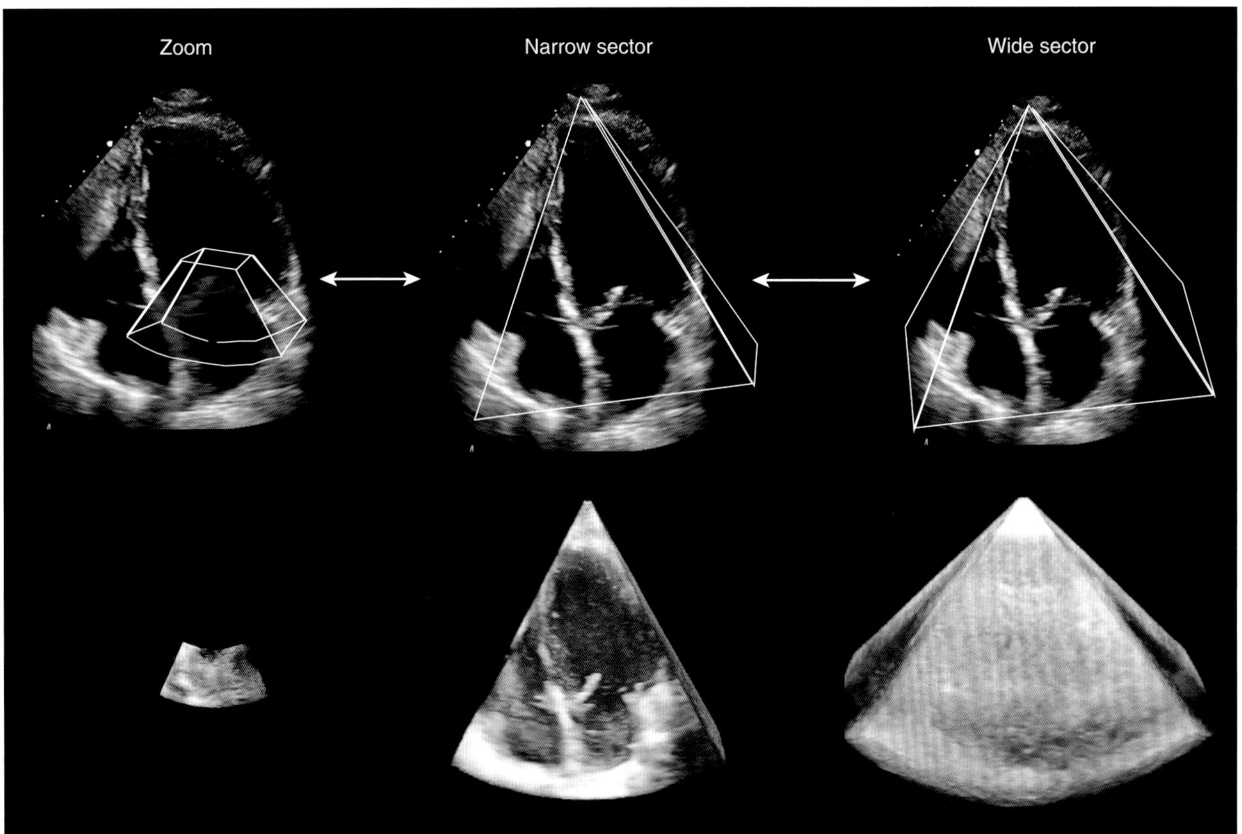

Fig. 1.12 Pyramidal volume size. Pyramidal sizes are a continuum from very small (zoom) to the largest size possible (wide sector). Zoom is ideal for 3D imaging acquisition of valves. Narrow sector is useful for percutaneous procedures, and wide sector is used for imaging larger structures such as the LV. The video demonstrates the loss in volume rate with changes in pyramid size using single-beat acquisition. With the smallest pyramid size (zoomed mode), the volume rate is highest at 38 Hz (Video 1.12A). With a larger pyramid size, the volume rate decreases to 22 Hz (Video 1.12B). With the largest pyramid size, the volume rate is only 9 Hz (Video 1.12C).

TABLE 1.3 Choice of 3D Pyramidal Volume Size Based on Cardiac Structure.

Pyramidal Size	*Cardiac Structure*	*Strengths*	*Weaknesses*
Zoom	• Valves • Interatrial septum • Interventricular septum	• Increased temporal resolution	• Loss of spatial resolution with excessive magnification • Loss of orientation
Narrow sector	• Interventional procedures	• Visualization of region of interest and adjacent related anatomy	• Insufficient size to cover an entire structure
Wide sector	• LV • RV • Entire heart	• Complete visualization of large cardiac structures and adjacent anatomy	• Low volume rate

TABLE 1.4 Choice of Temporal and Spatial Resolution Based on the Cardiac Issue Studied.

Issue	*Requirements*	*Reason*	*Possible Solutions*
Left and right cardiac chamber volumes	High temporal resolution with a large pyramidal size	To capture true end-diastole and end-systole	Multibeat acquisition High-volume-rate methods (e.g., parallel beamforming, virtual apex) Decreased line density
Small, highly mobile cardiac structure (e.g., valves, vegetation)	High spatial and temporal resolution	To visualize small mobile structures	Decreased pyramidal size Use high-volume-rate method (e.g., multibeat) Increased line density

COLOR-FLOW DOPPLER

Currently, 3DE color Doppler imaging can be acquired with one to six individual gated volumes. Volume rate differences between color Doppler and noncolor 3D volumes that are otherwise acquired with identical parameters may or may not be significant depending on the ultrasound machine vendor. Traditionally, there is a reduction in volume rate when 3D color Doppler imaging is used.

CHALLENGES WITH 3D ECHOCARDIOGRAPHY ACQUISITION

Temporal Versus Spatial Resolution

The main trade-off in 3DE imaging is between temporal resolution (volume rate) and spatial resolution (Table 1.4; see also Fig. 1.9). As discussed previously, improvements in spatial resolution can be achieved by increasing the scan-line density of the 3D volume. However, with this method it takes longer to acquire and process the image, limiting the overall volume rate. By decreasing the 3D volume size, volume rates can be increased while maintaining spatial resolution. Volume rates can also be increased through the use of ECG-gating (multibeat acquisition). To prevent artifacts secondary to ECG-gating, ultrasound companies have developed technology and methods that allow acquisition of single-beat, wide-sector 3D pyramidal data with high spatial and temporal resolution.

ECG-Gating and Breath-Hold

ECG-gated data sets are challenging in patients who are unable to hold their breaths or have arrhythmias, as this can result in stitch artifacts (see Fig. 1.5). Gating artifacts are best identified using multiplane viewing. Typically, subsectors are acquired in sweep planes parallel to the reference image. Thus, stitch lines are parallel to the reference imaging plane and therefore can only be identified from planes perpendicular to the sweep/reference plane. Gating artifacts can be also minimized by optimizing the ECG tracing so that a distinct R wave is present and by minimizing patient and probe motion.

TABLE 1.5 Challenges with 3D Image Optimization Options.

Option	*Increase*	*Decrease*
Gain	Loss of resolution Loss of 3D perspective/depth	Dropout
Brightness	White out, loss of depth	Image too dark
Smoothing	Loss of texture/details of the structure under study	Overidentification of abnormalities

3D IMAGE OPTIMIZATION

The goal of 3D image optimization should be to adjust the 3D rendering of the data set to give it a 3D appearance while simultaneously removing artifacts. Typically, these adjustments can be performed before or after the 3D data set acquisition. The settings available vary depending on the ultrasound vendor. However, core settings available across vendors that may need adjustments include gain, brightness, smoothing, colorization, and compression (Table 1.5). In practice, with current ultrasound systems, gain is the setting that most often requires adjustment because available presets provide adequate image quality.

GAIN

Gain is the amplification of the electronic signal generated from the echo that returns to the body. Low gain settings can result in echo dropout, which may artificially eliminate anatomic structures that cannot be recovered during postprocessing (Fig. 1.13). With excess gain there is a decrease in resolution and a loss of 3D perspective or depth within the data set. Gain can be adjusted using either overall gain or time gain compensation (TGC) settings. TGC alters the sensitivity at each depth, thereby allowing for compensation from uneven signal loss. Overall gain can be adjusted before or after acquisition, whereas TGC can be adjusted only before acquisition. Ideally, gain settings should be set in the midrange (50 Units) and optimized with slightly higher time gain controls to enable the greatest flexibility with postprocessing gain and compression. Therefore, it is recommended to slightly overcompensate the brightness of the image with the time gain controls rather than by using

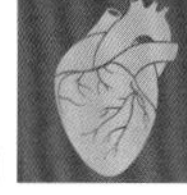

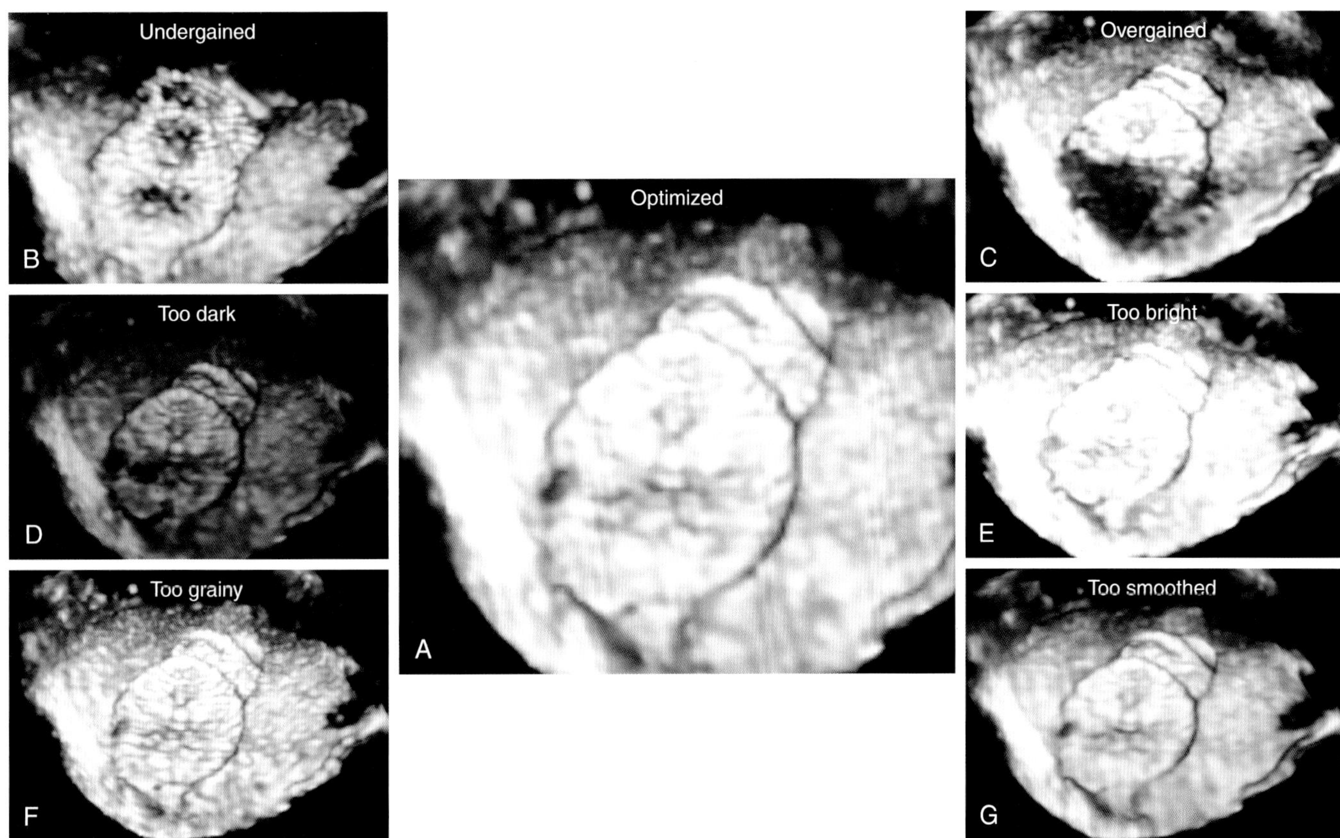

Fig. 1.13 3D volume-rendered settings. These images demonstrate the effects of brightness, gain, and smoothing rendering thresholds on a volume-rendered 3D TTE image of an undersized interatrial septal defect closure device in which both sides of the device are visible. (A) Optimized image. Low gain on the 3DE image (B) results in echo dropout, whereas excess gain (C) decreases resolution and obscures the structure of interest. When brightness is too low (D), the structure appears too dark, as if in a shadow. Conversely, if brightness is too high (E), the appearance of 3D depth is lost, similar to having a very bright light shining on an object. (F) When smoothing is decreased, more details of these atrial septal closure devices can be best appreciated, but this also increases graininess of the other structures. (G) Increasing smoothing excessively reduces the texture of the atrial septal closure device. Video 1.13A shows a volume-rendered 3D TTE data set of the tricuspid valve as viewed from the right ventricle, that has been undergained. The tricuspid valve leaflets have areas of dropout. When gain is too high, there is too much noise in the ventricle, and the leaflets cannot be seen (Video 1.13B). When gain is optimized, the edges and body of the leaflets are even and are seen well throughout the cardiac cycle (Video 1.13C).

the power-output gain. As with 2D imaging, the optimization of lateral and axial resolution is important during 3D image acquisition.

BRIGHTNESS

Brightness is the equivalent of having a spotlight on the cardiac structure of interest. If brightness is too high, then there is a loss of 3D depth appearance (see Fig. 1.13). If the brightness is set too low, then the structure appears too dark or in a shadow, resulting in an inadequate 3D appearance.

SMOOTHING

Smoothing adjusts the 3D rendering by altering the texture of the cardiac structure. When smoothing is increased, there is a loss of roughness, and the surface of the cardiac structure appears more regular (see Fig. 1.13). In contrast, when smoothing is decreased, irregularities in cardiac structures become more apparent. If the 3D rendering is too smoothed, it runs the risk of appearing artificial and losing the fine details of the structure under study. The appearance of small mobile irregularities may be missed. However, abnormalities may be overidentified if smoothing is decreased too much.

COLORIZATION

Changing the colorization setting results in changes to the predefined chroma maps, which are applied to the image to highlight the data. Typically, the default is a sepia-type tone, although some users prefer a grayscale appearance for color Doppler imaging.

3D ECHOCARDIOGRAPHIC IMAGE DISPLAY

DATA SET CROPPING

Cropping plays an important role in displaying a structure of interest that is located within the 3D pyramidal volume. It allows the cardiac structure of interest to be presented such that the viewer can appreciate its anatomy and how it relates to the surrounding structures. Cropping can be performed before or after 3D data acquisition. If it is performed before acquisition, the cropped image is immediately available without the need for post-processing; however, data that have been cropped are not recoverable after acquisition. Typically, cropping is performed after data acquisition, because acquisition modes such as zoom can be used to obtain a small data set of interest that can be displayed immediately after acquisition. However, a common error in cropping is

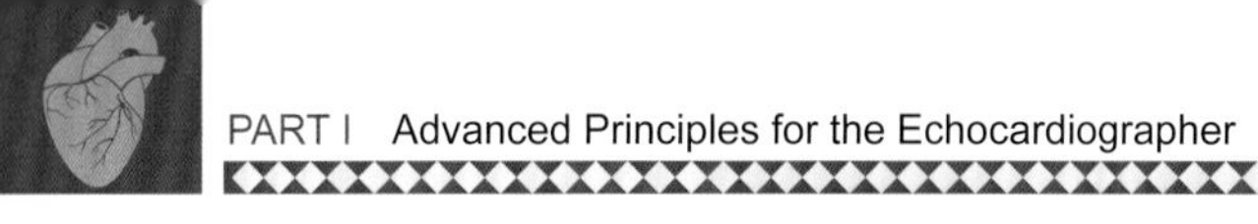

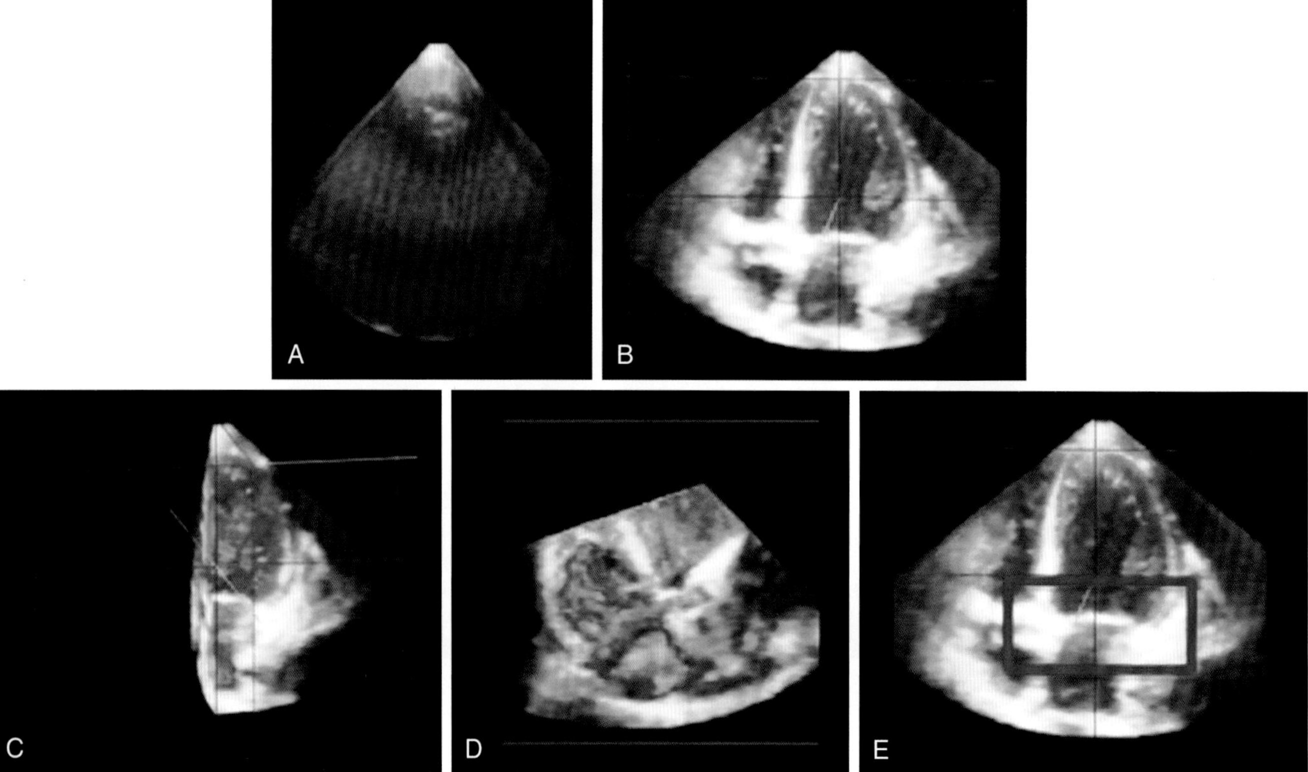

Fig. 1.14 Cropping methods. A 3DE data set (A) can be cropped by several methods. (B) Autocrop automatically cuts the pyramidal data set to the midpoint, with the cut plane parallel to the reference plane. In this case, the reference plane was the apical 4-chamber view. (C) In the box crop method, the crop plane cuts into the data set along the x-, y-, or z-axes, in this case the *red* and *green* planes. (D) The plane crop method allows cropping in any angle. In this example, the tops of the right and left ventricles have been removed with an off-axis cut plane. (E) Two-plane or quick crop methods simplify the number of steps required to crop around an object. In this example, the mitral valve was chosen as the object of interest and all structure outside the red planes will be removed.

to acquire a pyramidal data set that is cropped too tightly around the structure of interest. This results in a loss of perspective and a lessened ability to visualize the relationship with surrounding structures, which makes it difficult to orient a reader who is unfamiliar with the case when later reviewing the 3DE images.

The approach to cropping depends on what viewing perspective is required, which in turn depends on the structure under inspection. The viewing perspective for 3DE images is from the chamber that is in immediate continuity with the region of interest. For example, to visualize the MV en face, the data set needs to be cropped to remove the apex of the heart and half of the atria. By doing this, the MV can be visualized as if "looking down" from the surgeon's or left atrial (LA) perspective or "looking up" from the left ventricular (LV) apex. One of the greatest advantages of 3DE imaging is that the interpreter is not limited by the use of traditional cross-sectional visualization planes.

Cropping can be performed by several methods: autocrop, box crop, plane crop, and two-plane crop (Fig. 1.14 and Table 1.6). These methods may have different names according to the ultrasound system being used, but they are the ones most commonly available. Autocrop automatically crops the dataset to the center of the pyramid plane. It was used to quickly visualize the acquired 3DE dataset quality. While still available on some systems, it is not as widely used now with the ability to acquire in multiplane mode.

Box Crop

Box crop allows cropping of the pyramidal data set along the x-, y-, or z-axes with the center of these planes in the center of the pyramid. This cropping method is ideal when the structure of interest is aligned with the x-, y-, and z-axes. However, if the structure of interest is off-axis, then alignment of the crop plane is not parallel to it, making it difficult to adequately expose the structure of interest without removing essential parts.

TABLE 1.6 Cropping Methods.

Option	*Function*	*Use*
Autocrop	Crops to the middle of the acquired pyramid	• Evaluates 3D image quality • Displays structures that are centered in the pyramid
Box crop	Crops along the x-, y-, or z-axis with the center of these planes in the center of the pyramid	• Displays structures that are aligned along the x-, y-, or z-axis in the pyramid
Plane crop	Freehand cropping	• Displays structures that are not aligned in the x-, y-, or z-axis in the pyramid • Removes artifacts
Two-plane crop	Crops data on two sides of an object of interest	• Convenient for quick visualization • Useful for inexperienced croppers

Plane Crop

Plane crop is the one of the most flexible cropping tools available. This cropping method allows cropping to be performed in any angle, because the cropping plane is not limited in positioning. This method should be used to crop data sets if the structure

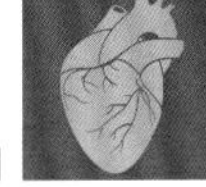

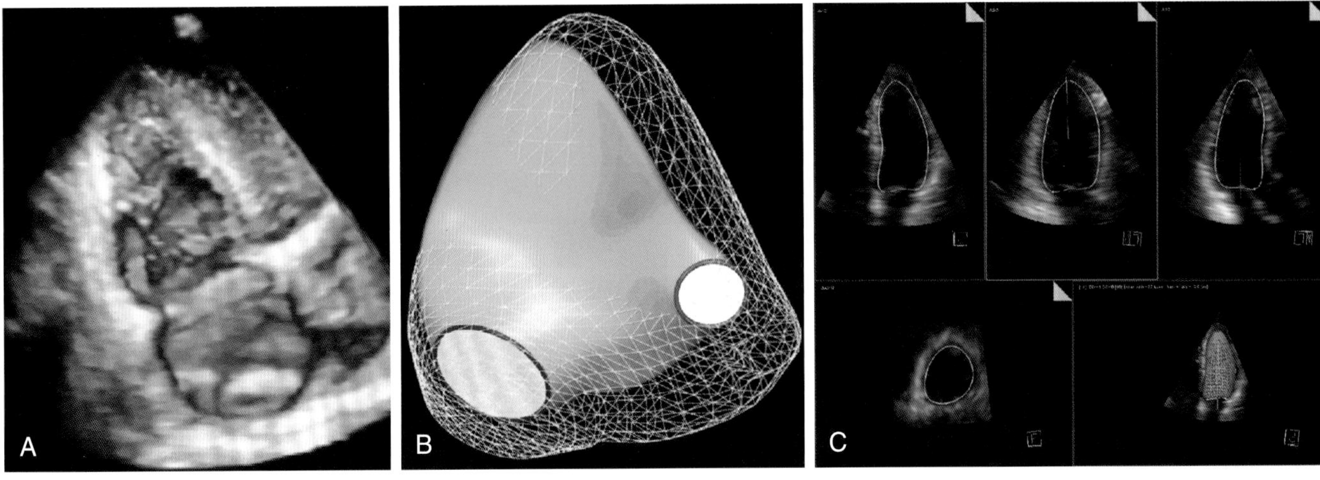

Fig. 1.15 3D image display. (A) Volume rendering of the RV. (B) Surface rendering of the RV with a wire frame appearance in diastole and a solid appearance in systole. (C) 2D tomographic 4-, 2-, and 3-chamber reconstructed slices from a 3D LV data set.

of interest is oddly positioned or if irregular artifacts need to be removed to visualize the structure of interest.

Quick Cropping Methods

Two-plane crop is also known on various ultrasound systems as *QuickVue* or *2-point crop.* This method simplifies the number of steps required to crop on two sides of an object of interest. Using this option, the user simply chooses two points on either side of the object of interest positioned within a large 3D pyramidal data set. This results in 2 planes with retention of only structures between the planes. Similarly, quick cropping can be done using pre-formed boxes (i.e., iCrop) that can be adjusted with elimination of all data outside the box. These methods are convenient for quick visualization of small structures such as valves.

POST-ACQUISITION DISPLAY

After the 3DE data set has been acquired, a number of 3D visualization and rendering software packages can be used to display the 3D data. These packages can be divided into three broad categories: (1) volume rendering, (2) surface rendering (including wire frame display), and (3) 2D tomographic slices (Fig. 1.15). The choice of display technique is generally determined by the clinical application.

Volume Rendering

3DE data are presented as volume-rendered images on 3D ultrasound machines. Volume rendering is the technique that preserves all the 3D information of the imaged structure when it is projected onto a 2D plane for viewing. Typically, it aims to make the structure of interest appear as lifelike as possible.[34] Volume rendering is achieved by using different types of algorithms (e.g., ray casting, shear-warp), all of which function essentially as follows. First, the algorithm "casts" a light beam through the collected voxels. Then, all voxels along each light beam are weighted to obtain a voxel gradient intensity that is integrated with different levels of opacification, shading, and lighting. This process allows an individual structure to appear solid (i.e., tissue) or transparent (i.e., blood pool). Last, a variety of shading techniques (distance shading, gray-level gradient coding, and texture shading) are used to generate a 3D display of the depths and textures of cardiac structures (Fig. 1.16).

Depending on the acquisition, volume-rendered data may or may not require cropping before presentation. If cropping is required, the user can manually crop and rotate the 3D data set or use the programs provided by some ultrasound systems that automatically crop and present the AV or MV in the correct orientation in both en face views. There are also options to automatically present the 2-, 3-, or 4-chamber views.

Surface Rendering

Surface rendering is a visualization technique that shows surfaces of structures in a solid or wire frame appearance. To use this technique, segmentation of the data set is needed to identify the structure of interest. Typically, manual, semiautomated, or fully automated border detection algorithms are used to trace the borders in cross-sectional images generated from the 3D data set to obtain contours of the structure of interest. These contours are combined to generate a 3D shape that can be visualized as either a solid or a wire frame object. Wire frame reconstruction is used to generate 3D images of subsets of the entire data set in a cagelike picture.

There are two advantages to using this technique. First, solid and wire frame surface rendering techniques provide a stereoscopic appearance that allows appreciation of the shape and extent of cardiac motion (i.e., cardiac chamber volume changes) during the cardiac cycle. This can improve the visual assessment of left and right ventricular shape and structure. Second, as the structures of interest are segmented, quantitative information is obtained and can be presented. Not only do models of the MV with color-encoded parametric maps of leaflet displacement demonstrate the anatomy and provide visual cues of the severity, but the measurements can be used for clinical decision making (Fig. 1.17).[35,36] One limitation to surface-rendered images is that they frequently fail to provide details of cardiac textures.

2D Tomographic Slices

3D data sets can be sliced or cropped to obtain multiple simultaneous 2D views of the same 3D structure. On various ultrasound systems this option is known as *multislice* or *iSlice.* With this presentation choice, a single 3D acquisition from any acoustic window can provide 2D cut planes in any traditional or nontraditional view desired. This is not only timesaving but also reduces the need to acquire multiple 2D images from multiple acoustic windows. Additionally, some of the unique 2D cut

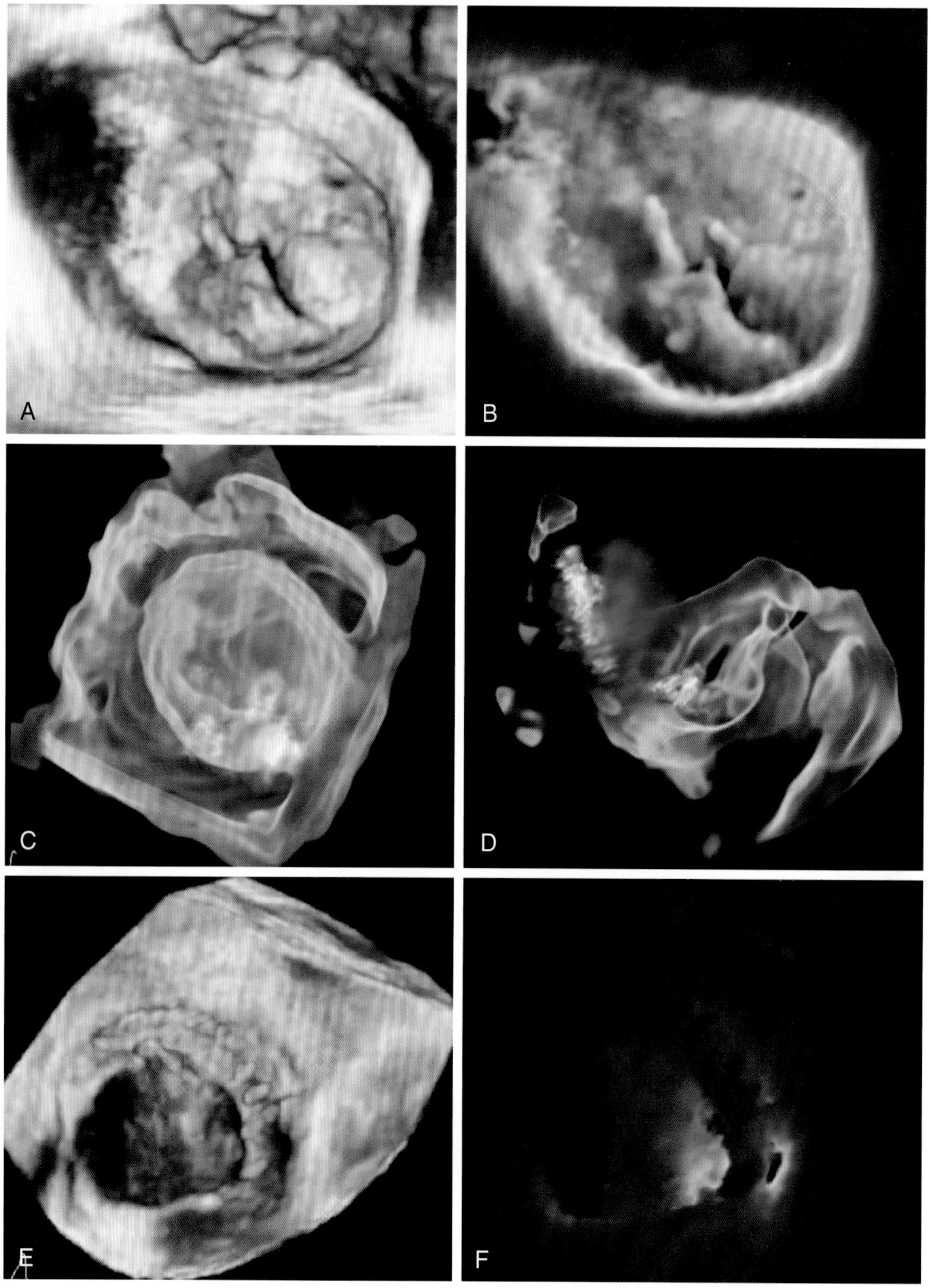

Fig. 1.16 3D mitral valve image display. (A: Video 1.16A) 3D volume-rendered transesophageal image of the mitral valve (MV) demonstrates flail P2 and P3 segments with a pseudo-cleft. (B; Video 1.16B) The same image visualized with the use of a photorealistic tissue mode with transillumination from the LA side. 3D transesophageal images of the MV en face (C; Video 1.16C) and in profile (D; Video 1.16D) rendered by using a mode in which the MV tissue appears transparent, improving visualization of the ischemic mitral regurgitant jet. (E; Video 1.16E) A 3D volume-rendered transesophageal image of a mechanical MV with a paravalvular leak. (F; Video 1.16F) The site of the paravalvular leak is better visualized using the photorealistic tissue mode with transillumination through a virtual light from the ventricular side of the MV.

planes obtained may be difficult or impossible to acquire using a 2D transducer.

Slicing methods that are available include arbitrary plane, simultaneous orthogonal (or arbitrary angle) slices, and parallel slice planes. The arbitrary plane cut allows the operator to orient the 2D plane in any direction for optimal viewing of the cardiac structures of interest. The simultaneous orthogonal 2D slice mode consists of two or three 2D planes (coronal, sagittal, and transverse) displayed simultaneously. Finally, it is possible to obtain multiple 2D parallel tomographic slices with uniformly spaced 2D parallel slices.

2D tomographic views improve measurements of cardiac chamber dimensions or valve or septal defect areas and evaluation of the morphology and function of cardiac structures. The simultaneous orthogonal 2D slice mode provides multiple visualization of the same segment within a single cardiac cycle, which can be useful for ventricular function analysis as well as for wall motion assessment.

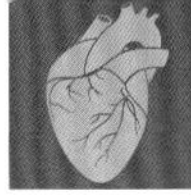

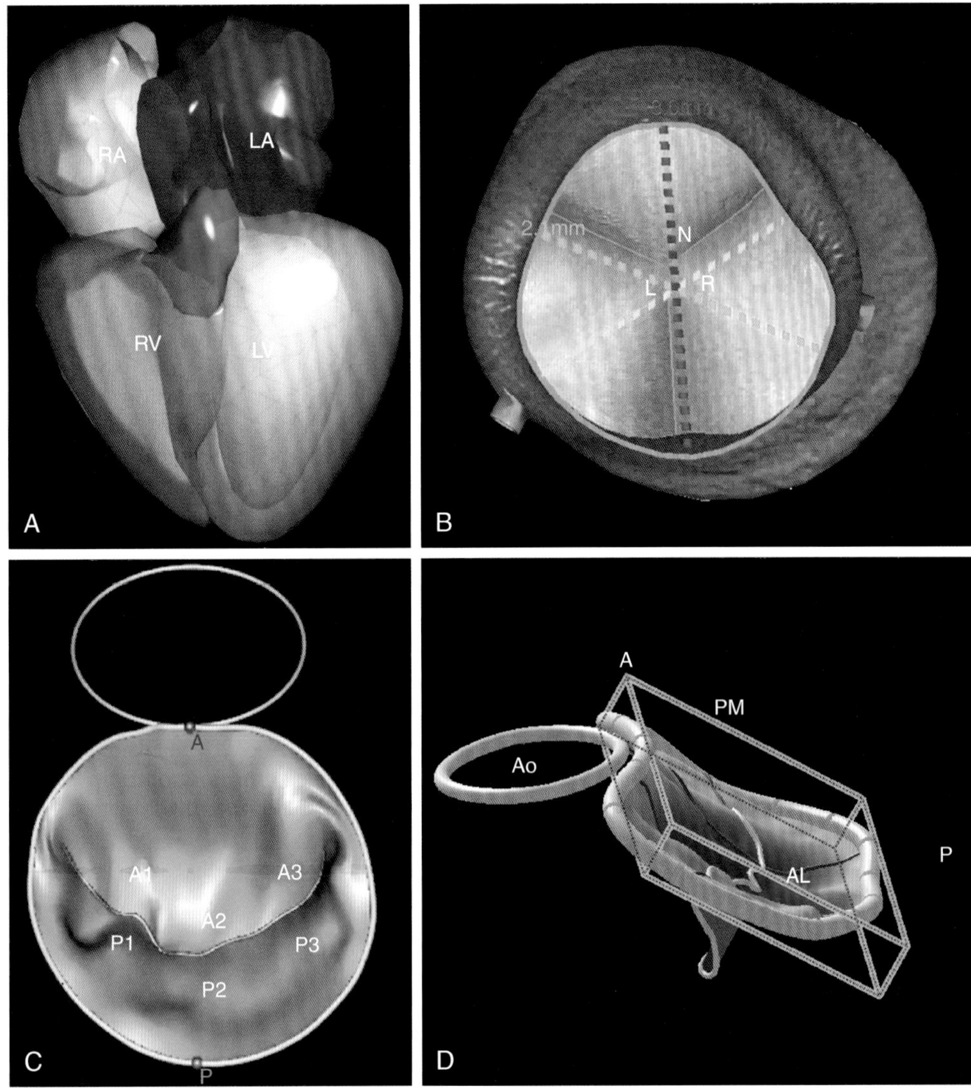

Fig. 1.17 3D models. Surface-rendered 3D models of the cardiac chambers (A), the aortic root (B), and the mitral valve (C and D). *A*, Anterior; *AL*, anterolateral; *Ao*, aorta; *L*, left coronary cusp; *N*, non-coronary cusp; *P*, posterior; *PM*, posteromedial; *R*, right coronary cusp.

3D ECHOCARDIOGRAPHIC ANALYSIS

Analysis of 3DE data depends not only on the cardiac structure under study (i.e., ventricle vs. valve) but also on the answer required (i.e., pathomorphology vs. quantification). However, methods for analysis generally fall into three categories: (1) multiplanar reconstruction (MPR), (2) modeling, and (3) color Doppler analysis.

MULTIPLANAR RECONSTRUCTION

MPR creates 2D images from the 3DE data set. With MPR, there are three planes that can be angulated in any direction and location with respect to each other and the structure under study. Typically, they are placed orthogonally to each other with one plane parallel to the structure of interest. This parallel plane allows measurement of regurgitant orifices, stenotic orifices, and atrial and ventricular septal defect sizes (see Fig. 1.11).

MODELING

Modeling involves the use of a surface-rendered image to obtain quantitative information. Modeling usually requires an analysis package with a manual, semiautomated, or fully automated tracing algorithm to contour the structure of interest. The resulting contours form a model from which measurements can be extracted. Programs currently exist to analyze chambers such as the LV, right ventricle (RV), and LA; the aortic root; the tricuspid valve annulus; and valves such as the MV or AV (see Fig. 1.17).

COLOR DOPPLER

Although color Doppler data can be analyzed using MPR of the 3D color Doppler jet, 3D color-flow data can also be analyzed using flow methods. In one method, a region of interest is chosen and color flow through that region of interest is measured. In this way, regurgitant volume can be determined from the difference between the flow through two valves. Alternatively, a newer technique involves direct measurement of the 3D proximal isovelocity surface area (PISA).

TRUE 3D VISUALIZATION

3DE data is typically visualized on a screen, which reduces the acquired 3D data to a 2D image that appears 3D through

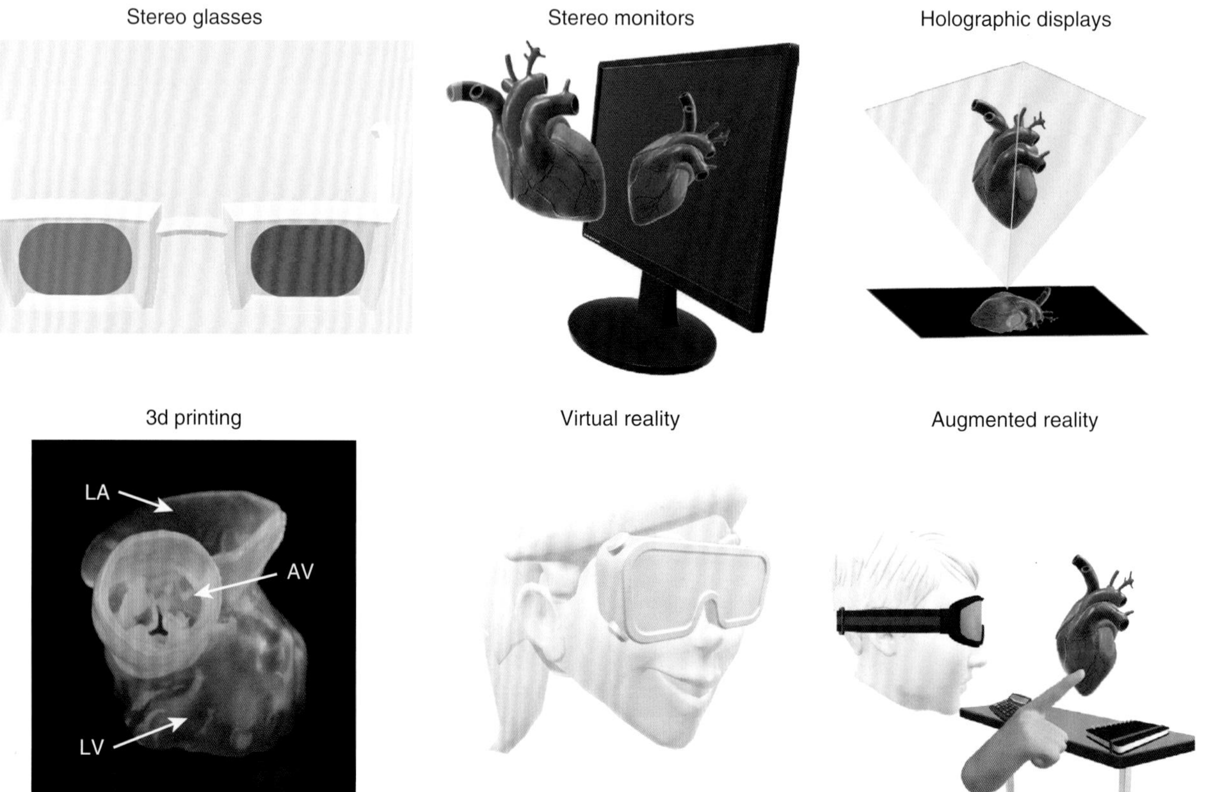

Fig. 1.18 Methods for true 3D visualization of 3DE data. 3DE data can be visualized in three dimensions with the use of stereo glasses, stereo monitors, holographic displays, 3D printing, virtual reality, or augmented reality. Video 1.18 demonstrates virtual reality visualization of a mechanical mitral valve. The mechanical valve is seen and manipulated in a virtual space.

renderings and shadows. This 2D visualization limits the value gained from acquiring and analyzing a 3D data set. True 3D visualization would enhance the value of 3DE data. There are many ways in which 3DE data sets can be fully visualized in three dimensions (Fig. 1.18). One of the oldest methods is the use of stereo glasses; other methods include stereo monitors with special glasses and holographic displays. More recently, the development of 3D printing has allowed the viewer to hold the 3D structure in their hands.[37–39] Virtual reality, traditionally used in computer gaming, has also entered the clinical workspace. With special headsets, which take over the wearer's vision, the wearer is placed in a virtual space with the 3DE structure.[1] Last, there has been the development of augmented reality, which allows visualization of the 3D structure in the wearer's environment.

3D ECHOCARDIOGRAPHIC ACQUISITION AND ANALYSIS PROTOCOLS

Early adoption of 3DE was driven by the ability to visualize the MV en face and the capability to obtain more accurate LV volumetric measurements. Current uses also now include the following: (1) assessment of native and prosthetic valve anatomy; (2) quantitation of valvular stenosis and regurgitation severity; (3) volumetric cardiac chamber measurements; and (4) assessment and guidance for before, during, and after percutaneous cardiac interventions for structural heart disease (Table 1.7).[40–43] The following sections discuss specific protocols for ventricular and valvular structures as recommended by the American Society of Echocardiography guidelines.[40,41]

LEFT VENTRICLE

Acquisition

To maximize volume rate, the smallest pyramidal size that covers the entire LV should be used for acquisition. High-volume-rate methods such as multibeat acquisition may be required to achieve volume rates greater than 20 Hz. Use of low-frame-rate data runs the risk of missing true end-systole, which results in an artificially larger end-systolic volume with a reduced ejection fraction. Typically, image acquisition begins with a 2D 4-chamber view. Multiplane views should be used to ensure that the entire LV is included in the 3D pyramidal volume.

Presentation

The LV can be presented using (1) multiple short-axis views (tomographic 2D views), which allows visualization of all the walls; (2) orthogonal slice plane views, which allows 2D planar visualization of the 2-, 3-, and 4-chamber views; (3) surface rendering, which allows visualization and quantitation of systolic function from the volumetric model; or (4) volume rendering, which is used to demonstrate LV thrombi, masses, and septal defects.

Analysis

LV volumes are obtained by using a 3D-guided biplane Simpson method or direct volumetric quantification based on semiautomated or fully automated LV volume analysis packages.[44–48] Landmarks used by these software packages include the mitral annulus and the LV apex, which are used to initiate edge detection by the software. Other anatomic features of importance are the LV trabeculae and papillary muscles, which should be included within the LV cavity for the calculation of LV volumes.

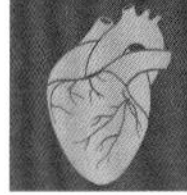

TABLE 1.7 Indications for 3D Echocardiography.

Structure	*Clinically Indicated*	*Promising Use*	*Under Study*
LV	• Volume measurement	• Mass measurement	• Shape measurement • Dyssynchrony assessment
RV	• Volume measurement		
LA		• Volume measurement	• Shape assessment
RA			• Volume measurement
Atrial/ventricular septal defects	• Localization of defect • Size measurement		
Mitral valve	• Native anatomy lesion localization • Rheumatic stenosis valve area • Prosthetic anatomy • Paravalvular regurgitation	• Regurgitation quantification	
Aortic root	• Root measurements	• Aortic valve stenosis quantification • Aortic valve anatomy	• Regurgitation quantification
Tricuspid valve	• Mechanism of regurgitation		
Percutaneous procedures	• Guidance of procedures		

Modified from Lang et al.[40]

The mitral annulus, the papillary muscles, the apical portion of the LV cavity, and the anterior and posterior RV insertion points of the septum are used to divide the LV into a 17-segment model. Regional LV volume is defined in most programs by the space between the endocardial border and a centerline through the LV cavity. This definition is problematic because this virtual landmark may shift with alterations of the LV mass and remodeling after myocardial infarction, leading to underestimation of serial regional volume changes.

Once the model is created, LV wall motion can be assessed and LV volumes obtained. 3DE-derived LV strain, shape, and mass can also be measured. 3DE-derived speckle-tracking strain imaging allows tracking of the speck along the x-, y-, and z-axes, unlike 2D imaging, in which the speckles may pass in and out of the imaging plane. 3D-derived LV shape imaging allows better characterization of global and regional LV remodeling, and the entire LV cavity is assessed.[49] In contrast, with 2D imaging, LV shape is assessed using the sphericity index, which fails to account for regional abnormalities. LV mass requires accurate detection of not only the endocardial but also the epicardial border. It is usually measured using either the 3DE-guided biplane technique or volumetric analysis. MPR should be used to obtain measurements of ventricular septal defects.

Limitations

The larger pyramidal volumes required for a larger heart result in lower volume rates. This can be addressed through the use of single-beat, high-volume-rate methods. Multibeat acquisition is helpful but introduces the risk of stitch artifact and is not reliable in patients with irregular heart rhythms or those who are unable to breath-hold.

RIGHT VENTRICLE

Acquisition

To maximize volume rate, the smallest pyramidal size that covers the entire RV should be used for acquisition. As with LV 3D image acquisition, the highest volume rate possible should be acquired. A dedicated RV view from the apical window should be the starting point for the acquisition. Multiplane views should be used to ensure that the entire RV is included in the 3D pyramidal volume, and in particular the apical RV free wall and the RV outflow tract. Usually, the reference plane is a dedicated RV view, whereas the orthogonal plane demonstrates the RV inflow and outflow.

Presentation

The RV can be presented using (1) multiple short-axis views (tomographic 2D views), which allow visualization of all the walls; (2) surface rendering, which allows visualization and quantitation of systolic function from the volumetric model; or (3) volume rendering, which is used to demonstrate RV wires, thrombi, masses, and septal defects.

Analysis

Semiautomated or fully automated RV volume analysis packages are available on some ultrasound systems. Landmarks used for this process are the tricuspid, aortic, and pulmonic annulus and the RV free wall. Once the model is created, RV volumes are obtained.

Limitations

As with the LV, the larger pyramidal volumes required for larger hearts result in lower volume rates.[50]

LEFT ATRIUM

Acquisition

To maximize volume rate, the smallest pyramidal size that covers the entire LA should be used for acquisition. High volume rates are possible because of the smaller overall size of the LA compared with the ventricles. Typically, a dedicated LA view from the apical 4-chamber window is used for acquisition. Multiplane viewing should be used to ensure that the entire LA is included in the 3D pyramidal volume.

Presentation

The LA can be presented using (1) surface rendering, which allows visualization and quantitation of systolic function from the volumetric model, or (2) volume rendering, which is used to demonstrate LA wires, thrombi, masses, and septal defects.

Analysis

Semiautomated LA volume analysis packages are not available on current ultrasound systems. Some laboratories have used LV programs to analyze the LA.[51] However, assumptions built into an LV analysis program may introduce errors when the LA is analyzed. Typical landmarks used for these programs include the mitral annulus. Once the model is created, LA volumes are provided. For atrial septal defects, MPR should be used to obtain accurate size measurements.

Limitations

Although there are abundant data supporting the prognostic value of 2D-derived LA volumes, limited data exist for 3D-derived LA volumes.

MITRAL VALVE

Acquisition

Acquisition of the MV during transthoracic imaging should start with either the parasternal long-axis view of the valve or the apical 4-chamber view. On transesophageal imaging, the long-axis (~120 degrees) view of the MV is preferred, but the view where the valve is best visualized on 2D TEE should be the starting point. Although transthoracic imaging of the MV has improved greatly, 3D MV assessment is still best performed with TEE. The multiplane mode should be used to ensure that the entire mitral annulus and leaflets are included in the 3D volume, and the smallest pyramidal volume (zoom mode) should be used. However, the volume should include the AV to allow for orientation of the valve after acquisition. For planning MV procedures such as the MitraClip procedure, the biplane mode, which demonstrates the long-axis view and the bicommissural view simultaneously, or a small pyramidal volume–sized surface rendering can be used to visualize the valve morphology and the regurgitant jet. Additionally, sweeping the valve with biplane mode may be helpful in confirming the pathology.[52] 3DE surface renderings are also useful for percutaneous paravalvular closure procedures.

Presentation

The MV can be presented using (1) surface rendering, which allows visualization and quantitation from the volumetric model, or (2) volume rendering, which is used to demonstrate the anatomy as well as surrounding structures during procedures. For presentation, the MV should be oriented en face, with the AV at the 12 o'clock position regardless of whether the LA or LV perspective is used.

Analysis

MV analysis is mainly based on the volume-rendered images. MPR is used to measure the MV orifice by planimetry.[53] Quantification for degenerative valve disease remains mainly in the research realm, although semiautomated or fully automated MV analysis packages exist on all ultrasound machines.[54] Once the model is created, leaflet displacement and other abnormalities can be assessed and measurements obtained.

Limitations

Often patients with MV disease are in atrial fibrillation, which limits the use of multibeat acquisition. High-volume-rate methods that do not rely on ECG-gating have been developed that address this weakness.

AORTIC VALVE

Acquisition

Images of the AV can be acquired from the long-axis (120–140 degrees) view with TEE or with the parasternal long-axis or the apical 5-chamber view on TTE. Multiplane views should be used to ensure that the entire aortic annulus is included in the 3D volume. Typically, a small pyramidal volume or zoom mode is used.

Presentation

The AV can be presented using (1) surface rendering, which allows visualization and quantitation from the volumetric model, or (2) volume rendering, which is used to demonstrate the anatomy as well as surrounding structures during interventional procedures. For presentation, the AV should be oriented en face with the noncoronary cusp in the 6 o'clock position regardless of whether the aortic or LV outflow tract perspective is used.

Analysis

AV pathology is mainly analyzed based on the volume-rendered images. MPR is used to measure the aortic annulus and area by planimetry.[55] Semiautomated or fully automated AV analysis packages exist on some ultrasound machines.[56–60] Although the size of the annulus is one of the many measurements that can be obtained, the clinical utility of the other 3D measurements is still under study.[55,61]

Limitations

In patients with thin, noncalcified, mobile cusps, it is difficult to capture the cusps without dropout using 3D imaging because of the parallel orientation between the ultrasound beam and the AV. On TEE, improved visualization and 3D acquisition could be achieved using transgastric views; from that perspective, the valve is more perpendicular to the ultrasound beam.

TRICUSPID VALVE

Acquisition

Because of the location of the tricuspid valve (TV) in the chest, visualization is feasible and optimal in most patients using TTE.[62,63] The TV can be acquired from the apical 4-chamber view on TTE. If TV image acquisition is required during TEE, a low esophageal view may improve visualization of the valve enough for acquisition of a high-quality 3D data set. The multiplane view should be used to ensure that the entire tricuspid annulus is included in the 3D volume. Typically, a small pyramidal volume or zoom mode is used.

Presentation

The TV can be presented using volume rendering to demonstrate the anatomy. For presentation, the TV should be oriented en face with the septal leaflet in the 6 o'clock position regardless of whether the RA or RV perspective is used.

Analysis

TV pathology is mainly analyzed based on the volume-rendered images.[63] No commercial software packages for analysis are currently available.

Limitations

In approximately 20% of patients, apical transthoracic windows are so poor that the TV cannot be seen well on 2D imaging, which also affects 3D visualization. Parasternal windows could be used in these circumstances to attempt visualization.

3D COLOR DOPPLER ACQUISITION

Acquisition

Similar to conventional 2D imaging, color Doppler imaging superimposes flow information onto 3D morphology. 3D color Doppler images can be acquired using single-beat or multibeat methods and are limited by the restrictions associated with these acquisition methods. Although 3D color Doppler data acquisition is feasible with TTE or TEE examinations, 3D TEE acquisition currently provides significantly better color Doppler image quality.

Presentation

Color Doppler data can be presented using (1) volume rendering or (2) MPR. Understanding the orientation of color Doppler flow within the displayed views is clinically important. To help with the orientation, it is recommended that the 3D color Doppler data be displayed in at least two different views with a known orientation to each other as indicated by different-colored cutting planes. It is also recommended that the 3D color Doppler data be displayed together with anatomic 3D information using standard views.

Analysis

Color-flow analysis includes the proximal flow convergence region of valvular regurgitation and flow-through heart defects such as ventricular or atrial septal defects. As discussed previously, color Doppler data can be analyzed using (1) MPR of the 3D color Doppler jet or (2) 3D color-flow methods.

Cropping of 3D color Doppler data sets follows the same principles as noncolor Doppler data set cropping and is mainly determined by the analysis intended. For MPR of regurgitant jets, it is recommended that the 3D color Doppler data set show two long-axis views of the jet, one with the narrowest and one with the broadest width of the jet. This display should also include a short-axis view of the jet at the level of the vena contracta, which can be measured.

Limitations

The limitations of 3D color Doppler acquisition include poor spatial and temporal resolution, both of which are expected to improve with the advancement of 3D technology.

SUMMARY Cardiac Structure Acquisition, Presentation, and Analysis.

Cardiac Structure	Transesophageal Acquisition View/ Window	Transthoracic Acquisition View/ Window	Pyramidal Size	Volume-Rendering Presentation Orientation	Analysis
LV	Midesophageal 0/90/120 degrees	Apical 4-chamber	Wide	Short-axis or 4-chamber view	MPR, dedicated LV analysis programs
RV	Midesophageal 0/45 degrees	Dedicated RV/ apical 4-chamber	Wide	Short-axis or 4-chamber view	MPR, dedicated RV analysis programs
LA	—	Dedicated apical 4-chamber Dedicated LA view	Zoom	From the LA perspective, the right upper pulmonary vein should be at the 1 o'clock position. From the RA perspective, the superior vena cava should be at the 11 o'clock position.	MPR, repurposed LV analysis programs
RA	Midesophageal 0–10/90 degrees	Dedicated RV/ apical 4-chamber	Zoom	Short-axis or 4-chamber view	MPR
Interatrial septum	Midesophageal 0/45/90/120 degrees	—	Zoom	Short-axis or 4-chamber view	MPR
Aortic valve	Midesophageal 60 or 120 degrees	Parasternal long- or short-axis views or apical 3- or 5-chamber view	Zoom	Right coronary cusp at the 6 o'clock position	MPR, dedicated analysis programs
Mitral valve	Midesophageal 0/45–60/90/120 degrees	Apical 4-chamber or parasternal long-axis view	Zoom	Aortic valve at the 12 o'clock position	MPR, dedicated analysis programs
Tricuspid valve	Midesophageal 0–30 degrees Transgastric 40 degrees	Dedicated RV/ apical 4-chamber	Zoom	Septal leaflet at the 6 o'clock position	MPR
Pulmonic valve	High esophageal 90 degrees Midesophageal 120 degrees	Parasternal RV outflow	Zoom	Anterior cusp at the 12 o'clock position	MPR

MPR, Multiplanar reconstruction.

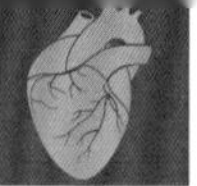

REFERENCES

1. Lang RM, et al. 3-Dimensional echocardiography: latest developments and future directions. *JACC Cardiovasc Imaging*. 2018;11(12):1854–1878.
2. Handke M, et al. Transesophageal real-time three-dimensional echocardiography methods and initial in vitro and human in vivo studies. *J Am Coll Cardiol*. 2006;48(10):2070–2076.
3. Sugeng L, et al. Live 3-dimensional transesophageal echocardiography initial experience using the fully-sampled matrix array probe. *J Am Coll Cardiol*. 2008;52(6):446–449.
4. Quien MM, Saric M. Ultrasound imaging artifacts: how to recognize them and how to avoid them. *Echocardiography*. 2018;35(9):1388–1401.
5. vonRamm OT, Thurstone FL. Cardiac imaging using a phased array ultrasound system. I. System design. *Circulation*. 1976;53(2):258–262.
6. Ota T, et al. Real-time, volumetric echocardiography: usefulness of volumetric scanning for the assessment of cardiac volume and function. *J Cardiol*. 2001;37(suppl 1):93–101.
7. Li X, et al. Preliminary work of real-time ultrasound imaging system for 2-D array transducer. *Bio Med Mater Eng*. 2015;26(suppl 1):S1579–S1585.
8. Light ED, et al. Progress in two-dimensional arrays for real-time volumetric imaging. *Ultrason Imaging*. 1998;20(1):1–15.
9. Vegas A. Three-dimensional transesophageal echocardiography: principles and clinical applications. *Ann Card Anaesth*. 2016;19(suppl):S35–S43.
10. Salgo IS. Three-dimensional echocardiographic technology. *Cardiol Clin*. 2007;25(2):231–239.
11. Badano LP. The clinical benefits of adding a third dimension to assess the left ventricle with echocardiography. *Scientifica (Cairo)*. 2014;2014:897431.
12. Chen C, et al. A prototype PZT matrix transducer with low-power integrated receive ASIC for 3-D transesophageal echocardiography. *IEEE Trans Ultrason Ferroelectr Freq Control*. 2016;63(1):47–59.
13. Yu Z, et al. Front-end receiver electronics for a matrix transducer for 3-D transesophageal echocardiography. *IEEE Trans Ultrason Ferroelectr Freq Control*. 2012;59(7):1500–1512.
14. Wygant IO, et al. An integrated circuit with transmit beamforming flip-chip bonded to a 2-D CMUT array for 3-D ultrasound imaging. *IEEE Trans Ultrason Ferroelectr Freq Control*. 2009;56(10):2145–2156.
15. Daeichin V, et al. Acoustic characterization of a miniature matrix transducer for pediatric 3D transesophageal echocardiography. *Ultrasound Med Biol*. 2018;44(10):2143–2154.
16. Bera D, et al. Dual stage beamforming in the absence of front-end receive focusing. *Phys Med Biol*. 2017;62(16):6631–6648.
17. Perrin DP, et al. Temporal enhancement of 3D echocardiography by frame reordering. *JACC Cardiovasc Imaging*. 2012;5(3):300–304.
18. Provost J, et al. 3D ultrafast ultrasound imaging in vivo. *Phys Med Biol*. 2014;59(19):L1–L13.
19. Sauvage J, et al. A large aperture row column addressed probe for in vivo 4D ultrafast Doppler ultrasound imaging. *Phys Med Biol*. 2018;63(21):215012.
20. Denarie B, Bjastad T, Torp H. Multi-line transmission in 3-D with reduced crosstalk artifacts: a proof of concept study. *IEEE Trans Ultrason Ferroelectr Freq Control*. 2013;60(8):1708–1718.
21. Bera D, et al. Fast volumetric imaging using a matrix transesophageal echocardiography probe with partitioned transmit-receive array. *Ultrasound Med Biol*. 2018;44(9):2025–2042.
22. Chen Y, et al. Feasibility of multiplane-transmit beamforming for real-time volumetric cardiac imaging: a simulation study. *IEEE Trans Ultrason Ferroelectr Freq Control*. 2017;64(4):648–659.
23. Skaug TR, et al. Quantification of mitral regurgitation using high pulse repetition frequency three-dimensional color Doppler. *J Am Soc Echocardiogr*. 2010;23(1):1–8.
24. Hergum T, et al. Quantification of valvular regurgitation area and geometry using HPRF 3-D Doppler. *IEEE Trans Ultrason Ferroelectr Freq Control*. 2009;56(5):975–982.
25. Skaug TR, et al. Quantification of aortic regurgitation using high-pulse repetition frequency three-dimensional colour Doppler. *Eur Heart J Cardiovasc Imaging*. 2014;15(6):615–622.
26. Punithakumar K, et al. Multiview three-dimensional echocardiography image fusion using a passive measurement Arm. *Conf Proc IEEE Eng Med Biol Soc*. 2018;2018:903–906.
27. Punithakumar K, et al. Multiview echocardiography fusion using an electromagnetic tracking system. *Conf Proc IEEE Eng Med Biol Soc*. 2016;2016:1078–1081.
28. Punithakumar K, et al. Multiview 3-D echocardiography fusion with breath-hold position tracking using an optical tracking system. *Ultrasound Med Biol*. 2016;42(8):1998–2009.
29. Rajpoot K, et al. Multiview fusion 3-D echocardiography: improving the information and quality of real-time 3-D echocardiography. *Ultrasound Med Biol*. 2011;37(7):1056–1072.
30. Bhave NM, et al. Three-dimensional modeling of the right ventricle from two-dimensional transthoracic echocardiographic images: utility of knowledge-based reconstruction in pulmonary arterial hypertension. *J Am Soc Echocardiogr*. 2013;26(8):860–867.
31. Raichlen JS, et al. Dynamic three-dimensional reconstruction of the left ventricle from two-dimensional echocardiograms. *J Am Coll Cardiol*. 1986;8(2):364–370.
32. Faletra FF, et al. Artifacts in three-dimensional transesophageal echocardiography. *J Am Soc Echocardiogr*. 2014;27(5):453–462.
33. Hung J, et al. 3D echocardiography: a review of the current status and future directions. *J Am Soc Echocardiogr*. 2007;20(3):213–233.
34. Genovese D, et al. First clinical experience with 3-dimensional echocardiographic transillumination rendering. *JACC Cardiovasc Imaging*. 2019;12(9):1868–1871.
35. Chandra S, et al. Characterization of degenerative mitral valve disease using morphologic analysis of real-time three-dimensional echocardiographic images: objective insight into complexity and planning of mitral valve repair. *Circ Cardiovasc Imaging*. 2011;4(1):24–32.
36. Tsang W, et al. The value of three-dimensional echocardiography derived mitral valve parametric maps and the role of experience in the diagnosis of pathology. *J Am Soc Echocardiogr*. 2011;24(8):860–867.
37. Olivieri LJ, et al. Three-dimensional printing of intracardiac defects from three-dimensional echocardiographic images: feasibility and relative accuracy. *J Am Soc Echocardiogr*. 2015;28(4):392–397.
38. Fan Y, et al. Device sizing guided by echocardiography-based three-dimensional printing is associated with superior outcome after percutaneous left atrial appendage occlusion. *J Am Soc Echocardiogr*. 2019;32(6):708–719 e1.
39. Muraru D, et al. 3D printing of normal and pathologic tricuspid valves from transthoracic 3D echocardiography data sets. *Eur Heart J Cardiovasc Imaging*. 2017;18(7):802–808.
40. Lang RM, et al. EAE/ASE recommendations for image acquisition and display using three-dimensional echocardiography. *J Am Soc Echocardiogr*. 2012;25(1):3–46.
41. Lang RM, et al. Recommendations for cardiac chamber quantification by echocardiography in adults: an update from the American Society of Echocardiography and the European Association of Cardiovascular Imaging. *J Am Soc Echocardiogr*. 2015;28(1):1–39 e14.
42. Tsang W, Lang RM. Three-dimensional echocardiography is essential for intraoperative assessment of mitral regurgitation. *Circulation*. 2013;128(6):643–652. discussion 652.
43. Chui J, et al. The trileaflet mitral valve. *Am J Cardiol*. 2018;121(4):513–519.
44. Nedadur R, Tsang W. Automated three-dimensional left ventricular volumes: rise of the machines? *J Am Soc Echocardiogr*. 2019;32(9):1116–1119.
45. Kitano T, et al. Accuracy of left ventricular volumes and ejection fraction measurements by contemporary three-dimensional echocardiography with semi- and fully automated software: systematic review and meta-analysis of 1,881 subjects. *J Am Soc Echocardiogr*. 2019;32(9):1105–1115 e5.
46. Tsang W, et al. Transthoracic 3D echocardiographic left heart chamber quantification using an automated adaptive analytics algorithm. *JACC Cardiovasc Imaging*. 2016;9(7):769–782.
47. Medvedofsky D, et al. Three-dimensional echocardiographic quantification of the left-heart chambers using an automated adaptive analytics algorithm: multicentre validation study. *Eur Heart J Cardiovasc Imaging*. 2018;19(1):47–58.
48. Sugeng L, et al. Quantitative assessment of left ventricular size and function: side-by-side comparison of real-time three-dimensional echocardiography and computed tomography with magnetic resonance reference. *Circulation*. 2006;114(7):654–661.
49. Salgo IS, et al. Geometric assessment of regional left ventricular remodeling by three-dimensional echocardiographic shape analysis correlates with left ventricular function. *J Am Soc Echocardiogr*. 2012;25(1):80–88.
50. Addetia K, et al. New directions in right ventricular assessment using 3-dimensional echocardiography. *JAMA Cardiol*. 2019;4(9):936–944.
51. Nemes A, et al. Normal reference values of three-dimensional speckle-tracking echocardiography-derived left atrial strain parameters (results from the MAGYAR-Healthy Study). *Int J Cardiovasc Imaging*. 2019;35(6):991–998.

52. Geyer M, et al. Advanced protocol for three-dimensional transesophageal echocardiography guidance implementing real-time multiplanar reconstruction for transcatheter mitral valve repair by direct annuloplasty. *J Am Soc Echocardiogr*. 2019.
53. Tsang W, Freed BH, Lang RM. The role of 3-dimensional echocardiography in the diagnosis and management of mitral valve disease: myxomatous valve disease. *Cardiol Clin*. 2013;31(2):203–215.
54. Calleja A, et al. Quantitative modeling of the mitral valve by three-dimensional transesophageal echocardiography in patients undergoing mitral valve repair: correlation with intraoperative surgical technique. *J Am Soc Echocardiogr*. 2015;28(9):1083–1092.
55. Ballocca F, et al. Aortic root changes before and after surgery for chronic aortic dilatation: a 3D echocardiographic study. *Echocardiography*. 2019;36(2):376–385.
56. Queiros S, et al. Assessment of aortic valve tract dynamics using automatic tracking of 3D transesophageal echocardiographic images. *Int J Cardiovasc Imaging*. 2019;35(5):881–895.
57. Stella S, et al. Accuracy and reproducibility of aortic annular measurements obtained from echocardiographic 3D manual and semi-automated software analyses in patients referred for transcatheter aortic valve implantation: implication for prosthesis size selection. *Eur Heart J Cardiovasc Imaging*. 2019;20(1):45–55.
58. Prihadi EA, et al. Feasibility, accuracy, and reproducibility of aortic annular and root sizing for transcatheter aortic valve replacement using novel automated three-dimensional echocardiographic software: comparison with multi-detector row computed tomography. *J Am Soc Echocardiogr*. 2018;31(4):505–514 e3.
59. Mediratta A, et al. 3D echocardiographic analysis of aortic annulus for transcatheter aortic valve replacement using novel aortic valve quantification software: comparison with computed tomography. *Echocardiography*. 2017;34(5):690–699.
60. Garcia-Martin A, et al. Accuracy and reproducibility of novel echocardiographic three-dimensional automated software for the assessment of the aortic root in candidates for thanscatheter aortic valve replacement. *Eur Heart J Cardiovasc Imaging*. 2016;17(7):772–778.
61. Calleja A, et al. Automated quantitative 3-dimensional modeling of the aortic valve and root by 3-dimensional transesophageal echocardiography in normals, aortic regurgitation, and aortic stenosis: comparison to computed tomography in normals and clinical implications. *Circ Cardiovasc Imaging*. 2013;6(1):99–108.
62. Muraru D, et al. 3-Dimensional echocardiography in imaging the tricuspid valve. *JACC Cardiovasc Imaging*. 2019;12(3):500–515.
63. Badano LP, et al. Morphological assessment of the tricuspid apparatus and grading regurgitation severity in patients with functional tricuspid regurgitation: thinking outside the box. *JACC Cardiovasc Imaging*. 2019;12(4):652–664.

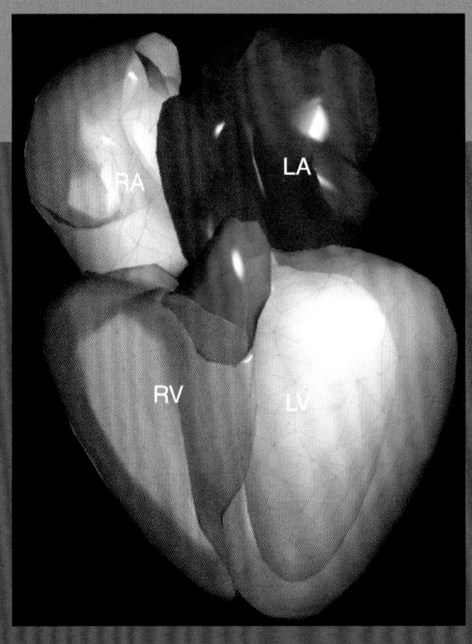

中文导读

第2章 心肌力学和应变成像原理

在日常临床实践中，通常采用二维超声心动图评估左心室功能，运用射血分数评估左心室整体收缩功能，通过肉眼观察室壁运动的状态，评价左心室局部功能。超声斑点追踪成像技术，可以获取左心室整体纵向应变，该指标相比于左室射血分数，对轻度收缩功能障碍的检测更加敏感。此外，通常应用组织多普勒成像技术，测量二尖瓣环纵向运动速度来评估左心室舒张功能。

本章阐述了组织多普勒成像和超声斑点追踪成像的技术原理、局限性及其各项参数的生理意义，主要介绍了其在心肌缺血、心室收缩同步性及右心室收缩功能评估中的应用价值。

吴伟春

2 Principles of Myocardial Mechanics and Strain Imaging

OTTO A. SMISETH, MD, PhD | THOR EDVARDSEN, MD, PhD | HANS TORP, DrTech

In daily clinical practice, left ventricular (LV) function is commonly evaluated by two-dimensional (2D) echocardiography. The most widely used measure of global LV function is ejection fraction (EF), and regional function is evaluated by visual assessment of wall motion. LV global longitudinal strain (GLS), as measured by speckle tracking echocardiography (STE), was introduced as a more sensitive parameter than LVEF to detect mild systolic dysfunction. Measurement of longitudinal mitral annular velocities by tissue Doppler imaging (TDI) is used in the evaluation of LV diastolic function. This chapter explains the technical principles behind TDI and STE and the physiologic meaning of the various parameters. The clinical applications of the methodologies are reviewed. Finally, synchrony of ventricular contraction is addressed.

VELOCITY IMAGING

Myocardial velocity imaging provides important insights into LV systolic and diastolic function. Peak LV shortening velocity measured by TDI is a parameter of contractile function, and early diastolic lengthening velocity measured at the mitral annulus is an important measure of diastolic function.

VELOCITIES BY COLOR DOPPLER

Myocardial velocity imaging was first introduced in the early 1990s.[1,2] Separation between velocities in the myocardium and in blood is possible because they have different signal amplitudes and Doppler frequencies, as illustrated in Fig. 2.1.

Like color-flow imaging, TDI uses an autocorrelator technique to calculate and display multigated points of color-coded velocities along a series of ultrasound scan lines within a 2D sector. As illustrated in Fig. 2.2, myocardial motion can be imaged as color-coded velocities superimposed on a 2D grayscale image in real time. The frame rate for 2D color Doppler imaging is typically 80 to 200 frames per second (fps), depending on the width of the ultrasound sector, and it is usually set higher than for the simultaneous grayscale images. Myocardial velocities are automatically decoded into numeric values, which can be stored digitally for later off-line analyses.[3] By convention, velocities toward the transducer are color-coded red and velocities away from the transducer are coded blue. Fig. 2.3 shows recordings from a healthy person and from a patient with acute myocardial infarction (MI).

Assessment of LV function by TDI in parasternal short-axis views is possible, but only a very limited number of segments can be imaged (Fig. 2.4). Therefore, apical views are usually preferred when assessing LV function by TDI.

VELOCITIES BY PULSED DOPPLER

Another approach is to use spectral TDI with pulsed Doppler activation, which is applied mainly to measure mitral annular velocities (Fig. 2.5). The velocity spectrum shows the distribution of velocities within the sample volume, and the myocardial velocity trace can easily be identified, even if clutter noise is present. It is important to be aware of spectral broadening (i.e., broadening of the velocity trace), which can lead to severe overestimation, depending on the gain setting (see Fig. 2.5B). For color-mode TDI, mean velocities are used (see Fig. 2.5A). The mean velocity trace is not affected by spectral broadening, but underestimation may result from clutter noise. This implies that velocities measured by the 2D color method described previously are lower than velocities measured by pulsed Doppler; a difference as high as 25% has been reported.[4] To minimize overestimation in spectral TDI, it is recommended to adjust the gain as low as possible. In the example shown in Fig. 2.5B, the second beat is close to the optimal gain setting.

Peak early diastolic mitral annular velocity (e') by pulsed Doppler is used in routine clinical practice as an index of

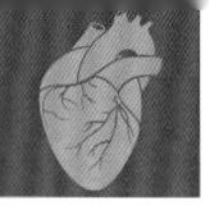

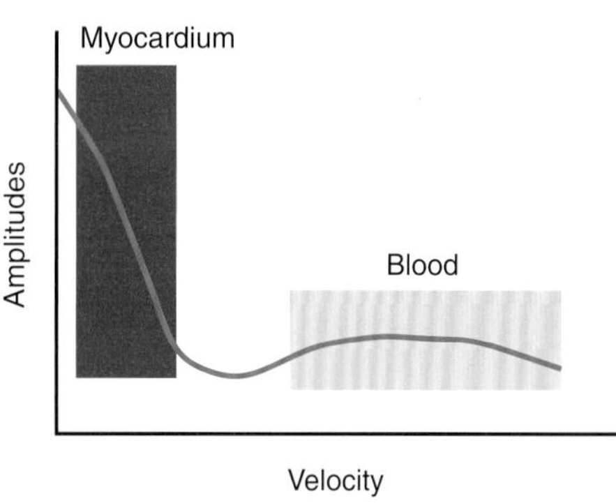

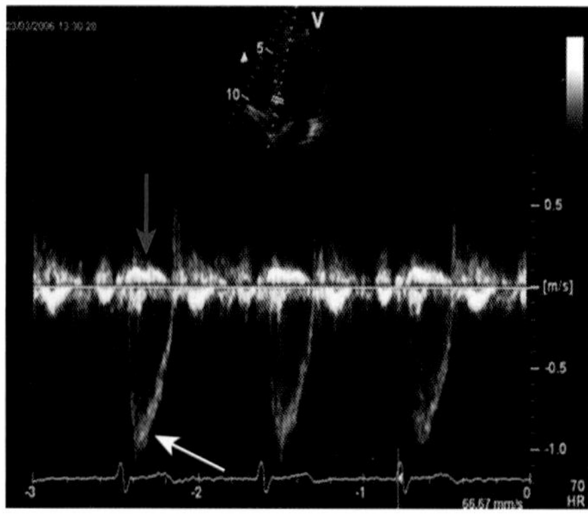

Fig. 2.1 **Myocardial velocities and blood flow.** Principle for separation of myocardial velocities from blood-flow velocities: The graph *(left)* illustrates the differences in velocity and amplitude between myocardium and blood. The myocardium is moving much more slowly than the blood, and therefore Doppler frequencies are lower. Furthermore, the amplitude of the myocardial signals is much higher than those for blood. The recording in the LV outflow tract *(right)* samples both myocardial and blood-flow velocities. The *red arrow* points to the high-intensity signals from the myocardium, and the *white arrow* indicates the low-intensity, high-velocity signals from the blood.

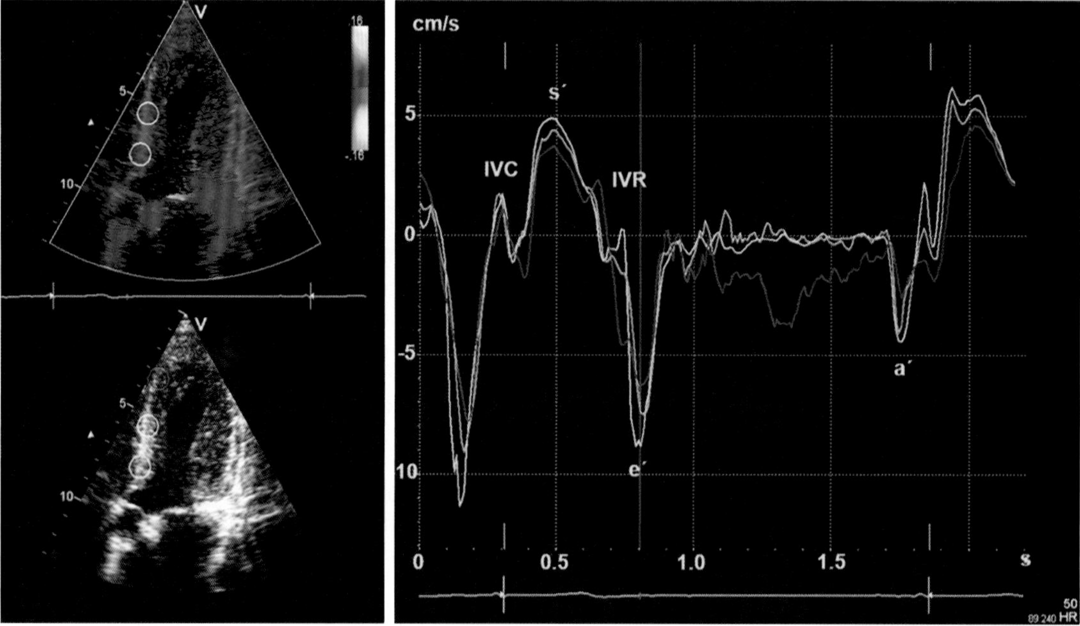

Fig. 2.2 **Normal myocardial velocities.** The *upper left panel* shows an apical long-axis view with color-coded LV myocardial velocities (*red* toward and *blue* away from the transducer), and the *lower left panel* shows sampling points for the velocities displayed in the *right panel.* Tissue Doppler imaging of velocities from the interventricular septum in a healthy individual. *a′,* Velocity during atrial-induced filling; *e′,* velocity during early diastolic filling; *IVC,* isovolumic contraction period; *IVR,* isovolumic relaxation period; *s′,* systolic ejection velocity.

myocardial relaxation and restoring forces.[5,6] Importantly, in adults, *e′* velocity decreases with age; therefore, age-based normal reference values should be used when applying these measures of LV diastolic function in clinical practice.

DEFORMATION IMAGING

BASIC CONCEPTS

Strain means deformation. It is an excellent parameter for quantification of myocardial function. In principle, strain may also be used to assess diastolic function, but this application has not been well developed and is not yet recommended for routine diagnostics.[5]

Quantification of myocardial function in terms of strain and strain rate has been available for a long time in cardiac physiology using implanted myocardial markers and for clinical research by magnetic resonance imaging with tissue tagging. Strain by echocardiography was first introduced as a TDI-based method[7,8] but was later replaced by 2-D strain using STE.[9] Strain by STE is a more robust clinical method than strain by TDI, so the former has become the preferred modality in diagnostic routine.

In echocardiography, the term *strain* is used to describe local shortening, thickening, and lengthening of the myocardium. The term originates from the field of continuum mechanics and is used to describe a general three-dimensional (3D) deformation of a small cube during a short time interval. The strain tensor has six components: three numbers express the shortening along three orthogonal axes (x, y, and z), and three shared strain numbers give the skew in the x-y, x-z, and y-z planes. By dividing the myocardium into a large number of cubes, complex and detailed deformation can be described by one strain tensor for each small cube at each time during the cardiac cycle.

This description is, however, too detailed for practical use in echocardiography, where there is a need for a limited number of measurable parameters representing the average deformation within a segment of the myocardium. It is more convenient to use an internal coordinate system aligned with the three cardiac

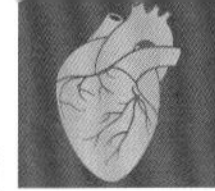

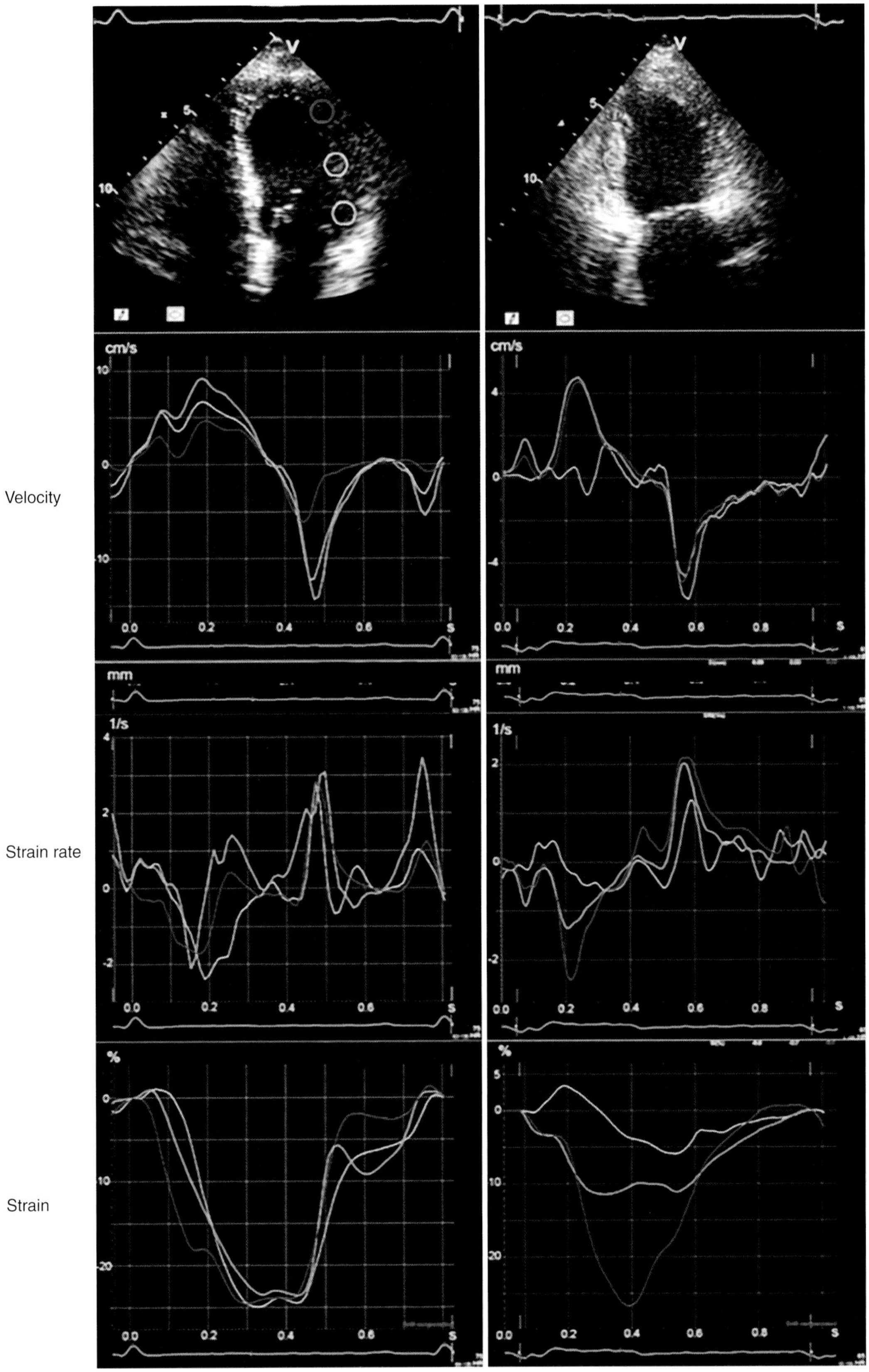

Velocity

Strain rate

Strain

Fig. 2.3 **Acute myocardial infarction.** Recordings from a healthy individual *(left)* and from a patient with posterior myocardial infarction *(right)*; notice the different scales. All tissue Doppler imaging modalities are sampled from three identical levels along the LV lateral wall in an apical 4-chamber view *(left panels)* and the posterior wall in an apical 2-chamber view *(right panels)*. In ischemic myocardium, systolic velocities are typically reduced *(right upper traces)*, and there are reductions in systolic strain rate *(right middle traces)* and strain *(right lower traces)*.

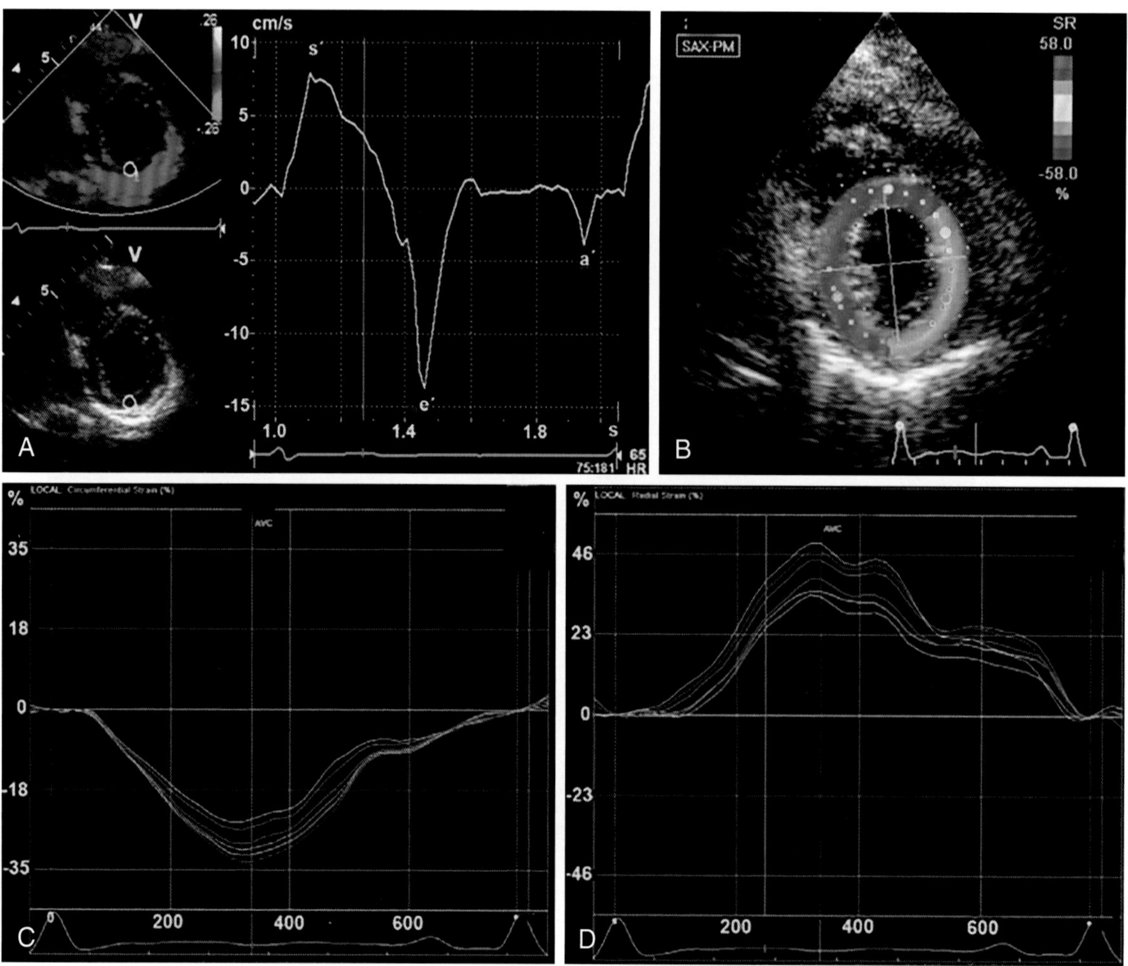

Fig. 2.4 **Deformation imaging from the short-axis view.** (A) Myocardial velocities from the posterior LV segment in a parasternal short-axis view. (B) Assessment of strain by STE from an LV parasternal short-axis view. (C) Circumferential strain in a healthy individual. (D) Radial strain in the same person as imaged in *B*. *a′*, Velocity during atrial-induced filling; *e′*, velocity during early diastolic filling; *s′*, systolic ejection velocity.

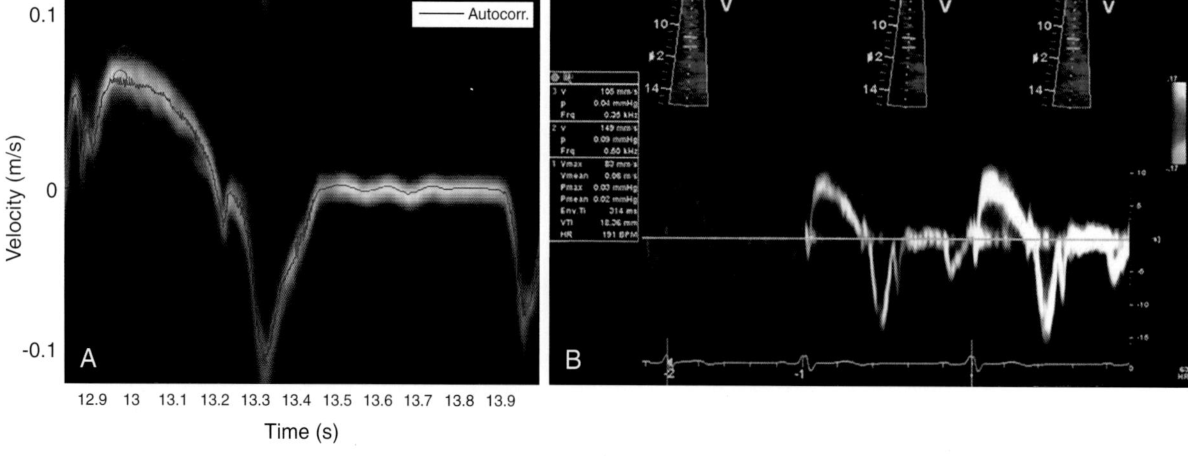

Fig. 2.5 **Spectral tissue Doppler imaging.** (A) Spectral TDI from the septal side of the mitral annulus. The overlay trace is the mean velocity as used in color TDI. (B) Effect of gain adjustment in spectral TDI. Three different gain settings, with increasing gain from left to right, result in different peak velocities. (Modified from Manouras A, Shahgaldi K, Winter R, et al. Comparison between colour-coded and spectral tissue Doppler measurements of systolic and diastolic myocardial velocities: effect of temporal filtering and offline gain setting. *Eur J Echocardiogr.* 2009;10:406–413.)

axes—longitudinal, circumferential, and radial—and to measure shortening and elongation in the three directions through the cardiac cycle, with reference to the size at the time of the QRS complex. If $L(t)$ denotes the segment length along one of these directions at any time t in the cardiac cycle, one-dimensional strain (ε) is defined as the ratio between the change in length and the initial length (L_0):

$$\varepsilon(t) = \frac{L(t) - L_0}{L_0} \qquad \text{(Eq. 2.1)}$$

This is also called *Lagrange strain.* It is measured by the distance between two material points in the myocardium measured after contraction and relaxation. Fig. 2.6 illustrates schematically the principles for calculation of Lagrange strain. By convention, lengthening and thickening strains are assigned positive values, and shortening and thinning strains are given negative values, reported as a percentage. This implies that systolic shortening results in negative strains, and systolic thickening results in positive strains.

When evaluating LV systolic function, strain can be measured as peak systolic strain (positive or negative), as peak strain at end-systole (at the time of aortic valve closure), or as peak strain regardless of timing (in systole or early diastole). When using data from multiple segments to estimate global strain, end-systolic strain is the preferred measure, because this is what determines stroke volume.

The slope of the strain curve, called the *strain rate* (SR) also carries important information. Because strain is dimensionless, SR has units of 1 per second. Of special interest is the maximum slope in systole, as well as in early and late diastole. SR can be calculated from the time derivative of strain, which is given by the velocity difference ($v_2[t] - v_1[t]$) between the end points of the segment $L(t)$:

$$SR_L(t) = \frac{v_2(t) - v_1(t)}{L_0} \qquad \text{(Eq. 2.2)}$$

This definition of strain rate is quite similar to the myocardial velocity gradient, also known as the *Euler strain rate:*

$$SR(t) = \frac{v_2(t) - v_1(t)}{L(t)} \qquad \text{(Eq. 2.3)}$$

The only difference is in the denominator; in the first formulation, the velocity difference is compared with the initial segment length, whereas the velocity gradient uses the segment length at the same time instant as the velocity difference is measured. Myocardial velocity gradient was first measured by M-mode TDI to determine the rate of wall thickening.[10] Later, velocity gradient measurement was combined with 2D TDI to image the longitudinal strain rate in the myocardium from apical views.[7]

Starting with the Euler strain rate, strain can be calculated by time integration of SR from end diastole ($t = 0$) to any time t in the cardiac cycle:

$$\begin{aligned} \varepsilon_N(t) &= \int_0^t SR(\tau)d\tau = \ln[1+\varepsilon(t)] \\ \varepsilon(t) &= \exp[\varepsilon_N(t)] - 1 \end{aligned} \qquad \text{(Eq. 2.4)}$$

This version of strain, ε_N, is usually called *natural strain,* probably because of its relation with *Langrange strain,* ε, given by the natural logarithm function, ln, and τ is the variable of integration. In echocardiography, Euler strain rate is preferred over Lagrange strain rate because it is easier to calculate as a direct spatial derivative of myocardial velocity, without the need to track segment end points through the cardiac cycle. For strain measurements, Lagrange strain is the preferred method because it can be directly interpreted as shortening or elongation, as opposed to natural strain, for which the conversion formula (Eq. 2.4) is needed.

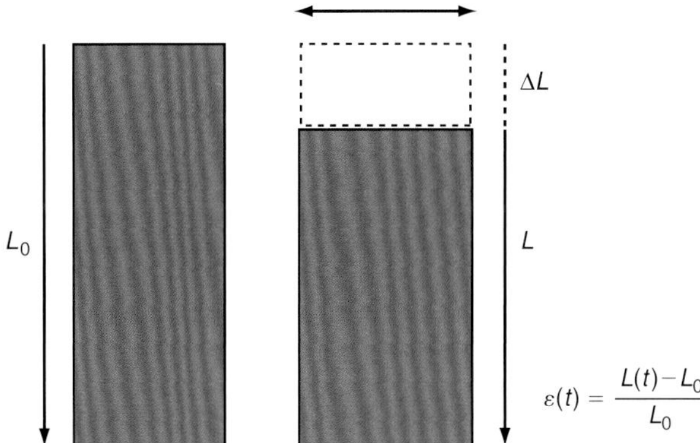

Fig. 2.6 Definition of myocardial strain. Lagrange strain (ε) at time t equals the change in length from original length divided by the original length. *L(t),* Segment length at a given time. (Courtesy Dr. Thomas Helle-Valle.)

STRAIN AND STRAIN RATE BY TISSUE DOPPLER IMAGING

In TDI, the velocity component along the ultrasound beam is measured at several spatial points simultaneously. By picking two velocity values, v_1 and v_2, along the beam with a spatial distance L, the Euler strain rate SR(t), or velocity gradient, can be calculated according to Eq. 2.3 for each TDI frame. The accuracy can be further improved by using several adjacent spatial points followed by linear regression. Using this concept, Heimdal et al.[7] introduced real-time strain rate imaging based on myocardial Doppler velocities. Temporal integration of the velocity gradient gives the logarithmic strain estimate denoted *natural strain* (ε_N) in Eq. 2.4. Lagrange strain (ε) can be derived from natural strain using the mathematical conversion in Eq. 2.4. To accurately determine strain, it is necessary to track and follow the motion of the material points (fixed particles) within the myocardium through time. This is not feasible with TDI, and therefore a small error is introduced, especially in the basal segments, where the motion relative to the ultrasound probe is highest.

The rationale for using spatial velocity gradient as a marker of myocardial function is that a velocity difference between two adjacent regions implies either compression or lengthening of the tissue in between, and the spatial velocity gradient equals the strain rate. When LV systolic function is studied in the LV long axis, strain rate measures the regional shortening rate, and strain measures the regional shortening fraction. In the LV short axis, strain rate measures the systolic thickening rate. During diastole, strain rate measures myocardial lengthening rate.

In principle, SR is not influenced by overall motion of the heart (translation) and only to a limited degree by motion caused by contraction in adjacent segments. This is in contrast to *velocity* within a myocardial segment, which is the net result of motion caused by contractions in that segment, motion due to tethering to other segments, and cardiac translation.[8,11] The effect of tethering explains why LV longitudinal velocities measured from an apical window increase progressively from the apex toward the base, whereas strains and strain rates are more similar.

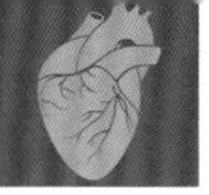

PHYSICAL PRINCIPLES OF SPECKLE TRACKING ECHOCARDIOGRAPHY

STE measures local myocardial displacement in echocardiographic images and may be used to quantify myocardial function in terms of velocity and strain. Furthermore, STE may be used to assess LV rotation and twist. The speckles are created by interference of ultrasound beams in the myocardium and are seen in grayscale B-mode images as a characteristic speckle pattern. The speckles are the result of constructive and destructive interference of ultrasound waves, which are back-scattered from structures smaller than a wavelength of ultrasound. Random noise is filtered out by the computer algorithm, yielding small segments of myocardium with temporarily stable and unique speckle patterns.[12] These segments, or *kernels*, serve as acoustic markers that can be tracked from frame to frame within an image plane using block matching.

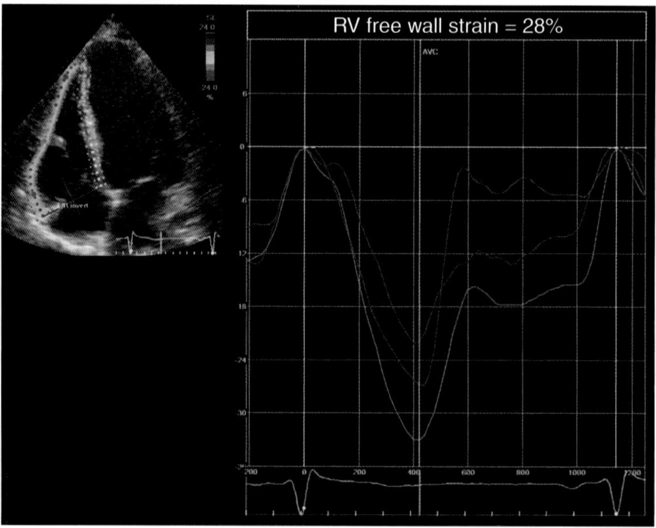

Fig. 2.7 Right ventricular strain imaging. RV strain from the lateral free wall in a healthy person. Global RV strain is approximately −27%. Video 2.7 demonstrates RV strain in a normal individual and the lower strain values in the septum compared with the RV lateral wall.

STRAIN AND STRAIN RATE BY SPECKLE TRACKING ECHOCARDIOGRAPHY

In contrast to TDI-based strain, which measures velocities from a fixed point in space with reference to an external probe, STE measures the instantaneous distance between two kernels. Therefore STE can measure strain in different directions in the same image. The ability of STE to measure strain had been documented in studies using both sonomicrometry and magnetic resonance imaging as reference methods.[9] Strain rate by STE can be calculated as the time derivative of the strain curve, followed by application of the conversion formula in Eq. 2.4 to obtain the Euler strain rate.

When applying STE, it is important to optimize the image quality of the grayscale image. This includes keeping the focus position at intermediate depth and adjusting the sector depth and width to include little but the region of interest. Assessment of 2D strain by STE is a semiautomatic method that requires a brief manual definition of a few points along the endocardial border. Furthermore, the sampling region of interest needs to be adjusted to ensure that most of the wall thickness is incorporated in the analysis and to avoid the pericardium. When automated tracking does not fit with the visual impression of wall motion, regions of interest need to be adjusted manually. End-systole is defined by aortic valve closure in the apical long-axis view, and this view should always be analyzed first.

Assessment of 2D strain by STE can be done successfully in multiple LV segments in most patients. Strain values are calculated for each segment (segmental strain) and as the average value of all segmental strains (global strain).[13] Feasibility is best for longitudinal and circumferential strain; it is more challenging for radial strain because fewer speckles are present in this direction and the measured values in a normal ventricle differ substantially between inner and outer layers of the wall, reflecting a geometric effect.[14] GLS is calculated as the average of the peak systolic longitudinal strain values from all LV segments in apical 4-, 3-, and 2-chamber views.[15] Because longitudinal strain is normally negative, reporting of values can be confusing. Therefore, it is recommended to report changes in strain in absolute values.[15]

In spite of different software in ultrasound machines from different vendors, GLS values are relatively similar.[16] However, there are small differences in strain values among vendors and among different software packages from the same vendor. Therefore, when doing serial studies, such as observing effects of chemotherapy on LV function, this limitation needs to be taken into account, and one should preferably use a machine from the same vendor and with similar software when repeating studies in an individual patient. In normal hearts, typical absolute values for GLS are about 20%. The lower limit for normal GLS was found to be 15.9% in a large meta-analysis[17] and 17.2% in a large multicenter study of healthy individuals.[18] Therefore, in clinical practice, absolute values of GLS less than 16% to 17% indicate reduced LV systolic function.

It is also feasible to measure right ventricular (RV) strain by STE (Fig. 2.7), but in some cases, speckle tracking of the thin RV lateral wall can be challenging. The same applies for the left atrium (LA), but here the signal quality is poorer due to low spatial resolution. A small structure in the image will blur out, with the amount of blurring given by the formula, ($\lambda \times$ depth)/probe aperture, where λ is the ultrasonic wavelength. Typical values for a 3-MHz cardiac probe are $\lambda = 0.5$ mm and aperture = 2 cm; this can result in a blurring of 3 mm in a 12-cm depth, and 4 mm in a 16-cm depth.

LA reservoir function (reservoir strain) by STE is measured from LV end-diastole (onset of QRS) to peak LA strain. LA reservoir strain is related to LA mean pressure and has been proposed as a supplementary index for estimating LV filling pressure (Fig. 2.8). The cutoff for LA reservoir strain as a marker of elevated LV filling pressure has so far not been defined in appropriately designed studies.

In contrast to 2D STE, which cannot track motion occurring out of plane, 3D STE can track motion of speckles within the scan volume, regardless of its direction (Figs. 2.9 and 2.10). One limitation of the 3D STE technique is its dependency on image quality and, in particular, its ability to define the endocardial border. Furthermore, 3D STE is limited by relatively low temporal and spatial resolution. Currently, technology for 3D STE strain imaging is developing rapidly, and it is expected to become an increasingly important modality.

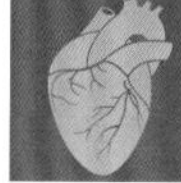

LV ROTATION AND TWIST

LV twist is the relative rotation of the apex around the LV long axis with respect to the base during the cardiac cycle; it can be measured by STE.[19,20] When viewed from apex to base, the apex rotates counterclockwise during systole, and the base rotates in the opposite direction. This is demonstrated in Fig. 2.11, which shows LV rotation by STE in a healthy individual.

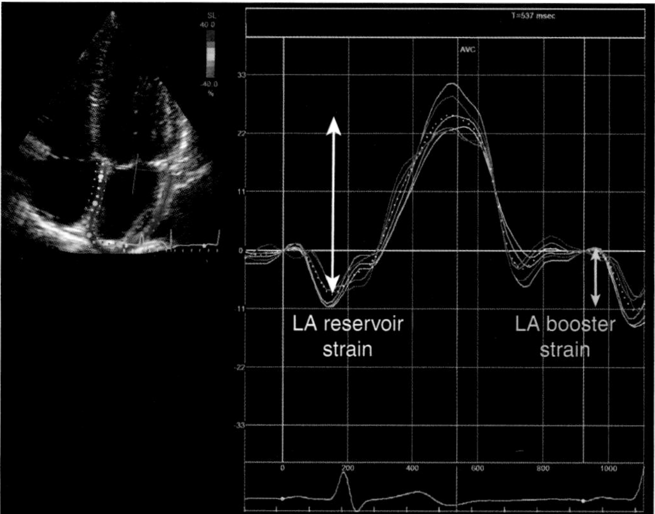

Fig. 2.8 Left atrial strain imaging. LA reservoir strain (also named LAS r) is calculated as the difference between onset of filling and end-diastole. LA booster strain (also named LAS ct) is calculated as the difference between end-diastole and onset of atrial filling. The zero strain reference point is at the onset of atrial contraction, but we recommend zero strain at end-diastole. *LAS*, Left atrial strain; *r*, reservoir; *ct*, contraction.

The *rotation* is expressed in degrees, and the apex-to-base difference in rotation is referred to as the *LV twist angle* (degrees). The term *torsion* is a normalized value and refers to the base-to-apex gradient in rotation angle, expressed in degrees per centimeter (°/cm) (see Fig. 2.11).

LIMITATIONS OF VELOCITY AND STRAIN IMAGING

ANGLE DEPENDENCY

TDI-based velocity and strain rate imaging are angle dependent because only velocity components in the beam direction are recorded. Because of the complex motion of the myocardium, angle correction is not feasible. Therefore it is essential to align the ultrasound beam parallel to the LV wall in long-axis imaging and perpendicular to the wall for radial measurements in the short axis. In longitudinal views, velocities should not be measured near the apex, because the apical curvature causes large angle problems.

Although STE can track speckles independent of angle, the measurements are still angle dependent because the polarity of radial strain is opposite that of the longitudinal and circumferential strains. If the image plane intersects the ventricular wall at an angle intermediate between the long and the short axis, the measurement will underestimate true strain in the main axis. This implies that foreshortening might affect the strain results and should be reduced to a minimum. Similarly, short-axis views should be circular to assess the deformation in the true circumferential or radial plane. Furthermore, because there is lower spatial resolution in the lateral direction, optimal performance is achieved in the direction of the ultrasound beam.

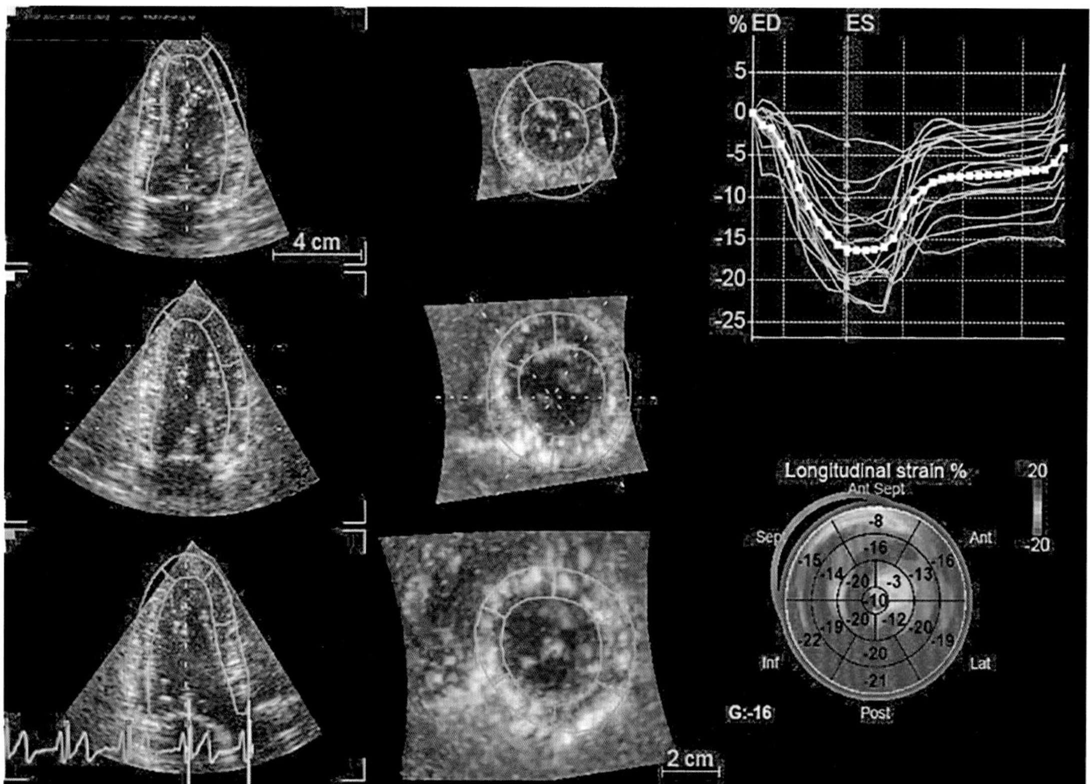

Fig. 2.9 3D strain from a patient before cancer treatment. Strain curves *(top right)* are assessed from a 3D longitudinal view and presented in a bull's-eye plot *(bottom right)*. (Courtesy Richard Massey, MSc.)

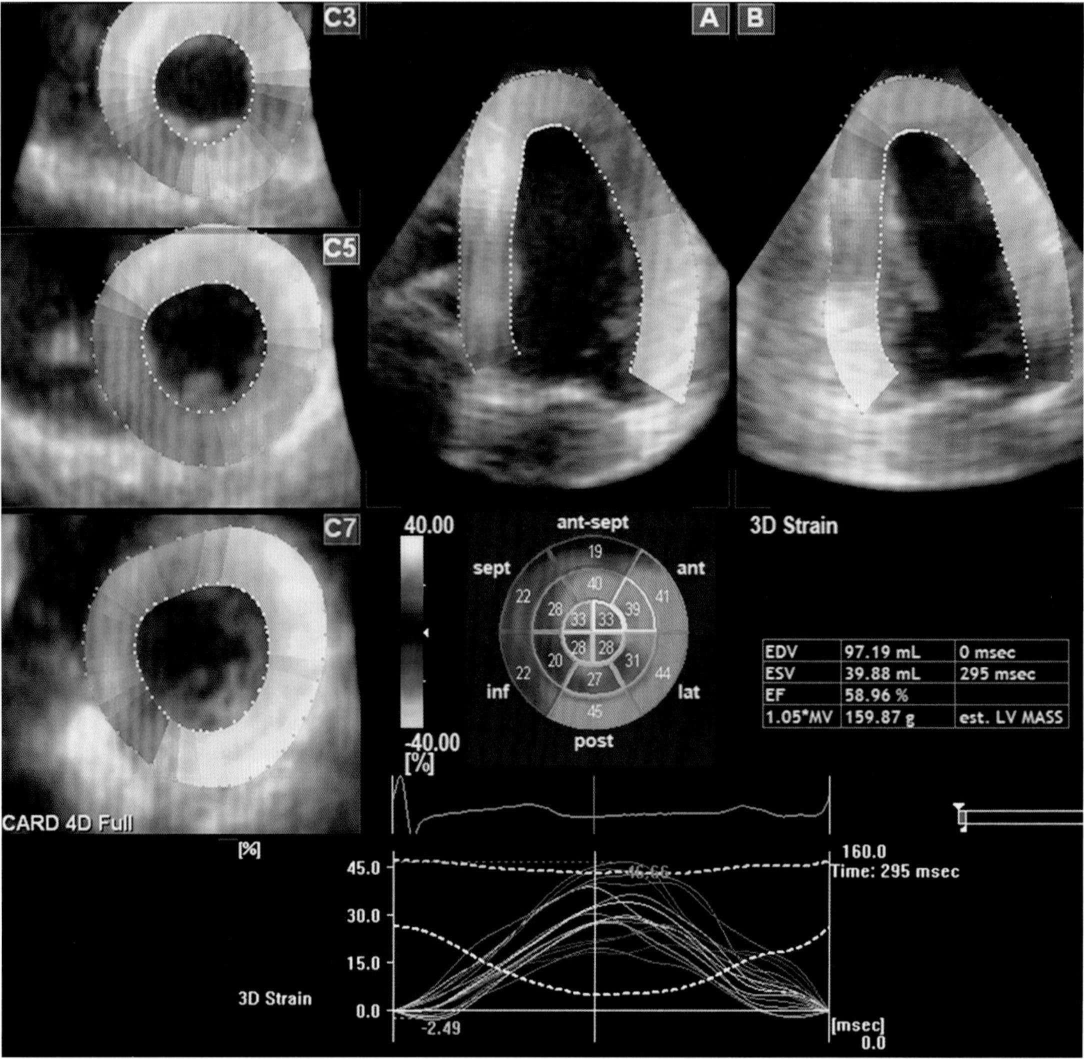

Fig. 2.10 **3D strain from a healthy individual.** The software calculates the 3D strain values from a combination of short-axis stacks and long-axis views. The values are presented in a bull's-eye plot in the middle of the figure, and the 3D strain curves are shown in the lower part of the figure. *EDV*, End-diastolic volume; *EF*, ejection fraction; *ESV*, end-systolic volume. (Courtesy Dr. Thomas Muri Stokke.)

INADEQUATE TRACKING

When strain traces appear unphysiologic, one should evaluate signal quality and suboptimal tracking as potential causes. The global strain might be misjudged if too many segmental strain values are discarded due to suboptimal tracking. This is particularly true in localized myocardial diseases where strain values are unevenly distributed.

NOISE REDUCTION VERSUS SPATIAL AND TEMPORAL RESOLUTION

The raw TDI/STE data are often quite noisy, so temporal and spatial averaging are needed to extract useful information. For TDI, smoothing is performed by local averaging of neighboring points in space and time. For STE, smoothing is often performed using a spline method, which gives a good fit to the raw data while preventing too rapid fluctuations. However, spline smoothing can also to a larger degree influence neighboring segments and reduce regional differences in strain.

Strain rate measurement is significantly affected by random noise. When using TDI, this reflects an effect of measuring a difference between velocities, because the error is the sum of the errors of the two velocities. The signal-to-noise ratio for TDI strain and strain rate can be improved by increasing the spatial offset (strain length) for the velocity points, which increases the velocity difference but will reduce the spatial resolution. The problem with random noise can also be reduced by temporal averaging within a heart cycle and by averaging multiple heart cycles. However, these methods for noise reduction represent compromises between optimal signal-to-noise ratio and requirements for high spatial and temporal resolution.

When using TDI, the spatial offset for measurement of longitudinal strain and strain rate is typically between 5 and 12 mm but can be defined by the operator. For transmural radial strain, wall thickness and translational motion restrict the range for adjustment of strain length. As a rule of thumb, the strain length should be set to approximately half the systolic thickness of the wall.[21] Strain rate imaging has relatively low lateral resolution, which limits the ability to measure separately from subendocardial and subepicardial wall layers in long-axis views. Furthermore, when the sample volume is at the inner or outer LV wall layer, the signal may in part represent velocities in the blood pool or pericardium, respectively. Fortunately, measurement of strain by TDI is associated with fewer noise problems than

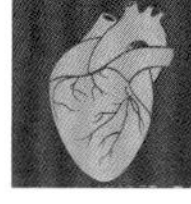

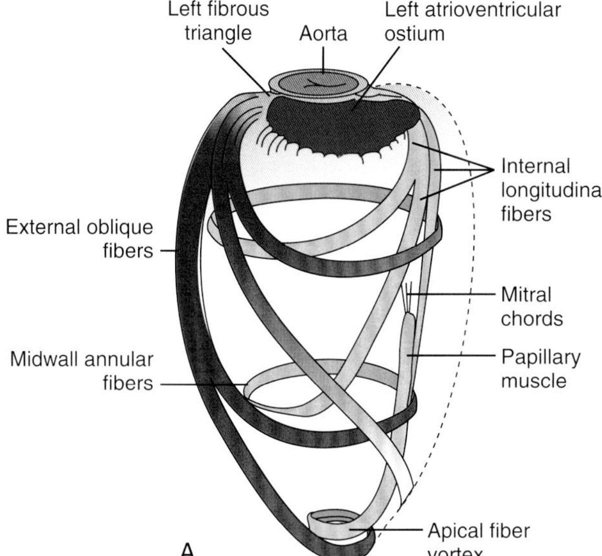

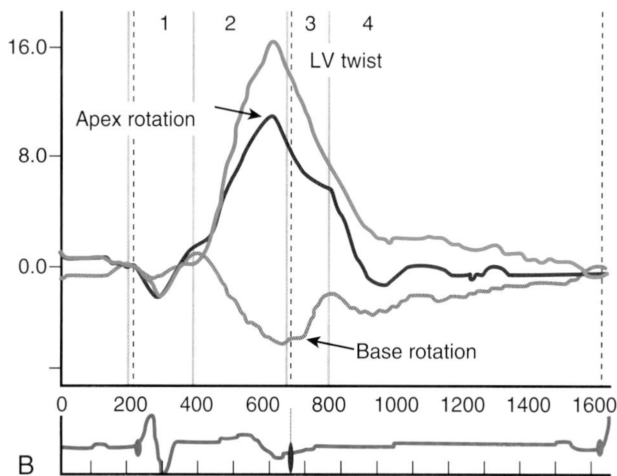

Fig. 2.11 Fiber orientation and LV twist. (A) Fiber orientation in the LV. The subendocardial fibers have an approximately longitudinal orientation, and the midwall fibers have an approximately circumferential orientation. The subepicardial fibers are oriented about 60 degrees relative to the circumferential direction. (B) LV twist calculated from the apical and basal rotations by STE in a normal healthy subject. The difference between the two rotations provides an estimate of net LV twist angle. During isovolumic contraction (phase 1), the apex shows a brief clockwise rotation and the base shows a brief counterclockwise rotation. During ejection (phase 2), the direction of rotation changes to counterclockwise at the LV apex and clockwise at the LV base. Untwisting occurs predominantly during isovolumic relaxation (phase 3) and early diastolic filling (phase 4). Animation of LV rotation as seen from a longitudinal view (Video 2.11A) and an apical view (Video 2.11B). The animation is based on a finite element simulation model of the LV. Notice the counterclockwise rotation of the LV apex. (A, Modified from Nakatani S. Left ventricular rotation and twist: why should we learn? *J Cardiovasc Ultrasound.* 2011;19(1):1–6. B, From Sengupta PP, Tajik AJ, Chandrasekaran K, Khandheria BK. Twist mechanics of the left ventricle: principles and application. *JACC Cardiovasc Imaging.* 2008;1:366–376. Videos courtesy E.W. Remme.)

measurement of strain rate because integration tends to reduce random noise in the strain rate signal. In the strain signal, however, there may be significant drift within a given heart cycle.

For STE, frame rates of 40 to 80 fps are recommended. Too low a frame rate may cause the speckles to move out of plane or beyond the search area in successive frames. Too high a frame rate can also be a problem, because this is normally achieved by reducing the number of ultrasound beams in each frame, thereby reducing the image quality. However, frame rates higher than 80 fps may be needed to prevent undersampling in tachycardia. The relatively low temporal resolution of STE is a limitation, particularly in regard to assessment of peak velocities and strain rates, because accurate measurement of these variables may require higher frame rates.

MOVEMENT OF SAMPLE VOLUME RELATIVE TO MYOCARDIUM

TDI measures velocity within a fixed area in space but not within a defined piece of myocardium. Because of cardiac motion, the difference between the two may be significant. This limitation, which applies to all TDI modalities, can in part be compensated for by using tracking algorithms that move the sample volume continuously or in steps during the heart cycle.

REVERBERATIONS

Reverberations are echoes caused by multiple reflections within the body, and in transthoracic imaging they are often caused by relatively motionless tissue layers close to the body surface. In grayscale imaging they are seen as false echoes or reduced contrast. For color TDI, the reverberations result in a bias toward zero velocity in the mean velocity estimate. The amount of bias depends on the intensity of the reverberation signal relative to the tissue velocity signal. Still, the sign of the velocity is seldom affected, so it might be difficult to detect reverberations when using the color display. For strain rate, however, imaging a small local bias in the velocity will cause large changes in the spatial velocity gradient and therefore in the strain rate, which will appear as random noise. The only way to avoid reverberation noise is to get a better scanning window. When analyzing the strain rate data, it is important to recognize the reverberation artifacts and to avoid the affected regions. Curved anatomic M-mode can be an effective tool to identify larger reverberation artifacts, and the experienced user can recognize them as unphysiologic color patterns.

With STE, reverberations increase the noise level in the strain values. For high reverberation levels, there can be substantial underestimation of strain. Furthermore, any artifact that resembles speckles will influence the speckle tracking quality, and care should be taken to prevent these.

LOAD DEPENDENCY

Similar to global EF, all regional ejection phase indices are load dependent.[8,22]

LIMITATIONS OF LV ROTATION AND TWIST

Because rotation increases progressively toward the apex, it is critical to include the distal apex in the image. The optimal distal cross-sectional image plane should include only a small part or no part of the RV. Furthermore, out-of-plane motion of the LV base caused by longitudinal motion is a significant limitation. Because 2D echocardiography does not provide accurate measures of distance between the two image planes, it is difficult to measure torsion. It is expected that several of these limitations will be improved with 3D STE, which is a promising, emerging technology.[23]

TRANSMURAL STRAIN GRADIENT

In a normal heart there are higher strains in the subendocardium than in the subepicardium; this effect is most pronounced for radial and circumferential strains. This is a purely geometric effect and does not mean that there is a difference in contractility between the inner and outer wall layers.[24]

INTERVENDOR VARIABILITY IN STRAIN

Because vendors use various methods for tracking speckles and in data processing, there are significant intervendor differences in strain values.[16] It is essential to keep this in mind when using reference values for normal strain. Furthermore, caution should be used when companies deliver upgrades of software, because this may lead to changes in measured strain values.

NORMAL LV PHYSIOLOGY

LV stroke volume is a result of longitudinal and circumferential myocardial shortening and twist, which cause LV wall thickening and thereby reduction in ventricular cavity volume.[25–28] In healthy people the systolic descent of the LV base is approximately 12 to 15 mm,[25,28] whereas the apex is relatively stationary, moving only a few millimeters. The myocardium lengthens during early diastole and during atrial-induced filling.

The structural basis for twisting is the spiral architecture of myocardial fibers, with subendocardial and subepicardial fibers arranged in a right-handed and left-handed helix, respectively[20,29,30] (see Fig. 2.11). Because of this architecture, contractions in the subepicardium and subendocardium produce opposite directions of twist: counterclockwise and clockwise, respectively. There is a larger lever arm and therefore larger torque in the subepicardium, so normal hearts have counterclockwise rotation of the apex in systole when seen from the LV apex toward the base. However, because the subendocardial fibers are activated earliest in systole, there is a brief clockwise twisting of small magnitude during isovolumic contraction, followed by counterclockwise twisting throughout ejection, reaching the maximum before the end of systole.[31] As illustrated in Fig. 2.11, rotation at the apex makes the largest contribution to LV twist.[29] The figure also illustrates that most of the untwisting is completed during isovolumic relaxation in the normal heart, whereas patients with diastolic dysfunction may have substantial untwisting after onset of transmitral filling.

LV torsion allows uniform distribution of fiber stress across the wall of the ventricle, which contributes to efficient systolic contraction. The twisting motion also contributes to diastolic filling by the sudden release of potential elastic energy, which causes rapid untwisting and leads to suction of blood from the atrium.[31–33]

A number of cardiac disorders are associated with reductions in systolic twist and reduction and delay in the untwisting velocity (Table 2.1). However, patients with LV hypertrophy and normal LVEF, aortic stenosis, or hypertrophic cardiomyopathy can have increased systolic twist,[34,35] probably because increased LV wall thickness results in an increase in the lever arm for subepicardial fibers and therefore larger torque. In the hypertrophic ventricle, delay in the onset of diastolic untwist contributes to diastolic dysfunction.[36] This untwisting may represent a means to differentiate between physiologic hypertrophy in elite athletes and pathologic hypertrophy in individuals with cardiomyopathies.

The magnitude of LV twist is sensitive to changes in both regional and global LV function.[34,37–45] Therefore, assessment

TABLE 2.1 LV Twist and Untwisting Velocity in Cardiac Disease.

Cardiac Disease	*Twist*	E_r
Systolic heart failure	↓	↓
Diastolic heart failure	N or ↑	N or ↓
Aortic stenosis	N or ↑	↓
Mitral regurgitation	↓	↓
Transmural infarction	↓	↓
Subendocardial ischemia	N	N or ↓
Dilated cardiomyopathy	↓	↓
Hypertrophic cardiomyopathy	N or ↑	↓
Restrictive cardiomyopathy	N or ↑	N
Constrictive pericarditis	↓	↓

↓, Reduced; ↑, increased; E_r, early diastolic untwisting velocity; *N*, normal.
From Sengupta PP, Tajik AJ, Chandrasekaran K, Khandheria BK. Twist mechanics of the left ventricle: principles and application. *JACC Cardiovasc Imaging*. 2008;1:366–376.

of LV twist represents an interesting approach for quantifying LV systolic and diastolic function. Assessment of LV twist by STE, however, is considered an emerging modality that is not yet ready for application in routine clinical settings.[5]

SYSTOLIC VELOCITIES

During LV isovolumic contraction there is a brief velocity spike caused by shortening before mitral valve closure. Isovolumic contraction displaces blood into the bulging mitral leaflets, and contraction is temporarily arrested when the mitral valve reaches its final closing position[46] (see Fig. 2.2). In some cases there is a small negative velocity component at the end of isovolumic contraction, which may reflect slight normal asynchrony in electromechanical activation.

Peak systolic ejection velocity (s') has proved to be a marker of regional systolic function.[46–48] Myocardial velocity reaches a peak during the early phase of ejection and then decreases gradually. In some cases a second, smaller peak occurs later during ejection. Longitudinal velocities are more reproducible than radial velocities and can be measured in virtually all vascular territories of the LV. For that reason, longitudinal velocities are recommended in the assessment of LV function. Table 2.2 presents normal ejection velocities from the LV long axis as assessed by TDI.

DIASTOLIC VELOCITIES

In the LV long axis there is a negative velocity spike during isovolumic relaxation; it starts near end-systole and is temporarily interrupted by aortic valve closure,[46] reflecting myocardial lengthening (see Fig. 2.2). This is analogous to the mechanism for the isovolumic contraction velocity and is attributed to a slight increase in LV volume associated with aortic valve closure and bulging of the valve leaflets into the LV. At the end of isovolumic relaxation there is normally a small positive velocity component that represents slight postsystolic shortening,[49] probably reflecting normal intraventricular asynchrony of relaxation.[50] In the diseased ventricle, and in particular during myocardial ischemia, there may be marked postsystolic shortening, and the postsystolic velocity may extend into the diastolic filling phase. Postsystolic velocities and strains in healthy subjects are of low amplitude and occur before mitral valve opening.[49]

Assessment of mitral annulus velocities by TDI plays an important role in the evaluation of suspected diastolic

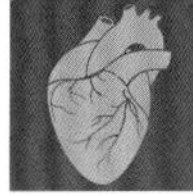

TABLE 2.2 **Normal Reference Ranges for Systolic Mitral Annular Velocities According to Age.**[a]

	Total							
	20–40 y		40–60 y		>60 y			
Parameters (cm/s)	*Mean ± SD*	*95% CI*	*Mean ± SD*	*95% CI*	*Mean ± SD*	*95% CI*	P^b	rP^c
Septal *s′* wave	8.6 ± 1.3	6.0–12.0	7.9 ± 1.4	5.9–11.0	7.5 ± 1.3	5.0–10.0	<0.001	−0.30; <0.001
Lateral *s′* wave	10.7 ± 2.3	6.1–16.0	9.4 ± 2.2	5.0–14.0	8.5 ± 2.5	4.0–15.0	<0.001	−0.37; <0.001
Average septal and lateral *s′* wave	9.6 ± 1.6	7.0–13.0	8.7 ± 1.5	6.0–12.0	8.1 ± 1.6	5.5–12.5	<0.001	−0.39; <0.001
Inferior *s′* wave	9.3 ± 1.5	7.0–12.0	8.8 ± 1.5	6.0–12.0	8.2 ± 1.5	5.0–12.0	<0.001	−0.26; <0.001
Anterior *s′* wave	10.0 ± 2.1	6.6–13.4	8.6 ± 2.0	5.0–13.0	7.6 ± 2.1	4.0–12.0	<0.001	−0.45; <0.001
Posterior *s′* wave	10.2 ± 1.8	7.0–14.0	9.2 ± 1.9	6.0–13.2	8.8 ± 2.7	5.6–18.6	<0.001	−0.27; <0.001
Average *s′* wave	9.7 ± 1.7	7.2–12.9	8.7 ± 1.4	6.2–11.9	8.1 ± 1.6	5.7–12.7	<0.001	−0.41; <0.001

[a]The study included 449 individuals (mean age: 45.8 ± 13.7 years, 198 men and 251 women).
[b]Probability difference *(P)* between groups according to age category by analysis of variance (two-way ANOVA).
[c]Probability *(P)* and correlation *(r)* with age for both genders (Pearson correlation test).
Modified from Caballero L, Kou S, Dulgheru R, et al. Echocardiographic reference ranges for normal cardiac Doppler data: results from the NORRE Study. *Eur Heart J Cardiovasc Imaging.* 2015;16:1031–1041.

TABLE 2.3 **Normal Reference Ranges for Parameters of Diastolic Filling According to Age.**[a]

	20–40 y		40–60 y		≥60 y		
Parameters	*Mean ± SD*	*95% CI*	*Mean ± SD*	*95% CI*	*Mean ± SD*	*95% CI*	P^b
Pulse Doppler at the Mitral Valve							
E wave velocity (cm/s)	0.82 ± 0.16	053–1.22	0.75 ± 0.17	0.46–1.13	0.70 ± 0.16	0.39–1.03	<0.001
A wave velocity (cm/s)	0.50 ± 0.13	0.30–0.87	0.62 ± 0.15	0.37–0.97	0.74 ± 0.16	0.40– 1.04	<0.001
E wave deceleration time (ms)	178.2 ± 43.1	105.2–269.0	187.6 ± 45.5	114.6–288.1	208.9 ± 62.7	114.0–385.9	<0.001
E/A ratio	1.71 ± 0.52	0.89–3.18	1.24 ± 0.39	0.71–2.27	0.98 ± 0.29	0.53–1.80	<0.001
Tissue Doppler Data							
Septal *e′* wave (cm/s)	12.1 ± 2.5	8.0–17.0	9.8 ± 2.6	5.0–16.0	7.6 ± 2.3	3.0–13.0	<0.001
Septal *a′* wave (cm/s)	8.5 ± 1.7	5.3–12.0	9.8 ± 2.0	6.9–14.0	10.5 ± 1.7	7.0–14.0	<0.001
Lateral *e′* wave (cm/s)	16.4 ± 3.4	10.0–23.0	12.5 ± 3.0	6.0–18.0	9.6 ± 2.8	4.0–17.0	<0.001
Lateral *a′* wave (cm/s)	8.2 ± 2.2	5.0–13.0	9.4 ± 2.6	5.0–15.0	10.6 ± 2.9	6.0–17.0	<0.001
Average septal and lateral *e′* wave	14.3 ± 2.7	9.1–19.5	11.1 ± 2.5	6.0–16.0	8.6 ± 2.3	3.5–15.0	<0.001
***E/e′* Ratio**							
Septal *E/e′*	6.9 ± 1.6	4.4–10.6	8.1 ± 2.3	4.3–13.2	9.7 ± 2.8	5.0–16.9	<0.001
Lateral *E/e′*	5.1 ± 1.3	3.1–8.5	6.3 ± 2.2	3.7–12.0	7.8 ± 2.2	4.2–12.8	<0.001
Average septal and lateral *E/e′*	5.8 ± 1.3	3.6–9.1	7.0 ± 2.1	4.2–11.5	8.5 ± 2.2	4.6–13.5	<0.001

[a]The study included 449 individuals (mean age: 45.8 ± 13.7 years, 198 men and 251 women).
[b]Probability difference *(P)* between groups according to age category by analysis of variance (one-way ANOVA).
Modified from Caballero L, Kou S, Dulgheru R, et al. Echocardiographic reference ranges for normal cardiac Doppler data: results from the NORRE Study. *Eur Heart J Cardiovasc Imaging.* 2015;16:1031–1041.

dysfunction. Measurements are taken from apical views, and velocities may be measured at the septal, lateral, anterior, and inferior mitral annular areas. There are two main diastolic velocities, reflecting early diastolic (*e′*) and atrial-induced (*a′*) myocardial lengthening, respectively (see Fig. 2.2). Mitral annulus velocities are measured from an apical 4-chamber view using either the septal velocity, the lateral velocity, or an average of the two. The *e′* wave is often followed by an oppositely directed wave of low amplitude (*e″*) during early diastasis, which reflects changes in geometry associated with redistribution of blood within the LV cavity.[48] Similar to systolic velocities, diastolic velocities decrease progressively from the base toward the apex.

Normal values for mitral annular diastolic velocities by pulsed-wave TDI are presented in Table 2.3. Velocities measured in 2D color mode are lower than those measured by pulsed-wave Doppler, and this needs to be taken into account when interpreting *e′* in a clinical context. In adults, *e′* velocity decreases with age; therefore, age-based normal values should be used when applying these measures of LV diastolic function in clinical practice.[5]

The magnitude of *e′* is closely related to active myocardial relaxation, as indicated by its correlation with the time constant of LV isovolumic relaxation.[51–54] In addition, *e′* is determined by LV restoring forces, which represent release of energy that is stored in the myocardium when the ventricle has contracted below its resting length[55] (Fig. 2.12). During early diastole, the restoring forces recoil the fibers back to their resting length, analogous to the recoil of a spring that has been compressed below its unstressed length. Restoring forces increase progressively when end-systolic volume is reduced and are therefore dependent on LV contractility. This illustrates the tight coupling between systolic shortening and diastolic lengthening and implies that *e′* is determined by systolic as well as diastolic function.

In addition to LV relaxation and restoring forces, *e′* is also determined by early diastolic load (LV lengthening load), which is represented by the LV transmural pressure at the onset of filling.[55] Therefore, the three main determinants of *e′* are rate of relaxation, restoring forces, and early diastolic

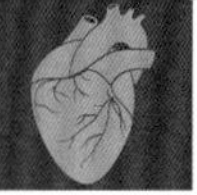

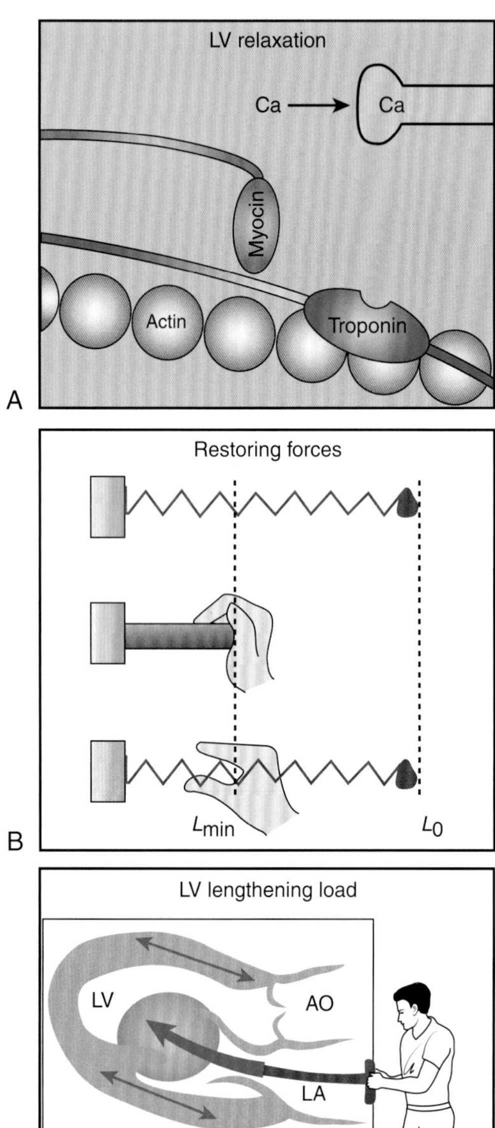

Fig. 2.12 Determinants of *e′*. (A) Myocardial relaxation is caused by decline of the intracellular calcium transient and inactivation of the myofilament. (B) Restoring forces can be illustrated as an elastic spring that is compressed to a dimension (L_{min}) less than its resting length (L_0); the spring recoils back to resting length when the compression is released. Similarly, when the LV contracts to a volume that is less than its unstressed resting volume, it recoils back in early diastole when the myocardium relaxes. (C) The LV lengthening load is the pressure in the LA at mitral valve opening, which "pushes" blood into the LV and thereby lengthens the ventricle. *AO*, Aorta; *Ca*, calcium. (Modified from Smiseth OA, Remme E, Opdahl A, et al. Heart failure with normal left ventricular ejection fraction: basic principles and clinical diagnostics. In: Bartunek J, Vanderheyden M, eds. *Translational Approach to Heart Failure*. New York, NY: Springer; 2013.)

pressure. In addition, LV diastolic stiffness may modulate *e′*. It is also possible to evaluate diastolic function by diastolic strain rates using TDI or STE, but this application needs more validation before recommendations can be made with regard to clinical use. Therefore, at the present time, it is recommended that TDI-derived mitral annulus velocities, calculated as the average of the septal and lateral velocities by pulsed-wave Doppler, be used for the routine clinical evaluation of LV relaxation and early diastolic function.[5,56]

MYOCARDIAL ISCHEMIA

Myocardial ischemia can be caused either by a reduction in coronary blood flow, as in acute coronary syndrome, or by an increase in myocardial oxygen demand during stress in patients with coronary artery stenosis. In either case, ischemia leads to a reduction in regional myocardial function that ranges from reduced systolic shortening (hypokinesia) to systolic lengthening (dyskinesia) (Figs. 2.13 and 2.14).

Furthermore, myocardial ischemia leads to postsystolic shortening—that is, segmental shortening after the end of LV ejection. Reduced systolic shortening, systolic lengthening, and postsystolic shortening, which are the three hallmarks of ischemic dysfunction, can be quantified by both velocity and deformation imaging.[7,8,47,57–60]

The most prominent velocity features in mild and moderate myocardial ischemia are reduced peak ejection velocity and increased postsystolic velocity (see Fig. 2.3). The dominantly positive velocity during isovolumic contraction diminishes, and with more marked ischemia the isovolumic contraction velocity becomes negative.[61] Furthermore, dyskinesia is associated with enhanced postsystolic velocity due to postsystolic shortening. Therefore a typical velocity trace from dyskinetic myocardium has a large negative velocity spike during isovolumic contraction and a large positive velocity during isovolumic relaxation, with velocities near zero during ejection.[22]

Postsystolic shortening by velocity or strain imaging (see Fig. 2.14) can be used as a marker of acute as well as stress-induced myocardial ischemia.[3,60–62] The mechanism of postsystolic shortening can be delayed active contraction, passive recoil of dyskinetic myocardium, or a combination of active contraction and passive recoil.[63,64] When postsystolic shortening occurs in entirely passive or necrotic myocardium, it is analogous to the behavior of a stretched elastic spring that recoils passively when the stretching force is removed. In moderately ischemic myocardium, postsystolic shortening is the result of delayed active contraction.[64] Because postsystolic shortening may occur in actively contracting myocardium as well as in necrotic myocardium, it is nonspecific with regard to tissue viability. At present, the clinical value of postsystolic shortening, measured as either postsystolic velocity or postsystolic strain, is that it serves as a marker of ischemia. One should also remember, however, that postsystolic shortening can be present in a normal ventricle but is then of small magnitude.[60]

CARDIAC SYNCHRONY

Normally, ventricular activation spreads rapidly through the conduction system, resulting in a synchronized ventricular contraction. In patients with severe heart failure, there is often prolonged intraventricular conduction, which leads to interventricular or intraventricular mechanical dyssynchrony, resulting in ineffective ventricular function. In addition, heart failure patients may have a prolonged atrioventricular (AV) interval and therefore AV dyssynchrony. It is LV intraventricular dyssynchrony that is the principal factor associated with the development of heart failure.

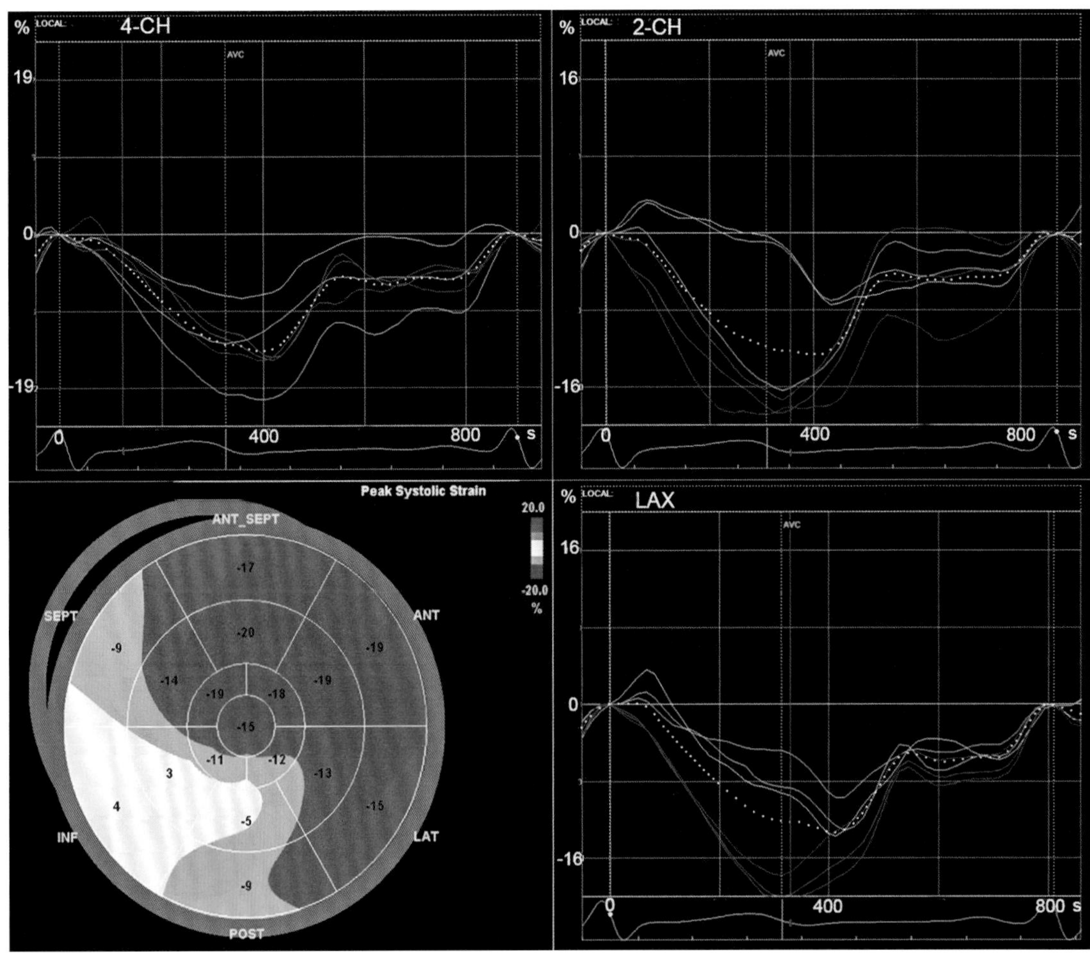

Fig. 2.13 **Bull's-eye plot in acute myocardial infarction.** STE in a patient with an occluded right coronary artery (RCA) who had an acute myocardial infarction. The LV strain curves from the LV segments perfused by the RCA show a typical pattern of acute ischemia with an early systolic stretch, reduced systolic strain, and postsystolic shortening.

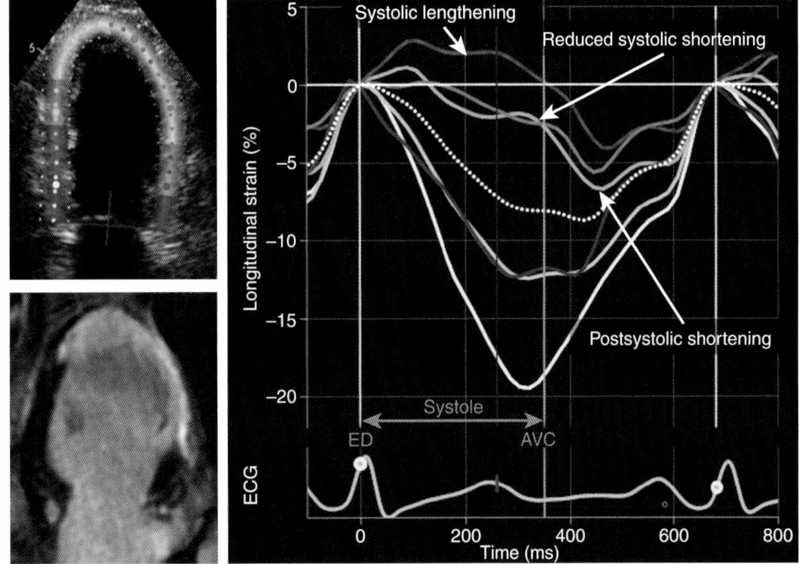

Fig. 2.14 **Acute myocardial infarction.** Longitudinal strain by STE (2-chamber view) in a patient with acute myocardial infarction the day after percutaneous coronary intervention (PCI) of an occluded left anterior descending coronary artery. Follow-up late enhancement by cardiac magnetic resonance imaging *(lower left)* showed myocardial scarring represented by the white area in the apex and anterior wall. Strain curves display typical features of ischemic dysfunction, with lengthening throughout systole in a segment with transmural infarction and different degrees of dysfunction in other segments. The *yellow curve* shows normal contraction in a noninfarcted segment. (From Smiseth OA, Torp H, Opdahl A, et al. Myocardial strain imaging: how useful is it in clinical decision making? *Eur Heart J.* 2016;37:1196–1207.)

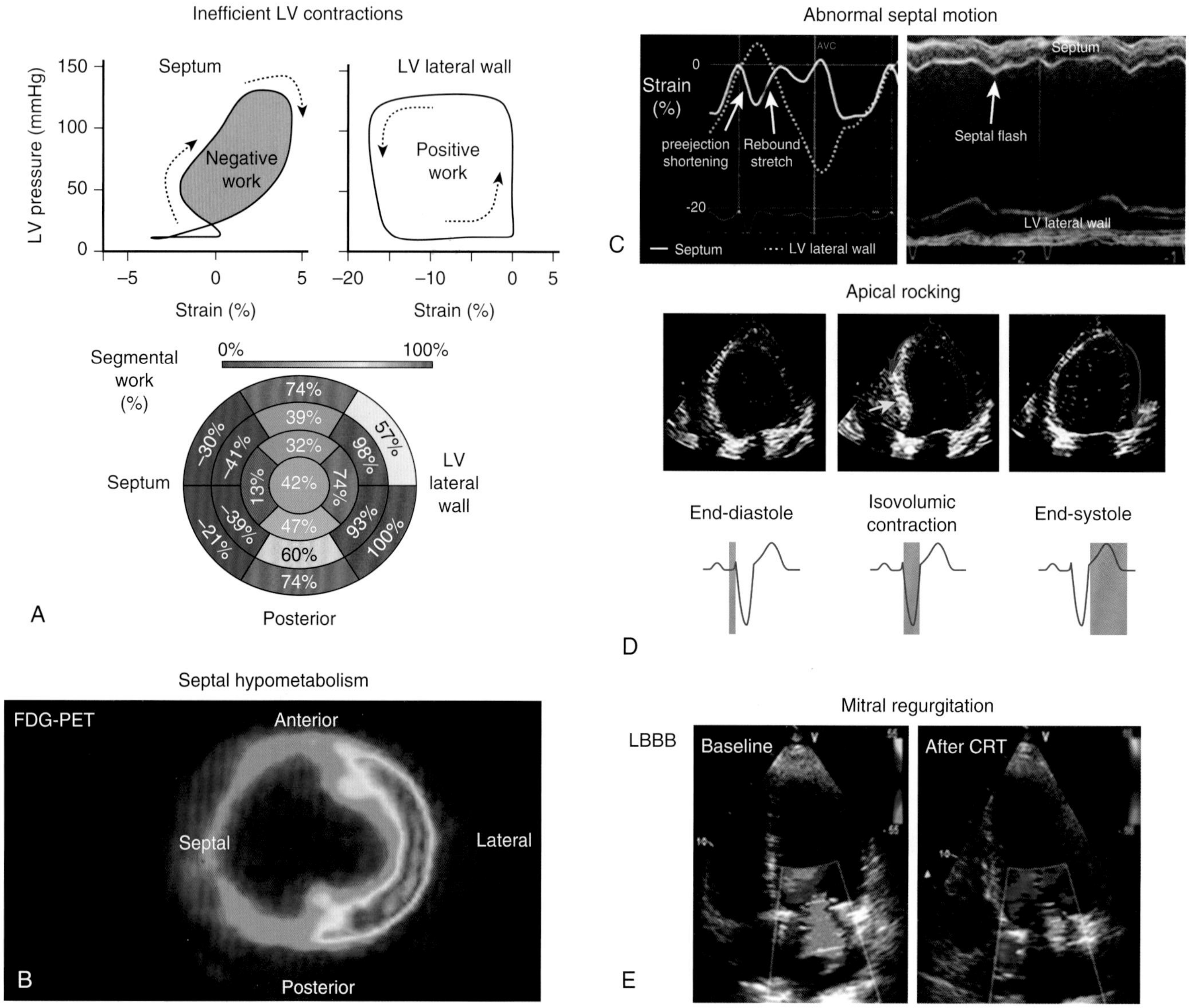

Fig. 2.15 Pathophysiology of left bundle branch block. (A) Contractile inefficiency: *Upper panels* display pressure-strain loops from the septum and LV lateral wall in a patient with LBBB and non-ischemic cardiomyopathy. Loop area reflects segmental work. The lateral wall shows normal counterclockwise rotation of the pressure-strain coordinates with shortening in systole. The septal pressure-strain loop rotates clockwise, which means lengthening in systole, and the result is negative (wasted) work, as indicated by the *red-colored* loop area. The *lower panel* displays segmental work distribution in the entire ventricle. Values are given as percentages of the segment with the highest work value. (B) Septal hypometabolism: ^{18}Fluorodeoxyglucose–positron emission tomographic (FDG-PET) LV short- and long-axis images from a representative patient with LBBB and non-ischemic cardiomyopathy. The point with the highest FDG uptake is used as reference (100%), and segmental values are reported as percentages of this value. *Green color* in septum indicates low metabolism relative to the lateral wall. The reduced septal work, illustrated in panel A, explains the reduced septal metabolism. *Red color* in the LV lateral wall indicates a high rate of glucose metabolism. (C) Abnormal septal motion: *Left panel,* Septal and LV lateral wall strain traces from a representative LBBB patient with non-ischemic cardiomyopathy. There is septal preejection shortening with corresponding LV lateral wall stretch. As the LV lateral wall starts to shorten, there is rebound stretch of the septum, and septal shortening at end-systole is reduced. *Right panel,* Parasternal M-mode image from the same patient. Preejection shortening and rebound stretch are visualized as septal flash. (D) Apical rocking: During isovolumetric contraction, the apex is pulled rightward by early septal and RV free wall contraction *(middle panel),* whereas later in systole it is pulled back by the forceful contraction in the late-activated LV lateral wall. (E) Mitral regurgitation: Echocardiographic recordings from a patient with congestive heart failure and LBBB. The *left panel* shows severe mitral regurgitation, as indicated by large color Doppler jet area. The *right panel* shows marked reduction of mitral regurgitation after cardiac resynchronization therapy (CRT). Video 2.15 ▶ shows left ventricular motion in a patient with a LBBB and typical rocking pattern. (Adapted from Smiseth OA, Aalen JM. Mechanism of harm from left bundle branch block. *Trends Cardiovasc Med.* 2019;29[6]:335–342.)

MECHANISMS OF LV INTRAVENTRICULAR DYSSYNCHRONY

It is a clinical challenge to differentiate between dyssynchrony that is caused by electrical conduction delay (electrical dyssynchrony) and dyssynchrony that is caused by load or ischemia (primary mechanical dyssynchrony). This differentiation is important because presumably only electrical dyssynchrony can be treated with biventricular pacing. At the present time, QRS width in electrocardiography (ECG) is the only routine method that is used to identify electrical dyssynchrony, and the left bundle branch block (LBBB) pattern is the QRS morphology that best predicts success of cardiac resynchronization therapy (CRT).

EFFECT OF LEFT BUNDLE BRANCH BLOCK ON LV FUNCTION

LBBB has several detrimental effects on LV function.[64a] Fig. 2.15 summarizes how LBBB modifies LV function and metabolism and may cause mitral regurgitation. The most prominent echocardiographic feature of LBBB is abnormal systolic

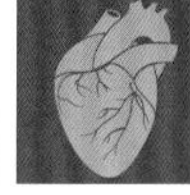

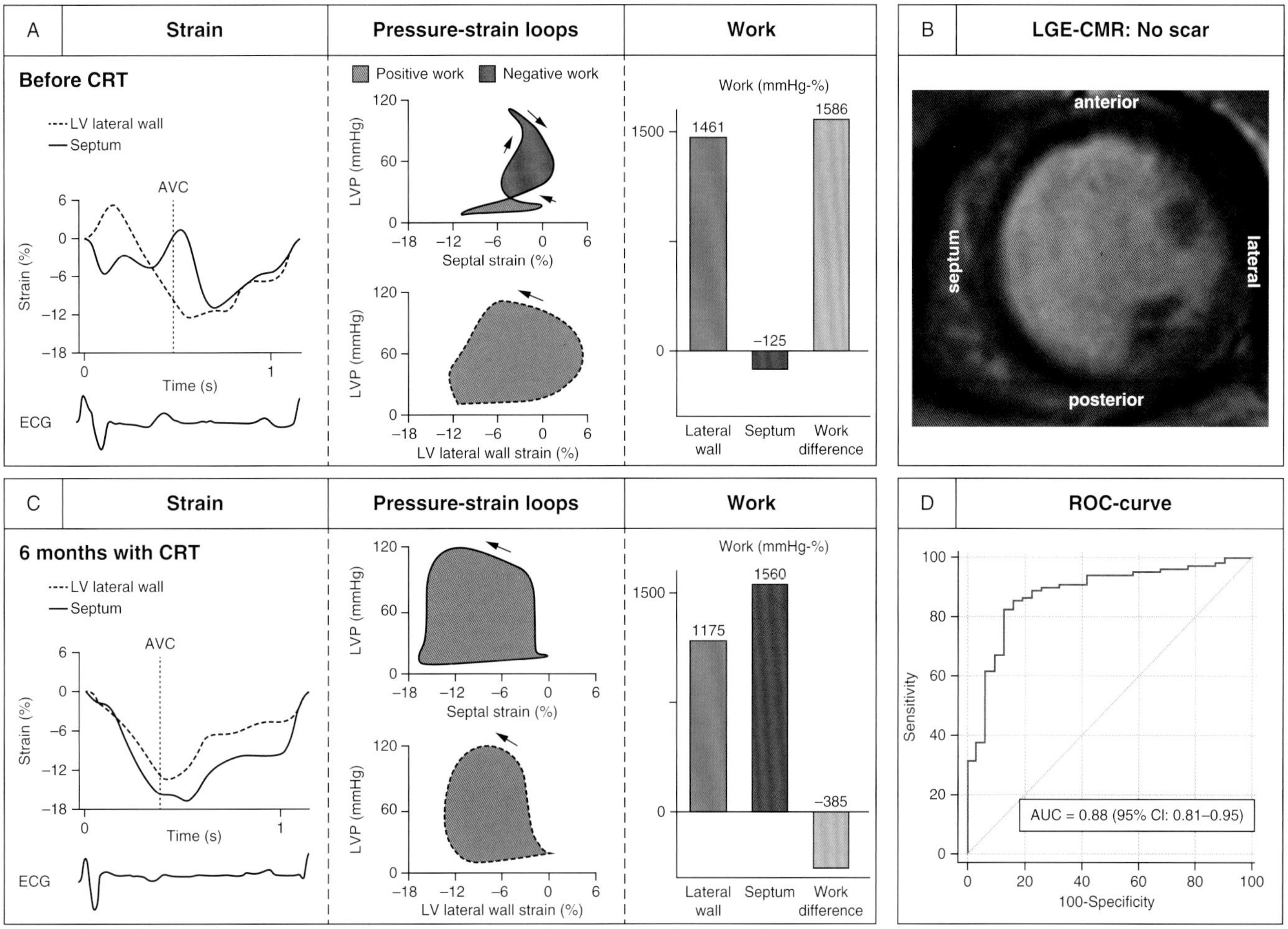

Fig. 2.16 LV work asymmetry combined with septal viability identifies CRT responders. (A–C) The panels are from the same patient and illustrate how the lateral-to-septal work difference is used in combination with viability by LGE-CMR to identify CRT responders. (A) Before CRT, there is dominantly negative septal work, as indicated by the red-colored pressure-strain loop area, but compensatory increase in LV lateral wall work, which gives a large lateral-to-septal work difference. (B) Viable septum indicates potential for recovery of septal function. (C) After 6 months with CRT, there is fine recovery of septal function. The highly inefficient septal contractions before CRT are converted to positive work throughout systole. The improvement in septal function is accompanied by reduced workload on the lateral wall. (D) ROC curve displaying combined assessment of work difference and septal viability for CRT response prediction (n = 123). *AUC*, Area under curve; *AVC*, aortic valve closure; *CI*, confidence interval; *LGE-CMR*, late gadolinium enhancement cardiac magnetic resonance; *LVP*, left ventricular pressure; *ROC*, receiver operating characteristic.

motion of the interventricular septum, starting with rapid leftward motion of the septum during preejection, followed by rightward (paradoxical) motion.[65] This motion was originally referred to as *septal beaking*[66] and more recently as *septal flash*[67] (see Fig. 2.15). Septal flash is caused predominantly by active contraction of the early-activated septum, but a passive push caused by elevation of RV pressure before the rise in LV pressure may contribute.[68–70] Another echocardiographic feature of hearts with LBBB is a rocking motion of the apex caused by an imbalance of forces generated by contractions in early- and late-activated parts of the LV wall.[71] The disturbed LV mechanical function in LBBB has a major impact on LV contractile efficiency.[72]

The research group of Smiseth et al. has introduced a clinical method for estimation of regional LV myocardial work by echocardiography.[72a] Similar to calculation of LV stroke work from pressure-volume loops, myocardial segmental work is calculated as the area of the pressure-strain loop. Pressure is assessed noninvasively based on brachial systolic pressure and valvular event timing, whereas strain is measured by STE (Fig. 2.16). The validity of this approach for assessing myocardial work is supported by good correlation between segmental work and the *regional* myocardial metabolic rate of glucose utilization measured by ^{18}fluorodeoxyglucose–positron emission tomography (FDG-PET). In patients with LBBB, septal segments typically shorten during early systole when pressure is low and thus perform just a small amount of positive work (constructive work). This is often followed by systolic lengthening of septal myocardium, which implies negative work (wasted work). Later in systole there is a variable degree of septal shortening and a component of positive work (constructive work). The net result is a marked reduction in septal work, and in some patients septal segments may show net negative work. As illustrated in Fig. 2.16, septal work can be markedly reduced in patients with LBBB and may improve with CRT. The wasted septal work is the result of contractions in the LV lateral wall and implies that the septum absorbs energy from the LV free wall. The increased work load on the free wall is a stimulus for remodeling, which contributes to the development or progression of global LV dysfunction and ultimately congestive heart failure. A recent prospective multicenter study showed that assessment of myocardial work improves prediction of response to CRT.[72b] A large difference in work between the LV lateral wall and septum predicted a positive response to CRT, as illustrated in Fig. 2.16. When work by echocardiography was combined with viability assessment by cardiac magnetic resonance and the septum was viable, prediction was even better.

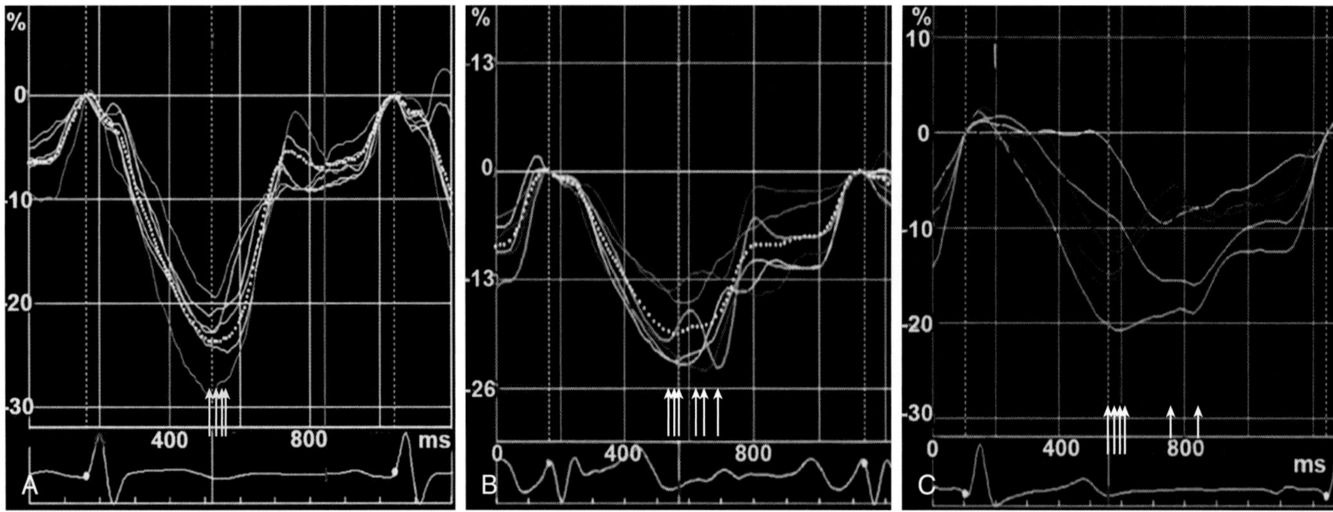

Fig. 2.17 **Mechanical dispersion.** (A) Strain curves from the apical 4-chamber view in a healthy individual. (B) Strain in a patient after myocardial infarction who died of ventricular fibrillation during follow-up. (C) LV strain in a patient with arrhythmogenic RV cardiomyopathy (ARVC) with episodes of ventricular tachycardia. *Vertical arrows* indicate the timing of peak negative strain.

DYSSYNCHRONY AND RISK OF VENTRICULAR ARRHYTHMIAS

LV dyssynchrony, defined as non-uniform timing of peak myocardial shortening, may have several underlying mechanisms, including defects in His-Purkinje conduction, disturbances in electromechanical coupling, and purely mechanical causes. The last group includes non-uniform wall stresses resulting from altered geometry and regional differences in contractility. Intramyocardial conduction delay due to fibrosis and scarring can lead to dyssynchrony. Furthermore, non-uniform electrical properties, such as in patients with long QT syndrome (LQTS), are associated with dyssynchrony.[73,74] It was proposed that dyssynchrony in LQTS is caused by dispersion in action potential duration, and the dyssynchrony was therefore named *mechanical dispersion* or *strain dispersion.* It was found that dyssynchrony was a predictor of risk of ventricular arrhythmias in LQTS patients[73,74] and in several diseases, including coronary artery disease. Furthermore, mechanical dispersion appears to serve as a marker of risk for ventricular arrhythmias and sudden death regardless of the level of EF, and also in some preclinical conditions with normal EF and normal GLS.[73,75] The clinical value of dyssynchrony as a risk marker remains to be determined.

Fig. 2.17 shows how mechanical dispersion is measured as the standard deviation (SD) of time from the onset of QRS in ECG to maximum myocardial shortening in 16 LV segments; data are shown for a healthy individual and for two patients who had experienced ventricular arrhythmias. In the healthy heart there is essentially similar timing of peak strain in all segments. In the patients, however, there is marked variability in timing of peak strain between segments. Various terms are used to describe dyssynchrony in hearts with intact His-Purkinje conduction, including dyscoordination, incoordination, and mechanical dispersion.

STRAIN IMAGING IN SUBCLINICAL LV DYSFUNCTION

Measurement of GLS has recently been incorporated in the clinical routine as a method to identify patients with mild systolic dysfunction that is not reflected in reduced EF. In patients with valvular heart disease, myocardial strain appears to be more sensitive than EF and can identify myocardial dysfunction before a fall in EF.[76] In heart failure with preserved EF, there may be reduction in GLS as a sign of reduced systolic function.[77]

Better sensitivity of GLS to detect mild systolic dysfunction is explained by the fact that EF is related predominantly to LV circumferential shortening, whereas GLS measures longitudinal shortening.[78,79] The principle that LV EF reflects predominantly circumferential shortening is illustrated in Fig. 2.18. Furthermore, the myofibers that account for longitudinal shortening are located mainly in the vulnerable subendocardium, so reduction in GLS often precedes reduction in EF.

Furthermore, because of the presence of small LV cavities in ventricles with concentric hypertrophy, even a small stroke volume caused by systolic dysfunction may result in normal or hypernormal EF. This is a significant limitation of the use of EF in patients with hypertrophic LV.[79] Typical examples of cardiac diseases in which EF may not reflect systolic function are aortic stenosis, hypertrophic cardiomyopathy, and amyloidosis.[80–84] In asymptomatic patients with aortic stenosis, GLS appears to be superior to EF as a parameter of systolic dysfunction and for risk stratification.[80,82]

In patients undergoing chemotherapy, reduction in myocardial strain precedes significant change in LVEF, and GLS by STE is recommended for early detection of subclinical LV dysfunction.[85,86] Importantly, the value of these changes in predicting the clinical outcome after chemotherapy remains to be determined. Strain imaging may also be used to detect subclinical LV dysfunction in specific cardiomyopathies such as hypertrophic cardiomyopathy. It has also been shown that GLS is an excellent marker of mortality after MI and in patients with known or suspected LV impairment.[85,87]

RV FUNCTION

The RV has a complex anatomic structure and is divided into two parts, the inflow tract and the outflow tract, which are separated by the crista supraventricularis.

Echocardiographic imaging of RV function and measurement of EF are difficult because of the complex shape and

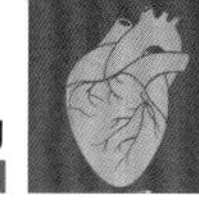

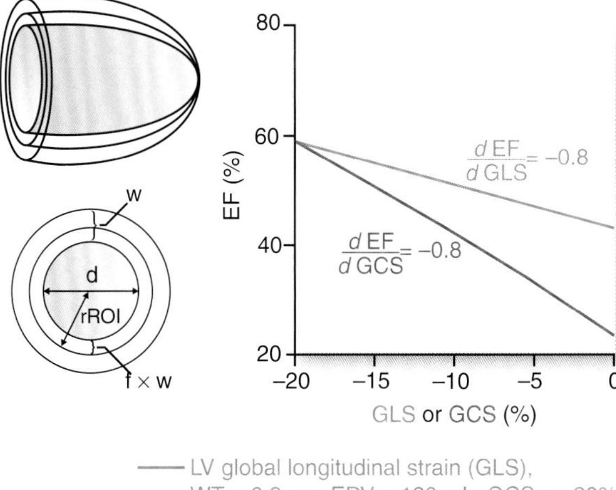

Fig. 2.18 Geometric model of the LV and relationships between EF and measurements of global strain. A truncated, thick-walled ellipsoid model of the LV is shown *(upper left)*. A short-axis view of the model *(lower left)* illustrates the internal diameter *(d)*, wall thickness *(w)*, and radius to the center of the speckle-tracking region of interest (rROI) where strain is measured. The distance from the endocardium to this center is the wall thickness *(w)* multiplied by a factor *(f)* that varies from 0 (endocardium) to 1 (epicardium), depending on ROI placement. The relationships between EF and GLS and between EF and GCS are shown on the right, demonstrating the flatter slope and lesser effect of GLS on EF. *EDV*, End-diastolic volume; *EF*, ejection fraction; *GCS*, global circumferential strain; *GLS*, global longitudinal strain; *WT*, wall thickness. (Modified from Stokke TM, Hasselberg NE, Smedsrud MK, et al. Geometry as a confounder when assessing ventricular systolic function: comparison between ejection fraction and strain. *J Am Coll Cardiol*. 2017;70[8]:942–954.)

motion pattern of the RV and problems with defining the endocardial surface of the thin RV free wall. Another important factor that complicates the interpretation of RV function is the varying loading conditions. In daily cardiology practice, RV function has traditionally been evaluated qualitatively by 2D echocardiography.

Normal RV lateral wall function causes approximately 25% to 30% longitudinal shortening, with the base descending toward the apex.[88,89] The apical part is relatively stationary. In addition, there is circumferential shortening that squeezes the ventricle. The interventricular septum contributes to RV as well as LV function, and the relative contributions can be different in the normal and the diseased heart.

RV fractional area change measured in a 4-chamber view can be used as a measure of RV function; values lower than 35% indicate reduced RV systolic function.[15] Furthermore, tricuspid annular plane systolic excursion by M-mode echocardiography (TAPSE) can be used to measure RV function, and a TAPSE value of less than 17 mm suggests reduced RV systolic function.[15,86–88] Global RV strain and free RV wall strain are measured as the average peak systolic strain from the three RV lateral wall segments in the apical 4-chamber view[90] (see Fig 2.7). The septal segments have less deformation compared with the free lateral wall, and this complicates interpretation of the results.[84] Normal absolute values for RV free wall strain have been reported to be 28.5% ± 4.8%.[91] It has been reported that these values decrease with aging,[92] but the lowest expected absolute value of RV free wall strain should still not be less than 20%.[15]

A reduced global RV strain predicts worse prognosis in a number of diseases affecting the RV: arrhythmogenic RV cardiomyopathy, pulmonary arterial hypertension, and congenital heart diseases.[89,90,93–97] Analyses of regional and global LV strain have been successfully implemented in many echocardiographic laboratories, but implementation of RV strain analysis has been slower.

SUMMARY Clinical Applications of Myocardial Velocity and Strain Imaging.

	Parameter	Views	Application	Interpretation
LV Systolic Function				
Velocities by pulsed wave TDI	Peak systolic mitral annular velocity (*s*′)	Apical 4-chamber	When GLS not feasible	Reduced *s*′ indicates systolic dysfunction.
Strain by STE	GLS	3 standard apical	May be used routinely	Reduced GLS indicates systolic dysfunction.
	Segmental LV strains	Standard	Mainly for research	Difficult to interpret due to lack of well-defined normal values.
Strain rate by STE	Longitudinal segmental or global strain rate	3 standard apical	Research only	Reduced peak systolic strain rate in systolic dysfunction.
Twisting by STE	Peak systolic twist	Short-axis at apex and base	Research only	Reduced twist in systolic dysfunction. Method not standardized.
LV Diastolic Function				
Velocities by pulsed-wave TDI	Early diastolic mitral annular velocity (*e*′)	Apical 4-chamber	Routine method for evaluation of diastolic function	Reduced *e*′ indicates impaired relaxation; use age-adjusted reference values.

Continued

SUMMARY Clinical Applications of Myocardial Velocity and Strain Imaging.—cont'd

	Parameter	Views	Application	Interpretation
Strain rate by STE	Longitudinal or radial strain rate	Apical	Research only	Reduced early diastolic strain rate in diastolic dysfunction.
Twisting motion by STE	Peak value and timing of untwisting rate	Short-axis at apex and base	Research only	Reduced rate or delay in peak untwisting in diastolic dysfunction. Method not standardized.
Synchrony				
Strain by STE	Longitudinal strain	Apical	Evaluation of CRT candidates	No proven added value in prediction of CRT response.
	Radial strain	Short-axis	To guide lead placement in CRT	Segment with latest contraction identifies latest activated myocardium.
	Mechanical dispersion	Apical	Research only	Variability in timing of peak strain predicts risk of ventricular arrhythmias.
Ischemia				
Strain by STE	Longitudinal or radial strain	Apical or short-axis	Supplement to other methods in acute ischemia and stress echocardiography Longitudinal strain preferred	Systolic lengthening, reduced systolic shortening, and postsystolic shortening are signs of ischemia. In short-axis, reduced systolic thickening is a sign of ischemia.
Pulsed-wave TDI	Peak systolic velocity (s')	Apical or short-axis	When strain not feasible	Reduced s' in ischemic segments.
RV Systolic Function				
Velocities by pulsed-wave TDI	Peak systolic tricuspid annular velocity (s')	Apical 4-chamber	Supplement to other methods	Reduced s' indicates RV dysfunction.
Strain by STE	RV free wall segmental strain	Apical 4-chamber	Research only	Reduced systolic strain in RV dysfunction.
LA Function				
Strain by STE	Speckle tracking of global LA reservoir strain from QRS onset to peak strain.	Apical views	Research only	Reduced peak LA reservoir strain is a marker of elevated atrial pressure.

CRT, Cardiac resynchronization therapy; *GLS,* global longitudinal strain; *LA,* left atrial; *STE,* speckle tracking echocardiography; *TDI,* tissue Doppler imaging.

REFERENCES

1. McDicken WN, Sutherland GR, Moran CM, Gordon LN. Colour Doppler velocity imaging of the myocardium. *Ultrasound Med Biol.* 1992;18(6–7):651–654.
2. Sutherland GR, Stewart MJ, Groundstroem KW, et al. Color Doppler myocardial imaging: a new technique for the assessment of myocardial function. *J Am Soc Echocardiogr.* 1994;7(5):441–458.
3. Edvardsen T, Aakhus S, Endresen K, et al. Acute regional myocardial ischemia identified by 2-dimensional multiregion tissue Doppler imaging technique. *J Am Soc Echocardiogr.* 2000;13(11):986–994.
4. Stoylen A, Heimdal A, Bjornstad K, et al. Strain rate imaging by ultrasonography in the diagnosis of coronary artery disease. *J Am Soc Echocardiogr.* 2000;13(12):1053–1064.
5. Nagueh SF, Smiseth OA, Appleton CP, et al. Recommendations for the evaluation of left ventricular diastolic function by echocardiography: an update from the American Society of Echocardiography and the European Association of Cardiovascular Imaging. *J Am Soc Echocardiogr.* 2016;29(4):277–314.
6. Opdahl A, Remme EW, Helle-Valle T, et al. Myocardial relaxation, restoring forces, and early-diastolic load are independent determinants of left ventricular untwisting rate. *Circulation.* 2012;126(12):1441–1451.
7. Heimdal A, Stoylen A, Torp H, Skjaerpe T. Real-time strain rate imaging of the left ventricle by ultrasound. *J Am Soc Echocardiogr.* 1998;11(11):1013–1019.
8. Urheim S, Edvardsen T, Torp H, et al. Myocardial strain by Doppler echocardiography. Validation of a new method to quantify regional myocardial function. *Circulation.* 2000;102(10):1158–1164.
9. Amundsen BH, Helle-Valle T, Edvardsen T, et al. Noninvasive myocardial strain measurement by speckle tracking echocardiography: validation against sonomicrometry and tagged magnetic resonance imaging. *J Am Coll Cardiol.* 2006;47(4):789–793.
10. Derumeaux G, Ovize M, Loufoua J, et al. Assessment of nonuniformity of transmural myocardial velocities by color-coded tissue Doppler imaging: characterization of normal, ischemic, and stunned myocardium. *Circulation.* 2000;101(12):1390–1395.

11. Uematsu M, Nakatani S, Yamagishi M, et al. Usefulness of myocardial velocity gradient derived from two-dimensional tissue Doppler imaging as an indicator of regional myocardial contraction independent of translational motion assessed in atrial septal defect. *Am J Cardiol.* 1997;79(2):237–241.
12. Leitman M, Lysyansky P, Sidenko S, et al. Two-dimensional strain—a novel software for real-time quantitative echocardiographic assessment of myocardial function. *J Am Soc Echocardiogr.* 2004;17(10):1021–1029.
13. Gjesdal O, Hopp E, Vartdal T, et al. Global longitudinal strain measured by two-dimensional speckle tracking echocardiography is closely related to myocardial infarct size in chronic ischaemic heart disease. *Clin Sci (Lond).* 2007;113(6):287–296.
14. Gjesdal O, Helle-Valle T, Hopp E, et al. Noninvasive separation of large, medium, and small myocardial infarcts in survivors of reperfused ST-elevation myocardial infarction: a comprehensive tissue Doppler and speckle-tracking echocardiography study. *Circ Cardiovasc Imaging.* 2008;1(3):189–196. 182 p following 196.
15. Lang RM, Badano LP, Mor-Avi V, et al. Recommendations for cardiac chamber quantification by echocardiography in adults: an update from the American Society of Echocardiography and the European Association of Cardiovascular Imaging. *J Am Soc Echocardiogr.* 2015;28(1):1–39. e14.
16. Farsalinos KE, Daraban AM, Unlu S, et al. Head-to-head comparison of global longitudinal strain measurements among nine different vendors: the EACVI/ASE inter-vendor comparison study. *J Am Soc Echocardiogr.* 2015;28(10):1171–1181. e1172.
17. Potter E, Marwick TH. Assessment of left ventricular function by echocardiography: the case for routinely adding global longitudinal strain to ejection fraction. *JACC Cardiovasc Imaging.* 2018;11(2 Pt 1):260–274.
18. Sugimoto T, Dulgheru R, Bernard A, et al. Echocardiographic reference ranges for normal left ventricular 2D strain: results from the EACVI NORRE study. *Eur Heart J Cardiovasc Imaging.* 2017;18(8):833–840.
19. Helle-Valle T, Crosby J, Edvardsen T, et al. New noninvasive method for assessment of left ventricular rotation: speckle tracking echocardiography. *Circulation.* 2005;112(20):3149–3156.
20. Notomi Y, Lysyansky P, Setser RM, et al. Measurement of ventricular torsion by two-dimensional ultrasound speckle tracking imaging. *J Am Coll Cardiol.* 2005;45(12):2034–2041.
21. Matre K, Fannelop T, Dahle GO, et al. Radial strain gradient across the normal myocardial wall in open-chest pigs measured with Doppler strain rate imaging. *J Am Soc Echocardiogr.* 2005;18(10):1066–1073.
22. Skulstad H, Urheim S, Edvardsen T, et al. Grading of myocardial dysfunction by tissue Doppler echocardiography: a comparison between velocity, displacement, and strain imaging in acute ischemia. *J Am Coll Cardiol.* 2006;47(8):1672–1682.
23. Lilli A, Baratto MT, Del Meglio J, et al. Left ventricular rotation and twist assessed by four-dimensional speckle tracking echocardiography in healthy subjects and pathological remodeling: a single center experience. *Echocardiography.* 2013;30(2):171–179.
24. Smiseth OA, Torp H, Opdahl A, et al. Myocardial strain imaging: how useful is it in clinical decision making? *Eur Heart J.* 2016;37(15):1196–1207.
25. Alam M, Hoglund C, Thorstrand C. Longitudinal systolic shortening of the left ventricle: an echocardiographic study in subjects with and without preserved global function. *Clin Physiol.* 1992;12(4):443–452.
26. Becker M, Hoffmann R, Kuhl HP, et al. Analysis of myocardial deformation based on ultrasonic pixel tracking to determine transmurality in chronic myocardial infarction. *Eur Heart J.* 2006;27(21):2560–2566.
27. Marwick TH, Leano RL, Brown J, et al. Myocardial strain measurement with 2-dimensional speckle-tracking echocardiography: definition of normal range. *JACC Cardiovasc Imaging.* 2009;2(1):80–84.
28. Pai RG, Bodenheimer MM, Pai SM, et al. Usefulness of systolic excursion of the mitral anulus as an index of left ventricular systolic function. *Am J Cardiol.* 1991;67(2):222–224.
29. Sengupta PP, Tajik AJ, Chandrasekaran K, Khandheria BK. Twist mechanics of the left ventricle: principles and application. *JACC Cardiovasc Imaging.* 2008;1(3):366–376.
30. Wu MT, Tseng WY, Su MY, et al. Diffusion tensor magnetic resonance imaging mapping the fiber architecture remodeling in human myocardium after infarction: correlation with viability and wall motion. *Circulation.* 2006;114(10):1036–1045.
31. Gibbons Kroeker CA, Ter Keurs HE, Knudtson ML, et al. An optical device to measure the dynamics of apex rotation of the left ventricle. *Am J Physiol.* 1993;265(4 Pt 2):H1444–H1449.
32. Rademakers FE, Buchalter MB, Rogers WJ, et al. Dissociation between left ventricular untwisting and filling. Accentuation by catecholamines. *Circulation.* 1992;85(4):1572–1581.
33. Wang J, Khoury DS, Yue Y, et al. Left ventricular untwisting rate by speckle tracking echocardiography. *Circulation.* 2007;116(22):2580–2586.
34. Stuber M, Scheidegger MB, Fischer SE, et al. Alterations in the local myocardial motion pattern in patients suffering from pressure overload due to aortic stenosis. *Circulation.* 1999;100(4):361–368.
35. van Dalen BM, Kauer F, Soliman OI, et al. Influence of the pattern of hypertrophy on left ventricular twist in hypertrophic cardiomyopathy. *Heart.* 2009;95(8):657–661.
36. Nagel E, Stuber M, Burkhard B, et al. Cardiac rotation and relaxation in patients with aortic valve stenosis. *Eur Heart J.* 2000;21(7):582–589.
37. Buchalter MB, Rademakers FE, Weiss JL, et al. Rotational deformation of the canine left ventricle measured by magnetic resonance tagging: effects of catecholamines, ischaemia, and pacing. *Cardiovasc Res.* 1994;28(5):629–635.
38. DeAnda Jr A, Komeda M, Nikolic SD, et al. Left ventricular function, twist, and recoil after mitral valve replacement. *Circulation.* 1995;92(9 Suppl):II458–II466.
39. Fuchs E, Muller MF, Oswald H, et al. Cardiac rotation and relaxation in patients with chronic heart failure. *Eur J Heart Fail.* 2004;6(6):715–722.
40. Hansen DE, Daughters 2nd GT, Alderman EL, et al. Effect of volume loading, pressure loading, and inotropic stimulation on left ventricular torsion in humans. *Circulation.* 1991;83(4):1315–1326.
41. Kroeker CA, Tyberg JV, Beyar R. Effects of ischemia on left ventricular apex rotation. An experimental study in anesthetized dogs. *Circulation.* 1995;92(12):3539–3548.
42. Maier SE, Fischer SE, McKinnon GC, et al. Evaluation of left ventricular segmental wall motion in hypertrophic cardiomyopathy with myocardial tagging. *Circulation.* 1992;86(6):1919–1928.
43. Sandstede JJ, Johnson T, Harre K, et al. Cardiac systolic rotation and contraction before and after valve replacement for aortic stenosis: a myocardial tagging study using MR imaging. *AJR Am J Roentgenol.* 2002;178(4):953–958.
44. Tibayan FA, Rodriguez F, Langer F, et al. Alterations in left ventricular torsion and diastolic recoil after myocardial infarction with and without chronic ischemic mitral regurgitation. *Circulation.* 2004;110(11 suppl 1):II109–II114.
45. Yun KL, Niczyporuk MA, Daughters 2nd GT, et al. Alterations in left ventricular diastolic twist mechanics during acute human cardiac allograft rejection. *Circulation.* 1991;83(3):962–973.
46. Remme EW, Lyseggen E, Helle-Valle T, et al. Mechanisms of preejection and postejection velocity spikes in left ventricular myocardium: interaction between wall deformation and valve events. *Circulation.* 2008;118(4):373–380.
47. Derumeaux G, Ovize M, Loufoua J, et al. Doppler tissue imaging quantitates regional wall motion during myocardial ischemia and reperfusion. *Circulation.* 1998;97(19):1970–1977.
48. Isaaz K, Munoz del Romeral L, Lee E, Schiller NB. Quantitation of the motion of the cardiac base in normal subjects by Doppler echocardiography. *J Am Soc Echocardiogr.* 1993;6(2):166–176.
49. Voigt JU, Lindenmeier G, Exner B, et al. Incidence and characteristics of segmental postsystolic longitudinal shortening in normal, acutely ischemic, and scarred myocardium. *J Am Soc Echocardiogr.* 2003;16(5):415–423.
50. Sengupta PP, Khandheria BK, Korinek J, et al. Apex-to-base dispersion in regional timing of left ventricular shortening and lengthening. *J Am Coll Cardiol.* 2006;47(1):163–172.
51. Firstenberg MS, Greenberg NL, Main ML, et al. Determinants of diastolic myocardial tissue Doppler velocities: influences of relaxation and preload. *J Appl Physiol (1985).* 2001;90(1):299–307.
52. Nagueh SF, Middleton KJ, Kopelen HA, et al. Doppler tissue imaging: a noninvasive technique for evaluation of left ventricular relaxation and estimation of filling pressures. *J Am Coll Cardiol.* 1997;30(6):1527–1533.
53. Ommen SR, Nishimura RA, Appleton CP, et al. Clinical utility of Doppler echocardiography and tissue Doppler imaging in the estimation of left ventricular filling pressures: a comparative simultaneous Doppler-catheterization study. *Circulation.* 2000;102(15):1788–1794.
54. Sohn DW, Chai IH, Lee DJ, et al. Assessment of mitral annulus velocity by Doppler tissue imaging in the evaluation of left ventricular diastolic function. *J Am Coll Cardiol.* 1997;30(2):474–480.
55. Opdahl A, Remme EW, Helle-Valle T, et al. Determinants of left ventricular early-diastolic lengthening velocity: independent contributions from left ventricular relaxation, restoring forces, and lengthening load. *Circulation.* 2009;119(19):2578–2586.
56. Nagueh SF, Bhatt R, Vivo RP, et al. Echocardiographic evaluation of hemodynamics in patients with decompensated systolic heart failure. *Circ Cardiovasc Imaging.* 2011;4(3):220–227.
57. Edvardsen T, Skulstad H, Aakhus S, et al. Regional myocardial systolic function during

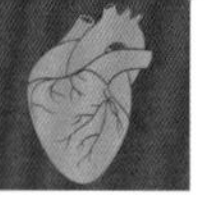

acute myocardial ischemia assessed by strain Doppler echocardiography. *J Am Coll Cardiol.* 2001;37(3):726–730.

58. Gorcsan 3rd J, Strum DP, Mandarino WA, Pinsky MR. Color-coded tissue Doppler assessment of the effects of acute ischemia on regional left ventricular function: comparison with sonomicrometry. *J Am Soc Echocardiogr.* 2001;14(5):335–342.
59. Madler CF, Payne N, Wilkenshoff U, et al. Non-invasive diagnosis of coronary artery disease by quantitative stress echocardiography: optimal diagnostic models using off-line tissue Doppler in the MYDISE study. *Eur Heart J.* 2003;24(17):1584–1594.
60. Voigt JU, Exner B, Schmiedehausen K, et al. Strain-rate imaging during dobutamine stress echocardiography provides objective evidence of inducible ischemia. *Circulation.* 2003;107(16):2120–2126.
61. Edvardsen T, Urheim S, Skulstad H, et al. Quantification of left ventricular systolic function by tissue Doppler echocardiography: added value of measuring pre- and postejection velocities in ischemic myocardium. *Circulation.* 2002;105(17):2071–2077.
62. Kukulski T, Jamal F, Herbots L, et al. Identification of acutely ischemic myocardium using ultrasonic strain measurements. A clinical study in patients undergoing coronary angioplasty. *J Am Coll Cardiol.* 2003;41(5):810–819.
63. Lyseggen E, Rabben SI, Skulstad H, et al. Myocardial acceleration during isovolumic contraction: relationship to contractility. *Circulation.* 2005;111(11):1362–1369.
64. Skulstad H, Edvardsen T, Urheim S, et al. Postsystolic shortening in ischemic myocardium: active contraction or passive recoil? *Circulation.* 2002;106(6):718–724.

64a. Smiseth OA, Aalen JM. Mechanism of harm from left bundle branch block. *Trends Cardiovasc Med.* 2019;29(6):335–342.

65. McDonald IG. Echocardiographic demonstration of abnormal motion of the interventricular septum in left bundle branch block. *Circulation.* 1973;48(2):272–280.
66. Dillon JC, Chang S, Feigenbaum H. Echocardiographic manifestations of left bundle branch block. *Circulation.* 1974;49(5):876–880.
67. Parsai C, Bijnens B, Sutherland GR, et al. Toward understanding response to cardiac resynchronization therapy: left ventricular dyssynchrony is only one of multiple mechanisms. *Eur Heart J.* 2009;30(8):940–949.
68. Gjesdal O, Remme EW, Opdahl A, et al. Mechanisms of abnormal systolic motion of the interventricular septum during left bundle-branch block. *Circ Cardiovasc Imaging.* 2011;4(3):264–273.
69. Little WC, Reeves RC, Arciniegas J, et al. Mechanism of abnormal interventricular septal motion during delayed left ventricular activation. *Circulation.* 1982;65(7):1486–1491.
70. Walmsley J, Huntjens PR, Prinzen FW, et al. Septal flash and septal rebound stretch have different underlying mechanisms. *Am J Physiol Heart Circ Physiol.* 2016;310(3):H394–H403.
71. Szulik M, Tillekaerts M, Vangeel V, et al. Assessment of apical rocking: a new, integrative approach for selection of candidates for cardiac resynchronization therapy. *Eur J Echocardiogr.* 2010;11(10):863–869.
72. Prinzen FW, Hunter WC, Wyman BT, McVeigh ER. Mapping of regional myocardial strain and work during ventricular pacing: experimental study using magnetic resonance imaging tagging. *J Am Coll Cardiol.* 1999;33(6):1735–1742.

72a. Russell K, Eriksen M, Aaberge L, et al. A novel clinical method for quantification of regional left ventricular pressure-strain loop area: a non-invasive index of myocardial work. *Eur Heart J.* 2012;33(6):724–733.

72b. Aalen JM, Donal E, Larsen CK, et al. Imaging predictors of response to cardiac resynchronization therapy: left ventricular work asymmetry by echocardiography and septal viability by cardiac magnetic resonance. *Eur Heart J.* 2020 Sep 11:ehaa603. Online ahead of print.

73. Haugaa KH, Amlie JP, Berge KE, et al. Transmural differences in myocardial contraction in long-QT syndrome: mechanical consequences of ion channel dysfunction. *Circulation.* 2010;122(14):1355–1363.
74. Haugaa KH, Edvardsen T, Leren TP, et al. Left ventricular mechanical dispersion by tissue Doppler imaging: a novel approach for identifying high-risk individuals with long QT syndrome. *Eur Heart J.* 2009;30(3):330–337.
75. Haugaa KH, Smedsrud MK, Steen T, et al. Mechanical dispersion assessed by myocardial strain in patients after myocardial infarction for risk prediction of ventricular arrhythmia. *JACC Cardiovasc Imaging.* 2010;3(3):247–256.
76. Witkowski TG, Thomas JD, Debonnaire PJ, et al. Global longitudinal strain predicts left ventricular dysfunction after mitral valve repair. *Eur Heart J Cardiovasc Imaging.* 2013;14(1):69–76.
77. Kraigher-Krainer E, Shah AM, Gupta DK, et al. Impaired systolic function by strain imaging in heart failure with preserved ejection fraction. *J Am Coll Cardiol.* 2014;63(5):447–456.
78. Aurigemma GP, Silver KH, Priest MA, Gaasch WH. Geometric changes allow normal ejection fraction despite depressed myocardial shortening in hypertensive left ventricular hypertrophy. *J Am Coll Cardiol.* 1995;26(1):195–202.
79. Stokke TM, Hasselberg NE, Smedsrud MK, et al. Geometry as a confounder when assessing ventricular systolic function: comparison between ejection fraction and strain. *J Am Coll Cardiol.* 2017;70(8):942–954.
80. Dahl JS, Magne J, Pellikka PA, et al. Assessment of subclinical left ventricular dysfunction in aortic stenosis. *JACC Cardiovasc Imaging.* 2019;12(1):163–171.
81. Haland TF, Hasselberg NE, Almaas VM, et al. The systolic paradox in hypertrophic cardiomyopathy. *Open Heart.* 2017;4(1):e000571.
82. Magne J, Cosyns B, Popescu BA, et al. Distribution and prognostic significance of left ventricular global longitudinal strain in asymptomatic significant aortic stenosis: an individual participant data meta-analysis. *JACC Cardiovasc Imaging.* 2019;12(1):84–92.
83. Phelan D, Collier P, Thavendiranathan P, et al. Relative apical sparing of longitudinal strain using two-dimensional speckle-tracking echocardiography is both sensitive and specific for the diagnosis of cardiac amyloidosis. *Heart.* 2012;98(19):1442–1448.
84. Pibarot P, Dumesnil JG. Improving assessment of aortic stenosis. *J Am Coll Cardiol.* 2012;60(3):169–180.
85. Ersboll M, Valeur N, Mogensen UM, et al. Prediction of all-cause mortality and heart failure admissions from global left ventricular longitudinal strain in patients with acute myocardial infarction and preserved left ventricular ejection fraction. *J Am Coll Cardiol.* 2013;61(23):2365–2373.
86. Plana JC, Galderisi M, Barac A, et al. Expert consensus for multimodality imaging evaluation of adult patients during and after cancer therapy: a report from the American Society of Echocardiography and the European Association of Cardiovascular Imaging. *Eur Heart J Cardiovasc Imaging.* 2014;15(10):1063–1093.
87. Stanton T, Leano R, Marwick TH. Prediction of all-cause mortality from global longitudinal speckle strain: comparison with ejection fraction and wall motion scoring. *Circ Cardiovasc Imaging.* 2009;2(5):356–364.
88. Fine NM, Chen L, Bastiansen PM, et al. Reference values for right ventricular strain in patients without cardiopulmonary disease: a prospective evaluation and meta-analysis. *Echocardiography.* 2015;32(5):787–796.
89. Forsha D, Risum N, Kropf PA, et al. Right ventricular mechanics using a novel comprehensive three-view echocardiographic strain analysis in a normal population. *J Am Soc Echocardiogr.* 2014;27(4):413–422.
90. Sarvari SI, Haugaa KH, Anfinsen OG, et al. Right ventricular mechanical dispersion is related to malignant arrhythmias: a study of patients with arrhythmogenic right ventricular cardiomyopathy and subclinical right ventricular dysfunction. *Eur Heart J.* 2011;32(9):1089–1096.
91. Morris DA, Krisper M, Nakatani S, et al. Normal range and usefulness of right ventricular systolic strain to detect subtle right ventricular systolic abnormalities in patients with heart failure: a multicentre study. *Eur Heart J Cardiovasc Imaging.* 2017;18(2):212–223.
92. Park JH, Choi JO, Park SW, et al. Normal references of right ventricular strain values by two-dimensional strain echocardiography according to the age and gender. *Int J Cardiovasc Imaging.* 2018;34(2):177–183.
93. Chowdhury SM, Hijazi ZM, Fahey JT, et al. Speckle-tracking echocardiographic measures of right ventricular function correlate with improvement in exercise function after percutaneous pulmonary valve implantation. *J Am Soc Echocardiogr.* 2015;28(9):1036–1044.
94. Kannan A, Poongkunran C, Jayaraj M, Janardhanan R. Role of strain imaging in right heart disease: a comprehensive review. *J Clin Med Res.* 2014;6(5):309–313.
95. La Gerche A, Claessen G, Dymarkowski S, et al. Exercise-induced right ventricular dysfunction is associated with ventricular arrhythmias in endurance athletes. *Eur Heart J.* 2015;36(30):1998–2010.
96. Vitarelli A, Mangieri E, Terzano C, et al. Three-dimensional echocardiography and 2D-3D speckle-tracking imaging in chronic pulmonary hypertension: diagnostic accuracy in detecting hemodynamic signs of right ventricular (RV) failure. *J Am Heart Assoc.* 2015;4(3):e001584.
97. Zahid W, Bergestuen D, Haugaa KH, et al. Myocardial function by two-dimensional speckle tracking echocardiography and activin A may predict mortality in patients with carcinoid intestinal disease. *Cardiology.* 2015;132(2):81–90.
98. Manouras A, Shahgaldi K, Winter R, et al. Comparison between colour-coded and spectral tissue Doppler measurements of systolic and diastolic myocardial velocities: effect of temporal filtering and offline gain setting. *Eur J Echocardiogr.* 2009;10(3):406–413.

中文导读

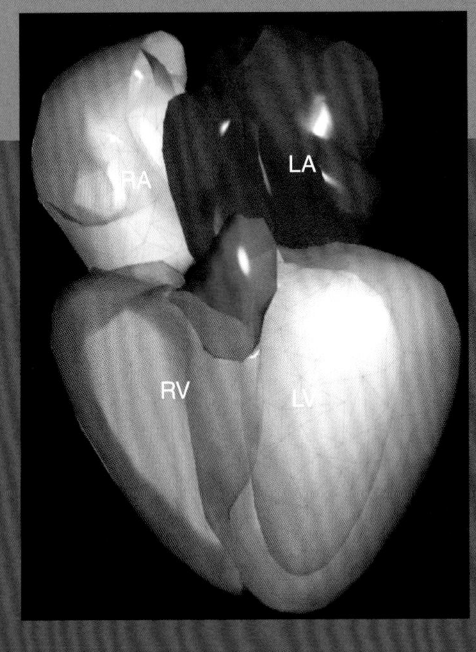

第3章 超声声学造影

超声声学造影主要目的是增强心脏显像，从而提高超声诊断的质量和准确性，其安全性、临床实用性和有效性已经得到证实。本章分别简要介绍了右心声学造影，以声振气泡作为造影媒介，气泡直径一般较大。其次重点介绍了左心声学造影。左心声学造影微泡为商用造影剂，目前主流有4种，气泡直径均较小，可以通过肺毛细血管滤过进入左心，最后通过呼吸代谢。

超声造影不仅可以提供诊断信息，还可以对特定组织进行靶向标记甚至发挥治疗作用。超声造影主要可以对心腔的血池和心肌显影，左心室造影的主要临床应用包括评价心腔容积、射血分数，评价局部室壁运动，联合负荷试验评估冠状动脉异常，左心室心尖部血栓的筛查，肥厚型心肌病、限制型心肌病及心肌致密化不全等心肌病的评估。对于微循环血流灌注的评估，是超声造影的另外一个优势，可以评价局部心肌的微循环灌注异常，从而检测缺血心肌、存活心肌，为患者的预后提供影像学证据。对于心脏占位性病变，超声造影有助于鉴别血栓、原发或转移性肿瘤等情况。通过常规超声成像与超声造影技术相结合，超声诊断的准确性明显提高。

权　欣

3 Contrast Echocardiography

JONATHAN R. LINDNER, MD

Contrast echocardiography describes an array of techniques that produce acoustic enhancement of the blood pool during cardiovascular ultrasound imaging in order to improve the accuracy of conventional echocardiography or to create new diagnostic capabilities.[1–3] A broad definition of contrast echocardiography extends to the use of rapidly dissolving air bubbles formed from hand agitation of fluid, such as saline, for detection of right-to-left shunt physiology, a technique that is described elsewhere. This chapter focuses on the application of stable, encapsulated contrast agents or ultrasound enhancing agents (UEAs) that are designed to transit through the pulmonary circulation after intravenous administration. A wide variety of UEAs and unique ultrasound imaging technology to detect them in the chambers of the heart or the vasculature have been developed. This chapter provides an overview of contrast agent composition, behavior, and safety; contrast-specific imaging modalities designed to maximize signal-to-noise ratio during imaging; and clinical applications for myocardial contrast echocardiography (MCE), including those that are approved and some that have not yet been approved by regulatory agencies.

ULTRASOUND ENHANCING AGENTS

Signal enhancement during contrast echocardiography is attributable to the dynamic compression and expansion of particles, usually microbubbles, exposed to the pressure fluctuations of an ultrasound field. The initial description of contrast enhancement was made when ultrasound signals were detected in the right heart after rapid, forceful intravenous injections of a water-soluble fluorophore used for cardiac output measurement during heart catheterization.[4] Over the ensuing decades, iterations of non-encapsulated microbubbles generated by hand agitation or by low-frequency sonication were created and injected by an intracoronary route in experimental studies to assess myocardial perfusion with MCE. The clinical use of these UEAs was limited by the inability to control and standardize microbubble size and an inability of most of these microbubbles to transit to the left heart and systemic circulation after intravenous injection.

The safety, efficacy, reproducibility, and widespread clinical feasibility of contrast echocardiography are contingent on the ability to administer these UEAs intravenously and then generate robust contrast enhancement of left-sided cardiac structures and portions of the systemic circulation. Safe, unimpeded transit through the pulmonary and systemic circulations requires UEAs to be smaller than the average functional capillary diameter of 5 to 7 μm when taking into account the intraluminal dimension of the endothelial glycocalyx. The expansion and compression of microbubbles during ultrasound pressure peaks and nadirs, respectively, produces volumetric oscillations of these particles, the primary source of signal generation during imaging.[5] Accordingly, contrast agents need to be suitably compressible/expandable in the pressure fluctuations of diagnostic ultrasound, smaller than the wavelength of ultrasound, and stable after intravenous injection.

CLINICAL AGENTS FOR CONTRAST ECHOCARDIOGRAPHY

Currently, several microbubble ultrasound contrast agents are being commercially produced, marketed, and used in patients in many countries (Table 3.1). These agents are stable, acoustically active, and size-controlled so that they are able to pass freely through pulmonary and systemic capillaries based on two major design features: (1) high-molecular-weight gas in the microbubble core, and (2) microbubble encapsulation.[1,3] Ambient air (nitrogen and oxygen) and the high-molecular-weight gases that have been used in UEA preparations are several orders of magnitude more compressible than water or tissue. The stability of a gas bubble in any given medium depends on its size, its surface tension, and the solubility and diffusion characteristics of the gas.[6] Microbubbles composed entirely of air are no longer manufactured because of their instability caused by rapid loss of gas through diffusion. Instead, UEAs have been composed with gases such as octafluoropropane (C_3F_8), decafluorobutane (C_4F_{10}), and sulfur hexafluoride (SF_6), which have low diffusion coefficients and low solubility in water or blood

TABLE 3.1 Commercially Produced Ultrasound Enhancing Agents With Regulatory Agency Approval

Commercial Name	*Generic Name*	*Bubble Diameter (μm)*	*Shell Composition*	*Gas Core*
Optison	perflutren protein-type A microspheres	3.0–4.5 (95% ≤10)	Human albumin	Perflutren (octafluoropropane C_3F_8)
Definity	perflutren lipid microspheres	1.1–3.3 (98% ≤10)	Phospholipid	Perflutren (octafluoropropane C_3F_8)
SonoVue/Lumason	sulfur hexafluoride lipid-type A microspheres	1.5–2.5 (99% ≤10)	Phospholipid	Sulfur hexafluoride (SF_6)
Sonazoid	perflubutane lipid microspheres	2.6 (99% ≤7)	Phospholipid	Decafluorobutane (C_4F_{10})

Storage and preparation
- ± Refrigeration
- ± Reconstitution (desiccated agents)
- ± Physical activation of an aqueous mixture

Size
- Average diameter
- Monodisperse vs. polydisperse

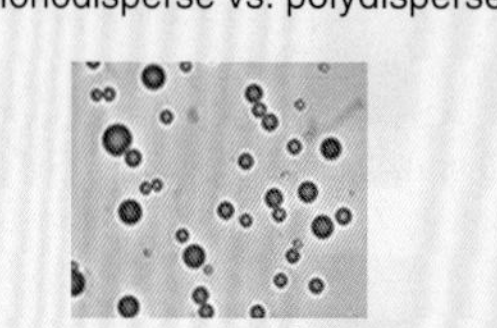

Administration
- Bolus only vs. infusion
- Amenability for dilution
- Noncardiac indications
- Clearance rate and susceptibility to US-mediated destruction

Fig. 3.1 Characteristics of ultrasound contrast agents. Characteristics that differentiate commercially produced ultrasound enhancing agents, apart from their chemical composition. *US*, Ultrasound.

(Ostwald coefficient), resulting in enhanced stability.[7] These gases are inert and safe for human use and are eventually cleared through respiration.

The encapsulation of the microbubbles using biocompatible shell materials such as albumin or lipid surfactants is a second common feature of contemporary UEAs that enhances in vivo stability by reducing outward diffusion of the gas core. Encapsulation also reduces surface tension of the microbubbles, thereby improving their shelf life and in vivo stability, and allows control of microbubble size distribution. Much of the albumin used in microbubble shells is predicted to exist in a denatured form resulting from the manufacturing process. When used in microbubbles, lipids generally are arranged as a monolayer with inner orientation of the hydrocarbon residues because of the hydrophobic nature of perfluorocarbons. The chemical nature and self-assembly of the components of the encapsulated microbubbles result in differences in not only contrast agent composition but also size distribution (polydisperse rather than monodisperse diameters), storage, and preparation protocols (Fig. 3.1). The shell composition is the dominant feature for determining the physical properties of microbubble volumetric resonation (cavitation) in an acoustic field.

TABLE 3.2 Investigational Uses for Conventional and Novel UEAs in Cardiovascular Medicine.

Investigational Agent or Approach	*Clinical Application*
Targeted UEAs for molecular imaging	Detection of atherosclerosis, thrombus, angiogenesis, inflammation (allograft rejection, myocarditis, ischemia)
Sonothrombolysis with UEA inertial cavitation	Treatment of acute coronary syndrome, microvascular no-reflow, venous/arterial thrombosis, stroke, pulmonary embolism
Payload-bearing UEAs for acoustically targeted delivery	Site-targeted delivery of DNA (gene therapy), therapeutic RNA (e.g., siRNA, microRNA), drugs
Shear-mediated vasodilation from inertial cavitation	Augmentation of tissue perfusion in CAD, peripheral artery disease, pulmonary embolism, stroke
Nanodroplets or phase-conversion UEAs	Transvascular drug/gene delivery, perfusion imaging without cavity attenuation
High-power or HIFU-mediated inertial cavitation for histotripsy	Tissue ablation for arrhythmias, HCM, palliative shunt formation, tumor reduction

CAD, Coronary artery disease; *HCM*, hypertrophic cardiomyopathy; *HIFU*, high-intensity focused ultrasound; *siRNA*, signal-interfering ribonucleic acid; *UEA*, ultrasound enhancing agent.

INVESTIGATIONAL AGENTS

Many different investigational contrast agents have been developed that are not currently in routine clinical use. These agents have been specially formulated for specific diagnostic or therapeutic purposes (Table 3.2). Nanoscale contrast agents (emulsions, nanodroplets, and acoustically active liposomes) that are less than 1 μm in diameter have been developed based on the potential of these agents to have longer intravascular circulation times, to potentially exit the vascular space in certain circumstances, and to be better matched with high-frequency ultrasound imaging based on the inverse relationship between bubble size and ideal resonant frequency. To improve the ordinarily low degree of ultrasound signal enhancement from submicron agents, phase-shifting nanodroplets have been developed that possess a condensed liquid-phase perfluorocarbon core that undergoes expansion and vaporization to gas phase during the negative-pressure phase of an acoustic field.[8]

There has been extensive investigation into the use of targeted microbubble contrast agents that bear binding ligands for performing ultrasound-based molecular imaging. Clinical areas of interest for this technology include imaging of tissue ischemia, vascular inflammation and atherosclerosis, thrombus formation, and angiogenesis.[9,10] Novel microbubble agents have also been formulated for therapeutic purposes, including payload-containing microbubbles for gene or drug delivery and agents designed specifically for sonothrombolysis (i.e., dissolution of thrombus through cavitation energy).[11] Full elaboration of these cutting-edge experimental agents is beyond the scope of this chapter, yet knowledge of their applications in contrast echocardiography is important for realizing their possible future role in improving patient care.

SAFETY AND MICROVASCULAR BEHAVIOR OF MICROBUBBLES

The UEAs that have been approved by regulatory authorities have been shown to be among the safest contrast agents used in all forms of cardiovascular noninvasive imaging.[3,12–14] The safety issues that are unique to microbubbles relate to three primary factors: (1) their microvascular behavior; (2) the physical and biochemical bioeffects from acoustic cavitation; and (3) interaction of microbubbles with components of the mammalian innate and adaptive immune processes.

The organ-specific vascular kinetic profile (rheology) of UEAs in the microcirculation is vital for understanding tracer kinetics and safety. Investigational studies using first-pass tracer kinetics or intravital microscopy have firmly established that albumin and lipid microbubbles transit the myocardial and muscle microcirculation unimpeded, do not coalesce or aggregate, and have a velocity profile similar to that of red blood cells (RBCs) in arterioles, venules, and capillaries (Fig. 3.2).[15,16] The similar rheology of UEAs and RBCs is a critical consideration when using MCE to assess microvascular perfusion. This rheologic profile and the ability to control microbubble size through encapsulation are important for minimizing capillary or pre-capillary lodging and ensuring that microbubbles will transit to the systemic circulation after intravenous injection. Because lodging in the pulmonary circulation is minimized, administration of UEAs (including full-dose administration of a polydisperse-sized microbubble agent) in patients with at least moderate preexisting pulmonary hypertension has been shown not to increase either pulmonary pressure or pulmonary vascular resistance.[17] Concern for possible systemic microvascular lodging in patients with a permanent or transient right-to-left shunt has been raised. However, only a small proportion of microbubbles are large enough to lodge in peripheral microvessels (see Table 3.1), and microscopy has indicated that any size-based retention is a transient event because of gradual deflation.[15] Accordingly, use of commercially produced UEAs in the presence of a right-to-left shunt has been demonstrated to be safe,[18] and the presence of known or suspected shunts is no longer a contraindication to their use.

Clearance of UEAs from the blood pool generally is performed by reticuloendothelial organs. The dominant removal mechanism for lipid-based agents is opsonization, whereby serum complement facilitates receptor-mediated uptake by monocytic/phagocytic cells such as Kupffer cells of the liver.[19] Complement-mediated interaction with phagocytic cells and microbubble removal are increased by specific lipids (e.g., phosphatidylserine) in the microbubble shell and by the use of other lipids that produce a larger net charge (zeta potential) on the shell surface. The rate of removal is decreased by the presence of polymeric moieties such as polyethylene glycol, which reduce opsonization and microbubble–cell interactions.[20] Although albumin-shelled microbubbles can be opsonized, other pathways may be involved, such as the ability of specific integrins on phagocytic cells to bind denatured albumin.[21]

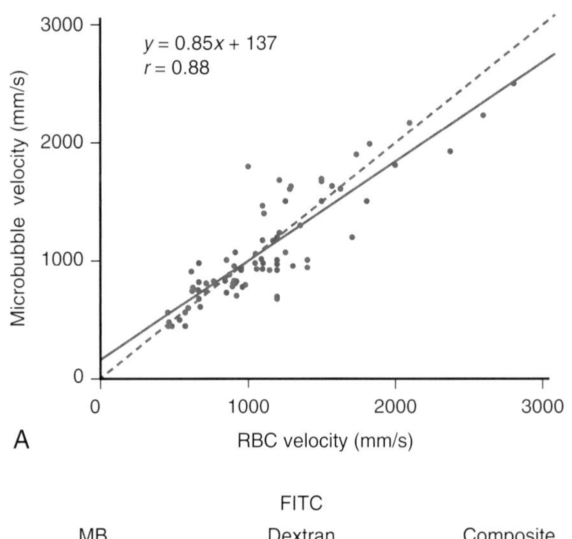

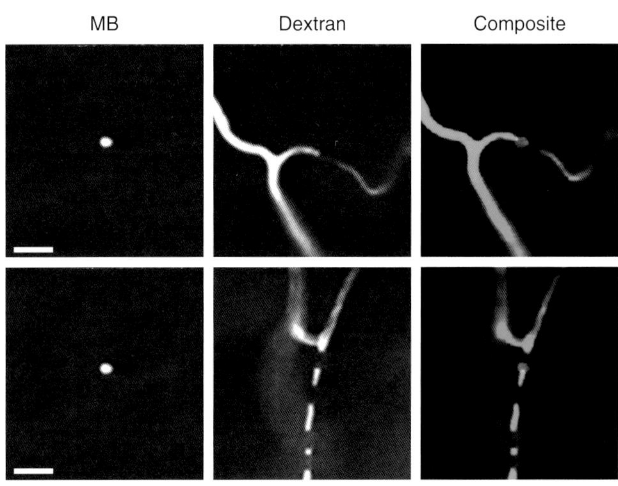

Fig. 3.2 Rheologic behavior of microbubbles used as ultrasound enhancing agents. (A) Relationship between capillary and non-capillary microvascular velocities for a lipid-shelled microbubble agent (Definity) and velocities of red blood cells (RBCs) determined by intravital microscopy of the cremaster muscle. (B) *Left panels,* Intravital microscopy shows two separate fluorescently labeled microbubbles (MB). *Middle panels,* The microcirculation is imaged by injection of fluorescein isothiocyanate (FITC)–labeled dextran (dark intravascular shadows represent RBCs). *Right panels,* The pseudo-colorized composite image (*red* = microbubble, *green* = intravascular dextran) illustrates microbubbles in the microvascular compartment. (Reproduced with permission from Lindner JR, Song J, Jayaweera AR, Sklenar J, Kaul S. Microvascular rheology of Definity microbubbles after intra-arterial and intravenous administration. *J Am Soc Echocardiogr.* 2002;15:396–403.)

Because complement can be activated by microbubble shell components,[22] pseudoanaphylactic reactions (i.e., not mediated by immunoglobulin E) are possible. For any lipid-based particles, these reactions are predicted to be influenced by the peak blood pool concentration of the lipid.[23] Fortunately, serious pseudoanaphylactic reactions for lipid-based agents are rare, with serious cardiopulmonary reactions occurring in only 0.01% of doses administered.[14,24] Lipid-shelled microbubbles can also produce back or flank pain; this may be attributable to a mild form of complement-mediated renal cortex retention whereby the generation of discomfort is more likely caused by mediators that activate pain receptors than by any tissue injury.[25]

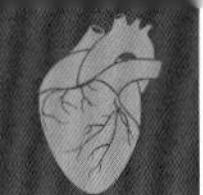

Microbubble resonance in an ultrasound field is categorized as either stable cavitation (volumetric oscillation without destruction) or inertial cavitation (exaggerated nonlinear oscillation that results in abrupt agent destruction).[26] In vitro and preclinical animal studies have indicated that inertial cavitation can cause transient endothelial microporation, vascular permeability, calcium-dependent cell activation, purinergic pathway activation, and even petechial hemorrhage.[27–29] However, the major deleterious effects of inertial cavitation occur at acoustic pressures and microbubble doses beyond the limits approved by regulatory agencies. Within the approved pressure ranges, bioeffects produced by microbubble inertial cavitation have been leveraged to enhance gene/drug delivery or to promote shear-mediated flow augmentation or lysis of blood clots.[11,29–31] Extensive safety studies performed in the course of regulatory approval and post-marketing studies in humans have not detected any evidence of tissue injury or vascular disruption. A large retrospective study of hospital inpatients demonstrated that the mortality rate was lower in those receiving UEAs during echocardiography, suggesting that the net beneficial impact of contrast echocardiography on diagnosis and management outweighed any safety concerns.[13] Because premature ventricular contractions have been reported during very-high-power imaging, regulatory guidelines for some agents caution that safety has not been established when imaging at the very high end of the mechanical index for clinical scanners.

With regard to special patient categories, most UEAs have been assigned a Category C classification in pregnancy, indicating lack of definitive data in humans. Several studies have established the safety of UEAs in pediatric populations,[32,33] although no agent is yet approved for left ventricular opacification (LVO) in these patients. Although there are warnings against intraarterial administration of commercially produced UEAs, some agents have been administered off-label into branches of the left anterior descending (LAD) coronary artery to define the perfusion territories in the course of planning for alcohol septal ablation in patients with hypertrophic cardiomyopathy (HCM).

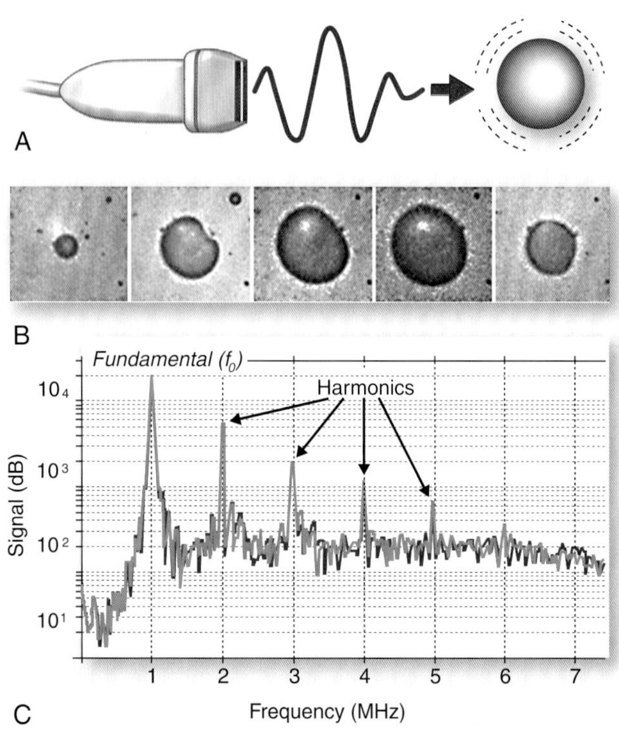

Fig. 3.3 Signal generation from microbubble ultrasound enhancing agents. (A) Pressure fluctuations of an ultrasound field stimulate vibration or volumetric oscillation of microbubbles. (B) High-speed video microscopy images show microbubble volumetric compression and expansion during the pressure fluctuations on ultrasound imaging. (Images courtesy Dr. Nico DeJong.) (C) Ultrasound frequency–amplitude spectra received from lipid-shelled decafluorobutane-containing microbubbles exposed to ultrasound at 1 MHz, an acoustic pressure sufficiently high to produce nonlinear stable cavitation of microbubbles, show returning ultrasound signals not only at the transmit (fundamental) frequency (f_0) but also with harmonic peaks (multiples of the fundamental) and some lower amplitude broadband signals (between harmonic frequencies).

MICROBUBBLE ULTRASOUND SIGNAL GENERATION

Signal generation from UEAs occurs because they are deformable and smaller than the wavelength of ultrasound, which results in their volumetric oscillation (resonance) in response to the pressure fluctuations of ultrasound (Fig. 3.3).[34] This resonance behavior and, secondarily, signal generation from microbubbles is complex but can be described by Rayleigh-Plesset laws, which describe how the magnitude of sound-producing oscillation is dependent on the compressibility and density of the gas core, the viscosity and density of the surrounding medium, the frequency and power of ultrasound applied, and microbubble radius.[6] Energy losses occur from thermal and viscous damping. For encapsulated microbubbles, viscous and viscoelastic damping from the shell is an important factor that influences bubble oscillation.[35] In practical terms, for any given ultrasound power and frequency, less oscillation and acoustic signal is generated from microbubbles that possess stiff shells.

Resonant frequency is another important determinant of UEA signal generation. Ideal resonant frequency is influenced by microbubble size through an inverse-square relationship and by the physical properties of the shell and gas.[35] When acoustic pressures near the resonant frequency are sufficiently high, nonlinear oscillation of microbubbles occurs. In this paradigm, microbubble size is not linearly related to the acoustic pressure, and alternate compression and expansion are asymmetric.[5] It is this nonlinear behavior that produces unique acoustic signatures that can be used to selectively detect microbubble signal. As pressure is increased, the first form of nonlinear signal is the production of harmonics, and there is a relative increase in signal at multiples of the transmit (fundamental) frequency (see Fig. 3.3).[32] Bandpass filtering for the harmonic frequency ranges enhances the signal of microbubbles relative to that of tissues, which produce relatively fewer harmonics at low to medium acoustic pressures. With further increases in acoustic pressure, microbubbles can undergo inertial cavitation, which leads to microbubble destruction, transient release of free gas bubbles, and the generation of strong broadband signals.[26] The acoustic power at which inertial cavitation occurs depends on the UEA composition, particularly shell composition,[36] and the ultrasound frequency. For most approved agents, nondestructive, very-low-power MCE imaging is performed at a mechanical index of 0.1 to 0.2, whereas purposeful destruction of microbubbles is performed at a mechanical index greater than 0.8.

CONTRAST-SPECIFIC IMAGING METHODS

State-of-the-art ultrasound imaging systems are equipped with technology for increasing the contrast agent signal-to-noise ratio by both detecting the nonlinear signals from microbubbles and suppressing signal from tissue.[1,37] When used during LVO, these contrast-specific techniques reduce variation in image quality by

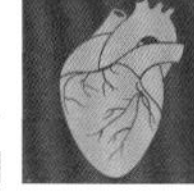

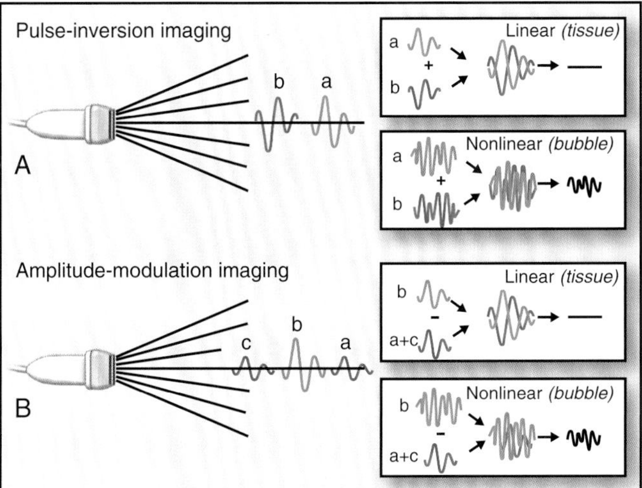

Fig. 3.4 Contrast-specific imaging protocols. Multipulse ultrasound imaging protocols are used to increase microbubble signal relative to background or tissue during contrast echocardiography using a very low mechanical index. (A) During pulse-inversion or phase-inversion imaging, each focused transmit line contains at least two pulses that are phase-inverted by 180 degrees (mirror images). Returning signals are then summed. Because tissue produces linear backscatter at a low mechanical index, returning signals are similar to transmit signals, and their summation results in signal cancellation. The nonlinear signals produced by microbubbles are encoded with many frequencies and therefore do not cancel on summation. (B) During amplitude-modulation imaging, alternating in-phase pulses are transmitted at full- and half-amplitude. Two received half-amplitude pulses are added together, then subtracted from the full-amplitude pulse. Tissue produces linear backscatter at both full- and half-amplitude, resulting in signal cancellation. For microbubbles, nonlinear signal generation is much greater for the full-amplitude pulse, resulting in incomplete cancellation when the summed half-amplitude signals are subtracted.

providing adequate LV border definition with minimal adjustment of system settings. Because myocardial tissue also generates backscatter, the application of these algorithms is essential when performing low-power real-time MCE perfusion imaging.[1]

With current technology, contrast echocardiography is almost always performed at a low mechanical index (<0.3), and almost all MCE perfusion studies are performed with a very low mechanical index (<0.2). At these pressures, harmonic imaging can be performed for the LVO based on the nonlinear microbubble signals that are generated with only a small amount of tissue signal. Signal processing techniques that completely eliminate tissue signals are commonly used to further optimize the contrast agent signal-to-tissue ratio and are vital for myocardial perfusion imaging protocols.[1,38] When pulse-inversion or phase-inversion imaging algorithms are used (Fig. 3.4A), successive focused transmit lines are sent in which pulses are phase-inverted (i.e., phase-shifted by 180 degrees).[38] Linear backscatter will return primarily at the fundamental frequency and can be eliminated by summing the two phase-shifted signals. The nonlinear signal with multiple encoded frequencies that comes from cavitation of microbubbles does not cancel by summation, and a signal is displayed according to the amplitude of this signal. For amplitude-modulation imaging (see Fig. 3.4B), alternating pulses with either low acoustic power or half-amplitude of that power are sent. Linear fundamental signals that return from tissue are similar in phase and frequency for each pulse and can be eliminated by doubling the half-amplitude signal and subtracting it from the low-power signal. Microbubbles produce little nonlinear signal at the half-amplitude pulse, but they produce broadband nonlinear signals at full amplitude. Hence, doubling of the low-power linear signal, even at the

TABLE 3.3 User-Defined Variables That Influence Contrast Echocardiography Image Quality.

User-Defined Factor	*Clinical Impact*
UEA dose	Insufficient dose → incomplete LV or myocardial opacification Excess dose → cavity attenuation or saturation of dynamic range during MCE perfusion imaging
UEA bolus versus infusion	Bolus → high concentration early after injection, resulting in attenuation and need to delay imaging until decay of blood pool concentration When administered by sonographer, bolus injection requires interruption of scanning. Some UEAs are poorly suited to dilution for continuous infusion.
Acoustic pressure or mechanical index	Microbubble destruction at high power → incomplete LV or myocardial opacification Insufficient power → poor myocardial opacification in the far field on MCE perfusion imaging
Transmit frequency	Contrast signal-to-noise is less robust at high frequencies (≥10 MHz). User-defined settings that adjust frequency can be used to optimize penetration and resolution balance.
Acoustic focus	Positioning in the far field → excessive line overlap and near-field microbubble destruction and swirling on apical views Positioning in the near field → inadequate myocardial opacification in the far field during MCE perfusion imaging
Dynamic range	Low dynamic range → reduction in ability to discriminate differences in perfusion High dynamic range → poor differentiation between cavity and myocardium
Multipulse tissue-subtraction techniques	Necessary for robust MCE perfusion imaging Reduce frame rate Can result in flash artifact at high heart rates during stress echocardiography due to incomplete cancellation of signal from rapidly moving tissue

LVO, Left ventricular opacification; *MCE*, myocardial contrast echocardiography; *UEA*, ultrasound-enhancing agent.

fundamental frequency, will not result in complete cancellation of signal. Some ultrasound systems have combined both phase inversion and amplitude modulation.

All of these multipulse techniques result in a reduction of the frame rate. This drawback is often addressed by automatic reduction in line density because current technologies for augmenting the frame rate by reducing the aperture on transmit and by temporal correlation of neighboring elements on receive (often called retrospective beamforming) have not yet been universally applied to contrast imaging.

Image quality during LVO, and in particular during MCE perfusion imaging, is highly dependent on technical aspects of imaging that are under operator control. Some of the variables that can be controlled to optimize image quality include UEA dose, UEA injection technique, mechanical index (or transmit power), transmit frequency, line density, contrast-specific algorithm selected, acoustic focus, and dynamic range (Table 3.3).[37]

CLINICAL APPLICATIONS OF LEFT VENTRICULAR OPACIFICATION

RESTING QUANTITATION OF LV VOLUMES AND EJECTION FRACTION

The most frequent clinical indication for MCE is the need to better delineate the endocardial contours of the LV cavity using LVO.[39] The intravenous administration of UEAs allows excellent discrimination between the LV blood pool and myocardium, improving the ability to assess LV chamber dimensions and systolic function (Fig. 3.5). Because only approximately

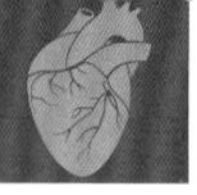

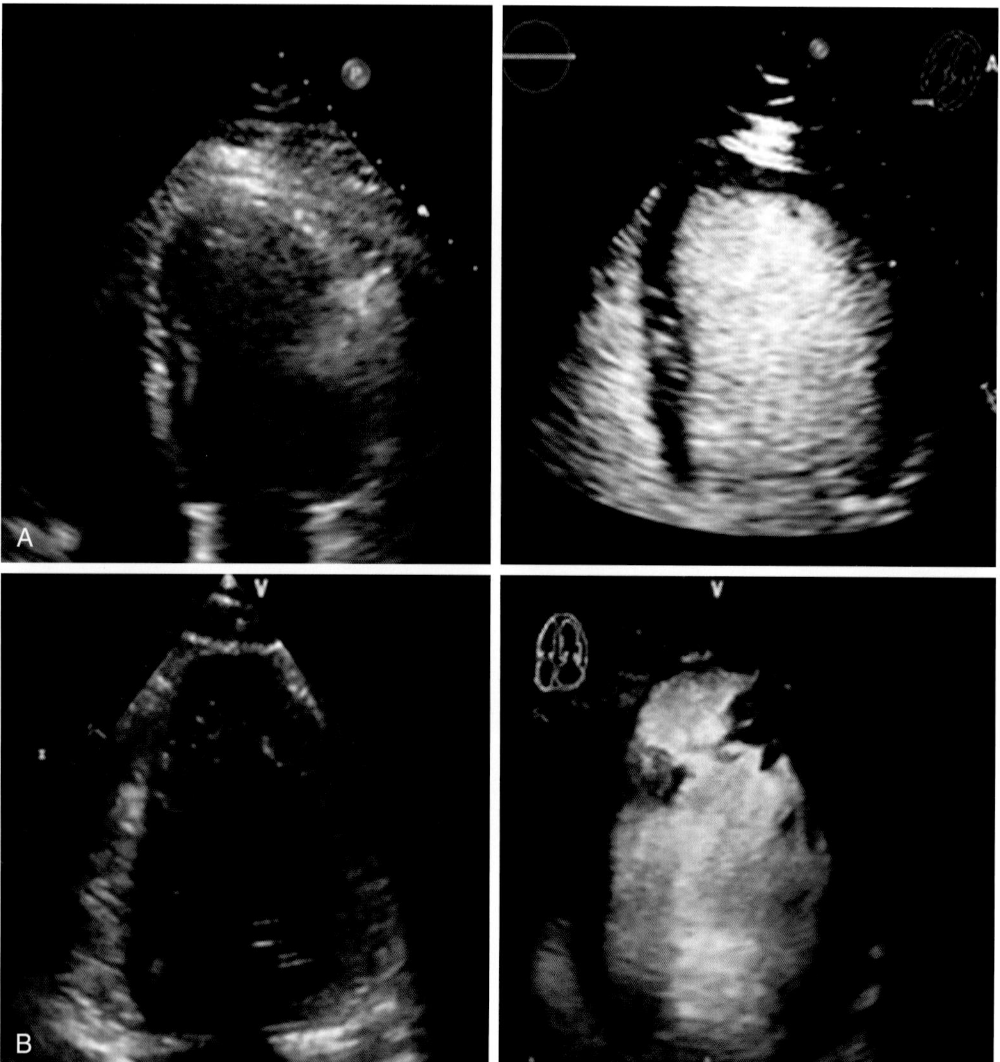

Fig. 3.5 Left ventricular opacification. (A and B) Non-contrast *(left)* and contrast-enhanced *(right)* images in two patients show that use of contrast increased the ability to delineate the myocardium and identify the true endocardial–blood pool interface, particularly in the lateral wall and apex. The contrast-enhanced image in B revealed the presence of prominent trabeculation and a false tendon. See Videos 3.5A, B, C, and D.

5% to 10% of the mass of the myocardium is attributable to its microvascular blood volume,[40] the contrast signal in the myocardium is a small fraction of that within the LV cavity, thereby providing selective cavity opacification. With sufficiently high doses of UEAs and multipulse contrast-specific imaging methods, myocardial opacification can occur, detracting from the ability to discriminate LV cavity and myocardium. Accordingly, LVO is usually performed with either small, repetitive intravenous boluses of contrast or a continuous infusion of contrast at a modest rate that results in full opacification of the blood pool without attenuation. Although LVO is useful for defining endocardial borders, it is important to recognize that, as in all forms of imaging, the quality is affected by rib attenuation and other beam-altering artifacts.

Clinical scenarios in which UEAs are commonly used for LVO include (1) the inability to otherwise fully examine LV myocardial dimensions; (2) the frequent use of echocardiography to guide management in critically ill patients who have difficult acoustic windows due to positive-pressure ventilation or the inability to cooperate with the ultrasound examination; and (3) the incorporation of echocardiography in critical decision making based on accurate quantification of systolic function or LV dimension or the presence of segmental wall motion when every myocardial region needs to be well seen with a high degree of reader confidence (i.e., during active chest pain). Clinical situations in which LVO has consistently been shown to have a positive impact in patient care are listed in Table 3.4.

RESTING LV REGIONAL WALL MOTION

Quantitative measurement of LV dimensions or LV ejection fraction (LVEF) is an important part of clinical decision making in cardiovascular medicine. Accurate and reproducible measurements are required to appropriately select patients for implantable defibrillators, cardiac resynchronization therapy, or valve intervention and to guide drug therapy in patients with heart failure or cardiotoxic cancer chemotherapies. When echocardiography is compared with either left ventriculography or cardiac magnetic resonance imaging (MRI) as a reference, echocardiographic measurement of LV volumes and LVEF have been shown to be more accurate and more precise with the use of intravenous UEA administration for LVO rather than non-enhanced echocardiography.[41–45] Contrast enhancement for

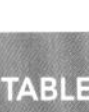

TABLE 3.4 Clinical Scenarios and Conditions in Which LV or Vascular Opacification Improves Diagnostic Yield.

Detection of segmental wall motion abnormalities (rest or stress)
Quantification of LV ejection fraction
Quantification of LV dimensions or volumes
Detection of LV or atrial thrombus
Detection and characterization of LV masses
Confirmation of the presence of apical hypertrophic cardiomyopathy
Evaluation of eosinophilic cardiomyopathy
Detection of ventricular pseudoaneurysm
Evaluation of ventricular noncompaction cardiomyopathy
Augmentation in Doppler signals
Detection of aortic thrombus or dissection

LVO results in larger dimensions and volumes compared with non-enhanced echocardiography (Fig. 3.6), largely because of the better ability to identify the true endocardial border, exclude trabeculae, and avoid foreshortening.[3,41,44] Contrast administration also improves interobserver variability when measuring LV volumes or LVEF, particularly when the images obtained with non-enhanced echocardiography are of poor quality.[42,43,46]

When applying echocardiography to evaluate for resting wall motion abnormalities, the use of LVO has consistently been shown to increase not only the number of interpretable studies but also the number of interpretable segments. In multicenter studies, the administration of UEAs during echocardiography improved the identification of wall motion abnormalities when MRI was used as a gold standard and resulted in the lowest interobserver variability for detection of regional wall motion abnormalities compared with MRI or unenhanced echocardiography.[41,42] In

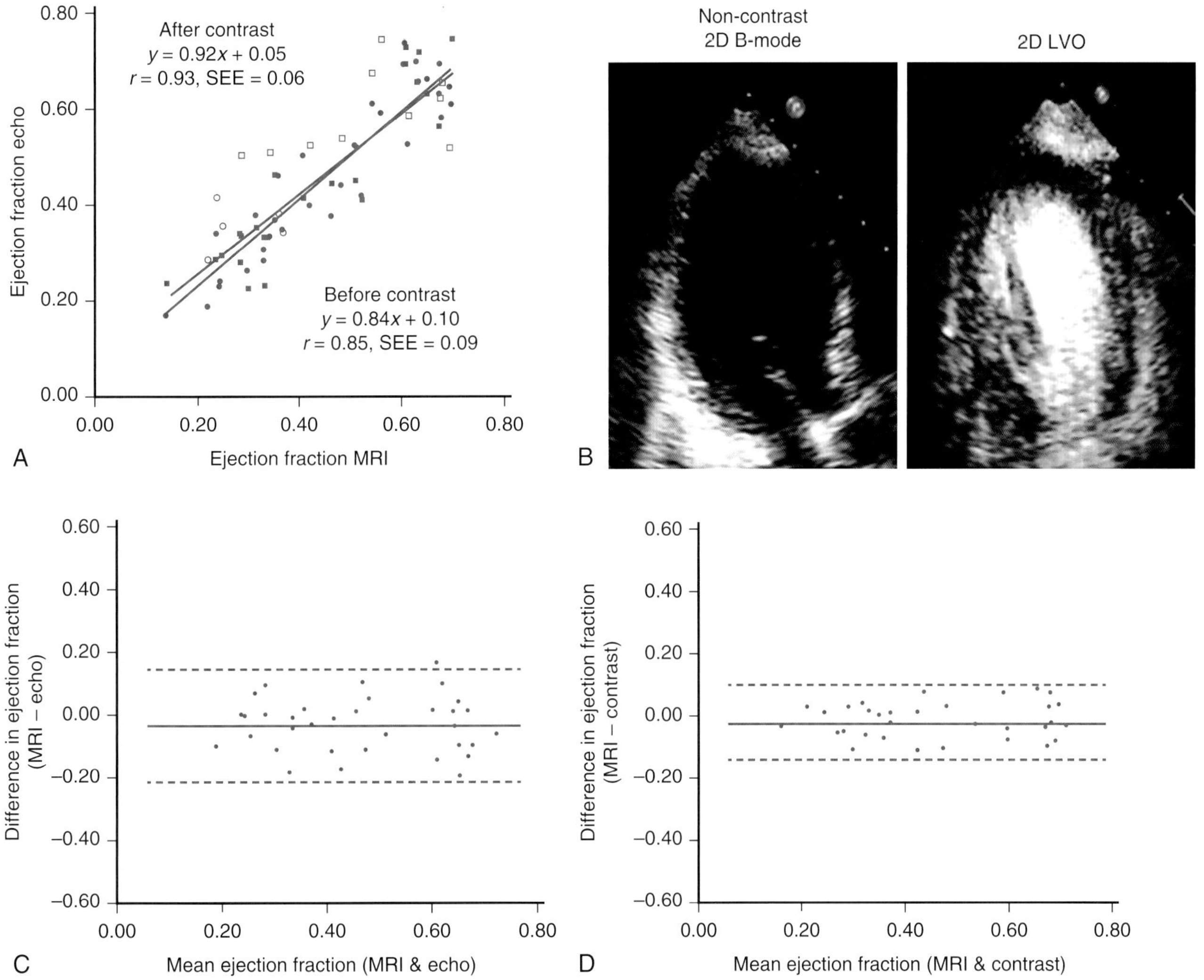

Fig. 3.6 Impact of left ventricular opacification on measurement of LV dimensions. (A) Correlation (*r*) between contrast-enhanced magnetic resonance imaging (MRI) and non-contrast echocardiography for measurement of LV ejection fraction (*filled squares* = before contrast; *filled circles* = after contrast; *open* symbols = 2 or more myocardial segments not seen). The standard error of the estimate *(SEE)* is smaller for measurements made with contrast. (B) In this example, the ability to evaluate true cavity dimensions is better during left ventricular opacification (LVO) compared with non-contrast echocardiography, in which image quality is good but endocardial borders are not well defined. Bland-Altman plots are used to compare values obtained by non-enhanced echocardiography (C) and contrast-enhanced MRI (D) in the same patient. The administration of contrast-reduced variability, as indicated by the more narrow limits of agreement (95% confidence interval; *dashed lines*). See also Videos 3.6A and B. (Graphs reproduced with permission from Hundley WG, Kizilbash AM, Afridi I, et al. Administration of an intravenous perfluorocarbon contrast agent improves echocardiographic determination of left ventricular volumes and ejection fraction: comparison with cine magnetic resonance imaging. *J Am Coll Cardiol*. 1998;32:1426–1432.)

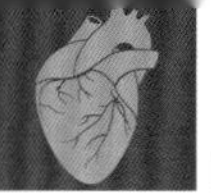

a study of 1017 patients presenting with symptoms suspicious for myocardial ischemia, implementation of LVO during point-of-care echocardiography to identify wall motion abnormalities was shown to add substantial incremental value to traditional risk assessment tools in identifying high-risk patients with ischemia.[47] When LVO is used for wall motion assessment, both endocardial and epicardial surfaces must be visualized for wall thickening evaluation; therefore, certain contrast-specific settings that completely eliminate the myocardial signal may not be advantageous if the epicardium cannot be defined.

Because use of LVO in certain populations can improve diagnostic accuracy, reproducibility, and confidence in the assessment of LV volumes and function, formal recommendations for its use have been made by American and European cardiovascular imaging societies.[3,48] The recommendations for use of LVO are based primarily on the inability to adequately visualize two or more segments with non-enhanced echocardiography. This approach, while simple, is limited in its ability to guide the use of UEAs in certain specific clinical scenarios in which impact of contrast addition may be particularly high or low. Accordingly, it is reasonable to consider the use of contrast based on two separate considerations: (1) What is the quality of non-contrast echocardiographic images? and (2) Will contrast have a major impact on answering the clinical question? With this paradigm (illustrated schematically in Fig. 3.7), UEAs should be used more liberally in situations in which accurate measurement of LV dimensions or function is important or when wall motion abnormalities must be excluded with confidence; contrast is unlikely to aid in evaluating conditions in which LVO is not of great benefit. When used in selected patients to better visualize the LV, UEAs have been shown to have a positive impact on management with regard to changes in therapy or subsequent procedures performed (Fig. 3.8), particularly for patients in intensive care units, in whom imaging is often difficult, and for those with reduced LVEF.[49,50] When used in selected patients, LVO has been shown to be cost-effective because it lowers downstream resource utilization needed to address limitations of technically inadequate non-enhanced imaging.[49,51,52]

LV OPACIFICATION DURING STRESS

Exercise or pharmacologic stress echocardiography for evaluation of coronary artery disease (CAD) relies on the regional assessment of contractile reserve and the detection of resting or stress wall thickening abnormalities. The diagnostic performance of stress echocardiography depends on the ability to adequately visualize all myocardial territories. In a study of 839 patients referred for stress echocardiography, the use of UEAs for LVO resulted in adequate images for interpretation at rest and during stress in more than 99% of patients.[53] Contrast echocardiography for LVO during stress has also been shown to increase the number of interpretable segments, subjective study quality, and reader confidence.[54,55] The use of LVO has the greatest impact in patients with suboptimal non-enhanced images; it results in diagnostic accuracy similar to that obtained in those with optimal image quality at baseline.[24] Contrast enhancement especially aids in the assessment of myocardial segments that commonly suffer from poor endocardial discrimination, such as the basal-lateral and basal-inferior segments on apical views, and in the assessment of the LV apex when there is foreshortening or near-field clutter artifact. Overall, the use of UEAs during

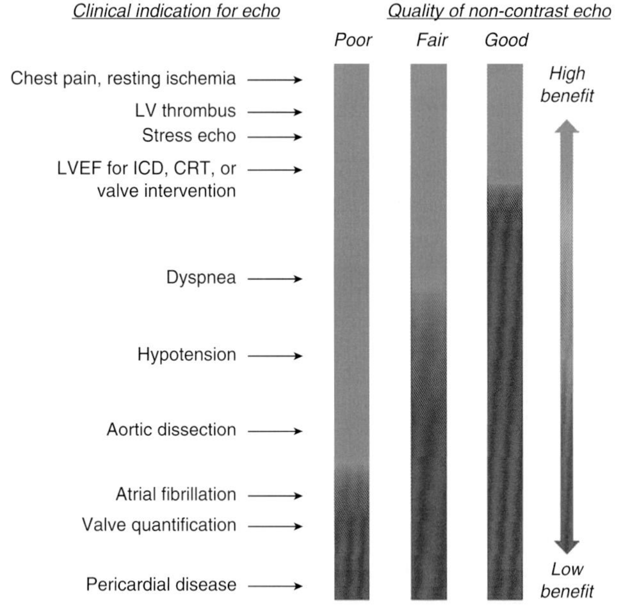

Fig. 3.7 Relative benefits of using a contrast agent. Schematic diagram illustrates the potential clinical impact of administration of a UEA for LVO according to both the clinical indication for transthoracic echocardiography and the quality of the baseline non-contrast images. *Green* hues denote situations where LVO is likely to have an impact on diagnosis, accuracy, and/or confidence, whereas *red* colors denote situations in which clinical impact is likely to be low. This diagram represents a more nuanced approach than guideline-based recommendations because it takes into account the indication for the study. *CRT*, Cardiac resynchronization therapy; *ICD*, implantable cardioverter defibrillator; *LVEF*, left ventricular ejection fraction; *LVO*, left ventricular opacification; *UEA*, ultrasound enhancing agent.

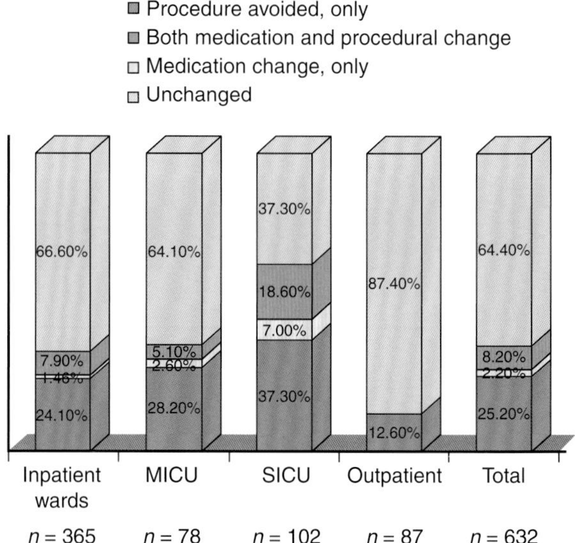

Fig. 3.8 Effect of contrast echocardiography on clinical decision making. Data from a large cohort of outpatients and inpatients (general wards and intensive care units) illustrate the impact of adding contrast echocardiography for LVO to non-enhanced echocardiography to aid clinical decisions on medications or procedures. Imaging with LVO may have been impactful even in those who did not have a change in management by confirming that no changes in medications or procedures were warranted. *LVO*, Left ventricular opacification; *MICU*, medical intensive care unit; *SICU*, surgical intensive care unit. (Reproduced by permission from Kurt M, Shaikh KA, Peterson L, et al. Impact of contrast echocardiography on evaluation of ventricular function and clinical management in a large prospective cohort. *J Am Coll Cardiol*. 2009;53:802–810.)

stress echocardiography increases the likelihood of achieving a positive study without compromising positive predictive value and improves overall diagnostic accuracy.[55,56]

LV OPACIFICATION FOR INTRACARDIAC ABNORMALITIES

Thrombus formation in the LV cavity most commonly occurs in the setting of severe global or segmental LV dysfunction. In those with myocardial infarction (MI), the presence of an LV thrombus on echocardiography is associated with a fivefold increased risk of embolic complication.[57] Thrombus formation often occurs at the LV apex which, based on its position in the near field on apical views, is subject to clutter and reverberation artifacts and weak harmonic signal generation.[58] The ability to accurately detect or exclude thrombus affects not only anticoagulation decisions but also risk assessment in those being evaluated for interventional valve procedures or LV assist devices. The sensitivity for detecting LV thrombus when using cine-MRI as a gold standard has been shown to be as low as 50% for non-enhanced echocardiography.[59] Diagnostic accuracy and interobserver variability for detecting LV thrombi with echocardiography are markedly improved by LVO (Fig. 3.9), resulting in a level of accuracy similar to that achieved with cardiac cine-MRI.[60–62] In a study of patients after MI whose non-contrast echocardiograms were inconclusive, LVO excluded thrombus and reversed recommendations for oral anticoagulation therapy in almost one third of patients with suspected thrombus and detected thrombus in 11% of patients in whom non-contrast echocardiography was indeterminate because of poor imaging quality.[60] Although contrast-specific beamforming and pulse schemes have not been routinely incorporated into conventional transesophageal echocardiography (TEE) technology, UEAs have been used during TEE to discriminate between artifact and thrombus, particularly in the left atrial appendage. The use of contrast with TEE improves interpreter confidence before TEE-guided cardioversion, and a negative study practically eliminates the risk for embolic complication of cardioversion.[63]

In patients with HCM, UEAs can improve the definition of endocardial borders and regional myocardial thickness, particularly in apical HCM, where non-enhanced echocardiography fails to identify disease in approximately 10% of cases.[64] Contrast echocardiography is helpful for detecting apical thickening and differentiating it from apical foreshortening. It is also helpful for detecting localized apical aneurysms, which occur in many of these patients (Fig. 3.10A). Accordingly, guidelines have recommended the use of contrast in the evaluation of suspected apical HCM.

Eosinophilic cardiomyopathy is manifested by eosinophilic infiltration, myonecrosis, and fibrosis, often culminating in a restrictive cardiomyopathy.[65] Thrombosis is a common feature and is thought to occur from eosinophilic degranulation and myocyte necrosis, which lead to loss of normal anti-thrombotic properties of the endocardium and release of pro-thrombotic substances. Contrast echocardiography is often helpful for clearly visualizing the apical filling of the LV or right ventricle (RV) created by inflammation and thrombosis.[3] It is also helpful

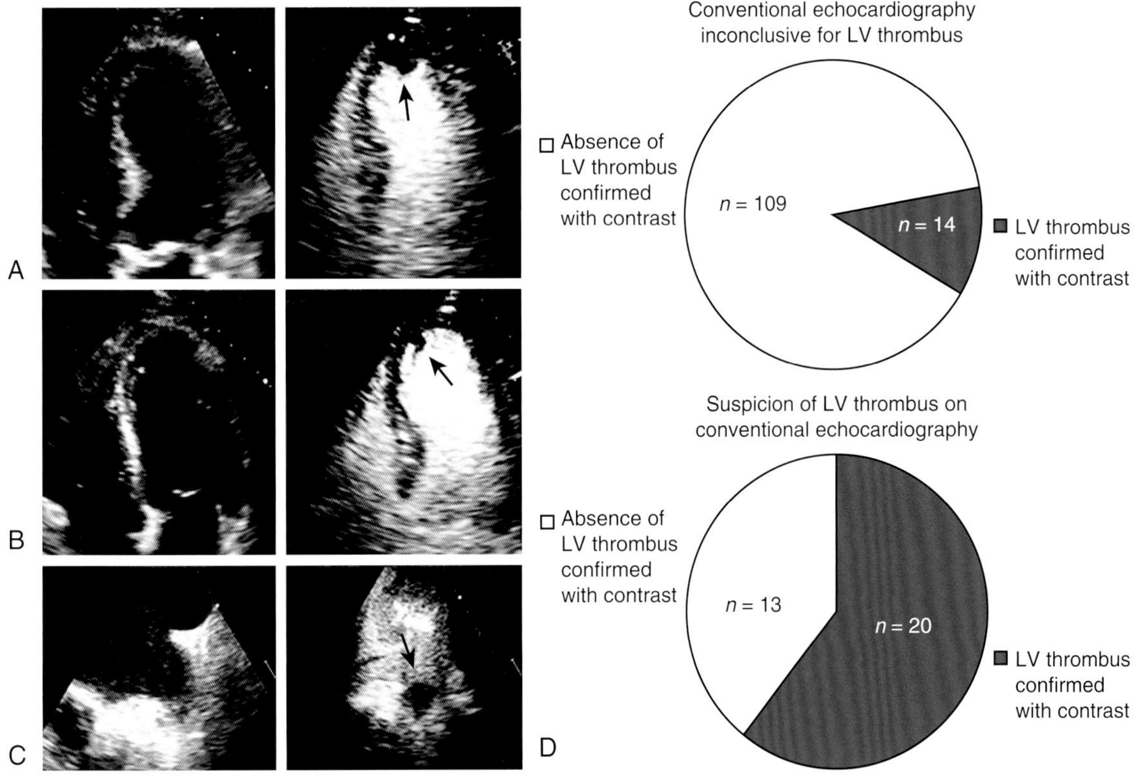

Fig. 3.9 Contrast echocardiography for detection of LV thrombus. Non-contrast *(left)* and corresponding contrast-enhanced *(right)* echocardiographic images illustrate the better ability to detect thrombus *(arrows)* when ultrasound enhancing agents (UEAs) are used. On transthoracic imaging in the apical 4-chamber view, contrast enhancement revealed the presence of (A) a mural sessile apical thrombus and (B) a pedunculated apical thrombus. (C) On TEE, thrombus at the apex of the left atrial appendage, suspected on non-contrast imaging, was confirmed by contrast enhancement. (D) Pie charts from a study of patients after myocardial infarction show the number of patients in whom the diagnosis of LV thrombus was reclassified based on administration of UEAs when the baseline non-contrast TTE results were either inconclusive *(top panel)* or suspicious *(bottom panel)* for thrombus. See also Videos 3.9A, B, C, and D. (Data from Siebelink HM, Scholte AJ, Van de Veire NR, et al. Value of contrast echocardiography for left ventricular thrombus detection postinfarction and impact on antithrombotic therapy. *Coron Artery Dis.* 2009;20:462–426.)

for differentiating eosinophilic from apical HCM by characterizing the shape of the LV cavity and through use of MCE perfusion imaging, which discriminates between myocardium and thrombus.

LV non-compaction cardiomyopathy has many different phenotypic manifestations and occurs secondary to incomplete consolidation of the myocardial trabecular network, which normally occurs by approximately 18 weeks of gestation. This leads to thinning of the compacted portion of the myocardium and a spongiform network of trabeculae with deep inter-trabecular recesses, most commonly involving the LV apex and distal lateral walls. Because other disease states can result in prominent LV trabeculation, echocardiographic criteria for diagnosis of non-compaction have been proposed.[66] Some of the major elements of these criteria are a systolic or diastolic ratio of non-compacted to compacted myocardium of at least 2:1, flow into trabecular recesses, and a compacted myocardial thickness of less than 8 mm. Administration of UEAs can reveal hypertrabeculation and inter-trabecular flow, and it can more accurately quantify the relative thicknesses of the compacted and non-compacted myocardial layers (see Fig. 3.10B).[3] Because flow into inter-trabecular recesses is slow, imaging at an intermediate mechanical index (0.2–0.5), to gradually destroy microbubbles, can be helpful for better characterizing regions with slow intra-trabecular flow.

Contrast echocardiography for LVO has been used to reveal several other clinically impactful findings in the LV. The detection of small, non-thrombus intracavitary masses has been improved when echocardiography is performed with UEAs. Detection of ventricular pseudoaneurysm and the presence of layered thrombus within an aneurysm are improved by LVO. Anatomic evaluation of extracardiac vascular structures can also be enhanced by the use of UEAs. High-impact vascular applications include enhanced delineation of carotid plaque dimension and ulceration, diagnosis and assessment (true vs. false lumen) of aortic dissection, diagnosis of arterial pseudoaneurysm, detection of endograft leaks, and evaluation of plaque neovascularization.[3,67]

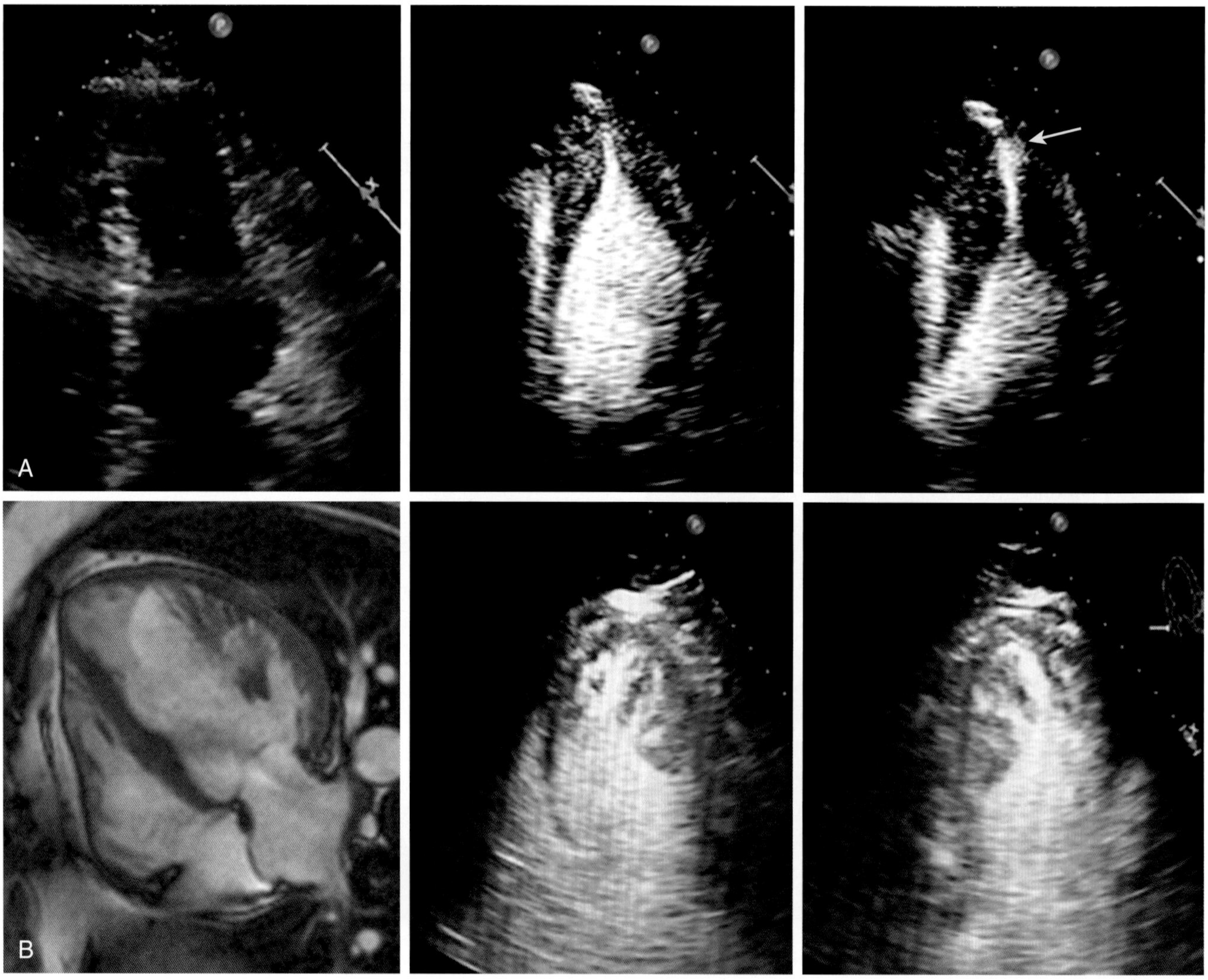

Fig. 3.10 Contrast echocardiography for evaluation of apical pathologies. (A) Example of the use of ultrasound enhancing agents (UEAs) to improve the diagnosis of apical hypertrophic cardiomyopathy on TTE from the apical 4-chamber view. Images show an unenhanced end-systolic image *(left)* and contrast-enhanced images during diastole *(center)* and systole *(right)*. On the end-systolic image, an apical region of dyskinesis from pressure overload *(arrow)* is shown. (B) Example of non-compaction cardiomyopathy seen on cardiac magnetic resonance imaging (steady-state free-precession imaging, *left panel*) and contrast echocardiography in the apical 4-chamber (*center panel*) and 3-chamber (*right panel*) views. UEAs reveal flow into the inter-trabecular recesses and the dimensions of both non-compacted and compacted myocardium. See also Videos 3.10A, B, and C.

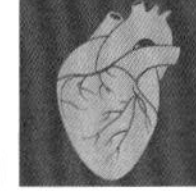

MYOCARDIAL PERFUSION IMAGING

The commercially available UEAs used during LVO are pure intravascular tracers. Accordingly, the degree of signal enhancement in any tissue is proportional to the relative blood volume within that tissue, provided that the contrast agent remains stable, that it is not destroyed through inertial cavitation, and that the concentration does not produce a degree of enhancement that is below or above the dynamic range of the imaging system.[1] The total coronary circulation in large mammals contains 10 to 12 mL of blood per 100 g of LV myocardium.[68] The bulk of blood volume in the coronary arteries and veins resides on the epicardial surface, whereas 80% to 90% of the intramyocardial blood volume is represented by the microcirculation, most of which is in capillaries. Accordingly, myocardial signal enhancement during MCE is dominated by signal from the capillary compartment.

Myocardial blood flow (MBF) is defined as the volume of blood transiting through tissue at a certain rate. Information on both microvascular blood volume and flux rate are needed for this calculation are measurable by MCE.[69] When myocardial contrast signal is obtained in steady state without destruction of UEAs, signal enhancement represents the relative myocardial blood volume (MBV); this can be further quantified in milliliters per mass (grams) of myocardium by normalizing to the LV cavity signal, provided that both measurements are within the dynamic range of the concentration–intensity relationship. Attenuation from microbubbles within the LV cavity can also influence this measurement. For assessment of MBF, the transit rate is derived from kinetic information after inertial cavitation of microbubbles by several high-power ultrasound frames; signal recovery is then assessed over time, representing the reappearance of contrast into the volume of myocardium in the imaging plane.[69] Generally, this kinetic information is achieved by low-power real-time imaging over the ensuing 5 to 15 cardiac cycles to capture microbubble re-entry into the microcirculation (Fig. 3.11). End-systolic frames gated to the T wave of the electrocardiogram (ECG) are used for this analysis because the signal from large intramyocardial vessels is minimized by systolic contraction.[70] The time-versus-intensity relation can then be fit to a monoexponential function:

$$y = A\left(1 - e^{-\beta t}\right)$$

where y is the intensity at time t, A is the plateau intensity representing MBV, and β is the rate constant of the curve, which represents the microvascular flux rate. The product of MBV and β represents MBF and can be quantified in mL/min per gram of tissue when MBV is normalized to the blood pool.[69] Quantification of MBF requires (1) a constant concentration of microbubbles within the blood pool during imaging, which is best accomplished by a constant intravenous infusion of contrast; (2) minimal destruction of microbubbles during replenishment imaging, which requires a low mechanical index (<0.2); and (3) system settings that provide a relatively linear relation between microbubble concentration and signal intensity.

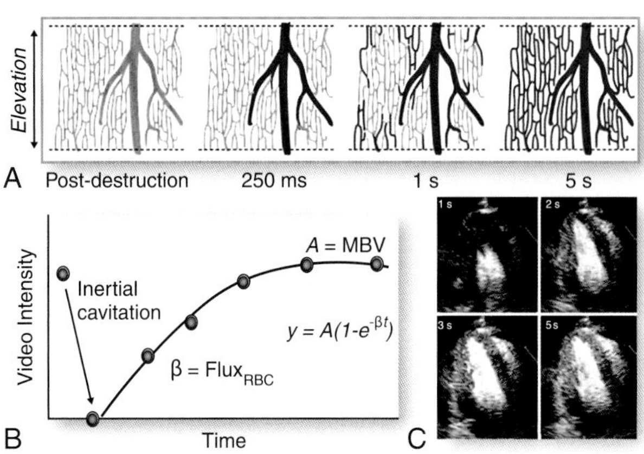

Fig. 3.11 Physiologic basis for assessing perfusion on myocardial contrast echocardiography. (A) Illustration of the myocardial microcirculation within the volume of the ultrasound elevational plane where microbubble replenishment *(blue)* occurs progressively after exposure to high mechanic index ultrasound to clear the contrast agent by inertial cavitation. Microbubble refill occurs first in larger vessels that have fast flow velocity but constitute a minority of the blood volume; later there is filling of capillaries that have slow flow velocities but dominate the signal intensity. The time–intensity graph (B) and end-systolic MCE images (C) obtained by low-power imaging in the apical 2-chamber view illustrate typical data obtained after inertial cavitation of microbubbles. Time–intensity data for myocardial contrast refill are fit to a monoexponential function for calculation of the A value (plateau intensity), reflecting microvascular blood volume (MBV), and the rate constant or β-value, reflecting the RBC flux rate (Flux$_{RBC}$). The images reveal normal time-related contrast replenishment which, under resting conditions, occurs over approximately 5 seconds at rest. Attenuation of the basal segments caused by high cavity contrast concentration is observed.

DETECTION OF ISCHEMIA

Because echocardiography is readily available for use at the bedside, it is increasingly used for point-of-care evaluation of patients who have active symptoms of angina. In this setting, its use is intended to address the limitations of clinical history, electrocardiography, and cardiac enzymes in either rapidly confirming or excluding myocardial ischemia. Echocardiography can rapidly detect segmental wall motion abnormalities at rest caused by ongoing or recently resolved ischemia. It can also be used to identify other cardiovascular problems that may be responsible for symptoms such as pericardial effusion, aortic dissection, or valve disease. The value of adding MCE perfusion imaging when there is already a wall motion abnormality is based on the ability to be able to identify the flow status as either (1) complete lack of perfusion; (2) hypoperfusion with some antegrade or collateral flow; or (3) stunning, in which perfusion has normalized but a wall motion abnormality persists (Fig. 3.12). Perfusion imaging may also be helpful to discern a pattern typical for conditions that may mimic acute coronary syndrome. For this reason, perfusion imaging with MCE has been shown not only to increase the predictive accuracy for the diagnosis of ischemia beyond clinical information, ECG, and early cardiac enzymes but also to provide prognostic information on the risk for short-term and long-term cardiac events.[47,71]

Mild resting hypoperfusion is manifested by a reduced microvascular flux rate (β-value or reappearance rate) on dynamic imaging, whereas severe hypoperfusion can result in subendocardial or transmural reduction in contrast enhancement even after full replenishment has occurred (i.e., reduced MBV). The high negative predictive value of normal function and myocardial perfusion during symptoms may be helpful as a way of streamlining care, although the value of this approach may be limited in those with prior events or when there is a long delay between resolution of ischemic symptoms and imaging. In those patients who have already been diagnosed with acute coronary syndromes, MCE perfusion imaging can provide

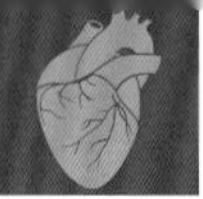

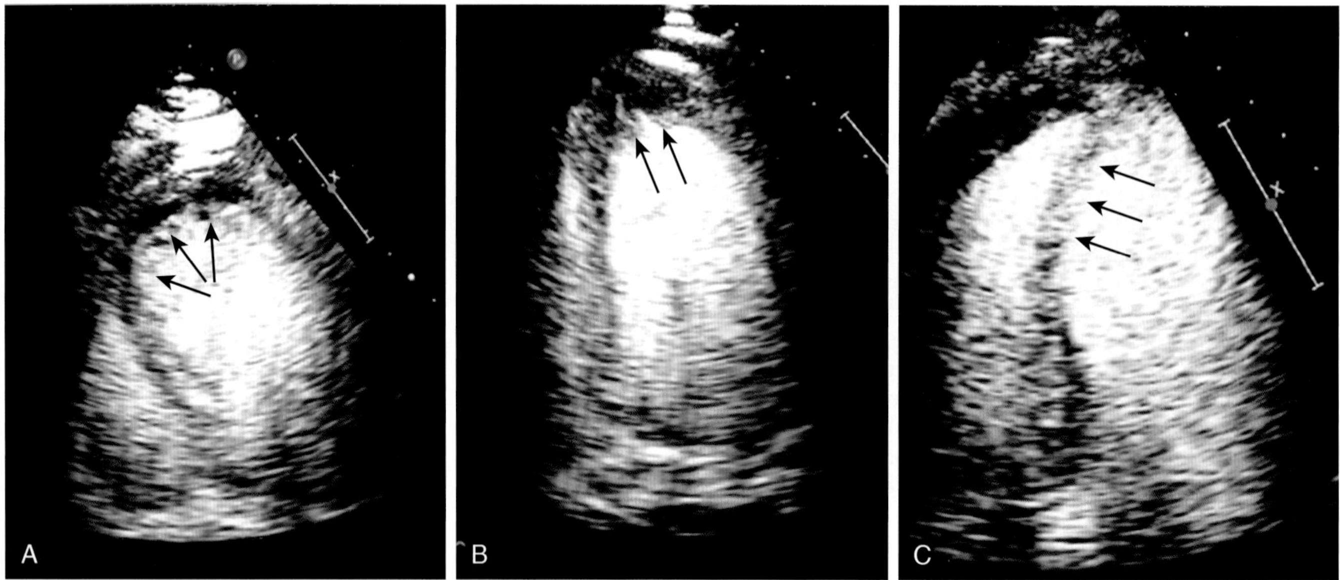

Fig. 3.12 Myocardial contrast echocardiography perfusion imaging. These examples show TTE images from three patients presenting with acute coronary syndromes related to left anterior descending (LAD) coronary artery disease. (A) Apical 4-chamber view obtained after full microbubble replenishment illustrates lack of perfusion in the distal anteroseptum and apex (*arrows*) in a patient with acute LAD occlusion. (B) Apical 2-chamber view obtained early after a high-power pulse illustrates a contrast defect in the apex (*arrows*) that showed partial refill later (late after destruction) in a patient with hypoperfusion from acute mid-LAD thrombosis but a small amount of residual antegrade flow on angiography. See also Video 3.12B. (C) Apical 4-chamber view obtained early after a high-power pulse illustrates hyperemic flow in the distal septum (*arrows*), which was akinetic, in a patient who achieved rapid reperfusion of the LAD after thrombolytic therapy.

information on the risk area.[1] However, the clinical value of risk area measurement has not been established; instead, this approach has been used in clinical trials of therapies designed to reduce infarct size as a percentage of the risk area.

MCE perfusion imaging has also been used to augment diagnostic performance of exercise or pharmacologic stress testing for the detection of CAD. Because MCE directly evaluates myocardial microvascular perfusion, it can be used in stress imaging protocols that involve either exercise, inotropic agents such as dobutamine, or vasodilators. Abnormalities in regional MBV, whether transmural or subendocardial, are thought to represent either lack of recruitment or active derecruitment of microvascular units produced by the lower precapillary perfusion pressure during stress.[72] With this approach, MCE provides comparable information to single-photon emission computed tomography (SPECT) perfusion imaging with regard to the spatial extent of defects and their reversibility.[1,73] Because reduction in MBV during stress is not linearly related to the degree of ischemia and occurs only with relatively severe stenosis,[74] measurement of the microvascular blood flux rate (β-value) or MBF (product of MBV and β) have more commonly been used to detect and quantify stress-induced perfusion defects. The relatively simple assessment of flux rate (β-value) alone correlates well with MBF as measured by other methods such as radiolabeled microspheres, intracoronary flow wires, and positron emission tomography.[69,75,76] A smaller degree of increase in the flux rate from rest to stress also has been shown to provide high sensitivity for detecting significant coronary stenosis.[77] A more common and practical approach has been to use semiquantitative visual analysis, whereby normal resting perfusion is defined as a complete post-destruction signal replenishment time of four to five cardiac cycles at rest and one to two cycles during stress (Fig. 3.13).[78–80]

Clinical studies using a variety of stress approaches have demonstrated that for the detection of ischemia, MCE is at least comparable to radionuclide SPECT imaging.[78] In a multicenter trial enrolling more than 600 subjects, MCE was found to be superior to SPECT for the detection of CAD regardless of whether stenosis severity was defined as severe (>70%) or moderate (>50%), although it had a somewhat lower specificity.[81] The higher sensitivity of MCE compared with SPECT is in part attributable to its ability to detect isolated subendocardial perfusion defects. Because of the quantitative or semiquantitative nature of MCE imaging, it has also been shown to be extremely sensitive for detecting the presence of multivessel CAD, which is a recognized weakness in other perfusion imaging techniques that rely on territorial heterogeneity in tracer uptake.[80,81]

On conventional stress echocardiography, the relationship between hyperemic blood flow during stress and radial thickening is not linear, and mild to moderate reductions in flow reserve may be manifested by minimal changes in visual wall thickening.[82] The semiquantitative analysis of myocardial perfusion with MCE during stress has been shown to be superior to wall motion assessment with regard to sensitivity for the detection of stenosis, particularly for moderate rather than severe stenosis, and for the detection of disease when the target work level is not achieved.[80,83] It has also been shown to be superior to wall motion assessment for determining the spatial extent of ischemia and for detecting multivessel CAD.[80,83] Perfusion may be particularly important in those with previous MI because the sensitivity of contractile reserve for the diagnosis of ischemia is particularly problematic in regions where there are preexisting wall motion abnormalities at rest. In symptomatic patients referred for angiography, stress perfusion on MCE, when compared with invasive coronary hemodynamics, is almost always abnormal in situations where the fractional flow reserve is abnormal (<0.8), but it is also frequently abnormal when the

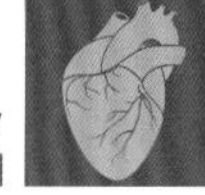

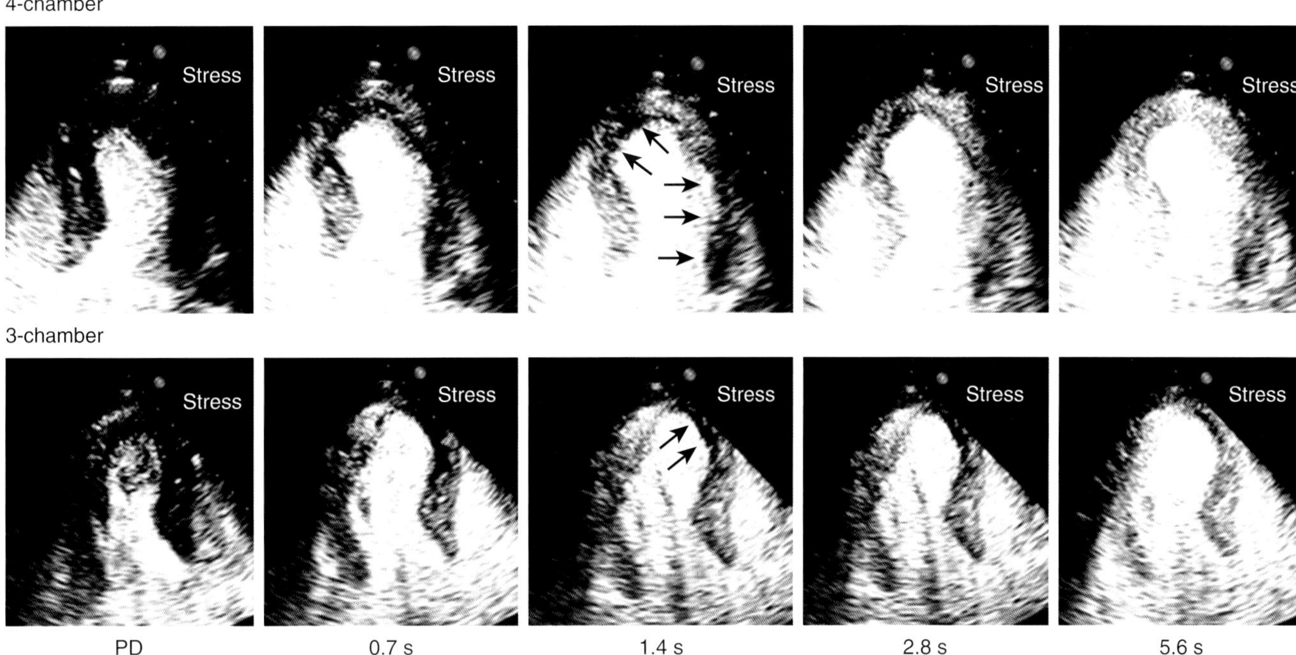

Fig. 3.13 Stress myocardial contrast echocardiography perfusion imaging. End-systolic images recorded in the apical 4- and 3-chamber views after stress testing with regadenoson infusion reveal multivessel coronary artery disease. Contrast replenishment early after contrast clearance (1.4 s) demonstrates delayed appearance in the distal anteroseptum, the apex, and the lateral wall (*arrows*), with particularly slow replenishment in the endocardial layer. By 5.6 s, most regions demonstrate refill except the basal-lateral wall on the 4-chamber view and the endocardial portion of the anteroseptum on the 3-chamber view. The patient was found to have greater than 70% stenosis in both the left anterior descending and left circumflex coronary arteries. *PD*, Post-destruction images.

fractional flow reserve is normal (>0.8), particularly when the invasively measured microvascular resistance is abnormal.[84]

With regard to long-term decision making and prognostic value, MCE at rest and with vasodilator stress is useful for distinguishing an ischemic versus non-ischemic etiology for new-onset heart failure.[85] MCE has also been shown to provide additional predictive value when compared with wall motion assessment for detecting higher risk for adverse clinical events (e.g., death, MI) and consequent need for clinically indicated revascularization (Fig. 3.14).[86,87]

MYOCARDIAL VIABILITY

The evaluation of myocardial viability by MCE can be performed at the bedside and is based on the ability of MCE to quantify the extent of an intact microcirculation. Under normal physiologic conditions, myocyte viability requires perfusion of approximately 0.20 to 0.25 mL/min per gram, below which myocellular necrosis occurs. This knowledge has led to the approach of assessing MBV, which reflects microvascular integrity, to detect viability by MCE. A simple, nonquantitative approach has been to visually examine for the presence of any myocardial contrast enhancement.[1] However, in patients with CAD and chronic LV dysfunction, the presence of *both* viability and ischemia, either at rest or during stress, is of key interest, and this has led to the use of destruction-replenishment kinetics.

When considering the performance of noninvasive imaging in chronic LV dysfunction, it is inaccurate to define viability as recovery of resting function after revascularization. Wall thickening at rest is determined primarily by the status of the endocardium.[88] Even if recovery of function does not occur due to subendocardial scar, revascularization of middle and epicardial regions can improve contractile reserve during exercise, reduce symptoms of angina and heart failure, and improve prognosis.[89] Because the transmural extent of viability is important, MCE has been compared with delayed enhancement on gadolinium-enhanced cardiac MRI and has been shown to provide similar transmural information on the extent of scar.[90] The distribution and extent of myocardial viability on MCE also correlates well with radionuclide SPECT techniques.[1] MCE is also at least as accurate as dobutamine stress echocardiography for assessing myocardial viability, and it may be even more sensitive in situations in which contractile response is influenced not only by viability but also by the presence of severe inducible ischemia.[91] When recovery of resting function is used as an end point, MCE has a higher sensitivity but lower specificity than dobutamine echocardiography because it detects viability in regions other than the endocardium that do not necessarily contribute to resting function.[92] The use of destruction-replenishment perfusion imaging algorithms rather than MBV assessment is particularly helpful for detecting situations in which there is resting hypoperfusion because of critical stenosis or coronary occlusion with collateral perfusion.

In the early post-MI period, MCE can provide information on both the success of reperfusion therapy and the spatial extent of myocardial salvage. The area lacking capillary perfusion predicts the infarct zone and lack of recovery of wall motion.[1] The presence of microvascular perfusion does not, however, guarantee recovery of contractile function in all patients because infarction that is patchy or confined to the subendocardial region often does not have normokinesia. Hence, segments that have partial myocardial opacification on MCE but lack recovery of wall motion after acute revascularization have been shown to have contractile reserve under low-dose dobutamine echocardiography.[93] In

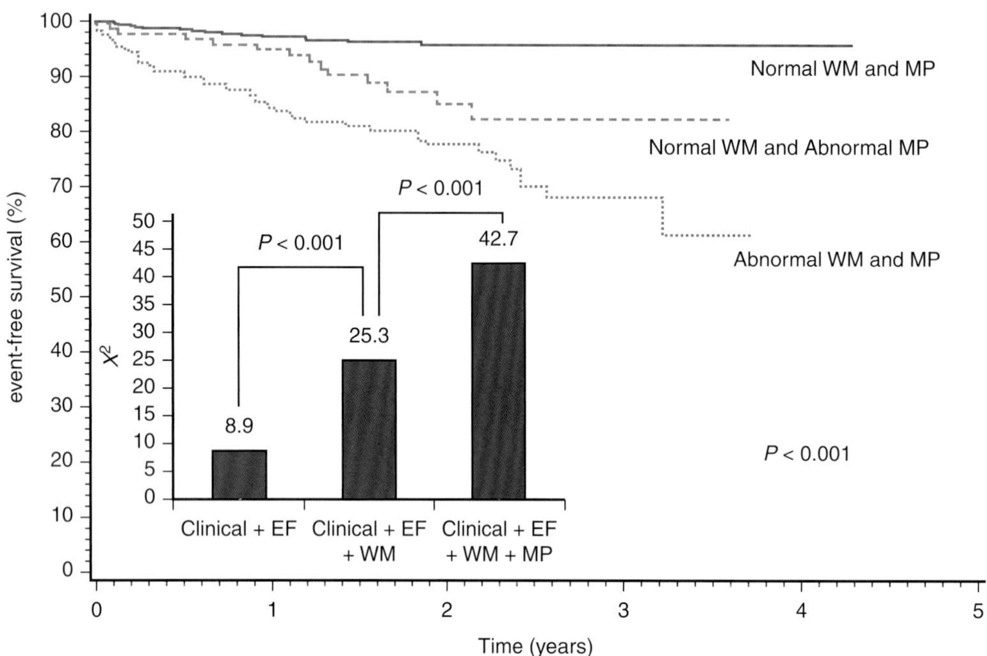

Fig. 3.14 Predictive value of myocardial contrast echocardiography perfusion imaging. Kaplan-Meier curves show event-free survival in 788 patients referred for dobutamine stress echocardiography according to results of wall motion (*WM*) and MCE-derived myocardial perfusion (*MP*) testing. The inset bar graph depicts χ^2 values (goodness of fit) as a measure of incremental prognostic value. Abnormal MP findings had significant incremental value over clinical factors, resting LV ejection fraction (*EF*), and WM response to dobutamine in predicting events (death and nonfatal myocardial infarction). (Reproduced with permission from Tsutsui JM, Elhendy A, Anderson JR, et al. Prognostic value of dobutamine stress myocardial contrast perfusion echocardiography. *Circulation.* 2005;112:1444–1450.)

patients with ST-elevation myocardial infarction (STEMI), MCE performed before revascularization can provide information on the likelihood of functional recovery. In this setting, the presence of perfusion in the risk area, whether from residual antegrade flow or from collateral supply, is highly predictive of maintenance of viability and recovery of function.[93]

OTHER PERFUSION IMAGING APPLICATIONS

Myocardial perfusion abnormalities can occur not only from epicardial artery stenosis but also from functional abnormalities of the coronary microcirculation. Because of its ability to assess perfusion at the microvascular level in response to various physiologic stressors, MCE has been used to detect microvascular dysfunction at rest or during hyperemic challenge and, in some cases, to assess response to therapies. In asymptomatic patients with diabetes mellitus, MCE has been shown to detect not only high-risk obstructive CAD but also perfusion abnormalities resulting from diffuse coronary narrowing or microvascular dysfunction.[94] MCE performed in patients referred for computed tomographic (CT)–guided coronary angiography for suspected CAD has detected the presence of microvascular dysfunction on vasodilator testing in approximately 40% of those without significant stenosis.[95] In symptomatic patients with presumed microvascular dysfunction, those who have MCE perfusion defects during stress without obstructive CAD show similar long-term prognosis as those with perfusion defects from CAD.[96]

Microvascular perfusion imaging with MCE has also been shown to be helpful in the evaluation of intracardiac masses, specifically for the differentiation of thrombus from primary or metastatic tumors (Fig. 3.15). Although avascularity can be found in certain tumors such as fibroelastomas, the presence of a functional microcirculation confirms that an intracardiac mass is a tumor. Highly vascularized tumors on MCE perfusion imaging have been demonstrated to be more likely consistent with malignant tumors, whereas certain stromal tumors including myxomas often demonstrate spatially heterogeneous perfusion.[97]

MCE has been used in specific clinical indications in which knowledge of myocardial perfusion can assist in either diagnosis or clinical decision making.[3,98] MCE perfusion imaging can aid in the diagnosis of eosinophilic cardiomyopathy by detecting the presence of viable apical myocardium surrounding an avascular luminal filling defect caused by thrombotic complications of the disease. MCE can also be helpful in diseases in which regional wall motion abnormalities result from conditions other than ischemic CAD. In sarcoidosis, MCE perfusion imaging is often complementary to LVO; it demonstrates normal perfusion in hypokinetic or akinetic regions that are atypical in their distribution for CAD. Similarly, normal perfusion can differentiate apical dyskinesia associated with apical forms of HCM from ischemic coronary disease. In stress-induced or takosubo cardiomyopathy, because microvascular perfusion is often abnormal, particularly early in the disease process, MCE does not by itself distinguish the condition from ischemic disease. However, studies have indicated that acute MI generally results in lower myocardial perfusion on MCE than does stress cardiomyopathy.[99] Contrast ultrasound perfusion imaging at rest and during contractile exercise has also been used with good success for the diagnosis and assessment of peripheral vascular disease. In this group of patients, it can provide incremental information on the degree of flow impairment to augment the findings of conventional methods such as the ankle-brachial index.[100]

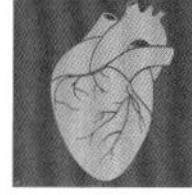

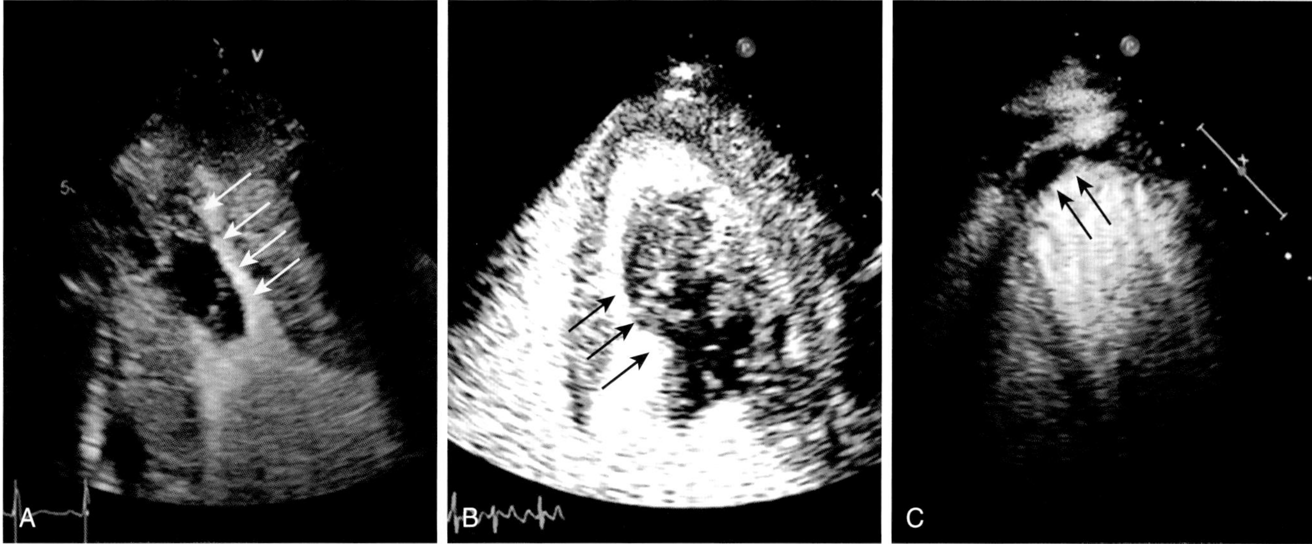

Fig. 3.15 MCE perfusion imaging for evaluation of intracardiac masses. (A) Apical 3-chamber view demonstrates partial perfusion at the base of a cardiac metastasis from soft tissue sarcoma (*arrows*). (B) Apical 4-chamber view demonstrates almost complete tumor perfusion from a metastatic melanoma (*arrows*). (C) Apical 4-chamber view demonstrates complete lack of perfusion in a thrombus (*arrows*) compared with portions of the perfused septum and lateral wall. See also Videos 3.15A, B, and C.

SUMMARY Contrast Echocardiography.

Clinical Applications	Contrast Modality	Imaging Methods	Comments
Resting LV volumes and LVEF	LV opacification	Low-MI, contrast-specific real-time imaging	Detection of endocardial borders
Regional wall motion at rest and during stress	LV opacification	Low-MI, contrast-specific real-time imaging	Detection of endocardial borders and regional thickening
Intracardiac abnormalities (e.g., masses, thrombi, non-compaction cardiomyopathy)	LV opacification; MCE perfusion imaging	Low-MI real-time imaging; low-MI multipulse imaging with destruction-replenishment imaging	Detection of masses, excluding artifacts, unusual LV geometry, differentiation of clot vs. tumor
Detection of ischemia in CAD (rest, stress)	MCE perfusion imaging	Low-MI multipulse imaging with destruction-replenishment imaging	Quantitative or semiquantitative perfusion assessment
Myocardial viability	MCE perfusion imaging	Low-MI multipulse imaging of microvascular blood volume	Quantitative or semiquantitative assessment of microvascular integrity
Detection of microvascular dysfunction	MCE perfusion imaging	Low-MI multipulse imaging with destruction-replenishment imaging	Quantitative or semiquantitative perfusion assessment

CAD, Coronary artery disease; *LV*, left ventricular; *LVEF*, left ventricular ejection fraction; *MCE*, myocardial contrast echocardiography; *MI*, mechanical index.

REFERENCES

1. Kaufmann BA, Wei K, Lindner JR. Contrast echocardiography. *Curr Probl Cardiol.* 2007;32:51–96.
2. Bhatia VK, Senior R. Contrast echocardiography: evidence for clinical use. *J Am Soc Echocardiogr.* 2008;21:409–416.
3. Porter TR, Mulvagh SL, Abdelmoneim SS, et al. Clinical applications of Ultrasonic enhancing agents in echocardiography: 2018 American Society of Echocardiography guidelines update. *J Am Soc Echocardiogr.* 2018;31:241–274.
4. Gramiak R, Shah PM. Echocardiography of the aortic root. *Invest Radiol.* 1968;3:356–366.
5. de Jong N, Frinking PJ, Bouakaz A, et al. Optical imaging of contrast agent microbubbles in an ultrasound field with a 100-MHz camera. *Ultrasound Med Biol.* 2000;26:487–492.
6. Epstein PSP MS. On the stability of gas bubbles in liquid-gas solutions. *J Chem Phys.* 1950;18:1505–1509.
7. Kabalnov A, Klein D, Pelura T, Schutt E, Weers J. Dissolution of multicomponent microbubbles in the bloodstream: 1. Theory. *Ultrasound Med Biol.* 1998;24:739–749.
8. Sheeran PS, Luois S, Dayton PA, Matsunaga TO. Formulation and acoustic studies of a new

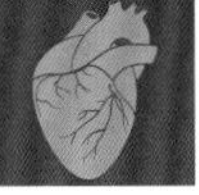

phase-shift agent for diagnostic and therapeutic ultrasound. *Langmuir*. 2011;27:10412–10420.

9. Lindner JR. Molecular imaging of cardiovascular disease with contrast-enhanced ultrasonography. *Nat Rev Cardiol*. 2009;6:475–481.
10. Villanueva FS, Wagner WR. Ultrasound molecular imaging of cardiovascular disease. *Nat Clin Pract Cardiovasc Med*. 2008;5(suppl 2):S26–S32.
11. Unger E, Porter T, Lindner J, Grayburn P. Cardiovascular drug delivery with ultrasound and microbubbles. *Adv Drug Deliv Rev*. 2014;72:110–126.
12. Main ML, Hibberd MG, Ryan A, et al. Acute mortality in critically ill patients undergoing echocardiography with or without an ultrasound contrast agent. *JACC Cardiovasc Imaging*. 2014;7:40–48.
13. Main ML, Ryan AC, Davis TE, et al. Acute mortality in hospitalized patients undergoing echocardiography with and without an ultrasound contrast agent (multicenter registry results in 4,300,966 consecutive patients). *Am J Cardiol*. 2008;102:1742–1746.
14. Wei K, Mulvagh SL, Carson L, et al. The safety of Definity and Optison for ultrasound image enhancement: a retrospective analysis of 78,383 administered contrast doses. *J Am Soc Echocardiogr*. 2008;21:1202–1206.
15. Lindner JR, Song J, Jayaweera AR, Sklenar J, Kaul S. Microvascular rheology of Definity microbubbles after intra-arterial and intravenous administration. *J Am Soc Echocardiogr*. 2002;15:396–403.
16. Jayaweera AR, Edwards N, Glasheen WP, et al. In vivo myocardial kinetics of air-filled albumin microbubbles during myocardial contrast echocardiography. Comparison with radiolabeled red blood cells. *Circ Res*. 1994;74:1157–1165.
17. Wei K, Main ML, Lang RM, et al. The effect of Definity on systemic and pulmonary hemodynamics in patients. *J Am Soc Echocardiogr*. 2012;25:584–588.
18. Kalra A, Shroff GR, Erlien D, Gilbertson DT, Herzog CA. Perflutren-based echocardiographic contrast in patients with right-to-left intracardiac shunts. *JACC Cardiovasc Imaging*. 2014;7:206–207.
19. Schneider M, Broillet A, Tardy I, et al. Use of intravital microscopy to study the microvascular behavior of microbubble-based ultrasound contrast agents. *Microcirculation*. 2012;19:245–259.
20. Lindner JR, Song J, Xu F, et al. Noninvasive ultrasound imaging of inflammation using microbubbles targeted to activated leukocytes. *Circulation*. 2000;102:2745–2750.
21. Lindner JR, Coggins MP, Kaul S, et al. Microbubble persistence in the microcirculation during ischemia/reperfusion and inflammation is caused by integrin- and complement-mediated adherence to activated leukocytes. *Circulation*. 2000;101:668–675.
22. Fisher NG, Christiansen JP, Klibanov A, et al. Influence of microbubble surface charge on capillary transit and myocardial contrast enhancement. *J Am Coll Cardiol*. 2002;40:811–819.
23. Szebeni J, Muggia F, Gabizon A, Barenholz Y. Activation of complement by therapeutic liposomes and other lipid excipient-based therapeutic products: prediction and prevention. *Adv Drug Deliv Rev*. 2011;63:1020–1030.
24. Dolan MS, Gala SS, Dodla S, et al. Safety and efficacy of commercially available ultrasound contrast agents for rest and stress echocardiography a multicenter experience. *J Am Coll Cardiol*. 2009;53:32–38.
25. Liu YN, Khangura J, Xie A, et al. Renal retention of lipid microbubbles: a potential mechanism for flank discomfort during ultrasound contrast administration. *J Am Soc Echocardiogr*. 2013;26:1474–1481.
26. Chomas JE, Dayton P, Allen J, Morgan K, Ferrara KW. Mechanisms of contrast agent destruction. *IEEE Trans Ultrason Ferroelectr Freq Control*. 2001;48:232–248.
27. Belcik JT, Davidson BP, Xie A, et al. Augmentation of muscle blood flow by ultrasound cavitation is mediated by ATP and purinergic signaling. *Circulation*. 2017;135:1240–1252.
28. Meijering BD, Juffermans LJ, van Wamel A, et al. Ultrasound and microbubble-targeted delivery of macromolecules is regulated by induction of endocytosis and pore formation. *Circ Res*. 2009;104:679–687.
29. Miller DL, Driscoll EM, Dou C, Armstrong WF, Lucchesi BR. Microvascular permeabilization and cardiomyocyte injury provoked by myocardial contrast echocardiography in a canine model. *J Am Coll Cardiol*. 2006;47:1464–1468.
30. Taniyama Y, Tachibana K, Hiraoka K, et al. Local delivery of plasmid DNA into rat carotid artery using ultrasound. *Circulation*. 2002;105:1233–1239.
31. Bekeredjian R, Grayburn PA, Shohet RV. Use of ultrasound contrast agents for gene or drug delivery in cardiovascular medicine. *J Am Coll Cardiol*. 2005;45:329–335.
32. Coleman JL, Navid F, Furman WL, McCarville MB. Safety of ultrasound contrast agents in the pediatric oncologic population: a single-institution experience. *AJR Am J Roentgenol*. 2014;202:966–970.
33. Kutty S, Xiao Y, Olson J, et al. Safety and efficacy of cardiac ultrasound contrast in Children and Adolescents for resting and stress echocardiography. *J Am Soc Echocardiogr*. 2016;29:655–662.
34. Qin S, Caskey CF, Ferrara KW. Ultrasound contrast microbubbles in imaging and therapy: physical principles and engineering. *Phys Med Biol*. 2009;54:R27–R57.
35. de Jong N, Hoff L, Skotland T, Bom N. Absorption and scatter of encapsulated gas filled microspheres: theoretical considerations and some measurements. *Ultrasonics*. 1992;30:95–103.
36. Seol SH, Davidson BP, Belcik JT, et al. Real-time contrast ultrasound muscle perfusion imaging with intermediate-power imaging coupled with acoustically durable microbubbles. *J Am Soc Echocardiogr*. 2015;28. 718–726 e2.
37. Porter TR, Abdelmoneim S, Belcik JT, et al. Guidelines for the cardiac sonographer in the performance of contrast echocardiography: a focused update from the American Society of Echocardiography. *J Am Soc Echocardiogr*. 2014;27:797–810.
38. Eckersley RJ, Chin CT, Burns PN. Optimising phase and amplitude modulation schemes for imaging microbubble contrast agents at low acoustic power. *Ultrasound Med Biol*. 2005;31:213–219.
39. Chahal NS, Senior R. Clinical applications of left ventricular opacification. *JACC Cardiovasc Imaging*. 2010;3:188–196.
40. Judd RM, Levy BI. Effects of barium-induced cardiac contraction on large- and small-vessel intramyocardial blood volume. *Circ Res*. 1991;68:217–225.
41. Hoffmann R, Barletta G, von Bardeleben S, et al. Analysis of left ventricular volumes and function: a multicenter comparison of cardiac magnetic resonance imaging, cine ventriculography, and unenhanced and contrast-enhanced two-dimensional and three-dimensional echocardiography. *J Am Soc Echocardiogr*. 2014;27:292–301.
42. Hoffmann R, von Bardeleben S, Kasprzak JD, et al. Analysis of regional left ventricular function by cineventriculography, cardiac magnetic resonance imaging, and unenhanced and contrast-enhanced echocardiography: a multicenter comparison of methods. *J Am Coll Cardiol*. 2006;47:121–128.
43. Hoffmann R, von Bardeleben S, ten Cate F, et al. Assessment of systolic left ventricular function: a multi-centre comparison of cineventriculography, cardiac magnetic resonance imaging, unenhanced and contrast-enhanced echocardiography. *Eur Heart J*. 2005;26:607–616.
44. Hundley WG, Kizilbash AM, Afridi I, et al. Administration of an intravenous perfluorocarbon contrast agent improves echocardiographic determination of left ventricular volumes and ejection fraction: comparison with cine magnetic resonance imaging. *J Am Coll Cardiol*. 1998;32:1426–1432.
45. Malm S, Frigstad S, Sagberg E, Larsson H, Skjaerpe T. Accurate and reproducible measurement of left ventricular volume and ejection fraction by contrast echocardiography: a comparison with magnetic resonance imaging. *J Am Coll Cardiol*. 2004;44:1030–1035.
46. Lindner JR, Dent JM, Moos SP, Jayaweera AR, Kaul S. Enhancement of left ventricular cavity opacification by harmonic imaging after venous injection of Albunex. *Am J Cardiol*. 1997;79:1657–1662.
47. Rinkevich D, Kaul S, Wang XQ, et al. Regional left ventricular perfusion and function in patients presenting to the emergency department with chest pain and no ST-segment elevation. *Eur Heart J*. 2005;26:1606–1611.
48. Senior R, Becher H, Monaghan M, et al. Clinical practice of contrast echocardiography: recommendation by the European Association of Cardiovascular Imaging (EACVI) 2017. *Eur Heart J Cardiovasc Imaging*. 2017;18:1205–1205af.
49. Kurt M, Shaikh KA, Peterson L, et al. Impact of contrast echocardiography on evaluation of ventricular function and clinical management in a large prospective cohort. *J Am Coll Cardiol*. 2009;53:802–810.
50. Zhao H, O'Quinn R, Ambrose M, et al. Contrast-enhanced echocardiography has the greatest impact in patients with reduced ejection fractions. *J Am Soc Echocardiogr*. 2018;31:289–296.
51. Yong Y, Wu D, Fernandes V, et al. Diagnostic accuracy and cost-effectiveness of contrast echocardiography on evaluation of cardiac function in technically very difficult patients in the intensive care unit. *Am J Cardiol*. 2002;89:711–718.
52. Shaw LJ, Gillam L, Feinstein S, Dent J, Plotnick G. Use of an intravenous contrast agent (Optison) to enhance echocardiography: efficacy and cost implications. Optison Multicenter Study Group. *Am J Manag Care*. 1998;4. Spec No:SP169-S176.
53. Shah BN, Balaji G, Alhajiri A, et al. Incremental diagnostic and prognostic value of contemporary stress echocardiography in a chest pain unit: mortality and morbidity outcomes from

a real-world setting. *Circ Cardiovasc Imaging.* 2013;6:202–209.
54. Rainbird AJ, Mulvagh SL, Oh JK, et al. Contrast dobutamine stress echocardiography: clinical practice assessment in 300 consecutive patients. *J Am Soc Echocardiogr.* 2001;14:378–385.
55. Plana JC, Mikati IA, Dokainish H, et al. A randomized cross-over study for evaluation of the effect of image optimization with contrast on the diagnostic accuracy of dobutamine echocardiography in coronary artery disease the OPTIMIZE Trial. *JACC Cardiovasc Imaging.* 2008;1:145–152.
56. Thomas D, Xie F, Smith LM, et al. Prospective randomized comparison of conventional stress echocardiography and real-time perfusion stress echocardiography in detecting significant coronary artery disease. *J Am Soc Echocardiogr.* 2012;25:1207–1214.
57. Vaitkus PT, Barnathan ES. Embolic potential, prevention and management of mural thrombus complicating anterior myocardial infarction: a meta-analysis. *J Am Coll Cardiol.* 1993;22:1004–1009.
58. Thomas JD, Rubin DN. Tissue harmonic imaging: why does it work? *J Am Soc Echocardiogr.* 1998;11:803–808.
59. Weinsaft JW KH, Crowley AL, Klem I, et al. LV thrombus detection by routine echocardiography: insights into performance characteristics using delayed enhancement CMR. *JACC Cardiovasc Imaging.* 2011;4(7):702–712.
60. Siebelink HM, Scholte AJ, Van de Veire NR, et al. Value of contrast echocardiography for left ventricular thrombus detection postinfarction and impact on antithrombotic therapy. *Coron Artery Dis.* 2009;20:462–466.
61. Weinsaft JW, Kim RJ, Ross M, et al. Contrast-enhanced anatomic imaging as compared to contrast-enhanced tissue characterization for detection of left ventricular thrombus. *JACC Cardiovasc Imaging.* 2009;2:969–979.
62. Wada H, Yasu T, Sakakura K, et al. Contrast echocardiography for the diagnosis of left ventricular thrombus in anterior myocardial infarction. *Heart Ves.* 2014;29:308–312.
63. Bansal M, Kasliwal RR. Echocardiography for left atrial appendage structure and function. *Indian Heart J.* 2012;64:469–475.
64. Eriksson MJ, Sonnenberg B, Woo A, et al. Long-term outcome in patients with apical hypertrophic cardiomyopathy. *J Am Coll Cardiol.* 2002;39:638–645.
65. Ogbogu PU, Rosing DR, Horne 3rd MK. Cardiovascular manifestations of hypereosinophilic syndromes. *Immunol Allergy Clin North Am.* 2007;27(3):457–475.
66. Kohli SK, Pantazis AA, Shah JS, et al. Diagnosis of left-ventricular non-compaction in patients with left-ventricular systolic dysfunction: time for a reappraisal of diagnostic criteria? *Eur Heart J.* 2008;29:89–95.
67. Coll B, Nambi V, Feinstein SB. New advances in noninvasive imaging of the carotid artery: CIMT, contrast-enhanced ultrasound, and vasa vasorum. *Curr Cardiol Rep.* 2010;12:497–502.
68. Kassab GS, Lin DH, Fung YC. Morphometry of pig coronary venous system. *Am J Physiol.* 1994;267(6 Pt 2):H2100–H2113.
69. Wei K, Jayaweera AR, Firoozan S, et al. Quantification of myocardial blood flow with ultrasound-induced destruction of microbubbles administered as a constant venous infusion. *Circulation.* 1998;97:473–483.
70. Wei K, Le E, Jayaweera AR, et al. Detection of noncritical coronary stenosis at rest without recourse to exercise or pharmacological stress. *Circulation.* 2002;105:218–223.
71. Tong KL, Kaul S, Wang XQ, et al. Myocardial contrast echocardiography versus Thrombolysis in Myocardial Infarction score in patients presenting to the emergency department with chest pain and a nondiagnostic electrocardiogram. *J Am Coll Cardiol.* 2005;46:920–927.
72. Jayaweera AR, Wei K, Coggins M, et al. Role of capillaries in determining CBF reserve: new insights using myocardial contrast echocardiography. *Am J Physiol.* 1999;277:H2363–H2372.
73. Kaul S, Senior R, Dittrich H, et al. Detection of coronary artery disease with myocardial contrast echocardiography: comparison with 99mTc-sestamibi single-photon emission computed tomography. *Circulation.* 1997;96:785–792.
74. Leong-Poi H, Rim SJ, Le DE, et al. Perfusion versus function: the ischemic cascade in demand ischemia: implications of single-vessel versus multivessel stenosis. *Circulation.* 2002;105:987–992.
75. Wei K, Ragosta M, Thorpe J, et al. Noninvasive quantification of coronary blood flow reserve in humans using myocardial contrast echocardiography. *Circulation.* 2001;103:2560–2565.
76. Vogel R, Indermuhle A, Reinhardt J, et al. The quantification of absolute myocardial perfusion in humans by contrast echocardiography: algorithm and validation. *J Am Coll Cardiol.* 2005;45:754–762.
77. Peltier MV, Vancraeynest D, Pasquet A, et al. Assessment of the physiologic significance of coronary disease with dipyridamole real-time myocardial contrast echocardiography. Comparison with technetium-99m sestamibi single-photon emission computed tomography and quantitative coronary angiography. *J Am Coll Cardiol.* 2004;43(2):257–264.
78. Jeetley P, Hickman M, Kamp O, et al. Myocardial contrast echocardiography for the detection of coronary artery stenosis: a prospective multicenter study in comparison with single-photon emission computed tomography. *J Am Coll Cardiol.* 2006;47:141–145.
79. Abdelmoneim SS, Mulvagh SL, Xie F, et al. Regadenoson stress real-time myocardial perfusion echocardiography for detection of coronary artery disease: feasibility and accuracy of two different ultrasound contrast agents. *J Am Soc Echocardiogr.* 2015;28:1393–1400.
80. Shah BN, Chahal NS, Bhattacharyya S, et al. The feasibility and clinical utility of myocardial contrast echocardiography in clinical practice: results from the incorporation of myocardial perfusion assessment into clinical testing with stress echocardiography study. *J Am Soc Echocardiogr.* 2014;27:520–530.
81. Senior R, Moreo A, Gaibazzi N, et al. Comparison of sulfur hexafluoride microbubble (SonoVue)-enhanced myocardial contrast echocardiography with gated single-photon emission computed tomography for detection of significant coronary artery disease: a large European multicenter study. *J Am Coll Cardiol.* 2013;62:1353–1361.
82. Leong-Poi H, Coggins MP, Sklenar J, et al. Role of collateral blood flow in the apparent disparity between the extent of abnormal wall thickening and perfusion defect size during acute myocardial infarction and demand ischemia. *J Am Coll Cardiol.* 2005;45:565–572.
83. Elhendy A, O'Leary EL, Xie F, et al. Comparative accuracy of real-time myocardial contrast perfusion imaging and wall motion analysis during dobutamine stress echocardiography for the diagnosis of coronary artery disease. *J Am Coll Cardiol.* 2004;44:2185–2191.
84. Barton D, Xie F, O'Leary E, et al. The relationship of capillary blood flow assessments with real time myocardial perfusion echocardiography to invasively derived microvascular and epicardial assessments. *J Am Soc Echocardiogr.* 2019;32:1095–1101.
85. Senior R, Janardhanan R, Jeetley P, Burden L. Myocardial contrast echocardiography for distinguishing ischemic from nonischemic first-onset acute heart failure: insights into the mechanism of acute heart failure. *Circulation.* 2005;112:1587–1593.
86. Tsutsui JM, Elhendy A, Anderson JR, et al. Prognostic value of dobutamine stress myocardial contrast perfusion echocardiography. *Circulation.* 2005;112:1444–1450.
87. Porter TR, Smith LM, Wu J, et al. Patient outcome following 2 different stress imaging approaches: a prospective randomized comparison. *J Am Coll Cardiol.* 2013;61:2446–2455.
88. Lieberman AN WJ, Jugdutt BI, et al. Two-dimensional echocardiography and infarct size: relationship of regional wall motion and thickening to the extent of myocardial infarction in the dog. *Circulation.* 1981;63(4):739–746.
89. Samady HE J, Abbott BG, Mattera JA, McPherson CA, Wackers FJ. Failure to improve left ventricular function after coronary revascularization for ischemic cardiomyopathy is not associated with worse outcome. *Circulation.* 1999;100(12):1298–1304.
90. Janardhanan R, Moon JC, Pennell DJ, Senior R. Myocardial contrast echocardiography accurately reflects transmurality of myocardial necrosis and predicts contractile reserve after acute myocardial infarction. *Am Heart J.* 2005;149:355–362.
91. Iliceto S, Galiuto L, Marchese A, et al. Analysis of microvascular integrity, contractile reserve, and myocardial viability after acute myocardial infarction by dobutamine echocardiography and myocardial contrast echocardiography. *Am J Cardiol.* 1996;77:441–445.
92. deFilippi CR, Willett DL, Irani WN, et al. Comparison of myocardial contrast echocardiography and low-dose dobutamine stress echocardiography in predicting recovery of left ventricular function after coronary revascularization in chronic ischemic heart disease. *Circulation.* 1995;92:2863–2868.
93. Balcells E, Powers ER, Lepper W, et al. Detection of myocardial viability by contrast echocardiography in acute infarction predicts recovery of resting function and contractile reserve. *J Am Coll Cardiol.* 2003;41:827–833.
94. Scognamiglio R, Negut C, Ramondo A, Tiengo A, Avogaro A. Detection of coronary artery disease in asymptomatic patients with type 2 diabetes mellitus. *J Am Coll Cardiol.* 2006;47:65–71.
95. Taqui S, Ferencik M, Davidson BP, et al. Coronary microvascular dysfunction by myocardial contrast echocardiography in nonelderly patients referred for computed tomographic coronary angiography. *J Am Soc Echocardiogr.* 2019;32:817–825.
96. Kutty S, Bisselou Moukagna KS, Craft M, et al. Clinical outcome of patients with inducible capillary blood flow abnormalities during

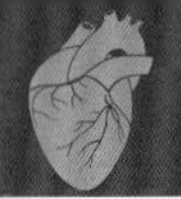

demand stress in the presence or absence of angiographic coronary disease. *Circ Cardiovasc Imaging*. 2018;11:e007483.

97. Kirkpatrick JN, Wong T, Bednarz JE, et al. Differential diagnosis of cardiac masses using contrast echocardiographic perfusion imaging. *J Am Coll Cardiol*. 2004;43:1412–1419.
98. Mulvagh SL, Rakowski H, Vannan MA, et al. American Society of Echocardiography Consensus statement on the clinical applications of ultrasonic contrast agents in echocardiography. *J Am Soc Echocardiogr*. 2008;21:1179–1201. quiz 1281.
99. Min SY, Song JM, Shin Y, et al. Quantitative segmental analysis of myocardial perfusion to differentiate stress cardiomyopathy from acute myocardial infarction: a myocardial contrast echocardiography study. *Clin Cardiol*. 2017;40:679–685.
100. Davidson BP, Hodovan J, Mason OR, et al. Limb perfusion during exercise assessed by contrast ultrasound Varies according to symptom severity in patients with peripheral artery disease. *J Am Soc Echocardiogr*. 2019;32. 1086-1094 e3.

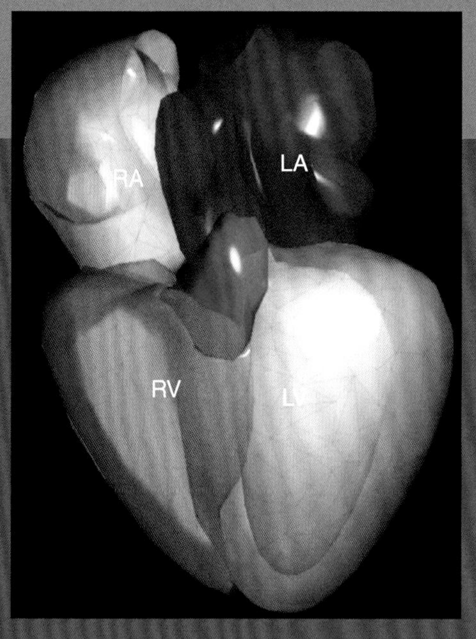

中文导读

第4章 左心室解剖和收缩功能的定量分析

在临床工作中，超声可以测量和分析左心室的解剖大小和收缩功能。首先，测量左心室大小的方法包括线性测量和体积测量。左心室的线性测量仅适用于大致判断其大小，不适用于评估其体积。左心室的体积可以通过二维或三维成像来确定，要求图像心内膜边界描述精确。目前二维方法是临床医师采用的主要方法，应用最多的是双平面Simpson法。左心室的质量可以通过计算体积获得，其与心血管预后密切相关。许多心脏病会导致心脏的形状以整体或局部的方式偏离理想的椭圆体，此时，三维超声心动图是计算体积和质量的最佳方法。

其次，左心室收缩功能是评价心脏的另一个重要组成部分。心脏的适当充盈和收缩取决于前负荷和后负荷。一些疾病会导致压力和容量过负荷，负荷在一定范围内，心脏可以通过调节来维持正常功能；如果心脏功能失代偿，就会导致相关测量指标的异常。左心室的收缩是一个复杂的过程，在临床实践中测量左心室收缩功能的参数通常是射血分数和整体纵向应变。

具体而言，左心室整体收缩功能可以通过射血分数、整体纵向应变、dp/dt、心肌做功指数和压力-容积环等指标来反映；左心室局部收缩功能可以通过心肌节段运动、短轴缩短率、二尖瓣环平面收缩期位移和组织多普勒成像等指标来反映。

吴伟春

4 Quantitative Analysis of Left Ventricular Anatomy and Systolic Function

FELIX C. TANNER, MD | PETROS NIHOYANNOPOULOS, MD

QUANTITATIVE ANALYSIS OF LV ANATOMY

LV SIZE

Linear Measurements

The shape of the normal left ventricle (LV) corresponds to a prolate ellipsoid.[1] Linear measurements of the LV therefore allow limited conclusions about its size and should not be used for determining its volume. Nevertheless, the diameter of the LV provides an estimation of LV size and may be useful in patients with limited echocardiographic windows, such as ventilated patients in the intensive care unit, who often have reduced image quality in the apical views. Linear measurements of the LV are supported by outcome data. For example, the LV end-diastolic short-axis diameter is associated with death for patients with dilated cardiomyopathy.[2]

The diameter of the LV should be determined in the parasternal long-axis view.[3] The line used for measurements should be oriented perpendicular to the LV long axis at the level of the mitral valve leaflet tips (Fig. 4.1). The calipers should be placed at the intersection points of this line with the myocardial wall on the edge of the compacted myocardium[4] (Table 4.1).

This measurement can be obtained by two-dimensional (2D) echocardiography or by a 2D-guided M-mode approach. The M-mode is technically more demanding in that it may be difficult to line up the correct orientation of the measurement line. However, M-mode has an excellent temporal resolution with a frame rate of several thousand scan lines per second with high interphase definition and consequently reproducible measurements.[5] In most patients, the M-mode orientation can be improved by tilting the patient forward and moving the transducer toward the upper sternum.

Because the LV diameter is a linear measurement, it is representative of LV size only for ventricles with a normal shape and for the anteroposterior diameter. Alterations in global shape such as elongation or truncation of the ventricular long axis and changes in regional shape such as aneurysm formation hamper its diagnostic accuracy. Extrapolation of LV volumes from such linear measurements using the Teichholz or Quinones method, each of which assumes a prolate ellipsoid LV shape, is no longer recommended.[3]

Volumetric Measurements

LV volumes can be determined by 2D or 3D imaging. Although the 2D method is still considered the standard approach by most clinicians, the 3D method is gaining popularity in clinical routine.[6]

The 2D and 3D methods for determining LV volumes are based on precise tracing of the endocardial border of the compacted myocardium. The tracing points are placed on the endocardial border, and all the noncompacted structures, such as papillary muscles, muscle bundles, and trabeculations, are excluded. The tracing line is closed by connecting the two tracing points at the mitral annulus by a straight line. The long axis of the ventricle is defined by a straight line between the mitral annulus and the most apical point of the LV (Fig. 4.2).

The recommended approach for 2D measurement of LV volumes is the biplane Simpson method. It is based on careful tracing of the endocardial border of the compacted myocardium in the 4-chamber and 2-chamber projections (see Fig. 4.2). This approach is not ideal with regard to ventricular geometry because the two views are separated by an angle of approximately 60 degrees rather than being perpendicular to each other. Moreover, the left ventricular outflow tract (LVOT) is excluded from the volume calculation because the 3-chamber projection is not included. Nevertheless, this method has acceptable reproducibility and associated outcomes.[7–10]

2D measurements of LV volumes are supported by strong prognostic data. The LV end-diastolic volume index is associated with mortality for patients with advanced heart failure caused by severely reduced systolic function. The LV end-systolic volume index is associated with hospitalization for heart failure in patients with coronary artery disease (Fig. 4.3).[12]

Optimal image quality with clear endocardial border definition is essential for accomplishing an accurate and reproducible tracing line. Image depth and width should be reduced so that only the LV from apex to annulus is depicted; with this LV-centered approach, a frame rate greater than 60 fps can easily be reached, ensuring an appropriate temporal resolution for LV border tracing and strain measurement. Care should be taken to visualize the maximal length of the LV without foreshortening of the apex.

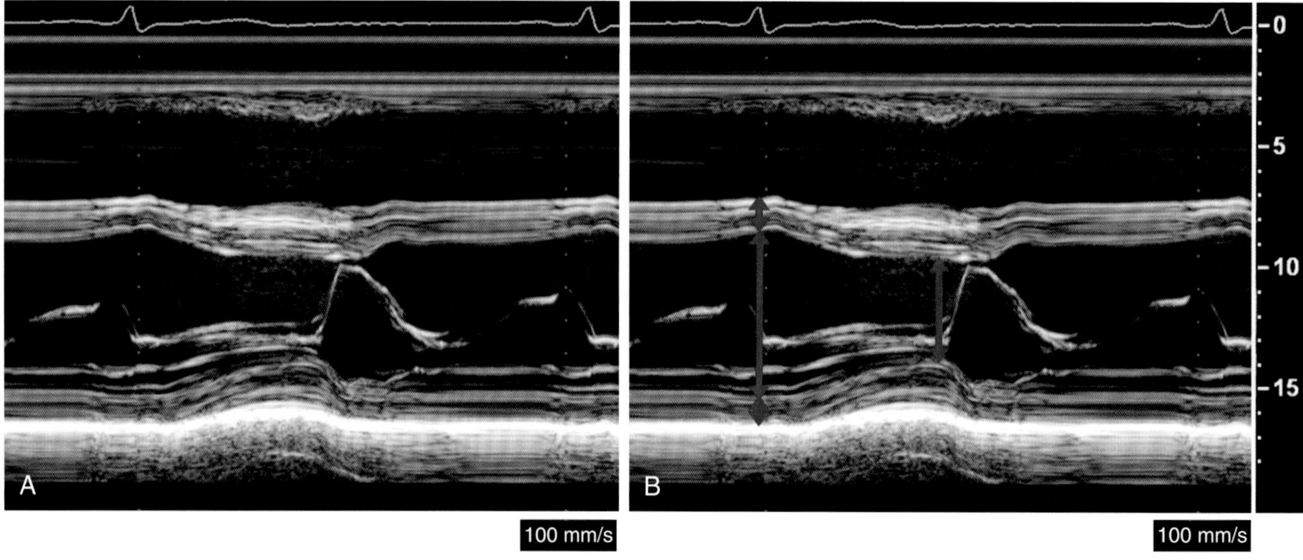

Fig. 4.1 LV M-mode tracing. (A) M-mode is applied in parasternal long-axis view perpendicular to the LV long axis at the level of the mitral leaflet tips. (B) The *red arrows* indicate measurements for septal and posterior wall thickness, as well as LV diameter at end-diastole and end-systole.

TABLE 4.1 Quantification of LV Size and Function: Checklist for Acquisition of Appropriate Views and Measurements.

1-Dimensional Method

- Anteroseptal wall: septomarginal band discernible from compacted myocardial wall?
- Inferolateral wall: accessory papillary muscle discernible from compacted myocardial wall?
- Measurement axis perpendicular to LV long axis?
- Measurement axis at the level of mitral valve leaflet tips?
- Calipers placed on the edge of the compacted myocardium?
- 2D instead of M-mode measurement: no correction required with yo-yo view?

2-Dimensional Method

- Endocardium of all LV segments visible, or contrast agent required?
- Apical morphology of LV in 4-chamber and 2-chamber view consistent?
- Difference in length of LV in 4-chamber and 2-chamber view less than 5%?
- Tracing line placed on the edge of the compacted myocardium with all trabeculations and the papillary muscles excluded?
- No correction required with yo-yo view?

3-Dimensional Method

- Image artifact in any LV segment, preventing appropriate reproduction of LV wall?
- Endocardium of all LV segments in reconstructed 2D-equivalent views (4-, 3-, 2-, and apical/mid/basal short-axis views) visible?
- Tracing line placed on the edge of the compacted myocardium with all trabeculations and the papillary muscles excluded?
- No correction required with enlarged reconstructed 2D-equivalent views?

Identification of the true apex is facilitated by two observations: (1) myocardial thickness decreases toward the apex, and (2) the apex does not move in a longitudinal direction during the cardiac cycle. To ensure that the true apex is depicted, it is useful to compare the apex as imaged in 4-chamber and 2-chamber projections. The left atrium (LA) should not be considered on such images; it appears shortened in most individuals because the atrial and ventricular long axes are usually not located in the same plane. Truncation of the LA on LV-centered images has an additional advantage in that the echocardiographer is not distracted by the atrial contours.

Even for experienced echocardiographers, it can be challenging to generate a correct tracing line throughout the LV endocardial border, and the lateral wall often is not clearly seen. The process can be facilitated by observing the LV borders for a few heartbeats in real time before tracing is initiated and can be further improved by letting several frames adjacent to the end-diastolic frame run back and forth (i.e., yo-yo view). After the tracing line in 4-chamber and 2-chamber views has been completed, LV length in both views should be compared, and the measurement should be repeated if there is a difference in length of more than 5%.

If the endocardial borders of two or more myocardial segments cannot be visualized, the use of an intravenous contrast agent is recommended.[13] Because it is easier to recognize the true border of the compacted myocardium in the presence of a contrast agent, the volumes measured under the latter conditions are somewhat larger than those measured without contrast. The normal values available for LV volumes should not be applied when contrast has been used; separate normal values have been developed for contrast-enhanced LV quantification[14] (Table 4.1).

Normal values for 2D LV volumes are well established[3] (Table 4.2). Even after indexing for body surface area, normal ranges differ for males and females. They are also influenced by age, which can be explained by the lifelong remodeling of the LV that occurs in the normal population and results in a progressive decrease in LV volumes with advancing age[15,15a] (Fig. 4.4).

Calculation of LV volumes with the use of 3D imaging is gaining popularity in clinical practice. The 3D approach has several advantages over 2D.[16] It depends less on geometric assumptions and is less prone to foreshortening, although the latter is not automatically excluded in a 3D volume data set, and it might escape the attention of the investigator that part of the LV was not included.

The LV volumes derived from 3D data sets are larger than those from 2D acquisitions and therefore closer to the volumes obtained by cardiac magnetic resonance (CMR) imaging.[17–19] This observation has been confirmed by several studies of different patient populations (Table 4.3). The 3D LV measurements seem to exhibit a stronger association with outcomes than the 2D parameters, suggesting that the 3D measurements are closer to reality.[20] The latest 3D applications have good accuracy and underestimate the CMR-derived LV volumes by less than 10% (Table 4.4).[21,22]

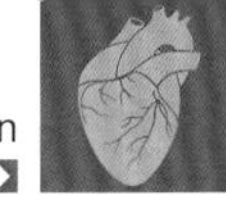

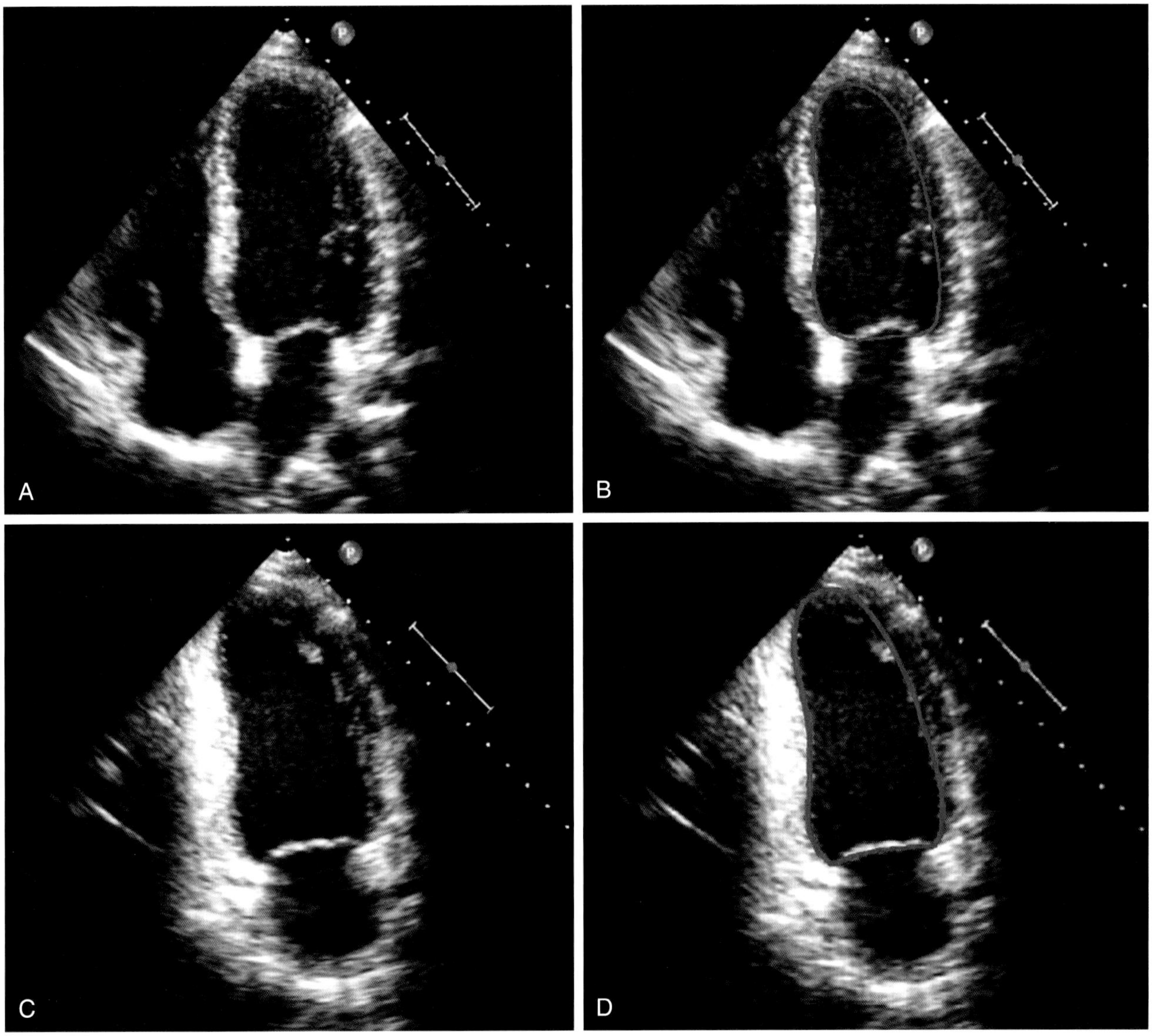

Fig. 4.2 2D Measurement of LV volumes and ejection fraction. Apical 4-chamber view (A) (see Video 4.2A) with tracing for measurement of LV biplane end-diastolic volume (B) (see Video 4.2B). Apical 2-chamber view (C) (see Video 4.2B) with tracing for measurement of LV biplane end-diastolic volume (D).

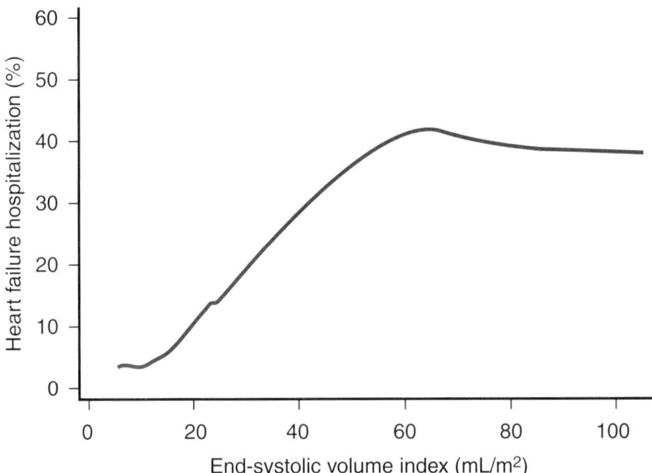

Fig. 4.3 Relationship between end-systolic volume index and outcome. Smoothed scatterplot of the proportion of patients hospitalized with heart failure during a 5.5-year follow-up. A modest increase in LV volume is accompanied by a sharp rise in congestive heart failure events.

To reach an optimal accuracy, LV volumes in a 3D data set are usually determined by a semi-automated approach involving automated border detection with manual contour adjustment. Multiple rounds of correction sometimes are required because the algorithm may not always accept the manual changes. Manual editing seems particularly important when image quality is poor because the accuracy of automated border detection is lower under such conditions. The quality of manual editing depends on operator experience, and automated border detection can be improved by experienced investigators.[23] In addition to manual correction, the accuracy of 3D LV measurements can be increased by a higher volume rate and by the application of echocardiographic contrast.[24]

Whereas manual measurements of 3D LV volumes exhibit moderate intraobserver and interobserver reproducibility, the latter is improved when automated border detection is combined with manual contour adjustment and improved even further when no manual correction is performed.[22] In these circumstances, however, the accuracy of the measurements usually decreases. This situation opens the possibility of applying 3D echocardiography for determining LV volumes in a patient-tailored approach.

TABLE 4.2 **Normal Values and Severity Partition Cutoff Values for 2D Echocardiography-Derived LV Size and Function.**

	Male				Female			
Measurement	*Normal Range*	*Mildly Abnormal*	*Moderately Abnormal*	*Severely Abnormal*	*Normal Range*	*Mildly Abnormal*	*Moderately Abnormal*	*Severely Abnormal*
LV Dimension								
LV diastolic diameter (cm)	4.2–5.8	5.9–6.3	6.4–6.8	>6.8	3.8–5.2	5.3–5.6	5.7–6.1	>6.1
LV diastolic diameter/ BSA (cm/m²)	2.2–3.0	3.1–3.3	3.4–3.6	>3.6	2.3–3.1	3.2–3.4	3.5–3.7	>3.7
LV systolic diameter (cm)	2.5–4.0	4.1–4.3	4.4–4.5	>4.5	2.2–3.5	3.6–3.8	3.9–4.1	>4.1
LV systolic diameter/ BSA (cm/m²)	1.3–2.1	2.2–2.3	2.4–2.5	>2.5	1.3–2.1	2.2–2.3	2.4–2.6	>2.6
LV Volume								
LV diastolic volume (mL)	62–150	151–174	175–200	>200	46–106	107–120	121–130	>130
LV diastolic volume/ BSA (mL/m²)	34–74	75–89	90–100	>100	29–61	62–70	71–80	>80
LV systolic volume (mL)	21–61	62–73	74–85	>85	14–42	43–55	56–67	>67
LV systolic volume/ BSA (mL/m²)	11–31	32–38	39–45	>45	8–24	25–32	33–40	>40
LV Function								
LVEF (%)	52–72	41–51	30–40	<30	54–74	41–53	30–40	<30

BSA, Body surface area; *LVEF*, LV ejection fraction.
From Lang RM, Badano LP, Mor-Avi V, et al. Recommendations for cardiac chamber quantification by echocardiography in adults: an update from the American Society of Echocardiography and the European Association of Cardiovascular Imaging. *J Am Soc Echocardiogr*. 2015;28(1):1–39.

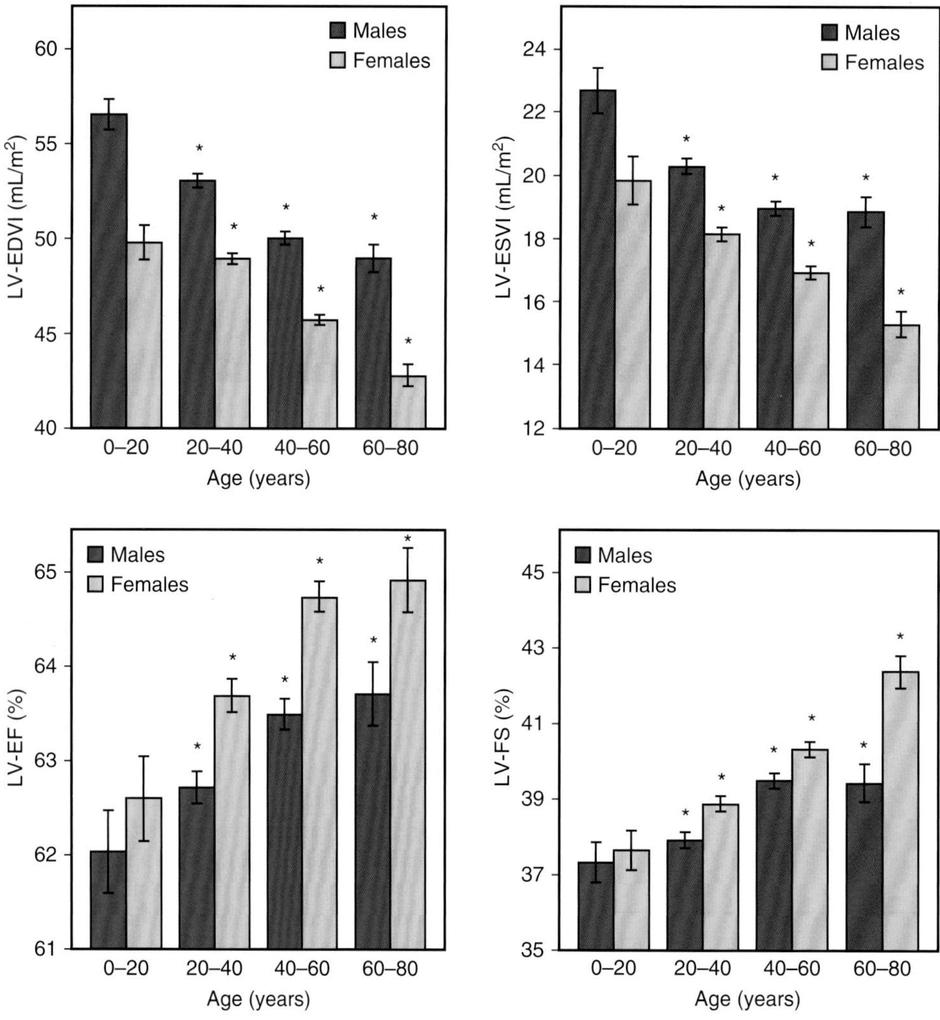

Fig. 4.4 Age-dependent changes in LV volumes and systolic function in a large population of normal individuals. LV end-diastolic volume index *(EDVI)* and end-systolic volume index *(ESVI)* decrease with age. LV ejection fraction *(EF)* and fractional shortening *(FS)* increase with age. Changes are more pronounced in females. (From Gebhard C, Stahli BE, Gebhard CE, et al. Age- and gender-dependent left ventricular remodeling. *Echocardiography*. 2013;30[10]:1143–1150.)

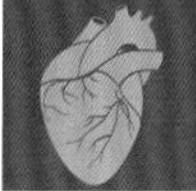

TABLE 4.3 Comparison of 2D and 3D Echocardiography–Derived Values for LV End-Diastolic Volume, End-Systolic Volume, and Ejection Fraction.

		LV EDV (mL)		LV ESV (mL)		LV EF (%)	
Study[a]	*Study Type*	*2D Echo*	*3D Echo*	*2D Echo*	*3D Echo*	*2D Echo*	*3D Echo*
Dorosz et al.[16]	Meta-analysis 1174 patients	ΔCMR = −48	ΔCMR = −16	ΔCMR = −28	ΔCMR = −10	ΔCMR = 0.1	ΔCMR = 0.0
Muraru et al.[42]	Single center 226 patients	97 ± 25	107 ± 25	35 ± 11	39 ± 11	65 ± 4	64 ± 4
Tamborini et al.[21]	Single center 189 patients	142 ± 58	175 ± 64	71 ± 49	102 ± 59	54 ± 15	45 ± 14
Medvedofsky et al.[20]	Single center 416 patients	166 ± 85	187 ± 89	88 ± 77	99 ± 84	52 ± 16	52 ± 17

[a]The first study (Dorosz et al.) is a meta-analysis, and the difference between echocardiographic- and cardiac magnetic resonance–derived values (ΔCMR) is indicated. For all the other studies, mean values and standard deviations of 2D and 3D echocardiographic measurements are listed.
EF, Ejection fraction; *EDF*, end-diastolic volume; *ESV*, end-systolic volume.

TABLE 4.4 Comparison of 3D Echocardiography Versus Cardiac Magnetic Resonance–Derived Values for LV End-Diastolic Volume, End-Systolic Volume, and Ejection Fraction.

		LV EDV (mL)		LV ESV (mL)		LV EF (%)	
Study[a]	*Study Type*	*3D Echo*	*CM*	*3D Echo*	*CMR*	*3D Echo*	*CMR*
Dorosz et al.[16]	Meta-analysis 1174 patients 3D manual or automated	Δ Echo-CMR = −19		Δ Echo-CMR = −10		Δ Echo-CMR = −1	
Tsang et al.[22]	Single center 159 patients 3D automated + manual adjustment	190 ± 64	201 ± 66	118 ± 60	122 ± 71	41 ± 12	43 ± 16
Tamborini et al.[21]	Single center 189 patients 3D automated + manual adjustment	175 ± 61	200 ± 74	108 ± 59	117 ± 73	42 ± 13	45 ± 17

[a]The first study (Dorosz et al.) is a meta-analysis, and the difference between echocardiographic- and CMR-derived values (ΔCMR) is indicated. For all the other studies, mean values and standard deviations of 3D echocardiographic and CMR measurements are listed.
CMR, Cardiac magnetic resonance; *EF*, ejection fraction; *EDF*, end-diastolic volume; *ESV*, end-systolic volume.

Automatic border detection should be corrected manually when accuracy is more important, but refraining from manual correction can be considered when changes in LV volumes or LVEF are essential for follow-up. When reproducibility is preferred, the maximal benefit of the automated approach can be achieved when images of good quality are examined by inexperienced echocardiographers, and application of echocardiographic contrast can improve interobserver reproducibility.[23,24]

The 3D LV volumes need to be recorded very carefully to avoid data sets that cannot be quantified. All LV measurements are obtained from a single data set in the 3D approach, and this is often not possible, particularly in very dilated ventricles. Control of the image quality of the 3D data set in reconstructed imaging planes derived from the data set being registered is recommended. These imaging planes should include the equivalent of the apical 4-chamber, 2-chamber, and 3-chamber views and short-axis views at the apical, mid-ventricular, and basal levels (Fig. 4.5). The 3D data set should be accepted only when the endocardial border of the compacted myocardium is visible in all segments.

3D can be applied for measurement of LV volumes in any patient in whom image quality is sufficient for appropriate acquisition of the LV. Important indications for routine clinical application include a need for frequent follow-up examinations for surveillance of LV systolic function, such as in patients undergoing cardiotoxic chemotherapy and those under optimization of medical therapy before implantation of a cardioverter-defibrillator or cardiac resynchronization therapy. Consequently, it becomes essential that the same method of LV volume quantification is maintained during serial assessment of LV function.[25,26]

Normal values for 3D-derived LV volumes are less well established than those for 2D volumes, and there are not enough data to allow clear definition of a normal range. However, several well-performed studies providing normal values for relatively small populations are available (Table 4.5). When an LV volume is determined in a 3D data set, it has to be documented in the echocardiography report because the normal values are larger than those measured in 2D due to systematic underestimation of LV volumes by the 2D approach.[3]

The advantages and disadvantages of various methods for measuring LV volumes are summarized in Table 4.6.

LV WALL THICKNESS AND MASS

LV mass shows a strong association with cardiovascular outcomes and independently predicts adverse events, including death.[27] LV mass determined by echocardiography provides information on outcomes independent of cardiovascular risk factors.[28] The Framingham Heart Study showed that LV mass measured by echocardiography was associated with total mortality, cardiovascular mortality, and cardiovascular morbidity rates.[29]

LV mass can be calculated by M-mode, 2D, or 3D imaging.[3] All of these methods determine myocardial volume, which is then converted into myocardial mass by multiplying the volume by the specific gravity of myocardial tissue (1.04 g/cm^3). Whereas myocardial volume has to be calculated when using M-mode or 2D imaging, it can be measured directly using 3D.[30] For all the methods mentioned, the recommendation is to place the tracing points on the endocardial border of the compacted myocardium.[3] This approach has become possible

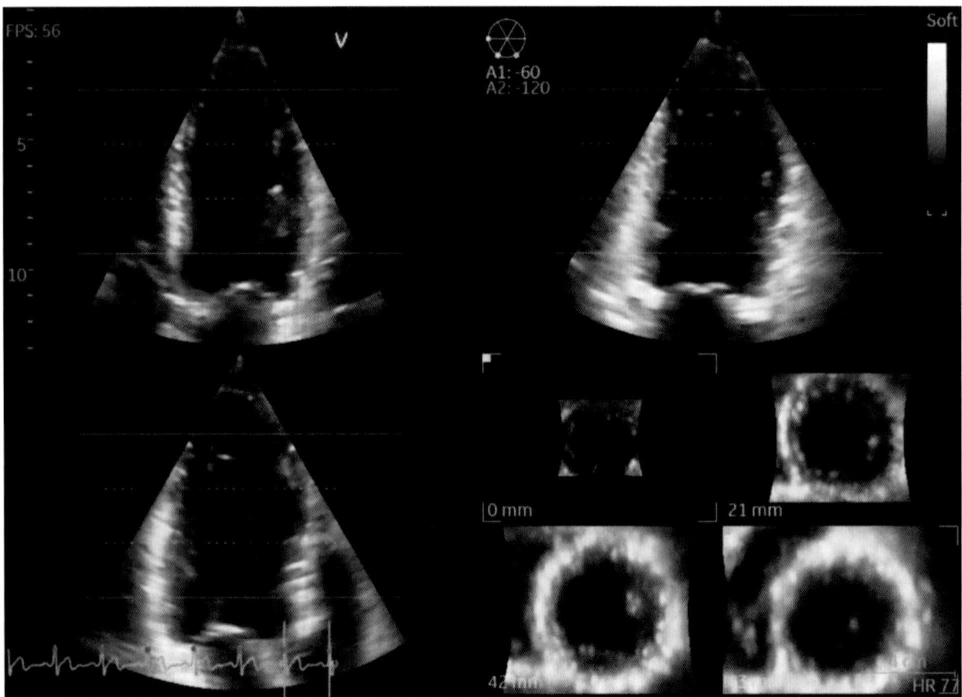

Fig 4.5 3D LV volume measurements. LV 3D full-volume acquisition with reconstructed apical 4-chamber view *(upper left)*, 2-chamber view *(upper right)*, 3-chamber view *(lower left)*, and short-axis views at the apical, mid-ventricular, and basal levels *(lower right)*. The endocardium should be visible in all segments before tracing is performed (see Video 4.5.)

TABLE 4.5 Normal Values for 3D Echocardiography–Derived LV End-Diastolic Volume Index and Ejection Fraction in Various Populations.[a]

Study	*Population*	*LV EDVI (mL/m²)*	*LV Ejection Fraction (%)*
Aune et al.[17]	Scandinavian men (n = 79) Scandinavian women (n = 87)	66 ± 10 58 ± 8	57 ± 4 61 ± 6
Fukuda et al.[41]	Japanese men (n = 222) Japanese women (n = 134)	50 ± 12 46 ± 9	61 ± 4 63 ± 4
Chahal et al.[18]	European White men (n = 338) European White women (n = 161)	49 ± 9 42 ± 8	61 ± 6 62 ± 5
	South Asian men (n = 290) South Asian women (n = 189)	41 ± 9 39 ± 8	62 ± 5 62 ± 5
Mararu et al.[42]	White men (n = 101) White women (n = 125)	63 ± 11 56 ± 8	62 ± 4 65 ± 4
Bernard et al.[19]	European men (n = 187) European women (n = 253)	69 ± 14 60 ± 11	59 ± 4 60 ± 5

[a]Individual data sources are indicated because there is no consensus on normal values.
EF, Ejection fraction; EDVI, end-diastolic volume index.

TABLE 4.6 Quantification of LV Size and Function: Advantages and Disadvantages of Various Methods.

Method	*Advantages*	*Disadvantages*
1D	High temporal resolution	Acquisition may be technically difficult
	Very good reproducibility	Obsolete for calculation of ejection fraction
	Many published data, outcome data	For calculation of muscle mass, accurate only in normally shaped ventricles with constant muscle thickness
2D	Reasonably good reproducibility	Accurate endocardial border detection may be technically difficult
	Fewer geometric assumptions	Real apex visualization may be technically difficult
	Many published data, outcome data	Blind to changes in shape or function not visualized in 4- and 2-chamber views
3D	Virtually no geometric assumptions	More dependent on image quality
	Less underestimation of volumes	Lower special and temporal resolution
	Higher reproducibility of measurements in some studies	Fewer published data, outcome data

because of refinements in echocardiographic technology that allow detection of the true border of the myocardium corresponding to the blood–tissue interface. Previously, the recommended approach was to measure from leading edge to leading edge because gain settings influence the trailing edge of the endocardial signal. This method resulted in inaccurate calculations at both ends of the LV size spectrum, with overestimation of LV mass in small ventricles and underestimation of mass in large ventricles.[31]

Use of M-mode for LV mass calculation requires measurement of the LV inner diameter and the anteroseptal and inferolateral diameters of the compacted myocardium, all in one line at the level of the mitral valve leaflet tips in end-diastole[1] (see Fig. 4.1). This approach is based on the assumption that the LV is a prolate ellipsoid with a ratio of 2:1 for its long versus short axis.[32] The following formula is applied for calculation of muscle mass and has been validated anatomically:

$$\text{LV mass} = 0.8 \times 1.04\left[\left(\text{SWT}_d + \text{LVID}_d + \text{PWT}_d\right)^3 - \text{LVID}_d^3\right] + 0.6\ \text{g}$$

SWT_d is the diastolic septal wall thickness; LVID_d the diastolic LV inner diameter; and PWT_d is the diastolic posterior wall thickness. Because these linear measurements are cubed, small measurement errors have a considerable effect on the accuracy of mass calculation.

The 2D method for LV mass calculation is based on measurement of LV length obtained from the apical 4-chamber projection and calculation of mean myocardial wall thickness at mid-ventricular level obtained from parasternal short-axis imaging in end-diastole. LV mass is then calculated by the area-length or the truncated ellipsoid method.[33] The formula applied for calculation of muscle mass based on the area-length method is as follows:

$$\text{LV mass} = 1.05 \left\{[5/6\ A_1\,(a + d + t)] - [5/6\ A_2\,(a + d)]\right\}$$

A_1 is the LV epicardial cross-sectional area in short-axis view; A_2 is the endocardial cross-sectional area in short-axis view; a is the distance of the LV minor radius to the LV apex, d is the distance to the LV mitral valve plane, and t is the LV mean wall thickness. Muscle volume is obtained as the difference between the epicardial and the endocardial shell.

Although there are fewer geometric assumptions with this approach compared with M-mode imaging, it is still assumed that the LV is an ellipsoid. The LV mass determined by M-mode is comparable to that obtained by both 2D methods, and all three methods show a moderate correlation with true LV mass measured at autopsy.[33]

Depending on the clinical situation, it may be indicated to give preference to a specific method. In patients with a normally shaped LV, the M-mode method is reasonable because it is simple and has low variability and good accuracy. In patients with a remodeled LV, the 2D method may be the better solution because it offers an improved analysis of LV shape and is better suited for follow-up.

The 3D method for LV mass calculation is based on tracing the endocardial borderline of the ventricular cavity and the epicardial border. This approach has the advantage of being independent of geometric assumptions because all of the ventricular borders are contained within the 3D data set. The 3D method is potentially more accurate than the 2D method and has a better agreement with CMR measurement. It also has lower intraobserver and interobserver variability under study conditions.[30,34] However, it critically depends on having very good image quality, particularly because the spatial and temporal resolution of 3D images are inferior to those of 2D.

A frequently encountered problem is subaortic septal hypertrophy (i.e., sigmoid septum), which can often be seen in elderly individuals.[35] M-mode measurements should not be used in this situation because the septal wall thickness is measured at the site of a localized hypertrophy and LV mass would be overestimated. The 2D method is more accurate because wall thickness is determined at the mid-ventricular level; however, localized hypertrophy would be ignored and LV mass underestimated with this approach. The best method for measuring LV mass in such individuals is probably the 3D method, as long as image quality allows accurate tracing of the compacted myocardium.

LV wall thickness relative to LV diameter in end-diastole is a simple parameter for assessing LV geometry.[36] It is determined by calculating the ratio of posterior wall thickness times 2 and the LV inner diameter obtained in end-diastole with the transducer in the parasternal long-axis position:

$$\text{Relative wall thickness} = 2 \times PWT_d / LVID_d$$

PWT_d is the diastolic posterior wall thickness, and $LVID_d$ is the diastolic LV inner diameter. A cutoff value of 0.42 separates

TABLE 4.7 Descriptors of LV Remodeling With Cutoff Values for Geometry and Hypertrophy.

Type of Remodeling	*Population*	*LV Mass Index (g/m^2)*	*Relative Wall Thickness*
Normal	Men	≤115	≤0.42
	Women	≤95	≤0.42
Concentric remodeling	Men	≤115	>0.42
	Women	≤95	>0.42
Eccentric hypertrophy	Men	>115	≤0.42
	Women	>95	≤0.42
Concentric hypertrophy	Men	>115	>0.42
	Women	>95	>0.42

Data from Lang RM, Badano LP, Mor-Avi V, et al. Recommendations for cardiac chamber quantification by echocardiography in adults: an update from the American Society of Echocardiography and the European Association of Cardiovascular Imaging. *J Am Soc Echocardiogr*. 2015;28(1):1–39.

normal geometry from concentric remodeling when LV mass is in the normal range and eccentric from concentric hypertrophy when LV mass is increased[37] (Table 4.7). Relative wall thickness is a ratio, so it should always be considered in the context of the absolute values for LV diameter and wall thickness (Fig. 4.6).

LV mass should be indexed to body surface area (BSA) because LV mass depends on body size.[3] Because of the difference between males and females in LV mass, separate reference ranges are required for the indexed values. Although indexing to body surface area is reasonable, it is not accurate for all groups of individuals and underestimates LV hypertrophy in obese patients. Like other echocardiographic parameters, indexing to BSA is particularly important for individuals with small body size. An alternative approach is indexing to height, but this is less well accepted than BSA.[38,39]

Normal values for 3D-derived LV mass are more difficult to define than for 2D because fewer studies are available.[3,40–42] Normal values for LV mass depend on body size, body mass, gender, age, and ethnic group.[36] The normal values for the M-mode and 2D methods are provided in Table 4.8, and those for the 3D approach are provided in Table 4.9. Advantages and disadvantages of the various methods are summarized in Table 4.6.

LV SHAPE AND ITS IMPLICATIONS FOR MEASUREMENTS

The normally shaped LV is a prolate ellipsoid with a ratio of the long axis to short axis of approximately 2:1.[1] The linear method for LV mass calculation is based on the assumption that the LV fulfills this criterion. In many individuals with cardiac disease, however, the LV undergoes remodeling, resulting in a shape that diverges from the ideal ellipsoid in a global or a regional manner.

Global aberration from the standard shape consists of an atypical ratio of LV short and long axes. In normal individuals, this ratio ranges from 0.45 to 0.62.[43,44] In hypertensive patients with normal LV ejection fraction (LVEF), the ratio tends to be higher, with values ranging from 0.52 ± 0.04 for those with concentric remodeling to 0.63 ± 0.03 for those with hypertrophy. Similarly, the LV undergoes a spherical remodeling in cardiomyopathies such as dilated cardiomyopathy or noncompaction cardiomyopathy.[45] In these patients, the remodeling seems to be particularly pronounced in the apical and septal regions of the LV.[46]

Spherical remodeling has also been observed in patients with mitral or aortic regurgitation.[47] In patients with acute myocardial infarction, LV sphericity predicts the extent of ventricular remodeling.[46] In a population with various cardiac diseases,

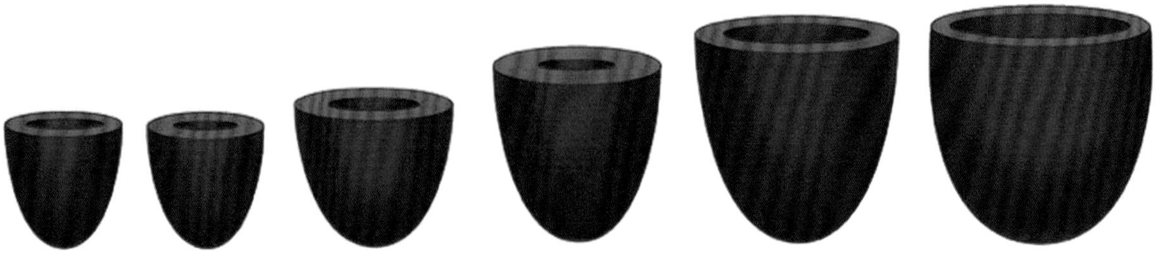

	Normal	Concentric Remodeling (Hypertension)	Concentric Hypertrophy (Hypertension/ Aortic Stenosis)	Hypertrophic Cardiomyopathy	Eccentric Hypertrophy (Aortic/Mitral Regurgitation)	Dilated Cardiomyopathy
Mass	N	N	↑	↑	↑↑	↑↑
Volume	N	N-↓	N	N-↓	↑↑	↑↑↑
RWT	N	↑	↑	↑↑	N-↓	↓
M/V	N	↑	↑	↑↑	N-↓	↓
Systolic stress	N	N-↓	V	↓	↑↑	↑↑↑
Systolic shortening						
Endocardial	N	N	N-↓	↑↑	N	↓
Midwall	N	N-↓	↓	–	N	↓

Fig. 4.6 LV volume, mass, geometry, stress, and systolic shortening in various cardiac disorders. LV mass, volume, relative wall thickness (RWT), and mass/volume (M/V) ratio are classified as normal (N), increased (↑ through ↑↑↑), or decreased (↓ through ↓↓↓). (Redrawn from Aurigemma GP, Gaasch WH, Villegas B, Meyer TE: Noninvasive assessment of left ventricular mass, chamber volume, and contractile function. *Curr Probl Cardiol.* 1995;20:385.)

TABLE 4.8 Normal Values and Severity Partition Cutoff Values for 2D Echocardiography-Derived LV Mass.

	Male				Female			
	Normal Range	*Mildly Abnormal*	*Moderately Abnormal*	*Severely Abnormal*	*Normal Range*	*Mildly Abnormal*	*Moderately Abnormal*	*Severely Abnormal*
LV Mass by Linear Method								
Septal wall thickness (cm)	0.6–1.0	1.1–1.3	1.4–1.6	>1.6	0.6–0.9	1.0–1.2	1.3–1.5	>1.5
Posterior wall thickness (cm)	0.6–1.0	1.1–1.3	1.4–1.6	>1.6	0.6–0.9	1.0–1.2	1.3–1.5	>1.5
LV mass (g)	88–224	225–258	259–292	>292	67–162	163–186	187–210	>210
LV mass/BSA (g/m^2)	49–115	116–131	132–148	>148	43–95	96–108	109–121	>121
LV Mass by 2D Method								
LV mass (g)	96–200	201–227	228–254	>254	66–150	151–171	172–193	>193
LV mass/BSA (g/m^2)	50–102	103–116	117–130	>130	44–88	89–100	101–112	>112

BSA, Body surface area.
From Lang RM, Badano LP, Mor-Avi V, et al. Recommendations for cardiac chamber quantification by echocardiography in adults: an update from the American Society of Echocardiography and the European Association of Cardiovascular Imaging. *J Am Soc Echocardiogr.* 2015;28(1):1–39.

global and regional alterations of LV shape are associated with cardiovascular mortality.[20] When LV systolic function is supported by a ventricular assist device, LV volume and sphericity progressively decrease with increasing speed of the assist device, and the LV regains a more conical shape.[48] Patients with mild heart failure with reduced ejection fraction (EF) undergoing cardiac resynchronization therapy develop an increase in LVEF accompanied by a decrease in sphericity, and improved sphericity is associated with fewer heart failure hospitalizations and lower mortality rates.[49] A similar reverse remodeling can be observed after surgical or percutaneous repair of mitral regurgitation.[50]

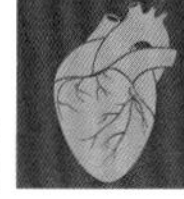

TABLE 4.9 Normal Values for 3D Echocardiography–Derived LV Mass in Various Populations.[a]

Study	*Population*	*3D LV Mass (g/m²)*
Fukuda et al.[41]	Japanese men (n = 222)	64 ± 12
	Japanese women (n = 134)	56 ± 11
Mararu et al.[42]	White men (n = 101)	77 ± 10
	White women (n = 125)	74 ± 8
Mizukoshi et al.[40]	Japanese men (n = 121)	70 ± 8
	Japanese women (n = 109)	61 ± 8
	American men (n = 78)	70 ± 10
	American women (n = 82)	60 ± 8

[a]Individual data sources are indicated because there is no consensus on normal values.

The LV may also undergo elongation during a global remodeling process such as occurs in individuals with an athlete's heart.[51] It is essential to recognize these alterations and to choose the method for calculation of LV sphericity, volumes, and mass accordingly. The linear method can be used for LV size in such situations, but the LV diameter should be reported as a diameter, and neither LV volume nor LV mass should be calculated from it. The area-length method is more useful for these patients, but it is still based on geometric assumptions. The Simpson method is not greatly affected by alterations in LV shape and is useful in these instances. The 3D method is certainly the best approach in patients with appropriate echocardiographic windows.

Regional deviations from the standard LV shape can occur for various reasons. Apical hypoplasia is a rare congenital abnormality, and endomyocardial fibrosis is an acquired pathology associated with a disturbed LV shape in the apical region.[52,53] Aneurysms usually occur from regional loss of myocardial tissue in coronary artery disease or myocarditis but may be congenital.[54] Similarly, large diverticula represent a problem for accurate quantification of LV volume.[55]

Whenever there are regional abnormalities of LV shape or regional thinning of the LV wall, neither LV volume nor LV mass should be calculated from the linear measurements. The area-length method and the Simpson rule likewise may not be accurate for quantification of LV volume. 3D echocardiography is the best method of calculating volumes and mass in these patients when they have appropriate echocardiographic windows.

QUANTITATIVE ANALYSIS OF LV SYSTOLIC FUNCTION

LV RESPONSE TO PRESSURE AND VOLUME OVERLOAD

The heart operates as a pump by converting chemical into mechanical energy. Blood flow results from ejection of stroke volume at the pressure required to overcome total peripheral resistance. Besides proper filling and sufficient contraction, LV function is determined by preload and afterload.

Preload corresponds to stretching of resting sarcomeres in end-diastole; it is limited by sarcomere length and corresponds to end-diastolic wall stress. Preload is analogous to the preload of a strip of isolated cardiac muscle measured by a myograph. The force exerting stretch on the myocardium is counteracted by the stiffness or compliance of the cardiac muscle. Preload can be determined in clinical practice as the end-diastolic diameter (EDD) or end-diastolic volume (EDV). When preload is enhanced, sarcomeres are stretched, leading to increased active muscle fiber tension and an increase in stroke volume with reduction of the higher EDV. This phenomenon operates on a beat-to-beat basis and is referred to as the Frank-Starling mechanism.[56]

The preload reserve of the ventricle depends on the baseline hemodynamic conditions and the compliance of the myocardium. In the upright position, normal people exhibit a substantial preload reserve; in the recumbent position, the preload reserve is small. This difference is related to the baseline EDV, which is larger in the recumbent position due to increased venous return.

When exercise studies are interpreted, the position of the individual is an important detail. In various cardiac disorders with reduced ventricular compliance and preload reserve, the ability to recruit the Frank-Starling mechanism and to increase LVEF is limited. This may be observed in patients with exercise intolerance due to hypertensive heart disease, aortic stenosis, or hypertrophic cardiomyopathy. In contrast, a dilated LV does not necessarily indicate that there is a reduced preload reserve. Patients with an athlete's heart and those with a compensated aortic or mitral regurgitation retain the ability to use preload reserve for augmenting stroke volume during exercise.

Afterload is the force developed by the myocardium to overcome all the factors counteracting the ejection of stroke volume, and it therefore corresponds to systolic wall stress. It is directly related to LV systolic pressure and LV radius and inversely related to wall thickness. Although systolic blood pressure and arterial compliance influence afterload, they are not equivalent with it. A slowly progressive increase in afterload, as occurs with aortic stenosis, induces an adaptive increase in LV muscle mass, and the afterload or force borne by each unit of cardiac muscle may remain near normal in these circumstances. In contrast, an acute increase in LV systolic pressure can result in increased afterload.

Changes in preload and afterload influence each other to some extent. Afterload does not affect preload per se, but an increase in afterload reduces the shortening velocity of myocyte fibers, resulting in a lower stroke volume and a higher preload with augmented EDV and end-diastolic pressure. When preload is enhanced, sarcomeres are stretched, leading to increased active muscle fiber tension and increased stroke volume with reduction of the higher EDV. Consistent with the interdependence of preload and afterload, there is virtually no situation of cardiac overload that results in a pure pressure or volume burden. For instance, aortic regurgitation induces LV volume overload but is always accompanied by some degree of pressure overload.

Contractility can be regarded as the property of cardiac muscle that determines performance independent of loading conditions. It corresponds to the inotropic state and is measured as extent and velocity of force development and muscle shortening. In many cardiac diseases, LV systolic function may be altered by loading conditions or contractility or both. Accordingly, a sensitive index of contractility unaffected by loading conditions would represent a very interesting parameter. Unfortunately, there is no load-independent descriptor of contractility, and it has not been possible to define a basal level of contractility in patients with chronic cardiac disease.

Pressure Overload

Pressure overload of the LV occurs with increased afterload. This includes all types of aortic stenosis and coarctation, increased peripheral resistance related to arterial hypertension, and decreased arterial compliance caused by atherosclerosis or arterial calcification. It can also result from high cardiac output, as in hyperthyroidism, and from high stroke volume, as in total atrioventricular block and other causes of severe bradycardia.

In chronic compensated pressure overload, stroke volume is normal or mildly reduced, and heart rate and cardiac output remain in the normal range. However, a characteristic adaptation is increased wall thickness, leading to concentric remodeling or hypertrophy. Although the latter is an important mechanism that allows the ventricle to eject the stroke volume against the abnormal peripheral resistance, it eventually causes decreased LV compliance, leading to diastolic dysfunction and enhanced diastolic pressure.[57,58]

Volume Overload

Volume overload of the LV occurs with increased preload. This occurs in valvular disease, such as mitral regurgitation and aortic regurgitation, but it can also be related to intracardiac shunts such as ventricular septal defect and extracardiac shunts such as aortopulmonary window, persistent ductus arteriosus, and arteriovenous fistula. Another important cause of volume overload is total atrioventricular block or other causes of severe bradycardia. Volume overload can result from systemic diseases such as anemia.

In chronic compensated volume overload, EDV and stroke volume are increased. Typically, the fraction of stroke volume in EDV is normal. In contrast to pressure overload, there is a mild increase in LV wall thickness. Nevertheless, muscle mass usually is increased because of dilation of the ventricle. LV compliance may remain in the normal range, leading to small increases or even normal values for diastolic pressure.

LV MECHANICS

The systolic function of the LV is a complex process involving a coordinated contraction of myocardial fibers. The fibers are arranged in a helical manner with different orientations of subendocardial, midwall, and subepicardial fibers.[58a] In the mid-ventricular region, midwall fibers are oriented circumferentially, and contraction of these fibers mediates the decrease in the minor axis of the ventricle during generation of stroke volume. Longitudinally oriented fibers in the subendocardial and subepicardial layers of the myocardium mainly contribute to shortening along the major axis of the ventricle and thereby to stroke volume. In addition to circumferential and longitudinal shortening, the apex of the LV rotates in a counterclockwise direction, and the base performs a clockwise rotation when observed from the apex (Fig. 4.7). The resulting twist of the LV is considered to contribute to effective ventricular contraction and vortex flow.[58a]

Different parameters applied for analysis of LV systolic function assess different aspects of ventricular mechanics. Parameters used for LV global function in clinical routine are EF and global longitudinal strain (GLS). LVEF mainly represents circumferential systolic shortening, whereas GLS measures longitudinal deformation. Other parameters, such as mitral

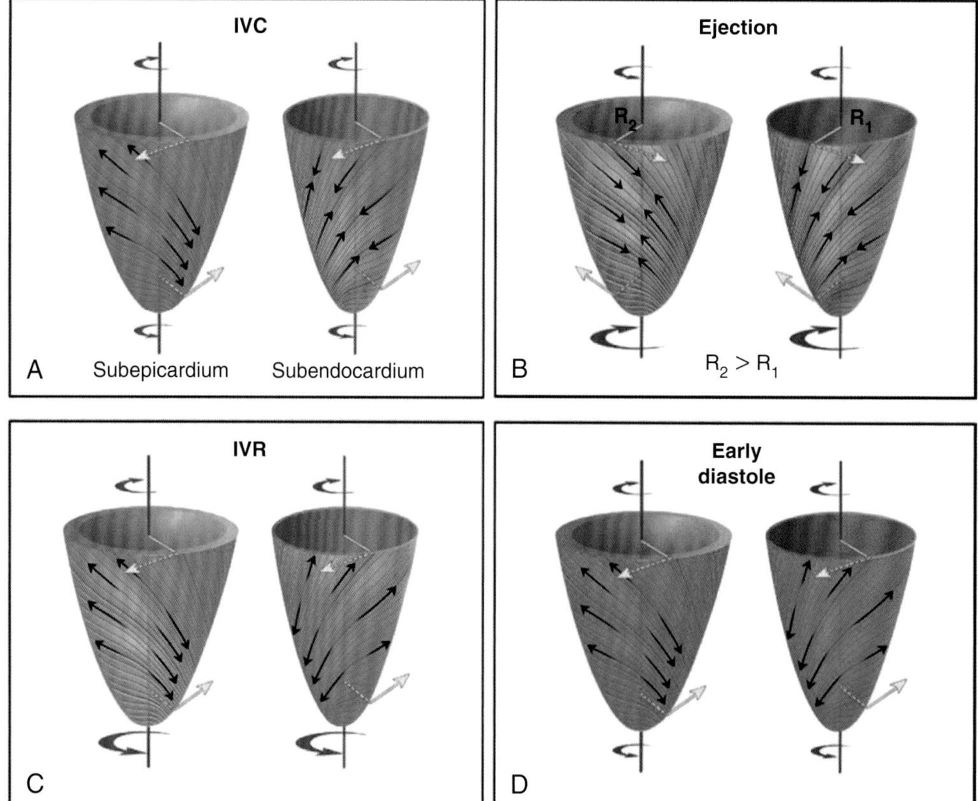

Fig. 4.7 LV mechanics during the cardiac cycle. Mechanical activation is initiated in the apical subendocardium. During the ejection phase, the base rotates in a clockwise direction and the apex in a counterclockwise direction, resulting in twist (A and B). During isovolumic relaxation and to a lesser extent during diastole, untwisting occurs (C and D). *IVC*, Isovolumic contraction period; *IVR*, isovolumic relaxation period; R, radius. (From Sengupta PP, Tajik AJ, Chandrasekaran K, Khandheria BK. Twist mechanics of the left ventricle: principles and application. *JACC Cardiovasc Imaging*. 2008;1[3]:366–376.)

annulus plane systolic excursion (MAPSE) and tissue Doppler *s′*, represent longitudinal function of a ventricular region only. Although all these parameters are valuable tools for the assessment of LV systolic function and are associated with outcomes for patients with cardiac disease, the only method to analyze LV mechanics in all its complexity is a complete 2D strain analysis or, even better, 3D strain analysis.

LV GLOBAL FUNCTION

Ejection Fraction

Global LV systolic function is typically expressed as EF. This parameter is obtained by calculating the difference between the EDV and the end-systolic volume (ESV) divided by its end-diastolic value.[3]

$$EF\,(\%) = [(EDV - ESV) \times 100] / EDV$$

End-diastole is defined as the first frame after mitral valve closure, and end-systole corresponds to the frame depicting the smallest LV dimension in the cardiac cycle or, alternatively, the first frame after aortic valve closure. It follows that a higher frame rate leads to more accurate quantification, and the recommended frame rate for measurement of LV systolic function is greater than 60 fps. This rule is also helpful for LV strain measurement because such a frame rate is a prerequisite for accurate strain quantification with current software programs.[59,60]

The most commonly used method for measurement of EDV and ESV is the biplane method of disks (i.e., Simpson rule). This approach requires apical 4-chamber and 2-chamber views of the LV. The endocardial border is traced in end-diastole and end-systole. The LV is then divided into a defined number of disks along its long axis; usually, 20 to 25 disks are defined for this purpose. The accuracy of the measurement is determined by the number of disks. The volume of each disk is calculated by multiplying disk area by disk height, and ventricular volume is obtained by addition of the individual disk volumes (Fig. 4.8).

The normal 2D LVEF is 60% to 65%, with a normal range of 52% to 72% for men and 54% to 74% for women (see Table 4.2). The age-dependent decline in diastolic and systolic LV volumes is more pronounced in females than in males. Because

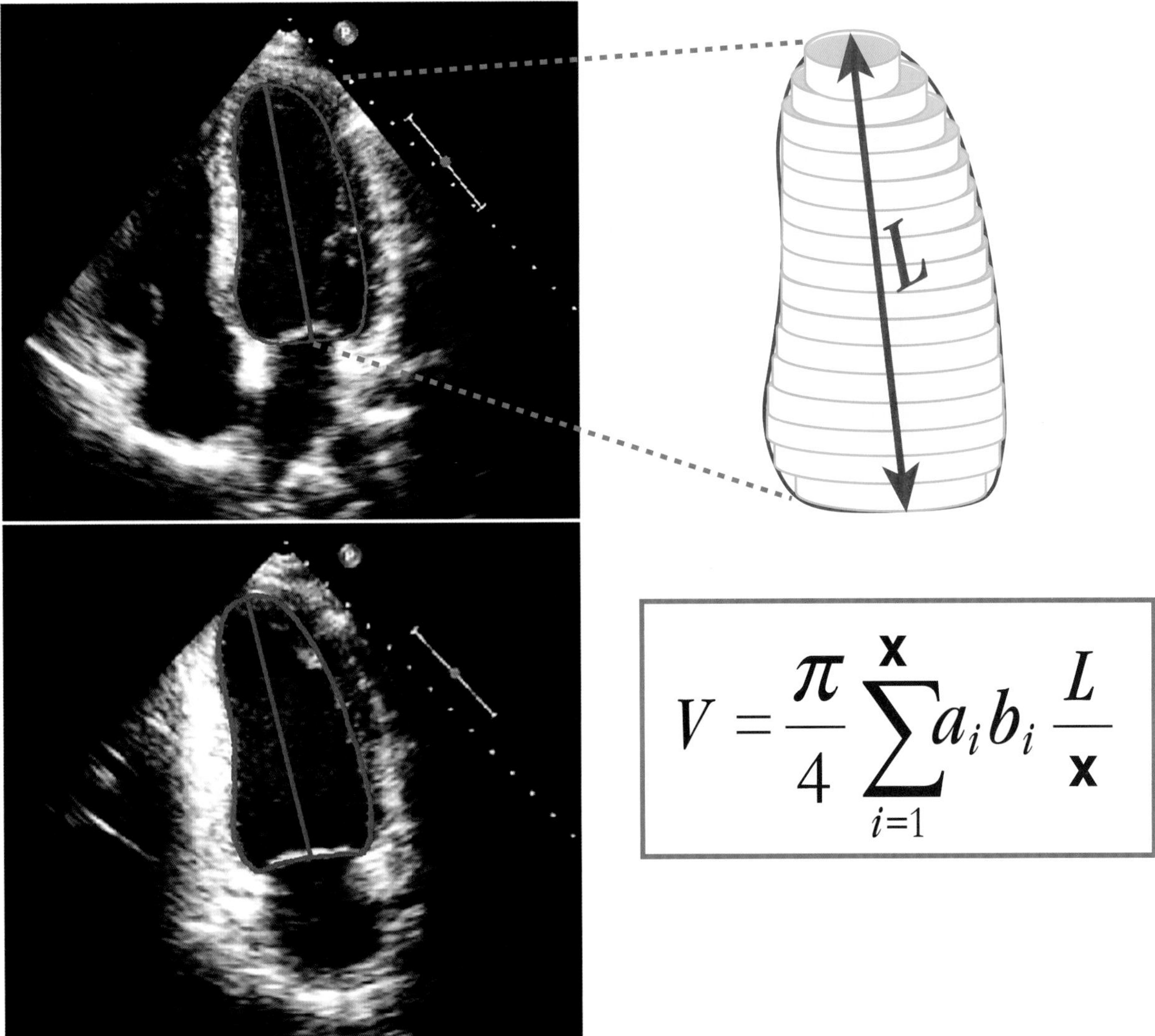

Fig. 4.8 The Simpson rule for calculation of LV ejection fraction. Apical 4-chamber view *(upper left)* and 2-chamber view *(lower left)* with endocardial border tracing and long-axis representation for calculation of LV volume. The principle of the method is depicted schematically at *upper right* and mathematically at *lower right*. In the formula, *a* is the disc diameter in 4-chamber view, *b* the disc diameter in 2-chamber view, *L* the length of the LV long axis, and x the number of discs.

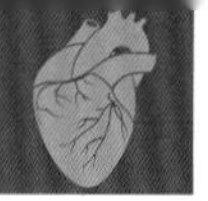

the age-dependent change is similar in EDV and ESV, EF does not decrease with age; to the contrary, LVEF slightly increases with increasing age of the population, particularly in women (see Fig. 4.4). This is considered to represent a compensatory mechanism because longitudinal function of the LV decreases with age. Normal age-dependent remodeling should be taken into account in clinical routine when very young or very old patients are examined.[3,15a,61]

In patients with hypertensive heart disease, coronary artery disease, or various cardiomyopathies, it is generally accepted that mildly reduced values for LVEF, between 40% and 50%, are of little clinical significance. In contrast, for patients with aortic regurgitation or aortic stenosis, an EF lower than 50% may indicate significant depression of contractile LV function, and this may be the case with an EF lower than 60% for those with mitral regurgitation.[63] It is important to keep this difference in mind because outcomes after valve intervention are reduced if a decrease in LVEF is ignored, even in asymptomatic patients.

An important question remains about whether LV function can recover after proper treatment has been conducted. The answer seems to depend mainly on whether there is a functional reason for the reduced EF (e.g., afterload mismatch) or structural changes of the LV have occurred.[64] When LVEF is reduced due to increased wall stress, recovery of LV function can be expected, but this is not the case when increased wall stress is out of proportion and structural alterations of the myocardium have developed. In the clinical setting, it can be very difficult to predict functional recovery of the LV in such situations.[65]

In patients exhibiting heart failure with reduced EF, LVEF is associated with all-cause mortality and cardiovascular hospitalizations. Symptomatic patients with dilated cardiomyopathy and a severely impaired LVEF have a worse outcome than those with less severe impairment of LV systolic function.[66] For a large patient population with a broad spectrum of symptomatic heart failure, the risk of all-cause mortality and cardiovascular death increases with decreasing LVEF (Fig. 4.9).[67] Similar findings are made in acute heart failure because patients with takotsubo cardiomyopathy exhibit higher rates of in-hospital complications when LVEF is reduced.[68]

LVEF determined by the Simpson method is a simple approach because only apical 4-chamber and 2-chamber views are required. However, these views must be obtained carefully by following the rules outlined previously and in Tables 4.1 and 4.6. This is particularly important for the 2-chamber view, which is sometimes acquired in an oblique manner (i.e., foreshortened projection).

Because the difference between EDV and ESV of the LV corresponds to stroke volume, cardiac output can be calculated by multiplying stroke volume and heart rate if aortic and mitral regurgitation are assumed to be absent. However, this method for determining cardiac output is not very accurate and may underestimate stroke volume because of foreshortening of the LV in apical projections.

If there are doubts regarding the measurement of stroke volume, it can also be calculated by multiplying the LVOT area by the velocity–time integral (VTI) acquired by pulsed-wave Doppler imaging at the same level as the outflow tract diameter is measured. The VTI can also be acquired at other locations in the heart, but accuracy seems to be best in the LVOT. Nevertheless, this alternative method may result in inaccurate stroke volume calculations.

Stroke volume may be underestimated due to the oval shape of the LVOT (rather than the assumed circular shape) because

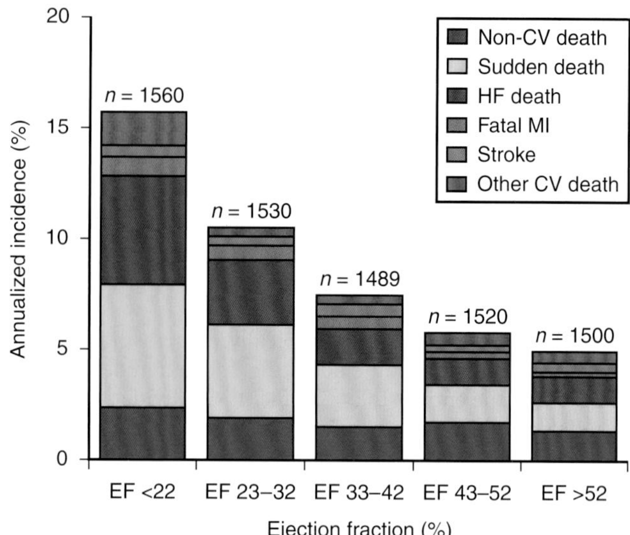

Fig. 4.9 Prognosis by ejection fraction in patients with heart failure. Ejection fraction *(EF)* is a powerful predictor of cardiovascular outcome in heart failure patients across a broad spectrum of LV function. *CV,* Cardiovascular; *HF,* heart failure; *MI,* myocardial infarction. (From Solomon SD, Anavekar N, Skali H, et al. Influence of ejection fraction on cardiovascular outcomes in a broad spectrum of heart failure patients. *Circulation.* 2005;112[24]:3738–3744.)

the diameter determined in the parasternal long-axis view effectively corresponds to the short diameter of the oval in many patients. When this problem is suspected, a 3D acquisition of the outflow tract allows determination of its real shape (Fig. 4.10).[69,70] However, stroke volume may be overestimated when the tracing of the VTI does not follow the modal velocity or, alternatively, when the flow velocity in the LVOT is too heterogeneous.[71] The latter is a particularly important problem when the LVOT is dilated. In that case, flow velocity in the center of the LVOT, where the Doppler sample volume is usually placed, can be considerably higher than in the more peripheral locations of the outflow tract, leading to overestimation of stroke volume.[72]

The Simpson method for LVEF is based on a simple principle, is reproducible, and is associated with numerous prognostic data. However, its value is limited by technical challenges during image acquisition and border tracing and by principle flaws such as the angle between 4-chamber and 2-chamber views and exclusion of the LVOT. The method is also blind to changes in LV shape and/or function not represented in apical 4-chamber or 2-chamber views. Many of these drawbacks can be avoided by acquisition of an LV 3D data set (see Fig. 4.5). This allows tracing of the border of the compacted myocardium around the circumference of the LV and virtually eliminates geometric assumptions.[42]

The 3D approach reduces shortening of the LV, and it may therefore be considered superior to the 2D method.[16] An incremental value of 3D-derived LVEF, compared with the 2D measurement with regard to outcome association, has been documented in patients at high cardiovascular risk.[73] This observation has been confirmed in a population with various cardiovascular diseases.[20]

To exploit the advantages of the 3D approach for LV quantification, it is essential to optimize image quality, particularly because the current 3D applications go along with a lower spatial and temporal resolution compared with 2D. The major problem during 3D volumes acquisition is the fact that an identical scanning point is used for all myocardial segments. It is not possible to eliminate artifacts originating from the lungs or the ribs by minimal translational movements of the transducer. It is strongly recommended to acquire the 3D volumes under visual control of all the apical and parasternal views used in 2D echocardiogram reconstructed from the 3D volume being recorded (see Fig. 4.5). Similarly, the tracking line generated for LV quantification should be reviewed in the reconstructed views.

Available 3D software programs offer automated border detection algorithms for determining LV volumes and LVEF. This is a time-saving feature and is therefore attractive for the clinical routine. However, the automated detection does not always recognize the true endocardial border, particularly in ventricles with an abnormal shape and in those with many apical trabeculations or muscle bundles. It is important to critically review the result of automated border detection and to correct the tracking line when necessary.

Some studies reported reduced interobserver variability for the 3D compared with the 2D method of LV quantification.[16] This interesting feature is primarily based on the automated border detection of the 3D software. Although it may be particularly important to optimize reproducibility of LV quantification in certain patient groups requiring frequent follow-up visits, the possibility of reduced accuracy should always be kept in mind and weighed against the possible advantage of better reproducibility.

Analysis of LV volumes by 3D imaging results in greater values compared with 2D echocardiography. This is largely related to reduced shortening of the LV by 3D quantification; however, differences in endocardial border tracing cannot be ruled out. In contrast to LV volumes, there is not much difference between LVEF determined by the 2D or 3D approach. This is related to the fact that LVEF is a percentage of LV volume; when a similar difference between 2D and 3D is assumed for EDV and ESV, the differences are eliminated during calculation of the LVEF.[15,17]

Normal values for 3D-derived LVEF are less well established than 2D-derived values, and there are not enough data to allow clear definition of a normal range (see Table 4.5). When LVEF

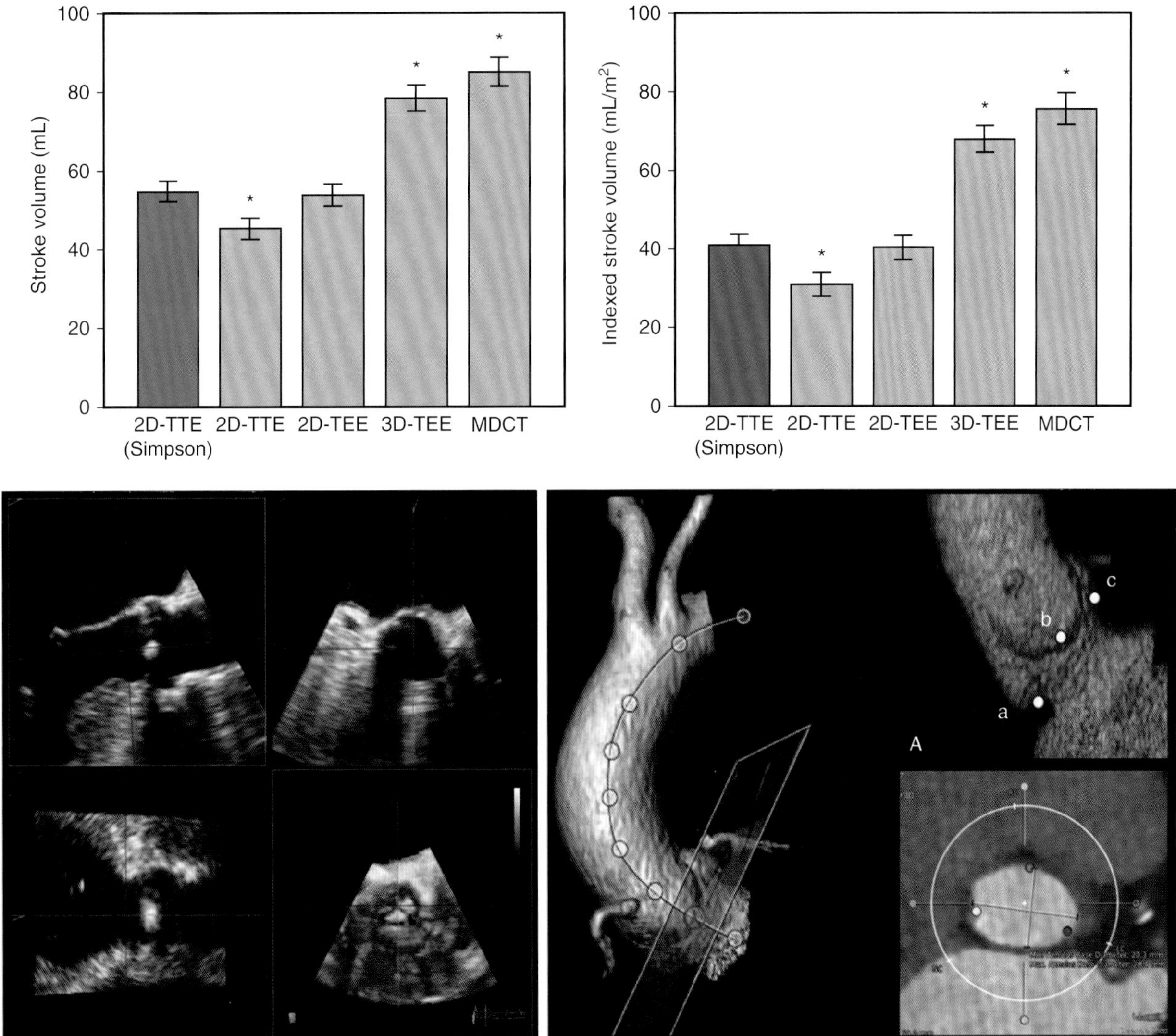

Fig. 4.10 Comparison of stroke volume measurement by 2D and 3D echocardiography. Stroke volume *(upper left)* and stroke volume index *(upper right)* are underestimated by the 2D Simpson method and the 2D left ventricular outflow tract (LVOT) method. In contrast, 3D TEE provides a more accurate stroke volume calculation *(lower left)* because it can assess the true shape of the LVOT, similar to cardiac computed tomography *(lower right)*. *MDCT*, Multidetector computed tomography. (From Stahli BE, Stadler T, Holy EW, et al. Impact of stroke volume assessment by integrating multi-detector computed tomography and Doppler data on the classification of aortic stenosis. *Int J Cardiol.* 2017;246:80–86.)

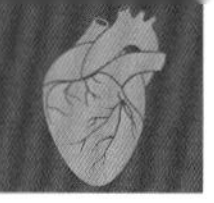

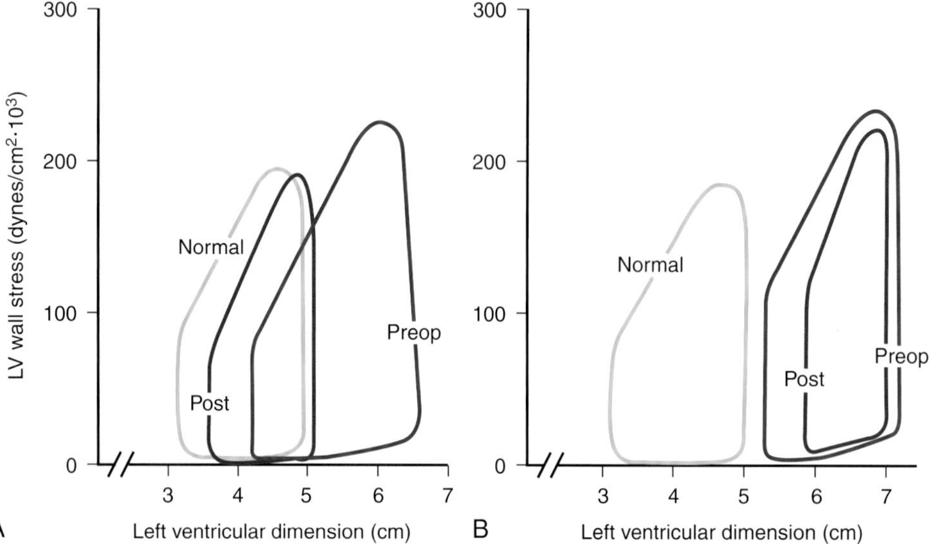

Fig. 4.11 Response to mitral valve replacement in compensated and decompensated mitral regurgitation. LV wall stress dimension loops in two cases of mitral regurgitation, before *(Preop)* and after *(Post)* valve replacement. (A) The preoperative loop indicates compensated ventricular function; the end-diastolic dimension is 6.5 cm, the end-systolic dimension is 4.2 cm, systolic wall stress is minimally elevated, and fractional shortening is normal (35%). After valve replacement, dimensions and wall stress return to normal, but fractional shortening decreases (29%). (B) The preoperative loop indicates a decompensated ventricle with markedly increased dimensions and low fractional shortening. After valve replacement, there is persistent ventricular dilatation and a further decline in fractional shortening. (From Aurigemma GP, Gaasch WH, Villegas B, Meyer TE. Noninvasive assessment of left ventricular mass, chamber volume, and contractile function. *Curr Probl Cardiol.* 1995;20[6]:361–440.)

is determined in a 3D data set, it has to be documented in the echocardiography report.

The use of intravenous injection of contrast in ultrasound reduces interobserver variability for quantification of LV volumes and LVEF.[24] As with the 2D approach, larger values for LV volumes, but not for LVEF, are measured in the presence of LV contrast.[14]

Strain

LV global function can be assessed by deformation imaging.[74,75] This approach determines LV deformation based on speckle tracking imaging or on tissue Doppler imaging. It can be performed by a 2D or 3D acquisition of the LV and provides data on longitudinal, circumferential, and radial deformation of each myocardial segment during the cardiac cycle.

In clinical practice, speckle tracking–derived longitudinal strain has been established as a solid parameter for analysis of LV function because it is easily acquired from the apical 4-chamber, 2-chamber, and 3-chamber views and because it is associated with outcomes for various patient groups.[76–78] It is complementary to LVEF in that it provides information on global longitudinal function, whereas LVEF depends more on radial function. It is also an excellent parameter for combination with MAPSE and tissue Doppler s′, which are well-established parameters for regional longitudinal function.[79] Chapter 2 offers in-depth information on LV strain.

dP/dt

The systolic performance of the LV can be evaluated by determining the rate at which ventricular pressure increases during systole (*dP/dt*). The major part of this increase occurs during the isovolumetric contraction period. It can be determined by two noninvasive methods using echocardiography. One approach is based on the steepness of the continuous-wave Doppler signal of the mitral regurgitation jet; the time required for the transmitral flow velocity to increase from 1 to 3 m/s is determined.[80] The other method is based on measurement of isovolumetric contraction time and diastolic blood pressure and estimation of LV end-diastolic pressure.[81]

Myocardial Work and Pressure-Volume Loops

LV wall stress is the force acting against the myocardium. It is proportional to LV pressure (P) and radius (r) and indirectly proportional to wall thickness (WT):

$$\text{Wall stress} = (P \times r)/(2 \times WT)$$

LV pressure can be determined invasively and combined with echocardiographic data, or it can be estimated by various noninvasive methods, at least the systolic pressure. The easiest of these methods assumes that LV systolic pressure can be approximated by the peak arterial blood pressure measured with a cuff. By plotting LV pressure or wall stress against LV volume throughout the cardiac cycle, pressure-volume loops can be generated.[82] The height of the loops is determined by systolic pressure and the width by stroke volume; therefore, the area within the loop is a measure of myocardial work or stroke work (Fig. 4.11).[83]

Modern approaches replace ventricular dimensions by strain and therefore plot pressure against deformation of the LV.[84] The loops can provide a comprehensive description of ventricular function and can be used for determining myocardial work under different afterload conditions. By manipulating pressure and dimension, the relationship of these parameters can be assessed systematically. They exhibit an almost linear direct relationship; the slope is relatively insensitive to acute changes in loading conditions but is affected by contractility.

LV REGIONAL FUNCTION

Myocardial Segments

The LV myocardium is divided into 16 (or 17 when the apical cap is included) standardized segments that exhibit comparable

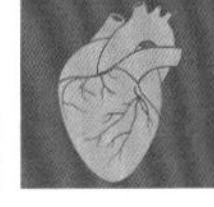

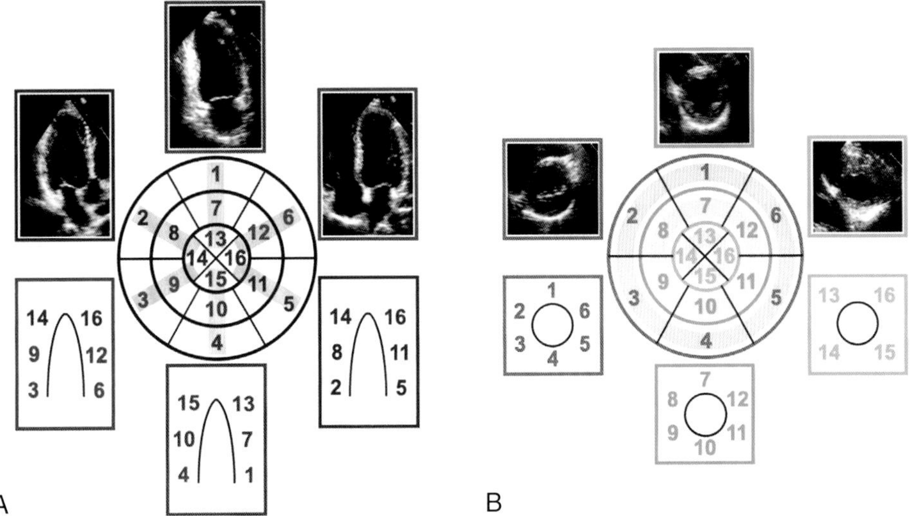

Fig. 4.12 **Myocardial segments (16-segment model).** (A) The 2-chamber view shows the anterior wall (segments 1, 7, and 13) and the inferior wall (segments 4, 10, and 15). In the apical long-axis view, the anterior septum (segments 2, 8, and 14) and the inferolateral wall (segments 5, 11, and 16) are seen. The 4-chamber view shows the inferior septum (segments 3, 9, and 14) and the anterolateral wall (segments 6, 12, and 16). (B) Short-axis views show the same segments at the LV base (segments 1–6), at the level of the papillary muscle (segments 7–12), and at the apex (segments 13–16). The target diagrams show the LV apex in the center with the base around the edge of the circle.

masses, which allows clear communication within echocardiography and with other imaging modalities. When the LV is depicted from the apex, the myocardial segments can be arranged as a bull's-eye model. The segments are numbered and labeled in a counterclockwise manner, starting at the anteroseptal position (Fig. 4.12). The segments can be related to the perfusion territories of the three major coronary arteries, which is particularly important in stress echocardiography and for understanding regional wall motion abnormalities.

Regional wall motion abnormalities are primarily quantified by visual assessment. Each segment should be analyzed separately in multiple views. The segments should first be evaluated in end-diastole for assessment of wall thinning, myocardial fibrosis, and aneurysm formation. The normal LV myocardial wall exhibits a minimal thickness of 6 mm in end-diastole. The apex is the exception to this rule because the normal myocardium thins out in the apical region.

Myocardial fibrosis cannot be detected directly by echocardiography, but it can be recognized as a region with enhanced echocardiographic density. The diagnosis of regional fibrosis can usually be made when myocardial morphology is studied in the context of myocardial function and patient history.

An LV aneurysm is defined as an outward bulging of the ventricular contour that involves all the tissue layers of the wall. It is usually caused by myocardial necrosis resulting from ischemia or inflammation and leads to myocardial fibrosis and scar formation (Fig. 4.13). Alternatively, it can be congenital, in which case it most often consists of hypokinetic myocardium.[85]

An LV aneurysm should be differentiated from a myocardial diverticulum and a myocardial cleft. A myocardial diverticulum is a fingerlike, saclike, or hooklike protrusion occurring in any LV wall. It is typically surrounded by hypokinetic myocardium and can be associated with thoracoabdominal midline defects[86] (see Fig. 4.13). LV diverticula may cause ventricular arrhythmia and/or thromboembolic events.

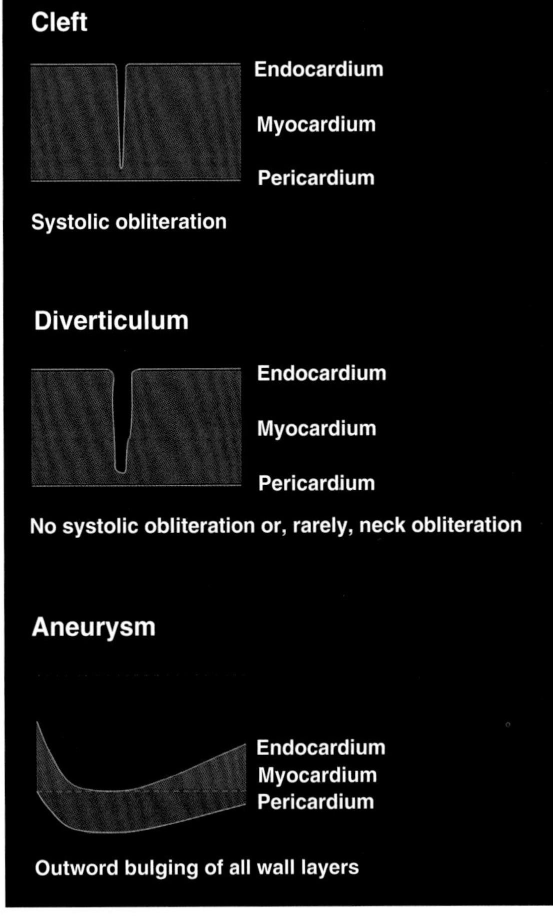

Fig. 4.13 **Schematic representation of myocardial cleft, diverticulum, and aneurysm.** A cleft *(upper panel)* is defined as a narrow, deep indentation in the myocardium that is obliterated with contraction. A diverticulum *(middle panel)* is wider but remains open during systole. An aneurysm *(lower panel)* is defined as a diastolic contour abnormality with akinesia or dyskinesia and thinning and scarring of the myocardium.

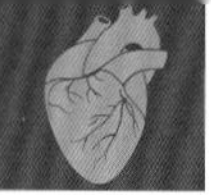

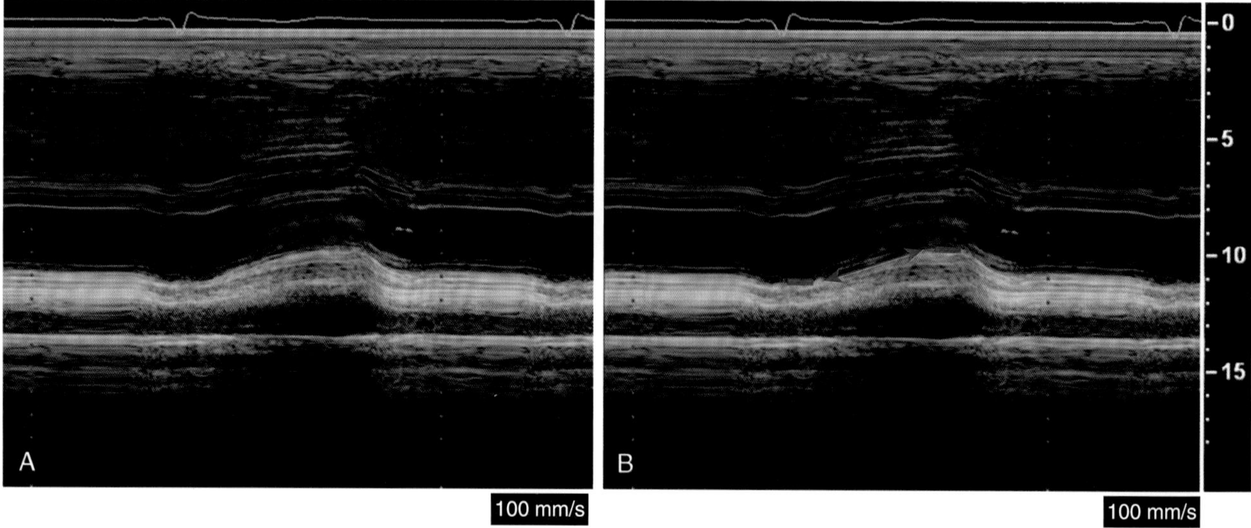

Fig. 4.14 Mitral annular plane systolic excursion (MAPSE). (A) The M-mode is positioned through the lateral annulus of the LV and oriented parallel to the direction of movement of the annulus. (B) The vertical distance between the positions at isovolumetric contraction and at endsystole is measured.

A myocardial cleft is a V-shaped protrusion occurring most often in the inferior and septal LV wall. It is typically surrounded by normokinetic myocardium and is associated with arterial hypertension and hypertrophic cardiomyopathy.[86] LV clefts probably have no clinical significance.[87]

After the myocardial segments have been evaluated at end-diastole, each segment should be studied during the cardiac cycle to understand regional wall motion during systole. The latter is determined by myocardial thickening, inward movement, and the time point of thickening and inward movement. All these aspects should be considered to evaluate regional wall motion and establish a wall motion score. The score is based on the following system:

- 1 point: normokinesis or hyperkinesis (normal or high normal thickening/movement)
- 2 points: hypokinetic (reduced and/or delayed thickening/movement)
- 3 points: akinetic (absent thickening/movement)
- 4 points: dyskinetic (systolic stretching/outward movement)

The wall motion score is determined by adding the scores from all segments and dividing by the number of segments. The same score can also be used for stress echocardiography.

Fractional Shortening

Fractional shortening (FS) can provide information on LV regional systolic function. It is obtained from the M-mode method by calculating the difference between the end-diastolic diameter (EDD) and end-systolic diameter (ESD) divided by the end-diastolic value:

$$FS\,(\%) = [(EDD - ESD) \times 100] \,/\, EDD$$

Because this is a 1-dimensional measurement, it is representative of LV systolic function only in the basal region in an anteroposterior direction. In consideration of this limitation, it can be applied as a marker of LV systolic function in individuals without regional wall motion abnormalities (see Fig. 4.1). Because it is mainly determined by circumferential fiber shortening, it correlates well with LVEF. The use of FS may be particularly reasonable when the apical views do not allow accurate measurements of LVEF due to poor image quality. Even under these conditions, it should be used for FS only, and global functional extrapolations such as the Teichholz method should be avoided.

Mitral Annulus Plane Systolic Excursion

MAPSE quantifies the systolic displacement of the mitral annulus toward the apex and is a marker of longitudinal ventricular systolic function.[79] It is determined by M-mode in the apical projection, typically in a 4-chamber view for measuring the displacement of the lateral annulus, but it can be acquired in all the apical views (Fig. 4.14). MAPSE is hardly influenced by image quality, and it can be acquired in most patients. However, it is angle dependent, and the movement of the annulus should therefore be parallel to the M-mode line, which often requires atypical apical views.

There is a good correlation between MAPSE and LVEF in patients with normal or dilated ventricles. A MAPSE value of 10 mm or greater is associated with a normal LVEF, whereas a value lower than 8 mm suggests an impaired LVEF.[88] In contrast, the correlation of MAPSE with LVEF is poor for patients with aging or hypertrophic ventricles; this is related to the decline in longitudinal systolic function that occurs with increasing age or hypertrophic myocardium and that is often compensated by increased radial and circumferential contraction.[89,90] For these patients, the MAPSE value may be particularly valuable because it can complement LVEF as an early marker of decreased longitudinal function.

MAPSE is an integrative assessment of longitudinal myocardial function and does not provide information on regional heterogeneity of the LV. MAPSE should be interpreted with caution in patients who have very small or very large hearts because the MAPSE value depends on cardiac size. Severe calcification of the mitral annulus also influences longitudinal function of the myocardium, and a reduced MAPSE value is not specific for a depressed longitudinal function in these conditions.

MAPSE is useful to detect subtle myocardial dysfunction even before LVEF is affected in various forms of cardiovascular disease such as arterial hypertension,[91] coronary artery disease,[92] and severe aortic stenosis.[93] It has also been recognized

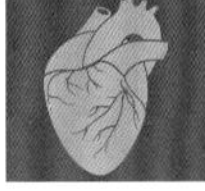

TABLE 4.10 Characteristics, Advantages, and Disadvantages of Various Methods for Evaluation of LV Longitudinal Function

Characteristic	*MAPSE*	*S′*	*GLS*
Method	M-mode	Tissue Doppler imaging	Speckle tracking imaging
Parameter	Annulus displacement	Tissue velocity	Tissue deformation
Extension	Regional	Regional	Global
Analyzer experience dependence	+	++	+++
Time for acquisition and analysis	+	++	+++
Reproducibility of acquisition and analysis	+++	++	++
Image quality dependence	+	++	+++
Cardiac size dependence	++	+	–
Angle dependence	+++	+++	+
Temporal resolution	+++	++	+

GLS, Global longitudinal strain; *MAPSE*, mitral annulus plane systolic excursion; *S′*, systolic tissue velocity.

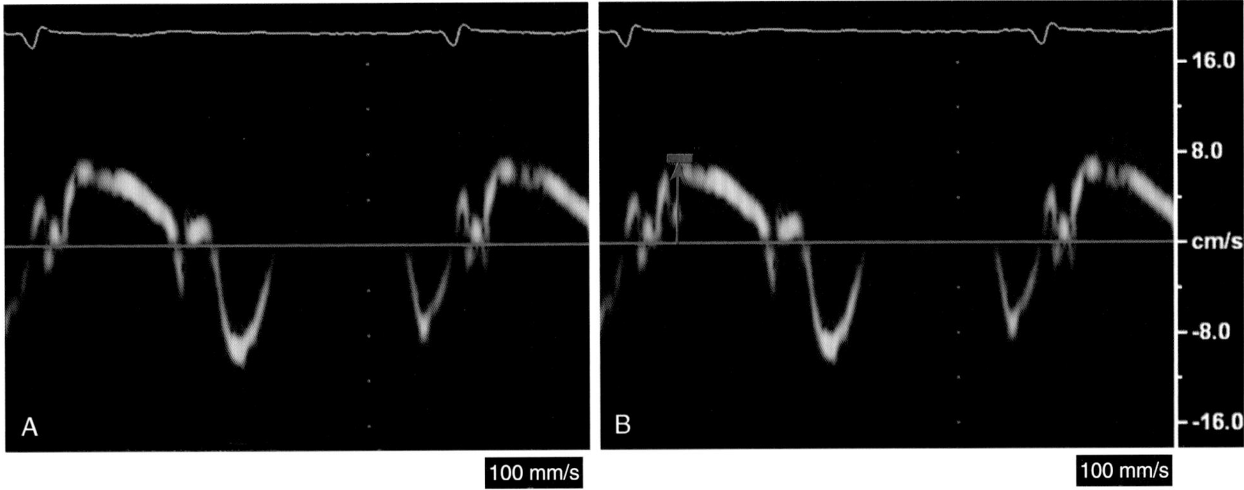

Fig. 4.15 Tissue Doppler imaging of the mitral anulus. (A) The pulsed-wave Doppler sample volume is placed on the basal myocardium so that it is at the mitral anulus level at endsystole. The sample volume is oriented parallel to the direction of movement of the annulus. (B) The maximal systolic tissue velocity is measured.

to be helpful in the diagnosis of heart failure with preserved EF[94] (Table 4.10).

Tissue Doppler Imaging

Tissue Doppler imaging allows measurement of the velocity of the myocardium throughout the cardiac cycle. Apart from systolic and diastolic peak velocity, the respective myocardial acceleration (time to peak) can be determined.

Tissue Doppler is another method for examining longitudinal ventricular systolic function.[95] It is usually measured by placing the pulsed-wave Doppler sample volume in the myocardial region close to the mitral annulus and ascertaining that the sample volume remains just within the ventricular myocardium rather than the atrial wall at end-systole (Fig. 4.15). Alternatively, it can be determined with color tissue Doppler imaging, which allows measurement of myocardial velocities in any ventricular segment. Similar to MAPSE, it can be acquired in all the apical views but is typically measured in apical 4-chamber view in the lateral and septal basal segment. It is angle dependent, and therefore the movement of the annulus should be parallel to the M-mode line, which often requires atypical apical views.

There is a good correlation between MAPSE and tissue Doppler *s′* for healthy individuals and for those with cardiovascular disease (e.g., obese individuals).[95,96] LVEF and tissue Doppler *s′* display a reasonable correlation for patients with normal LVEF and those with systolic dysfunction.[97,98] An *s′* value lower than 8 cm/s has good sensitivity and specificity for LVEF values between 30% and 50%, as does an *s′* value lower than 6 cm/s for LVEF values less than 30%.[98]

Similar to MAPSE, tissue Doppler *s′* is not specific for a depressed longitudinal systolic function in patients with severe mitral annulus calcification. In contrast to MAPSE, regional heterogeneity of longitudinal function in the involved LV sector may be explored by placing the pulsed-wave Doppler sample volume on various levels of the myocardium from base to apex or by applying color tissue Doppler imaging, which has the advantage of being applicable off-line as well.[99]

Like MAPSE, tissue Doppler *s′* is useful for detection of subtle myocardial dysfunction even before LVEF is affected in arterial hypertension,[100] coronary artery disease,[101] diabetes mellitus,[102] and hypertrophic cardiomyopathy.[103] It can also be applied to provide prognostic information, such as for patients with coronary artery disease or heart failure[101] (see Table 4.10).

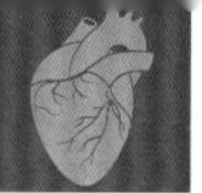

SUMMARY Summary Quantification of LV Size, Mass, and Function.

Parameter	Method	Technique	Advantages	Limitations	Importance
LV Mass					
Mass	M-mode	Linear measurement at end-diastole in parasternal long-axis view at the level of the mitral valve leaflet tips; perpendicular beam alignment to LV long axis	Simple method Good reproducibility High temporal resolution	Single dimension Angle dependent Accurate only for normally shaped ventricles with constant muscle thickness	Many outcome data
	2D	Area length or truncated ellipsoid method Epicardial and endocardial cross-sectional area in parasternal short-axis view at the papillary muscle level to obtain mean wall thickness LV length measured in 4-chamber view from center to apex and base.	Fewer geometric assumptions than for linear measurement	Many measurements required Normal values less established than for linear measurements	Some outcome data
	3D	Automatic border detection with different 3D software programs and manual adjustment if needed Alternatively, multiplanar reconstruction	Virtually no geometric assumptions	Lower temporal and spatial resolution than 2D and much lower than linear measurement Normal values to be established	Few outcome data
LV Size					
EDDI	M-Mode	Linear measurement at end-diastole in parasternal long-axis view at the level of the mitral valve leaflet tips; perpendicular beam alignment to LV long axis	Simple method Good reproducibility High temporal resolution	Single dimension Angle dependent	Some outcome data
2D Volume	2D	Tracing of endocardial border in apical 4-chamber and 2-chamber views at end-diastole. Modified Simpson rule (biplane method of disks)	Fewer geometric assumptions than for linear measurement Improved border detection with LV contrast	Foreshortening often occurs 3-Chamber view not represented Different normal values with LV contrast	Many outcome data
3D Volume	3D	Automated border detection with different 3D software programs and manual adjustment if needed Alternatively, multiplanar reconstruction	Virtually no geometric assumptions Low interstudy variation Improved border detection with LV contrast Validation against MRI	Lower temporal and spacial resolution than 2D and much lower than linear measurement Normal values to be established	Few outcome data
LV Function					
Fractional shortening	M-mode	Linear measurement at end-diastole and end-systole in parasternal long-axis view at the level of the mitral valve leaflet tips; perpendicular beam alignment to LV long axis	Simple method Good reproducibility High temporal resolution Useful when 2D image quality is poor in apical views	Angle dependent Regional function only	Some outcome data

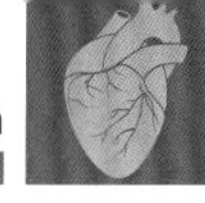

SUMMARY Summary Quantification of LV Size, Mass, and Function.—cont'd

Parameter	Method	Technique	Advantages	Limitations	Importance
MAPSE	M-mode	Measurement of mitral annular longitudinal displacement from isovolumetric contraction to peak systole in 4-chamber view M-mode oriented parallel to direction of annulus movement	Easy to perform Good reproducibility High temporal resolution Useful when 2D image quality is poor	Angle dependent Size dependent Load dependent Regional function only Tissue displacement	Some outcome data
Pulsed-tissue Doppler *s*′	Tissue Doppler	Measurement of peak systolic tissue velocity obtained by placing the sample volume at the mitral annulus level Beam oriented parallel to direction of annulus movement	Easy to perform Fair reproducibility Fair temporal resolution	Angle dependent Size dependent Load dependent Regional function only Tissue velocity	Many outcome data
Ejection fraction	2D	Tracing of endocardial border in apical 4-chamber and 2-chamber views at end-diastole and end-systole Modified Simpson rule (biplane method of disks)	Fewer geometric assumptions than for linear measurement Improved border detection with LV contrast No need for body size adjustment Well-established normal values Comparable values for adults of various sizes and ages	Load dependent Adequate image quality required Foreshortening often occurs 3-Chamber view not represented Different normal values with LV contrast	Many outcome data
Ejection fraction	3D	Automated border detection with different 3D software programs and manual adjustment if needed Alternatively, multiplanar reconstruction	Virtually no geometric assumptions Low interstudy variation Improved border detection with LV contrast No need for body size adjustment Validation against MRI	Load dependent Good image quality required Lower temporal and spatial resolution than 2D and much lower than linear measurement Normal values to be established	Few outcome data May provide superior outcome prediction than 2D ejection fraction
Global longitudinal strain	Speckle tracking	Automated border detection with different software programs and manual adjustment if needed Segmental myocardial deformation measured in 16- or 17-segment model	Largely angle independent Sensitive parameter for functional damage Useful when patient is used as own control	Load dependent Vendor dependent Good image quality required Severity partition values to be established	Many outcome data May provide more sensitive outcome prediction than 2D ejection fraction

Continued

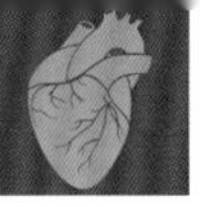

SUMMARY Summary Quantification of LV Size, Mass, and Function.—cont'd

Parameter	Method	Technique	Advantages	Limitations	Importance
Stroke volume	VTI (2D or 3D) method	LVOT area calculated from 2D LVOT diameter or traced in 3D LVOT view Stroke volume calculated by multiplying LVOT area with velocity–time integral obtained by placing the pulsed-wave Doppler sample volume in the LVOT in 5- or 3-chamber view Multiply stroke volume by heart rate to obtain cardiac output	Simple method Available in 2D and 3D	Load dependent Beat-to-beat variability in patients with abnormal rhythm LVOT area often underestimated by 2D method	Useful especially in ICU setting to adapt treatment
Stroke volume	Simpson method	Tracing of endocardial border in apical 4-chamber and 2-chamber views at end-diastole and end-systole Modified Simpson rule (biplane method of disks) for determining end-diastolic and end-systolic LV volume Stroke volume calculated by subtracting end-systolic from end-diastolic volume Multiply stroke volume by heart rate to obtain cardiac output	Simple method Available in 2D and 3D	Load dependent Beat-to-beat variability in patients with abnormal rhythm LV volumes often underestimated by 2D method	Useful especially in ICU setting to adapt treatment

EDDI, Indexed end-diastolic diameter; *ICU*, intensive care unit; *LVOT*, left ventricular outflow tract; *MAPSE*, mitral annulus plane systolic excursion; *MRI*, magnetic resonance imaging; *VTI*, velocity–time integral.

REFERENCES

1. Armstrong AC, Gidding S, Gjesdal O, Wu C, Bluemke DA, Lima JAC. LV mass assessed by echocardiography and CMR, cardiovascular outcomes, and medical practice. *JACC Cardiovasc Imaging.* 2012;5(8):837–848. https://doi.org/10.1016/j.jcmg.2012.06.003.
2. Douglas PS, Morrow R, Ioli A, Reichek N. Left ventricular shape, afterload and survival in idiopathic dilated cardiomyopathy. *J Am Coll Cardiol.* 1989;13(2):311–315. https://doi.org/10.1016/0735-1097(89)90504-4.
3. Lang RM, Badano LP, Mor-Avi V, et al. Recommendations for cardiac chamber quantification by echocardiography in adults: an update from the American Society of Echocardiography and the European Association of Cardiovascular Imaging. *J Am Soc Echocardiogr.* 2015;28(1):1–39. https://doi.org/10.1016/j.echo.2014.10.003. e14.
4. Ganau A, Devereux RB, Pickering TG, et al. Relation of left ventricular hemodynamic load and contractile performance to left ventricular mass in hypertension. *Circulation.* 1990;81(1):25–36. https://doi.org/10.1161/01.cir.81.1.25.
5. Feigenbaum H. Role of M-mode technique in today's echocardiography. *J Am Soc Echocardiogr.* 2010;23(3):240–247. https://doi.org/10.1016/j.echo.2010.01.015.
6. Marwick TH. The role of echocardiography in heart failure. *J Nucl Med.* 2015;56(suppl 4): 31S–38S. https://doi.org/10.2967/jnumed.114.150433.
7. McGowan JH, Cleland JGF. Reliability of reporting left ventricular systolic function by echocardiography: a systematic review of 3 methods. *Am Heart J.* 2003;146(3):388–397. https://doi.org/10.1016/S0002-8703(03)00248-5.
8. Moss AJ, Hall WJ, Cannom DS, et al. Cardiac-resynchronization therapy for the prevention of heart-failure events. *N Engl J Med.* 2009;361(14):1329–1338. https://doi.org/10.1056/NEJMoa0906431.
9. Somaratne JB, Berry C, McMurray JJV, Poppe KK, Doughty RN, Whalley GA. The prognostic significance of heart failure with preserved left ventricular ejection fraction: a literature-based meta-analysis. *Eur J Heart Fail.* 2009;11(9):855–862. https://doi.org/10.1093/eurjhf/hfp103.
10. Bristow MR, Kao DP, Breathett KK, et al. Structural and functional phenotyping of the failing heart: is the left ventricular ejection fraction obsolete? *JACC Heart Fail.* 2017;5(11):772–781. https://doi.org/10.1016/j.jchf.2017.09.009.
11. Deleted in review.
12. McManus DD, Shah SJ, Fabi MR, Rosen A, Whooley MA, Schiller NB. Prognostic value of left ventricular end-systolic volume index as a predictor of heart failure hospitalization in stable coronary artery disease: data from the Heart and Soul Study. *J Am Soc Echocardiogr.* 2009;22(2):190–197. https://doi.org/10.1016/j.echo.2008.11.005.
13. Shah BN, MacNab A, Lynch J, Hampson R, Senior R, Steeds RP. Stress echocardiography in contemporary clinical cardiology: practical considerations and accreditation. *Echo Res Pract.* 2018;5(1):E1–E6. https://doi.org/10.1530/ERP-17-0032.
14. Senior R, Becher H, Monaghan M, et al. Clinical practice of contrast echocardiography: recommendation by the European Association of Cardiovascular Imaging (EACVI) 2017. *Eur Heart J Cardiovasc Imaging.* 2017;18(11):1205. https://doi.org/10.1093/ehjci/jex182.
15. Kaku K, Takeuchi M, Otani K, et al. Age- and gender-dependency of left ventricular geometry assessed with real-time three-dimensional transthoracic echocardiography. *J Am Soc Echocardiogr.* 2011;24(5):541–547. https://doi.org/10.1016/j.echo.2011.01.011.

15a. Gebhard C, Stahli BE, Gebhard CE, et al. Age- and gender-dependent left ventricular remodeling. *Echocardiography.* 2013;30(10):1143–1150. https://doi.org/10.1111/echo.12264.

16. Dorosz JL, Lezotte DC, Weitzenkamp DA, Allen LA, Salcedo EE. Performance of 3-dimensional echocardiography in measuring left ventricular volumes and ejection frac-

tion: a systematic review and meta-analysis. *J Am Coll Cardiol*. 2012;59(20):1799–1808. https://doi.org/10.1016/j.jacc.2012.01.037.

17. Aune E, Baekkevar M, Rodevand O, Otterstad JE. Reference values for left ventricular volumes with real-time 3-dimensional echocardiography. *Scand Cardiovasc J*. 2010;44(1): 24–30. https://doi.org/10.3109/14017430903114446.
18. Chahal NS, Lim TK, Jain P, Chambers JC, Kooner JS, Senior R. Population-based reference values for 3D echocardiographic LV volumes and ejection fraction. *JACC Cardiovasc Imaging*. 2012;5(12):1191–1197. https://doi.org/10.1016/j.jcmg.2012.07.014.
19. Bernard A, Addetia K, Dulgheru R, et al. 3D echocardiographic reference ranges for normal left ventricular volumes and strain: results from the EACVI NORRE study. *Eur Heart J Cardiovasc Imaging*. 2017;18(4):475–483. https://doi.org/10.1093/ehjci/jew284.
20. Medvedofsky D, Maffessanti F, Weinert L, et al. 2D and 3D echocardiography-derived indices of left ventricular function and shape: relationship with mortality. *JACC Cardiovasc Imaging*. 2018;11(11):1569–1579. https://doi.org/10.1016/j.jcmg.2017.08.023.
21. Tamborini G, Piazzese C, Lang RM, et al. Feasibility and accuracy of automated software for transthoracic three-dimensional left ventricular volume and function analysis: comparisons with two-dimensional echocardiography, three-dimensional transthoracic manual method, and cardiac magnetic resonance imaging. *J Am Soc Echocardiogr*. 2017;30(11): 1049–1058. https://doi.org/10.1016/j.echo.2017.06.026.
22. Tsang W, Salgo IS, Medvedofsky D, et al. Transthoracic 3D echocardiographic left heart chamber quantification using an automated adaptive Analytics algorithm. *JACC Cardiovasc Imaging*. 2016;9(7):769–782. https://doi.org/10.1016/j.jcmg.2015.12.020.
23. Medvedofsky D, Mor-Avi V, Byku I, et al. Three-dimensional echocardiographic automated quantification of left heart chamber volumes using an adaptive analytics algorithm: feasibility and impact of image quality in nonselected patients. *J Am Soc Echocardiogr*. 2017;30(9):879–885. https://doi.org/10.1016/j.echo.2017.05.018.
24. Hoffmann R, Barletta G, von Bardeleben S, et al. Analysis of left ventricular volumes and function: a multicenter comparison of cardiac magnetic resonance imaging, cine ventriculography, and unenhanced and contrast-enhanced two-dimensional and three-dimensional echocardiography. *J Am Soc Echocardiogr*. 2014;27(3):292–301. https://doi.org/10.1016/j.echo.2013.12.005.
25. Kolla BC, Roy SS, Duval S, Weisdorf D, Valeti U, Blaes A. Cardiac imaging methods for chemotherapy-related cardiotoxicity screening and related radiation exposure: current practice and Trends. *Anticancer Res*. 2017;37(5):2445–2449. https://doi.org/10.21873/anticanres.11584.
26. Stahlberg M, Braunschweig F, Gadler F, Mortensen L, Lund LH, Linde C. Cardiac resynchronization therapy: results, challenges and perspectives for the future. *Scand Cardiovasc J*. 2016;50(5–6):282–292. https://doi.org/10.1080/14017431.2016.1221530.
27. Verdecchia P, Carini G, Circo A, et al. Left ventricular mass and cardiovascular morbidity in essential hypertension: the MAVI study. *J Am Coll Cardiol*. 2001;38(7):1829–1835.
28. Gardin JM, McClelland R, Kitzman D, et al. M-mode echocardiographic predictors of six- to seven-year incidence of coronary heart disease, stroke, congestive heart failure, and mortality in an elderly cohort (the Cardiovascular Health Study). *Am J Cardiol*. 2001;87(9):1051–1057. https://doi.org/10.1016/s0002-9149(01)01460-6.
29. Levy D, Garrison RJ, Savage DD, Kannel WB, Castelli WP. Prognostic implications of echocardiographically determined left ventricular mass in the Framingham Heart Study. *N Engl J Med*. 1990;322(22):1561–1566. https://doi.org/10.1056/NEJM199005313222203.
30. Mor-Avi V, Sugeng L, Weinert L, et al. Fast measurement of left ventricular mass with real-time three-dimensional echocardiography: comparison with magnetic resonance imaging. *Circulation*. 2004;110(13):1814–1818. https://doi.org/10.1161/01.CIR.0000142670.65971.5F.
31. Deague JA, Wilson CM, Grigg LE, Harrap SB. Discrepancies between echocardiographic measurements of left ventricular mass in a healthy adult population. *Clin Sci (Lond)*. 1999;97(3):377–383.
32. Devereux RB, Reichek N. Echocardiographic determination of left ventricular mass in man. Anatomic validation of the method. *Circulation*. 1977;55(4):613–618. https://doi.org/10.1161/01.cir.55.4.613.
33. Park SH, Shub C, Nobrega TP, Bailey KR, Seward JB. Two-dimensional echocardiographic calculation of left ventricular mass as recommended by the American Society of Echocardiography: correlation with autopsy and M-mode echocardiography. *J Am Soc Echocardiogr*. 1996;9(2):119–128.
34. Chuang ML, Beaudin RA, Riley MF, et al. Three-dimensional echocardiographic measurement of left ventricular mass: comparison with magnetic resonance imaging and two-dimensional echocardiographic determinations in man. *Int J Card Imaging*. 2000;16(5):347–357.
35. Canepa M, Malti O, David M, et al. Prevalence, clinical correlates, and functional impact of subaortic ventricular septal bulge (from the Baltimore Longitudinal Study of Aging). *Am J Cardiol*. 2014;114(5):796–802. https://doi.org/10.1016/j.amjcard.2014.05.068.
36. Marwick TH, Gillebert TC, Aurigemma G, et al. Recommendations on the use of echocardiography in adult hypertension: a report from the European Association of Cardiovascular Imaging (EACVI) and the American Society of Echocardiography (ASE). *Eur Heart J Cardiovasc Imaging*. 2015;16(6):577–605. https://doi.org/10.1093/ehjci/jev076.
37. Ganau A, Devereux RB, Roman MJ, et al. Patterns of left ventricular hypertrophy and geometric remodeling in essential hypertension. *J Am Coll Cardiol*. 1992;19(7):1550–1558.
38. Gaasch WH, Zile MR. Left ventricular structural remodeling in health and disease: with special emphasis on volume, mass, and geometry. *J Am Coll Cardiol*. 2011;58(17):1733–1740. https://doi.org/10.1016/j.jacc.2011.07.022.
39. Chirinos JA, Segers P, De Buyzere ML, et al. Left ventricular mass: allometric scaling, normative values, effect of obesity, and prognostic performance. *Hypertens (Dallas, Tex 1979*. 2010;56(1):91–98. https://doi.org/10.1161/HYPERTENSIONAHA.110.150250.
40. Mizukoshi K, Takeuchi M, Nagata Y, et al. Normal values of left ventricular mass index assessed by transthoracic three-dimensional echocardiography. *J Am Soc Echocardiogr*. 2016;29(1):51–61. https://doi.org/10.1016/j.echo.2015.09.009.
41. Fukuda S, Watanabe H, Daimon M, et al. Normal values of real-time 3-dimensional echocardiographic parameters in a healthy Japanese population: the JAMP-3D Study. *Circ J*. 2012;76(5):1177–1181. https://doi.org/10.1253/circj.cj-11-1256.
42. Muraru D, Badano LP, Peluso D, et al. Comprehensive analysis of left ventricular geometry and function by three-dimensional echocardiography in healthy adults. *J Am Soc Echocardiogr*. 2013;26(6):618–628. https://doi.org/10.1016/j.echo.2013.03.014.
43. St John Sutton MG, Plappert T, Crosby L, Douglas P, Mullen J, Reichek N. Effects of reduced left ventricular mass on chamber architecture, load, and function: a study of anorexia nervosa. *Circulation*. 1985;72(5):991–1000. https://doi.org/10.1161/01.cir.72.5.991.
44. Byrd 3rd BF, Wahr D, Wang YS, Bouchard A, Schiller NB. Left ventricular mass and volume/mass ratio determined by two-dimensional echocardiography in normal adults. *J Am Coll Cardiol*. 1985;6(5):1021–1025. https://doi.org/10.1016/s0735-1097(85)80304-1.
45. Oechslin E, Jenni R. Left ventricular non-compaction revisited: a distinct phenotype with genetic heterogeneity? *Eur Heart J*. 2011;32(12):1446–1456. https://doi.org/10.1093/eurheartj/ehq508.
46. Salgo IS, Tsang W, Ackerman W, et al. Geometric assessment of regional left ventricular remodeling by three-dimensional echocardiographic shape analysis correlates with left ventricular function. *J Am Soc Echocardiogr*. 2012;25(1):80–88. https://doi.org/10.1016/j.echo.2011.09.014.
47. Enache R, Popescu BA, Piazza R, et al. Left ventricular shape and mass impact torsional dynamics in asymptomatic patients with chronic aortic regurgitation and normal left ventricular ejection fraction. *Int J Cardiovasc Imaging*. 2015;31(7):1315–1326. https://doi.org/10.1007/s10554-015-0684-0.
48. Addetia K, Uriel N, Maffessanti F, et al. 3D Morphological changes in LV and RV during LVAD Ramp studies. *JACC Cardiovasc Imaging*. 2018;11(2 Pt 1):159–169. https://doi.org/10.1016/j.jcmg.2016.12.019.
49. St John Sutton M, Linde C, Gold MR, et al. Left ventricular architecture, long-term reverse remodeling, and clinical outcome in mild heart failure with cardiac resynchronization: results from the REVERSE trial. *JACC Heart Fail*. 2017;5(3):169–178. https://doi.org/10.1016/j.jchf.2016.11.012.
50. Gripari P, Tamborini G, Bottari V, et al. Three-dimensional transthoracic echocardiography in the comprehensive evaluation of right and left heart chamber remodeling following percutaneous mitral valve repair. *J Am Soc Echocardiogr*. 2016;29(10):946–954. https://doi.org/10.1016/j.echo.2016.06.009.
51. Schiros CG, Ahmed MI, Sanagala T, et al. Importance of three-dimensional geometric analysis in the assessment of the athlete's heart. *Am J Cardiol*. 2013;111(7):1067–1072. https://doi.org/10.1016/j.amjcard.2012.12.027.
52. Meng H, Li J-R, Sun X. Left ventricular apical hypoplasia: a case series and review of the literature. *Acta Cardiol*. 2013;68(3):339–342. https://doi.org/10.2143/AC.68.3.2983433.
53. Duraes AR, de Souza Lima Bitar Y, Roever L, Neto MG. Endomyocardial fibrosis: past, pre-

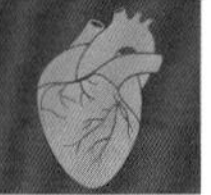

sent, and future. *Heart Fail Rev*. August 2019. https://doi.org/10.1007/s10741-019-09848-4.

54. Ikonomidis I, Varounis C, Paraskevaidis I, Parissis J, Lekakis J, Anastasiou-Nana M. Congenital left ventricular aneurysm: a cause of impaired myocardial torsion and peripheral thrombo-embolic events. *Eur J Echocardiogr*. 2011;12(2):E7. https://doi.org/10.1093/ejechocard/jeq103.
55. Megevand P, Vincenti GM, Carballo D, et al. A palpable source of stroke. *Circulation*. 2011;124(9):e232–e233. https://doi.org/10.1161/CIRCULATIONAHA.110.014431.
56. Sequeira V, van der Velden J. Historical perspective on heart function: the Frank-Starling Law. *Biophys Rev*. 2015;7(4):421–447. https://doi.org/10.1007/s12551-015-0184-4.
57. Crozatier B, Hittinger L. Mechanical adaptation to chronic pressure overload. *Eur Heart J*. 1988;9(Suppl E):7–11. https://doi.org/10.1093/eurheartj/9.suppl_e.7.
58. Nadruz W. Myocardial remodeling in hypertension. *J Hum Hypertens*. 2015;29(1):1–6. https://doi.org/10.1038/jhh.2014.36.

58a. Sengupta PP, Tajik AJ, Chandrasekaran K, Khandheria BK. Twist mechanics of the left ventricle: principles and application. *JACC Cardiovasc Imaging*. 2008;1(3):366–376. https://doi.org/10.1016/j.jcmg.2008.02.006.

59. Voigt J-U, Pedrizzetti G, Lysyansky P, et al. Definitions for a common standard for 2D speckle tracking echocardiography: consensus document of the EACVI/ASE/Industry Task Force to standardize deformation imaging. *Eur Heart J Cardiovasc Imaging*. 2015;16(1):1–11. https://doi.org/10.1093/ehjci/jeu184.
60. Stanton T, Leano R, Marwick TH. Prediction of all-cause mortality from global longitudinal speckle strain: comparison with ejection fraction and wall motion scoring. *Circ Cardiovasc Imaging*. 2009;2(5):356–364. https://doi.org/10.1161/CIRCIMAGING.109.862334.
61. Kou S, Caballero L, Dulgheru R, et al. Echocardiographic reference ranges for normal cardiac chamber size: results from the NORRE study. *Eur Heart J Cardiovasc Imaging*. 2014;15(6):680–690. https://doi.org/10.1093/ehjci/jet284.
62. Deleted in review.
63. Baumgartner H, Falk V, Bax JJ, et al. ESC/EACTS Guidelines for the management of valvular heart disease. *Eur Heart J*. 2017;38(36):2739–2791. https://doi.org/10.1093/eurheartj/ehx391. 2017.
64. Carabello BA, Green LH, Grossman W, Cohn LH, Koster JK, Collins JJJ. Hemodynamic determinants of prognosis of aortic valve replacement in critical aortic stenosis and advanced congestive heart failure. *Circulation*. 1980;62(1):42–48. https://doi.org/10.1161/01.cir.62.1.42.
65. Sutton M, Plappert T, Spiegel A, et al. Early postoperative changes in left ventricular chamber size, architecture, and function in aortic stenosis and aortic regurgitation and their relation to intraoperative changes in afterload: a prospective two-dimensional echocardiographic study. *Circulation*. 1987;76(1):77–89. https://doi.org/10.1161/01.cir.76.1.77.
66. Rihal CS, Nishimura RA, Hatle LK, Bailey KR, Tajik AJ. Systolic and diastolic dysfunction in patients with clinical diagnosis of dilated cardiomyopathy. Relation to symptoms and prognosis. *Circulation*. 1994;90(6):2772–2779. https://doi.org/10.1161/01.cir.90.6.2772.
67. Solomon SD, Anavekar N, Skali H, et al. Influence of ejection fraction on cardiovascular outcomes in a broad spectrum of heart failure patients. *Circulation*. 2005;112(24):3738–3744. https://doi.org/10.1161/CIRCULATIONAHA.105.561423.
68. Templin C, Ghadri JR, Diekmann J, et al. Clinical features and outcomes of takotsubo (stress) cardiomyopathy. *N Engl J Med*. 2015;373(10):929–938. https://doi.org/10.1056/NEJMoa1406761.
69. Stahli BE, Stadler T, Holy EW, et al. Impact of stroke volume assessment by integrating multi-detector computed tomography and Doppler data on the classification of aortic stenosis. *Int J Cardiol*. 2017;246:80–86. https://doi.org/10.1016/j.ijcard.2017.03.112.
70. Kamperidis V, van Rosendael PJ, Katsanos S, et al. Low gradient severe aortic stenosis with preserved ejection fraction: reclassification of severity by fusion of Doppler and computed tomographic data. *Eur Heart J*. 2015;36(31):2087–2096. https://doi.org/10.1093/eurheartj/ehv188.
71. Zhou YQ, Faerestrand S, Matre K. Velocity distributions in the left ventricular outflow tract in patients with valvular aortic stenosis. Effect on the measurement of aortic valve area by using the continuity equation. *Eur Heart J*. 1995;16(3):383–393. https://doi.org/10.1093/oxfordjournals.eurheartj.a060922.
72. Baumgartner HC, Hung JC-C, Bermejo J, et al. Recommendations on the echocardiographic assessment of aortic valve stenosis: a focused update from the European Association of Cardiovascular Imaging and the American Society of Echocardiography. *Eur Heart J Cardiovasc Imaging*. 2017;18(3):254–275. https://doi.org/10.1093/ehjci/jew335.
73. Stanton T, Jenkins C, Haluska BA, Marwick TH. Association of outcome with left ventricular parameters measured by two-dimensional and three-dimensional echocardiography in patients at high cardiovascular risk. *J Am Soc Echocardiogr*. 2014;27(1):65–73. https://doi.org/10.1016/j.echo.2013.09.012.
74. Reisner SA, Lysyansky P, Agmon Y, Mutlak D, Lessick J, Friedman Z. Global longitudinal strain: a novel index of left ventricular systolic function. *J Am Soc Echocardiogr*. 2004;17(6):630–633. https://doi.org/10.1016/j.echo.2004.02.011.
75. Yingchoncharoen T, Agarwal S, Popovic ZB, Marwick TH. Normal ranges of left ventricular strain: a meta-analysis. *J Am Soc Echocardiogr*. 2013;26(2):185–191. https://doi.org/10.1016/j.echo.2012.10.008.
76. Tadic M, Pieske-Kraigher E, Cuspidi C, et al. Left ventricular strain and twisting in heart failure with preserved ejection fraction: an updated review. *Heart Fail Rev*. 2017;22(3):371–379. https://doi.org/10.1007/s10741-017-9618-3.
77. Amano M, Izumi C, Nishimura S, et al. Predictors of prognosis in light-chain amyloidosis and chronological changes in cardiac morphology and function. *Am J Cardiol*. 2017;120(11):2041–2048. https://doi.org/10.1016/j.amjcard.2017.08.024.
78. Nagata Y, Takeuchi M, Wu VC-C, et al. Prognostic value of LV deformation parameters using 2D and 3D speckle-tracking echocardiography in asymptomatic patients with severe aortic stenosis and preserved LV ejection fraction. *JACC Cardiovasc Imaging*. 2015;8(3):235–245. https://doi.org/10.1016/j.jcmg.2014.12.009.
79. Hu K, Liu D, Herrmann S, et al. Clinical implication of mitral annular plane systolic excursion for patients with cardiovascular disease. *Eur Heart J Cardiovasc Imaging*. 2013;14(3):205–212. https://doi.org/10.1093/ehjci/jes240.
80. Bargiggia GS, Bertucci C, Recusani F, et al. A new method for estimating left ventricular dP/dt by continuous wave Doppler-echocardiography. Validation studies at cardiac catheterization. *Circulation*. 1989;80(5):1287–1292. https://doi.org/10.1161/01.cir.80.5.1287.
81. Rhodes J, Udelson JE, Marx GR, et al. A new noninvasive method for the estimation of peak dP/dt. *Circulation*. 1993;88(6):2693–2699. https://doi.org/10.1161/01.cir.88.6.2693.
82. McKay RG, Aroesty JM, Heller GV, et al. Left ventricular pressure-volume diagrams and end-systolic pressure-volume relations in human beings. *J Am Coll Cardiol*. 1984;3(2 Pt 1):301–312. https://doi.org/10.1016/s0735-1097(84)80013-3.
83. Aurigemma GP, Gaasch WH, Villegas B, Meyer TE. Noninvasive assessment of left ventricular mass, chamber volume, and contractile function. *Curr Probl Cardiol*. 1995;20(6):361–440.
84. Manganaro R, Marchetta S, Dulgheru R, et al. Echocardiographic reference ranges for normal non-invasive myocardial work indices: results from the EACVI NORRE study. *Eur Heart J Cardiovasc Imaging*. 2019;20(5):582–590. https://doi.org/10.1093/ehjci/jey188.
85. Ohlow M-A, von Korn H, Lauer B. Characteristics and outcome of congenital left ventricular aneurysm and diverticulum: analysis of 809 cases published since 1816. *Int J Cardiol*. 2015;185:34–45. https://doi.org/10.1016/j.ijcard.2015.03.050.
86. Cresti A, Cannarile P, Aldi E, et al. Multimodality imaging and clinical significance of congenital ventricular outpouchings: recesses, diverticula, aneurysms, clefts, and crypts. *J Cardiovasc Echogr*. 2018;28(1):9–17. https://doi.org/10.4103/jcecho.jcecho_72_17.
87. Cagli K, Golbasi Z, Turak O, Ozeke O, Ekizler FA. 3D echocardiographic imaging of a septal myocardial cleft in hypertrophic cardiomyopathy. *Echocardiography*. 2016;33(12):1929–1930. https://doi.org/10.1111/echo.13343.
88. Simonson JS, Schiller NB. Descent of the base of the left ventricle: an echocardiographic index of left ventricular function. *J Am Soc Echocardiogr*. 1989;2(1):25–35.
89. Wandt B, Bojo L, Hatle L, Wranne B. Left ventricular contraction pattern changes with age in normal adults. *J Am Soc Echocardiogr*. 1998;11(9):857–863.
90. Aurigemma GP, Silver KH, Priest MA, Gaasch WH. Geometric changes allow normal ejection fraction despite depressed myocardial shortening in hypertensive left ventricular hypertrophy. *J Am Coll Cardiol*. 1995;26(1):195–202.
91. Xiao HB, Kaleem S, McCarthy C, Rosen SD. Abnormal regional left ventricular mechanics in treated hypertensive patients with "normal left ventricular function". *Int J Cardiol*. 2006;112(3):316–321. https://doi.org/10.1016/j.ijcard.2005.10.001.
92. Willenheimer R, Rydberg E, Stagmo M, Gudmundsson P, Ericsson G, Erhardt L. Echocardiographic assessment of left atrioventricular plane displacement as a complement to left ventricular regional wall motion evaluation in the detection of myocardial dysfunction. *Int J Cardiovasc Imaging*. 2002;18(3):181–186.
93. Weidemann F, Herrmann S, Stork S, et al. Impact of myocardial fibrosis in patients with symptomatic severe aortic stenosis. *Circulation*. 2009;120(7):577–584. https://doi.org/10.1161/CIRCULATIONAHA.108.847772.

94. Wenzelburger FWG, Tan YT, Choudhary FJ, Lee ESP, Leyva F, Sanderson JE. Mitral annular plane systolic excursion on exercise: a simple diagnostic tool for heart failure with preserved ejection fraction. *Eur J Heart Fail.* 2011;13(9):953–960. https://doi.org/10.1093/eurjhf/hfr081.
95. Nikitin NP, Witte KKA, Thackray SDR, de Silva R, Clark AL, Cleland JGF. Longitudinal ventricular function: normal values of atrioventricular annular and myocardial velocities measured with quantitative two-dimensional color Doppler tissue imaging. *J Am Soc Echocardiogr.* 2003;16(9):906–921. https://doi.org/10.1016/S0894-7317(03)00279-7.
96. Mondillo S, Galderisi M, Ballo P, Marino PN. Left ventricular systolic longitudinal function: comparison among simple M-mode, pulsed, and M-mode color tissue Doppler of mitral annulus in healthy individuals. *J Am Soc Echocardiogr.* 2006;19(9):1085–1091. https://doi.org/10.1016/j.echo.2006.04.005.
97. Gulati VK, Katz WE, Follansbee WP, Gorcsan 3rd J. Mitral annular descent velocity by tissue Doppler echocardiography as an index of global left ventricular function. *Am J Cardiol.* 1996;77(11):979–984. https://doi.org/10.1016/s0002-9149(96)00033-1.
98. Duzenli MA, Ozdemir K, Aygul N, Altunkeser BB, Zengin K, Sizer M. Relationship between systolic myocardial velocity obtained by tissue Doppler imaging and left ventricular ejection fraction: systolic myocardial velocity predicts the degree of left ventricular dysfunction in heart failure. *Echocardiography.* 2008;25(8):856–863. https://doi.org/10.1111/j.1540--8175.2008.00694.x.
99. Kadappu KK, Thomas L. Tissue Doppler imaging in echocardiography: value and limitations. *Heart Lung Circ.* 2015;24(3):224–233. https://doi.org/10.1016/j.hlc.2014.10.003.
100. Dini FL, Galderisi M, Nistri S, et al. Abnormal left ventricular longitudinal function assessed by echocardiographic and tissue Doppler imaging is a powerful predictor of diastolic dysfunction in hypertensive patients: the SPHERE study. *Int J Cardiol.* 2013;168(4):3351–3358. https://doi.org/10.1016/j.ijcard.2013.04.122.
101. Correale M, Totaro A, Ieva R, Ferraretti A, Musaico F, Di Biase M. Tissue Doppler imaging in coronary artery diseases and heart failure. *Curr Cardiol Rev.* 2012;8(1):43–53.
102. Fang ZY, Schull-Meade R, Leano R, Mottram PM, Prins JB, Marwick TH. Screening for heart disease in diabetic subjects. *Am Heart J.* 2005;149(2):349–354. https://doi.org/10.1016/j.ahj.2004.06.021.
103. Nagueh SF, Bachinski LL, Meyer D, et al. Tissue Doppler imaging consistently detects myocardial abnormalities in patients with hypertrophic cardiomyopathy and provides a novel means for an early diagnosis before and independently of hypertrophy. *Circulation.* 2001;104(2):128–130. https://doi.org/10.1161/01.cir.104.2.128.

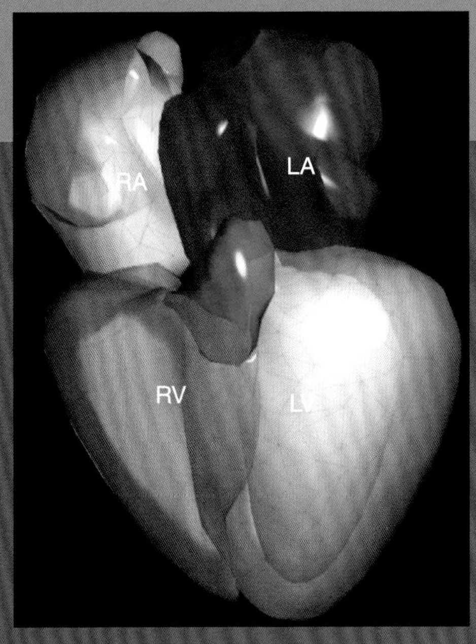

中文导读

第5章 左心室舒张功能

正常左心室舒张功能被定义为无论在静息或运动状态下，正常左心室充盈压状态下左心室能够充分充盈，并提供正常每搏容量的能力。左心室松弛、顺应性和左心房收缩是左心房和左心室之间驱动压力和左心室充盈的关键决定因素。左心室舒张功能不全的机制非常复杂，评估左心室舒张功能要同时考虑各个参数受年龄、血流动力学状态和伴发病变的影响，从而对特定情况下各个参数值进行综合及个体化的解读。

左心室舒张功能不全在心力衰竭的病理生理过程中起重要作用，是诊断左室射血分数保存型心力衰竭的重要依据，对有呼吸困难或心力衰竭的患者来说，评估左心室舒张功能是整个心脏功能评估中至关重要的环节。作为评估左心室舒张功能的一线影像学手段，超声心动图能够为左心室舒张功能评估提供相关的结构和功能信息。常规二维超声及多普勒超声可以反映心脏结构和功能异常，斑点追踪超声、负荷超声、三维超声和人工智能等新技术的发展为左心室舒张功能的评估提供了进一步的信息和更广阔的前景。

吴伟春

5 Left Ventricular Diastolic Function

BOGDAN A. POPESCU, MD, PhD | CARMEN C. BELADAN, MD, PhD

Left ventricular diastolic dysfunction (LVDD) plays a major role in the pathophysiology of heart failure (HF). From a practical perspective, LV diastolic function assessment is particularly useful when evaluating patients with dyspnea of suspected or known cardiac origin.

In patients with dyspnea and preserved LV ejection fraction (EF), the identification of LVDD offers the pathophysiologic basis for diagnosing HF with preserved ejection fraction (HFpEF), which is believed to account for about half of all HF cases and to have similar or even worse prognosis than HF with reduced ejection fraction (HFrEF).[1] Furthermore, noninvasive estimates of LV filling pressures (LVFPs) can be used to determine the hemodynamic status, provide prognostic information, and guide therapy in all patients with HF, irrespective of LVEF.

Echocardiography is the noninvasive diagnostic method that is most widely available, safe, and cost-effective; it is able to provide structural and functional information relevant to assessment of diastolic function (i.e., markers of LVDD and/or elevated LVFP).

This chapter summarizes the current status and role of echocardiography in assessment of diastolic function and discusses gaps in evidence and future perspectives.

PHYSIOLOGY OF DIASTOLE

Diastole is defined as the time interval between aortic valve closure and mitral valve (MV) closure. It comprises four phases: isovolumic relaxation, rapid filling, diastasis (with slow filling), and filling during atrial contraction[2] (Fig. 5.1).[3]

Normal diastolic function is defined as the ability of the LV to fill adequately to provide a normal stroke volume at normal LVFP, both at rest and during exercise. LV relaxation, compliance, and left atrial (LA) contraction are key determinants of the driving pressure between the LA and the LV and of LV filling. In young, healthy individuals, most LV filling occurs in early diastole, during the rapid filling period.[4]

With impaired LV relaxation and increased wall stiffness, filling progressively shifts to late diastole, and therefore the atrial contribution to cardiac output increases. The atrial contribution to LV filling may increase from about 20% in young, healthy individuals with robust LV suction to about 40% in elderly subjects with alterations of LV relaxation and compliance.[5]

Separation of the cardiac cycle into two distinct phases—systole and diastole—may be well suited for academic purposes, but studies of cardiac mechanics emphasize that diastolic filling cannot be separated from the previous systole, and the two phases are linked with each other. Myocardial relaxation starts in systole, before aortic valve closure, and continues through isovolumic relaxation and early filling. Release of the potential energy stored during systolic twisting promotes subsequent elastic recoil and untwisting.[6]

Apical clockwise rotation, which is mainly responsible for early diastolic filling, begins in late systole and extends into the first third of diastole.[7] Ventricular untwisting precedes diastolic lengthening and expansion of myocardial fibers; it is responsible for the early diastolic base-to-apex pressure gradients and for diastolic suction. The brisk untwist leads to a rapid decrease in early diastolic LV pressure and to MV opening with rapid filling.[8] Blood flows into the LV until the pressures in the left chambers equalize, resulting in diastasis.

In normal hearts, increased LV contractility and smaller end-systolic volume (e.g., with exercise, inotropes) lead to a stronger recoil that begets more rapid early diastolic filling.[6,8] Alterations of the temporal sequence between twisting and recoil that result in prolonged systolic twisting and delayed and shortened recoil are associated with impaired LV filling in patients with aortic stenosis, hypertrophic cardiomyopathy (HCM), ischemia, and age-related changes.[7,9–11]

The traditional concept that diastolic dysfunction precedes systolic dysfunction has been questioned and replaced with the more likely hypothesis that LV systolic and diastolic dysfunction usually coexist. Consequently, it is recommended that LV systolic function parameters be considered when assessing diastolic function.

In conclusion, LVDD is usually the result of abnormal LV relaxation, with or without reduced restoring forces (responsible for early diastolic suction), and increased LV chamber stiffness.[12]

INVASIVE EVALUATION OF LV DIASTOLIC FUNCTION

Cardiac catheterization is the gold standard for demonstrating abnormalities of LV relaxation, compliance, and filling by direct measurements of the LV relaxation time constant (τ), stiffness modulus, and LVFP.

The term "LV filling pressures" has been widely and indiscriminately used in cardiology with respect to any of the following invasive measurements: mean pulmonary capillary wedge pressure (PCWP), mean LA pressure (LAP), LV pre-A pressure (before atrial contraction), mean LV diastolic pressure (M-LVDP), and LV end-diastolic pressure (LVEDP) (Fig. 5.2).[13] Although these pressures correlate with each other, there are important pathophysiologic differences between them.[12] These differences need to be acknowledged when assessing different echocardiographic parameters in relation to diastolic abnormalities. Moreover, significant effects on the performance of various diagnostic algorithms for LVDD evaluation are expected when using a specific filling pressure as a reference.

In the clinical setting, the LVFPs most often measured invasively are the LVEDP, which is obtained by left heart catheterization, and the PCWP (an indirect estimate of mean LAP), which is obtained by right heart catheterization. Filling pressure is considered to be elevated when the mean PCWP is >12 mmHg or the LVEDP is >16 mmHg.[14]

Invasive measurements are impractical for daily routine. However, catheterization remains the gold standard whenever noninvasive measurements are inconclusive.

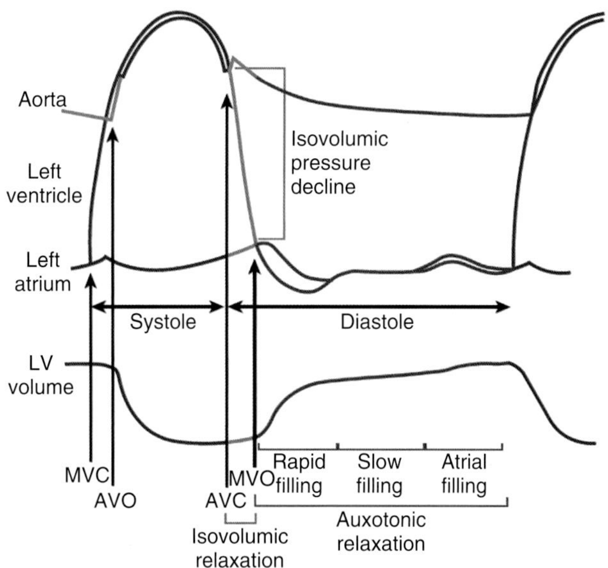

Fig. 5.1 Physiology of diastole. Changes in LV pressure and volume during the cardiac cycle. Diastole represents the time from AVC to MVC. It comprises isovolumic LV relaxation (period from AVC to MVO), during which LV pressure declines without a change in volume, and auxotonic relaxation (period from MVO to MVC), during which LV filling occurs and LV volume increases at variable pressure. The period of LV filling has three subphases: (1) early rapid filling, which occurs as a result of the pressure gradient between the LA and the LV; (2) diastasis (slow filling), in which relatively equal LA and LV pressures result in minimal to no flow across the mitral valve; and (3) atrial filling, during which LV filling occurs as a result of atrial contraction. *AVC,* Aortic valve closure; *AVO,* aortic valve opening; *MVC,* mitral valve closure; *MVO,* mitral valve opening. (Adapted from Bonnema DD, Baicu C, Zile MR. Pathophysiology of diastolic heart failure: relaxation and stiffness. In: Klein AL, Garcia MJ, eds. *Diastology: Clinical Approach to Diastolic Heart Failure.* Philadelphia, PA: Saunders; 2008.)

ECHOCARDIOGRAPHIC ASSESSMENT OF DIASTOLIC FUNCTION

BASIC PRINCIPLES

Echocardiography is the first-line imaging modality for assessment of LV diastolic function in clinical practice. A large number of echocardiographic parameters have been tested and validated for their correlation with invasively measured diastolic function determinants, but none of them is accurate enough to be used as a single diagnostic marker for LVDD.

The assessment of diastolic function should always be placed in the clinical context of the individual patient. Attention should be directed to any clinical information that is relevant for the diagnosis of LVDD or HF (e.g., signs or symptoms of HF, obesity, history of hypertension, coronary artery disease, diabetes, chronic kidney disease), including specific settings that may require personalization of the general algorithm for diastolic function evaluation (e.g., atrial fibrillation [AF], conduction abnormalities, paced rhythm).

Two-dimensional (2D) echocardiography may identify structural abnormalities of the heart (e.g., LV hypertrophy, LA dilation) that represent either the cause or the consequence of LVDD and reflect its severity and/or duration. The presence of such abnormalities increases the likelihood of LVDD, and these parameters are generally more stable than Doppler parameters.

Doppler echocardiography can identify functional abnormalities, providing further information regarding LV diastolic properties and LVFP. Discerning whether the main driver of LVDD is abnormal LV relaxation or decreased compliance is relevant with respect to LVDD etiology.

LV volumes and LVEF, measured according to current recommendations,[15] provide key information when assessing LV diastolic function. In patients with dilated ventricles and reduced LVEF, LVDD is presumed to be present, and the main question relates to the level of LVFP. In patients with normal LV

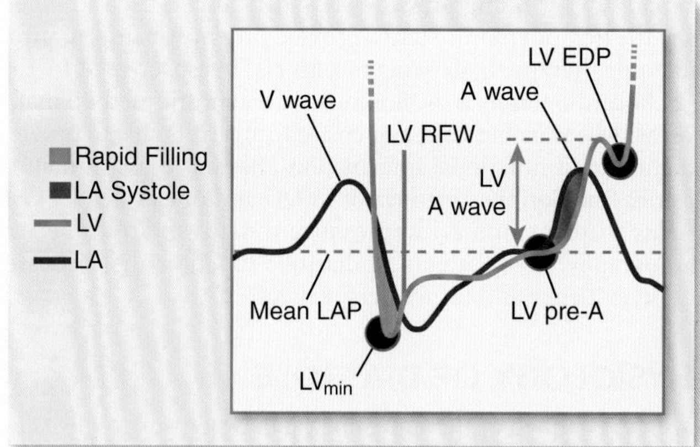

Fig. 5.2 Left ventricular filling pressures. Recording of LV diastolic pressures *(pink line)* shows LV minimal pressure *(LV_{min})*, LV rapid filling wave *(RFW)*, LV pre-A pressure *(pre-A)*, the LV A-wave rise with atrial contraction *(arrows)*, and LV end-diastolic pressure *(EDP)*. Recording of left atrial pressures (LAP; *dark blue line*) shows the peak *V wave* (highest LAP at end-systole) and peak *A wave* (rise of LV pressure when the LA contracts). In a normal LV, the early diastolic pressure gradient *(blue area)* leads to peak early diastolic mitral inflow velocity (E). In late diastole, the LA contracts with the rise in LAP (A wave), and another positive pressure gradient occurs *(orange area)*, leading to mitral inflow A velocity. Mean LAP is lower than the V-wave and A-wave pressures. (Adapted from Nagueh SF. Left ventricular diastolic function: understanding pathophysiology, diagnosis, and prognosis with echocardiography. *JACC: Cardiovasc Imag.* 2020;13[1 Pt 2]:228–244.)

volumes and normal LVEF, a comprehensive evaluation of all the structural and functional abnormalities relevant for LVDD is necessary.

The Doppler echocardiographic parameters used to assess LV diastolic function perform differently in patients with reduced LVEF than in those with preserved LVEF.

CONVENTIONAL ECHOCARDIOGRAPHIC PARAMETERS OF DIASTOLIC FUNCTION

Mitral Inflow Parameters

The mitral inflow signal recorded by pulsed-wave (PW) echocardiography represented for many years the cornerstone of diastolic function assessment.[16]

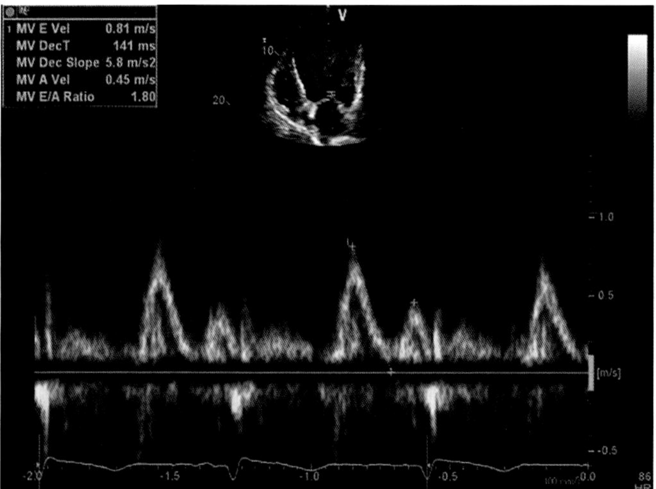

Fig. 5.3 Mitral inflow by pulsed-wave Doppler echocardiography. Recording of mitral inflow shows a short E-wave deceleration time (141 ms) in a patient with reduced LV ejection fraction. This combination (i.e., a pseudonormal filling pattern) is highly suggestive for increased LV filling pressure.

Mitral Inflow Patterns

In young, healthy individuals, the peak velocity of the E wave exceeds that of the A wave because most of the LV filling occurs during the rapid filling phase and is driven by ventricular suction (E/A ratio >1). With delayed relaxation (e.g., in elderly patients), the early diastolic pressure gradient is reduced and the contribution of atrial contraction to LV filling is increased (E/A ratio <1), leading to an *impaired relaxation* pattern, with prolonged isovolumic relaxation time (IVRT) and E-wave deceleration time (EDT). Further alteration of LV relaxation requires a compensatory increase in LAP to preserve cardiac output. In such cases, the E/A ratio appears normal again (E/A ratio >1): this is the *pseudonormal* (PN) filling pattern.

Progression of LVDD results in a tall E wave with marked shortening of the EDT (i.e., early filling driven by elevated LAP with rapid equilibration of LA and LV diastolic pressures in the noncompliant LV) and a reduced A wave (i.e., high LV diastolic pressure). The *restrictive* filling pattern (E/A ratio >2) is a negative prognostic marker in patients with HF[17] (Fig. 5.3).

The opposing effects of impaired relaxation and increased LVFP on the E/A ratio explain its parabolic distribution (U-shaped curve) along the transition from normal function to severe LVDD[18] (Fig. 5.4). Deciding whether a patient is on the "good" left side (normal pattern) or on the "bad" right side (PN pattern) of the curve sometimes requires additional information.[19]

Because of their high load dependency, mitral inflow parameters reflect a snapshot of the hemodynamic relationship between LA and LV pressures rather than an evolutive stage of LVDD.

Loading conditions and aging are important factors that influence the mitral inflow parameters and need to be taken into account when evaluating diastolic function. The reference values of mitral inflow parameters according to age and gender are presented in Table 5.1.[20,21]

The load dependency of mitral inflow parameters can be overcome by performing a standardized *Valsalva maneuver*. This can effectively unload the heart, helping to distinguish

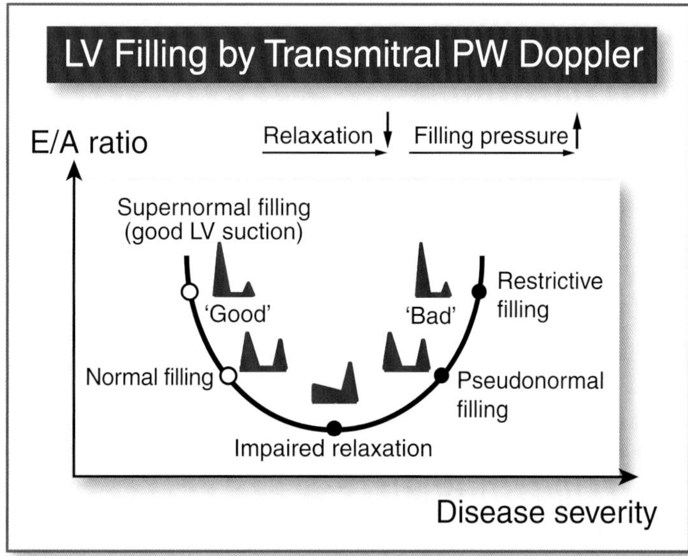

Fig. 5.4 Changes in mitral inflow pattern during progression of LVDD. The mitral inflow pattern describes a parabolic distribution (U-shaped curve) during progression from normal LV diastolic function to severe diastolic dysfunction. *E/A ratio*, Ratio of E-wave to A-wave peak velocity; *LVDD*, LV diastolic dysfunction; *PW*, pulsed-wave.

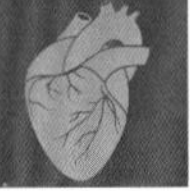

TABLE 5.1 **Reference Ranges for Conventional Doppler Flow Parameters of LV Diastolic Function.**[a]

	Mitral E (cm/s)	*Mitral A (cm/s)*	*E/A Ratio*	*EDT (ms)*	*IVRT (ms)*	*Pulm S (cm/s)*	*Pulm D (cm/s)*	*Pulm S/D Ratio*
Female								
Feasibility, no. (%)	657 (99)	657 (99)	657 (99)	657 (99)	653 (98)	646 (98)	637 (96)	635 (96)
<40 yr (*n* = 208)	80 ± 16	48 ± 15	1.85 ± 0.76	212 ± 55	85 ± 16	58 ± 12	55 ± 11	1.09 ± 0.31
40–60 yr (*n* = 336)	74 ± 15	59 ± 15	1.32 ± 0.40	220 ± 66	95 ± 20	59 ± 12	48 ± 12	1.29 ± 0.35
>60 yr (*n* = 119)	69 ± 16	75 ± 18	0.96 ± 0.32	244 ± 79	105 ± 23	62 ± 12	43 ± 11	1.51 ± 0.39
All (*n* = 663)	75 ± 16	58 ± 18	1.42 ± 0.62	218 ± 66	93 ± 21	59 ± 12	49 ± 12	1.26 ± 0.37
Male								
Feasibility, no. (%)	599 (99)	599 (99)	599 (99)	599 (99)	597 (99)	583 (97)	583 (97)	578 (96)
<40 yr (*n* = 126)	75 ± 15	44 ± 14	1.86 ± 0.64	217 ± 65	91 ± 17	52 ± 11	55 ± 12	0.99 ± 0.29
40–60 yr (*n* = 327)	64 ± 15	52 ± 14	1.30 ± 0.42	232 ± 81	100 ± 21	55 ± 11	47 ± 11	1.22 ± 0.31
>60 yr (*n* = 150)	61 ± 14	65 ± 18	0.99 ± 0.34	269 ± 97	118 ± 29	62 ± 13	43 ± 11	1.50 ± 0.40
All (*n* = 603)	66 ± 15	54 ± 17	1.34 ± 0.54	238 ± 85	103 ± 24	56 ± 12	48 ± 12	1.23 ± 0.37

[a]Data are presented as mean ± SD for Doppler flow velocities from 1266 healthy individuals by sex and age, unless otherwise indicated.

E/A ratio, Ratio of early to atrial peak filling velocity; *EDT,* E-wave deceleration time; *IVRT,* isovolumic relaxation time; *Pulm D,* peak diastolic pulmonary velocity; *Pulm S,* peak systolic pulmonary velocity.

Data from Dalen H, Thorstensen A, Vatten LJ, et al. Reference values and distribution of conventional echocardiographic Doppler measures and longitudinal tissue Doppler velocities in a population free from cardiovascular disease. *Circ Cardiovasc Imaging.* 2010;3:614–622; Hurrell DG, Nishimura RA, Ilstrup DM, Appleton CP. Utility of preload alteration in assessment of left ventricular filling pressure by Doppler echocardiography: a simultaneous catheterization and Doppler echocardiographic study. *J Am Coll Cardiol.* 1997;30:459–467.

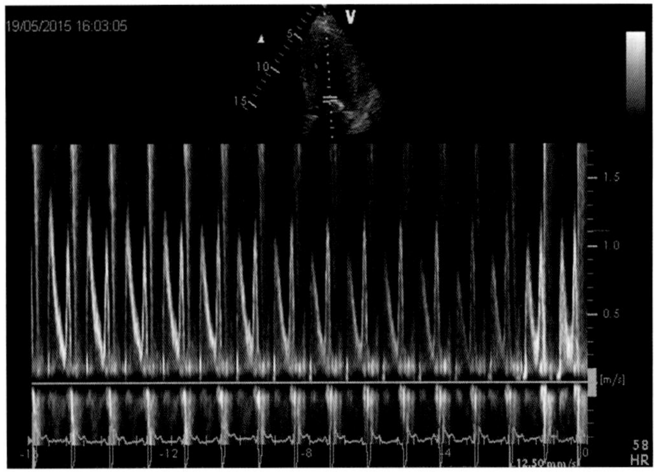

Fig. 5.5 Changes in mitral inflow pattern during the Valsava maneuver. Continuous recording of mitral inflow with pulsed-wave Doppler imaging during Valsalva maneuver. The E/A ratio decreases from 1.2 at baseline to 0.7, and the A-wave velocity increases, both of which are highly suggestive for elevated LV filling pressures.

normal LV filling from PN filling (Fig. 5.5), reveal whether restrictive LV filling is reversible or not, and unmask high LVFP in patients with an impaired relaxation pattern at baseline.[22,23]

A decrease in E/A ratio of ≥50% during Valsalva maneuver is highly specific for increased LVFP.[24] The procedure should be standardized by continuous recording of the mitral inflow using PW Doppler echocardiography during the straining phase of the maneuver, with the patient blowing into a sphygmomanometer to raise the pressure to 40 mmHg and keep it stable at that level for 10 seconds.[25] Valsalva maneuver is not easy to perform in every patient and cannot be applied in critically ill or intubated patients.

The utility, advantages, and limitations of mitral flow parameters for evaluation of LV diastolic function are summarized in Table 5.2.[12]

Pulmonary Venous Flow Parameters

Evaluation of pulmonary venous (PV) flow provides further information about LV diastolic function. Normal PV flow has two forward waves, S (systolic) and D (diastolic), and a reversal wave (Ar) at the time of atrial contraction. In normal subjects, the systolic-to-diastolic flow ratio (S/D) is usually >1, and the Ar wave is usually small (Fig. 5.6).

With LVDD, as LV compliance decreases and LAP increases, there is blunting of the S wave and a decrease the systolic filling fraction. Conversely, the D wave becomes more prominent, with shortened deceleration time, while Ar duration and velocity increase.[26–28] A D-wave deceleration time >220 msec has excellent accuracy in predicting a normal PCWP in patients with AF.[29]

PV flow parameters are also influenced by loading conditions and aging. The reference values for PV flow parameters according to age and gender are presented in Table 5.1, and their advantages and limitations are shown in Table 5.2.

Color M-Mode Echocardiography

Color M-mode echocardiography allows interrogation of the flow filling the LV in diastole, from LV base to the apex. Normally, patients in sinus rhythm have two waves of color flow in diastole. The first wave (E), from the mitral annulus to the apex, represents the early LV filling driven by the basal-apical intraventricular diastolic pressure gradient, and the second wave (A) corresponds to atrial contraction and normally does not exceed the middle portion of the LV.

The propagation velocity (Vp) of the E wave has emerged as an index of LV relaxation: the slower the relaxation, the lower the Vp.[30] It can be assessed by measuring the slope of the early filling wave (Fig. 5.7). A Vp <50 cm/s suggests the presence of LVDD. Vp decreases progressively with LVDD and does not undergo the phenomenon of pseudonormalization.

The propagation velocity can be falsely normal despite LVDD in patients with preserved LVEF and LVH/small LV volume. Because of these limitations and a lower reproducibility,

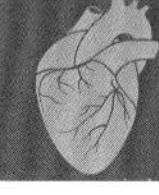

TABLE 5.2 Utility, Advantages, and Limitations of Parameters Used to Assess LV Diastolic Function.

Parameter	*Utility and Physiologic Background*	*Advantages*	*Limitations*
Mitral E velocity (PW Doppler)	E-wave velocity reflects the LA–LV pressure gradient during early diastole and is affected by alterations in rate of LV relaxation and LAP.	1. Feasible and reproducible. 2. In patients with DCM and reduced LVEF, mitral velocities correlate better with LVFPs, functional class, and prognosis than LVEF does.	1. In patients with CAD and patients with HCM in whom LVEF is >50%, mitral velocities correlate poorly with LVFPs. 2. More challenging to apply in patients with arrhythmias. 3. Directly affected by alterations in LV volumes and elastic recoil. 4. Age-dependent (decreases with aging).
Mitral A velocity (PW Doppler)	A-wave velocity reflects the LA–LV pressure gradient during late diastole, which is affected by LV compliance and LA contractile function.	Feasible and reproducible	1. Sinus tachycardia, first-degree AV block, and paced rhythm can result in fusion of the E and A waves. If mitral flow velocity at the start of atrial contraction is >20 cm/s, A velocity may be increased. 2. Not applicable in patients with AF or atrial flutter. 3. Age-dependent (increases with aging).
Mitral E/A ratio	Mitral inflow E/A ratio and EDT are used to identify the filling patterns: normal, impaired relaxation, PN, or restrictive filling.	1. Feasible and reproducible. 2. Provides diagnostic and prognostic information. 3. In patients with DCM, filling patterns correlate better with LVFPs, functional class, and prognosis than LVEF does. 4. A restrictive filling pattern in combination with LA dilation in patients with normal EF is associated with a poor prognosis, similar to a restrictive pattern in DCM.	1. The U-shaped relation with LV diastolic function makes it difficult to differentiate normal from PN filling, particularly in patients with normal LVEF, without measuring additional variables. 2. If mitral flow velocity at the start of atrial contraction is >20 cm/s, E/A ratio will be reduced due to fusion. 3. Not applicable in patients with AF or atrial flutter. 4. Age-dependent (decreases with aging).
Mitral EDT (PW Doppler)	EDT is influenced by LV relaxation, LV diastolic pressures after MV opening, and LV stiffness.	1. Feasible and reproducible. 2. A short EDT in patients with reduced LVEF indicates increased LVFP with high accuracy both in sinus rhythm and in AF.	1. EDT does not relate to LVEDP when LVEF is normal. 2. EDT should not be measured in patients with E and A fusion due to potential inaccuracy. 3. Not applicable in atrial flutter. 4. Age-dependent (increases with aging).
Changes in mitral inflow with Valsalva maneuver	Helps distinguish normal from PN filling patterns. A decrease in E/A ratio of ≥50% or an increase in A-wave velocity during the maneuver, not caused by E and A fusion, are highly specific for increased LVFP.	When performed adequately under standardized conditions (e.g., keeping 40 mmHg intrathoracic pressure constant for 10 s), accuracy in diagnosing increased LVFP is good.	1. Not every patient can perform this maneuver adequately. The patient must generate and sustain a sufficient increase in intrathoracic pressure, and the examiner needs to maintain the correct sample volume location between the mitral leaflet tips during the maneuver. Not applicable in critically ill or intubated patients. 2. Difficult to assess if the procedure is not standardized.
Mitral "L" velocity	Markedly delayed LV relaxation in the setting of elevated LVFP allows for ongoing LV filling in mid-diastole and thus L velocity. The heart rate needs to be low enough for the L wave to be seen.	When present in patients with known cardiac disease (e.g., LVH, HCM), it is specific for elevated LVFP. However, its overall sensitivity is low.	Rarely seen in normal LV diastolic function when the subject has bradycardia. In such cases, the L velocity is usually <20 cm/s.
IVRT	IVRT is prolonged in patients with impaired LV relaxation but normal LVFP. When LAP increases, IVRT shortens, and its duration is inversely related to LVFP in patients with cardiac disease.	1. Overall, feasible and reproducible. 2. IVRT can be combined with other mitral inflow parameters such as E/A ratio to estimate LVFP in patients with HFrEF. 3. It can be combined with LV end-systolic pressure to estimate the time constant of LV relaxation (τ). 4. It can be applied in patients with mitral stenosis, in whom the same relation with LVFP described above holds. 5. In patients with MR or after MV replacement or repair, it can be combined with $T_{E-e'}$ to estimate LVFP.	1. IVRT duration is in part affected by heart rate and arterial pressure. 2. It is more challenging to measure and interpret with tachycardia. 3. Results differ based on using CW or PW Doppler for acquisition.
TDI-derived mitral annular early diastolic velocity *e′* (PW Doppler)	A significant association is present between *e′* and τ; this was shown in both animals and humans. The hemodynamic determinants of *e′* velocity include LV relaxation, restoring forces, and LVFP.	1. Feasible and reproducible. 2. LVFP has a minimal effect on *e′* in the presence of impaired LV relaxation. 3. Less load-dependent than conventional blood-pool Doppler parameters.	1. Limited accuracy in patients with CAD and regional dysfunction in the sampled segments, significant mitral annular calcification, surgical rings or prosthetic MVs, or pericardial disease. 2. Need to sample at least two sites with precise location and adequate size of sample volume. 3. Different cutoff values depending on the sampling site for measurement. 4. Age-dependent (decreases with aging).
Mitral E/*e′* ratio	The *e′* velocity can be used to correct for the effect of LV relaxation on mitral E velocity, and the E/*e′* ratio can be used to estimate LVFP.	1. Feasible and reproducible. 2. Values for average E/*e′* ratio <8 usually indicate normal LVFP; values >14 have high specificity for increased LVFP.	1. E/*e′* ratio is not accurate in normal subjects, patients with heavy mitral annular calcification, MV disease, or pericardial disease. 2. There is a "gray zone" of values (8–14) in which LVFP is indeterminate. 3. Accuracy is reduced in patients with CAD and regional dysfunction at the sampled segments. 4. Different cutoff values depending on the site used for measurement.

TABLE 5.2 Utility, Advantages, and Limitations of Parameters Used to Assess LV Diastolic Function.—cont'd

Parameter	Utility and Physiologic Background	Advantages	Limitations
$T_{E-e'}$ time interval	Can identify patients with LVDD due to delayed onset of *e'* velocity compared with onset of mitral E velocity in these patients.	1. Ratio of IVRT to $T_{E-e'}$ can be used to estimate LVFP in normal subjects and in patients with MV disease. 2. $T_{E-e'}$ can be used to differentiate patients with restrictive cardiomyopathy (who have a prolonged time interval) from those with pericardial constriction (in whom it is usually not prolonged).	More challenging to acquire satisfactory signals; close attention to location, gain, and filter settings and matching of RR intervals are required.
LAVi	LA volume reflects the cumulative effects of increased LVFP over time. Increased LA volume is an independent predictor of death, heart failure, AF, and ischemic stroke.	1. Feasible and reproducible. 2. Provides diagnostic and prognostic information about LVDD and chronicity of disease. 3. Apical 4-chamber view provides visual estimate of LA and RA size confirming that LA is enlarged.	1. LA dilation is seen in patients with bradycardia, high-output states, AF or atrial flutter, significant MV disease, or heart transplant with biatrial technique despite normal LV diastolic function. 2. LA dilatation occurs in well-trained athletes who have bradycardia and are well hydrated. 3. Suboptimal image quality and/or scanning technique, including LA foreshortening, precludes accurate measurements. 4. It can be difficult to measure LA volumes properly in patients with ascending or descending aortic aneurysm and in those with large interatrial septal aneurysm.
Pulmonary veins: peak systolic (S) velocity, peak diastolic (D) velocity, and S/D ratio (PW Doppler)	S-wave velocity is influenced by changes in LAP, LA contractility, and LV and RV contractility. D-wave velocity is mainly influenced by early diastolic LV filling and compliance, and it changes in parallel with mitral E velocity. Decrease in LA compliance and increase in LAP is associated with decrease in S velocity and increase in D velocity.	1. Reduced S velocity, S/D ratio <1, and systolic filling fraction (systolic VTI/total forward flow VTI) <40% indicate increased mean LAP in patients with reduced LVEF. 2. In patients with AF, DDT can be used to estimate mean PCWP.	1. Feasibility of recording PV inflow can be suboptimal, particularly in ICU patients. 2. The relationship between PV systolic filling fraction and LAP has limited accuracy in patients with normal LVEF, AF, MV disease, or HCM.
Ar – A duration	The time difference between Ar duration and mitral A duration during atrial contraction is associated with LV pressure rise due to atrial contraction and correlates with LVEDP: the longer the time difference, the higher the LVEDP.	1. PV Ar > mitral A duration by 30 ms indicates an increased LVEDP. 2. Independent of age and LVEF. 3. Accurate in patients with MR and patients with HCM.	1. Adequate recordings of Ar duration may not be feasible by TTE in some patients. 2. Not applicable in patients with AF. 3. Difficult to interpret in patients with sinus tachycardia or first-degree AV block with E and A fusion.
TR peak jet velocity (CW Doppler)	A significant correlation exists between systolic PA pressure and noninvasively derived LAP. In the absence of pulmonary disease, increased systolic PA pressure suggests elevated LAP.	Systolic PA pressure can be used as an adjunctive parameter of mean LAP. Evidence of pulmonary hypertension has prognostic implications.	1. Indirect estimate of LAP. 2. Adequate recording of a full envelope is not always possible in unenhanced studies, but intravenous agitated saline increases the yield. 3. With severe TR and low systolic RV–RA pressure gradient, accuracy of calculation depends on reliable estimation of RA pressure.
Color M-mode Vp and E/Vp ratio	Vp correlates with τ and can be used as a parameter of LV relaxation. E/Vp ratio correlates with LAP.	1. Vp is reliable as an index of LV relaxation in patients with depressed LVEF and dilated LV but not in patients with normal LVEF. 2. E/Vp ≥2.5 predicts PCWP >15 mmHg with reasonable accuracy in patients with depressed LVEF.	1. There are different methods for measuring mitral-to-apical flow propagation. 2. In patients with normal LV volumes and LVEF but elevated LVFP, Vp can be misleadingly normal. 3. Lower reproducibility. 4. Angulation between M-mode cursor and flow results in erroneous measurements.

AF, Atrial fibrillation; *Ar*, atrial reversal velocity in pulmonary veins; A_{dur}, mitral A wave duration; *AV*, atrioventricular; *CAD*, coronary artery disease; *CW*, continuous-wave; *DCM*, dilated cardiomyopathy; *DDT*, deceleration time of pulmonary vein D wave; *e'*, mitral annulus early diastolic velocity; *E/A ratio*, ratio of early to atrial peak filling velocity; *EDT*, deceleration time of mitral E velocity; *HCM*, hypertrophic cardiomyopathy; *HFrEF*, heart failure with reduced ejection fraction; *ICU*, intensive care unit; *IVRT*, isovolumic relaxation time; *LAP*, left atrial pressure; *LAVi*, LA maximum volume index; *LVDD*, left ventricular diastolic dysfunction; *LVEDP*, left ventricular end-diastolic pressure; *LVEF*, left ventricular ejection fraction; *LVFP*, left ventricular filling pressure; *LVH*, left ventricular hypertrophy; *MR*, mitral regurgitation; *MV*, mitral valve; *PA*, pulmonary artery; *PCWP*, pulmonary capillary wedge pressure; *PN*, pseudonormal; *PV*, pulmonary vein; *PW*, pulsed-wave; *τ*, time constant of LV relaxation; *TDI*, pulsed-wave tissue Doppler imaging; $T_{E-e'}$, time interval between onset of mitral E velocity and onset of annular *e'* velocity; *TR*, tricuspid regurgitation; *TTE*, transthoracic echocardiography; *Vp*, flow propagation velocity; *VTI*, velocity–time integral.

Adapted from Nagueh SF, Smiseth OA, Appleton CP, et al. Recommendations for the evaluation of left ventricular diastolic function by echocardiography: an update from the American Society of Echocardiography and the European Association of Cardiovascular Imaging. *J Am Soc Echocardiogr*. 2016;29:277–314.

Vp is not currently recommended as a first-line parameter for evaluation of LV diastolic function evaluation.[12]

In combination with peak E velocity, Vp can also be used to assess LVFP. Thus, the E/Vp ratio is a predictor of the PCWP.[31,32]

The advantages and limitations of color M-mode in assessing LV diastolic function are shown in Table 5.2.

Tissue Doppler Echocardiography

PW tissue Doppler imaging (TDI) allows the assessment of diastolic function by measuring peak diastolic velocities of the mitral annulus (Fig. 5.8).

The early diastolic velocity, *e'*, is a marker of ventricular relaxation (Fig. 5.9). It is inversely related to the relaxation constant, τ, and is less load-dependent than conventional Doppler flow parameters.[33,34] The late diastolic velocity, *a'*, corresponds to atrial contraction and is correlated with transmitral A-wave velocity and atrial function.

Of note, TDI-derived velocities are highly age dependent, and this should be taken into account when using them to evaluate diastolic function.[35]

With the progression of LVDD, there is a continuous decline of *e'* because this parameter is less affected by the progressive increase in LVFP compared with the mitral E wave (Fig. 5.10).[18] The combination of mitral E velocity (which increases with LVDD severity) and TDI-derived *e′* velocity (which decreases with LVDD severity) provides a parameter, the E/*e′* ratio, that is directly related to LVFP.[34]

The correlation between E/*e′* and LVFP has been confirmed in patients with both HFrEF and HFpEF, using different cutoff values for E/*e′* ratio according to the site of *e′* measurement. The current recommendation is to measure both the septal and lateral sides of the mitral annulus and to average the values when calculating E/*e′* ratio to predict LVFP.[12]

The reference values for TDI parameters of diastolic function according to age and gender are presented in Table 5.3,[35] and their advantages and limitations are shown in Table 5.2.

ECHOCARDIOGRAPHIC FINDINGS SUPPORTING THE PRESENCE OF DIASTOLIC DYSFUNCTION

Pathologic left ventricular hypertrophy (LVH) is a marker of impaired myocardial relaxation and increased myocardial stiffness, and it is a predictor of cardiovascular events.[36] Echocardiographic evidence of increased LV mass detected in subjects who are not trained athletes strongly suggests the presence of LVDD.

The reference values for LV mass are gender specific. Using the 2D guided linear dimension method, which is recommended in patients without major cardiac geometry distortions, LVDD should be suspected if the LV mass index is >95 g/m² in women or >115 g/m² in men.[15] Echocardiographic 2D methods are less dependent on geometric assumptions and more accurate than M-mode estimates in the setting of asymmetric hypertrophy. However, current use of 2D methods is limited by methodological issues, low reproducibility, and limited prognostic data.

Three-dimensional echocardiography (3DE) is free of geometric assumptions and provides more accurate measurements of LV mass in patients with remodeled ventricles. There are still insufficient data available from normal subjects to recommend reference values for LV mass assessed by 3DE, and prognostic data are scarce.[15]

Echocardiographic evidence of LVH in patients with HF symptoms and normal LVEF favors the diagnosis of HFpEF; however, its absence cannot rule out the diagnosis.

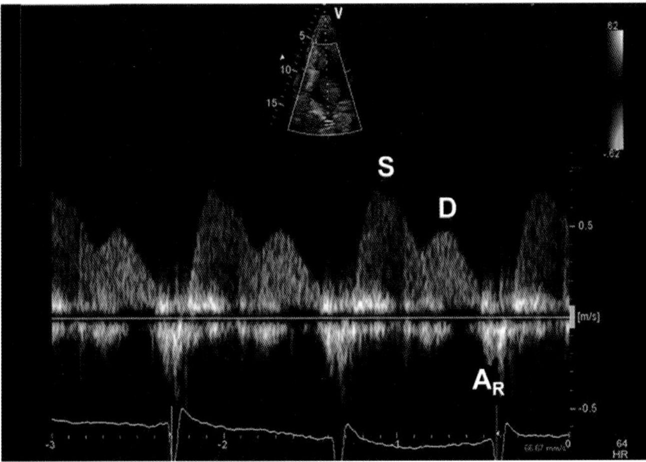

Fig. 5.6 Pulmonary venous flow by pulsed-wave Doppler echocardiography. Doppler recording of pulmonary venous flow in a healthy subject shows a higher systolic (S) than diastolic (D) forward flow wave with a small reversal of flow at the time of atrial contraction (Ar).

Left Atrial Dilation

LA dilation is an established marker for LVDD with the ability to provide information about the presence and chronicity of elevated LVFP and to characterize global cardiovascular risk.[37]

LA enlargement is non-uniform, and the anteroposterior diameter often underestimates the true LA size. Measuring LA volume with 2D echocardiography at end-systole, when the LA reaches maximum expansion, allows an accurate assessment of LA remodeling and provides superior prognostic information compared with LA diameter or area.[38] It is very important to use apical views optimized for LA recording; these maximize the size of the LA to avoid foreshortening and underestimation of LA volume (Fig. 5.11).

3DE overcomes the limitations of 2D echocardiography in estimating LA volume because of the lack of geometric assumptions, and it has better prognostic value.[39] However, the variability of 3DE measurements of LA volume and the limited normative data have prevented wider use of 3DE for LA size assessment.

Indexing of the maximal LA volume to body surface area (LAVi) is currently recommended when assessing LA size. A

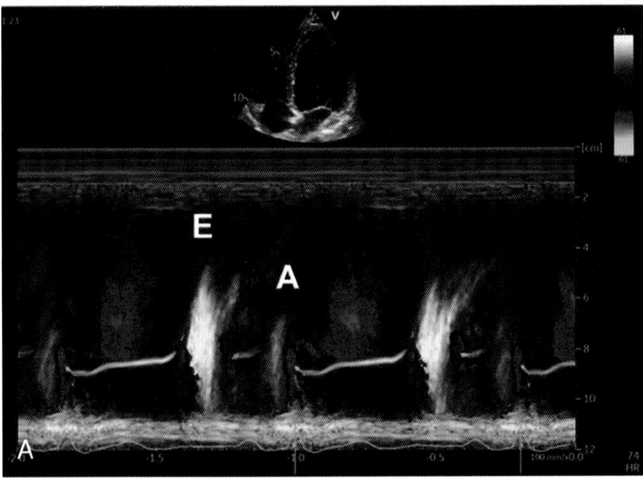

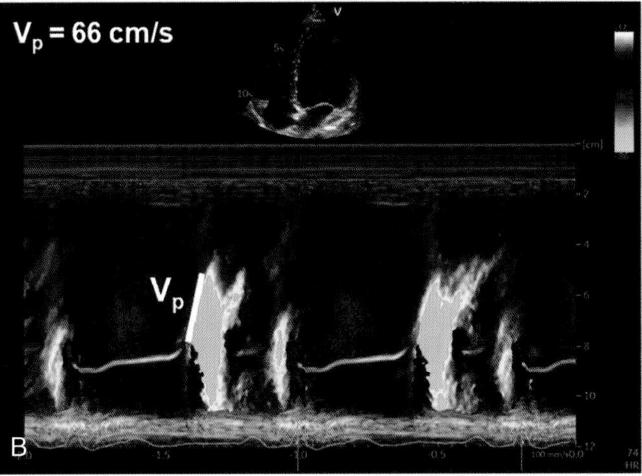

Fig. 5.7 Velocity of flow propagation by color M-mode echocardiography. (A) Color M-mode echocardiography from the apical 4-chamber view in a normal subject. Two diastolic flow waves are seen: an early filling wave (E wave), and a late filling wave at atrial contraction (A wave). The velocity propagation of flow (Vp) can be measured as the slope of the color–no color interface of the early filling wave. (B) To make the measurement of this slope easier, the color flow baseline was shifted, making the interface clearly visibile. The slope of the first aliasing velocity during early filling is measured from the mitral valve plane into the left ventricle, resulting in a normal Vp value of 66 cm/s.

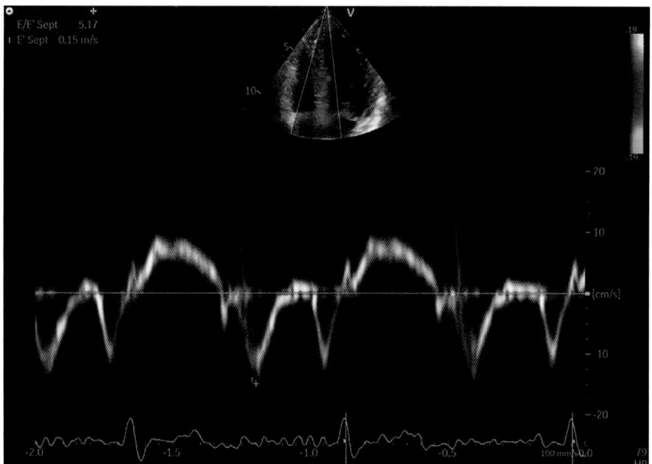

Fig. 5.8 **Pulsed-wave tissue Doppler echocardiographid recording of mitral annular velocities in a normal subject.** Normal myocardial velocities are seen, with a septal *e′* velocity of 15 cm/s.

cutoff value of 34 mL/m^2 has been set as the upper limit of the normal range and as the reference value for diastolic function and LVFP assessment.[12] It should be noted that LA volume reflects the cumulative effects of increased LVFP over time, but it is an insensitive biomarker of the early phases of LVDD.[40]

Left atrial minimum volume ($LAVi_{min}$) measured at end-diastole (when the LA is directly exposed to the LV pressure) was recently reported to better reflect LVFP increase even at early stages of LVDD, with greater prognostic value than maximum LA volume.[41]

In a study comparing echocardiographic features in hypertensive patients with and without HFpEF, the product of LV mass index and LAV emerged as the most accurate parameter in predicting HFpEF.[42] Therefore, the presence of LVH and LA dilation in a patient with dyspnea increases the likelihood of HFpEF.

Pulmonary Hypertension

Pulmonary hypertension is highly prevalent and often severe in patients with HFpEF, and when present, it is associated with worse exercise capacity and prognosis.[43,44] A significant correlation was demonstrated between pulmonary artery systolic pressure (PASP) and noninvasively derived LVDP.[43] In the absence of pulmonary disease, pulmonary hypertension suggests LVDD with elevated LAP, and PASP can be used as a surrogate of LVFP.[12]

PASP can be estimated by measuring the peak velocity of tricuspid regurgitation (TR) and adding an estimate of RA pressure. A TR peak velocity >2.8 m/s in the absence of primary pulmonary disease supports the presence of elevated LVFP.[12]

CONSIDERATIONS ABOUT THE ASSESSMENT OF DIASTOLIC FUNCTION IN THE ELDERLY

Assessment of diastolic function may be difficult in elderly individuals due to age-related changes in LV structure and function (e.g., delayed LV relaxation, increased LV stiffness) and the increased prevalence of comorbidities (e.g., hypertension, coronary artery disease). These features are usually associated with changes in mitral flow and TDI parameters, including reduction of E and *e′* velocities and reduced E/A ratio.[35]

In normal elderly subjects, the mitral filling patterns may be similar to those seen in younger patients with mild LVDD.[12] However, an *E/e′* >15 is extremely unlikely in the presence of normal diastolic function. In a study reporting normal values for Doppler echocardiographic parameters in healthy volunteers, 55.4% of patients ≥60 years of age had a septal *e′* <8 cm/s, and 19.0% had a lateral *e′* <8 cm/s, but none of them had an averaged *E/e′* >15 or a lateral *E/e′* >13.35.

Similarly, a significant change in mitral inflow pattern during the Valsalva maneuver (>50% decrease in the E/A ratio) or an increased difference between PV Ar duration and mitral A wave duration (Ar – A duration) suggests the presence of increased LVEDP regardless of the patient's age. The presence of pulmonary hypertension in the absence of primary causes (i.e., pre-capillary pulmonary hypertension) is suggestive of LVDD at any age.

Other features suggesting the presence of LVDD independent of age are LA dilation (in the absence of MV disease or atrial arrhythmias) and pathologic LV hypertrophy.

NEW TECHNOLOGIES FOR THE ASSESSMENT OF DIASTOLIC FUNCTION

Diastolic Stress Echocardiography

Diastolic stress echocardiography is recommended in patients who have exercise-related symptoms and when resting echocardiography shows impaired LV relaxation but not elevated LVFP. There is no indication to perform the test in patients who have normal results on resting 2D echocardiography and normal *e′* velocities because there is a very low likelihood that they will develop an exercise-induced increase in LVFP. Similarly, there is no indication to perform a diastolic stress test in patients who have Doppler findings consistent with increased LAP already evident at rest.[12]

Normal individuals have enhanced LV relaxation during exercise, which increases the LV suction effect, allowing LVFP to remain normal even with the shortened diastole. This is reflected by an increase in both E and *e′* velocities during exercise. Hence, the E/*e′* ratio remains virtually unchanged as LVFP remains normal during exertion.

By contrast, patients with HFpEF have impaired LV relaxation at rest (i.e., low *e′* velocity) that fails to improve (remains reduced) during exercise, leading to increased LAP (increased E velocity). As a consequence, the E/*e′* ratio increases during stress. A cutoff value of E/*e′* ratio >13 during exercise was associated with an increased LVEDP >15 mmHg, whereas an E/*e′* ratio ≥10 at stress was the best predictor of reduced exercise capacity (≤7 metabolic equivalents [METs]).[45]

Diastolic stress echocardiography has a diagnostic and prognostic role in patients with HFpEF.[46,47] A PASP ≥45 mmHg during exercise identified patients with HFpEF in another study.[48]

Exercise echocardiography is preferred to pharmacologic stress echocardiography because it is safer and provides further insight on functional status. The diastolic stress testing should be performed by measuring mitral E, septal annular *e′*, and TR peak velocities at baseline, during each stage including peak exercise, and during recovery.[12]

In patients with normal diastolic reserve, the averaged E/*e′* (or septal E/*e′*) ratio remains <10, and TR velocity remains ≤2.8 m/s. The test is considered abnormal, indicating increased LVFP, when all of the following conditions are met during exercise: averaged E/*e′* >14 or septal E/*e′* >15, TR peak velocity >2.8 m/s, and septal *e′* velocity <7 cm/s (Fig. 5.12). Unless all three criteria are met, the test should be considered nondiagnostic.[12]

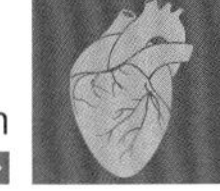

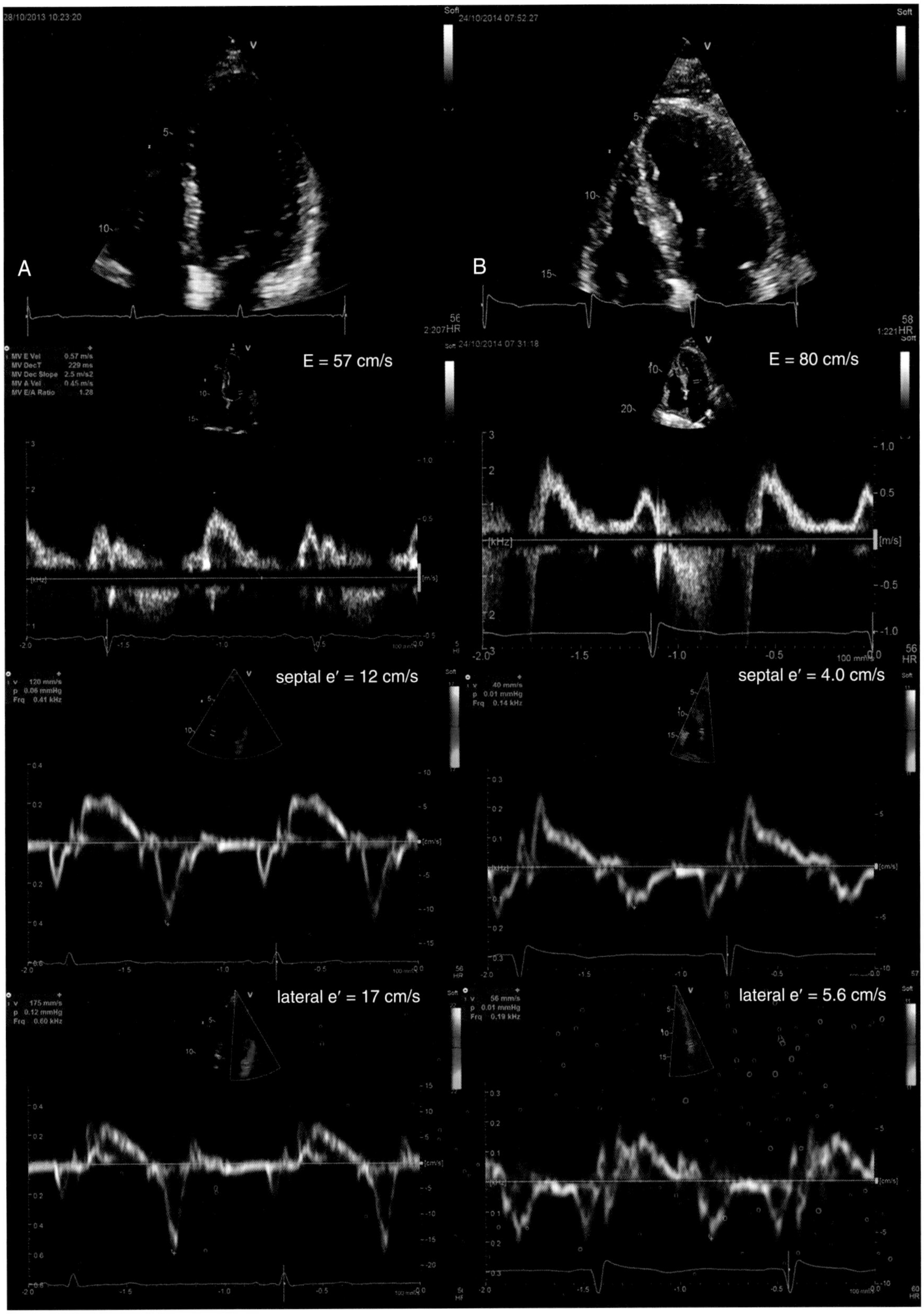

Fig. 5.9 LV long-axis function in health and disease. (A) Echocardiographic images of a 58-year-old healthy subject with normal left ventricular ejection fraction (LVEF) (Video 5.9A). He has a normal mitral inflow pattern with an E/A ratio >1. Both septal *e′* and lateral *e′* velocities are normal, at 12 and 17 cm/s, respectively. (B) Echocardiographic images of a 54-year-old patient who has hypertrophic cardiomyopathy with a normal LVEF (Video 5.9B). He has markedly reduced septal *e′* and lateral *e′* velocities (4 and 5.6 cm/s, respectively), consistent with severely impaired LV relaxation. The mitral flow pattern is pseudonormal in this case (E/A ratio = 1.52), with an average E/*e′* ratio >14, consistent with elevated LV filling pressure.

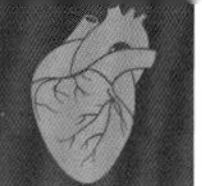

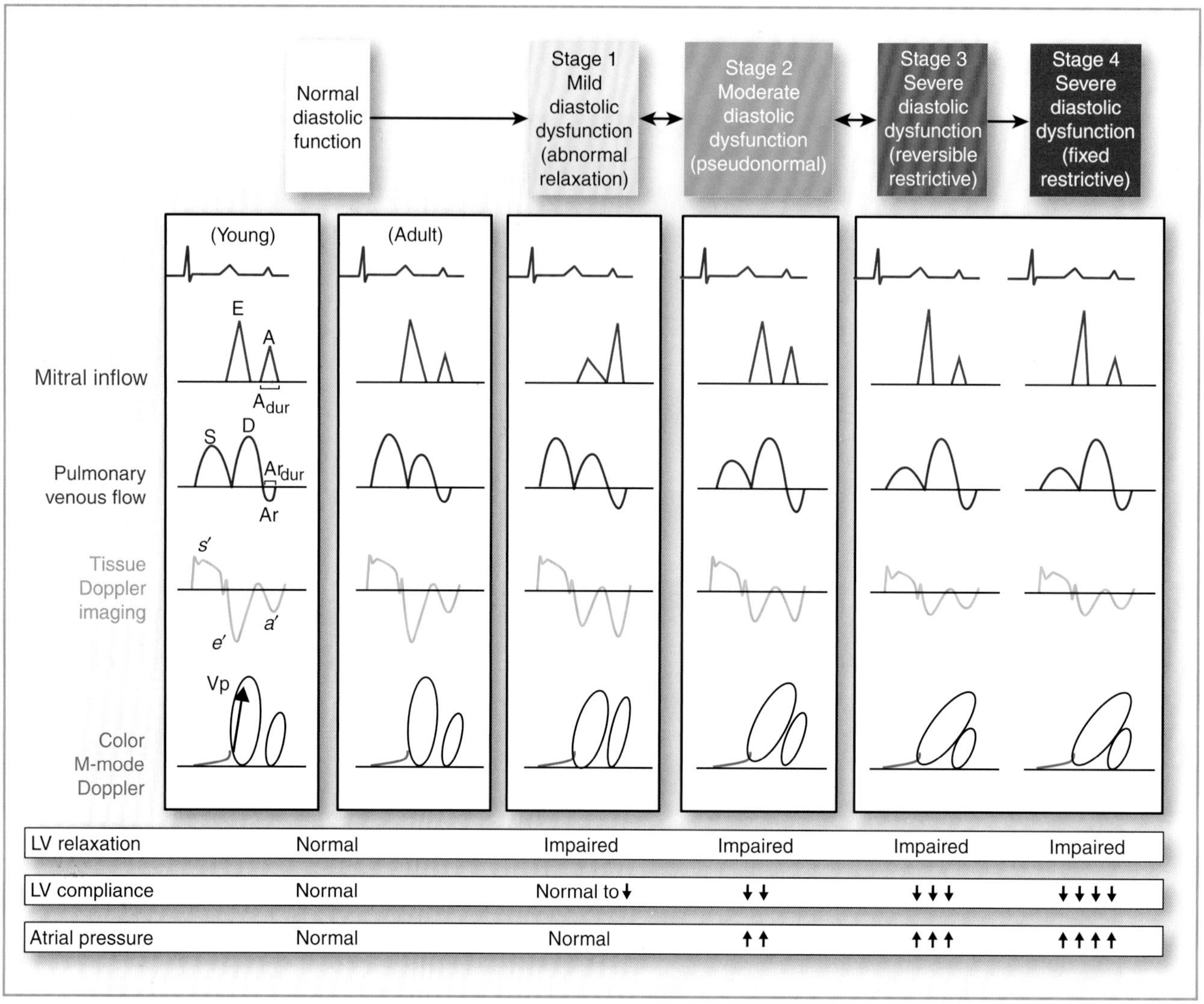

	Normal diastolic function (Young)	Normal diastolic function (Adult)	Stage 1 Mild diastolic dysfunction (abnormal relaxation)	Stage 2 Moderate diastolic dysfunction (pseudonormal)	Stage 3 Severe diastolic dysfunction (reversible restrictive)	Stage 4 Severe diastolic dysfunction (fixed restrictive)
LV relaxation	Normal		Impaired	Impaired	Impaired	Impaired
LV compliance	Normal		Normal to ↓	↓↓	↓↓↓	↓↓↓↓
Atrial pressure	Normal		Normal	↑↑	↑↑↑	↑↑↑↑

Fig. 5.10 Changes in echocardiographic parameters during the progression of LV diastolic dysfunction. Integration of Doppler echocardiographic parameters into normal LV diastolic function and diastolic dysfunction grades. *, xxx; *A*, Mitral filling wave at atrial contraction; *a′*, tissue Doppler mitral annular late diastolic velocity; A_{dur}, duration of mitral filling wave at atrial contraction; *Ar*, pulmonary venous reverse flow velocity at atrial contraction; Ar_{dur}, duration of pulmonary venous reverse flow velocity at atrial contraction; *D*, pulmonary venous diastolic flow; *E*, mitral early filling wave; *e′*, tissue Doppler mitral annular early diastolic tissue velocity; *S*, pulmonary venous systolic flow; *s′*, tissue Doppler mitral annular systolic velocity; *Vp*, color M-mode velocity propagation. (Adapted from Garcia MJ, Thomas JD, Klein AL. New Doppler echocardiographic applications for the study of diastolic function. *J Am Coll Cardiol*. 1998;32:865–875.)

Left Ventricular Strain

Assessment of global and regional LV deformation (myocardial strain or strain rate, twisting and untwisting) can be performed by speckle tracking echocardiography (STE). The assessment of LV strain may confer important diagnostic information. This evaluation is especially useful in patients with suspected HF and normal LVEF.[49] The finding of LV longitudinal systolic dysfunction reflected by reduced LV global longitudinal strain (GLS) provides evidence supporting the diagnosis of HFpEF. Lower absolute values for GLS denote more impaired LV global longitudinal function. Values of GLS below 16% are definitely abnormal.[50] Moreover, the pattern of regional strain abnormalities seen on the bull's-eye plot may provide important hints as to the cause of LV dysfunction. An apical-sparing pattern of GLS has been described as an accurate and reproducible method of identifying patients with cardiac amyloidosis[51] (Fig. 5.13).

Ventricular untwisting plays a major role in normal LV filling; it is responsible for the early diastolic base-to-apex pressure gradients and for diastolic suction.[8] In normal hearts, a brisk untwisting leads to a rapid decrease in early diastolic LV pressure and to MV opening with rapid filling at normal pressure.

LV early diastolic strain rate and LV untwisting velocity provide diagnostic information similar to that provided by *e′* (reflecting both LV relaxation and restoring forces) and can be derived from STE data sets. However, methodological challenges limit their practical applicability, and their assessment is not recommended for routine clinical use at present.[12]

Left Atrial Strain

The assessment of LA function is very important in identifying elevated LVFP. LAP is related to LA size and function, and a long-standing increase in LAP will be reflected by changes in both LA size and function. Many studies have suggested that measurements of LA function may be superior to measurements of LA size and may provide useful information even when the LA is not dilated.[52]

LA longitudinal strain is a promising LA function parameter for the assessment of LV diastolic function. 2D STE is now the

TABLE 5.3 Tissue Doppler-Derived LV Diastolic Function Parameters According to Age and Gender.

	20–40 years				40–60 years				≥60 years				P^a				
Parameters	*Total Mean ± SD*	*Total 95% CI*	*Male Mean ± SD*	*Female Mean ± SD*	*Total Mean ± SD*	*Total 95% CI*	*Male Mean ± SD*	*Female Mean ± SD*	*Total Mean ± SD*	*Total 95% CI*	*Male Mean ± SD*	*Female Mean ± SD*	*Total*	*Male*	*Female*	*Male[b] r (P)*	*Female[b] r (P)*
Pulse Doppler at the Miral Value																	
E wave velocity (cm/s)	0.82 ± 0.16	0.53–1.22	0.79 ± 0.14	0.84 ± 0.17	0.75 ± 0.17	0.46–1.13	0.72 ± 0.16	0.77 ± 0.17	0.70 ± 0.16	0.39–1.03	0.67 ± 0.15	0.72 ± 0.17	<0.001	<0.001	<0.001	−031; <0.001	−029; <0.001
A wave velocity (cm/s)	0.50 ± 0.13	0.30–0.87	0.50 ± 0.13	0.51 ± 0.12	0.62 ± 0.15	0.37–0.97	0.61 ± 0.15	0.63 ± 0.14	0.74 ± 0.16	0.40–1.04	0.73 ± 0.16	0.76 ± 0.16	<0.001	<0.001	<0.001	0.49; <0.001	052; <0.001
E wave deceleration time (ms)	178.2 ± 43.1	105.2–269.0	179.8 ± 46.4	176.7 ± 40.1	187.6 ± 45.5	114.6–288.1	186.6 ± 52.8	188.2 ± 39 .8	208.9 ± 62.7	114.0–385.9	217.5 ± 69.7	201.5 ± 55.7	<0.001	0.002	0.008	0.23; 0.001	0.18; 0.006
E/A ratio	1.71 ± 0.52	0.89–3.18	1.69 ± 0.52	1.72 ± 0.52	1.24 ± 0.39	0.71–2.27	1.22 ± 0.31	1.26 ± 0.43	0.98 ± 0.29	0.53–1.80	0.96 ± 0.27	0.99 ± 0.31	<0.001	<0.001	<0.001	−0.61; <0.001	−0.54 <0.001
Tissue Doppler Data (cm/s)																	
Septal *e′* wave	12.1 ± 2.5	8.0–17.0	11.9 ± 2.7	12.3 ± 2.3	9.8 ± 2.6	5.0–16.0	9.8 ± 2.6	9.7 ± 2.5	7.6 ± 2.3	3.0–13.0	7.3 ± 2.2	7.9 ± 2.3	<0.001	<0.001	<0.001	−0.58 (<0.001)	−0.58 (<0.001)
Septal *a′* wave	8.5 ± 1.7	5.3–12.0	8.9 ± 1.6	8.1 ± 1.8	9.8 ± 2.0	6.9–14.0	10.6 ± 2.0	9.1 ± 1.8	10.5 ± 1.7	7.0–14.0	10.6 ± 1.9	10.4 ± 1.6	<0.001	<0.001	<0.001	0.40 (<0.001)	0.44 (<0.001)
Lateral *e′* wave	16.4 ± 3.4	10.0–23.0	16.2 ± 3.6	16.6 ± 3.2	12.5 ± 3.0	6.0–18.0	12.6 ± 3.0	12.4 ± 3.0	9.6 ± 2.8	4.0–17.0	9.5 ± 2.1	9.7 ± 3.2	<0.001	<0.001	<0.001	−0.65 (<0.001)	−0.65 (<0.001)
Lateral *a′* wave	8.2 ± 2.2	5.0–13.0	8.5 ± 2.0	8.0 ± 2.3	9.4 ± 2.6	5.0–15.0	9.8 ± 2.7	9.2 ± 2.5	10.6 ± 2.9	6.0–17.0	10.9 ± 3.0	10.4 ± 2.8	<0.001	<0.001	<0.001	0.36 (<0.001)	0.33 (<0.001)
Average septal and lateral *e′* wave	14.3 ± 2.7	9.1–19.5	14.0 ± 2.9	14.5 ± 2.4	11.1 ± 2.5	6.0–16.0	11.2 ± 2.4	11.1 ± 2.5	8.6 ± 2.3	3.5–15.0	8.5 ± 1.9	8.8 ± 2.6	<0.001	<0.001	<0.001	−0.66 (<0.001)	−0.66 (<0.001)
Inferior *e′* wave	14.2 ± 3.1	8.0–20.3	13.6 ± 3.0	14.7 ± 3.1	11.0 ± 2.9	6.0–17.0	10.5 ± 2.8	11.4 ± 2.9	8.4 ± 2.4	2.7–14.0	8.2 ± 2.6	8.6 ± 2.3	<0.001	<0.001	<0.001	−0.65 (<0.001)	−0.65 (<0.001)
Inferior *a′* wave	8.9 ± 1.8	5.0–13.0	9.3 ± 1.8	8.5 ± 1.7	10.5 ± 2.3	6.0–16.0	11.1 ± 2.2	10.1 ± 2.2	11.8 ± 2.0	7.7–16.0	11.8 ± 2.0	11.8 ± 2.1	<0.001	<0.001	<0.001	0.49 (<0.001)	0.49 (<0.001)
Anterior *e′* wave	14.5 ± 2.9	9.0–20.0	14.0 ± 3.0	15.0 ± 2.8	11.0 ± 2.8	6.0–18.0	11.1 ± 2.8	10.9 ± 2.8	8.0 ± 2.3	3.0–14.0	8.2 ± 2.8	7.9 ± 1.8	<0.001	<0.001	<0.001	−0.66 (<0.001)	−0.75 (<0.001)
Anterior *a′* wave	7.6 ± 1.7	4.0–11.0	8.1 ± 1.7	7.2 ± 1.6	8.7 ± 2.2	5.0–15.0	9.0 ± 2.3	8.5 ± 2.1	9.9 ± 2.4	5.0–14.3	9.9 ± 2.3	9.9 ± 2.4	<0.001	<0.001	<0.001	0.36 (<0.001)	0.39 (<0.001)
Posterior *e′* wave	15.9 ± 3.1	10.0–23.0	15.9 ± 3.5	15.9 ± 2.6	12.3 ± 2.9	7.0–18.1	12.3 ± 3.0	12.3 ± 2.8	9.8 ± 2.7	3.6–15.8	9.9 ± 2.7	9.7 ± 2.6	<0.001	<0.001	<0.001	−0.65 (<0.001)	−0.67 (<0.001)
Posterior *a′* wave	8.2 ± 2.0	4.0–13.0	8.6 ± 1.9	7.9 ± 2.1	10.0 ± 2.7	6.0–17.0	10.6 ± 2.7	9.7 ± 2.7	11.5 ± 2.8	6.3–20.1	11.7 ± 3.3	11.4 ± 2.3	<0.001	<0.001	<0.001	0.46 (<0.001)	0.45 (<0.001)
Average *e′* wave	14.5 ± 2.3	10.2–19.4	14.5 ± 2.6	14.9 ± 2.0	11.2 ± 2.3	6.5–15.5	11.0 ± 2.2	11.3 ± 2.3	8.6 ± 1.9	3.5–12.6	8.9 ± 2.0	8.3 ± 1.7	<0.001	<0.001	<0.001	−0.73 (<0.001)	−0.78 (<0.001)
E/e′ Ratio																	
Septal E/*e′*	6.9 ± 1.6	4.4–10.6	6.9 ± 1.7	6.9 ± 1.6	8.1 ± 2.3	4.3–13.2	7.8 ± 2.4	8.2 ± 2.2	9.7 ± 2.8	5.0–16.9	9.8 ± 3.0	9.7 ± 2.6	<0.001	<0.001	<0.001	0.42 (<0.001)	0.41 (<0.001)
Lateral E/*e′*	5.1 ± 1.3	3.1–8.5	5.0 ± 1.3	5.2 ± 1.3	6.3 ± 2.2	3.7–12.0	6.1 ± 2.2	6.5 ± 2.3	7.8 ± 2.2	4.2–12.8	7.6 ± 2.1	7.9 ± 2.2	<0.001	<0.001	<0.001	0.43 (<0.001)	0.44 (<0.001)
Average septal and lateral E/*e′*	5.8 ± 1.3	3.6–9.1	5.8 ± 1.4	5.9 ± 1.3	7.0 ± 2.1	4.2–11.5	6.7 ± 2.1	7.2 ± 2.0	8.5 ± 2.2	4.6–13.5	8.4 ± 2.2	8.6 ± 2.2	<0.001	<0.001	<0.001	0.45 (<0.001)	0.46 (<0.001)
Average E/*e′*	5.6 ± 1.1	3.7–7.9	5.6 ± 1.2	5.5 ± 1.0	6.8 ± 1.8	4.0–11.6	6.7 ± 1.8	6.9 ± 1.9	8.3 ± 2.2	4.4–14.8	8.1 ± 2.3	8.6 ± 2.2	<0.001	<0.001	<0.001	0.50 (<0.001)	0.55 (<0.001)

CI, Confidence interval; *F*, female; *M*, male; *P*, differences between groups according to age category (one-way ANOVA); *r (P)*, correlation with age for both sexes (Pearson correlation test).
From Caballero L, Kou S, Dulgheru R, et al. Echocardiographic reference ranges for normal cardiac Doppler data: results from the NORRE Study. *Eur Heart J Cardiovasc Imaging*. 2015;16:1031–1041.
[a]*P* differences between groups according to age category (one-way ANOVA).
[b]P and r correlation with age for both genders (Pearson correlation test).

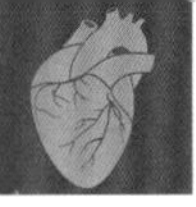

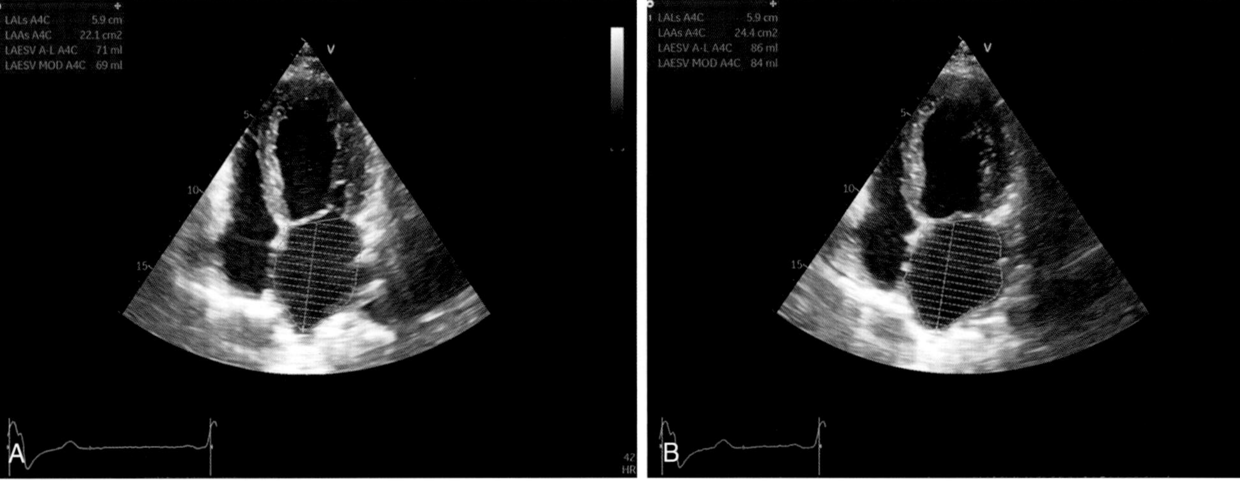

Fig. 5.11 **2D echocardiographic acquisition of left atrial volume.** Echocardiographic images from a 58-year-old man (body surface area [BSA] of 2.2 m^2). (A) Suboptimal acquisition of the LA from the apical 4-chamber view, with LA foreshortening and a measured LA volume of 71 mL (Video 5.11A). (B) Dedicated acquisition of the LA from the apical 4-chamber view for optimal LA volume measurements (Video 5.11B). LA size is maximized, and the LA maximal volume is 86 mL. Because the longitudinal axes of the LV and LA lie in different planes, a dedicated 4-chamber apical view is needed to maximize LA size and avoid LA foreshortening. In this case, the incorrect acquisition of the LA would have led to an 18% underestimation of maximal LA volume and to the erroneous conclusion that the patient had a normal LA volume (32 mL/m^2), when in fact his LA was dilated (39 mL/m^2).

main method used to measure LA strain (Fig. 5.14). A significant correlation between invasively measured PCWP and LA peak longitudinal strain was found: the higher the pressure, the lower the strain.[53] The relationship between LA strain and LVFP appears to be stronger in patients with HFrEF than in patients with normal LVEF. The assessment of LA reservoir function by LA peak strain provides prognostic information independent of LA volume and LV longitudinal function in HFrEF.[54]

In a study of 329 healthy subjects, normal LA reservoir strain was 45.5% ± 11.4% with a lowest cutoff value of 23%.[55] When this cutoff was applied to a group of 377 patients with LVDD, LA strain was found to be reduced in 23% of patients with a normal LAVi and in 27% of patients with a normal LA emptying fraction.[55] Similar findings were reported in patients with hypertension or diabetes or both, who had reduced LA strain despite a normal LA volume.[52]

Importantly, the measurement of LA strain needs to be properly standardized.[56] Issues such as intervendor variability and the lack of validation in larger cohorts of specific cutoff values to be used for LVDD assessment limit the use of LA strain on a larger scale in daily practice. Therefore, current recommendations do not include LA strain in the algorithms proposed to evaluate LVDD and LVFP.

However, LA strain could play a practical role in the assessment of LVDD and LVFP (Fig. 5.15),[40] particularly in patients with borderline or indeterminate readings.[40] The LA is an important compensatory mechanism in the initial stages of LVDD, compensating for the impaired LV relaxation to preserve cardiac output. Therefore, LA dysfunction or failure could be the main factor responsible for the progression from asymptomatic LVDD to HFpEF.

ECHOCARDIOGRAPHIC ASSESSMENT OF LV FILLING PRESSURE

Increased LVFP is the ultimate consequence of LVDD, representing the final pathway for HF regardless of etiology. Therefore, assessing LVFP is a key objective for diagnostic, prognostic, and therapeutic reasons.

In the early stages of LVDD, the patient is asymptomatic at rest and LVFP is normal. With further worsening of LV diastolic function, LVEDP increases but mean LAP may initially remain normal. The increase in LVEDP leads to a decrease in the late-diastolic transmitral pressure gradient. The abnormalities in end-diastolic Doppler signals associated with elevated LVEDP are reduced A-wave velocity and duration, decreased fraction of LV filling due to LA contraction, and shortened mitral A deceleration time. The mitral annulus late-diastolic velocity (*a′*) is also reduced in patients with elevated LVEDP.[57]

When LVEDP is increased, the proportion of blood sent by LA contraction back into the PV increases. Therefore, the higher the LVEDP, the more prominent the PV flow Ar wave. An Ar wave duration that is >30 ms longer than the mitral A wave duration is a good indicator of elevated LVEDP (Fig. 5.16), irrespective of LVEF and age.[58–60]

Conditions that make late-diastolic Doppler signals unavailable or unreliable for LVEDP assessment are LA systolic dysfunction; AF, atrial flutter, or tachycardia; and atrioventricular block.

In patients with more advanced LVDD, dyspnea with exercise reflects increased mean LAP. In such cases, the MV opens at a high LAP, early diastolic filling becomes dominant despite the impaired LV relaxation, and the IVRT is shortened. The combination of an increased E/A ratio (≥2) with a short EDT in patients with myocardial disease reflects increased LVFP[61,62] (see Fig. 5.3).

Another consequence of increased mean LAP is a lower PV–LA pressure gradient in systole than in diastole. This leads to a blunted S wave, with a lower S/D velocity ratio of the PV flow, and a taller D wave, with a shorter deceleration time.[63]

However, the age and load dependency of E velocity, E/A ratio, EDT, IVRT, and S/D ratio limit their use as stand-alone parameters to predict invasively measured LVFP.

The role of Valsalva maneuver for LVFP assessment is based on the preload reduction that occurs during the maneuver, which allows one to distinguish a normal from a PN filling pattern[12] (see Fig. 5.5). A decrease in E/A ratio ≥50% or an increase in A-wave velocity during the maneuver is highly suggestive for increased LVFP.[22–24]

The flow propagation velocity, Vp, can be used in combination with mitral E velocity to assess LVFP: the higher the

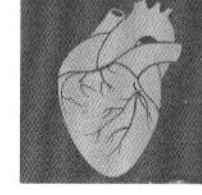

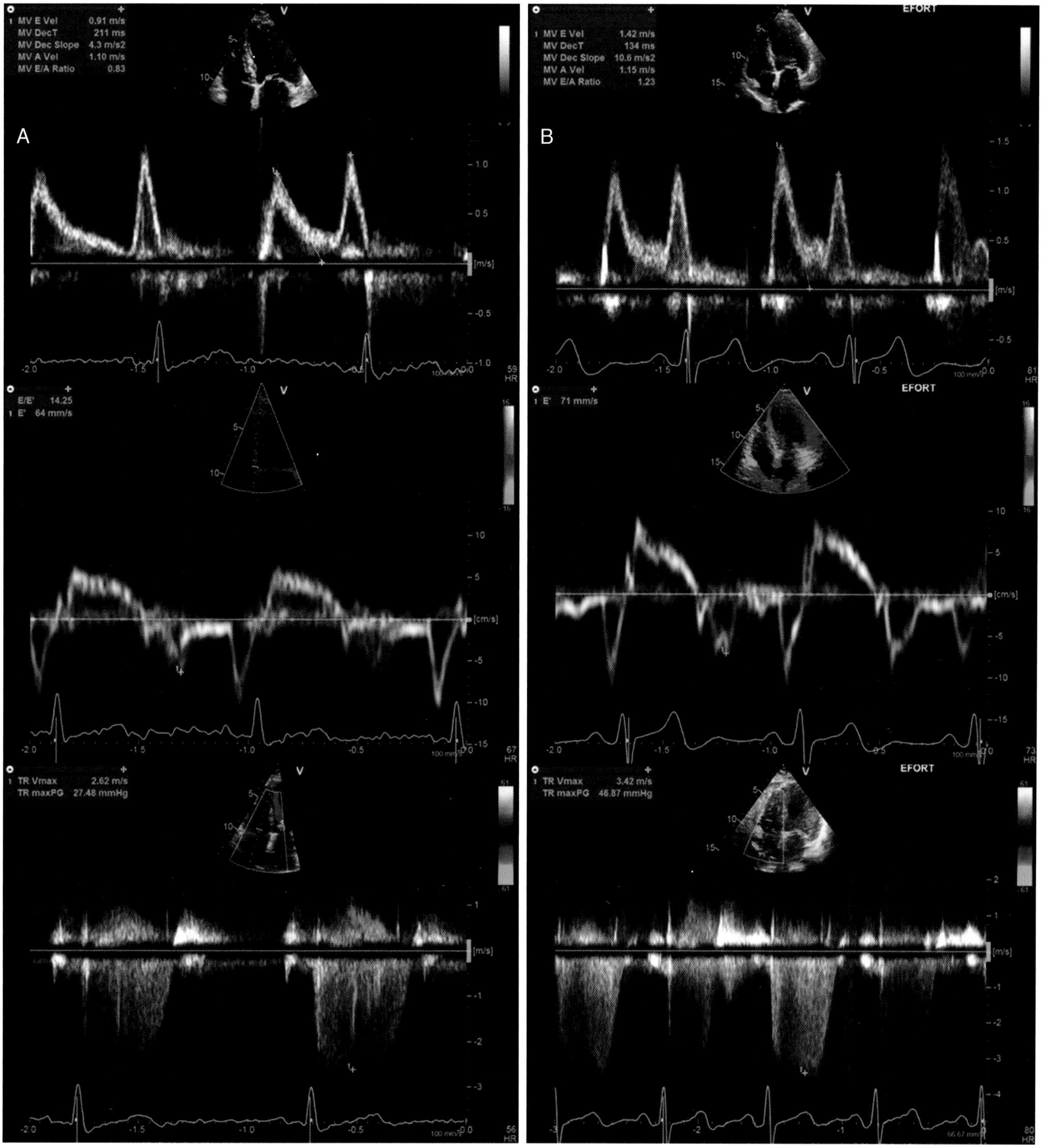

Fig. 5.12 Diastolic stress echocardiography. Diastolic stress testing performed in an 81-year-old woman with dyspnea and fatigue at mild to moderate exertion. Resting 2D echocardiography revealed LV hypertrophy, LA dilation, and normal LV ejection fraction. (A) Pulsed-wave Doppler echocardiography at rest showed the following: E = 91 cm/s, E/A = 0.83, septal e' (e'_{sep}) = 6.4 cm/s, E/e'_{sep} ratio = 14, and maximum TR velocity ($V_{max}TR$) = 2.6 m/s. During exercise the patient's symptoms were reproduced, and significant changes were noted even at mild effort (80 beats/min). (B) The following parameters were recorded during stress testing: E = 142 cm/s, e'_{sep} = 7.1 cm/s (exercise E/e' ratio = 20), and $V_{max}TR$ = 3.42 m/s, suggesting increased left ventricular filling pressure (LVFP) with exercise and confirming the diagnosis of heart failure with preserved ejection fraction (HFpEF) in clinical context.

E/Vp, the higher the LVFP.[31,32] An increased E/Vp ratio (>1.5) also carries prognostic information in patients after myocardial infarction.[64] The E/Vp ratio should be used with caution in patients with preserved LVEF because it can be normal despite elevated LVFP, especially in patients with normal LV volumes.[12]

The mitral E/e' ratio is often used to assess LVFP. Mitral E velocity is increased both in young healthy subjects and in patients with LVDD and elevated LAP; e' is decreased only in patients with LVDD. Therefore, because the mitral E/e' ratio adjusts the mitral E velocity for LV relaxation, it better reflects the LVFP.

An average E/e' >14 is highly specific for elevated LVFP, regardless of the patient's age, and it provides convincing evidence of LVDD.[24] When E/e' is <8, LAP is usually normal. When E/e' is intermediate (between 8 and 15), other parameters are necessary to estimate LVFP.[24]

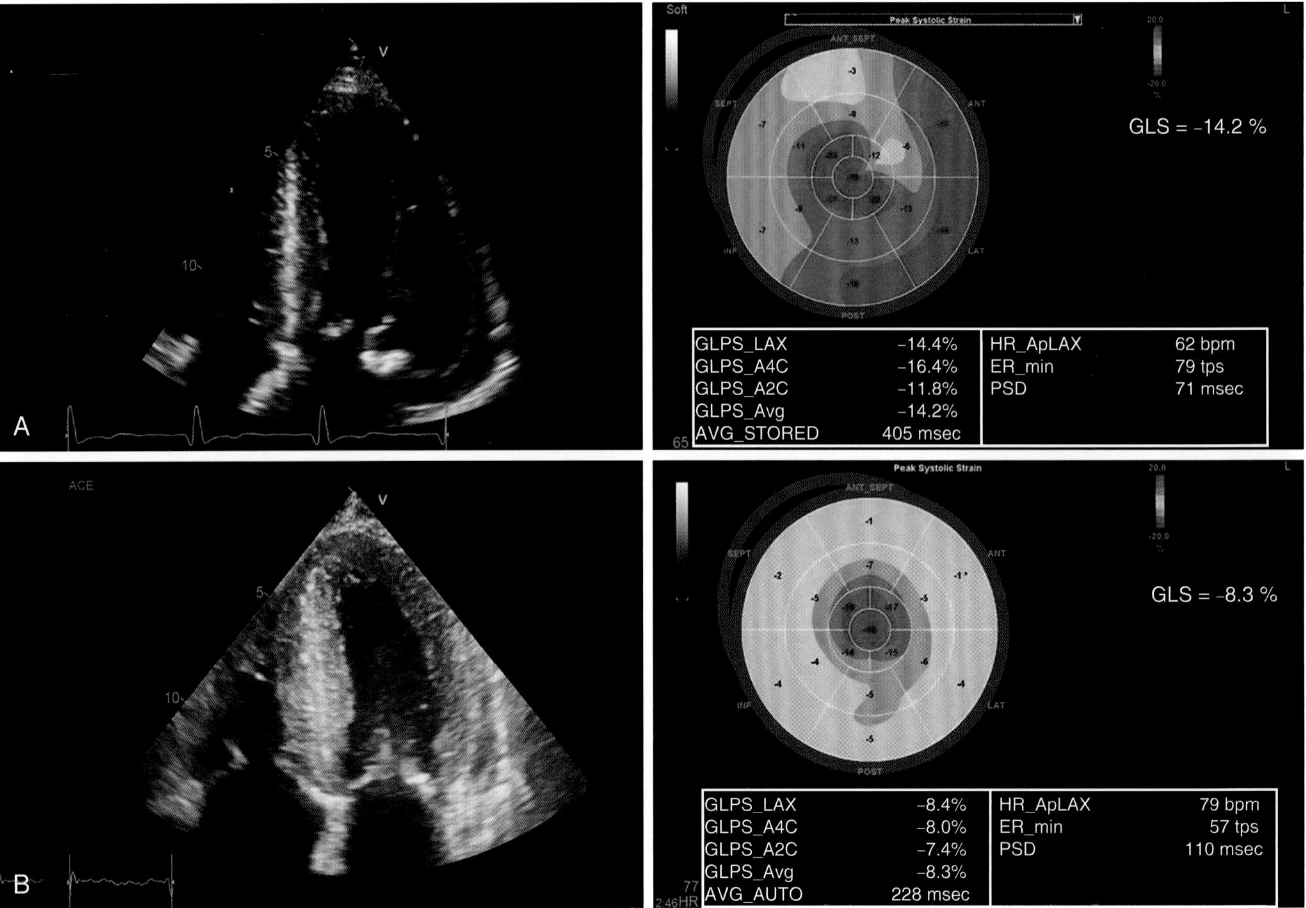

Fig. 5.13 LV longitudinal strain in heart failure with preserved ejection fraction. Representative 2D images and speckle tracking longitudinal strain patterns (bull's-eye plots) in two patients with LV hypertrophy (LVH) and preserved left ventricular ejection fraction (LVEF). (A) In a patient with hypertrophic obstructive cardiomyopathy, LVEF is normal with severe LVH and limited longitudinal excursion of the mitral annulus (Video 5.13A). (B) A patient with cardiac amyloidosis also has severe LVH, a normal LVEF, and very limited longitudinal excursion of the mitral annulus (Video 5.13B). Although both patients have reduced LV global longitudinal strain (GLS), the bull's-eye plots have different patterns. The patient in A has mild to moderate reduction of GLS (−14.2%) with regional impairment of longitudinal strain mainly in the basal and mid-interventricular septum, corresponding to the location of LVH. The patient in B has severe reduction of GLS (−8.3%) with an apical-sparing regional pattern, suggestive of cardiac amyloidosis.

Although E/*e*′ is specific, it is a less sensitive indicator of increased LVFP. Many patients with increased LVFP have an E/*e*′ ratio <14, especially when LVEF is preserved. Clinical settings in which the E/*e*′ ratio is a less reliable measure of increased LVFP include MV disease, surgical ring or prosthetic MV, more-than-mild mitral annulus calcification, left bundle branch block, ventricular pacing, pericardial disease, and normal hearts.[12]

Other echocardiographic signs of elevated LAP include the presence of a transmitral mid-diastolic L wave. This is a consequence of a prolonged transmitral gradient during mid-diastole caused by delayed LV relaxation with continued forward PV flow into middle to late diastole.[65]

Increased PASP in the absence of pulmonary disease can also be used to identify patients with increased LAP.[12] A summary of the echocardiographic parameters used to assess LVFP is presented in Table 5.4.[22,23,26,32,34,58,59,61,66–70]

ALGORITHMS TO DIAGNOSE LV DIASTOLIC DYSFUNCTION AND ESTIMATE LV FILLING PRESSURE BY ECHOCARDIOGRAPHY

No single parameter is accurate enough to diagnose LVDD or to estimate LVFP in isolation. Therefore, a multiparametric approach is needed for this purpose. The 2009 recommendations for diastolic function assessment, including a large number of echocardiographic parameters, were perceived as too complex.[71] In 2016, the American Society of Echocardiography (ASE) and the European Association of Cardiovascular Imaging (EACVI) recommended a streamlined approach to make use of these parameters easier in daily clinical practice.[12]

According to this approach, the evaluation of LV diastolic function should always start by assessing the presence of clinical risk factors known to be associated with LVDD (e.g., hypertension, coronary artery disease, diabetes), by looking for the presence of structural cardiac abnormalities (e.g., LV hypertrophy, LA dilation), and by measuring LVEF.

If clinical and 2D echocardiographic findings do not indicate myocardial disease and LVEF is normal, the measurement of four first-line parameters is proposed for the diagnosis of LVDD: *e*′, E/*e*′ ratio, LAVi, and TR velocity. The following abnormal cutoff values are proposed: septal *e*′ <7 or lateral *e*′ <10 cm/s; mean E/*e*′ >14, LAVi >34 mL/m^2; and peak TR velocity >2.8 m/s. Diastolic function is interpreted as normal if <50% of the measured values meet these criteria and abnormal if >50% of these criteria are met; the study is inconclusive if half of the parameters are normal and half are abnormal[12] (Fig. 5.17).

In patients with structural heart abnormalities or LV systolic dysfunction (reduced LVEF or impaired GLS), LVDD is assumed to be present and the echocardiographic examination should focus on the assessment of LVFP.[12] For this, it is

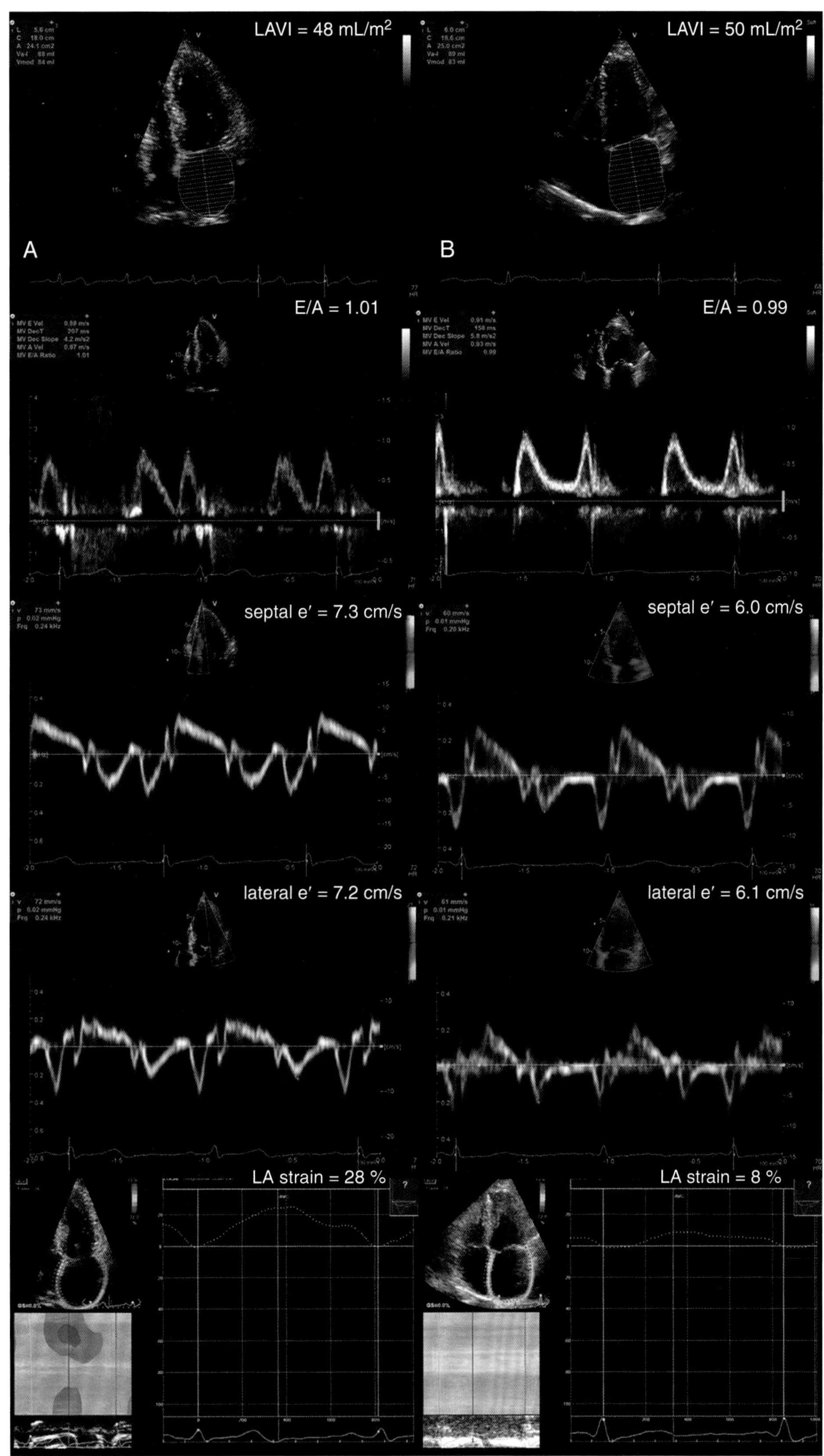

Fig. 5.14 **Role of LA strain in assessing LV diastolic dysfunction.** Echocardiographic measurements of LV diastolic function (including LA peak systolic strain by speckle tracking echocardiography from apical 4-chamber view) in two different patients. (A) A 57-year-old man, New York Heart Association (NYHA) class I, in sinus rhythm, with no history of atrial fibrillation. (B) A 75-year-old man, NYHA class III, in sinus rhythm, with a history of paroxysmal atrial fibrillation. Despite similar values for LA maximal volume, E/A ratio, and e′ velocities at both septal and lateral sites, the asymptomatic patient in A has only a mild reduction in LA peak systolic strain (28%), whereas the symptomatic patient in B has severely reduced LA strain (8%), consistent with more severe disease.

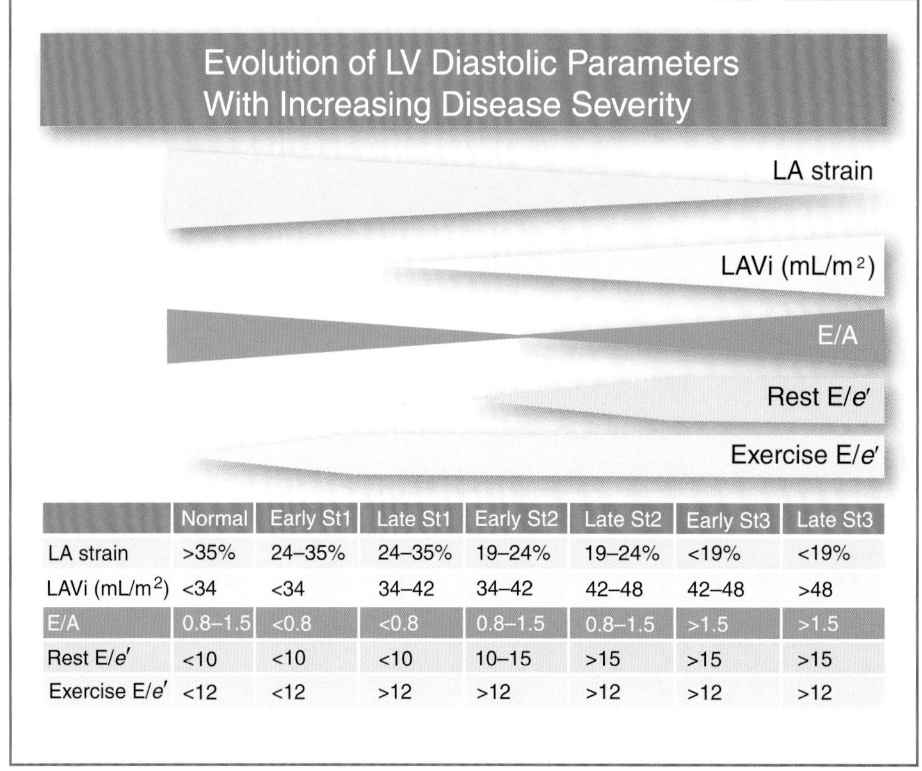

	Normal	Early St1	Late St1	Early St2	Late St2	Early St3	Late St3
LA strain	>35%	24–35%	24–35%	19–24%	19–24%	<19%	<19%
LAVi (mL/m²)	<34	<34	34–42	34–42	42–48	42–48	>48
E/A	0.8–1.5	<0.8	<0.8	0.8–1.5	0.8–1.5	>1.5	>1.5
Rest E/*e*′	<10	<10	<10	10–15	>15	>15	>15
Exercise E/*e*′	<12	<12	>12	>12	>12	>12	>12

Fig. 5.15 Evolution of LA strain values with increasing disease severity. A continuous decrease in LA strain with increasing severity of LV diastolic dysfunction may improve the assessment of the disease stage since other parameters pseudonormalize, or change late in the disease, or change early and do not progress. (From Thomas L, Marwick TH, Popescu BA, et al. Left atrial structure and function, and left ventricular diastolic dysfunction: JACC State-of-the-Art Review. *J Am Coll Cardiol.* 2019;73:1961–1977.)

recommended to start from the mitral inflow pattern and follow the algorithm presented in Fig. 5.18.[12]

- Patients with a mitral E/A ratio <0.8 and a peak E velocity ≤50 cm/s are diagnosed with grade I LVDD (normal mean LAP).
- Patients with a mitral E/A ratio ≥2 are diagnosed with grade III LVDD (elevated mean LAP).
- If the E/A is ≤0.8 with an E velocity >50 cm/s, or the E/A is between 0.8 and 2, the recommendation is to determine the following three parameters: E/*e*′, peak TR velocity, and LAVi.

If >50% of these parameters are normal, LAP is likely normal; if >50% of these parameters are abnormal, LAP is likely elevated. If only two of these three parameters can be determined and they give conflicting results, LAP is considered indeterminate and additional parameters should be determined.

In patients with dyspnea on exertion and preserved LVEF, the echocardiographic diagnosis of grade I LVDD with normal resting LAP should not exclude the presence of cardiac dyspnea, and stress echocardiography is recommended in this setting.

Attention should be paid to identifying specific settings in which the general algorithm does not apply; they require specific adjustments in the manner in which LV diastolic function is evaluated. Such settings include AF or atrial flutter; cardiomyopathies; pericardial constriction; MV disease, MV prosthesis, or significant mitral annular calcification; and conduction abnormalities or paced rhythm.[12]

ASSESSMENT OF DIASTOLIC FUNCTION IN SPECIFIC GROUPS OF PATIENTS

Atrial Fibrillation

LVDD causes LA enlargement that can lead to AF.[72,73] There is a close relationship between AF and HF, and they can cause and exacerbate each other.[74] The correct assessment of LV diastolic function and early diagnosis of HF in patients with AF are extremely important to stop the progression of HF. However, several factors, including cycle length variability, loss of synchronized atrial contraction, and the frequent finding of LA enlargement independent of LVFP increase make the noninvasive assessment of LV diastolic function more challenging in patients with AF.

Measurements from 10 consecutive cardiac cycles, or averaging from three nonconsecutive beats with cycle lengths within 10% to 20% of the average heart rate, is recommended.[12] However, cardiac cycle length and equivalence seem more important than the number of averaged beats. Accordingly, the reproducibility of measurements is higher when the two preceding cardiac cycles have similar RR intervals and the heart rate is controlled (<100 beats/min).[75]

Estimation of PASP, which is related to LAP, may be used to evaluate LVFP. A peak TR velocity >2.8 m/s is suggestive of elevated LAP.

In AF patients with an incomplete TR jet, other Doppler echocardiographic measurements that can be applied to predict increased LVFP include EDT (≤160 ms in patients with reduced LVEF), peak acceleration rate of mitral E velocity (≥1.900 cm/sec^2), IVRT (≤65 msec), deceleration time of the PV D wave (<220 ms), E/Vp ratio (≥1.4), and E/*e*′ ratio (≥11).[12] The delay in annular *e*′ velocity detected by measuring the time interval between the onset of mitral E velocity and that of annular *e*′ velocity can also be used to predict LVFP. All these Doppler parameters have been validated against the invasive measurement of LVFP in patients with AF, with adequate reproducibility.[75]

Last but not least, the variability of mitral E velocity in relation to the RR cycle length should be examined because patients with AF and increased LVFP have less beat-to-beat variation.[76]

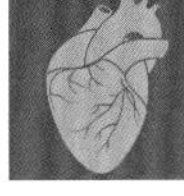

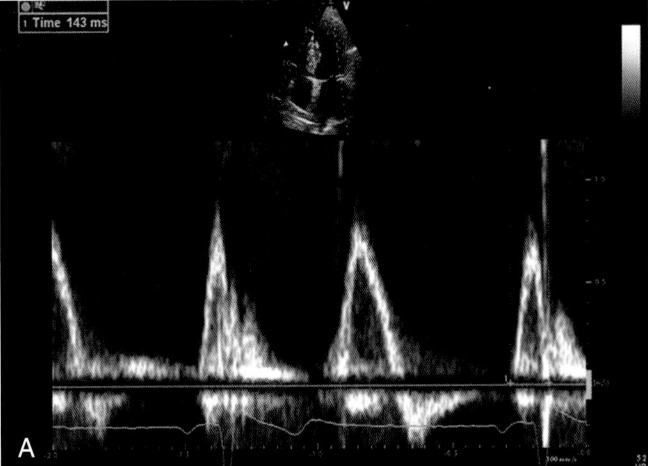

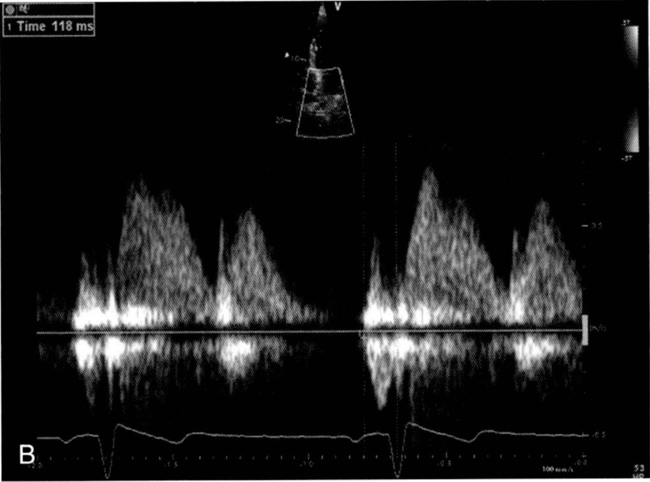

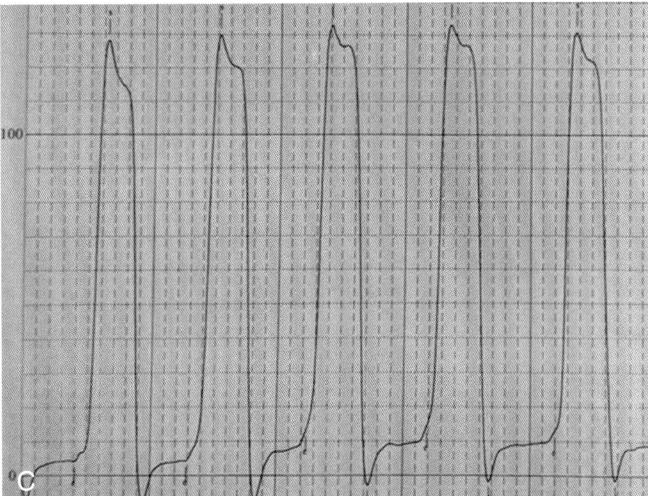

Fig. 5.16 Comparison of atrial wave durations to estimate LV end-diastolic pressure. Pulsed-wave Doppler recordings of mitral inflow (A) and pulmonary vein flow (B) in a 52-year-old man. The duration of flow reversal into the pulmonary veins (Ar_{dur}) was 118 ms, shorter than the mitral flow A-wave duration (A_{dur}) of 143 ms, which is consistent with normal LV end-diastolic pressure (LVEDP). This was confirmed at left heart catheterization (C), with a measured LVEDP of 9 mmHg.

Hypertrophic Cardiomyopathy

The assessment of LVFP in patients with HCM is useful for evaluation of symptoms and disease staging. Different combinations of altered LV relaxation and compliance and LVFP can occur in this clinical setting. Individual measurements have modest correlations with LVFP because of phenotype variability, differences in both LV mass and myocardial fiber disarray, and the presence or absence of the obstructive physiology. Therefore, a comprehensive evaluation of LV diastolic function is recommended as part of the routine assessment of HCM and includes the following parameters and cutoff values[12]:

- Average E/*e*′ ratio >14;
- LAVi >34 mL/m²;
- PV Ar duration – transmitral A duration (Ar – A duration) ≥30 ms;
- CW Doppler-derived TR jet peak velocity >2.8 m/s.

If more than half of these parameters meet the threshold values, then LVFPs are elevated. Normal LVFP can be assumed when <50% of these measurements are abnormal. If 50% of these variables are normal and 50% are abnormal, findings are inconclusive to estimate LVFP. Grade III LVDD is diagnosed when both a restrictive filling pattern and an abnormally reduced *e*′ velocity (septal, <7 cm/s; lateral, <10 cm/s) are present.

This comprehensive approach can be applied regardless of the obstructive physiology or the presence of mitral regurgitation. However, for HCM patients with associated significant mitral regurgitation, Ar – A difference and TR jet velocity remain the only valid parameters for assessing LV diastolic function.

More recent studies using STE have demonstrated the association between LV systolic and LV diastolic strain rates and the relation of LV twisting and untwisting with diastolic function in HCM.[77] Furthermore, their results have linked LV function, including torsion and untwisting, and LA function to exercise tolerance.[78,79] However, additional prospective studies are needed before these parameters can be endorsed as routine measurements in patients with HCM.

Constrictive Pericarditis

Constrictive pericarditis represents a potentially reversible cause of HF, and its pathophysiologic mechanisms include dissociation of intrathoracic and intracardiac pressures along with enhanced ventricular interaction.[80]

Echocardiography provides important tools for the clinically relevant distinction between constriction and restriction.[81] Abnormalities in ventricular septal motion with respiration often provide the first clue to the diagnosis of constrictive pericarditis. Moreover, the inferior vena cava is dilated, the E/A ratio is >0.8, and the septal *e*′ velocity is preserved or increased (usually >8 cm/s). When septal *e*′ velocity ranges between 6 and 8 cm/s, a lateral *e*′ velocity lower than the septal *e*′ velocity (annulus reversus) and a ratio of ≥0.8 between hepatic vein respiratory end-diastolic reversal velocity and forward flow velocity are consistent with constriction.[12]

In patients with constrictive pericarditis, E/*e*′ ratio should not be used to estimate LVFP.

The advanced stages of restrictive cardiomyopathies are usually characterized by a mitral inflow E/A ratio >2.5, EDT <150 ms, IVRT <50 ms, and decreased mitral annular *e*′ velocities (<6 cm/s). Unlike constrictive pericarditis, in restrictive cardiomyopathy the lateral *e*′ velocity is higher than the septal *e*′ velocity. Moreover, the ratio of LV lateral wall strain to septal strain by STE is ≥1 in patients with restrictive cardiomyopathy, whereas it is usually <1 in patients with constrictive pericarditis because of less deformation of the anterolateral wall compared with the LV septum.[12,82]

Other parameters in favor of restriction are an E/*e*′ ratio >15, PV systolic fraction <40%, and LAVi >48 mL/m².[12]

TABLE 5.4 **Echocardiographic Predictors of LV Filling Pressures in Patients With Sinus Rhythm.**

Echo Correlate of LVFP	*Study Population*	*LVEF of Study Population*	*LVFP Used as Invasive Reference (mmHg)*	*Optimal Cutoff Values of Echo Indices for Predicting Elevated LVFP*	*Correlations of Echo Indices With LVFP*	*Sn (%)*	*Sp (%)*	*AUC*
Mitral E/A ratio	61 patients with acute decompensated HF[61]	<50%	PCWP >15	>1.37	$r = 0.64$ $P < 0.001$	82	82	0.87
	140 patients post-MI[66]	<35%	PCWP >20	≥2	$r = 0.65$ $P < 0.01$	43	99	
EDT (ms)	178 consecutive patients with LV dysfunction and a wide range of LVEF[67]	All range	PCWP >15	<150		83	98	—
	140 patients post-MI[66]	<35%	PCWP >20	<120	$r = -0.91$ $P < 0.001$	100	99	
Response of mitral flow pattern to Valsalva maneuver	20 consecutive patients referred for cardiac catheterization[23]	All range	LVEDP >25	A wave increase by >9 cm/s	$r = 0.85$			
	100 consecutive patients referred for clinically indicated left heart catheterization[24]		M-LVDP >15	Decrease in E/A with the Valsalva maneuver ≥0.5	$r = 0.43$			0.80
Systolic fraction of pulmonary venous flow – VTI	116 consecutive patients undergoing elective cardiac catheterization for various cardiac abnormalities[26]	All range	PCWP >18	<36%	$r = -0.88$	90	85	—
A – Ar duration (ms)	50 consecutive patients undergoing diagnostic cardiac catheterization[59]	All range	LVEDP >15	Ar > A duration	$r = 0.68$	85	79	—
	178 consecutive patients with LV dysfunction and a wide range of LVEF[67]		PCWP >15	≥30		73	80	
	70 consecutive patients referred for cardiac catheterization[58]		LVEDP >12	≥20	$r = 0.77$	74	95	
Septal E/e′ ratio	100 consecutive patients referred for clinically indicated left heart catheterization[24]	All range	M-LVDP >15	>15	$r = 0.64$		86	0.81
Lateral E/e′ ratio	60 patients referred for right heart catheterization[34]	All range	PCWP >15	>10	$r = 0.87$	97	78	—
Average E/e′ ratio	159 patients referred for cardiac catheterization[68]	All range	LVEDP >15	>14	$r = 0.31$	13	93	—
LAVi (mL/m²)	159 patients referred for cardiac catheterization[68]	All range	LVEDP >15	>34	$r = 0.28$	46	64	—
Peak atrial longitudinal strain (%)	76 patients with a spectrum of LV function referred for clinically indicated left-heart catheterization[69]	All range	Pre–A-wave LV diastolic pressure >15	<20				0.76
	80 stable patients undergoing cardiac catheterization[70]		M-LVDP >12	<18		96	92	0.87
E/Vp	70 patients admitted to the intensive care department with a balloon-tipped pulmonary artery catheter[32]	All range	PCWP >15	>2.6		74	95	0.90

A, Mitral A wave; *Ar*, peak pulmonary vein reversal wave; *AUC*, area under the curve; *E/A ratio*, ratio of early to atrial peak filling velocity; *Echo*, echocardiographic; *EDT*, deceleration time of mitral E velocity; *E/e′*, ratio between early mitral inflow velocity and mitral annular early diastolic velocity; *E/Vp*, ratio between early diastolic filling velocity and flow propagation velocity; *HF*, heart failure; *LAVi*, LA volume index; *LVEDP*, LV end-diastolic pressure; *LVEF*, LV ejection fraction; *LVFP*, LV filling pressure; *MI*, myocardial infarction; *M-LVDP*, mean LV diastolic pressure; *P*, statistical probability; *PCWP*, pulmonary capillary wedge pressure; *r*, correlation coefficient; *Sn*, sensitivity; *Sp*, specificity; *VTI*, velocity-time integral.

VALIDATION OF THE 2016 ASE/EACVI RECOMMENDATIONS

Hemodynamic Validation

The algorithm proposed by expert consensus for the echocardiographic assessment of LVFP was tested in several studies against invasively measured LVFP. These studies showed that the 2016 recommendations are fairly accurate and superior to the previous ones. All studies have shown the superiority of the integrated multiparametric approach over each single parameter used alone. They have also shown differences in the correlations of the recommended echocardiographic parameters with invasively measured LVFP. The results of these studies are summarized in Table 5.5.[68,83,84]

Prognostic Validation

Other studies have reported on the relationship between LVDD diagnosed using the 2016 ASE/EACVI recommendations and clinical outcomes. These studies, summarized in Table 5.6,[85–89] were conducted in various clinical settings (e.g., acute myocardial infarction, suspected HF, patients with severe aortic

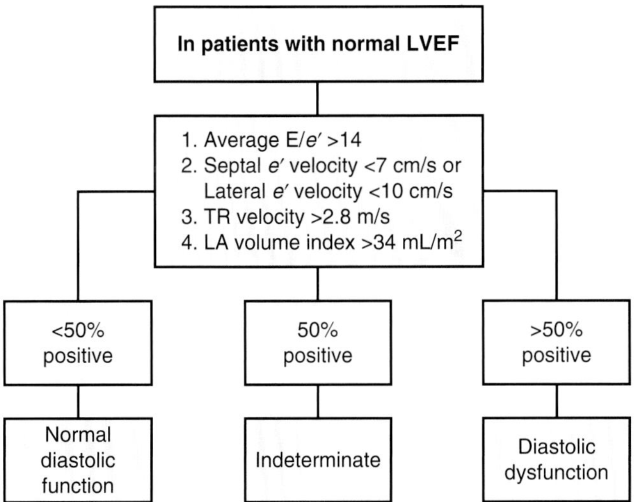

Fig. 5.17 Algorithm for the assessment of LV diastolic function in subjects with normal LV ejection fraction. Four parameters are measured in patients who have normal LVEF and no myocardial disease. LV diastolic dysfunction is diagnosed if >50% of the measured values are abnormal. (From Nagueh SF, Smiseth OA, Appleton CP, et al. Recommendations for the evaluation of left ventricular diastolic function by echocardiography: an update from the American Society of Echocardiography and the European Association of Cardiovascular Imaging. *J Am Soc Echocardiogr.* 2016;29:277–314, Fig. 8.)

stenosis undergoing transcatheter aortic valve implantation [TAVI]). They have all shown the 2016 recommendations to provide superior prognostic information (on all-cause mortality or combined major adverse cardiac events) compared with the 2009 version. Again, not all the recommended echocardiographic parameters have an equal correlation with the outcome measure, and the integrated approach is superior to each individual parameter taken alone.

Clinical Implications

The clinical implications of the 2016 recommendations on the calculated prevalence of LVDD and on interobserver variability have also been evaluated. The prevalence of LVDD in a general population of 1000 patients with LVEF >50% was only 1.6% using the 2016 recommendations, compared with 38.1% using the 2009 version.[90] However, this retrospective study did not apply the 2016 recommendations in detail (including clinical data and specific signals) but rather focused on the algorithms. Another study analyzed 1485 patients with LVEF >50% from a community-based cohort and diagnosed LVDD in only 1.3% of patients using the 2016 recommendations, compared with 5.9% using the 2009 version.[91] This raised concerns about differences in the calculated prevalence of LVDD and about interobserver variability in making the diagnosis.

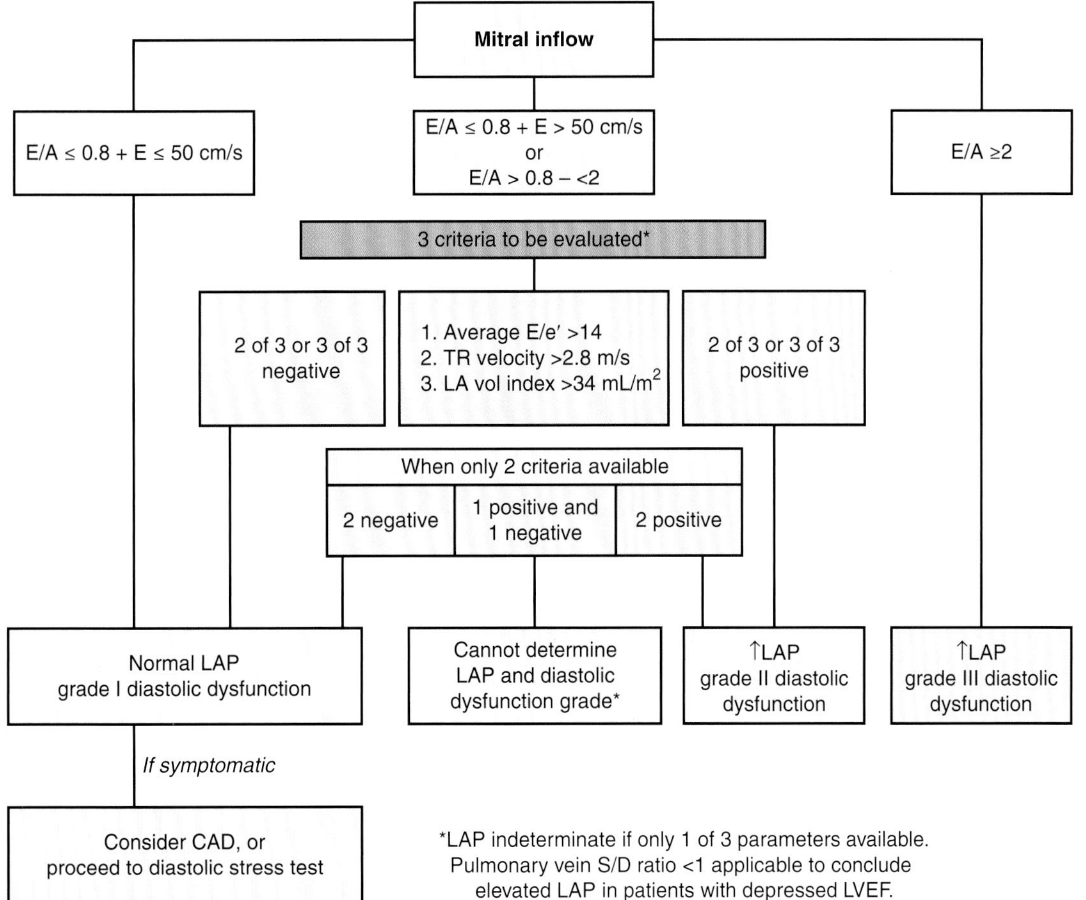

Fig. 5.18 Algorithm for estimating LV filling pressures and grading LVDD in patients with reduced LVEF and in those with myocardial disease and normal LVEF. The echocardiographic examination focuses on the assessment of LV filling pressure. *CAD*, Coronary artery disease; *E velocity*, early diastolic LV filling velocity; *E/A ratio*, ratio of early to atrial peak filling velocity; *E/e′*, ratio between early mitral inflow velocity and mitral annular early diastolic velocity; *LAP*, LA pressure; *LAVi*, LA volume index; *LVDD*, LV diastolic dysfunction; *LVEF*, LV ejection fraction; *TR*, tricuspid regurgitation. (From Nagueh SF, Smiseth OA, Appleton CP, et al. Recommendations for the evaluation of left ventricular diastolic function by echocardiography: an update from the American Society of Echocardiography and the European Association of Cardiovascular Imaging. *J Am Soc Echocardiogr.* 2016;29:277–314, Fig. 8.)

TABLE 5.5 **Hemodynamic Studies Validating the 2016 ASE/EACVI Recommendations for Echocardiographic Assessment of LV Filling Pressure.**

Study	*N*	*LVEF*	*Invasive LVFP Used*	*Sensitivity (%)*	*Specificity (%)*	*PPV (%)*	*NPV (%)*
Lancellotti et al. (2017)[68]	159	≥50%, *n* = 120 <50%, *n* = 39	LVEDP >15 mmHg (echo simultaneous with catheterization)	75	74	39	93
Andersen et al. (2017)[83]	450	≥50%, *n* = 243 <50%, *n* = 207	PCWP or LV pre-A pressure >12 mmHg (echo either during or immediately after catheterization)	87	88	91	83
Balaney et al. (2018)[84]	90	≥50%, *n* = 56 <50%, *n* = 34	LV pre-A pressure >12 mmHg (echo just before catheterization)	69	81	77	77

ASE, American Society of Echocardiography; *EACVI*, European Association of Cardiovascular Imaging; *echo*, echocardiography; *LVEF*, LV ejection fraction; *LVFP*, LV filling pressure; *LVEDP*, LV end-diastolic pressure; *NPV*, negative predictive value; *PCWP*, pulmonary capillary wedge pressure; *PPV*, positive predictive value, *pre-A pressure*, pressure before atrial contraction.

TABLE 5.6 **Studies Investigating the Relationship Between Diastolic Dysfunction Assessed by 2016 ASE/EACVI Diagnostic Algorithms and Clinical Outcomes.**

Study	*N*	*Study Population*	*Main Outcome Measure*	*Median Follow-up*	*Results*
Sato et al. (2017)[86]	460	Patients undergoing elective cardiac catheterization and echo within 24 h	All-cause mortality	419 days	2016 ASE/EACVI guideline algorithms predicted all-cause mortality better than either 2009 ASE/EAE algorithms or individual guideline-recommended parameters.
Prasad et al. (2018)[87]	419	Patients with first-ever MI; echo within 24 h after admission	MACE (death, MI, HF)	2 yr	2016 ASE/EACVI guideline algorithms predicted MACE (and all-cause mortality) better than either 2009 ASE/EAE algorithms or individual guideline-recommended parameters.
Sanchis et al. (2018)[88]	157	Patients with suspected HF attending a "one-stop" HF clinic	MACE (death, HF readmission)	65 mo	When higher event rates were classified using 2016 ASE/EACVI guidelines compared with 2009 ASE/EAE guidelines, Kaplan-Meier curves showed significant differences in survival curves with the 2016 classification but not with the 2009 classification.
Asami et al. (2018)[89]	777	Patients with severe aortic stenosis undergoing TAVR	All-cause mortality	12 mo	LVDD grades I–III classified according to 2016 ASE/EACVI guidelines were independent predictors of 1-year mortality and showed increasing hazard with increasing grade.

ASE, American Society of Echocardiography; *EACVI*, European Association of Cardiovascular Imaging; *EAE*, European Association of Echocardiography; *echo*, echocardiography; *HF*, heart failure; *LVDD*, LV diastolic dysfunction; *MACE*, major adverse cardiac events; *MI*, myocardial infarction; *TAVR*, transcatheter aortic valve replacement.
From Prasad SB, Holland DJ, Atherton JJ, Whalley G. New diastology guidelines: evolution, validation and impact on clinical practice. *Heart Lung Circ.* 2019;28:1411–1420.

The impact of applying the 2016 recommendations on accuracy and interobserver variability was assessed in four groups of observers with different experiences, using invasively acquired LVFP as the gold standard. Observers were provided with clinical and echocardiographic measurements but not with invasive hemodynamic data. The sensitivity to detect elevated LVFP was high (between 88% for experienced sonographers and 92% for senior cardiologists), and there was also very good interobserver agreement.[92]

Patients with suspected HF were screened with brain natriuretic peptide (BNP) measurement and echocardiography. A high proportion (49%) of those initially diagnosed with grade I LVDD using the 2009 algorithms were reclassified as having normal diastolic function by the 2016 recommendations. Importantly, patients reclassified as having normal diastolic function had lower BNP levels, and a lower proportion had a clinical HF diagnosis.[88] Although LVDD is not equivalent to HF, and BNP is a measure of HF and not of LVDD, the result is clinically relevant. It shows that the 2016 recommendations allow a more accurate classification of patients in relation to the HF diagnosis.

Limitations

The 2016 recommendations propose four key parameters and give them equal weight in the algorithms, whereas studies have shown this not to be the case—that is, not all of the four recommended echocardiographic parameters demonstrated an equal predictive value for the presence or severity of LVDD. A sizeable proportion of cases are labeled as indeterminate, and more specific guidance about how to further proceed is needed. This happens mainly because one of the four key parameters, TR velocity, is often unavailable, especially in patients with normal LVEF. TR velocity was not measurable in 40% to 60% of patients included in two of the validation studies.[68,84]

Single cutoff values are proposed for each of the parameters, even for those that are highly age dependent. Although this is easier to apply in practice, it may have a cost in terms of accuracy. Newer promising parameters, such as LA strain or GLS, are not yet included in the current algorithms.

FUTURE PERSPECTIVES

Diastole is a very complex process. It is challenging to find the right balance between accuracy (for proper patient management) on the one hand and simplicity and practicality (for widespread use) on the other hand. The current recommendations are clearly more accurate and easier to use than the previous ones, but a number of issues remain to be improved.

Some of the classic diastology parameters (e.g., PV flow, Valsalva maneuver) could be used to adjudicate the indeterminate cases. Some of the newer markers of LVDD (e.g., LA strain, LV strain) should be tested prospectively in a new algorithm to further improve accuracy.

Finally, the use of artificial intelligence for assessment of diastolic function was recently proposed. An unsupervised machine-learning algorithm focused on large volumes of data may be able to separate similar cases by revealing cluster analysis patterns and correlations without the constraint of an a priori model.[93,94]

Turning from an expert-based assessment to data-driven analysis is a paradigm shift and opens a new field of research. Such developments may have the potential to reduce interobserver variability and to improve the quality of interpretation as well as efficiency and workload. However, more prospective studies are needed to test these promising approaches.

Ultimately, any new proposal needs proper validation by both direct comparison with invasive gold standard measurements and, more importantly, by testing of its correlations against outcomes to confirm their clinical usefulness for patient management.

SUMMARY Acquisition, Analysis, and Interpretation of Echocardiographic Parameters of Diastolic Function

Echocardiographic Parameter[a]	2D Imaging View for Acquisition	Analysis and Measurement	Clinical Interpretation
Mitral inflow Doppler parameters • E-wave velocity (cm/s) • A-wave velocity (cm/s) • A-wave duration (ms) • E/A ratio	• Use an apical 4-chamber view with color-flow imaging. • Align the Doppler beam with the inflow direction. • Place a PW Doppler sample volume (1–3 mm axial size) at mitral leaflet tips. • Use a low wall filter setting (100–200 MHz). • Reduce/adjust Doppler gain so that modal frequency is seen and spectral waveforms do not display signal spikes or feathering.	E-wave: Peak modal velocity in early diastole (after ECG T wave) at the leading edge of spectral waveform A-wave duration: Time interval from A-wave onset to end of A wave at zero baseline If E and A are fused, A-wave onset is determined at the end of E-wave deceleration. E/A ratio: E velocity divided by A-wave velocity	Normal filling pattern: E/A ratio 1–2 Deceleration time is 150–240 ms Impaired relaxation: E/A ratio <1 Deceleration time ≥240 ms Pseudonormal pattern: E/A ratio 1–1.5 Deceleration time is 150–200 ms Restrictive pattern: E/A ratio >1.5 Deceleration time is <150 ms Increased E/A ratio (>2) usually predicts elevated LVFP in patients with myocardial disease but is not useful for this purpose in normal subjects.
• E-wave deceleration time (EDT) (ms)		EDT: Time interval from peak E-wave along the slope of LV filling extrapolated to the zero-velocity baseline	
• Mitral "L" velocity (L wave)		Peak modal velocity in mid-diastole	L-wave velocities >20 cm/s help identify a pseudonormal pattern. L-wave velocities, usually <20 cm/s, may be seen in patients with normal LV diastolic function and low heart rates.

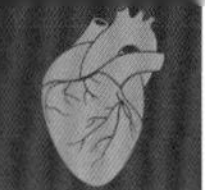

SUMMARY Acquisition, Analysis, and Interpretation of Echocardiographic Parameters of Diastolic Function—cont'd

Echocardiographic Parameter[a]	2D Imaging View for Acquisition	Analysis and Measurement	Clinical Interpretation
• Valsalva maneuver	Mitral inflow recording (as above) is obtained continuously as the patient performs forced expiration for 10 s with mouth and nose closed.	Change in E/A ratio and in A-wave velocity during peak strain and after release	In normal subjects, preload reduction with Valsalva maneuver lowers both E-wave velocity and, to a lesser extent, A-wave velocity. A 20 cm/s decrease in E velocity during the maneuver (assuming that the position of the PW Doppler sample did not change) indicates adequate respiratory effort in patients with a non-restrictive Doppler profile.
• IVRT		IVRT: Time between aortic valve closure and MV opening.	Normal IVRT is 90–100 ms IVRT prolongation (>110 ms) is an early manifestation of impaired LV relaxation. A short IVRT (<60 ms) indicates that mean LAP is elevated.
PV flow Doppler parameters • S wave (cm/s) • D wave (cm/s)	• Apical 4-chamber view with color-flow imaging • "Open-up" the right upper pulmonary vein (RUPV) by angulating the transducer superiorly (such that the aortic valve is seen) • Align the Doppler cursor with the PV flow direction (by color Doppler) • Place a pulsed Doppler sample volume (1–3 mm axial size) at 1–2 cm depth into RUPV • Use low wall filter setting (100–200 MHz) and low signal gain. • Spectral waveforms should not display signal spikes or feathering. • Decrease velocity scale (low pulse repetition frequency). • Record tracings during apnea.	S wave: Peak modal velocity in systole at the leading edge of spectral waveform D wave: Peak modal velocity in early diastole after MV opening at leading edge of spectral waveform	S/D is >1 in normal adults. Young adults <40 years of age may have S/D <1 due to enhanced LV suction. In the presence of a long PR interval, both components of the systolic flow, atrial relaxation (S1) and longitudinal apical displacement of the mitral annulus (S2) become visible; in this situation, S2 will be used to calculate the S/D ratio.
• Peak atrial reversal velocity (Ar) (cm/ms)		Ar: Peak modal velocity in late diastole before MV closure at leading edge of spectral waveform	Normal Ar is <35 cm/s. Values ≥35 cm/s suggest elevated LVEDP.
• Duration of atrial reversal (Ar_{dur}) (ms)		Ar_{dur}: Time interval from Ar wave onset to end of Ar at zero baseline	

Continued

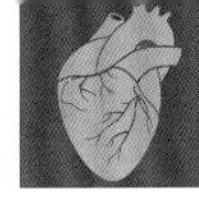

SUMMARY Acquisition, Analysis, and Interpretation of Echocardiographic Parameters of Diastolic Function—cont'd

Echocardiographic Parameter[a]	2D Imaging View for Acquisition	Analysis and Measurement	Clinical Interpretation
• S/D ratio		S/D ratio: Peak S-wave velocity divided by peak D-wave velocity	Severe mitral regurgitation can cause blunting of the S wave and a decrease in the S/D ratio independent of LAP. In patients immediately after cardioversion, the S-wave and Ar peak velocities may be reduced due to atrial stunning.
PW TDI diastolic velocities of the mitral annulus • *e′* velocity (cm/s) • E/*e′* ratio	• Apical 4-chamber view • Align the PW Doppler cursor as parallel as possible to the longitudinal annular motion. • Place a PW TDI sample volume (3–5 mm axial size) at the septal or lateral sites of the mitral annulus. • Check that the annulus is moving through the sample volume during the whole cardiac cycle. • Use ultrasound system presets for wall filter and lowest signal gain. • The velocity scale should be set at about ±20 cm/s to avoid velocity aliasing. • Set the sweep speed at 50–100 mm/s. • Spectral waveforms should not display signal spikes or feathering.	*e′*: Peak modal velocity in early diastole at the leading edge of spectral waveform E/*e′* ratio: Mitral valve peak E velocity divided by mitral annulus peak *e′* velocity	PV flow velocities can be increased in patients after radiofrequency ablation due to PV. Normal lateral *e′* is usually >10 cm/s, whereas septal *e′* is >7 cm/s. *e′* velocities are highly age dependent, and the patient's age needs to be considered when evaluating diastolic function using *e′*. Average E/*e′* ratio <8 usually indicates normal LVFP. When only the lateral *e′* or septal *e′* velocity is available, a lateral E/*e′* ratio >13 or a septal E/*e′* >15 is considered abnormal.
Color M-mode echocardiography • Flow propagation velocity (Vp) (cm/s)	• Apical 4-chamber view with color-flow imaging for M-mode cursor position • Shift color baseline upward to lower velocity scale for red/yellow inflow velocity profile.	Vp: Slope of inflow from MV plane into LV chamber during early diastole at 4 cm distance	Normal Vp ≥50 cm/s With delayed relaxation, the slope becomes prolonged with Vp <50 cm/s. Vp is most accurate in patients with dilated ventricles and LV dysfunction.
• LA maximum volume index (LAVi) (mL/cm^2)	Apical 4- and 2-chamber views. LA volume should be recorded in apical views dedicated for the LA in which LA size is maximized	LA contour should be traced at the end of systole where the LA is largest, usually one frame before MV opening. Exclude the entrance of PVs, LA appendage, and the area under the mitral valve annulus. Length of LA should be similar in apical 4- and 2-chamber views. Use the biplane method of disks or the area–length method.	Upper limit of normal of LAVi for both men and women is 34 mL/m^2.

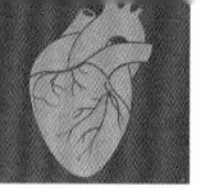

SUMMARY Acquisition, Analysis, and Interpretation of Echocardiographic Parameters of Diastolic Function—cont'd

Echocardiographic Parameter[a]	2D Imaging View for Acquisition	Analysis and Measurement	Clinical Interpretation
• CW Doppler TR jet peak systolic velocity (m/s)	Parasternal and apical 4-chamber view with color-flow imaging aligned with CW Doppler cursor to obtain the highest velocity Adjust gain and contrast to display complete spectral envelope without signal spikes or feathering.	Peak modal velocity during systole at leading edge of spectral waveform	In the absence of pulmonary disease, a PASP >35 mmHg suggests the presence of diastolic dysfunction.
• Peak atrial longitudinal strain (%)	Non-foreshortened apical 4-chamber view of the LA.	Speckle-tracking measurement of atrial strain: The LA is contoured, extrapolating across the PVs and LA appendage orifice. Once the ROI has been defined, the user should visually check the quality of tracking. A dedicated mode for atrial analysis should be used if available. Ventricular end-diastole is recommended as the time reference to define the zero baseline for LA strain curves.	Normal value of LA strain is >35%. Increased LVFP was predicted optimally by peak LA strain <20%. The relationship between LA strain and LVFP appears to be stronger in patients with HF and reduced EF than in patients with normal EF.

[a]All Doppler variables should be measured at end-expiration at a spectral display speed of 75–100 mm/s.

A, Atrial filling; *Ar*, atrial reversal velocity in pulmonary veins; *CW*, continuous wave; *D*, diastolic velocity; *E*, early filling; *e'*, mitral annulus early diastolic velocity; *E/A*, ratio of early to atrial peak filling velocity; *ECG*, electrocardiographic; *EDT*, E-wave deceleration time; *EF*, ejection fraction; *HF*, heart failure; *IVRT*, isovolumic relaxation time; *LA*, left atrium; *LAP*, left atrial pressure; *LVFP*, left ventricular filling pressure; *MV*, mitral valve; *PASP*, pulmonary artery systolic pressure; *PV*, pulmonary vein; *PW*, pulse wave; *ROI*, region of interest; *S*, systolic velocity; *TDI*, pulsed-wave tissue Doppler imaging; *TR*, tricuspid regurgitation; *Vp*, flow propagation velocity.

Data from Nagueh SF, Smiseth OA, Appleton CP, et al. Recommendations for the evaluation of left ventricular diastolic function by echocardiography: an update from the American Society of Echocardiography and the European Association of Cardiovascular Imaging. *J Am Soc Echocardiogr*. 2016;29:277–314; Abraham TP, Mayer SA. Left ventricular diastolic function. In: Catherine M. Otto, ed. *The Practice of Clinical Echocardiography*. 5th ed. Philadelphia, PA: Elsevier; 2016:147–165.

REFERENCES

1. Pfeffer MA, Shah AM, Borlaug BA. Heart failure with preserved ejection fraction in perspective. *Circ Res*. 2019;124:1598–1617.
2. Little WC, Downes TR. Clinical evaluation of left ventricular diastolic performance. *Prog Cardiovasc Dis*. 1990;32:273–290.
3. Bonnema DD, Baicu C, Zile MR. Pathophysiology of diastolic heart failure: relaxation and stiffness. In: Klein AL, Garcia MJ, eds. *Diastology: Clinical Approach to Diastolic Heart Failure*. Philadelphia: Saunders; 2008.
4. Remme EW, Opdahl A, Smiseth OA. Mechanics of left ventricular relaxation, early lengthening, and suction investigated in a mathematical model. *Am J Physiol Heart Circ Physiol*. 2011;300:H1678.
5. Kuo LC, Quinones MA, Rokey R, et al. Quantification of atrial contribution to left ventricular filling by pulsed Doppler echocardiography and the effect of age in normal and diseased hearts. *Am J Cardiol*. 1987;59:1174–1178.
6. Esch BT, Scott JM, Haykowsky MJ, et al. Changes in ventricular twist and untwisting with orthostatic stress: endurance athletes versus normally active individuals. *J Appl Physiol. (1985)*. 2010;108:1259–1266.
7. Buckberg GD, Nanda NC, Nguyen C, Kocica MJ. What is the heart? Anatomy, function, pathophysiology, and misconceptions. *J Cardiovasc Dev Dis*. 2018;5(2):33.
8. Notomi Y, Martin-Miklovic MG, Oryszak SJ, et al. Enhanced ventricular untwisting during exercise: a mechanistic manifestation of elastic recoil described by Doppler tissue imaging. *Circulation*. 2006;113:2524–2533.
9. Stuber M, Scheidegger MB, Fischer SE, et al. Alterations in the local myocardial motion pattern in patients suffering from pressure overload due to aortic stenosis. *Circulation*. 1999;100:361–368.
10. Kroeker CA, Tyberg JV, Beyar R. Effects of ischemia on left ventricular apex rotation. An experimental study in anesthetized dogs. *Circulation*. 1995;92:3539–3548.
11. Zile MR, Brutsaert DL. New concepts in diastolic dysfunction and diastolic heart failure: Part I: diagnosis, prognosis, and measurements of diastolic function. *Circulation*. 2002;105:1387–1393.
12. Nagueh SF, Smiseth OA, Appleton CP, et al. Recommendations for the evaluation of left ventricular diastolic function by echocardiography: an update from the American Society of Echocardiography and the European Association of Cardiovascular Imaging. *J Am Soc Echocardiogr*. 2016;29:277–314.
13. Nagueh SF. Left ventricular diastolic function: understanding pathophysiology, diagnosis, and prognosis with echocardiography. *JACC Cardiovasc Imaging*. 2020;13(1 Pt 2):228–244.https://doi.org/10.1016/j.jcmg.2018.10.038.
14. Paulus WJ, Tschöpe C, Sanderson JE, et al. How to diagnose diastolic heart failure: a consensus statement on the diagnosis of heart failure with normal left ventricular ejection fraction by the Heart Failure and Echocardiography Associations of the European Society of Cardiology. *Eur Heart J*. 2007;28:2539–2550.
15. Lang RM, Badano LP, Mor-Avi V, et al. Recommendations for cardiac chamber quantification by echocardiography in adults: an update from the American Society of Echocardiography and the European Association of Cardiovascular Imaging. *Eur Heart J Cardiovasc Imaging*. 2016;17:412.
16. Nishimura RA, Tajik AJ. Evaluation of diastolic filling of left ventricle in health and disease: Doppler echocardiography is the clinician's Rosetta stone. *J Am Coll Cardiol*. 1997;30:8–18.

17. Whalley GA, Gamble GD, Doughty RN. The prognostic significance of restrictive diastolic filling associated with heart failure: a meta-analysis. *Int J Cardiol.* 2007;116:70–77.
18. Garcia MJ, Thomas JD, Klein AL. New Doppler echocardiographic applications for the study of diastolic function. *J Am Coll Cardiol.* 1998;32:865–875.
19. Popescu BA. Assessment of diastolic function. In: Lancellotti P, Cosyns B, eds. *The EACVI Echo Handbook.* Oxford University Press; 2016:161–185.
20. Abraham TP, Mayer SA. Left ventricular diastolic function. In: Otto CM, ed. *The Practice of Clinical Echocardiography.* 5th ed. Elsevier; 2016:147–165.
21. Dalen H, Thorstensen A, Vatten LJ, et al. Reference values and distribution of conventional echocardiographic Doppler measures and longitudinal tissue Doppler velocities in a population free from cardiovascular disease. *Circ Cardiovasc Imaging.* 2010;3:614–622.
22. Hurrell DG, Nishimura RA, Ilstrup DM, Appleton CP. Utility of preload alteration in assessment of left ventricular filling pressure by Doppler echocardiography: a simultaneous catheterization and Doppler echocardiographic study. *J Am Coll Cardiol.* 1997;30:459–467.
23. Schwammenthal E, Popescu BA, Popescu AC, et al. Noninvasive assessment of left ventricular end-diastolic pressure by the response of the transmitral A-wave velocity to a standardized Valsalva maneuver. *Am J Cardiol.* 2000;86:169–174.
24. Ommen SR, Nishimura RA, Appleton CP, et al. Clinical utility of Doppler echocardiography and tissue Doppler imaging in the estimation of left ventricular filling pressures: a comparative simultaneous Doppler-catheterization study. *Circulation.* 2000;102:1788–1794.
25. Agarwal SK. A new device to perform a standardized Valsalva's maneuver. *Chest.* 1979;75:208–209.
26. Brunazzi MC, Chirillo F, Pasqualini M, et al. Estimation of left ventricular diastolic pressures from precordial pulsed-Doppler analysis of pulmonary venous and mitral flow. *Am Heart J.* 1994;128:293–300.
27. Kuecherer HF, Kusumoto F, Muhiudeen IA, et al. Pulmonary venous flow patterns by transesophageal pulsed Doppler echocardiography: relation to parameters of left ventricular systolic and diastolic function. *Am Heart J.* 1991;122:1683–1693.
28. Pozzoli M, Capomolla S, Pinna G, et al. Doppler echocardiography reliably predicts pulmonary artery wedge pressure in patients with chronic heart failure with and without mitral regurgitation. *J Am Coll Cardiol.* 1996;27:883–893.
29. Chirillo F, Brunazzi MC, Barbiero M, et al. Estimating mean pulmonary wedge pressure in patients with chronic atrial fibrillation from transthoracic Doppler indexes of mitral and pulmonary venous flow velocity. *J Am Coll Cardiol.* 1997;30:19–26.
30. Brun P, Tribouilloy C, Duval AM, et al. Left ventricular flow propagation during early filling is related to wall relaxation: a color M-mode Doppler analysis. *J Am Coll Cardiol.* 1992;20:420–432.
31. Firstenberg MS, Levine BD, Garcia MJ, et al. Relationship of echocardiographic indices to pulmonary capillary wedge pressures in healthy volunteers. *J Am Coll Cardiol.* 2000;36:1664–1669.
32. González-Vilchez F, Ayuela J, Ares M, et al. Comparison of Doppler echocardiography, color M-mode Doppler, and Doppler tissue imaging for the estimation of pulmonary capillary wedge pressure. *J Am Soc Echocardiogr.* 2002;15:1245–1250.
33. Sohn DW, Chai IH, Lee DJ, et al. Assessment of mitral annulus velocity by Doppler tissue imaging in the evaluation of left ventricular diastolic function. *J Am Coll Cardiol.* 1997;30:474–480.
34. Nagueh SF, Middleton KJ, Kopelen HA, et al. Doppler tissue imaging: a noninvasive technique for evaluation of left ventricular relaxation and estimation of filling pressures. *J Am Coll Cardiol.* 1997;30:1527–1533.
35. Caballero L, Kou S, Dulgheru R, et al. Echocardiographic reference ranges for normal cardiac Doppler data: results from the NORRE Study. *Eur Heart J Cardiovasc Imaging.* 2015;16:1031–1041.
36. Lorell BH, Carabello BA. Left ventricular hypertrophy: pathogenesis, detection, and prognosis. *Circulation.* 2000;102:470–479.
37. Hoit BD. Left atrial size and function: role in prognosis. *J Am Coll Cardiol.* 2014;63:493–505.
38. Tsang TS, Abhayaratna WP, Barnes ME, et al. Prediction of cardiovascular outcomes with left atrial size: is volume superior to area or diameter? *J Am Coll Cardiol.* 2006;47:1018–1023.
39. Mor-Avi V, Yodwut C, Jenkins C, et al. Real-time 3D echocardiographic quantification of left atrial volume: multicenter study for validation with CMR. *JACC Cardiovasc Imaging.* 2012;5:769–777.
40. Thomas L, Marwick TH, Popescu BA, et al. Left atrial structure and function, and left ventricular diastolic dysfunction: JACC state-of-the-art review. *J Am Coll Cardiol.* 2019;73:1961–1977.
41. Russo C, Jin Z, Homma S, et al. LA phasic volumes and reservoir function in the elderly by real-time 3D echocardiography: normal values, prognostic significance, and clinical correlates. *J Am Coll Cardiol Img.* 2017;10:976–985.
42. Melenovsky V, Borlaug BA, Rosen B, et al. Cardiovascular features of heart failure with preserved ejection fraction versus nonfailing hypertensive LVH in the urban Baltimore community: the role of atrial remodeling/dysfunction. *J Am Coll Cardiol.* 2007;49:198–207.
43. Lam CS, Roger VL, Rodeheffer RJ, et al. Pulmonary hypertension in heart failure with preserved ejection fraction: a community-based study. *J Am Coll Cardiol.* 2009;53:1119–1126.
44. Obokata M, Olson TP, Reddy YNV, et al. Haemodynamics, dyspnoea, and pulmonary reserve in heart failure with preserved ejection fraction. *Eur Heart J.* 2018;39:2810–2821.
45. Burgess MI, Jenkins C, Sharman JE, et al. Diastolic stress echocardiography: hemodynamic validation and clinical significance of estimation of ventricular filling pressure with exercise. *J Am Coll Cardiol.* 2006;47:1891–1900.
46. Holland DJ, Prasad SB, Marwick TH. Contribution of exercise echocardiography to the diagnosis of heart failure with preserved ejection fraction (HFpEF). *Heart.* 2010;96:1024–1028.
47. Kosmala W, Przewlocka-Kosmala M, Rojek A, et al. Association of abnormal left ventricular functional reserve with outcome in heart failure with preserved ejection fraction. *JACC Cardiovasc Imaging.* 2017;11:1747–1749.
48. Borlaug BA, Nishimura RA, Sorajja P, et al. Exercise hemodynamics enhance diagnosis of early heart failure with preserved ejection fraction. *Circ Heart Fail.* 2010;3:588–595.
49. Kraigher-Krainer E, Shah AM, Gupta DK, et al. Impaired systolic function by strain imaging in heart failure with preserved ejection fraction. *J Am Coll Cardiol.* 2014;63:447–456.
50. Pieske B, Tschöpe C, de Boer RA, et al. How to diagnose heart failure with preserved ejection fraction: the HFA-PEFF diagnostic algorithm: a consensus recommendation from the Heart Failure Association (HFA) of the European Society of Cardiology (ESC). *Eur Heart J. pii.* 2019. https://doi.org/10.1093/eurheartj/ehz641. ehz641. ([Epub ahead of print]).
51. Phelan D, Collier P, Thavendiranathan P, et al. Relative apical sparing of longitudinal strain using two-dimensional speckle-tracking echocardiography is both sensitive and specific for the diagnosis of cardiac amyloidosis. *Heart.* 2012;98:1442–1448.
52. Mondillo S, Cameli M, Caputo ML, et al. Early detection of left atrial strain abnormalities by speckle-tracking in hypertensive and diabetic patients with normal left atrial size. *J Am Soc Echocardiogr.* 2011;24:898–908.
53. Cameli M, Lisi M, Mondillo S, et al. Left atrial longitudinal strain by speckle tracking echocardiography correlates well with left ventricular filling pressures in patients with heart failure. *Cardiovasc Ultrasound.* 2010;8:14.
54. Carluccio E, Biagioli P, Mengoni A, et al. Left atrial reservoir function and outcome in heart failure with reduced ejection fraction. *Circ Cardiovasc Imaging.* 2018;11:e007696.
55. Morris DA, Takeuchi M, Krisper M, et al. Normal values and clinical relevance of left atrial myocardial function analysed by speckle-tracking echocardiography: multicentre study. *Eur Heart J Cardiovasc Imaging.* 2015;16:364–372.
56. Badano LP, Kolias TJ, Muraru D, et al. Standardization of left atrial, right ventricular, and right atrial deformation imaging using two-dimensional speckle tracking echocardiography: a consensus document of the EACVI/ASE/Industry Task Force to standardize deformation imaging. *Eur Heart J Cardiovasc Imaging.* 2018;19:591–600.
57. Yamamoto T, Oki T, Yamada H, et al. Prognostic value of the atrial systolic mitral annular motion velocity in patients with left ventricular systolic dysfunction. *J Am Soc Echocardiogr.* 2003;16:333–339.
58. Appleton CP, Galloway JM, Gonzalez MS, et al. Estimation of left ventricular filling pressures using two-dimensional and Doppler echocardiography in adult patients with cardiac disease. Additional value of analyzing left atrial size, left atrial ejection fraction and the difference in duration of pulmonary venous and mitral flow velocity at atrial contraction. *J Am Coll Cardiol.* 1993;22:1972–1982.
59. Rossvoll O, Hatle L. Pulmonary venous flow velocities recorded by transthoracic Doppler ultrasound: relation to left ventricular diastolic pressures. *J Am Coll Cardiol.* 1993;21:1687–1696.

60. Nagueh SF. Non-invasive assessment of left ventricular filling pressure. *Eur J Heart Fail.* 2018;20:38–48.
61. Nagueh SF, Bhatt R, Vivo RP, et al. Echocardiographic evaluation of hemodynamics in patients with decompensated systolic heart failure. *Circ Cardiovasc Imaging.* 2011;4:220–227.
62. Dokainish H, Nguyen JS, Bobek J, et al. Assessment of the American Society of Echocardiography–European Association of Echocardiography guidelines for diastolic function in patients with depressed ejection fraction: an echocardiographic and invasive haemodynamic study. *Eur J Echocardiogr.* 2011;12:857–864.
63. Kuecherer HF, Muhiudeen IA, Kusumoto FM, et al. Estimation of mean left atrial pressure from transesophageal pulsed Doppler echocardiography of pulmonary venous flow. *Circulation.* 1990;82:1127–1139.
64. Møller JE, Søndergaard E, Seward JB, et al. Ratio of left ventricular peak E-wave velocity to flow propagation velocity assessed by color M-mode Doppler echocardiography in first myocardial infarction: prognostic and clinical implications. *J Am Coll Cardiol.* 2000;35:363–370.
65. Silbiger JJ. Pathophysiology and echocardiographic diagnosis of left ventricular diastolic function. *J Am Soc Echocardiogr.* 2019;32:216–232.e2.
66. Giannuzzi P, Imparato A, Temporelli PL, et al. Doppler-derived mitral deceleration time of early filling as a strong predictor of pulmonary capillary wedge pressure in postinfarction patients with left ventricular systolic dysfunction. *J Am Coll Cardiol.* 1994;23:1630–1637.
67. Dini FL, Ballo P, Badano L, et al. Validation of an echo-Doppler decision model to predict left ventricular filling pressure in patients with heart failure independently of ejection fraction. *Eur J Echocardiogr.* 2010;11:703–710.
68. Lancellotti P, Galderisi M, Edvardsen T, et al. Echo-Doppler estimation of left ventricular filling pressure: results of the multicentre EACVI Euro-Filling study. *Eur Heart J Cardiovasc Imaging.* 2017;18:961–968.
69. Singh A, Medvedofsky D, Mediratta A, et al. Peak left atrial strain as a single measure for the non-invasive assessment of left ventricular filling pressures. *Int J Cardiovasc Imaging.* 2019;35:23–32.
70. Cameli M, Sparla S, Losito M, et al. Correlation of left atrial strain and Doppler measurements with invasive measurement of left ventricular end-diastolic pressure in patients stratified for different values of ejection fraction. *Echocardiography.* 2016;33:398–405.
71. Nagueh SF, Appleton CP, Gillebert TC, et al. Recommendations for the evaluation of left ventricular diastolic function by echocardiography. *J Am Soc Echocardiogr.* 2009;22:107–133.
72. Tsang TS, Gersh BJ, Appleton CP, et al. Left ventricular diastolic dysfunction as a predictor of the first diagnosed nonvalvular atrial fibrillation in 840 elderly men and women. *J Am Coll Cardiol.* 2002;40:1636–1644.
73. Vasan RS, Larson MG, Levy D, et al. Doppler trans-mitral flow indexes and risk of atrial fibrillation (the Framingham Heart Study). *Am J Cardiol.* 2003;91:1079–1083.
74. Wang TJ, Larson MG, Levy D, et al. Temporal relations of atrial fibrillation and congestive heart failure and their joint influence on mortality: the Framingham Heart Study. *Circulation.* 2003;107:2920–2925.
75. Kotecha D, Mohamed M, Shantsila E, et al. Is echocardiography valid and reproducible in patients with atrial fibrillation? A systematic review. *Europace.* 2017;19:1427–1438.
76. Nagueh SF, Kopelen HA, Quiñones MA. Assessment of left ventricular filling pressures by Doppler in the presence of atrial fibrillation. *Circulation.* 1996;94:2138–2145.
77. Pasipoularides A. LV twisting and untwisting in HCM: ejection begets filling. Diastolic functional aspects of HCM. *Am Heart J.* 2016;162:798–810.
78. Rosca M, Popescu BA, Beladan CC, et al. Left atrial dysfunction as a correlate of heart failure symptoms in hypertrophic cardiomyopathy. *J Am Soc Echocardiogr.* 2010;23:1090–1098.
79. Wang J, Buergler JM, Veerasamy K, et al. Delayed untwisting: the mechanistic link between dynamic obstruction and exercise tolerance in patients with hypertrophic obstructive cardiomyopathy. *J Am Coll Cardiol.* 2009;54:1326–1334.
80. Welch TD. Constrictive pericarditis: diagnosis, management and clinical outcomes. *Heart.* 2018;104:725–731.
81. Welch TD, Ling LH, Espinosa RE, et al. Echocardiographic diagnosis of constrictive pericarditis. *Circ Cardiovasc Imaging.* 2014;7:526–534.
82. Kusunose K, Dahiya A, Popovic ZB, et al. Biventricular mechanics in constrictive pericarditis comparison with restrictive cardiomyopathy and impact of pericardiectomy. *Circ Cardiovasc Imaging.* 2013;6:399–406.
83. Andersen OS, Smiseth OA, Dokainish H, et al. Estimating left ventricular filling pressure by echocardiography. *J Am Coll Cardiol.* 2017;69:1937–1948.
84. Balaney B, Medvedofsky D, Mediratta A, et al. Invasive validation of the echocardiographic assessment of left ventricular filling pressures using the 2016 diastolic guidelines: head-to-head comparison with the 2009 guidelines. *J Am Soc Echocardiogr.* 2018;31:79–88.
85. Prasad SB, Holland DJ, Atherton JJ, Whalley G. New diastology guidelines: evolution, validation and impact on clinical practice. *Heart Lung Circ.* 2019;28:1411–1420.
86. Sato K, Grant ADM, Negishi K, et al. Reliability of updated left ventricular diastolic function recommendations in predicting elevated left ventricular filling pressure and prognosis. *Am Heart J.* 2017;189:28–39.
87. Prasad SB, Lin AK, Guppy-Coles KB, et al. Diastolic dysfunction assessed using contemporary guidelines and prognosis following myocardial infarction. *J Am Soc Echocardiogr.* 2018;31:1127–1136.
88. Sanchis L, Andrea R, Falces C, et al. Differential clinical implications of current recommendations for the evaluation of left ventricular diastolic function by echocardiography. *J Am Soc Echocardiogr.* 2018;31:1203–1208.
89. Asami M, Lanz J, Stortecky S, et al. The impact of left ventricular diastolic dysfunction on clinical outcomes after transcatheter aortic valve replacement. *J Am Coll Cardiol Cardiovasc Interv.* 2018;26:593–601.
90. Almeida JG, Fontes-Carvalho R, Sampaio F, et al. Impact of the 2016 ASE/EACVI recommendations on the prevalence of diastolic dysfunction in the general population. *Eur Heart J Cardiovasc Imaging.* 2018;19:380–386.
91. Huttin O, Fraser AG, Coiro S, et al. Impact of changes in consensus diagnostic recommendations on the echocardiographic prevalence of diastolic dysfunction. *J Am Coll Cardiol.* 2017;69:3119–3121.
92. Nagueh SF, Abraham TP, Aurigemma GP, et al. Interobserver variability in applying American Society of Echocardiography/European Association of Cardiovascular Imaging 2016 guidelines for estimation of left ventricular filling pressure. *Circ Cardiovasc Imaging.* 2019; 12(1):e008122.
93. Omar AMS, Narula S, Abdel Rahman MA, et al. Precision phenotyping in heart failure and pattern clustering of ultrasound data for the assessment of diastolic dysfunction. *J Am Coll Cardiol Cardiovasc Imaging.* 2017;10:1291–1303.
94. Lancaster MC, Omar AMS, Narula S, et al. Phenotypic clustering of left ventricular diastolic function parameters: patterns and prognostic relevance. *JACC Cardiovasc Imaging.* 2019;12(7 Pt 1):1149–1161.

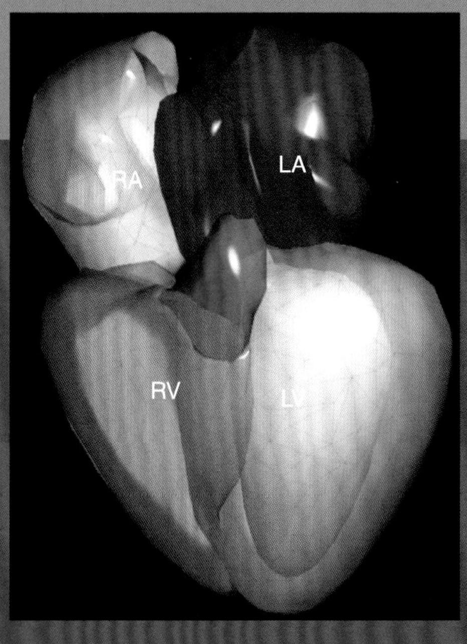

中文导读

第6章 右心室解剖和功能

右心室解剖结构的复杂性，导致其一度成为超声心动图评估的技术难点。现今的超声心动图技术，具有高时间分辨率、无放射性和简便快捷等特点，加之新技术层出不穷，可以全面评价右心室的解剖和功能。以此为基础，本章还详细阐述了右心室的生理功能。

2010年美国超声心动图学会出台了第一部右心功能评估指南，2015年对该指南进行了更新。结合指南，本章重点介绍了右心室外部结构、毗邻关系，包括三尖瓣、上下腔静脉、肺动脉瓣和肺动脉等右心室内部的解剖结构。规范化的评估是建立在标准化切面基础之上的，文中通过图片和表格，详细列举了经胸及经食管超声评估右心室的切面及相关评估参数，对右心室的大小、形态、功能和血流动力学进行准确的定性和定量超声评价。右心室的重要参数，已经广泛常规应用于临床并协助进行快速临床决策，如肺栓塞。三维成像虽然能够真实还原右心室解剖结构改变，但是仍有耗时、分辨率低等技术局限。但在未来，随着软件技术的急速更新，右心室的超声技术会有更好的前景。

权　欣

6 Right Ventricular Anatomy and Function

JAMES LEE, MD | DEE DEE WANG, MD

The right ventricle (RV) is a complex but critical structure for normal cardiovascular function. Descriptions of the role of the RV in normal cardiovascular physiology have evolved throughout history. Some of the earliest documented studies of cardiac anatomic structures were performed by Leonardo da Vinci in his cadaveric dissections.[1] His interest in the RV structure is catalogued in notebook sketches of an anatomic study of an ox heart, with careful detailing of RV papillary muscles, chordae tendineae, and the tricuspid valve.

The 20th century was a period of increased understanding of modern cardiovascular physiology. Initial human in vivo cardiac catheterization procedures in the 1920s first visualized dynamic RV function with invasive right ventriculography using iodinated contrast media.[2] This laid the foundation for work in the 1940s and 1950s in which the technique of right heart catheterization was refined and extensively used for the in vivo study of cardiac and pulmonary physiology. Much of this work was done in canine studies, which showed that an extensively injured RV led to no significant acute increase in central venous filling pressure or decrease in RV systolic pressures.[3,4] This finding was later reinforced by the use of the Fontan procedure to provide a direct passive conduit of venous flow to the pulmonary arteries.[5]

From these and other studies, it was concluded that normal RV contractility played a minor role in normal cardiovascular function. Although this concept has had extraordinary resilience, there has been increasing recognition that it is an incomplete simplification of a complex issue.

With improved availability of echocardiographic imaging and rapid percutaneous intervention techniques, isolated RV ischemia has become recognized as a unique and potentially catastrophic clinical entity. Although the adverse hemodynamics of acute RV myocardial infarction can potentially be reversed with acute coronary reperfusion, acute mortality rates remain high.[6–9] This clinical point has become further relevant due to the high risk of death from left or right coronary obstruction as a complication of transcatheter aortic valve replacement (TAVR).[10,11]

If patients survive beyond the acute phase of cardiogenic shock, those with right heart failure may have improved survival rates compared with those with left-sided pump failure.[12] However, persistent perturbations in normal RV function have important prognostic implications for a wide variety of cardiovascular conditions, and there is renewed interest in better understanding the nuances of RV function. Whereas early tools for the interrogation of RV physiology were invasive, current noninvasive imaging techniques can provide high-quality and reproducible assessments of the RV.

Echocardiography is the first-line modality for imaging the RV, and it has well-established guidelines for application (Table 6.1).[13,14] The advantages of echocardiography lie in its wide availability, high temporal resolution, integrative Doppler physiologic assessments, lack of ionizing radiation, rapid improvements in image quality, and new technologies such as strain and three-dimensional (3D) imaging. They provide a comprehensive toolset for the integrative assessment of RV anatomy and physiology.

This chapter provides an in-depth review of advanced echocardiographic topics regarding RV anatomy and function and focuses on the technical aspects of image acquisition and data prognostication. It also discusses the specific advantages, limitations, and correlations of echocardiography with complementary imaging technologies.

TABLE 6.1 Echocardiography Guidelines for RV Assessment.

Year	*Title*	*Authors*	*Journal*
2010	Guidelines for the echocardiographic assessment of the right heart in adults: A report from the American Society of Echocardiography endorsed by the European Association of Echocardiography, a registered branch of the European Society of Cardiology, and the Canadian Society of Echocardiography	Rudski et al.[14]	*Journal of the American Society of Echocardiography*
2015	Recommendations for cardiac chamber quantification by echocardiography in adults: An update from the American Society of Echocardiography and the European Association of Cardiovascular Imaging	Lang et al.[13]	*Journal of the American Society of Echocardiography*

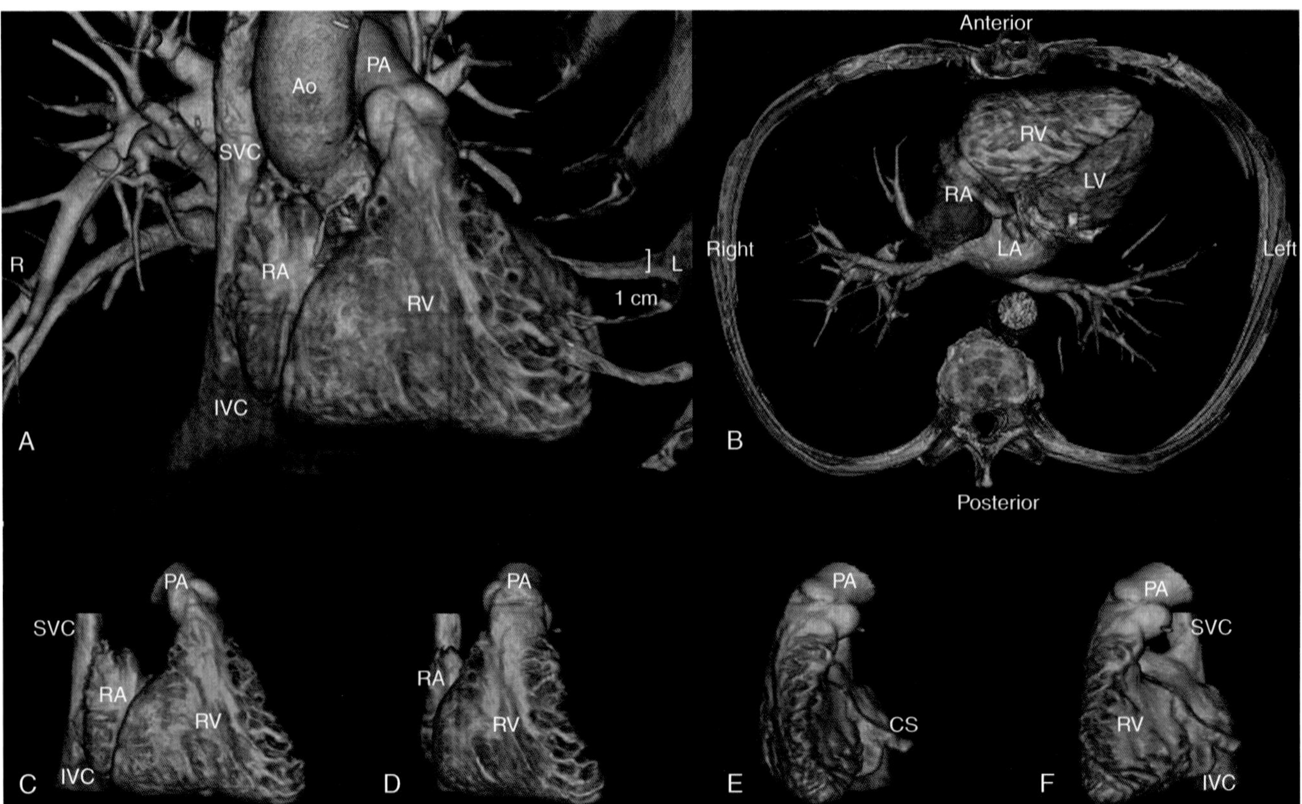

Fig. 6.1 RV external anatomic structure. ECG-gated computed tomography angiography (CTA) volume-rendered images demonstrate the complex shape of the RV and its relation to nearby anatomic structures. (A) Direct anterior projection as seen in a radiologic coronal imaging plane shows the RV and nearby structures (Video 6.1A). (B) CTA volume-rendered image in an inferior projection as seen in a radiologic axial projection. This image demonstrates the proximity of the RV free wall to the sternum (Video 6.1B). (C–F) CTA volume-rendered visualization of the RV from multiple anterior projections demonstrates the complex shape of the RV (Videos 6.1C and 6.1D). *Ao*, Aorta; *CS*, coronary sinus; *ECG*, electrocardiogram; IVC, inferior vena cava; *L*, left; *PA*, pulmonary artery; *R*, right; *SVC*, superior vena cava.

RV ANATOMY AND PHYSIOLOGY

RV EXTERNAL ANATOMY

The RV is the most anterior cardiac chamber, lying immediately posterior to the sternum (Fig. 6.1). The RV rests inferiorly on the diaphragm; posteriorly, it wraps the obliquely oriented left ventricle (LV). This oblique orientation aligns the RV apex anteriorly and inferiorly. The base of the RV is the tricuspid annular plane, which lies posteriorly and to the right as it communicates with the right atrium (RA). Superiorly, the RV outflow tract (RVOT) tapers at the muscular infundibulum as it gives rise to the pulmonic valve and pulmonary artery.

The RV structure is complex and does not readily conform to common geometric shapes. From the short-axis view, the RV has the appearance of an asymmetric crescent. When viewed in a horizontal or vertical long-axis projection, the RV has a more triangular appearance. The full 3D structure of the RV can be conceptualized as a flexible triangular pouch wrapped around the LV.

RV INTERNAL ANATOMY

The internal anatomy of the RV can be roughly divided into an inflow region, an outflow region, and a main body (Fig. 6.2). These regions have distinct morphologic characteristics and can provide helpful localization of pathology, such as a ventricular septal defect (VSD). Membranous or perimembranous VSDs are located in the inflow region. Supracrystal or outflow tract VSDs are located in the outflow region. Muscular VSDs are located in the main body of the RV.

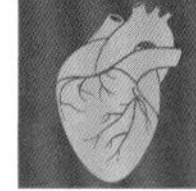

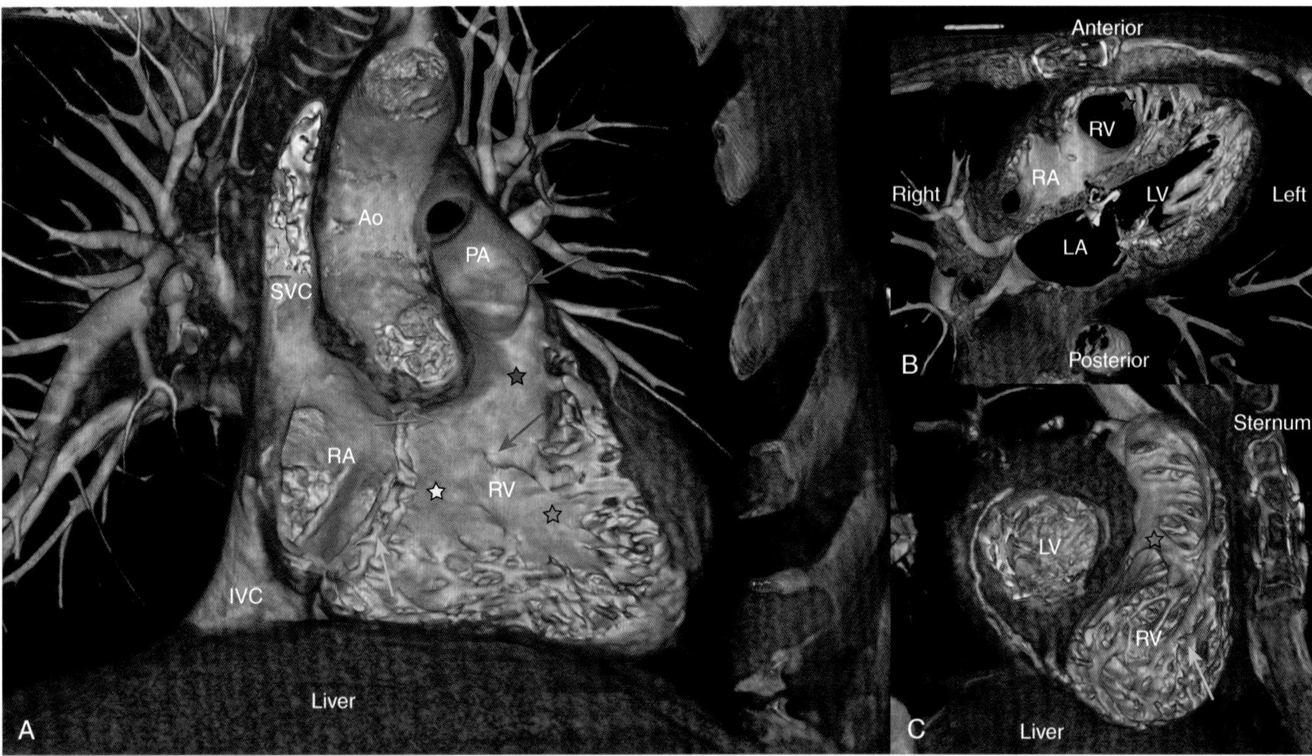

Fig. 6.2 **RV internal anatomic structure.** ECG-gated computed tomography angiography volume-rendered imaging with transparent blood pool shading allows for visualization of the internal structure of the RV and nearby anatomy. (A) The RV can be divided into inflow, outflow, and main body regions. The inflow region *(yellow star)* is bordered posteriorly and to the right by the tricuspid valve *(yellow arrow)*. Superiorly, the inflow region is demarcated by the crista supraventricularis *(red arrow)*, which extends toward the apex of the RV as it forms the moderator band (also called the *septomarginal trabecula*). The membranous portion of the interventricular septum is also located in the inflow region *(blue arrow)*. The infundibulum or smooth outflow portion of the RV *(purple star)* is superior to the crista supraventricularis and inferior to the pulmonic valve *(purple arrow)*. The main body of the RV *(green star)* is highly trabeculated and contains the muscular portion of the interventricular septum (Video 6.2A). (B) Inferior projection of the RV demonstrates the course of the moderator band *(red star)* (Video 6.2B). (C) View of the RV from the perspective of the RA. Within the rich trabecular structure of the RV, the moderator band *(red star)* and tricuspid valve papillary muscles *(yellow arrow)* are visualized (Video 6.2C). *Ao*, Aorta; *ECG*, electrocardiogram; *IVC*, inferior vena cava; *PA*, pulmonary artery; *SVC*, superior vena cava.

The inflow region of the RV borders the tricuspid annulus and is demarcated superiorly by the crista supraventricularis, a muscular ridge that is contractile and extends from the tricuspid annulus along the interventricular septum (IVS) before forming the moderator band near the apex. The outflow region (i.e., infundibulum) of the RV is a smooth and cylindrical muscular structure. Overdevelopment of this musculature can lead to pulmonary stenosis as an isolated entity or as part of the tetralogy of Fallot. The main body of the RV is highly trabeculated and includes a network of tricuspid chordae and associated tricuspid papillary muscles. Hypertrophied anomalous muscle bundles in the main body of the RV can lead to a dual-chambered RV physiology.

TRICUSPID VALVE

The tricuspid valve and its supporting apparatus are inexorably tied to the internal structure of the RV (Table 6.2). Although the tricuspid valve often comprises a varied number of leaflets and scallops, it is classically described as having septal, anterior, and posterior leaflets.[15] Given the compliant nature of the RV cavity and the tricuspid annulus, right-sided volume loads readily lead to tricuspid annular dilation and secondary tricuspid regurgitation (TR) (Fig. 6.3).

TABLE 6.2 Tricuspid Valve Anatomy.

Papillary Muscles	*Tricuspid Valve Leaflets*	*Associated Structures in the RV*
Anterior	Anterior, posterior	Moderator band, anterior wall
Posterior	Septal	Posterior free wall
Septal	Anterior, septal	Interventricular septum

The base of the tricuspid valve leaflets inserts into the tricuspid annulus, which is anteriorly displaced compared with the mitral annulus. The anterior tricuspid annular displacement and identification of the moderator band and extensive RV trabeculation can help in distinguishing the morphologic RV from the LV in congenital heart disorders. Failure of delamination of the septal and posterior leaflets of the tricuspid valve can cause

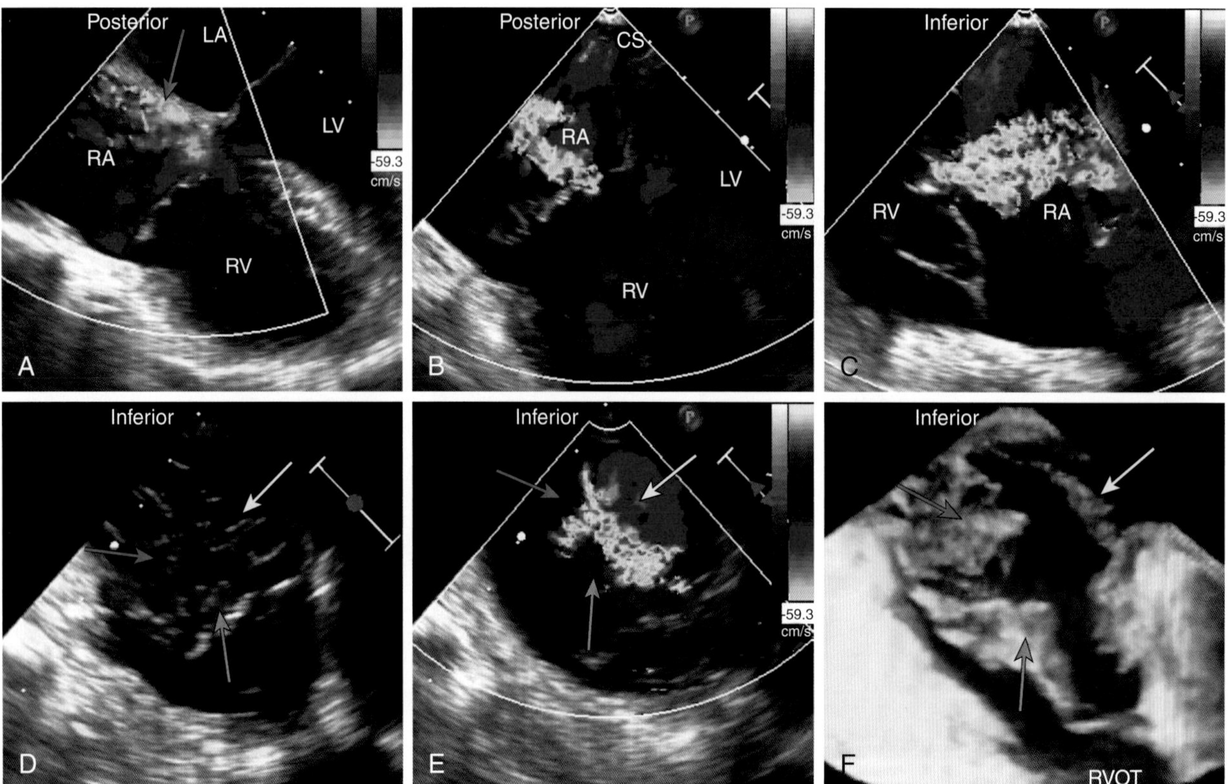

Fig. 6.3 Tricuspid valve evaluation with TEE. The tricuspid valve has a complex, star-shaped regurgitant orifice that requires multiple imaging planes for a comprehensive evaluation on TEE. (A) TEE mid-esophageal view at 0 degrees with an RV-focused orientation shows only a small amount of tricuspid regurgitation (TR) on color Doppler imaging *(red arrow)* (Video 6.3A). (B) Improved visualization of eccentric jets of TR can often be obtained by advancing the TEE probe near the gastroesophageal junction. Visualization of the coronary sinus *(CS)* confirms deeper and more posterior probe positioning (Video 6.3B). (C) Transgastric view of the tricuspid valve at approximately 90 degrees demonstrates a broader jet of tricuspid regurgitation (Video 6.3C). In D through F, the anterior leaflet is indicated by an *orange arrow*, the septal leaflet by a *yellow arrow*, and the posterior leaflet by a *blue arrow*. (D) The tricuspid valve short axis on TEE can be seen in the transgastric view with anteflexion at an angle of 0 to 20 degrees (Video 6.3D). (E) Color Doppler view of the tricuspid valve short axis further highlights the star-shaped tricuspid regurgitant orifice (Video 6.3E). (F) 3D TEE can provide additional understanding of the tricuspid valve leaflet morphology.

an apparent apical displacement of the tricuspid annulus (i.e., Ebstein anomaly).

RIGHT ATRIUM AND INFERIOR VENA CAVA

The RA and RV are anatomic neighbors whose functions are closely intertwined. The RV receives blood from the RA by passive flow, active RV relaxation, and right atrial contraction. The RA is filled by the superior and inferior vena cavae and the coronary sinus. Isolated RA dilation can be a sign of TR or restrictive RV filling. Conversely, a large volume load from an atrial septal defect can cause RV and RA dilation. Because of the close physiologic relationship of these structures, an abnormality of either one warrants a comprehensive evaluation of all right-sided cardiac structures (Fig. 6.4).

PULMONIC VALVE AND PULMONARY ARTERY

The pulmonic valve connects the RVOT with the pulmonary arteries. The pulmonic valve is a tricuspid structure with leaflets that are thinner than the aortic valve leaflets. The anterior and superior location of the pulmonic valve and the thin pulmonic leaflets render the valve challenging to image with almost all imaging modalities (Fig. 6.5).

The pulmonary artery is a thin-walled, high-flow, low-pressure system that provides flow from the RV into the pulmonary vascular bed. The normally low-pressured nature of the pulmonary vascular system means that the RV is poorly suited for increases in pulmonary pressures resulting from pulmonary hypertension (Table 6.3).

RV BLOOD SUPPLY

The RV blood supply predominantly arises from the right coronary artery (RCA), with accessory contribution along the IVS from the left coronary artery (LCA) system (Fig. 6.6). The RCA ostium normally arises in an anterior direction from the right coronary cusp of the sinus of Valsalva. It has proximal, middle, and distal segments, which are delineated by the superior and inferior margins of the RV. The proximal portion of the RCA commonly provides an atrioventricular nodal branch and a conus branch that supplies blood to the RVOT or infundibulum.

The midportion of the RCA gives off multiple RV acute marginal branches that supply blood to the RV free wall. In most individuals, the RCA is dominant and gives rise to a right posterior descending artery (rPDA) branch and a right posterolateral branch. The rPDA typically supplies the basal and mid-inferoseptum, and the LCA supplies the remainder of the IVS, primarily through septal perforators from the left anterior descending coronary artery.[16]

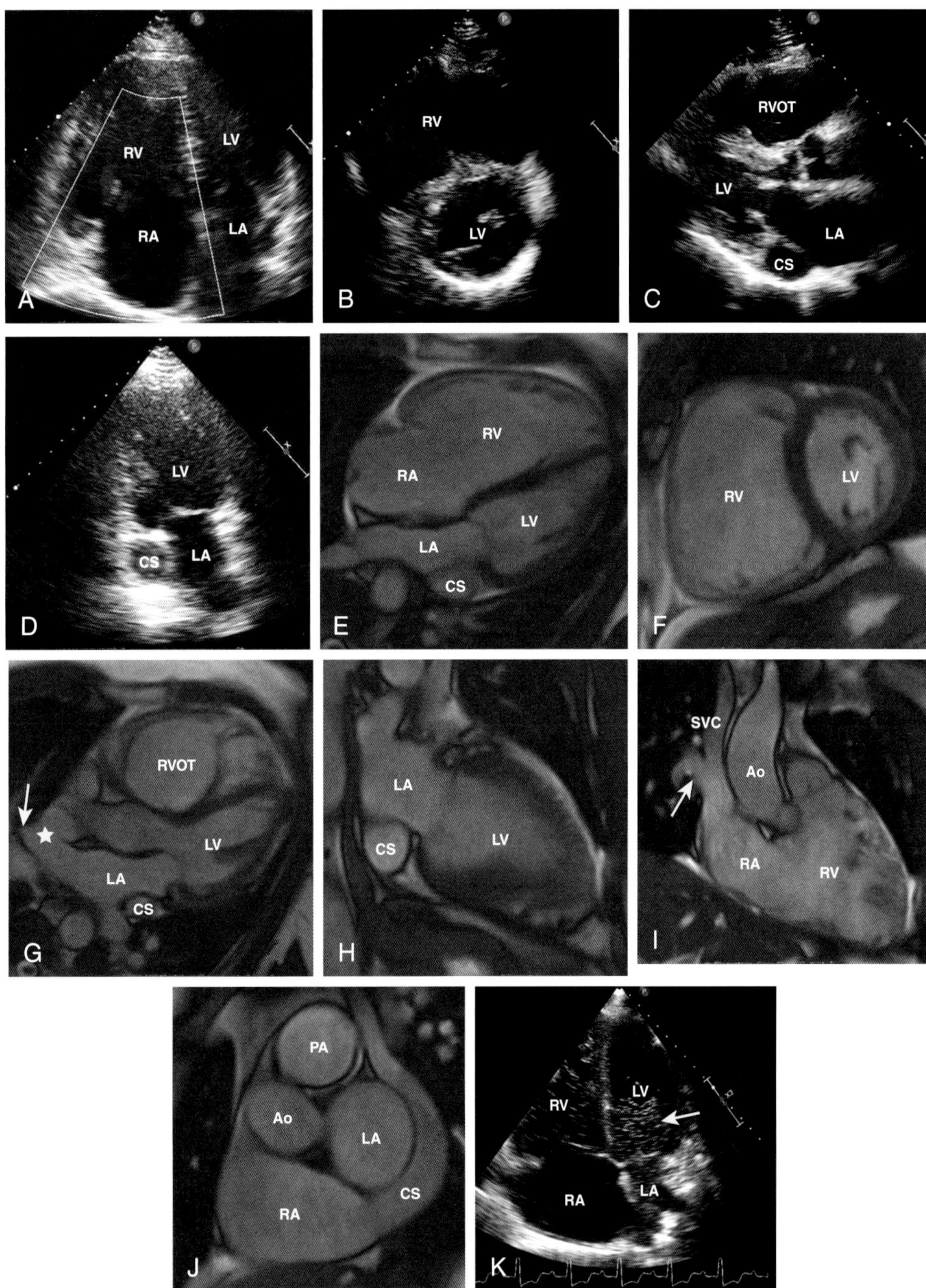

Fig. 6.4 **Multimodality imaging of the sinus venosus atrial septal defect.** Unexplained RV dilation can be caused by left-to-right shunts from an atrial septal defect (ASD) due to an increased RV volume load. (A) TTE apical RV-focused view shows severely dilated right-sided cardiac chambers with a corresponding cardiac magnetic resonance (CMR) image (E) that is notable for additional visualization of a dilated coronary sinus *(CS)* (Videos 6.4A and E). (B) TTE parasternal short-axis image with a corresponding CMR image (F) further demonstrates severe RV chamber dilation (Videos 6.4B and F). (C) TTE parasternal long-axis image shows a dilated RV outflow tract and the dilated CS. The corresponding CMR image (G) shows an anomalous pulmonary venous return *(yellow arrow)* at the confluence of the superior vena cava with the RA and LA, causing a sinus venosus ASD *(yellow star)*. This confluence *(yellow arrow)* is also shown in a secondary CMR view (I) (Videos 6.4C, G, and I). (D) A TTE apical 2-chamber view and corresponding CMR image (H) show the dilated CS. Its full extent is seen by CMR (J) where it communicates superiorly as a persistent left subclavian vein (Videos 6.4D, H, and J). (K) A left-sided agitated saline injection may help distinguish between a sinus venosus ASD and an unroofed CS. In a patient with an unroofed CS, bubbles *(yellow arrow)* from a left arm agitated saline injection first appear in the LA rather than the RA (Video 6.4K). *Ao*, Aorta; *PA*, pulmonary artery; *RVOT*, right ventricular outflow tract; *SVC*, superior vena cava.

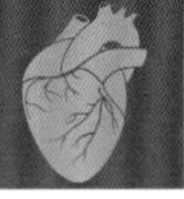

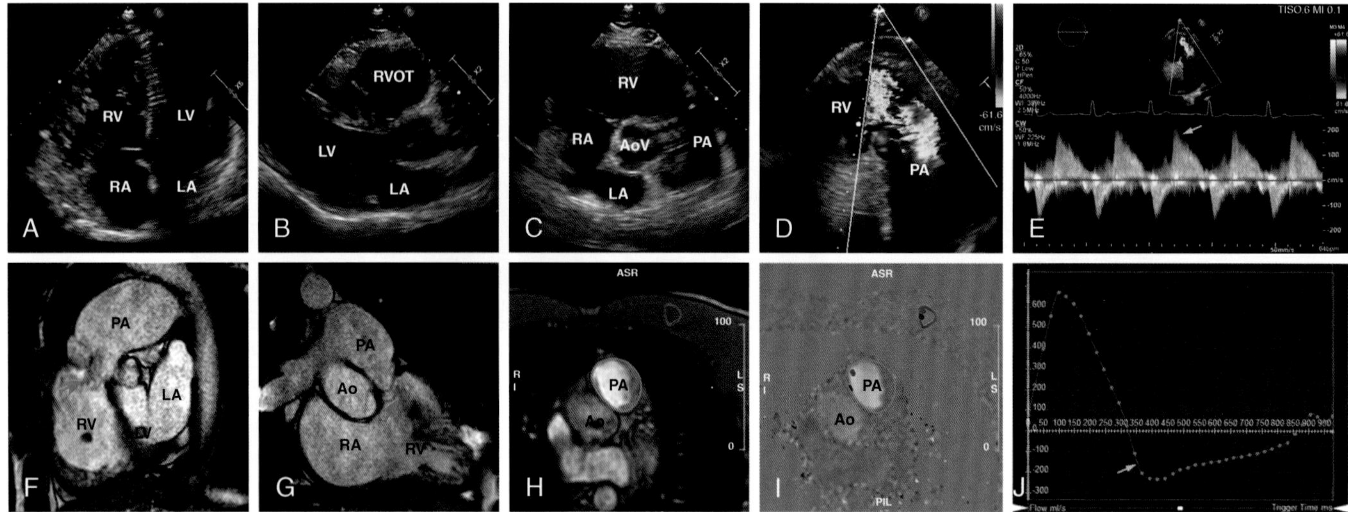

Fig. 6.5 Multimodality imaging of pulmonary regurgitation. TTE can provide an anatomic and functional interrogation of unexplained RV dilation. (A) TTE apical 4-chamber RV-focused view shows RV dilation. The interventricular septum is bowed toward the LV in diastole, suggesting right-sided volume overload (Video 6.5A). (B) TTE parasternal long-axis view shows dilation of the right ventricular outflow tract *(RVOT)* (Video 6.5B). (C) RV dilation is seen in parasternal short-axis view at the level of the AV (Video 6.5C). (D) TTE color Doppler with focus on the pulmonic valve shows a large regurgitant jet consistent with severe pulmonic regurgitation (Video 6.5D). (E) CW spectral Doppler can be helpful in severe pulmonary regurgitation by demonstrating a dense envelope of pulmonary regurgitation with a triangular shape caused by the rapid diastolic pressure equalization between the pulmonary artery and right ventricle *(yellow arrow)* (Video 6.5E). (F and G) Two oblique views of the RVOT on cardiac magnetic resonance imaging (CMR) with steady-state free precession (SSFP) intrinsic bright blood cine imaging (Video 6.5F). Pulmonary regurgitant jets can be seen on CMR SSFP images *(orange arrows)* due to proton dephasing from turbulent flow. This can be difficult to appreciate and is not an ideal technique for quantification of regurgitant flow. Evaluation of pulmonary regurgitation on CMR is better performed with phase-contrast imaging (Qflow, Medis Medical Imaging Systems, Raleigh, NC), which allows the quantitative assessment of flow through an imaging plane that has been prescribed in a double-oblique fashion just superior to the valve plane. (H) Qflow magnitude anatomic localizer image. (I) Qflow phase-contrast, through-plane image in which blood flowing through the plane is encoded as *black* or *white*, depending on direction. A region of interest *(green circle)* can be prescribed to quantitate this flow. (J) Graph of flow quantitated by Qflow imaging. Forward flow is the area of the curve above the baseline. Regurgitant flow is the area of the curve below the baseline *(yellow arrow)*. In this patient, the forward flow was 134 mL and regurgitant volume was 76 mL, yielding a regurgitant fraction of 56.7%. *Ao*, Aorta; *AoV*, aortic valve; *LA*, left atrium; *LV*, left ventricle; *PA*, pulmonary artery.

TABLE 6.3 Classification of Pulmonary Hypertension.

Type of Pulmonary Hypertension	*Subtypes and Associations*
Pulmonary arterial hypertension (PAH)	• Idiopathic PAH • Heritable PAH • Drug and toxin induced • Associated with connective tissue, HIV infection, portal hypertension, congenital heart disease, schistosomiasis • Pulmonary veno-occlusive disease and/or pulmonary capillary hemangiomatosis • Persistent pulmonary hypertension of the newborn • LV systolic dysfunction • LV diastolic dysfunction • Valvular disease • Congenital/acquired left heart inflow/outflow tract obstruction and congenital cardiomyopathies • Chronic obstructive pulmonary disease • Interstitial lung disease • Other pulmonary diseases with mixed restrictive and obstructive pattern • Sleep-disordered breathing • Alveolar hypoventilation disorders • Chronic exposure to high altitude • Developmental lung diseases
Chronic thromboembolic pulmonary hypertension (CTEPH)	• No subcategories
Pulmonary hypertension with unclear multifactorial mechanisms	• Hematologic disorders: chronic hemolytic anemia, myeloproliferative disorders, splenectomy • Systemic disorders: sarcoidosis, pulmonary histiocytosis, lymphangioleiomyomatosis • Metabolic disorders: glycogen storage disease, Gaucher disease, thyroid disorders • Others: tumoral obstruction, fibrosing mediastinitis, chronic renal failure, segmental pulmonary hypertension

HIV, Human immunodeficiency virus.
Adapted from Simonneau G, Robbins IM, Beghetti M, et al. Updated clinical classification of pulmonary hypertension. *J Am Coll Cardiol.* 2009;30;54(1 suppl):S43–S54.

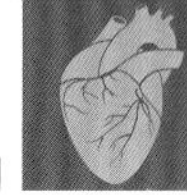

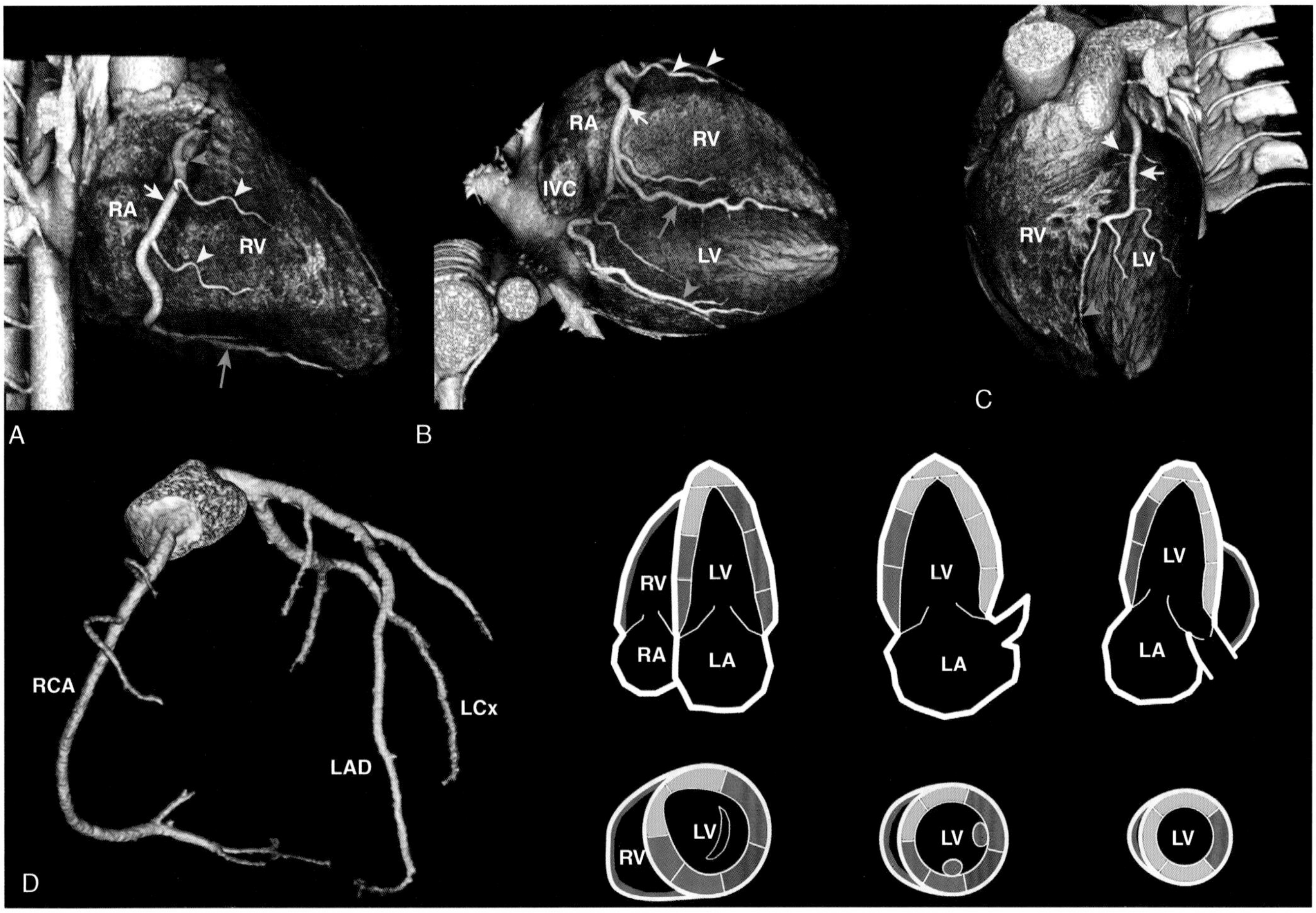

Fig. 6.6 RV blood supply. The RV receives its blood supply predominantly from the RCA, as visualized with ECG-gated coronary tomography angiography (CTA) volume-rendered images. (A) Right anterior oblique view shows the RCA *(yellow arrow)* originating anteriorly off the right coronary cusp and traversing the AV groove while giving off RV acute marginal branches *(yellow arrowheads)*. A small conus branch feeding the RV outflow tract is frequently the first vessel branching from the RCA *(orange arrowhead)*. In a right-dominant coronary artery system, the RCA distally gives off a right posterior descending artery (rPDA) branch *(orange arrow)*, which feeds much of the infraseptal portion of the interventricular septum. (B) Right anterior oblique and caudal view. After the exit of the RV acute marginal branches *(yellow arrowheads)*, the RCA *(yellow arrow)* gives off a large rPDA *(orange arrow)* and right posterolateral branch *(orange arrowhead)*. (C) Left anterior oblique and cranial view. Due to the shared interventricular septum, the blood supply to the interventricular septum is important to RV function. The left anterior descending coronary artery *(LAD) (yellow arrow)* largely supplies the basal and mid-regions of the anteroseptum via septal perforator branches (*yellow arrowhead*). As the LAD traverses distally along the AV groove, it provides blood to the distal septum (*orange arrowhead*). (D) Diagrams of normal myocardial segments fed by the coronary arteries as identified on the *left*. *AV*, Atrioventricular; *ECG*, electrocardiogram; *IVC*, inferior vena cava; *LAD*, left anterior descending coronary artery; *LCx*, left circumflex coronary artery; *RCA*, right coronary artery.

Acute RV ischemia can lead to cardiogenic shock that is associated with a high mortality rate. Historically, the RV was thought to tolerate ischemia better than the LV. This was attributed to the lower metabolic demands of the RV, greater thickness of the LV myocardium, and differences in coronary physiology, with RCA flow being less phasic and augmented in systole compared with LCA flow, which occurs primarily in diastole.[17,18] However, in TAVR patients, early coronary occlusion of the RCA or LCA leads to acute ischemia and a combined hospital mortality rate of 50%.[11] This suggests that the adverse outcomes from acute RCA occlusion may be related more to the territory of myocardial involvement than to differences in coronary and myocardial physiology. This is further supported by data in patients with acute RV infarctions who underwent late gadolinium enhancement imaging by cardiac magnetic resonance imaging (CMR). In these patients, evidence of RV injury was noted in 57% of patients, which persisted at 13 months[18a] (Fig. 6.7).

RV PHYSIOLOGY

In anatomically normal hearts, RV and LV systolic functions mirror each other. Differences in appearance of the RV size on traditional 2D imaging results from the anatomic location of the RV in the thoracic cavity and the inability of a planar 2D ultrasound beam to capture a 3D structure. Although the RV appears smaller than the LV in most 2D projections, the total RV volume is larger than the LV in normal individuals.[19] This means that the RV ejection fraction must be lower than the LV ejection fraction for any given cardiac output. These relationships are defined by the following formulas:

$$\text{Cardiac output} = \text{Stroke volume} \times \text{Heart rate}$$

$$\text{Stroke volume} = \text{End diastolic volume} - \text{End systolic volume}$$

$$\text{Ejection fraction} = \text{Stroke volume} \div \text{End diastolic volume}$$

RV and LV functions have direct interactions, called *ventricular interdependence*. Ventricular interdependence is multifactorial, but a primary contributor is the shared space in

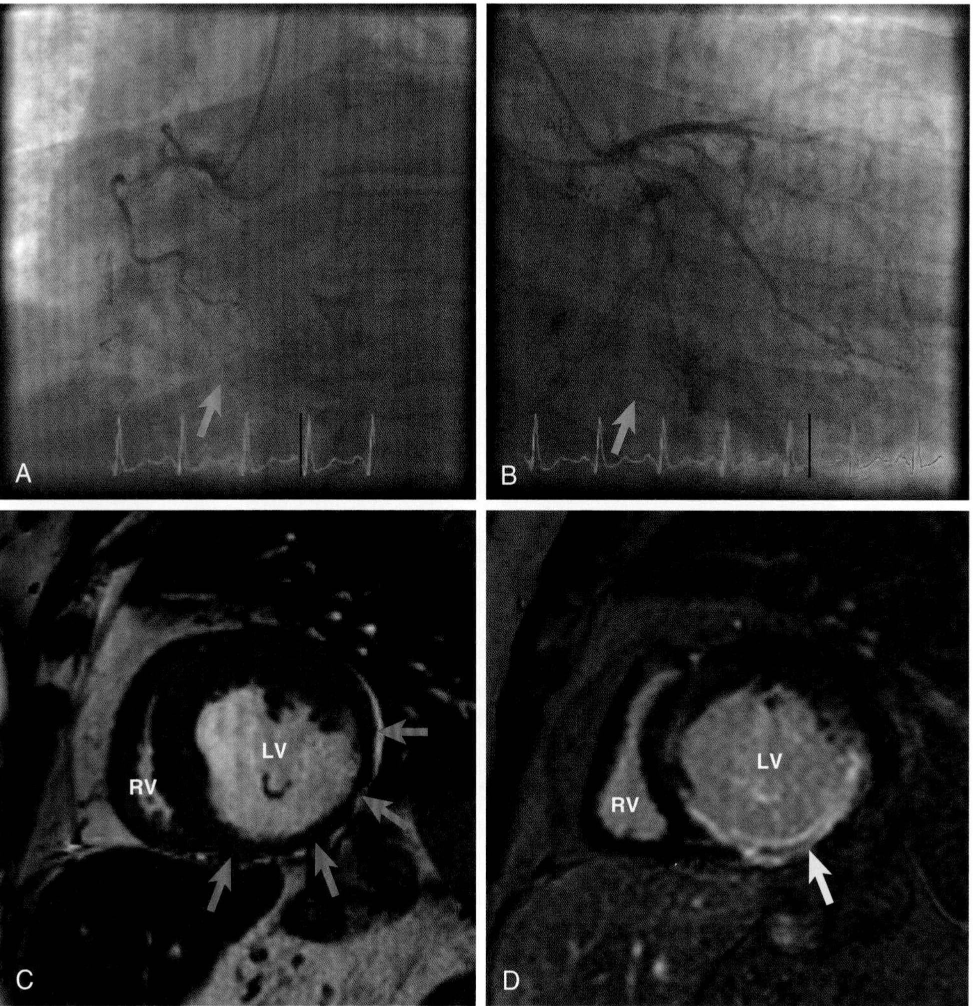

Fig. 6.7 RV and ischemic insults. The RV is not immune to ischemic insults, and cases in which there is no apparent RV dysfunction or infarct may be related to robust collateral development from chronic ischemic heart disease or incorrect identification of the culprit vessel. (A) Right coronary artery (RCA) injection on invasive coronary angiography shows total occlusion of the RCA *(orange arrow)* (Video 6.7A). (B) Left coronary artery injection on invasive coronary angiography shows left-to-right collateral flow *(orange arrow)* (Video 6.7B). (C) Cardiovascular magnetic resonance (CMR) steady-state free precession cine imaging demonstrates thinning of the myocardium *(orange arrows)* in the shared distribution of the RCA and the left circumflex coronary artery (Video 6.7C). (D) CMR late gadolinium-enhanced image demonstrates dense late gadolinium enhancement in the endocardium of the corresponding region of wall thinning, consistent with an almost transmural myocardial infarction *(yellow arrow)*.

the pericardial cavity[20] (Fig. 6.8). During normal inspiration, decreased intrathoracic pressure augments flow into the RV. As the RV preload increases, RV cardiac output is augmented by normal Frank-Starling interactions.[21–23] Although the pericardium is a tough fibrous structure, there is a normal physiologic capacity that can accommodate this additional flow.[24] Loss of this normal pericardial capacity in pathologic states such as pericardial constriction or pericardial tamponade can lead to an inspiratory RV septal shift that impinges on normal LV filling. Other situations of significant RV pressure and/or volume overload due to factors such as pulmonary hypertension, pulmonary embolism, or RV infarction can also displace the IVS and similarly affect LV filling (Fig. 6.9).

Another contributor to ventricular interdependence is the shared ventricular muscle fibers. The LV has three distinct layers of muscle fibers, whereas the RV contains only a superficial and an endocardial layer. The superficial layer of the RV myocardial fibers is circumferential and is contiguous with the LV; the thicker RV endocardial layer of muscle fibers is longitudinally oriented and forms the RV side of the shared IVS. The difference in myocardial fiber orientation contributes to a unique RV contractile pattern that is more reliant on longitudinal shortening than on free wall motion.[25]

In addition to normal ventricular interactions, the RV is highly sensitive to small changes in preload and afterload, likely related to its thin walls. This may lead to perturbations in RV diastolic function. Although RV diastolic function is less well described than that of the LV, it is driven by same parameters of active relaxation, passive filling, and ventricular chamber compliance.

BASIC PRINCIPLES OF IMAGE ACQUISITION

RV imaging should use an integrative approach that includes multiple echocardiographic and Doppler techniques to evaluate all right-sided cardiac structures (Fig. 6.10). Transthoracic

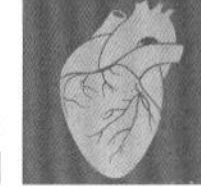

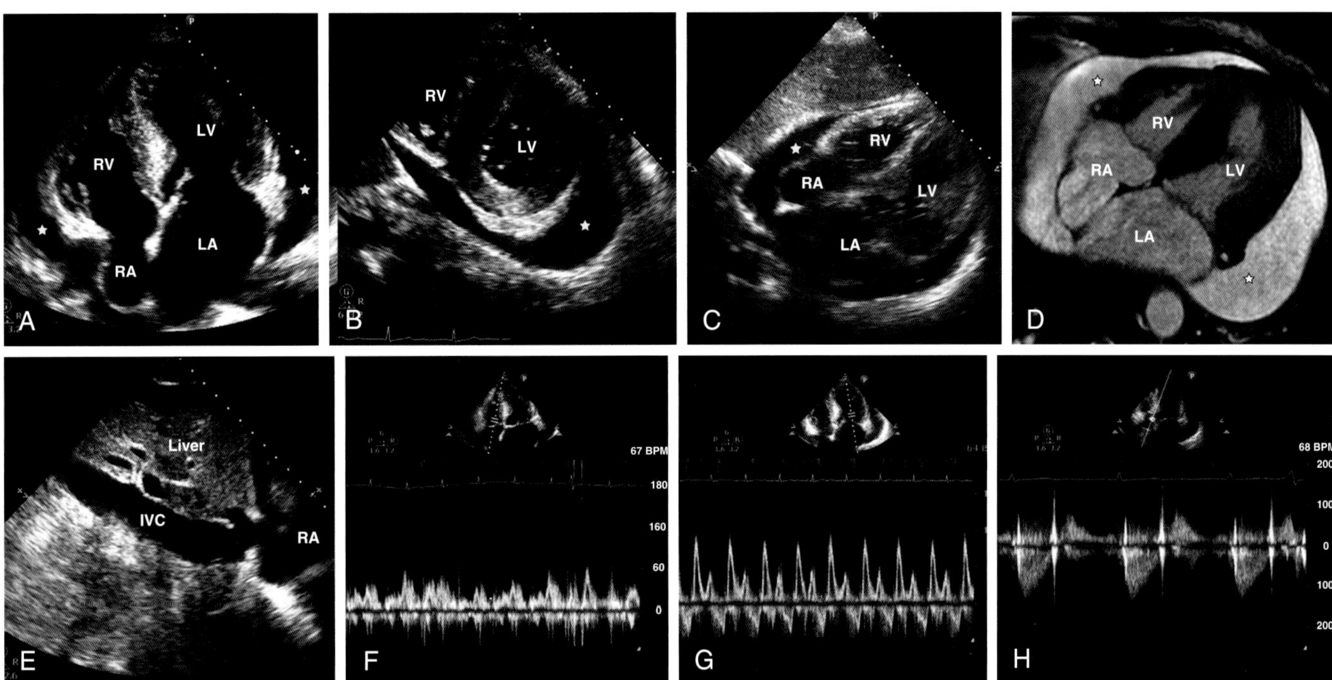

Fig. 6.8 **Relationship of the RV and pericardium.** Because of its lower intrinsic filling pressures, the RV is sensitive to changes from pericardial effusions. The high temporal resolution of TTE is ideal for interrogation of the RV for physiologic signs of pericardial tamponade such as diastolic free wall collapse of the RV or systolic free wall collapse of the RA. The RV free wall can be difficult to image with TTE, but larger effusions may enhance RV imaging through displacement of air-filled lung or posterior displacement of the RV into a more favorable imaging window. A pericardial effusion *(yellow stars)* is evaluated by TTE in apical 4-chamber (A), parasternal short-axis (B), and subcostal 4-chamber (C) views (Videos 6.8A, B, and C). (D) Cardiac magnetic resonance (CMR) steady-state free precession cine imaging has intrinsic bright blood imaging and a large field of view that aid in understanding the full extent of a pericardial effusion (yellow stars) (Video 6.8D). (E) Identification of a plethoric inferior vena cava that does not collapse with an inspiratory sniff maneuver indicates elevated RA pressures, which can be caused by poor RV filling due to the high pericardial pressures in pericardial tamponade (Video 6.8E). Spectral Doppler imaging of the tricuspid (F) and mitral (G) inflows and the aortic outflow (H) can identify respirophasic changes in flow caused by the exaggerated ventricular interdependence that characterize pericardial tamponade. This patient has no significant variation despite a large circumferential effusion, which suggests that no tamponade physiology is present (Video 6.8F). Spectral Doppler evaluation for tamponade is ideally performed with a respirometer and a slow sweep speed. If there is excessive cardiac motion due to a large effusion or exaggerated respiration, a changing angle of incidence to the probe may confound this evaluation.

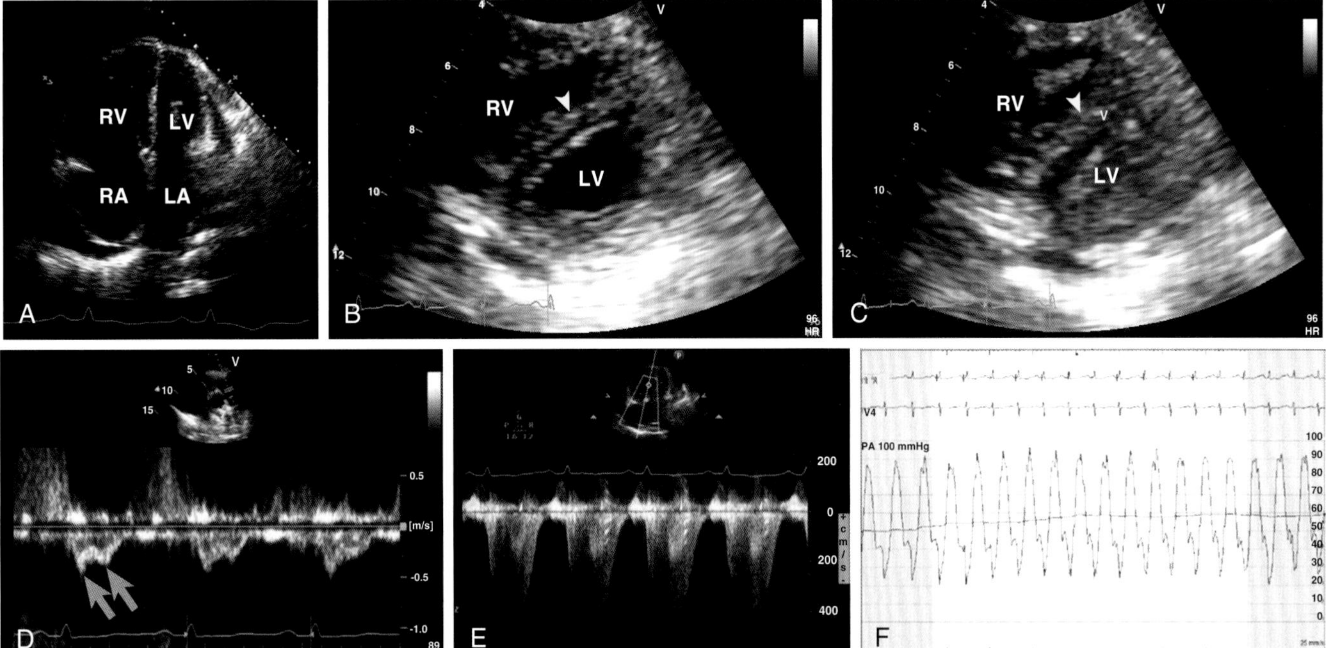

Fig. 6.9 **Pulmonary hypertension and RV function.** The RV normally pumps against a low-pressure system and is highly susceptible to the increase in afterload caused by pulmonary hypertension. (A) TTE apical 4-chamber view shows severe RV dilation. Rather than dilation, some patients may respond to pulmonary hypertension with chamber hypertrophy (Video 6.9A). (B and C) TTE parasternal short-axis view shows a D-shaped interventricular septum *(yellow arrowheads)* shifted toward the LV in diastole (B) (Video 6.9B) and in systole (C), suggesting RV pressure and volume overload. (D) Pulmonic outflow pulsed-wave Doppler has a notched appearance indicative of early pulmonic valve closure due to severe pulmonary hypertension. A similar finding can be seen with the use of M-mode imaging through the pulmonic valve and is known colloquially as the *flying W sign.* (E) CW Doppler of a tricuspid regurgitant jet with a peak velocity greater than 4 m/s suggests severely elevated RV pressure and, by correlation, severely elevated pulmonary artery systolic pressure. (F) Severe pulmonary hypertension confirmed by invasive right heart catheterization.

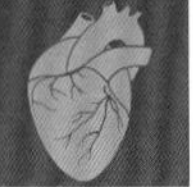

Right ventricle diagnostic approach

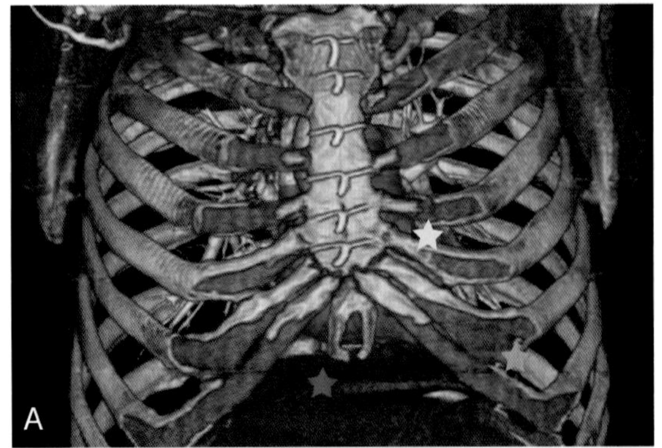

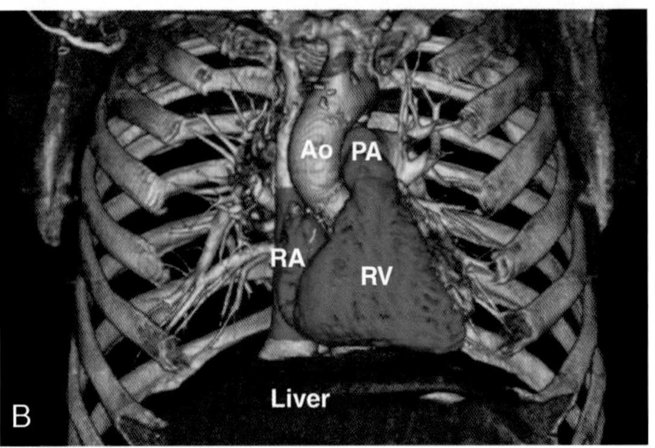

	View / Technique	Evaluation
Parasternal Windows	PLAX	• RVOT Prox
	PSAX basal	• RVOT Prox • RVOT distal
	PSAX mid ventricle	• RV/LV relative size
	RVIT/RVOT + color Doppler/CW	• Tricuspid and pulmonic valve morphology and function
Apical Window	4-chamber RV focus	• FAC • RVD1 • RVD2 • Right atrial size
	M-Mode	• TAPSE
	Tissue Doppler lateral tricuspid annulus	• S' • RIMP
	PW tricupid annulus	• RIMP
	CW tricuspid valve	• Tricuspid regurgitation • *dP/dt*
	Color Doppler	• Tricuspid regurgitation
Subcostal Window	4-chamber	• RV wall thickness • RV function
	Color Doppler	• Interatrial septum

Fig. 6.10 **RV diagnostic approach with TTE.** The RV is the most anterior cardiac chamber and lies immediately posterior to the sternum, as visualized with this ECG-gated computed tomography volume-rendered image without (A) and with (B) sternum segmentation. The RV position, in combination with its complex shape, leads to challenging imaging for the typical TTE windows. The parasternal imaging windows *(yellow star in upper image)* are limited due to the small imaging field of view of proximal structures, near-field clutter artifact, and available imaging windows between rib spaces. The apical views *(green star)* are better able to capture the full length of the RV. However, the location of ribs and lungs may limit the ability to fully visualize the RV free wall. In some patients with difficult windows, imaging may rely on the subcostal windows *(purple star)* for adequate visualization of the RV. *Ao*, Aorta; *dP/dt*, instantaneous rate of RV pressure rise in early systole; *ECG*, electrocardiogram; *FAC*, fractional area change; *PA*, pulmonary artery; *PLAX*, parasternal long-axis view; *PSAX*, parasternal short-axis view; *PW*, pulsed-wave; *RIMP*, right ventricular index of myocardial performance; *RVD1*, the widest portion (dimension) of the basal one third of the RV; *RVD2*, the width of the middle one third of the RV; *RVIT*, right ventricular inflow tract; *RVOT*, right ventricular outflow tract; *S′*, tricuspid annular systolic velocity; *TAPSE*, tricuspid annular plane systolic excursion.

echocardiographic (TTE) imaging of the RV can be challenging because of its location in the anterior chest. In parasternal views, the sternum and ribs may limit the available echocardiographic windows, and the proximity of the RV to the transducer probe may degrade image quality due to near-field clutter artifact. From the parasternal imaging windows, a standard phased array ultrasound transducer has a triangular beam that is unable to provide full visualization of the entire RV in a single field of view and may require apical or subcostal windows for improved visualization.

RV ANATOMIC EVALUATION

QUALITATIVE EVALUATION

Evaluation of RV size begins with a qualitative impression of the RV relative to the LV. Although the RV volume is normally larger than the LV, it is accepted that from a standard apical 4-chamber view, the RV should not exceed two thirds of the LV size or total length.[14] When the RV size is equivalent to that of the LV, it is considered to be moderately dilated, and when the RV appears larger than the LV, it is considered to be severely dilated. These qualitative assessments are primarily derived from expert opinion.[13,14]

2D MEASUREMENTS OF RV SIZE

The quantitative assessment of RV size is performed with multiple 2D linear measurements of size and wall thickness, 2D area measurements, 3D volumetric measurements, and evaluation of the relative sizes of associated structures (Table 6.4).

The *apical 4-chamber* view allows a cross-sectional plane of the entire RV long axis to be seen in a single field of view. When optimized to an RV-focused view, it provides a window to evaluate the RV and other right-sided cardiac structures such as the RA and tricuspid valve. Three linear measurements are performed in this view. RVD1 is the widest portion (dimension) of the basal one third of the RV. RVD2 is the width of the middle one third of the RV. RVD3 is the length of the RV measured from the tricuspid valve annulus to the RV apex[13,14] (Fig. 6.11A).

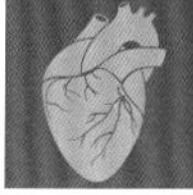

TABLE 6.4 RV Normative Measurements.

Region	*Mean*	*Upper Reference Value (+2 SD)*
RV basal diameter (mm)	33	41
RV mid-cavity diameter (mm)	28	35
RV longitudinal diameter (mm)	71	83
RVOT diameter (PLAX) (mm)	25	30
RVOT proximal (PSAX) (mm)	28	35
RVOT distal (PSAX) (mm)	22	27
RV subcostal wall thickness (mm)	3	5
RV end-diastolic area (cm^2)		
Men	17	24
Women	14	20
RV end-systolic area (cm^2)		
Men	9	15
Women	7	11
3D RV end-diastolic volume index (mL/m^2)		
Men	61	87
Women	53	74
3D RV end-systolic volume index (mL/m^2)		
Men	27	44
Women	22	36

PLAX, Parasternal long-axis; *PSAX*, parasternal short-axis; *RVOT*, right ventricular outflow tract; *SD*, standard deviation.

Adapted from Lang RM, Badano LP, Mor-Avi F, et al. Recommendations for cardiac chamber quantification by echocardiography in adults: an update from the American Society of Echocardiography and the European Association of Cardiovascular Imaging. *J Am Soc Echocardiogr*. 2015;28:1–39.

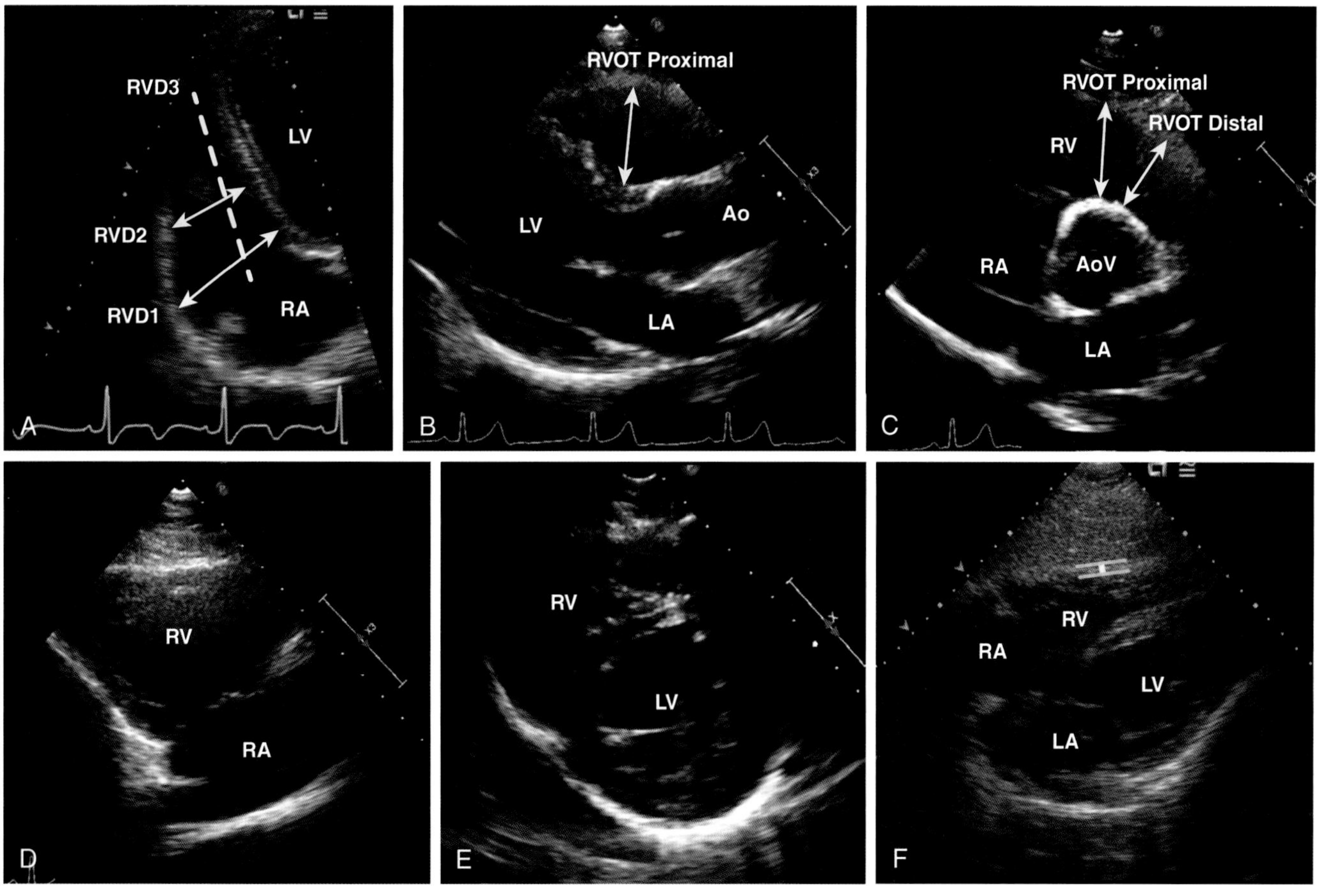

Fig. 6.11 RV imaging windows and linear measurements. TTE views that are most helpful for RV evaluation and the performance of linear measurements *(double-headed arrows)*. (A) TTE apical 4-chamber view with RV focus. Measurements are performed in the widest portion of the basal one third *(RVD1)* and in the middle one third *(RVD2)* of the RV. The RV length is measured from the mid-annular plane to the RV apex *(RVD3)*. RV trabeculae must be excluded to avoid underestimation of RV size. (B) TTE parasternal long-axis view with RVOT measurement. (C) TTE parasternal short-axis view with proximal and distal measurements of the RVOT. (D) Parasternal long-axis view of the RV inflow. (E) TTE parasternal short-axis view at the mid-ventricular level. (F) TTE subcostal 4-chamber view. Measurements of RV wall thickness are best performed in this view *(yellow line between orange lines)*. *Ao*, Aorta; *AoV*, aortic valve; *RVOT*, right ventricular outflow tract.

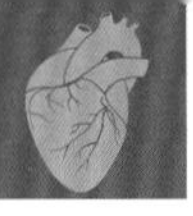

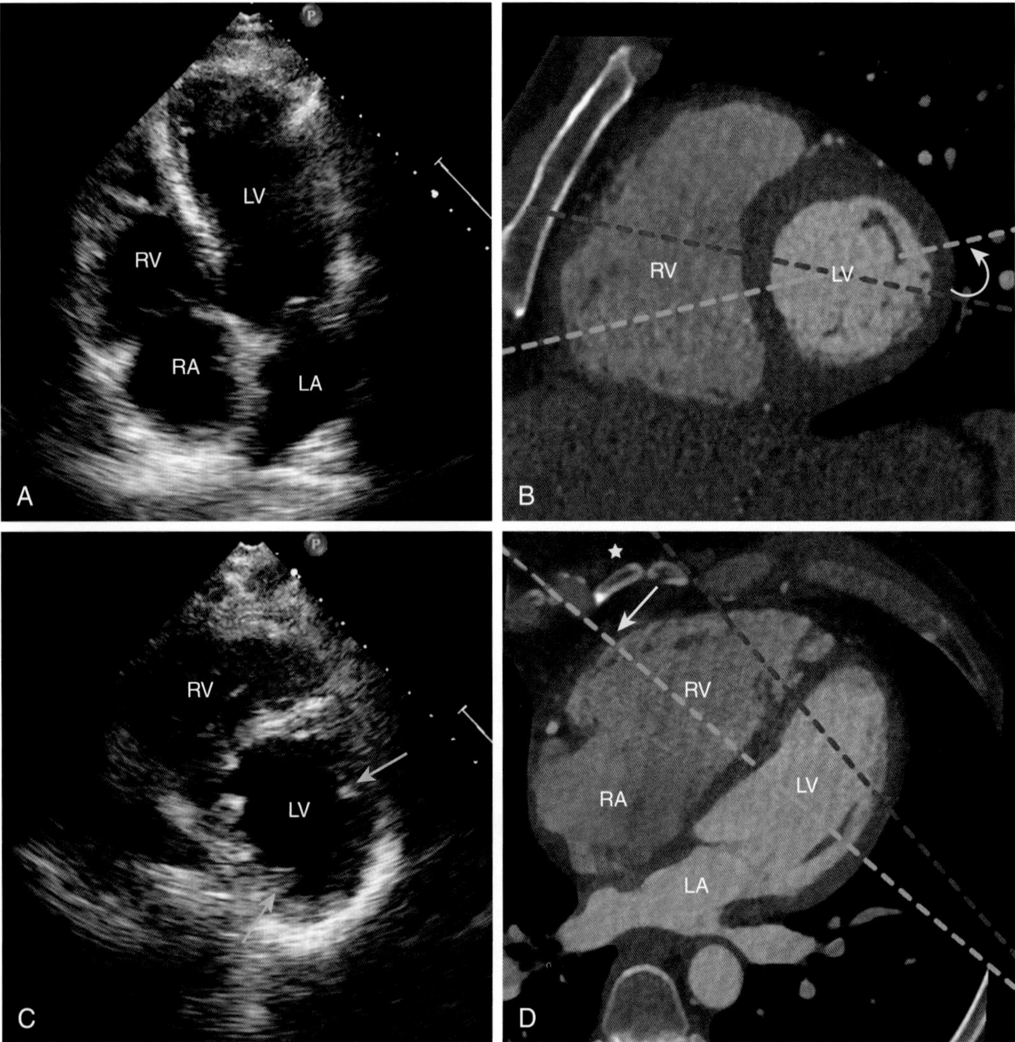

Fig. 6.12 Techniques to optimize visualization of the RV with TTE. Optimization of the RV by TTE requires sonographer experience and in-depth understanding of cardiac anatomy. This image series uses ECG-gated computed tomography angiography (CTA) to demonstrate the importance of careful optimization of RV-focused images. (A) TTE apical 4-chamber RV-focused view with acceptable delineation of the RV free wall and an RV size that appears normal (Video 6.12A). (B) The RV when seen on CTA is dilated, demonstrating the difficulty of RV assessment in suboptimal angles and TTE imaging planes that would have benefitted from additional counterclockwise probe rotation *(yellow arrow)* from the *dotted red line* to the *dotted green line* (Video 6.12B). (C) Similarly, the TTE parasternal short-axis view did not show RV dilation. A foreshortened image should be suspected because of the oval appearance of the LV and the distal insertion points of the LV papillary muscles *(orange arrows)* (Video 6.12C). (D) The *dotted red line* is the likely plane of acquisition for the short-axis image in C. Correct true short-axis image acquisition would require moving the probe to the right of the patient *(yellow arrow)*, shifting the imaging plane from the *dotted red line* to the *dotted green line*. Given the location of the sternum *(orange star)*, this may not have been an achievable imaging plane (Video 6.12D). *ECG*, Electrocardiogram.

The standard apical 4-chamber view is obtained by placing the transducer at the left midclavicular line in the space between the 4th and 5th ribs. The transducer index marker is pointed posteriorly toward the bed. The transducer head has a slightly superior tilt with the tail of the probe toward the feet. Tilting the probe anteriorly with a slight counterclockwise rotation brings out the RV-focused view. The size of the RV is easily underestimated if the plane of acquisition does not cross the widest portion of the inferior margin of the RV (Fig. 6.12).

The RV-focused apical 4-chamber view has some limitations. The apex of the RV may not be easily visualized due to near-field clutter artifact, or the RV free wall may not be well visualized due to adjacent lung tissue and artifact generated from the fluid–air interface. The use of contrast may improve visualization of the RV (Fig. 6.13A).

The *parasternal long-axis* (PLAX) view should transect the center of the LV outflow tract and the anteroseptal and inferolateral walls of the LV. In this view, a portion of the RVOT can be seen and measured from the free wall of the RV to the crux between the aorta and the LV (see Fig. 6.11B).

The PLAX view is obtained with the transducer at the left sternal border in the 3rd or 4th intercostal space and with the transducer index marker pointed at the patient's right shoulder. If the imaging window is too inferior, the RV free wall will be seen rather than the RVOT.

The *parasternal short axis* provides multiple views of the RV. Images are obtained by performing an approximately 90-degree clockwise rotation from the PLAX view. On completion of this rotation, the marker should point toward the patient's left shoulder. The basal views can be obtained by angulation of the head of the probe slightly toward the right shoulder and with the tail down toward the left hip. The mid-ventricle can be seen by angulation of the probe slightly away from the right shoulder and may require translation of the probe more apically or movement to a lower rib space. The lack of landmarks to readily identify

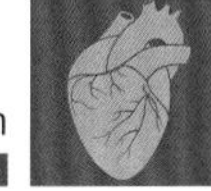

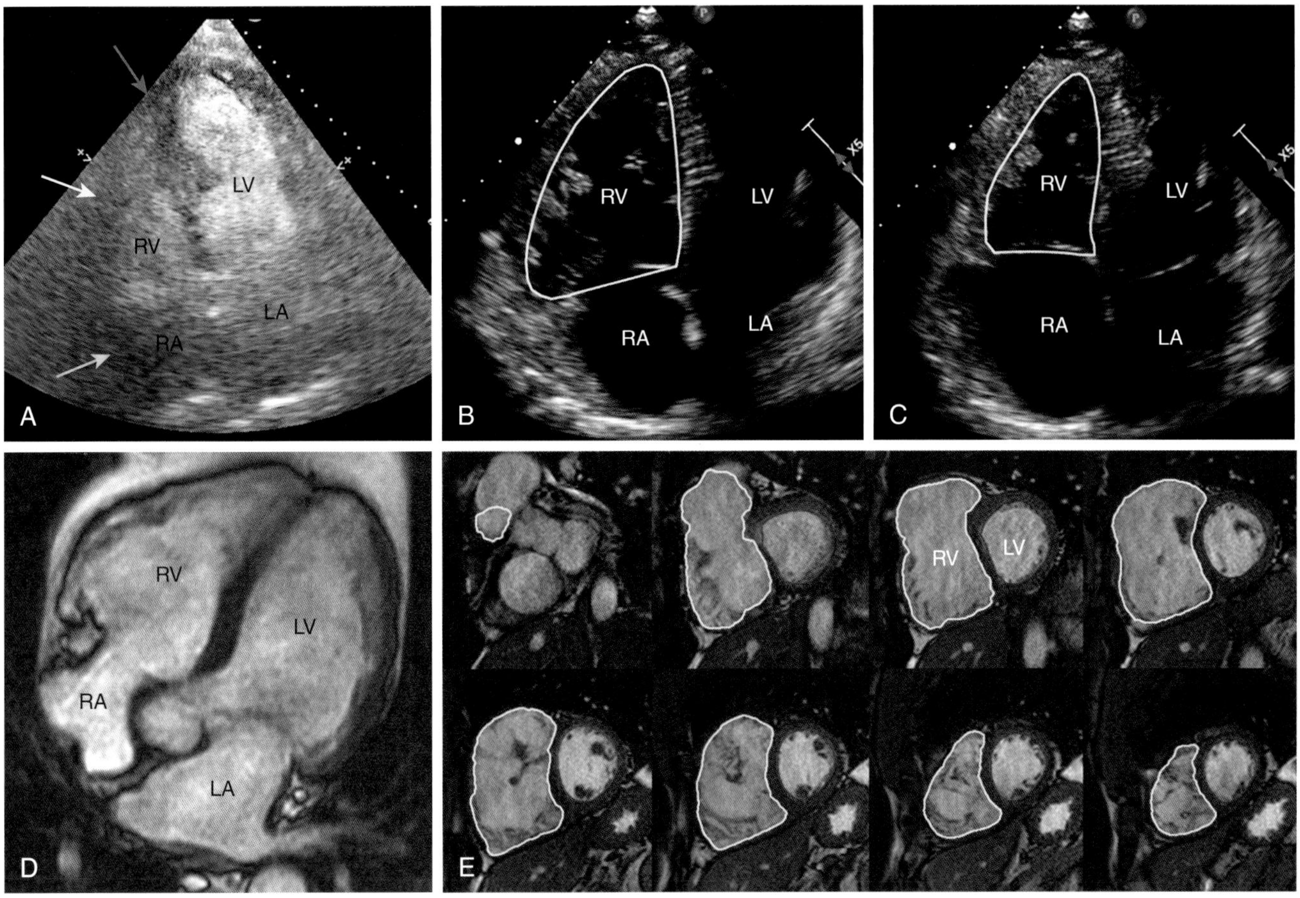

Fig. 6.13 Multimodality evaluation of RV size and function. The apical 4-chamber RV-focused projection allows qualitative assessments and several linear and area-based measurements. (A) In some patients, particularly those with severe pulmonary disease, the RV free wall is difficult to image. Microbubble echocardiographic contrast can be helpful, particularly for visualization of the RV apex *(blue arrow)*. However, there may be limited improvement in visualization of the RV free wall *(yellow arrow)*, and the contrast may obscure distal structures such as the inferior margin of the RV free wall and the RA *(orange arrow)* (Video 6.13A). When the RV can be well visualized, the fractional area change (FAC) may be calculated by tracing the RV endocardium in diastole (B) and in systole (C). The FAC is a directional 2D measurement with no 3D assumptions, in contrast to the biplane technique used to derive the LV ejection fraction. When tracing the RV endocardium, care must be taken to exclude the dense trabecular network and to not trace the inner edge of the moderator band rather than the true RV apex (Video 6.13B and C). (D) Cardiac magnetic resonance (CMR) steady-state free precession cine image with intrinsic bright blood contrast can improve visualization of the RV free wall. (E) The CMR approach to quantifying RV size and function involves tracing the RV endocardium in systole and diastole and generating volumes from the summed image thicknesses.

the midbody of the RV renders this view prone to oblique cuts that may overestimate or underestimate the RV size.

The most basal view is at the level of the aortic valve, where the RV free wall is seen extending into the RVOT. Proximal and distal measurements of the RVOT can be well visualized in this view (see Fig. 6.11C). This view helps to distinguish an inflow-tract from an outflow-tract VSD and allows assessment of the pulmonic valve, tricuspid valve, and RA.

The short-axis view at the mid-ventricular level provides a cross-sectional image of both ventricles (see Fig. 6.11E). This view is helpful for assessment of RV size, evaluation of ventricular wall motion and ventricular interdependence, and screening for muscular VSDs.

The *parasternal long-axis RV inflow* view is obtained by starting with the parasternal long-axis view in the 3rd or 4th intercostal space and then angling the transducer head toward the right hip with the tail of the transducer moving toward the left shoulder. Structures such as the tricuspid leaflet coaptation plane, the coronary sinus, and the inferior vena cava are visualized in this window (see Fig. 6.11D),

The *parasternal long-axis RV outflow* view optimizes interrogation of the RVOT, the pulmonic valve, and the proximal portion of the pulmonary artery. This view is obtained by starting with the parasternal long axis. The transducer head is then angled toward the left shoulder with the tail moving toward the right hip. This window assists evaluation of pulmonic valve pathophysiology, screening for a patent ductus arteriosus, and assessment of a massive pulmonary embolus.

The *subcostal 4-chamber* view is commonly acquired as an alternative view for evaluation of RV size, function, and wall thickness (see Fig. 6.11F). The subcostal 4-chamber view is obtained by placing the probe just inferior to the xyphoid process with the marker toward the patient's left side. The transducer head is then angled superiorly with the tail of the transducer moving toward the patient's body. Because of the perpendicular axis of the interatrial septum in this view, it commonly assists in detection of interatrial shunts.

Pertinent to assessment of the RV and RA, the IVC is routinely interrogated from the subcostal view with a 60- to 90-degree counterclockwise rotation of the ultrasound probe and with the marker directed toward the head of the patient. Further lateral translation and rotations may be required to visualize the entire long axis of the IVC. Imaging should positively confirm identification of the IVC by clearly demonstrating its anastomosis with the RA. M-mode or 2D imaging can be used to estimate RA filling pressures with techniques such as the rapid sniff maneuver for evaluation of IVC compliance (Table 6.5).

3D VOLUMETRIC MEASUREMENTS OF RV SIZE

With 3D echocardiographic imaging capabilities, RV volumes can be measured with accuracy that compares favorably to CMR as a reference standard.[26] Although there are many advantages to using 3D echocardiography to perform a full volumetric measurement of RV size, barriers for its adoption into routine clinical practice include the increased cost and lower availability of 3D-capable TTE transducers, availability of and expertise with 3D postprocessing software, time constraints and reimbursement for performance of 3D quantification, and expertise in acquisition of the high-quality data sets required for 3D analysis[19,27–29] (Table 6.6).

RV FUNCTIONAL EVALUATION

QUALITATIVE EVALUATION

Evaluation of RV systolic function begins with a visual impression. This visual assessment is difficult and requires experience to perform in a reproducible fashion. Quantitative data can then be added to form a complete integrative impression of RV function (Table 6.7). The initial review should include global assessment of RV contractility and identification of focal abnormalities that may not be well characterized in single quantitative metric. An example is RV dysfunction in the setting of an acute pulmonary embolism, in which case there can be mid–free wall akinesis with preservation of RV apical contraction, perhaps as a result of tethering from LV contraction.[30] Other relevant pathology includes arrhythmogenic RV dysplasia/cardiomyopathy (ARVD/C), for which major and minor imaging criteria rely on the qualitative identification of regional RV akinesia or dyskinesia[31] (Table 6.8). Qualitative evaluations of RV function also help in identifying the abnormalities of interventricular septal motion seen in pericardial pathology or various states of RV pressure and/or volume overload.

TABLE 6.5 Inferior Vena Cava Hemodynamics for Estimation of RA Pressure.

IVC Diameter (cm)	*% Collapse with Sniff*	*Estimated RA Pressure (mmHg)*
≤2.1	>50	0–5
≤2.1	<50	5–10
>2.1	>50	5–10
>2.1	<50	10–20

Adapted from Rudski LG, Lai WW, Afilalo J, et al. Guidelines for the echocardiographic assessment of the right heart in adults: a report from the American Society of Echocardiography endorsed by the European Association of Echocardiography, a registered branch of the European Society of Cardiology, and the Canadian Society of Echocardiography. *J Am Soc Echocardiogr.* 2010;23:685–713.

FRACTIONAL AREA CHANGE

The RV fractional area change (FAC) is a 2D metric for evaluation of RV function, and there is a wealth of evidence to support its use[32–39] (see Fig. 6.13B and C). The FAC measurement is performed by tracing the RV endocardium in an apical 4-chamber RV-focused view in diastole and in systole. The change in area is divided by the RV diastolic area, producing the percentage reported as the FAC. Unlike the biplane method of disk summation, which is commonly used for LV volumetric and ejection fraction calculations, this is a pure fractional calculation of areas with no geometric assumptions of 3D shape built into the analysis:

RV FAC = (RV end-diastolic area − RV end-systolic area) ÷ RV end-diastolic area

Although the concept is straightforward, the practical performance of an FAC measurement can be challenging because its accuracy and reproducibility rely on high-quality imaging of the RV free wall. Even when the RV is well visualized, experience and care are required when excluding the complex and prominent network of RV trabeculations. This is particularly true at the RV apex because of the confluence of trabeculations with the moderator band and the apical near-field clutter artifact.

TRICUSPID ANNULAR PLANE SYSTOLIC EXCURSION

The tricuspid annular plane systolic excursion (TAPSE) is a linear metric for evaluation of RV function that uses M-mode imaging. TAPSE is one of the quantitative metrics most commonly used for RV function, and it has a large base of supporting evidence[34,38,40–43] (Fig. 6.14A). The success of TAPSE likely reflects the large contribution of the RV longitudinal myocardial fibers to normal RV function.[44]

The TAPSE measurement is performed by setting up an apical 4-chamber RV-focused view so that the anterolateral tricuspid annulus is ideally centered in the imaging sector. The M-mode imaging plane is then prescribed from the RV apex through the anterolateral tricuspid annulus. As the RV contracts, the dynamic movement of the tricuspid annulus is plotted over time with high temporal resolution. The distance traveled by the tricuspid annulus is reported as the TAPSE measurement. If M-mode imaging is not performed or is of poor

TABLE 6.6 Normative RV Reference Volumes by Modality.

	Men			Women		
Modality	*EDV (Mean ± SD)*	*EDVi (Mean ± SD)*	*N*	*ESV (Mean ± SD)*	*ESVi (Mean ± SD)*	*N*
3D TTE	99 ± 14 mL	52 ± 8 mL/m²	119	74 ± 14 mL	46 ± 8 mL/m²	126
CMR	173 ± 36 mL	88 ± 17 mL/m²	576	130 ± 24 mL	76 ± 13 mL/m²	760
CTA	145 ± 29 mL	70 ± 13 mL/m²	188	105 ± 20 mL	59 ± 10 mL/m²	381

CMR, Cardiac magnetic resonance imaging; *CTA*, cardiac computed tomography angiography; *EDV*, end-diastolic volume; *EDVi*, end-diastolic volume index; *ESV*, end-systolic volume; *ESVi*, end-systolic volume index; *N*, sample size; *SD*, standard deviation.

Data from Foppa M, Arora G, Gona P, et al. Right ventricular volumes and systolic function by cardiac magnetic resonance and the impact of sex, age, and obesity in a longitudinally followed cohort free of pulmonary and cardiovascular disease: The Framingham Heart Study. *Circ Cardiovasc Imaging.* 2016;9(3):e003810; Fuchs A, Mejdahl MR, Kühl JT, et al. Normal values of left ventricular mass and cardiac chamber volumes assessed by 320-detector computed tomography angiography in the Copenhagen General Population Study. *Eur Heart J Cardiovasc Imaging.* 2016;17(9):1009–1017; Tamborini G, Marsan NA, Gripari P, et al. Reference values for right ventricular volumes and ejection fraction with real-time three-dimensional echocardiography: evaluation in a large series of normal subjects *J Am Soc Echocardiogr.* 2010;23(2):109–115.

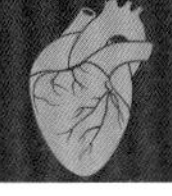

quality, a similar longitudinal shortening measurement can be performed on any 4-chamber cine image in which the lateral tricuspid annulus is adequately visualized.

The major limitation of the TAPSE measurement is that it assumes all movement of the anterolateral tricuspid annulus originates from RV longitudinal shortening. This does not take into account cardiac movement not related to the RV, such as tethered movement from LV contraction, cardiac translational movement in large pericardial effusions, or patient respiratory movement during image acquisition.

THE *dP/dt* FUNCTION FOR ASSESSING MYOCARDIAL WORK

The *dP/dt* function is used to assess RV myocardial work by employing the TR spectral Doppler jet to quantify the RV systolic change in pressure over time (see Fig. 6.14B). This technique requires a well-defined envelope of TR on spectral Doppler.

The traditional method is to quantify the amount of time it takes for the TR velocity to increase from 1 m/s to 2 m/s. Using the modified Bernoulli equation, this can be restated as the time it takes for the RV to generate a pressure change of 12 mmHg. A *dP/dt* value of less than 400 mmHg/s is considered abnormal. Because the *dP/dt* function is an indirect derivation, its accuracy relies on a well-defined TR envelope and may be confounded by the rapid pressure equalization found in severe TR.

TABLE 6.7 RV Function Reference Values.

Metrics	*Measurement*	*Mean*	*Abnormality Threshold (2 SD)*
Systolic	TAPSE (mm)	24	<17
	Pulsed-wave Doppler S wave (cm/s)	14.1	<9.5
	Color Doppler S wave (cm/s)	9.7	<6.0
	Pulsed Doppler MPI	0.26	>0.43
	Tissue Doppler MPI	0.39	>0.54
	RV fractional area change	49	<35
	3D RV ejection fraction	58	<45
Diastolic	E-wave deceleration time (ms)	180	<119 or >242
	E/a	1.4	<0.8 or >2.0
	e′/a′	1.18	<0.52
	e′	14.0	<7.8
	E/*e′*	4	>6.0

MPI, Myocardial performance index; *TAPSE*, tricuspid annular plane systolic excursion.
Adapted from Lang RM, Badano LP, Mor-Avi F, et al. Recommendations for cardiac chamber quantification by echocardiography in adults: an update from the American Society of Echocardiography and the European Association of Cardiovascular Imaging. *J Am Soc Echocardiogr*. 2015;28:1–39.

TISSUE DOPPLER TRICUSPID ANNULAR SYSTOLIC VELOCITY

Another technique used to identify normal RV function is the tissue Doppler–derived lateral tricuspid annular systolic velocity (*S′*) (see Fig. 6.14C). This measurement is obtained in the same RV-focused 4-chamber view as TAPSE and can be performed with pulsed-wave (PW) and color modes. With PW tissue Doppler, the sample volume is placed at the RV myocardium adjacent to the lateral tricuspid annulus. This plots the velocity of the lateral tricuspid annulus over time, and the peak tricuspid annular velocity in systole is reported. With color tissue Doppler, samples of the phase shift of two successive pulses in the entire sector are acquired. This allows velocities to be simultaneously sampled across the entire imaging sector, but the technique requires off-line analysis and has lower reference values compared with the PW tissue Doppler technique.

With both techniques, data may be difficult to obtain if image quality of the lateral tricuspid annulus is poor. As with TAPSE, the measurements are angle dependent, and results may be confounded by movement not related exclusively to the RV.

RV INDEX OF MYOCARDIAL PERFORMANCE

The *r*ight ventricular *i*ndex of *m*yocardial *p*erformance (RIMP), also called the *Tei index* after the researcher who proposed modifications, is an indirect method of quantifying RV systolic function (see Fig. 6.14D). The RIMP is a ratio of non-ejection time to ejection time. The non-ejection time is the sum of the isovolumic contraction time (IVCT) and the isovolumic relaxation time (IVRT). This value can also be obtained by taking the total tricuspid valve closure (opening time) interval (TCO) and subtracting the systolic ejection time (ET):

$$\text{Non-contraction time (NCT)} = \text{IVCT} + \text{IVRT} = \text{TCO} - \text{ET}$$

$$\text{RIMP} = \text{NCT} \div \text{ET}$$

The RIMP is helpful as a global metric of RV function, but it requires high image quality for accuracy. When calculating an RIMP, the fidelity of the data from tissue Doppler or spectral Doppler imaging often does not yield a distinct enough separation to distinguish between the IVCT and the IVRT. The cutoff values are different for tissue Doppler and spectral Doppler methods.

3D VOLUMETRIC ASSESSMENT OF RV FUNCTION

The 3D assessment of RV function has considerable appeal because it addresses the complexities of RV shape with few assumptions (Fig. 6.15). This can be of significant utility for

TABLE 6.8 2010 Imaging Criteria for Arrhythmogenic RV Cardiomyopathy/Dysplasia (ARVC/D).

Modality	*Major Criteria*	*Minor Criteria*
Echocardiography	Regional RV akinesia, dyskinesia, or aneurysm and one of the following: 1. Parasternal long-axis RVOT ≥32 mm (19 mm/m²) 2. Parasternal short-axis RVOT ≥36 mm (21 mm/m²) 3. Fractional area change ≤33%	Regional RV akinesia, dyskinesia, or aneurysm and one of the following: 1. Parasternal long-axis RVOT 29–32 mm (16–19 mm/m²) 2. Parasternal short-axis RVOT 32–36 mm (18–21 mm/m²) 3. Fractional area change 33%–40%
Cardiac magnetic resonance imaging	Regional RV akinesia, dyskinesia, or aneurysm and one of the following: 1. RV end-diastolic volume index ≥110 mL/m² (male) 2. RV end-diastolic volume index ≥100 mL/m² (female) 3. RV ejection fraction ≤40%	Regional RV akinesia, dyskinesia, or aneurysm and one of the following: 1. RV end-diastolic volume index 100–110 mL/m² (male) 2. RV end-diastolic volume index 90–100 mL/m² (female) 3. RV ejection fraction 40%–45%

RVOT, Right ventricular outflow tract.
Data from Marcus FI, McKenna WJ, Sherrill D, et al. Diagnosis of arrhythmogenic right ventricular cardiomyopathy/dysplasia (ARVC/D). *Circulation*. 2010;121(13):1533–1541.

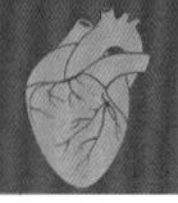

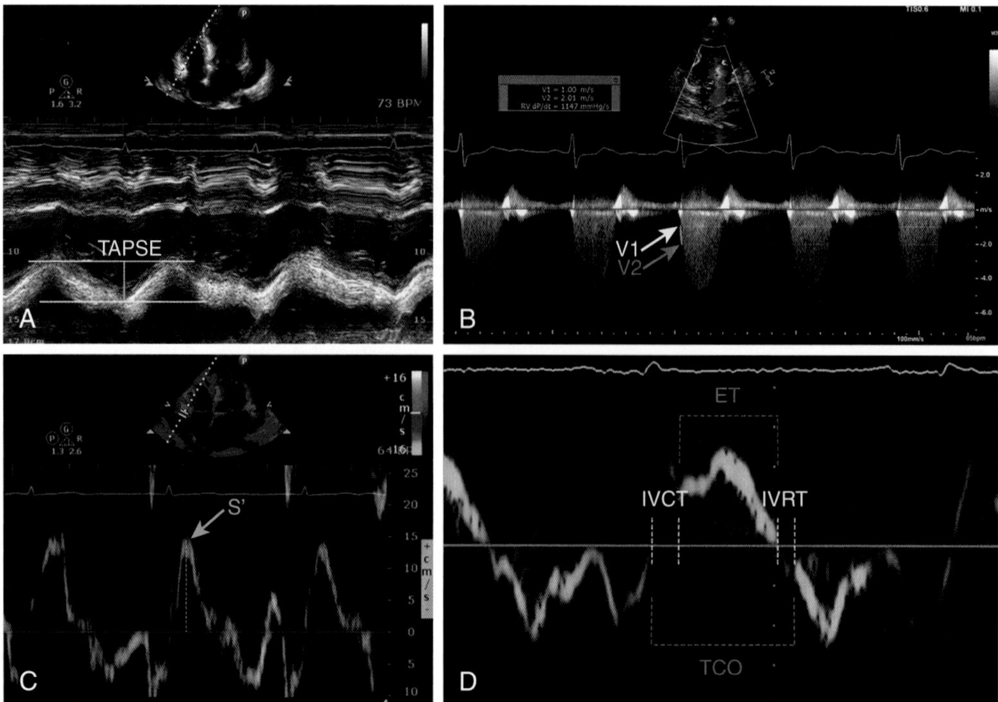

Fig. 6.14 Specialized echocardiographic and Doppler techniques for quantifying RV function. TTE has several unique modes and techniques that allow for a comprehensive physiologic interrogation of RV mechanics that go beyond the volumetric- or area-based approaches used by most other imaging modalities. (A) The tricuspid annular plane systolic excursion *(TAPSE)* method is performed with M-mode acquisition, which provides a linear sample of tricuspid annular translation plotted over time. (B) The spectral Doppler technique can provide an indirect measure of RV work by evaluating the change in pressure divided by the change in time (*dP/dt*) of tricuspid regurgitant flow. (C) Tissue Doppler techniques allow direct measurement of the velocity of the lateral tricuspid annulus (*S'*) over time. (D) The RV myocardial performance index (RIMP) is determined by using tissue Doppler or spectral Doppler techniques with differing cutoffs. The RIMP is calculated as the non-contractile time (IVCT + IVRT) divided by the systolic ejection time *(ET)*. *IVCT*, Isovolumic contraction time; *IVRT*, isovolumic relaxation time; *TCO*, tricuspid valve closure time; *V1*, velocity at 1 m/s; *V2*, velocity at 2 m/s.

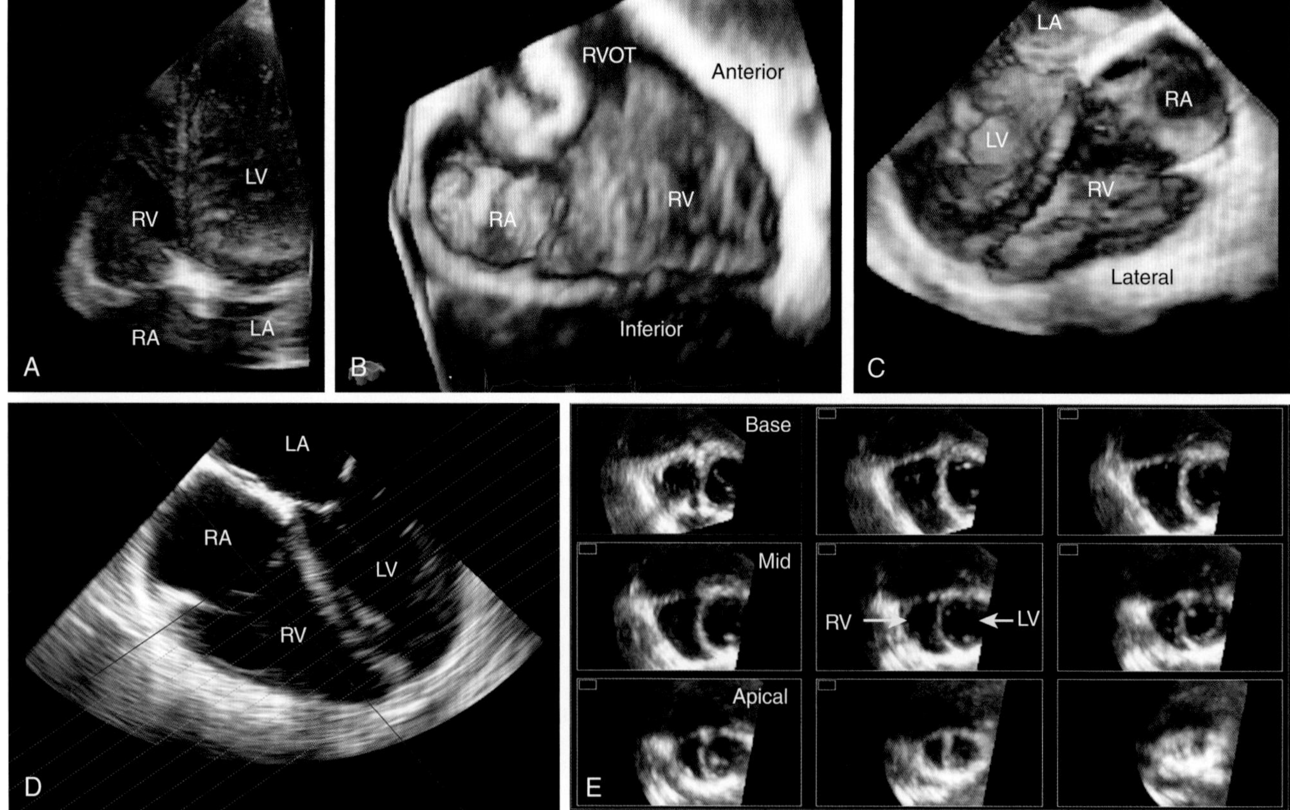

Fig. 6.15 3D Echocardiography for RV assessment. 3D echocardiography holds promise for improving the accuracy and reproducibility of RV function assessment. Increasingly, this technology is available for TTE (A) and TEE (B and C) investigations. Regardless of which modality is used, 3D quantification of the RV depends on a complete data set in which good-quality images are achieved in the entire imaging sector. (D and E) Example of a good-quality 3D TEE data set with multiple planes cut through the entirety of the ventricle. To achieve adequate frame rates, 3D data sets have decreased spatial resolution compared with dedicated 2D imaging, compounding the difficulties in distinguishing the RV endocardial border. *RVOT*, right ventricular outflow tract.

patients with LV assist devices, for whom accurate detection of RV failure has significant clinical and prognostic implications.[45] When acquiring 3D echocardiography data sets, ensuring that all structures of interest are well visualized within two biplane-imaging sectors can minimize artifacts. If an image is not adequately seen in 2D before 3D volumetric acquisition, dropout of key structures will occur.

Current 3D probe technology remains limited in its ability to provide an adequate frame rate for the large imaging sector required to visualize the entire RV in a single heartbeat. Use of multibeat acquisitions can increase spatial or temporal resolution, but they require breath-holding maneuvers to avoid data set misregistration. To maintain adequate frame rates, 3D echocardiography data sets should use the smallest field of view possible to adequately visualize the structure of interest. This can produce a limited field of view and generally poor imaging of extracardiac landmarks, leading to difficulty with manipulation of 3D echocardiography data sets. Because of the thin wall and highly trabeculated nature of the RV, its endocardial border may be difficult to appreciate in a 3D data set.

RV STRAIN AND STRAIN RATE

The limitations of many current techniques for RV function have led to interest in the use of myocardial deformation imaging or myocardial strain. Myocardial strain imaging has long been available as a research tool, and its clinical use for the evaluation of LV function is growing. As for the LV, use of strain imaging techniques such as speckle tracking for the RV provides a quantitative metric for the intrinsic tissue deformation of the myocardium, which is relatively angle independent and not affected by noncardiac translational movement.

Evaluation of RV strain (or the related metric of strain rate) is confounded by a relative lack of outcome data or normative values and difficulties with interobserver and intervendor reproducibility. Further heterogeneity exists for the technique and technology used to obtain strain values, the use of global versus regional metrics, algorithms that evaluate in the endocardium versus the midwall, and the high-quality imaging required to perform RV strain measurements.[46]

Despite these challenges, there is considerable enthusiasm for the use of RV strain and increasing evidence supporting the use of myocardial strain imaging for the RV. This technique will likely play a growing role in the evaluation of RV function.[45–50]

RV DIASTOLIC FUNCTION

Metrics of normal RV diastolic function are less well characterized than those of LV diastolic function.[13,14] RV diastolic dysfunction is therefore less commonly recognized, and limited data are available to guide diagnosis or prognostication, but it is commonly seen in patients with heart failure.[51] The physiologic implications of RV diastolic dysfunction may be clinically important, particularly when RV filling becomes restrictive and becomes an impediment to overall cardiac function. RV diastolic dysfunction may be more commonly recognized in congenital heart disease or RV-specific myopathy states such ARVD/C, acute RV infarction, pulmonary hypertension, or hypertrophic cardiomyopathy.[52,53]

BEYOND SURFACE ECHOCARDIOGRAPHY

TRANSESOPHAGEAL ECHOCARDIOGRAPHY

When imaging windows with TTE are suboptimal, characterization of the RV and other right-sided cardiac structures can sometimes be improved with the use of transesophageal echocardiography (TEE) (Fig. 6.16). The basic imaging planes in TEE are generally the same as TTE views, but evaluation of the RV by TEE can have limitations due to available imaging windows and the location of the RV in the far field of the TEE imaging sector in the mid-retroesophageal view. This leads to worse temporal and spatial resolution and to frequent shadowing of the RV from more proximal structures.

Some of the limitations of TEE can be overcome with skillful use of alternative high and deep retroesophageal views. When a right-sided cardiac structure of interest is not seen well in these views, transgastric views may be helpful because the RV is in the near field of the TEE probe's imaging field.

INTRACARDIAC ECHOCARDIOGRAPHY

Intracardiac echocardiography (ICE) is primarily used in the cardiac catheterization laboratory in conjunction with valvular interventions or electrophysiology procedures. The ICE catheter is typically introduced through central venous vasculature and is advanced into the RA. The close proximity of the ICE catheter to the right-sided cardiac structures allows for evaluation of patients who may have poor TTE or TEE imaging windows. However, given the limited ICE technology, 2D and 3D TEE remains the mainstay of valvular imaging due to higher frame rates, larger imaging field, and 3D imaging capabilities.

CARDIAC MAGNETIC RESONANCE IMAGING

Because of its high degree of accuracy, reproducibility, and intrinsic bright blood imaging, CMR imaging is frequently cited as a reference standard for assessing RV size and function. The CMR technique for quantification of RV size and function relies on a stack of images obtained throughout the entire heart. This is commonly performed in short axis, although some RV-focused protocols use an axial stack of images. The endocardium of the RV is then traced in every frame, in diastole and systole.

This concept is similar to the derived echocardiographic method of disks technique, except it is performed in a stack through the whole heart with actual summation of disk volumes projected from the thickness of each traced slice. The accuracy of CMR volumetric measurements can be internally validated by comparison of volumetric stroke volumes with flow values derived from phase-contrast flow imaging because the stroke volume determined by both techniques should be equivalent in the absence of shunts or regurgitant valve lesions. Limitations to CMR scanning include lengthy image acquisition times, need for frequent breath-holds, need for steady rhythm on the ECG, and an experienced technician to properly prescribe cardiac imaging planes.

CARDIAC COMPUTED TOMOGRAPHY ANGIOGRAPHY

ECG-gated computed tomography angiography (CTA) is another technique that can be used to accurately quantify RV size and function with adequate temporal resolution. CTA has a high spatial resolution, and the image voxel size of modern scanners is isotropic or near isotropic, allowing images to be essentially true volumetric measurements. Despite its theoretical advantages, CTA is not widely used for evaluation of RV function. Reasons include a lack of commercially available

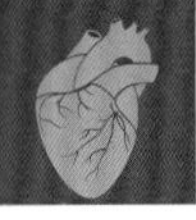

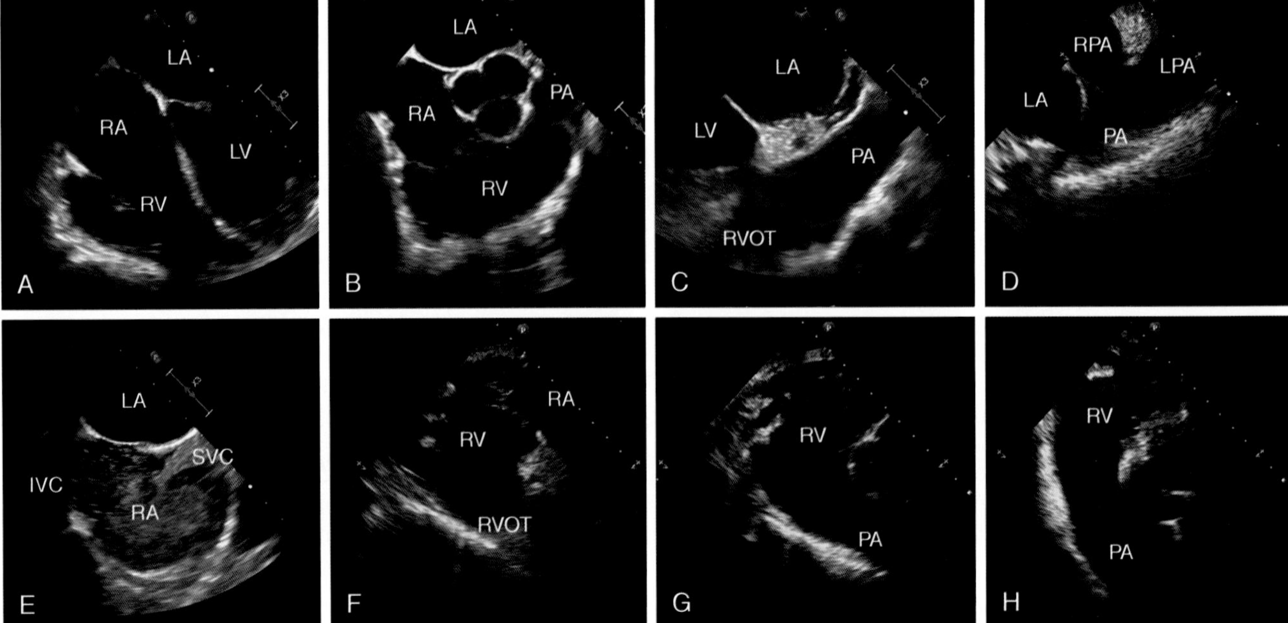

Fig. 6.16 Key TTE views of the RV. TEE can help visualize the RV and other right-sided cardiac structures. (A) TEE retroesophageal 4-chamber view with RV focus (Video 6.16A). (B) TEE retroesophageal short-axis view. This window is usually acquired at 45 to 60 degrees with a clockwise rotation of the probe handle (Video 6.16B). (C) The RVOT, pulmonic valve, and proximal pulmonary artery can be visualized from the retroesophageal view. This can be achieved with the omniplane at approximately 60 degrees and withdrawal of the probe to a high retroesophageal window. If shadowing from the left mainstem bronchus occurs, further withdrawal of the probe above the bronchus may yield an excellent view of the pulmonic valve (Video 6.16C). (D) The right and left branches of the pulmonary artery can be seen in the high retroesophageal view using a low omniplane angle of 0 to 20 degrees (Video 6.16D). (E) The bicaval view is an ideal window for interrogating the interatrial septum for the presence or absence of interatrial shunts. This is usually achieved with an omniplane angle of 90 to 135 degrees and a clockwise rotation of the probe handle. The IVC can be carefully tracked into the transgastric view if Doppler imaging of the hepatic vein is desired for assessment of tricuspid regurgitation (Video 6.16E). (F) The RV can be seen in the transgastric view with an omniplane angle of 60 to 90 degrees. At its basal level, the tricuspid valve is well seen. (G) Advancing the probe to the midbody of the RV may provide a view of the entire long axis of the RV. (H) Further advancement of the probe combined with anteflexion can improve visualization of the pulmonic valve in a plane with an angle of incidence favorable for color and spectral Doppler. At this apical view and with a low omniplane angle of 0 to 20 degrees, a 4-chamber view of the RV can sometimes be achieved with additional careful anteflexion and probe advancement. *IVC*, Inferior vena cava; *LPA*, left pulmonary artery; *PA*, pulmonary artery; *RPA*, right pulmonary artery; *RVOT*, right ventricular outflow tract.

postprocessing tools to quickly, accurately, and reproducibly segment the RV; lack of specific reimbursement for specialized functional analysis from 3D CTA data sets; lack of normalization data; use of ionizing radiation; and the need for potentially nephrotoxic iodinated contrast.

RADIONUCLEOTIDE ANGIOGRAPHY

RV radionucleotide angiography (i.e., multigated acquisition [MUGA] scanning) uses the patient's radiolabeled red blood cells and ECG-gated cardiac scintigraphy. Imaging data are collected with a planar gamma camera in multiple standard orientations. This technique uses imaging data from hundreds of cardiac cycles leading to a high degree of precision, but its use is limited due to radiation exposure and inadequate imaging projections. Like invasive RV ventriculography and CTA, this technique is rarely used given the radiation-free alternatives of TTE and CMR.

CLINICAL UTILITY

DISEASE STATES AND OUTCOME DATA

The role of the RV and its various qualitative and quantitative metrics are studied in most disease states, with continued interest in quantification as new technologies and therapies are developed. For instance, the lack of RV contractile reserve on exercise TAPSE predicts adverse outcomes for patients with mitral regurgitation.[38] The RV may be involved in 16.5% of takotsubo syndrome (i.e., stress cardiomyopathy) cases, and RV involvement is an independent predictor of acute heart failure and of a composite end point that includes adverse events such as acute heart failure, cardiogenic shock, and increased in-hospital mortality.[54]

The use of tools for assessing RV function follows a pattern similar to that for other imaging technologies, with a slow but steady progression from inception to identification of interobserver and intraobserver reproducibility, clinical implementation for diagnosis, and ultimately, application for prognostication. Each of the tools used for evaluating RV function has been studied in a variety of settings, both in isolation and in aggregate[32–34,36,37,39–42,48–50,55–60] (Table 6.9). This has produced a large and increasing body of work that validates the utility of echocardiography as a prognostic tool for RV assessment.

The reproducible evaluation of RV function may provide clues for the identification of undiagnosed systemic diseases. Many systemic diseases that affect the right heart may be downstream of the RV and difficult to identify by direct visualization. In these cases, abnormalities in RV size or function may be the primary clue to the existence of other pathology. Causes of RV failure that may play a role in clinical diagnosis fall into a few main categories: (1) extrinsic extracardiac factors, (2) intrinsic RV myopathies, (3) increases in RV afterload, and (4) increases in RV preload. Each category is associated with a number of pathologic states (Table 6.10).

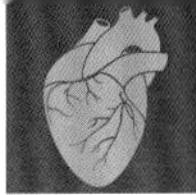

TABLE 6.9 Selected Studies Showing Association of Clinical Outcomes With Echocardiographic Parameters of RV Size and Systolic Function.

Year	*Study*	*N*	*Population*	*Follow-Up*	*End Point*	*Results*	*Adjusted For*
2002	Samad et al.[55]	194	First MI	24 mo	Death	TAPSE < 15 mm → increased mortality ($P < 0.02$)	Age, LVEF
2002	Zornoff et al.[39]	416	LVEF ≤ 40%, 11 days post-MI	31 mo	Death	RV FAC < 32% → HR = 2.6, adjusted	Age, LVEF, sex, MI, DM, HTN, infarct size, smoking, treatment
2005	Scridon et al.[56]	141	Acute PE	1 mo	Death	RVEDd/LVEDd > 0.9 → higher mortality rate (9% vs. 5% for no TnI leak, 38% vs. 23% for TnI > 0.1 ng/mL)	Age, sex, hypotension
2005	Skali et al.[36]	291	1 year post-MI	22 mo	Death	RV FAC < 32% → HR = 9.7, adjusted	Age, LVEF, sex, DM, blood pressure
2006	Forfia et al.[41]	63	PH (47 with PAH)	19 mo	Death	Adjusted HR = 1.16 for every 1-mm decrease in TAPSE in PAH cohort	Effusion, WHO class
2008	Anavekar et al.[32]	522	LVSD or HF, 0.5–10 days post-MI	25 mo	Composite	Every 5% decrease in RV FAC → HR = 1.53, adjusted; RV FAC independently associated with all-cause and CV mortality, HF, stroke	Age, LVEF, HF, Killip class, prior MI, first MI, angina, DM, AF, COPD, GFR
2008	Dini et al.[34]	142	LVEF ≤ 45%, MR VC ≥ 5 mm	20 mo	Death	TAPSE < 16 mm → HR = 2.6, adjusted	Age, LVEF, sex, CAD, NYHA class
2013	Vivo et al.[57]	109	LVAD	1 mo	RV failure	RVEDd/LVEDd > 0.75 → higher RV failure (OR = 5.40, $P = 0.012$)	Matthews and Kormos scores
2014	Ameloot et al.[40]	78	PAH, CTEPH	42 mo	Death	RV dP/dt < 410 mmHg/s, TAPSE < 15 mm predicted mortality (HR = 2.67, 95% CI: 1.3–5.5, $P = 0.007$)	TAPSE
2014	Mohammed et al.[59]	562	HF with preserved LVEF	10 yr	Death	Semiquantitative RV function (all-cause mortality HR = 1.35; $P = 0.03$; CV mortality HR = 1.85; $P = 0.006$)	Age, sex, pulmonary artery systolic pressure, and comorbidities
2014	Shimony et al.[58]	768	CABG	96 h	AF	RV MPI predicted AF (OR = 1.50, 95% CI: 1.01–2.24)	Age, gender, BMI, arrhythmia history, PAD, CVA, Cr
2015	Galli et al.[42]	200	TAVR	16 mo	Death	TAPSE ≤ 17 and LVEF ≤ 50% (HR = 4.08, $P = 0.012$)	CAD, AVA, and sPAP
2017	Bartko et al.[60]	240	ECMO	27 mo	Death	RV free wall strain < −14%, (HR = 0.48, $P = 0.001$)	Age, sex, SAPS 3, TR, type of CV surgery, and procedure duration
2017	Couperus et al.[33]	139	Surgical LV restoration	30 days	Death	RV free wall peak longitudinal strain of > −20% (HR = 1.15; $P < 0.01$)	LVEF and aortic cross-clamping time
2018	Risum et al.[50]	790	Acute MI	898 days	SCD, admit with ventricular arrhythmias, appropriate ICD shock	RV free wall strain > −22% (HR = 9.8, $P = 0.002$), for each 1% reduction in strain (HR = 1.15, $P = 0.038$)	Age, LV GLS
2018	Nochioka et al.[49]	1004	Community-based elderly cohort	4.1 yr	Incident HF or death	3D RVEF (HR = 1.20 per 5% decrease in RVEF; $P = 0.03$)	Age, sex, and race/ethnicity
2019	Terluk et al.[37]	233	Acute PE	3 yr	Death	RV PLAX > 37 mm (HR = 2.3, $P = 0.016$), TR velocity > 2.9 m/s (HR = 1.9, $P = 0.021$); RA area > 20 cm^2 (HR = 2.0, $P = 0.016$); combined HR = 16.9, $P < 0.001$	Age

AF, Atrial fibrillation; *AVA,* aortic valve area; *BMI,* body mass index; *CAD,* coronary artery disease; *CABG,* coronary artery bypass grafting; *CI,* confidence interval; *COPD,* chronic obstructive pulmonary disease; *Cr,* creatinine; *CTEPH,* chronic thromboembolic pulmonary hypertension; *CV,* cardiovascular; *CVA,* cerebral vascular accident; *DM,* diabetes mellitus; *ECMO,* extra corporal membrane oxygenation; *FAC,* fractional area change; *GFR,* glomerular filtration rate; *GLS,* global longitudinal strain; *HF,* heart failure; *HR,* hazard ratio; *HTN,* hypertension; *ICD,* implantable cardioverter-defibrillator; *LVAD,* left ventricular assist device; *LVEDd,* left ventricular internal diastolic dimension; *LVEF,* left ventricular ejection fraction; *LVSD,* left ventricular systolic dysfunction; *MI,* myocardial infarction; *MPI,* myocardial performance index; *MR,* mitral regurgitation; *NYHA,* New York Heart Association; *OR,* odds ratio; *PAD,* peripheral artery disease; *PE,* pulmonary embolism; *PH,* pulmonary hypertension; *PAH,* pulmonary arterial hypertension; *PLAX,* parasternal long-axis view; *RVEDd,* right ventricular diastolic dimension; *RVEF,* right ventricular ejection fraction; *SAPS 3,* Simplified Acute Physiology Score 3; *SCD,* sudden cardiac death; *sPAP,* systolic pulmonary artery pressure; *TAVR,* transcatheter aortic valve replacement; *TAPSE,* tricuspid annular plane systolic excursion; *TnI,* troponin I; *TR,* tricuspid regurgitation; *VC,* vena contracta; *WHO,* World Health Organization.

TABLE 6.10 Pathologic States Associated With RV Failure.

Causes of RV Failure	*Associated Pathology*
Extrinsic factors	• Pericardial effusion, tamponade • Pericardial constriction • Isolated RV pacing, bundle branch block, dyssynchrony
Intrinsic myopathy	• Ischemia, infarction • ARVD • Myocarditis • Hypertrophic cardiomyopathy
Increases in afterload	• Pulmonary stenosis • Pulmonary embolism • Acute lung injury • Left heart failure
Increases in preload	Tricuspid regurgitation • Functional regurgitation • Endocarditis • Pacemaker lead • Ebstein anomaly • Rheumatic heart disease • Carcinoid • Iatrogenic injury (e.g., right heart biopsy, PA catheter) Pulmonary regurgitation • Primary pulmonary regurgitation • Tetralogy of Fallot • Carcinoid • Iatrogenic injury (e.g., PA catheter) Shunts • Atrial septal defect • Ventricular septal defect

ARVD, Arrhythmogenic right ventricular dysplasia; *PA*, pulmonary artery.

TRANSCATHETER PROCEDURES

The state of RV function is important when considering transcatheter valve procedures. For instance, in left-sided valve procedures such as TAVR or transcatheter mitral valve repair, the presence of RV dysfunction portends a worse prognosis.[61,62] Given the rapid developments in transcatheter valve technologies, more techniques for treating right-sided valve pathology are becoming available, and there will be continued interest in how the RV responds to the hemodynamic changes created by these technologies.

MECHANICAL SUPPORT DEVICES

The traditional concept of heart failure has focused on the LV, with little attention paid to specific medical or procedure-based therapies.[63,64] Although RV failure frequently occurs as a consequence of left-sided heart failure, acute RV failure from ischemia or acute RV pressure/volume overload states may manifest in certain clinical situations as a primary cause of cardiogenic shock. Initial hemodynamic support can often be provided by medical therapy with inotropic agents.

The decision to initiate mechanical right-sided support begins with a careful echocardiographic evaluation but frequently requires confirmation with invasive right heart catheterization. Right-sided mechanical support includes percutaneous technologies (e.g., extracorporeal membrane oxygenation) for temporary support and right-sided ventricular assist devices for long-term support.[65–67] Right-sided support devices are frequently technically difficult to image, and echocardiographers should be well versed in the echocardiographic appearances of and imaging parameters needed for specific devices.[68,69]

FUTURE DIRECTIONS

Progress in RV evaluation will revolve around improving education in RV assessment, incorporation of software-based workflow improvements, hardware developments that advance image quality, and large-scale validation of these emerging technologies. Development of point-of-care ultrasound is being driven by improvements in image quality and lower hardware costs, allowing more health care providers to access this technology. The bedside use of this technology for rapid clinical decision making in conditions such as acute pulmonary embolism is spreading.[70] Particularly for structures such as the RV, which can be difficult to image even by experienced sonographers, this is driving the need for education in high-quality image acquisition and interpretation.

Other advancements in evaluation of the RV will involve workflow improvements of current technology, such as RV strain analysis and 3D volumetric evaluation of RV size and function. These technologies have long been available but have had slow adoption into clinical practice. It is estimated that these technologies are routinely used in only 3% and 1% of cases, respectively.[71] This is in part related to available expertise, interobserver reproducibility, intervendor reproducibility, reimbursement challenges, availability of postprocessing tools, and ease of use of advanced dedicated software packages. Emerging technologies such as artificial intelligence and machine learning may lead to increased efficiency in imaging processing and improvements in measurement reproducibility.[72]

Improved imaging technology continues to generate insights into the normal and pathologic states of RV function. As the importance of the RV continues to be validated by prognostic data derived from larger patient cohorts, translation of these techniques to routine clinical practice will be key.

ACKNOWLEDGMENTS

The authors wish to acknowledge Anjali Vaidya, MD, and James N. Kirkpatrick, MD, the authors of related chapters in previous editions of *The Practice of Clinical Echocardiography.*

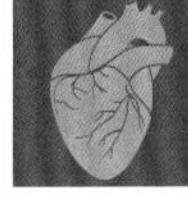

SUMMARY A Practical Approach to Echocardiographic Data Acquisition, Measurement, and Interpretation.

Imaging Approaches and Techniques	Applications
Transthoracic Echocardiography	
Parasternal long-axis	• Limited view of high RVOT • Evaluate for membranous VSD
Parasternal RV/tricuspid inflow	• Tricuspid valve morphology and function
Parasternal RVOT	• Pulmonic valve morphology and function • PA size • RVOT VTI (systolic function, Qp:Qs for shunt) • RVOT diameter (Qp:Qs for shunt)
Parasternal short-axis (mid-ventricle)	• Interventricular septal position and motion (volume/pressure overload of RV) • Evaluate muscular VSD
Parasternal short-axis (aortic valve)	• TV morphology, stenosis, regurgitation • Pulmonic valve morphology and function • IAS (PFO, ASD) • RVOT VTI (systolic function, Qp:Qs) • RVOT diameter (Qp:Qs for shunt) • Localize inflow and outflow VSDs
Standard apical 4-chamber	• RV function • TV morphology and function • RA size • Interventricular septal position and motion (volume/pressure overload of RV)
RV-focused apical 4-chamber	• RV size and function • RV FAC • RV free wall assessment • TV morphology and function
Subcostal views (4-chamber and IVC)	• RV free wall thickness • Evaluation for ASD • Evaluation for VSD • IVC dynamics
Transesophageal Echocardiography	
Mid-esophageal 4-chamber 0 degrees (Optimization tip: RV is usually foreshortened at apex and requires retroflexion to optimize.)	• RV size and function • TV morphology and function
Mid-esophageal bicaval 90–135 degrees (Optimization tip: Withdraw or advance probe to interrogate for superior and inferior sinus venosus defects. Sweep image to distinguish coronary sinus from IVC.)	• RA size and morphology • SVC • IVC and associated structures (eustachian valve, Chiari network) • IAS (PFO/ASD) • Agitated saline bubble study • Right atrial appendage • Coronary sinus • TV on imaging sweep
Mid-esophageal short-axis 45–60 degrees (Optimization tip: If pulmonic valve is shadowed, withdraw probe to high esophageal window. Pulmonary bifurcation can be seen at this level.)	• TV morphology and function • Pulmonic valve morphology and function • RVOT and PA size • VSD localization
Mid-esophageal inverted 4-chamber 130–150 degrees (equivalent to −30 degrees) (Optimization tip: If prominent, aortic sinus may require probe retroflexion or advancement.)	• TV morphology and function

SUMMARY A Practical Approach to Echocardiographic Data Acquisition, Measurement, and Interpretation.—cont'd

Imaging Approaches and Techniques	Applications
Transgastric IVC 60–90 degrees (Optimization tip: Maintain visualization of the IVC while advancing probe from RA into transgastric views.)	• IVC size and flow dynamics by PWD and color Doppler
Basal mid-transgastric short-axis 0–20 degrees (Optimization tip: In the mid-transgastric position with mild anteflexion, a 15–20 degree increase in angle can help.)	• TV valve morphology and function • Pulmonic valve morphology and function
Mid-transgastric long-axis 60–90 degrees (Optimization tip: A parallel angle of incidence with the pulmonic outflow may require advancement to the apex with anteflexion.)	• TV valve morphology and function • Pulmonic valve morphology and function • RVOT size, RVOT VTI
Deep transgastric 0 degrees (foreshortened 4-chamber view) (Optimization tip: Careful sequential advancement of the probe and anteflexion can help.)	• TV valve morphology and function • RV function
Intracardiac Echocardiography	
RA	• TV morphology and function • IAS (PFO/ASD) • SVC
RV	• RVOT • PA size
RV Quantification	
Size: subcostal 4-chamber	• Free wall > 5 mm
Size: RV-focused apical 4-chamber	• Enlarged RV is > ⅔ of LV size • Basal, middle, and longitudinal diameters • Diastolic area
Size: parasternal short-axis (mid-ventricle)	• Mid-ventricular dimension
Size: parasternal short-axis (AoV)	• RVOT
Systolic function: apical 4-chamber	• FAC • TAPSE • Anterolateral annular S′ by TDI • *dP/dt* from TR CWD • Isovolumic acceleration by TDI • MPI by PWD or TDI (RVH may falsely shorten IVRT)
Diastolic function: apical 4-chamber	• E/A TV inflow by PWD • E DT by PWD • Lateral annular e′ by TDI • RA enlargement
Diastolic function: subcostal	• IVC size and collapsibility • Hepatic vein S/D ratio
3D evaluation of RV volumes and function	• No geometric assumptions • Requires adequate endocardial definition
RV free wall peak longitudinal systolic strain	• Highest strain in midwall • Requires adequate endocardial definition

ASD, Atrial septal defect; *AoV,* aortic valve; *CWD,* continuous-wave Doppler; *dP/dt,* change in pressure over change in time; *DT,* deceleration time; *E/A,* ratio of early to atrial peak filling velocity; *FAC,* fractional area change; *IAS,* interatrial septum; *IVC,* inferior vena cava; *IVRT,* intraventricular relaxation time; *MPI,* myocardial performance index; *PA,* pulmonary artery; *PFO,* patent foramen ovale; *PWD,* pulsed-wave Doppler; *Qp:Qs,* ratio of pulmonic flow to systemic flow; *RA,* right atrium; *RVH,* right ventricular hypertrophy; *RVOT,* RV outflow tract; *S′,* tricuspid annular systolic velocity; *S/D ratio,* systolic VTI/diastolic VTI; *SVC,* superior vena cava; *TAPSE,* tricuspid annular plane systolic excursion; *TDI,* tissue Doppler imaging; *TR,* tricuspid regurgitation; *TV,* tricuspid valve; VSD, ventricular septal defect; *VTI,* velocity–time integral.

REFERENCES

1. Sterpetti AV. Cardiovascular Research by Leonardo da Vinci (1452–1519). *Circ Res.* 2019;124(2):189–191.
2. Meyer JA. Werner Forssmann and catheterization of the heart, 1929. *Ann Thorac Surg.* 1990;49(3):497–499.
3. Starr I, Jeffers WA, Meade RH. The absence of conspicuous increments of venous pressure after severe damage to the right ventricle of the dog, with a discussion of the relation between clinical congestive failure and heart disease. *Am Heart J.* 1943;26(3):291–301.
4. Bakos ACP. The question of the function of the right ventricular myocardium: an experimental study. *Circulation.* 1950;1(4):724–732.
5. Fontan F, Baudet E. Surgical repair of tricuspid atresia. *Thorax.* 1971;26(3):240–248.
6. Cohn JN, Guiha NH, Broder MI, Limas CJ. Right ventricular infarction. Clinical and hemodynamic features. *Am J Cardiol.* 1974;33(2):209–214.
7. Moreyra AE, Suh C, Porway MN, Kostis JB. Rapid hemodynamic improvement in right ventricular infarction after coronary angioplasty. *Chest.* 1988;94(1):197–199.
8. Inohara T, Kohsaka S, Fukuda K, Menon V. The challenges in the management of right ventricular infarction. *Eur Heart J Acute Cardiovasc Care.* 2013;2(3):226–234.
9. Gumina RJ, Murphy JG, Rihal CS, Lennon RJ, Wright RS. Long-term survival after right ventricular infarction. *Am J Cardiol.* 2006;98(12):1571–1573.
10. Ramirez R, Ovakimyan O, Lasam G, Lafferty K. A very late presentation of a right coronary artery occlusion after transcatheter aortic valve replacement. *Cardiol Res.* 2017;8(3):131–133.
11. Jabbour RJ, Tanaka A, Finkelstein A, et al. Delayed coronary obstruction after transcatheter aortic valve replacement. *J Am Coll Cardiol.* 2018;71(14):1513–1524.
12. Brodie BR, Stuckey TD, Hansen C, Bradshaw BH, Downey WE, Pulsipher MW. Comparison of late survival in patients with cardiogenic shock due to right ventricular infarction versus left ventricular pump failure following primary percutaneous coronary intervention for ST-elevation acute myocardial infarction. *Am J Cardiol.* 2007;99(4):431–435.
13. Lang RM, Badano LP, Mor-Avi V, et al. Recommendations for cardiac chamber quantification by echocardiography in adults: an update from the American Society of Echocardiography and the European Association of Cardiovascular Imaging. *J Am Soc Echocardiogr.* 2015;28(1):1–39 e14.
14. Rudski LG, Lai WW, Afilalo J, et al. Guidelines for the echocardiographic assessment of the right heart in adults: a report from the American Society of Echocardiography endorsed by the European Association of Echocardiography, a registered branch of the European Society of Cardiology, and the Canadian Society of Echocardiography. *J Am Soc Echocardiogr.* 2010;23(7):685–713. quiz 786-688.
15. Athavale S, Deopujari R, Sinha U, Lalwani R, Kotgirwar S. Is tricuspid valve really tricuspid? *Anat Cell Biol.* 2017;50(1):1–6.
16. Kini S, Bis KG, Weaver L. Normal and variant coronary arterial and venous anatomy on high-resolution CT angiography. *AJR Am J Roentgenol.* 2007;188(6):1665–1674.
17. Marcus JT, Smeenk HG, Kuijer JP, Van der Geest RJ, Heethaar RM, Van Rossum AC. Flow profiles in the left anterior descending and the right coronary artery assessed by MR velocity quantification: effects of through-plane and in-plane motion of the heart. *J Comput Assist Tomogr.* 1999;23(4):567–576.
18. Goodwill AG, Dick GM, Kiel AM, Tune JD. Regulation of coronary blood flow. *Compr Physiol.* 2017;7(2):321–382.
18a. Kumar A, Abdel-Aty H, Kriedemann I, et al. Contrast-enhanced cardiovascular magnetic resonance imaging of right ventricular infarction. *J Am Coll Cardiol.* 2006;48(10):1969-1976.
19. Foppa M, Arora G, Gona P, et al. Right ventricular volumes and systolic function by cardiac magnetic resonance and the impact of sex, age, and obesity in a longitudinally followed cohort free of pulmonary and cardiovascular disease: the Framingham heart study. *Circ Cardiovasc Imaging.* 2016;9(3):e003810.
20. Naeije R, Badagliacca R. The overloaded right heart and ventricular interdependence. *Cardiovasc Res.* 2017;113(12):1474–1485.
21. Omoto T, Tanabe H, LaRia PJ, Guererro J, Vlahakes GJ. Right ventricular performance during left ventricular unloading conditions: the contribution of the right ventricular free wall. *Thorac Cardiovasc Surg.* 2002;50(1):16–20.
22. Pinsky MR. The right ventricle: interaction with the pulmonary circulation. *Crit Care.* 2016;20(1):266.
23. Berlin DA, Bakker J. Starling curves and central venous pressure. *Crit Care.* 2015;19(1):55.
24. Ivens EL, Munt BI, Moss RR. Pericardial disease: what the general cardiologist needs to know. *Heart (British Cardiac Society).* 2007;93(8):993–1000.
25. Sanz J, Sanchez-Quintana D, Bossone E, Bogaard HJ, Naeije R. Anatomy, function, and dysfunction of the right ventricle: JACC state-of-the-art review. *J Am Coll Cardiol.* 2019;73(12):1463–1482.
26. Nagata Y, Wu VC, Kado Y, et al. Prognostic value of right ventricular ejection fraction assessed by Transthoracic 3D echocardiography. *Circ Cardiovasc imaging.* 2017;10(2).
27. Fuchs A, Mejdahl MR, Kuhl JT, et al. Normal values of left ventricular mass and cardiac chamber volumes assessed by 320-detector computed tomography angiography in the Copenhagen General Population Study. *Eur Heart J Cardiovasc Imaging.* 2016;17(9):1009–1017.
28. Tamborini G, Marsan NA, Gripari P, et al. Reference values for right ventricular volumes and ejection fraction with real-time three-dimensional echocardiography: evaluation in a large series of normal subjects. *J Am Soc Echocardiogr.* 2010;23(2):109–115.
29. Maffessanti F, Muraru D, Esposito R, et al. Age-, body size-, and sex-specific reference values for right ventricular volumes and ejection fraction by three-dimensional echocardiography: a multicenter echocardiographic study in 507 healthy volunteers. *Cir Cardiovasc imaging.* 2013;6(5):700–710.
30. McConnell MV, Solomon SD, Rayan ME, Come PC, Goldhaber SZ, Lee RT. Regional right ventricular dysfunction detected by echocardiography in acute pulmonary embolism. *Am J Cardiol.* 1996;78(4):469–473.
31. Marcus FI, McKenna WJ, Sherrill D, et al. Diagnosis of arrhythmogenic right ventricular cardiomyopathy/dysplasia: proposed modification of the task force criteria. *Circulation.* 2010;121(13):1533–1541.
32. Anavekar NS, Skali H, Bourgoun M, et al. Usefulness of right ventricular fractional area change to predict death, heart failure, and stroke following myocardial infarction (from the VALIANT ECHO Study). *Am J Cardiol.* 2008;101(5):607–612.
33. Couperus LE, Delgado V, Palmen M, et al. Right ventricular dysfunction affects survival after surgical left ventricular restoration. *J Thorac Cardiovasc Surg.* 2017;153(4):845–852.
34. Dini FL, Fontanive P, Panicucci E, Andreini D, Chella P, De Tommasi SM. Prognostic significance of tricuspid annular motion and plasma NT-proBNP in patients with heart failure and moderate-to-severe functional mitral regurgitation. *Eur J Heart Fail.* 2008;10(6):573–580.
35. Puwanant S, Hamilton KK, Klodell CT, et al. Tricuspid annular motion as a predictor of severe right ventricular failure after left ventricular assist device implantation. *J Heart Lung Transplant.* 2008;27(10):1102–1107.
36. Skali H, Zornoff LA, Pfeffer MA, et al. Survival, Ventricular Enlargement I. Prognostic use of echocardiography 1 year after a myocardial infarction. *Am Heart J.* 2005;150(4):743–749.
37. Terluk AD, Trivedi SJ, Kritharides L, et al. Echocardiographic predictors of long-term mortality in patients presenting with acute pulmonary embolism. *Am J Cardiol.* 2019;124(2):285–291.
38. Vitel E, Galli E, Leclercq C, et al. Right ventricular exercise contractile reserve and outcomes after early surgery for primary mitral regurgitation. *Heart (British Cardiac Society).* 2018;104(10):855–860.
39. Zornoff LA, Skali H, Pfeffer MA, et al. Right ventricular dysfunction and risk of heart failure and mortality after myocardial infarction. *J Am Coll Cardiol.* 2002;39(9):1450–1455.
40. Ameloot K, Palmers PJ, Vande Bruaene A, et al. Clinical value of echocardiographic Doppler-derived right ventricular dp/dt in patients with pulmonary arterial hypertension. *European heart journal cardiovascular Imaging.* 2014;15(12):1411–1419.
41. Forfia PR, Fisher MR, Mathai SC, et al. Tricuspid annular displacement predicts survival in pulmonary hypertension. *Am J Respir Crit Care Med.* 2006;174(9):1034–1041.
42. Galli E, Guirette Y, Feneon D, et al. Prevalence and prognostic value of right ventricular dysfunction in severe aortic stenosis. *European heart journal cardiovascular Imaging.* 2015;16(5):531–538.
43. Ghio S, Recusani F, Klersy C, et al. Prognostic usefulness of the tricuspid annular plane systolic excursion in patients with congestive heart failure secondary to idiopathic or ischemic dilated cardiomyopathy. *Am J Cardiol.* 2000;85(7):837–842.
44. Brown SB, Raina A, Katz D, Szerlip M, Wiegers SE, Forfia PR. Longitudinal shortening accounts for the majority of right ventricular contraction and improves after pulmonary vasodilator therapy in normal subjects and patients with pulmonary arterial hypertension. *Chest.* 2011;140(1):27–33.
45. Magunia H, Dietrich C, Langer HF, et al. 3D echocardiography derived right ventricular function is associated with right ventricular failure and mid-term survival after left ventricular assist device implantation. *Int J Cardiol.* 2018;272:348–355.
46. Badano LP, Cucchini U, Muraru D, Al Nono O, Sarais C, Iliceto S. Use of three-dimensional

speckle tracking to assess left ventricular myocardial mechanics: inter-vendor consistency and reproducibility of strain measurements. *Eur Heart J Cardiovasc Imaging*. 2013; 14(3):285–293.

47. Lisi M, Cameli M, Righini FM, et al. RV longitudinal deformation Correlates with myocardial fibrosis in patients with end-stage heart failure. *JACC Cardiovasc Imaging*. 2015;8(5):514–522.
48. Carluccio E, Biagioli P, Alunni G, et al. Prognostic value of right ventricular dysfunction in heart failure with reduced ejection fraction: Superiority of longitudinal strain over tricuspid annular plane systolic excursion. *Circulation Cardiovascular imaging*. 2018;11(1):e006894.
49. Nochioka K, Querejeta Roca G, Claggett B, et al. Right ventricular function, right ventricular-pulmonary artery coupling, and heart failure risk in 4 US communities: the atherosclerosis risk in communities (ARIC) study. *JAMA Cardiol*. 2018;3(10):939–948.
50. Risum N, Valeur N, Sogaard P, Hassager C, Kober L, Ersboll M. Right ventricular function assessed by 2D strain analysis predicts ventricular arrhythmias and sudden cardiac death in patients after acute myocardial infarction. *European heart journal cardiovascular Imaging*. 2018;19(7):800–807.
51. Yu CM, Sanderson JE, Chan S, Yeung L, Hung YT, Woo KS. Right ventricular diastolic dysfunction in heart failure. *Circulation*. 1996;93(8):1509–1514.
52. Pagourelias ED, Efthimiadis GK, Parcharidou DG, et al. Prognostic value of right ventricular diastolic function indices in hypertrophic cardiomyopathy. *Eur J Echocardiogr*. 2011;12(11):809–817.
53. Gan CT, Holverda S, Marcus JT, et al. Right ventricular diastolic dysfunction and the acute effects of sildenafil in pulmonary hypertension patients. *Chest*. 2007;132(1):11–17.
54. Citro R, Bossone E, Parodi G, et al. Independent impact of RV involvement on in-hospital outcome of patients with takotsubo syndrome. *JACC Cardiovasc Imaging*. 2016;9(7):894–895.
55. Samad BA, Alam M, Jensen-Urstad K. Prognostic impact of right ventricular involvement as assessed by tricuspid annular motion in patients with acute myocardial infarction. *Am J Cardiol*. 2002;90(7):778–781.
56. Scridon T, Scridon C, Skali H, Alvarez A, Goldhaber SZ, Solomon SD. Prognostic significance of troponin elevation and right ventricular enlargement in acute pulmonary embolism. *Am J Cardiol*. 2005;96(2):303–305.
57. Vivo RP, Cordero-Reyes AM, Qamar U, et al. Increased right-to-left ventricle diameter ratio is a strong predictor of right ventricular failure after left ventricular assist device. *J Heart Lung Transplant*. 2013;32(8):792–799.
58. Shimony A, Afilalo J, Flynn AW, et al. Usefulness of right ventricular dysfunction to predict new-onset atrial fibrillation following coronary artery bypass grafting. *Am J Cardiol*. 2014;113(6):913–918.
59. Mohammed SF, Hussain I, AbouEzzeddine OF, et al. Right ventricular function in heart failure with preserved ejection fraction: a community-based study. *Circulation*. 2014;130(25):2310–2320.
60. Bartko PE, Wiedemann D, Schrutka L, et al. Impact of right ventricular performance in patients Undergoing extracorporeal membrane oxygenation following cardiac surgery. *J Am Heart Assoc*. 2017;6(8):e005455.
61. Cremer PC, Zhang Y, Alu M, et al. The incidence and prognostic implications of worsening right ventricular function after surgical or transcatheter aortic valve replacement: insights from PARTNER IIA. *Eur Heart J*. 2018;39(28):2659–2667.
62. Kaneko H, Neuss M, Weissenborn J, Butter C. Prognostic significance of right ventricular dysfunction in patients with functional mitral regurgitation Undergoing MitraClip. *Am J Cardiol*. 2016;118(11):1717–1722.
63. Yancy CW, Jessup M, Bozkurt B, et al. 2017 ACC/AHA/HFSA focused update of the 2013 ACCF/AHA guideline for the management of heart failure: a report of the American College of Cardiology/American Heart Association task force on clinical practice guidelines and the Heart Failure Society of America. *Circulation*. 2017;136(6):e137–e161.
64. Yancy CW, Jessup M, Bozkurt B, et al. American College of Cardiology F, American Heart Association task force on practice G. 2013 ACCF/AHA guideline for the management of heart failure: a report of the American College of Cardiology Foundation/American Heart Association task force on practice guidelines. *J Am Coll Cardiol*. 2013;62(16):e147–239.
65. Haneya A, Philipp A, Puehler T, et al. Temporary percutaneous right ventricular support using a centrifugal pump in patients with postoperative acute refractory right ventricular failure after left ventricular assist device implantation. *Eur J Cardio Thorac Surg*. 2012;41(1):219–223.
66. Kapur NK, Esposito ML, Bader Y, et al. Mechanical circulatory support devices for acute right ventricular failure. *Circulation*. 2017;136(3):314–326.
67. Anderson M, Morris DL, Tang D, et al. Outcomes of patients with right ventricular failure requiring short-term hemodynamic support with the Impella RP device. *J Heart Lung Transplant*. 2018;37(12):1448–1458.
68. Jain A, Al-Ani M, Arnaoutakis G, Alviar C, Vilaro J. Troubleshooting right ventricular failure: role of transesophageal echocardiography in assessing Impella Rp® position. *J Am Coll Cardiol*. 2019;73(9):2636.
69. Schmack B, Weymann A, Popov AF, et al. Concurrent left ventricular assist device (LVAD) implantation and percutaneous temporary RVAD support via CardiacAssist Protek-Duo TandemHeart to preempt right heart failure. *Med Sci Monit Basic Res*. 2016;22:53–57.
70. Filopei J, Acquah SO, Bondarsky EE, et al. Diagnostic accuracy of point-of-care ultrasound performed by pulmonary critical care physicians for right ventricle assessment in patients with acute pulmonary embolism. *Crit Care Med*. 2017;45(12):2040–2045.
71. Schneider M, Aschauer S, Mascherbauer J, et al. Echocardiographic assessment of right ventricular function: current clinical practice. *Int J Cardiovasc Imaging*. 2019;35(1):49–56.
72. Genovese D, Rashedi N, Weinert L, et al. Machine learning-based three-dimensional echocardiographic quantification of right ventricular size and function: validation against cardiac magnetic resonance. *J Am Soc Echocardiogr*. 2019;32(8):969–977.

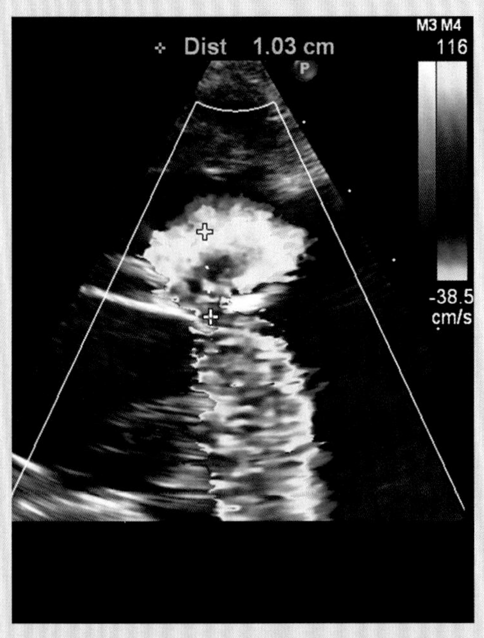

PART Ⅱ

第二部分

Echocardiography Best Practices

超声心动图实践优化

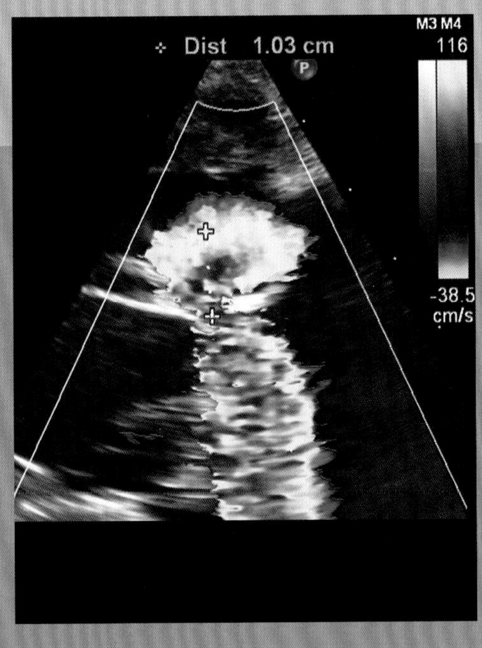

中文导读

第7章 超声心动图诊断科室：结构、标准和质量改进

高质量的医疗服务意味着在现有的技术条件下尽可能为患者带来最佳的医疗产出，同时兼顾效率和公平。现代高质量的超声心动图科室的结构包括：经行业认证委员会认证的科室设施；获得相应资质并保证继续教育的员工（医师和技师）；具备经胸超声心动图、经食管超声心动图和负荷超声心动图的检查能力；配备有图像存储系统和超声报告系统等设置的超声仪器；应定期维护仪器以保证其精确的检查能力。

高质量的超声心动图检查离不开适当地选择患者、标准的图像采集流程和检查流程。同时应保证员工和患者的安全，包括减少可能受到的核医学辐射，控制院内感染的发生，尤其是新型冠状病毒感染流行期间患者的选择、防护，仪器探头的消毒等；高质量的超声心动图检查同样离不开标准的超声图像采集、图像解读、报告出具，以及医师之间的良好沟通；超声诊断质量控制及持续改进需要进行定期病例回顾分析，并与其他影像及临床结果进行对照以及时改进。

以上内容应制定具体而详细的工作制度以便于科室日常管理，在主管负责人变动的情况下，谨慎且恰当地存档和修订制度有利于科室质量管理保持稳定发展和传承。

朱振辉

Diagnostic Echocardiography Laboratory: Structure, Standards, and Quality Improvement

RAYMOND F. STAINBACK, MD

Echocardiography has evolved dramatically, starting with initial M-mode and two-dimensional (2D) imaging in the 1970s and growing with the addition of spectral and color Doppler in the 1980s. Since then, the breadth and sophistication of echocardiography's clinical applications, as detailed elsewhere in this textbook, have exploded and continue to evolve.

To manage this growth, echocardiography laboratories must establish and maintain an appropriate environment of care encompassing the physical, technical, and human resources necessary for supporting the services their institution aspires to provide. Beyond traditional routine workloads, examples of evolving subspecialized multidisciplinary programs requiring readily available and often sophisticated levels of echocardiography services include heart valve teams,[1] adult congenital heart disease programs,[2] hypertrophic cardiomyopathy centers,[3] heart failure programs,[4] advanced heart failure and mechanical circulatory support teams,[5,6] and cardio-oncology services.[5] Do the patients being served by these subspecialty teams have access to an appropriately calibrated echocardiography laboratory such that proper protocols for diagnosis, procedural guidance, and follow-up surveillance can be performed routinely at a high level? Are specialized services well incorporated into the laboratory's routine work, or do they hamper its efficiency? Updated clinical practice guidelines and improved methods of data handling for imaging, transmission, analysis, archiving, and reporting, along with the availability of online continuing education, make it possible to achieve exceptional quality in both complex and basic laboratory structures. For even moderately complex laboratories, a formal analysis of structure may be needed to avoid the potential quality-undermining effects of unbalanced physical plant, technologic assets, and human resources.

Although the terms *continuous quality improvement* (QI) and *quality assurance* (QA) are sometimes used interchangeably, QI is preferred herein to avoid implying that quality can at some point be truly assured. This chapter preserves a notable historical "quality in context" discussion from this text's previous (5th) edition. Most of the updated echocardiography-related quality documents cited herein include a stated assumption of laboratory accreditation. Therefore, selected accreditation topics are highlighted, but the coverage of that subject here is not comprehensive, and readers should consult the standards published by the Intersocietal Accreditation Commission (IAC) Echocardiography division for detailed information.[7]

Echocardiographers are on the front line of patient care, and they must be prepared to adequately protect themselves and their patients from infectious disease transmission. Late in the preparation of this chapter, the novel coronavirus (COVID-19) pandemic emerged, precipitating a need to rethink the meaning of appropriate use criteria (AUC) under the conditions of a widespread respiratory pathogen and the need for additional safety measures beyond what laboratories should typically deploy to contain contagion.[8]

Whereas the focus of this chapter is adult echocardiography, laboratory accreditation standards are also available for pediatric and fetal echocardiography, and perioperative transesophageal echocardiography (TEE) standards are under development. Suggestions and tools for real-world laboratory management are provided here (e.g., staff turnover, physical plant layout, machine and staff rosters and competencies, analysis of obstacles to productivity). Every laboratory represents a unique environment serving a select patient population, so a "one size fits all" approach is not valid.

Defining interactions between clinical echocardiography laboratories and echocardiography core laboratories (ECLs) has not been addressed in the context of laboratory accreditation. However, continuous QI interactions between these two types of laboratories can be synergistic, improving both the rigor of clinical cardiovascular research and the day-to-day diagnostic accuracy of clinical site laboratories. As a local cornerstone of the diagnosis and management of cardiovascular disease, each echocardiography laboratory deserves a well-thought-out (and well-documented) structural analysis and implementation strategy to provide a high-quality work environment and a high-value product, even in the event of leadership or staff turnover.

QUALITY IN CONTEXT

Quality of care has been defined by the Institute of Medicine as "the degree to which health care systems, services, and supplies for individuals and populations increase the likelihood for desired health outcomes in a manner consistent with current professional knowledge."[9] Furthermore, health care should be safe, effective, patient-centered, timely, efficient, and equitable.[10] Similarly, in this "volume-to-value" transition period in medicine,[11] there is an increasing focus on value in health care, defined as health outcomes achieved per dollar spent.[12] Specific to echocardiography, several professional societies[13–17] have taken the lead in setting minimum standards and also in defining QA practices that diagnostic echocardiography laboratories should follow.

Continuous QI initiatives provide the framework for a team of physicians, sonographers, administrators, and other health care professionals to deliver high-quality care. Implementation of a Plan-Do-Study-Act (PDSA) cycle, also known as the Deming Cycle,[18] can provide a useful framework for ensuring continuous improvement. The focus of this chapter is the existing and evolving components of echocardiography laboratory quality, structure, and standards. Setting quality goals helps ensure sustainable, high-value, accessible, and cost-effective delivery of echocardiographic services to cardiovascular patients, now and in the future.

STRUCTURE AND STANDARDS

An initial step in achieving quality in echocardiography is to define a taxonomy and model of the *dimensions of care*, which then makes it possible to measure quality and identify areas for improvement. A dimensions of care framework has been developed for echocardiography,[14,15] and this model divides the process of clinical echocardiography into two principal components: the laboratory structure and the imaging process (Fig. 7.1).

LABORATORY STRUCTURE

The laboratory structure can be divided into a minimum of four components: the physical laboratory, equipment, personnel (sonographers and physicians), and the imaging and reporting process (Table 7.1). For each of these components, standards have been defined.[15] For the physical laboratory, accreditation by the IAC is recommended for existing laboratories; new facilities should initiate the process for submitting applications within 2 years after beginning operation.

LABORATORY ACCREDITATION

The IAC is an independent, not-for-profit organization formed in the 1990s by a consortium of medical subspecialty stakeholder societies that recognized that patient care would benefit from an organization whose sole mission was laboratory accreditation. In 1996, the IAC's sponsoring organizations commissioned the Intersocietal Commission for the Accreditation of Echocardiography Laboratories (ICAEL). The ICAEL name was retired in 2006 after all the IAC's divisions merged, and the commission's echocardiography division was renamed IAC Echocardiography.[19] This division now accredits laboratories performing adult transthoracic, adult transesophageal, adult stress, pediatric transthoracic, pediatric transesophageal, fetal, and (in the near future) perioperative transesophageal echocardiography. The IAC's accreditation model is centered on laboratory standards that were written by the IAC Echocardiography's board of directors (content knowledge experts) and accepted after a public comment period. Standards are derived from the appropriate peer-reviewed clinical practice guidelines and consensus documents, including AUC.

IAC Echocardiography's laboratory standards are publicly available on the organization's website.[7] The IAC accreditation process includes an objective quality review of a laboratory's submitted actual work (complete images and reports) and laboratory protocols and verification that the ongoing internal QI practices are such that any deficiencies become self-correcting within a laboratory. The IAC's minimum-standards format can be used by very small laboratories with limited goals or as an invaluable foundation on which more complex laboratories can build as needed. The standards are updated approximately every 2 years or when dictated by major changes in the field.[7]

The IAC Adult Echocardiography Standards are divided into the following domains:

- Personnel and supervision (medical staff, technical staff, support services)
- Facility (examination and interpretation areas, storage, instrument maintenance)
- Examination reports and records
- Facility safety
- Quality Improvement program

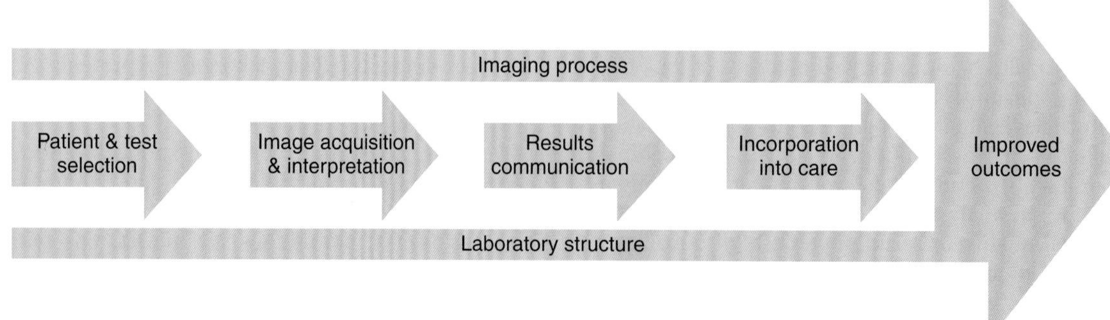

Fig. 7.1 Dimensions of care for evaluating quality in an echocardiography laboratory. The imaging process consists of patient and test selection, image acquisition, image interpretation, communicating the results, and incorporating the results into care. The goal is to maximize quality in the imaging process and laboratory structure, thereby improving patient outcomes.

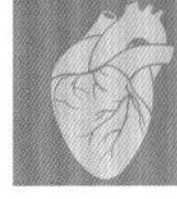

TABLE 7.1 Components of Echocardiography Laboratory Structure.

Component	*Requirements*
Physical laboratory	• IAC accreditation (and reaccreditation every 3 years) • Sufficient support staff (to assist with scheduling and disseminating reports to ordering clinicians) • Sanitizing equipment (capability for high-level disinfection of TEE probes; cleansing products for TTE transducers, ultrasound machines, and beds; readily available sinks and approved hand cleaners)
Equipment	• Machines capable of performing 2D, M-mode, and color and spectral (both flow and tissue) Doppler • Machine display that identifies the institution, patient's name, and date and time of study • Electrocardiogram and depth or flow velocity calibrations present on all displays; capability to display other physiologic signals (e.g., respiration) • Stress echocardiogram machines with software for split-screen and quad-screen display • TTE transducers that can provide high- and low-frequency imaging and dedicated nonimaging CW Doppler • Machines with harmonic imaging capabilities and settings to optimize standard and contrast-enhanced examinations • Capability for 3D and strain imaging • Multiplane TEE probes • Machines with a digital image storage method • Availability of contrast agents and intravenous supplies • Patient beds that include a drop-down portion of the mattress to facilitate apical imaging • Equipment required to treat medical emergencies (e.g., oxygen suction, code carts) • Adherence to manufacturers' recommendations for preventive maintenance and accuracy testing; service records maintained in the laboratory
Sonographer	• Minimum standards in education and credentialing achieved and maintained (provisional staff: credential within 1 year of graduation for new graduates) • Credentialing as a Registered Diagnostic Cardiac Sonographer through ARDMS or Registered Cardiac Sonographer through CCI • Fulfillment of any local or state requirements, including licensure
Physician	• Minimum of level II training in TTE imaging for all physicians independently interpreting echocardiograms, and meeting annual criteria to maintain that competence • Physicians who trained before this level of training in fellowship programs: achievement of adequate training through an experience-based pathway • Special competency and board certification by passing NBE examination (recommended) • Physician director who has completed level III training • Adequate supervision of studies as determined by the Centers for Medicare and Medicaid Services: general supervision (general oversight, not on site), direct supervision (physician in the office suite and immediately available), or personal supervision (physician in the room)

ARDMS, American Registry of Diagnostic Medical Sonographers; *CCI*, Cardiovascular Credentialing International; *CW*, continuous wave; *IAC*, Intersocietal Accreditation Commission; *NBE*, National Board of Echocardiography.

From Picard MH, Adams D, Bierig SM, et al: American Society of Echocardiography recommendations for quality echocardiography laboratory operations. *J Am Soc Echocardiogr*. 2011;24:1–10.

LABORATORY STAFF

Experience and dedication at the administrative, medical, and technical staff levels are critical for laboratory quality and productivity (value). Employee turnover in each of these areas has accelerated in recent years, and this alone can challenge laboratory operations for extended periods, particularly if laboratory structure is not clearly and consistently defined and supported. Because of the aging of the population, many seasoned echocardiography doctors, nurses, and sonographers have recently retired or will soon retire from the workforce. In some geographic areas, there are too few adequately trained and experienced replacement workers to succeed them. Simultaneously, laboratories are expected to provide more sophisticated, higher-value services to a patient population with unprecedented longevity and, as a result, an elevated prevalence of accumulated chronic illnesses (e.g., palliated heart failure; coronary artery disease, congenital conditions, valvular heart disease).

Since 2015, millennial-generation workers (born 1981–1996)[20] have come to dominate the workforce, and this shift has been cited, perhaps inappropriately, as a cause of the increased staff turnover observed in recent years. In general, the following positive traits can be applied to younger millennial workforce members[21] and bode well for laboratory operations if fostered: tech savvy; enjoyment of teamwork and being associated with a strong brand; strong loyalty when placed in a positive and supportive learning environment that fosters skill improvement; a desire for work–life balance (i.e., not driven solely by financial concerns); enjoyment of frequent feedback, open communication, and working closely *with* superiors as opposed to working *for* them; and social advocacy and diversity acceptance. Laboratories with well-defined but flexible team structures (Fig. 7.2) that also foster a lifelong learning environment, adequate staffing levels, and the rewards of patient service are likely to have low staff turnover and high efficiency.

PHYSICIAN TRAINING

Physicians who interpret echocardiograms are required to have considerable training and expertise. The Accreditation Council for Graduate Medical Education (ACGME) provides regulatory oversight for internal medicine subspecialty training programs. The American Board of Internal Medicine (ABIM) certifies individual specialists and subspecialists. The American College of Cardiology (ACC) has aligned with the ACGME and ABIM to provide curricular content detailed by the Core Cardiology Training Symposium (COCATS) documents for proficiency and competency (levels I, II, and III) in the various cardiovascular disciplines, including adult echocardiography.

Unlike prior COCATS documents, the 2015 COCATS 4 training statement[22] focuses on level I and level II echocardiography training and addresses competency and outcomes-based training, as opposed to focusing solely on time spent in a laboratory and on procedural volumes. Level I training covers transthoracic echocardiography (TTE) only; it is required for all cardiology fellows and is a prerequisite for level II training. Level II includes TTE, contrast, TEE, and stress echocardiography; it is the minimal requirement for independently performing and interpreting echocardiograms. This level of competency can be achieved in many standard 3-year cardiology fellowship programs, depending on the trainee's career interests and the use of available elective time.

Level III echocardiography training was the focus of the 2019 Advanced Training Statement on Echocardiography published by the ACC, the American Heart Association (ASA), and the American Society of Echocardiographers (ASE).[23] It consists of training beyond level II that includes

- acquiring additional expertise in advanced imaging techniques (3D, strain, contrast, stress echocardiography for structural heart disease);

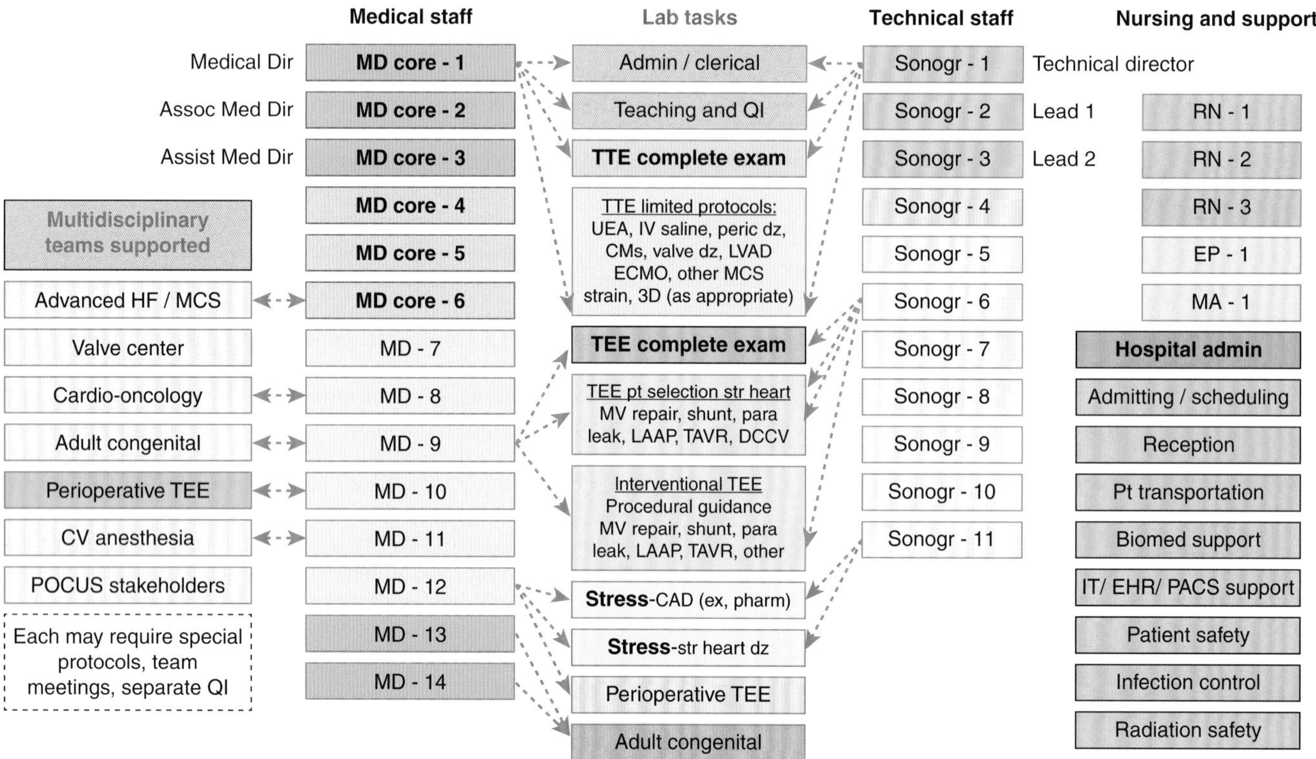

Fig. 7.2 Organizational chart. Staff member categories and individuals have different assignments *(blue arrows)* based on their competencies. The number and types of boxes will obviously vary greatly among laboratories. This type of graphic can be helpful for showing a laboratory's actual scope of work and for appropriately matching staff and equipment to the expected work to be performed. The laboratory should maintain an up-to-date, comprehensive staff roster that includes contact information and a daily laboratory coverage schedule that can be shared with appropriate parties, including patient coordinators and ordering physicians. Other essential support staff *(purple boxes*, plus members of the various multidisciplinary teams) may not be wholly dedicated to the echocardiography laboratory. To avoid confusion and to ensure efficient laboratory operations, each of these personnel and the multidisciplinary team liaisons should be formally identified as having an important support role, and they should be included in echocardiography laboratory meetings and pertinent communications whenever possible. *Admin*, Administration; *Assist*, assistant; *Assoc*, associate; *biomed*, biomedical; *CAD*, coronary artery disease; *CMs*, cardiomyopathies; *CV*, cardiovascular; *DCCV*, direct current cardioversion; *Dir*, director; *dz*, disease; *ECMO*, extracorporeal membrane oxygenation; *EHR*, electronic health record; *EP*, exercise physiologist; *ex*, exercise; *HF*, heart failure; *IV*, intravenous; *IT*, information technology; *LAAP*, left atrial appendage; *LVAD*, left ventricular assist device; *MA*, medical assistant; *MCS*, mechanical circulatory support; *MD*, medical doctor; *MV*, mitral valve; *PACS*, picture archiving and communication system; *para*, paravalvular; *peric*, pericardial; *pharm*, pharmacologic; *POCUS*, point-of-care ultrasonography; *pt*, patient; *QI*, quality improvement; *RN*, registered nurse; *Sonogr*, sonographer; *str*, structural; *surg*, surgery; *TAVR*, transcatheter aortic valve replacement; *UEA*, ultrasound enhancing agents.

- treating specialized populations (adult patients with congenital conditions, advanced heart failure, or complex valve disease), mechanical circulatory support device evaluation, and cardio-oncology;
- performing TTE and TEE during cardiovascular interventions (pericardiocentesis, endomyocardial biopsy, structural heart interventions);
- adequate exposure to emergency echocardiography; and
- data analysis and reporting.

Level III training should occur in an accredited laboratory so that trainees can understand the importance of laboratory structure, including the implementation and maintenance of QI processes.[15]

Whether a laboratory intends to operate as an ACGME-accredited training facility has implications with regard to laboratory structure as defined by the COCATS 4, Task Force 5 statement.[24] The IAC does not provide a separate, more advanced accreditation standard for teaching laboratories aspiring to provide advanced (level III) ACGME-approved physician training or for laboratories that could be described as providing comprehensive echocardiography services, although training laboratories should be IAC-accredited. Advanced and teaching laboratory leaders should review the facility and staff training recommendations provided in the recent COCATS 4, Task Force 5 statement[24] and the ACC/AHA/ASE Advanced Training Statement on Echocardiography[23] because a variety of additional resources (beyond minimal laboratory accreditation standards) must be available, including level III-trained mentors, an environment of scholarship and learning, and teaching sonographers with both the time and the ability to provide hands-on instruction in scanning and image-optimization techniques as specified in Table 7.2 for each physician trainee.

MEDICAL DIRECTOR

The medical director of an IAC-accredited laboratory is a licensed physician who ensures that both medical and technical staff members comply with the laboratory's standards. The medical director must actively participate in interpretation of studies performed in the laboratory. Although the medical director may delegate supervision of specific laboratory operations, he or she is ultimately responsible for all clinical services provided by the laboratory, including determining examination appropriateness and quality. For recent trainees with level II or level III initial training and National Board of Echocardiography (NBE)[25] Testamur status, assuming the medical directorship

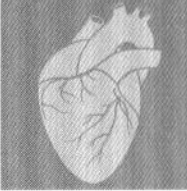

TABLE 7.2 **Summary of Training Requirements for Echocardiography.**

Level	*Duration of Training*[a] *(mo)*	*Cumulative Duration of Training*[a] *(mo)*	*Minimum No. of TTE Examinations Performed (Cumulative)*	*Minimum No. of TTE Examinations Interpreted (Cumulative)*	*TEE and Special Procedures*
I	3	3	75	150	Yes[b]
II	3	6	150	300	Yes[c]
III	3	9	300	750	Yes

[a]Typical duration assuming acceptable progress toward milestones and demonstrated competency.
[b]Exposure to TEE and other special procedures.
[c]Level II and additional special training must be completed to achieve full competence in TEE and other special procedures.

must be preceded by at least 18 months of qualifying echocardiography practice experience; trainees without NBE Testamur status must have qualifying clinical practice experience over the preceding 24 months, as outlined in the standards.[26] The medical director standards are designed to accommodate physicians who completed their initial training in years past and have no level II or level III training documentation but who have maintained an ongoing robust clinical echocardiography practice experience (≥1800 examinations) and qualifying practice experience over the previous 36 months. Medical directors must have completed a program of at least 30 hours of echocardiography-relevant continuing medical education (CME) activity over the preceding 3 years. This CME requirement is considered fulfilled when a physician obtains the NBE Testamur certificate or when a physician's initial echocardiography COCATS level II or level III training has been completed within 3 years of joining the laboratory.

TABLE 7.3 **Credentialing Organizations for Sonographers.**

Credential	*Issuer*	*Web Address*
Registered Diagnostic Cardiac Sonographer (RDCS)	ARDMS	https://www.ardms.org/get-certified/rdcs/
Adult Echocardiography (AE)	ARDMS	
Pediatric Echocardiography (PE)	ARDMS	
Registered Cardiac Sonographer (RCS)	CCI	http://www.cci-online.org/CCI/Certifications/RCS.aspx
Registered Congenital Cardiac Sonographer (RCCS)	CCI	http://www.cci-online.org/CCI/Certifications/RCCS.aspx
Advanced Cardiac Sonographer (ACS)	CCI	http://www.cci-online.org/CCI/Certifications/ACS.aspx
Canadian Registered Cardiac Sonographer (CRCS)	Sonography Canada	https://sonographycanada.ca/certification/credentials

ARDMS, American Registry of Diagnostic Medical Sonography; *CCI*, Cardiovascular Credentialing International.

MEDICAL STAFF

Members of the medical staff must also be licensed physicians who meet at least one of three criteria: (1) documented initial level II or III COCATS training, (2) unable to provide evidence of initial level II or III training but with active NBE Testamur status and qualifying clinical practice experience over the preceding 12 months, and (3) cumulative practice experience of at least 600 echocardiography examination interpretations and qualifying practice experience over the preceding 12 months. All medical staff members must perform and/or interpret at least 150 TTE examinations, 25 TEE examinations, and 25 stress echocardiography examinations per year (on average over 3 years), and these need not all be performed in the same IAC-accredited laboratory. All regular medical staff members must participate in the laboratory's QI program and obtain at least 15 hours of echocardiography-related CME over a 3-year period.

TECHNICAL DIRECTOR

Technical director is a full-time, on-site position, although provisions can be made for supervision of additional sites when a credentialed technical staff member is available to perform the technical director's duties at each site. Laboratory technical directors must have an active credential issued by one of the organizations listed in Table 7.3.

The technical director is responsible for overseeing day-to-day laboratory operations—including equipment inventory and maintenance and compliance with the standardized scanning protocols—and ensuring the proper function of the laboratory's ordering, imaging, online and offline analysis, reporting, and data archival infrastructure. The technical director and medical director, as a team, ensure that the medical and technical human resources are appropriate for the laboratory's intended scope of practice. The technical director works closely with the appropriate facility administrator and ancillary nursing staff to support patients' experience, safety, and confidentiality and to ensure compliance with local, state, and federal regulations. Other laboratory organizational duties include coordinating information technology (IT) and biomedical support teams and implementing and maintaining the laboratory's QI program.

A technical director should allocate time for actively participating in the laboratory's daily clinical work to spot problem areas and to serve as a role model, "second pair of hands," and an educational resource for junior sonographers and other trainees. The diagrams in Figs. 7.2, 7.3, and 7.4 can be modified as appropriate to illustrate a given technical director's purview. Dedicated administrative time may vary with the facility's size, complexity, and supporting resources. The newly available Advanced Cardiac Sonographer (ACS) credential (see Table 7.3), although not required, has enabled sonographers to demonstrate their experience and mastery of the exceptional skills needed in an advanced or comprehensive teaching echocardiography laboratory.[27]

TECHNICAL STAFF

All accredited laboratory technical staff members must have one of the credentials listed in Table 7.3. Prerequisites for taking a credentialing examination typically include graduation from a Council on Accreditation of Allied Health Education Programs (CAAHEP)-accredited ultrasonography training

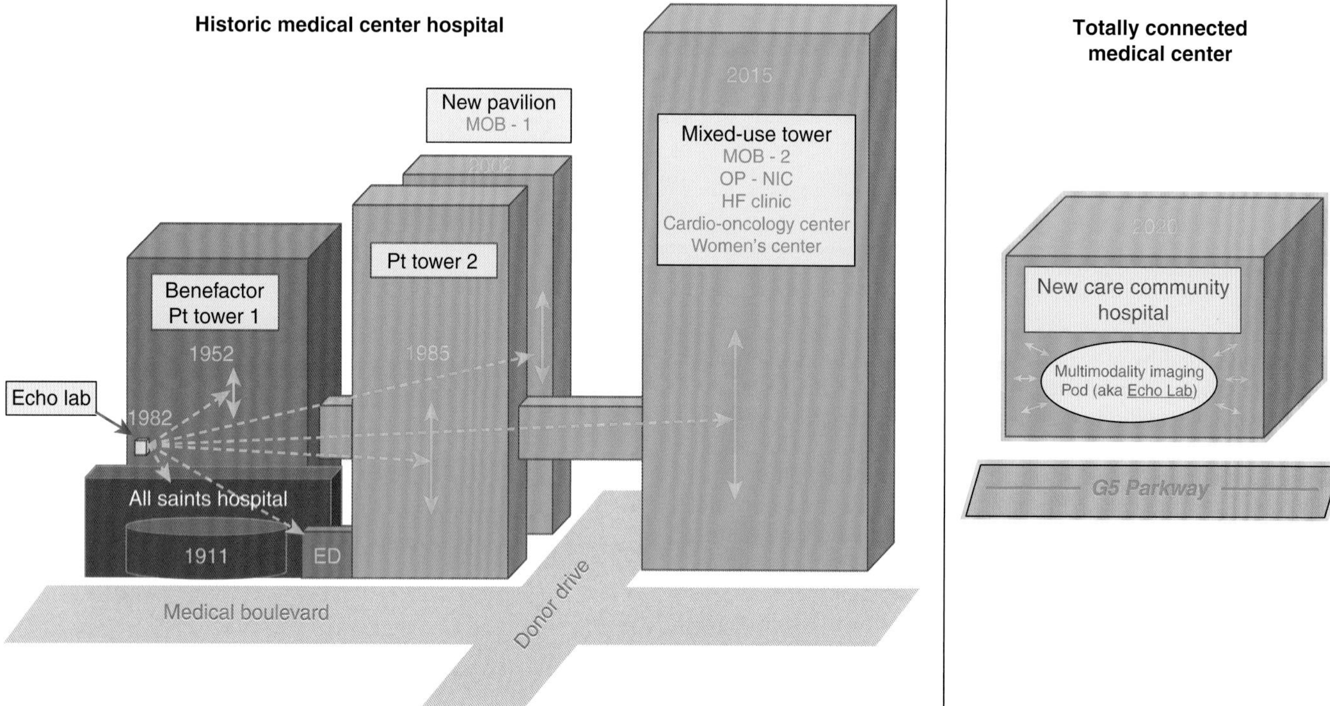

Fig. 7.3 Facility design impacts lab productivity. An echocardiography laboratory's productivity benchmarks should be evaluated in the context of both facility design and case complexity. Many still-operating historic teaching and referral hospitals were founded between the early 19th and early 20th centuries (a few are much older) and have grown by expansion. (A) After the advent of hospital echocardiography laboratories (echo labs) in the 1980s, certain architectural and data connectivity obstacles sometimes arose as the echo lab provided services throughout an expanding facility. (B) Newer facilities are typically designed around current technology, may serve special populations, and have different echocardiography productivity benchmarks than older facilities. *Echo*, Echocardiography; *ED*, emergency department; *HF*, heart failure; *MOB*, medical office building; *NIC*, noninvasive cardiology; *OP*, outpatient; *pt*, patient.

school.[28] When a laboratory employs new ultrasonography program graduates who are not yet credentialed, these employees must be listed in the laboratory's IAC accreditation application as "provisional" technical staff members with a plan to pass their credentialing examination within 1 year of their graduation date. Individuals employed in an accredited facility who are cross-training to fulfill the clinical experience prerequisites required for eventual adult echocardiography certification (to be obtained within 2 years) are also listed as provisional technical staff members. Provisional technical staff members must operate under the supervision of appropriately credentialed sonographers. All technical staff members, including the technical director, must earn 15 hours of echocardiography-related CME credits over 3 years; this requirement is automatically fulfilled when sonographers remain in good standing with their credentialing organization.

ANCILLARY PERSONNEL

Laboratories require enough clerical and administrative support staff members to ensure efficient operation and record keeping. Nursing and other ancillary clinical support personnel (e.g., medical assistants, exercise physiologists) working under the supervision of medical staff should be formal members of the echocardiography team (see Fig. 7.2) with clearly defined roles and availability, particularly if they are working in shared arrangements with other departments and not as full-time laboratory employees. Levels of supportive care vary according to a laboratory's scope of practice but may include placing and managing peripheral intravenous (IV) access, administering IV saline contrast or ultrasound enhancing agents, managing conscious sedation protocols (for TEE) and pharmacologic and exercise testing protocols (for stress echocardiography), and ensuring the appropriate level of ongoing care (e.g., oxygen delivery, telemetry monitoring, continuous IV drug delivery) for patients transported to the echocardiography laboratory. The laboratory should follow appropriate facility transportation, monitoring, and handoff procedures.

Some laboratories have formal relationships with nurse anesthetists or anesthesiologists for delivering moderate or higher levels of sedation for TEE procedures. Stress echocardiography testing protocols should be managed by appropriately trained individuals (e.g., exercise physiologists, nurses, physicians). If patients with mechanical circulatory support devices are studied, the appropriate care team, a supervising knowledgeable echocardiography medical staff member, or both should be present when device-setting changes are made by the heart failure team or by circulatory support technical staff members under their supervision.

PHYSICAL SPACE

FACILITY

By the IAC's definition, the most basic echocardiography facility is "an entity located at one postal address, composed of at least one ultrasound instrument and a Medical Director and a Technical Director performing and/or interpreting transthoracic echocardiography (TTE)."[26] Whereas many laboratories are basic, such as those in a physician's office, hospital laboratories are typically more complex. Some physical spaces

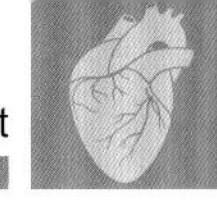

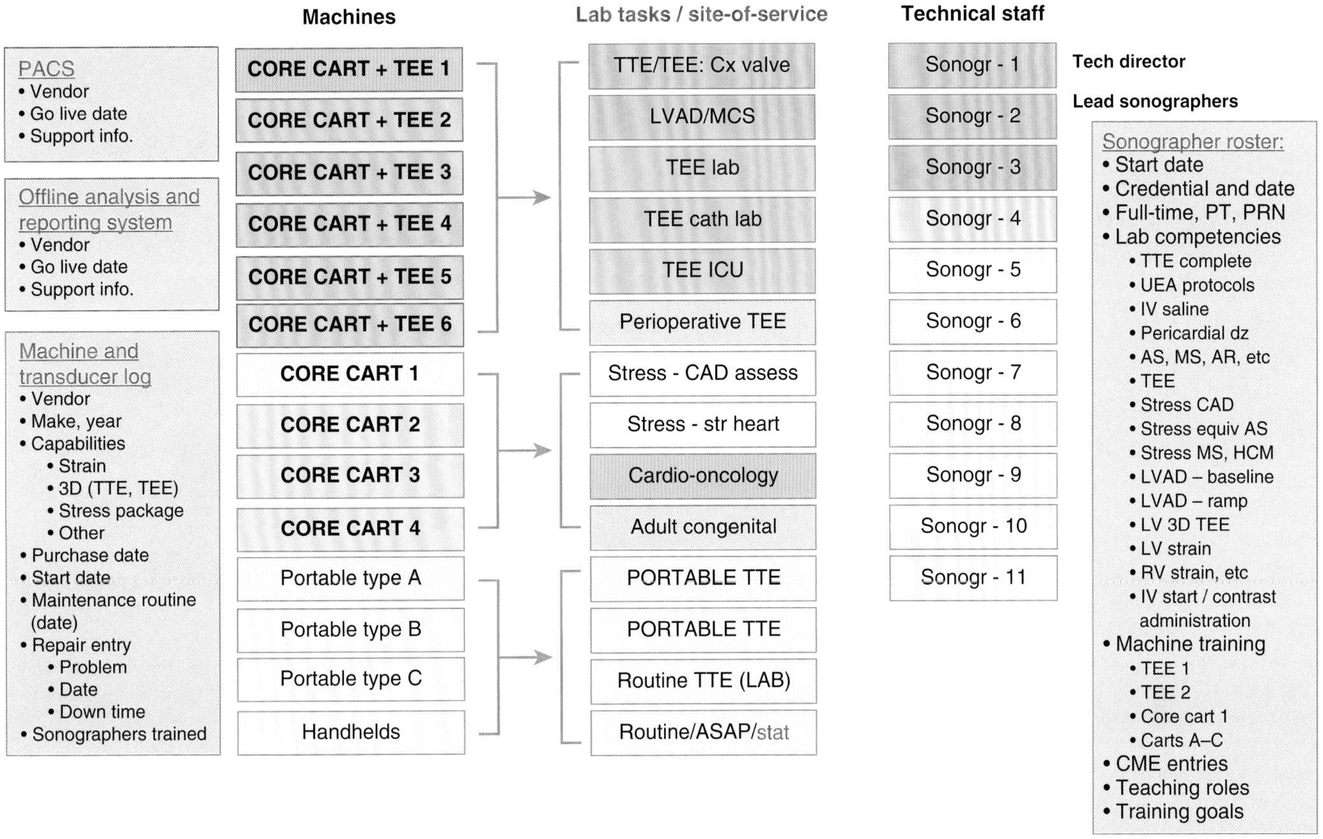

PACS
- Vendor
- Go live date
- Support info.

Offline analysis and reporting system
- Vendor
- Go live date
- Support info.

Machine and transducer log
- Vendor
- Make, year
- Capabilities
  - Strain
  - 3D (TTE, TEE)
  - Stress package
  - Other
- Purchase date
- Start date
- Maintenance routine (date)
- Repair entry
  - Problem
  - Date
  - Down time
- Sonographers trained

Machines	Lab tasks / site-of-service
CORE CART + TEE 1	TTE/TEE: Cx valve
CORE CART + TEE 2	LVAD/MCS
CORE CART + TEE 3	TEE lab
CORE CART + TEE 4	TEE cath lab
CORE CART + TEE 5	TEE ICU
CORE CART + TEE 6	Perioperative TEE
CORE CART 1	Stress - CAD assess
CORE CART 2	Stress - str heart
CORE CART 3	Cardio-oncology
CORE CART 4	Adult congenital
Portable type A	PORTABLE TTE
Portable type B	PORTABLE TTE
Portable type C	Routine TTE (LAB)
Handhelds	Routine/ASAP/stat

Technical staff

Sonogr - 1	Tech director
Sonogr - 2	Lead sonographers
Sonogr - 3	
Sonogr - 4	
Sonogr - 5	
Sonogr - 6	
Sonogr - 7	
Sonogr - 8	
Sonogr - 9	
Sonogr - 10	
Sonogr - 11	

Sonographer roster:
- Start date
- Credential and date
- Full-time, PT, PRN
- Lab competencies
  - TTE complete
  - UEA protocols
  - IV saline
  - Pericardial dz
  - AS, MS, AR, etc
  - TEE
  - Stress CAD
  - Stress equiv AS
  - Stress MS, HCM
  - LVAD – baseline
  - LVAD – ramp
  - LV 3D TEE
  - LV strain
  - RV strain, etc
  - IV start / contrast administration
- Machine training
  - TEE 1
  - TEE 2
  - Core cart 1
  - Carts A–C
- CME entries
- Teaching roles
- Training goals

Fig. 7.4 **Equipment list for an echocardiography laboratory.** The technical director should maintain an accurate list of all equipment, including the picture archiving and communication system (PACS), offline analysis and reporting systems, and a "fleet list" with data on each individual imaging machine, transducer, and TEE probe. This inventory is needed to ensure that properly functioning machines with the necessary imaging capabilities are available when and where they are needed. (Note: "Core cart" refers to an echocardiography machine that is stationed primarily in the laboratory.) Some procedures (e.g., interventional TEE) tie up machines for longer-than-expected periods, creating the need for equipment redundancy in some centers. Resource allocation may be facilitated by linking specialized machines to a site-of-service type (e.g., stress echocardiography laboratory, catheterization laboratory [cath lab]). The equipment inventory list (or spreadsheet) can be used to spot accumulated outdated technology or excessive machine downtime. This inventory can inform a proactive technology replacement cycle. A detailed sonographer roster is equally valuable when it includes the sonographers' machine-specific scanning and/or data analysis competencies. A sonographer competency "report card" can be a source of pride and motivation for sonographers and can be used to identify career goal preferences, including those of capable individuals who require learning pathways for pursuing advanced credentialing (e.g., congenital conditions, advanced cardiac sonography). *AR*, Aortic regurgitation; *AS*, aortic stenosis; *ASAP*, as soon as possible; *CAD*, coronary artery disease; *CME*, continuing medical education; *Cx*, complex; *dz*, disease; *HCM*, hypertrophic cardiomyopathy; *ICU*, intensive care unit; *IV*, intravenous; *LVAD*, left ventricular assist device; *MCS*, mechanical circulatory support; *MS*, mitral stenosis; *PRN*, when necessary; *PT*, part-time; *Sonogr*, sonographer; *stat*, immediately (urgent); *str*, structural; *UEA*, ultrasound enhancing agent.

(e.g., reception, administration, interpretation) can be either dedicated or shared, depending on the whether the laboratory stands alone or is located in a multimodality imaging department or adjacent to a related patient-care area. However, a dedicated echocardiography examination room is required; it must accommodate a specialized echocardiography bed (to enable proper patient positioning), an echocardiography machine, and a sonographer's physical workspace. The room (or rooms) must comply with infection control and ergonomic standards to ensure patient safety and to avoid sonographer injury. TEE or stress echocardiography rooms can be used for routine TTE examinations, but they must additionally have a fully supplied crash cart, IV access equipment, oxygen supply, and wall suction.

It is understood that many hospital examinations will be performed on a portable basis and that the laboratory's reach extends throughout a facility (see Fig. 7.3). However, portable examinations incur a quality and efficiency cost. The number of dedicated echocardiography examination rooms and the availability of patient transportation services should be appropriate for the facility's size so that unnecessary portable examinations are minimized. If there is continuous high demand, a satellite dedicated echocardiography examination room can be considered for remote patient areas within the same facility.

PATIENT SAFETY

Infection Control

The movement of patients into the laboratory and of echocardiography machines, cables, and transducers throughout a facility creates a high risk of contamination and infection spread. All laboratory personnel should be well versed in the hospital's infection prevention and control program. Laboratory leaders should demonstrate proper technique and should provide educational resources, which may include inviting internal reviews by the facility's infection control professionals to ensure compliance with facility standards, both because the facility may be subject to external audit[29] and out of sincere concern for their patients' and laboratory staff members' well-being. All staff must routinely practice proper hand and respiratory hygiene and injection safety and attend to all appropriate environmental and equipment-cleaning standards.[30] Facilities engineers may be needed to ensure that all clinical care surfaces and scanning furniture are appropriate and intact for routine decontamination. TEE probes must go through the proper special decontamination procedures outlined by the facility's standards for deep decontamination and appropriate storage.

The COVID-19 pandemic revealed an acute need for consensus among echocardiographers and facilities on how to protect patients and frontline care providers when echocardiograms are required. New recommendations, first published in April 2020, highlight policies to mitigate further potential laboratory-related spread of a dangerous respiratory pathogen while providing essential care. These recommendations (some of which are departures from usual care) are summarized in Table 7.4 (Figs. 7.5 and 7.6).[8,31,32] Many of them may be appropriate for future emergent pathogens and for the more common highly infectious organisms already familiar to echocardiographers (e.g., seasonal influenza, active tuberculosis, *Clostridium difficile*).

Time-Out

Although the procedural risks of echocardiography procedures (including TEE and stress echocardiography) are low, instances of performing the wrong procedure on the wrong patient are well documented in the patient safety literature.[33] An immediate preprocedure "time-out" exercise (patient at procedure, team member verbal verification of the patient's identity and planned procedure) can improve the detection of clerical errors such as patient misidentification and wrong procedure order. The absolute and relative contraindications for TEE[34] and stress testing should be familiar to staff members and incorporated into pretesting checklists.

Moderate Sedation

Moderate sedation (previously called *conscious sedation*) is defined as "a drug-induced depression of consciousness during which patients respond purposefully to verbal commands either given alone or accompanied by light tactile stimulation"[35] and do not require interventions to maintain adequate spontaneous ventilation. Moderate sedation is used in various practice settings by a wide variety of care providers, including physicians performing TEE. Therefore, appropriately credentialed TEE medical and nursing support staff members should be well versed in moderate sedation protocols and should follow their facility's internal moderate sedation policies. A designated individual other than the person performing the TEE must be continuously available to monitor level of consciousness, respiratory status, and hemodynamics; to administer oxygen and any appropriate medications; and to ensure a contemporaneous recording of monitored parameters. Sedation and analgesia for TEE patients were reviewed in detail by Hahn et al.,[34] and practice guidelines for moderate procedural sedation and analgesia have been updated.[35]

Radiation Safety

After decades of use, there continues to be no scientific evidence that exposure to diagnostic medical instrument ultrasound energy has adverse biologic effects on patients or sonographers.[36] However, in some practice settings, sonographers may be exposed to low-level ionizing radiation when examining patients who were recently injected with radioisotopes for diagnostic imaging purposes.[37] Risk to sonographers from this type of diagnostic radioisotope exposure is very low, but it can be further mitigated by scheduling echocardiography examinations in advance of nuclear imaging studies whenever possible, waiting a short period of time for adequate radioisotope decay, and providing accommodations for at-risk employees such as pregnant women. The echocardiography laboratory's technical director should consult with the facility's radiation safety officer to establish best practice policies and employee education and to ensure regulatory compliance.

Many contemporary laboratories must manage the inherent risk of radiation exposure to individuals performing interventional TEE in fluoroscopic laboratories.[38] Interventional TEE operators providing TEE guidance during certain percutaneous cardiac interventions can receive a scattered radiation dose equivalent to that received by the primary interventional

TABLE 7.4 Summary Recommendations for Policies and Procedures During COVID-19 Outbreak.[a]

Defer/Reschedule Options

- Identify and defer elective examinations
- Identify and perform urgent/emergency examinations

Assess patient COVID-19 status (low risk vs. suspected vs. confirmed)

Provide Appropriate Levels of Self-Protection

TEEs are high-risk—defer whenever possible; perform in suspected/confirmed cases with airborne PPE precautions

Institutional PPE Conservation

- Defer nonurgent/emergency examinations in suspected/confirmed cases
- POCUS—imaging by trained clinician already caring for patient

Limiting Exposure During Examinations

- Problem-focused, limited examinations that are guided by prior studies, other imaging including POCUS findings
- One-person examinations (sonographer or physician; limit trainees)[b,c]
- Defer ECG recordings (remove ECG leads and cables; use timed acquisition)[b]
- Ultrasound system modifications to limit cross-contamination[b,c]
- Remove nonessential material from carts (e.g., paperwork, multiple-use gel containers, linens, ECG cables, extra probes)
- Single-use gel packets, or gel-filled syringes for single use (no bottles)
- For airborne pathogen environments (e.g., ventilated patients, high-flow oxygen, TEEs), drape ultrasound systems to avoid unnecessary contamination of touchable surfaces (see Figs. 7.5 and 7.6)

Reading-Room Methods To Reduce Transmission

- Facilitate remote report generation and echocardiography consultation
- Frequent disinfection of computer keyboard, mouse, surfaces, chairs, doorknobs
- Discourage congregation in the echocardiography laboratory reading room
- Hand hygiene stations widely available

Hand Hygiene Stations Widely Available

Identify and appropriately reassign personnel with special risk factors (e.g., age >60 y, immunosuppression, chronic disease, cardiopulmonary conditions, pregnancy)

[a]These recommendations were developed in response to the COVID-19 pandemic. Some elements may be subject to change, although many will be useful for honing a laboratory's policies when it comes to mitigating the spread of many other types of infectious diseases. Please refer to the source documents and your facility's policies and procedures for disinfection of personal protective devices.

[b]From Mitchell C, Collins K, Hua L, et al. Specific considerations for sonographers when performing echocardiography during the 2019 novel coronavirus outbreak: supplement to the American Society of Echocardiography statement. *J Am Soc Echocardiogr.* 2020;33(6):654–657.

[c]From Nicoara A, Maldonado Y, Kort S, Swaminathan M, Mackensen GB. Specific considerations for the protection of patients and echocardiography service providers when performing perioperative or periprocedural transesophageal echocardiography during the 2019 novel coronavirus outbreak: Council on Perioperative Echocardiography Supplement to the Statement of the American Society of Echocardiography Endorsed by the Society of Cardiovascular Anesthesiologists. *J Am Soc Echocardiogr.* 2020;33(6):666–669.

ECG, Electrocardiogram; *POCUS*, point-of-care ultrasonography; *PPE*, personal protective equipment; *TEE*, transesophageal echocardiography.

Adapted from Kirkpatrick JN, Mitchell C, Taub C, Kort S, Hung J, Swaminathan M. ASE statement on protection of patients and echocardiography service providers during the 2019 novel coronavirus outbreak. *J Am Soc Echocardiogr.* 2020;33(6):648–653.

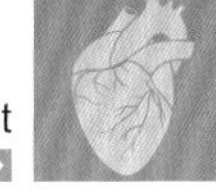

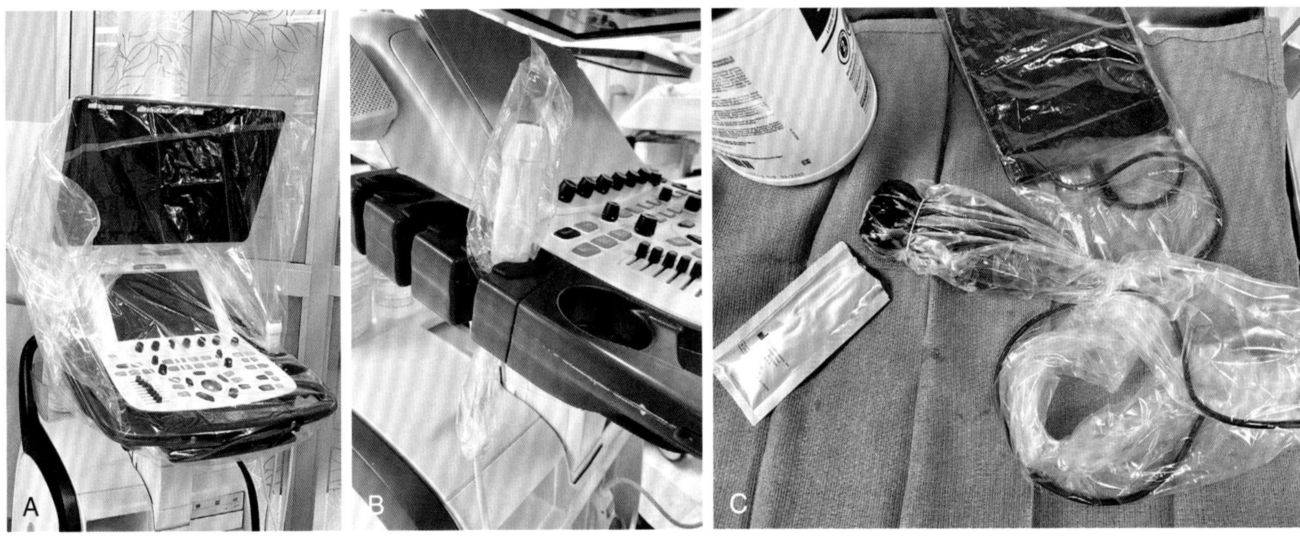

Fig. 7.5 **Infection control approaches to ultrasound systems.** (A) Partial draped ultrasound system (knob, console, and screen). (B) Draped probe. Draping indicates that it is decontaminated and safe for next use. (C) Completely draped handheld system (probe, cable, and imaging platform).

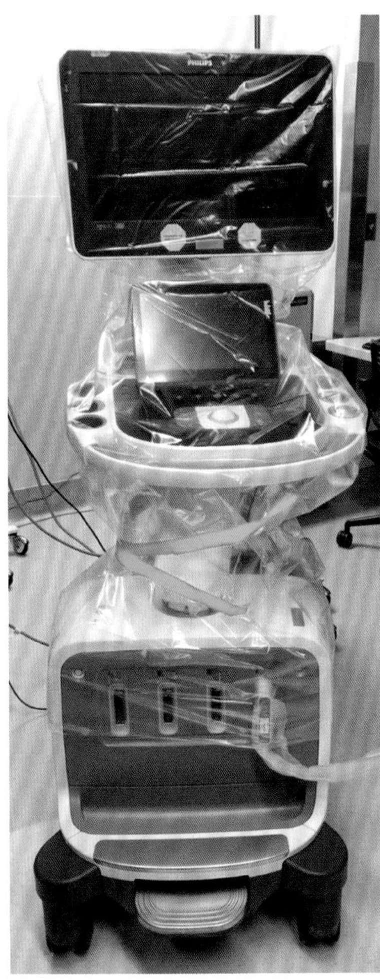

Fig. 7.6 **Draping of ultrasound system for TEE studies.** Near-complete draping of the ultrasound system (knobs, screen, cart, and probe cable) to avoid unnecessary contamination of touchable surfaces before TEE. (From Nicoara A, Maldonado Y, Kort S, Swaminathan M, Mackensen GB. Specific considerations for the protection of patients and echocardiography service providers when performing perioperative or periprocedural transesophageal echocardiography during the 2019 novel coronavirus outbreak: Council on Perioperative Echocardiography supplement to the statement of the American Society of Echocardiography Endorsed by the Society of Cardiovascular Anesthesiologists. *J Am Soc Echocardiogr.* 2020;33[6]:666–669.)

cardiologist, and higher doses are possible during procedures with a primary right anterior oblique fluoroscopic projection when the TEE equipment is placed at the patient's left side (the typical arrangement). Exposure of TEE operators can be greatly reduced (up to 82%) by a dedicated ceiling-suspended acrylic lead shielding device.[39] Interventional echocardiographers should be included in the facility's radiation safety program, accommodated by adequate fluoroscopy laboratory shielding design strategies, and issued appropriately fitted lead shielding garments.

Instrument Maintenance

Diagnostic instruments must be kept in good operating condition for test accuracy and patient safety. Instrument maintenance logs should include documentation of routine electrical safety, surface and filter cleaning, and accuracy testing according to the manufacturers' recommendations. Probes for TEE must be checked for structural and electrical integrity after each use with an electrical current tester; the "passed" or "failed" result should be documented in the TEE probe cleaning and maintenance log, and action should be taken on "failed" results.[26]

Instrument Inventory

An important aspect of laboratory management is creating an instrument inventory (see Fig. 7.4). A "fleet list" can be used to ensure that appropriate machines are available when needed for protocols requiring specialized or advanced features (e.g., stress, 3D, strain imaging), to identify faulty equipment, and to establish a proactive technology replacement cycle. Inventory entries include instrument type (e.g., ultrasonography cart, TEE probe, transducer), vendor, key features, manufacture date, service entry date, routine maintenance history, repair history (including out-of-service dates), and usage time. Prolonged maintenance of outdated equipment is not uncommon in laboratories with stringent cost-containment policies or when equipment oversight is simply lacking. If left unchecked, this situation can eventually result in patient care costs related to overall substandard image quality, unplanned downtime, and the potential for unplanned urgent purchases as opposed to strategic technology upgrades. Additionally, wide variation in imaging platform vintages and user interface types may impair sonographers' ability to consistently optimize images

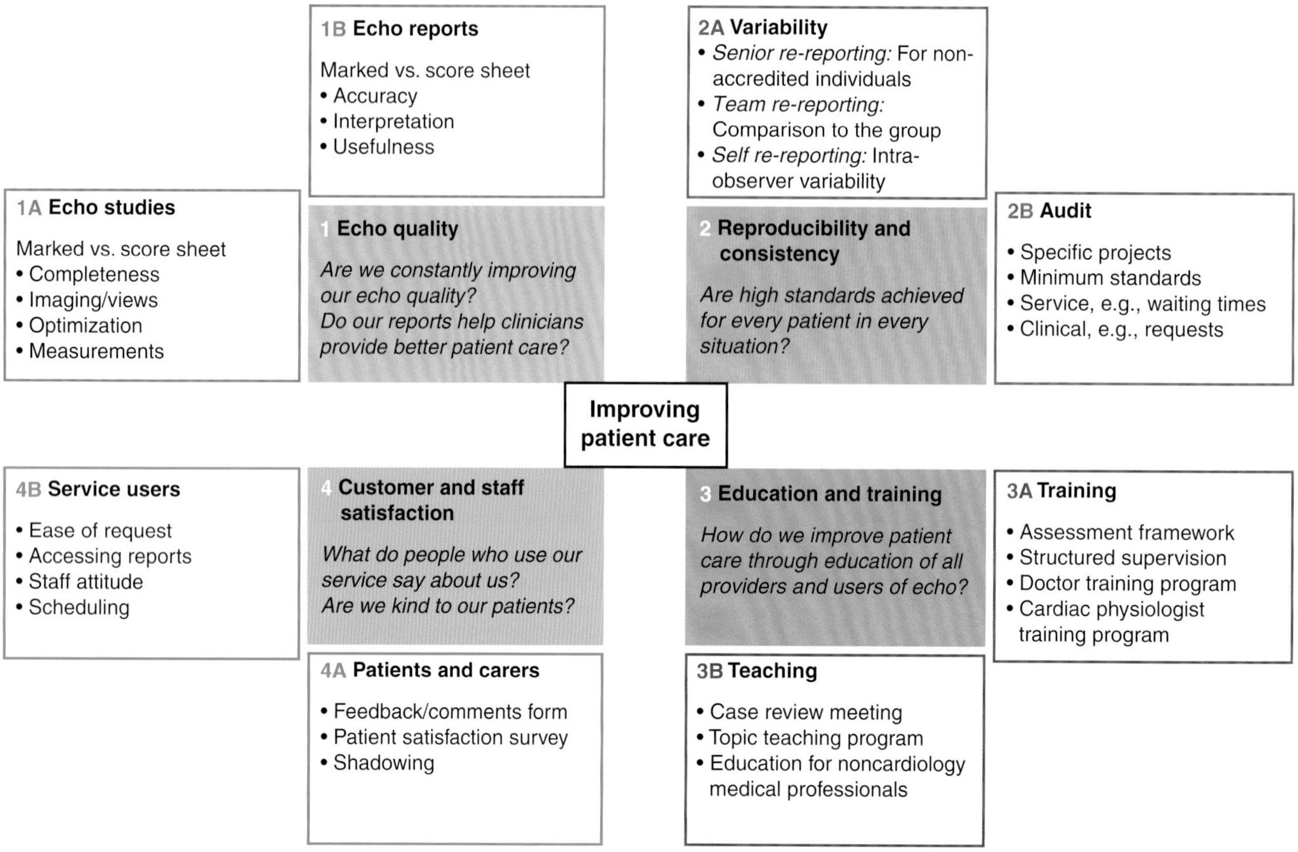

1B Echo reports
Marked vs. score sheet
- Accuracy
- Interpretation
- Usefulness

2A Variability
- *Senior re-reporting:* For non-accredited individuals
- *Team re-reporting:* Comparison to the group
- *Self re-reporting:* Intra-observer variability

1A Echo studies
Marked vs. score sheet
- Completeness
- Imaging/views
- Optimization
- Measurements

1 Echo quality
Are we constantly improving our echo quality?
Do our reports help clinicians provide better patient care?

2 Reproducibility and consistency
Are high standards achieved for every patient in every situation?

2B Audit
- Specific projects
- Minimum standards
- Service, e.g., waiting times
- Clinical, e.g., requests

Improving patient care

4B Service users
- Ease of request
- Accessing reports
- Staff attitude
- Scheduling

4 Customer and staff satisfaction
What do people who use our service say about us?
Are we kind to our patients?

3 Education and training
How do we improve patient care through education of all providers and users of echo?

3A Training
- Assessment framework
- Structured supervision
- Doctor training program
- Cardiac physiologist training program

4A Patients and carers
- Feedback/comments form
- Patient satisfaction survey
- Shadowing

3B Teaching
- Case review meeting
- Topic teaching program
- Education for noncardiology medical professionals

Fig. 7.7 The Echocardiography Quality Framework. This EQF for implementing quality improvement was developed by the British Society of Echocardiography. *echo*, Echocardiography. (From Ingram TE, Baker S, Allen J, et al.: A patient-centred model to quality assure outputs from an echocardiography department: consensus guidance from the British Society of Echocardiography. *Echo Res Pract.* 2018;5:G25–G33.)

on all of the different platforms, although this possibility has not been formally studied.

QUALITY IMPROVEMENT PROGRAM

Quality improvement can be defined as a systematic and continuous set of actions using specific techniques to improve process and quality, ideally leading to measurable improvements in health care services. The quality premise behind IAC accreditation is that feedback from an objective external review of facility structure and submitted "best work" is an important starting point for a laboratory's self-assessment and a quality evaluation.

The most important and ongoing step in obtaining and maintaining laboratory accreditation (and quality) is the development of a QI plan. The IAC laboratory accreditation standards require that facilities develop a written QI program of recurrent internal evaluation in four areas. A fifth item, correlation, is strongly recommended but not required because some facilities may not have the means to do so routinely.

1. Appropriate use (according to the AUC guidelines)
2. Technical quality (and safety when applicable, such as with TEE or stress imaging)
3. Quality of analysis and interpretation
4. Completeness and timeliness of reports
5. Correlation of findings with those from other imaging modalities

The laboratory's medical director, a QI committee, or both must provide QI program oversight, including reviewing QI evaluations, documenting any deficiencies, planning and implementing corrective action, and performing follow-up assessment. QI parameters must be assessed on a quarterly basis, and facilities must conduct at least two QI meetings per year.

Historically, implementing and maintaining a laboratory QI program was viewed as time-consuming and requiring additional resources. With advances in digital technology and streamlined processes for case reviews, QI management and documentation have become less labor intensive. The IAC recommends use of an online QI tool[40] for laboratory self-assessment. The QI tool includes analytic features to show progress and automatically fulfill the ongoing accreditation requirement by reporting the QI analysis and follow-up initiatives. QI record keeping includes case review data from laboratory QI meetings, meeting minutes, and the staff attendance list. Although the medical and technical directors and key staff must review the laboratory's QI data at least quarterly, a formal gathering of the laboratory staff must occur at least semiannually. Few peer-reviewed publications have examined how best to perform continuous QI in echocardiography laboratories. The British Society of Echocardiography put forth an echocardiography quality framework (EQF)[41] as a means for implementing QA, and this was further developed by Ingram et al.[42] The EQF, illustrated in Fig. 7.7, is a holistic, patient-centered approach that includes all aspects of IAC-recommended quality metrics. The EQF highlights the need for laboratory self-evaluation and active engagement in QA processes that support an echocardiography laboratory's historic central role as a place for staff improvement through ongoing learning and technical training while providing compassionate care and efficient service.

APPROPRIATE USE CRITERIA: A BRIEF HISTORY AND GUIDELINE UPDATES

As the cornerstone of diagnosis, risk-stratification, and management of cardiovascular disease, echocardiography is the most frequently ordered imaging test. To safeguard the quality and availability of this valuable resource, laboratories should demonstrate that the studies they perform are in general, clinically indicated. The American College of Cardiology Foundation initially published appropriateness criteria for TTE and TEE (in 2007)[43] and for stress echocardiography (in 2008)[44] to provide physician-driven guidance for improving the use of these modalities. The appropriateness methodology employs a rating system that is used by a panel of experts and other stakeholders (in a modified Delphi process) to achieve consensus on appropriate use of echocardiography in specific clinical scenarios (i.e., indications), particularly in situations in which clinical outcome studies are lacking.[45]

Beginning in 2011, revised AUC for echocardiography[46] incorporated methodology refinements and a more comprehensive approach, including 202 indications for TTE, TEE, and stress echocardiography.[47,48] The initial panel of modality-specific AUC documents were focused on nuclear medicine procedures (e.g., single-photon emission computed tomography [SPECT], positron emission tomography [PET]), cardiac computed tomography (CCT) and cardiac magnetic resonance (CMR) imaging, adult echocardiography, and diagnostic heart catheterization. They provided validation data for the AUC method, but cross-referencing of each document for similar clinical indications proved unwieldly for practitioners in their daily work. The AUC have now been updated (2018) to prescribe a multimodality imaging approach.[49] Tables listing consistent clinical indications for various disease states across the commonly available imaging modalities (including echocardiography) are more easily used by busy clinicians. The multimodality format can potentially be incorporated into decision-support tools, mobile point-of-care applications, and outcomes research.[49]

The AUC for echocardiography are found in the following companion documents:

- *Stable Ischemic Heart Disease*—2013 Multimodality AUC (stress echocardiography)[50]
- *Valvular Heart Disease*—2017 Multimodality AUC (TTE, TEE, stress echocardiography)[51]
- *Cardiac Structure and Function (Nonvalvular Heart Disease)*—2019 Multimodality AUC (TTE, TEE, stress echocardiography)[52]
- *Congenital Heart Disease, Follow-up Care*—2019 Multimodality AUC (TTE, TEE, stress echocardiography)[53]

In the AUC documents, clinical indications are broken down into disease state categories, whether the test is initial or follow-up, the presence or absence of symptoms, and whether the examination is or is not indicated for screening or surveillance purposes. To apply the AUC, certain general assumptions must be made, including (1) the indication is based on a nonurgent clinical circumstance and (2) a clinical history and physical examination have been performed by a qualified clinician.[52] The appropriate use categories are A, appropriate; M, may be appropriate (formerly called "unsure"); and R, rarely appropriate (formerly called "inappropriate").

Appropriate Indications

Echocardiography is rated "appropriate" most often for symptomatic patients with known or suspected cardiovascular disease. In hospitalized patients, particularly those with high-risk comorbidities, initial complete TTEs are frequently appropriate and are potentially underutilized.[54] Repeat echocardiography examinations during the same hospitalization may be appropriate after a phase-of-care change (e.g., after cardiac surgery or other intervention) or after the development of unexplained new symptoms. It is important to emphasize that echocardiography does not have to be performed whenever an appropriate indication is identified. The echocardiogram should be viewed as an appropriate option when the clinician determines that it could be clinically useful.

Rarely Appropriate Indications

Clinical indications rated as "rarely appropriate" most often involve outpatients with mild heart disease who are undergoing repeat examinations for routine surveillance less than 3 years after diagnosis. Programs to reduce inappropriate use often focus on these and the other indications listed in Table 7.5.[46] Clinical judgment is essential for determining the best course of care for a specific patient; the AUC documents are not intended to be rigidly applied but to be used as a tool for identifying patterns of excessive use. Providers should be able to explain the additional clinical circumstances that justified the use of echocardiography in certain cases with "may be appropriate" or "rarely appropriate" indications. Investigators have shown that the number of rarely appropriate outpatient echocardiograms ordered by academic cardiologists can be significantly reduced by applying focused educational tools and an auditing process that provides constructive feedback.[55] This educational intervention process has also proved successful across different ordering physician types and payment environments.[56]

Appropriate Use In Practice

To determine the extent of an echocardiographic examination needed for a complete interpretation and summary report, a sonographer must know precisely why the examination has been requested. If the laboratory's available medical record or order-entry process systematically omits clinical information needed to support the examination indication (e.g., comorbidities, known

TABLE 7.5 Most Common "Rarely Appropriate"[a] Indications for Transthoracic Echocardiography in Clinical Practice.

- Lightheadedness/presyncope when there are no other symptoms or signs of cardiovascular disease
- Routine surveillance of ventricular function in a patient with known coronary artery disease and no change in clinical status or cardiac examination
- Routine preoperative evaluation of ventricular function in a patient with no symptoms or signs of cardiovascular disease
- Routine surveillance (<3 y) of mild valvular stenosis without a change in clinical status or cardiac examination findings
- Routine surveillance (<3 y after valve implantation) of a prosthetic valve if there is no known or suspected valve dysfunction
- Suspected endocarditis in a patient with transient fever but no evidence of bacteremia or new murmur
- Routine evaluation of a patient with systemic hypertension but no symptoms or signs of heart disease
- Routine surveillance (<1 y) of heart failure (systolic or diastolic) when there is no change in clinical status or cardiac examination findings

[a]Formerly termed "inappropriate."

Data from Douglas PS, Garcia MJ, Haines DE, et al. ACCF/ASE/AHA/ASNC/HFSA/HRS/SCAI/SCCM/SCCT/SCMR 2011 Appropriate use criteria for echocardiography: a report of the American College of Cardiology Foundation Appropriate Use Criteria Task Force, American Society of Echocardiography, American Heart Association, American Society of Nuclear Cardiology, Heart Failure Society of America, Heart Rhythm Society, Society for Cardiovascular Angiography and Interventions, Society of Critical Care Medicine, Society of Cardiovascular Computed Tomography, and Society for Cardiovascular Magnetic Resonance. Endorsed by the American College of Chest Physicians. *J Am Soc Echocardiogr*. 2011;24:229–267.

or suspected disease states), examination quality can be adversely affected. Laboratory efficiency is reduced whenever these clinical data elements must be tracked down before an examination can be started or, even worse, after the examination has been performed. Laboratories should have reference copies of the current AUC document tables on hand. An IAC-accredited QI program requires an appropriate use evaluation of at least two examinations quarterly for each accredited area (i.e., TTE, TEE, and stress echocardiography). Although this may seem like a small number, there is no validated correct number for QI purposes, and laboratories may evaluate larger sample sizes.

In practice, the responsible laboratory personnel should review the clinical data and indication fields of selected examination reports and then assign a rating (A, M, or R) as described in the most recent AUC documents. This exercise can detect ordering patterns that may need to be investigated to reduce "rarely appropriate" use. Some examination indications may be so vague that the rating assignment must be "unable to determine" (e.g., a notation of "aortic regurgitation" without any information on time course, severity, or symptoms). Detection of frequent "unable to determine" appropriateness cases should prompt an evaluation of the laboratory's ordering and clinical documentation process. Depending on the amount of information omitted, corrective actions could include AUC education for ordering clinicians, revising open electronic order-entry tools for examinations, and retraining of clerical scheduling and technical personnel with the goal of measurably improving performance.

The COVID-19 pandemic, and presumably any regional epidemic, may necessitate rethinking the AUC and, perhaps, temporarily changing them. When community or facility disease-transmission risk is high, there may be an inordinate risk for disease spread among patients and health care workers, including sonographers, who must work in close proximity to patients. In such situations, there is consensus that only urgently needed examinations should be performed. Examination urgency can be determined on a case-by-case basis by consultation between ordering physicians and members of the laboratory's key medical staff or programmatically by postponing otherwise appropriate surveillance testing or diagnostic testing that will not immediately affect patient care (see Table 7.4).[31]

PROTOCOL CONSISTENCY

A set of protocols defines the scope of work performed in a laboratory (e.g., TTE, stress imaging, TEE). For IAC accreditation purposes, the laboratory's comprehensive examination protocol must define the components of the standard examination. An examination protocol at its most basic is the examination sequence (i.e., the order of views). An evaluation of examination quality includes assessing the sonographer's ability to capture the proper number of cardiac cycles, employ scanning maneuvers and machine adjustments for image optimization, and perform appropriate measurements and analysis according to protocol details and the patient's disease state.

Published guidelines for minimum protocol standards purposefully lack certain specific details. However, all examinations conducted at the same facility should include the same sequence of views, extent of data obtained, and any special imaging techniques to be used for given specific indications by all staff members (including temporary or new staff). Ability to follow laboratory-specific protocols is the basis for sonographer and trainee competency assessment (Figs. 7.4 and 7.8) and QI programs (e.g., case reviews).

Transthoracic Echocardiography Protocol

New guidelines for performing a comprehensive TTE examination (Table 7.6) have been published by the ASE.[57] This document provides recommendations for examination content (image acquisition windows, 2D, M-mode, color Doppler, spectral Doppler) and recommendations for image optimization techniques, which are also detailed elsewhere in this book. Protocols for using ultrasound enhancing agents, longitudinal strain, and three-dimensional (3D) imaging for left ventricular (LV) size, as well as functional assessment when indicated and feasible, can be considered new standards for certain patient populations. Sonographers should know when to selectively apply protocols for assessing pericardial disease (i.e., pericardial effusion) and intracardiac shunts (IV saline contrast imaging) with Valsalva maneuver when appropriate.

ANALYSIS AND INTERPRETATION QUALITY

Numerous operator- and patient-dependent variables interact to determine echocardiography quality outcomes. Image quality can be undermined by improper measurement, interpretation, or reporting. By the same token, even the best analysis and interpretation techniques will be undermined by poor image quality. The quality (i.e., diagnostic accuracy) of clinical echocardiography examination interpretation depends on whether medical staff have an appropriate level of baseline training and experience and participate in CME. Laboratory interpretive quality may benefit if all medical staff members know they are allowed to consult with peers and senior or more experienced medical staff members when needed. A formal or informal arrangement for consultation expertise can be made between independent facilities, as well.

A laboratory's QI program must include a process for case reviews. Minimal case review criteria (as prescribed for IAC laboratory accreditation) can be helpful for identifying problem areas to discuss and potentially address with a more comprehensive action program during the laboratory's QI meetings. Case review programs involve a system for retrospective colleague over-reads to ensure consistency within the laboratory. This is usually a nonblinded evaluation performed to determine whether the reviewer and the initial interpreter agree or disagree on the reported cardiac structure and function statements regarding the four heart valves, all four cardiac chambers, the great vessels, and the pericardium. When patterns or specific examples of disagreement are found (regarding valve regurgitation or stenosis severity, left or right ventricular size and function, segmental wall motion, or other hemodynamic data), corrective action can include appropriate constructive feedback, discussion and learning segments during quarterly QI meetings, and refinements of laboratory reporting standards.

Case correlations with other imaging modalities, when available, are recommended; these correlations can become an important teaching component in QI meetings. Formal programs for reducing interobserver variability in clinical echocardiography laboratories[58–64] are ideal. Efforts to develop rigorous, novel QI methods are ongoing.[65] However, validating a laboratory's internal interobserver and intraobserver variability can become a time-consuming project, reliant on local subject-matter expertise and cumbersome traditional methodologies.

Recent developments in the field of artificial intelligence, derived from a growing array of machine deep-learning systems that use mathematical algorithmic analysis of large data sets, promise to eventually revolutionize laboratory quality assessment and workflow.[66–69] For the time being, significant

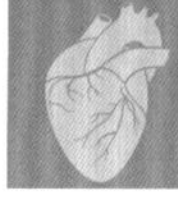

Checklist for IAC adult echocardiography laboratory accreditation

Lab type and location

- ❑ Single site – single address
- ❑ Multi-site – single address (fixed and / or mobile)

Services provided

- ❑ Adult TTE
- ❑ Adult Stress
- ❑ Adult TEE (must be TTE-accredited)

Medical staff[a]

- ❑ Medical director
  - ❑ Training
  - ❑ Clinical practice experience
- ❑ Medical staff
  - ❑ Training
  - ❑ Clinical practice experience

Technical staff[a]

- ❑ Technical director
  - ❑ Training (appropriate credential)
  - ❑ Exam performance, participation, and oversight responsibilities
- ❑ Technical staff
  - ❑ Training (appropriate credential)
- ❑ Provisional staff
  - ❑ Appropriate credential within 1 y of graduation
- ❑ Updated semianually (subject to audit)

Continuing medical education (CME)[b]

❑ Medical director	30 hours
❑ Medical staff	15 hours
❑ Technical director	15 hours
❑ Technical staff	15 hours

Obtained during 3 years before application

Ancillary staff support

- ❑ Adequate nursing, administrative, biomedical, infection control, medical staff services, etc.

Workspace (facility)

- ❑ Procedure rooms, interpretation, cleaning, and storage areas compliant with regulatory standards

Instrument quality and maintenance

- ❑ Adequate capabilities (state-of-the art)
- ❑ Similar device quality across all sites
- ❑ Methods and frequency of routine maintenance and safety checks – assign individual(s) for log updates

Patient and staff safety

- ❑ Compliance with facility-wide regulatory standards
- ❑ Infection control policies and compliance (inherent risk)
  - ❑ Low-level disinfection (LLD) indications
  - ❑ High-level disinfection (HLD) indications
  - ❑ Personal protective equipment (PPE) use

❑ Tools for assessing patient satisfaction

Exam performance, analysis, interpretation, and reporting

- ❑ Scheduling
  - ❑ Policy to accommodate routine, urgent, and stat exams
  - ❑ Appropriate use policy tool
- ❑ Protocol development
  - ❑ Create lab's protocol inventory for each modality / test type
  - ❑ Briefly list required views *in sequence*, noting any required data elements and required online analysis capture
  - ❑ [Detailed "how to" instructions not needed]
  - ❑ Include ECG cycle capture rules (when to use timed capture)
  - ❑ Create additional imaging and analysis subprotocols (e.g., for tamponade, MR, AS, agitated IV saline, ultrasound-enhancing agent use) to be applied when appropriate
  - ❑ Apply uniformly — all sonographers and testing sites
- ❑ Establish data analysis workflow
  - ❑ Online, offline, or both
  - ❑ Pre-analysis and interpretation by trainees / technical staff
  - ❑ Final interpretation by medical staff
- ❑ Reporting policy
  - ❑ Consistent report elements — all readers and all sites
  - ❑ Processes for ensuring both timely final interpretation and results communication appropriate for patient diagnosis and acuity
  - ❑ Policy for critical results communication
- ❑ Track exam turnaround times
- ❑ Accreditation case submissions
  - ❑ Gather best work for required case types (e.g., MR, AS), which differs according to modality (TTE, TEE, stress)
  - ❑ Numbers required vary with lab staff size [consult IAC standard]

Quality improvement

- ❑ Establish quarterly QI review and QI meeting standing agenda: Volumes, turnaround times, appropriate use, case reviews (technical quality, analysis, reporting), and updates (e.g., staff, equipment, protocols)
- ❑ QI meeting minutes available for random audit / reaccreditation

Fig. 7.8 Checklist for IAC adult echocardiography laboratory accreditation. According to the 2017 IAC Adult Echocardiography Standards, "An echocardiography facility is defined as an entity located at one postal address, composed of at least one ultrasound instrument and a Medical Director and a Technical Director performing and/or interpreting transthoracic echocardiography. There may be additional physicians and sonographers. The facility may also perform transesophageal or stress echocardiography" (https://www.intersocietal.org/echo/standards/IACAdultEchocardiographyStandards2017.pdf). With a practice of quarterly information updates, a laboratory should be fully prepared on a continual basis for reaccreditation or an audit without additional efforts. Similar checklists can be developed for pediatric and perioperative laboratories; complex and teaching laboratories will require additional elements, and these can be added to assist with additional resource allocations and oversight assignments. [a], A policy must be in place for facility *primary source verification* of appropriate medical education, training, licensing, credentialing, and CME status; [b], Medical Staff CME requirements are considered fulfilled if formal training or National Board of Echocardiography (NBE) Testamur status is obtained or renewed within 3 years of the application. *AS*, Aortic stenosis; *ECG*, electrocardiogram; *IV*, intravenous; *MR*, mitral regurgitation.

TABLE 7.6 Brief Standard TTE Imaging Windows Protocol and Provisos for Limited TTE Follow-Up Examinations and Additional Views.

Standard TTE Examination Views	**Limited TTE—May Follow A Comprehensive Examination**
Parasternal long-axis (PLAX) • LV/LVOT • RVIT/RVOT Parasternal short-axis (PSAX) • Great vessels/valves • LV Apical • 4-chamber • 4-chamber—RV focused • 5-chamber—LVOT (RVOT with tilt) • 4-chamber—posterior (coronary sinus) • 2-chamber • 3-chamber (apical long-axis) Subcostal • 4-chamber • IVC/hepatic vein Suprasternal notch	Whenever the comprehensive TTE interpretation is inconclusive (return for further imaging), or When known abnormalities must be reassessed (e.g., pericardial fluid, PAP, LVEF) • Extra pair of hands for standard views • Need for add-on (e.g., UEA, IV saline, 3D, strain) • Pericardial effusion • LV function • RV and pulmonary hypertension **A Standard Comprehensive TTE Protocol** May include additional views and procedures depending on the reason for the examination and the underlying and possibly previously undetected disease • LV assessment (strain, UEA, 3D, LVEF) • Pericardial disease assessment • Valve disease • Atrial septal communications (IV saline, Valsalva) • Intrapulmonary shunt (IV saline) • Dynamic LVOT obstruction (Valsalva) • LA pressure (Valsalva)

IVC, Inferior vena cava; *LVEF*, left ventricular ejection fraction; *LVOT*, left ventricular outflow tract; *PAP*, pulmonary artery pressure; *RVIT*, right ventricular inflow tract; *RVOT*, right ventricular outflow tract; *UEA*, ultrasound enhancing agent.

Adapted from Mitchell C, Rahko PS, Blauwet LA, et al. Guidelines for performing a comprehensive transthoracic echocardiographic examination in adults: recommendations from the American Society of Echocardiography. *J Am Soc Echocardiogr*. 2019;32:1-64.

limitations on embedding artificial intelligence–assisted analysis and interpretation include the need for further validation studies, lack of source data standardization, and legacy technology.

Echocardiography Core Laboratory

The QI responsibilities of ECLs are inherently different from those of clinical echocardiography laboratories, although they are related. The ASE 2009 expert consensus statement[70] noted that "[echocardiography] is an essential element of cardiovascular clinical research. The noninvasive assessment of cardiac structure and function and of hemodynamics using echocardiography can provide essential data on the safety and efficacy of drugs and devices, as well as insight into mechanisms of disease and therapeutic benefit." The ECL must design enrollment criteria for participating clinical echocardiography laboratories (sites) to ensure the accuracy and reproducibility of submitted data, although this can be difficult to achieve.[71] In addition, the ECL must develop internal processes for continually following QI practices that will optimize all aspects of internal data analysis and adherence to client and regulatory agency standards. Quality standards for ECLs are not specifically addressed by the IAC. However, ECLs often require that clinical sites be IAC-accredited at a minimum. If chosen to participate in clinical trials managed by an ECL, clinical echocardiography laboratory sites must receive appropriate training, approval, and ongoing monitoring and feedback. This iterative relationship

TABLE 7.7 **Steps Taken to Ensure Optimal Study Quality.**[a]

Optimizing Structure		Optimizing Processes	
Protocol Design	*Site Selection and Initial Training*	*ECL Structure and Processes*	*Image Acquisition Continuous Quality Improvement Initiatives*
The ECL Principal Investigator served on the trial steering committee and had input to the original protocol and all protocol revisions.	A survey was sent to potential sites assessing key personnel and resources including the ability to acquire 3D echocardiographic images. Completion of the survey identifying key staff and resources was required for site participation.	Each ECL sonographer underwent an initial determination of acceptable IIR using the study-specific analysis protocol before analyzing study echoes and then annually.	The site MD echocardiographer reviewed and approved the 3D images before the subject left the site.
An imaging-specific manual of procedures was developed that specified certification of the sonographer (rather than the site alone), image acquisition and transfer protocols, ECL review of site images, and multiple feedback processes.	All sites underwent online training to review the protocol and to provide instructions on 2D and 3D image acquisition. Training slides were available to all sites, and satisfactory quiz completion was required for initial sonographer certification.	Dedicated ECL research sonographers with acceptable IIR reviewed and performed the initial measurements on the site-submitted echocardiograms.	An ECL sonographer assessed the adequacy of each 2D and 3D study reviewed for the required critical views to measure LV volume, LVEDV, and LVEF. Sites were asked to resubmit inadequate studies and, in some cases, to rescan the subjects (queries).
The primary trial end point of change in LVEDV from baseline to 6 mo was selected a priori. Paired 3D echocardiographic data were preferred, but if not present, 2D echocardiographic data were used.	Sites were invited to attend two live training sessions that included didactics, a live demonstration, and vendor-specific hands-on training for 3D acquisition; 33% of sites attended the live training sessions. A survey was sent to sites to assess the value of the live investigator training sessions.	All study sonographers underwent quarterly group reads to review and improve reproducibility and harmonize reads across the group.	The ECL provided quarterly feedback to each site via a scorecard detailing the site's echo quarterly measurability score benchmarked to other sites.
To minimize interobserver variability, only certified MD cardiologists/sonographers were acceptable to scan the baseline, postdeployment, and 6-month protocol echocardiograms.	MD cardiologists/sonographers at each site were required to submit test 2D and 3D images for approval/certification by the ECL before studies were performed.	NBE-certified, level 3–trained ECL cardiologist echocardiographers with at least 5 y of experience overread sonographer data.	Follow-up retraining was offered to sites achieving <85% measurability on the site quarterly scorecard. Retraining involved a 30-min web-based conference call between an ECL sonographer and the site to review adequate and inadequate echocardiographic studies and the protocol, including suggestions to improve image quality.
—	Site certification occurred after two MD cardiologist echocardiographer/sonographers were certified.	Each ECL MD cardiologist reader underwent an initial determination of acceptable IIR before analyzing study images, and then biannually.	Echocardiography investigator meetings were held at the ASE scientific sessions for two consecutive years to assess enrollment and answer site questions.

[a]Example of an echocardiography core laboratory process for improving endocardial definition among site laboratories participating in a clinical research trial in which left ventricular size and function were examined after an intervention.

ASE, American Society of Echocardiography; *echo*, echocardiogram; *ECL*, echocardiography core laboratory; IIR, intra- and interreader reproducibility; LVEDV, left ventricular end-diastolic volume; LVEF, left ventricular ejection fraction; *MD*, medical doctor; *NBE*, National Board of Echocardiography.

From Crowley AL, Yow E, Rabineau D, et al. The impact of a rigorous quality program on 3D echocardiography data quality in an international multisite randomized trial. *JACC Cardiovasc Imaging*. 2018;11:1918–1920.

should improve quality in participating clinical laboratories, which is also critical for ensuring the rigor of clinical research.

Statistical analyses have been published regarding several important quality parameters of clinical investigation laboratories. These include whether enrolled sites can submit examinations with complete endocardial border definition in two apical views for calculations of LV volume and ejection fraction. When laboratories with a high experience level were certified as imaging sites after a training process and qualifying test echocardiography submissions, subsequent clinical trial examinations showed low rates of acceptable endocardial definition in two apical views: 43.5%[72] and 47.9%.[73] However, when an experimental intervention was implemented that targeted a key variable (diastolic LV volume), measurements taken before and after the intervention revealed dramatic improvement.[73] Interventions to improve image-acquisition skills included post-training quizzes, individual sonographer certification, monthly quality updates, scorecards, and on-site physician approval of submitted examinations (Table 7.7). Although this type of detailed, day-to-day oversight could be burdensome for a clinical laboratory's daily operations, some of these concepts can be applied in a sustainable way to improve practice in clinical laboratories.

REPORTING

Report Completeness and Consistency

Echocardiography can improve patient outcomes only when critical data elements are accurately recorded, analyzed, interpreted, and communicated to care providers in a timely manner and in a format that can be readily understood and translated into patient-care decisions. An echocardiogram report is also frequently linked to billing systems, and because it documents a discrete episode of care, a report may become legal evidence. Therefore, the report itself represents the final critical link in a chain of quality.

The concept of structured reporting has been promoted as an important mechanism for improving patient care.[74,75] A structured reporting process organizes data into consistent demographic, anatomic, hemodynamic, and interpretation data elements in a standardized fashion, which can facilitate its use clinically and in QI initiatives. Such initiatives can include tracking of internal quality indicators such as appropriate use, timeliness, completeness, and diagnostic accuracy (as determined by multimodality correlation), as well as participation in data registry programs designed to foster clinical care outcomes research.[76,77] In current practice, most commercially available laboratory analysis and reporting systems are in compliance with the IAC's minimum structured reporting standards.

TABLE 7.8 Echocardiography Examination Demographic Data.[a]

- Study date (and time)
- Facility name and/or identifier
- Patient name and/or identifier
- Patient date of birth and/or age
- Indication for the study
- Sonographer name or initials
- Ordering physician name and/or identifier
- Height, weight, gender
- Blood pressure (systolic and diastolic blood pressure must be obtained at or around the time of the study and displayed on the report)

[a]The information must be sufficient to allow the identification and retrieval of previous studies on the same patient.
Adapted from the Intersocietal Accreditation Commission Standards and Guidelines (available at https://www.intersocietal.org/echo/seeking/echo_standards.htm),

For IAC accreditation, all reports must contain the demographic data elements noted in Table 7.8.

The IAC Echocardiography standards and 2019 ACC/AHA/ASE key data elements and definitions for TTE reporting[76] include use of the standard 17-segment LV model and broad categories of left and right heart structure, left and right heart function, aorta, pulmonary artery, right heart hemodynamics, congenital heart disease, and heart valves. A report summary must include pertinent positive and negative findings, particularly as they relate to the indication for examination.

Expected quantitative and anatomic descriptions of TTE and TEE examinations[34] will be different because of the inherent strengths and limitations of each modality. Adult TEE reports must include medications used, ease of transducer insertion, complications (yes/no, describe), and procedure components (Doppler modalities and contrast administration, if any).

Stress echocardiography accreditation at this time pertains to protocols for assessing coronary artery disease.[78] The IAC's standards for stress echocardiography reporting components are shown in Table 7.9. Guidelines have been published regarding the reporting elements for performance and interpretation of stress echocardiography protocols in the assessment of non-ischemic structural heart disease.[79]

Stress testing for non-ischemic heart disease has not been formally incorporated into IAC accreditation standards for stress echocardiography laboratories. Laboratories performing these tests are encouraged to develop internal QI programs in parallel with coronary artery disease stress testing.

Report Timeliness

Echocardiography can improve patient outcomes only when the interpreting physician's findings are communicated to care providers in a safe and timely manner. Once an echocardiogram has been performed, the sonographer's worksheets, comments, or unedited data can be provided only to a qualified interpreting physician. For the purposes of this discussion, a *preliminary report* is one that has been generated by a qualified interpreting physician after review and analysis of the data, before the final report is produced in a standardized format in the laboratory's reporting system. Only the interpreting physician may provide a preliminary report to care providers, with the understanding that this same information will soon be translated into a finalized report.

Routine *inpatient* examinations must be interpreted by a qualified physician within 24 hours after completion of the examination. Findings from a stat (or urgent) echocardiogram or "critical results" of any examination must be communicated immediately by the interpreting physician to the appropriate care provider. In the absence of any critical results detected by the sonographer, outpatient studies must be interpreted by the end of the next business day. Final reports should always be completed in the system within 48 hours, even if the information in them has already been documented in a preliminary report in the medical record.[7]

TABLE 7.9 IAC Stress Echocardiography for Coronary Artery Disease: Required Reporting Components.

- Exercise time, or maximum dose of pharmacologic agent (if used)
- Target heart rate
- Maximum heart rate achieved
- Whether target heart rate was achieved and/or stress was adequate
- Resting blood pressure and blood pressure response to exercise stress
- Reason for termination of the examination
- Patient's cardiac symptoms, if any, during the examination
- Summary of stress ECG findings
- Image description must include
  - Pre-exercise segmental wall motion and global systolic function
  - Post-exercise wall motion comparison and global systolic function
- Summary results statements: any pertinent positive findings (e.g., ischemia, viability and coronary distribution, LV cavity size, EF response) and pertinent negative findings

ECG, Electrocardiogram; *EF*, ejection fraction.
Adapted from the Intersocietal Accreditation Commission Standards and Guidelines (available at https://www.intersocietal.org/echo/seeking/echo_standards.htm),

Examination Status and Turnaround Times

Echocardiography is a potentially life-saving procedure when it is performed with appropriate urgency. Laboratories must have provisions to perform urgent examinations in the next available time period; stat examinations must be performed as soon as possible, preempting other studies,[7] with the understanding that a life-threatening condition may exist. Ordering personnel should ideally transmit urgent and stat examination requests by standard order entry, with an additional direct verbal communication to the appropriate laboratory personnel because detection of a computer-only order entry may be significantly delayed, depending on the sophistication of the facility's work order list. The laboratory should provide appropriate hospital personnel with a daily coverage schedule and direct contact information for technical and medical staff members assigned to handle urgent and stat echocardiography requests.

In a hospital environment, one of the most important quality indicators is TTE turnaround time, which is matched to study status (i.e., routine, urgent, or stat). The total turnaround time is the time from study order to study report. However, this information is useful for QI purposes only when two components are evaluated individually: (1) the time from order entry to examination performance (technical staff) and (2) the time from examination performance to examination interpretation (medical staff).

In general, a hospital laboratory should be able to perform and interpret most non-urgent examinations within 24 hours after the order is placed. If this cannot be achieved most of the time, productivity barriers should be examined (Table 7.10). When most routine examinations cannot be performed within 24 hours, examination "status upgrades" may be made (i.e., from routine to urgent or from urgent to stat) that are unrelated to the patient's actual clinical status. Significantly delayed routine echocardiograms can become urgent or even stat in the minds of ordering physicians when subsequent care, including length-of-stay decision making, is thought to depend on echocardiography results.

Echocardiograms ordered as stat without supportive evidence of high patient acuity have been called "pseudo stat" examinations. Pseudo stat examinations can represent a patient safety issue if they crowd out the resources needed for actual stat examinations, particularly when multiple stat orders are

TABLE 7.10 Echocardiography Laboratory Productivity Barriers.[a]

Facility-Related
In-laboratory delays
- Patient transportation lacking
- Patient "no shows," late arrivals, registration delays
- Portable examination delays (see Fig. 7.2)
- Sonographer transit time (elevators and hallways)
- Poor connectivity—examination results cannot be transmitted back to laboratory (transit time)
- Worklist inadequacies (undetected orders or analysis)

Equipment-related downtime (inadequate inventory—more sonographers than machines)
- Equipment failures
- Needed equipment in use (competing procedures)

Technical Staff–Related (Time From Examination Order To Performance)
Experienced staff
- Proficient but understaffed for workload
- Teaching responsibilities (trainees, temporary staff, inexperienced staff [second pair of hands])

Inexperienced staff
- Longer scanning times
- Sendbacks—incomplete examinations (e.g., needed contrast, IV saline, special protocols [e.g., pericardial effusion])
- Poor images—requires second pair of hands by experienced staff
- Comprehensive examinations performed (to be safe) when tailored limited examinations are appropriate

Patient-Related (Time From Examination Order To Performance)
Complex patient population—expected added times for the following:
- Contrast administration (IV saline or UEAs)
- Other extended protocols (complex valve, LVAD, procedural guidance [e.g., pericardiocentesis, endomyocardial biopsy])
  Competing procedures (patients unavailable—in other departments)

Medical Staff–Related (Time From Examination Performance To Interpretation)
Experienced staff
- Proficient but understaffed for given workload
- Proficient but unavailable
  - Poorly scheduled
  - Competing clinical, teaching, or administrative work

Inexperienced staff—longer read times
Analysis and/or reporting systems slow (interpretation bottleneck)

[a]Note: When determining appropriate staffing levels, decision-makers must consider sonographer productivity benchmarks in the context of facility design and type (see Fig. 7.2) and sonographer experience. Does the laboratory have major teaching responsibilities and serve a large, possibly outdated, distant referral center (poor connectivity) with complex patients? Or is the facility very new, with superior data connectivity and centralized services, and serving a more general or focused patient population?
LVAD, Left ventricular assist device.

received in rapid succession. The echocardiography laboratory's medical staff and ordering physicians should consider adopting a written hospital policy for conditions and diagnoses that warrant true stat echocardiography examination status. The stat echocardiography status assignment would typically activate a direct stat communication pathway and not simply a computerized order entry. A spike in the number of stat echocardiography orders in a facility requires evaluation because it may be related to lengthy turnaround times for routine examinations.

SUMMARY

A modern echocardiography laboratory may be either simple, consisting of one echocardiography machine and one sonographer and/or physician in an outpatient setting, or complex, operating within a quaternary facility. Regardless of the laboratory's scope and size, laboratory accreditation can be used as a starting point for implementing an ongoing QI process. Fig. 7.8 provides a detailed adult echocardiography laboratory accreditation checklist. Creating detailed, laboratory-specific documents for daily laboratory management can be very useful; these documents may include an organizational chart, facility description, key personnel and equipment lists, work schedules, policies, protocols, and a list of potential obstacles to productivity that need to be addressed. Artificial intelligence holds the potential for transformational advancements in QI management, but this can be accomplished only in the context of a well-structured laboratory. Hallmarks of laboratory success include developing and regularly engaging in the QI of laboratory structure and processes that is centered on compassionate and excellent patient care. Careful archiving of a laboratory's structure and process documentation can help to ensure appropriate handoffs and stability despite the inevitable expected or unexpected leadership changes that can occur gradually or abruptly.

SUMMARY Quality Goals and Action Items for Echocardiography Laboratories.

Dimension of Care	Quality Goals	Recommended Approach
Laboratory structure	• Ensure standards for equipment and staff proficiency	• Mandate laboratory accreditation (IAC). • Support physician training and certification. • Support sonographer credentialing. • Retain machines capable of performing complete echocardiograms.
Patient selection	• Minimize inappropriate echocardiograms	• Apply and track AUC for all echocardiographic modalities. • Educate staff and referring physicians about AUC. • Implement processes to reduce inappropriate echocardiograms (physician education, decision support tools).
Image acquisition	• Diagnostic-quality images • Patient safety • Staff safety	• Develop and adhere to imaging protocols and sequences. • Use contrast appropriately to minimize nondiagnostic studies. • Adhere to SE safety protocols for exercise and pharmacologic stress. • Adhere to hospital infection control and radiation safety policies (interventional TEE).
Image interpretation	• Reproducibility • Accuracy	• Develop and test methods for determining interreader and intrareader variability. • Allocate sufficient time for physician interpretation. • Include all structures and measurements required for complete interpretation. • Include a summary and/or synthesis of findings to highlight key abnormalities. • Compare findings with those from the most recent prior study.

Continued

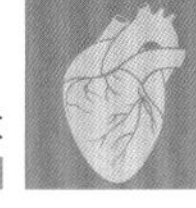

SUMMARY Quality Goals and Action Items for Echocardiography Laboratories.—cont'd

Dimension of Care	Quality Goals	Recommended Approach
Results communication	• Clarity • Completeness • Timeliness	• Develop and track timeliness criteria. • Adhere to standards for completeness of reports. • Use key structured reporting data elements. • Include all demographic information on reports. • Document physician-to-physician communication of critical values.
Improved patient care and outcomes	• Satisfaction • Effect on clinical management • Morbidity • Mortality • Acceptable wait times for routine echocardiograms	• Standardize methods for determining cross-modality correlation. • Develop methods for measuring patient outcomes and effects on medical decision-making. • Assess patient satisfaction with surveys and respond to suggestions for improving the patient experience. • Develop a mechanism to track wait times for inpatient and outpatient studies.

AUC, Appropriate use criteria; *IAC*, Intersocietal Accreditation Commission; *SE*, stress echocardiography.

REFERENCES

1. Nishimura RA, Otto CM, Bonow RO, et al. 2014 AHA/ACC guideline for the management of patients with valvular heart disease: a report of the American College of cardiology/American heart association task force on practice guidelines. *J Am Coll Cardiol.* 2014;63:e57–185.
2. Stout KK, Daniels CJ, Aboulhosn JA, et al. 2018 AHA/ACC Guideline for the management of adults with congenital heart disease: a report of the American College of Cardiology/American Heart Association task force on clinical practice guidelines. *J Am Coll Cardiol.* 2019; 73:e81-e192.
3. Gersh BJ, Maron BJ, Bonow RO, et al. ACCF/AHA guideline for the diagnosis and treatment of hypertrophic cardiomyopathy: a report of the American College of Cardiology Foundation/American Heart Association Task Force On Practice Guidelines. Developed in collaboration with the American Association for Thoracic Surgery, American Society of Echocardiography, American Society of Nuclear Cardiology, Heart Failure Society of America, Heart Rhythm Society, Society for Cardiovascular Angiography and Interventions, and Society of Thoracic Surgeons. *J Am Coll Cardiol.* 2011;58:e212–260.
4. Yancy CW, Jessup M, Bozkurt B, et al. 2013 ACCF/AHA guideline for the management of heart failure: a report of the American College of Cardiology Foundation/American Heart Association Task Force on practice guidelines. *J Am Coll Cardiol.* 2013;62:e147–239.
5. Jessup M, Drazner MH, Book W, et al. ACC/AHA/HFSA/ISHLT/ACP Advanced training statement on advanced heart failure and transplant cardiology (Revision of the ACCF/AHA/ACP/HFSA/ISHLT 2010 Clinical Competence Statement on management of patients with advanced heart failure and cardiac transplant): a report of the ACC Competency Management Committee. *J Am Coll Cardiol.* 2017;69:2977–3001.
6. Stainback RF, Estep JD, DA Agler, et al. Echocardiography in the management of patients with left ventricular assist devices: recommendations from the American Society of Echocardiography. *J Am Soc Echocardiogr.* 2015;28:853–909.
7. Intersocietal Accreditation Commission. IAC standards and guidelines. Accessed 23 September, 2019. Available at: https://www.intersocietal.org/echo/seeking/echo_standards.htm.
8. Kirkpatrick JN, Mitchell C, Taub C, Hung J, Swaminathan M. ASE statement on protection of patients and echocardiography service providers during the 2019 novel coronavirus outbreak. *J Am Soc Echocardiogr.* 2020 Apr, 75 (24) 3078–3084.
9. Lohr KN, Schroeder SA. A strategy for quality assurance in Medicare. *N Engl J Med.* 1990;322:707–712.
10. The National Academies of Sciences. Crossing the quality chasm: the IMO health care quality initiative. Accessed 23 September, 2019. Available at: http://www.nationalacademies.org/hmd/Global/News%20Announcements/Crossing-the-Quality-Chasm-The-IOM-Health-Care-Quality-Initiative.aspx.
11. VanLare JM, Conway PH. Value-based purchasing—national programs to move from volume to value. *N Engl J Med.* 2012;367:292–295.
12. Porter ME. What is value in health care? *N Engl J Med.* 2010;363:2477–2481.
13. American Society of Echocardiography. Recommendations for continuous quality improvement in echocardiography. *J Am Soc Echocardiogr.* 1995;8:S1–S28.
14. Douglas P, Iskandrian AE, Krumholz HM, et al. Achieving quality in cardiovascular imaging: proceedings from the American College of Cardiology-Duke University Medical Center Think Tank on Quality in Cardiovascular Imaging. *J Am Coll Cardiol.* 2006;48:2141–2151.
15. Picard MH, Adams D, Bierig SM, et al. American Society of Echocardiography recommendations for quality echocardiography laboratory operations. *J Am Soc Echocardiogr.* 2011;24:1–10.
16. Popescu BA, Andrade MJ, Badano LP, et al. European Association of Echocardiography recommendations for training, competence, and quality improvement in echocardiography. *Eur J Echocardiogr.* 2009;10:893–905.
17. Popescu BA, Stefanidis A, Nihoyannopoulos P, et al. Updated standards and processes for accreditation of echocardiographic laboratories from the European Association of Cardiovascular Imaging. *Eur Heart J Cardiovasc Imaging.* 2014;15:717–727.
18. The W. Edwards Deming Institute. PDSA cycle. Accessed 23 September, 2019. Available at: https://deming.org/explore/p-d-s-a.
19. Intersocietal Accreditation Commission. Echocardiography. Accessed 23 September, 2019. Available at: https://www.intersocietal.org/echo/.
20. Dimock M. Defining generations: where Millennials end and Generation Z begins. Accessed 23 September, 2019. Available at: https://www.pewresearch.org/fact-tank/2019/01/17/where-millennials-end-and-generation-z-begins/.
21. Myers KK, Sadaghiani K. Millennials in the workplace: a communication perspective on millennials' organizational relationships and performance. *J Bus Psychol.* 2010;25:225–238.
22. Halperin JL, Williams ES, Fuster V, et al. ACC 2015 core cardiovascular training statement (COCATS 4) (revision of COCATS 3). *J Am Coll Cardiol.* 2015;65:1721–1723.
23. Wiegers SE, Ryan T, Arrighi JA, et al. 2019 ACC/AHA/ASE Advanced training statement on echocardiography (revision of the 2003 ACC/AHA clinical competence statement on echocardiography): a report of the ACC Competency Management Committee. *J Am Coll Cardiol.* 2019;74:377–402.
24. Ryan T, Berlacher K, Lindner JR, Mankad SV, Rose GA, Wang A. COCATS 4 task force 5: training in echocardiography. *J Am Coll Cardiol.* 2015;65:1786–1799.
25. National Board of Echocardiography Inc. Echoboards.org. Accessed 23 September, 2019. Available at: https://www.echoboards.org/.
26. IAC Intersocietal Accreditation Commission - Echocardiography. *IAC Standards and Guidelines for Adult Echocardiography Accreditation.* Intersocietal Accreditation Commission; 2017.
27. Mitchell C, Miller FA Jr, Bierig SM, et al. Advanced cardiovascular sonographer: a proposal of the American society of echocardiography advanced practice sonographer task force. *J Am Soc Echocardiogr.* 2009;22:1409–1413.
28. American Society of Echocardiography. Sonographer training. Accessed 23 September, 2019. Available at: https://www.asecho.org/clinical-information/sonographer-training/.

29. Centers for Medicare & Medicaid Services. Hospital infection control worksheet. Accessed 23 September, 2019. Available at: https://www.cms.gov/Medicare/Provider-Enrollment-and-Certification/SurveyCertificationGenInfo/Downloads/Survey-and-Cert-Letter-15-12-Attachment-1.pdf.
30. Association for Medical Ultrasound. Official Statements: Guidelines for cleaning and preparing external- and internal-use ultrasound transducers between patients & safe handling and use of ultrasound coupling gel. Accessed 23 September, 2019. Available at: https://www.aium.org/officialStatements/57.
31. Mitchell C, Collins K, Hua L, et al. Specific considerations for sonographers when performing echocardiograms during the 2019 novel coronavirus outbreak: supplement to the American Society of Echocardiography Statement. *J Am Soc Echocardiogr*. 2020;33(6):647–778.
32. Nicoara A, Maldonado Y, Kort S, Swaminathan M, Mackensen GB. Specific considerations for the protection of patients and echocardiography service providers when performing perioperative or periprocedural transesophageal echocardiography during the 2019 novel coronavirus outbreak: Council on Perioperative Echocardiography Supplement to the Statement of the American Society of Echocardiography: endorsed by the Society of Cardiovascular Anesthesiologists. *J Am Soc Echocardiogr*. 2020;33(6):666–669.
33. Naidu SS, Rao SV, Blankenship J, et al. Clinical expert consensus statement on best practices in the cardiac catheterization laboratory: society for Cardiovascular Angiography and Interventions. *Catheter Cardiovasc Interv*. 2012;80:456–464.
34. Hahn RT, Abraham T, Adams MS, et al. Guidelines for performing a comprehensive transesophageal echocardiographic examination: recommendations from the American Society of Echocardiography and the Society of Cardiovascular Anesthesiologists. *J Am Soc Echocardiogr*. 2013;26:921–964.
35. Practice guidelines for moderate procedural sedation and analgesia 2018: a report by the American Society of Anesthesiologists Task Force on Moderate Procedural Sedation and Analgesia, the American Association of Oral and Maxillofacial Surgeons, American College of Radiology, American Dental Association, American Society of Dentist Anesthesiologists, and Society of Interventional Radiology. *Anesthesiology*. 2018;128: 437–479.
36. American Institute of Ultrasound in Medicine. Official statements: Prudent clinical use and safety of diagnostic ultrasound. Accessed 23 September, 2019. Available at: https://www.aium.org/officialStatements/34.
37. McIlwain EF, Coon PD, Einstein AJ, et al. Radiation safety for the cardiac sonographer: recommendations of the Radiation Safety Writing Group for the Council on Cardiovascular Sonography of the American Society of Echocardiography. *J Am Soc Echocardiogr*. 2014;27:811–816.
38. Klein LW, Goldstein JA, Haines D, et al. SCAI Multi-society position statement on occupational health hazards of the catheterization laboratory: Shifting the paradigm for healthcare workers' protection. *J Am Coll Cardiol*. 2020;75:1718–1724.
39. Crowhurst JA, Scalia GM, Whitby M, et al. Radiation exposure of operators performing transesophageal echocardiography during percutaneous structural cardiac interventions. *J Am Coll Cardiol*. 2018;71:1246–1254.
40. Intersocietal Accreditation Commission. The new IAC QI tool. Accessed 23 September, 2019. Available at: https://www.intersocietal.org/QITool/.
41. Masani N. The Echocardiography Quality Framework: a comprehensive, patient-centered approach to quality assurance and continuous service improvement. *Echo Res Pract*. 2018;5:G35–G41.
42. Ingram TE, Baker S, Allen J, et al. A patient-centred model to quality assure outputs from an echocardiography department: consensus guidance from the British Society of Echocardiography. *Echo Res Pract*. 2018;5:G25–G33.
43. Douglas PS, Khandheria B, Stainback RF, et al. ACCF/ASE/ACEP/ASNC/SCAI/SCCT/SCMR 2007 appropriateness criteria for transthoracic and transesophageal echocardiography: a report of the American College of Cardiology Foundation Quality Strategic Directions Committee Appropriateness Criteria Working Group, American Society of Echocardiography, American College of Emergency Physicians, American Society of Nuclear Cardiology, Society for Cardiovascular Angiography and Interventions, Society of Cardiovascular Computed Tomography, and The Society for Cardiovascular Magnetic Resonance. endorsed By the American College of Chest Physicians and the Society of Critical Care Medicine. *J Am Coll Cardiol*. 2007;50:187–204.
44. Douglas PS, Khandheria B, Stainback RF, et al. ACCF/ASE/ACEP/AHA/ASNC/SCAI/SCCT/SCMR 2008 appropriateness criteria for stress echocardiography: a report of the American College of Cardiology Foundation Appropriateness Criteria Task Force, American Society of Echocardiography, American College of Emergency Physicians, American Heart Association, American Society of Nuclear Cardiology, Society for Cardiovascular Angiography and Interventions, Society of Cardiovascular Computed Tomography, and Society for Cardiovascular Magnetic Resonance: endorsed by the Heart Rhythm Society and the Society of Critical Care Medicine. *Circulation*. 2008;117:1478–1497.
45. Stainback RF. Overview of quality in cardiovascular imaging and procedures for clinicians: focus on appropriate-use-criteria guidelines. *Methodist Debakey Cardiovasc J*. 2014;10:178–184.
46. Douglas PS, Garcia MJ, DE Haines, et al. ACCF/ASE/AHA/ASNC/HFSA/HRS/SCAI/SCCM/SCCT/SCMR 2011 appropriate use criteria for echocardiography: a report of the American College of Cardiology Foundation Appropriate Use Criteria Task Force, American Society of Echocardiography, American Heart Association, American Society of Nuclear Cardiology, Heart Failure Society of America, Heart Rhythm Society, Society for Cardiovascular Angiography and Interventions, Society of Critical Care Medicine, Society of Cardiovascular Computed Tomography, and Society for Cardiovascular Magnetic Resonance. Endorsed by the American College of Chest Physicians. *J Am Soc Echocardiogr*. 2011;24:229–267.
47. Mansour IN, Razi RR, Behave NM, Ward RP. Comparison of the updated 2011 appropriate use criteria for echocardiography to the original criteria for transthoracic, transesophageal, and stress echocardiography. *J Am Soc Echocardiogr*. 2012;25:1153–1161.
48. Singh A, Ward RP. Appropriate use criteria for echocardiography: evolving applications in the era of value-based healthcare. *Curr Cardiol Rep*. 2016;18:93.
49. Hendel RC, Lindsay BD, Allen JM, et al. ACC appropriate use criteria methodology: 2018 update: a report of the American College of Cardiology Appropriate Use Criteria Task Force. *J Am Coll Cardiol*. 2018;71:935–948.
50. Wolk MJ, Bailey SR, Doherty JU, et al. ACCF/AHA/ASE/ASNC/HFSA/HRS/SCAI/SCCT/SCMR/STS 2013 multimodality appropriate use criteria for the detection and risk assessment of stable ischemic heart disease: a report of the American College of Cardiology Foundation Appropriate Use Criteria Task Force, American Heart Association, American Society of Echocardiography, American Society of Nuclear Cardiology, Heart Failure Society of America, Heart Rhythm Society, Society for Cardiovascular Angiography and Interventions, Society of Cardiovascular Computed Tomography, Society for Cardiovascular Magnetic Resonance, and Society of Thoracic Surgeons. *J Am Coll Cardiol*. 2014;63:380–406.
51. Doherty JU, Kort S, Mehran R, Schoenhagen P, Soman P. ACC/AATS/AHA/ASE/ASNC/HRS/SCAI/SCCT/SCMR/STS 2017 appropriate use criteria for multimodality imaging in valvular heart disease: a report of the American College of Cardiology Appropriate Use Criteria Task Force, American Association for Thoracic Surgery, American Heart Association, American Society of Echocardiography, American Society of Nuclear Cardiology, Heart Rhythm Society, Society for Cardiovascular Angiography and Interventions, Society of Cardiovascular Computed Tomography, Society for Cardiovascular Magnetic Resonance, and Society of Thoracic Surgeons. *J Am Coll Cardiol*. 2017;70:1647–1672.
52. Doherty JU, Kort S, Mehran R, et al. ACC/AATS/AHA/ASE/ASNC/HRS/SCAI/SCCT/SCMR/STS 2019 appropriate use criteria for multimodality imaging in the assessment of cardiac structure and function in nonvalvular heart disease: a report of the American College of Cardiology Appropriate Use Criteria Task Force, American Association for Thoracic Surgery, American Heart Association, American Society of Echocardiography, American Society of Nuclear Cardiology, Heart Rhythm Society, Society for Cardiovascular Angiography and Interventions, Society of Cardiovascular Computed Tomography, Society for Cardiovascular Magnetic Resonance, and the Society of Thoracic Surgeons. *J Am Soc Echocardiogr*. 2019;32:553–579.
53. Sachdeva R, Valente AM, Armstrong AK, et al. ACC/AHA/ASE/HRS/ISACHD/SCAI/SCCT/SCMR/SOPE 2020 appropriate use criteria for multimodality imaging during the follow-up care of patients with congenital heart disease: a report of the American College of Cardiology Solution Set Oversight Committee and Appropriate Use Criteria Task Force, American Heart Association, American Society of Echocardiography, Heart Rhythm Society, International Society for Adult Congenital Heart Disease, Society for Cardiovascular Angiography and Interventions, Society of Cardiovascular Computed Tomography, Society for Cardiovascular Magnetic Resonance, and Society of Pediatric Echocardiography. *J Am Coll Cardiol*. 2020;75:657–703.
54. Chiriac A, Kadkhodayan A, Pislaru SV, et al. Clinical importance of transthoracic echocardiography with direct input from treating physicians. *J Am Soc Echocardiogr*. 2016;29:195–204.

55. Dudzinski DM, Bhatia RS, Mi MY, Isselbacher EM, Picard MH, Weiner RB. Effect of educational intervention on the rate of rarely appropriate outpatient echocardiograms ordered by attending academic cardiologists: a randomized clinical trial. *JAMA Cardiol.* 2016;1:805–812.
56. Bhatia RS, Ivers NM, Yin XC, et al. Improving the appropriate use of transthoracic echocardiography: the Echo WISELY trial. *J Am Coll Cardiol.* 2017;70:1135–1144.
57. Mitchell C, Rahko PS, Blauwet LA, et al. Guidelines for performing a comprehensive transthoracic echocardiographic examination in adults: recommendations from the American Society of Echocardiography. *J Am Soc Echocardiogr.* 2019;32:1–64.
58. Thavendiranathan P, Popovic ZB, Flamm SD, Dahiya A, Grimm RA, Marwick TH. Improved interobserver variability and accuracy of echocardiographic visual left ventricular ejection fraction assessment through a self-directed learning program using cardiac magnetic resonance images. *J Am Soc Echocardiogr.* 2013;26:1267–1273.
59. Grant AD, Thavendiranathan P, Rodriguez LL, Kwon D, Marwick TH. Development of a consensus algorithm to improve interobserver agreement and accuracy in the determination of tricuspid regurgitation severity. *J Am Soc Echocardiogr.* 2014;27:277–284.
60. Dahiya A, Bolen M, Grimm RA, et al. Development of a consensus document to improve multireader concordance and accuracy of aortic regurgitation severity grading by echocardiography versus cardiac magnetic resonance imaging. *Am J Cardiol.* 2012;110:709–714.
61. Ling LF, Obuchowski NA, Rodriguez L, Popovic Z, Kwon D, Marwick TH. Accuracy and interobserver concordance of echocardiographic assessment of right ventricular size and systolic function: a quality control exercise. *J Am Soc Echocardiogr.* 2012;25:709–713.
62. Johnson TV, Symanski JD, Patel SR, Rose GA. Improvement in the assessment of diastolic function in a clinical echocardiography laboratory following implementation of a quality improvement initiative. *J Am Soc Echocardiogr.* 2011;24:1169–1179.
63. Barnhart HX, Yow E, Crowley AL, et al. Choice of agreement indices for assessing and improving measurement reproducibility in a core laboratory setting. *Stat Methods Med Res.* 2016;25:2939–2958.
64. Johri AM, Picard MH, Newell J, Marshall JE, King ME, Hung J. Can a teaching intervention reduce interobserver variability in LVEF assessment: a quality control exercise in the echocardiography lab. *JACC Cardiovasc Imaging.* 2011;4:821–829.
65. Minter S, Armour A, Tinnemore A, et al. Crowdsourcing consensus: proposal of a novel method for assessing accuracy in echocardiography interpretation. *Int J Cardiovasc Imaging.* 2018;34:1725–1730.
66. Narula S, Shameer K, Salem Omar AM, Dudley JT, Sengupta PP. Machine-learning algorithms to automate morphological and functional assessments in 2D echocardiography. *J Am Coll Cardiol.* 2016;68:2287–2295.
67. Tsay D, Patterson C. From machine learning to artificial intelligence applications in cardiac care. *Circulation.* 2018;138:2569–2575.
68. Madani A, Arnaout R, Mofrad M, Arnaout R. Fast and accurate view classification of echocardiograms using deep learning. *NPJ Digit Med.* 2018;1.
69. Kusunose K, Abe T, Haga A, et al. A deep learning approach for assessment of regional wall motion abnormality from echocardiographic images. *JACC Cardiovasc Imaging.* 2020;13:374–381.
70. Douglas PS, DeCara JM, Devereux RB, et al. Echocardiographic imaging in clinical trials: American Society of Echocardiography Standards for echocardiography core laboratories: endorsed by the American College of Cardiology Foundation. *J Am Soc Echocardiogr.* 2009;22:755–765.
71. Crowley AL, Yow E, Barnhart HX, et al. Critical review of current approaches for echocardiographic reproducibility and reliability assessment in clinical research. *J Am Soc Echocardiogr.* 2016;29:1144–1154. e1147.
72. Oh JK, Pellikka PA, Panza JA, et al. Core lab analysis of baseline echocardiographic studies in the STICH trial and recommendation for use of echocardiography in future clinical trials. *J Am Soc Echocardiogr.* 2012;25:327–336.
73. Crowley AL, Yow E, Rabineau D, et al. The impact of a rigorous quality program on 3D echocardiography data quality in an international multisite randomized trial. *JACC Cardiovasc Imaging.* 2018;11:1918–1920.
74. Douglas PS, Hendel RC, Cummings JE, et al. ACCF/ACR/AHA/ASE/ASNC/HRS/NASCI/RSNA/SAIP/SCAI/SCCT/SCMR 2008 Health policy statement on structured reporting in cardiovascular imaging. *J Am Coll Cardiol.* 2009;53:76–90.
75. Hendel RC, Budoff MJ, Cardella JF, et al. ACC/AHA/ACR/ASE/ASNC/HRS/NASCI/RSNA/SAIP/SCAI/SCCT/SCMR/SIR 2008 key data elements and definitions for cardiac imaging: a report of the American College of Cardiology/American Heart Association Task Force On Clinical Data Standards (writing committee to develop clinical data standards for cardiac imaging). *Circulation.* 2009;119:154–186.
76. Douglas PS, Carabello BA, Lang RM, et al. 2019 ACC/AHA/ASE key data elements and definitions for transthoracic echocardiography: a report of the American College of Cardiology/American Heart Association Task Force On Clinical Data Standards (writing committee to develop cardiovascular endpoints data standards) and the American Society of Echocardiography. *Circ Cardiovasc Imaging.* 2019;12:e000027.
77. Hendel RC, Bozkurt B, Fonarow GC, et al. ACC/AHA 2013 methodology for developing clinical data standards: a report of the American College of Cardiology/American Heart Association Task Force on Clinical Data Standards. *Circulation.* 2014;129:2346–2357.
78. Pellikka PA, Nagueh SF, Elhendy AA, Kuehl CA, Sawada SG. American Society of Echocardiography recommendations for performance, interpretation, and application of stress echocardiography. *J Am Soc Echocardiogr.* 2007;20:1021–1041.
79. Lancellotti P, Pellikka PA, Budts W, et al. The clinical use of stress echocardiography in non-ischaemic heart disease: recommendations from the European Association of Cardiovascular Imaging and the American Society of Echocardiography. *J Am Soc Echocardiogr.* 2017;30:101–138.

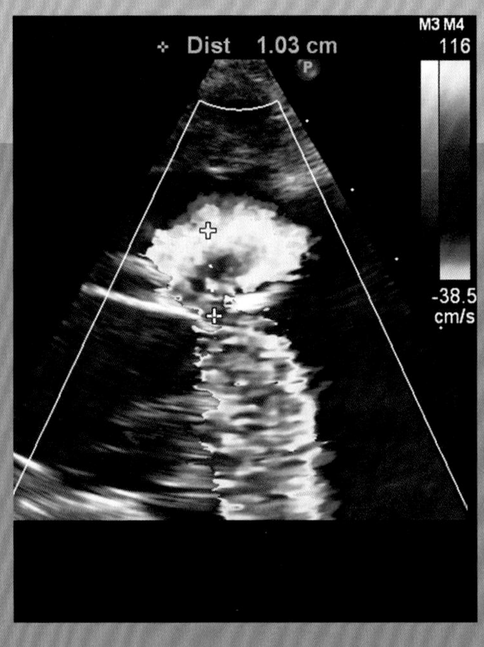

中文导读

第8章 综合诊断性经胸和经食管超声心动图

超声心动图是评估心脏解剖、功能和血流动力学的最常用影像学方法，对于心脏、肺和大血管的各种疾病诊断和评估有着广泛的临床应用。本章讲述了综合性经胸超声心动图和经食管超声心动图的基础知识，主要为以下几个方面：①经胸超声心动图各标准切面的名称、内容和获取方法；②经胸超声心动图的常用模式方法包括M型、多普勒（连续多普勒、脉冲多普勒、多普勒血流图和组织多普勒）的概念及其临床应用方法；③综合经胸超声心动图诊断的规范化检查流程以避免漏诊误诊；④经食管超声心动图是一种侵入性检查，可作为经胸超声心动图的互补和补充，可以提供更清晰的图像和补充视角。经食管超声心动图的适应证、风险和并发症等；⑤掌握经食管超声心动图的规范化培训内容；⑥经食管超声心动图患者的准备和镇静；⑦经食管超声心动图检查的操作方法、标准切面的获取方法和解读；⑧特定心脏结构的经食管超声心动图成像方法：心房、左心耳、主动脉和主动脉瓣、二尖瓣、三尖瓣和肺动脉瓣等；⑨三维经食管超声心动图方法学；⑩经食管超声心动图的常见临床应用场景，包括卵圆孔的右心声学造影诊断、左心耳及心内血栓和肿物的诊断、自体和人工心脏瓣膜病变的评价、感染性心内膜炎的诊断、急性主动脉疾病的诊断等；⑪最后介绍了综合经食管超声心动图的规范化检查流程建议。

朱振辉

8 Comprehensive Diagnostic Transthoracic and Transesophageal Echocardiography

GARY HUANG, MD | ROSARIO V. FREEMAN, MD, MS

Echocardiography is the most commonly used imaging modality for the evaluation of cardiac anatomy and function; it allows comprehensive evaluation of left ventricular (LV) and right ventricular (RV) function, regional wall motion, valvular heart disease, and pericardial disease, as well as estimation of pulmonary pressures and central venous pressure. Comprehensive transthoracic echocardiography (TTE) consists of a combination of two-dimensional (2D), M-mode, and Doppler imaging, with three-dimensional echocardiography (3DE; see Chapter 1) increasingly being incorporated into imaging protocols.[1] Appropriate use criteria for multimodality imaging address the use of TTE in the diagnosis and management of valvular and structural heart disease (Table 8.1).[2,3] Echocardiography is appropriate for the diagnosis and clinical management of cardiac diagnoses but is rarely indicated when results would not likely alter the course of treatment.

Transesophageal echocardiography (TEE) is a semi-invasive procedure that is widely used for a range of clinical applications, including diagnostic, intraprocedural, and real-time cardiac monitoring. Compared with TTE, TEE allows improved visualization of most cardiac structures and is indicated when TTE imaging is likely to be nondiagnostic or when highly detailed images are needed (e.g., imaging of prosthetic valves). Advances in image processing and display, the addition of 3DE, and the relative portability of ultrasound systems have dramatically increased the availability and utility of TEE in a variety of clinical settings, including the cardiac catheterization laboratory, operating room, and intensive care unit.

THE DIAGNOSTIC TRANSTHORACIC ECHOCARDIOGRAM

NOMENCLATURE

Echocardiographic *acoustic windows* are transducer positions that allow ultrasound access to the heart, and *views* are cardiac imaging planes that are transected by the transducer beam. Transthoracic images are typically obtained from four primary acoustic windows: left parasternal, apical, subcostal, and suprasternal notch (Fig. 8.1).[4]

Standard imaging planes are used as reference for each echocardiographic view:

1. The long-axis plane lies parallel to the long axis of the LV, transects the LV apex and the center of the aortic valve (AV), and is aligned with the anteroposterior diameter of the mitral valve (MV).
2. The short-axis plane is perpendicular to the LV long axis and allows visualization of cross-sections of the LV, MV, and AV, depending on the level along the long axis that is transected.
3. The 4-chamber plane is oriented orthogonal to the long- and short-axis views of the LV; this plane transects both atria and ventricles and is aligned with the mediolateral diameter of the MV and tricuspid (TV) valves.
4. The 2-chamber plane is oriented from apex to base and lies orthogonal to the short-axis view of the LV.

TABLE 8.1 Common Appropriate Indications for TTE as a Diagnostic Test.

Appropriate
Valvular heart disease (VHD) or structural heart disease
Pulmonary arterial hypertension
Presyncope or syncope
Hypotension or hemodynamic instability
Hypertensive heart disease
Respiratory failure or shortness of breath of uncertain etiology
Infective endocarditis (IE)
Cardiac mass, tumor, or thrombus; potential cardiac source of emboli
Arrhythmia or conduction disorder
Complications of myocardial ischemia or infarction
Candidacy for and optimization of implantable cardioverter-defibrillator/cardiac resynchronization therapy and ventricular assist device
Pericardial disease
Acute aortic pathology including acute aortic syndrome
Re-evaluation (3–5 years) of stage A (bicuspid aortic valve or aortic sclerosis) VHD or stage B (mild) VHD
Re-evaluation (1–2 years) of stage B (moderate) VHD
Re-evaluation (6–12 months) of stage C1 (asymptomatic and severe) VHD
Follow-up testing of new or worsening symptoms in VHD, IE, or structural heart disease
Preoperative, perioperative, and postoperative evaluation of surgical valve replacement or repair
Preprocedural, periprocedural, and postprocedural evaluation of structural heart disease intervention procedures
Rarely Appropriate
Transient fever and pathogen not typically associated with IE, a documented nonendovascular source of infection, no bacteremia, and/or no evidence of a new murmur
Preparticipation athletics assessment in a patient with no symptoms, normal examination findings, and no family history of congenital heart disease

Adapted from Doherty JU, Kort S, Mehran R, Schoenhagen P, Soman P. ACC/AATS/AHA/ASE/ASNC/HRS/SCAI/SCCT/SCMR/STS 2017 appropriate use criteria for multimodality imaging in valvular heart disease: a report of the American College of Cardiology Appropriate Use Criteria Task Force, American Association for Thoracic Surgery, American Heart Association, American Society of Echocardiography, American Society of Nuclear Cardiology, Heart Rhythm Society, Society for Cardiovascular Angiography and Interventions, Society of Cardiovascular Computed Tomography, Society for Cardiovascular Magnetic Resonance, and Society of Thoracic Surgeons. *J Am Coll Cardiol.* 2017;70:1647–1672; and Doherty JU, Kort S, Mehran R, et al. ACC/AATS/AHA/ASE/ASNC/HRS/SCAI/SCCT/SCMR/STS 2019 appropriate use criteria for multimodality imaging in the assessment of cardiac structure and function in nonvalvular heart disease: a report of the American College of Cardiology Appropriate Use Criteria Task Force, American Association for Thoracic Surgery, American Heart Association, American Society of Echocardiography, American Society of Nuclear Cardiology, Heart Rhythm Society, Society for Cardiovascular Angiography and Interventions, Society of Cardiovascular Computed Tomography, Society for Cardiovascular Magnetic Resonance, and the Society of Thoracic Surgeons. *J Am Coll Cardiol.* 2019;73:488–516.

PATIENT AND TRANSDUCER POSITION

TTE is performed by a physician or cardiac sonographer. Time needed to perform a TTE examination ranges from minutes for rapid assessment of a critically ill patient to a lengthier study for a comprehensive evaluation, such as in patients with complex valvular heart disease (VHD) or congenital heart disease. The sonographer is typically sitting at the patient's left side, with the patient lying in a supine or left lateral decubitus position; this improves ultrasound windows by bringing the heart anteriorly and lateral to the sternum. Adjustments of the transducer on the chest wall, obtained by tilting, sweeping, rotating, sliding, rocking, and angling the transducer, produce different imaging views as the ultrasound beam is directed through the heart at different angles (Fig. 8.2). Guidelines for the performance of a comprehensive TTE examination were published by the American Society of Echocardiography in 2019.[4]

Parasternal Window

Parasternal Long-Axis View. For the left parasternal window, the patient is placed in a left lateral decubitus position with the transducer in the third or fourth left intercostal space. The LV long-axis view is obtained with the transducer index marker facing toward the patient's right shoulder at approximately the 10-o'clock position (see Fig. 8.2C). This view allows visualization of the LV, left atrium (LA), MV, AV, and proximal ascending aorta (Fig. 8.3).[5] The LV should lie perpendicular to the ultrasound beam, with the anterior (AMVL) and posterior (PMVL) mitral valve leaflets and the right and noncoronary cusps of the AV visualized (Table 8.2). With increased depth in the imaging sector, the parasternal long-axis view (PLAX) allows differentiation of pericardial and pleural effusions: the oblique pericardial sinus lies between the LA and the descending thoracic aorta, and a pericardial effusion lies between these two structures, whereas a pleural effusion tracks posterior to the descending thoracic aorta (see Fig. 8.3B). The size of a pericardial effusion does not necessarily correlate with hemodynamic impact. In this view, the true LV apex is not visualized; rather, the "apex" is typically an oblique image plane through the anterolateral wall.

RV Inflow View. The RV inflow view is obtained by tilting the transducer inferomedially from the PLAX and rotating it slightly clockwise. In this view, the right atrium (RA), TV, and RV are visualized in a long-axis plane. The TV anterior leaflet is present along with the posterior leaflet. The coronary sinus enters the RA adjacent to the posterior tricuspid annulus, and the inferior vena cava (IVC) enters the RA inferior to the coronary sinus (Fig. 8.4).

Parasternal Short-Axis Views. The parasternal short-axis (PSAX) views are obtained by rotating the transducer 90 degrees clockwise from the PLAX, with the transducer index marker pointed toward the left supraclavicular fossa at approximately the 2-o'clock position, placing the ultrasound beam perpendicular to the LV long-axis plane. By tilting the transducer superiorly or inferiorly, different cross-sectional views of the heart may be visualized.

When the transducer is tilted superiorly, a transverse view of the heart is recorded at the level of the great vessels. In this view, the AV, LA, interatrial septum (IAS), RA, TV, and RV outflow tract (RVOT) are visualized. The right, left, and noncoronary cusps of the AV are seen, with the IAS attached just adjacent to the noncoronary cusp. The right coronary cusp is positioned anteriorly and abuts the RVOT; the left coronary cusp is adjacent to the proximal pulmonary artery (see Table 8.2). The origins of the left main and right coronary arteries can often be identified in this view.

For the MV short-axis view, the transducer is tilted inferiorly so that the ultrasound beam transects the heart at the level of the mitral leaflets. In this view, the AMVL and PMVL are seen en face. Each leaflet is segmented into three major scallops, called *lateral* (A1 and P1), *middle* (A2 and P2), and *medial* (A3 and P3), respectively (Fig. 8.5A). If the transducer is tilted further inferiorly, a cross-sectional view is obtained at the midventricular (papillary muscle) level. In this view, a normal LV appears circular in shape, and the anterolateral and posteromedial papillary muscles are present at approximately the 3- and 8-o'clock positions, respectively (see Fig. 8.5B).

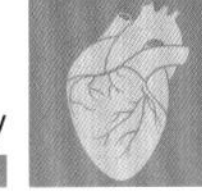

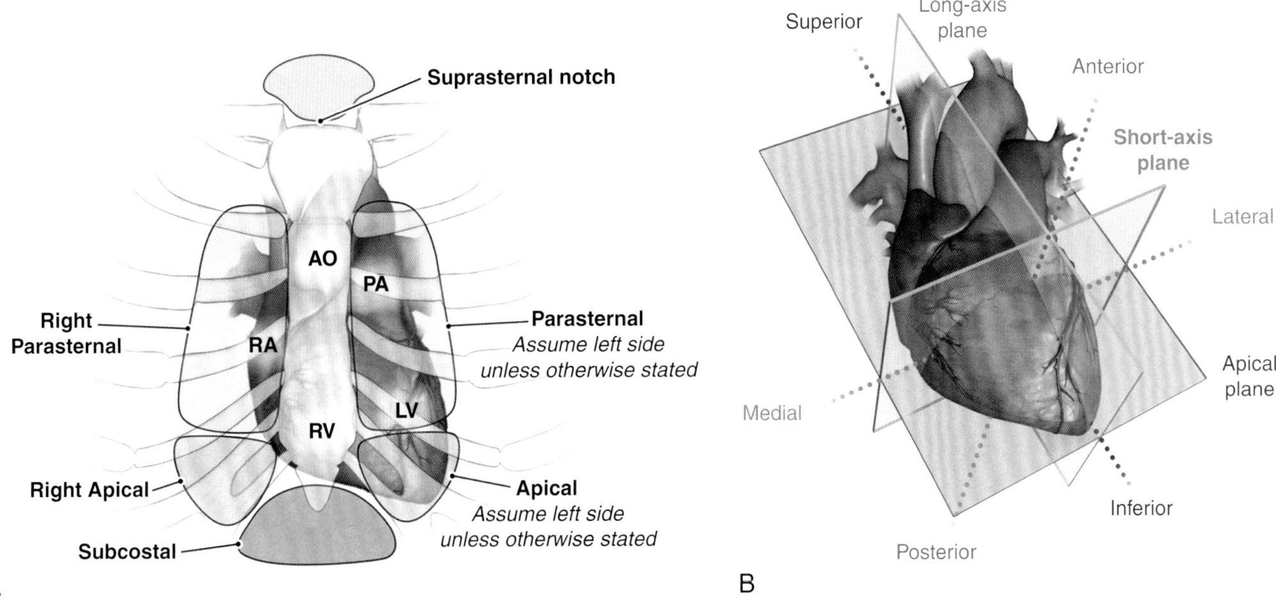

Fig. 8.1 Echocardiographic windows and standard imaging planes of the heart. (A) The four primary echocardiographic windows used to obtain images are the left parasternal window, the apical window, the subcostal window, and the suprasternal notch window. (B) The long-axis plane lies parallel to the long axis of the LV. The short-axis plane is perpendicular to the long-axis plane, allowing for visualization of cross-sectional views of the heart, depending on the level of transection of the long axis. *AO*, Aorta; *PA*, pulmonary artery. (From Mitchell C, Rahko PS, Blauwet LA, et al. Guidelines for performing a comprehensive transthoracic echocardiographic examination in adults: recommendations from the American Society of Echocardiography. *J Am Soc Echocardiogr.* 2019;32:1–64.)

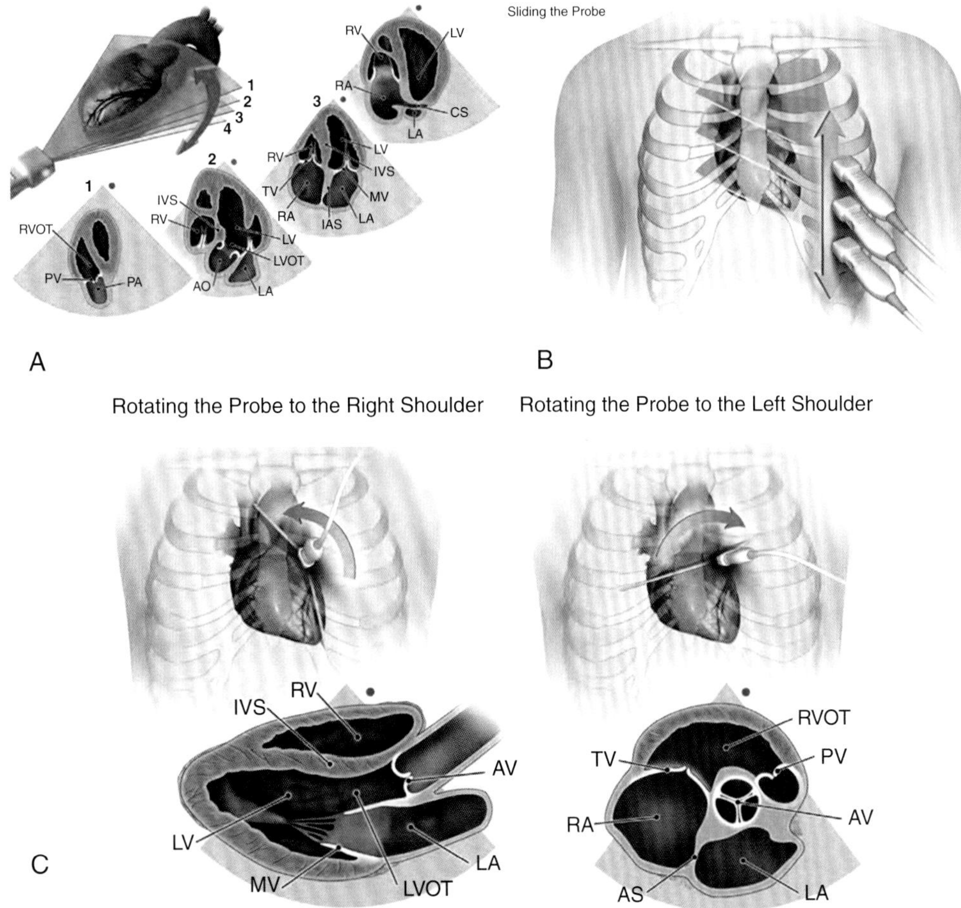

Fig. 8.2 Transducer movements. Adjustments of the transducer on the chest wall produces different imaging views as the ultrasound beam is directed through the heart at different angles. *Blue dot* represents the orientation of the transducer index marker in each view. (A) Tilting the transducer in place through the heart at different angles redirects the ultrasound beam. Similarly, different imaging views are obtained by sliding the transducer along the chest wall (B) and by rotating the transducer in place (C). *AO*, Aorta; *CS*, coronary sinus; *IAS*, interatrial septum; *IVS*, interventricular septum; *LVOT*, left ventricular outflow tract; *MV*, mitral valve; *PA*, pulmonary artery; *RVOT*, right ventricular outflow tract; *TV*, tricuspid valve. (From Mitchell C, Rahko PS, Blauwet LA, et al. Guidelines for performing a comprehensive transthoracic echocardiographic examination in adults: recommendations from the American Society of Echocardiography. *J Am Soc Echocardiogr.* 2019;32:1–64.)

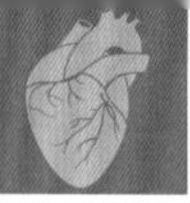

TABLE 8.2 Components and Proposed Sequence of a Comprehensive TTE Study.

Sequence	*Window*	*View*	*Modality*	*Structures Evaluated and Measurements*
1.	Parasternal	PLAX (maximum depth)	2D	Overview of the heart and pericardial and pleural spaces
			2D	Descending aorta, coronary sinus
2.		PLAX (standard depth)	2D	LV, aorta, AV, MV
3.			2D	Cardiac dimensions: LA: anterior-posterior diameter at end-systole
4.			2D	Cardiac dimensions: LV, interventricular septum
5.			2D guided M-mode (M-mode cursor at MV leaflet tips)	Cardiac dimensions: maximum LV dimension (end-diastole), minimum LV dimension (end-systole)
6.			2D	Ascending aorta maximum diameter (end-diastole)
7.			Color Doppler	MV, AV
8.		RV inflow	2D	RA, TV, RV
9.			Color, CW Doppler	TR jet
10.		PSAX	2D	LV (papillary muscle sweep to apex)
11.			2D, color Doppler	MV, AV
12.			2D, color, CW Doppler	RVIT/TV/TR jet (peak velocity)
13.			2D, color, PW, CW Doppler	RVOT, PV/PA bifurcation
14.	Apical	4- and 5-chamber (maximum depth)	2D	Descending aorta
15.		4- and 5-chamber (standard depth)	2D	LV, RV
16.			2D	Coronary sinus, LA (area, height in 4-chamber view), RA
17.			2D	AV (5-chamber view)
18.		4-chamber (decrease depth or zoom)	2D	LV endocardial border tracing (end-systole, end-diastole), biplane EF
19.		4-chamber (decrease depth or zoom)	2D	LA height and volume tracing (end-systole), biplane volume
20.		2-chamber (standard depth)	2D	
21.		2-chamber (decrease depth or zoom)	2D	LV endocardial border tracing (end-systole, end-diastole), biplane EF
22.		2-chamber (decrease depth or zoom)	2D	LA volume tracing (end-systole), biplane volume
23.		LAX (standard depth)	2D	
24.		RV (standard depth)	2D	
25.			Color, CW Doppler	TV (TR, peak velocity)
26.		RV focused (standard depth)	2D	RV diameter (distal to the TV annulus)
27.			M-mode	RV systolic function (TAPSE)
28.			Tissue Doppler	RV systolic function (systolic excursion at the basal RV free wall)
29.		4- and 5-chamber	2D, color Doppler	MV, TV, LVOT, AV, interatrial septum
30.		4-chamber	PW Doppler	Diastology: MV E- and A-wave velocities (leaflet tips, MV deceleration time, and MV annulus a wave duration
31.		4-chamber	Tissue Doppler	Septum, lateral wall (maximum *e′* velocity 1 cm distal to the MV annulus)
32.			PW Doppler	Pulmonary vein: peak velocity, A-wave duration, systolic and diastolic waves
33.			PW Doppler	IVRT
34.			PW Doppler	LVOT peak velocity
35.			CW Doppler, Pedof probe	Valvular anatomy and function: MV (MR), AV (AI), TV (TR, peak velocity)
36.	Subcostal		2D, M-mode	LV, RV, LA, RA, IVC diameter
37.			PW	TR severity: IVC/HV confluence
38.			2D, color, PW Doppler	Abdominal aorta
39.	Suprasternal notch	LAX	2D	Aorta and take-off of the great vessels
40.			Color, PW or CW Doppler	Descending thoracic aorta

AI, Aortic insufficiency; *AV*, aortic valve; *CW*, continuous wave; *EF*, ejection fraction; *HV*, hepatic vein; *IVC*, inferior vena cava; *IVRT*, isovolumic relaxation time; *LAX*, long-axis view; *LVOT*, left ventricular outflow tract; *MR*, mitral regurgitation; *MV*, mitral valve; *PA*, pulmonary artery; *PLAX*, parasternal long-axis view; *PSAX*, parasternal short-axis view; *PV*, pulmonic valve; *PW*, pulsed wave; *RVIT*, right ventricular inflow tract; *RVOT*, right ventricular outflow tract; *TAPSE*, tricuspid annular plane systolic excursion; *TR*, tricuspid regurgitation; *TV*, tricuspid valve.

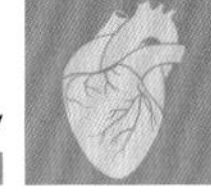

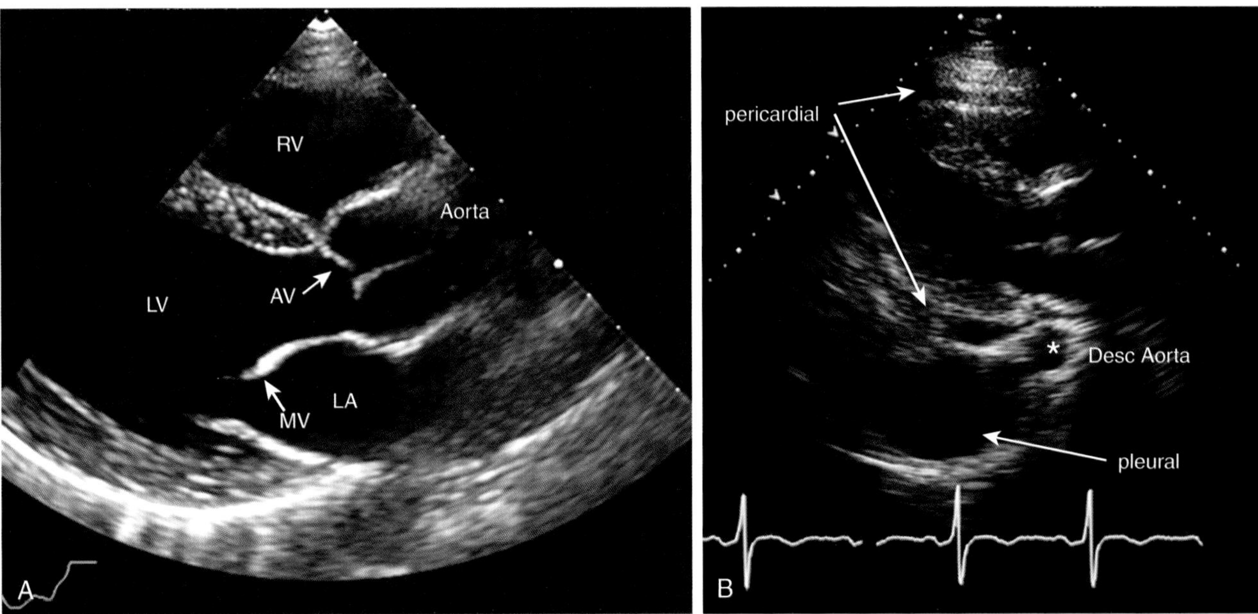

Fig. 8.3 Parasternal long-axis view. (A) At standard imaging depth, the RV is an anterior structure, and the LA is posterior. In diastole, the mitral valve *(MV)* is open. (B) Increased depth allows visualization of structures posterior to the heart, such as pleural and pericardial effusions, both of which are shown. Pericardial fluid tracks anterior to the descending thoracic aorta *(*)*, and pleural fluid tracks posterior to the descending thoracic aorta (Video 8.3). *AV*, Aortic valve.

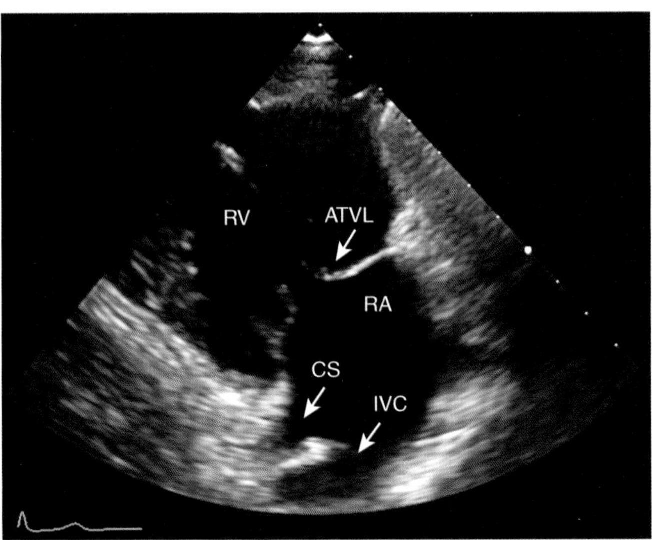

Fig. 8.4 RV inflow view. The RA, tricuspid valve, and RV are well visualized in this view. The os of the coronary sinus *(CS)* is superior to the opening of the inferior vena cava *(IVC)* as they enter the RA. In this view, the anterior tricuspid valve leaflet *(ATVL)* and posterior tricuspid valve leaflet are visualized.

Apical Window

Apical 4-Chamber View. The apical window is obtained by placing the transducer at the point of maximal impulse, with the patient in the left lateral decubitus position. Rotation of the transducer allows for acquisition of the apical views. For the apical 4-chamber view, the ultrasound beam is directed medially and superiorly toward the patient's right scapula, with the transducer index marker at approximately 3 o'clock. In this view, all four chambers of the heart, the IAS, and the interventricular septum (IVS) are visualized (Fig. 8.6; see Table 8.2). The LV appears as a truncated ellipse with visualization of the anterolateral wall, apex, and inferoseptum. The AMVL is adjacent to the septum, and the PMVL is adjacent to the lateral wall.

The tricuspid annulus is more apically positioned than the mitral annulus, with insertion of the septal TV leaflet up to 1 cm displaced relative to the AMVL insertion. This anatomic distinction aids in the identification of cardiac chambers if there is ambiguity in the orientation of the heart. The atria[6] and the IAS are also visualized in this view; however, ultrasound resolution is often limited due to their distal positions relative to the transducer. Rotation of the transducer from the apical window allows visualization of all 17 myocardial segments (Fig. 8.7). Slight counterclockwise rotation of the transducer produces the RV-focused view (Fig. 8.8).[7] RV size and function parameters obtained from the RV-focused view are more reproducible than those measured from the apical 4-chamber view.[8]

Apical 2-Chamber and Long-Axis Views. Rotating the transducer counterclockwise approximately 60 degrees from the apical 4-chamber view provides the apical 2-chamber view. The anterior LV wall and the P1 scallop of the MV are seen on the right of the display, whereas the inferior wall and P3 scallop are seen on the left (see Fig. 8.7). Ejection fraction is calculated with the use of geometric assumptions based on the areas traced from end-diastolic and end-systolic frames in the apical 4-chamber and 2-chamber views (Fig. 8.9).

Longitudinal strain is another measurement used for the evaluation of LV function (Fig. 8.10; see Chapter 2).[9] By convention, strain percentages are reported as negative for shortening. Averaged values from multiple regions provide global measures of LV function such as global longitudinal strain (GLS) (see Fig. 8.10B).

An additional 60 degrees counterclockwise rotation of the transducer yields the apical long-axis view, which is analogous to the image plane for the PLAX but with the transducer now positioned at the point of maximal impulse (see Figs. 8.6 and 8.7). Although the LV apex is now visualized in the apical long-axis view, image resolution for the AV, MV, and LV outflow tract (LVOT) is now relatively poorer because of the greater imaging depth from the transducer.

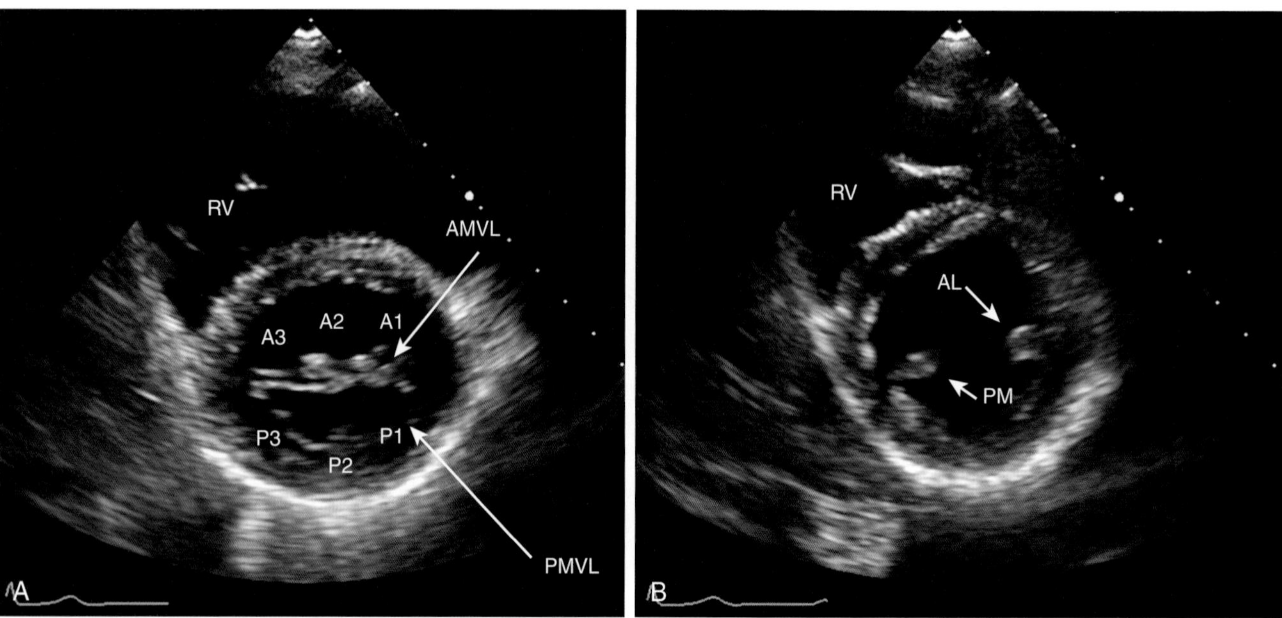

Fig. 8.5 Parasternal short-axis views. (A) Short-axis view at the mitral valve level displays the RV and LV with the anterior *(AMVL)* and posterior *(PMVL)* mitral valve leaflets. The mitral valve scallops are designated, from lateral to medial, as *A1, A2,* and *A3* for the anterior leaflet and *P1, P2,* and *P3* for the posterior leaflet (Video 8.5A ▶). (B) Short-axis plane at the papillary muscle level demonstrates the anterolateral *(AL)* and posteromedial *(PM)* papillary muscles (Video 8.5B ▶).

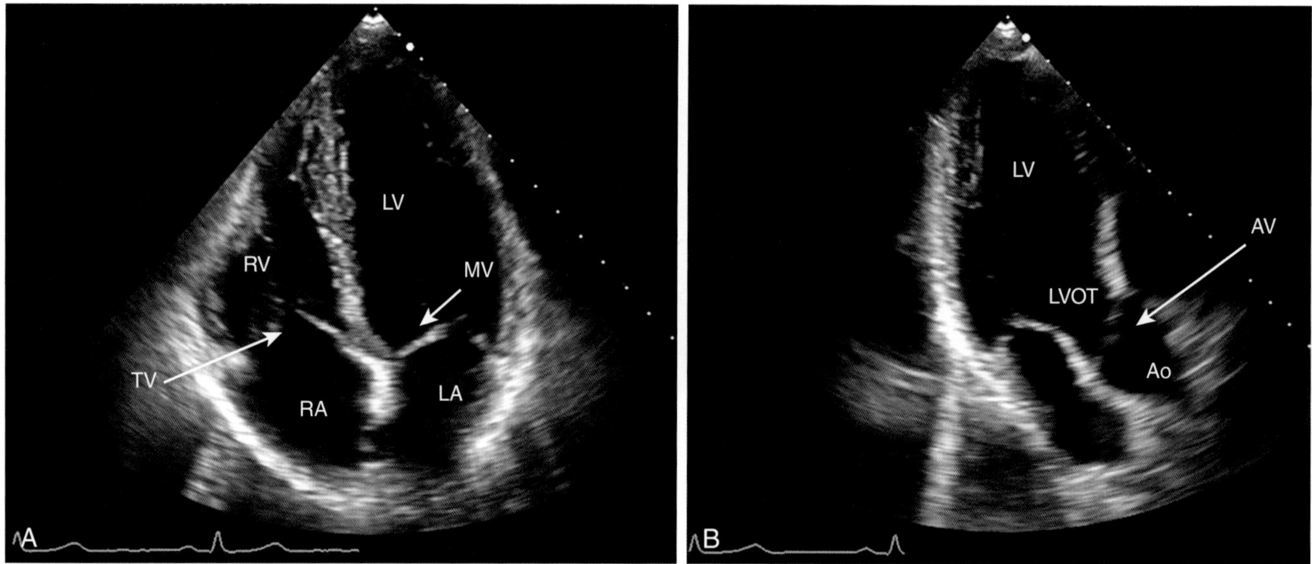

Fig. 8.6 Apical views. The apical views are obtained with the transducer at or near the point of maximal apical impulse. (A) The apical 4-chamber view shows the relationships of all four cardiac chambers. In this view, the anterolateral wall and the inferoseptum of the LV are visualized. Rotation of the transducer provides the apical long-axis view (Video 8.6A ▶). (B), which allows visualization of the left ventricular outflow tract *(LVOT)*, aortic valve *(AV)*, and proximal ascending aorta *(Ao)*. In this view, the inferolateral wall and anteroseptum are visualized (Video 8.6B ▶). *TV*, Tricuspid valve.

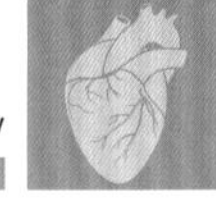

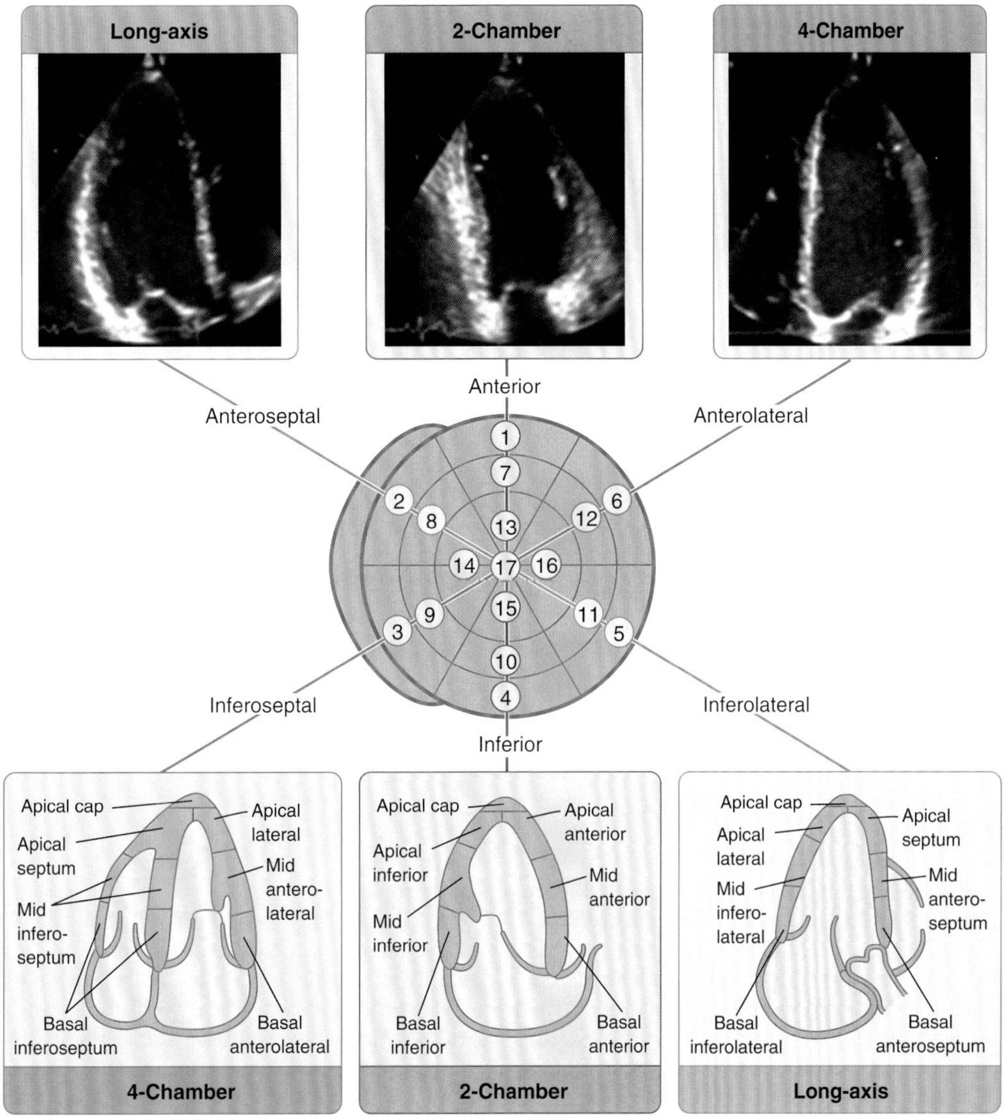

Fig. 8.7 Standard echocardiographic imaging planes and the standard 17-segment model. Standard echocardiographic imaging planes for the apical 4-chamber, 2-chamber, and long-axis views relative to the bull's-eye schematic depicting the LV segments from the standard 17-segment model. Nomenclature of the myocardial segments is shown in the bottom panels. (From Lang R, Badano L, Mor-Avi V, et al. Recommendations for cardiac chamber quantification by echocardiography in adults: an update from the ASE and EACI. *J Am Soc Echocardiogr.* 2015;28:1–39.)

Subcostal Window

Subcostal imaging is performed with the patient in a supine position and knees flexed to relax the abdominal muscles and minimize patient discomfort during optimal transducer placement in the subxiphoid region. The transducer index marker should be pointed toward the patient's left shoulder. Analogous to the apical 4-chamber view, all four chambers of the heart are visualized, including the RV free wall, inferoseptal LV wall, and anterolateral LV wall (Fig. 8.11; see Table 8.2). However, because of increased distance between the cardiac apex and the transducer, the LV apex is commonly foreshortened or poorly visualized. One benefit of this view is the perpendicular orientation of the imaging plane relative to the interatrial and interventricular septa, which allows for visualization of atrial and ventricular septal defects. This view is particularly useful for the detection of sinus venosus atrial septal defects because it enables visualization of the superior portion of the IAS. Counterclockwise 90-degree rotation of the transducer yields the subcostal LV short-axis view.

From the subcostal 4-chamber view, rotating the transducer counterclockwise with angulation to the patient's left side yields a long-axis view of the IVC as it enters the RA. The dimensions of the IVC and its change in size in response to negative intrathoracic pressure produced by respiration and intentional sniff allow estimation of right atrial pressure (RAP). The IVC should be evaluated 1 to 2 cm proximal to the junction of the RA. In normal individuals (RAP = 3 mmHg), the diameter perpendicular to the IVC long axis should be less than 2.1 cm and should have greater than 50% collapse with an inspiratory sniff. An elevated RAP of 15 mmHg is estimated when the IVC diameter is greater than 2.1 cm and there is insufficient inspiratory collapse. The proximal abdominal aorta may be imaged from the subcostal view by angulating the probe toward the patient's right side; this is an important evaluation for incidental abdominal aortic aneurysm.[10]

Suprasternal Notch Window

To facilitate imaging from the suprasternal notch window, the patient's neck should be comfortably hyperextended to create space for transducer placement. This may be achieved by

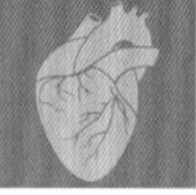

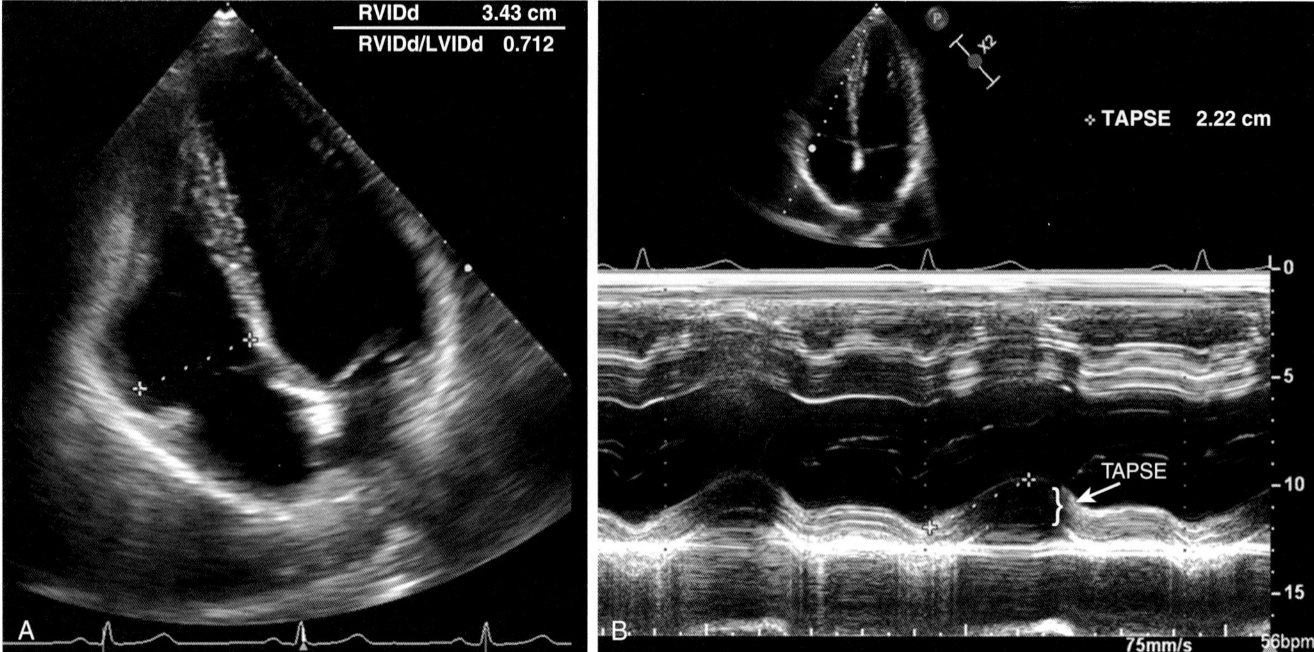

Fig. 8.8 RV size and function measurements. (A) The basal RV linear dimension is obtained from an optimized apical 4-chamber view at end-diastole, measuring 3.43 cm. (B) Tricuspid annular planar systolic excursion *(TAPSE)*, a measure of RV systolic function, is obtained by M-mode echocardiography with the cursor placed across the tricuspid lateral annulus in the apical 4-chamber view. It is defined as the total excursion of the tricuspid annulus toward the transducer during systole (i.e., the distance indicated by "}"); in this case, TAPSE was 2.2 cm.

placing a pillow behind the patient's shoulders with the patient lying supine. The suprasternal long-axis view is recorded with the transducer index marker directed toward the left supraclavicular region (approximately the 2-o'clock position). In this view, the aortic arch, the origin of the brachiocephalic arteries, and the descending thoracic aorta are visualized. A cross-sectional view of the right pulmonary artery (RPA) is just under the aortic arch (see Fig. 8.11B). Rotating the transducer clockwise, perpendicular to the long-axis view, shows the aortic arch in cross-section and the RPA in long axis. Although they are not easily visualized due to their distance from the transducer, the suprasternal short-axis view is the only view in which all four pulmonary veins entering the LA may be concurrently imaged.

M-MODE ECHOCARDIOGRAPHY

M-mode echocardiography plays an important role in comprehensive cardiac assessment.[11] M-mode tracings are displayed as a single scan line from the transducer located in a selected position within the sector width. Depth is displayed on the vertical axis against time on the horizontal axis. The rapid sampling rate of M-mode echocardiography yields excellent temporal resolution, providing precise measurements of cardiac dimensions, and allows the sonographer to more accurately evaluate highly mobile structures and assess the timing of motion in these structures. M-mode recordings should be obtained with guidance from 2D echocardiographic imaging for optimal placement of the M-mode cursor.[5]

In the PLAX view, M-mode tracings are obtained for the evaluation of LV chamber size (measured at the level of MV tip coaptation), MV, AV, and LA. Although measurements of the LV from M-mode are limited because of their one-dimensional spatial representation, they are typically accurate and reproducible in evaluating disease processes that result in symmetric changes to the LV, such as volume overload and hypertrophy.

A 2D-guided M-mode recording at the MV level is useful in the evaluation of LV systolic function, aortic insufficiency, and hypertrophic obstructive cardiomyopathy. For example, an increased E-point septal separation, which is the distance between the septal wall and the E-point (point of maximum excursion of the AMVL toward the IVS in early diastole) indicates LV dilation and systolic dysfunction. Abnormal motion of the AMVL may suggest an underlying pathology (e.g., fluttering of the leaflet in the setting of aortic insufficiency). M-mode recordings through the proximal ascending aorta at the level of the AV leaflet tip are useful for evaluating AV pathologies. For example, thickened cusps and reduced AV opening during systole suggests valve stenosis, and thin cusps with early closure indicate prevalve systolic obstruction, which can occur in hypertrophic cardiomyopathy (Fig. 8.12A).

M-mode examination is also used in the evaluation of pulmonary hypertension, RV dysfunction, and pericardial effusion and tamponade. A classic finding in pulmonary hypertension is mid-systolic closure (i.e., notching) of pulmonic valve motion, which produces a characteristic flying W shape (see Fig. 8.12B). RV systolic function is gauged by the evaluation of tricuspid annular plane systolic excursion (TAPSE) on apical M-mode recording.[12] In patients with hemodynamically significant pericardial effusions, directing the M-mode scan line through the RV free wall can demonstrate early diastolic collapse and respiratory variability in cardiac chamber size.

DOPPLER ECHOCARDIOGRAPHY

Doppler echocardiography and color-flow Doppler are essential parts of the complete echocardiographic examination. Doppler echocardiography complements 2D and M-mode assessments of cardiac structure, providing important hemodynamic information.[13]

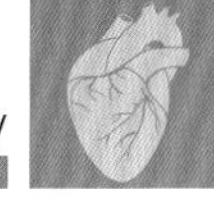

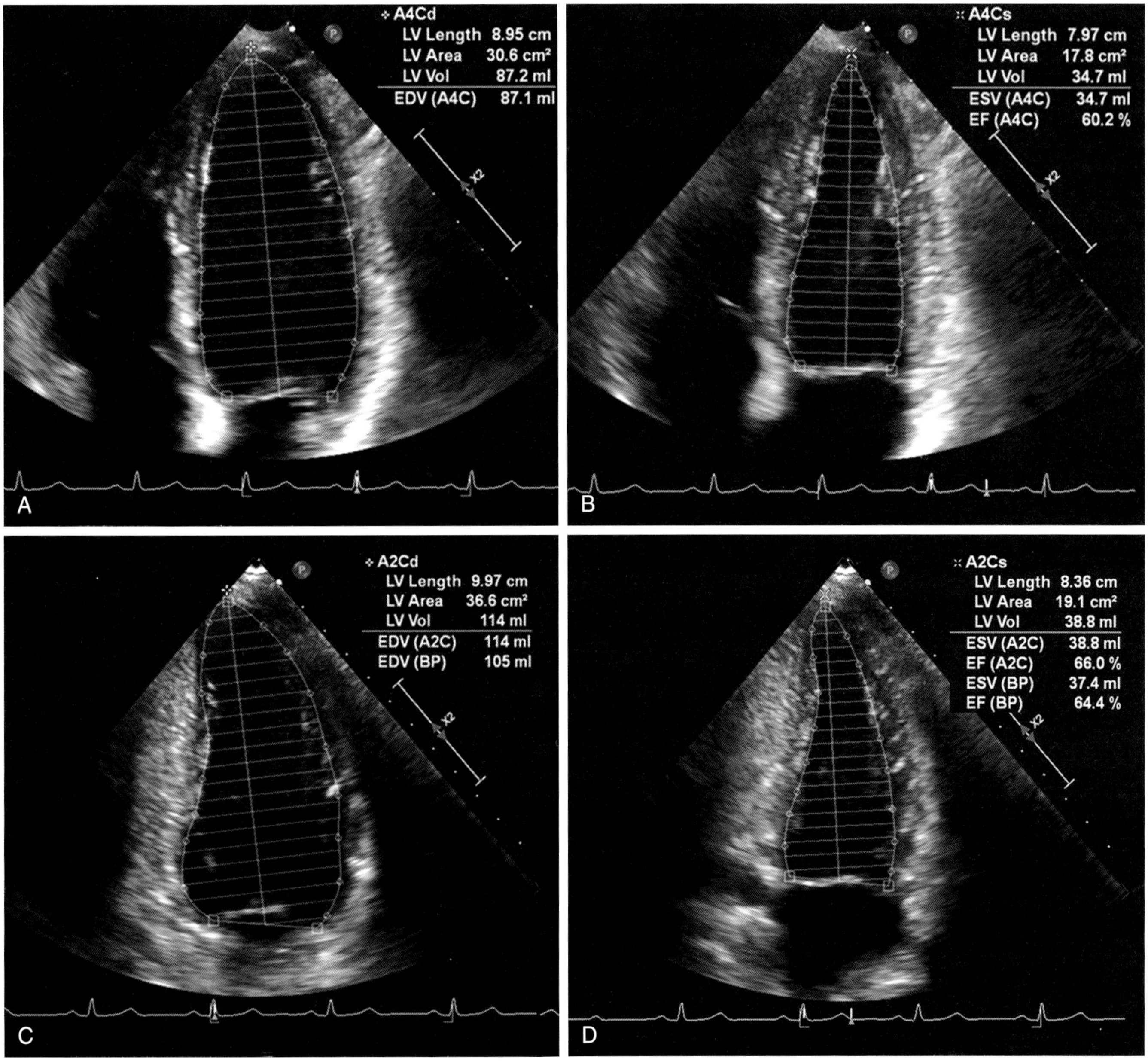

Fig. 8.9 Apical biplane LV volumes. Biplane LV volumes are obtained by tracing endocardial borders at the blood–tissue interface from apical 4-chamber views at end-diastole (A) and end-systole (B) and from apical 2-chamber views at end-diastole (C) and end-systole (D). Careful attention is required to avoid apical foreshortening with resultant underestimation of LV volumes. Biplane LV diastolic and systolic volumes (105 mL and 37.4 mL, respectively, in this example) are then used to calculate the ejection fraction (64.4%).

PRINCIPLES OF DOPPLER ECHOCARDIOGRAPHY

Doppler imaging allows evaluation of cardiac blood flow and tissue motion to provide hemodynamic data. The term *Doppler effect* describes the change in frequency of an ultrasound wave in relation to a moving target, either a red blood cell or myocardial tissue, as its distance from the transducer changes. A red blood cell or myocardial tissue moving toward the transducer will appear to shift the transmitted frequency upward on reflection of the ultrasound, resulting in a higher observed frequency. In contrast, the frequency of reflected ultrasound waves decreases when the object is moving away from the transducer. The difference between the emitted frequency and the reflected frequency is called the *Doppler shift*.

The Doppler shift (Δf) is related to the transmitted frequency (f_0), the velocity of blood flow (v), the speed of sound in blood (c = 1540 m/s), and the angle between the ultrasound beam and the direction of blood flow (θ), as expressed in the Doppler equation:

$$\Delta f = 2f_0 \times [(v \times \cos\theta)/c]$$

The highest calculated velocity is obtained by positioning the ultrasound beam parallel to flow. Measurement of the maximal frequency shift is inversely related to the angle of incidence between the ultrasound beam and the direction of motion. Imperfect alignment of the interrogation beam will result in a θ angle greater than 0 degrees and underestimation of peak velocity. Echocardiographic applications of Doppler ultrasound include continuous-wave (CW) Doppler, pulsed-wave (PW) Doppler, and color-flow imaging. Proper placement of sample volumes and appropriate adjustment of Doppler gains and display variables should be performed to ensure accurate measurements.

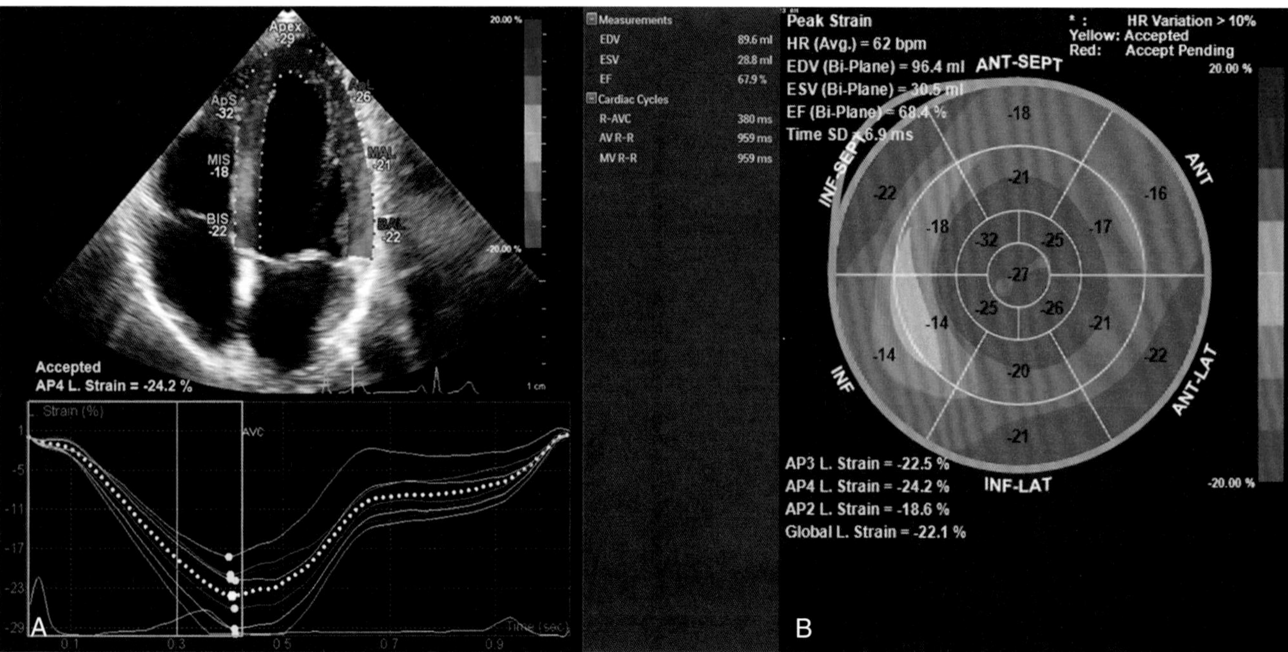

Fig. 8.10 Speckle tracking strain imaging. Apical 4-chamber view of a normal LV strain pattern with color display (A) (Video 8.10A) and a corresponding composite bull's-eye plot (B) show global longitudinal strain from the apical long-axis (3-chamber) view (–22.5%), the apical 4-chamber view (–24.2%), and the apical 2-chamber view (–18.6%), for an average longitudinal strain of –22.1%, which is in the normal range.

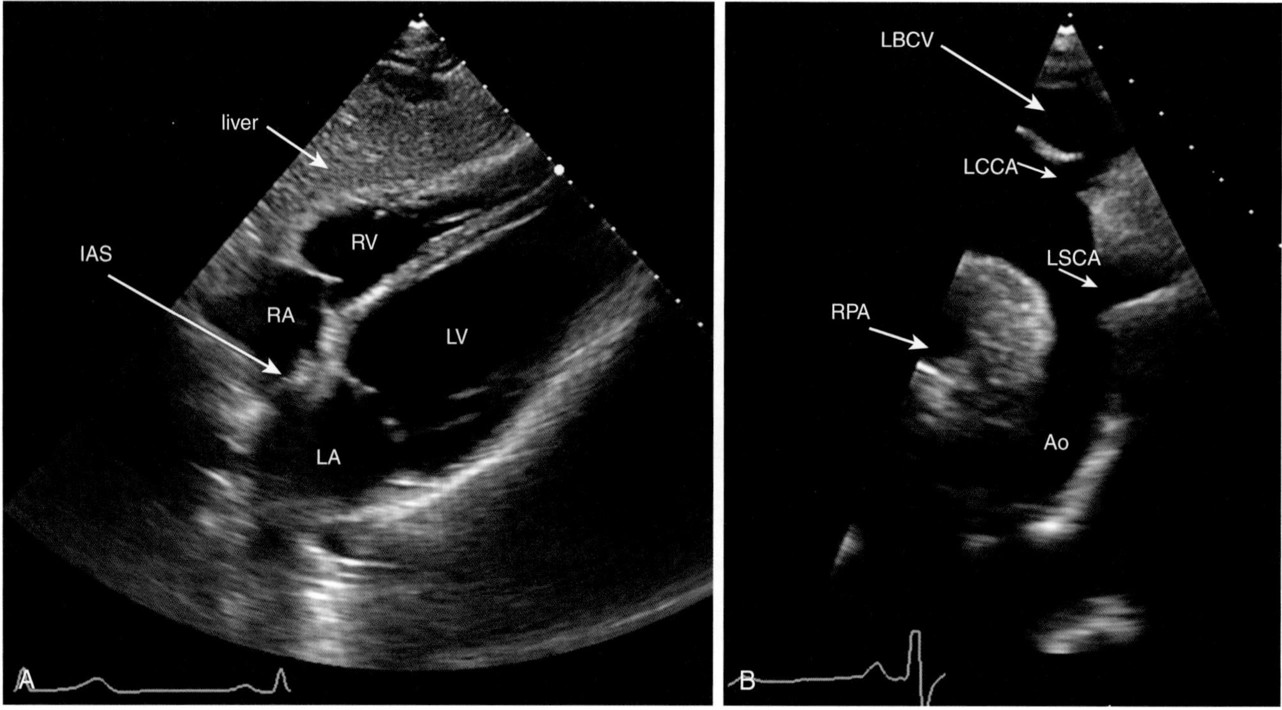

Fig. 8.11 Subcostal 4-chamber view and suprasternal notch view. (A) The ultrasound beam is perpendicular to the interatrial septum *(IAS)* and the interventricular septum in the subcostal 4-chamber view, allowing for evaluation of atrial and ventricular septal defects. In this view, the right heart is adjacent to the liver, which is in the near field. Pericardial effusion, if present, is easily visualized as an echolucent space between the liver and the RV (Video 8.11A). (B) In the suprasternal notch view, the aortic arch, the proximal descending thoracic aorta *(Ao)*, and origins of the left common carotid *(LCCA)* and left subclavian *(LSCA)* arteries are shown. The left brachiocephalic vein *(LBCV)* is in the near field, and a segment of the right pulmonary artery *(RPA)* is visualized in short axis beneath the aortic arch (Video 8.11B).

CONTINUOUS-WAVE DOPPLER ECHOCARDIOGRAPHY

CW Doppler ultrasound is used to detect and record high-velocity flows along the ultrasound beam. CW Doppler employs the use of two crystals in the transducer, one continuously transmitting and the other continuously receiving ultrasound signals. Continuous sampling along the ultrasound beam allows for the highest velocity obtainable to be measured. However, with continuous emission of the transmitted signal and simultaneous sampling of all signals along the beam path, range resolution along the ultrasound beam is impossible. Velocities obtained from CW Doppler are used to calculate intracardiac pressures, intrapulmonary pressures, and pressure gradients across stenotic or regurgitant valves.

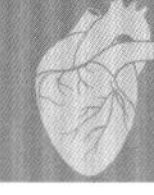

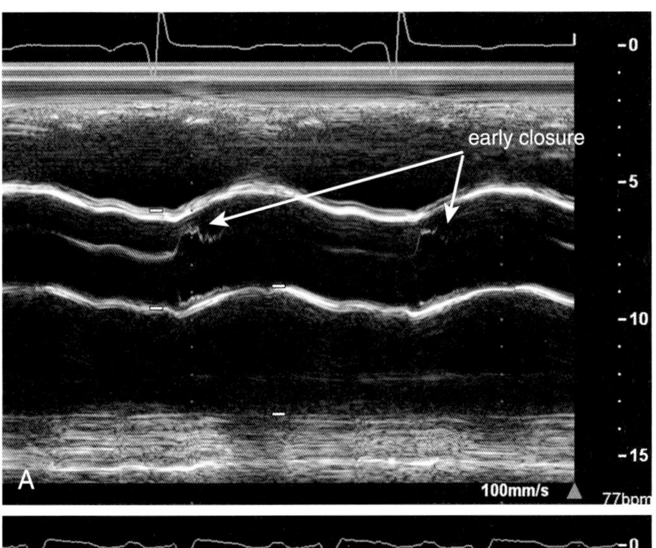

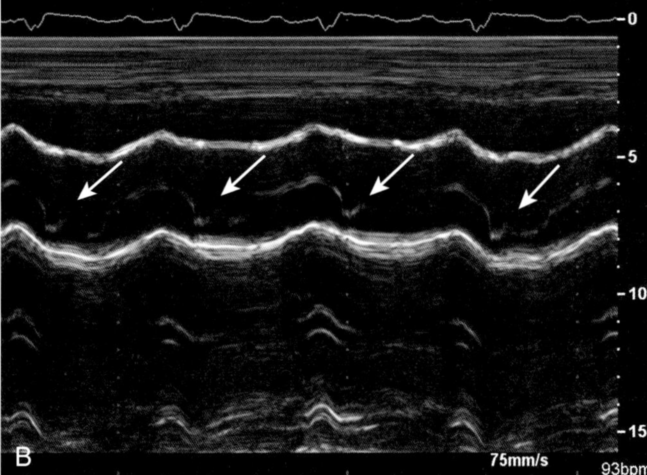

Fig. 8.12 M-mode imaging. (A) In hypertrophic cardiomyopathy, M-mode imaging at the level of the aortic valve *(AV)* shows early closure of the AV *(arrows)*, followed by fluttering of the AV leaflets. (B) In pulmonary hypertension, M-mode imaging of the pulmonic valve demonstrates mid-systolic closure, creating the characteristic flying W motion *(arrows)*.

PULSED-WAVE DOPPLER ECHOCARDIOGRAPHY

PW Doppler ultrasound allows sampling of blood flow velocity information at specific points along the transmitted beam. A pulse of ultrasound energy is transmitted, after which the transducer "listens" for the returning signal. The time interval required for the signal to return is determined by the depth of interest. The frequency of this send-wait-receive cycle is called the *pulse repetition frequency* (PRF); it is depth dependent, higher at shallower depths and lower at more distant points. To accurately characterize the frequency of an ultrasound waveform, the signal must be sampled at least twice per wavelength. Therefore, the maximum detectable frequency shift (i.e., Nyquist limit) is one-half of the PRF; below that limit, the sampling rate is insufficient to identify the Doppler frequency. Therefore, the greater the depth of the point of interest, the lower the PRF, and the lower the Nyquist limit.

If the velocity of interest exceeds the Nyquist limit, the maximum velocity cannot be resolved due to ambiguity in the speed and direction of the Doppler signal, a phenomenon known as *signal aliasing*. Methods by which aliasing can be avoided include using CW Doppler ultrasound, increasing the Nyquist limit, activating high-PRF mode, and using a lower-frequency transducer.

APPLICATION OF DOPPLER ECHOCARDIOGRAPHY: LV OUTFLOW TRACT

The apical long-axis view is used to obtain a parallel angle between the transducer beam and blood flow through the LVOT. The PW Doppler sample volume should be placed in the LVOT within 5 mm of the aortic annulus to avoid flow acceleration. Normal LVOT peak velocities range between 0.7 and 1.1 m/s. CW Doppler interrogation of the AV from the apex is used for evaluation of aortic regurgitation and aortic stenosis. Normal peak transaortic velocities range between 1.0 and 1.7 m/s. For regurgitant lesions, qualitative evaluation of Doppler jet density is concordant with severity of flow: higher-density jets correspond to higher flow volumes. Higher-severity aortic regurgitant jets show increased density, with a steeper deceleration slope, indicative of more rapid equalization of the aorta-to-LV pressure gradient; concordantly, severe or acute aortic regurgitation is suggested by a shortened pressure half-time (i.e., time required for the aorta-to-LV pressure gradient to decrease by one half).

APPLICATION OF DOPPLER ECHOCARDIOGRAPHY: PULMONARY PRESSURE ESTIMATION

An integral part of the right heart assessment is estimation of pulmonary pressures. Using the simplified Bernoulli principle, the peak tricuspid regurgitant velocity (V_{TR}) provides the pressure gradient between the RV and the RA. RAP is estimated by evaluating the IVC. Assuming there is no pressure gradient between the RV and the pulmonary artery (i.e., no pulmonary stenosis), the pulmonary artery systolic pressure (PASP) is equal to $4(V_{TR})^2$ + RAP. Pulmonary artery peak diastolic pressure (PADP) can similarly be estimated from the end-diastolic pulmonary regurgitation velocity (V_{PI}) with the following equation: PADP = $4(V_{PI})^2$ + RAP.

APPLICATION OF DOPPLER ECHOCARDIOGRAPHY: DIASTOLIC FUNCTION

Assessment of diastolic LV function requires integration of multiple parameters. PW Doppler imaging of mitral inflow velocities at the mitral leaflet tips from an apical 4-chamber view categorizes LV filling patterns as early diastolic filling (E wave) and atrial contribution to LV filling (A wave). The E/A ratio is greater than 1 in normal, young individuals, but with increasing age and impaired LV relaxation, there is increased reliance on atrial contraction to fill the LV, decreasing the ratio to less than 1. Worsening diastolic dysfunction leads to elevated LV filling pressures with rapid equalization of the LA-to-LV pressure gradient, resulting in *pseudonormalization* of the E/A ratio.

Tissue Doppler measurements of the septal and lateral mitral annulus obtained from the apical 4-chamber view during early diastolic filling (*e′*) correlate with myocardial relaxation; an elevated E/*e′* ratio greater than 14 provides a good surrogate for elevated filling pressures (Fig. 8.13; see Chapter 5).[14] Additional indices suggesting decreased ventricular compliance and increased LA pressure include shorter MV E-wave deceleration time and prolongation of the pulmonary venous atrial wave duration (PVa) relative to the mitral inflow A-wave duration (A_{dur}).

COLOR DOPPLER FLOW IMAGING

Color Doppler flow imaging is based on PW Doppler principles. However, in contrast to spectral Doppler imaging, multiple sample volumes along transducer beams are used to record Doppler shifts. Data are combined from multiple adjacent ultrasound beams and superimposed on an M-mode, 2D, or 3D template to generate a color-flow image. The Doppler

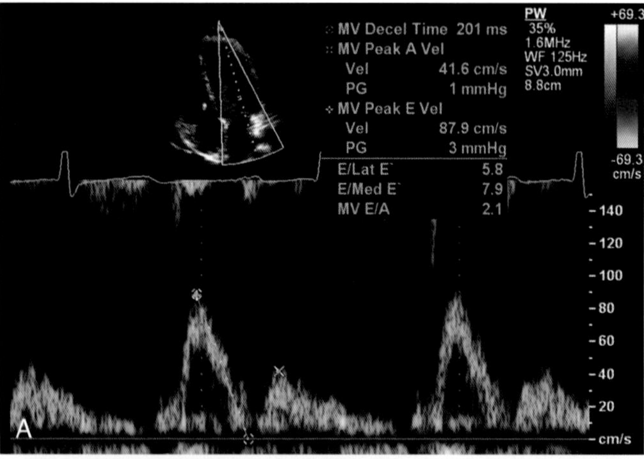

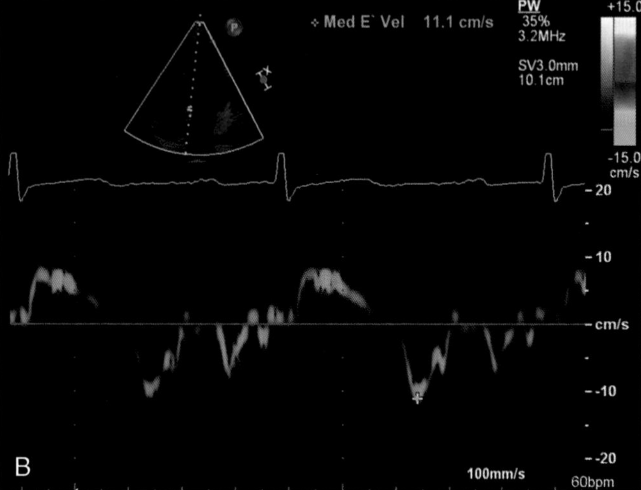

Fig. 8.13 Normal LV diastolic filling pattern and tissue Doppler velocities. (A) Pulsed-wave Doppler recording at the mitral leaflet tips during diastole in an apical 4-chamber view is used to measure early diastolic velocity (E), late diastolic velocity with atrial contraction (A), and deceleration time to characterize diastolic filling. (B) Tissue Doppler recording of the basal septum adjacent to the mitral annulus. The peak early tissue velocity (*e'*) of 11.1 cm/s is in the normal range. The ratio of peak early diastolic mitral inflow velocity (E) to peak early tissue Doppler velocity (*e'*) is an indicator of LV filling pressure.

shift at each sampling site is measured and displayed using a preset color algorithm in which blood flow directed toward the transducer is conventionally color-coded in red and flow away from the transducer is shown in blue. Lighter shades of color denote higher velocities within the Nyquist limit. Turbulence, or high variance, is coded in shades of green. Abnormal blood flow can therefore be identified by a mosaic appearance of colors, depending on the direction and velocity of flow and the degree of turbulence.

To optimize visualization of intracardiac flow patterns, the color velocity scale (or color Nyquist limit) should typically be set as high as possible to avoid detection of lower-velocity flow at the periphery of the jet. The color sector size should be adjusted to be as narrow and shallow as possible to maximize the imaging frame rate.

PROPOSED SEQUENCE OF A COMPREHENSIVE TTE STUDY

A comprehensive TTE incorporates elements from 2D, 3D, M-mode, and Doppler flow imaging to evaluate cardiac anatomy and function. Similar to point-of-care cardiac ultrasound (see Chapter 11), the diagnostic TTE examination should be directed toward answering the particular clinical question posed for each study. However, a systematic and consistent format should be followed in performing a comprehensive TTE to ensure that important pathologies are not overlooked. A proposed standard TTE imaging protocol is summarized in Table 8.2. The best views for the evaluation of specific cardiac structures are shown in Table 8.3. A set of core diagnostic elements that should be included in every TTE examination is shown in the Summary table at the end of this chapter.

TABLE 8.3 TTE: Best Views for Specific Cardiac Structures.

Anatomic Structures	*Best Views*
Cardiac Chambers	
LV	PLAX, PSAX, apical 4-chamber, apical 2-chamber, apical long-axis, subcostal 4-chamber, subcostal short-axis
RV	PLAX, RV inflow, PSAX (MV and LV levels), apical 4-chamber, subcostal 4-chamber
LA	PLAX, PSAX (AV level), apical 4-chamber, apical 2-chamber, apical long-axis, subcostal 4-chamber
RA	PSAX (AV level), apical 4-chamber, subcostal 4-chamber, subcostal short-axis
Vessels	
Aorta: ascending	PLAX (one interspace above standard view)
Aorta: arch	Suprasternal notch
Aorta: descending thoracic	Suprasternal notch, parasternal with angulation, modified apical 2-chamber, subcostal
Coronary sinus	PLAX to RV inflow (sweep), posterior angulation from apical 4-chamber
Valves	
Aortic valve	PLAX, PSAX, apical long-axis, anteriorly angulated apical 4-chamber
Mitral valve	PLAX, PSAX, apical 4-chamber, apical long-axis
Pulmonic valve	PSAX (AV level), RV outflow, subcostal short-axis (AV level)
Tricuspid valve	RV inflow, apical 4-chamber, subcostal 4-chamber and short axis

AV, Aortic valve; *MV*, mitral valve; *PLAX*, parasternal long-axis view; *PSAX*, parasternal short-axis view.

THE DIAGNOSTIC TRANSESOPHAGEAL ECHOCARDIOGRAM

INDICATIONS FOR TEE

Information acquired from TEE is complementary and supplemental to TTE findings. Relative contraindications for TEE include clinical diagnoses that may impede safe probe placement, such as esophageal varices, severe bleeding diathesis, prior upper gastrointestinal surgery, and restriction of neck mobility. Absolute contraindications for TEE include perforated viscus and active upper GI bleeding. If necessary, preprocedural evaluation by a gastroenterologist may aid in risk stratification for the procedure.

A comprehensive diagnostic TEE encompasses 2D and 3D imaging, color-flow Doppler, and spectral Doppler. TEE provides improved acoustic windows because of the absence of intervening structures (ribs) and air (lungs), as well as improved visualization of posterior structures such as the LA, MV, and descending thoracic aorta. Appropriate use criteria for echocardiography describe clinical scenarios for TEE and emphasize consideration of whether results would alter treatment. Appropriate indications may include evaluation when there is a high likelihood of a nondiagnostic TTE, evaluation of acute aortic pathology, diagnosis of infective endocarditis, evaluation for a cardiac source of embolus, and facilitation of decision making in patients undergoing cardioversion (Table 8.4).[2,3]

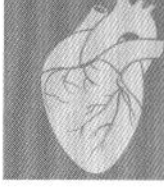

TABLE 8.4 Appropriate Indications for TEE as a Diagnostic Test.

Appropriate

Use of TEE when there is a high likelihood of a nondiagnostic TTE due to patient characteristics or inadequate visualization of relevant structures

Re-evaluation of prior TEE finding for interval change when a change in therapy is anticipated

Guidance during percutaneous noncoronary cardiac interventions, including but not limited to closure device placement, radiofrequency ablation, and percutaneous valve procedures

Suspected acute aortic pathology, including but not limited to dissection/transection

Evaluation of valve structure and function to assess suitability for, and assist in planning of, an intervention

Diagnosis of infective endocarditis when there is a moderate or high pretest probability

Evaluation for a cardiovascular source of embolus when there is no identified noncardiac source

Evaluation to facilitate clinical decision making with regard to anticoagulation, cardioversion, or radiofrequency ablation

May Be Appropriate

Evaluation for cardiovascular source of embolus when there is a previously identified noncardiac source

Rarely Appropriate

Routine use of TEE when a diagnostic TTE is reasonably anticipated to resolve all diagnostic and management concerns

Surveillance of prior TEE finding for interval change when no change in therapy is anticipated

Routine assessment of pulmonary veins in an asymptomatic patient after pulmonary vein isolation

Diagnosis of infective endocarditis with a low pretest probability

Evaluation for a cardiovascular source of embolus when there is a known cardiac source and a TEE would not change management

Evaluation when a decision has been made to anticoagulate and not to perform cardioversion

Adapted from Doherty JU, Kort S, Mehran R, Schoenhagen P, Soman P. ACC/AATS/AHA/ASE/ASNC/HRS/SCAI/SCCT/SCMR/STS 2017 appropriate use criteria for multimodality imaging in valvular heart disease: a report of the American College of Cardiology Appropriate Use Criteria Task Force, American Association for Thoracic Surgery, American Heart Association, American Society of Echocardiography, American Society of Nuclear Cardiology, Heart Rhythm Society, Society for Cardiovascular Angiography and Interventions, Society of Cardiovascular Computed Tomography, Society for Cardiovascular Magnetic Resonance, and Society of Thoracic Surgeons. *J Am Coll Cardiol.* 2017;70:1647–1672; and Doherty JU, Kort S, Mehran R, et al. ACC/AATS/AHA/ASE/ASNC/HRS/SCAI/SCCT/SCMR/STS 2019 appropriate use criteria for multimodality imaging in the assessment of cardiac structure and function in nonvalvular heart disease: a report of the American College of Cardiology Appropriate Use Criteria Task Force, American Association for Thoracic Surgery, American Heart Association, American Society of Echocardiography, American Society of Nuclear Cardiology, Heart Rhythm Society, Society for Cardiovascular Angiography and Interventions, Society of Cardiovascular Computed Tomography, Society for Cardiovascular Magnetic Resonance, and the Society of Thoracic Surgeons. *J Am Coll Cardiol.* 2019;73:488–516.

TRAINING AND PERSONNEL

Providers should complete the appropriate training and credentialing needed within their specialty for independent practice in TEE. Suggested minimum requirements for TEE procedures from the American College of Cardiology's Core Training Symposium include interpretation of 300 complete TTE examinations and performance of at least 50 supervised TEE studies, including 25 esophageal intubations.[15] These recommendations are concordant with most published guidelines and competency statements, but they also acknowledge the need for an understanding of surgical and interventional cardiology procedures by practitioners performing intraprocedural TEE, as well as additional advanced training in echocardiography.[15–18] Clinical competence statements in echocardiography detail technical skills in which providers must be proficient to safely perform TEE (Table 8.5).[18] Laboratory processes for continuous quality improvement review should be in place.[19]

TABLE 8.5 Technical Skills Necessary for Performance of TEE.

Uses conscious sedation safely and effectively

Exhibits proficiency in performing a complete TTE examination, using all echocardiographic modalities relevant to the case

Safely passes TEE probe into the esophagus and stomach and adjusts probe position to obtain necessary tomographic images and Doppler data

Operates ultrasonographic instrumentation correctly, including controls affecting the quality of displayed data

Recognizes abnormalities of cardiac structure and function detected from TEE images, distinguishes normal from abnormal findings, and recognizes artifacts

Performs qualitative and quantitative analyses of echocardiographic data

Produces a cogent written report of echocardiographic findings and their clinical implications

Adapted from Quiñones MA, Douglas PS, Foster E, et al. ACC/AHA clinical competence statement on echocardiography: a report of the ACC/AHA/ACP/ASIM Task Force on Clinical Competence. *J Am Soc Echocardiogr.* 2003;16:379–402.

TABLE 8.6 Clinical Features Associated With Increased Risk of Respiratory Compromise During Moderate Conscious Sedation.

Airway patency—prior history of airway management problems, obstructive sleep apnea, small mouth opening, significant malocclusion

Elderly patient—increased sensitivity to sedatives and higher incidence of interactions with other medications

Congestive heart failure—severe LV systolic dysfunction, critical aortic stenosis

Underlying respiratory disease—oxygen dependency, severe pulmonary hypertension, or cor pulmonale

Neurologic or neuromuscular disorders that compromise respiration or swallowing; inability to follow commands

Nonfasting state

TABLE 8.7 Risk of Complications of TEE.

Complication	*Incidence (%)*
Mortality	<0.01–0.02
Esophageal perforation	<0.01
Major bleeding	<0.01
Minor bleeding	0.01–0.2
Bronchospasm	0.07
Dental injury	0.1
Arrhythmia	0.06–0.3
Dysphagia	1.8
Hoarseness	12
Lip injury	13

Adapted from Hilberath J, Oakes D, Shernan S, Bulwer B, D'Ambra M, Eltzschig H. Safety of transesophageal echocardiography. *J Am Soc Echocardiogr.* 2010;23:1115–1127.

PATIENT PREPARATION AND SEDATION

A brief history should be taken to document symptoms, identify current medications, and review indications for TEE. For patients who are deemed to be at higher risk for respiratory compromise during moderate sedation, anesthesia support may be necessary (Table 8.6).[20] Endocarditis prophylaxis is not indicated for TEE.[21] On the day of the procedure, patients should refrain from oral intake for 6 hours preceding TEE.[22] Written informed consent should be obtained. Overall, the risk of TEE is low, with dysphagia occurring in 1% to 2% of cases and more severe complications (e.g., esophageal trauma, oropharyngeal bleeding, arrhythmia) occurring in less than 1% of cases (Table 8.7).[23–26]

Intravenous access is obtained for administration of medications during the procedure. Electrocardiographic telemetry, pulse oximetry, an automated blood pressure cuff, and, in some facilities, capnography, are applied continuously for patient

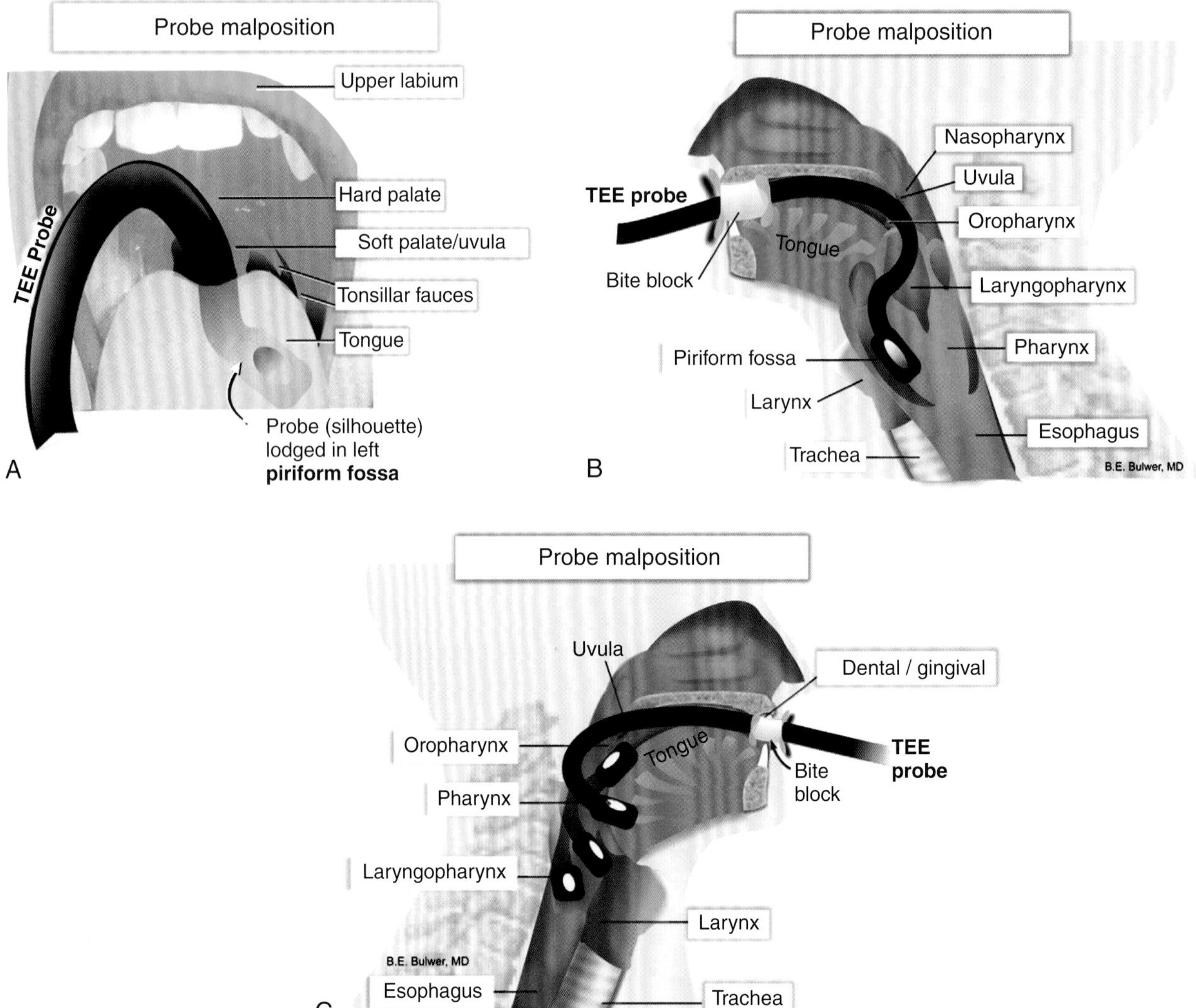

Fig. 8.14 TEE probe malposition. (A and B) Difficulty during probe insertion can be encountered if the TEE probe is lodged into one of the piriform sinuses. (C) In addition to causing mucosal injury to the oropharynx, the TEE probe can occasionally become distorted in extreme flexion. (From Hilberath J, Oakes D, Shernan S, Bulwer B, D'Ambra M, Eltzschig H. Safety of transesophageal echocardiography. *J Am Soc Echocardiogr* 2010;23:1115–1127.)

monitoring. Local anesthesia of the palate, tonsils, and posterior pharynx with a topical anesthetic (e.g., lidocaine) diminishes the gag reflex, facilitating patient comfort. Dosing of agents for moderate conscious sedation should be adjusted to the minimum amount necessary to avoid patient confusion or hemodynamic instability. Medications that reverse the effects of agents, such as naloxone (for opioid agents) or flumazenil (for benzodiazepine agents), should be readily available.

ESOPHAGEAL INTUBATION

In preparation for esophageal intubation, patients should be advised that they may experience mild abdominal discomfort and that pharyngeal spasm (gag reflex) may be triggered during probe placement. Dentures should be removed, and a bite block should be placed before initiation of sedation. The probe should be maintained in an unlocked, central position because locking of flexion controls inhibits maximal flexibility of the probe.

Patients are placed in a left lateral decubitus position to decrease the likelihood of aspiration during the procedure. After adequate sedation is achieved, after application of ultrasound gel to the transducer, the probe is advanced through the bite block. Resting the probe tip on the posterior tongue while the patient acclimates to the sensation decreases reflexive laryngeal spasm. Maintaining a neutral, central position decreases lateral deviation into the piriform fossa (Fig. 8.14). The patient's head should be slightly flexed with the probe mildly anteflexed to decrease the likelihood of tracheal intubation. Tracheal intubation is a noxious stimulant and should be suspected if the patient develops persistent coughing or agitation. Intubated patients should have larger-bore orogastric or nasogastric tubes removed because poor ultrasound penetration through air-filled tubes hinders image acquisition. During probe placement, the tip should be positioned posterior to the endotracheal tube while the mandible is pulled forward.

PROBE MANIPULATION AND STANDARD IMAGING VIEWS

Guidelines published by the American Society of Echocardiography (ASE) and the Society of Cardiovascular Anesthesiologists (SCA) established TEE views for standard examinations, comprising 28 standard views (Table 8.8).[27] TEE imaging uses a steerable, multiplane TEE transducer probe, allowing for operator-manipulable controls to adjust and rotate the imaging plane. Optimal TEE probe placement within the esophagus varies among individuals because of differences in esophageal location relative to the heart.

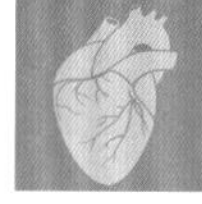

TABLE 8.8 Standard TEE Views.

View	*Transducer Angle in Degrees (±10 Degrees Each View)*
Mid-esophageal (ME) Views	
[1] ME 5-chamber view	0
[2] ME 4-chamber view	10
[3] ME mitral commissural view	60
[4] ME 2-chamber view	90
[5] ME LV long-axis view	130
[6] ME AV long-axis view	130
[7] ME right pulmonary vein view	10
[8] ME AV short-axis view	40
[9] ME RV inflow-outflow view	70
[10] ME bicaval TV view	70
[11] ME bicaval view	100
[12] ME left atrial appendage	90
Upper-esophageal (UE) Views	
[13] UE ascending aorta long axis view	100
[14] UE ascending aorta short-axis view	30
[15] UE pulmonary veins view	90
Transgastric (TG) Views	
[16] TG LV basal short-axis view	0
[17] TG LV mid-papillary short-axis view	0
[18] TG LV apical short-axis view	0
[19] TG RV basal view	0
[20] TG RV inflow-outflow view	0
[21] TG 2-chamber view	90
[22] TG LV long-axis view	120
[23] TG RV inflow view	90
[24] Deep TG LV view	0
Aortic Views	
[25] ME aorta descending short-axis view	0
[26] ME aorta descending long-axis view	90
[27] UE aortic arch long-axis view	0
[28] UE aortic arch short-axis view	90

AV, Aortic valve.

Advancing and *withdrawing* the probe moves the transducer tip to different positions within the esophagus and stomach. Probe placement sites include *upper-esophageal, mid-esophageal, transgastric*, and *deep transgastric* positions. At each position, manipulation of the probe allows various image views. Manual *turning* of the probe turns the probe tip toward the patient's right side (clockwise turn) or left side (counterclockwise turn). Because there are no articulating components between the probe tip and controls, turning should simultaneously include the handle and transducer to reduce probe torsion. Flexion of the probe tip *rightward* or *leftward* within the esophagus is controlled by the small control knob on the probe handle. The larger control knob allows for anterior flexion of the transducer tip (*anteroflexion*) or posterior flexion (*retroflexion*). The button controls on the probe handle allow rotational steering of the imaging plane between 0 and 180 degrees (Fig. 8.15).

IMAGE FORMATTING AND DISPLAY

By convention, because of the posterior placement of the probe relative to the heart, anterior structures are displayed in the far field. At 0 degrees of rotation, left-sided cardiac structures are shown on the right side of the display. Matrix array transducers allow acquisition of a 3D-image volume data set rather than a single-plane image acquisition. 3D volume data sets allow concurrent display of two image slices from different rotational positions in the imaging field. Typically, the secondary image is 90 degrees offset from the primary image (Fig. 8.16).

Sequencing of TEE imaging should be initially focused on the primary study indication, given that the procedure may be truncated due to patient discomfort, hemodynamic instability, or respiratory difficulties during sedation. After this, the goal of TEE should be to complete a comprehensive study. Imaging protocols typically start in the mid-esophageal position because probe placements in the upper esophagus and in transgastric positions tend to be more uncomfortable. Imaging depth should be adjusted throughout the examination to optimize imaging.

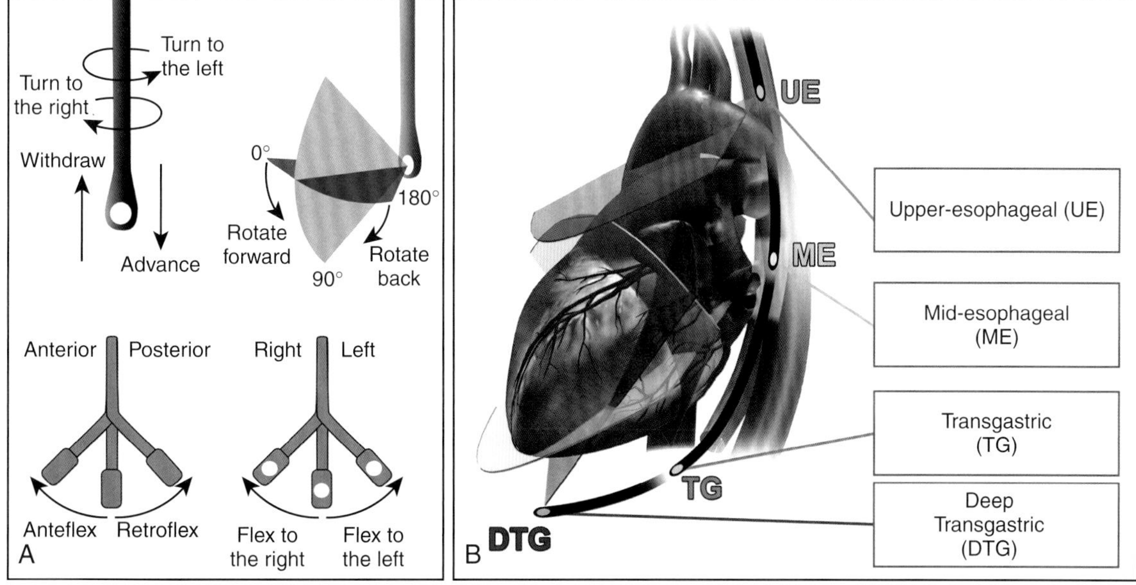

Fig. 8.15 TEE probe manipulation and esophageal position. (A) A button on the probe handle electronically controls the transducer angle. Controls on the handle allow manipulation of the probe tip with anteflextion /retroflextion (larger control knob), and right/left flexion (smaller control knob). (B) Probe placement positions. (From Hahn R, Abraham T, Adams M, et al. Guidelines for performing a comprehensive transesophageal echocardiographic examination: recommendations from the American Society of Echocardiography and the Society of Cardiovascular Anesthesiologists. *J Am Soc Echocardiogr.* 2013;26:921–964.)

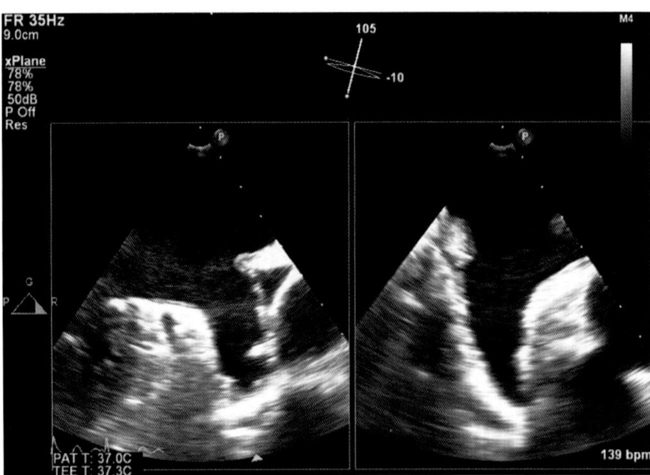

Fig. 8.16 Biplane image of the left atrial appendage. The primary image (view 12; *left side*) and the secondary image in a perpendicular plane (*right side*) are simultaneously displayed (Video 8.16).

TRANSESOPHAGEAL IMAGING VIEWS

LEFT AND RIGHT VENTRICLES

The mid-esophageal 4-chamber view provides an excellent overview of biventricular systolic function and chamber size and is obtained by advancing the transducer to a depth of approximately 30 cm, at a transducer angle of 0 degrees, with retroflexion and mild flexion of the tip toward the LV apex (Table 8.9 and Fig. 8.17A [view 2]). The long axis of the RV and LV should be vertical in the imaging sector. This view allows evaluation of the inferoseptal and anterolateral walls.[5] Anteflexion from this view produces the mid-esophageal 5-chamber view, with visualization of the LVOT and AV (see Fig. 8.17B [view 1]). The LV apex tends to be foreshortened because of the challenge of aligning the transducer tip with the true long axis.

From the 4-chamber view, the 2-chamber view is obtained by rotating to a transducer angle of approximately 90 degrees. Before the 2-chamber view is reached, the mitral commissural view (see Fig. 8.17C [view 3]) is obtained at approximately 60 degrees. As in TTE, the LV anterior and inferior walls are visualized with the 2-chamber view (see Fig. 8.17D [view 4]).[5] The long-axis view is obtained by further rotating the transducer to approximately 120 degrees, allowing visualization of the anteroseptum, inferolateral wall, LVOT, and AV (Fig. 8.18A [view 5]).[5]

Transgastric views are excellent for the assessment of biventricular systolic function; they are obtained by advancing the probe past the gastroesophageal sphincter in a neutral position (see Table 8.9). In the stomach, the probe tip should be anteflexed for an LV short-axis view. In this view, the image is flipped compared with TTE, with the inferior wall closer to the transducer and the anterior wall in the far field. Higher in the stomach, the LV short-axis view is at the base of the heart with an en face view of the MV (Fig. 8.19A [view 16]); the AMVL is on the left side of the image. With slight advancement of the probe, the anterolateral papillary muscle is seen in the far field (see Fig. 8.19C [view 17]). Turning of the probe clockwise moves the probe toward the right side of the patient, with visualization of the RV at the basal level (view 19), and with slight advancement of the probe, the inflow-outflow level is reached (view 20). Further advancement of the probe to the distal stomach allows visualization of a deep transgastric 4-chamber view with the LV apex in the near field (see Fig. 8.19D [view 24]). From the transgastric LV short-axis view, rotation of the transducer angle to approximately 90 degrees produces a 2-chamber view (view 21), and rotation to 120 degrees produces a long-axis view (view 22). Clockwise rotation of the probe from the long-axis view allows visualization of RV inflow and assessment of TV function (see Fig. 8.19B [view 23]).

TABLE 8.9 Standard TEE Views for Cardiac Structures: Cardiac Chambers and Great Vessels.

Structure	*View*	*Transducer Angle (Degrees) and Probe Position*
Cardiac Chambers		
Left ventricle	[2] ME 4-chamber view	10, tip leftward and retroflexed
	[4] ME 2-chamber view	90
	[5] ME LV long-axis view	130
	[17] TG LV mid-papillary short-axis view	0, anteflexed
	[21] TG 2-chamber view	90
	[24] Deep TG LV view	0
	3D echocardiography	Entire LV in imaging sector
Left atrium	[2] ME 4-chamber view	10, decreased depth
	[4] ME 2-chamber view	90
	[5] ME LV long-axis view	130
Left atrial appendage	[12] ME left atrial appendage	90, biplane imaging
Pulmonary veins	[15] UE pulmonary veins view	90, tip rightward for right PV
	[7] ME right pulmonary vein view	10, or tip leftward for left PV
Right ventricle	[2] ME 4-chamber view	10, tip rightward
	[9] ME RV inflow-outflow view	70
	[20] TG RV inflow-outflow view	0, tip rightward
	[23] TG RV inflow view	90
Right atrium	[2] ME 4-chamber view	10, decreased depth
	[23] TG RV inflow view	90
Interatrial	[11] ME bicaval view	100, tip rightward
	3D echocardiography	100, decreased depth
Great Vessels		
Ascending aorta	[6] ME AoV long-axis view	130
	[13] UE ascending aorta long-axis view	100, tip rightward
	[14] UE ascending aorta short-axis view	30
Descending aorta	[25] ME aorta descending short-axis view	0
	[26] ME aorta descending long-axis view	90
	[27] UE aortic arch long-axis view	0
	[28] UE aortic arch short-axis view	90
Pulmonary artery	[9] ME RV inflow-outflow view	70, probe to UE, tip rightward
	[28] UE aortic arch short-axis view	90

AoV, Aortic valve; *ME*, mid-esophageal; *PV*, pulmonary veins; *TG*, transgastric; *UE*, upper-esophageal.

ATRIA AND LEFT ATRIAL APPENDAGE

The pulmonary veins, left atrial appendage (LAA), and MV are well visualized by TEE. The LAA is best visualized from the

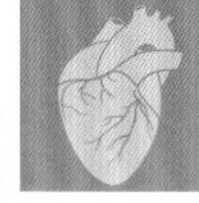

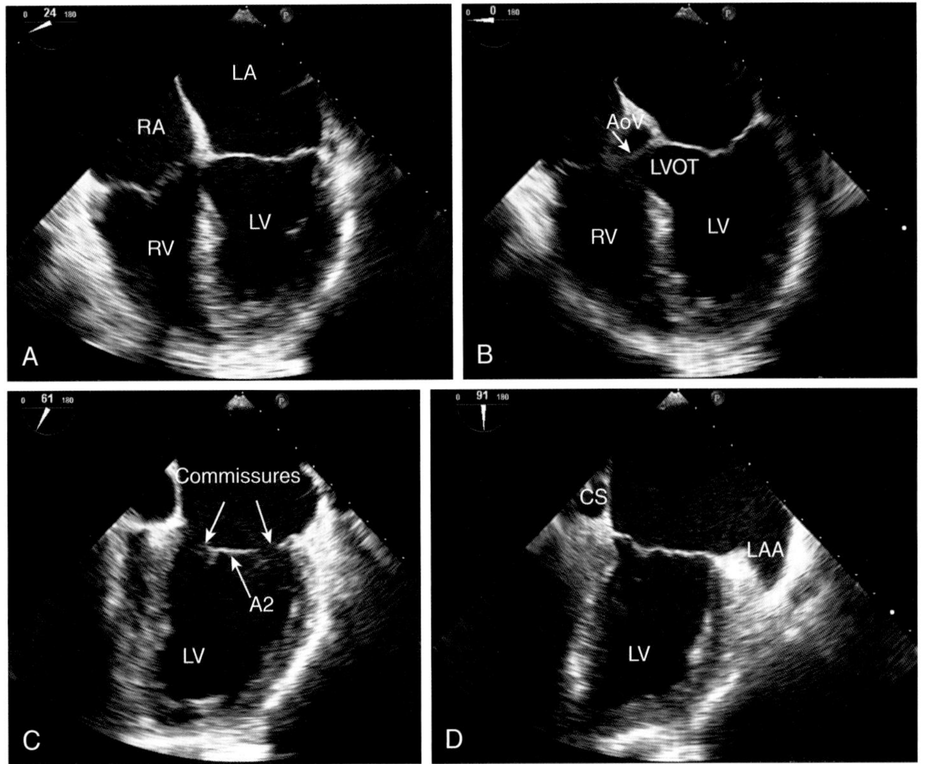

Fig. 8.17 The left ventricular views. (A) Mid-esophageal 4-chamber view (view 2): the atria are in the near field, and the ventricles are in the far field (Video 8.17A). (B) Mid-esophageal 5-chamber view (view 1) with the probe tip slightly anteflexed: the left ventricular outflow tract *(LVOT)* and aortic valve *(AoV)* are seen (Video 8.17B). (C) Mid-esophageal mitral commissural view (view 3): the midportion of the anterior mitral valve leaflet (A2 segment) is seen with commissures on either side of the segment (Video 8.17C). (D) Mid-esophageal 2-chamber view (view 4): the left atrial appendage *(LAA)* is on the right side of the display, and the coronary sinus *(CS)* is on the left side (Video 17D).

mid-esophageal position, at a transducer angle of approximately 90 degrees. Simultaneous biplane imaging of an orthogonal view of the LAA aids in excluding appendage thrombi before cardioversion procedures (see Fig. 8.16 [view 12]).

The bicaval view is obtained from the mid-esophageal position, at a transducer angle of approximately 100 degrees, with the probe turned toward the patient's right side. In this view, the IAS bisects the sector horizontally (see Fig. 8.18C [view 11]). Just below the septum, the superior vena cava enters the RA from the right side of the image. The septum is well aligned in this view for 3D volume acquisition to assess for a patent foramen ovale (PFO) or atrial septal defects. Clockwise turning of the probe tip further allows visualization of the right upper pulmonary vein entering the LA (view 15; see Fig. 8.20). For visualization of the TV below the IAS, the transducer angle should be moved to approximately 60 degrees (view 10).

The left pulmonary veins are visualized from the LAA view at approximately 80 to 90 degrees (Fig. 8.20A [view 12]) by withdrawing and turning the probe counterclockwise. The os of the left lower pulmonary vein is seen with mild advancement of the probe (see Fig. 8.20B [view 15]).

AORTIC VALVE AND AORTA

A short-axis view of the AV is obtained from the mid-esophageal view with anteflexion of the probe tip at a transducer angle of approximately 40 degrees (Fig. 8.21A[view 8] and Table 8.10). Care should be taken to have an en face view of the valve. With slight advancement of the probe at a transducer angle of approximately 70 degrees, the RV inflow-outflow view is accessed, with the TV on the left side, and the pulmonic valve on the right (see Fig. 8.21B [view 9]). Rotation of the transducer angle to the long-axis view of the AV (approximately 120 degrees) allows visualization of the LVOT and the proximal ascending aorta (see Fig. 8.18B [view 6]). Color Doppler flow interrogation of the AV should be performed for short- and long-axis views. 3DE imaging of the AV may be helpful in evaluating calcification for stenosis severity assessment. By convention, when displaying 3D images from the aorta side of the valve, the AV is shown with the right coronary cusp at the bottom of the image.

Optimized long-axis views of the ascending aorta are obtained starting from the mid-esophageal long-axis view of the AV and LVOT (see Table 8.9). With clockwise rotation and slight withdrawal of the probe, the ascending aorta is visualized (see Fig. 8.18D [view 13]). Rotation of the transducer angle to 90 degrees produces the ascending aorta short-axis view [view 14]. These views are excellent for exclusion of a proximal ascending aortic dissection or aneurysm. Aortic dimensions should be measured at end-diastole from several locations, typically at the level of the sinuses, the sinotubular junction, and the mid-ascending aorta. As the probe is withdrawn, poor ultrasound penetration through the air-filled trachea obscures visualization of the distal ascending aorta. To image this region, other tomographic imaging modalities, such as magnetic resonance angiography (MRA) or computed tomography (CT), should be used.

Anatomically, the esophagus lies between the heart and the descending aorta. Manual turning of the probe to image from the opposite side of the esophagus allows visualization of the descending thoracic aorta and proximal abdominal aorta. This view is excellent when evaluating for aortic dissection,

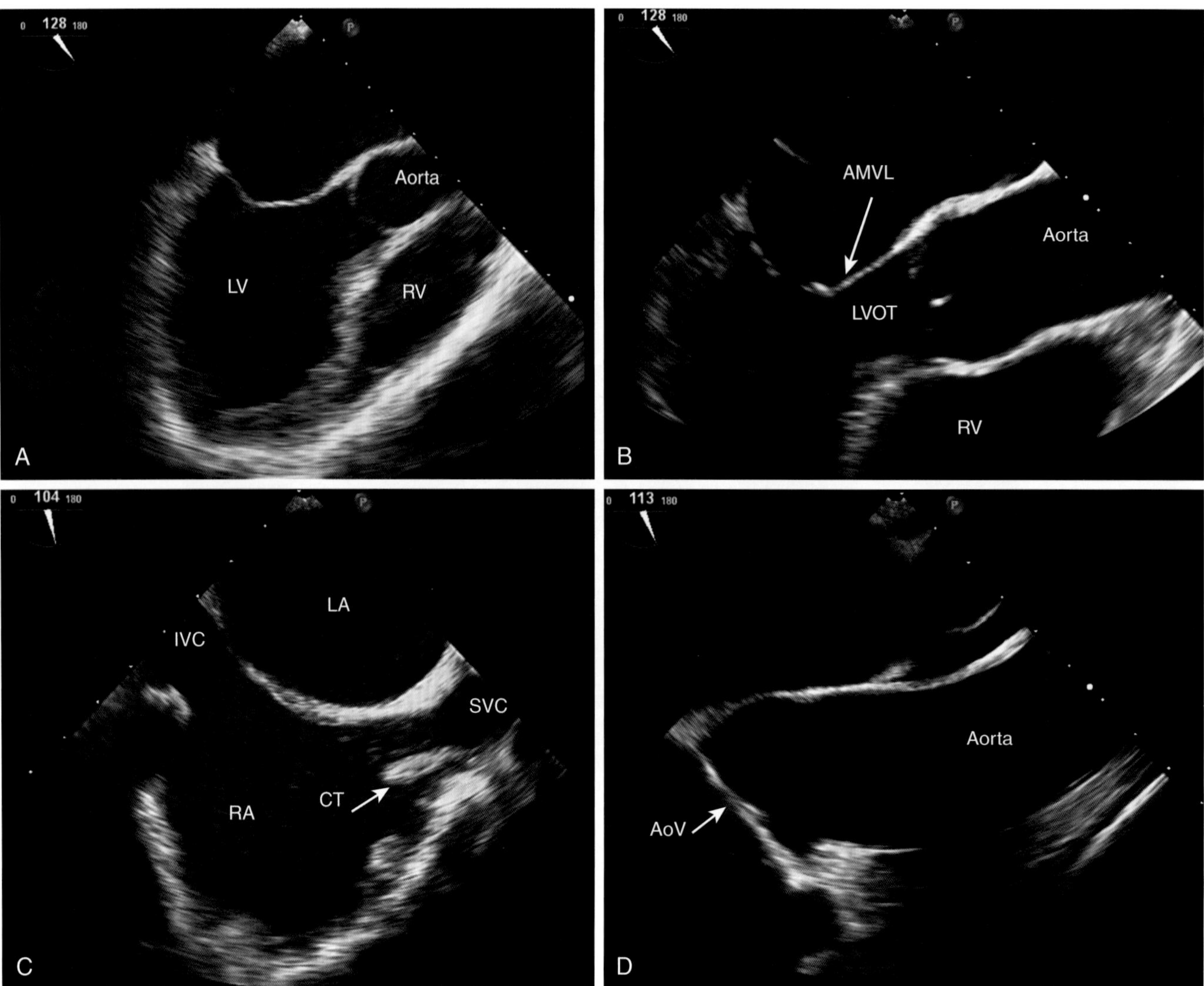

Fig. 8.18 LV long-axis, bicaval, and proximal aorta views. (A) Mid-esophageal LV long-axis view (view 5): the *LV* and the ascending aorta *(Aorta)* are seen, with a portion of the *RV* in the far field, toward the right side of the image (Video 8.18A). (B) Mid-esophageal ascending aorta long-axis view (view 6): the anterior mitral valve leaflet *(AMVL)* is adjacent to the posterior aspect of the *aortic valve (AoV)*; this view is obtained by decreasing the depth from the LV long-axis view and rotating the probe slightly so that the *AoV* is in the center of the sector (Video 8.18B). (C) Mid-esophageal bicaval view (view 11): the LA is in the near field with the interatrial septum bisecting the imaging sector. The superior vena cava *(SVC)* drains on the right side of the display; adjacent to the SVC is the crista terminalis *(CT)*. The AoV is visualized on the left side of the display (Video 18C). (D) Upper-esophageal ascending aorta long-axis view (view 13) (Video 18D). *IVC*, Inferior vena cava; *LVOT*, LV outflow tract.

atheroma, and periaortic hematoma (Fig. 8.22 [views 25 and 26]). As the probe is withdrawn to the distal aortic arch, the os of the left subclavian artery (on the right side of the image display) and the aortic arch are visualized (view 27).

MITRAL VALVE

Comprehensive evaluation of the MV should be performed from a range of transducer positions and angles (see Table 8.10). Anatomically, the MV is saddle shaped, with leaflet coaptation running along the major axis of the valve and the AMVL having a smaller circumferential attachment relative to the PMVL. The AV lies anterior to the AMVL, and the os of the LAA lies lateral to the valve. Each of the two mitral leaflets (A, anterior, and P, posterior) is subdivided into three segments—lateral (A1 and P1), middle (A2 and P2), and medial (A3 and P3) (Fig. 8.23).[27]

Anatomic orientation of the MV leaflets during imaging is critical, particularly for intraprocedural and surgical planning. At a transducer angle of 0 degrees (see Fig. 8.17A [view 2]), the image plane bisects through the center point of the MV, with the A2 segment seen on the left side of the display and the P2 segment on the right side. As the transducer angle is increased, the imaging plane rotates in the plane perpendicular to the MV plane (see Fig. 8.23). At the mitral commissural view (see Fig. 8.17C [view 3]), the medial (A3/P3) and lateral (A1/P1) commissures are seen on either side of the midportion of the AMVL (A2). With the AV long-axis view (transducer angle, 130 degrees; see Fig. 8.18B [view 6]), A2 is displayed on the right side of the image, just adjacent to the AV.

3D echocardiography of the MV allows detailed visualization of leaflet anatomy and the subvalvular apparatus.[28] By convention, en face views are displayed from the atrial side of the valve with an orientation in which the AV is at the top of the display and the PMVL is at the bottom. In this orientation, the medial side of the MV is on the right of the display.

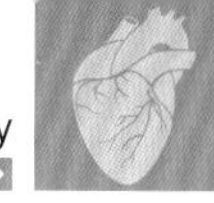

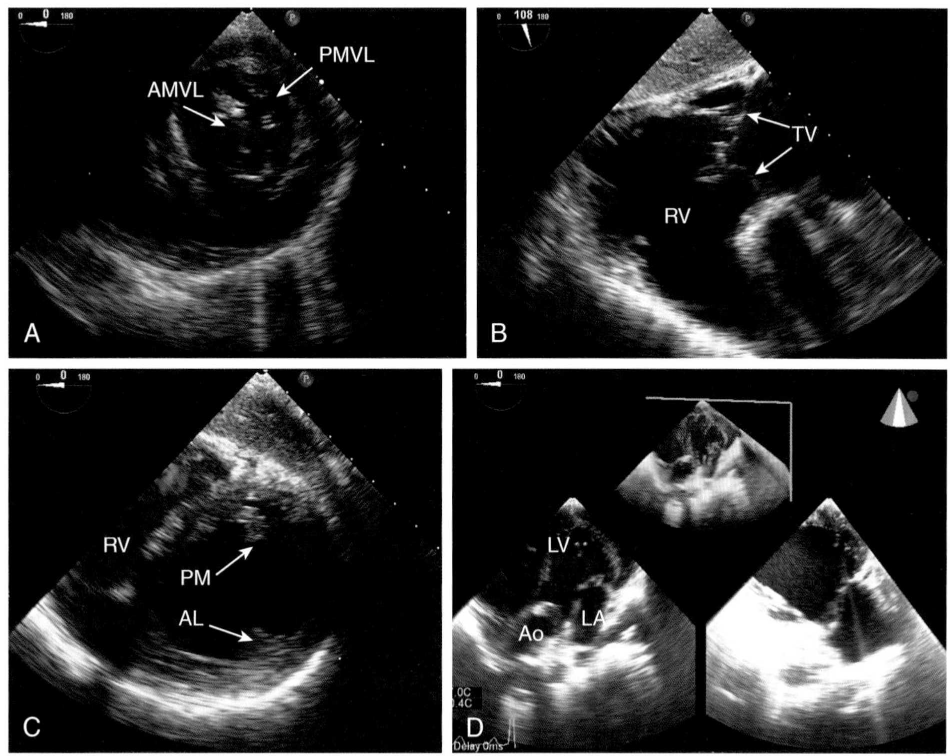

Fig. 8.19 Transgastric views. (A) Transgastric LV basal short-axis view (view 16). The anterior mitral valve leaflet *(AMVL)* is on the left side of the display, and the posterior mitral valve leaflet *(PMVL)* is on the right (Video 19A). (B) Transgastric RV inflow view (view 23). The RV is on the left side of the display, and the RA is on the right side of the display (Video 8.19B). (C) Transgastric LV mid-papillary short-axis view (view 17). The inferior wall and the posteromedial *(PM)* papillary muscle are in the near field, and the anterior wall and anterolateral *(AL)* papillary muscle are in the far field (Video 8.19C). (D) Biplane imaging of the LV from a deep gastric position (view 24). The LV is in the near field, with the AV in the far field. The orthogonal view of the LV is concurrently displayed on the right side of part D (Video 8.19D). *Ao*, Aorta; *TV*, tricuspid valve.

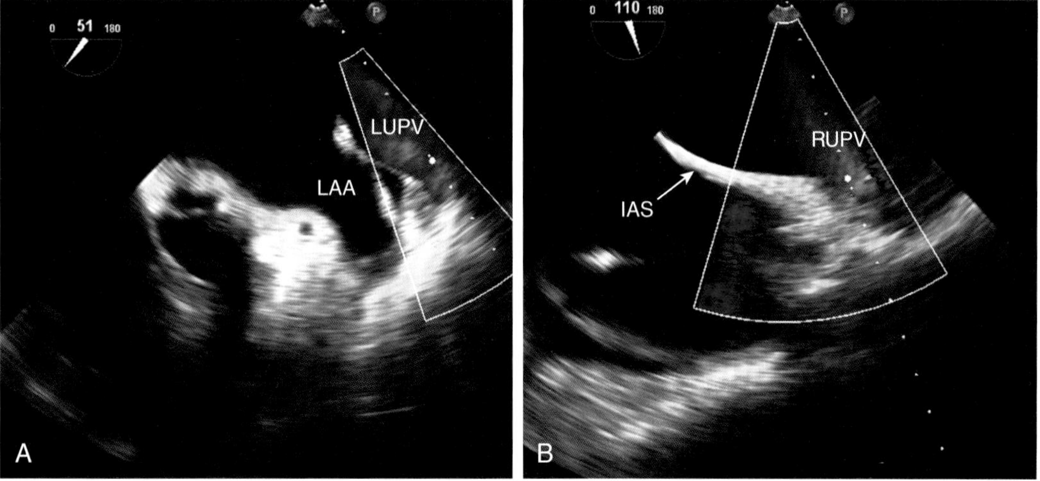

Fig. 8.20 Visualization of the pulmonary veins. (A) The left upper pulmonary vein *(LUPV)* (view 12) is adjacent to the left atrial appendage *(LAA)* and in some cases may be better visualized at a lower transducer angle than 90 degrees (in this case, at 51 degrees) (Video 8.20A). (B) The right upper pulmonary vein *(RUPV)* (view 15) is adjacent to the interatrial septum *(IAS)* (Video 8.20B).

TRICUSPID AND PULMONIC VALVES

The TV is an anterior cardiac structure and therefore is in the TEE imaging far field. The three leaflets of the TV (anterior, posterior, and septal leaflets) are challenging to visualize en face. 3DE en face images of the TV, when available, may be valuable for evaluating leaflet anatomy and motion, such as during assessment for leaflet impingement by cardiac device leads and wires.

From the mid-esophageal 4-chamber view (see Fig. 8.17A [view 2]), the septal and anterior leaflets are usually seen. Increasing the transducer angle to 60 degrees with slight clockwise rotation of the probe produces the RV inflow-outflow view (see Fig. 8.21B [view 9]). Because the TV is a larger valve, portions of leaflet coaptation may be out of plane in standard views. Therefore, color Doppler imaging should be performed at multiple image planes with different probe orientations to ensure

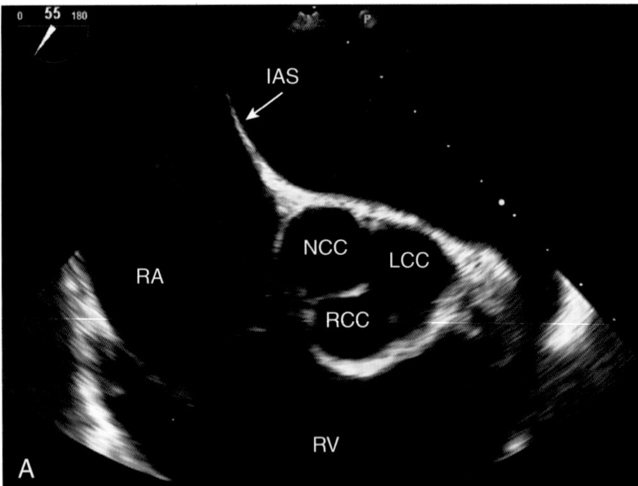

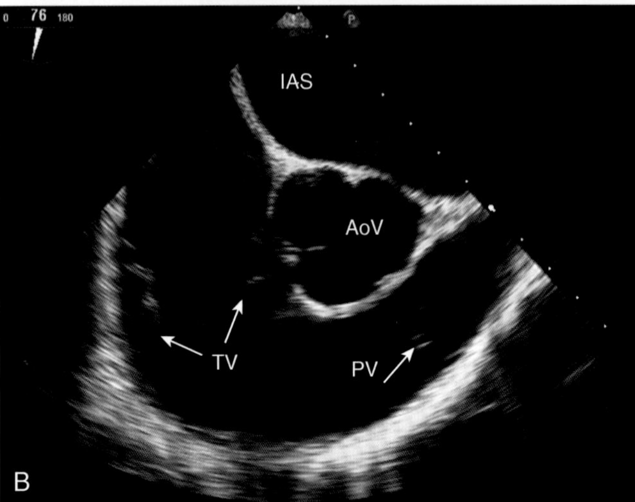

Fig. 8.21 Short-axis aortic valve and RV outflow views. (A) Mid-esophageal aortic valve short-axis view (view 8). The noncoronary cusp *(NCC)* is bisected by the interatrial septum *(IAS)*, and the right coronary cusp *(RCC)* is adjacent to the RV (Video 8.21A). (B) Mid-esophageal RV inflow-outflow view (view 9). The pulmonic valve *(PV)* is in the far field at the right side of the display (Video 8.21B). *AoV*, Aortic valve; *LCC*, left coronary cusp; *TV*, tricuspid valve.

that the full regurgitant jet is visualized. The TV is also well visualized from a transgastric RV inflow view (transducer angle moved to approximately 90 degrees, probe rotated clockwise) (see Fig. 8.19B [view 23]). In this view, the tricuspid posterior leaflet is in the near field.

The valve plane of the pulmonic valve and pulmonary artery is orthogonal to that of the AV and ascending aorta. In the RV inflow-outflow view (see Fig. 8.21B [view 9]), the pulmonic valve is seen in long axis in the far field, to the right side of the display.

3-DIMENSIONAL ECHOCARDIOGRAPHY

Technologic advances in matrix array transducers and computer processing allow high-quality 3DE imaging. With 3DE, there is relative loss in temporal and imaging resolution, compared with 2D imaging, although with improved assessment of spatial relationships between cardiac structures (Fig. 8.24).

With real-time 3DE, pyramidal volume data sets may be acquired over a single cardiac cycle, but because of relative constraints in data processing, the volume data set comprises a narrower imaging sector. For a wider sector, data from several narrower pyramidal volumes must be obtained over several cardiac cycles and then stitched together to create the larger-volume data set. Relative limitations of full-volume data sets include stitching artifacts between the volumes, which can occur with irregular rhythms or patient movement during image acquisition.

Comprehensive 3DE requires considerable operator time and expertise to manipulate the data sets and optimize image display. Given infinite imaging cropping planes and display options with volume data sets, optimal 3DE should be focused to address specific clinical questions. Current guidelines recommend integration of 3DE into diagnostic assessment of LV volumes and LV ejection fraction (Fig. 8.25), evaluation of MV stenosis, and guidance in transcatheter procedures. However, with increasingly widespread use and general expertise in 3DE among TEE operators, use of 3DE is expanding, particularly in catheterization laboratory–based procedures.[27,29]

Evaluation of LV function by standard 2D TEE is relatively limited because of the challenges in visualizing the true LV apex. 3DE allows visualization of the entire LV and quantitation of LV chamber volumes and function using automated endocardial border tracking algorithms. Reliance on endocardial border tracking, rather than on geometric assumptions, results in larger end-diastolic and end-systolic measurements but a comparable overall ejection fraction calculation. For qualitative evaluation of RV size and function by 3DE, the TEE probe should be turned toward the patient's right side from the mid-esophageal 4-chamber view (see Fig. 8.17A [view 2]), with the RV in the center of the imaging sector to ensure that it is captured in the acquired data set.[30]

The impact of 3DE has been significant in the evaluation of MV anatomy and function. 3DE allows en face views of the MV leaflets, which aids in the anatomic definition of leaflet

TABLE 8.10 Standard TEE Views for Cardiac Structures: Cardiac Valves.

Structure	View	Transducer Angle (Degrees) and Probe Position
Mitral valve	[2] ME 4-chamber view	10
	[3] ME mitral commissural view	60
	[5] ME LV long-axis view	130
	[16] TG LV basal short-axis view	0, en face image, anteflexed
	3D echocardiography	Zoomed en face image, rotate to AV at top of display
Aortic valve	[1] ME 5-chamber view	0, anteflexed
	[6] ME AoV long-axis view	130
	[8] ME AoV short-axis view	40, anteflexed
	[22] TG LV long-axis view	120
	3D echocardiography	Zoomed en face image, rotate to right cusp at bottom of display
Tricuspid valve	[2] ME 4-chamber view	10
	[9] ME RV inflow-outflow view	70
	[10] ME bicaval TV view	70
	[19] TG RV basal view	0, en face image
	[23] TG RV inflow view	90
	3D echocardiography	Zoomed en face image
Pulmonic valve	[9] ME RV inflow-outflow view	70

AoV, Aortic valve; *ME*, mid-esophageal; *TG*, transgastric.

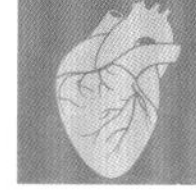

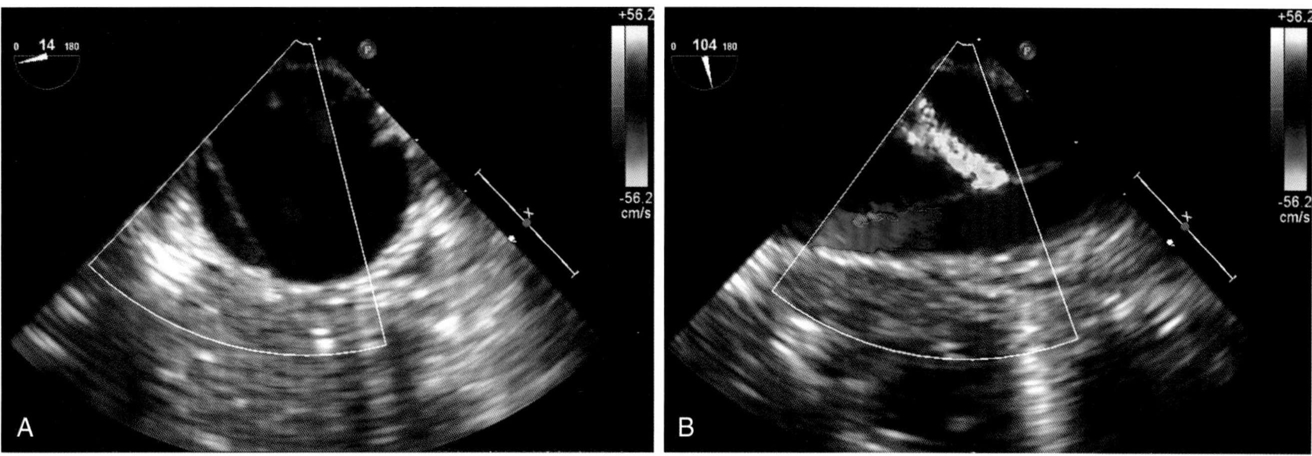

Fig. 8.22 **Descending thoracic aortic dissection.** (A) Mid-esophageal descending aorta short-axis view (14 degrees; view 25) shows a dissection flap (Video 8.22A). (B) The mid-esophageal descending aorta long-axis view (104 degrees; view 26) shows an orthogonal view of the dissection flap, with color Doppler allowing visualization of the communication between the true and false lumens (Video 8.22B).

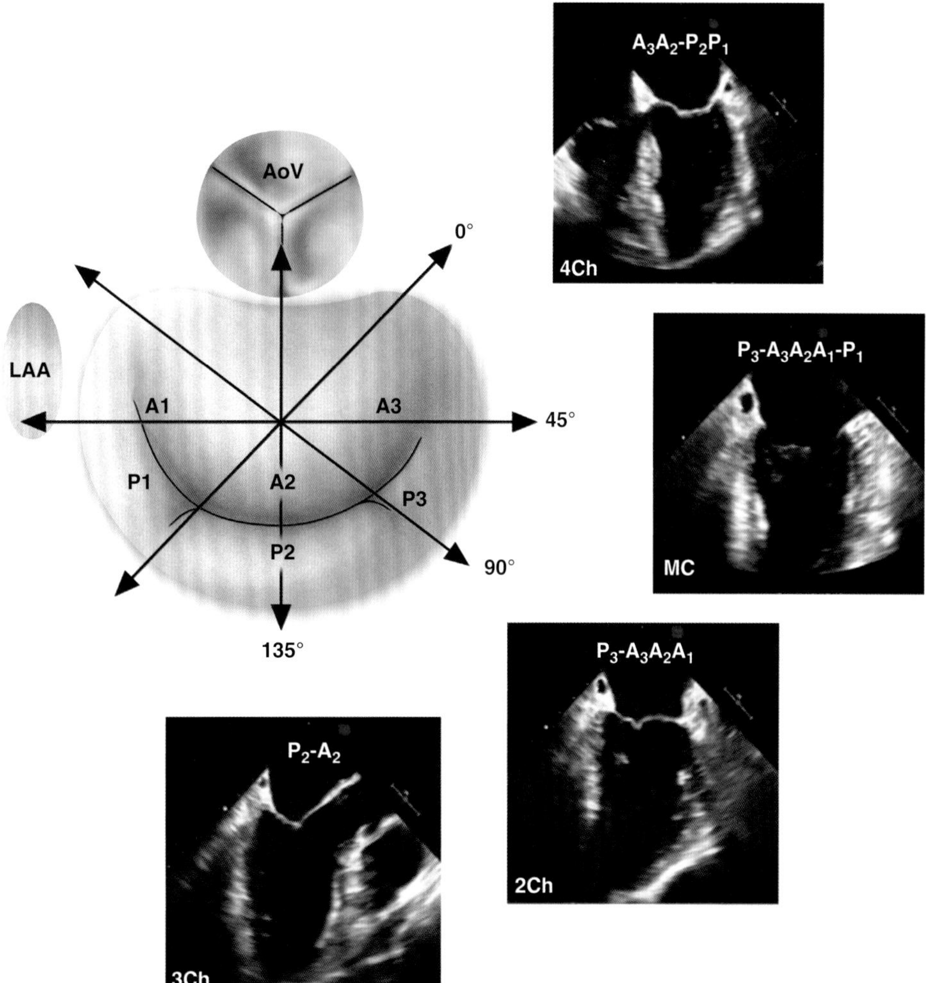

Fig. 8.23 **Schematic diagram of the mitral valve with labeled segments.** At each transducer angle, a corresponding image from that view is shown. Anatomic variation and probe placement may slightly vary the exact mitral segment imaged. *AoV*, Aortic valve; *Ch*, chamber; *LAA*, left atrial appendage; *MC*, mitral commissural. (From Hahn R, Abraham T, Adams M, et al. Guidelines for performing a comprehensive transesophageal echocardiographic examination: recommendations from the American Society of Echocardiography and the Society of Cardiovascular Anesthesiologists. *J Am Soc Echocardiogr.* 2013;26:921–964.)

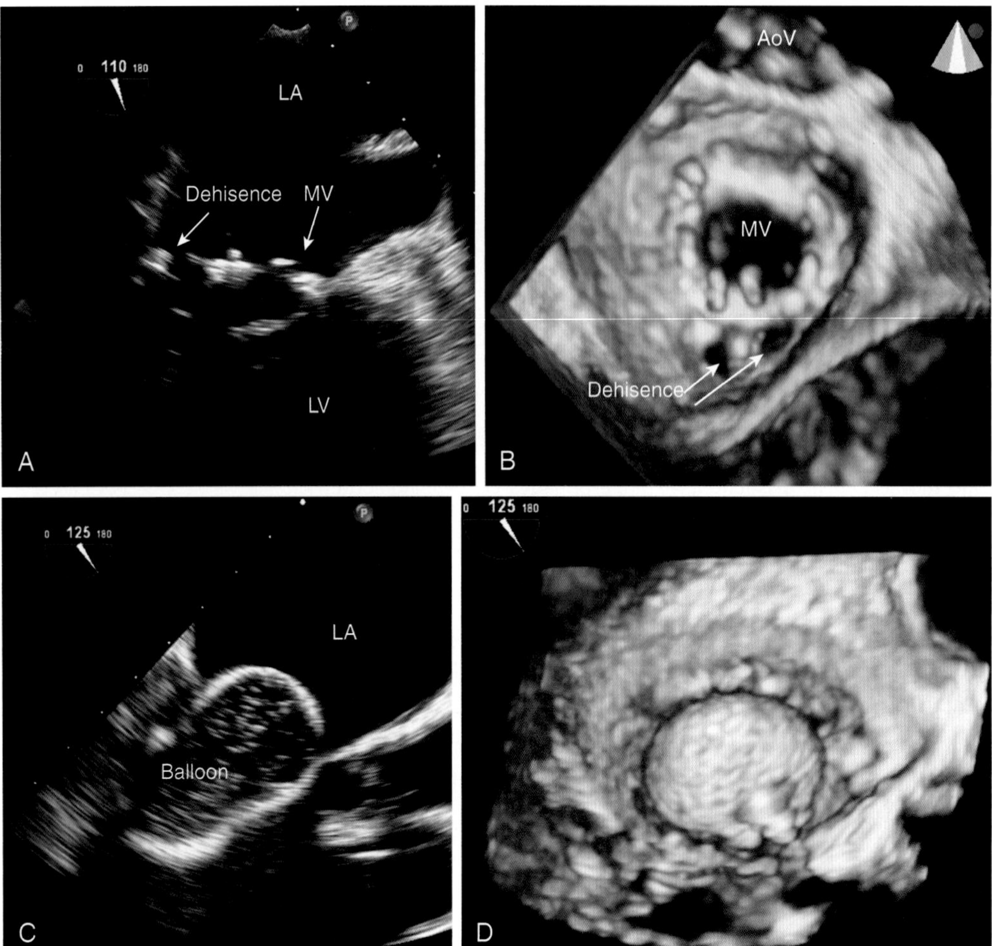

Fig. 8.24 Mitral valve prosthesis dehiscence. (A) 2D TEE image demonstrates a valve dehiscence adjacent to the MV prosthesis (Video 8.24A). (B) 3D imaging in the same patient enables improved spatial resolution with visualization of two defects adjacent to the lateral portion of the valve annulus (Video 8.24B). (C) In a different patient, TEE guidance (2D) allows optimal placement of an MV valvuloplasty balloon during the procedure (Video 8.24C). (D) 3D image of the patient shown in C (Video 8.24D). *AV*, Aortic valve; *MV*, mitral valve.

anatomy and assessment of the mechanism of MV dysfunction. In patients with mitral stenosis, 3DE en face views of the valve orifice allow valve area planimetry and intraprocedural monitoring of percutaneous balloon mitral valvuloplasty, including guidance of valvuloplasty balloon placement and assessment for postprocedural mitral regurgitation (see Fig. 8.24). For surgical and nonsurgical MV repair procedures, intraprocedural 3DE is used to guide the procedure and gauge the efficacy of repair.[13] In the case of nonsurgical MV edge-to-edge repair, 3DE is used first to visualize the atrial septum for optimal placement of the transseptal puncture for left atrial access, and then for catheter guidance and positioning during grasping of the MV leaflets for device placement (see Chapter 26).[13,31–33]

3D echocardiography has demonstrated increasing utility for other catheterization-based laboratory procedures. For intracardiac closure procedures (e.g., atrial and ventricular septal defects), 3DE allows sizing of the defect and optimization of device placement, including seating of the device and evaluation for residual communication.[34] Percutaneous transcatheter AV replacement is another catheterization-based procedure for which 3DE has shown utility; it allows visualization of the minor and major axes of a cross-section of the LVOT to avoid undersizing of the transcatheter AV prosthesis and to minimize postprocedural paravalvular regurgitation.[13,35–37]

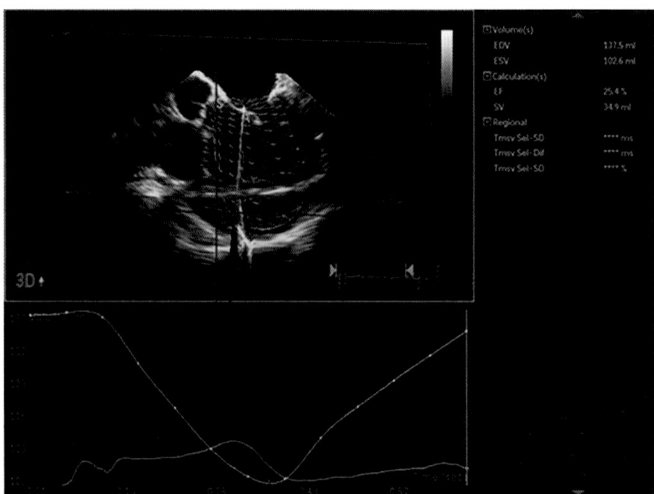

Fig. 8.25 Three-dimensional evaluation of LV function. 3D end-diastolic volume (EDV) is 137 mL and end-systolic volume (ESV) is 103 mL, with a stroke volume of 35 mL and a calculated ejection fraction (EF) of 25% (Video 8.25).

Transcatheter LAA device exclusion is a newer technique for the prevention of cardioembolism. 3DE is used to assess the amenability of appendage anatomy for device placement before the procedure and intraprocedurally during device placement for catheter guidance and evaluation of device positioning.[38]

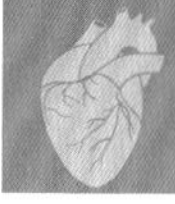

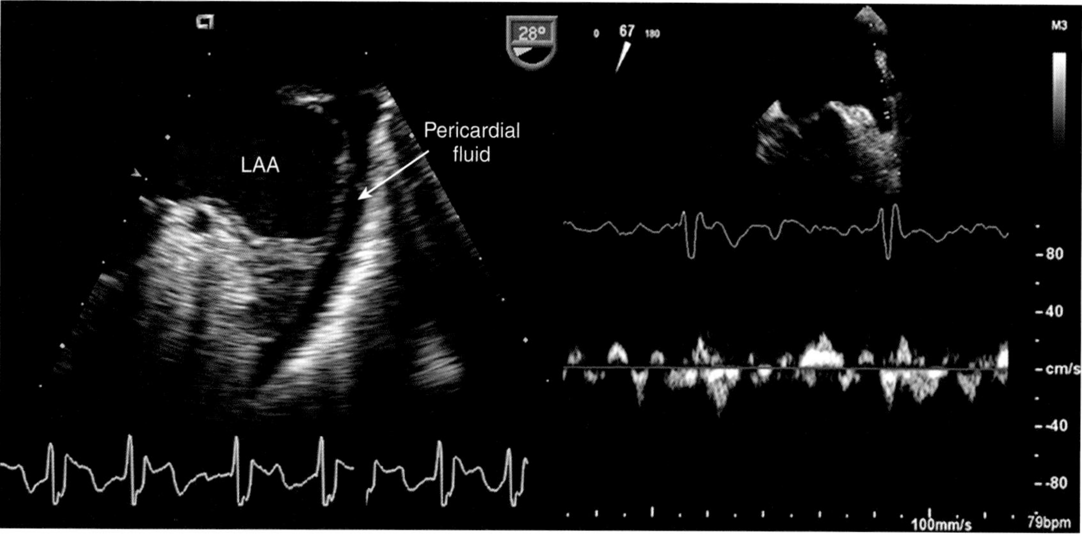

Fig. 8.26 Left atrial appendage thrombus filling the distal third of the appendage. Echolucent pericardial fluid adjacent to the left atrial appendage *(LAA)* provides contrast between the pericardium and the thrombus-filled appendage (left side of display). Pulsed-wave Doppler interrogation from the body of the LAA is shown on the right. The electrocardiogram (ECG) tracing shows atrial fibrillation. Velocities in the appendage are decreased at a peak of approximately 20 cm/s (Video 8.26).

CLINICAL APPLICATIONS OF TEE IMAGING

ATRIAL FIBRILLATION AND CARDIAC SOURCE OF EMBOLUS

In patients with cerebral vascular events, TEE is appropriate for evaluation of a cardiovascular source of embolus when no clear noncardiac source of stroke has been identified.[39] TEE is also indicated to exclude a potential cardiac source of embolus in patients who are under consideration for direct current cardioversion (see Table 8.4).[40] In addition to intracardiac masses, increased risk for cardioembolism is seen in conditions associated with increased likelihood of thrombus formation, such as the presence of prosthetic valves or device leads, or with low-velocity blood flow, as can occur with atrial fibrillation and flow stasis in the LAA (see Fig. 8.26).

LAA anatomy varies in shape, depth, and size among individuals. Therefore, it is important to evaluate the appendage and the LA from multiple views.[41] Spectral Doppler evaluation of emptying velocity aids in determining relative stasis in the appendage, with velocities of less than 0.20 m/s suggestive of a lower flow state and thrombus formation (see Fig. 8.26). Spontaneous echocardiographic contrast is an indicator of low flow and is often concurrently seen when thrombi are present. A prominent tissue ridge between the LAA and the left upper pulmonary vein may cause acoustic shadowing or reverberations and hinder complete appendage visualization.

To reduce the risk of cardioembolic stroke in patients with atrial fibrillation lasting longer than 48 hours who are under consideration for direct current cardioversion, clinical guidelines recommend that anticoagulation begin at least 3 weeks before cardioversion and continue for at least 4 weeks after the procedure (class I recommendation).[40] To shorten the period of anticoagulation, an alternative strategy is to perform a TEE to exclude left atrial thrombus at the time of cardioversion, provided that a therapeutic level of anticoagulation is achieved before TEE (class IIa recommendation).[40] In patients with nonvalvular atrial fibrillation, transcatheter LAA exclusion is a newer catheterization laboratory–based technique intended to prevent cardioembolism. TEE is used throughout the procedure to assess the amenability of appendage anatomy for device placement, provide catheter guidance, and evaluate the effectiveness of appendage occlusion.[31,38,42]

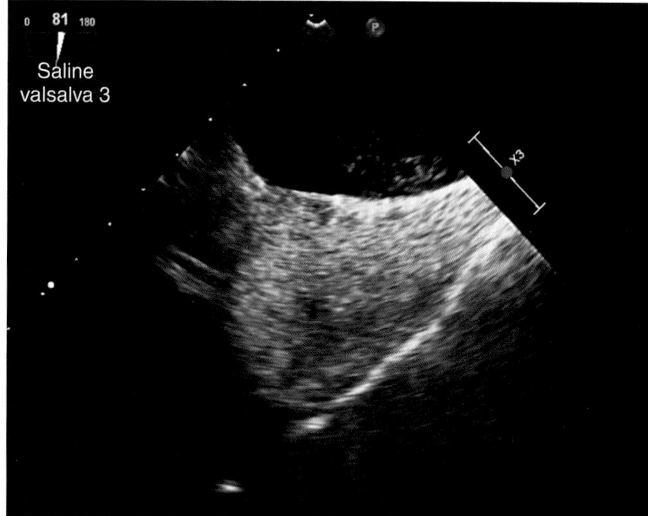

Fig. 8.27 Agitated saline contrast study. Mid-esophageal bicaval view (view 11). Agitated saline enters the LA from the superior vena cava. Following the Valsalva maneuver, a small number of bubbles are seen just above the interatrial septum in the LA on the right-hand side of the image after crossing a patent foramen ovale (Video 8.27).

A PFO may be visualized with 2D TEE from multiple views and with 3DE en face imaging of the IAS using color Doppler. Venous injection of agitated saline contrast may be diagnostic, with bubbles entering through the superior vena cava on the right side of the display and then crossing to the LA through the PFO.[43] Visualization of the septum during saline contrast studies tends to be best from the mid-esophageal bicaval view (see Figs. 8.18C and 8.27 [view 11]), although a transient increase in RAP (e.g., after Valsalva maneuver) may be needed to overcome the relative pressure gradient between the left and right atria (Fig. 8.27).

The presence of atherosclerotic plaque in the ascending aorta and aortic arch proximal to the take-off of the great vessels poses a potential source of cerebral embolic stroke. Atherosclerotic

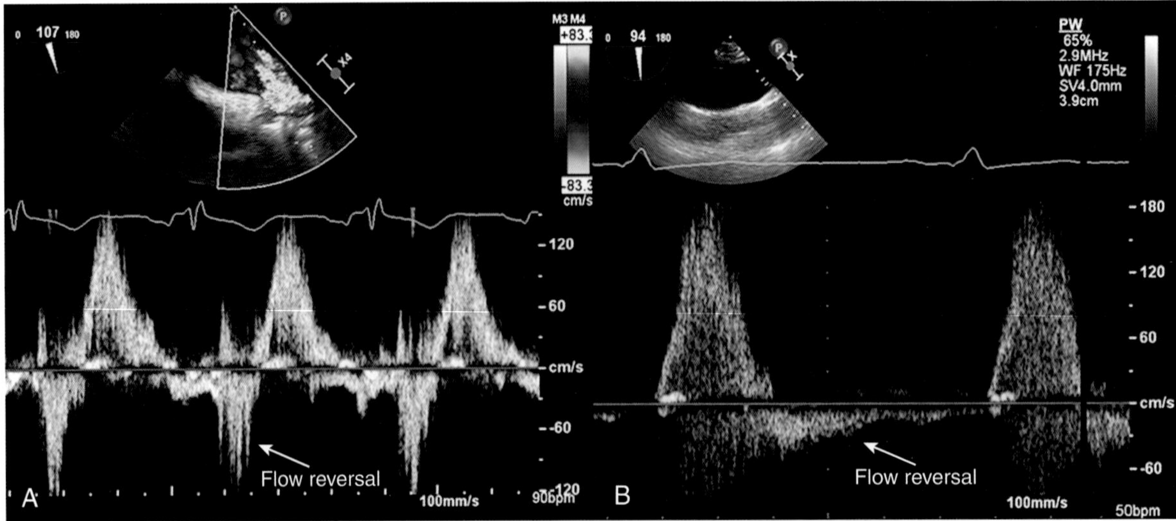

Fig. 8.28 **Reversal of flow in mitral and aortic regurgitation.** (A) Spectral Doppler interrogation of the right upper pulmonary vein in a patient with severe mitral regurgitation demonstrates systolic reversal of flow (as shown in the accompanying electrocardiographic tracing), with signal directed away from the transducer. (B) In a patient with severe aortic regurgitation, Doppler interrogation of the thoracic aorta shows reversal of flow during diastole.

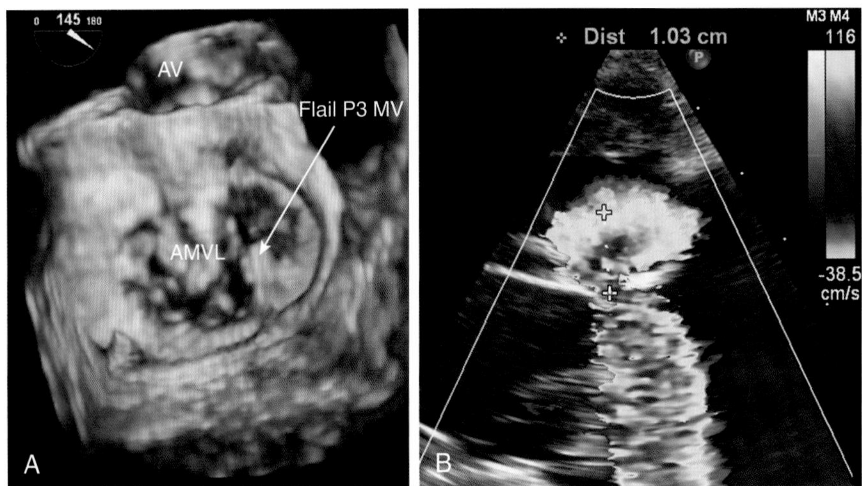

Fig. 8.29 **Severe mitral regurgitation.** (A) En face view of the mitral valve (MV) by 3DE shows flail of the medial portion of the posterior MV leaflet in the P3 segment (Video 8.29A). (B) With the color baseline moved in the direction of flow, away from the transducer, the aliasing velocity is 38.5 cm/s. At this aliasing velocity, the radius of the proximal isovelocity surface area measured 1.03 cm (Video 8.29B). *AMVL*, Anterior mitral valve leaflet; *AV*, atrial valve.

plaque may be associated with ulceration, superimposed thrombi, or a heavy calcification burden.

NATIVE AND PROSTHETIC VALVE EVALUATION

Echocardiography is the recommended diagnostic test for a comprehensive evaluation of valve anatomy and function. Assessment of the hemodynamic effects of valve lesions, such as on pulmonary pressures or cardiac function, is more easily accomplished with TTE compared with TEE because of the superiority of TTE in optimizing transducer placement and aligning Doppler interrogation. However, TEE provides improved image quality and anatomic visualization for en face imaging of the cardiac valves. Assessing the severity of regurgitant lesions is challenging and requires the integration of many variables using qualitative and quantitative measures.[13] Color Doppler imaging allows assessment of regurgitant jet origin and flow convergence. Semiquantitative assessment of the narrowest section of the jet (vena contracta) is a surrogate for the regurgitant orifice diameter and correlates with regurgitation severity. With significant regurgitation, spectral Doppler interrogation samples from an upstream chamber should demonstrate reversal of flow (Fig. 8.28).

Quantitative assessment of regurgitant volumes and effective regurgitant orifice area is important when qualitative or semiquantitative measures are inconclusive. The proximal isovelocity surface area (PISA) method relies on the continuity equation and the principle of flow convergence. As regurgitant flow accelerates uniformly toward an orifice, isovelocity hemispheres form. Measurement of the radius (r) of the hemispherical shell at its corresponding Nyquist limit allows calculation of the effective regurgitant orifice area, regurgitant volume, and regurgitant fraction (Figs. 8.29 and 8.30).

For suspected prosthetic valve dysfunction or thrombosis, TTE is the preferred initial diagnostic procedure because it allows assessment of valve function, pulmonary pressures, and ventricular size and function. However, if the valve is not well visualized, TEE should be performed (class I recommendation) (see Chapter 31).[44,45] Prosthetic valves in the mitral position are challenging to evaluate by TTE because of acoustic shadowing of the LA by prosthetic material (Fig. 8.31). With mechanical prostheses, if a thrombus is identified and the patient is under consideration for thrombolytic therapy, TEE should be performed to assess thrombus burden.[46] Thrombus size (area measurement by TEE) is an independent predictor of complications after administration of thrombolytic agents, with an area smaller than 0.8 cm^2 associated with a lower risk of complications (e.g., stroke).[44] After thrombolysis therapy, repeat echocardiography should be performed to assess for resolution of the thrombus and improved valve hemodynamics.[39]

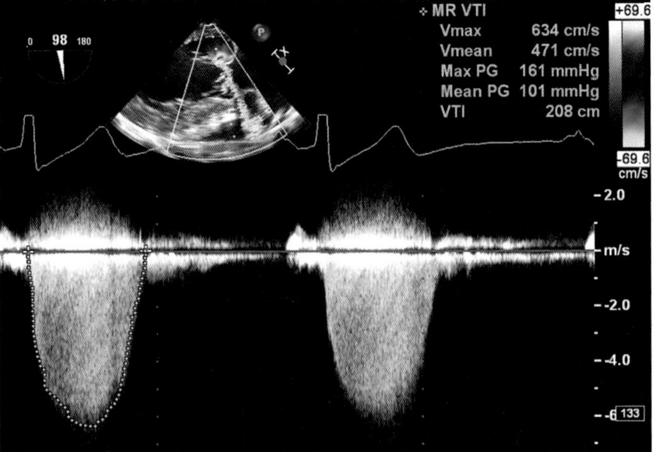

Fig. 8.30 **Severe mitral regurgitation.** CW spectral Doppler tracing of the mitral regurgitant jet. Optimal alignment of the regurgitant jet was obtained from the transgastric long-axis view (98 degrees). The peak velocity was 634 cm/s, with the velocity–time integral (VTI) measuring 208 cm. The effective regurgitant orifice area (EROA) calculation based on Fig. 8.29 is ($2\pi r^2$ × aliasing velocity)/peak regurgitant velocity. (2π[1.03 cm]^2 x 38.5 cm/s) = 0.4 cm^2, consistent with severe mitral regurgitation. The EROA multiplied by the mitral regurgitant VTI provides a regurgitant volume of 84 mL.

INFECTIVE ENDOCARDITIS

Modified Duke major criteria for diagnosis of infective endocarditis (IE) include positive blood cultures or evidence of endocardial involvement, such as diagnosis of new valve regurgitation or characteristic echocardiographic findings (i.e., vegetation, abscess, or new partial dehiscence of a prosthetic valve).[47,48] TTE is the preferred initial procedure because it is often diagnostic in advanced cases; however, the image resolution of TTE is relatively limited with smaller vegetation lesions (<3 mm), and it tends to provide inadequate visualization of paravalvular extension and complications such as abscess and leaflet destruction (see Fig. 8.31). Sensitivity for IE diagnosis by TTE is 70% to 90% for native valve IE but lower (≈50%) for IE-associated abscess or prosthetic valve IE. Sensitivity for IE diagnosis by TEE is significantly higher, more than 90%.[44,48,49]

Current clinical guidelines recommend TEE for all patients with known or suspected IE when transthoracic imaging is nondiagnostic, for patients with prosthetic valves or intracardiac device leads (implantable cardioverter-defibrillator/pacemaker), and for those with suspected complications of endocarditis such as abscess or valve dehiscence (class I recommendation).[44,49] False-positive TEE findings for IE may occur in patients with preexisting leaflet calcification, sclerotic changes, or prosthetic material such as a sewing ring or sutures. A false-negative study may occur if TEE imaging is performed too early in the disease course, when complications have not yet fully developed. TEE should also be considered in patients with infection by more virulent organisms, such as staphylococcal or fungal species, given that these organisms are associated with significant morbidity and mortality and carry a higher incidence of paravalvular abscess and systemic embolization compared with other species.

Prosthetic material is highly reflective, and acoustic shadowing in the far field obscures visualization of distal cardiac structures, particularly with posterior abnormalities (see Fig. 8.31). Prosthetic valve IE tends to manifest with paravalvular extension of infection (abscess) rather than the vegetative lesions more

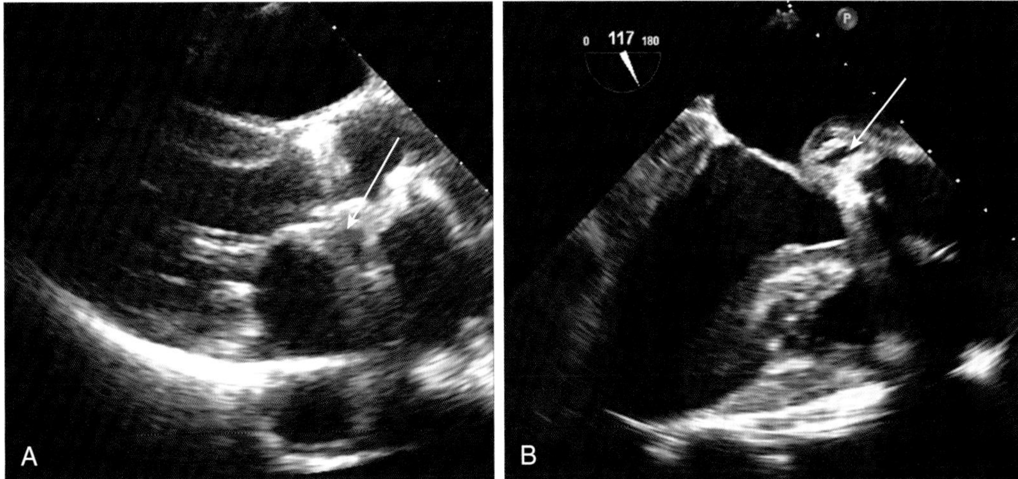

Fig. 8.31 **Paravalvular abscess.** Transthoracic imaging of a mechanical aortic valve (AV) prosthesis from the parasternal long-axis view in a patient presenting with fatigue and an elevated white blood cell count. Acoustic shadowing from the prosthesis precludes definitive evaluation of the posterior portion of the AV annulus *(arrow)* (Video 8.31A). (B) Subsequent TEE imaging from the mid-esophageal long-axis view at 117 degrees (view 5) clearly demonstrates abnormal thickening adjacent to the prosthetic valve with a central echolucency concerning for abscess *(arrow)* (Video 8.31B).

commonly seen in native valve IE. In one prospective study of patients with 114 suspected IE episodes who underwent both TTE and TEE imaging, TEE aided in reclassification of IE diagnosis in 11% of patients with suspected native valve IE and in 34% of those with prosthetic valve IE; overall, TEE had a positive predictive value of 90%.[50] Given the challenge in diagnosing prosthetic valve IE with TTE alone, TEE is recommended for patients with prosthetic valves and clinical suspicion for IE (class I recommendation) and for patients with persistent fever, even in the absence of bacteremia (class IIA recommendation).[44,49]

ACUTE AORTIC SYNDROMES

TEE allows high-resolution imaging of most of the ascending aorta, aortic arch, and descending thoracic aorta. TEE is highly sensitive and specific for the diagnosis of acute aortic syndromes and can concurrently assess for associated complications of these diagnoses, such as aortic regurgitation, coronary artery involvement, LV dysfunction, and pericardial effusion. Mechanisms of aortic regurgitation in patients with acute ascending aortic dissection include poor leaflet coaptation due to aortic dilation, propagation of the dissection flap to the AV plane with prolapse through the valve, and preexisting valve disease.[51] In patients with a suspected acute ascending (type A) aortic dissection, TEE is an appropriate initial study because image resolution for TTE is relatively limited and TEE allows diagnosis and evaluation of the extent of dissection, complications, and possible extension of the dissection plane to the carotid arteries or to the coronary arteries (see Chapter 32).[2,3,52,53] During TEE imaging, care should be taken to exclude a reverberation artifact mimicking the dissection flap.[54,55]

Advantages of TEE over other tomographic imaging modalities include the ability to perform the study at the bedside in hemodynamically unstable patients without the need for iodinated contrast or ionizing radiation exposure (compared with MRA or CT).[54] Color Doppler flow interrogation may aid in identifying the entry and/or exit points of the dissection and may differentiate the true and false lumens (see Fig. 8.22). Intramural hematoma, a focal separation of the intimal layer due to hemorrhage into the medial layer of the aorta, presents echocardiographically as a focal, circumferential, crescentic echodensity along the aortic wall edge and can progress to aortic dissection or rupture.

Traumatic aortic rupture is typically the result of abrupt shear forces with rupture at the aortic isthmus; it is commonly fatal. For patients who survive the initial rupture, TEE can aid in rapid diagnosis.[54,56,57] The echocardiographic appearance of traumatic aortic rupture is disruption of the aortic wall, most commonly at the proximal descending aorta, with an intraluminal dissection flap and absence of laminar flow in the aortic lumen.

PROPOSED SEQUENCE OF A COMPREHENSIVE TEE STUDY

A structured sequence for TEE imaging ensures a comprehensive evaluation of cardiac anatomy and function. Because of the semi-invasive nature of TEE, sequencing should start with evaluation of the primary indication for the study. Although protocols for TEE sequencing vary among echocardiography laboratories, key components should be included in all protocols to provide a complete evaluation while minimizing patient discomfort and the time needed to perform the procedure. A proposed sequence for a comprehensive TEE study is provided in the Summary table at the end of this chapter. This proposed sequence starts in the mid-esophageal position at an increased imaging depth to assess biventricular chamber size and function, including 3D evaluation of the LV. Next, detailed evaluation of the cardiac valves is performed, including 3D imaging, with attention to anatomic and functional assessment from various imaging views. If more than mild valve stenosis or regurgitation is present, additional quantitation of severity is warranted. The bicaval view allows evaluation of the IAS and pulmonary veins; then, after assessment of the pericardial space, the probe is advanced to the transgastric position for further evaluation. Last, the probe is rotated to view the descending thoracic aorta as it is withdrawn.

SUMMARY Core Elements of a Diagnostic TTE Examination and Proposed Sequence of a Comprehensive TEE Study.

Diagnostic TTE: Core Elements

Sequence	Window	View/Signal	Measurements
2D Imaging			
1.	Parasternal	Long-axis	LV ED and ES dimensions, LV ED wall thickness, aortic ED sinus dimension, LA dimension
		RV inflow	
		Short-axis aortic valve	
		Short-axis mitral valve	
		Short-axis LV (papillary muscle level)	
2.	Apical	4-chamber	Visually estimated or quantitative EF
		Anteriorly angulated 4-chamber	
		2-chamber	Visually estimated or quantitative EF
		Long-axis	

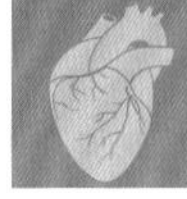

SUMMARY Core Elements of a Diagnostic TTE Examination and Proposed Sequence of a Comprehensive TEE Study.—cont'd

Diagnostic TTE: Core Elements

Sequence	Window	View/Signal	Measurements
3.	Subcostal	4-chamber	IVC diameter
		IVC with respiration	
		Proximal abdominal aorta	
4.	Suprasternal	Aortic arch	
Pulsed-Wave Doppler			
5.	Parasternal	Pulmonary artery flow	Pulmonary artery velocity
6.	Apical	LV inflow	E velocity, A velocity
		LV outflow	LV outflow velocity
Continuous-Wave Doppler			
7.	Parasternal	Tricuspid valve	TR-jet velocity (pulmonary pressures)
		Pulmonic valve	
8.	Apical	Aortic valve	Aortic velocity
		Mitral valve	
		Tricuspid valve	TR-jet velocity
Color-Flow Doppler			
9.	Parasternal	Long-axis: aortic and mitral valves	
		RV inflow: tricuspid valve	
		Short-axis: aortic, pulmonic, and tricuspid valves	
10.	Apical	4-chamber: mitral and tricuspid valves	
		Long-axis: aortic and mitral valves	

Comprehensive TEE: Proposed Sequence

Sequence	Structure	Comments
Mid-esophageal Views		
1.	Evaluate primary study indication	Endocarditis evaluation, cardiac source of embolus, acute aortic syndrome, other indications.
2.	LV size and function	Depth to include entire LV. Transducer angle, 0–130 degrees. Global and regional function, 3DE LV volumes, and EF.
3.	RV size and function	Depth to include entire RV. Transducer angle, 0–70 degrees.
4.	Left atrium	Decrease depth to below MV. Sweep across the atrium at transducer angles between 0 and 90 degrees.
5.	Left atrial appendage	Biplane imaging. Adjust position to decrease artifact from ridge between LUPV and LAA. Pulsed-wave Doppler of velocities for atrial fibrillation.
6.	Right atrium	Decrease depth to just below MV. Sweep across the atrium at transducer angles between 0 and 90 degrees.
7.	Mitral valve	2D imaging and color Doppler from multiple views; transducer angle, 0–130 degrees. Quantitation of regurgitation severity, vena contracta, and PISA EROA calculation for more than mild regurgitation. Mitral inflow gradient for stenosis. 3DE en face view of valve rotated to aortic valve at top of display.

Continued

SUMMARY Core Elements of a Diagnostic TTE Examination and Proposed Sequence of a Comprehensive TEE Study.—cont'd

Diagnostic TTE: Core Elements

Sequence	Window	View/Signal Measurements
8.	Aortic valve	2D imaging and color Doppler from multiple views; transducer angle, 0–130 degrees. Vena contracta for more than mild regurgitation. 3DE en face view of valve rotated to right coronary cusp at bottom of display.
9.	Ascending aorta (upper esophageal)	Transducer angle, 100 degrees. Measure if dilated (sinuses, sinotubular junction, mid-ascending aorta).
10.	Tricuspid valve	2D imaging and color Doppler from multiple views; transducer angle, 0–60 degrees.
11.	Pulmonic valve	2D imaging and color Doppler; transducer angle, 70 degrees.
12.	Interatrial septum and bicaval view	2D imaging and color Doppler at lower Nyquist setting; transducer angle, 100 degrees. If shunt is suspected, 3DE en face view and agitated saline contrast study; if present, evaluate.
13.	Pulmonary veins	2D imaging and color Doppler; transducer angle, 0 and 100 degrees for left and right pulmonary veins. Pulsed-wave Doppler if significant MR is present, to evaluate for flow reversal.
15.	Pericardial space	Sweep across the heart at a transducer angle of 0 degrees.
Transgastric Views		
16.	Ventricular function	Evaluate biventricular size and function; transducer angle, 0 and 120 degrees. Rotate probe tip rightward for RV and tricuspid valve. En face view of MV with color Doppler if significant MR is present.
17.	Deep transgastric view	Advance probe from transgastric view. Visualize LV outflow for Doppler interrogation if needed.
Aorta View		
18.	Descending thoracic aorta	Image from the diaphragm to the aortic arch. Biplane imaging, 0 and 90 degrees. Pulsed-wave Doppler if significant AR is present, to evaluate for flow reversal. Image atherosclerotic plaque.

AR, Aortic regurgitation; *ED*, end-diastolic; *EF*, ejection fraction; *EROA*, effective regurgitant orifice area; *ES*, end-systolic; *IVC*, inferior vena cava; *LAA*, left atrial appendage; *LUPV*, left upper pulmonary vein; *MR*, mitral regurgitation; *MV*, mitral valve; *PISA*, proximal isovelocity surface area; *TR*, tricuspid regurgitation.

REFERENCES

1. Lang RM, Badano LP, Tsang W, et al. EAE/ASE recommendations for image acquisition and display using three-dimensional echocardiography. *J Am Soc Echocardiogr.* 2012;25:3–46.
2. Doherty JU, Kort S, Mehran R, Schoenhagen P, Soman P. ACC/AATS/AHA/ASE/ASNC/HRS/SCAI/SCCT/SCMR/STS 2017 appropriate use criteria for multimodality imaging in valvular heart disease: a report of the American College of Cardiology Appropriate Use Criteria Task Force, American Association for Thoracic Surgery, American Heart Association, American Society of Echocardiography, American Society of Nuclear Cardiology, Heart Rhythm Society, Society for Cardiovascular Angiography and Interventions, Society of Cardiovascular Computed Tomography, Society for Cardiovascular Magnetic Resonance, and Society of Thoracic Surgeons. *J Am Coll Cardiol.* 2017;70:1647–1672.
3. Doherty JU, Kort S, Mehran R, et al. ACC/AATS/AHA/ASE/ASNC/HRS/SCAI/SCCT/SCMR/STS 2019 appropriate use criteria for multimodality imaging in the assessment of cardiac structure and function in nonvalvular heart disease: a report of the American College of cardiology appropriate use criteria Task force, American Association for Thoracic Surgery, American Heart Association, American Society of Echocardiography, American Society of Nuclear Cardiology, Heart Rhythm Society, Society for Cardiovascular Angiography and Interventions, Society of CardioVascular Computed Tomography, Society for Cardiovascular Magnetic Resonance, and the Society of Thoracic Surgeons. *J Am Coll Cardiol.* 2019;73:488–516.
4. Mitchell C, Rahko PS, Blauwet LA, et al. Guidelines for performing a comprehensive transthoracic echocardiographic examination in adults: recommendations from the American Society of Echocardiography. *J Am Soc Echocardiogr.* 2019;32:1–64.
5. Lang R, Badano L, Mor-Avi V, et al. Recommendations for cardiac chamber quantification by echocardiography in adults: an update from the ASE and EACI. *J Am Soc Echocardiogr.* 2015;28:1–39.
6. Vyas H, Jackson K, Chenzbraun A. Switching to volumetric left atrial measurements: impact on routine echocardiographic practice. *Eur J Echocardiogr.* 2011;12:107–111.
7. Rudski LG, Lai WW, Afilalo J, et al. Guidelines for the echocardiographic assessment of the right heart in adults: a report from the American Society of Echocardiography endorsed by the European Association of Echocardiography, a registered branch of the European Society of Cardiology, and the Canadian Society of Echocardiography. *J Am Soc Echocardiogr.* 2010;23:685–713; quiz 86-8.
8. Genovese D, Mor-Avi V, Palermo C, et al. Comparison between four-chamber and right ventricular-focused views for the quantitative evaluation of right ventricular size and function. *J Am Soc Echocardiogr.* 2019;32:484–494.
9. Potter E, Marwick TH. Assessment of left ventricular function by echocardiography: the case for routinely adding global longitudinal strain to ejection fraction. *JACC Cardiovascular imaging.* 2018;11:260–274.
10. Lee SH, Chang SA, Jang SY, et al. Screening for abdominal aortic aneurysm during transthoracic echocardiography in patients with significant coronary artery disease. *Yonsei Medical Journal.* 2015;56:38–44.

11. Feigenbaum H. Role of M-mode technique in today's echocardiography. *J Am Soc Echocardiogr*. 2010;23:240–257. 335-7.
12. Aloia E, Cameli M, D'Ascenzi F, Sciaccaluga C, Mondillo S. TAPSE: an old but useful tool in different diseases. *Int J Cardiol*. 2016;225:177–183.
13. Zoghbi WA, Asch FM, Bruce C, et al. Guidelines for the evaluation of valvular regurgitation after percutaneous valve repair or replacement: a report from the American Society of Echocardiography developed in collaboration with the Society for Cardiovascular Angiography and Interventions, Japanese Society of Echocardiography, and Society for Cardiovascular Magnetic Resonance. *J Am Soc Echocardiogr*. 2019;32:431–475.
14. Nagueh SF, Smiseth OA, Appleton CP, et al. Recommendations for the evaluation of left ventricular diastolic function by echocardiography: an update from the American Society of Echocardiography and the European Association of Cardiovascular Imaging. *J Am Soc Echocardiogr*. 2016;29:277–314.
15. Ryan T, Berlacher K, Lindner J, et al. COCATS 4 Task force 5: training in echocardiography. *J Am Coll Cardiol*. 2015;65:1786–1799.
16. Mathew J, Glas K, Troianos C, et al. ASE/SCA recommendations and guidelines for continuous quality improvement in perioperative echocardiography. *J Am Soc Echocardiogr*. 2006;19:1303–1313.
17. Reeves S, Finley A, Skubas N, et al. Basic perioperative transesophageal echocardiography examination: a consensus statement of the American Society of Echocardiography and the Society of Cardiovascular Anesthesiologists. *J Am Soc Echocardiogr*. 2013;26:443–456.
18. Wiegers SE, Ryan T, Arrighi JA, et al. 2019 ACC/AHA/ASE advanced training statement on echocardiography (Revision of the 2003 ACC/AHA clinical competence statement on echocardiography): a report of the ACC Competency Management Committee. *J Am Coll Cardiol*. 2019;74:377–402.
19. Picard M, Adams D, Bierig S, et al. American Society of Echocardiography recommendations for quality echocardiography laboratory operations. *J Am Soc Echocardiogr*. 2011;24:1–10.
20. Gross J, Bailey P, Connis R, et al. Practice guidelines for sedation and analgesia by non-anesthesiologists. *Anesthesiology*. 2002;96:1004–1017.
21. Wilson W, Taubert K, Gewitz M, et al. Prevention of infective endocarditis: guidelines from the American Heart Association: a guideline from the American Heart Association Rheumatic Fever, Endocarditis, and Kawasaki Disease Committee, Council on Cardiovascular Disease in the Young, and the Council on Clinical Cardiology, Council on Cardiovascular Surgery and Anesthesia, and the Quality of Care and Outcomes Research Interdisciplinary Working Group. *Circulation*. 2007;116:1736–1842.
22. Apfelbaum J, Caplan R, Connis R, et al. Practice guidelines for preoperative fasting and the use of pharmacologic agents to reduce the risk of pulmonary aspiration: application to healthy patients undergoing elective procedures. American Society of Anesthesiologists Committee on Standards and Practice Parameters. *Anesthesiology*. 2011;114:495–511.
23. Hilberath J, Oakes D, Shernan S, Bulwer B, D'Ambra M, Eltzschig H. Safety of transesophageal echocardiography. *J Am Soc Echocardiogr*. 2010;23:1115–1127.
24. Kallmeyer I, Collard C, Fox J, Body S, Shernan S. The safety of intraoperative transesophageal echocardiography: a case series of 7200 cardiac surgical patients. *Anesth Analg*. 2001;92:1126–1130.
25. Min J, Spencer K, Furling K, et al. Clinical features of complications from transesophageal echocardiography: a single-center case series of 10,000 consecutive examinations. *J Am Soc Echocardiogr*. 2005;18:925–929.
26. Piercy M, McNichol L, Dinh D, Story D, Smith J. Major complications related to the use of transesophageal echocardiography in cardiac surgery. *J Cardiothorac Vasc Anesth*. 2009;23:62–65.
27. Hahn R, Abraham T, Adams M, et al. Guidelines for performing a comprehensive transesophageal echocardiographic examination: recommendations from the American Society of Echocardiography and the Society of Cardiovascular Anesthesiologists. *J Am Soc Echocardiogr*. 2013;26:921–964.
28. Chandra S, Salgo I, Sugeng L, et al. Characterization of degenerative mitral valve disease using morphologic analysis of real-time three-dimensional echocardiographic images: objective insight into complexity and planning of mitral valve repair. *Circ Cardiovasc Imaging*. 2011;4:24–32.
29. Zamorano J, Badano L, Bruce C, et al. EAE/ASE recommendations for the use of echocardiography in new transcatheter interventions for valvular heart disease. *J Am Soc Echocardiogr : Official Publication of the American Society of Echocardiography*. 2011;24:937–965.
30. Lang R, Badano L, Tsang W, et al. EAE/ASE recommendations for image acquisition and display using three-dimensional echocardiography. *J Am Soc Echocardiogr*. 2012;25:3–46.
31. Ho S, McCarthy K, Faletra F. Anatomy of the left atrium for interventional echocardiography. *Eur J Echocardiogr*. 2011;12:i11–i15.
32. Lang R, Adams D. 3D echocardiographic quantification in functional mitral regurgitation. *JACC Cardiovascular imaging*. 2012;5:346–347.
33. McCarthy K, Ring L, Rana B. Anatomy of the mitral valve: understanding the mitral valve complex in mitral regurgitation. *Eur J Echocardiogr*. 2010;11:i3–19.
34. Mullen M, Dias B, Walker F, Siu S, Benson L, McLaughlin P. Intracardiac echocardiography guided device closure of atrial septal defects. *J Am Coll Cardiol*. 2003;41:285–292.
35. Kasel A, Cassese S, Bleiziffer S, et al. Standardized imaging for aortic annular sizing: implications for transcatheter valve selection. *JACC Cardiovascular imaging*. 2013;6:249–262.
36. Bloomfield G, Gillam L, Hahn R, et al. A practical guide to multimodality imaging of transcatheter aortic valve replacement. *JACC Cardiovascular imaging*. 2012;5:441–455.
37. Gripari PES, Fusini L, Muratori M, Ng AC, Cefalu C, et al. Intraoperative 2D and 3D transoesophageal echocardiographic predictors of aortic regurgitation after transcatheter aortic valve implantation. *Heart*. 2012;98:1229–1236.
38. Wunderlich N, Beigel R, Swaans M, et al. Percutaneous interventions for left atrial appendage exclusion. Options, assessment, and imaging using 2D and 3D echocardiography. *J Am Coll Cardiol Img*. 2015;8:472–488.
39. Saric M, Armour A, Arnaout M, et al. Guidelines for the use of echocardiography in the evaluation of a cardiac source of embolism. *J Am Soc Echocardiogr*. 2016;29:1–42.
40. January C, Wann L, Alpert J, et al. AHA/ACC/HRS guideline for the management of patients with atrial fibrillation: executive summary. A report of the American College of Cardiology/American Heart Association Task Force on Practice Guidelines and the Heart Rhythm Society. *J Am Coll Cardiol*. 2014;64:2246–2280.
41. Donal E, Yamada H, Leclercq C, Herpin D. The left atrial appendage, a small, blind-ended structure: a review of its echocardiographic evaluation and its clinical role. *Chest*. 2005;128:1853–1862.
42. Qamruddin S, Shinbane J, Shriki J, Naqvi T. Left atrial appendage: structure, function, imaging modalities and therapeutic options. *Expert Rev Cardiovasc Ther*. 2010;8:65–75.
43. Marriott K, Manins V, Forshaw A, Wright J, Pascoe R. Detection of right-to-left atrial communication using agitated saline contrast imaging: experience with 1162 patients and recommendations for echocardiography. *J Am Soc Echocardiogr*. 2013;26:96–102.
44. Nishimura R, Otto C, Bonow R, et al. AHA/ACC guideline for the management of patients with valvular heart disease. A report of the American College of Cardiology/American Heart Association Task force on Practice Guidelines. *J Am Coll Cardiol*. 2014;63:e57–185.
45. Zoghbi W, Chambers J, Dumesnil J, et al. Recommendations for evaluation of prosthetic valves with echocardiography and Doppler ultrasound: a report from the American Society of Echocardiography's Guidelines and Standards Committee and the Task Force on Prosthetic Valves. *J Am Soc Echocardiogr*. 2009;22:975–1014.
46. Barbetseas J, Nagueh S, Pitsavos C, et al. Differentiating thrombus from pannus formation in obstructed mechanical prosthetic valves: an evaluation of clinical, transthoracic and transesophageal echocardiographic parameters. *J Am Coll Cardiol*. 1998;32:1410–1417.
47. Li J, Sexton D, Mick N, et al. Proposed modifications to the Duke criteria for the diagnosis of infective endocarditis. *Clin Infect Dis*. 2000;30:633.
48. Baddour L, Wilson W, Bayer A, et al. Infective endocarditis in adults: diagnosis, Antimicrobial therapy, and management of complications: a scientific statement for healthcare professionals from the American Heart Association. *Circulation*. 2015;132:1435–1486.
49. Habib G, Lancellotti P, Antunes M, et al. ESC guidelines for the management of infective endocarditis: the Task Force for the Management of Infective Endocarditis of the European Society of Cardiology (ESC). Endorsed by: European Association for Cardio-Thoracic Surgery (EACTS), the European Association of Nuclear Medicine (EANM). *Eur Heart J*. 2015;36:3075–3128. 2015.
50. Roe M, Abramson M, Li J, et al. Clinical information determines the impact of transesophageal echocardiography on the diagnosis of infective endocarditis by the Duke criteria. *Am Heart J*. 2000;139:945.
51. Movsowitz H, Levine R, Hilgenberg A, Isselbacher E. Transesophageal echocardiographic description of the mechanisms of aortic regurgitation in acute type A aortic dissection: implications for aortic valve repair. *J Am Coll Cardiol*. 2000;36:884–890.
52. Goldstein S, Evangelista A, Abbara S, et al. Multimodality imaging of diseases of the thoracic aorta in adults: from the American Society of Echocardiography and the European Association of Cardiovascular Imaging: Endorsed by the Society of Cardiovascular Computed tomography and Society for Cardiovascular Magnetic Resonance. *J Am Soc Echocardiogr*. 2015;28:119–182.

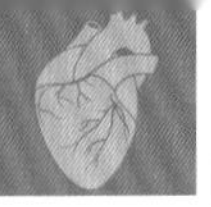

53. Hiratzka LFBG, Beckman JA, et al. ACCF/AHA/AATS/ACR/ASA/SCA/SCAI/SIR/STS/SVM guidelines for the diagnosis and management of patients with thoracic aortic disease: executive summary. A report of the American College of Cardiology Foundation/American Heart Association Task Force on Practice Guidelines, American Association for Thoracic Surgery, American College of Radiology, American Stroke Association, Society of Cardiovascular Anesthesiologists, Society for Cardiovascular Angiography and Interventions, Society of Interventional Radiology, Society of Thoracic Surgeons, and Society for Vascular Medicine. *J Am Coll Cardiol.* 2010;55:e27–129. 2010.
54. Goldstein S, Evangelista A, Abbara S, et al. Multimodality imaging of diseases of the thoracic aorta in adults: from the American Society of Echocardiography and the European Association of Cardiovascular Imaging: Endorsed by the Society of Cardiovascular Computed Tomography and Society for Cardiovascular Magnetic Resonance. *J Am Soc Echocardiogr.* 2015;28:119.
55. Vignon P, Spencer K, Rambaud G, et al. Differential transesophageal echocardiographic diagnosis between linear artifacts and intraluminal flap of aortic dissection or disruption. *Chest.* 2001;119:1778–1790.
56. Hiratzka L, Bakris G, Beckman J, et al. ACCF/AHA/AATS/ACR/ASA/SCA/SCAI/SIR/STS/SVM guidelines for the diagnosis and management of patients with thoracic aortic disease. *J Am Coll Cardiol.* 2010;55:e27–129.
57. Cinnella G, Dambrosio M, Brienza N, et al. Transesophageal echocardiography for diagnosis of traumatic aortic injury: an appraisal of the evidence. *J Trauma.* 2004;57:1246–1255.
58. Quinones M, Douglas P, Foster E, et al. ACC/AHA clinical competence statement on echocardiography: a report of the ACC/AHA/ACP/ASIM Task Force on Clinical Competence. *J Am Soc Echocardiogr.* 2003;16:379–402.

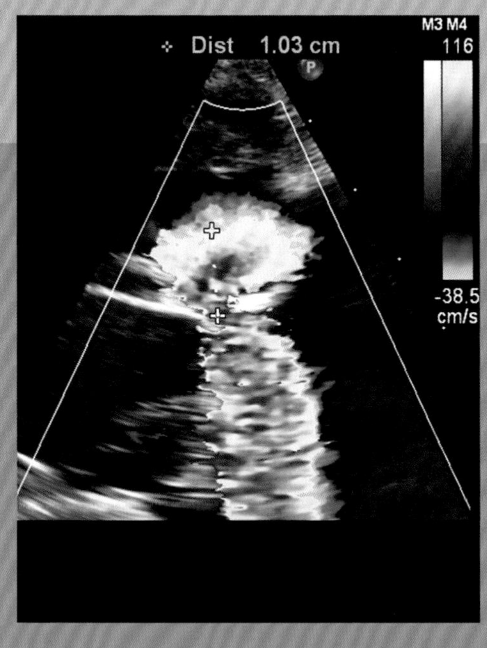

中文导读

第9章 术中超声心动图

心脏外科手术或非心脏外科手术中应用术中经食管超声心动图进行监测已经有了很大的进展和普遍应用，既往单纯应用于心室壁运动的观察，现在广泛应用于左、右心功能和容积，节段性室壁运动的定量评估。本章详细讲述了其具体测量方法及多样化的技术手段，包括血流多普勒、组织多普勒、斑点追踪成像技术评价应变和应变率等方法的应用。

此外，详细阐述了术中经食管超声心动图在不同的临床环境下发挥特定的作用：体外循环撤机后的心腔排气指导；非体外循环不停跳冠状动脉旁路移植术中的室壁运动观察和监测；心血管内装置如肺动脉漂浮导管、主动脉内球囊反搏、左心室辅助、右心室辅助、全人工心脏、静脉-静脉体外膜肺、冠状静脉插管、股静脉插管等置入的定位引导等的具体应用方法；在心脏、肺脏、肝脏等移植手术中也发挥作用。术中经食管超声心动图的风险和禁忌证主要是食道和上消化道疾病。除经食管超声心动图外，配有消毒护膜的普通探头在心外膜或主动脉外膜监测也可作为经食管超声心动图的替代方法。

本章最后阐述了术中经食管超声心动图应用的临床产出和成本效益：不同研究表明，术中经食管超声心动图将会有新的诊断发现，并在不同程度上改变手术计划和策略，因此而带来可观的卫生经济效益。

朱振辉

9 Intraoperative Echocardiography

MICHAEL L. HALL, MD | DONALD C. OXORN, MD

The use of transesophageal echocardiography (TEE) in the operating room has evolved from a simple tool to look at ventricular wall motion to a powerful diagnostic modality for examining every facet of cardiac[1] and noncardiac surgery.[2] Its use has improved the quality of perioperative care. Intraoperative assessments of valvular function, chamber size, masses, and great vessels are covered in other chapters of this textbook.

The milieu of the operating room is unique and not always conducive to obtaining TEE images of high quality. Image quality can be improved by dimming the lights in the room as much as possible to avoid the necessity for overgaining, completing the important parts of the study before the surgical incision is made, and setting the loop cycle to a time-based rather than a beat-based mode to prevent premature looping when electrocautery is used. The TEE probe is placed under general anesthesia, making understanding of the difficulties of probe insertion and manipulation especially important.

ECHOCARDIOGRAPHY

PROCEDURAL AND TECHNICAL EXPERIENCE

General standards and training requirements are necessary to ensure competency and the quality of echocardiography in any institution.[3] Trainees perform and interpret studies under supervision from certified faculty and must meet certain criteria for their own certification.

Echocardiography is a growing field in terms of technology and its use for assessing diseases and confirming diagnoses. There is opportunity for lifelong learning and continued mastering of skills. The American Society of Echocardiography, Society of Cardiovascular Anesthesiologists, Canadian Cardiovascular Society, and European Society of Cardiology require continuing medical education (CME) and a minimum number of yearly TEE studies for maintenance of certification. Competency and certification are maintained by governing bodies, and a minimum number of procedures ensures adequate familiarity with the techniques. Proficiency in TEE includes the ability to perform the examination safely, manipulate the probe in a variety of domains, adjust controls to optimize images, recognize abnormalities in cardiac structures or function, perform qualitative and quantitative analysis, and accurately report findings.

RISKS AND CONTRAINDICATIONS

Risks and contraindication for TEE are listed in Table 9.1. TEE is contraindicated for patients with esophageal disease (e.g., esophageal stricture), tumor, active upper gastrointestinal (GI) bleeding, and perforated viscous.[4] The risks associated with TEE are rare but can cause serious morbidity and mortality. Each case should be evaluated based on a risk-benefit analysis, with special attention to the absolute and relative contraindications to TEE.[4]

EVALUATION OF INTRAOPERATIVE VENTRICULAR FUNCTION

LV DIASTOLIC FUNCTION

In patients with impaired diastolic function, left ventricular (LV) filling in the period after separation from cardiopulmonary bypass is especially tenuous. Diastolic function is often further reduced, and depending on the degree, it may portend an increased incidence of adverse myocardial events.[5–8] In addition to the standard parameters of mitral inflow and pulmonary venous flow velocities, newer techniques may be used to better define problems with ventricular filling.[9,10]

Tissue Doppler imaging (TDI) of the mitral annulus has been proposed as a descriptor of LV relaxation that is less affected by changes in loading conditions and ventricular function than more traditional Doppler parameters.[11] Because the E′ velocity relates directly to LV relaxation, this parameter has been used to correct for LV relaxation and render the E wave of mitral inflow more accurate in the estimation of LV filling pressure (E/e′ ratio). This approach has been validated using transthoracic echocardiography (TTE) and also with TEE in the nonoperative ICU setting; however, results obtained with TEE in patients undergoing cardiac surgery have not been replicated.[12] Kumar et al., using filling pressures derived from pulmonary artery (PA) catheters as the standard, showed that TDI of the lateral mitral annulus was unable to accurately predict LV filling

TABLE 9.1 Relative and Absolute Contraindications to TEE.

Absolute Contraindications[a]	Relative Contraindications
Previous esophagectomy or esophagogastrectomy	Esophageal varices
Active upper GI bleed	Active esophagitis or peptic ulcer disease
Esophageal	Restricted neck mobility
Stricture	Barrett esophagus
Tumor	Recent upper GI bleed
Injury	History of GI surgery
Diverticulum	Dysphagia
	Vocal cord paralysis or injury
	Coagulopathy
	Severe thrombocytopenia
	Symptomatic hiatal hernia

[a]There is debate among experts about what constitutes absolute contraindications; risks and benefits must be weighed for each patient.
GI, Gastrointestinal.
Data from Hahn RT, Abraham T, Adams MS, et al. Guidelines for performing a comprehensive transesophageal echocardiographic examination: recommendations from the American Society of Echocardiography and the Society of Cardiovascular Anesthesiologists. *J Am Soc Echocardiogr*. 2013;26:921–964; Reeves ST, Glas KE, Eltzschig H, et al. Guidelines for performing a comprehensive epicardial echocardiography examination: recommendations of the American Society of Echocardiography and the Society of Cardiovascular Anesthesiologists. *J Am Soc Echocardiogr*. 2007;20):427–437; Flachskampf FA, Badano L, Daniel WG, et al. Recommendations for transoesophageal echocardiography: update 2010. *Eur J Echocardiogr*. 2010;11:557–576.

pressures.[13] Many conditions other than left atrial (LA) pressure that influence the E/E′ ratio[14] are present in the intraoperative population, limiting the usefulness of this parameter.[9,10]

Color M-mode flow propagation velocity is another less load-dependent measure of diastolic function and is attractive in that it examines simultaneous pulsed-wave (PW) Doppler measurements throughout the LV cavity. Djaiani et al.[15] showed that in patients undergoing coronary artery bypass grafting (CABG), a value less than 50 cm/s identifies abnormal diastolic function. Color M-mode has shown dependability as a simple method to quickly and reliably evaluate LV diastolic function.[16] The numerous parameters available and their lack of validity in the intraoperative setting limit the usefulness of diastolic dysfunction evaluation after cardiac surgery.[13,17]

SYSTOLIC FUNCTION

LV Systolic Function

The American Society of Echocardiography's guidelines and standards committee published recommendations for chamber quantification by TTE and TEE. The normal ranges for dimension and volume are comparable for the two techniques.[18,19]

Several investigators have examined the intraoperative relationship between end-diastolic area or end-systolic area measured at the transgastric mid-papillary level and cardiac volume status. Cheung et al.[20] performed an elegant study examining the effect of graded hypovolemia produced by autologous blood collection on hemodynamic- and TEE-derived indices of LV preload in patients undergoing coronary artery bypass surgery. Patients with valvular insufficiency, rhythms other than sinus, or overt congestive heart failure were excluded. End-diastolic area, end-systolic area, pulmonary capillary wedge pressure, and measures of end-diastolic and end-systolic wall stress decreased linearly as blood volume was reduced by 0% to 15% in all patients; however, in patients with impaired LV function, only the TEE-derived indices maintained linearity. As the study authors acknowledged, estimation of ventricular volume in patients with asymmetric ventricular dysfunction can be problematic because hypokinetic or akinetic areas may not be represented in the area of the two-dimensional (2D) cut.

The presence of a small end-diastolic area or end-systolic area does not always reflect decreased intravascular volume. Small LV volumes can be seen with restrictions to filling (e.g., pericardial disease) or decreased right-sided heart function (Fig. 9.1), such as with a right ventricular (RV) infarction or a large pulmonary embolus. Other causes of a small LV volume include increased inotropy or redistribution of blood out of the thoracic cavity.

LV Volumes

The accepted approach for volume measurement is the biplane method of disks (i.e., Simpson's rule). Studies using multiplane probes[21] have shown that volumetric data obtained by 2D TTE and 2D TEE show minor or no differences.

3D TTE has proved to be a useful tool in the measurement of LV volumes, and normal ranges of values have been published.[22,23] Notwithstanding the fact that 3D echocardiography-derived volumes tend to be underestimated compared with cardiac magnetic resonance (CMR) imaging,[24] the data obtained are significantly closer to those of CMR than 2D, and they are more robust when tested for intraobserver and interobserver variability and for test-retest reproducibility.[25] Compared with magnetic resonance imaging (MRI), echocardiography slightly underestimates (by 4%) volumes and ejection fractions (EFs) and is less sensitive for detection of wall motion abnormalities.[26]

The use of real-time 3D TEE in the operating room has increased dramatically, particularly for mitral valve assessment and periprocedural monitoring. Meris et al.[27] compared intraoperative 2D and 3D TEE measurements of ventricular volumes and EFs. The 2D data were obtained using automated border detection, followed by manual tracing in the 2- and 4-chamber views and application of the Simpson rule. The 3D data were acquired in full-volume mode and subsequently analyzed with the use of Philips Q-lab 3D-Advanced quantification software (Philips Medical Systems, Boston, MA).[28]

The results are shown in Table 9.2. The EF was the same using both modalities. Ventricular volumes were greater in the 3D group, but although the difference was statistically significant, it did not lead to any differences in LV classification as normal, mildly to moderately dilated, or severely dilated. Data acquisition times were similar, but analysis of the data took longer in the 3D group and was predicated on a stable rhythm, a necessity for multiple beat acquisition.

Conclusions

Assessment of preload with intraoperative TEE is in most cases a semiquantitative estimate based on visual inspection of end-diastolic area and end-systolic area and supported by an array of Doppler indices. The use of 2D TEE to quantitate ventricular volumes is feasible, but the use of 3D TEE is limited by beat acquisition difficulties and long analysis times. Confounding conditions, such as RV failure, vasodilation, or the administration of inotropic agents, must be considered.

GLOBAL SYSTOLIC FUNCTION

Cardiac Output

Doppler TEE has the potential for use in the intraoperative setting for the continuous measurement of cardiac output. These methods are based on the concept that the cross-sectional area of a conduit in the cardiovascular system multiplied by the

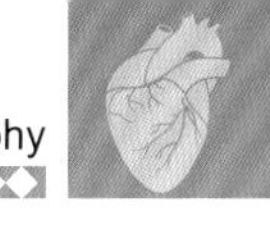

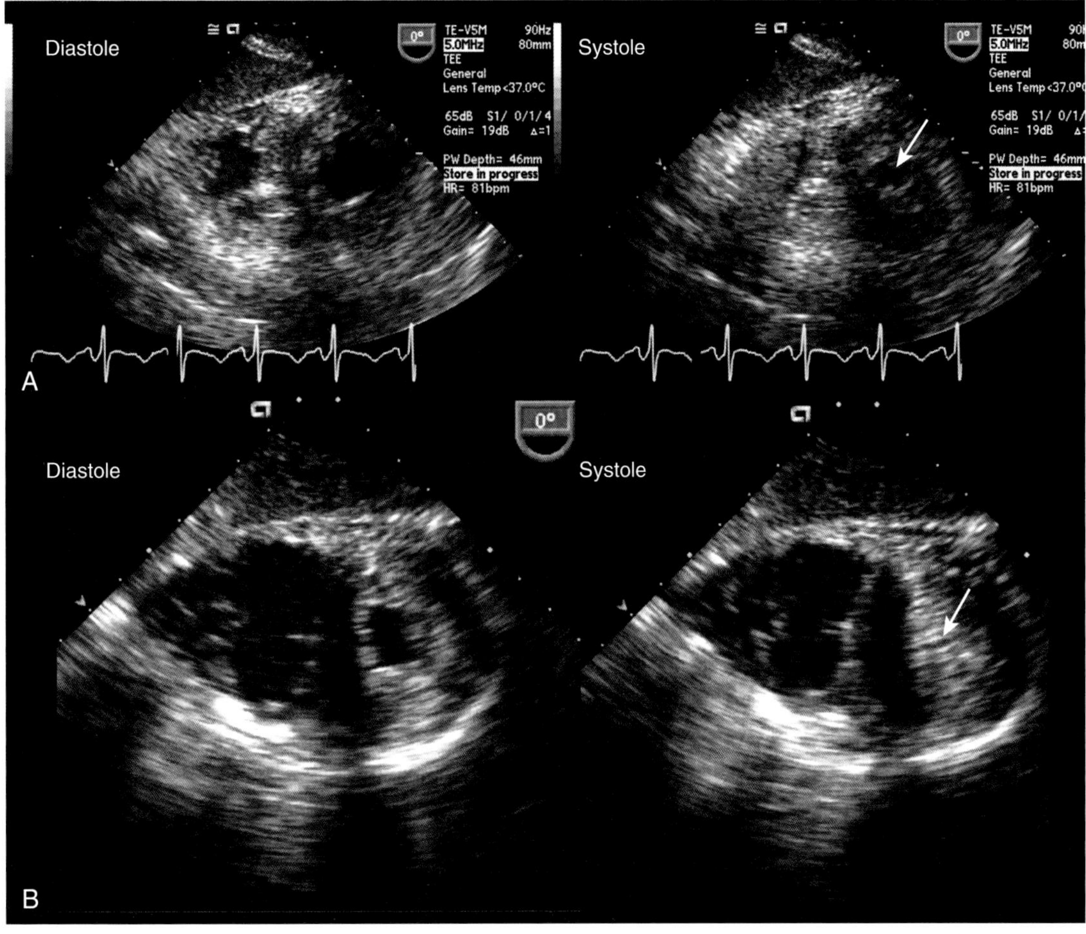

Fig. 9.1 **Decreased LV end-systolic volume.** Transgastric TEE scans were obtained for two patients with decreased end-systolic volume in the LV. (A) Two scans show decreased volume in the right and left ventricles *(arrow)*, which is consistent with hypovolemia or profound peripheral vasodilation (see Video 9.1A). (B) The patient had pulmonary hypertension due to cystic fibrosis. Although the end-systolic area of the LV is exceedingly small *(arrow)*, this condition was caused by right-sided heart failure, not absolute hypovolemia (see Video 9.1B).

Doppler-derived time–velocity integral yields the stroke volume through that conduit. When the result is multiplied by heart rate, the product is cardiac output.

Several important assumptions are inherent in this approach. Valid area formulas must be applicable to the anatomic site being analyzed. The velocity profile across the valve must be flat and devoid of skew.[29,30] Whichever anatomic area is chosen, the ability to consistently obtain the image and to interrogate parallel to flow is mandatory.

Cardiac output can also be calculated from 2D or 3D volumetric measurements by subtracting the systolic volume from the diastolic volume and multiplying by the heart rate to obtain cardiac output. This process is more time-consuming than Doppler-derived data, less accurate in the setting of mitral regurgitation or arrhythmia, and seldom used in the operating room.

LV Outflow Tract

Use of Doppler technique in regard to the left ventricular outflow tract (LVOT) has been extensively studied and found to be extremely accurate when applied to a group of patients before and after cardiopulmonary bypass.[31] With the probe in the stomach, turned leftward, in the flexed position, and at low imaging frequency, the aortic valve and LVOT can usually be imaged between 0 and 140 degrees (Fig. 9.2). Imaging from the stomach allows parallel pulsed-Doppler interrogation of the LVOT; its diameter can be obtained from the stomach or from the mid-esophageal long-axis view. Calculations of the cross-sectional area and cardiac output follow the standard formula (see Fig. 9.2). To avoid contamination of the Doppler signal by the region of flow acceleration adjacent to the aortic valve orifice, the sample volume must be placed precisely in the LVOT. In the setting of outflow tract obstruction, the validity of the measurement may be compromised.

Lodato et al.[32] measured LVOT area using 2D and 3D TTE with color Doppler in the assessment of stroke volume and compared the values with thermodilution-acquired stroke volumes. Although they correlated well, there was less bias with 3D measurements, which was attributed by the study authors to 3D's independence from geometric assumptions. Similar findings with TTE were observed by Shahgaldi et al.,[33] who found that stroke volume measurements using a 3D planimetered LVOT area (Fig. 9.3) were more accurate than traditional 2D measurements and the biplane method of disks (i.e., Simpson's rule), although CMR remains the true gold standard for measurement of LV volumes.

Montealegre-Gallegos et al. compared cardiac output measurements made with 2D and 3D TEE.[34] They posited that the assumption of a circular LVOT could introduce error because of its actual ellipsoid shape.[35] Using 3D TEE and multiplanar reconstruction, they substituted a planimetered measurement of the LVOT area. Although the 2D and 3D measurements were highly correlated, the 2D method was on average 10% lower. The main limitation was that there was no comparison with a gold standard.

TABLE 9.2 3D and 2D TEE Indexed Volumes and Function for a Study Population (N = 152) and Its Subgroups.

Parameter	*3D TEE*	*2D TEE*	*P Value*	*Median Pairwise Difference (99% CI)*
EF (%)	55 ± 14	55 ± 14	0.227	−0.4 (−1.2 to 0.3)
iEDV (mL/m²)	54 ± 21	51 ± 21	<0.001	3.3 (2.5 to 4.2)
iESV (mL/m²)	26 ± 18	24 ± 17	<0.001	1.4 (1.0 to 2.0)
3D and 2D iEDV (mL/m²)[a]				
Systolic Function				
Normal (62%)	47 ± 16	43 ± 15	<0.001	3.2 (2.3 to 4.4)
Mildly abnormal (16%)	53 ± 14	51 ± 12	0.794	3.6 (−3.8 to 5.8)
Moderately abnormal (14%)	71 ± 23	67 ± 23	0.001	3.3 (1.6 to 6.2)
Severely abnormal (8%)	89 ± 23	85 ± 24	0.023	3.9 (0.7 to 6.9)
Ventricular Volume				
Normal (86%)	48 ± 12	45 ± 12	<0.001	3.5 (2.4 to 4.2)
Dilated (14%)	101 ± 19	96 ± 17	0.002	3.2 (1.2 to 5.6)

[a]Subgroups of patients are reported as a percentage (in parentheses) of the whole population (N = 152).
CI, Confidence interval; *EF*, ejection fraction; *iEDV*, indexed end-diastolic volume; *iESV*, indexed end-systolic volume; *TEE*, transesophageal echocardiography.
From Meris A, Santambrogio L, Casso G. Intraoperative three-dimensional versus two-dimensional echocardiography for left ventricular assessment. *Anesth Analg.* 2014;118:711–720.

Pulmonary Artery

With the probe at 0 degrees and retroflexed, the main PA and pulmonic valve can be imaged at the base of the heart. In a study by Gorcsan et al.[36] using PW and continuous-wave (CW) methods and with the PA diameter measured just distal to the pulmonic valve, intraoperative cardiac output was calculated. Interobserver variability was low in all studies, and correlation with thermodilution cardiac output was strong. Alternatively, the main PA may be imaged at 60 to 90 degrees using the aortic arch as a window (Fig. 9.4).

RV Outflow Tract

From the transgastric approach, the probe is turned rightward and flexed to image the RV outflow tract at a rotation angle between 0 and 120 degrees. Imaging frequency is usually reduced to ensure optimal penetration. Maslow et al.[37] found excellent correlation between cardiac output calculated with PW Doppler and with thermodilution. Patients with pulmonary hypertension, significant tricuspid regurgitation, and nonsinus rhythms were excluded. In a significant percentage (16%) of patients, the 2D image was not suitable.

Practical Considerations

For intraoperative transesophageal Doppler calculation of cardiac output, the LVOT method is the most reproducible. Adjustments in the degree of probe flexion and imaging angle should be made to ensure that the aortic valve and ascending aorta are clearly visualized and that the Doppler intercept angle is small (see Fig. 9.2).

Several measurements should be made and then averaged; this is especially important with rhythms other than sinus. In

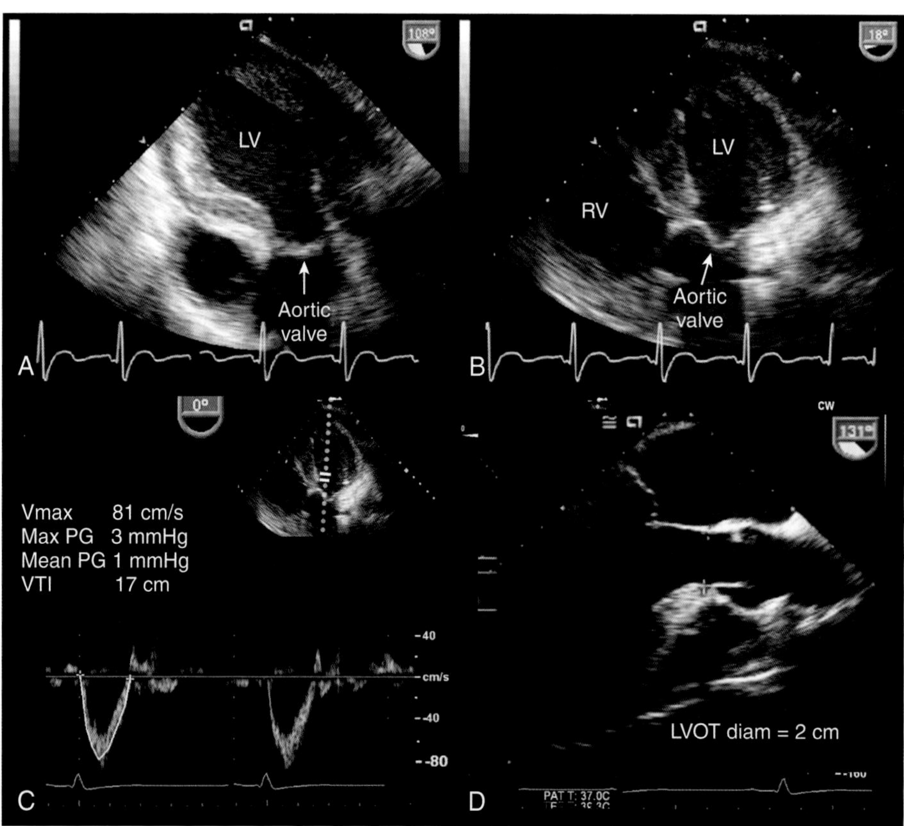

Fig. 9.2 Doppler interrogation of the LV outflow tract *(LVOT)* and ascending aorta. TEE imaging from the stomach allows parallel alignment with the LVOT and ascending aorta. Images were obtained from a transgastric long-axis view (A) and a deep transgastric long-axis view (B). (C) A pulsed-Doppler sample volume with a small intercept angle has been placed into the LVOT, yielding a velocity–time integral *(VTI)* of 17 cm. (D) A mid-esophageal long-axis view enables measurement of the LVOT diameter *(diam)* and calculation of the LVOT area, which allows calculation of the stroke volume. *Mean PG*, mean pressure gradient; *Vmax*, maximum velocity.

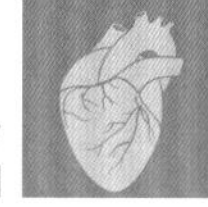

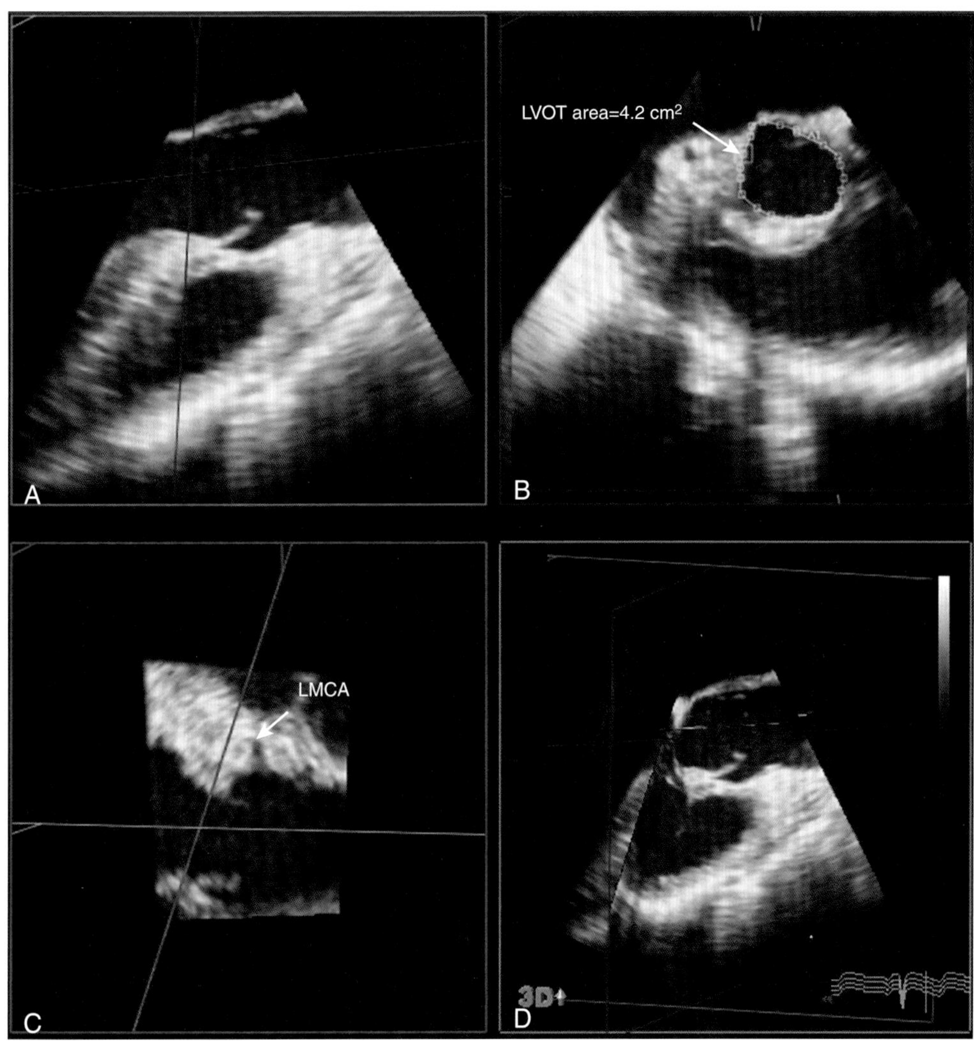

Fig. 9.3 Multiplanar reconstruction of the LV outflow tract *(LVOT)*. (A–D) The LVOT area can be measured using 3D TEE and multiplanar reconstruction. Orthogonal cuts through the LVOT *(red lines)* yield a 2D cross-sectional area that is suitable for planimetry. *LMCA*, Left main coronary artery.

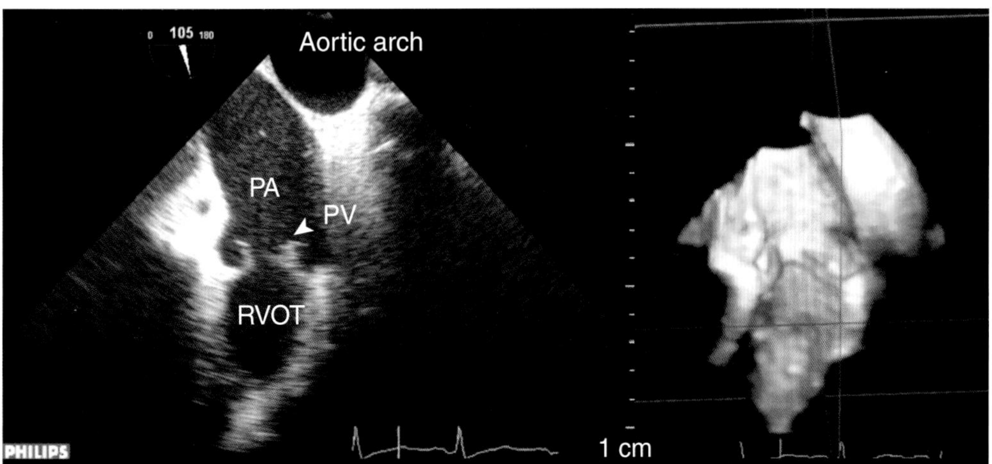

Fig. 9.4 Imaging of the main pulmonary artery from the upper esophagus in 2D and 3D. Using the aortic arch as a window, the high esophageal aortic arch short-axis view is obtained, followed by slight turning of the probe to the patient's right. The main pulmonary artery *(PA)*, pulmonic valve *(PV)*, and RV outflow tract *(RVOT)* are seen. This view is suitable for Doppler interrogation (see Video 9.4).

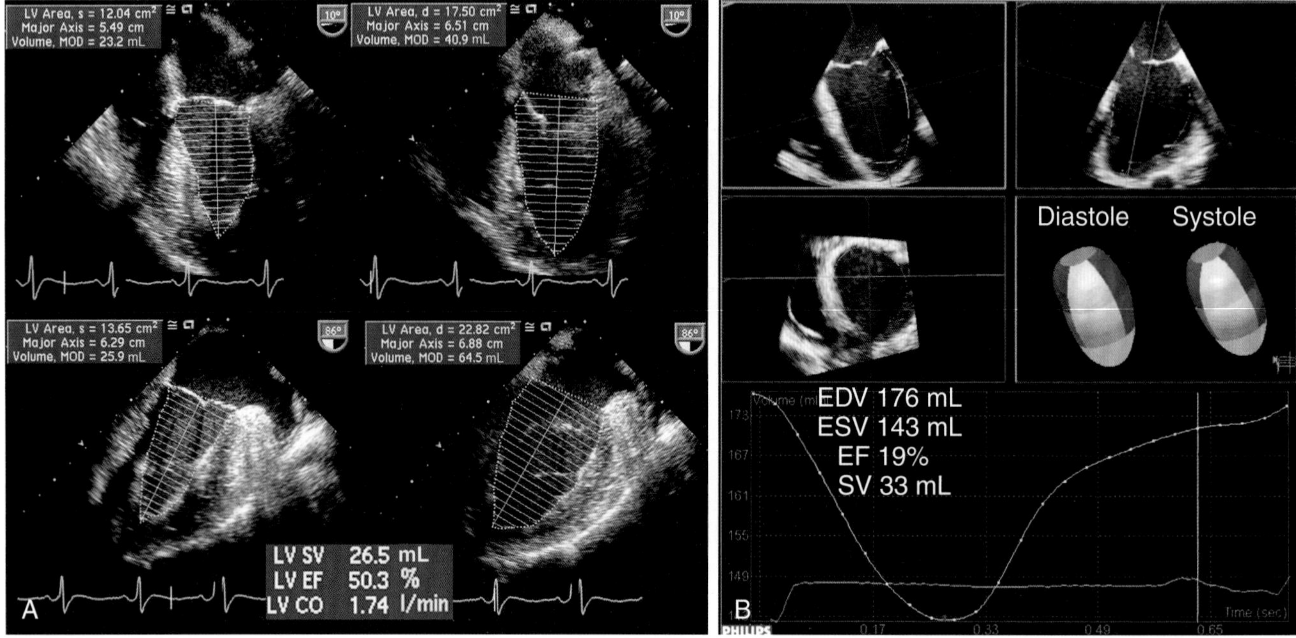

Fig. 9.5 2D and 3D TEE calculation of the ejection fraction. (A) Measurements of the systolic *(left)* and diastolic *(right)* areas made with the 4-chamber *(top panels)* and 2-chamber *(bottom panels)* views to obtain volumetric data by the method of disks *(MOD)*. From these measurements, the stroke volume *(SV)*, ejection fraction *(EF)*, and cardiac output *(CO)* can be calculated. (B) 3D TEE is used to calculate the EF in an patient with a cardiomyopathy (see Video 9.5). *EDV*, End-diastolic volume; *ESV*, end-systolic volume.

practical terms, Doppler measurement of cardiac output is used when a PA catheter is not in place or when conditions (e.g., severe tricuspid regurgitation) render thermodilution inaccurate. When right- and left-sided outputs are obtained simultaneously, the shunt fraction may be calculated.

There is a need for further validation of this approach in patients with a spectrum of cardiovascular diseases. 3D TEE has intuitive appeal because it may circumvent the geometric assumptions inherent in 2D measurement, but it has yet to be validated against a gold standard such as thermodilution or CMR.[38] Limitations of 3D TEE for cardiac output measurement in the operating room are the interference with multibeat acquisition by electrocautery, cardiac manipulation by the surgical team, and the frequent presence of rhythms other than sinus.

Ejection Fraction and Stroke Volume

Although it is load dependent and therefore not a pure index of contractility, the EF is often assumed to reflect ventricular contractility. During intraoperative TEE, the fractional area of change (FAC) measured at the transgastric mid-papillary level is often used interchangeably with EF, although gauging volume in a potentially asymmetric chamber based on a measure of area has obvious limitations.

In an elegant study, Royse et al.[39] demonstrated that FAC, when corrected for afterload, was closely related to preload recruitable stroke work, a relatively load-independent measure of contractility. The *dP*/*dt* value was more load dependent and less reliable. The patient group was quite diverse in terms of overall ventricular function. The most commonly accepted method for volume measurement is the biplane method of disks (i.e., Simpson's rule) (Fig. 9.5).

Practically, the intraoperative EF is still most often visually estimated or measured by single-plane FAC. Concern remains that FAC underestimates the EF in patients in whom hypokinetic areas are not represented in the measurement. For the technical reasons alluded to previously, real-time 3D TEE is not routinely used for determination of EF or ventricular volumes intraoperatively.

Tissue Doppler Imaging

The use of TDI to record systolic myocardial velocity at the lateral mitral annulus is a measure of longitudinal systolic function that correlates with EF; however, the velocity and direction assessments may be affected by translation, rotation, tethering, and the necessity for parallel intercept of annular motion by the Doppler signal.[40,41] The annulus is frequently calcified in surgical patients, and this may also limit usefulness.[42]

To circumvent these issues, the use of strain and strain rate imaging in the assessment of LV function has been extensively studied and is discussed in several excellent reviews[43–45] (see Chapter 4). In essence, strain rate represents the local rate of myocardial deformation and is estimated by spatial velocity gradients obtained by TDI. Unfortunately, the necessity for parallel alignment of the Doppler signal limits the use of intraoperative TDI for strain analysis.[44]

Speckle Tracking Imaging

Speckle tracking imaging is an angle- and translational-independent tool for measuring strain and strain rate (Fig. 9.6).[44] Speckle tracking evaluation of global longitudinal strain can effectively quantify LV function and remains accurate in the setting of wall motion abnormalities.[46] Impaired LV strain has been associated with increased 30-day mortality and hospital re-admission rates.[47] By acquiring high-quality 2D echocardiographic images and identifying unique acoustic markers in the image to track specific areas of myocardium over time, strain and strain rate can be calculated.

Several investigators have done feasibility studies of intraoperative strain analysis using TDI[48] and speckle tracking.[49] Kukucka et al.[49] found that when speckle tracking was used in

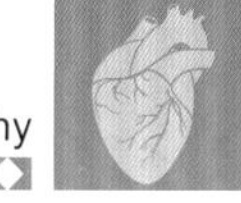

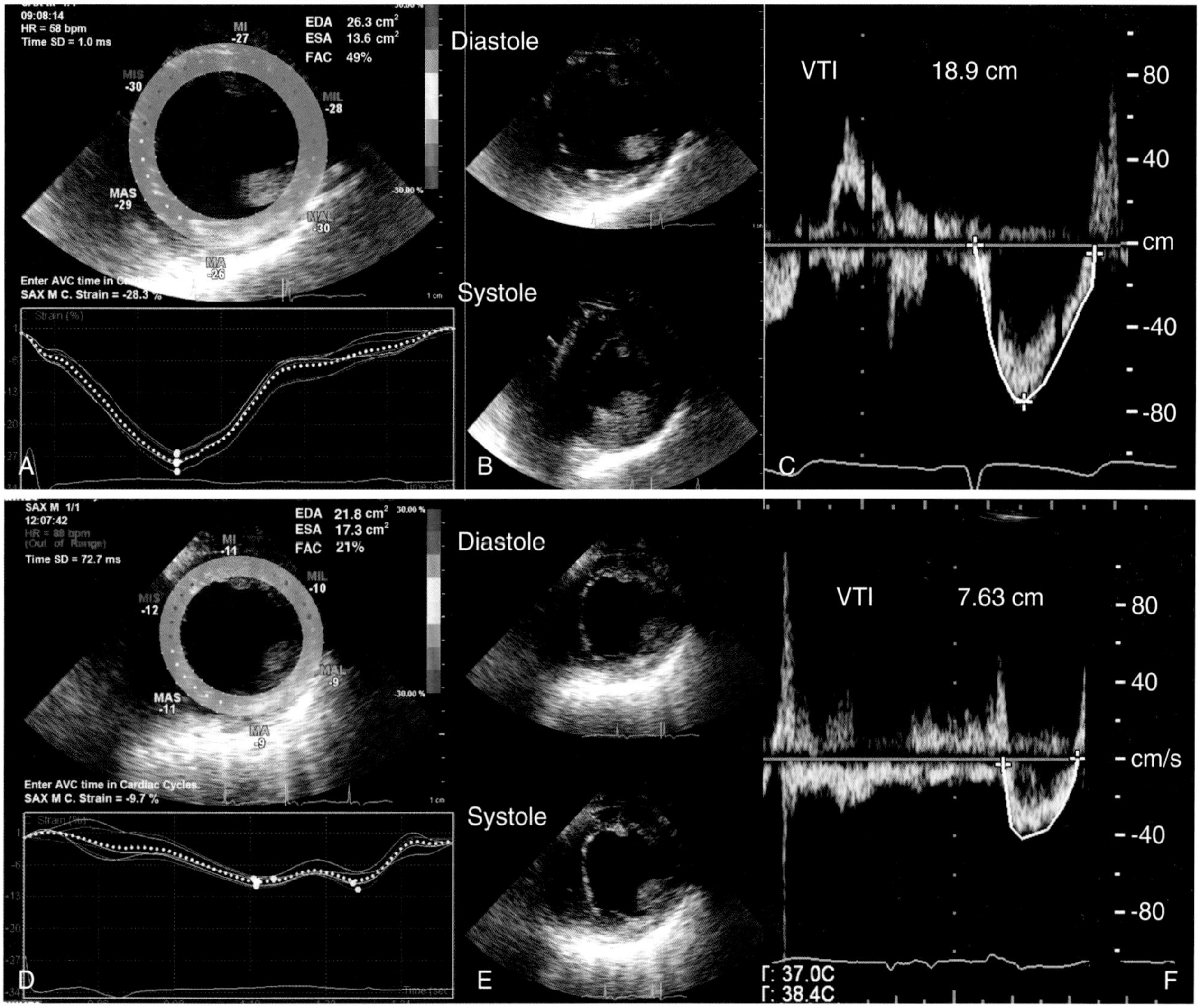

Fig. 9.6 **Assessment of LV function.** Surrogates for LV function are shown for a patient before and after cardiopulmonary bypass. (A–C) Circumferential strain (A), end-diastolic and end-systolic areas (B), and LV outflow tract velocity–time integrals *(VTIs)* (C) are obtained before bypass in a patient undergoing mitral valve replacement (see Videos 9.6A and B). (D–F) The same measurements are made after a long pump run and aortic cross-clamping time. Decrements in all three parameters are seen. The values returned toward baseline with time and after institution of resuscitative measures (see Videos 9.6C and D). *EDA*, End-diastolic area; *ESA*, end-systolic area; *FAC*, fractional area of change.

the setting of cardiac surgery, interobserver and intraobserver variability in the assessment of longitudinal and radial strain was acceptable and wall motion scores correlated best with radial strain.

These results must be tempered with the realities of the operating room, where decisions are often made in seconds by necessity. The practical techniques used to define the regions of interest are exacting and are prone to error if done improperly.[50] The different components of strain correspond to the orientation of myocardial fibers (i.e., longitudinal, radial, and circumferential) and are affected by underlying disease processes.[51] With TEE, global strain measurements are more robust than regional strain measurements.[44] Measurements must be made off-line, which is time-consuming. Although intraoperative strain analysis shows promise for the analysis of global and regional systolic function, better validation in the setting of cardiac surgery must be demonstrated.

RV

In the setting of cardiopulmonary bypass, the evaluation of RV function is important. RV dysfunction often occurs because of inadequate delivery of cardioplegia,[52] the development or worsening of left-sided pathology with pulmonary hypertension and tricuspid regurgitation, or embolization of intracardiac air down the right coronary artery after separation from cardiopulmonary bypass (Figs. 9.7 and 9.8). Numerous techniques described for TTE have been extrapolated to TEE. The triangular shape of the RV makes its global function hard to quantitate with TEE, although the modified method of disks has been used in off-line analysis in the setting of CABG.[53]

Tricuspid annular velocity (i.e., tricuspid annular plane systolic excursion [TAPSE]) measured by TDI has been used to quantitate RV function, with excursions less than 1.5 cm associated with a poor prognosis in a variety of cardiovascular diseases.[54] The technique employed during cardiac surgery uses a modified transgastric imaging view to facilitate parallel alignment with the lateral tricuspid annulus[55] (Fig. 9.9). TDI of the lateral tricuspid annulus is another technique that has been validated against CMR. Transgastric imaging facilitates parallel alignment of the Doppler signal with the movement of the annulus.

RV free wall strain imaging by speckle tracking compares well with RV function determined by CMR.[56] It was shown to be

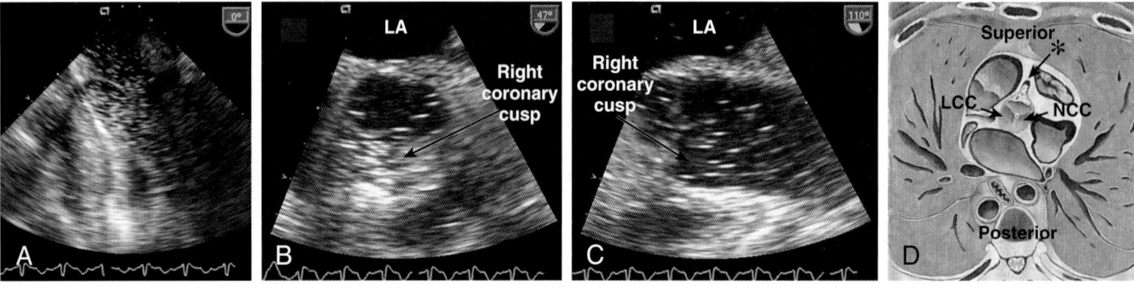

Fig. 9.7 Air emboli in the right coronary artery. (A) The LV and LA cavities are full of bubbles after release of the aortic cross-clamp (see Video 9.7A). Short-axis (B) and long-axis (C) views of the aortic valve show the bubbles coalescing in the vicinity of the right coronary cusp (see Video 9.7B). (D) The cross-sectional view with the patient supine shows that the right coronary cusp *(asterisk)* is most superior. Bubbles collect in the right coronary sinus of Valsalva and may embolize down the right coronary artery. *LCC*, Left coronary cusp; *NCC*, noncoronary cusp.

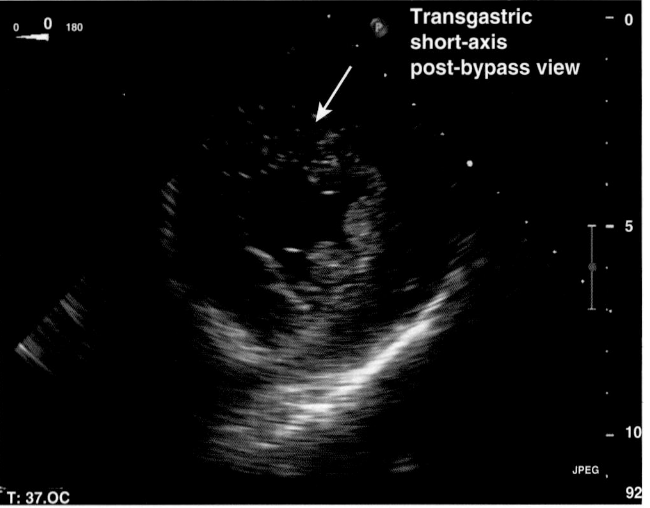

Fig. 9.8 Decreased RV function after air embolization. Inferior wall function decreases after air embolization down the right coronary artery. A new wall motion defect is seen in the inferior wall in the transgastric short-axis view and the mid-esophageal 2-chamber view, with apparent intramyocardial air *(arrow)*. In real time, a normal pre-bypass 2-chamber view is followed by segmental wall motion defects in the right coronary distribution (see Video 9.8).

feasible in the operating room[53] and compared well with other indices, such as TAPSE and FAC. There are no guidelines for reference values, but a low strain rate has predicted adverse cardiac events.[57]

3DE is an accurate and reproducible method of measuring RV function compared with MRI and radionuclide ventriculography.[57] Semi-automated border detection can be used for RV function and volume measurements. TEE assessment of intraoperative RV function is best accomplished by visual inspection and semiquantitative assessment in the transgastric and the 4-chamber views.[57]

REGIONAL WALL MOTION

The link between perioperative myocardial ischemia and cardiac morbidity[58] has led to an intensive search for accurate methods for its intraoperative detection (Fig. 9.10). TEE detection of segmental wall motion abnormalities (SWMAs) is a sensitive indicator of ischemia and can identify abnormalities before electrocardiographic (ECG), PA catheter, or hemodynamic changes are seen.[59]

The paucity of contraindications to TEE means that it can be used in most patients undergoing general anesthesia. The mid-papillary view is easy to obtain and demonstrates areas of myocardium subtended by the three major coronary arteries. Interpretation is rarely confounded by rhythm disturbances, in contrast to automated ST-segment analysis by ECG.

The prognostic implications of regional wall motion abnormalities for cardiac and noncardiac surgery have been published. London et al.[60] studied 156 patients undergoing noncardiac surgery who were at high risk for coronary artery disease. Specific clinical, ECG, or hemodynamic events prompted analysis of stored images. The number of new wall motion abnormalities detected was low, and discordance with ECG findings was significant. The number of postoperative cardiac complications was low, limiting the routine use of TEE in noncardiac surgery patients. In the study by Leung et al.,[61] patients undergoing CABG were examined with ECG and TEE. Although pre-bypass ischemia was rare, post-bypass ischemia was more common, and postoperative cardiovascular complications were associated more closely with TEE findings than with ECG alone.

It is now accepted that regional wall motion abnormalities, although often the result of myocardial ischemia, may result from hypovolemia, tethering of non-ischemic myocardium, and myocardial stunning after cardiopulmonary bypass. Abnormal interventricular septum abnormalities are seen after cardiopulmonary bypass, with right-sided chamber overload, ventricular pacing, and bundle branch blocks. Regional wall motion abnormalities that subtend the anatomic distribution of coronary artery flow are more often a result of ischemia than those that do not. Individual myocardial segments can be described with 2D tomographic cuts and the use of a bull's-eye display. There is variability in the distribution of coronary artery flow.

Comunale et al.[62] documented the poor concordance between TEE and ECG results and attributed this finding to the lack of standard definitions of significant regional wall motion abnormalities and ischemic ST-segment changes, the exclusion of longitudinal TEE views, and the use of different models of segment nomenclature. The overall concordance between ECG and TEE remains controversial.

TEE is the most sensitive test for intraoperative myocardial ischemia and has therefore been adapted by many practitioners. Conditions that lead to its lack of specificity must be taken into account. The ability to monitor additional tomographic planes; the use of cine loops for comparison; and the advent of new technologies, such as TDI and speckle tracking with strain imaging and real-time 3D TEE, should improve

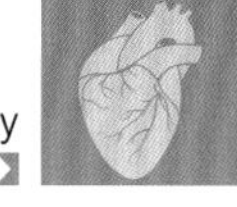

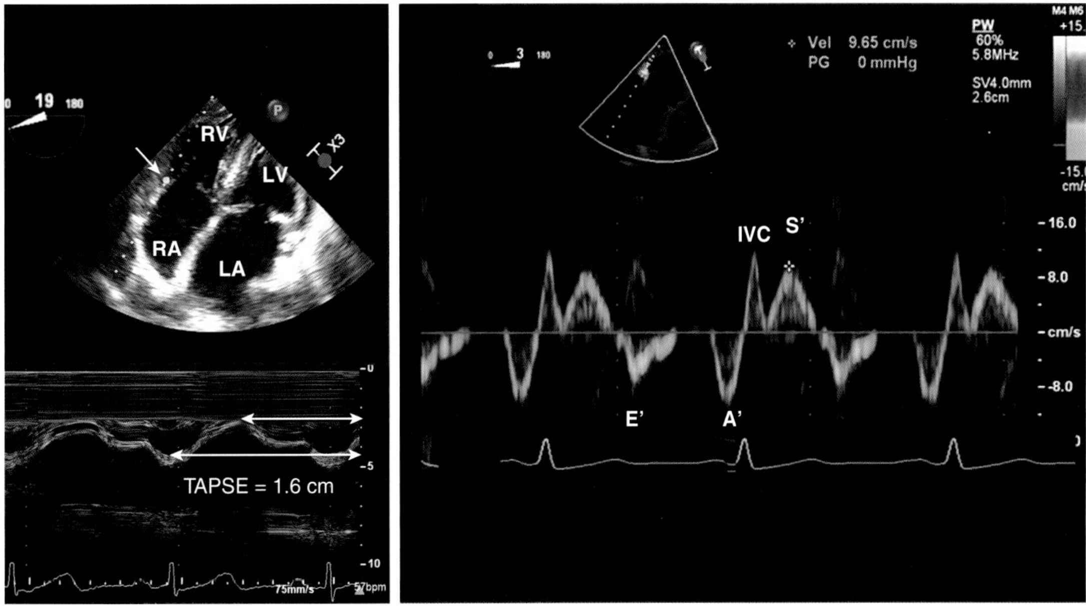

Fig. 9.9 **Assessment of RV function.** From a deep transgastric position with anteflexion, a reverse 4-chamber view is used, to identify the lateral tricuspid annulus *(arrow)*. In this view, the tricuspid annular plane systolic excursion *(TAPSE)* is measured with M-mode echocardiography and found to be 1.6 cm, consistent with normal RV function *(left)*. 2D is also well suited to tissue Doppler imaging of the tricuspid annulus because Doppler interrogation is parallel to the direction of annular movement. The *S′* velocity of 9.65 cm/s is consistent with normal RV function *(right)* (see Video 9.9).

accuracy. Regional longitudinal strain shows promise for detecting areas of ischemia,[63] but larger studies are needed before it can be used in routine clinical practice. Regional wall motion abnormalities precede ECG changes,[64] and after ischemia is diagnosed, TEE can be used to directly monitor the effects of intervention.

TEE MONITORING OF INTRAOPERATIVE CARDIAC FUNCTION IN SPECIFIC CLINICAL ENTITIES

The use of TEE has improved management of instability after cardiopulmonary bypass. It has elucidated the intraoperative changes that occur with some techniques used for coronary revascularization, and it can guide the placement of numerous intracardiac and intravascular devices. Its use in monitoring of cardiac function during noncardiac surgery is most advantageous in the diagnosis of sudden and unexplained hemodynamic instability.

SEPARATION FROM CARDIOPULMONARY BYPASS

At the time of separation of the patient from cardiopulmonary bypass, TEE helps guide the anesthesiologist in the use of pharmacologic and nonpharmacologic therapies such as volume resuscitation, and it can maximize the likelihood of smooth weaning from cardiopulmonary bypass.

Intracardiac Air

Left-sided intracardiac air is ubiquitous after procedures in which left-sided chambers have been open to the atmosphere. It is identified by its characteristic firefly appearance. Air is often seen entering the LA from the pulmonary veins or enmeshed in the mitral subvalvular apparatus (see Fig. 9.7). Echocardiographic inspection is carried out in the 2-chamber, 4-chamber, and transgastric long-axis views. Careful evacuation by the surgeon is important and involves suctioning of the aortic root vent or needle aspiration of the LV apex to evacuate trapped pockets. In addition to guiding evacuation, TEE is useful in diagnosing the consequences of embolization through the right coronary ostium, which results in ventricular dysfunction in a right coronary distribution (see Fig. 9.8).

Cardiac Output

Perioperative myocardial infarction is the primary cause of low cardiac output immediately after cardiopulmonary bypass.[65,66] The pre-bypass TEE-derived wall motion score index was found to independently predict the need for post-bypass inotropic support.[65]

OFF-PUMP CORONARY BYPASS SURGERY

One of the major controversies in cardiac surgery is the performance of coronary revascularization without cardiopulmonary bypass (i.e., off-pump bypass or beating heart operation). The major criticism is that incomplete revascularization leads to repeat interventions and that coexistent pathology such as mitral regurgitation cannot be dealt with. The pivotal study by Shroyer et al.[66] showed that at 1 year, the off-pump strategy led to worse composite outcomes, although the accompanying editorial emphasized that for certain patient subsets, benefits may still exist,[67] such as for those with atheromatous disease of the aorta.[68] The cardiac surgeon's learning curve for off-pump revascularization and center experience have been criticized in studies, and the debate continues.[68]

Hemodynamic instability can occur from intraoperative ischemia or cardiovascular deformation caused by the device used to stabilize the heart during coronary anastomoses.[69] Although the number of interpretable myocardial segments decreases during cardiac displacement, TEE can adequately detect regional wall motion abnormalities in most patients[70] and may help guide revascularization strategy.[71] It has been suggested that displacing the heart with a saline bag posteriorly improves transgastric image quality.[72]

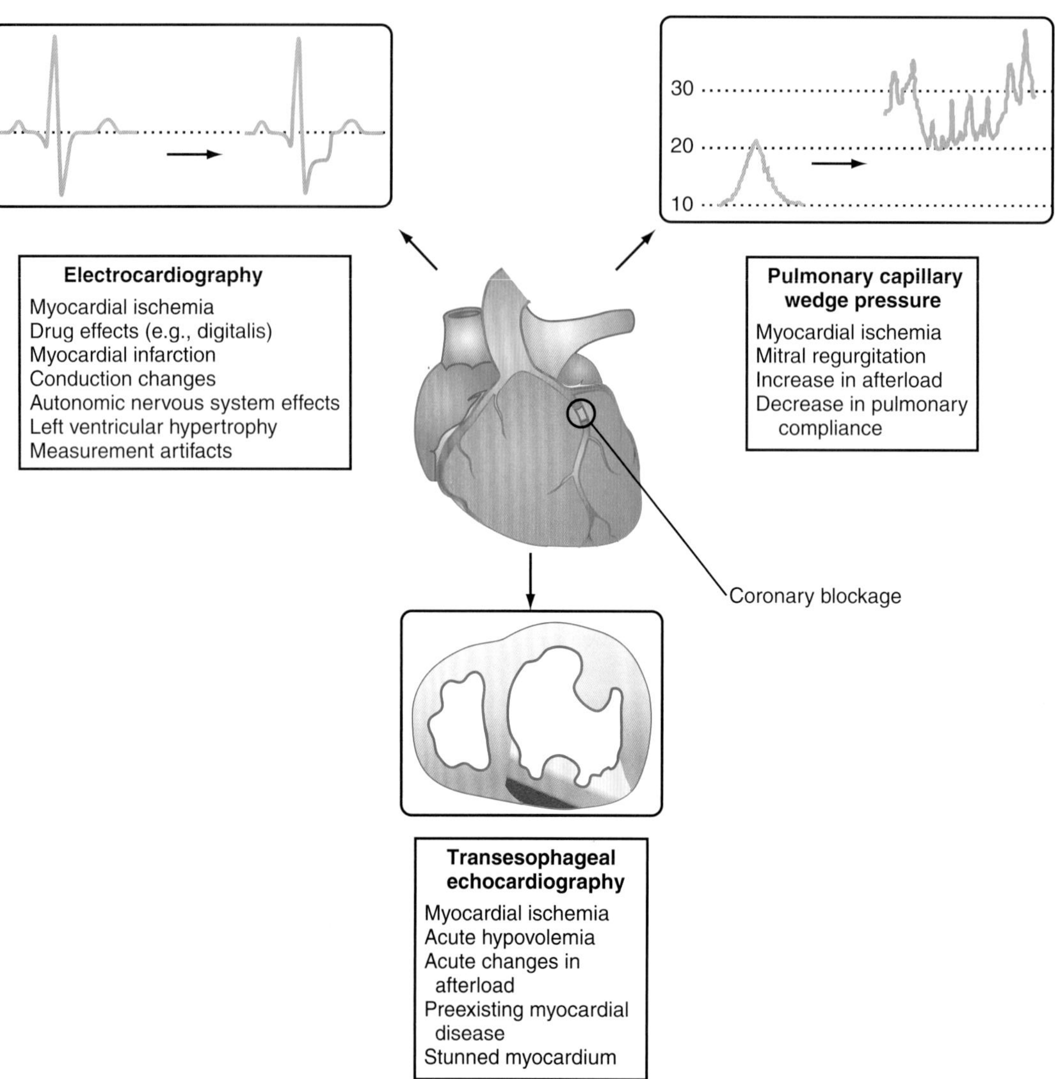

Fig. 9.10 Causes of ischemic changes detected by intraoperative monitors. TEE, pulmonary artery catheterization, and electrocardiography are used for monitoring perioperative myocardial ischemia. (From Fleisher LA, Weiskopf RB. Real-time intraoperative monitoring of myocardial ischemia in non-cardiac surgery. *Anesthesiology*. 2000;92(4):1183–1188.)

POSITIONING OF INTRAVASCULAR DEVICES

Intraoperative TEE can be used to guide the positioning of intravascular devices and to help to identify complications related to malposition or other cardiac injuries.

Pulmonary Artery Catheters

Proper placement of a PA catheter may be challenging in cases of right heart dysfunction, tricuspid regurgitation, or atrial fibrillation. Guidance with TEE facilitates passage through the tricuspid valve. It also allows determination of the depth of advancement into the PA, which can be important when the PA may be transected, such as in lung transplantation. Use of biplane imaging and temporarily filling of the PA catheter balloon can assist in verification of the tip of the catheter.

Intraaortic Balloon Pump

The intraaortic balloon pump is best imaged in the descending aorta in a vertical TEE plane. Correct positioning of the catheter tip is at the inferior border of the transverse aortic arch.[58] After the tip of the balloon is visualized at a transducer angle of approximately 90 degrees, the probe marking at the teeth is noted. The probe is slowly withdrawn until the left subclavian artery orifice is seen, and the marking is again noted. The distance between the balloon and the subclavian orifice should be approximately 5 cm (Fig. 9.11).

LV Assist Device

As the LV assist device (LVAD) withdraws blood from the LV, LA pressure falls below RA pressure. A patent foramen ovale (PFO) may become unmasked after LVAD placement as the left-sided pressure decreases compared with preoperative values.[73] It is important to determine whether a PFO is present because right-to-left shunting will invariably occur.

Any thrombi detected on the left side of the heart must be dealt with before instituting flow through the device. A mechanical aortic valve, even if functional, should be replaced with a bioprosthetic valve to minimize the increased risk of valvular thrombosis and possible embolization.

Mitral stenosis, if significant, may limit the ability of blood to be removed to the device by the inflow cannula. The orifice

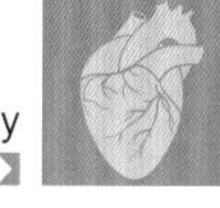

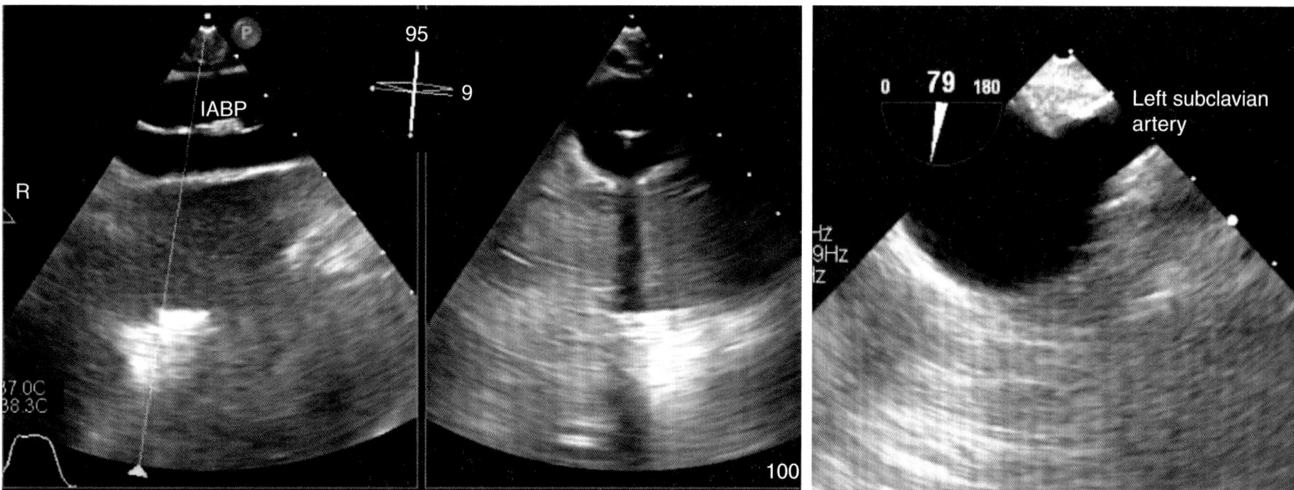

Fig. 9.11 Intraaortic balloon pump monitoring. The intraaortic balloon pump *(IABP)* is positioned in the descending thoracic aorta. The left subclavian artery *(right)* is visualized to ensure that the IABP does not encroach on the vessel orifice (see Video 9.11).

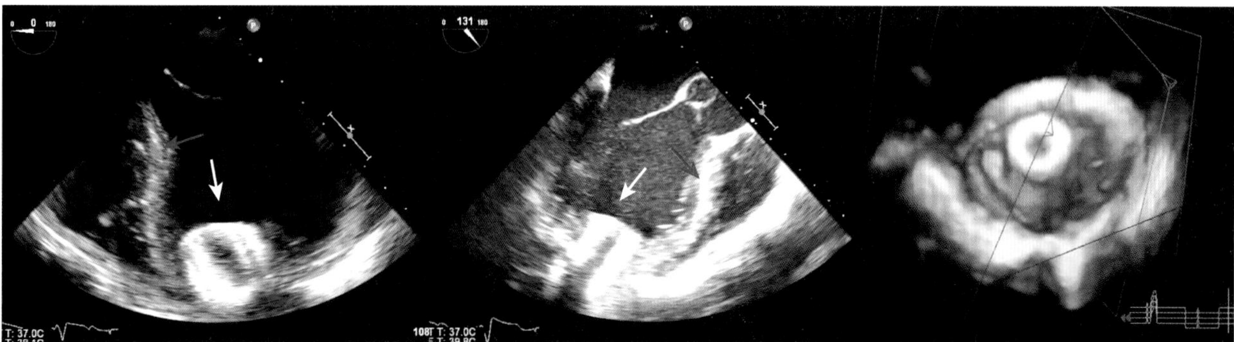

Fig. 9.12 LV assist device inflow cannula positioning. The inflow cannula *(white arrow)* of the left ventricular assist device (LVAD) freely enters the apical region of the LV and does not abut the interventricular septum *(red arrow)*, as seen in the mid-esophageal 4-chamber view *(left)* and the mid-esophageal long-axis view *(center)*. The 3D TEE image *(right)* shows the LV after cropping from the mitral valve to the mid-ventricular cavity. The orifice of the inflow cannula is completely unobstructed (see Videos 9.12A and B).

of the ventricular apical cannula (inflow cannula) should be imaged in the 4- and 2-chamber views and, if available, a 3D image showing the cannula tip sitting in the ventricular cavity. Lack of obstruction by adjacent walls should be ascertained (Fig. 9.12). Because the outflow cannula terminates in the ascending aorta (Fig. 9.13), it is important to rule out significant aortic regurgitation, which would lead to LV distention during aortic flow and diminished blood flow to the body due to recirculation through the pump.

If the intravascular volume is too low or the RV function diminishes to a critical level, a suction event may occur in which the walls of the LV are drawn inward, blocking the inflow cannula (Fig. 9.14). Treatment involves turning down the speed of the pump drawing blood out of the LV, increasing intravascular volume, and supporting RV function. Patients may return to the operating room because of LVAD malfunction. The TEE examination should focus on possible causes such as intracardiac thrombi or problems with the cannulas.[74]

Newer percutaneous or centrally placed axial flow assist devices are available for temporary ventricular support. The Impella RP (Abiomed, Danvers, MA) is placed retrograde through the aortic valve. These devices offer temporary support for a failing heart as a bridge to recovery, transplantation, surgical decision making, or a more durable device. They are also placed during some high-risk procedures, such as a high-risk percutaneous coronary intervention and ventricular tachycardia ablation procedures.[75] Echocardiographic guidance can aid in appropriate placement into the LV and evaluation of impingement on the mitral valve apparatus leading to mitral valve dysfunction. The aortic valve long-axis view is typically the best for measuring depth, and evaluation at multiple angles may be necessary to rule out mitral valve dysfunction caused by the device (Fig. 9.15).

RV Assist Device

In positioning the RV assist device (RVAD), it is preferable to avoid impingement on the tricuspid valve. RV dysfunction after LVAD is common and occurs in up to 40% of patients; a small percentage of these patients may need mechanical RV support.[76] A temporary centrally cannulated RVAD is most commonly used in those who require support, but the Impella RP and ProtekDuo (CardiadAssist, Inc., Pittsburgh, PA) are percutaneous options for temporary support of RV failure.

Total Artificial Heart

Options for end-stage biventricular heart failure include biventricular assist devices (BI-VADs), LVADs with medical optimization of the RV, and total artificial hearts. Echocardiographic imaging of a total artificial heart is limited due to four mechanical valves and poor echocardiographic penetration through the total artificial heart device. The native atrium in

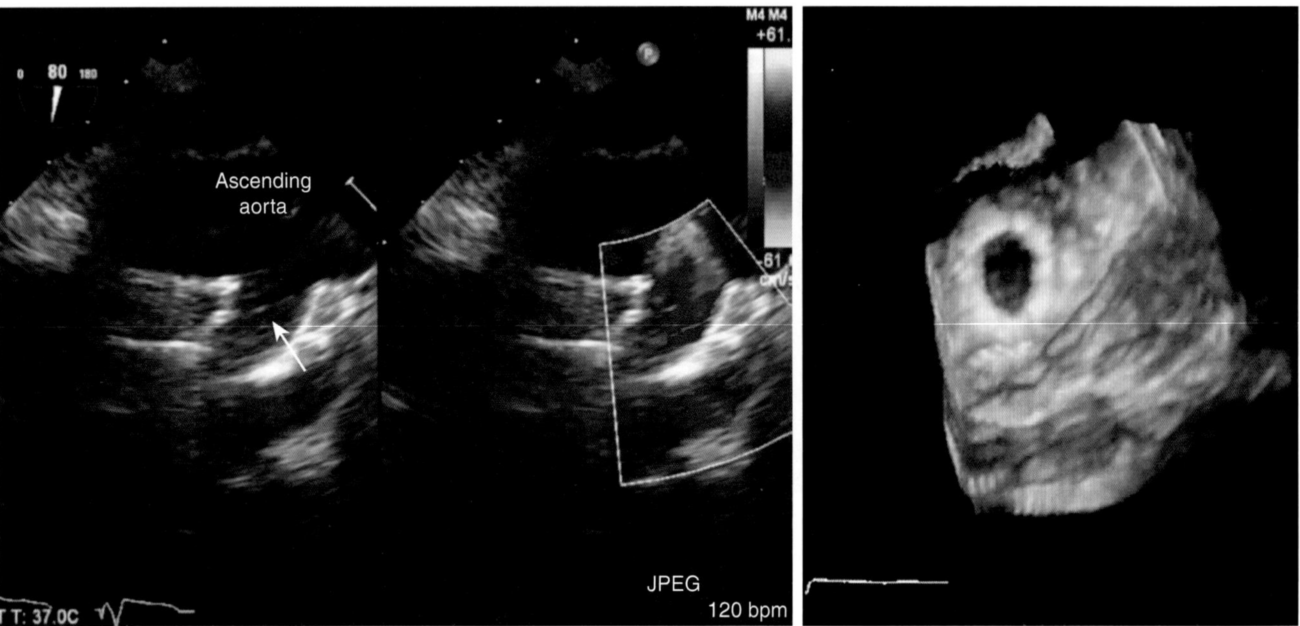

Fig. 9.13 LV assist device outflow cannula positioning. The outflow cannula of the left ventricular assist device (LVAD) terminates in the ascending aorta. The 3D image *(right)* highlights the anastomosis between the end of the synthetic graft and the side of the ascending aorta (see Video 9.13).

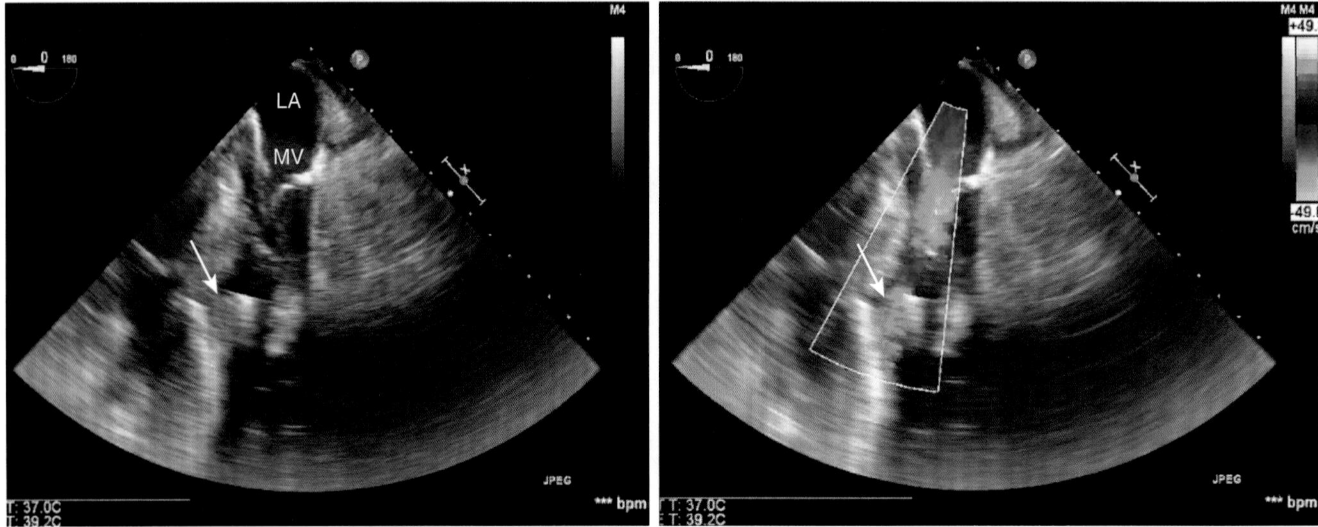

Fig. 9.14 Hypotension after LV assist device placement. A suction event manifested as hypotension is seen in mid-esophageal 4-chamber view. On the left, the LV cavity *(arrow)* is extremely small, and the lateral and septal walls of the LV impede flow through the inflow cannula and to the device. On the right, there is color turbulence of flow to the inflow cannula *(arrow)*. Administering intravascular volume and temporarily reducing the pump speed rectified the situation (see Video 9.14).

these patients remains intact, and tamponade can occur. TTE may have limited ability to visualize the heart, and TEE or computed tomography often is necessary to rule out impaired filling of the atrium due to pericardial fluid (Fig. 9.16).

Venovenous Extracorporeal Membrane Oxygenation

In patients with respiratory failure refractory to ventilator management in whom cardiac function is adequate, venovenous extracorporeal membrane oxygenation (VV ECMO) can be used to support lung function. A double-lumen cannula is placed through the internal jugular vein into the RA and inferior vena cava (IVC). Venous blood exits the patient to the device, oxygenation and carbon dioxide are removed, and the blood is pumped back into the RA. TEE is used to position the latter orifice opposite the tricuspid valve to ensure that the oxygenated blood enters the RV and does not recirculate through the device (Fig. 9.17). An alternative cannulation strategy involves separate cannulas inserted into the superior vena cava (SVC) and IVC, with the oxygenated blood flowing into the SVC cannula. Echocardiography can verify cannula positioning and decrease the amount of recirculation if cannulas are positioned too close together.[77]

Coronary Sinus Cannulation

The coronary sinus is cannulated through a blind RA puncture for the purpose of administering retrograde cardioplegia. Occasionally, TEE guidance is required, especially in minimally invasive surgical procedures, and it can also verify correct placement of the cannula (Fig. 9.18).

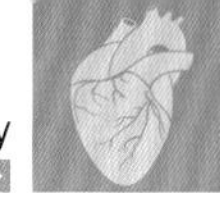

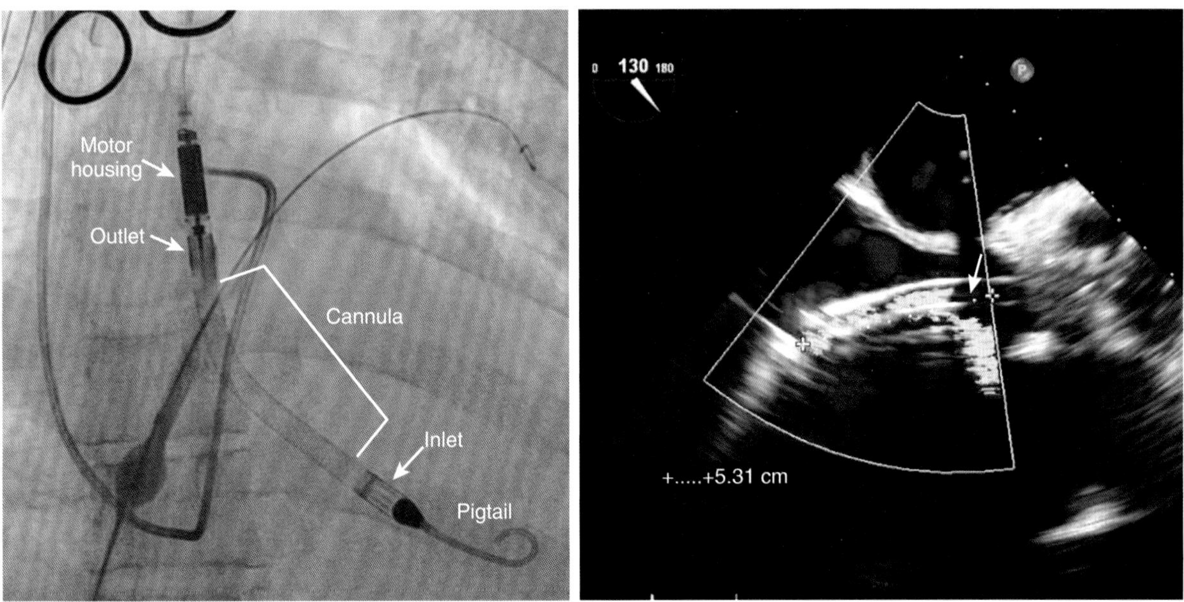

Fig. 9.15 **Assessment of Impella positioning.** X-ray view *(left)* of an Impella RV assist device identifies its components. Blood is aspirated from the LV *(inlet)* and pumped in the supravalvular aorta *(outlet)*. Mid-esophageal long-axis view *(right)* shows that the outlet is above the aortic valve *(arrow)* and the device is 5.3 cm into the LV cavity.

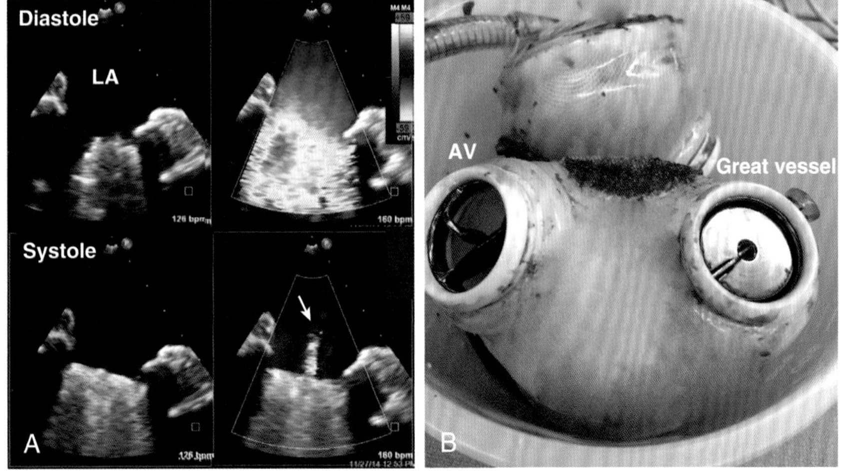

Fig. 9.16 **Imaging of the total artificial heart.** In the total artificial heart, the ventricles are excised with the atrioventricular valves, and the atria are connected to the artificial heart. (A) TEE image shows adequate function of the tilting-disc prosthetic mitral valve, with a cleaning jet seen during systole *(arrow)*. (B) The left side of the artificial heart was explanted before heart transplantation; the mitral valve is on the *left*, and the aortic prosthetic valve is on the *right* (see Video 9.16). *AV*, Atrioventricular valve.

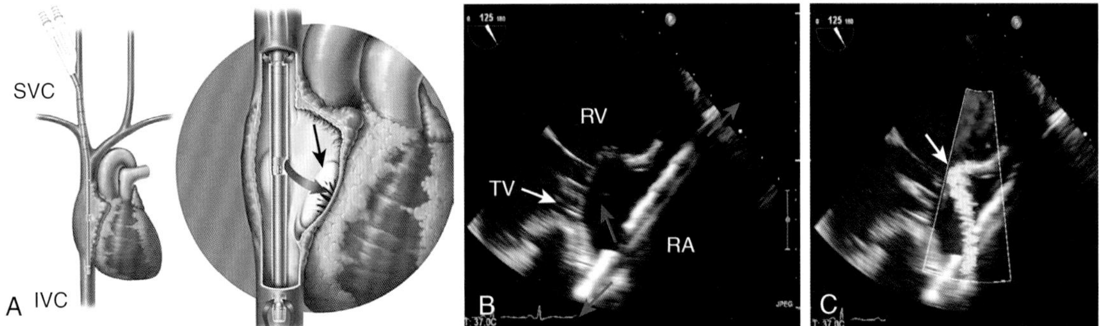

Fig. 9.17 **Venovenous extracorporeal membrane oxygenation cannula positioning.** (A) Avalon (Maquet, Rastatt, Germany) bicaval dual-lumen cannula for venovenous extracorporeal membrane oxygenation (ECMO). The catheter enters the internal jugular vein and is advanced to facilitate drainage of venous blood from the inferior vena cava *(IVC)* and superior vena cava *(SCV)*, with the outflow lumen placed opposite the tricuspid valve *(TV) (black arrow)*. (B) Transgastric long-axis view of the RA and RV shows venous blood leaving the patient *(blue arrow)* and oxygenated blood exiting the cannula *(red arrow)* and directed to the TV *(white arrow)*. (C) Color Doppler illustrates flow from the cannula through the TV *(white arrow)* (see Video 9.17). (A, From Souilamas R, Souilamas J, Alkhamees K, et al. Extracorporeal membrane oxygenation in general thoracic surgery: a new single veno-venous cannulation. *J Cardiothorac Surg*. 2011;6:52–54.)

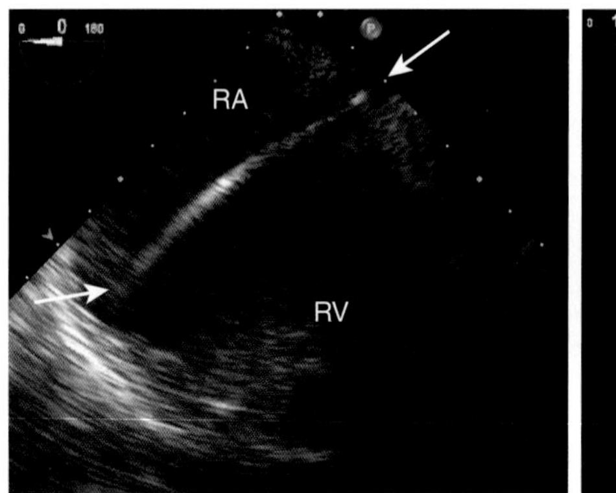

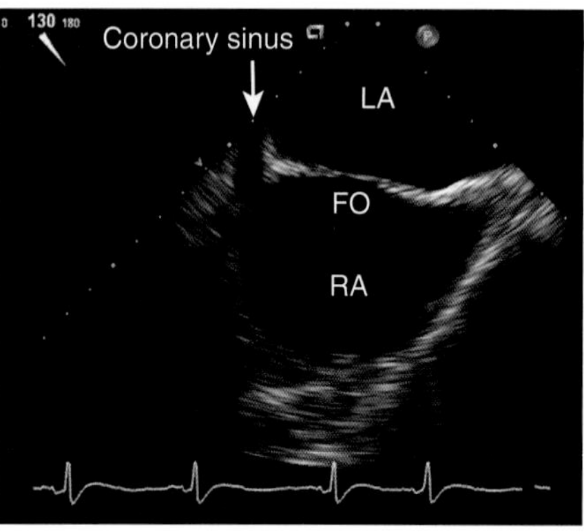

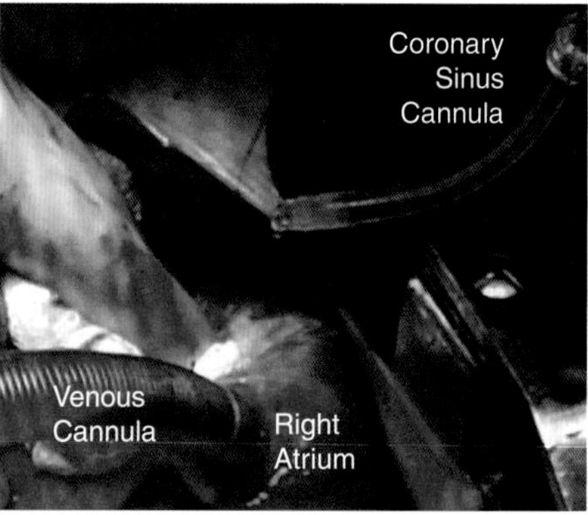

Fig. 9.18 Coronary sinus cannula positioning. The coronary sinus is visualized in a low esophageal view *(left)* and a bicaval view *(middle)*. The catheter traverses the RA and enters the coronary sinus orifice *(arrows)*. The surgeon introduces the cannula through a small incision in the posterior RA *(right)*. *FO*, Foramen ovale.

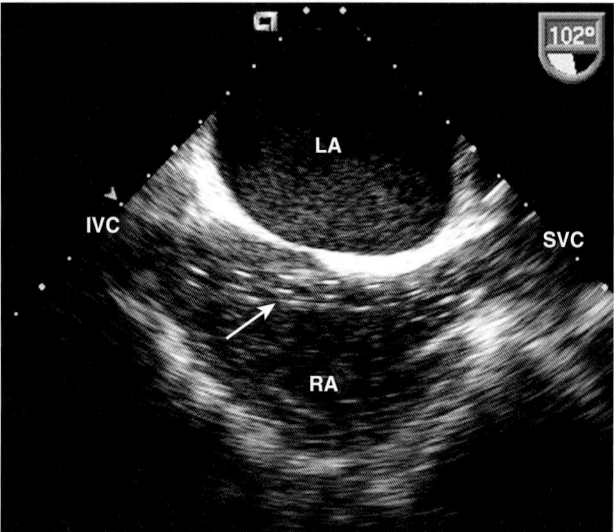

Fig. 9.19 Femoral venous cannula positioning. The multiorifice femoral venous cannula *(arrow)* enters the RA from the inferior vena cava *(IVC)*. *SVC*, Superior vena cava.

Femoral Venous Cannula

Occasionally, venous drainage on bypass is achieved through femoral venous cannulation with advancement into the RA and SVC (Fig. 9.19). Appropriate positioning reveals the cannula in the SVC and without tenting or pressure on the interatrial septum.

TRANSPLANT SURGERY

Heart Transplantation

TEE is used to examine the native heart for LV thrombi and to assess the function of the donor heart before procurement and after the recipient is separated from cardiopulmonary bypass, when the effects of the ischemic time may become evident. The anastomoses may be examined if obstruction is suspected.

Lung Transplantation

TEE has been used to evaluate vascular anastomoses during lung transplantation. The pulmonary venous anastomoses typically are well seen, and velocities are usually less than 1 m/s in the absence of significant obstruction.[78,79]

The right PA anastomoses (and, less likely, the left) may be visualized in the mid-esophageal ascending aortic short-axis view, although the angle of flow usually precludes Doppler interrogation of the anastomosis. If the recipient's heart exhibits RV hypertrophy, RV outflow tract obstruction may develop when the new lungs are reperfused.

Liver Transplantation

During reperfusion of the transplanted liver, significant right-sided embolization can occur, with resultant hemodynamic instability. TEE can aid in this diagnosis and guide treatment.

ALTERNATIVE TECHNIQUES

EPICARDIAL AND EPIAORTIC ECHOCARDIOGRAPHY

Occasionally, there may be contraindications to TEE, or the images obtained may be suboptimal. Using a high-frequency ultrasound probe in a sterile sheath, the cardiac surgeon can image the heart by placing it on the epicardial surface and obtaining standard surface echocardiographic images.[80] Similarly, the ascending aorta can be scanned for regions of atheromatous disease, which should be avoided during aortic cross clamping.[81]

INTRAOPERATIVE TEE: IMPACT ON POSTOPERATIVE OUTCOMES AND COST-EFFECTIVENESS

The recommendations of the American Society of Anesthesiologists and the Society of Cardiovascular Anesthesiologists Task Force for the use of perioperative TEE[82] and the European Association of Echocardiography for the use of intraoperative TEE in cardiac and noncardiac surgery[83] are presented in Table 9.3. Contraindications for TEE must be considered along with equipment and expertise for evaluation of the study.[82] In all instances, benefits must be weighed against the reported complication rate of TEE of approximately 0.2%.[84] TTE and other diagnostic modalities should be considered as alternatives to TEE.

In a series of unselected and consecutive cardiac surgical patients having exclusively CABG with TEE monitoring, Qaddoura et al,[85] reported pre-bypass findings for 52 (10%) patients that resulted in alterations of the surgical procedure for 21 (3.4%) of them; the most common finding was a previously undiagnosed PFO (Table 9.4). After bypass, there were 19 new findings for 15 patients that resulted in 15 surgical interventions in 10 of the patients (see Table 9.4).

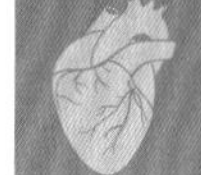

TABLE 9.3 Recommendations for the Use of Perioperative TEE in Adults.

Clinical Situation	*ASA/SCA Task Force Recommendations*	*European Association of Echocardiography Recommendations*
Cardiac (non-CABG) and thoracic aortic surgery	Should be used in all adults without contraindications to TEE	TEE should be used in adult patients undergoing cardiac surgery or thoracic aorta surgery under general anesthesia, particularly valvular repair procedures.
CABG	Should also be considered in CABG operations • To confirm and refine the preoperative diagnosis • To detect new or unsuspected pathology • To adjust the anesthesia and surgical plan accordingly • To assess the results of surgical intervention	—
Transcatheter intracardiac procedures	May be used	—
Noncardiac surgery	TEE may be used when the nature of the planned surgery or the patient's known or suspected cardiovascular pathology might result in severe hemodynamic, pulmonary, or neurologic compromise. If equipment and expertise are available, TEE should be used when unexplained life-threatening circulatory instability persists despite corrective therapy.	TEE may be used in patients undergoing specific types of major surgery for which its value has been repeatedly documented, including neurosurgery with risk of venous thromboembolism, liver transplantation, lung transplantation, and major vascular surgery (including vascular trauma). TEE may be used in patients undergoing major noncardiac surgery in whom severe or life-threatening hemodynamic disturbance exists or is threatened. TEE may be used in major noncardiac surgery in patients who are at high cardiac risk, including severe cardiac valve disease, severe coronary heart disease, and heart failure.
Critical care	For critical care patients, TEE should be used when diagnostic information that is expected to alter management cannot be obtained by transthoracic echocardiography or other modalities in a timely manner.	TEE may be used in the critical care patient in whom severe or life-threatening hemodynamic disturbance is present and unresponsive to treatment, or in patients in whom new or ongoing cardiac disease is suspected and who are not adequately assessed by transthoracic imaging or other diagnostic tests.

ASA, American Society of Anesthesiologists; *CABG*, coronary artery bypass grafting; *SCA*, Society of Cardiovascular Anesthesiologists.

Data from Practice guidelines for perioperative transesophageal echocardiography. An updated report by the American Society of Anesthesiologists and the Society of Cardiovascular Anesthesiologists Task Force on Transesophageal Echocardiography. *Anesthesiology*. 2010;112:1084–1096; Flachskampf FA, Badano L, Daniel WG, et al. Recommendations for transoesophageal echocardiography: update 2010. *Eur J Echocardiogr*. 2010;11:557–576.

In a retrospective review of 2343 unselected patients having cardiac surgery, Forrest et al.[86] determined a surgical impact score of 4.5% for the TEE findings. When the data for CABG patients were analyzed, the surgical impact score was 6.7% for high-risk patients versus 2.8% for low-risk patients. Because of the designs of these two studies, it would be difficult to determine whether the additional procedures performed led to an improved outcome.

In studies from Australia,[87] Europe,[88,59] Canada,[89] and India,[90] the real-time accrual of information with TEE was demonstrated to be of value in the management of hemodynamic perturbations and planning for CABG and other cardiac surgical procedures. The effect of intraoperative TEE monitoring on patient outcomes was not assessed. These studies and others are summarized in Table 9.5.

Bergquist and colleagues[91,92] studied the concordance between real-time intraoperative TEE interpretation by five cardiac anesthesiologists and offline analysis by two blinded investigators in the assessment of LV filling, EF area, and regional wall motion. Results obtained by the two methods were within 10% of each other 75% of the time with respect to EF and filling. The accuracy of regional assessment varied; it was more accurate for normal than for abnormal wall motion and better when conducted by anesthesiologists with more advanced echocardiographic training. In the second part of the study, TEE was found to be the most important factor in guiding hemodynamic interventions in 17% of the cases examined.

Lacking is a clear demonstration that the TEE assessments were correct and that the same interventions would not have been undertaken if guided by more traditional monitors. Cost and outcomes were not examined. Mathew et al.[93] demonstrated that cardiac anesthesiologists interpret TEE examinations at a level comparable to that of physicians whose primary practice is echocardiography.

Cost-effectiveness was demonstrated by studies of the use of TEE in congenital cardiac surgery,[94] preparation for elective cardioversion,[95] and determination of antibiotic treatment duration for endocarditis.[99] Similar data for routine TEE monitoring of CABG are lacking.

Fanshawe et al.[96] showed substantial savings with the routine use of TEE for cardiac surgical patients, although not specifically CABG patients.[97] In some instances, surgery was cancelled, or new procedures were recommended based on the findings of intraoperative TEE; whether these alterations of treatment were beneficial was not determined during follow-up. The claim of improved patient outcomes must be tempered by the fact that most surgical changes involved closure of an asymptomatic PFO. These findings are summarized in Table 9.6.

In the largest series considering the impact of intraoperative TEE on decision making in cardiac surgery, Eltzschig et al.[98] retrospectively examined 12,566 patients. From 1990 to 2004, the frequency with which intraoperative TEE was performed increased steadily. The major findings, presented in Table 9.7, reveal that a large number of procedures were affected by TEE findings before and after cardiopulmonary bypass. As pointed out in the accompanying commentary,[99] changes in therapeutic management are not (as end points) as convincing as morbidity, mortality, and cost, but nonetheless, the study and its magnitude were commended as an "excellent resource for the design of future, randomized, controlled trials examining the potential benefits of intraoperative TEE on clinical outcome."[99]

The impact of monitoring ventricular function during noncardiac surgery has not been studied as closely. Hofer et al.[100] prospectively examined patients at high risk for myocardial ischemia who were having major noncardiac surgery. A large number of patients had therapeutic changes based on TEE findings (Table 9.8), but outcome data were lacking. Other

TABLE 9.4 New Findings for 474 CABG Patients and Surgical Impact of Intraoperative TEE.

New Pre-Bypass Findings (46 Patients)	*n*	*Surgical Impact of Pre-Bypass Findings (16 Patients)*	*n*	*New Post-Bypass Findings (15 Patients)*	*n*	*Surgical Impact of Post-Bypass Findings (10 Patients)*	*n*
PFO	22	PFO closed	7	Significant MR	3	MV repair	2
MVP with MR	3	No surgical impact	—	Altered cardiac function		Graft flow evaluation	3
Significant MR (5), TR (4), AR (3)	12	MV (2), TV (2), aortic valve (1) repair	5	Depressed LVF	6	Graft revision	5
Aortic valve disease (Lambl, mild AS)	2	Aortic valve explored (Lambl excised)	2	New RWMA	7	IABP inserted	5
Subvalvular AS	1	Myomectomy	1	New RWMA and depressed LV or RV function	2	—	—
Improved LVF	4	No IABP	4	Dynamic obstruction	1	Medical treatment	—
Aortic atheroma	5	OPCAB	2	Total	19	Total	15
Depressed LVF and RVF	2	No surgical impact	—	—	—	—	—
New RWMA	1	No surgical impact	—	—	—	—	—
Total	52	Total	21	—	—	—	—

AR, Aortic regurgitation; *AS*, aortic stenosis; *AV*, aortic valve; *EF*, ejection fraction; *IABP*, intraaortic balloon pump; *Lambl*, Lambl excrescence; *LVF*, left ventricular function; *MR*, mitral regurgitation; *MV*, mitral valve; *MVP*, mitral valve prolapse; *OPCAB*, off-pump coronary artery bypass; *PFO*, patent foramen ovale; *RVF*, right ventricular function; *RWMA*, regional wall motion abnormality; *TR*, tricuspid regurgitation; *TV*, tricuspid valve.

From Qaddoura FE, Abel MD, Mecklenburg KL, et al. Role of intraoperative transesophageal echocardiography in patients having coronary artery bypass graft surgery. *Ann Thorac Surg.* 2004;78:1586–1590.

TABLE 9.5 Studies Examining Alterations in Therapy During Cardiac Surgery With the Use of Intraoperative TEE.

Study	*Study Population*	*Surgery*	*Altered Therapy (n/%)*	*Outcome Reported*
Bergquist et al.[91,106]	N = 75, 584 interventions	C-revasc	98/17% of all interventions	No
Savage et al.[107]	N = 82, high risk	C-revasc	Surgical change: 27/33% of pts	Compared with historical controls
Savage et al.[107]	N = 82, high risk	C-revasc	Hemodynamic change: 42/51% of pts	Compared with historical controls
Sutton and Kluger[87]	N = 120	C-revasc	16/13% of all patients	No
Kolev et al.[59]	N = 224, 2232 interventions	C-all NC	560/25% of all interventions	No
Couture et al.[108]	N = 851	C-all	125/15% of all pts	No
Mishra et al.[90]	N = 5016	C-all	1146/23% of all pts	No
Click et al.[109]	N = 3245	C-all	441/14% of all pts pre-bypass 121/4% of all pts post-bypass	No
Qaddoura et al.[85]	N = 474	C-revasc	21/4% of all pts pre-bypass	No
Forrest et al.[86]	N = 1785: Low risk (*n* = 821) Medium risk (*n* = 696) High risk (*n* = 268)	C-revasc	62/3.5% of all pts 2.8% 2.9% 6.7%	No

C-all, Coronary and noncoronary cardiac surgery; *C-revasc*, coronary revascularizations; *NC*, noncardiac surgery; *pts*, patients.

TABLE 9.6 Alterations in Cardiac Surgery Based on Routine Intraoperative EE Findings.[a]

Procedure Proposed	*Procedure Performed*	*TEE Findings*	*Number of Patients*
CABG	CABG + TVR	TR +4	1
MVR	MV repair	P2 prolapse	1
CABG	CABG + MVR	MR +4	1
CABG + MVR	CABG	MR +1	1
MVR	—	MR +1	2

[a]Other than for patent foramen ovale procedures. Estimated costs (US$) for yearly TEE service per four operating rooms: machine, 100,000; service contract, 25,000; probe replacement/repair, 64,000; cleaning, 1200; storage/video, 3600; total cost, 193,800.

CABG, Coronary artery bypass grafting; *MR*, mitral regurgitation; *MV* repair, mitral valve repair; *MVR*, mitral valve replacement; *P2*, middle scallop of posterior mitral valve leaflet; *PFO*, patent foramen ovale; *TR*, tricuspid regurgitation; *TVR*, tricuspid valve replacement.

Adapted from Fanshawe M, Ellis C, Habib S, et al. A retrospective analysis of the costs and benefits related to alterations in cardiac surgery from routine intraoperative transesophageal echocardiography. *Anesth Analg.* 2002;95:824–827.

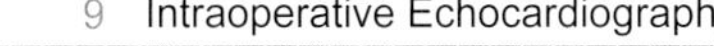

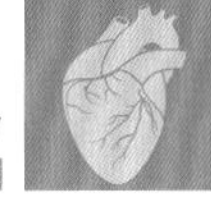

TABLE 9.7 Influence of TEE on Surgical Decision Making.

Surgical Subset	*Surgical Decisions (%) Influenced by Pre-CPB TEE*	*Surgical Decisions (%) Influenced by Post-CPB TEE*
All patients (N = 12,566)	7	2.2
CABG only (n = 3835)	5.4	1.5
Valve only (n = 3840)	6.3	3.3
CABG + valve (n = 2944)	12.3	2.2

CABG, Coronary artery bypass grafting; *CPB*, cardiopulmonary bypass.
From Eltzschig HK, Rosenberger P, Loffler M, et al. Impact of intraoperative transesophageal echocardiography on surgical decisions in 12,566 patients undergoing cardiac surgery. *Ann Thorac Surg*. 2008;85:845–853.

TABLE 9.8 Preoperative Cardiovascular Diagnoses and Intraoperative TEE: Incidence of Therapeutic Consequences.[a]

Diagnosis	*Total Patients N*	*Vasodilator n (%)*	*Vasopressor n (%)*	*Fluid n (%)*
CAD	61	36 (59)	28 (46)	11 (18)
CAD + valve	13	7 (54)	5 (39)	5 (39)
Valve	11	4 (36)	3 (27)	2 (18)
SWMA	28	26 (93)[b]	20 (71)[b]	9 (32)
EF < 40%	15	8 (53)	6 (40)	1 (7)
LHF	10	8 (80)[b]	3 (30)	1 (10)
PAH	11	8 (73)[b]	8 (73)[b]	4 (36)
RHF	10	7 (70)[b]	5 (50)	2 (20)
Total[c]	99	54 (55)	43 (43)	24 (24)

[a]Vasodilator/vasopressor/fluid, new therapy, or changes of therapy with respect to vasodilator/vasopressor and fluid management.
[b]$P < 0.05$.
[c]This table identifies changes or initiation of therapy. They can be included in more than one therapy, and the total and percentage can be more than 100%.
CAD, Coronary artery disease; *EF*, ejection fraction; *LHF*, left-sided heart failure; *PAH*, pulmonary arterial hypertension; *RHF*, right-sided heart failure; *SWMA*, systolic wall motion abnormality; *valve*, valve diseases.
From Hofer CK, Zollinger A, Rak M, et al. Therapeutic impact of intra-operative transoesophageal echocardiography during noncardiac surgery. *Anaesthesia*. 2004;59:3–9.

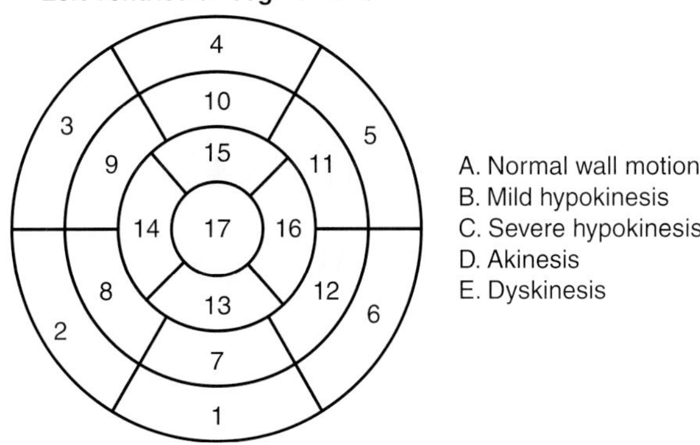

Fig. 9.20 Important components of a perioperative TEE report. The 17-segmented model of the heart allows for accurate and descriptive identification of localized and global wall motion abnormalities.

studies have described the changes in intraoperative management during noncardiac surgery,[101,102] but cost-effectiveness and outcome data were not provided. The study authors acknowledged that randomized, controlled clinical trials to evaluate outcomes with intraoperative TEE are difficult to perform.

Although data showing improved outcomes are lacking, intraoperative TEE has become an essential tool in the assessment of ventricular and valvular function during cardiac surgery and for monitoring specific clinical entities, such as device placement and organ transplantation. It must be emphasized that appropriate physician training and quality assurance are crucial for the correct interpretation of data. Numerous technologic advances are on the horizon and may improve intraoperative applicability. Fig. 9.20 shows important components of a perioperative TEE report.

SUMMARY Intraoperative Echocardiography

Parameter	Echocardiographic View	Additional Imaging	Clinical Pointers	Comments
Diastolic function	Image mitral valve in mid-esophageal (ME) 4-chamber view to acquire (preferably) PW Doppler inflow	Image pulmonary vein to acquire PW Doppler flow	Image mitral valve in ME 4-chamber view to facilitate TDI of lateral mitral annulus, and calculate E/E′ ratio	—
LV volumes	Image LV in ME 4-chamber and 2-chamber views, trace at end-systole and end-diastole to allow calculations (method of disks)	—	—	—
Cardiac output	Calculate LVOT area using the LVOT diameter obtained in the ME long-axis view	Alternatively, use the 3D zoom or full-volume mode to allow multiplanar reconstruction of the LVOT and planimetry to measure its area	LVOT measurements should be made in systole	—
Ejection fraction	Calculate fractional area of change using mid-papillary transgastric short-axis views of the LV and planimeter in systole and diastole; recognize the limitations of this technique	Perform similar calculations using the method of disks	Image mitral valve in ME 4-chamber view and acquire a multibeat full-volume loop of the LV	Use 3D software to calculate volumes; the software should calculate the ejection fraction
Other measures of global systolic function	Visual assessment of endocardial and myocardial thickening in the various ventricular segments	Image mitral valve in ME 4-chamber view to facilitate TDI of lateral mitral annulus	Measure S′	—
Strain	Measure strain using speckle tracking in the ME views and the transgastric mid-papillary view; recognize that properly identifying the region of interest is crucial	—	—	—
RV function	Using the transgastric window, align M-mode parallel to the lateral tricuspid annulus for TAPSE	Using the transgastric window, align tissue Doppler gate parallel to the lateral tricuspid annulus to assess S′	—	—

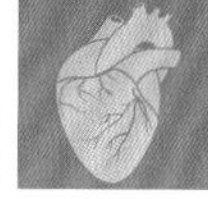

SUMMARY Intraoperative Echocardiography—cont'd

Parameter	Echocardiographic View	Additional Imaging	Clinical Pointers	Comments
Regional wall motion	Visual assessment of endocardial and myocardial thickening	Measure strain using speckle tracking	Acquire 3D volumes	—
Position of IABP	Image the descending thoracic aorta	Identify the tip of the balloon (suspending its inflation temporarily may help)	Image left subclavian artery	Assess distance between balloon tip and left subclavian artery
LVAD inflow cannulas	Image LV in ME 4-chamber and 2-chamber views	Assess position of the cannula tip relative to the ventricular walls	May also use 3D to assess cannula position	Color Doppler to assess velocities
LVAD outflow cannula	Image the ME long axis, and look for cannula entering the ascending aorta	Use color Doppler to assess velocities	—	—
Impella RVAD	Image ME long axis	Assess aortic valve pathology	Assess depth of device into LV	Assess mitral valve function
Total artificial heart	Use ME 4-chamber view to assess atrioventricular valves	ME long-axis views to look at aortic and pulmonic prosthetic valves	Look for central cleaning jets	Be vigilant for atrial compression from effusions
VV ECMO	Image the cavae and the tricuspid valve using a bicaval view of a transgastric long-axis view of the right heart	Use color Doppler to ensure that outflow from the device goes through tricuspid valve into the RV	—	—
Coronary sinus cannula	View in low ME 4-chamber view with retroflexion	View in bicaval with medial turn of probe	—	—
Femoral venous cannula	Bicaval view	—	—	—
Heart and lung transplantation	Image anastomoses, use Doppler if possible	—	—	—
Epicardial or epiaortic imaging	Have surgeon use sterile sheath to accept surface probe	Ensure adequate standoff is used to avoid near-field dropout	—	—

LVAD, left ventricular assist device; *IABP*, Intraaortic balloon pump; *LVOT*, left ventricular outlet tract; *ME*, mid-esophageal; *PW*, pulsed-wave; *TAPSE*, tricuspid annular plane systolic excursion; *TDI*, tissue Doppler imaging; *VV ECMO*, venovenous extracorporeal membrane oxygenation.

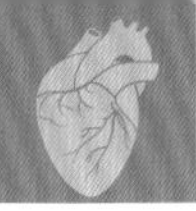

REFERENCES

1. Mahmood F, Shernan SK. Perioperative transoesophageal echocardiography: current status and future directions. *Heart (British Cardiac Society)*. 2016;102(15):1159–1167. https://doi.org/10.1136/heartjnl-2015-307962.
2. Fayad A, Shillcutt SK. Perioperative transesophageal echocardiography for non-cardiac surgery. *Can J Anaesth.* 2018;65(4):381–398. https://doi.org/10.1007/s12630-017-1017-7.
3. Committee SEWMFFCW, Committee TRMF FVCW, Member JAAMFWC, et al. 2019 ACC/AHA/ASE advanced training statement on echocardiography (Revision of the 2003 ACC/AHA clinical competence statement on echocardiography): a report of the ACC competency management committee. *J Am Coll Cardiol.* 2019;74(3):377–402. https://doi.org/10.1016/j.jacc.2019.02.003.
4. Hahn RT, Abraham T, Adams MS, et al. Guidelines for performing a comprehensive transesophageal echocardiographic examination: recommendations from the American Society of Echocardiography and the Society of Cardiovascular Anesthesiologists. *J Am Soc Echocardiogr*. 2013;26:921–964.
5. Denault AY, Couture P, Buithieu J, et al. Left and right ventricular diastolic dysfunction as predictors of difficult separation from cardiopulmonary bypass. *Can J Anaesth.* 2006;53(10):1020–1029.
6. Pauliks LB, Undar A, Clark JB, Myers JL. Segmental differences of impaired diastolic relaxation following cardiopulmonary bypass surgery in children: a tissue Doppler study. *Artif Organs*. 2009;33(11):904–908.
7. Tsang MW, Davidoff R, Korach A, et al. Diastolic dysfunction after coronary artery bypass grafting—the effect of glucose-insulin-potassium infusion. *J Card Surg.* 2007;22(3):185–191. https://doi.org/10.1111/j.1540-8191.2007.00382.x.
8. Swenson JD, Bull D, Stringham J. Subjective assessment of left ventricular preload using transesophageal echocardiography: corresponding pulmonary artery occlusion pressures. *J Cardiothorac Vasc Anesth*. 2001;15(5):580–583. https://doi.org/10.1053/jcan.2001.26535.
9. Sharifov OF, Gupta H. What is the evidence that the tissue Doppler index E/e′ reflects left ventricular filling pressure changes after exercise or pharmacological intervention for evaluating diastolic function? A systematic review. *J Am Heart Assoc*. 2017;6(3):546–28. https://doi.org/10.1161/JAHA.116.004766.
10. Nagueh SF, Smiseth OA, Appleton CP, et al. Recommendations for the evaluation of left ventricular diastolic function by echocardiography: an update from the American Society of Echocardiography and the European Association of Cardiovascular Imaging. *J Am Soc Echocardiogr*. 2016;29(4):277–314. https://doi.org/10.1016/j.echo.2016.01.011.
11. Ho CY, Solomon SD. A clinician's guide to tissue Doppler imaging. *Circulation.* 2006;113(10):e396–e398.
12. Sheu R, Ferreira R. Is intraoperative strain analysis for left ventricular diastolic function practical?; J Cardiothorac Vasc Anesth. 2019;33(6):1492–1494. https://doi.org/10.1053/j.jvca.2018.07.035.
13. Kumar K, Nepomuceno RG, Chelvanathan A, et al. The role of tissue Doppler imaging in predicting left ventricular filling pressures in patients undergoing cardiac surgery: an intraoperative study. *Echocardiography.* 2013;30(3):271–278. https://doi.org/10.1111/echo.12049. Mount Kisco, NY.
14. Masutani S. Restrictive left ventricular filling pattern does not result from increased left atrial pressure alone. *Circulation*. 2008;117:1550–1554. LWCHHCHJCCP.
15. Djaiani GN, McCreath BJ, Ti LK, et al. Mitral flow propagation velocity identifies patients with abnormal diastolic function during coronary artery bypass graft surgery. *Anesth Analg.* 2002;95(3):524–530.
16. Hernandez-Suarez DF, Kim Y, Lo′pez-FM, et al. Qualitative assessment of color M-mode signals in the evaluation of left ventricular diastolic function: a proof of concept study. *J Cardiothorac Vasc Anesth.* June 2019:1–5. https://doi.org/10.1053/j.jvca.2019.05.047.
17. McIlroy DR, Lin E, Durkin C. Intraoperative transesophageal echocardiography: a critical appraisal of its current role in the assessment of diastolic dysfunction. *J Cardiothorac Vasc Anesth.* 2015;29(4):1033–1043. https://doi.org/10.1053/j.jvca.2015.01.009.
18. Lang RM, Badano LP, Mor-Avi V, et al. Recommendations for cardiac chamber quantification by echocardiography in adults: an update from the American Society of Echocardiography and the European Association of Cardiovascular Imaging. *Eur Heart J Cardiovasc Imaging.* 2015;16(3):233–270. https://doi.org/10.1093/ehjci/jev014.
19. Lang RM, Bierig M, Devereux RB, et al. Recommendations for chamber quantification: a report from the American Society of Echocardiography's Guidelines and Standards Committee and the Chamber Quantification Writing Group, developed in conjunction with the European Association of Echocardiography, a branch of the European Society of Cardiology. *J Am Soc Echocardiogr.* 2005;18(12):1440–1463. https://doi.org/10.1016/j.echo.2005.10.005.
20. Cheung AT, Savino JS, Weiss SJ, Aukburg SJ, Berlin JA. Echocardiographic and hemodynamic indexes of left ventricular preload in patients with normal and abnormal ventricular function. *Anesthesiology.* 1994;81(2):376–387.
21. Colombo PC, Municino A, Brofferio A, et al. Cross-sectional multiplane transesophageal echocardiographic measurements: comparison with standard transthoracic values obtained in the same setting. *Echocardiography.* 2002;19(5):383–390. (Mount Kisco, NY).
22. Shiota T. Clinical application of 3-dimensional echocardiography in the USA. *Circ J.* 2015;79(11):2287–2298. https://doi.org/10.1253/circj.CJ-15-0982.
23. Chahal NS, Lim TK, Jain P, Chambers JC, Kooner JS, Senior R. Population-based reference values for 3D echocardiographic LV volumes and ejection fraction. *JACC Cardiovasc Imaging*. 2012;5(12):1191–1197. https://doi.org/10.1016/j.jcmg.2012.07.014.
24. Ruddox V, Edvardsen T, Bækkevar M, Otterstad JE. Measurements of left ventricular volumes and ejection fraction with three-dimensional echocardiography: feasibility and agreement compared to two-dimensional echocardiography. *Int J Cardiovasc Imaging.* 2014;30(7):1325–1330. https://doi.org/10.1007/s10554-014-0478-9.
25. Muraru D, Badano LP, Peluso D, et al. Comprehensive analysis of left ventricular geometry and function by three-dimensional echocardiography in healthy adults. *J Am Soc Echocardiogr.* 2013;26(6):618–628. https://doi.org/10.1016/j.echo.2013.03.014.
26. Gardner BI, Bingham SE, Allen MR, Blatter DD, Anderson JL. Cardiac magnetic resonance versus transthoracic echocardiography for the assessment of cardiac volumes and regional function after myocardial infarction: an intrasubject comparison using simultaneous intrasubject recordings. *Cardiovasc Ultrasound.* 2009;7(1). https://doi.org/10.1186/1476-7120-7-38. 29–7.
27. Meris A, Santambrogio L, Casso G, Mauri R, Engeler A, Cassina T. Intraoperative three-dimensional versus two-dimensional echocardiography for left ventricular assessment. *Anesth Analg.* 2014;118(4):711–720. https://doi.org/10.1213/ane.0000000000000093.
28. Corsi C, Lang RM, Veronesi F, et al. Volumetric quantification of global and regional left ventricular function from real-time three-dimensional echocardiographic images. *Circulation.* 2005;112(8):1161–1170. https://doi.org/10.1161/circulationaha.104.513689.
29. Samstad SO, Torp HG, Linker DT, et al. Cross sectional early mitral flow velocity profiles from colour Doppler. *Brit Heart J.*1989;62(3):177–184.
30. Savino JS, Troianos CA, Aukburg S, Weiss R, Reichek N. Measurement of pulmonary blood flow with transesophageal two-dimensional and Doppler echocardiography. *Anesthesiology*. 1991;75(3):445–451.
31. Parra V, Fita G, Rovira I, Matute P, Gomar C, Pare C. Transoesophageal echocardiography accurately detects cardiac output variation: a prospective comparison with thermodilution in cardiac surgery. *Eur J Anaesthesiol.* 2008;25(2):135–143.
32. Lodato JA, Weinert L, Baumann R, et al. Use of 3-dimensional color Doppler echocardiography to measure stroke volume in human beings: comparison with thermodilution. *J Am Soc Echocardiogr.* 2007;20(2):103–112. https://doi.org/10.1016/j.echo.2006.07.010.
33. Shahgaldi K, Manouras A, Brodin LA, Winter R. Direct measurement of left ventricular outflow tract area using three-dimensional echocardiography in biplane mode improves accuracy of stroke volume assessment. *Echocardiography.* 2010;27(9):1078–1085. https://doi.org/10.1111/j.1540-8175.2010.01197.x. (Mount Kisco, NY).
34. Montealegre-Gallegos M, Mahmood F, Owais K, Hess P, Jainandunsing JS, Matyal R. Cardiac output calculation and three-dimensional echocardiography. *J Cardiothorac Vasc Anesth.* 2014;28(3):547–550. https://doi.org/10.1053/j.jvca.2013.11.005.
35. Silva CD, Pedro F, Deister L, Sahlen A, Manouras A, Shahgaldi K. Two-dimensional color Doppler echocardiography for left ventricular stroke volume assessment: a comparison study with three-dimensional echocardiography. *Echocardiography.* 2012;29(7):766–772. https://doi.org/10.1111/j.1540-8175.2012.01695.x. (Mount Kisco, NY).
36. Gorcsan JD, Diana P, Ball BA, Hattler BG. Intraoperative determination of cardiac output

by transesophageal continuous wave Doppler. *Am Heart J*. 1992;123(1):171–176.
37. Maslow A, Comunale ME, Haering JM, Watkins J. Pulsed wave Doppler measurement of cardiac output from the right ventricular outflow tract. *Anesth Analg*. 1996;83(3):466–471.
38. Canty DJ MBBS Hons FPP, Kim M MBBS FMEP, Guha R BSc Hons MFFA, et al. Comparison of cardiac output of both 2-dimensional and 3-dimensional transesophageal echocardiography with transpulmonary thermodilution during cardiac surgery. *J Cardiothorac Vasc Anesth*. August 2019:1–10. https://doi.org/10.1053/j.jvca.2019.06.007.
39. Royse CF, Connelly KA, MacLaren G, Royse AG. Evaluation of echocardiography indices of systolic function: a comparative study using pressure-volume loops in patients undergoing coronary artery bypass surgery. *Anaesthesia*. 2007;62(2):109–116. https://doi.org/10.1111/j.1365-2044.2006.04911.x.
40. Galiuto L, Ignone G, DeMaria AN. Contraction and relaxation velocities of the normal left ventricle using pulsed-wave tissue Doppler echocardiography. *Am J Cardiol*. 1998;81(5):609–614.
41. Adel W, Roushdy AM, Nabil M. Mitral annular plane systolic excursion-derived ejection fraction: a simple and valid tool in adult males with left ventricular systolic dysfunction. *Echocardiography*. 2015;33(2):179–184. https://doi.org/10.1111/echo.13009. (Mount Kisco, NY).
42. Tousignant C. CON: intraoperative Doppler tissue imaging is a valuable addition to cardiac anesthesiologists' armamentarium. *Anesth Analg*. 2009;108(1):41–47. https://doi.org/10.1213/ane.0b013e31818a6c64.
43. Simmons LA, Weidemann F, Sutherland GR, et al. Doppler tissue velocity, strain, and strain rate imaging with transesophageal echocardiography in the operating room: a feasibility study. *J Am Soc Echocardiogr*. 2002;15(8):768–776.
44. MacLaren G, Kluger R, Connelly KA, Royse CF. Comparative feasibility of myocardial velocity and strain measurements using 2 different methods with transesophageal echocardiography during cardiac surgery. *J Cardiothorac Vasc Anesth*. 2011;25(2):216–220. https://doi.org/10.1053/j.jvca.2010.05.011.
45. Mondillo S, Galderisi M, Mele D, et al. Speckle-tracking echocardiography: a new technique for assessing myocardial function. *J Ultrasound Med*. 2011;30(1):71–83.
46. Brown J, Jenkins C, Marwick TH. Use of myocardial strain to assess global left ventricular function: a comparison with cardiac magnetic resonance and 3-dimensional echocardiography. *Am Heart J*. 2009;157(1):102.e1–102.e5. https://doi.org/10.1016/j.ahj.2008.08.032.
47. Saito M, Negishi K, Eskandari M, et al. Association of left ventricular strain with 30-day mortality and Readmission in patients with heart failure. *J Am Soc Echocardiogr*. 2015;28(6):652–666. https://doi.org/10.1016/j.echo.2015.02.007.
48. Lee CH, Yang MM, Ho AC, et al. Evaluation of the longitudinal contraction of the ventricle septum in patients undergoing off-pump coronary artery bypass graft surgery by strain rate imaging. *Acta Anaesthesiol Taiwan*. 2006;44(1):11–18.
49. Kukucka M, Nasseri B, Tscherkaschin A, Mladenow A, Kuppe H, Habazettl H. The feasibility of speckle tracking for intraoperative assessment of regional myocardial function by transesophageal echocardiography. *J Cardiothorac Vasc Anesth*. 2009;23(4):462–467.
50. Negishi K, Negishi T, Kurosawa K, et al. Practical guidance in echocardiographic assessment of global longitudinal strain. *JACC Cardiovascular imaging*. 2015;8(4):489–492. https://doi.org/10.1016/j.jcmg.2014.06.013.
51. Hung CL, Verma A, Uno H, et al. Longitudinal and circumferential strain rate, left ventricular remodeling, and prognosis after myocardial infarction. *J Am Coll Cardiol*. 2010;56(22):1812–1822. https://doi.org/10.1016/j.jacc.2010.06.044.
52. Winkelmann J, Aronson S, Young CJ, Fernandez A, Lee BK. Retrograde-delivered cardioplegia is not distributed equally to the right ventricular free wall and septum. J Cardiothorac Vasc Anesth. 9(2):135-139.
53. Samad BA, Alam M, Jensen-Urstad K. Prognostic impact of right ventricular involvement as assessed by tricuspid annular motion in patients with acute myocardial infarction. *Am J Cardiol*. 2002;90(7):778–781.
54. David J-S, Tousignant CP, Bowry R. Tricuspid annular velocity in patients undergoing cardiac operation using transesophageal echocardiography. *J Am Soc Echocardiogr*. 2006;19(3):329–334. https://doi.org/10.1016/j.echo.2005.09.013.
55. David JS, Tousignant CP, Bowry R. Tricuspid annular velocity in patients undergoing cardiac operation using transesophageal echocardiography. *J Am Soc Echocardiogr*. 2006;19(3):329–334.
56. Focardi M, Cameli M, Carbone SF, et al. Traditional and innovative echocardiographic parameters for the analysis of right ventricular performance in comparison with cardiac magnetic resonance. *Eur Heart J Cardiovasc Imaging*. 2015;16(1):47–52. https://doi.org/10.1093/ehjci/jeu156.
57. Kossaify A. Echocardiographic assessment of the right ventricle, from the conventional approach to speckle tracking and three-dimensional imaging, and insights into the "right way" to explore the forgotten chamber. *Clin Med Insights Cardiol*. 2015;9:65–75. https://doi.org/10.4137/CMC.S27462. 2015 CMC.S27462.
58. Swaminathan M, Morris RW, De Meyts DD, et al. Deterioration of regional wall motion immediately after coronary artery bypass graft surgery is associated with long-term major adverse cardiac events. *Anesthesiology*. 2007;107(5):739–745.
59. Kolev N, Brase R, Swanevelder J, et al. The influence of transoesophageal echocardiography on intra-operative decision making. A European multicentre study. European Perioperative TOE Research Group. *Anaesthesia*. 1998;53(8):767–773.
60. London MJ, Tubau JF, Wong MG, et al. The "natural history" of segmental wall motion abnormalities in patients undergoing noncardiac surgery. S.P.I. Research Group. *Anesthesiology*. 1990;73(4):644–655.
61. Leung JM, O'Kelly B, Browner WS, Tubau J, Hollenberg M, Mangano DT. Prognostic importance of postbypass regional wall-motion abnormalities in patients undergoing coronary artery bypass graft surgery. SPI Research Group. *Anesthesiology*. 1989;71(1):16–25.
62. Comunale ME, Body SC, Ley C, et al. The concordance of intraoperative left ventricular wall-motion abnormalities and electrocardiographic S-T segment changes: association with outcome after coronary revascularization. Multicenter Study of Perioperative Ischemia (McSPI) Research Group. *Anesthesiology*. 1998;88(4):945–954.
63. Norum IB, Ruddox V, Edvardsen T, Otterstad JE. Diagnostic accuracy of left ventricular longitudinal function by speckle tracking echocardiography to predict significant coronary artery stenosis. A systematic review. *BMC Med Imaging*. 2015;15:25.
64. Hauser AM, Gangadharan V, Ramos RG, Gordon S, Timmis GC. Sequence of mechanical, electrocardiographic and clinical effects of repeated coronary artery occlusion in human beings: echocardiographic observations during coronary angioplasty. *J Am Coll Cardiol*. 1985;5(2 Pt 1):193–197.
65. McKinlay KH, Schinderle DB, Swaminathan M, et al. Predictors of inotrope use during separation from cardiopulmonary bypass. *J Cardiothorac Vasc Anesth*. 2004;18(4):404–408.
66. Shroyer AL, Grover FL, Hattler B, et al. On-pump versus off-pump coronary-artery bypass surgery. N Engl J Med.2009;361(19):1827–1837.
67. Peterson ED. Innovation and comparative-effectiveness research in cardiac surgery. N Engl J Med. 2009;361(19):1897–1899. https://doi.org/10.1056/NEJMe0907887.
68. Mishra M, Malhotra R, Karlekar A, Mishra Y, Trehan N. Propensity case-matched analysis of off-pump versus on-pump coronary artery bypass grafting in patients with atheromatous aorta. *Ann Thorac Surg*. 2006;82(2):608–614. https://doi.org/10.1016/j.athoracsur.2006.03.071.
69. Kapoor PM, Chowdhury U, Mandal B, Kiran U, Karnatak R. Trans-esophageal echocardiography in off-pump coronary artery bypass grafting. *Ann Card Anaesth*. 2009;12(2):167.
70. Wang J, Filipovic M, Rudzitis A, et al. Transesophageal echocardiography for monitoring segmental wall motion during off-pump coronary artery bypass surgery. *Anesth Analg*. 2004;99(4):965–973.
71. Gurbuz AT, Hecht ML, Arslan AH. Intraoperative transesophageal echocardiography modifies strategy in off-pump coronary artery bypass grafting. *Ann Thorac Surg*. 2007;83(3):1035–1040.
72. Kim SH, Yeo JS, Yoon TG, Kim TY, Chee HK. Placing a saline bag underneath the displaced heart enhances transgastric transesophageal echocardiographic imaging during off-pump coronary artery bypass surgery. *Anesth Analg*. 2009;109(4):1038–1040.
73. Bartoli CR, McCants KC, Birks EJ, et al. Percutaneous closure of a patent foramen ovale to prevent paradoxical thromboembolism in a patient with a continuous-flow LVAD. J Invasive Cardiol. 2013;25(3):154–156.
74. Chumnanvej S, Wood MJ, MacGillivray TE, Melo MFV. Perioperative echocardiographic examination for ventricular assist device implantation. *Anesth Analg*. 2007;105(3):583–601. https://doi.org/10.1213/01.ane.0000278088.22952.82.
75. Lazkani M, Murarka S, Kobayashi A, Seibolt L, Yang T, Pershad A. A retrospective analysis of Impella use in all-comers: 1-year outcomes. *J Intervent Cardiol*. 2017;30(6):577–583. https://doi.org/10.1111/joic.12409.
76. Lampert BC, Teuteberg JJ. Right ventricular failure after left ventricular assist devices. *HEALUN*. 2015;34(9):1123–1130. https://doi.org/10.1016/j.healun.2015.06.015.
77. Pavlushkov E, Berman M, Valchanov K. Cannulation techniques for extracorporeal life support. *Ann Transl Med*. 2017;5(4):70–70. https://doi.org/10.21037/atm.2016.11.47.

78. Huang YC, Cheng YJ, Lin YH, Wang MJ, Tsai SK. Graft failure caused by pulmonary venous obstruction diagnosed by intraoperative transesophageal echocardiography during lung transplantation [In Process Citation]. *Anesth Analg.* 2000;91(3):558–560.
79. Michel-Cherqui M, Brusset A, Liu N, et al. Intraoperative transesophageal echocardiographic assessment of vascular anastomoses in lung transplantation. A report on 18 cases. *Chest.* 1997;111(5):1229–1235.
80. Reeves ST, Glas KE, Eltzschig H, et al. Guidelines for performing a comprehensive epicardial echocardiography examination: recommendations of the American Society of Echocardiography and the Society of Cardiovascular Anesthesiologists. *J Am Soc Echocardiogr.* 2007;20:427–437.
81. Glas KE, Swaminathan M, Reeves ST, et al. Guidelines for the performance of a comprehensive intraoperative epiaortic ultrasonographic examination: recommendations of the American Society of Echocardiography and the Society of Cardiovascular Anesthesiologists; endorsed by the Society of Thoracic Surgeons. *J Am Soc Echocardiogr.* 2007;20(11):1227–1235. https://doi.org/10.1016/j.echo.2007.09.001.
82. Practice guidelines for perioperative transesophageal echocardiography. An updated report by the American Society of Anesthesiologists and the Society Of Cardiovascular Anesthesiologists task force on transesophageal echocardiography. *Anesthesiology.* 2010;112:1084–1096.
83. Flachskampf FA, Badano L, Daniel WG, et al. Recommendations for transoesophageal echocardiography: update 2010. *Eur J Echocardiogr.* 2010;11:557–576.
84. Kallmeyer IJ, Collard CD, Fox JA, Body SC, Shernan SK. The safety of intraoperative transesophageal echocardiography: a case series of 7200 cardiac surgical patients. *Anesth Analg.* 2001;92(5):1126–1130.
85. Qaddoura FE, Abel MD, Mecklenburg KL, et al. Role of intraoperative transesophageal echocardiography in patients having coronary artery bypass graft surgery. *Ann Thorac Surg.* 2004;78(5):1586–1590.
86. Forrest AP, Lovelock ND, Hu JM, Fletcher SN. The impact of intraoperative transoesophageal echocardiography on an unselected cardiac surgical population: a review of 2343 cases. *Anaesth Intensive Care.* 2002;30(6):734–741.
87. Sutton DC, Kluger R. Intraoperative transoesophageal echocardiography: impact on adult cardiac surgery. *Anaesth Intensive Care.* 1998;26(3):287–293.
88. Mahdy S, Brien BO, Buggy D, Griffin M. The impact of intraoperative transoesophageal echocardiography on decision-making during cardiac surgery. *Middle East J Anesthesiol.* 2009;20(2):199–206.
89. Couture P, Denault AY, McKenty S, et al. Impact of routine use of intraoperative transesophageal echocardiography during cardiac surgery. *Can J Anaesth.* 2000;47(1):20–26.
90. Mishra M, Chauhan R, Sharma KKHP, et al. Real-time intraoperative transesophageal echocardiography—how useful? Experience of 5,016 cases. *J Cardiothorac Vasc Anesth.* 1998;12(6):625–632.
91. Bergquist BD, Leung JM, Bellows WH. Transesophageal echocardiography in myocardial revascularization: I. Accuracy of intraoperative real-time interpretation. *Anesth Analg.* 1996;82(6):1132–1138.
92. Bergquist BD, Bellows WH, Leung JM. Transesophageal echocardiography in myocardial revascularization: II. Influence on intraoperative decision making. *Anesth Analg.* 1996;82(6):1139–1145.
93. Mathew JP, Fontes ML, Garwood S, et al. Transesophageal echocardiography interpretation: a comparative analysis between cardiac anesthesiologists and primary echocardiographers. *Anesth Analg.* 2002;94(2):302–309.
94. Bettex DA, Pretre R, Jenni R, Schmid ER. Cost-effectiveness of routine intraoperative transesophageal echocardiography in pediatric cardiac surgery: a 10-year experience. *Anesth Analg.* 2005;100(5):1271–1275.
95. Seto TB, Taira DA, Tsevat J, Manning WJ. Cost-effectiveness of transesophageal echocardiographic-guided cardioversion: a decision analytic model for patients admitted to the hospital with atrial fibrillation. *J Am Coll Cardiol.* 1997;29(1):122–130.
96. Fanshawe M, Ellis C, Habib S, Konstadt SN, Reich DL. A retrospective analysis of the costs and benefits related to alterations in cardiac surgery from routine intraoperative transesophageal echocardiography. *Anesth Analg.* 2002;95(4):824–827.
97. Fanshawe M, Ellis C, Habib S, Konstadt SN, Reich DL. A retrospective analysis of the costs and benefits related to alterations in cardiac surgery from routine intraoperative transesophageal echocardiography. *Anesth Analg.* 2002;95(4):824–827.
98. Eltzschig HK, Rosenberger P, Loffler M, Fox JA, Aranki SF, Shernan SK. Impact of intraoperative transesophageal echocardiography on surgical decisions in 12,566 patients undergoing cardiac surgery. *Ann Thorac Surg.* 2008;85(3):845–852. https://doi.org/10.1016/j.athoracsur.2007.11.015.
99. Greilich PE. Invited commentary. *Ann Thorac Surg.* 2008;85(3):852–853.
100. Hofer CK, Zollinger A, Rak M, et al. Therapeutic impact of intra-operative transoesophageal echocardiography during noncardiac surgery. *Anaesthesia.* 2004;59(1):3–9.
101. Schulmeyer MC, Santelices E, Vega R, Schmied S. Impact of intraoperative transesophageal echocardiography during noncardiac surgery. *J Cardiothorac Vasc Anesth.* 2006;20(6):768–771.
102. Canty DJ, Royse CF. Audit of anaesthetist-performed echocardiography on perioperative management decisions for non-cardiac surgery. *Br J Anaesth.* 2009;103(3):352–358.
103. Fleisher LA, Weiskopf RB. Real-time intraoperative monitoring of myocardial ischemia in noncardiac surgery. *Anesthesiology.* 2000;92(4):1183–1188.
104. Souilamas R, Souilamas JI, Alkhamees K, et al. Extra corporal membrane oxygenation in general thoracic surgery: a new single veno-venous cannulation. *J Cardiothorac Surg.* 2011;6(1):52–53.
105. Brandt RR, Oh JK, Abel MD, Click RL, Orszulak TA, Seward JB. Role of emergency intraoperative transesophageal echocardiography. *J Am Soc Echocardiogr.* 1998;11(10):972–977.
106. Bergquist BD, Bellows WH, Leung JM. Transesophageal echocardiography in myocardial revascularization: II. Influence on intraoperative decision making. *Anesth Analg.* 1996;82(6):1139–1145.
107. Savage RM, Lytle BW, Aronson S, et al. Intraoperative echocardiography is indicated in high-risk coronary artery bypass grafting [see comments]. *Ann Thorac Surg.* 1997;64(2):368–373; discussion 373–374.
108. Couture P, Denault AY, McKenty S, et al. Impact of routine use of intraoperative transesophageal echocardiography during cardiac surgery. *Can J Anaesth.* 2000;47(1):20–26.
109. Click RL, Abel MD, Schaff HV. Intraoperative transesophageal echocardiography: 5-year prospective review of impact on surgical management. *Mayo Clin Proc.* 2000;75(3):241–247. https://doi.org/10.4065/75.3.241.

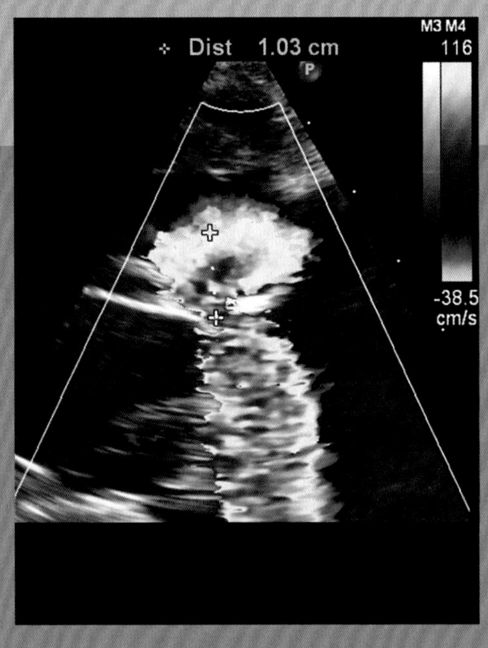

中文导读

第10章
介入超声心动图

随着结构性心脏病介入治疗技术的日新月异，超声心动图以其实时、便捷的优势发挥着重要作用。经食管超声心动图仍然是术中最常用的技术，可在术中监测引导，并以高清的二维、三维图像进行血流动力学评估。

具体应用：①经导管主动脉瓣置换术：术前准确测量主动脉瓣环直径及评估主动脉根部解剖可有效减少术后瓣周漏，术中观察并发症的发生并及时与导管医师交流；②经导管二尖瓣缘对缘修复术：术前准确评估反流量，术中辅助房间隔穿刺-导管和夹子的定位-瓣叶抓捕-夹子释放的每一个步骤，术后效果评估及预防并发症；③经导管二尖瓣置换术：术前评估二尖瓣器解剖、评估夹子的着陆区，术中辅助房间隔穿刺-导管的路径-经导管瓣膜释放-释放后效果评估等每一步骤，同时可及时评估左心室流出道狭窄等并发症并协助LAMPOON（预防左室流出道狭窄而切开二尖瓣前叶）解决方案；④经皮瓣周漏封堵术：超声对瓣周漏的形状、大小、位置等关键信息的准确评估至关重要，需要多切面多角度来综合判断，术中可协助导管定位，封堵器释放及术后效果评估；⑤左心耳封堵术：通常以0°、45°、90°和135°这4个角度观察左心耳的分叶形状并测量口径和深度，术中可引导房间隔穿刺，导管定位及封堵器释放。

朱振辉

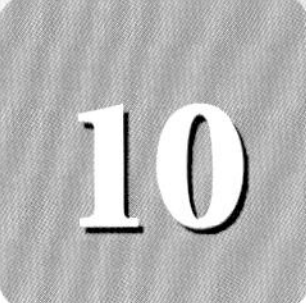

Interventional Echocardiography

RICHARD SHEU, MD | G. BURKHARD MACKENSEN, MD, PhD

Structural heart disease involves pathology of the valves and various other cardiac structures. Many of these defects can be treated by image-guided transcatheter procedures, often involving rapidly evolving technologies that present new challenges and opportunities for the echocardiographer. As novel catheter-based procedures and technologies are developed, more interventional procedures are being performed, improving outcomes for patients with previously untreatable conditions. Ongoing periprocedural cardiovascular imaging plays a critical role in the success of these delicate interventions.

ECHOCARDIOGRAPHIC IMAGING MODALITIES

Echocardiography offers many advantages in guiding transcatheter procedures. The real-time aspect of visualizing cardiac motion and flow dynamics by echocardiography cannot be achieved by imaging modalities such as computed tomography (CT) or magnetic resonance imaging (MRI). Although fluoroscopy provides live imaging, most thin, pliable, and dynamically moving intracardiac structures are not visible. Precise locations of minute pathology such as paravalvular defects are also extremely difficult to determine solely by fluoroscopy. In a single-center retrospective study, the addition of intraprocedural transesophageal echocardiography (TEE) to standard fluoroscopy for transcatheter patent foramen ovale closure was associated with reductions in postprocedural residual shunt, need for reintervention, and overall radiation exposure.[1]

Among echocardiographic imaging modalities, TEE has been the mainstay of procedural guidance because of its exceptional imaging quality. Its esophageal position allows concurrent fluoroscopy during the procedure because the TEE operator is often situated at the head or slightly to the side of the patient with his or her hands away from the chest and out of the fluoroscopic imaging field. In contrast, intraprocedural transthoracic echocardiography (TTE) often can be performed only intermittently because of the need to avoid interference with fluoroscopy. Nonetheless, successful transcatheter procedures guided by TTE instead of TEE have been reported.[2–4]

Like TEE, intracardiac echocardiography (ICE) can be used simultaneously with fluoroscopy, and it has recently gained traction as a reasonable alternative.[5] However, ICE requires additional vascular access, has a shallower imaging field, and provides inferior three-dimensional (3D) imaging resolution. The high cost for ICE-capable echocardiography platforms and disposable ICE transducers has prohibited its routine use for procedural guidance.[6]

Another reason favoring TEE over ICE for procedural guidance is familiarity with TEE among the structural heart team. Properly trained interventional echocardiographers, including cardiologists and cardiac anesthesiologists, are experienced in performing and interpreting procedural TEE studies. Interventional proceduralists are also well accustomed to TEE images, and procedural flow is often based on a routine sequence of expected TEE images. In short, TEE acts as a common language that facilitates communication among all team members.

Even though some studies suggest that TTE and ICE are safe, efficacious, and potentially superior imaging modalities,[7,8] TEE is accepted as the gold standard for optimal guidance of transcatheter procedures. This chapter provides an overview of interventional echocardiography focused mainly on TEE-related topics. Various imaging modalities are not mutually exclusive but rather complementary to one another, all based on specific intraprocedural imaging needs. The pros and cons of TEE, TTE, and ICE for transcatheter imaging guidance are summarized in Table 10.1.

TABLE 10.1 Advantages and Disadvantages of Echocardiographic Modalities for Transcatheter Procedural Guidance.

TEE	*TTE*	*ICE*
Advantages		
• Superior image quality • 3D imaging available • Allows comprehensive examination • Relatively low cost • Continuous procedural guidance • Well recognized by all structural heart team members	• 3D imaging available • Allows comprehensive examination • Relatively low cost • No need for general anesthesia • Noninvasive • Few absolute contraindications • Well recognized by all structural heart team members	• High image quality • Continuous procedural guidance • Need for only local anesthesia • Minimal personnel involvement if operated by procedural team
Disadvantages		
• Relatively invasive • Patient factors may present absolute contraindications • Need for general anesthesia with endotracheal intubation • Requires separate imaging team	• Imaging quality affected by patient body habitus and position • Intermittent procedural guidance • Cannot be performed during fluoroscopic imaging • Need for separate imaging team	• Limitations of 3D imaging with current technology • Narrow and shallow imaging window • High cost • Need for invasive vascular access • Patient factors may present absolute contraindications • Less recognized by structural heart team members and may require additional training

ICE, Intracardiac echocardiography.

ECHOCARDIOGRAPHIC IMAGING MODES

This section presents practical two-dimensional (2D) and 3D TEE imaging modes commonly used to guide transcatheter interventional procedures. Vendor-neutral terminology is used for description of specific 3D modes.

2D TEE

Conventional 2D TEE provides a quick overview of cardiac structures and motion, and it offers better spatial and temporal resolution than 3D TEE. It has been used extensively, along with Doppler techniques, during transcatheter interventional procedures to confirm preprocedural diagnoses, establish anatomic baseline details, identify morphologic contraindications, assess potential structural challenges, exclude iatrogenic complications, and evaluate midprocedural and final results.[9]

Patient loading conditions are significantly altered under general anesthesia, which is required for many structural heart interventions to enable extensive TEE imaging. The severity of valvular pathology must therefore be graded based on preprocedural imaging. Some have proposed augmentation of patient afterload with intravenous vasoconstrictive agents to push hemodynamic factors to baseline for more accurate assessment[10]; however, this practice does not fully mitigate other factors associated with general anesthesia, such as negative inotropic effects or reduction in preload due to positive-pressure ventilation. Even though patient physiologic variables can theoretically be pharmacologically adjusted to match their baseline hemodynamic values, there is an inherent risk of overestimation or underestimation of pathologic severity.[11] Nonetheless, preprocedural structural abnormalities, including causes and mechanisms of valvular disease, should be confirmed during comprehensive baseline TEE examination in the procedural setting.

3D TEE

Real-time 3D TEE has played an essential role in the exponential growth and innovation of transcatheter heart procedures in recent years. With the added dimension of elevation in 3D TEE, complex delivery of transcatheter devices can be accurately tracked within the cardiac cavity.[12] Most importantly, 3D TEE overcomes the major limitation of geometric assumptions often made during quantitative echocardiography. Like 2D TEE, 3D TEE imaging suffers from ultrasound artifacts such as dropout, blurring, blooming, reverberation, and shadowing artifacts.[13] Stitch artifacts, exclusive to gated 3D echocardiography, have become less of a hindrance with improvements in ultrasound transducer technology and machine computational power.

Ideal intraprocedural 3D TEE imaging used for transcatheter procedural guidance should include properties such as single-beat acquisition, large volumetric data set, high volume rate, and superb spatial resolution. Current modes of 3D TEE include live narrow-sector imaging, focused zoom, multibeat gated full-volume acquisition, and simultaneous biplane or multiplane imaging. The most valuable 3D TEE modes specific for structural heart imaging are the focused zoom and simultaneous biplane modes. Interventional echocardiographers must be proficient in using and switching among these different imaging modes.

Zoom mode is achieved by adjusting orthogonal imaging sector sizes that focus on the region of interest. When a smaller volumetric data set is selected, the region of interest is visualized with increased spatial and temporal resolution.[14] However, sufficient surrounding structures should be included in the imaging sector to serve as anatomic landmarks. In the absence of anatomic landmarks, the 3D structure of interest should be rotated and displayed in a conventional manner to facilitate communication (Fig. 10.1).[15] Real-time cropping of the 3D image is occasionally necessary to better appreciate the cardiac structure or pathology. Image cropping tools include fixed plane, flexible plane, multiplane, two-click crop, and box crop (Fig. 10.2). Cropping of 3D data sets before acquisition may further improve overall image resolution.

Postacquisition analysis of a 3D data set can be performed on-cart or off-cart in vendor-specific multiplanar reconstruction (MPR) software packages. All 2D imaging cut planes can be tilted and moved to numerous angles and positions around the region of interest, permitting accurate quantitative measurements of 3D structures. However, measurements made directly on 3D images may be subject to parallax error and should be performed with caution (Fig. 10.3).[14]

Depending on the reason for using 3D TEE, multibeat gated and single-beat real-time imaging can be applied to 3D zoom mode. In situations in which optimal resolution is prioritized, such as confirming preprocedural pathology or grading postprocedural results, multibeat acquisition is more appropriate to maximize image quality and volume rate. However, when 3D zoom mode is used for real-time visualization and guidance of the procedure, single-beat live imaging is more appropriate to allow for instantaneous response of the 3D image to transducer manipulation.

Live 3D TEE images have been superimposed on fluoroscopic images to form so-called fusion images (Fig. 10.4).[16] Fiducial markers placed on TEE images are immediately integrated into the fluoroscopic fused data set, facilitating communication between the echocardiographer and the interventionalist. Easier identification of precise locations by fusion imaging may improve overall procedural safety and completion time.[17]

Simultaneous biplane mode is another valuable 3D imaging mode for transcatheter procedural guidance. Its usefulness lies in the ability to concurrently visualize orthogonal sectors at various omniplane angles. Unlike other 3D TEE modes that require

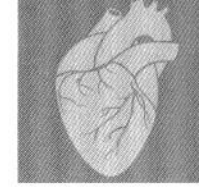

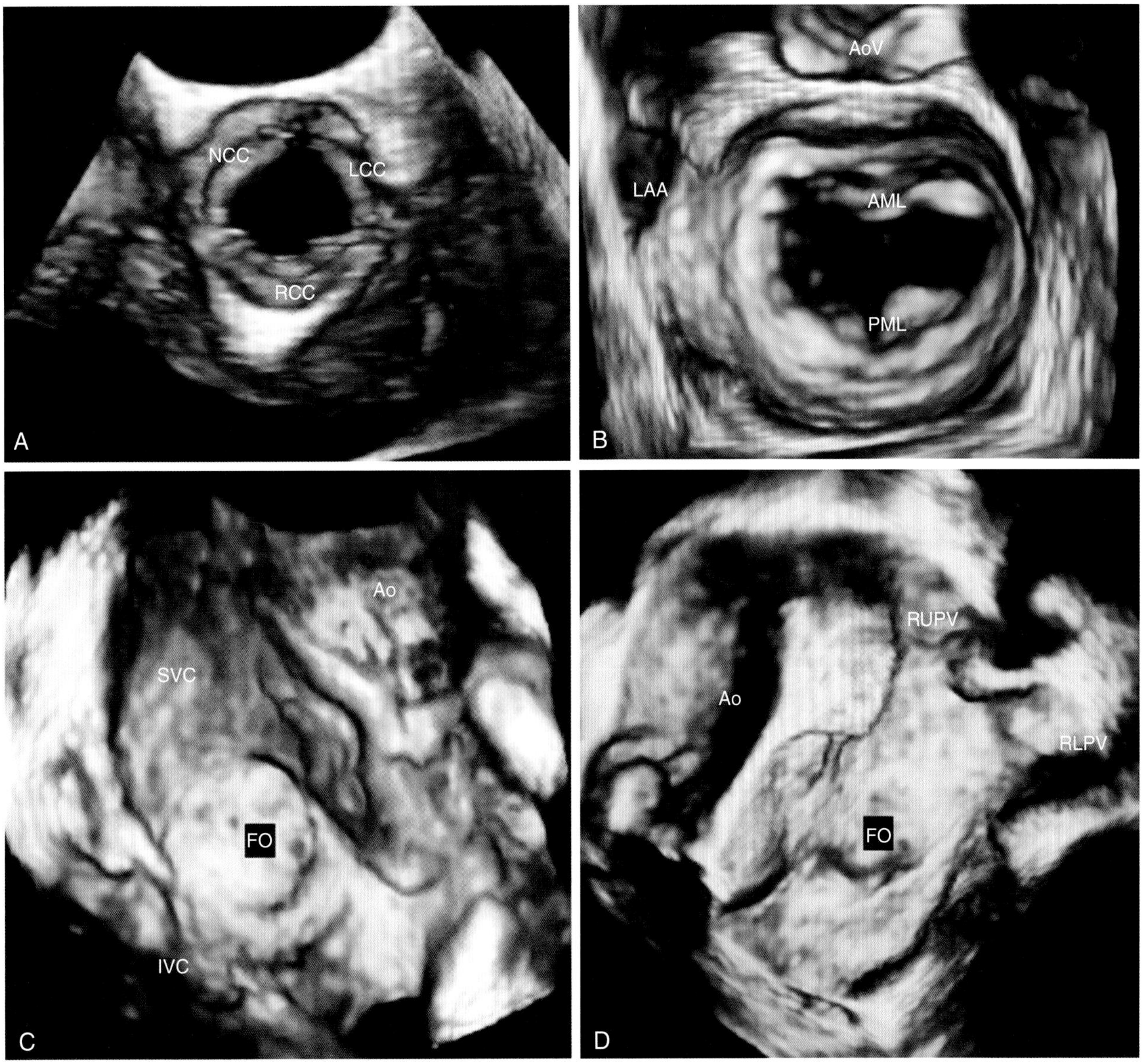

Fig. 10.1 **Conventional display of cardiac structures imaged by 3D TEE.** (A) Aortic valve. (B) Mitral valve. (C) Interatrial septum viewed from the LA. (D) Interatrial septum viewed from the RA. *Ao*, Aorta; *AML*, anterior mitral leaflet; *AoV*, aortic valve; *FO*, fossa ovalis; *IVC*, inferior vena cava; *LAA*, left atrial appendage; *LCC*, left coronary cusp; *NCC*, noncoronary cusp; *PML*, posterior mitral leaflet; *RCC*, right coronary cusp; *RLPV*, right lower pulmonary vein; *RUPV*, right upper pulmonary vein; *SVC*, superior vena cava.

tremendous computational power to process large volumetric data sets, this mode obtains only two perpendicular imaging planes, producing exceptional overall resolution. As an additional feature, the imager can use a flexible tilt plane to interrogate a specific structure or determine the precise location of a catheter or wire based on an exact perpendicular image plane. Because the superior-inferior and anterior-posterior rims of the fossa ovalis can be visualized simultaneously by this imaging mode, a major application is for procedures performed on the interatrial septum (IAS), including transseptal punctures and device placement for occlusion of atrial septal defects. The optimal transseptal locations for various left-sided interventions are summarized in Table 10.2.[18]

INTRAPROCEDURAL TEE FOR TRANSCATHETER AORTIC VALVE REPLACEMENT

The number of patients presenting for transcatheter aortic valve replacement (TAVR) has grown exponentially.[19] Although there is a significant trend for TAVR patients to receive minimal sedation and TTE postprocedural assessment, general anesthesia with intraprocedural real-time TEE guidance remains essential in certain situations.[20] This section focuses on practical aspects of intraprocedural TEE, such as sizing the aortic annulus, for TAVR in native and bioprosthetic valves.

Multiple studies have retrospectively associated undersized and oversized transcatheter heart valves (THVs) with postprocedural paravalvular leakage (PVL).[21,22] Accurate and reliable aortic annular measurements by appropriate imaging may reduce the overall incidence of these events. Contrast-enhanced multidetector computed tomography (MDCT) is considered the primary imaging modality for preprocedural characterization of valvular morphology and annular size. However, when contrast-enhanced MDCT is unavailable or contraindicated (e.g., emergent case, patient with advanced renal disease), 3D TEE is an appropriate alternative. Compared with 2D echocardiography, 3D TEE provides better appreciation of the noncircular annular plane. In a comparison with 3D TEE, 2D echocardiography was shown to

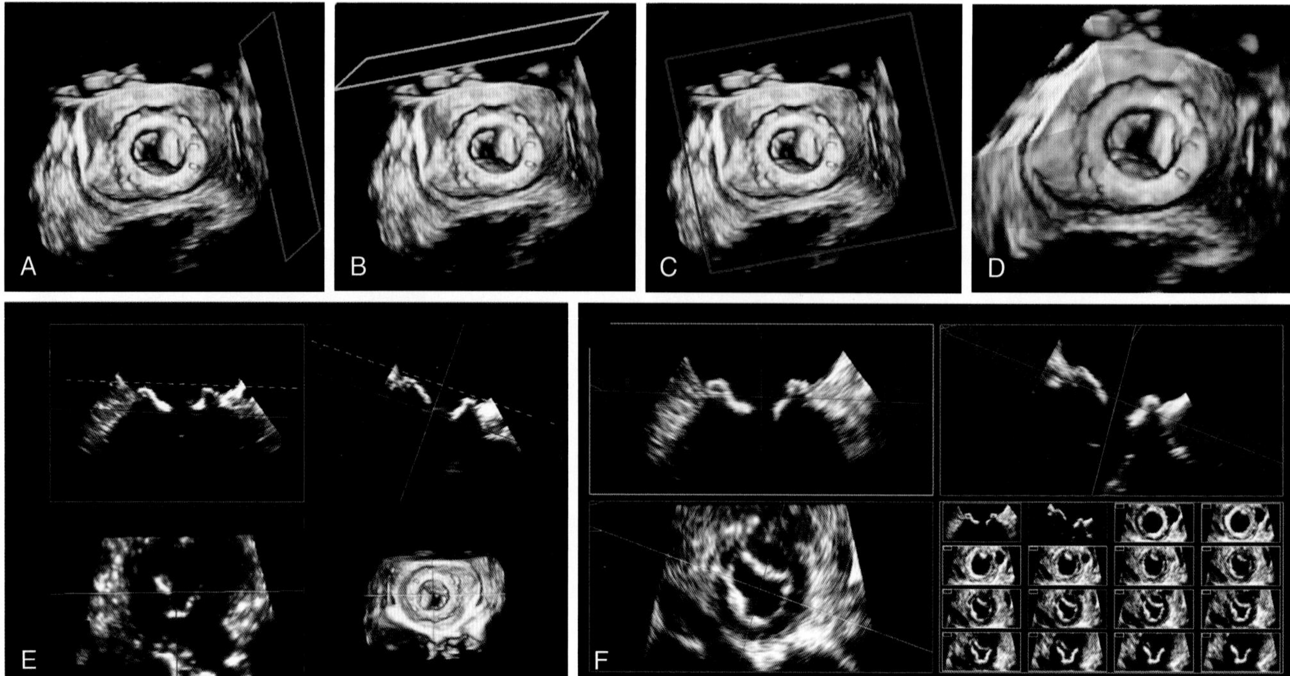

Fig. 10.2 Vendor-specific methods of cropping and trimming 3D-rendered images. (A–C) Crop planes *(red, green, and blue boxes)* with fixed angulation and orientation. (D) Flexible crop plane *(purple plane)* that can be moved freely according to the viewer's specific needs. (E) Multiplanar reconstruction of the 3D image, which can be performed in real time or after acquisition. (F) Multiplanar reconstruction of the 3D image with multiple 2D slices (planes) displayed simultaneously *(bottom right panel)* allows for detailed examination of the cardiac structure of interest.

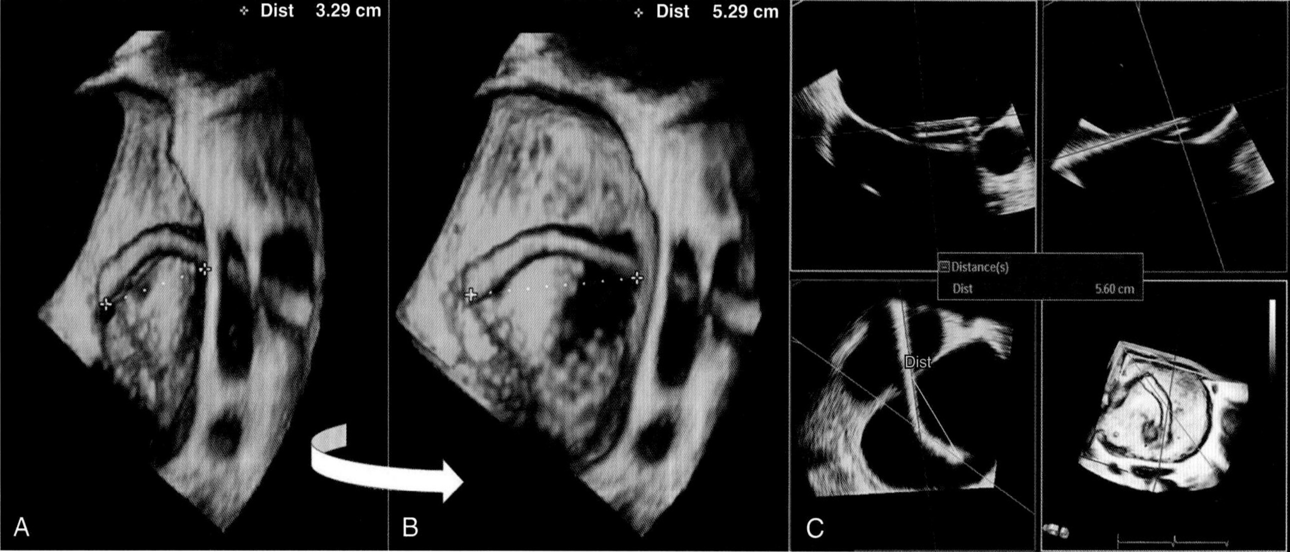

Fig. 10.3 Parallax effect with 3D echocardiography. (A and B) Depth is not well appreciated when 3D objects are displayed on 2D surfaces. Direct distance measurements from the catheter tip to the interatrial septum yield different results depending on the viewing angle. (C) Multiplanar reconstruction of the 3D object with proper alignment of the imaging planes eliminates the viewing bias and permits the true distance between two points to be measured. *White arrow* indicates the rotation of panel A around the y-axis to produce panel B.

consistently underestimate aortic annular dimensions, leading to a change in THV size selection in 23% of the patients.[23] A meta-analysis of 13 observational studies examined the agreement between measurements of the aortic annulus obtained by 3D TEE and by MDCT.[24] A significant linear correlation was established between the two imaging modalities, although annular area was found to be slightly smaller when measured by 3D TEE (mean difference, -2.22 mm^2; 95% limits of agreement: -12.79 to 8.36). This finding did not alter THV size selection or likelihood of procedural success. Because of its eccentricity, the mean diameter of the aortic annulus is often calculated by the measured area or circumference instead of by direct linear measurements from one cusp insertion (hinge-point) to another. Circumference-derived diameters have been shown to result in a lower incidence of post-procedural PVL, compared with area-derived diameters.[25] This could be a result of the larger diameter (23.4 ± 2.3 mm vs. 22.9 ± 2.3 mm; $P < 0.001$) calculated by measured circumference compared with area.

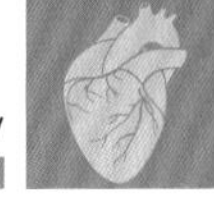

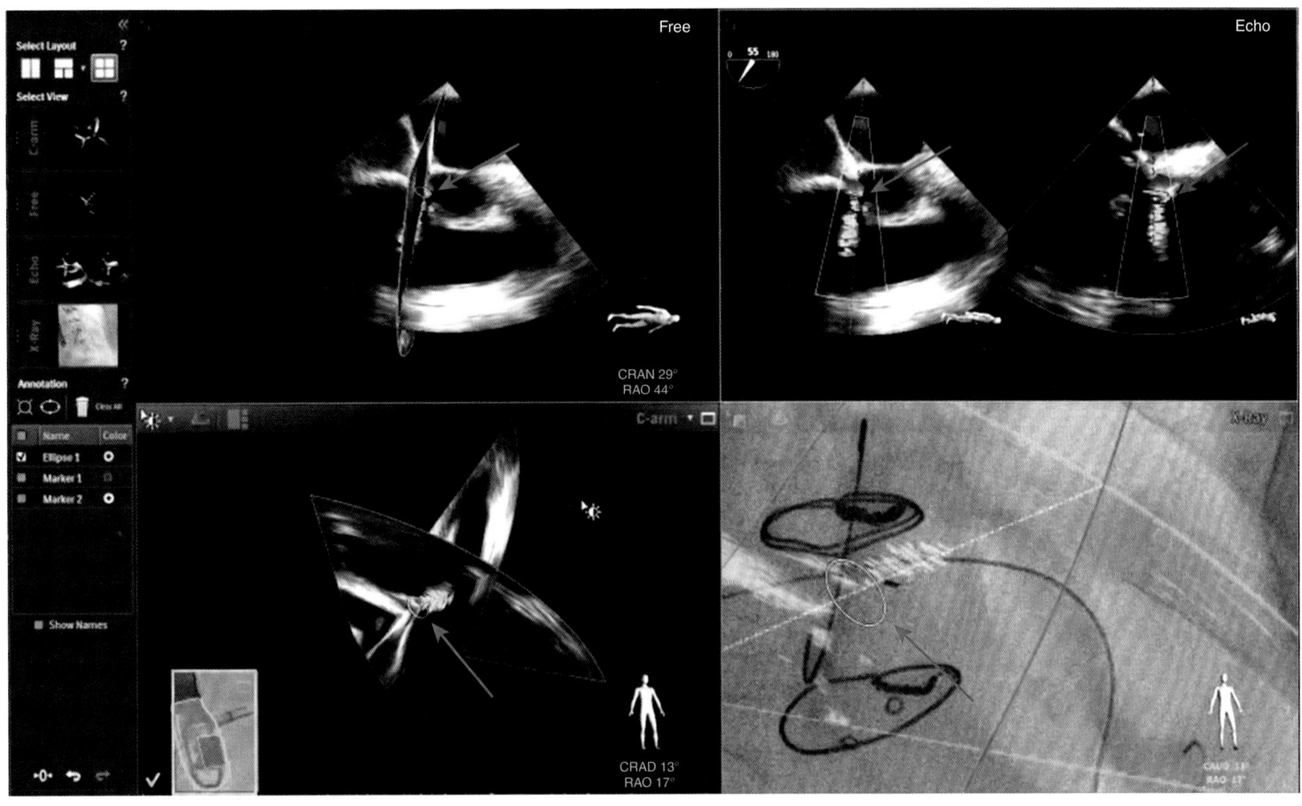

Fig. 10.4 Echocardiographic and fluoroscopic fusion imaging. Real-time fusion imaging is used to locate the paravalvular defect near a bioprosthetic tricuspid valve (Video 10.4). Conventional simultaneous biplane TEE imaging of the right ventricular inflow and outflow tract is displayed together (*top left panel*) and separated into side-by-side images (*top right panel*) in the software. TEE images are rotated to mimic fluoroscopy orientation (*bottom left panel*) and superimposed directly on fluoroscopic images (*bottom right panel*). Markers (*red arrow*) manually placed on TEE images are transferred automatically to fluoroscopic images. Green color of TEE transducer in the inset image signifies coregistration and real-time fusion imaging.

TABLE 10.2 Transseptal Location for Transcatheter Interventions.

Transcatheter Procedure	*ME Bicaval View (Superior/Inferior)*	*ME AoV SAX View (Anterior/Posterior)*
Balloon mitral valvuloplasty	Mid	Posterior
Mitral valve edge-to-edge repair	Superior	Posterior
Mitral valve replacement (valve-in-valve, valve-in-ring, valve-in-calcified annulus)	Mid	Posterior
Mitral paravalvular defect occlusion	Mid	Posterior
Left atrial appendage closure	Inferior	Posterior
Percutaneous LV assist device	Mid	Mid
Atrial septal defect/patent foramen ovale repair	Through defect	Through defect

AoV, Aortic valve; *ME*, mid-esophageal; *Mid*, middle; *SAX*, short axis.

Commercial software, using MPR of the 3D TEE data set, is often used for off-line analysis of the complex aortic root anatomy (Fig. 10.5). It is important to understand the concept of finding three aortic valve (AoV) anchoring sites, one from each cusp, to obtain an accurate cross-sectional plane of the aortic annulus (i.e., three points form a plane). This principle can be applied to any 3D volume, regardless of which TEE view is used to acquire the data set. A guide for attaining the aortic annulus cross-sectional plane, modified from the turnaround technique,[26] is described in Table 10.3.

The aortic annular area, circumference, and diameters can be measured manually on the transverse plane (see Fig. 10.5D). Semi-automated and fully automated measurements of these parameters have also been described with excellent and reliable results.[27,28] As with any measurements, cyclic variation may occur with respiration or cardiac contraction. It may be necessary to average several results. If a patient presents with a previously placed bioprosthetic valve of unknown size, the internal valvular diameter can be measured with the same technique as described for sizing of the aortic annulus.

Immediately after THV deployment, intraprocedural TEE can be used to detect potential complications, including coronary artery occlusion, THV malposition, residual aortic regurgitation, mitral valve (MV) impingement, THV embolization, pericardial effusion, and aortic rupture and dissection.[29,30] If preprocedural imaging analysis suggests a potential risk of coronary obstruction, several preventive strategies may be considered, including the newly described *b*ioprosthetic or native *a*ortic *s*callop *i*ntentional *l*aceration to prevent *i*atrogenic *c*oronary *a*rtery obstruction (BASILICA) procedure.[31]

The BASILICA procedure involves laceration of the AoV leaflet to create a triangular space in front of the coronary ostia, mitigating the risk of obstruction after TAVR.[32] Intraprocedural TEE plays a vital role for the success of this technically demanding procedure (Fig. 10.6). Simultaneous biplane mode is often used to guide the location, position, direction, and orientation of the leaflet traversal system in the aortic sinus (Table 10.4). After leaflet puncture, a wire is advanced into the left ventricular outflow tract (LVOT) and captured by a transvalvular snare, forming a loop around the targeted leaflet. Distinguishing catheters from one another by TEE may be difficult due to shadowing from native calcification or prosthetic valve cages and stents. After the targeted leaflet is lacerated by electrocautery, significant hemodynamic instability may occur with transition from a stenotic physiology to that of regurgitation. If severe aortic regurgitation is not appreciated on TEE, the leaflet puncture site should be re-examined.

INTRAPROCEDURAL TEE FOR PERCUTANEOUS MITRAL VALVE EDGE-TO-EDGE REPAIR

Favorable outcome of surgical repair for degenerative MV disease has been well documented.[33] Unfortunately, up to 49% of patients with symptomatic severe mitral regurgitation (MR) are denied surgical options due to unacceptable risk factors.[34] In recent years, percutaneous approaches to MV repair have been proposed for these patients with high or prohibitive risk.[35] Numerous large clinical trials have demonstrated a significant positive impact on clinical outcomes, such as reduced hospitalizations and reduced mortality.[36,37] Practical recommendations for intraprocedural TEE imaging of the most commonly used technology approved by the U.S. Food and Drug Administration, the MitraClip system (Abbott Vascular, Santa Clara, CA) are discussed later in this section. Improved real-time 3D TEE imaging technology has facilitated exponential growth in the use of this edge-to-edge clip (E-EC) system.

MV repair with E-EC therapy involves leaflet edge-to-edge approximation, drawing comparison to the surgical technique described by Alfieri et al.[38] Differences between these two methods are summarized in Table 10.5. In addition to improving leaflet coaptation, the E-EC system creates a tissue bridge that restricts mitral annular dilation and facilitates left ventricular (LV) remodeling. A reduction in mitral annular dimensions, including circumference and anteroposterior and bicommissural diameters, was documented by 3D TEE immediately after E-EC implantation.[39] Patients with functional MR were also found to have a reduction in mitral annular sphericity index (ratio between anteroposterior and mediolateral distances) and in anatomic MV orifice area after E-EC.[40] Interestingly, the mechanism of MR reduction by E-EC therapy in these patients seemed to depend on MR jet directionality. Those with central functional MR seemed to benefit most from the shortening of anteroposterior diameter and increase in coaptation area, whereas those with eccentric functional MR benefited from a decrease in average leaflet tethering angle.[41] Further, patients who received the E-EC therapy were found to have significant biventricular volume reduction and

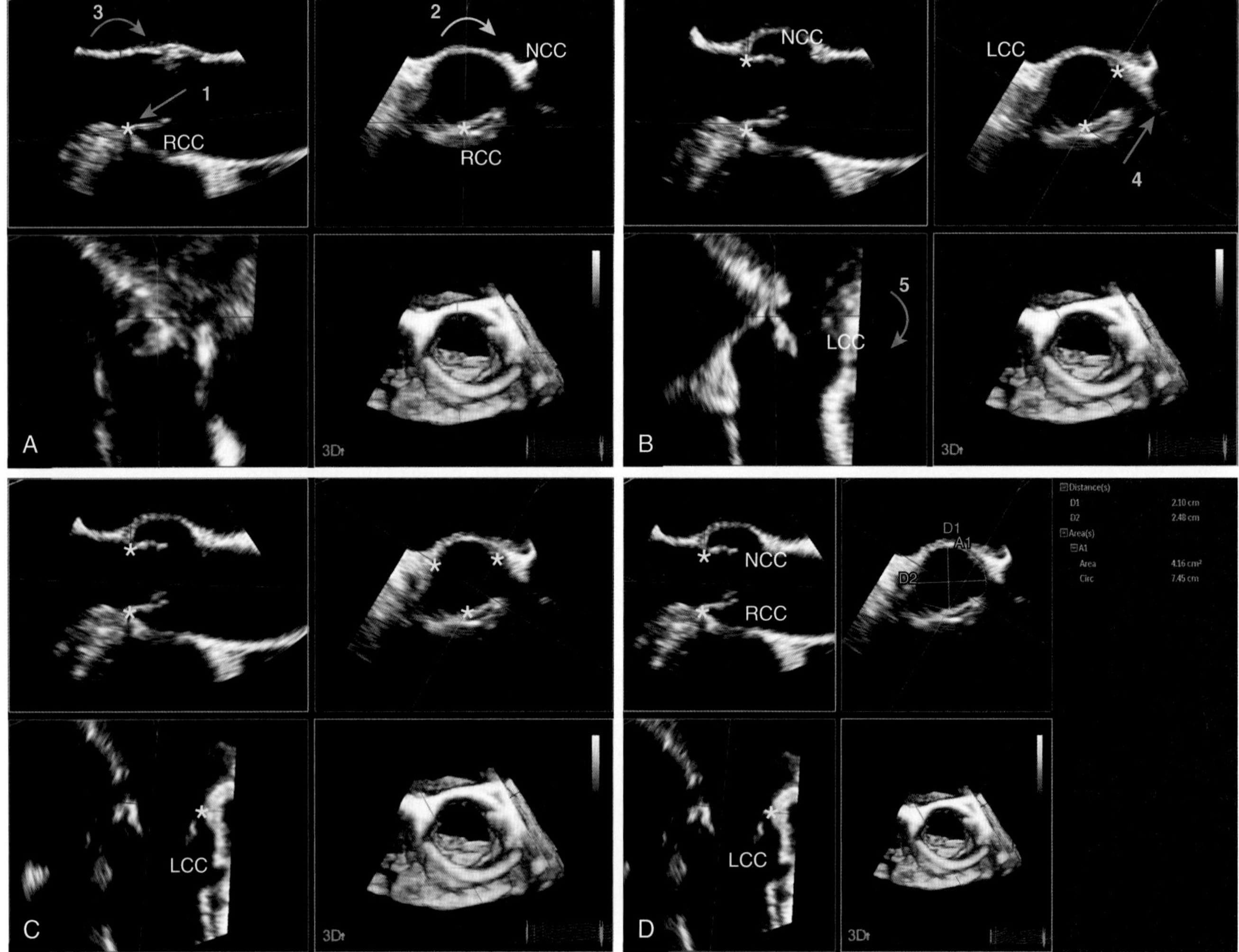

Fig. 10.5 **Aortic annular measurements in 3D multiplanar reconstruction.** Accurate measurement of the aortic annulus is obtained by sequential identification of the coronary cusp insertion sites *(asterisks)*. Numbers in the figure indicate the necessary movements (Video 10.5), but they do not correspond to the numbered steps described in Table 10.3. *LCC*, Left coronary cusp; *NCC*, noncoronary cusp; *RCC*, right coronary cusp.

functional improvement based on myocardial strain assessments after the procedure.[42,43] Because many of these beneficial effects are seen immediately or relatively soon after device implantation, some have proposed E-EC therapy as a reasonable solution to stabilize patients who are in acute cardiogenic shock from MR.[44]

TEE plays a pivotal role in preprocedural patient selection, intraprocedural guidance, postprocedural assessment, and complication exclusion. Numerous articles have reviewed the procedural steps and corresponding imaging sequence.[45–47]

TABLE 10.3 Step-by-Step Guide for Attaining the Aortic Annulus Cross-Sectional Plane.

1. Acquire a TEE volume data set of the aortic root using a focused 3D mode. While minimizing the pyramidal box size, ensure that the LVOT, the proximal ascending aorta, and the entire width of the aortic annulus are captured in the short and long axes. The ideal volume rate should be >10 Hz to allow accurate assessment of the annulus during mid-systole.
2. Open the 3D data set with a commercially available multiplanar reconstruction software program for off-line analysis. Fix (lock) the three orthogonal planes at 90 degrees from each other.
3. In mid-systole, with aortic valve leaflets open, move the crosshair formed by the transverse (short-axis) plane *(red)* and the coronal plane *(blue)* to the hinge-point where the right coronary cusp (RCC) attaches to the annulus on the sagittal (long-axis) plane *(green)* (Fig. 10.5A, *purple arrow*).
4. In the transverse plane, rotate the sagittal plane clockwise or counterclockwise along the noncoronary cusp (NCC) (Fig. 10.5A, *green arrow*) until the nadir of its annular insertion site is clearly visualized on the sagittal plane (Fig. 10.5B).
5. In the sagittal plane, rotate the transverse plane (Fig. 10.5A, *red arrow*), with the crosshair still at the base of the RCC, until it intersects the NCC insertion site (Fig. 10.5B).
6. Return to the transverse plane. Slide the coronal plane along the sagittal plane (Fig. 10.5B, *blue arrow*) until the nadir of the left coronary cusp (LCC) insertion site is seen in the coronal plane (Fig. 10.5C).
7. In the coronal plane, without moving the crosshair, rotate the transverse plane (Fig. 10.5B, *red arrow*) until it intersects the LCC insertion site (Fig. 10.5C).
8. The transverse plane then aligns with the short axis of the aortic annulus at the level where the RCC (step 3), NCC (step 5), and LCC (step 7) intersect with the annulus (Fig. 10.5D)

LCC, Left coronary cusp; *LVOT*, left ventricular outflow tract; *NCC*, noncoronary cusp; *RCC*, right coronary cusp.

TABLE 10.4 TEE Guidance and Confirmation Before Leaflet Puncture: BASILICA Leaflet Traversal System.

Location	Predetermined coronary cusp (left, right, or both)
Position	Leaflet base (closer to annulus) Directly in front of the coronary ostial opening (excellent results have also been reported in the middle of the cusp regardless of ostial site)
Direction	Coaxial to the aortic root for optimal angle
Orientation	Curved tip pointed inward (toward the center of the aortic valve) to avoid catastrophic aortic wall perforation

BASILICA, *B*ioprosthetic or native *a*ortic *s*callop *i*ntentional *l*aceration to prevent *i*atrogenic *c*oronary *a*rtery obstruction.

TABLE 10.5 Differences Between Transcatheter Mitral Valve Edge-to-Edge Repair and Alfieri Stitch Repair.

E-EC Therapy	*Alfieri Stitch Repair*
Percutaneous approach	Sternotomy with cardiopulmonary bypass
Indirect visualization of the diseased MV by TEE	Direct inspection of the diseased MV by surgeon
Isolated therapy	Can be easily combined with other MV repair strategies such as annuloplasty ring
Repair under dynamic (beating heart) conditions	Repair under static (arrested heart) conditions
Real-time evaluation of procedural results	Post-repair evaluation of surgical results after separation from cardiopulmonary bypass
Results in smooth MV atrial surface	Results in rough MV atrial surface

E-EC, Edge-to-edge clip; *MV*, mitral valve.

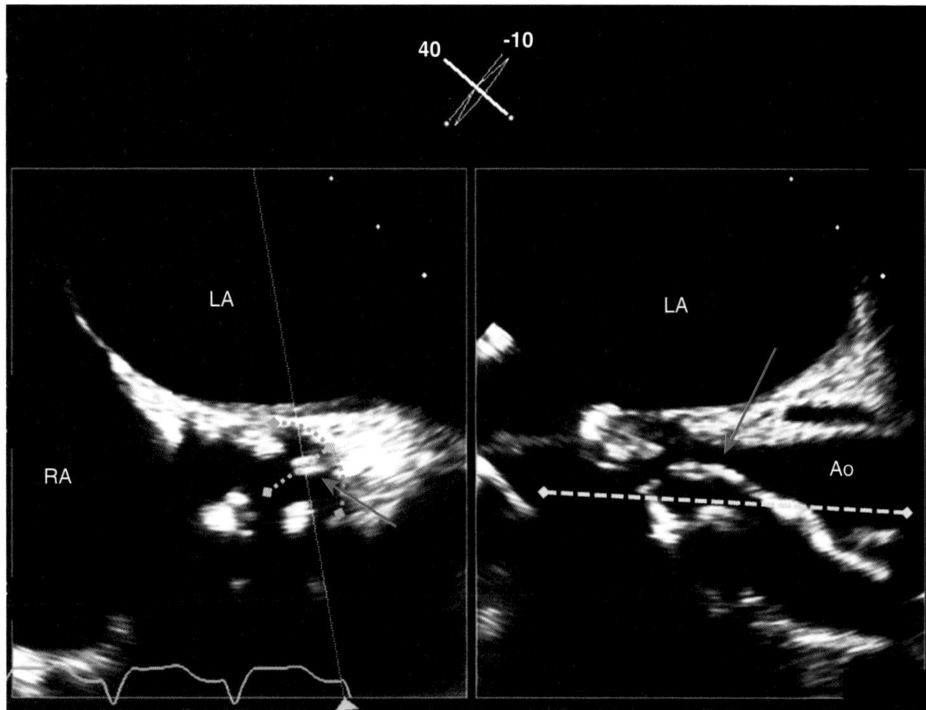

Fig. 10.6 **Optimal leaflet traversal system position and orientation for BASILICA procedure.** Simultaneous biplane imaging of the aortic root in the shortaxis *(left)* and longaxis *(right)* shows the position of the traversal system *(red arrow)* in the center of two prosthetic valve struts *(blue dotted line)* and at the base of the leaflet *(green dotted line)*. The tip of the traversal system is oriented toward the center of the aortic root axis *(yellow dashed line)* to avoid iatrogenic aortic injury. *Ao*, Aorta.

MITRAL VALVE AND REGURGITANT JET EVALUATION

Compared with MR severity grading during preprocedural screening echocardiography, grading of MR severity by TEE is less important during the procedure because of the significant physiologic effects of general anesthesia and mechanical ventilation. However, intraprocedural quantitative assessment of MR at baseline and throughout the procedure still plays a role because it is necessary to objectively assess the relative impact that the intervention has on MR reduction. Importantly, intraprocedural TEE should focus on comprehensive understanding of the morphologic nature of valvular disease and structural components of the MV apparatus. With improvements in operator experience and device technology, many MV features that were previously considered contraindications are today seen as challenging yet acceptable (Table 10.6).[48]

TABLE 10.6 Optimal and Challenging Mitral Valve Morphologic Features for Edge-to-Edge Clip Intervention.

Optimal Morphology	*Challenging Morphology*
Central A2/P2 lesion	Peripheral A1/P1, A3/P3, or commissural lesion
Posterior leaflet length >10 mm	Short posterior leaflet length 7–10 mm
Tenting height <11 mm	Tenting height ≥11 mm
Coaptation length >2 mm	Coaptation length ≤2 mm or noncoapting leaflets
Flail gap <10 mm	Flail gap ≥10 mm
Flail width <15 mm	Flail width ≥15 mm
Calcification absent	Calcification present in non-grasping zones
MV area >4 cm^2	MV area <4 cm^2 but >3 cm^2

A/P1–3, Anterior and posterior mitral leaf segments; *MV*, mitral valve.
Adapted from Nyman CB, Mackensen GB, Jelacic S, Little SH, Smith TW, Mahmood F. Transcatheter mitral valve repair using the edge-to-edge clip. *J Am Soc Echocardiogr.* 2018;31(4):434–453.

The mid-esophageal (ME) bicommissural view is extensively used for guidance during this procedure. It is of utmost importance to establish an accurate view that transects the commissures precisely. Because the 3D image obtained by narrow-angle real-time 3D mode with backward elevation tilt is rendered by adding 10 to 30 degrees of elevation angle to the 2D imaging plane, this unique 3D mode may help verify any 2D views (Fig. 10.7). After the true ME bicommissural view is attained, simultaneous biplane mode imaging with color-flow Doppler (CFD) can be activated with the scan line systematically sweeping through the MV from medial to lateral. The origins of the MR jet or jets can be individually identified and interrogated by this method (Fig. 10.8).

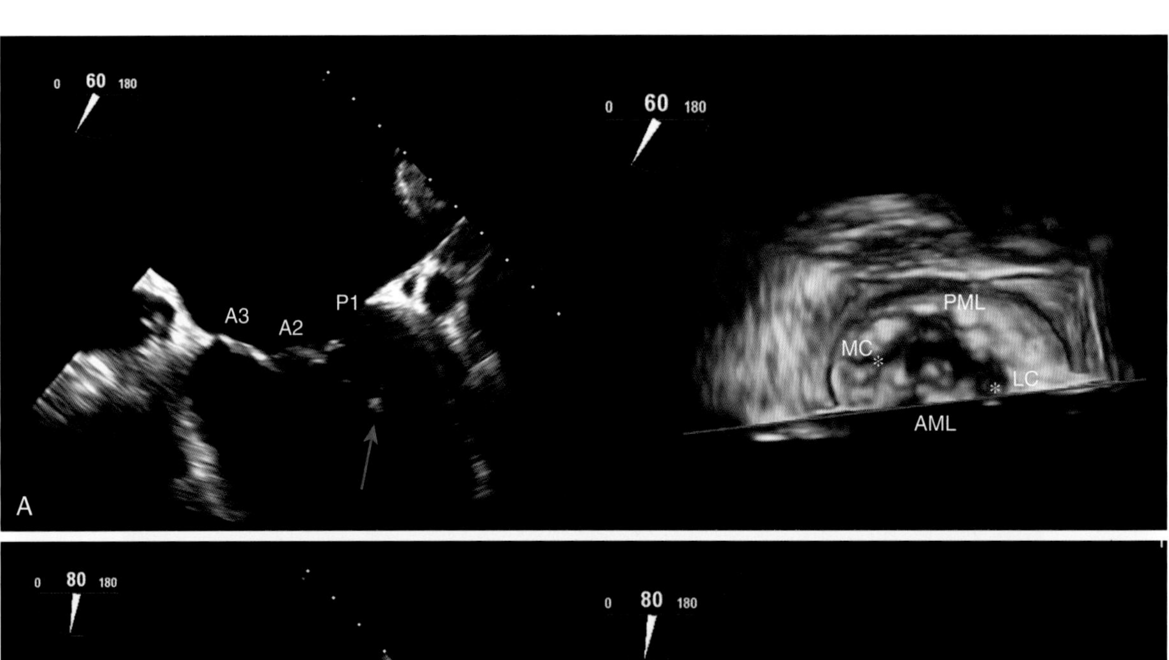

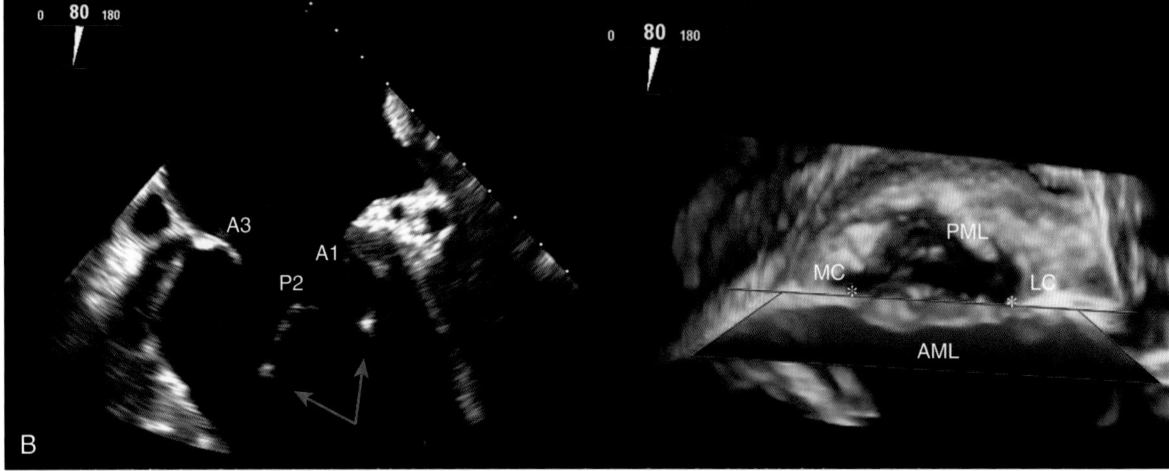

Fig. 10.7 Narrow-angle real-time 3D imaging mode to confirm true bicommissural view. (A) At the conventional bicommissural omniplane angle of 60 degrees, the imaging cut plane *(red line, right image)* transects only the lateral commissure and anterolateral papillary muscle head *(red arrow, left image)*. (B) With an increase in omniplane angle to 80 degrees, the imaging cut plane *(red plane, right image)* transects both medial and lateral commissures and both papillary muscle heads *(red arrows, left image)*. *A/P1–3*, Anterior and posterior mitral leaf segments; *AML*, anterior mitral leaflet; *LC*, lateral commissure; *MC*, medial commissure; *PML*, posterior mitral leaflet; *yellow asterisks*, mitral valve commissures.

The MR jet width in the ME bicommissural view may shed light on the potential number of devices needed to treat the pathology. For instance, if the width of the MR jet is 15 mm or greater, two or more E-EC devices may be needed to facilitate leaflet approximation. With the scan line cutting through the MR jet, CFD is suppressed to reveal the underlying valvular pathology. On the corresponding long-axis view window, anterior and posterior leaflet length, coaptation defect, flail or prolapse gap, calcification, tenting angle, and ventricular chordae attachments can be closely examined (Fig. 10.9). The overall MV anatomy and MR jet characteristics can be appreciated, with or without CFD, in 3D-rendered volume acquisition.

TRANSSEPTAL PUNCTURE

The ideal location for transseptal puncture for the E-EC system is in the superior and posterior portion of the thin fossa ovalis. This is best visualized in the ME bicaval view for superior-inferior positioning and in the ME AoV short-axis (SAX) view for anterior-posterior positioning. Simultaneous biplane mode is often used to display both views concurrently. Bear in mind that if this mode is activated in the ME bicaval view, the corresponding orthogonal view is the mirror image of the ME AoV SAX view, with left- and right-sided structures inverted (Fig. 10.10). A fibrotic, lipomatous, aneurysmal, or defective septum may pose difficulties for the proceduralist and should be communicated if discovered. Once the ideal location is identified, the distance between the IAS tenting site and the MV leaflet coaptation is measured in the ME 4-chamber view or in the inverted ME 4-chamber view at a 180-degree omniplane angle. The optimal distance is approximately 4.5 to 5 cm but heavily depends on factors such as E-EC type, MR etiology, and jet origin location.

POSITIONING OF STEERABLE GUIDE CATHETER AND CLIP DELIVERY SYSTEM

The steerable guide catheter and clip delivery system are crossed into the left atrium (LA) after the IAS is punctured. The trajectory of these devices needs to be visualized continuously to avoid injury to nearby structures such as the left atrial appendage (LAA) and the AoV. Single-beat 3D zoom mode with a large-volume sector encompassing the entire LA is often used for this step. As the clip and clip delivery system is being advanced, the TEE transducer is often rotated toward the patient's left side to follow along (Fig. 10.11).

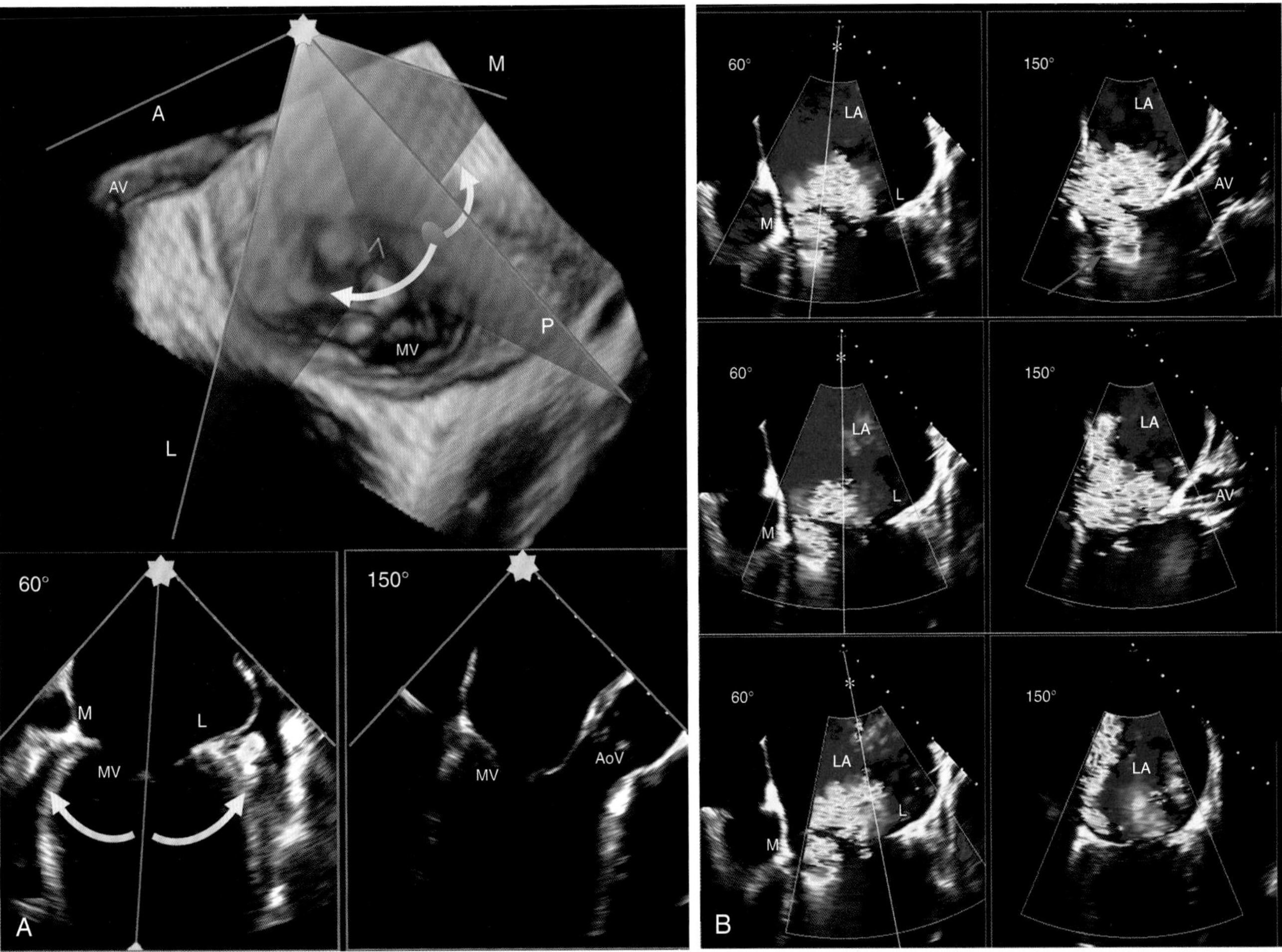

Fig. 10.8 Systematic evaluation of the mitral valve by simultaneous biplane imaging. (A) Simultaneous biplane imaging mode is activated on the main imaging plane *(red plane, bottom left panel)*; a concurrent orthogonal imaging plane *(blue plane, bottom right panel)* is generated by the ultrasound transducer *(orange star)*. The orthogonal imaging plane may be manually swept along the main imaging plane *(yellow arrows)* to interrogate various anatomic structures (medially and laterally in this instance). (B) Flow convergence *(red arrow)* is present only in the long-axis view *(right panels)* when the scan line is positioned medially, suggesting a focal medial origin of mitral regurgitation. *A*, Anterior; *AoV*, aortic valve; *L*, lateral; *M*, medial; *MV*, mitral valve; *P*, posterior.

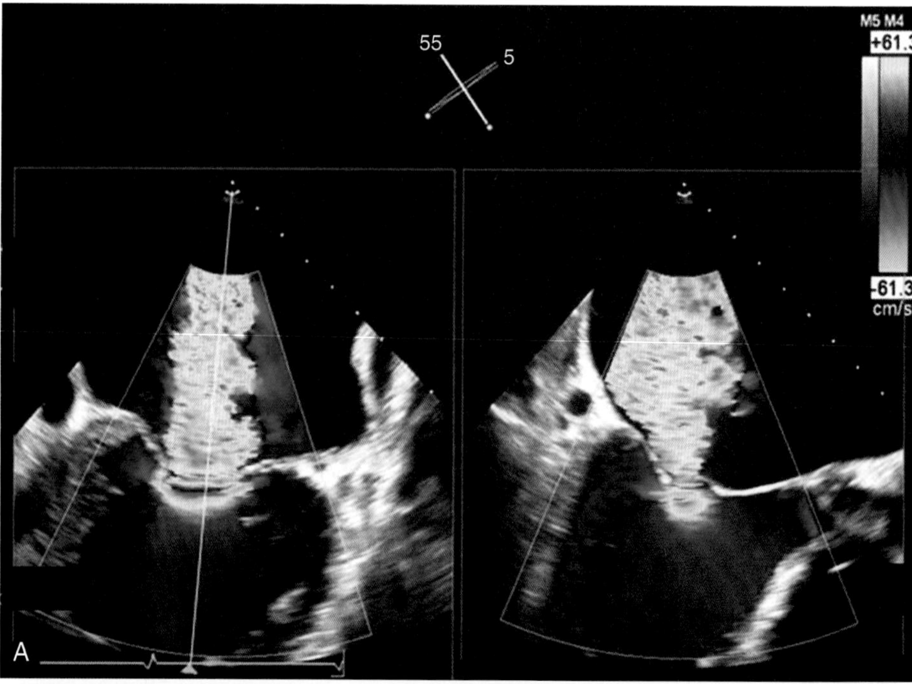

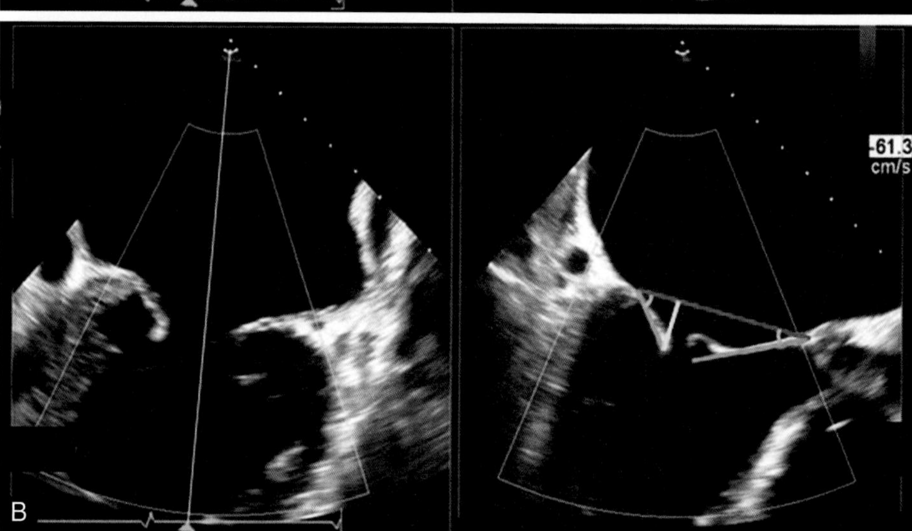

Fig. 10.9 **Color suppression reveals underlying pathology for comprehensive assessment.** (A) Simultaneous biplane mode with color-flow Doppler imaging of the bicommissural view *(left)* and its orthogonal long-axis view *(right)*. (B) The same view as in A, but with color-flow Doppler hidden or suppressed, reveals the underlying pathology of the mitral regurgitation. The anterior-posterior annular distance *(red line)*, anterior and posterior leaflet tenting angles *(green curves)*, anterior and posterior leaflet lengths *(blue lines)*, tenting height *(yellow line)*, and area (defined by *red and blue lines*), may all be examined in detail. The complex coaptation defect in this example is the result of both a restrictive posterior leaflet and relative prolapse of the anterior leaflet tip.

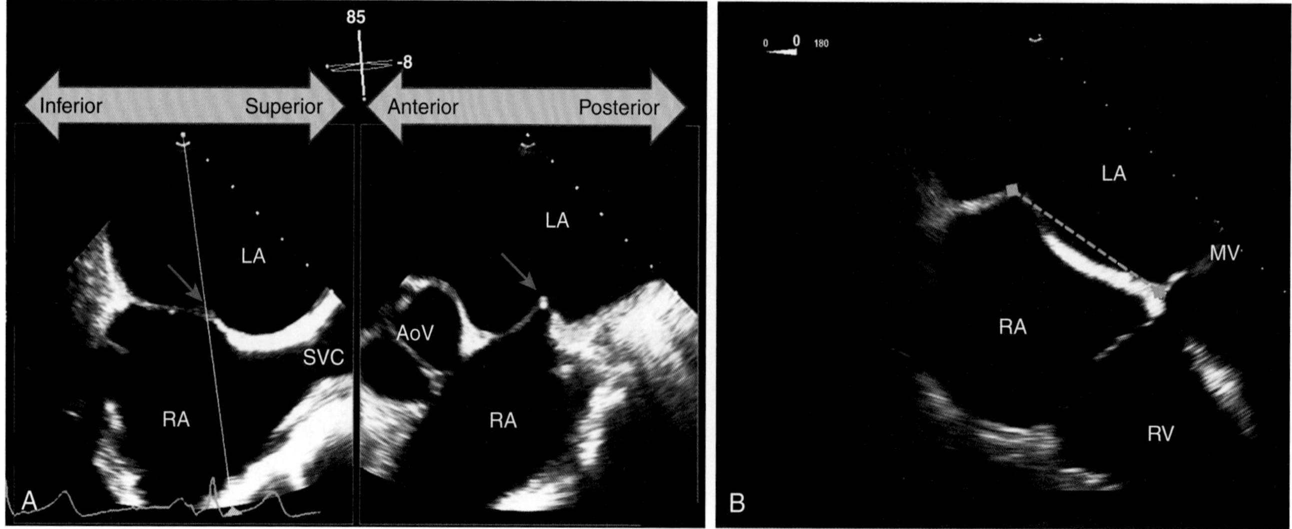

Fig. 10.10 **Transseptal puncture for transcatheter mitral valve edge-to-edge repair.** (A) Simultaneous biplane imaging is used to visualize the tented focal point *(red arrows)*, created by the transseptal needle, on the interatrial septum in the bicaval *(left panel)* and inverted AV short-axis *(right panel)* views. (B) The optimal distance between the transseptal puncture site and the mitral annulus *(blue dashed line)* is measured in the mid-esophageal 4-chamber view. *AoV*, Aortic valve; *MV*, mitral valve; *SVC*, superior vena cava.

The clip delivery system is then lowered and steered toward the MV, monitored by simultaneous biplane mode imaging of the ME bicommissural view and the corresponding ME long-axis (LAX) view to ensure that the device is positioned directly above the MR origin. The clip arms are then opened to check for orientation by 3D zoom mode. The perpendicularity of the E-EC device and the MV line of coaptation is confirmed. The omniplane angle may need to be adjusted in the bicommissural plane, depending on the laterality of the lesion, to maintain its parallel alignment to the coaptation line (Fig. 10.12).

ADVANCEMENT OF CLIP DEVICE INTO LV AND MITRAL LEAFLET GRASPING

After the E-EC position and orientation are satisfactory, the clip arms are closed, and the device is advanced into the LV under continuous imaging. The medial-lateral position often changes during this step due to the natural curvature of the delivery system. Clip orientation and location can be reconfirmed in the LV by simultaneous biplane and 3D zoom modes. 3D rendering is often undergained to eliminate the thin mitral leaflets that may conceal the echogenic E-EC arms in the LV.

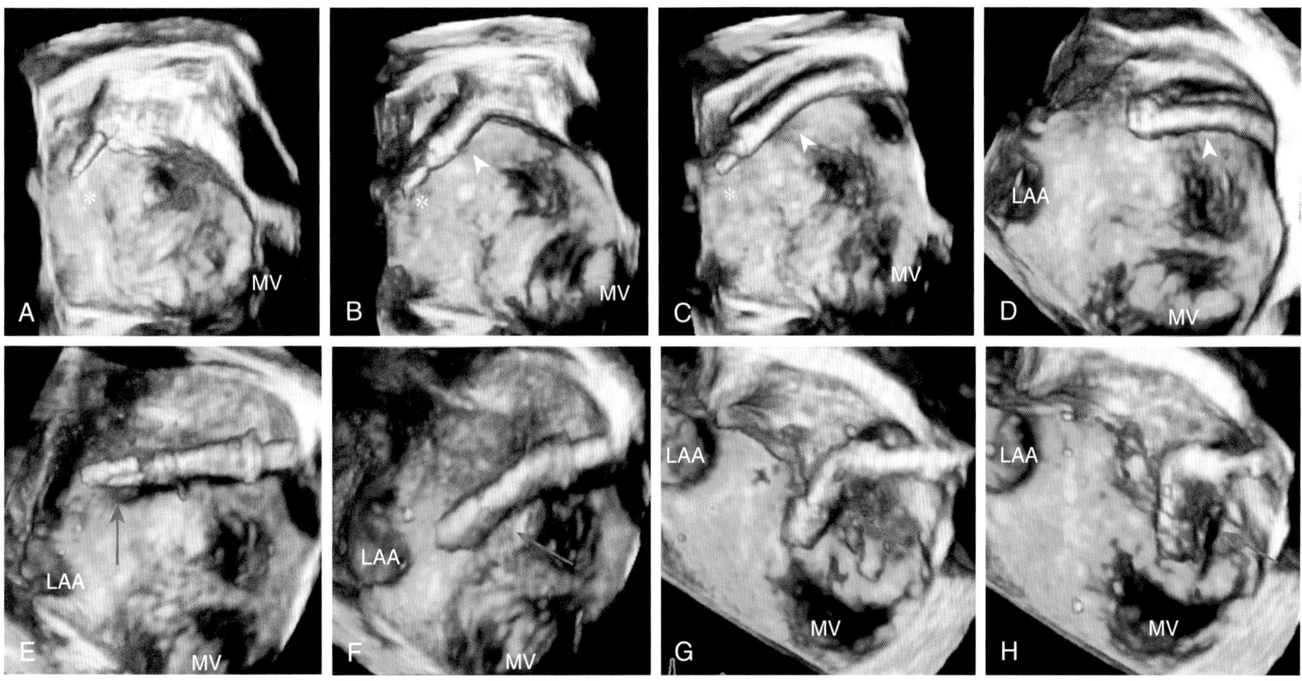

Fig. 10.11 **Advancement and positioning of the transcatheter mitral valve edge-to-edge repair system.** (A) The dilator tip *(asterisk)* crosses the interatrial septum and is seen in the LA. (B) The steerable guide catheter (SGC, *yellow arrowhead*) is advanced into the LA along with the dilator. (C) The SGC continues to advance along the anterior wall of the LA. (D) The dilator is withdrawn, leaving only the SGC in place. (E–H) The edge-to-edge clip device *(red arrow)* is advanced through the SGC into the LA and flexed apically toward the MV, steering past crucial structures such as the LAA (Video 10.11). The progress of the clip device is monitored by rotating the TEE transducer toward the patient's left side. Notice that the MV gradually comes into view with this imaging maneuver. *LAA*, Left atrial appendage; *MV*, mitral valve.

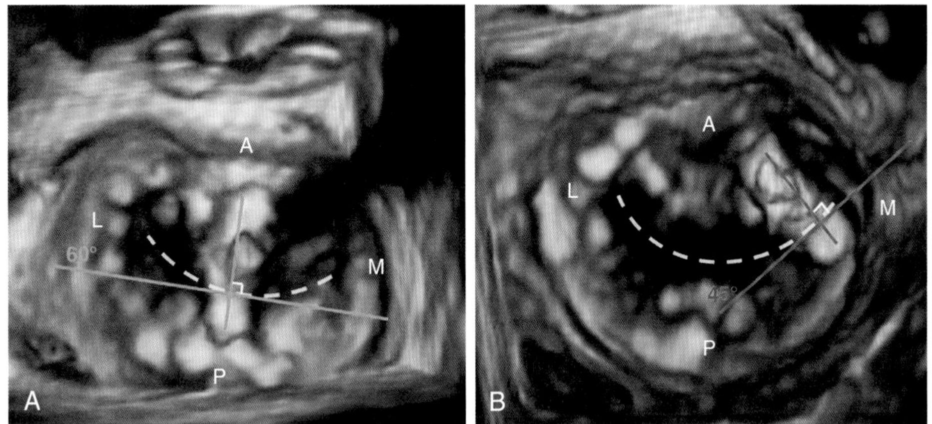

Fig. 10.12 **Edge-to-edge clip device positioning and orientation for mitral valve repair.** The device, with the clip arms opened, is positioned and rotated to achieve perpendicularity with the MV coaptation line *(yellow dashed line)* directly on the A2–P2 axis (A) and in the medial commissure (B). The omniplane angle must be decreased slightly *(from blue line to purple line)* to properly align the imaging plane with medial MV coaptation line if simultaneous biplane mode is used. *A*, Anterior; *L*, lateral; *M*, medial; *MV*, mitral valve.

The E-EC is slowly withdrawn toward the LA until the anterior and posterior MV leaflets fall between the opened clip arms and the delivery system shaft. Leaflet tips should insert directly at the base of the clip arms, and the operator should confirm this on the ME LAX view before lowering the grippers and partially closing the device arms (Fig. 10.13). Slight leaflet tethering should be appreciated on 2D imaging with partial clip arm closure. During complete closure of the clip arm, CFD is activated to assess, in real time, the change in MR severity. Several other echocardiographic parameters, such as pulmonary vein flow pattern and MR spectral Doppler density and contour, are evaluated to determine residual MR severity. Mean MV diastolic gradient is measured to confirm the absence of mitral stenosis. Before device release, with the E-EC arms fully closed, simultaneous biplane mode is used to scan through the MV to confirm adequate leaflet insertion and grasping. With the scan line on either side of the E-EC in the bicommissural view, the anterior and posterior leaflets should be seen moving freely in the corresponding ME LAX view. When the scan line is placed directly on the device, the leaflets should be firmly tethered with significant reduction of motion.

ASSESSMENT OF POSTPROCEDURAL RESULTS AND COMPLICATIONS

The E-EC should be released under continuous TEE monitoring to ensure device stability after full deployment. The MV and any residual MR should be thoroughly re-evaluated after clip release.[49] Severity, origin, and direction of residual MR may be different from before clip release because the delivery system is now completely dissociated from the E-EC. Consideration should be given to invasive hemodynamic parameters such as peak LA v-wave pressure, mean LA pressure, systolic blood pressure, pulmonary artery pressure, cardiac output, and cardiac index when deciding whether further intervention is needed.[50]

Immediate complications after E-EC deployment should be assessed. Early single-leaflet detachment may require additional E-EC devices to stabilize the failed device. Surgical repair, although undesirable, should remain an option for these high-risk patients.[51] Overall integrity of the MV apparatus should be examined, and the presence of a pericardial effusion should be excluded. Whether the iatrogenic atrial septal defect (iASD) should be closed after the procedure remains controversial.

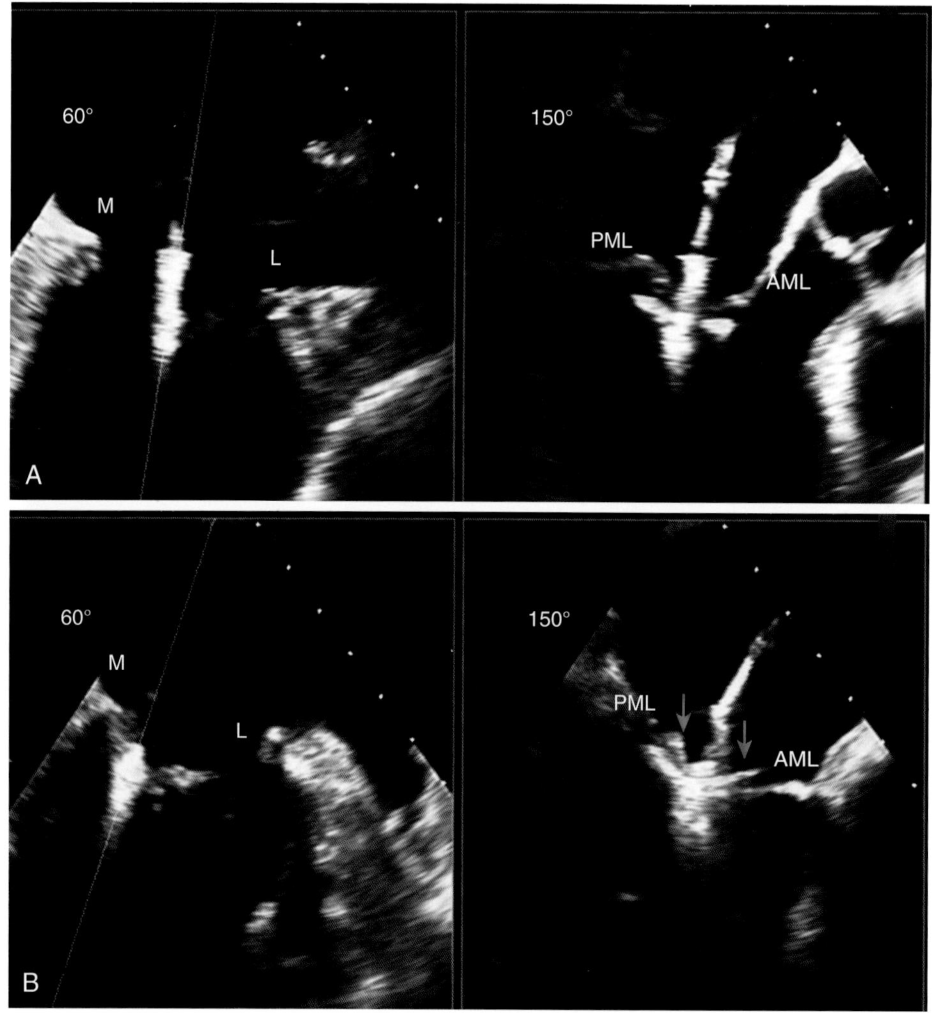

Fig. 10.13 Grasping of mitral valve leaflet by edge-to-edge clip device. (A) Simultaneous biplane view of the E-EC shows insertion of both anterior and posterior mitral leaflets into the base of the device *(right panel)* (Video 10.4). (B) Device grippers *(red arrows)* are lowered after anterior and posterior leaflets are fully inserted into the device. *AML*, Anterior mitral leaflet; *E-EC*, edge-to-edge clip; *L*, lateral; *M*, medial; *PML*, posterior mitral leaflet.

Schueler et al. showed that persistent iASD is associated with increased mortality after E-EC therapy.[52] Even though most iASDs close spontaneously within 1 year after the procedure, an elevated LA pressure has been associated with persistent iASD.[53] Some common opinion-based indications for iASD closure after the E-EC therapy include large defect size, significant shunting, right-sided heart failure, and pulmonary hypertension.[54]

INTRAPROCEDURAL TEE FOR TRANSCATHETER MITRAL VALVE REPLACEMENT

Following the wide success of TAVR and percutaneous MV edge-to-edge repair, transcatheter mitral valve replacement (TMVR) has gained substantial interest.[55] Although E-EC therapy is preferred for those with severe MR, a fair portion of these patients may be excluded for various reasons. For this subset, a viable alternative such as TMVR should be considered. As with MV surgical replacement versus repair, TMVR has the theoretical benefit of a more complete resolution of MV pathology compared with E-EC therapy. However, early outcome data on the off-label use of a balloon-expandable THV for TMVR were only moderately encouraging. TMVR in cases of failed surgical annuloplasty ring (valve-in-ring [ViR]) or severely calcified native mitral annulus (valve-in-mitral annular calcification [ViMAC]), although feasible, resulted in elevated procedural morbidity and mortality rates.[56,57] Several anatomic challenges, such as a dynamic annulus, various bioprosthetic sizes and shapes, complex subvalvular supporting structures, and questionable anchoring sites, may contribute to the risk of adverse events in TMVR. A one-size-fits-all universal THV for all clinical scenarios is impractical and unrealistic.[58] No dedicated TMVR systems are commercially available, and many of the procedures are performed off-label with THVs intended for TAVR. A plethora of devices designed specifically for the MV are being investigated in the preclinical or clinical phase.[55]

The preprocedural workup for TMVR is more complex than simply identifying the cause and severity of the pathology. Complete characterization of the THV landing zone is crucial for procedural success.[59] Dimensions of the mitral annulus, annuloplasty ring, and surgical bioprosthetic valve are needed for THV size selection. The true inner diameter of the degenerative surgical valve is obtained from the manufacturer. However, because pannus and calcification form over time, measurements obtained by MDCT are theoretically more accurate. Other details regarding the TMVR landing zone are also acquired by MDCT. For example, the extent and thickness of annular calcification are evaluated for ViMAC; completeness and rigidity of the annuloplasty ring are assessed for ViR; and stent height, radiopacity, position, and orientation of the surgical valve are obtained for valve-in-valve (ViV) replacement. The risk of LVOT obstruction is determined by simulating THV placement in MDCT reconstructed models (Fig. 10.14A).[60] Preprocedural TEE plays an important role in complementing MDCT for assessment of concomitant valve diseases, thin and pliable IAS, LA and LV geometry, LAA thrombus, and biventricular diastolic function. Potential technical challenges or anatomic contraindications can also be evaluated and excluded by comprehensive TEE.[61]

EVALUATION OF MITRAL VALVE PATHOLOGY

The goals of intraprocedural TEE are to confirm preprocedural findings, establish baseline images, address unanswered concerns, and anticipate potential complications. 3D zoom mode encompassing the entire mitral apparatus is often used for a quick overview of the valve. A 3D model of the acquired volume data set allows for automated or semi-automated measurements of mitral annular parameters. These measurements could be considered complementary to MDCT-derived dimensions and have been shown to closely correlate with them.[62] However, because the THV landing zone is frequently plagued by blooming artifacts caused by heavy calcification, 2D measurements obtained manually (as opposed to computer-generated borders based on the 3D MPR data set) may be more accurate. Regardless of the modality used for THV size selection, the risk of late THV migration or embolization may increase with significant size underestimation.

Unlike MDCT still images, 3D TEE renderings demonstrate dynamic interaction between the LVOT and mitral leaflets, chordae tendineae, and papillary muscles throughout the cardiac cycle. Any factors that reduce the post-TMVR residual LVOT area, also known as the neo-LVOT area, may increase the risk of obstruction. Some proposed risk factors include a long or redundant anterior mitral leaflet, perpendicular aortomitral angulation, small LV size, basal interventricular septum hypertrophy, ventricular protrusion, and flaring of THV.[63] Although minimal values for these risk factors have not been established, it is thought that an estimated neo-LVOT area of 1.7 cm^2 or less predicts LVOT obstruction with 96.2% sensitivity and 92.3% specificity.[64]

Currently, 3D TEE full-volume MPR is used in conjunction with the preprocedural MDCT data for LVOT obstruction risk assessment (see Fig. 10.14B and C). Bailout strategies such as placement of a percutaneous mechanical circulatory support device or septal alcohol ablation should be planned or executed in advance for patients with a high risk of LVOT obstruction.[65]

TRANSSEPTAL PUNCTURE AND ADVANCEMENT OF THE TRANSCATHETER HEART VALVE

TEE is used extensively to guide transseptal puncture at the mid-inferior and posterior fossa. It is important to obtain adequate height from the MV with the transseptal puncture so that the delivery system can steer acutely toward the LV apex. Balloon septostomy is often performed to enlarge the iASD for the bulky THV delivery system. Correct positioning of the balloon can be confirmed by TEE, with the IAS at the waist of the balloon, to ensure maximal stability during balloon inflation. Advancing and maneuvering the relatively large THV delivery system in the LA may cause wall perforation. The delivery system is followed closely by real-time TEE in 3D zoom or simultaneous biplane mode. Pericardial effusion should be excluded if injuries arise.

POSITIONING AND DEPLOYMENT OF THE TRANSCATHETER HEART VALVE

The final position of the THV at the landing zone depends on several patient and device factors. Ideal delivery height and angulation should aim for minimal LVOT obstruction and maximal anchoring stability (Fig. 10.15). The THV delivery system may initially cross the landing zone obliquely. However, the angle can be subtly adjusted to achieve optimal coaxiality during slow and controlled THV deployment. 3D zoom or simultaneous biplane TEE mode can be used to recognize canting or tilting of the THV.

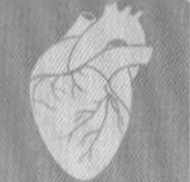

Valve size (mm)	Position (V/A%)	LVOT area without valve (mm²)	LVOT area with valve (mm²)
26	60/40	339.8	219.6
	80/20	315.6	147.4

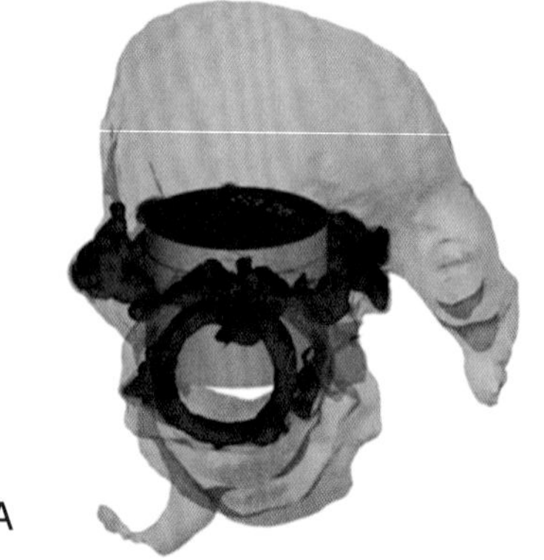

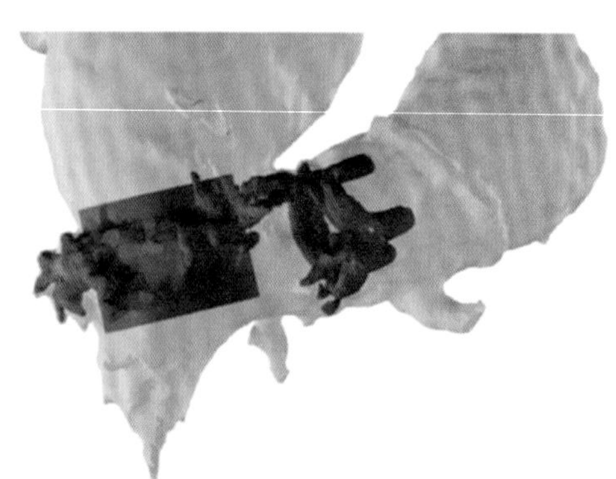

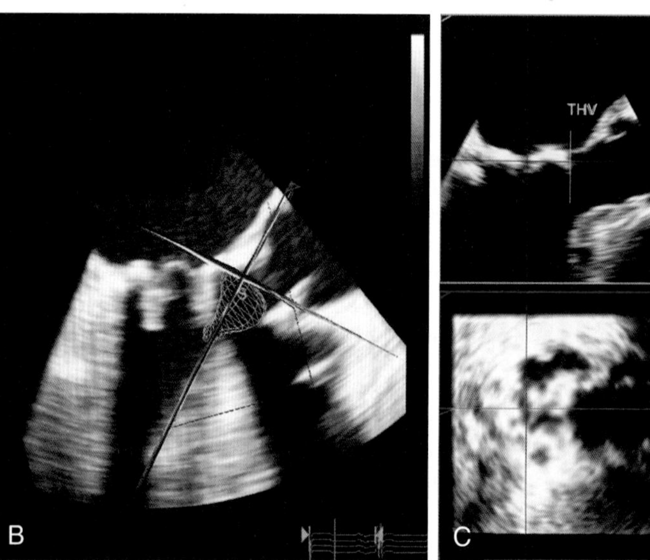

Fig. 10.14 **Multimodal evaluation of the risk of left ventricular outflow tract obstruction.** (A) Preprocedural simulation of a transcatheter heart valve (*THV*) placed at various depths in relation to the mitral annulus. Risk of LVOT obstruction can be estimated by tracing the sizes of the neo-LVOT areas. (B) Dynamic changes in LVOT 3D volume and its interaction with the preexisting THV are visualized using a semi-automated software package before valve-in-valve TMVR. (C) Multiplanar reconstruction of the LVOT before TMVR, with simulation of a 29-mm balloon-expandable THV with 22.5-mm height placed in the native mitral annulus, shows grossly acceptable distance between the THV frame and the interventricular septum. *A*, Atrial; *LVOT*, left ventricular outflow tract; *TMVR*, transcatheter mitral valve replacement; *V*, ventricular. (A, Images courtesy Dr. Dee Dee Wang, Henry Ford Health System, Detroit, MI.)

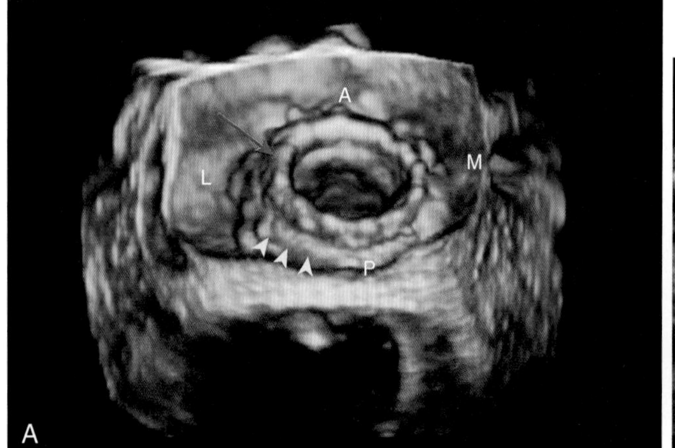

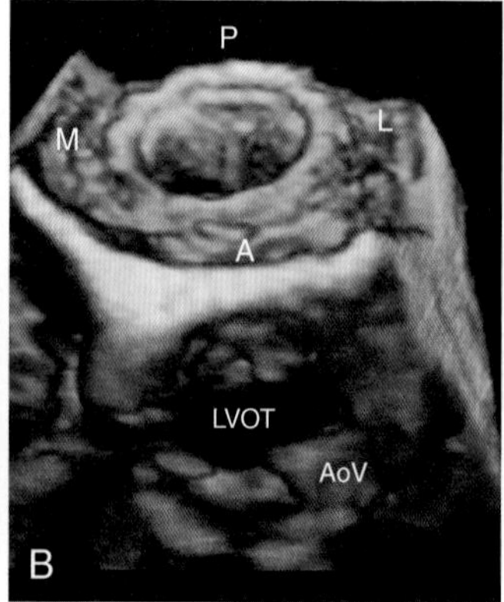

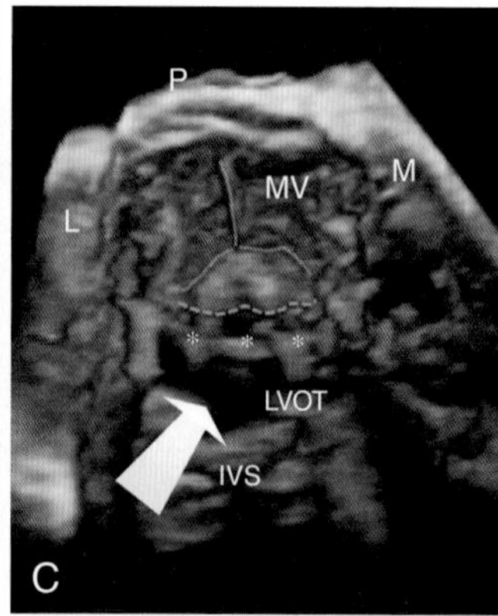

Fig. 10.15 **Ideal positioning of a transcatheter heart valve placed within a bioprosthetic mitral valve.** (A) Slight angulation of the 3D mitral en face view shows approximately one third of the THV skirt *(red arrow)* embedded in the preexisting bioprosthetic valve sewing ring *(yellow arrowheads)*, providing maximal stability and minimal risk of intervalvular regurgitation after deployment. (B) Wide-open LVOT viewed from the aortic side into the LV during systole after transcatheter mitral valve-in-valve placement. (C) Same wide-open LVOT as in B but viewed from the LV up into the aorta. Exposed THV open cells *(yellow asterisks)* are seen between the edge of the preexisting bioprosthetic valve *(blue dotted line)* and the rim of the metal frame, further allowing forward flow *(yellow gradient arrow)* during systole and valve closure (*green line* depicts valve coaptation lines). *A*, Anterior; *AoV*, aortic valve; *IVS*, interventricular septum; *L*, lateral; *LVOT*, left ventricular outflow tract; *M*, medial; *MV*, mitral valve; *P*, posterior; *THV*, transcatheter heart valve.

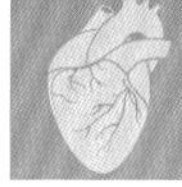

ASSESSMENT OF POSTPROCEDURAL RESULTS AND COMPLICATIONS

After final THV deployment, valve stability needs to be immediately assessed by 2D and 3D TEE. Flow and gradients through the LVOT should be assessed by spectral Doppler because 2D and CFD appearances may be misleading (Fig. 10.16). LV systolic function and regional wall motion should be evaluated. Other important surveys include THV integrity, PVL, and shunting through the iASD. Intravalvular regurgitation can happen with overexpansion or underexpansion of the THV (Fig. 10.17A). PVL is not uncommon in TMVR because of poor approximation between the THV and calcified landing zone surfaces (see Fig. 10.17B). The precise location and severity of PVL should be identified and quantified.

The iASD often needs to be addressed after retraction of the delivery system due to the resultant shunt. An appropriate percutaneous closure device can be selected based on 2D or 3D TEE defect sizing.[66] Small residual flow through the ASD closure device is expected; however, flow around the device suggests incorrect sizing.[66]

INTENTIONAL LACERATION OF THE ANTERIOR MITRAL VALVE LEAFLET TO PREVENT LV OUTFLOW TRACT OBSTRUCTION (LAMPOON PROCEDURE)

The native MV anterior leaflet is permanently displaced and forms a continuous screen around the cylindrical THV open cells after ViMAC or ViR TMVR. This decreases the native LVOT cross-sectional area and increases the risk of flow reduction and high gradients. The LAMPOON technique involves transcatheter incision of the anterior mitral leaflet A2 scallop before THV deployment (Fig. 10.18).[67] The lacerated anterior mitral leaflet is then pulled to the side by intact chordae attached medially and laterally, creating a triangular-shaped opening to the neo-LVOT. This technically challenging technique has been

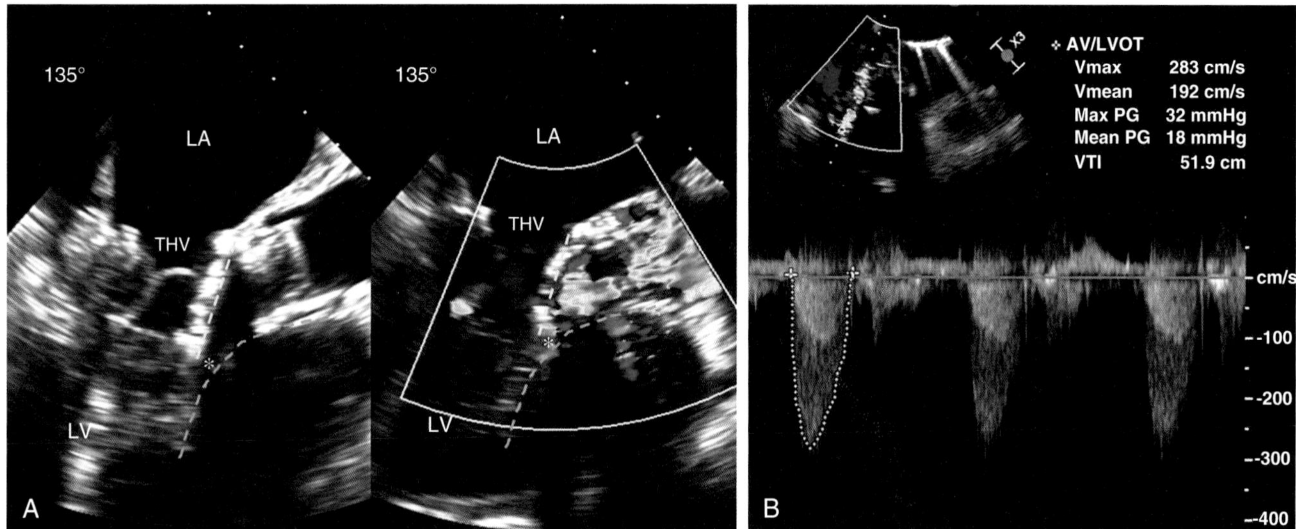

Fig. 10.16 Evaluation for LVOT obstruction after transcatheter mitral valve replacement. (A) Short distance between the anterior edge of the THV frame *(yellow dashed line)* and the interventricular septum *(blue dashed line)* suggests potential LVOT obstruction *(yellow asterisk)*. Turbulence in the LVOT on color-flow Doppler imaging *(right panel)* also suggests obstruction. (B) However, in this case, CW Doppler through the LVOT and aortic valve demonstrates normal peak velocity and mean gradient, indicative of a non-obstructed LVOT. *CW*, Continuous-wave; *LVOT*, left ventricular outflow tract; *THV*, transcatheter mitral valve.

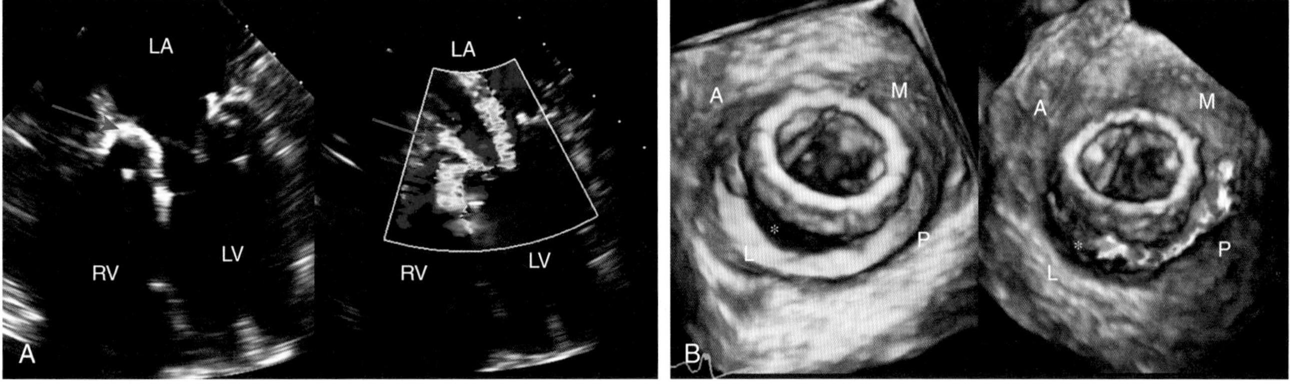

Fig. 10.17 Complications after transcatheter mitral valve replacement. (A) Mid-esophageal 4-chamber view of an underexpanded transcatheter heart valve *(red arrow)* that resulted in significant intravalvular regurgitation. (B) Atrial migration of the transcatheter heart valve resulted in regurgitation through a paravalvular defect *(asterisk)* between the valve fabric skirt and the calcified annulus. *A*, anterior; *P*, posterior; *M*, medial; *L*, lateral.

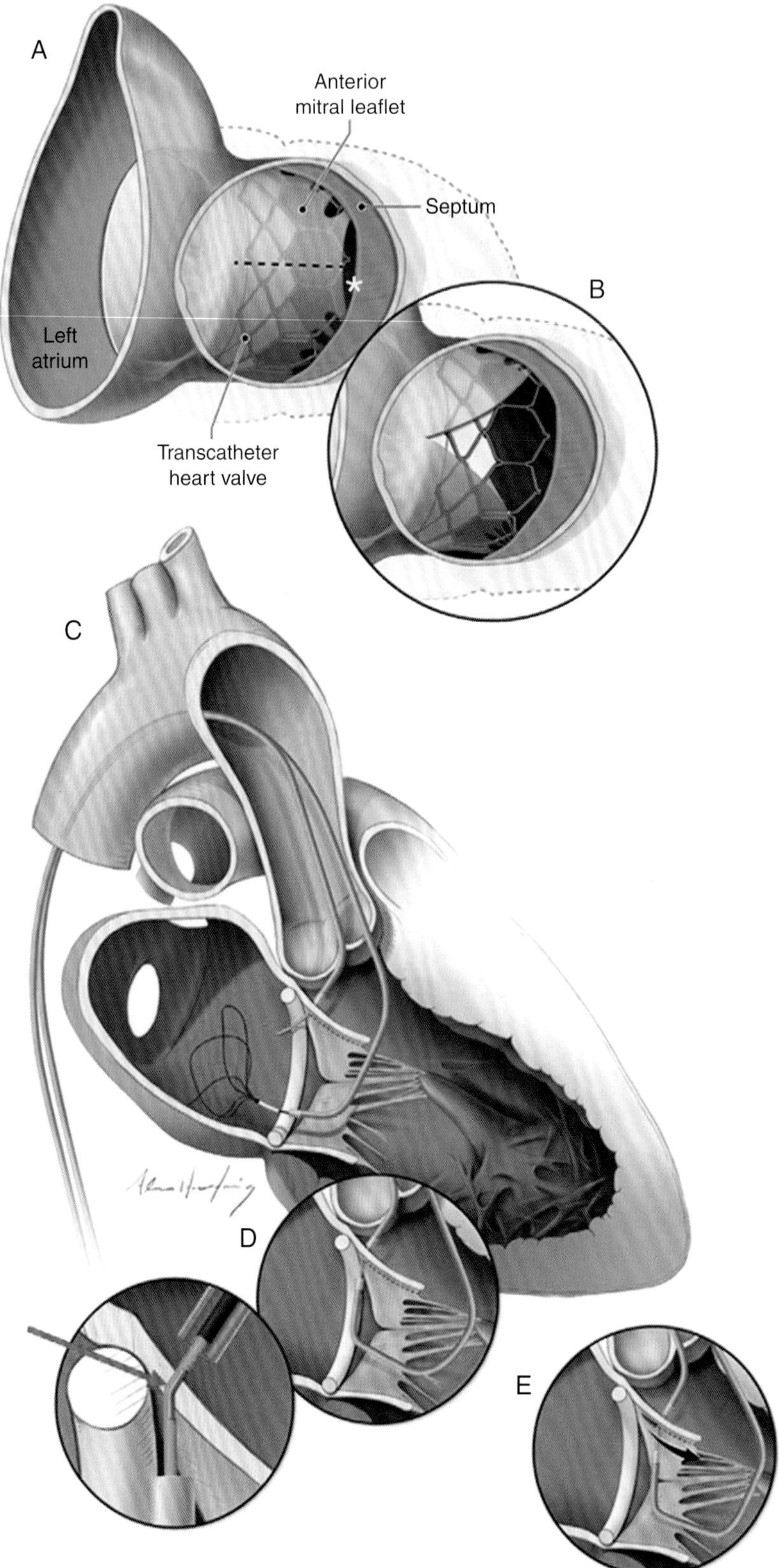

Fig. 10.18 LAMPOON procedure. (A) The anterior mitral leaflet is displaced by the transcatheter heart valve, resulting in significant left ventricular outflow tract obstruction *(yellow asterisk)*. (B) Lacerated anterior mitral leaflet is pulled to both sides, analogous to opening a curtain, which relieves the obstruction. (C–E) Illustration of the LAMPOON procedure shows (C) transcatheter retrograde puncture of the anterior mitral leaflet toward a multi-loop snare, (D) looped wire around the mitral leaflet, and (E) laceration of the mitral leaflet by brief electrocautery pulses and withdrawal of the catheters simultaneously. *Inset* depicts denuded and kinked guide wire *(red arrow)* that allows for electrocautery energy transmission. (Adapted from Babaliaros VC, Greenbaum AB, Khan JM, et al. Intentional percutaneous laceration of the anterior mitral leaflet to prevent outflow obstruction during transcatheter mitral valve replacement: first-in-human experience. *JACC Cardiovasc Interv.* 2017;10:798–809.)

shown to be feasible and safe in patients who are ineligible for stand-alone TMVR.[68]

The LAMPOON procedure is heavily guided by a combination of 2D and 3D TEE (Fig. 10.19). Simultaneous biplane mode imaging in the ME bicommissural view is used to direct the positioning of the guiding catheter in the LVOT. Alternative transgastric views may be needed if LVOT shadowing by the severely calcified annulus or leaflet is too profound in ME views. A multi-loop snare is placed across the AoV and into the LA through another retrograde guiding catheter. After both guiding catheters have been appropriately positioned and confirmed on TEE, the A2 scallop is punctured by brief electrocautery, and a guide wire is advanced into the LA. TEE is used to verify leaflet traversal and to exclude complications such as pericardial effusion or aortic perforation. The guide wire is then captured by the multi-loop snare under 3D TEE visualization. Gentle tension is applied on the guide wire loop to lacerate the anterior mitral leaflet with electrocautery. Immediately after leaflet laceration, the MV is carefully examined by TEE with the expectation of acutely exacerbated MR. TMVR is then performed expeditiously.

INTRAPROCEDURAL TEE FOR PERCUTANEOUS PARAVALVULAR LEAK OCCLUSION

PVL after surgical or transcatheter valve replacement is not uncommon. It results from an incomplete seal between the valvular prosthesis and the annulus. Patients with PVL may develop congestive heart failure, hemolytic anemia, or both over time.[69] Percutaneous closure of PVL is technically feasible and has acceptable rates of clinical success.[70] Whether it is a true alternative to surgical correction is debatable.[71,72] Refinement of transcatheter technology, advancement of 3D TEE imaging, and improvements in operator performance from accrued experience in recent years may result in different conclusions.[73] Regardless, percutaneous PVL closure offers the benefits of minimally invasive procedures: lower in-hospital morbidity, faster recovery, and shorter hospital stay.

Echocardiography is the primary imaging modality for PVL evaluation. Although TTE is used for initial screening and PVL diagnosis, TEE is used to further characterize the size, shape, location, and severity of PVL. Most paravalvular defects are

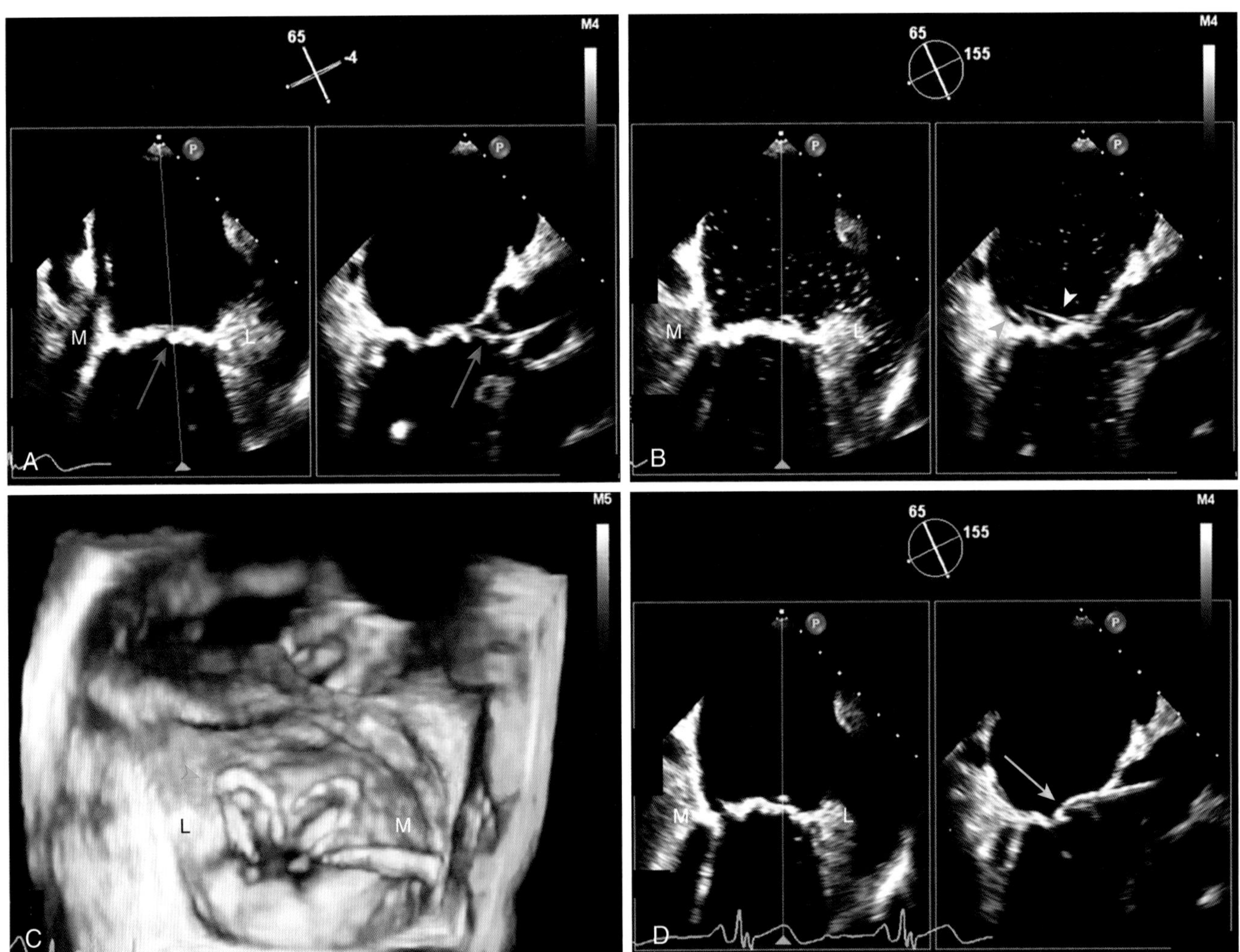

Fig. 10.19 TEE guidance of LAMPOON procedure. (A) Tip of guiding catheter *(red arrow)* is placed retrogradely through the aortic valve against the ventricular side of the mitral A2 scallop. (B) Electrocautery puncture with guide wire advancement into the LA *(yellow arrowhead)* is performed at the mitral A2 scallop (Video 10.19). Multi-loop snare *(blue arrowhead)* is in the LA and ready for guide wire capture. (C) Multi-loop snare *(blue arrow)*, visualized by real-time 3D TEE, facilitates guide wire capture in the LA. (D) Captured guide wire forms a loop *(orange arrow)* around the anterior mitral leaflet, ready for electrocautery laceration. *L*, Lateral; *M*, medial.

crescent-shaped, with serpiginous tracks instead of tube-like tunnels. Currently, transcatheter delivery systems and devices specifically for PVL repair are not commercially available in the United States. Most PVLs are treated with off-label use of circular vascular plugs or occluders. These devices typically consist of a cylindrical waist with or without circular disks at either end.[74] Mismatch between the paravalvular defect and the shape of the transcatheter device may lead to residual PVL after device placement. Precise location of the PVL is often described using a clock-face approach. It is important to establish common terminology with the interventionalist before the procedure to facilitate efficient communication.[75]

PARA-AORTIC DEFECT REPAIR

Diagnosis of PVL should be confirmed and the presence of active endocarditis excluded. Despite improvements in THV design to target better annular apposition, PVL is still more common after TAVR than after surgical replacement because of fundamental differences in implantation techniques.[76] PVL occurs more frequently with self-expanding valves than with balloon-expandable valves.[77]

Para-aortic defects are usually small and narrow. With acoustic shadowing and signal dropouts from the valve prosthesis or nearby structures, an irregular regurgitant jet path along the valve stent or cage can be extremely challenging to visualize by CFD; most often, only proximal flow convergence and eccentric jet tail can be appreciated. Multiple conventional and unconventional views may be needed to examine the valve. Occasionally, a combination of intraprocedural TEE and TTE may be needed to fully visualize the anterior and posterior portions of the AoV. Multibeat 3D TEE can provide enough spatial and temporal resolution to identify PVL origins.[78] Location of the PVL can be described with the IAS placed at the 10-o'clock position.

Although tactile feel and fluoroscopy can suggest defect crossing by the guide wire, TEE with simultaneous biplane imaging of the AoV in SAX and LAX is used to guide and confirm the paravalvular location of the wire through the defect (Fig. 10.20A and B). CFD can be turned on and suppressed to ensure that the guide wire is positioned correctly. Live narrow-sector 3D TEE in the ME AoV LAX view can add elevation perspective. Multiple wire and catheter exchanges may be needed, including stiff anchoring or support wires. Unintentional cardiac or aortic perforation can occur during this step and should be closely monitored by TEE.

After the final delivery sheath has been advanced through the defect, an appropriately sized occluder device is deployed under TEE and fluoroscopic visualization (see Fig. 10.20C). A slit-like defect that occupies a sizeable circumferential length may require multiple small devices deployed side by side. Alternatively, a single large device may be used, with the caveat that the wide disk may inadvertently interfere with the motion of the prosthetic valve leaflet. Aortic stenosis or worsening aortic regurgitation may suggest leaflet impingement and require retraction of the device. The TEE operator should be informed about the device or devices chosen to facilitate better recognition of subsequent echocardiographic findings.

The severity of a residual PVL after device deployment is frequently even more challenging to quantify than before deployment. Occluder devices often split the original PVL into multiple small jets, which may seem deceivingly large by CFD. Occluder devices may also redirect residual regurgitation eccentrically. If the procedure is being done to treat hemolysis, near-complete obliteration of PVL may be needed.[75] Immediate postprocedural complications such as device embolization, iatrogenic aortic injury, or coronary artery occlusion should be ruled out. The patient should undergo long-term follow-up after the procedure because new PVLs may emerge over time.[79]

PARA-MITRAL DEFECT REPAIR

Diagnosis of para-mitral defects should be confirmed, and valve dehiscence due to active endocarditis should be excluded. The clock-face system, with the MV oriented in standard en face view by 3D TEE, is commonly used to describe the location of the PVL. Alternatively, anatomic descriptions such as anterior-posterior, medial-lateral, or some combination thereof can be used. 3D zoom mode is used to identify the number and locations of PVLs. CFD can be used to differentiate true defects from acoustic dropout. If an adequate 3D image is obtained, off-line MPR of the defect can be performed (see Fig. 10.21A and B). The cross-sectional area and diameters of the defect may then be measured accurately.

The preferred approach to para-mitral defects is through the IAS. Simultaneous biplane TEE is used in combination with fluoroscopy for transseptal puncture. The ideal location for transseptal puncture is less important for para-mitral defect repairs than for other procedures that require transseptal puncture, except for para-mitral defects that are close to the IAS at the medial portion of the mitral annulus. Because an acute bend is needed in the LA for the delivery sheath to reach such defects, adequate transseptal puncture height is extremely important. A superior and posterior location within the fossa ovalis is ideal.[74] Another consideration before transseptal puncture is the need for a comprehensive LAA examination to exclude thrombus.[80]

Real-time fluoroscopy and TEE fusion imaging may be helpful in pinpointing the exact location of the defect. The presence of a guide wire in the LV suggests adequate paravalvular defect traversal. Because imaging of the LV can be difficult in ME views due to significant acoustic shadowing of far-field structures, this confirmatory finding is often visualized in TG views. An appropriately sized occluder device is chosen and deployed based on TEE measurements (see Fig. 10.21C and D). Larger devices may impinge on the prosthetic leaflet and affect its function, whereas smaller devices may not fully treat the PVL and risk tilting or embolization.

INTRAPROCEDURAL TEE FOR LEFT ATRIAL APPENDAGE OCCLUSION

The LAA is well established as a key thromboembolic source in patients with nonvalvular atrial fibrillation. Transcatheter devices that occlude the LAA were developed to reduce stroke risks in patients with contraindications to oral anticoagulants.[81] Although various devices are being deployed globally, this section focuses on the Watchman device (Boston Scientific, Plymouth, MA) as an example to highlight the practical aspects of TEE imaging for LAA exclusion procedural guidance.

PERIPROCEDURAL MULTIMODALITY IMAGING

LAA morphology varies widely among individuals. There is significant variation in depth, dimension, shape, and number of lobes.[82] MDCT is considered the gold standard for detailed preprocedural LAA evaluation and sizing.[83] 3D-printed heart models based on patient-specific MDCT can facilitate LAA

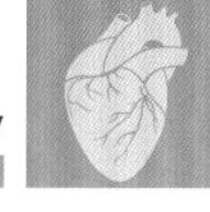

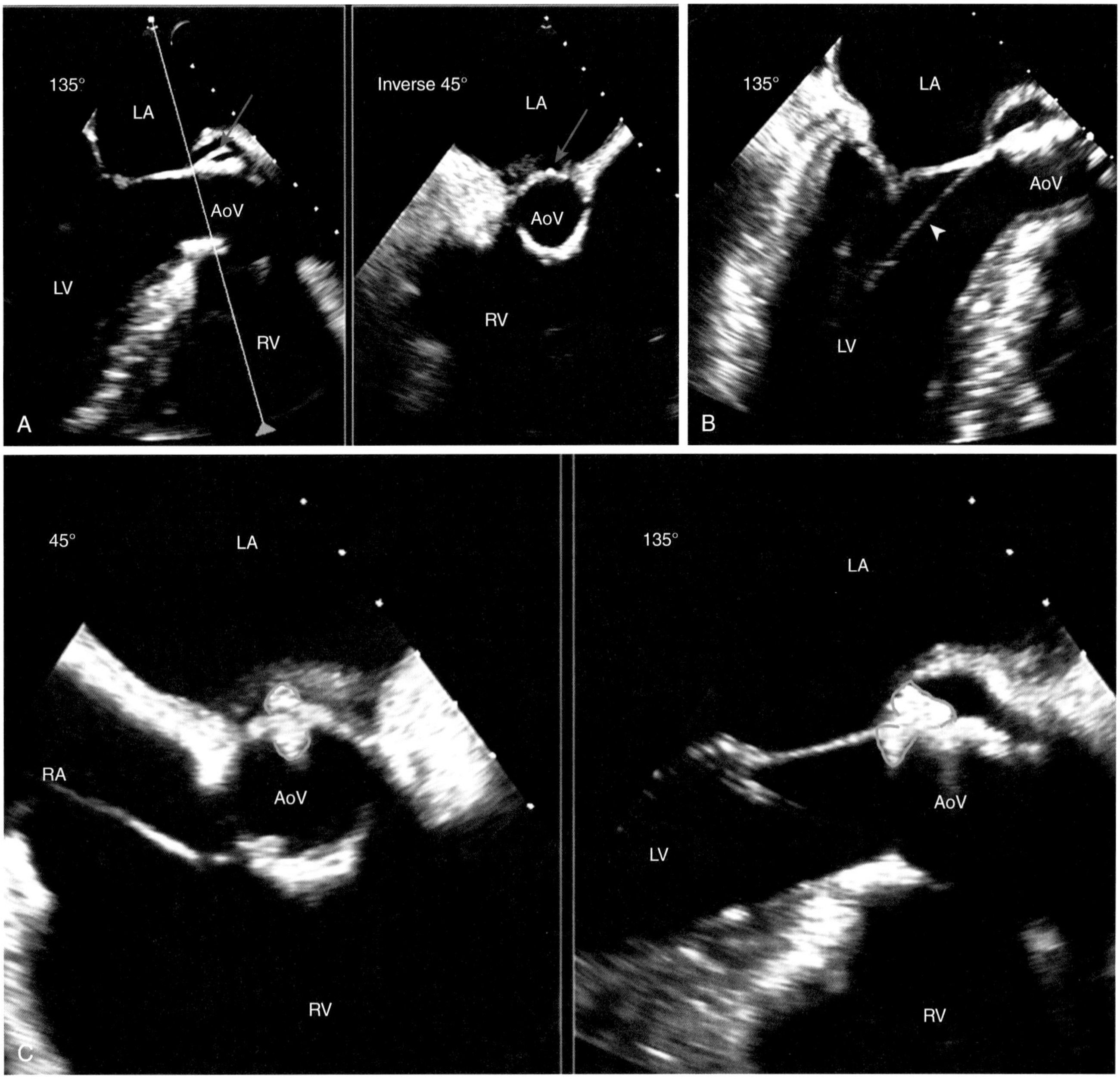

Fig. 10.20 **TEE guidance of para-aortic valve defect occlusion.** (A) Simultaneous biplane mode shows percutaneous delivery sheath *(red arrow)* in long-axis *(left panel)* and short-axis *(right panel)* views near the paravalvular defect at 12 o'clock. (B) Thin wire *(yellow arrowhead)* traverses the paravalvular defect in preparation for percutaneous occluder device deployment. (C) The paravalvular defect is treated by placement of a percutaneous occluder device *(blue line)*. *AoV*, Bioprosthetic aortic valve.

occluder implantation by accurately predicting device size and reducing overall procedural time.[84]

Intraprocedural guidance of LAA occluder implantation is traditionally performed with TEE. Although ICE was shown to be a feasible and effective alternative to TEE for procedural guidance, the associated longer procedural time and need for special imaging equipment and trained personnel have made this option less prevalent.[85] However, because use of ICE for procedural guidance precludes the need for general anesthesia, it may become the imaging modality of choice in the future.

INTRAPROCEDURAL TEE ASSESSMENT

Baseline TEE is performed meticulously to confirm preprocedural MDCT findings, exclude intracardiac thrombus, and uncover potential procedural challenges. The LAA ostia, neck, and body are identified and measured at 0-, 45-, 90-, and 135-degree omniplane angles by 2D TEE.[86] The LAA at 0 degrees is often the most challenging view to obtain. To view the LAA at 0 degrees, the ultrasound probe should be withdrawn past the MV, slightly anteflexed, and rotated counterclockwise.

The LAA at 45 and 90 degrees is easier to recognize because the adjacent ligament of Marshall and left upper pulmonary vein serve as distinct landmarks. Full visualization of the LAA at 135 degrees may also be difficult, especially in patients with a prominent ligament of Marshall. The tissue ridge often appears as a roof and spans the LAA. Although it is inevitably underestimated, the widest LAA ostial diameter should be measured at 135 degrees.

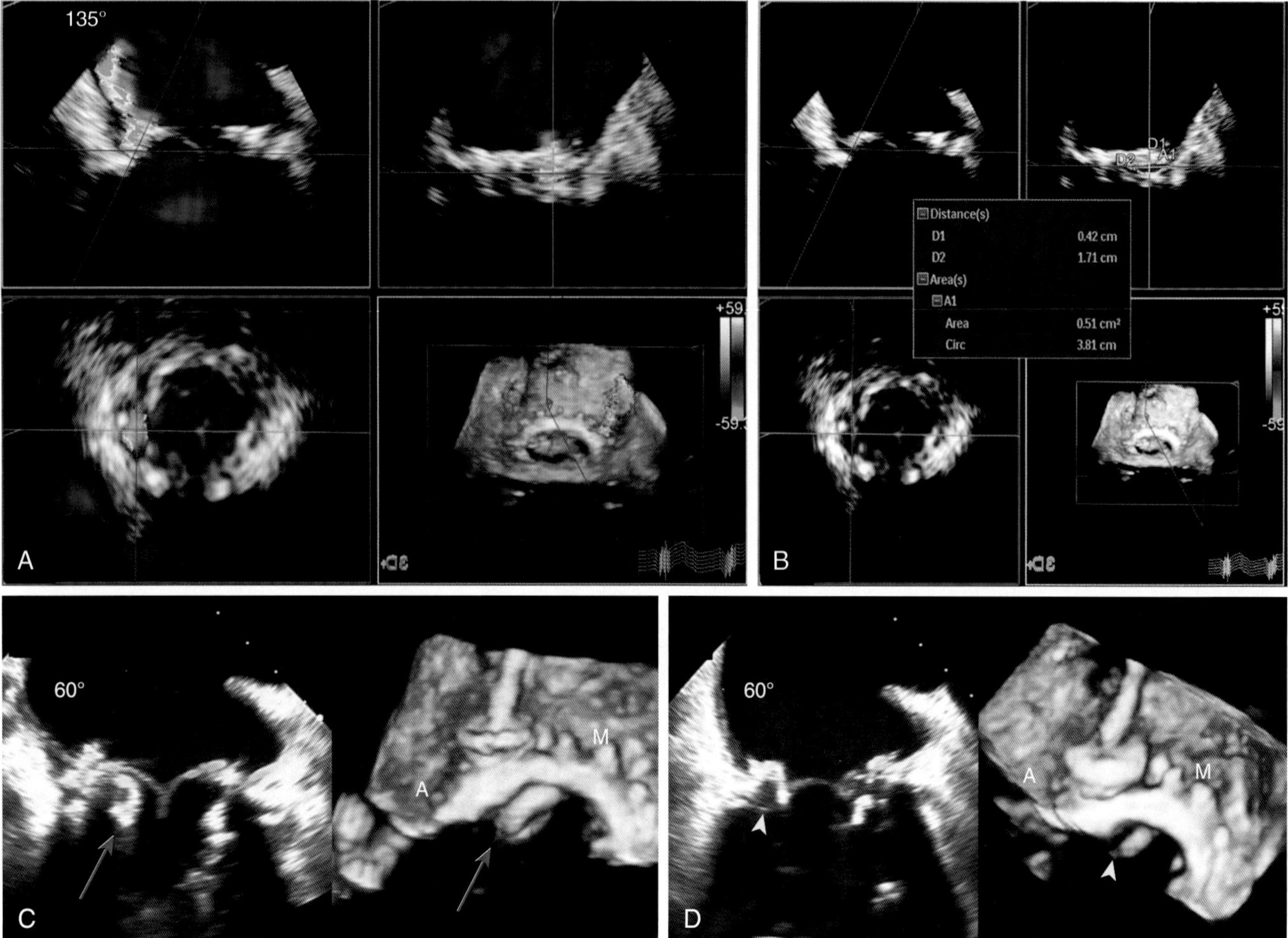

Fig. 10.21 Para-mitral valve defect evaluation by 3D multiplanar reconstruction. (A) Multiplanar reconstruction of bioprosthetic mitral paravalvular regurgitation by 3D zoom mode with color-flow Doppler. (B) Color suppression reveals the paravalvular defect, allowing for size and diameter measurements. (C) The large occluder disk *(red arrow)* protrudes into the bioprosthetic mitral valve inlet and affects normal leaflet opening. (D) A smaller occluder disk is tucked behind the bioprosthetic valve stent *(yellow arrowhead)* and does not affect the mitral leaflet opening. *A*, Anterior; *M*, medial.

The main LAA lobe is commonly foreshortened when imaged by 2D TEE, and 3D TEE is a better imaging technique to accurately size the LAA.[83] Multibeat-gated 3D acquisition is seldom practical because stitch artifacts from irregular heart rhythm commonly occur in this patient population. Simultaneous biplane mode has the advantage of circumventing this limitation. Another major advantage of simultaneous biplane imaging is its capability of acquiring images in pairs at 90-degree orthogonal angles. The challenging LAA angles at 135 and 0 degrees can be simply acquired by adjusting scan planes through the more easily visualized 45- and 90-degree angles.

When sizing the LAA by 3D MPR, all scan plane crosshairs should be moved to the center of the LAA ostia. Coronal and sagittal scan planes should be tilted to transect the tip of the LAA main lobe, permitting the depth to be fully visualized and measured. The cross-sectional plane can be moved more proximal or distal along the LAA axis, depending on the predetermined device implantation depth. The cross-sectional plane can also be tilted in various angles to simulate final device orientation. Landing-zone diameters are measured along this cross-sectional plane to ensure that all measurements are made at the same level (Fig. 10.22).

The LAA should be measured at ventricular end-systole to obtain its largest diameter. Because LAA size highly depends preload conditions, LA pressure should be obtained by direct catheterization and supported by intravenous volume loading before TEE sizing.[87]

TRANSSEPTAL PUNCTURE AND ADVANCEMENT OF THE LEFT ATRIAL APPENDAGE ACCESS SHEATH

The ideal location for transseptal puncture is at the inferior and posterior edge of the fossa ovalis. This provides the most direct route to the anterolaterally located LAA.[88] Occasionally, the LAA body is visualized steeply downward along the LA in the ME 2-chamber view. In these instances, the transseptal puncture should be made more toward the mid-fossa than inferior for better alignment.[89] An access sheath is guided by TEE into the LA over a support wire anchored in the left upper pulmonary vein and is advanced into the deepest LAA lobe over a pigtail catheter.

DEVICE DEPLOYMENT AND RELEASE

The self-expanding LAA occluder device is deployed in the LAA under fluoroscopic and TEE visualization. LAA views at 45 and 135 degrees are the TEE equivalent of the right anterior oblique cranial and caudal fluoroscopic views, respectively (Fig. 10.23).[88] After the device is fully deployed, a gentle backward pull (i.e., tug test) should be performed to confirm stability of the device.

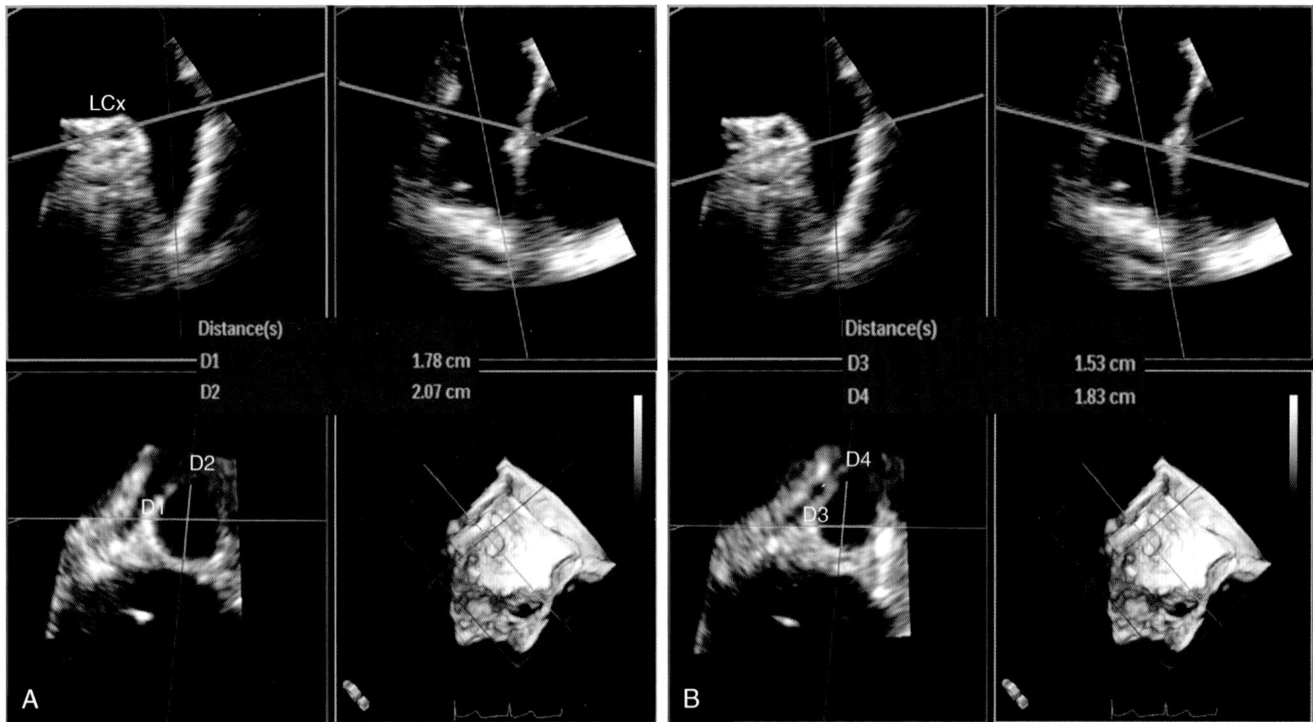

Fig. 10.22 Multiplanar reconstruction and analysis of the left atrial appendage. The occluder device landing-zone depth and tilt can be simulated by adjustment of the cross-sectional plane *(blue)*. Depending on the targeted implantation depth, landing-zone diameters (D1–D4) are different at the level of (A) the left circumflex artery and (B) the denser tissue ridge *(red arrow)*. *LCx*, Left circumflex artery.

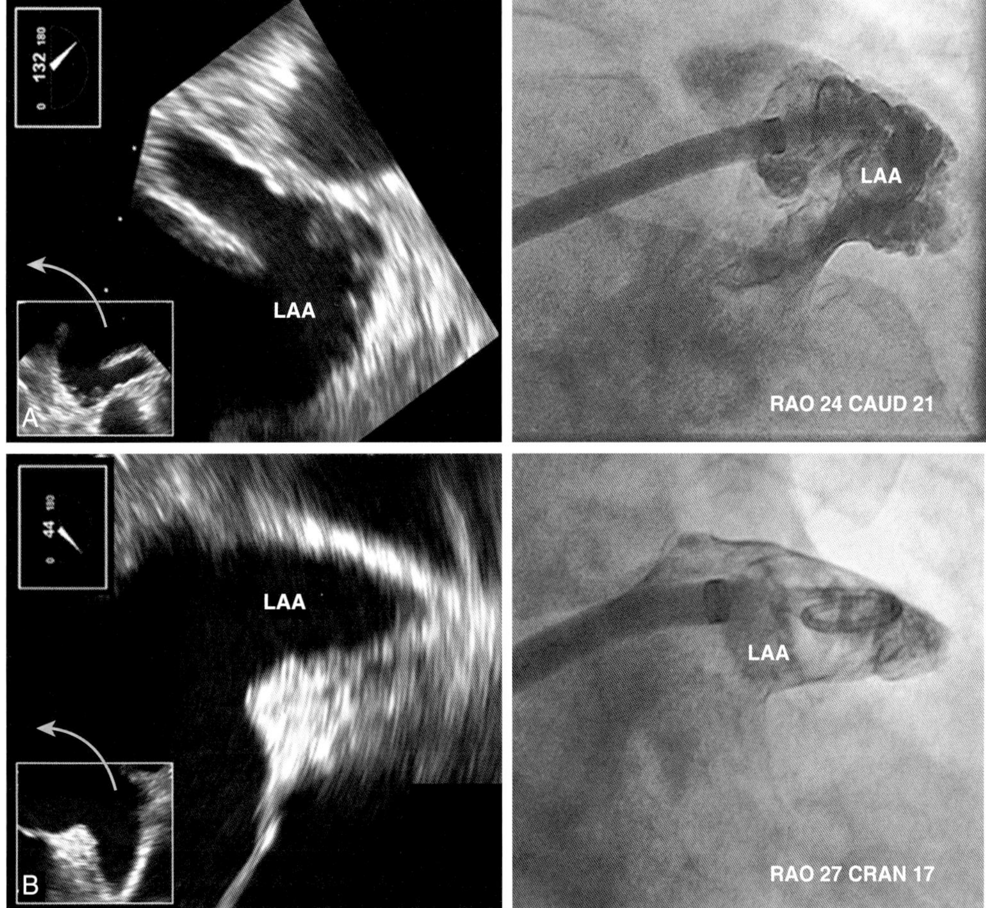

Fig. 10.23 TEE and fluoroscopic views of the left atrial appendage. TEE views of the left atrial appendage at 135- and 45-degree omniplane angles are the equivalent of fluoroscopic right anterior oblique caudal (A) and cranial (B) views, respectively, when turned counterclockwise 90 degrees *(orange arrow)*. *CAUD*, Caudal; *CRAN*, cranial; *LAA*, left atrial appendage; *RAO*, right anterior oblique. (Adapted from Vainrib AF, Harb SC, Jaber W, et al. Left atrial appendage occlusion/exclusion: procedural image guidance with transesophageal echocardiography. *J Am Soc Echocardiogr.* 2018;31:454–474.)

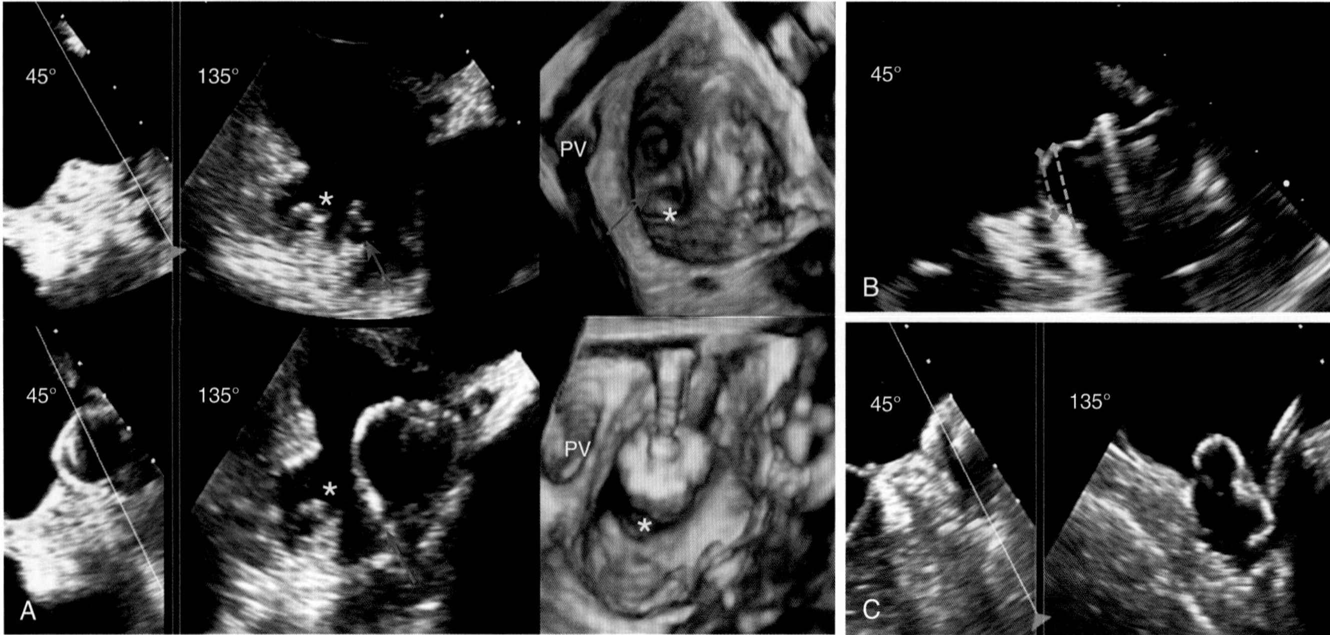

Fig. 10.24 Left atrial appendage occluder placement evaluation. (A) The LAA is divided into anterior and posterior *(yellow asterisk)* lobes by a prominent pectinate muscle *(red arrow)*. The distal anchors of the LAA occluder device are fixed to the pectinate muscle, leaving the posterior lobe uncovered. (B) The LAA occluder device shows a large shoulder height *(blue dashed line)* compared with the total device height *(green dashed line)* that protrudes into the LA. (C) Although it is not apparent on the 45-degree view, the LAA occluder device is severely canted with the anterior portion deep in the LAA in the 135-degree view. *LAA*, Left atrial appendage; *PV*, pulmonary vein.

For the Watchman device, a peridevice leakage of 5 mm or more by CFD, an uncovered secondary lobe, and a significant protrusion of the device into the LA (>40% of device height) should be excluded (Fig. 10.24).[88] Maximal device width is measured at 0, 45, 90, and 135 degrees to calculate the compression ratio. It is important to visualize the center of the device, indicated by the threaded insert, when measuring device width to ensure accurate results (Fig. 10.25). The PASS criteria (Table 10.7) must be met before the device is released.[88]

The post-deployment TEE examination should assess final position and tilt of the LAA occluder device. Device integrity should also be assessed for any deformities. Iatrogenic ASD and associated shunt direction should be evaluated and addressed after sheath withdrawal. Procedural and technical success is defined by device deployment and exclusion of the LAA with no para-device leak or complications.[90]

CHALLENGES AND HAZARDS

Dedicated structural heart interventional suites, unlike traditional catheterization laboratories, are fully capable of functioning as operating rooms (ORs) with surgical equipment available on standby. These hybrid ORs confer challenges for the interventional proceduralist and the echocardiographer. Integration of components from the catheterization laboratory and OR may overcrowd an already limited space. Anesthesia ventilators and fluoroscopic C-arms may be difficult to maneuver in an emergency, ultrasound machines and surgical trays may block vital pathways, connection wires and power cords may trip unsuspecting personnel, and ceiling-mounted lead shields and monitor screens may result in head injuries. Input from all multidisciplinary structural heart team members must be carefully considered when designing a hybrid OR.[91]

Interventional echocardiographers are most often situated at the head of the bed while performing TEE under surgical drapes. Distance from the patient, ambient noise, bright room lights, and inconsistent team members may be disorienting to the echocardiographer. Clear and close communication with the team is critical to thrive in this challenging environment.

As transcatheter interventions have become more sophisticated and complex, overall procedural times have lengthened. Occupational health hazards such as musculoskeletal pain are reportedly more prevalent among health care employees who work in interventional laboratories.[92] Risk of excessive radiation exposure is also a concern. Studies have shown that radiation doses to interventional echocardiographers are as high as those received by their procedural counterparts.[93] The addition of ceiling-suspended lead shields reduced radiation dose to echocardiographers by 81.7% ($P < 0.001$). Whether higher radiation doses to interventional echocardiographers lead to an increased risk of cataracts or cancer is unknown because of the paucity of data. However, efforts should be made to reduce radiation exposure as much as possible by applying additional protective gear.[94]

Prolonged TEE manipulation for procedural guidance may result in iatrogenic injuries to the patient, especially in the frail patient population.[95] Risk factors associated with major complications are low body weight, prior history of gastrointestinal bleeding, longer hospital stay, and use of immunosuppressive medication. Procedural time under TEE manipulation is an independent predictor of complications such as persistent dysphagia or odynophagia, bleeding requiring transfusion, and esophageal perforation (odds ratio = 1.13, 95% CI: 1.01–1.25, for each 10-minute increment in imaging time).[95] Extra care should be given when performing intraprocedural TEE to avoid excessive transducer manipulation and movement. Strategies to minimize imaging time and facilitate procedural progress, such as fusion imaging, should be considered, if available.

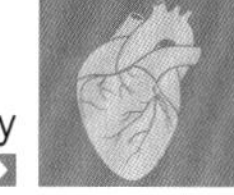

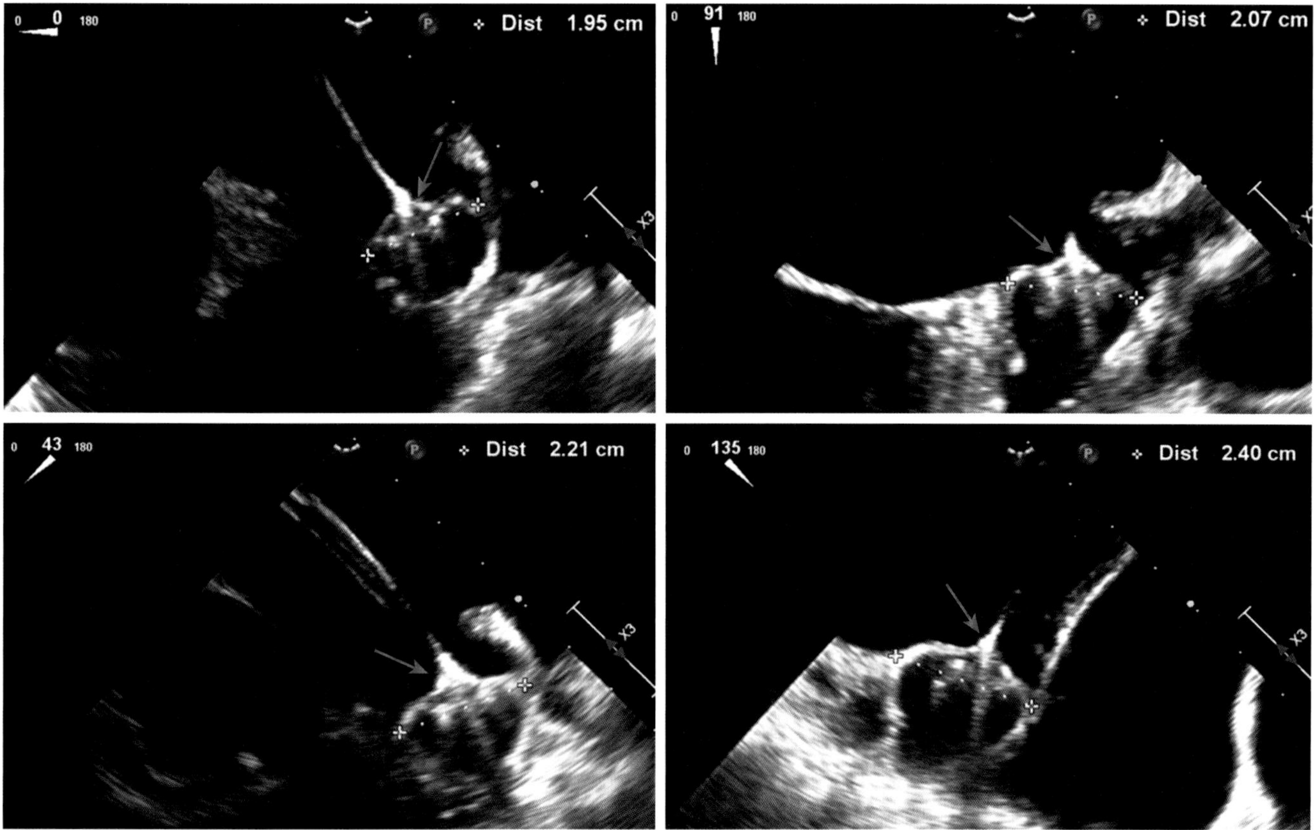

Fig. 10.25 **Measurement of left atrial appendage occluder diameter after deployment.** The compression ratio of the occluder device is calculated by measuring the device diameter in 0-, 45-, 90-, and 135-degree views divided by the selected device size. Notice that the center of the occluder device, denoted by the threaded insert *(red arrows)*, should be obtained to ensure accurate measurements.

TABLE 10.7 PASS Criteria for Watchman Release.

PASS Criteria	*Echocardiographic Findings*
Position	The plane with the maximal diameter of the device should be at or just distal to the plane of the ostium in the majority of views.
Anchor	The device and the LAA should move in unison during the tug test.
Size	Compression ratio is calculated from postdeployment measurement of maximal device width and is considered adequate if between 8% and 20%.
Seal	CFD with a low Nyquist limit (20–30 cm/s) is used to sweep around the device to assess for residual leak.[90] A peridevice leak of <5 mm is considered acceptable.

CFD, Color-flow Doppler; *LAA*, left atrial appendage.

FUTURE DIRECTIONS

Percutaneous treatment of structural heart disease is an exponentially growing field. This presents new challenges and opportunities for the interventional echocardiographer responsible for procedural guidance.[96] Future developments will include focus on enhanced safety and workplace ergonomics for the echocardiographer. Further advances will see increased integration and improvements in all procedural imaging modalities. Combining CT and/or MRI technology with 3D echocardiography will likely provide the most significant progress in facilitating preprocedural planning and intraprocedural guidance.

The evolving technology of 3D printing of cardiovascular structures and virtual reality platforms will enhance preprocedural planning for the structural heart team. Challenges for widespread 3D printing include lack of materials that mimic human tissue, the cost and time required to achieve high-quality point-of-care printing, and the need for single time-point selection.[97] However, virtual and augmented reality techniques will most likely have an even more significant clinical impact on 3D echocardiographic image comprehension. Substantial computing innovations will permit further improvements in volume rendering, user friendliness, display resolution, and the viewing experience, opening the door for this technology to enter clinical stages.[98]

Significant efforts are underway to optimize structural heart device development for echocardiographic imaging. Transcatheter device companies are joining forces with echocardiography platform companies to develop catheters and devices with ultrasound-friendly properties.

SUMMARY Interventional Echocardiography

Structural Heart Intervention	Preprocedural Evaluation	Intraprocedural Guidance	Postprocedural Assessment

Transcatheter aortic valve replacement (TAVR)	• Confirm pathology
	• Aortic root
	  • Annular and leaflet calcification
	  • Coronary height
	  • Leaflet length
	• Aortic annular sizing
	  • Ideally by 3D multiplanar reconstruction (MPR)
	  • Major and minor diameters
	  • Circumference
	  • Area
	• Establish semiquantitative and quantitative baseline parameters
		• Often not needed because deployment depends heavily on fluoroscopy
		• Increased value in valve-in-valve TAVR implantations
			• Transcatheter heart valve (THV)
			  • Function
			  • Location
			  • Stability
			• Paravalvular regurgitation
			  • Location
			  • Extent
			  • Overall severity
			• Biventricular function and regional wall motion
			• Compare semiquantitative and quantitative parameters to baseline
			• Exclude iatrogenic complications

Transcatheter mitral valve (MV) edge-to-edge repair	• Confirm cause of mitral regurgitation (MR)
	  • Degenerative
	  • Functional
	  • Combination
	• MV morphology
	  • Leaflet length
	  • Coaptation gap width
	  • Tenting height or angle
	  • Cleft or perforation
	• MR
	  • Origin
	  • Number of jets
	  • Width
	• Mitral apparatus
	  • Annular area
	  • Calcification
	  • Prominent chordae or papillary muscles
	• Establish semiquantitative and quantitative baseline parameters
		• Exclude unfavorable anatomy or presence of intracardiac thrombus
		• Determine accurate bicommissural view
		• Transseptal puncture
		• Advancement of steerable guide catheter
		• Positioning and orientation of clip delivery system
		• Advancement of clip device into LV
		• Insertion and grasping of mitral leaflet
		• After device closure but before release
		  • Residual MR
		  • Mitral diastolic gradient
		  • Compare semiquantitative and quantitative parameters to baseline
			• Confirm device stability
			• Check for changes in residual MR severity
			  • Compare semiquantitative and quantitative parameters to baseline
			• Assess mitral inflow gradient and remaining valve area
			• Exclude iatrogenic complications

Transcatheter MV replacement	• Confirm pathology
	• Mitral structure
	  • Native annulus
	  • Annular ring
	  • Preexisting bioprosthetic valve
	• Landing zone sizing
	  • Ideally by 3D MPR
	  • Major and minor diameters
	  • Circumference
	  • Area
	• Risk of left ventricular outflow tract (LVOT) obstruction
	  • Mitral anterior leaflet length
	  • Aortomitral angle
	  • LV size
	  • Basal interventricular septal thickness
	  • Ventricular positioning of THV
	• Establish semiquantitative and quantitative baseline parameters
		• Exclude unfavorable anatomy or presence of intracardiac thrombus
		• Transseptal puncture
		  • Potentially followed by balloon septostomy
		• Advancement of THV
		• Positioning and deployment of THV
			• Confirm adequate LV function and aortic valve opening
			• Quantitative assessment of LVOT gradient
			• THV
			  • Function
			  • Location
			  • Stability
			• Paravalvular regurgitation
			  • Location
			  • Extent
			  • Overall severity
			• Compare semiquantitative and quantitative parameters to baseline
			• Exclude iatrogenic complications

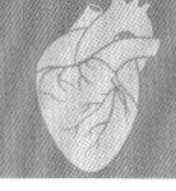

SUMMARY Interventional Echocardiography—cont'd

Structural Heart Intervention	Preprocedural Evaluation	Intraprocedural Guidance	Postprocedural Assessment

Percutaneous paravalvular leak occlusion	• Confirm pathology
	  • Location
	  • Extent
	  • Overall severity
	• Paravalvular defect sizing
	  • Ideally by 3D MPR
	  • Major and minor diameters
	  • Circumference
	  • Area
	• Establish semiquantitative and quantitative baseline parameters
		• Exclude unfavorable anatomy or presence of intracardiac thrombus
		• Transseptal puncture for paramitral defects
		• Confirm guide wire and delivery sheath traversal of paravalvular defect
		• Positioning and deployment of occluder device
			• Confirm device stability
			• Reassess residual paravalvular regurgitation severity
			  • Compare semiquantitative and quantitative parameters to baseline
			• Exclude iatrogenic complications

Percutaneous left atrial appendage (LAA) occlusion	• LAA
	  • Ideally by 3D MPR
	  • Overall shape
	  • Ostia, neck, and body diameter and length for sizing
	  • Number of lobes
	  • Prominent pectinate muscles
		• Exclude unfavorable anatomy and presence of intracardiac thrombus
		• Transseptal puncture
		• Advancement of LAA access sheath
		• After device deployment but before release
		  • Implantation depth
		  • Device tilt
		  • Compression ratio
		  • LAA coverage
		  • Device stability
		  • Para-device flow
			• Reassess device stability
			• Reassess para-device flow
			• Exclude iatrogenic complications

REFERENCES

1. Scacciatella P, Meynet I, Giorgi M, et al. Angiography vs transesophageal echocardiography-guided patent foramen ovale closure: a propensity score matched analysis of a two-center registry. *Echocardiography*. 2018;35(6):834–840.
2. Hart EA, Teske AJ, Voskuil M, et al. Transthoracic echocardiography guided MitraClip placement under conscious sedation. *JACC Cardiovasc Interv*. 2017;10(3):e27–e29.
3. Sengupta PP, Wiley BM, Basnet S, et al. Transthoracic echocardiography guidance for TAVR under monitored anesthesia care. *JACC Cardiovasc Imaging*. 2015;8(3):379–380.
4. Wang S, Ouyang W, Liu Y, et al. Transcatheter perimembranous ventricular septal defect closure under transthoracic echocardiographic guidance without fluoroscopy. *J Thorac Dis*. 2018;10(9):5222–5231.
5. Alkhouli M, Hijazi ZM, Holmes DR Jr, et al. Intracardiac echocardiography in structural heart disease interventions. *JACC Cardiovasc Interv*. 2018;11(21):2133–2147.
6. Bartel T, Müller S, Biviano A, et al. Why is intracardiac echocardiography helpful? Benefits, costs, and how to learn. *Eur Heart J*. 2014;35(2):69–76.
7. Bartakian S, El-Said HG, Printz B, et al. Prospective randomized trial of transthoracic echocardiography versus transesophageal echocardiography for assessment and guidance of transcatheter closure of atrial septal defects in children using the Amplatzer septal occluder. *JACC Cardiovasc Interv*. 2013;6(9):974–980.
8. Ribeiro JM, Teixeira R, Puga L, et al. Comparison of intracardiac and transoesophageal echocardiography for guidance of percutaneous left atrial appendage occlusion: a meta-analysis. *Echocardiography*. 2019;36(7):1330–1337.
9. Zamorano J, Gonçalves A, Lancellotti P, et al. The use of imaging in new transcatheter interventions: an EACVI review paper. *Eur Heart J Cardiovasc Imaging*. 2016;17(8):835. 835af.
10. Mihalatos DG, Gopal AS, Kates R, et al. Intraoperative assessment of mitral regurgitation: role of phenylephrine challenge. *J Am Soc Echocardiogr*. 2006;19(9):1158–1164.
11. Sanfilippo F, Johnson C, Bellavia D, et al. Mitral regurgitation grading in the operating room: a systematic review and meta-analysis comparing preoperative and intraoperative assessments during cardiac surgery. *J Cardiothorac Vasc Anesth*. 2017;31(5):1681–1691.
12. Khalique OK, Hahn RT. Role of echocardiography in transcatheter valvular heart disease interventions. *Curr Cardiol Rep*. 2017;19(12):128.
13. Faletra FF, Ramamurthi A, Dequarti MC, et al. Artifacts in three-dimensional transesophageal echocardiography. *J Am Soc Echocardiogr*. 2014;27(5):453–462.
14. Mahmood F, Jeganathan J, Saraf R, et al. A practical approach to an intraoperative three-dimensional transesophageal echocardiography examination. *J Cardiothorac Vasc Anesth*. 2016;30(2):470–490.
15. Lang RM, Badano LP, Tsang W, et al. EAE/ASE recommendations for image acquisition and display using three-dimensional echocardiography. *J Am Soc Echocardiogr*. 2012;25(1):3–46.
16. Thaden JJ, Sanon S, Geske JB, et al. Echocardiographic and fluoroscopic fusion imaging for procedural guidance: an overview and early clinical experience. *J Am Soc Echocardiogr*. 2016;29(6):503–512.
17. Biaggi P, Fernandez-Golfín C, Hahn R, et al. Hybrid imaging during transcatheter structural heart interventions. *Curr Cardiovasc Imaging Rep*. 2015;8(9):33.
18. Alkhouli M, Rihal CS, Holmes DR Jr. Transseptal techniques for emerging structural heart interventions. *JACC Cardiovasc Interv*. 2016;9(24):2465–2480.
19. Goldsweig AM, Tak HJ, Chen LW, et al. The evolving management of aortic valve disease: 5-year trends in SAVR, TAVR, and medical therapy. *Am J Cardiol*. 2019;124(5):763–771.
20. Hyman MC, Vemulapalli S, Szeto WY, et al. Conscious sedation versus general anesthesia for transcatheter aortic valve replacement: insights from the National Cardiovascular Data Registry Society of Thoracic Surgeons/American College of Cardiology Transcatheter Valve Therapy Registry. *Circulation*. 2017;136(22):2132–2140.
21. Athappan G, Patvardhan E, Tuzcu EM, et al. Incidence, predictors, and outcomes of aortic regurgitation after transcatheter aortic valve replacement: meta-analysis and systematic review of literature. *J Am Coll Cardiol*. 2013;61(15):1585–1595.
22. Shibayama K, Mihara H, Jilaihawi H, et al. 3D assessment of features associated with transvalvular aortic regurgitation after TAVR: a real-time 3D TEE study. *JACC Cardiovasc Imaging*. 2016;9(2):114–123.

23. Smith LA, Dworakowski R, Bhan A, et al. Real-time three-dimensional transesophageal echocardiography adds value to transcatheter aortic valve implantation. *J Am Soc Echocardiogr*. 2013;26(4):359–369.
24. Elkaryoni A, Nanda NC, Baweja P, et al. Three-dimensional transesophageal echocardiography is an attractive alternative to cardiac multi-detector computed tomography for aortic annular sizing: systematic review and meta-analysis. *Echocardiography*. 2018;35(10):1626–1634.
25. Papachristidis A, Papitsas M, Roper D, et al. Three-dimensional measurement of aortic annulus dimensions using area or circumference for transcatheter aortic valve replacement valve sizing: does it make a difference? *J Am Soc Echocardiogr*. 2017;30(9):871–878.
26. Kasel AM, Cassese S, Bleiziffer S, et al. Standardized imaging for aortic annular sizing: implications for transcatheter valve selection. *JACC Cardiovasc Imaging*. 2013;6(2):249–262.
27. Hahn RT, Khalique O, Williams MR, et al. Predicting paravalvular regurgitation following transcatheter valve replacement: utility of a novel method for three-dimensional echocardiographic measurements of the aortic annulus. *J Am Soc Echocardiogr*. 2013;26(9):1043–1052.
28. Prihadi EA, van Rosendael PJ, Vollema EM, et al. Feasibility, accuracy, and reproducibility of aortic annular and root sizing for transcatheter aortic valve replacement using novel automated three-dimensional echocardiographic software: comparison with multi-detector row computed tomography. *J Am Soc Echocardiogr*. 2018;31(4):505–514.e3.
29. Hahn RT, Kodali S, Tuzcu EM, et al. Echocardiographic imaging of procedural complications during balloon-expandable transcatheter aortic valve replacement. *JACC Cardiovasc Imaging*. 2015;8(3):288–318.
30. Hahn RT, Gillam LD, Little SH. Echocardiographic imaging of procedural complications during self-expandable transcatheter aortic valve replacement. *JACC Cardiovasc Imaging*. 2015;8(3):319–336.
31. Khan JM, Greenbaum AB, Babaliaros VC, et al. The BASILICA trial: prospective multicenter investigation of intentional leaflet laceration to prevent TAVR coronary obstruction. *JACC Cardiovasc Interv*. 2019;12(13):1240–1252.
32. Komatsu I, Mackensen GB, Aldea GS, et al. Bioprosthetic or native aortic scallop intentional laceration to prevent iatrogenic coronary artery obstruction. Part 2: how to perform BASILICA. *EuroIntervention*. 2019;15(1):55–66.
33. Coutinho GF, Antunes MJ. Mitral valve repair for degenerative mitral valve disease: surgical approach, patient selection and long-term outcomes. *Heart*. 2017 Nov;103(21):1663–1669.
34. Mirabel M, Lung B, Baron G, et al. What are the characteristics of patients with severe, symptomatic, mitral regurgitation who are denied surgery? *Eur Heart J*. 2007;28(11):1358–1365.
35. Sorajja P, Leon MB, Adams DH, et al. Transcatheter therapy for mitral regurgitation clinical challenges and potential solutions. *Circulation*. 2017;136(4):404–417.
36. Feldman T, Foster E, Glower DD, et al. Percutaneous repair or surgery for mitral regurgitation. *N Engl J Med*. 2011;364(15):1395–1406.
37. Stone GW, Lindenfeld J, Abraham WT, et al. Transcatheter mitral-valve repair in patients with heart failure. *N Engl J Med*. 2018 13;379(24):2307–2318.
38. Alfieri O, Maisano F, De Bonis M, et al. The double-orifice technique in mitral valve repair: a simple solution for complex problems. *J Thorac Cardiovasc Surg*. 2001;122(4):674–681.
39. Donmez E, Salcedo EE, Quaife RA, et al. The acute effects of edge-to-edge percutaneous mitral valve repair on the shape and size of the mitral annulus and its relation to mitral regurgitation. *Echocardiography*. 2019;36(4):732–741.
40. Noack T, Kiefer P, Mallon L, et al. Changes in dynamic mitral valve geometry during percutaneous edge-edge mitral valve repair with the MitraClip system. *J Echocardiogr*. 2019;17(2):84–94.
41. Utsunomiya H, Itabashi Y, Kobayashi S, et al. Comparison of mitral valve geometrical effect of percutaneous edge-to-edge repair between central and eccentric functional mitral regurgitation: clinical implications. *Eur Heart J Cardiovasc Imaging*. 2019;20(4):455–466.
42. Gripari P, Tamborini G, Bottari V, et al. Three-dimensional transthoracic echocardiography in the comprehensive evaluation of right and left heart chamber remodeling following percutaneous mitral valve repair. *J Am Soc Echocardiogr*. 2016;29(10):946–954.
43. Vitarelli A, Mangieri E, Capotosto L, et al. Assessment of biventricular function by three-dimensional Speckle-Tracking echocardiography in secondary mitral regurgitation after repair with the MitraClip system. *J Am Soc Echocardiogr*. 2015;28(9):1070–1082.
44. Flint K, Brieke A, Wiktor, et al. Percutaneous edge-to-edge mitral valve repair may rescue select patients in cardiogenic shock: findings from a single center case series. *Catheter Cardiovasc Interv*. 2019;94(2):E82–E87.
45. Nyman CB, Mackensen GB, Jelacic S, et al. Transcatheter mitral valve repair using the edge-to-edge clip. *J Am Soc Echocardiogr*. 2018;31(4):434–453.
46. Bushari LI, Reeder GS, Eleid MF, et al. Percutaneous transcatheter edge-to-edge MitraClip technique: a practical "Step-by-Step" 3-dimensional transesophageal echocardiography guide. *Mayo Clin Proc*. 2019;94(1):89–102.
47. Wunderlich NC, Beigel R, Ho SY, et al. Imaging for mitral interventions: methods and efficacy. *JACC Cardiovasc Imaging*. 2018;11(6):872–901.
48. Mackensen GB and Reisman M. Edge-to-Edge repair of the mitral valve with the Mitraclip system: evolution of leaflet grasping technology. *Structural Heart*. 2019;3(4):341–347.
49. Zoghbi WA, Asch FM, Bruce C, et al. Guidelines for the evaluation of valvular regurgitation after percutaneous valve repair or replacement: a report from the American Society of Echocardiography developed in collaboration with the Society for Cardiovascular Angiography and Interventions, Japanese Society of Echocardiography, and Society for Cardiovascular Magnetic Resonance. *J Am Soc Echocardiogr*. 2019;32(4):431–475.
50. Kuwata S, Taramasso M, Czopak A, et al. Continuous direct left atrial pressure: intraprocedural measurement predicts clinical response following MitraClip therapy. *JACC Cardiovasc Interv*. 2019;12(2):127–136.
51. Kreidel F, Alessandrini H, Wohlmuth P, et al. Is surgical or catheter-based interventions an option after an unsuccessful mitral clip? *Semin Thorac Cardiovasc Surg*. 2018 Summer;30(2):152–157.
52. Schueler R, Öztürk C, Wedekind JA, et al. Persistence of iatrogenic atrial septal defect after interventional mitral valve repair with the MitraClip system: a note of caution. *JACC Cardiovasc Interv*. 2015;8(3):450–459.
53. Ikenaga H, Hayashi A, Nagaura T, et al. Left atrial pressure is associated with iatrogenic atrial septal defect after mitral valve clip. *Heart*. 2019;105(11):864–872.
54. Beri N, Singh GD, Smith TW, et al. Iatrogenic atrial septal defect closure after transseptal mitral valve interventions: indications and outcomes. *Catheter Cardiovasc Interv*. 2019;94(6):829–836.
55. Regueiro A, Granada JF, Dagenais F, et al. Transcatheter mitral valve replacement: insights from early clinical experience and future challenges. *J Am Coll Cardiol*. 2017;69(17):2175–2192.
56. Guerrero M, Dvir D, Himbert, et al. Transcatheter mitral valve replacement in native mitral valve disease with severe mitral annular calcification: results from the first multicenter global registry. *JACC Cardiovasc Interv*. 2016;9(13):1361–1371.
57. Eleid MF, Whisenant BK, Cabalka AK, et al. Early outcomes of percutaneous transvenous transseptal transcatheter valve implantation in failed bioprosthetic mitral valves, ring annuloplasty, and severe mitral annular calcification. *JACC Cardiovasc Interv*. 2017;10(19):1932–1942.
58. Wyler von Ballmoos MC, Kalra A, Reardon MJ. Complexities of transcatheter mitral valve replacement (TMVR) and why it is not transcatheter aortic valve replacement (TAVR). *Ann Cardiothorac Surg*. 2018;7(6):724–730.
59. Urena M, Himbert D, Brochet E, et al. Transseptal transcatheter mitral valve replacement using balloon-expandable transcatheter heart valves: a step-by-step approach. *JACC Cardiovasc Interv*. 2017;10(19):1905–1919.
60. Wang DD, Eng M, Greenbaum A, et al. Predicting LVOT obstruction after TMVR. *JACC Cardiovasc Imaging*. 2016;9(11):1349–1352.
61. Mackensen GB, Lee JC, Wang D, et al. Role of echocardiography in transcatheter mitral valve replacement in native mitral valves and mitral rings. *J Am Soc Echocardiogr*. 2018;31(4):475–490.
62. Mak GJ, Blanke P, Ong K, et al. Three-dimensional echocardiography compared with computed tomography to determine mitral annulus size before transcatheter mitral valve implantation. *Circ Cardiovasc Imaging*. 2016;9(6).
63. Blanke P, Naoum C, Dvir D, et al. Predicting LVOT obstruction in transcatheter mitral valve implantation: concept of the neo-LVOT. *JACC Cardiovasc Imaging*. 2017;10(4):482–485.
64. Yoon SH, Bleiziffer S, Latib A, et al. Predictors of left ventricular outflow tract obstruction after transcatheter mitral valve replacement. *JACC Cardiovasc Interv*. 2019;12(2):182–193.
65. Wang DD, Guerrero M, Eng MH, et al. Alcohol septal ablation to prevent left ventricular outflow tract obstruction during transcatheter mitral valve replacement: first-in-man study. *JACC Cardiovasc Interv*. 2019;12(13):1268–1279.
66. Rana BS. Echocardiography guidance of atrial septal defect closure. *J Thorac Dis*. 2018;10(suppl 24):S2899–S2908.
67. Babaliaros VC, Greenbaum AB, Khan JM, et al. Intentional percutaneous laceration of the anterior mitral leaflet to prevent outflow obstruction during transcatheter mitral valve replacement: first-in-human experience. *JACC Cardiovasc Interv*. 2017;10(8):798–809.
68. Khan JM, Babaliaros VC, Greenbaum AB, et al. Anterior leaflet laceration to prevent ventricular outflow tract obstruction during transcatheter mitral valve replacement. *J Am Coll Cardiol*. 2019;73(20):2521–2534.

69. Kliger C, Eiros R, Isasti G, et al. Review of surgical prosthetic paravalvular leaks: diagnosis and catheter-based closure. *Eur Heart J*. 2013 Mar;34(9):638–649.
70. Ruiz CE, Jelnin V, Kronzon I, et al. Clinical outcomes in patients undergoing percutaneous closure of periprosthetic paravalvular leaks. *J Am Coll Cardiol*. 2011;58(21):2210–2217.
71. Millán X, Bouhout I, Nozza A, et al. Surgery versus transcatheter interventions for significant paravalvular prosthetic leaks. *JACC Cardiovasc Interv*. 2017;10(19):1959–1969.
72. Wells JA 4th, Condado JF, Kamioka N, et al. Outcomes after paravalvular leak closure: transcatheter versus surgical approaches. *JACC Cardiovasc Interv*. 2017;10(5):500–507.
73. Sorajja P, Cabalka AK2, Hagler D, et al. The learning curve in percutaneous repair of paravalvular prosthetic regurgitation: an analysis of 200 cases. *JACC Cardiovasc Interv*. 2014;7(5):521–529.
74. Kliger C, Eiros R, Isasti G, et al. Review of surgical prosthetic paravalvular leaks: diagnosis and catheter-based closure. *Eur Heart J*. 2013;34(9):638–649.
75. Rihal CS, Sorajja P, Booker JD, et al. Principles of percutaneous paravalvular leak closure. *ACC Cardiovasc Interv*. 2012;5(2):121–130.
76. Hamm CW, Arsalan M, Mack MJ. The future of transcatheter aortic valve implantation. *Eur Heart J*. 2016;37(10):803–810.
77. Van Belle E, Juthier F, Susen S, et al. Postprocedural aortic regurgitation in balloon-expandable and self-expandable transcatheter aortic valve replacement procedures: analysis of predictors and impact on long-term mortality: insights from the France2 Registry. *Circulation*. 2014;129(13):1415–1427.
78. Holmes M, Sheu R. The use of intraoperative three-dimensional echocardiography to evaluate origin of bioprosthetic aortic valve regurgitant jets. *J Cardiothorac Vasc Anesth*. 2019.
79. Al-Hijji MA, Alkhouli M, Sarraf M, et al. Characteristics and outcomes of re-do percutaneous paravalvular leak closure. *Catheter Cardiovasc Interv*. 2017;90(4):680–689.
80. Okutucu S, Mach M, Oto A. Mitral paravalvular leak closure: transcatheter and surgical solutions. *Cardiovasc Revasc Med*. 2020;21(3):422–431.
81. Holmes DR Jr, Schwartz RS, Latus GG, et al. A history of left atrial appendage occlusion. *Interv Cardiol Clin*. 2018;7(2):143–150.
82. Beigel R, Wunderlich NC, Ho SY, et al. The left atrial appendage: anatomy, function, and noninvasive evaluation. *JACC Cardiovasc Imaging*. 2014;7(12):1251–1265.
83. Morcos R, Al Taii H, Bansal P, et al. Accuracy of commonly-used imaging modalities in assessing left atrial appendage for interventional closure: review article. *J Clin Med*. 2018;7(11).
84. Obasare E, Mainigi SK, Morris DL, et al. CT based 3D printing is superior to transesophageal echocardiography for pre-procedure planning in left atrial appendage device closure. *Int J Cardiovasc Imaging*. 2018;34(5):821–831.
85. Frangieh AH, Alibegovic J, Templin C, et al. Intracardiac versus transesophageal echocardiography for left atrial appendage occlusion with watchman. *Catheter Cardiovasc Interv*. 2017;90(2):331–338.
86. Wunderlich NC, Beigel R, Swaans MJ, et al. Percutaneous interventions for left atrial appendage exclusion: options, assessment, and imaging using 2D and 3D echocardiography. *JACC Cardiovasc Imaging*. 2015;8(4):472–488.
87. Spencer RJ, DeJong P, Fahmy P, et al. Changes in left atrial appendage dimensions following volume loading during percutaneous left atrial appendage closure. *JACC Cardiovasc Interv*. 2015;8(15):1935–1941.
88. Vainrib AF, Harb SC, Jaber W, et al. Left atrial appendage occlusion/exclusion: procedural image guidance with transesophageal echocardiography. *J Am Soc Echocardiogr*. 2018;31(4):454–474.
89. Price MJ. The WATCHMAN left atrial appendage closure device: technical considerations and procedural approach. *Interv Cardiol Clin*. 2018;7(2):201–212.
90. Tzikas A, Holmes DR Jr, Gafoor S, et al. Percutaneous left atrial appendage occlusion: the Munich consensus document on definitions, endpoints and data collection requirements for clinical studies. *EuroIntervention*. 2016;12(1):103–111.
91. Kaneko T, Davidson MJ. Use of the hybrid operating room in cardiovascular medicine. *Circulation*. 2014;130(11):910–917.
92. Orme NM, Rihal CS, Gulati R, et al. Occupational health hazards of working in the interventional laboratory: a multisite case control study of physicians and allied staff. *J Am Coll Cardiol*. 2015;65(8):820–826.
93. Crowhurst JA, Scalia GM, Whitby M, et al. Radiation exposure of operators performing transesophageal echocardiography during percutaneous structural cardiac interventions. *J Am Coll Cardiol*. 2018;71(11):1246–1254.
94. McIlwain EF, Coon PD, Einstein AJ, et al. Radiation safety for the cardiac sonographer: recommendations of the Radiation Safety Writing Group for the Council on Cardiovascular Sonography of the American Society of Echocardiography. *J Am Soc Echocardiogr*. 2014;27(8):811–816.
95. Freitas-Ferraz AB, Rodés-Cabau J, Junquera Vega, et al. Transesophageal echocardiography complications associated with interventional cardiology procedures. *Am Heart J*. 2020;221:19–28.
96. Wang DD, Geske J, Choi A, et al. Interventional imaging for structural heart disease: challenges and new frontiers of an emerging multi-disciplinary field. *Structural Heart*. 2019;3(3):187–200.
97. Levin D, Mackensen GB, Reisman M, et al. 3D printing applications for transcatheter aortic valve replacement. *Curr Cardiol Rep*. 2020;22(4):23.
98. Lang RM, Addetia K, Narang A. 3-Dimensional echocardiography: latest developments and future directions. *JACC Cardiovasc Imaging*. 2018;11(12):1854–1878.

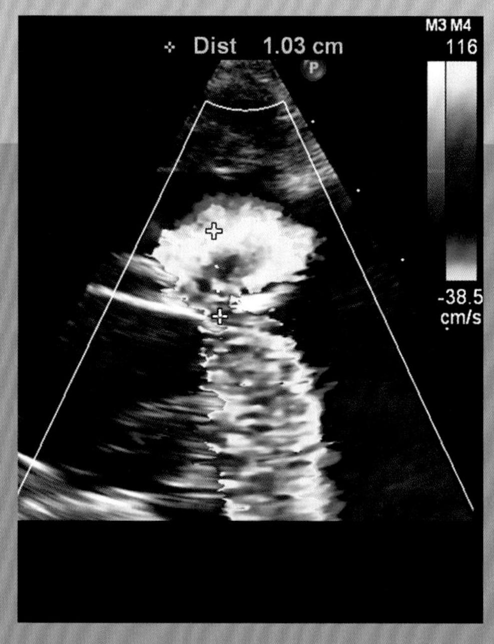

中文导读

第11章 床旁聚焦心脏超声

聚焦心脏超声主要用于床旁紧急情况下心脏疾病的基本诊断，从而快速做出临床决策。由于其方便、快捷，比常规查体更加可靠、精确，因此越来越广泛应用于临床，特别是在急危重症医学中。

聚焦心脏超声是由家庭医师在床旁进行，主要是定性检查，也可以对心脏结构和功能进行半定量评估，从而进一步评估具体的临床发现和诊断，其目标是评估左心室和右心室功能、容量状态和心包积液情况，但聚焦心脏超声常常无法诊断出更复杂的解剖或生理异常，因此其不能代替体格检查及更为先进、全面的诊断方法，如常规超声心动图。在紧急情况下，有时探头通常很难找到最佳的位置来获得完美的切面，本章给出了聚焦心脏超声检查的建议方法。在一些紧急的临床情况下，如不明原因低血压和休克、穿透性胸部损伤、大面积肺栓塞、心脏压塞和心脏骤停，聚焦心脏超声是快速诊断和处理的关键方法。相关文献提示，聚焦心脏超声可以降低诊断的不确定性，改变治疗计划，并提高临床医师在不同临床决策中的处理速度。然而，临床医师须接受图像采集、质量评估和图像解读方面的特别培训后才能使用聚焦心脏超声。

本章阐述了聚焦心脏超声的基础知识、实践范围和诊断目标、对患者结局的影响、目前的培训和认证实践，以及培训质量的挑战。

赵　莹

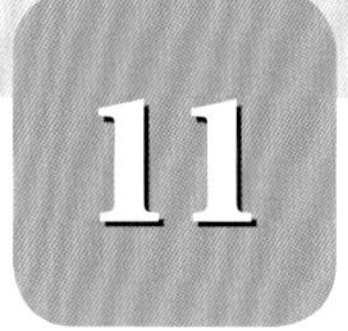

Focused Cardiac Ultrasound at the Bedside

SHANNON MCCONNAUGHEY, MD | CATHERINE M. OTTO, MD

Focused cardiac ultrasound (FoCUS) is a readily accessible and widely used tool for the bedside diagnosis of basic cardiac pathology. Long championed by emergency room and critical care physicians, point-of-care ultrasound (POCUS) in general, including FoCUS, is increasingly utilized by a range of providers, including physicians and advanced practice providers in both inpatient and outpatient settings across many specialties. FoCUS is emerging as a fundamental clinical tool that is taught to many medical students across the country in their preclinical years, and it may eventually be considered a core competency for all physicians.

As technology has evolved, ultrasound machines have become more portable and affordable and offer improved image quality. Handheld devices are now financially attainable for many individuals or small provider groups. In addition to providing high-resolution images of cardiovascular structures, these devices are generally equipped with M-mode and color Doppler modalities. A range of products are available on the market, including wireless and smartphone-compatible devices and probes (Fig. 11.1). Given the progressive miniaturization of ultrasound, it is conceivable that these same devices may eventually include spectral and tissue Doppler capabilities. With these increases in availability, portability, and quality, many medical providers now routinely use FoCUS in their daily practice. This chapter reviews the basics of performing a focused cardiac ultrasound examination, scope of practice and diagnostic targets of FoCUS, impact on patient outcomes, current training and certification practices, and quality assurance challenges.

SCOPE OF PRACTICE

Although cardiac ultrasound is a powerful tool for directly assessing anatomy and physiology at the point of care, its accuracy and utility are highly dependent on user skill. The safe and successful application of FoCUS depends on recognition by the user of both her or his personal limitations and the limitations of the technology. Given the expanding availability of portable ultrasound machines, it is important to define the purpose and scope of FoCUS. Multiple specialty, subspecialty, and imaging societies have published guidelines on the appropriate usage of FoCUS.[1–6] Although these recommendations vary on specific details, there is overarching agreement on the general role and scope of FoCUS.

FoCUS is a targeted examination that is performed at the bedside by the primary care provider with the goal of answering a specific clinical question. FoCUS is primarily a qualitative examination and includes only basic semiquantitative assessments of cardiac structure and function. This is distinctly different from limited echocardiography, which involves a limited number of images but is still a comprehensive diagnostic test that is performed by a trained sonographer using a multimodality ultrasound machine and interpreted by an echocardiographer. Even in limited echocardiography, sonographers record additional views and data for full quantitative metrics as needed.[1] Limited echocardiography studies must also be interpreted by a physician who is credentialed in echocardiography, typically a cardiologist. This limits its utility as the initial test in many critical care and emergency settings. As a problem-focused bedside examination performed by the primary care provider, FoCUS is well suited for use in clinically urgent cases in which there is an explicit diagnostic or management question that can be answered with ultrasound, and the findings can be immediately incorporated into patient management. Serial FoCUS examinations can also be performed to assess evolving clinical status, which is not practical for limited echocardiography.

Portable ultrasound machines are simpler to use and have a more focused suite of features compared with traditional echocardiogram machines. In the hands of expert users, these portable machines have the capacity to diagnose a wide range of cardiac pathologies (Table 11.1).[7–21] However, there is a clear gap between the diagnostic capacity of FoCUS in the hands of experts compared with less experienced users.[12] Although the capacity of these machines is quite broad, it is important to consider what is appropriate and within the diagnostic scope for most users.

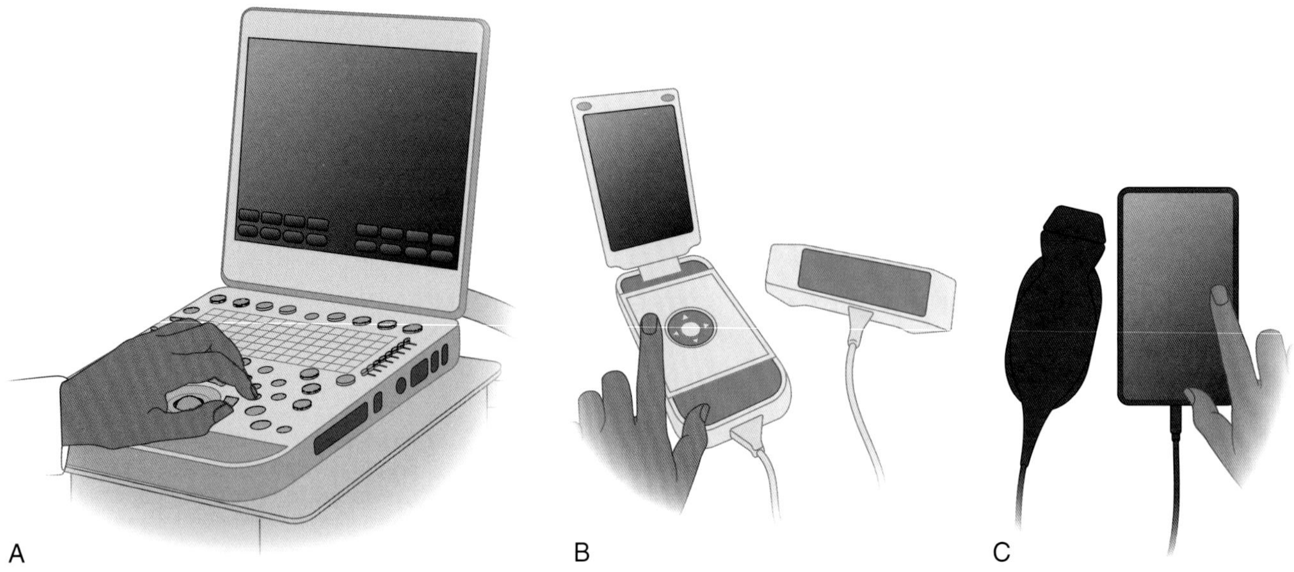

Fig. 11.1 Types of ultrasound machines used for FoCUS. Focused cardiac ultrasound (FoCUS) can be performed using portable machines (A), all-in-one handheld machines (B), or USB/wireless transducers that connect with tablets or smartphones (C).

TABLE 11.1 Diagnostic Capacity of Portable and Handheld Ultrasound Machines in the Hands of Experts.

Cardiovascular Anatomy	*Assessment Method*	*Published Examples (References)*
LV size	End-diastolic dimension	7, 8, 9, 14, 15, 17
LV hypertrophy	Interventricular septum and posterior wall diameter	7, 12, 16, 17, 21
Global LV function	Visual estimate	7, 9, 10, 12, 14, 15, 17, 18, 21
Left atrial enlargement	Parasternal long-axis dimension Visual estimate	8, 10 12
RV size	Visual estimate	10, 11, 12, 17, 18
Global RV function	Visual estimate	10, 11, 14, 18, 21
Inferior vena cava size	Subcostal long-axis diameter	9, 12
Pericardial effusion	Visually present vs. absent	9, 10, 12, 14, 18, 21

ECHOCARDIOGRAPHY AS AN ADJUNCT TO THE PHYSICAL EXAMINATION

FoCUS has proved to be clearly superior to the physical examination for several cardiovascular findings when used by both cardiologists and noncardiologists (Table 11.2).[12,19–46] Examples include left ventricular (LV) systolic dysfunction, increased LV filling pressures, and increased right atrial (RA) pressure. Compared to the traditional physical examination signs such as displaced cardiac point of maximal impulse, the presence of an S3 or S4 heart sound, and elevated jugular venous pressure, direct visualization of cardiac anatomy under ultrasound offers increased sensitivity for detection of these abnormalities.[25] FoCUS is also more accurate than a physical examination at localizing the source of a murmur in patients with valvular pathology, although such findings are not necessarily clinically significant.

DIAGNOSTIC TARGETS OF FoCUS

Beyond serving as an adjunct to the physical examination, FoCUS is a valuable diagnostic tool to further evaluate a number of specific clinical findings and diagnoses. The potential consequences of using FoCUS as a diagnostic test rather than just an extension of the physical examination have been detailed and debated in the literature and in clinical practice.[25] Potential diagnostic targets for FoCUS include LV and right ventricular (RV) function, volume status, and pericardial effusion.

LV Size and Function

FoCUS allows reliable and accurate assessment of global LV systolic function, even for novice users with only basic training.[12,24,46,47] The LV has a relatively simple hemi-ellipsoid shape and can be imaged from multiple views. An assessment of global function is made based on the degree of myocardial motion and thickening through systole. End systolic chamber size is also observed because patients with septic shock typically have hyperdynamic LV function with a small LV chamber and near-obliteration of the LV cavity at end-systole. Such visual assessments are a reasonable approximation of quantitative measurements of ejection fraction by formal echocardiography.[24] However, whereas quantitative estimates of LV function are possible with a complete echocardiographic study, with FoCUS, a qualitative approach is used to designate LV function as either normal or significantly abnormal.[5] When image quality is poor or LV function is uncertain, a formal echocardiogram is recommended to determine appropriate clinical management.

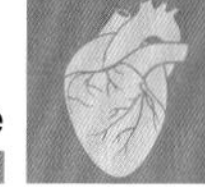

TABLE 11.2 Cardiac Bedside Examination: Traditional Versus FoCUS Findings.

Entity	*Physical Finding (SN%/SP%)*	*FoCUS Finding (SN%/SP%)*	*Notes*
LVSD	S3 in ED (11–51/85–98)[27]; rales in ED (13/98)[5] Displaced apical impulse (5–66/93–99)[27]; 15% incidence in symptomatic HFrEF cohort[28]	Subjective estimation of contraction and/or EPSS >1 cm (69–94/88–94)[12,19–23,26,29–35]	US criteria vary among studies but are easily learned and are reproducible by noncardiologists. Prevalence of physical findings in LVSD is <20%, and even lower in asymptomatic LVSD.
Elevated LA filling pressures	S4 (35–71/50–70)[27]	LAE (53–75/72–94)[19,22,36,37]	LAE is prognostic and not found by physical examination. US learned after brief training.
Pulmonary edema or interstitial disease	Rales (19–64/82–94)[27]; (62/68) in ED[5]	B lines (85–98/83–93)[35,38,41]	B lines are US artifacts and potentially vary among devices. US easily learned by novices. Prevalence of 13% in HFrEF cohort.[22]
Pleural effusion	Dullness to percussion (73–89/81–91)[27,39]	Fluid in thorax (64–90/72–95)[35,40]	Studies of physical findings used chest radiography as gold standard, whereas US used computed tomography. Significant increase in SN with US, especially for small effusions.
RVE or pulmonary hypertension	Sustained left parasternal lift (71/80)[27]	RV/LV > 1 (55/69)[42]	Nonspecific finding of RVE is seen in RVMI, submassive pulmonary embolism, chronic cor pulmonale. Expert US practice needed to use spectral Doppler.
Elevated central venous pressures	JVP (47–92/93–96)[27]; (37/87) in ED[35]; 22% incidence in HFrEF cohort[28]	IVC plethora (73/85)[43]	FoCUS is advantageous in the supine ICU patient. FoCUS data include nonexpert users. JVP by US correlates with physical estimates but underestimates catheter-confirmed pressure.
Valve regurgitation	Murmur for mild-or-worse mitral regurgitation (56–75/89–93) or aortic insufficiency (54–87/75–98)[27]	Color Doppler (82/93) for mild severity[45]	Color Doppler jet area limitations apply. Expert practice likely necessary to quantify severity.
Severe aortic stenosis	Late-peaking murmur (83–90/72–88)[27]	Restricted cusp mobility (85/89)[44]	Expert auscultation coupled with FoCUS may be the best screening method.

ED, Emergency department; *EPSS*, E-point septal separation; *FoCUS*, focused cardiac ultrasound; *HFrEF*, heart failure with reduced ejection fraction; *ICU*, intensive care unit; *IVC*, inferior vena cava; *JVP*, jugular venous pulsations; *LAE*, left atrial enlargement; *LVSD*, left ventricular systolic dysfunction; *POCUS*, point-of-care ultrasound; *RVE*, right ventricular enlargement; *RVMI*, right ventricular myocardial infarction; *S3*, third heart sound; *S4*, fourth heart sound; *SN%*, percent sensitivity; *SP%*, percent specificity; *US*, ultrasound.
Adapted from Kimura B. Point-of-care cardiac ultrasound techniques in the physical examination: better at the bedside. *Heart*. 2017;103:987–994, Table 2.

RV Size and Function

The RV has a less axially symmetric geometry than the LV. The base of the RV (tricuspid annulus) is in the same plane as the mitral annulus, whereas the body of the RV wraps around the LV in a U shape and connects to the RV outflow tract, which lies anterior to the aortic valve. As a result, it is more difficult to systematically image and assess the RV than the LV. Despite this, FoCUS can be a valid tool to assess RV size and function in clinically urgent situations.[48,49] The RV is significantly enlarged if it is larger than the LV (RV:LV size ratio >1:1). Other signs of RV pressure or volume overload include interventricular septal bowing toward the LV. However, FoCUS users must recognize that these are not specific or sensitive findings and do not necessarily indicate acute pathology because the same signs are present in chronic RV dysfunction. RV function normally appears as dynamic as that of the LV; any reduction in the RV dynamic motion raises concern for RV systolic dysfunction.

Pericardial Effusion

FoCUS is highly sensitive and specific for the detection of pericardial effusion.[12,50] Fluid in the pericardial space appears as a dark space between the myocardium and pericardium. Identification of pericardial fluid does not require the same careful attention to image quality as does the assessment of biventricular function or volume status, making FoCUS an accurate assessment tool even for less experienced users. As with ventricular function, multiple views are obtained to ensure that focal or loculated pockets of fluid are not missed. Pericardial fluid must also be carefully differentiated from pleural fluid, especially in the parasternal views, where the descending aorta serves as a dividing marker between fluid in the pericardial. space (superficial to the aorta) and fluid in the pleural space (deep to the aorta).

Intravascular Volume Status

Although a variety of ultrasound parameters have been studied for the assessment of intravascular volume status, assessment of inferior vena cava (IVC) size and respiratory variation is the most appropriate technique for FoCUS users in the spontaneously breathing patient. The IVC should be visualized in the long axis as it crosses the diaphragm into the RA. As intrathoracic pressure drops with spontaneous inspiration, blood is drawn into the thoracic cavity and the diameter of the intraabdominal IVC decreases. RA pressure is estimated by measuring the maximal diameter of the IVC 2 to 3 cm before it passes through the diaphragm and calculating the percentage change with inspiration.[51] M-mode can cause significant errors and should not be used to make IVC measurements because there is no way to visually ensure that the true long axis of the IVC is maintained throughout the respiratory cycle. In the spontaneously breathing patient, a dilated IVC with diminished inspiratory collapse indicates an elevated RA pressure.[52,53]

Notably, this method is not a reliable estimate of RA pressure in patients on positive-pressure ventilation because of alterations in intrathoracic pressure.[54] Additional potential confounding factors include baseline RV dysfunction, significant tricuspid regurgitation, and cardiac arrhythmias such as heart block. Other ultrasound parameters of volume status, such as stroke volume variation and aortic flow velocities, are more technically difficult and require a level of quantitative assessment that is beyond the ability of most FoCUS users.

LIMITATIONS OF FoCUS

More complex anatomic or physiologic abnormalities are typically beyond the scope of what FoCUS can reliably diagnose. FoCUS does not include quantitative assessment of blood flow or tissue velocities, so any diagnosis that relies on these metrics is outside the purview of FoCUS. This includes grading the severity of valvular abnormalities, determining the hemodynamic effects of a pericardial effusion, and diagnosing diastolic dysfunction. These limits should be especially respected in regard to valve assessment. Although obvious valve dysfunction may be observed, especially in extreme cases such as a severely calcified aortic valve or flail mitral valve leaflet, such findings should quickly be followed up with a formal echocardiogram.

Grading of valve dysfunction by ultrasound is a technically demanding task that incorporates complex quantitative assessments from multiple windows and is beyond the capacity of FoCUS. Despite this, FoCUS may be the only readily available tool in resource-limited areas and has been used as an effective screening tool for cardiac pathology, including valve disease, under these circumstances.[55] Utilizing remote review by experts, nonphysicians working in a low-resource area and trained in FoCUS were able to follow a screening protocol that included valve assessment (Fig. 11.2) to identify both mitral and aortic valve pathology (Fig. 11.3); the results were confirmed by formal echocardiography in 79% of cases.

Additionally, FoCUS is not sensitive enough to reliably diagnose regional wall motion abnormalities, aortic dissection, or LV thrombus.[1,5] If initial FoCUS findings suggest any of these diagnoses, additional studies are recommended to avoid diagnostic error. For example, image acquisition for regional wall motion assessment requires multiple apical views (4-chamber, 2-chamber, long-axis), with adequate endocardial definition to clearly see each of 17 wall segments. Contrast administration is often necessary for adequate visualization. Images that are off-axis or of insufficient quality can lead to misdiagnosis of regional myocardial dysfunction via both false-positive and false-negative findings. Identifying abnormal wall segment motion is also a high-level skill that requires extensive experience in echocardiographic interpretation and can be confounded by prior intrathoracic surgery, interventricular conduction delays, and ventricular interdependence.

Similarly, intimal flaps that might indicate aortic dissection can be confounded by image artifacts. This is not to say that such findings can never be captured by FoCUS; indeed, one small retrospective study indicated that patients with aortic dissection identified on initial FoCUS examination were ultimately diagnosed much faster and had higher survival rates than those who were not assessed with FoCUS.[56] However, FoCUS is not a sufficient test in these cases, and suspicion for any of these more complex abnormalities should lead to formal echocardiography or other imaging for confirmation of the diagnosis.

BASIC APPROACH TO THE FoCUS EXAMINATION

Under ideal circumstances, the mechanics of performing a FoCUS examination are similar to those of a sonographer performing standard echocardiography. However, it is often difficult to achieve optimal positioning and attain complete views in clinically urgent scenarios. This section presents a suggested approach to the FoCUS examination. A comprehensive curriculum is beyond the scope of this chapter, but numerous online resources are available for self-study (Table 11.3). After a standard approach to the FoCUS examination is implemented, positioning and views can be adjusted as needed based on the clinical setting.

Views are obtained from one of three acoustic windows, areas where the heart can be visualized with minimal interference from the lungs or ribs. These are the parasternal, the apical, and the subcostal windows (Fig. 11.4). There are standard starting points for each window that should be fairly consistent from patient to patient. From these standard locations, larger initial adjustments with the transducer are often needed to localize the anatomy because the orientation and position of the heart vary slightly for each patient. This may involve moving up or down between rib spaces as needed. Finer adjustments are then made with the transducer to achieve the desired view.

POSITIONING

Parasternal and apical views are best obtained with the patient in the left lateral decubitus position. If possible, have the patient raise the left arm above the head. This will widen the intercostal spaces and create a larger ultrasound window. If the patient is unable to roll into a left lateral decubitus position, the parasternal views can be obtained from a supine position. However, quality apical views are often difficult to obtain in supine patients.

Subcostal views are best obtained with the patient supine. If necessary, have the patient bend the knees up to relax the abdominal wall and allow for more maneuverability of the probe.

Before beginning the examination, drape the patient's chest with a towel. In female patients, the towel can be used to both cover and lift breast tissue when obtaining apical views.

STANDARD VIEWS

There are five standard views for a FoCUS examination, and they are typically obtained in the following order: parasternal long-axis, parasternal short-axis at the mid-ventricle, apical 4-chamber, subcostal 4-chamber, and subcostal IVC views. For less experienced users, the parasternal and subcostal views are the easiest to obtain and are less susceptible to errors in acquisition that can lead to inaccurate interpretation. Additional views may be learned over time, but the five views described here form the basis of a standard examination.

Parasternal Long-Axis View

The parasternal long-axis view is usually the best view to begin an examination because it is the easiest and often fastest view to obtain. To obtain the view, the transducer is placed in the 3rd or 4th intercostal space just left of the sternal border, with the notch of the probe pointed toward the patient's right shoulder (Fig. 11.5A). Adjustment to lower intercostal spaces may be needed to find the optimal acoustic window. The image sector should be roughly parallel to a line running between the patient's right shoulder and left hip, creating a slice through the long axis of the heart (Fig. 11.5B). This view can give an initial impression of LV function, although the apical segments are usually not visible, and it provides a quick screen of the mitral and aortic valves and aortic root.

Parasternal Short-Axis View at the Mid-Ventricle

An optimal parasternal axis view is best obtained by starting from a quality parasternal long-axis view and rotating the

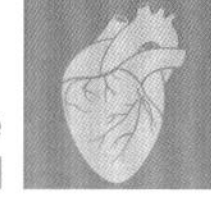

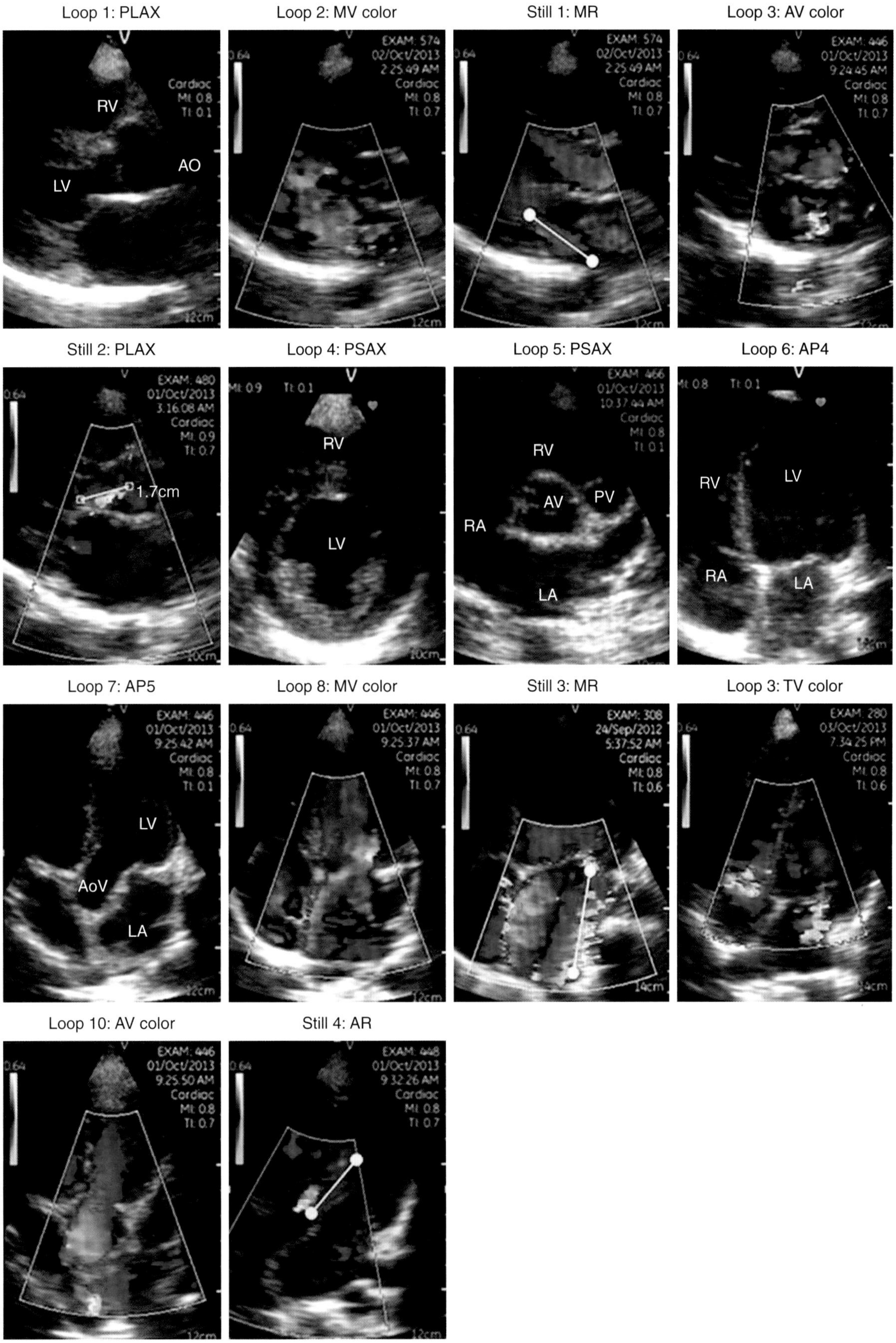

Loop 1: PLAX — RV, AO, LV

Loop 2: MV color

Still 1: MR

Loop 3: AV color

Still 2: PLAX — 1.7cm

Loop 4: PSAX — RV, LV

Loop 5: PSAX — RV, AV, PV, RA, LA

Loop 6: AP4 — RV, LV, RA, LA

Loop 7: AP5 — LV, AoV, LA

Loop 8: MV color

Still 3: MR

Loop 3: TV color

Loop 10: AV color

Still 4: AR

Fig. 11.2 FoCUS screening protocol used in a resource-limited area. Simplified screening protocol using handheld devices for evaluation of heart diseases in adults consists of 14 images (seven views): 10 loops and 4 still frames. *AoV*, Aortic valve; *AP4*, apical four chambers; *AP5*, apical five chambers; *AR*, aortic regurgitation; *MR*, mitral regurgitation; *MV*, mitral valve; *PLAX*, parasternal long-axis; *PSAX*, parasternal short-axis; *TV*, tricuspid valve. (From Nascimento B, Beaton A, Nunes MCP, et al. Integration of echocardiographic screening by non-physicians with remote reading in primary care. *Heart*. 2019;105:283–290.)

transducer 90 degrees clockwise. The transducer notch then points toward the patient's left shoulder. If starting de novo, the transducer is placed in the 3rd or 4th intercostal space with the notch of the probe pointed toward the patient's left shoulder (Fig. 11.5C). Depending on the angle of the probe, there are a number of possible short-axis views, moving from the apex of the LV to the aortic valve. The most useful view for FoCUS is at the level of the papillary muscles, or mid-ventricle; this position allows for the best assessment of LV size and systolic function (Fig. 11.5D). It also shows the RV size relative to the LV chamber.

Apical 4-Chamber View

The apical 4-chamber view is the most difficult to obtain because the acoustic window and location of the apex can vary widely among patients. However, if a quality image can be obtained, the apical 4-chamber view is the most helpful view for assessment of biventricular size and systolic function because it provides the best global view of the ventricles. When obtaining this view, palpation for the apical impulse can provide a starting place for probe position. If the apical impulse is not palpable, the transducer is initially placed in the 5th intercostal space, slightly lateral to the mid-clavicular line. The notch on the probe is pointed toward the patient's left side (Fig. 11.6A).

A true apical 4-chamber view captures all four cardiac chambers. The interventricular and interatrial septa should appear as a continuous vertical line. The tricuspid and mitral valves are also visible and form a continuous horizontal line (Fig. 11.6B). Importantly, the image sector cuts through the LV at its maximal long-axis diameter, called the *true apex*. If the sector cuts either above or below the true apex, the apex of the LV will appear to be rounded and more mobile, and the LV chamber size will appear falsely shortened (*foreshortening*). It is important to avoid foreshortening because it can cause significant error in the evaluation of both LV size and LV function.

Subcostal 4-Chamber View

The subcostal views are important to master for FoCUS because they may be the only obtainable views in critically ill patients due to the fixed positioning and interference of lung tissue in patients on positive-pressure ventilation. It is also particularly useful in ambulatory patients with underlying obstructive lung disease, in whom hyperinflation of the lungs can obscure both the parasternal and the apical views. For many providers, the subcostal views are the most commonly used views because

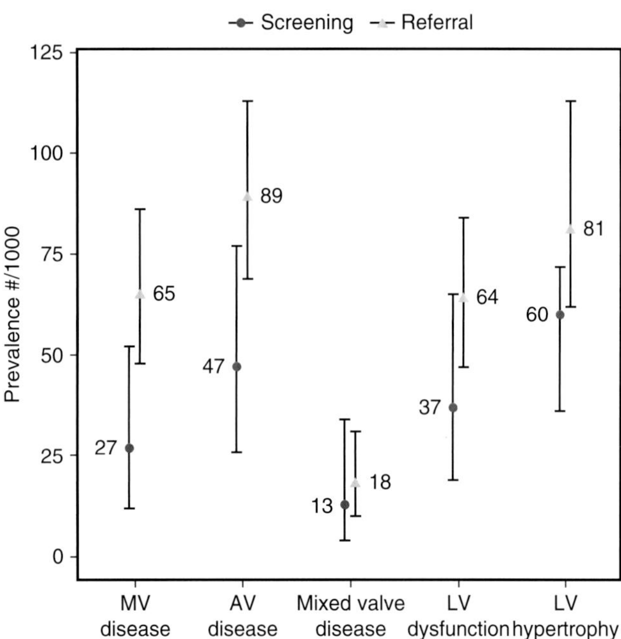

Fig. 11.3 Prevalence of cardiac pathology diagnosed by remote expert review of FoCUS images. Echocardiographic prevalence of major heart disease requiring priority referral based on the final conclusion of the expert readers, according to study group. *AV*, aortic valve; *MV*, mitral valve. (From Nascimento B, Beaton A, Nunes MCP, et al. Integration of echocardiographic screening by non-physicians with remote reading in primary care. *Heart* 2019;105:283–290.)

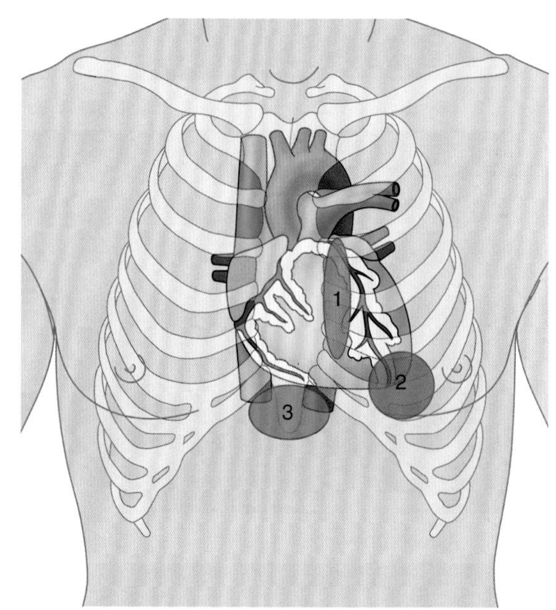

Fig. 11.4 Transthoracic echocardiographic windows. *(1)* Parasternal window, *(2)* apical window, and *(3)* subcostal window.

TABLE 11.3 Recommended Open-Access Online Resources for Learning FoCUS.

Publisher	*Title of Online Course/Modules*	*Website at the Time of Publication*
American Society of Echocardiography	Cardiovascular point-of-care imaging for the medical student and novice user	https://aselearninghub.org/topclass/topclass.do?expand-OfferingDetails-Offeringid=138217
American Society of Emergency Physicians	Echocardiography for emergency physicians	https://www.acep.org/sonoguide/cardiac.html
Stanford University	Focused bedside TTE and ultrasound	https://www.edx.org/course/focused-bedside-tte-and-ultrasound
University of Toronto	Virtual transthoracic echocardiography: Focused cardiac ultrasound	https://pie.med.utoronto.ca/TTE/TTE_content/focus.html
University of Utah	Perioperative echocardiography education (includes some noncardiac topics)	https://echo.anesthesia.med.utah.edu/tee/focus-content/

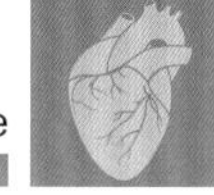

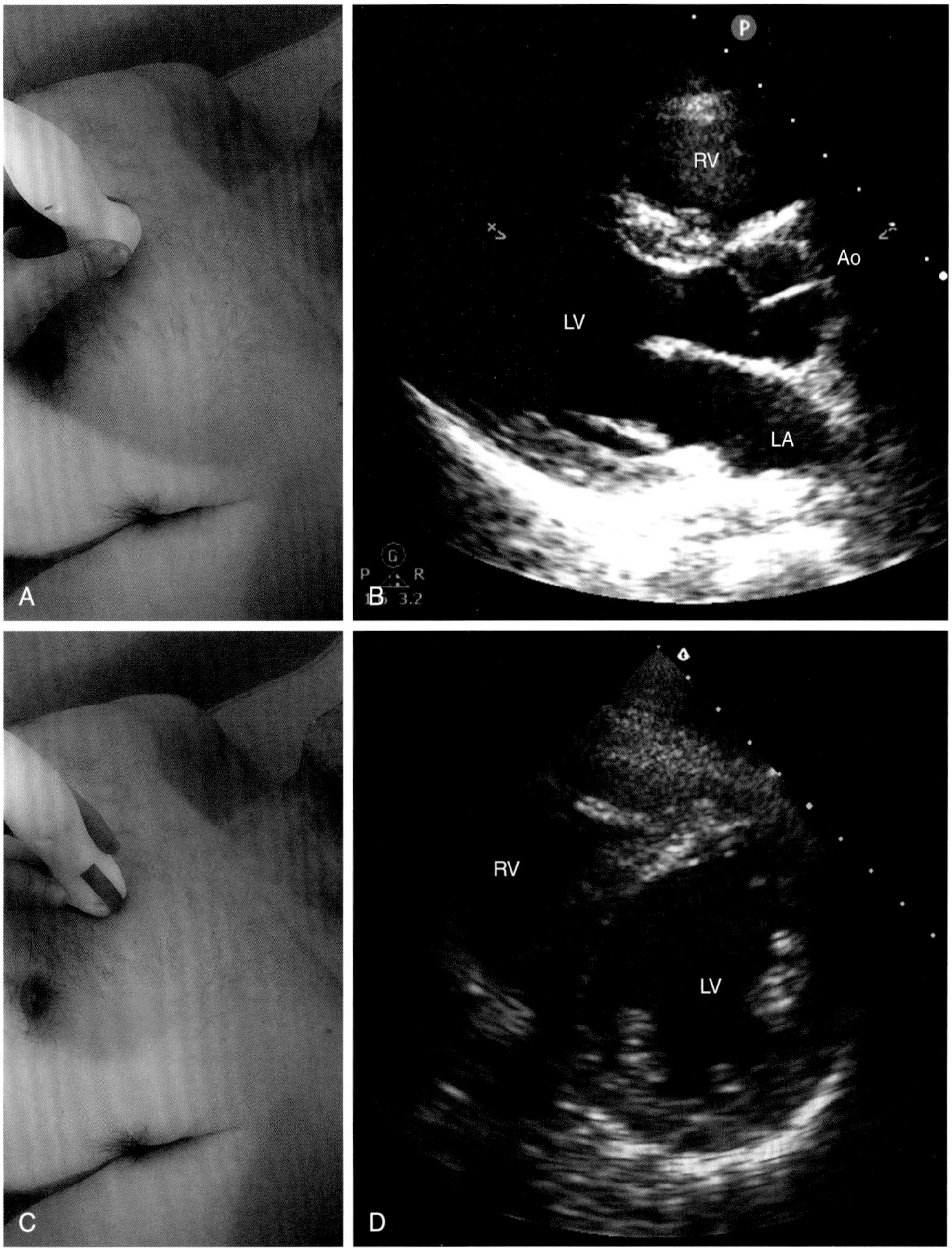

Fig. 11.5 Parasternal views. (A) Probe position for the parasternal long-axis (PLAX) view: in the 3rd or 4th intercostal space with the probe notch pointed toward the patient's right shoulder. (B) Normal anatomy of the PLAX view (Video 11.5B). *Ao,* Aorta. (C) Probe position for the parasternal short-axis (PSAX) view: rotated 90-degrees clockwise from the PLAX view, with the probe notch pointed toward the patient's left shoulder. (D) Normal anatomy of the PSAX view (Video 11.5D).

they provide a rapid assessment of biventricular function and volume status.

To obtain the subcostal 4-chamber view, the transducer is placed in the epigastric region, just below the xyphoid process. The notch on the transducer points toward the patient's left side (Fig. 11.7A). The subcostal 4-chamber view is similar to the apical 4-chamber view except that the probe is centered over the right side of the heart rather than the apex. As in the apical 4-chamber view, both ventricles, both atria, and both atrioventricular valves are seen (Fig. 11.7B). The ventricles may be slightly foreshortened and the LV apex is often not visible, but this view gives a good sense of global biventricular function.

Subcostal Inferior Vena Cava View

The easiest way to obtain an optimal view of the IVC is to start from a quality subcostal 4-chamber view that is centered on the RA. Keeping the RA centered, the transducer is rotated counterclockwise by approximately 90 degrees until the IVC is visualized crossing the diaphragm and draining into the RA. The transducer notch is pointed approximately toward the patient's head (Fig. 11.7C). Once the IVC is visualized entering the RA, the transducer can then be rotated or angled slightly as needed to bring the IVC into a full long-axis view (Fig. 11.7D).

If starting de novo, the transducer is placed in the epigastric region, just below the xiphoid process, with the transducer notch pointed toward the patient's head. The transducer is then

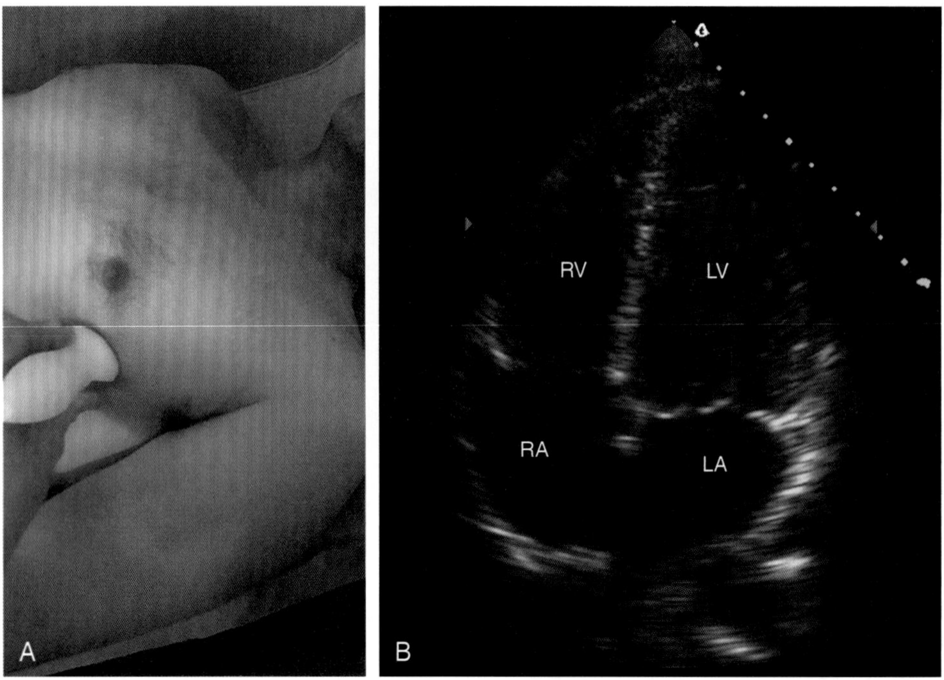

Fig. 11.6 **Apical views.** (A) Probe position for the apical 4-chamber (A4C) view: probe notch pointed toward the patient's left side. (B) Normal anatomy of the A4C view (Video 11.6B).

angled slowly in the lateral direction, toward the patient's right side, until the IVC comes into view. The transducer often needs to be rotated slightly clockwise or counterclockwise to bring the vessel into a long-axis view. It is important to trace the IVC to the point where it enters the RA. This ensures that you are seeing the IVC rather than the aorta, which runs just deep and parallel to the IVC, or one of the hepatic veins.

DOCUMENTATION

At a minimum, representative FoCUS images used for clinical decision making should be stored locally on the machine with which they were obtained. Ideally, images should also be stored in the same central repository as formal echocardiographic images so that providers can make direct comparison with past or future studies. This allows for image quality assurance and allows FoCUS users to get feedback on their images from others for ongoing education and skills improvement.

The provider performing FoCUS should document the examination in the electronic medical record. FoCUS results are typically reported along with the physical examination findings, with the text specifying the views obtained, impression of the study quality, image interpretation (with still frame images if possible), and the storage location of saved cine images.

EMERGENCY DIAGNOSES

There are many potential diagnoses that can be made using FoCUS, and a full review of specific diagnoses is beyond the scope of this chapter. However, there are several emergent clinical scenarios in which FoCUS can be key to rapid diagnosis and management.

UNDIFFERENTIATED HYPOTENSION AND SHOCK

FoCUS allows a direct visualization of cardiac anatomy and can provide valuable insight into potential causes of shock.[57] The primary role of FoCUS in this setting is to assess for potential cardiogenic shock by identifying abnormal LV systolic function and a dilated IVC consistent with elevated RA pressure. It is important to identify cardiogenic shock early because the treatment immediately diverges from the treatment of other types of shock. Standard initial treatment for most causes of hypotension, including fluids and vasopressors, can be severely detrimental to patients with cardiogenic shock. Other clues to shock etiology can also be identified through FoCUS, including hyperdynamic LV function in some cases of septic shock, pericardial effusion in a clinical setting consistent with tamponade, and a completely collapsible IVC in hypovolemic or hemorrhagic shock.

PENETRATING CHEST TRAUMA

In trauma patients, cardiac ultrasound is incorporated as part of a more comprehensive examination that includes lung and abdominal ultrasound, known as the Focused Assessment with Sonography in Trauma (FAST) examination.[58] The FAST examination is designed to look for sources of hemorrhage after trauma. From a cardiac standpoint, this entails assessing for pericardial effusion, which would suggest hemopericardium, or a hyperdynamic LV with a completely collapsible IVC, which might indicate hemorrhagic shock.

MASSIVE PULMONARY EMBOLUS

Pulmonary embolus (PE) is a relatively common diagnosis and cause of cardiovascular mortality in both emergency and critical care settings. Whereas computed tomographic (CT) angiography is the best diagnostic test for pulmonary embolus, FoCUS can be used to assess for indirect signs of PE when patients are too unstable for CT. In patients who have already been diagnosed with PE, FoCUS can be used to screen for evidence of right heart strain.[49] Signs of clinically

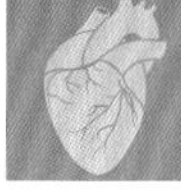

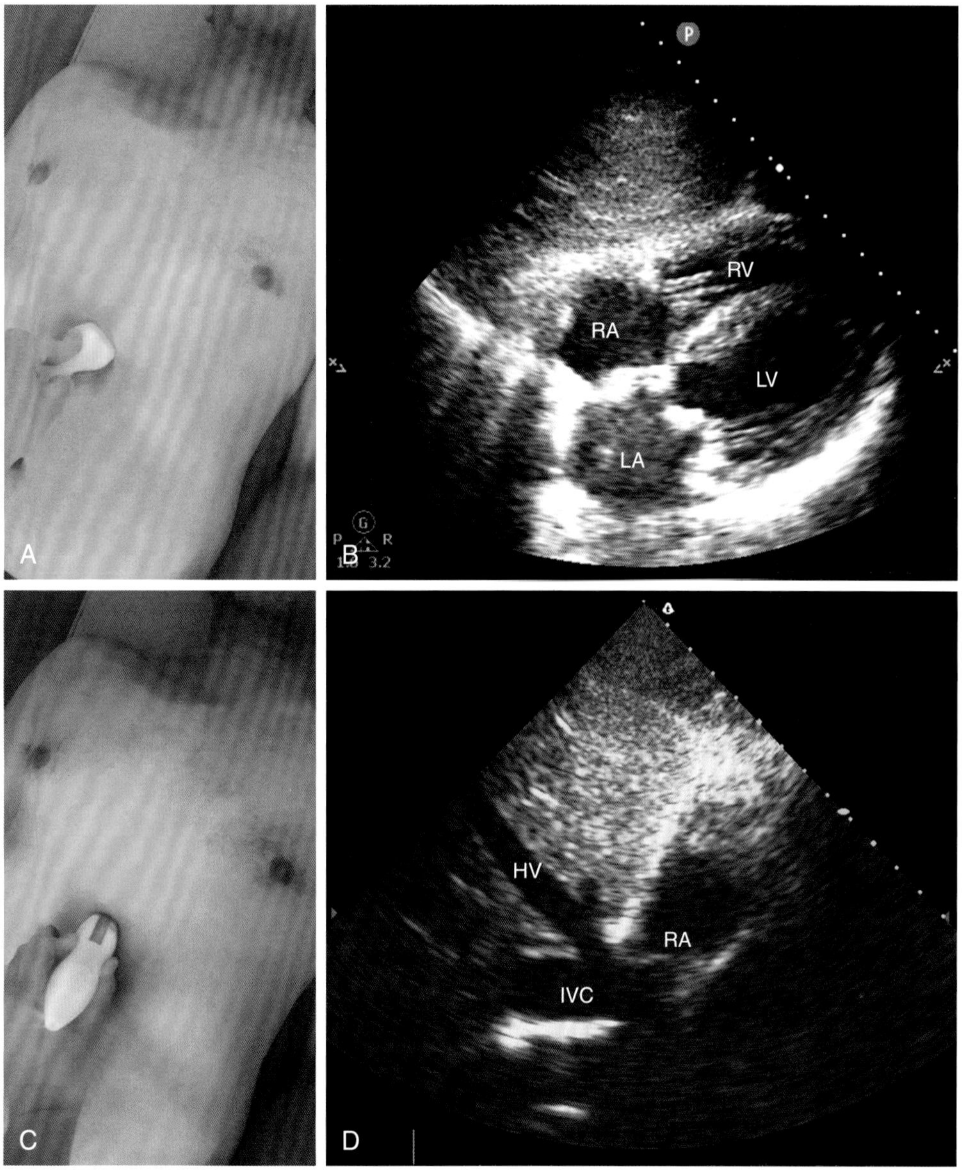

Fig. 11.7 **Subcostal views.** (A) Probe position for the subcostal 4-chamber (4C) view: probe beneath the xiphoid process with notch pointed toward the patient's left side. (B) Normal anatomy of the subcostal 4C view (Video 11.7B). (C) Probe position for the subcostal inferior vena cava view: probe notch pointed toward the patient's head. (D) Normal anatomy of the PSAX view (Video 11.7D). *HV*, Hepatic vein; *IVC*, inferior vena cava.

significant PE include significant RV enlargement with an RV:LV size ratio >1:1, RV hypokinesis, bowing of the interventricular septum into the LV, and a dilated IVC consistent with elevated RV filling pressures. FoCUS is neither sensitive nor specific in this setting because these ultrasound findings may be absent in patients with massive PE or present in patients with chronic RV dysfunction.[59,60] Suspected abnormalities should be confirmed with formal echocardiography. However, FoCUS remains a valuable tool to rapidly triage patients with possible or proven PE. In patients with severe hemodynamic instability or arrest, it may be the only available imaging tool to support management decisions such as administration of thrombolytics.

CARDIAC TAMPONADE

Cardiac tamponade is ultimately a clinical diagnosis and should not be made based on ultrasound alone. However, in patients with pericardial effusion, FoCUS can be used to assess for signs of tamponade.[58] FoCUS users should primarily look for diastolic collapse of the RA and RV, which occurs when intrapericardial pressure is elevated above intracardiac pressure. Additional supporting evidence includes interventricular septal shifting to the left with inspiration and a dilated IVC. Notably, the amount of pericardial fluid does not necessarily correlate with the presence or absence of tamponade. Acute pericardial effusions can be hemodynamically significant with relatively little intrapericardial volume, and chronic effusions that accumulate slowly can build up to a large volume without causing symptoms or hemodynamic effect. When tamponade is suspected, a formal echocardiogram should be obtained immediately if the clinical scenario allows. Echocardiography produces additional quantitative measurements that can support the diagnosis of tamponade and provides ultrasound guidance during pericardiocentesis. In emergency situations when echocardiography is not immediately available, FoCUS can also be used for ultrasound-guided pericardiocentesis.

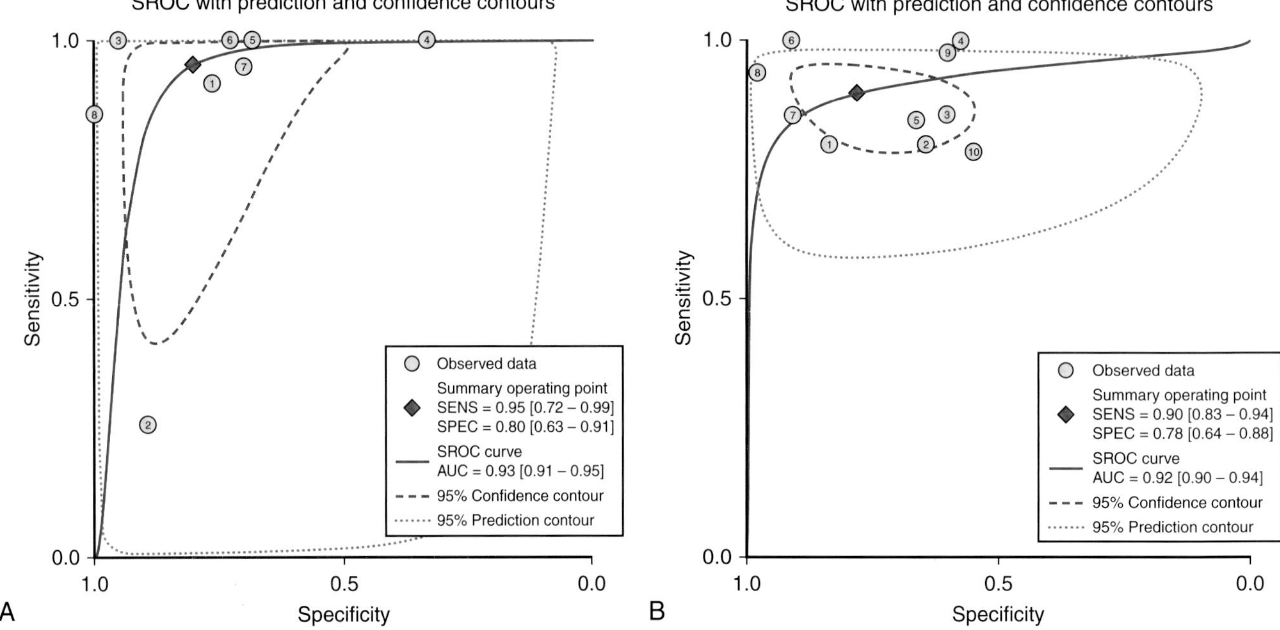

Fig. 11.8 Accuracy of outcome prediction in cardiac arrest with pulseless electrical activity using FoCUS. (A) Hierarchical summary receiver operating characteristic (SROC) model for prediction of return of spontaneous circulation using focused echocardiography. (B) Hierarchical SROC model for prediction of survival to hospital admission using focused echocardiography. *AUC*, Area under the curve; *SENS*, sensitivity; *SPEC*, specificity. (From Tsou Y, Kurbedin J, Chen Y-S, et al. Accuracy of point-of-care focused echocardiography in predicting outcome of resuscitation in cardiac arrest patients: a systematic review and meta-analysis. *Resuscitation*. 2017;114:92–99.)

CARDIAC ARREST

In cases of arrest with pulseless electrical activity (PEA), patients with organized cardiac contraction have improved survival compared to those with electromechanical dissociation.[61] In cases of cardiac arrest, FoCUS is used to assess for coordinated ventricular contraction and to identify reversible causes of arrest. Successful protocols generally focus on targeted imaging from the subcostal window between rounds of chest compressions to minimize interruption of cardiopulmonary resuscitation (CPR). In addition to aiding prognosis during resuscitation attempts by differentiating between patients with asystole and those with cardiac contraction, FoCUS can impact management by identifying reversible causes of PEA arrest (e.g., signs of tamponade or massive pulmonary embolism). It can also guide emergency procedures during resuscitation.

PATIENT OUTCOMES

Although the effect of FoCUS on outcomes such as patient mortality is difficult to quantify in most cases, it clearly has potential to impact physician decision making and patient care. Research studies on the impact of FoCUS have largely used clinical reasoning and management decisions as surrogate outcomes. There is a growing body of literature to suggest that FoCUS can decrease diagnostic uncertainty, change treatment plans, and improve the speed of patient disposition in a variety of clinical settings. For example, routine FoCUS screening of inpatients can alter the suspected diagnosis and management in approximately 20% of cases.[11]

In patients with undifferentiated hypotension, a number of studies have demonstrated that FoCUS decreases diagnostic uncertainty. In one randomized controlled trial, clinicians using FoCUS identified the correct cause of hypotension as the most likely cause in 80% of cases, compared with 50% of cases without the use of FoCUS.[57] The use of FoCUS also significantly impacts management[61,62] and decreases the time to disposition when used during initial patient evaluation.[63] Potential alterations in management include administering intravenous fluids or diuretics, starting inotropes or vasopressors, and moving toward pericardiocentesis. Retrospective data suggest that FoCUS-guided management of undifferentiated shock may lead to improved patient survival and lower rates of renal injury.[64]

In PEA arrest, the identification of coordinated ventricular contractility using FoCUS has been shown to have prognostic value.[61,65] Patients with cardiac contractility have a significantly better outcome than those with cardiac standstill, and FoCUS can rapidly differentiate between these two states. By identifying those with cardiac contractility, FoCUS has 92% to 95% sensitivity and 80% specificity for predicting the return of spontaneous circulation[66,67] (Fig. 11.8). Additionally, the use of FoCUS alters management in up to 89% of PEA arrest cases[10] by identifying possible causes of the arrest.

In patients with heart failure, the use of FoCUS to assess volume status helps guide the adjustment of diuretic dosing in the outpatient setting[68] (Fig. 11.9).

In specific clinical scenarios, FoCUS has been shown to directly impact patient outcomes. For patients with penetrating chest trauma, FoCUS decreases the time to diagnosis and disposition and has been shown to improve survival.[69] FoCUS can rapidly and accurately identify pericardial effusion after chest trauma, leading to decreased time from presentation to operative intervention. For patients with systolic heart failure, FoCUS measurement of IVC size and collapsibility before discharge proved to be predictive of the risk for hospital readmission[70,71] (Fig. 11.10).

TRAINING AND CERTIFICATION

Any provider who uses FoCUS in their clinical practice should have appropriate training in image acquisition, quality

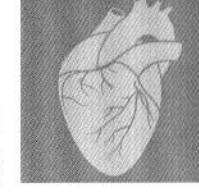

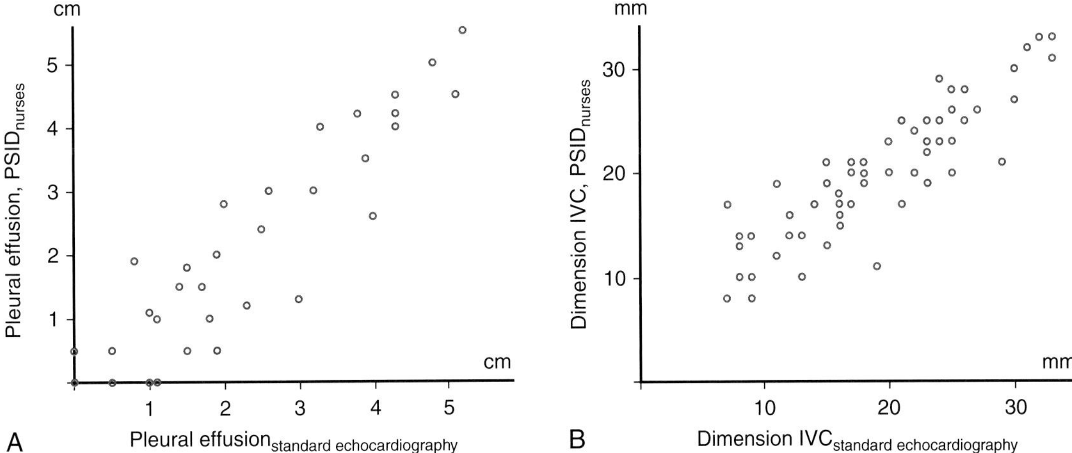

Fig. 11.9 Correlation between FoCUS findings and findings from formal echocardiography. Ultrasound indices to assess volume status were obtained by reference echocardiography and compared with (A) quantification of pleural effusion measured as centimeters of fluid between the diaphragm and the lung surface when the patient was in a sitting position and (B) end-expiratory dimension of the inferior vena cava (IVC). Both comparison measurements were obtained by nurses performing FoCUS examinations using a pocket-sized imaging device (PSID). In A, the finding of no effusion, as measured by both the nurse and the reference study, is represented at the coordinates (0,0), and the point at (0.5,0.5) refers to effusion in the costodiaphragmatic recess only, as measured by both users. (From Gundersen G, Norekval T, Haug HH, et al. Adding point of care ultrasound to assess volume status in heart failure patients in a nurse let outpatient clinic: a randomized study. *Heart.* 2016;102:29–34.)

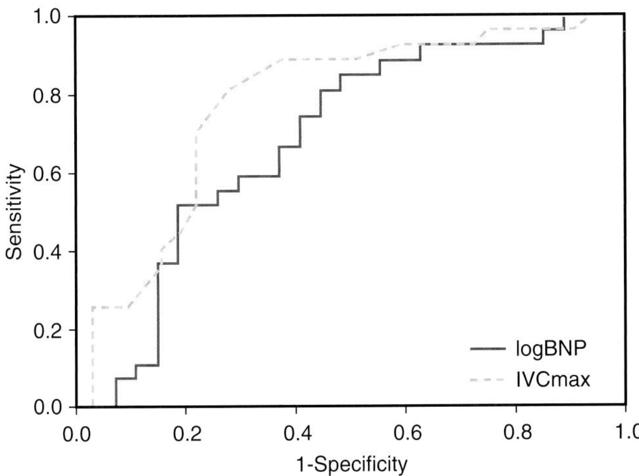

Fig. 11.10 Prognostic value of FoCUS-measured inferior vena cava diameter to predict hospital readmission. Receiver-operator curves for log-transformed values for brain natriuretic peptide (logBNP; *solid line*) and maximum diameter of the inferior vena cava (IVCmax; *dashed line*) to predict hospital readmission. The area under the curve is greater for IVCmax, indicating a greater likelihood of correctly predicting the need for repeat hospitalization after inpatient therapy for acutely decompensated congestive heart failure. (From Goonewardena S, Gemignani A, Ronan A, et al. Comparison of hand-carried ultrasound assessment of the inferior vena cava and N-terminal probrain natriuretic peptide for predicting readmission after hospitalization for acute decompensated heart failure. *JACC Cardiovasc Imaging.* 2008;1:595–601.)

assessment, and image interpretation before using the tool for clinical decision making. Current education practices are highly variable across specialties and institutions. Structured training in POCUS is required for emergency and critical care medicine residents, but outside of these specialties, the onus typically remains on individual programs and practitioners to establish formalized training. Although there is emerging interest in standardizing practices, there are currently no FoCUS education guidelines in the United States.

CURRENT TRAINING PRACTICES

Increasingly, FoCUS training is incorporated into medical school education.[72] Numerous curricula have been published that effectively incorporate ultrasound training into pathophysiology, anatomy, and physical examination courses longitudinally through the medical school years. An online curriculum has also been published by the American Society of Echocardiography that is freely available for medical students and other novice users.[73] Some residency programs in specialties outside emergency and critical care medicine have also instituted POCUS training, although resident surveys indicate that there is still a relative paucity of formal training compared to learner demand.[74]

Given the growing ubiquity of ultrasound and the shift toward emphasizing ultrasound skills earlier in training, FoCUS may ultimately be included as a core competency for all physicians, similar to the physical examination or basic skills in interpretation of chest radiographs. Currently, the lack of universal training opportunities poses a barrier to novice users without ready access to formal FoCUS education. Practitioners interested in FoCUS may use published resources to obtain didactic education and work locally with trained ultrasound practitioners for hands-on practice.

Current published training programs typically include a blend of didactic and hands-on learning.[72] Didactics can successfully be delivered through online modules, text, independent learning, or lecture. Strategies for incorporating hands-on learning vary and may be limited by instructor availability. These include one-on-one proctored scanning with an ultrasound expert, small groups wherein learners rotate between observation and practice scanning under the guidance of an ultrasound expert, and independent scanning followed by expert review and adjudication. Simulation is a frequently utilized tool to allow for basic hands-on practice in a nonthreatening, nonurgent environment.[75,76]

TRAINING RECOMMENDATIONS

All FoCUS users should go through formalized training to develop a basic foundation of knowledge.[1] Best practices for ultrasound training are unclear. Heterogeneity in published studies of successful training protocols makes it difficult to formulate generalizable, evidence-based training practices. Studies have included a range of learner populations, from medical students to attending physicians, as well as variable training length, methods, and learning targets. However, there are several generally agreed-upon principles for ultrasound training.[1,77]

1. Structured Training Should Include Didactic and Hands-On Learning

FoCUS is a complex task that requires both cognitive and psychomotor skills. The cognitive skills can be attained through a variety of didactic modalities, including lectures, reading, and videos.[78] There are numerous online modules, books, and other freely available resources for didactic learning in FoCUS. Although this builds a theoretical knowledge base and can be attained through independent learning, it is essential to also learn the technical skills of FoCUS through practice scanning. This requires instruction from a trained ultrasound practitioner. Ideally, hands-on practice is performed with real-time coaching from a sonographer or other trained expert in cardiac ultrasound. Simulation has proved to be a valuable and effective tool for building basic scanning skills, but it does not supplant the need to scan live patients.[78] The difficulty of FoCUS should not be underestimated. Although FoCUS is a directed examination using portable equipment with less complex functions than formal echocardiography machines, FoCUS examinations are often performed under the most arduous and demanding clinical circumstances. It takes a significant amount of technical skill to scan critically ill patients who are suboptimally positioned, often ventilated, and with various bandages, chest tubes, and other barriers to scanning. Being able to obtain quality images in such a setting is difficult even for trained sonographers and requires dedicated practice and coaching for aspiring FoCUS users.

2. Training Should Address Image Acquisition, Quality Assessment, and Image Interpretation

FoCUS practitioners must be able to acquire and interpret quality images in order to safely incorporate cardiac ultrasound into clinical care. As stated earlier, image acquisition requires practice to build technical skill. Published FoCUS curricula that have demonstrated success typically include instruction on image acquisition and interpretation. However, another important step in performing FoCUS is identifying images that are not of diagnostic quality. Although it is generally implied that only quality images will be used for interpretation, the step of assessing image quality should be explicitly included as a routine part of the FoCUS examination.

3. Ongoing Practice Is Required for Skills Retention

Although there are no standards for maintenance of competency, FoCUS providers should continue regular practice to maintain their skills after achieving initial proficiency. Well-trained residents who demonstrated competency in FoCUS at the end of their graduate medical education showed a loss of skill in just 1 to 2 years of nonuse after training.[79]

CERTIFICATION, CREDENTIALING, AND COMPETENCY

There is no required certification process for POCUS, but a variety of certification programs are available that vary widely in length and rigor of training. The idea of mandated certification is controversial because certification does not guarantee competency and places an additional financial burden on individual practitioners. Multiple subspecialties have identified FoCUS as an integral part of training, including emergency and critical care medicine. These trainees are expected to develop basic competency in FoCUS through their graduate medical education program and therefore should not need additional certification.

However, this issue is complicated by the lack of consistent training and competency standards. Competency standards are currently based on a minimum number of proctored scans performed, although the average number of scans needed to achieve competency is not well defined and likely varies widely among individuals. Studies on FoCUS training and assessment are very heterogeneous in methodology, study population, and target outcomes. For views that are easier to obtain, such as the parasternal long-axis view,[80] and simple clinical targets such as the presence or absence of pericardial effusion, it is possible to attain proficiency with relatively few scans.[81] However, to perform a full FoCUS examination on a critically ill patient and be able to diagnose a full range of pathologies, more training is needed. The recommended number of scans for presumed competency currently varies widely by society and specialty (Table 11.4).[1,2,6,82,83]

Individual institutions also vary in their credentialing requirements for FoCUS. Some hospitals have no formal credentialing procedure for POCUS, leaving individual providers to incorporate FoCUS into their practice as they choose. Other institutions require formal privileging and credentialing before allowing providers to perform, document, and in some cases bill for FoCUS. These institutions may require either internal or external certification before granting privileges, and they may expect credentialed providers to perform a minimum number of scans annually to maintain privileges. Credentialing procedures may change over time as FoCUS becomes more ubiquitous. The American College of Emergency Medicine recommends that every emergency medicine resident be provided with a credentialing letter on completion of their training.[2]

QUALITY ASSURANCE

As with training practices and competency maintenance, there is no published standard for quality assurance in FoCUS. This is an important issue because image misinterpretation, the use of poor-quality images for clinical decision making, or failure to refer patients for formal echocardiography when appropriate can lead to adverse patient outcomes. Some institutions have created systems that allow for basic quality assurance mechanisms, including automatic digital storage of FoCUS images in the same location as echocardiographic images and periodic expert review of FoCUS images. FoCUS users ultimately benefit from such practices because they allow other providers to verify their findings and provide ongoing learning and skills acquisition through expert feedback and correlation of FoCUS findings with the formal echocardiogram. Even with such systems in place, however, there is currently no mechanism for ensuring image quality at the point of care. Therefore, individual providers should be trained in image quality assessment and should always check image quality at the time of acquisition, before interpretation.

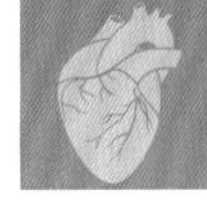

TABLE 11.4 Competency Standards for Performing Focused Cardiac Ultrasound.

Professional Society	*Recommended Training*	*Comments*
American College of Emergency Physicians	25–50 scans performed and interpreted[2]	• Training examinations should include a range of pathologies and patient types • All training examinations should be faculty reviewed • Some form of individualized assessment of competency after training
Society of Critical Care Medicine	30 scans performed, 50 scans interpreted[82]	• At least 20 hours of didactics during critical care fellowship
Canadian Cardiovascular Society, Canadian Society of Echocardiography	40 scans performed, 90 scans interpreted[83]	• Half of scans performed should contain some cardiac pathology • All performed scans should be under supervision of an ultrasound expert
American Society of Echocardiography	No recommended minimum[1]	—
European Society of Cardiovascular Imaging	No recommended minimum[6]	• Number of required scans should be adjusted for each individual based on ongoing competency assessments

SUMMARY Focused Cardiac Ultrasound at the Bedside.

Diagnostic Target	Goals of FoCUS	Imaging Views	Limitations
LV size and function	• Estimate overall LV systolic function (normal or mildly, moderately, or severely reduced). • Estimate LV size (relative to size of aortic root).	• Parasternal long- and short-axis views of LV • Apical 4-chamber view	• Quantitative measurement of LV ejection fraction is rarely possible. • Evaluation of regional wall motion requires considerable expertise but may be suggested by FoCUS findings.
RV size and function	• Estimate RV systolic function. • Detect RV dilation.	• Apical 4-chamber view • Subcostal view	• Complex RV shape limits evaluation of size and systolic function.
Pericardial effusion	• Detect pericardial effusion. • Estimate effusion size (small, moderate, or large).	• Parasternal • Apical • Subcostal	• Loculated effusions may be missed. • Tamponade physiology is a clinical diagnosis that should be considered for all moderate or large effusions.
Volume status	• Evaluate central venous pressure.	• Inferior vena cava size and respiratory variation from subcostal view (RA pressure)	• Unreliable in ventilated patients.
Other	• More complex anatomic and physiologic abnormalities may be suspected on a FoCUS study.	• All views	• A diagnostic echocardiogram is recommended when regional wall motion abnormalities are a concern, to evaluate for aortic disease, for valve stenosis or regurgitation, or to estimate pulmonary pressures.

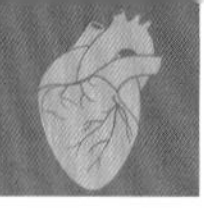

REFERENCES

1. Spencer K, Kimura B, et al. Focused cardiac ultrasound: recommendations from the American Society of Echocardiography. *J Am Soc Echocardiogr*. 2013;26:567–581.
2. Tayal V, Raio C, et al. Ultrasound guidelines: emergency, point-of-care, and clinical ultrasound guidelines in medicine. *Ann Emerg Med*. 2017;69:e27–e54.
3. Levitov A, Frankel H, et al. Guidelines for the appropriate use of bedside general and cardiac ultrasonography in the evaluation of crucially ill patients – Part II: cardiac ultrasound. *Crit Care Med*. 2016;44:1206–1227.
4. Via G, Hussain A, et al. International evidence-based recommendations for focused cardiac ultrasound. *J Am Soc Echocardiogr*. 2014;27:e1–e33. 683.
5. Labovitz A, Noble V, et al. Focused cardiac ultrasound in the emergent setting: a consensus statement of the American Society of Echocardiography and American College of Emergency Physicians. *J Am Soc Echocardiogr*. 2010;23:1225–1230.
6. Neskovic A, Edvardsen T, et al. Focus cardiac ultrasound: the European association of cardiovascular imaging viewpoint. *Eur Heart J Cardiovasc Imaging*. 2014;15:956–960.
7. Prinz C. Voigt J. Diagnostic accuracy of a hand-held ultrasound scanner in routine patients referred for echocardiography. *J Am Soc Echocardiogr*. 2011;24:111–116.
8. Fukuda S, Shimada K, et al. Pocket-sized transthoracic echocardiography device for the measurement of cardiac chamber size and function. *Circ J*. 2009;73:1092–1096.
9. Liebo M, Israel R, et al. Is pocket mobile echocardiography the next-generation stethoscope? A cross-sectional comparison of rapidly acquired images with standard transthoracic echocardiography. *Ann Intern Med*. 2011;155:33–38.
10. Andersen G, Haugen B, et al. Feasibility and reliability of point-of-care pocket-sized echocardiography. *Eur J Echo*. 2011;12:665–670.
11. Mjolstad O, Dalen H, et al. Routinely adding ultrasound examinations by pocket-sized ultrasound devices improves inpatient diagnostics in a medical department. *Eur J Intern Med*. 2012;23:185–191.
12. Galderisi M, Santoro A, et al. Improved cardiovascular diagnostic accuracy by pocket size imaging device in non-cardiologic outpatients: the NaUSiCa (Naples Ultrasound Stethoscope in Cardiology) study. *Cardiovasc Ultrasound*. 2010;8:51.
13. Chamsi-Pasha M, Sengupta P, et al. Handheld echocardiography – current state and future perspectives. *Circulation*. 2017;136:2178–2188.
14. Testuz A, Müller H, et al. Diagnostic accuracy of pocket-size handheld echocardiography used by cardiologists in the acute care setting. *Eur Heart J Cardiovasc Imaging*. 2013;14:38–42.
15. Giusca S, Jurcut R, et al. Accuracy of handheld echocardiography for bedside diagnostic evaluation in a tertiary cardiology center: comparison with standard echocardiography. *Echocardiography*. 2011;28:136–141.
16. Senior R, Galasko G, et al. Community screening for left ventricular hypertrophy in patients with hypertension using hand-held echocardiography. *J Am Soc Echocardiogr*. 2004;17:56–61.
17. Xie T, Chamoun AJ, et al. Rapid screening of cardiac patients with a miniaturized hand-held ultrasound imager: comparisons with physical examination and conventional two-dimensional echocardiography. *Clin Cardiol*. 2004;27:241–245.
18. Rugolotto M, Hu BS, et al. Rapid assessment of cardiac anatomy and function with a new hand-carried ultrasound device (OptiGo): a comparison with standard echocardiography. *Eur J Echocardiogr*. 2001;2:262–269.
19. Kimura B, Yogo N, et al. Cardiopulmonary limited ultrasound examination for "quick-look" bedside application. *Am J Cardiol*. 2011;108:586–590.
20. Mehta M, Jacobson T, et al. Handheld ultrasound versus physical examination in patients referred for transthoracic echocardiography for a suspected cardiac condition. *J Am Coll Cardiol Img*. 2014;7:983–990.
21. Panoulas V, Daigeler A, et al. Pocket-size hand-held cardiac ultrasound as an adjunct to clinical examination in the hands of medical students and junior doctors. *Eur Heart J Cardiovasc Imaging*. 2013;14:323–330.
22. Stokke T, Ruddox V, et al. Brief group training of medical students in focused cardiac ultrasound may improve diagnostic accuracy of physical examination. *J Am Soc Echocardiogr*. 2014;27:1238–1246.
23. DeCara J, Kirkpatrick J, et al. Use of hand-carried ultrasound devices to augment the accuracy of medical student bedside cardiac diagnoses. *J Am Soc Echocardiogr*. 2005;18:257–263.
24. Moore C, Rose G, et al. Determination of left ventricular function by emergency physician echocardiography of hypotensive patients. *Acad Emerg Med*. 2002;9:186–193.
25. Kimura B. Point-of-care cardiac ultrasound techniques in the physical examination: better at the bedside. *Heart*. 2017;103:987–994.
26. Kobal S, Trento L, et al. Comparison of effectiveness of hand-carried ultrasound to bedside cardiovascular physical examination. *Am J Cardiol*. 2005;96:1002–1006.
27. McGee S. *Evidence-based Physical Diagnosis*. 3rd ed. Philadelphia, PA: Elsevier Saunders; 2012.
28. Caldentey G, Khairy P, et al. Prognostic value of the physical examination in patients with heart failure and atrial fibrillation: insights from the AF-CHF trial (atrial fibrillation and chronic heart failure). *JACC Heart Fail*. 2014;2:15–23.
29. Kimura BJ, Amudnson S, et al. Usefulness of a hand-held ultrasound device for bedside examination of left ventricular function. *Am J Cardiol*. 2002;90:1038–1039.
30. Martin L, Howell E, et al. Hand-carried ultrasound performed by hospitalists: does it improve the cardiac physical exam? *Am J Med*. 2009;122:35–41.
31. Spencer KT, Anderson AS, Bhargava A, et al. Physician-performed point-of-care echocardiography using a laptop platform compared with physical examination in the cardiovascular patient. *J Am Coll Cardiol*. 2001;37. 2013– 2018.
32. Cardim N, Fernandez Golfin C, Ferreira D, et al. Usefulness of a new miniaturized echocardiographic system in outpatient cardiology consultations as an extension of physical examination. *J Am Soc Echocardiogr*. 2011;24:117–124.
33. Di Bello V, La Carrubba S, Conte L, et al. SIEC (Italian Society of Cardiovascular Echography). Incremental value of pocket-sized echocardiography in addition to physical examination during inpatient cardiology evaluation: a multicenter Italian study (SIEC). *Echocardiography*. 2015;32:1463–1470.
34. Johnson BK, Tierney DM, Rosborough TK, et al. Internal medicine point-of-care ultrasound assessment of left ventricular function correlates with formal echocardiography. *J Clin Ultrasound*. 2016;44:92–99.
35. Martindale JL, Wakai A, Collins SP, et al. Diagnosing acute heart failure in the emergency department: a systematic review and meta-analysis. *Acad Emerg Med*. 2016;23:223–242.
36. Kimura BJ, Fowler SJ, Fergus TS, et al. Detection of left atrial enlargement using hand-carried ultrasound devices: implications for bedside examination. *Am J Med*. 2005;118:912–916.
37. Kimura BJ, Kedar E, Weiss DE, et al. A bedside ultrasound sign of cardiac disease: the left atrium-to-aorta diastolic diameter ratio. *Am J Emerg Med*. 2010;28:203–207.
38. Miglioranza MH, Gargani L, Sant'Anna RT, et al. Lung ultrasound for the evaluation of pulmonary congestion in outpatients: a comparison with clinical assessment, natriuretic peptides, and echocardiography. *JACC Cardiovasc Imaging*. 2013;6:1141–1151.
39. Wong CL, Holroyd-Leduc J, Straus SE. Does this patient have a pleural effusion? *J Am Med Assoc*. 2009;301:309–317.
40. Kataoka H, Takada S. The role of thoracic ultrasonography for evaluation of patients with decompensated chronic heart failure. *J Am Coll Cardiol*. 2000;35:1638–1646.
41. Lichtenstein D, Goldstein I, Mourgeon E, et al. Comparative diagnostic performances of auscultation, chest radiography, and lung ultrasonography in acute respiratory distress syndrome. *Anesthesiology*. 2004;100:9–15.
42. Mansencal N, Vieillard-Baron A, Beauchet A, et al. Triage patients with suspected pulmonary embolism in the emergency department using a portable ultrasound device. *Echocardiography*. 2008;25:451–456.
43. Brennan JM, Blair JE, Goonewardena S, et al. Reappraisal of the use of inferior vena cava for estimating right atrial pressure. *J Am Soc Echocardiogr*. 2007;20:857–861.
44. Abe Y, Ito M, Tanaka C, et al. A novel and simple method using pocketsized echocardiography to screen for aortic Stenosis. *J Am Soc Echocardiogr*. 2013;26:589–596.
45. Kobal SL, Tolstrup K, Luo H, et al. Usefulness of a hand-carried cardiac ultrasound device to detect clinically significant valvular regurgitation in hospitalized patients. *Am J Cardiol*. 2004;93:1069–1072.
46. Razi R, Estrada J, et al. Bedside hand-carried ultrasound by internal medicine residents versus traditional clinical assessment for the identification of systolic dysfunction in patients admitted with decompensated heart failure. *J Am Soc Echocardiogr*. 2011;24:1319–1324.
47. Melamed R, Sprenkle M, et al. Assessment of left ventricular function by intensivists using hand-held echocardiography. *Chest*. 2009;135:1416–1420.
48. Dresden S, Mitchell P, et al. Right ventricular dilation on bedside echocardiography performed by emergency physicians aids in the diagnosis of pulmonary embolism. *Ann Emerg Med*. 2014;63:16–24.
49. Taylor R, Davis J, et al. Point-of-care focused cardiac ultrasound for prediction of pulmonary embolism adverse outcomes. *J Emerg Med*. 2013;45:392–399.

50. Mandavia D, Hoffner R, et al. Bedside echocardiography by emergency physicians. *Ann Emerg Med*. 2001;38:377–382.
51. Beigel R, Cercek B, et al. Noninvasive evaluation of right atrial pressure. *J Am Soc Echocardiogr*. 2013;26:1033–1042.
52. Cciozda W, Kedan I, et al. The efficacy of sonographic measurement of inferior vena cava diameter as an estimate of central venous pressure. *Cardiovasc Ultrasoun*. 2016;14:33.
53. Stawicki S, Braslow B, et al. Intensivist use of hand-carried ultrasound to measure IVC collapsibility in estimating intravascular volume status: correlations with CVP. *J Am Coll Surg*. 2009;209:55–61.
54. Jue J, Chung W, et al. Does inferior vena cava size predict right atrial pressures in patients receiving mechanical ventilation? *J Am Soc Echocardiogr*. 1992;5:613–619.
55. Nascimento B, Beaton A, et al. Integration of echocardiographic screening by non-physicians with remote reading in primary care. *Heart*. 2019;105:283–290.
56. Pare J, Liu R, et al. Emergency physician focused cardiac ultrasound improves diagnosis of ascending aortic dissection. *Am J Em Med*. 2016;34:486–492.
57. Jones A, Tayal V, et al. Randomized, controlled trial of immediate versus delayed goal-directed ultrasound to identify the cause of nontraumatic hypotension in emergency department patients. *Crit Care Med*. 2004;32:1703–1708.
58. Hall M, Coffey E, et al. The "5Es" of emergency physician-performed focused cardiac ultrasound: a protocol for rapid identification of effusion, ejection, equality, exit, and entrance. *Acad Emerg Med*. 2015;22:583–593.
59. Miniati M, Monti S, et al. Diagnosis of pulmonary embolism: results of a prospective study in unselected patients. *Am J Med*. 2001;110:528–535.
60. Bova C, Greco F, et al. Diagnostic utility of echocardiography in patients with suspected pulmonary embolism. *Am J Emerg Med*. 2003;21:180–183.
61. Breitkreutz R, Price S, et al. Focused echocardiographic evaluation in life support and peri-resuscitation of emergency patients: a prospective trial. *Resuscitation*. 2010;81:1527–1533.
62. Shokoohi H, Boniface K, et al. Bedside ultrasound reduces diagnostic uncertainty and guides resuscitation in patients with undifferentiated hypotension. *Crit Care Med*. 2015;43:2562–2569.
63. Hall M, Taylor R, et al. Impact of point-of-care ultrasonography on ED time to disposition for patients with nontraumatic shock. *Am J Em Med*. 2016;34:1022–1030.
64. Kanji H, McCallum J, et al. Limited echocardiography-guided therapy in subacute shock is associated with change in management and improved outcomes. *J Crit Care*. 2014;29:700–705.
65. Gaspari R, Weekes A, et al. A retrospective study of pulseless electrical activity, bedside ultrasound identifies interventions during resuscitation associated with improved survival to hospital admission. *Resuscitation*. 2017;120:103–107.
66. Blyth L, Atkinson P, et al. Bedside focused echocardiography as predictor of survival in cardiac arrest patients: a systematic review. *Acad Em Med*. 2012;19:1119–1126.
67. Tsou Y, Kurbedin J, et al. Accuracy of point-of-care focused echocardiography in predicting outcome of resuscitation in cardiac arrest patients: a systematic review and meta-analysis. *Resuscitation*. 2017;114:92–99.
68. Gundersen G, Norekval T, et al. Adding point of care ultrasound to assess volume status in heart failure patients in a nurse let outpatient clinic. A randomized study. *Heart*. 2016;102:29–34 (d).
69. Plummer D, Brunette D, et al. Emergency department echocardiography improves outcome in penetrating cardiac injury. *Emerg Med June*. 1992;21:709–712.
70. Goonewardena S, Gemignani A, et al. Comparison of hand-carried ultrasound assessment of the inferior vena cava and N-terminal pro-brain natriuretic peptide for predicting readmission after hospitalization for acute decompensated heart failure. *JACC Cardiovasc Imaging*. 2008;1:595–601.
71. Laffin L, Patel A, et al. Focused cardiac ultrasound as a predictor of readmission in acute decompensated heart failure. *Int J Cardiovasc Imaging*. 2018;34:1075–1079.
72. Johri A, Durbin, et al. Cardiac point-of-care ultrasound: state-of-the-art in medical school education. *J Am Soc Echocardiogr*. 2018;31:749–760.
73. Johri A. *Cardiovascular point of care imaging for the medical student and novice user*. American Society of Echocardiography; 2018. Retrieved from. https://aseuniversity.org/ase/lessons/47.
74. Conlin F, Connely N, et al. Focused transthoracic cardiac ultrasound: a survey of training practices. *J Cardiothor Vasc An*. 2016;30:102–106.
75. Lewiss R, Hoffmann B, et al. Point of care ultrasound education: the increasing role of simulation and multimedia resources. *J Ultrasound Med*. 2014;33:27–32.
76. Clau-Terre F, Sharma V, et al. Can simulation help to answer the demand for echocardiography education? *Anesthesiology*. 2014;120:32–41.
77. Soni N, Schnobrich D, et al. Point-of-care ultrasound for hospitalists: a position statement of the Society of Hospital Medicine. *J Hosp Med*. 2019;14:E1–E6.
78. Cawthorn T, Nickel C, et al. Development and evaluation of methodologies for teaching focused cardiac ultrasound skills to medical students. *J Am Soc Echocardiogr*. 2014;27:302–309.
79. Kimura BJ, Sliman S, et al. Retention of ultrasound skills and training. *J Am Soc Echocardiogr*. 2016;29:992–997.
80. Bowcock E, Morris I, et al. Basic critical care echocardiography: how many studies equate to competence? A pilot study using high fidelity echocardiography simulation. *J Intensive Care Soc*. 2017;18:198–205.
81. Chisholm C, Dodge W, et al. Focused cardiac ultrasound training: how much is enough? *J Emerg Med*. 2013;44:818–822.
82. Pustavoitau A, Blaivas M, Brown SM, et al. Ultrasound Certification Task Force on behalf of the Society of Critical Care Medicine. Official Statement of the Society of Critical Care Medicine: recommendations for achieving and maintaining competence and credentialing in critical care ultrasound with focused cardiac ultrasound and advanced critical care echocardiography. http://journals.lww.com/ccmjournal/Documents/Critical%20Care%20Ultrasound.pdf. Accessed August 18, 2019.
83. Burwasha I, Tamb J, et al. 2010 CCS/CSE guidelines for physician training and maintenance of competence in adult echocardiography. Can J Cardiol. 2011;27:862–864.

PART III
第三部分

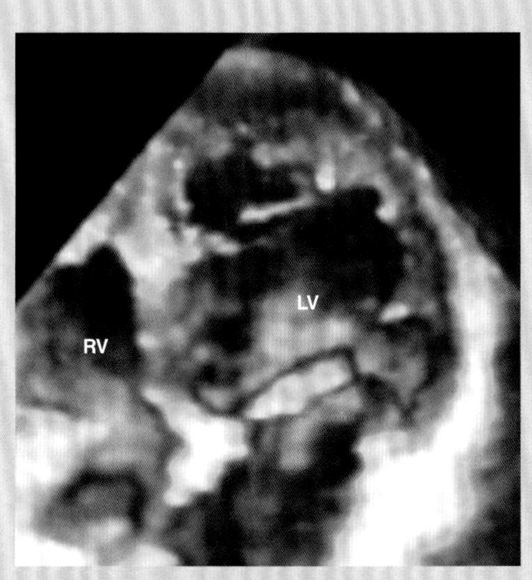

Cardiomyopathies, Tumors, and Pericardial Disease
心肌病、肿瘤和心包疾病

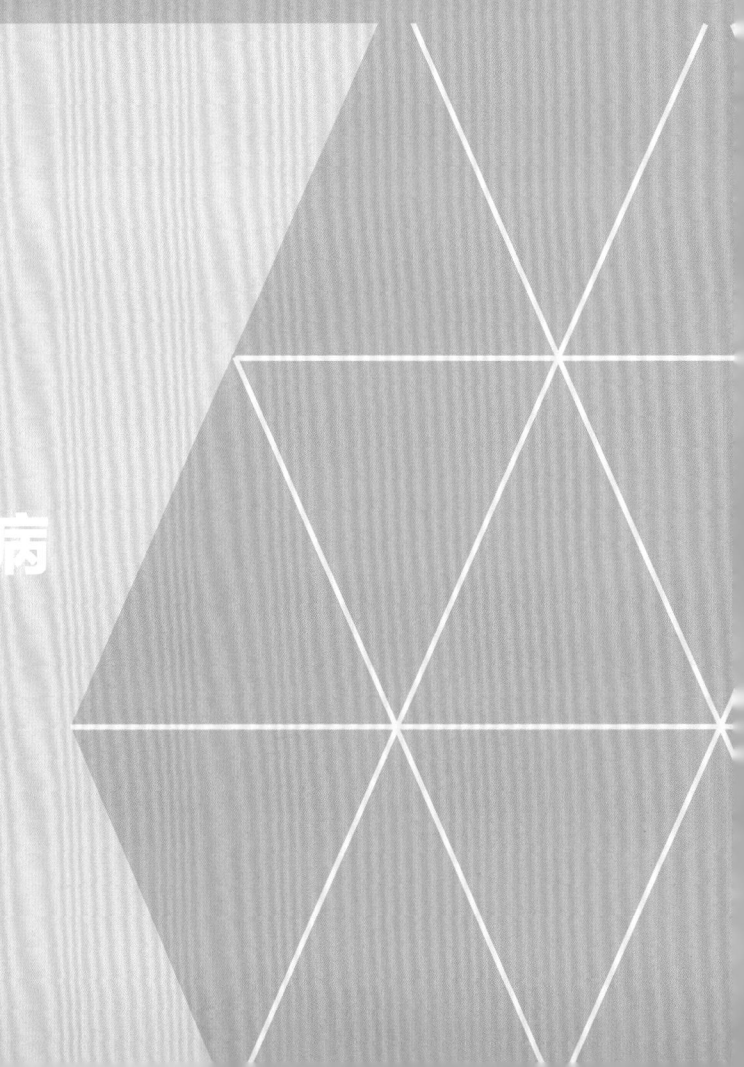

中文导读

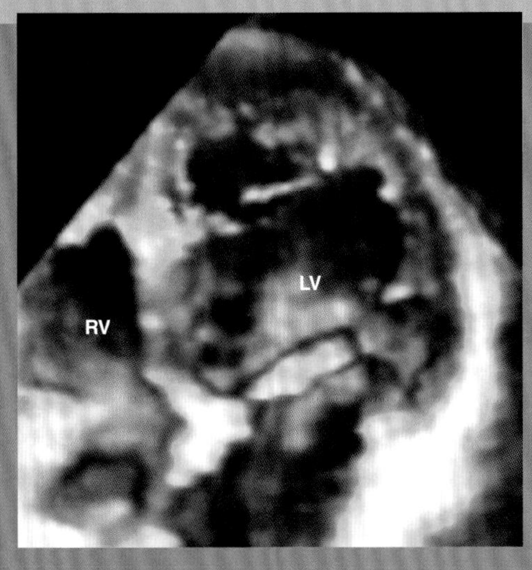

第12章 扩张型心肌病

扩张型心肌病是一类以不明原因的左心室扩大和收缩功能减低为特征的心肌受累疾病。扩张型心肌病的传统诊断标准：左心室射血分数<45%，左心室缩短分数<25%，矫正性别、年龄和体表面积的条件下，左心室舒张末期内径>112%。左心室的重构在短轴方向较长轴方向更显著，使得左心室从正常的椭圆形变成近球形，不仅左心室收缩功能更差，且更易造成二尖瓣反流；同时，左心室内血流速度减慢，增加其血栓的风险。

经胸超声心动图是首选检查方法，其在以下方面发挥重要作用：①左心室大小、形态和收缩功能的评价；②预后判断，如猝死风险评估等；③组织多普勒成像：左心室功能的评估和风险分层；④应变技术：无角度依赖，扩张型心肌病表现为各个维度（纵向、环形、径向应变和扭转）应变的减低。目前，三维斑点追踪成像技术也越来越多的应用于临床；⑤左心室舒张功能的评价；⑥继发性二尖瓣反流的评估；⑦左心室收缩储备的评估（非常规检查）方法：运动负荷和药物负荷超声（指标：心输出量、左室射血分数和应变等）；⑧右心功能评估：34%的患者合并右心受累；⑨鉴别诊断：心肌炎、Chagas病、左心室致密化不全、应激性心肌病、冠心病和瓣膜病导致的左心室扩大、高血压等。经胸超声心动图还在心脏再同步治疗方面发挥重要作用。

肖明虎

12 Dilated Cardiomyopathy

RICHARD K. CHENG, MD | SOFIA CAROLINA MASRI, MD

CLASSIFICATION OF DILATED CARDIOMYOPATHY

Precise designation of the cardiomyopathies can be challenging. The World Health Organization (WHO) 1995 classification introduced the following broad categories of cardiomyopathy based on pathophysiology and clinical cause: dilated (DCM), hypertrophic, restrictive, arrhythmogenic RV, and unclassified.[1] The WHO classification remains commonplace in clinical practice, and cases are efficiently stratified on the basis of imaging and descriptive parameters. The classification was revised by the American Heart Association (AHA) in 2006 to integrate genomic and molecular findings[2] and by the European Society of Cardiology (ESC) in 2008[3] to emphasize the morphofunctional phenotype while incorporating genetic data from the AHA paradigm. The 2013 MOGE(S) classification uses a nosology that synthesizes five attributes of a cardiomyopathic disorder (i.e., *m*orphofunctional characteristic, *o*rgan involvement, familial *g*enetic inheritance pattern, *e*tiologic annotation, functional *s*tatus) in a single nomenclature.[4]

In this chapter, *DCM* is used as a descriptive term, aligned with the clinical presentation and diagnostic patterns seen on echocardiography, to focus on those cardiomyopathies characterized by LV dilation and LV systolic dysfunction that cannot be explained by abnormal loading conditions (e.g., hypertension, valvular heart disease), and that correspond most closely with the WHO classification.

EPIDEMIOLOGY

Historically, the estimate for age-adjusted prevalence of DCM in the United States was 36 cases per 100,000 people.[5] An updated estimate in 2013 suggested a higher prevalence of 1 in 250 individuals.[6] Among patients without a clinically identifiable cause of DCM, approximately 25% to 35% have a positive genetic screening result.

Familial DCM is a phenotypic diagnosis that is made when DCM occurs in two closely related family members.[7] The mode of inheritance for familial DCM varies, with most mutations being autosomal dominant, but other inheritance patterns are possible, and there is genetic heterogeneity in disease states. More than 50 single genes are linked to a DCM phenotype, including mutations in genes encoding cytoskeletal, nucleoskeletal, mitochondrial, and calcium-handling proteins.[8]

CLINICAL PRESENTATION

DCM includes a heterogeneous group of myocardial disorders characterized by LV dilation and a depressed LV ejection fraction (LVEF) in the absence of other conditions causing increased afterload or volume overload. Myocardial disease is associated with abnormal pressure-volume relationships that result in LV dilation and eccentric remodeling (Fig. 12.1), with increases in total cardiac mass. Traditional diagnostic criteria include an LVEF less than 45%, fractional shortening less than 25%, and an LV end-diastolic dimension greater than 112% of that expected for body size.[9]

LV remodeling is a dynamic process that is triggered by an imbalance between myocardial wall stress and the normal restraining forces exerted by the viscoelastic collagen matrix. As wall stress increases, cell surface mechanoreceptors activate myocardial matrix metalloproteinases, leading to degradation of the extracellular collagen matrix, and resultant LV dilation. A gradual increase in LV size, disproportionately more in the short axis relative to the long axis, results in alterations of

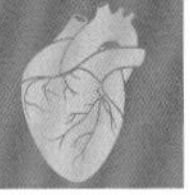

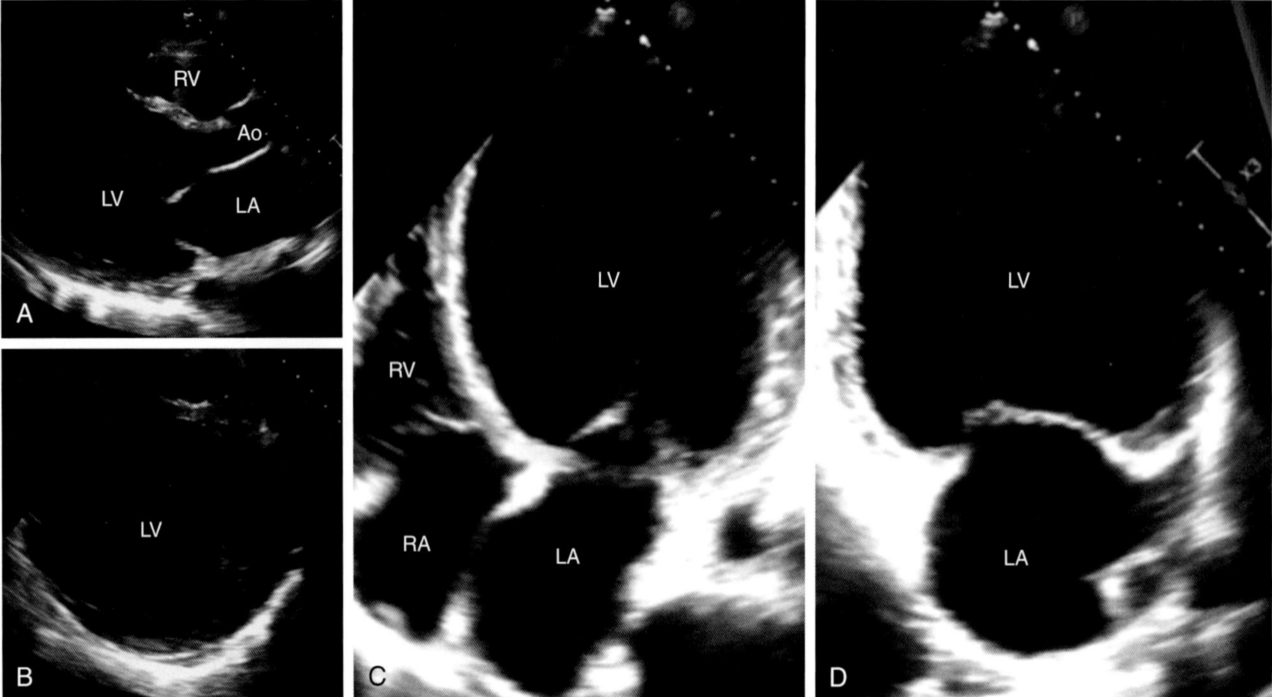

Fig. 12.1 Dilated cardiomyopathy. Parasternal long-axis (A), parasternal short-axis (B), apical 4-chamber (C), and apical 2-chamber (D) views of a patient with idiopathic dilated cardiomyopathy demonstrate reduced LV systolic function and LV dilation (see Videos 12.1A–D). This is caused by primary volume overload with a compensatory increase in wall thickness that fails to parallel the increase in cavity radius, resulting in eccentric hypertrophy. *Ao*, Aorta.

LV geometry from the normal prolate ellipse into a spherical shape. This remodeling can be characterized by the sphericity index (long-axis dimension/short-axis dimension, >1.5 in healthy individuals), which approaches 1 in cases of advanced DCM.

The more spherical LV shape affects other aspects of LV dynamics, most notably an increase in LV end-diastolic wall stress that interferes with contractile efficiency. In addition to larger LV volumes, LV wall thinning leads to further increases in loading conditions and decline of contractile function. Increased spherical geometry and eccentric remodeling result in a distortion of the mitral annulus and subvalvular apparatus, which prevents proper coaptation of the mitral valve (MV) leaflets and contributes to development of secondary mitral regurgitation (MR). Apart from the loss of forward flow, MR results in further escalation of loading conditions.

Alterations in the remodeling ventricle beget further LV dilation. A strong inverse relationship exists between end-systolic LV wall stress and LVEF, such that the greater the wall stress, the lower the LVEF. With the progressive decrease in contractility and increased LV volumes, there are decreased blood flow velocities within the LV and relative stasis, which is sometimes visualized as spontaneous contrast on echocardiography. This combination of factors predisposes to formation of LV thrombus (Fig. 12.2).

DCM results from myriad causes, and many other cardiac conditions resemble DCM (Table 12.1). Individuals with DCM develop signs and symptoms of left-sided heart failure (HF). Patients complain of limited functional capacity due to dyspnea on exertion. They have orthopnea and paroxysmal nocturnal dyspnea from volume overload. With right-sided involvement, lower extremity edema and abdominal bloating with evidence of renal dysfunction are common.

Cardiac imaging is paramount for the diagnosis of DCM and provides clues to a causative mechanism. Early evaluation of affected individuals shows subtle LV dilation and a slightly decreased LVEF. As the disease progresses, there is further LV dilation, thinning of the LV walls, and further decreases in systolic function. Regional variation in wall motion suggests that an ischemic cause is more likely than DCM, particularly if the abnormalities correspond to an isolated coronary artery distribution. With prior infarction, the scarred myocardium is thin, echogenic and aneurysm formation can occur (Fig. 12.3). Patients with non-ischemic causes may likewise have some regional variation in wall motion because the basal posterior segments often demonstrate better preservation of function compared with other walls. In cases of concurrent LV hypertrophy with LV dilation and LV dysfunction, the differential diagnosis includes end-stage hypertensive disease and infiltrative causes of cardiomyopathy with advanced remodeling.

FAMILIAL SCREENING

All first-degree relatives (including parents) of individuals with idiopathic DCM should be considered for echocardiographic and electrocardiographic (ECG) screening.[10] Challenges to routine screening include the problematic task of deciding whether subtle echocardiographic findings represent early signs of DCM; the earliest sign of preclinical disease is LV enlargement.[11] Family members with an initially normal screening result remain at increased risk for future disease. Repeat echocardiography every 3 to 5 years is recommended. For family members with identifiable mutations corresponding to DCM, screening should be more frequent, every 1 to 3 years.[12]

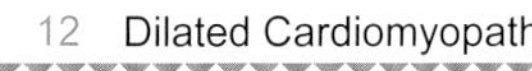

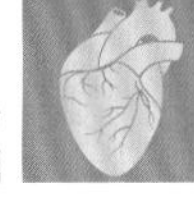

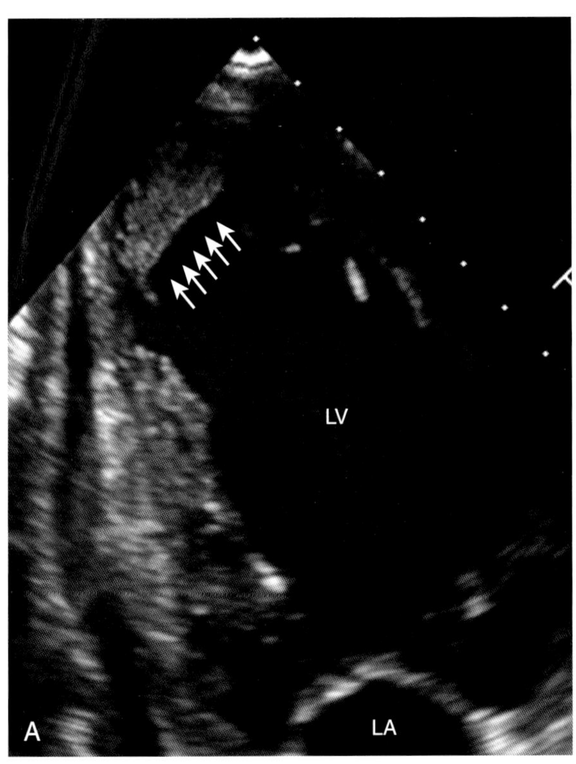

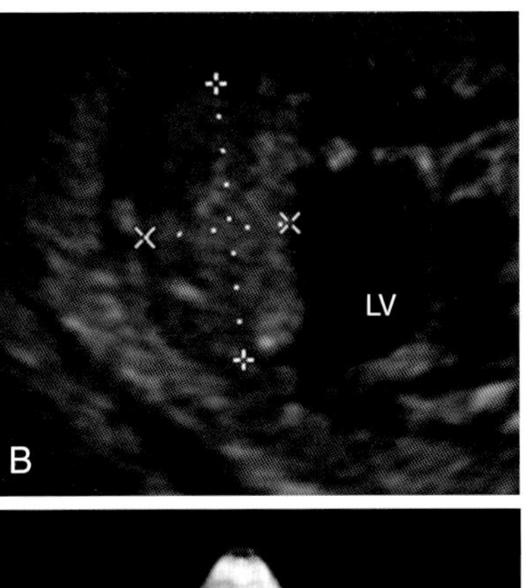

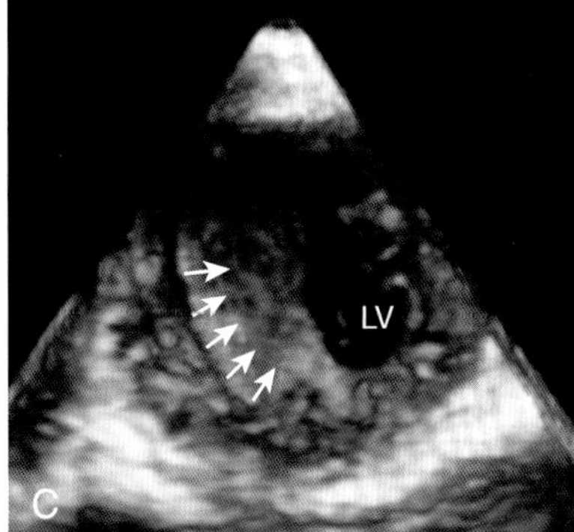

Fig. 12.2 LV apical thrombus. (A) Apical 2-chamber view with LV thrombus at the apex *(arrows)* (see Video 12.2A). (B) Sweep through the parasternal short-axis view demonstrates the LV thrombus (see Video 12B). (C) 3D echocardiographic imaging of the short-axis view shows the LV thrombus *(arrows)* (see Video 12.2C).

TABLE 12.1 Differential Diagnoses for Dilated Cardiomyopathy.

Diagnosis	*Echocardiographic Imaging Features and Comments*
Typically Considered a Form of DCM	
Chemotherapy (e.g., doxorubicin, trastuzumab, TKIs)	May appear similar to idiopathic DCM.
Connective tissue disease (autoimmune) (e.g., scleroderma, systemic lupus erythematosis, Marfan syndrome, polyarteritis nodosum, dermatomyositis, ankylosing spondylitis, rheumatoid arthritis, relapsing polychondritis, Wegener's granulomatosis, mixed connective tissue disease)	Findings vary and are nonspecific and depend on the condition. Valves, pericardium, myocardium, and/or coronary arteries can be involved.
Hypereosinophilic syndrome	Findings vary and are based on stage. Early presentation can have an almost normal-appearing echocardiogram. More advanced disease typically manifests with laminar thrombus at areas of damaged endocardium, valvular abnormalities from fibro-inflammatory remodeling, and increased endomyocardial echogenicity from fibrosis, particularly that affecting the posterior wall.
Idiopathic DCM, including familial (genetic) types	Classic findings include LV dilation, increased sphericity index, and LV systolic dysfunction.
Metabolic or endocrine conditions, including thyroid disease and nutritional deficiencies	May appear similar to idiopathic DCM.
Myocarditis, including infection	Wall motion can be diffuse or regional, LV dilation can vary, myocardium may be thickened from edema, and pericardial effusion may occur.
Neuromuscular diseases, including muscular dystrophy	May appear similar to idiopathic DCM.
Peripartum cardiomyopathy	May appear similar to idiopathic DCM. Diagnosis is often made based on the time course relative to recent pregnancy.
Toxins (e.g., alcohol, cocaine, amphetamines, heavy metals, carbon monoxide)	May appear similar to idiopathic DCM. Alcoholic cardiomyopathy often has marked LV dilation and increased sphericity; changes can reverse remodel with cessation of alcohol.
Not Typically Considered DCM but May Appear Similar on Imaging	
Hemochromatosis	Advanced cases may have mild or no LV dilation, mildly increased wall thickness, and abnormal diastolic parameters.
Hypertensive heart disease	End-stage hypertensive disease can manifest with LV dilation and systolic dysfunction. Most cases have LV hypertrophy. May be difficult to differentiate from advanced cases of infiltrative heart disease.
Ischemic heart disease	Regional wall motion abnormalities, echogenic and thinned walls due to scarring, and possible aneurysm formation in areas of prior infarct.
LV noncompaction	Prominent LV trabeculae with exaggerated intertrabecular recesses. More advanced disease has LV dilation and reduced LVEF.
Sarcoidosis	Advanced cases are characterized by LV dilation, septal thinning, reduced LVEF, and ventricular aneurysms. Cardiac tissue may appear echogenic due to scar formation, and there are often regional wall motion abnormalities in noncoronary distributions.
Stress-induced cardiomyopathy (takotsubo syndrome)	Apical hypokinesis with preserved basal segments is classic, although involvement of segments varies. Often there is a clearly identifiable stressor. Most cases resolve with normalization of LV function.

DCM, Dilated cardiomyopathy, *LVEF*, left ventricular ejection fraction; *TKIs*, tyrosine kinase inhibitors
Adapted from Thomas D, Wheeler R, Yousef ZR, Masani ND. The role of echocardiography in guiding management in dilated cardiomyopathy. *Eur J Echocardiogr*. 2009;10:iii15–iii21.

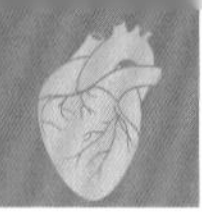

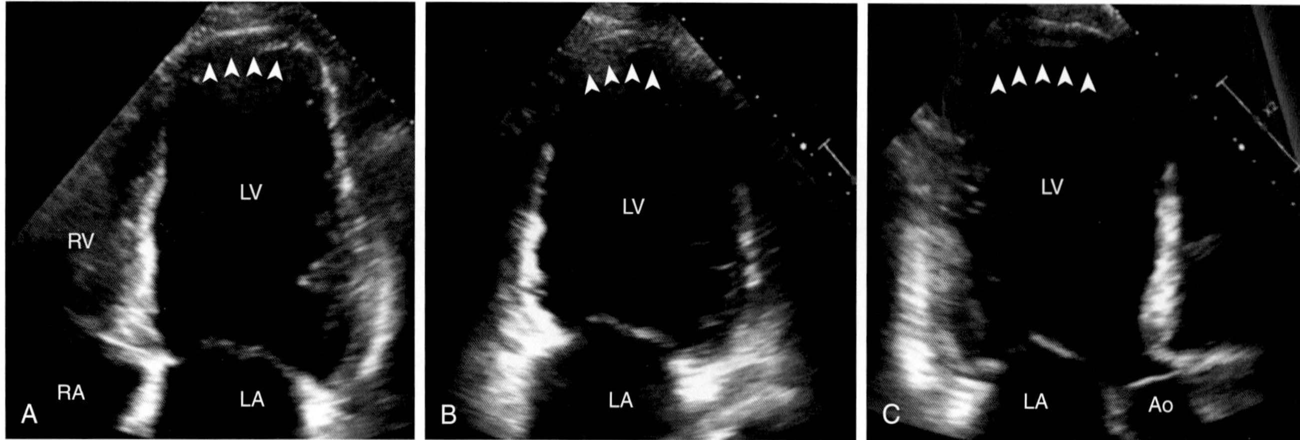

Fig. 12.3 Ischemic heart disease. Apical 4-chamber (A), apical 2-chamber (B), and apical 3-chamber (C) views (see Videos 12.3A–12.3C). The patient has a history of left anterior descending artery and right coronary artery infarct with multiple wall motion abnormalities, including myocardial thinning and echogenic scar of the anteroseptum and entire inferior wall, dyskinesis of the inferoseptum, and an aneurysmal-appearing apex *(arrowheads).*

APPROPRIATENESS CRITERIA FOR ECHOCARDIOGRAPHY

The American College of Cardiology Foundation (ACCF) and AHA provide a class I recommendation for echocardiographic imaging to characterize LV structure and other abnormalities that facilitate understanding of a clinical presentation with HF. Repeat imaging should be obtained for individuals with clinical changes and those who are being considered for treatments specific to systolic dysfunction, such as device therapy with implantable cardioverter-defibrillators (ICDs).[10]

The ACCF, American Society of Echocardiography (ASE), and AHA provide specific criteria for the appropriate use of echocardiography for cardiomyopathies, with applicable recommendations shown in Table 12.2.[13] A statement regarding appropriate use criteria for multimodality imaging was released in May 2019,[14] and relevant additional recommendations for DCM are shown in Table 12.3.

ECHOCARDIOGRAPHIC FEATURES OF DILATED CARDIOMYOPATHY

LV SYSTOLIC FUNCTION

Evaluation of LV systolic parameters should be performed for all patients with DCM. Chapter 4 describes a comprehensive evaluation of LV systolic function. The most common method for quantification of LVEF is by 2D imaging using the biplane method of disk summation (i.e., modified Simpson's rule) (Fig. 12.4A). LV apical foreshortening and lateral resolution on 2D images can be significant limitations. 3D echocardiography (see Fig. 12.4B) provides a more accurate determination of LV volume, mass, and LVEF, largely because the need for geometric assumptions is eliminated.

Some specific M-mode findings remain relevant to the assessment of patients with DCM. The E-point septal separation (EPSS; normal value < 6 mm) (Fig. 12.5) is an indirect indicator of reduced LVEF; progressive increases in EPSS are associated with worse systolic function. A more gradual closure of the aortic valve is a sign of decreased forward flow and low stroke volume. An older index of LV long-axis systolic function is the mitral annular displacement by M-mode (normal value > 10 mm). There is a direct relationship between annular excursion and LVEF, with lower excursion corresponding to decreasing LVEF. However, this is valid only when global systolic dysfunction is present because annular excursion does not detect distal or focal regional abnormalities.

Stroke volume and cardiac output can be calculated from the velocity–time integral obtained by a pulsed-wave Doppler recording of the LV outflow tract. Accurate estimation of the LV outflow tract diameter is crucial because small errors are magnified due to squaring of the radius in the calculation of stroke volume. Stroke volume and cardiac output are reduced in DCM. For patients with severe systolic dysfunction, there may be beat-to-beat variability in peak velocity and the velocity–time integral of the LV outflow tract, corresponding to clinical pulsus alternans (Fig. 12.6).

The rate of LV pressure change during isovolumic contraction (*dP/dt* max) is another index of LV contractility. The *dP/dt* value estimates the rate of increase in LV pressure, with the expectation that greater contractile forces will translate into higher rates. Normal values for *dP/dt* max are 1000 to 1200 mmHg/s, and there is often a marked reduction of these values in DCM. Estimates of *dP/dt* are extrapolated from the MR jet, and eccentric jets result in poor estimates. The *dP/dt* value also depends on preload, afterload, and heart rate, which vary with different loading conditions.

The myocardial performance index (MPI)[15] is a Doppler parameter that provides global assessment of systolic and diastolic performance. Advantages are that it is independent of heart rate and blood pressure and does not depend on ventricular geometry. MPI reflects disease severity and adds incremental prognostic value to other parameters in DCM at a cutoff of approximately 0.4,[16] with increasing values implying worse cardiac performance.

LV SYSTOLIC FUNCTION AND PROGNOSIS

LV systolic dysfunction is a robust determinant of functional capacity and overall prognosis. It can be assessed with various imaging modalities (Table 12.4). LVEF is often used as the main predictor of outcomes in clinical settings, with numerous studies confirming that as LVEF decreases, risk of death increases.[17,18] LVEF allows identification of patients with an increased risk of sudden death and is considered to be the most important parameter in guiding the decision to use an implantable cardioverter-defibrillator.

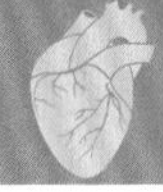

TABLE 12.2 2011 Appropriate Use Criteria for Echocardiography in Heart Failure and Dilated Cardiomyopathy.[a]

Appropriate Use

7. Clinical symptoms or signs consistent with a cardiac diagnosis known to cause lightheadedness, presyncope, or syncope (including but not limited to aortic stenosis, hypertrophic cardiomyopathy, or HF) (9, A)
70. Initial evaluation of known or suspected HF (systolic or diastolic) based on symptoms, signs, or abnormal test results (9, A)
71. Re-evaluation of known HF (systolic or diastolic) with a change in clinical status or cardiac examination without a clear precipitating change in medication or diet (8, A)
73. Re-evaluation of known HF (systolic or diastolic) to guide therapy (9, A)
76. Initial evaluation or re-evaluation after revascularization and/or optimal medical therapy to determine candidacy for device therapy and/or to determine optimal choice of device (9, A)
78. Known implanted pacing device with symptoms possibly due to device complication or suboptimal pacing device settings (8, A)
81. To determine candidacy for ventricular assist device (9, A)
86. Initial evaluation of known or suspected cardiomyopathy (e.g., restrictive, infiltrative, dilated, hypertrophic, or genetic cardiomyopathy) (9, A)
87. Re-evaluation of known cardiomyopathy with a change in clinical status or cardiac examination or to guide therapy (9, A)
90. Screening evaluation of structure and function in first-degree relatives of a patient with an inherited cardiomyopathy (9, A)

Uncertain Use

72. Re-evaluation of known HF (systolic or diastolic) with a change in clinical status or cardiac examination with a clear precipitating change in medication or diet (4, U)
75. Routine surveillance (≥1 y) of HF (systolic or diastolic) when there is no change in clinical status or cardiac examination (6, U)
77. Initial evaluation for CRT device optimization after implantation (6, U)
89. Routine surveillance (≥1 y) of known cardiomyopathy without a change in clinical status or cardiac examination (5, U)

Inappropriate Use

74. Routine surveillance (<1 y) of HF (systolic or diastolic) when there is no change in clinical status or cardiac examination (2, I)
88. Routine surveillance (<1 y) of known cardiomyopathy without a change in clinical status or cardiac examination (2, I)

[a]Use criteria: *A*, Appropriate; *I*, inappropriate; *U*, uncertain; *1–9*, appropriate use score. (After 2011, the A, U, and I categories were renamed Appropriate, May be appropriate, and Rarely appropriate, respectively.)

Adapted from Douglas PS, Garcia MJ, Haines DE, et al. 2011 Appropriate use criteria for echocardiography: a report of the American College of Cardiology Foundation Appropriate Use Criteria Task Force, American Society of Echocardiography, American Heart Association, American Society of Nuclear Cardiology, Heart Failure Society of America, Heart Rhythm Society, Society for Cardiovascular Angiography and Interventions, Society of Critical Care Medicine, Society of Cardiovascular Computed Tomography, Society for Cardiovascular Magnetic Resonance American College of Chest Physicians. *J Am Soc Echocardiogr*. 2011;24:229–267.

TABLE 12.3 2019 Appropriate Use Criteria for Multimodality Imaging in Nonvalvular Heart Disease (Heart Failure and Dilated Cardiomyopathy).[a]

Appropriate Use

3. Initial evaluation before exposure to medications/radiation that could result in cardiotoxicity/heart failure (9, A)
31. Evaluation of LV function in patients who are scheduled for or who have received chemotherapy (9, A)
58. Re-evaluation (<1 y) in a patient previously or currently undergoing therapy with potentially cardiotoxic agents (7, A)
73. Periodic re-evaluation in a patient undergoing therapy with cardiotoxic agents and worsening symptoms (9, A)
75. Re-evaluation for CRT device optimization in a patient with worsening HF (8, A)

[a]Use criteria: *A*, Appropriate; *M*, may be appropriate; *R*, rarely appropriate; *1–9*, appropriate use score.

Adapted from Doherty JU, Kort S, Mehran R, et al. 2019 Appropriate use criteria for multimodality imaging in the assessment of cardiac structure and function in nonvalvular heart disease: a report of the American College of Cardiology Appropriate Use Criteria Task Force, American Association for Thoracic Surgery, American Heart Association, American Society of Echocardiography, American Society of Nuclear Cardiology, Heart Rhythm Society, Society for Cardiovascular Angiography and Interventions, Society of Cardiovascular Computed Tomography, Society for Cardiovascular Magnetic Resonance, and the Society of Thoracic Surgeons. *J Am Coll Cardiol*. 2019;73:488–516.

Other methods of estimating cardiac function, such as *dP/dt* and MPI, correlate with poor survival when they are abnormal. In a study of HF patients, a *dP/dt* value of <600 mmHg/s conferred an increased risk of death or need for cardiac transplantation.[19] In another study of 285 patients undergoing cardiac resynchronization therapy (CRT) for chronic HF, a baseline *dP/dt* < 650 mmHg/s or a post-CRT *dP/dt* < 900 mmHg/s was associated with adverse clinical outcomes at 1 year, including all-cause mortality, heart transplantation, or placement of an LV assist device (LVAD).[20] In patients with DCM, an MPI > 0.77 predicts significantly lower survival rates at 1, 3, and 5 years.[16,21]

LV SIZE AND SHAPE

Increased LV size in end-systolic and end-diastolic diameters is strongly associated with poor outcomes. An analysis of the Studies of Left Ventricular Dysfunction (SOLVD) trial showed that an end-systolic diameter greater than 5.0 cm predicted an increased mortality rate.[22] In a series of patients with idiopathic DCM, the threshold for increased mortality risk appeared to be an end-diastolic dimension greater than 7.6 cm.[23] Similarly, increased systolic and diastolic LV volumes are associated with increased risk. A study evaluating echocardiographic parameters in patients with advanced HF found that LV end-diastolic volume index of 120 mL/m^2 was strongly predictive of mortality.[24] Moreover, serial changes in LV remodeling predict clinical outcomes for patients with LV dilation or decreased LVEF.[25]

An increase in LV mass due to myocyte hypertrophy in DCM independently confers a worse prognosis.[22,25] A change of one standard deviation in LV mass (mean, 298 ± 103 g) can increase the relative risk of death by as much as 1.3.[22] As the LV remodels in DCM, it increasingly loses its elliptical shape and becomes more spherical. End-systolic and end-diastolic sphericity indices lower than 1.5 are predictors of decreased exercise capacity and poor long-term outcomes.[26]

TISSUE DOPPLER IMAGING

The mechanics of LV systole involve complex, coordinated actions that include an integration of longitudinal contraction,

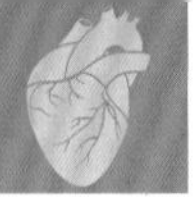

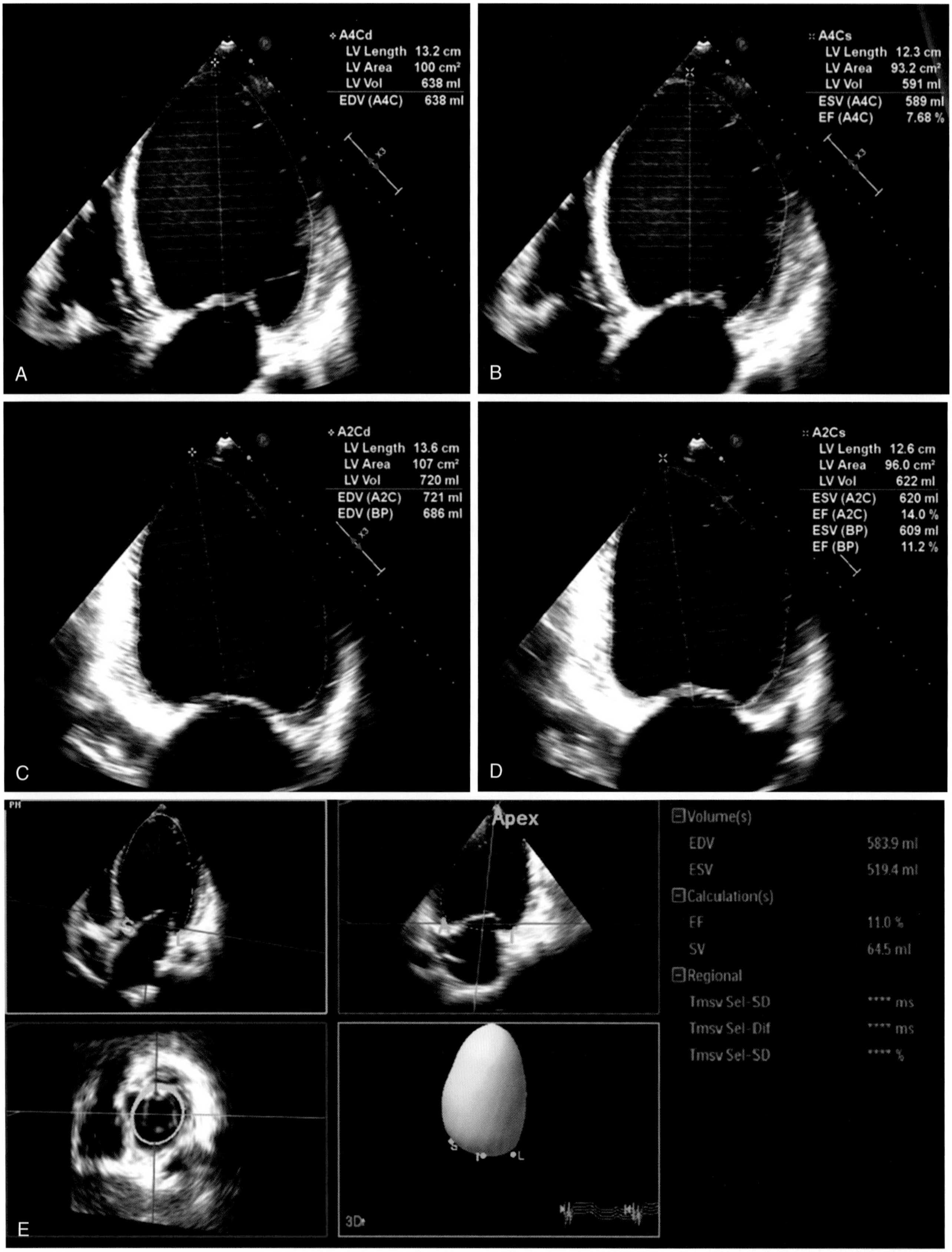

Fig. 12.4 Quantification of the ejection fraction for a patient with dilated cardiomyopathy. The biplane disk method is shown in the apical 4-chamber view for diastole and systole (A and B) and the apical 2-chamber view for diastole and systole (C and D). (E) 3D provides a more accurate determination of the LV volume and LV ejection fraction (LVEF) because it does not make any geometric assumptions. In this case, there is excellent correlation of LVEF by 2D biplane and 3D methods, both with an estimated LVEF of 11% (see Video 12.4E). *EDV*, End-diastolic volume; *EF*, ejection fraction; *ESV*, end-systolic volume; *SV*, stroke volume.

circumferential shortening, and radial thickening. Tissue velocities, strain, and strain rates are reduced in DCM and provide insight into the mechanics of LV dysfunction. Chapters 2 and 4 provide full details regarding these measurements.

If image quality is poor, tissue Doppler imaging (TDI) is useful for risk stratification because there is less dependence on image quality compared with LVEF. Longitudinal systolic mitral annular velocity (S_m) is reproducible, with interobserver variability of about 4% to 8%.[27] In chronic HF, low S_m predicts death or cardiac transplantation, with a cutoff of 2.8 cm/s.[28]

The combined use of spectral and tissue Doppler echocardiography has been referred to as an echo-based right heart catheterization to evaluate cardiac hemodynamics.[29] The integration of echo-based parameters provides noninvasive estimates of filling pressures and cardiac output.

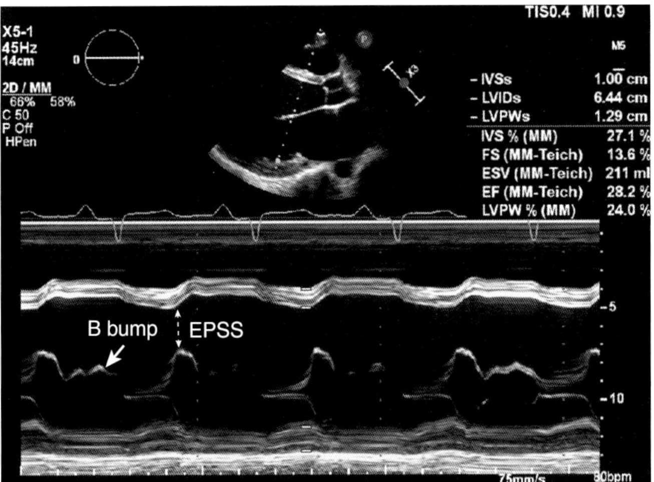

Fig. 12.5 M-mode findings in dilated cardiomyopathy. M-mode was obtained at the level of the mitral valve in the parasternal long-axis view. Increased LV dimensions, decreased fractional shortening, and increased E-point septal separation *(EPSS; double-headed arrow)* are present. The B bump *(arrow)* corresponds to elevated LV end-diastolic pressure. *EF*, Ejection fraction; *FS*, fractional shortening; *ESV*, end-systolic volume; *IVS*, interventricular septum; *LVPW*, LV posterior wall.

STRAIN IMAGING

Over the past decade, strain imaging has emerged as a sensitive and reproducible technique of assessing myocardial mechanics. Although TDI is useful, myocardial velocities measured by TDI are affected by tethering and translational motion of the heart and are angle dependent. This limitation can be overcome by measuring myocardial deformation using speckle-tracking strain and strain rate imaging. Myocardial velocities and displacement are higher in the basal segments compared with the apex, reflecting the contraction of the base toward a relatively fixed apex. Chapter 2 provides full details regarding strain imaging.

DCM is associated with a reduction of all deformational parameters, including longitudinal (Fig. 12.7), circumferential, and radial strain and torsion. Studies have shown that global longitudinal strain (GLS) assessed by speckle-tracking analysis is superior to LVEF for risk stratification.[30] GLS is most often used clinically because of its excellent reproducibility and the incremental addition of prognostic information to LVEF. Selected studies for strain imaging are summarized in Table 12.5.

In addition to 2D speckle tracking, 3D strain imaging has been used for the assessment of mitral annular displacement over its entire circumference, providing a more precise evaluation of complex annular excursion and deformation.[31] Global area strain has been shown to be a sensitive parameter for

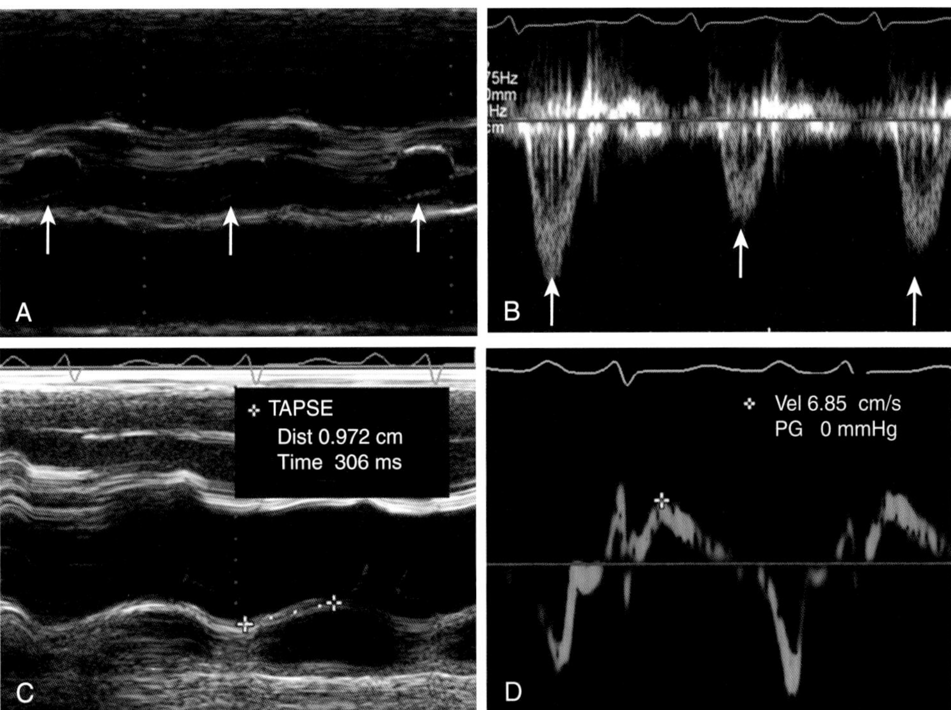

Fig. 12.6 Pulsus alternans and RV dysfunction in dilated cardiomyopathy. (A) Rounding of the aortic valve profile *(arrows)* on M-mode. (B) Example of pulsus alternans shows variation in stroke volume with each beat *(arrows)*. (C and D) The patient also has reduced RV function with a low tricuspid annular plane systolic excursion *(TAPSE)* and RV systolic wave velocity *(S')*. *PG*, Pressure gradient.

TABLE 12.4 **Imaging Modalities for Evaluation of LV Systolic Function.**

Imaging Modality	*Limitations*
2D Echocardiography (2DE)	
• Quantitative methods of LVEF assessment are preferred, such as biplane method of disks.	• Transducer position and angulation can result in foreshortening. • Geometric assumptions are required for quantitative estimates of LVEF. • There can be errors in tracing borders; consider contrast administration if endocardial borders are not well defined. • Poor reproducibility due to variation in image acquisition techniques.
3D Echocardiography	
• Improved image quality and simultaneous biplane imaging compared with 2DE • Automated detection of LV endocardial surface is less constrained by geometric assumptions; may be better than 2DE when the LV shape is distorted	• Lower temporal and spatial resolution than 2DE • Motion artifact can interfere with image acquisition.
Myocardial Strain Echocardiography	
• Assesses longitudinal contraction, circumferential shortening, and radial thickening • Can perform with tissue Doppler imaging or speckle tracking • Most commonly, LV global longitudinal strain with speckle tracking is used.	• Angle dependent if tissue Doppler imaging is used for strain • Signal noise and reverberation can create artifact and limit speckle tracking. • Out-of-plane cardiac motion may not be captured with either modality. • Postprocessing may be required in some cases, which can be time-consuming.
Nuclear Imaging	
• Multigated radionuclide angiography (MUGA) • Single-photon emission computed tomography (SPECT) • Positron emission tomography (PET) has better spatial and temporal resolution than SPECT	• Requires stable, regular heart rhythm for SPECT and PET • Need to correct for attenuation • Does not provide information on other cardiac parameters such as diastolic function or valves • Radiation exposure
Cardiac Computed Tomography (CT)	
• Multiphase acquisition can provide assessment of LVEF; retrospective gating is used to reconstruct images throughout cardiac cycle • Can provide volumetric assessment of LVEF • Higher spatial resolution than cardiac MRI or echocardiography	• Need slow heart rate for appropriate gating • Poor temporal resolution; may be difficult to accurately determine accurate portions of the cardiac cycle • Use of contrast for patients with renal disease • Radiation exposure
Cardiac Magnetic Resonance Imaging (MRI)	
• Higher spatial resolution than 2DE • Temporal resolution similar to 2DE • Less interference from adjacent bone or air compared with echocardiography • Fewer geometric constraints; volumetric analysis performed in small segments • Can accurately assess RV function • Superior border detection between blood pool and endocardium • No radiation (compared with CT or nuclear studies)	• Multiple breath-holds are required to obtain continuous slices for entire LV. • Discontinuous coverage or misalignment of LV slices can occur with varied breath-holds. • Image postprocessing is required. • Relatively long acquisition time is needed. • Incompatible with certain medical devices that contain metallic components

LVEF, Left ventricular ejection fraction.

detection of subtle LV systolic dysfunction. In a study that included healthy individuals and patients with HF, there was a progressive decrease in 3D strain with each progressive ACCF/AHA stage of HF from A through D.[32]

LV TORSION

The myocardium is composed of complex helical patterns, with longitudinal fibers forming a right-handed helix in the subendocardium and a left-handed helix in the subepicardium.[29] In DCM, there is an attenuation of LV rotation at the base and apex, which reduces LV twisting and untwisting velocities.[33] As a consequence of LV remodeling in DCM, the mechanical advantage of subepicardial myofibers is reduced, and LV twist is decreased as the LV cavity volume increases. Paradoxical reverse rotation of the LV (i.e., base with counterclockwise rotation and apex with clockwise end-systolic rotation) occurs in advanced cases of DCM.

LV DIASTOLIC FUNCTION

Almost all patients with systolic dysfunction have impaired relaxation and decreases in ventricular compliance. The assessment of LV diastolic function should be an integral part of the routine evaluation of patients with DCM (see Chapter 5). Abnormalities of LV diastolic filling are intimately related to functional status and prognosis, and patients with systolic function have drastically different hemodynamics based on the degree of diastolic dysfunction.

Most of the echocardiographic diastolic evaluation is performed by Doppler interrogation. However, one M-mode finding that remains relevant is the B bump (see Fig. 12.5), which is caused by delayed closure of the mitral leaflets that results in a small notch between the leaflet coaptation points. This finding correlates with an elevated LV end-diastolic pressure that typically exceeds 20 mmHg.

Patients with HF and abnormal diastolic dysfunction, particularly those who have a restrictive filling pattern, as characterized by high E/A ratios, rapid deceleration times, increased E/e′, and low e′ (Fig. 12.8), have increased mortality rates. A mitral E/A greater than 1.5 is associated with a twofold increased all-cause mortality rate and a threefold increased cardiac mortality rate even after adjustment for comorbidities.[34] A deceleration time of less than 150 ms predicted the combined end point of death, HF hospitalization, and heart transplantation in a trial of patients with advanced HF.[24] When HF patients were stratified on the basis of LVEF and the E/e′ ratio, those with LVEF of 40% or less and an E/e′ of 15 or greater were at the highest risk for readmission and cardiac death.[35] A restrictive filling pattern is associated with high mortality rates and the need for transplantation.[36]

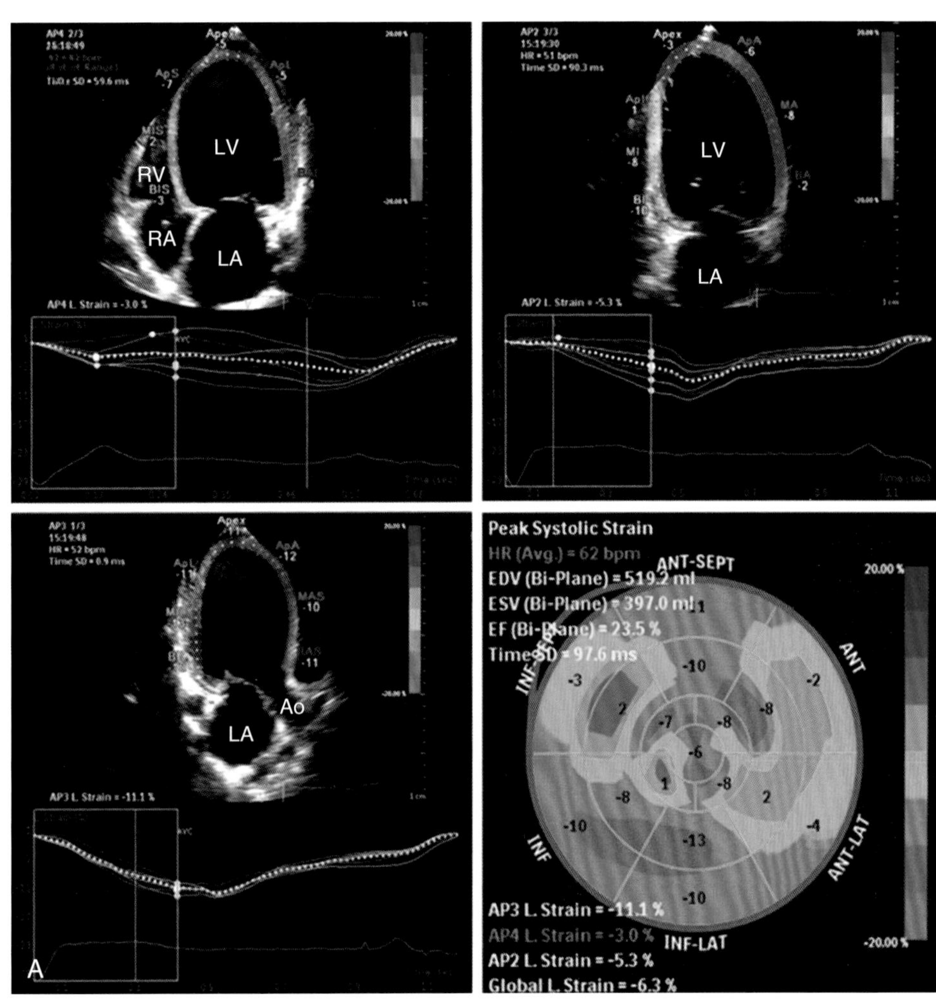

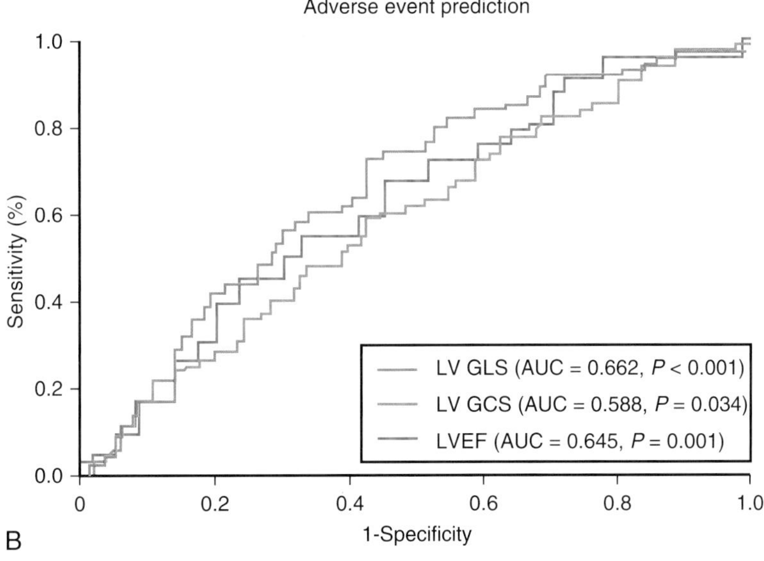

Fig. 12.7 **Reduced global longitudinal strain in dilated cardiomyopathy.** (A) Estimation of global longitudinal strain (GLS) in dilated cardiomyopathy in the apical 4-chamber *(upper left)*, apical 2-chamber *(upper right)*, and apical 3-chamber *(lower left)* views. In all views, the longitudinal strain is markedly abnormal, with a GLS of −6.3% correlating with a biplane LV ejection fraction (LVEF) of 23.5% *(lower right)*. (B) Receiver operating characteristic (ROC) curves for prediction of death, cardiac transplantation, or heart failure admission with LV GLS, global circumferential strain (GCS), and LVEF. The area under the curve (AUC) of GLS was the greatest, with an optimal ROC cutoff of −6.95%. *Blue line* indicates LV GLS; *orange line* indicates LV GCS; *red line* indicates LVEF. (From Motoki H, Borowski AG, Shrestha K, et al. Incremental prognostic value of assessing left ventricular myocardial mechanics in patients with chronic systolic heart failure. *J Am Coll Cardiol.* 2012;60:2074–2081.)

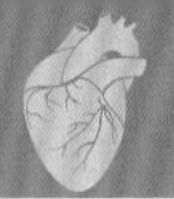

TABLE 12.5 Studies Evaluating LV Strain in Heart Failure With Reduced Ejection Fraction.

Study	*Cohort*	*Findings*
Motoki et al. (2012)[102]	194 patients with chronic systolic heart failure	LV GLS ≥ −6.95% was an independent predictor of death, cardiac transplantation, and HF-related admissions at 5 years in HF of ischemic or nonischemic cause, regardless of age, LVEF, and E/e′, and it had greater prognostic power than LVEF. LV GCS ≥ −7.15 % predicted adverse events only in patients with nonischemic HF.
Zhang et al. (2014)[104]	416 patients with chronic systolic heart failure	LV longitudinal, circumferential, and radial strain; addition of strain to LVEF improved AUC at 1 year (from 0.633 to 0.697) and at 5 years (from 0.638 to 0.700) for an end point of death, cardiac transplantation, or ventricular assist device.
Sengelov et al. (2015)[106]	1102 patients with chronic systolic heart failure	GLS was an independent predictor for death (hazard ratio = 1.15 per 1% decrease) and was superior to LVEF but did not appear to be a predictor for patients with atrial fibrillation or for women.
Park et al. (2018)[107]	4172 patients with acute heart failure, included reduced and preserved LVEF	Each 1% increase in GLS was associated with a 5% decreased risk of death. Moderate (8.1% < GLS < 12.5%) and severe GLS reductions (GLS ≤ 8.0%) predicted death, but LVEF was not a predictor of death.

AUC, Area under the curve; *GCS*, global circumferential strain; *GLS*, global longitudinal strain; *HF*, heart failure; *LVEF*, LV ejection fraction.

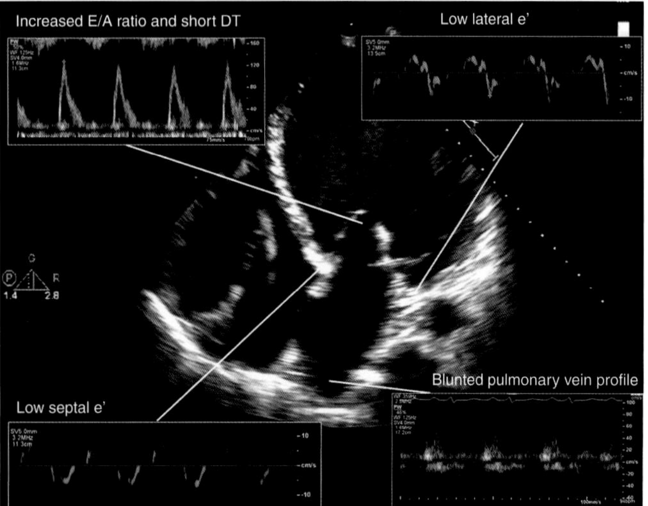

Fig. 12.8 Restrictive filling pattern in a patient with dilated cardiomyopathy. A markedly increased ratio of early to atrial *(E/A)* peak filling velocity, short deceleration time *(DT)*, reduced septal and lateral wall peak early tissue Doppler velocities *(e′)*, and blunting of the pulmonary vein systolic profile are present. In this case, there is also spontaneous echocardiographic contrast in the LV chamber, suggesting a low-flow state (see Video 12.8).

LA size is an important prognostic marker for patients with HF and DCM. In patients with significant HF, the LA contributes to stroke volume. LA dilation can compromise hemodynamics and is associated with higher mortality and cardiovascular hospitalization rates. For patients with DCM, an LA volume greater than 68.5 mL/m^2 was associated with increased risk compared with smaller LA volumes and was independently predictive even after accounting for the presence of atrial fibrillation, LV volume, LVEF, MR, and E/A ratio.[22,37]

There is growing interest in the use of speckle-tracking LA strain for assessment of diastolic function. LA systolic strain can quantitate atrial function, predict cardiovascular events,[38] and correlate with LV end-diastolic pressure. LA reservoir strain decreases linearly as LV diastolic dysfunction worsens, which is unusual among diastolic variables with its consistent direction of change (other parameters, such as E/A ratio are nonlinear with progressive severity). LA strain has been proposed as an adjunctive measurement, particularly for patients with indeterminate diastolic function.[39] LA strain is inversely correlated with LV filling pressures, with a peak LA reservoir strain cutoff of less than 20% providing a receiver operating characteristic (ROC) of 0.76 for a pre–A-wave LV diastolic pressure greater than 15 mmHg.[40]

SECONDARY MITRAL REGURGITATION

With progression of DCM, secondary MR (Fig. 12.9) results from a combination of LV remodeling with LV enlargement and increased sphericity, decreased closing forces from systolic dysfunction, mitral annular dilation and flattening, apical and lateral displacement of papillary muscles, and intraventricular dyssynchrony of the LV lateral and septal walls[41] (Fig. 12.10).

Because of LV remodeling, the mitral apparatus is deformed, resulting in tenting of the leaflets. Tenting area can be calculated in the parasternal long-axis view at mid-systole by measuring the area enclosed by the annular plane and coaptation point of the mitral leaflets. MV tenting area correlates with the severity of secondary MR, and a value of 3.4 cm^2 or greater is associated with an increased risk of death or HF hospitalization.[42] For individuals with HF, progressive severity of MR is a stepwise independent predictor of adverse outcomes.[24] In one study of HF patients with an LVEF of 35% or less, severe MR was associated with a relative risk of 1.8 for death.[43]

The evaluation of MR is covered in Chapter 24. Accurate assessment of secondary MR can be challenging. Conventional 2D evaluation relies on measurement of the MR jet at its vena contracta or proximal convergence zone, but these measurements assume a circular orifice. Instead, the secondary MR orifice is usually elliptical. 3D echocardiographic measurement (Fig. 12.11) can overcome this limitation by direct planimetry of the vena contracta. The severity of secondary MR varies during the cardiac cycle, which adds another layer of complexity to an accurate evaluation. Several studies have suggested that lower quantitative measures of MR correlate with increased severity of secondary MR compared with primary MR.[44] Accepted values consistent with severe secondary MR include an effective regurgitant orifice area (EROA) of 20 mm^2 or greater, a regurgitant volume of 30 mL or greater, and a regurgitant fraction of 50% or greater.[45]

Management of secondary MR is challenging, with efforts directed toward improving symptoms, reducing hospitalizations, and improving survival. Guideline-directed therapy for HF should be instituted with the hope of reverse remodeling that can lead to reduction in MR severity. CRT can be effective

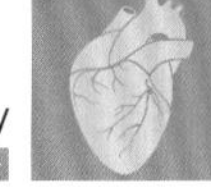

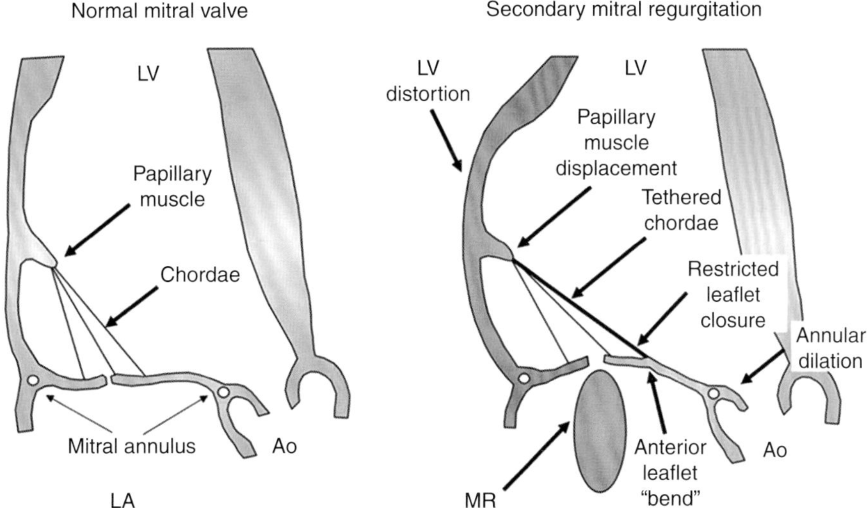

Fig. 12.9 Mechanism of secondary mitral regurgitation. Spatial relationship between the mitral valve apparatus and LV in a normal condition *(left)* and in the pathologic condition *(right)* of secondary mitral regurgitation *(MR). Ao*, Aorta. (From Iung J, Capoulade R. Therapy for secondary mitral regurgitation: time to 'cut the chord'? *Heart.* 2015;101:996–997.)

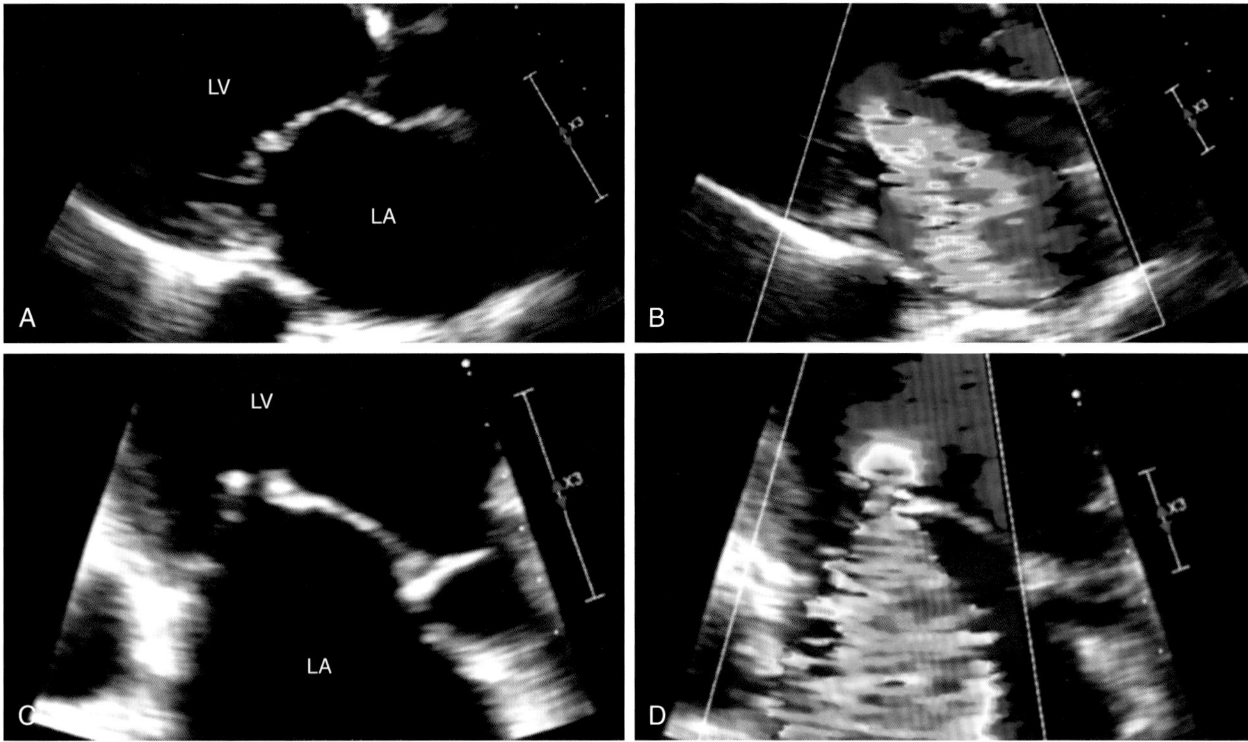

Fig. 12.10 Secondary mitral regurgitation. In a patient with dilated cardiomyopathy, there is distortion of the mitral annulus with displacement of the papillary muscles, resulting in a central mitral regurgitation (MR) jet. Transthoracic parasternal long-axis view shows tented mitral valve leaflets (A) and a central MR jet (B) (see Videos 12.10A and B). (C) Transthoracic 2-chamber view shows tented mitral valve leaflets (C) and a central MR jet (D) (see Videos 12.10C and D).

in selected individuals by restoring synchronous ventricular contraction, and it contributes to reverse remodeling, particularly in patients with non-ischemic cardiomyopathy. Severe secondary MR improves in about 40% to 50% of affected individuals treated with CRT.[46]

Although MV repair for secondary MR can lead to improvement in symptoms and LV function, there is no clear survival benefit.[47] In the absence of other cardiac surgery, the 2017 ACCF/AHA guidelines for the management of valvular heart disease provide a class IIb recommendation for MV repair or replacement in patients who remain severely symptomatic (New York Heart Association [NYHA] class III–IV) with chronic severe secondary MR (stage D) despite optimal medical therapies.[48]

Trials have evaluated the use of transcatheter MV repair with MitraClip to reduce the severity of secondary MR. The Mitra-FR

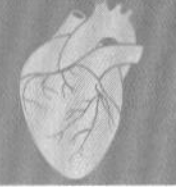

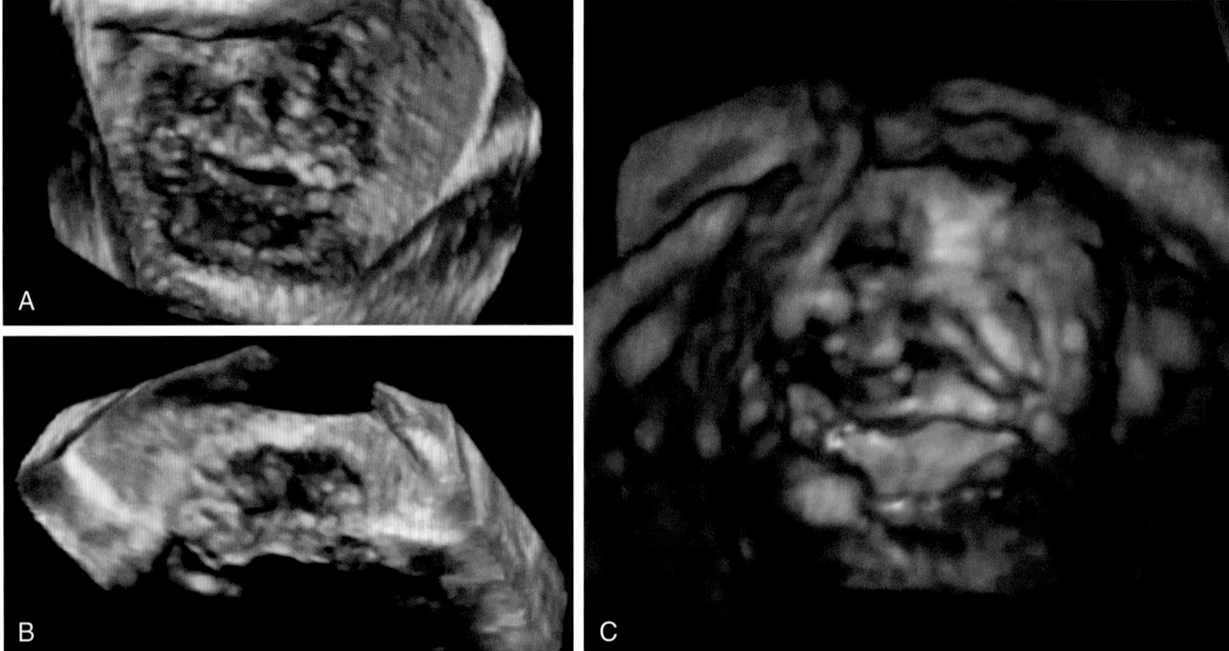

Fig. 12.11 3D TEE assessment of secondary mitral regurgitation. Elliptical orifice of the vena contracta jet without (A and B) and with (C) color Doppler (see Videos 12.11A–C). There is distortion of the mitral annulus and incomplete coaptation of the leaflets with resultant mitral regurgitation.

trial[49] randomized patients with severe secondary MR, an LVEF of 15% to 40%, and an EROA of greater than 20 mm^2 to guideline-directed medical therapy (GDMT) versus GDMT plus MitraClip. At 1 year, there was no benefit for the end point of HF-related hospitalization or all-cause mortality. The COAPT trial[50] randomized patients with an LVEF of 20% to 50%, grade 3 or 4 secondary MR, and ongoing symptoms (NYHA class II–IVa) to GDMT versus GDMT plus MitraClip. At 2 years, there was a reduction in HF-related hospitalization and lower all-cause mortality for patients receiving MitraClip. Both trials showed that MitraClip reduced MR volume, although the reduction was greater in COAPT. Patients in COAPT had more severe MR and less LV dilation. Correcting secondary MR may be more beneficial when it is disproportionate to the severity of LV dysfunction.[51] These data support the idea that carefully selected patients with functional MR may benefit from transcatheter MV repair.

LV CONTRACTILE RESERVE

A fraction of patients with DCM can augment systolic function in response to stress. This ability is directly correlated with survival.[52] Although it is not routinely performed in all individuals with DCM, contractile reserve can be estimated with stress echocardiography with low-dose dobutamine infusion while assessing changes in stroke volume. Other methods of contractile reserve determination have included the parameters of cardiac output, LVEF, wall motion stress index, and strain analysis. When LV contractile reserve was measured in DCM patients, there was an adequate specificity of 89% but poor sensitivity of 65% for predicting adverse events.[53] Common cutoffs include an increase in LVEF of 5% or greater at peak stress or a percentage change from baseline of 20% or greater.

RIGHT-SIDED INVOLVEMENT

Approximately 34% of patients with DCM have RV involvement.[54] RV dysfunction is not needed for the diagnosis of DCM but is a marker of poor prognosis when present. RV function is more difficult to quantitate than LV function because of the complex RV anatomy and shape. Patients with predominant LV involvement have better overall survival and less severe MR and TR compared with patients who have bilateral involvement.[55]

Tricuspid annular plane systolic excursion (TAPSE), as part of an echocardiographic evaluation of DCM (see Fig. 12.6), provides incremental prognostic information to the commonly used parameters of functional class, LVEF, and mitral Doppler variables for patients with DCM.[56] TDI assessment of RV function is prognostic. When evaluating various systolic and diastolic RV functional parameters, a tricuspid systolic annular velocity of less than 10.8 cm/s and an RV Tei index of greater than 1.20 predicts the lowest rate of event-free survival.[57]

Many DCM patients develop tricuspid regurgitation (TR) due to distortion of tricuspid valve anatomy and annular dilation from RV remodeling. TR is an independent predictor of poor clinical outcomes,[43] with a peak TR velocity greater than 2.5 m/s associated with increased mortality rates. DCM patients can develop elevated pulmonary artery pressures from abnormal LV filling or secondary MR, and this is associated with a worse prognosis.[58]

Similar to the uptake of LV GLS in clinical practice, RV strain is gaining traction as another method for quantifying RV function. RV strain of −14.8% or greater provides incrementally prognostic information for death, cardiac transplantation, and HF hospitalization.[59] For acute HF patients, RV strain is associated with death independent of LV GLS, and patients with biventricular GLS reduction have the worst prognosis.[60] In a cohort of advanced HF patients undergoing LV assist device

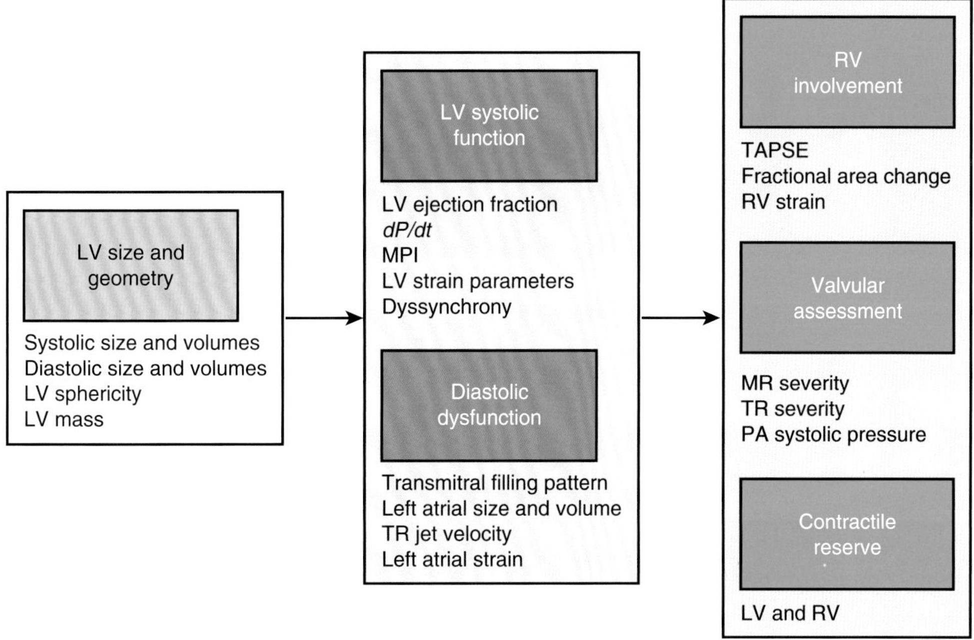

Fig. 12.12 Simplified approach to the echocardiographic evaluation of dilated cardiomyopathy. Flow chart shows an echocardiographic approach to dilated cardiomyopathy. *dP/dt,* Ratio of pressure change in the ventricular cavity during the isovolumic contraction period; *MPI,* myocardial performance index; *MR,* mitral regurgitation; *PA,* pulmonary artery; *TAPSE,* tricuspid annular plane systolic excursion; *TR,* tricuspid regurgitation.

implantation, RV free wall longitudinal strain with a cutoff of −9.6% was an independent predictor of post-implantation RV failure and incrementally additive to RV failure risk scores.[61] Fig. 12.12 summarizes a typical comprehensive echocardiographic assessment of DCM.

CONDITIONS THAT LEAD TO DILATED CARDIOMYOPATHY

MYOCARDITIS

There are many causes of myocarditis, with viral infection being the most common. Myocardial inflammation can be diffuse or focal and can involve any cardiac chamber. Findings on echocardiography are nonspecific; cases appear similar to DCM, but there is rapid progression in individuals without a known cardiac history. There is often a degree of LV dilation, increased sphericity, and focal or diffuse wall motion abnormalities. Affected individuals have abnormal diastolic findings, which can range from abnormal relaxation to advanced restrictive filling patterns. Myocytolysis causes changes in echocardiographic texture, and cell infiltration alters myocardial density, resulting in increased backscatter. Interstitial edema increases the interval between the reflecting surfaces. In combination, these changes produce higher average brightness, heterogeneity, and contrast.[62]

Depending on whether the myocarditis is fulminant or acute, cardiac parameters vary. Fulminant myocarditis manifests without significant LV dilation, but it frequently produces thickened LV walls and a marked decrease in systolic function. Conversely, acute myocarditis usually demonstrates LV dilation, normal LV wall thickness, and a more indolent decease in systolic function.

Echocardiographic features for myocarditis are nonspecific, and it is challenging to noninvasively confirm the diagnosis (Fig. 12.13A–D). Myocardial strain imaging is useful in guiding diagnosis because strain is diffusely and globally abnormal in myocarditis.[63] Cardiac MRI can assist with validation of the diagnosis by demonstrating increases in T2 intensity due to edema, early myocardial gadolinium enhancement from hyperemia and capillary leak, and late gadolinium enhancement involvement of the subepicardium due to necrosis and fibrosis[64] (see Fig. 12.13E and F).

The prognostic implications vary, with some individuals regaining normal function but others progressing to chronic DCM. A multicenter study demonstrated that fulminant myocarditis leads to increased rates of cardiac death and heart transplantation compared with nonfulminant myocarditis in the short- and long-term settings.[65]

CHAGAS HEART DISEASE

Chagas disease is caused by the protozoan *Trypanosoma cruzi*, and it is transmitted to humans by insect vectors. When involving the myocardium, it leads to inflammation, cell death, and fibrosis in a segmental or regional manner. Although traditionally found in Central America and South America, Chagas disease affects many residents in the United States. The acute form usually manifests as flu-like symptoms. However, 5% of patients present with myopericarditis. Chronic cases progress to DCM with HF, ventricular arrhythmias, and conduction abnormalities.

The most common echocardiographic findings are regional wall motion abnormalities in the apical and inferolateral walls, globally reduced systolic function, and pericardial effusion. Apical aneurysm is common in Chagas heart disease in patients with moderate to severe myocardial involvement (Fig. 12.14). Aneurysm morphology can vary from small, localized lesions to large areas of extensive wall thinning similar to ischemic aneurysm.

The ASE guideline on Chagas disease[66] recommends the use of 3D echocardiography for detection of small LV aneurysms that would otherwise be overlooked by 2D

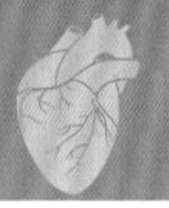

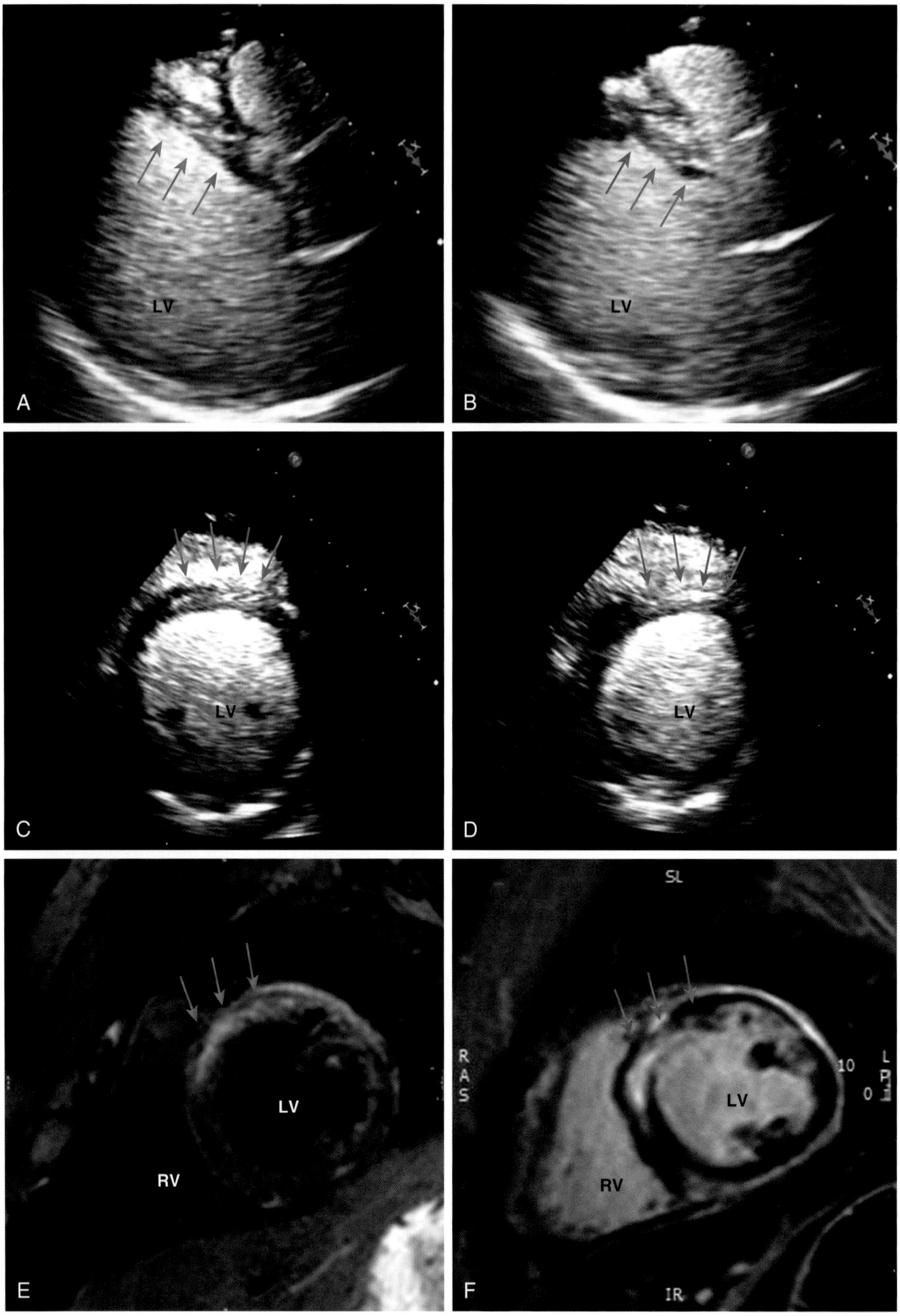

Fig. 12.13 Contrast echocardiography and cardiac magnetic resonance imaging of acute myocarditis. (A and B) Parasternal long-axis echocardiographic views (*left*, diastole; *right*, systole) with contrast enhancement. The region of active inflammation (i.e., basal anteroseptum) is echogenic on these images *(arrows)*. There is akinesis of the basal anteroseptum corresponding with the area of echogenicity (see Videos 12.13A and B). (C and D) Parasternal short-axis echocardiographic views (*left*, diastole; *right*, systole) with contrast enhancement. The region of active inflammation (i.e., mid-anterior wall) is echogenic on these images *(arrows)* with corresponding akinesis (see Videos 12.13C and D). (E) Cardiac MRI T2-weighted spin-echo image with high signal intensity of the mid-anterior wall and anteroseptum *(arrows)* is consistent with regional edema. (F) Cardiac MRI late gadolinium-enhanced image shows regional subepicardial enhancement *(arrows)* of the corresponding wall segments.

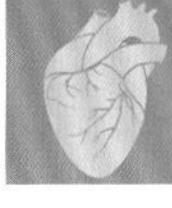

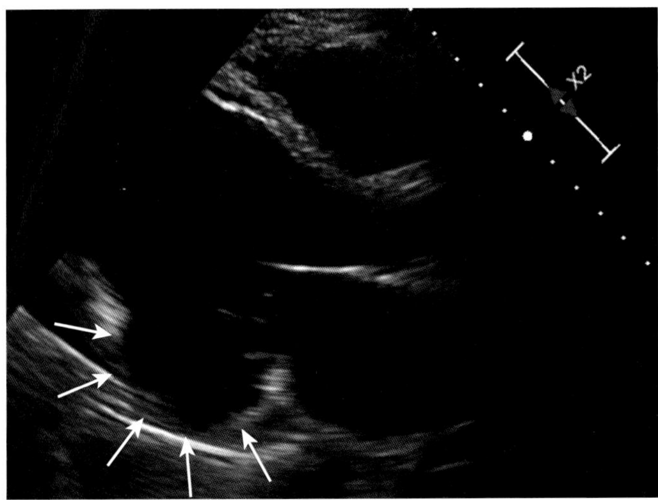

Fig. 12.14 **Chagas cardiomyopathy.** Parasternal long-axis view of a patient with Chagas heart disease shows a focal basal inferolateral aneurysm *(arrows)* (see Video 12.14).

echocardiography due to foreshortening. 3D echocardiography is more accurate than the 2D Simpson biplane method for assessing LV volume and LVEF in patients with significant wall motion abnormalities, including aneurysms with distorted LV geometry.

Speckle-tracking strain can detect subclinical myocardial dysfunction in Chagas heart disease, although the role of early changes in predicting disease progression is not well defined. Speckle tracking can also quantify the heterogeneity of systolic contraction, which is associated with risk of ventricular arrhythmia.[67]

OTHER CARDIAC CONDITIONS THAT MIMIC DILATED CARDIOMYOPATHY

LV NONCOMPACTION

Although not traditionally grouped with DCM, LV noncompaction (LVNC) bears discussion because advanced stages manifest with LV dilation and reduced LVEF. On echocardiography, noncompaction is distinct because it exhibits prominent LV trabeculae (Fig. 12.15) with exaggerated intertrabecular recesses. Noncompaction occurs due to an arrest of normal embryogenesis of the endocardium and myocardium, preventing compaction of the spongy meshwork of fibers and intertrabecular recesses that form the myocardium during embryonic life. Acquired LVNC has also been described in athletes, during pregnancy, and with chronic renal failure.

The most commonly used echocardiographic criteria for noncompaction are those proposed by Jenni et al.[68] and include a thickened LV wall with two layers having a ratio of noncompacted to compacted myocardium greater than 2:1 in the parasternal short-axis view at end-systole, intertrabecular spaces filling with blood flow on color Doppler, and the absence of coexisting cardiac abnormalities.

The bilayered myocardium should be assessed in multiple imaging windows in the short-axis views between the level of the papillary muscles and the apex because of the variation in appearance by level. There should be a thin, compacted epicardial layer with a thicker, noncompacted endocardial layer. Off-axis images can misrepresent bilayer thickness. Frequently, pathology is localized to the mid-lateral, mid-inferior, and apical segments. Administration of echocardiographic contrast improves resolution between the compacted and noncompacted layers of myocardium.

It is essential to exclude other causes that appear similar to noncompacted myocardium, including LV thrombus, false tendons, and apical hypertrophic cardiomyopathy. Systolic strain, strain rate, and LV rotation are reduced in noncompaction.[69] Cardiac MRI should be considered for confirmation (see Fig. 12.15).

There can be significant variation in LV trabecular anatomy. The prevalence of LVNC is increasingly reported in large series, but there is a lack of consensus about diagnostic standards. False-positive results can be avoided with meticulous technique and ensuring that the short-axis views are perpendicular to the long-axis views and not oblique.[29]

STRESS-INDUCED CARDIOMYOPATHY

Acute-onset stress-induced cardiomyopathy usually manifests with transient systolic dysfunction of the LV middle and apical segments. Proposed mechanisms include exaggerated sympathetic stimulation with adrenergic excess, coronary spasm, and microvascular dysfunction. The syndrome occurs more frequently in women than in men and typically in individuals older than 50 years of age.[70]

The Mayo Clinic criteria for diagnosis of stress-induced cardiomyopathy[71] include (1) transient akinesis or dyskinesis of the LV apical and mid-ventricular segments with regional wall motion abnormalities that involve more than a single coronary distribution; (2) absence of obstructive coronary artery disease; (3) new ECG abnormalities; and (4) absence of recent significant head trauma, pheochromocytoma, myocarditis, and hypertrophic cardiomyopathy.

Echocardiography frequently demonstrates LV apical ballooning (Fig. 12.16) with akinesis of the mid-apical one half of the LV, although regional abnormalities can occur in other patterns and distributions.[72] LV outflow tract obstruction can occur due to hyperkinesis of the basal segments relative to the more distal segments.[70] Speckle tracking shows reduced LV strain in a segmental territory that does not correlate with any single coronary territory,[73] LV thrombus formation can occur due to regional akinesis or dyskinesis. Most patients recover normal LV function in 1 to 4 weeks, but there is a risk of recurrence of 1.8% per patient-year.[74]

CARDIAC RESYNCHRONIZATION THERAPY

Contraction of the normal LV occurs synchronously and by a similar degree throughout the chamber. This contraction pattern can be disrupted by left bundle branch block (LBBB) or when the LV is electrically stimulated at a single site. In both instances, contraction becomes inefficient, because one side moves inward before the other and is then stretched as the latter continues contracting. This shifts a portion of blood volume back and forth in the chamber rather than ejecting it, resulting in a net decline of systolic performance. Interventricular dyssynchrony, especially in the setting of paradoxical septal motion in systole, may adversely affect RV function, further impeding venous return to the LV. Consequently, the efficiency of pump function is approximately 30% lower in dyssynchronous hearts (Fig. 12.17).

Conventionally, mechanical dyssynchrony (Fig. 12.18) is defined as an increased time delay between the various LV wall regions, most commonly the LV lateral and septal walls. The

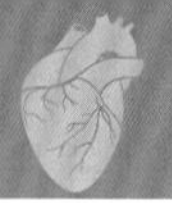

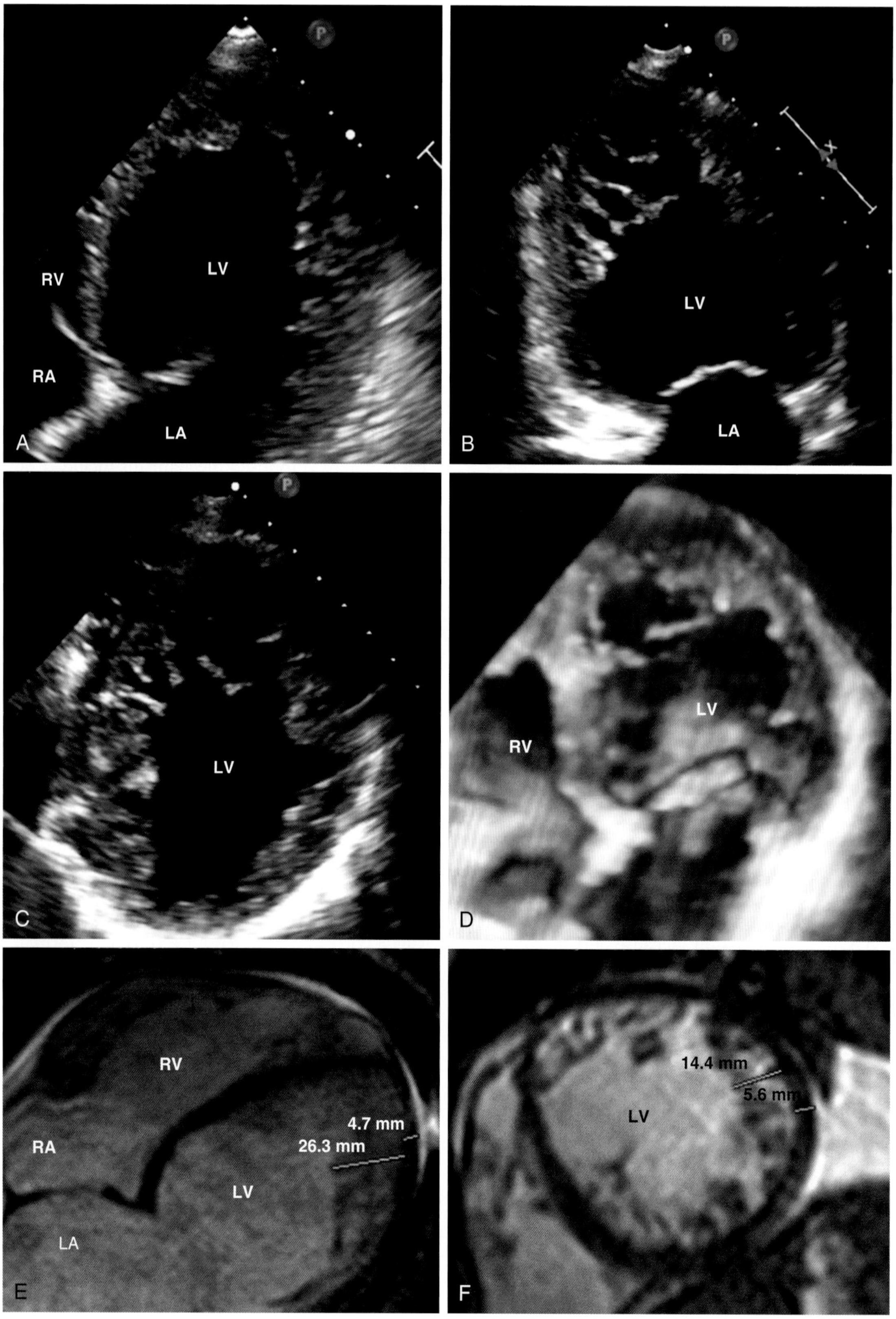

Fig. 12.15 Left ventricular noncompaction. (A) Apical 4-chamber view. There are prominent LV trabeculae and intertrabecular recesses at the LV apex (see Video 12.15A). (B) Apical 2-chamber view (see Video 12.15B). (C) Parasternal short-axis view (see Video 12.15C). (D) Apical 4-chamber view in 3D (see Video 12.15D). (E and F) Cardiac MRI correlation of noncompaction for the patient in Fig. 12.15 in the 4-chamber (A) and short-axis (B) view of the LV. The ratio of noncompacted to compacted myocardium is greater than 2:3, which is the MRI cutoff for noncompaction.

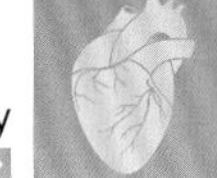

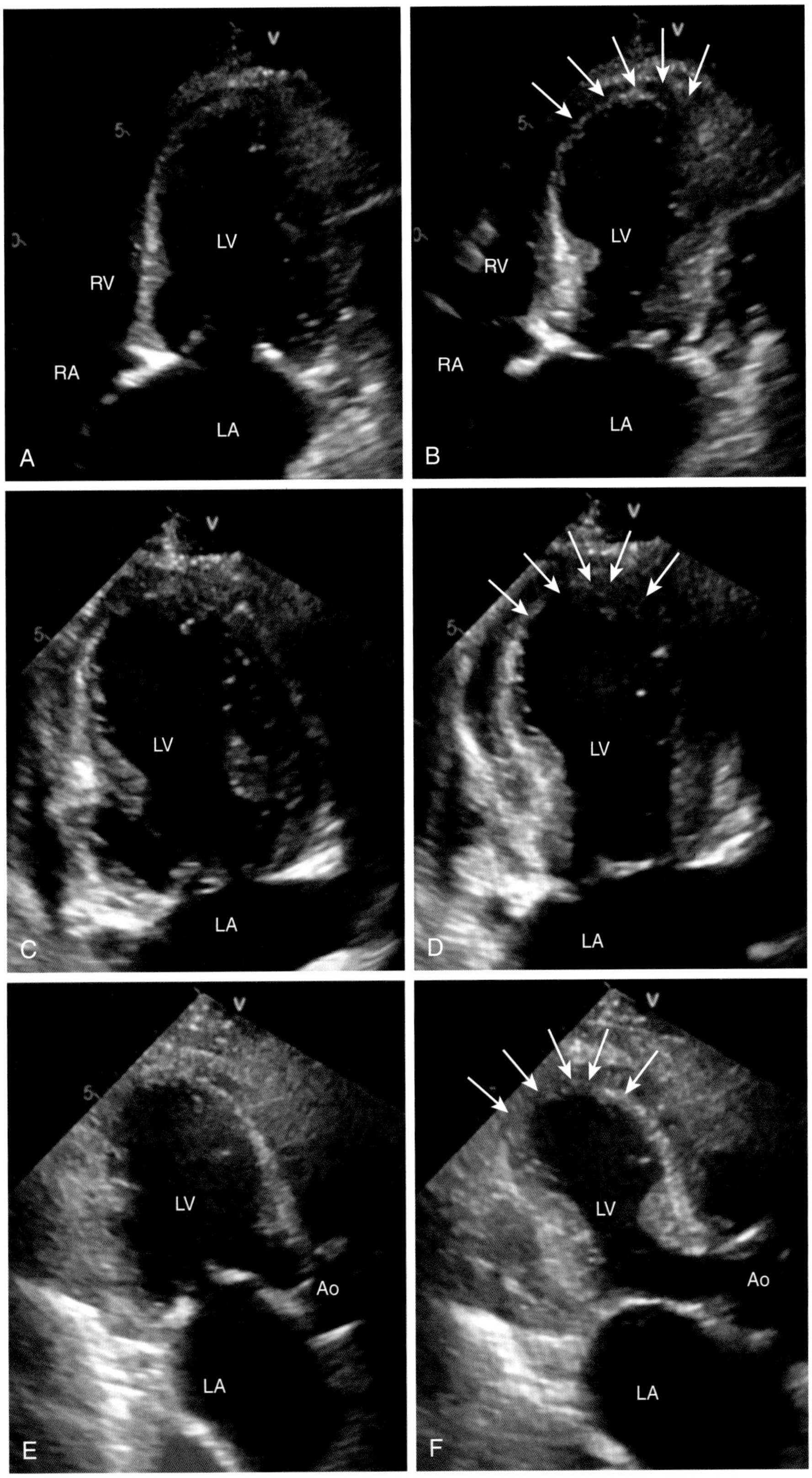

Fig. 12.16 Apical ballooning in a patient with stress-induced cardiomyopathy. *Left* panels show end-diastole, and *right* panels show end-systole, with *arrows* pointing to the apical ballooning and akinesis. (A and B) Apical 4-chamber view (see Videos 12.16A and B ▶). (C and D) Apical 2-chamber view (see Videos 12.16C and D ▶). (E and F) Apical 3-chamber view (see Videos 12.16E and F ▶). *Ao*, Aorta.

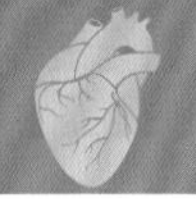

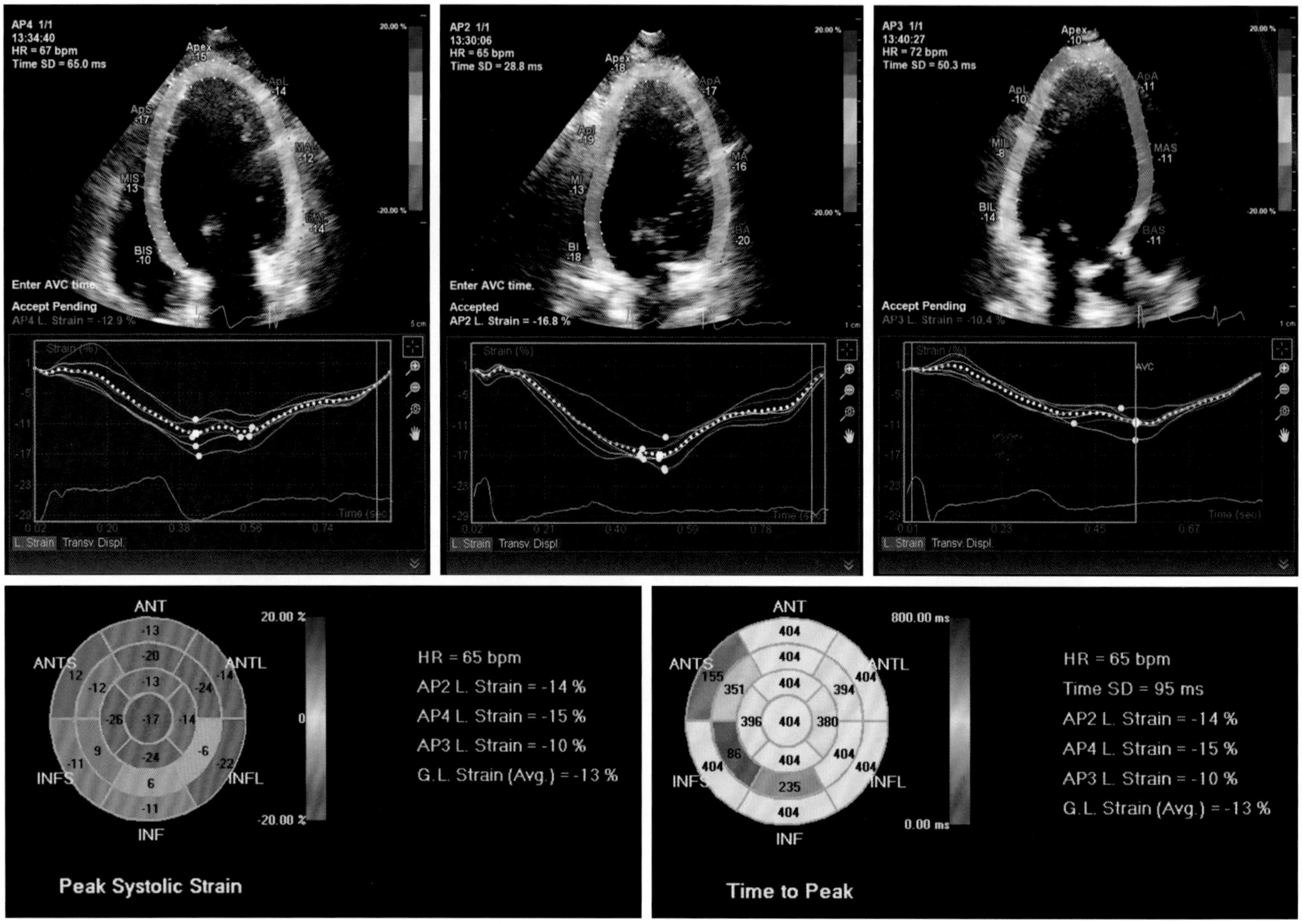

Fig. 12.17 Global longitudinal strain in a patient with dyssynchrony. *Top* panels demonstrate global longitudinal strain for apical 4-chamber, 2-chamber, and 3-chamber *(left to right)* views. *Bottom* panels demonstrate reduced global longitudinal strain of −13% *(left)* and increased standard deviation of 95 ms for time-to-peak *(right)*, which is consistent with significant dyssynchrony (see Video 12.17).

purpose of CRT in HF patients with LV dyssynchrony is to optimize atrioventricular conduction and LV filling, coordinate LV contraction by minimizing interventricular and intraventricular mechanical delay, and facilitate interventricular dependence. The improved synchrony and reduction in LV volumes decrease LV wall stress and stimulate reverse remodeling. This leads to decreased LV mass, restoration of mitral annular and subvalvular geometry, and reduction in secondary MR. Ultimately, the goals include alleviation of symptoms and improvement in functional capacity.

Randomized trials have established the role of CRT in patients with an LVEF of 35% or less, symptomatic HF (NYHA class II–IV), and abnormal QRS duration (>120 ms) and morphology. Guidelines have been updated to stratify patients according to their likelihood of benefiting from CRT. All cardiac societies concur that the greatest benefit is for patients with LBBB and a QRS duration of 150 ms or longer. However, for patient subgroups for whom evidence is limited, such as those with functional class NYHA I or IV, those with moderate QRS interval (120–149 ms), and those patients without LBBB, there are variations in guideline recommendations.[75,76] Unfortunately, even for patients meeting established criteria for CRT implantation, the CRT nonresponder rate remains high at 20% to 40%.[77]

ECHOCARDIOGRAPHY AND CARDIAC RESYNCHRONIZATION THERAPY

During the past decade, there have been discussions regarding whether assessment of dyssynchrony by echocardiography provides incremental value to QRS duration and morphology when assessing patients for CRT (Table 12.6). In the Predictors of Response to Cardiac Resynchronization (PROSPECT) trial, 12 echocardiographic parameters were simultaneously evaluated. This trial showed large variations in the predictive ability of echocardiography-based parameters regarding clinical outcomes, with limited sensitivity and specificity.[78] More recently, the EchoCRT trial found that in patients with NYHA class III or IV HF, a narrow QRS complex (<130 ms), and echocardiographic evidence of dyssynchrony, CRT does not reduce the rate of death and may increase mortality rates due to the onset of new delayed mechanical activation.[79]

Since the PROSPECT[78] and EchoCRT trials,[79] the role for echocardiography in selection of CRT candidates has been controversial. In both studies, the mechanical delay in contraction was addressed by methods that relied on the time-to-peak principle. This approach is limited in that it can detect dyssynchrony in the setting of heterogeneous intraventricular activation due to fibrosis or reduced contractility but does not necessarily represent a true activation delay

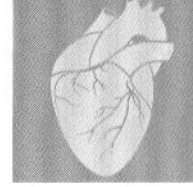

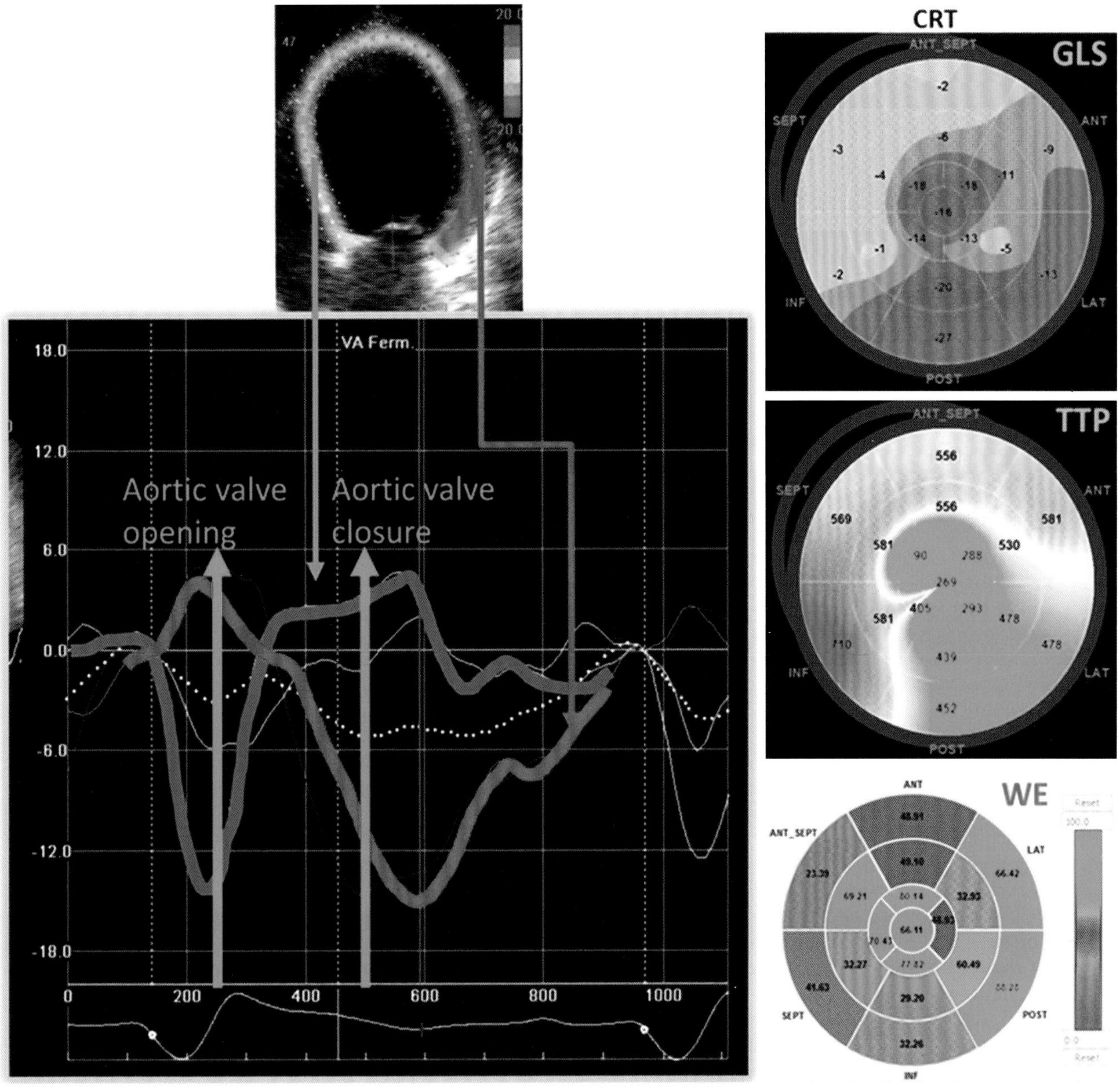

Fig. 12.18 **Mechanical dyssynchrony.** Impact of mechanical dyssynchrony on longitudinal strain curves: the septum with a too early contraction *(blue)*; the lateral wall with a delayed contraction *(red)*. *CRT*, Cardiac resynchronization therapy; *GLS*, Global longitudinal strain; *TTP*, time-to-peak; *WE*, wasted energy. (From Donal E, Delgado V, Magne J, et al. Rational and design of EuroCRT: an international observational study on multi-modality imaging and cardiac resynchronization therapy. *Eur Heart J Cardiovasc Imaging.* 2017;18:1120–1127.)

in substrate amenable to CRT response. Mechanical dyssynchrony based solely on segmental contraction does not incorporate viability or contractility of the underlying myocardial segments. If the underlying dyssynchronous myocardium does not have myocardial viability, correction of dyssynchrony will not improve cardiac function. Subsequent studies have focused on abnormal wall motion patterns typical in LBBB using strain imaging and may more reliably measure LV dyssynchrony.

The Heart Rhythm Society 2012 consensus statement[80] on CRT recognized that comprehensive assessment of mechanical dyssynchrony parameters can identify patients with a higher likelihood of CRT response but that echocardiography findings alone should not be used to exclude any patients from CRT. The ESC 2016 guidelines[81] for the diagnosis and treatment of HF stated that imaging tests for dyssynchrony have not been shown to be of value in selecting patients for CRT. Although patients with extensive scarring have an intrinsically worse prognosis, there is little evidence that they obtain less benefit from CRT. The value of trying to optimize the atrioventricular (AV) or ventriculoventricular (VV) intervals after implantation using echocardiographic or ECG criteria or blood pressure response is uncertain, but it may be considered for patients with a disappointing response to CRT.

INTRAVENTRICULAR DYSSYNCHRONY

Three types of cardiac dyssynchrony may occur: intraventricular, interventricular (i.e., VV), and AV. Abnormalities in the timing of regional mechanical LV activation (i.e., intraventricular

TABLE 12.6 Representative Echocardiographic Measures for Dyssynchrony.

Parameter	*Description of Method*	*Modality*	*Cutoff*
Apical rocking	Visual assessment of apical transverse motion	2D	Qualitative parameter
Septal flash	Visual assessment of short inward septal motion during beginning of systole	2D or M-mode	Large SF: marked fast motion, displacement > 50% of the septum Small SF: limited displacement
Interventricular delay	Difference between the onset of aortic and pulmonary artery flow	PW Doppler of LVOT and RVOT	>40 ms
Dyssynchrony index	SD of time-to-peak systolic velocity in all 12 basal and mid-LV segments	Tissue Doppler imaging	>32 ms
SD of time-to-peak strain	SD of time-to-peak strain in the 12 basal and mid-LV segments	Tissue Doppler imaging strain	>60 ms
Time-to-peak systolic radial strain	Difference between anteroseptal and posterior wall, from mid-short-axis view	Speckle tracking echo	>130 ms
Systolic stretch index	Sum of posterolateral systolic prestretch and septal systolic rebound stretch using radial strain	Speckle tracking echo	≥9.7%
Strain delay index	Sum of difference between end-systolic and peak strain across the 16 segments	Speckle tracking echo	>25%
RV strain	RV global longitudinal strain	Speckle tracking echo	<10%
Systolic dyssynchrony index	Standard deviation of time taken to reach minimum regional volume for each of 16 segments divided by RR interval	3D echo	>5.6%
LV discoordination index	Percentage of stretch/shortening or thinning/thickening during ejection	Speckle tracking echo	>38%

echo, Echocardiography; *LVOT*, LV outflow tract; *PW*, pulsed-wave; *RVOT*, RV outflow tract; *SD*, standard deviation; *SF*, septal flash.

dyssynchrony) appears to be the principal factor associated with contractile impairment and is most affected by CRT.

Septal Flash and Apical Rocking

Septal flash and apical rocking measure the direct mechanical consequences of dyssynchronous contraction and are highly reproducible. Septal flash is a premature contraction of the septum during the QRS and then before opening of the aortic valve. Apical rocking is a displacement of the LV apex toward the lateral wall. Whereas septal flash focuses on the isovolumic contraction phase, apical rocking focuses on the systolic phase. In a study of the relationship of visually assessed apical rocking and septal flash with response and long-term survival after CRT (PREDICT-CRT), researchers found that apical rocking and septal flash were associated with volumetric response and survival of HF patients after CRT.[82] The ongoing EuroCRT trial, an international observational study of multimodality imaging and CRT, is incorporating these parameters into quantification of mechanical dyssynchrony.[83]

Speckle-Tracking Imaging

LV dyssynchrony can be assessed by measuring the time difference in peak strain values between opposing segments (most frequently the anteroseptal and posterolateral walls). Radial strain is the least influenced by abnormal wall motion caused by ischemic disease, in which passive motion can be an important confounder. In the Speckle Tracking and Resynchronization (STAR) study, lack of baseline radial or transverse dyssynchrony appeared to be associated with increased risk of death, transplantation, or need for LVAD compared with dyssynchrony in NYHA class III or IV HF patients who underwent CR.[84]

Evaluation of longitudinal strain in different LV segments allows estimation of residual myocardial contractility, a variable that predicts CRT response.[85,86] In dyssynchronous ventricles, delayed segments do not fully contribute to end-systolic function because their contraction lasts after aortic valve closure.

More recent studies have focused on abnormal wall motion patterns that are typical for LBBB using strain imaging, including (1) early systolic shortening and rebound stretch in the septum, combined with early systolic lengthening; (2) early septal peak shortening (within the first 70% of the ejection phase); and (3) peak shortening after aortic valve closure in the LV lateral wall. A typical LBBB contraction pattern in CRT candidates was associated with a markedly improved response to CRT compared with lack of a typical pattern.[86,87]

It remains to be determined whether these insights can improve the CRT response. Speckle-tracking techniques have automated calculation of indices that should lead to high reproducibility and are more robust than previous approaches. The EuroCRT study will incorporate combined measures of LV dyssynchrony with myocardial scar estimated from cardiac MRI to determine whether the combination is beneficial for patient selection for CRT.[83]

INTERVENTRICULAR DELAY

The interventricular delay estimates mechanical dyssynchrony between the right and left ventricles and is determined by measuring the delay between the onset of RV and LV ejection as derived from pulsed-wave Doppler in the RV and LV outflow tracts, respectively. The pre-ejection intervals are measured from the onset of QRS to the onset of the RV and LV ejection flows. Interventricular delay of more than 40 ms is associated with increased reverse remodeling after CRT[88]; delays of 49 ms or more yield greater survival benefit from CRT compared with shorter delays.[89] RV function appears to mediate CRT response because an RV strain of less than 18% predicts a poor response to biventricular pacing.[90]

CHANGES IN DIASTOLIC FUNCTION WITH CARDIAC RESYNCHRONIZATION THERAPY

CRT can improve diastolic dysfunction by prolonging the duration of LV filling, separating the rapid filling phase from atrial systolic contraction, shortening interventricular delay, and coordinating global contraction and relaxation. It does not have the ability to normalize transmitral peak flow velocities during passive filling (E wave) or atrial contraction (peak A wave), the E/A ratio, or isovolumic relaxation time. After CRT, the E-wave deceleration time and MPI improve within 3 months and appear progressively better at 12 months. However, patients with restrictive LV filling exhibit little or no diastolic response to CRT.[91]

RESPONSE TO CARDIAC RESYNCHRONIZATION THERAPY

Approximately 60% to 65% of patients respond to CRT and exhibit LV reverse remodeling, characterized by a reduction in LV volumes, improved systolic function, normalization of diastolic function, and decreased severity of MR. The structural and functional changes associated with CRT occur as early as 3 months, typically become more pronounced by 6 months, and are sustained at 1 year.[92] Reduction in LV volumes and improvement in MR is two to three times greater in non-ischemic compared with ischemic cardiomyopathy. The decreased response to CRT for patients with ischemic cardiomyopathy is related to the presence of scar, which is not amenable to resynchronization.

An analysis of the Multicenter Automatic Defibrillator Implantation Trial-Cardiac Resynchronization Therapy (MADIT-CRT) trial found that female gender, a non-ischemic cause of HF, LBBB, QRS 150 ms or greater, prior HF hospitalization, LV end-diastolic volume 125 mL/m^2 or greater, and LA volume less than 40 mL/m^2 were associated with reverse remodeling with CRT as assessed by echocardiographic parameters.[93]

MANAGEMENT OF NONRESPONDERS

Mechanisms contributing to a lack of response include less LV radial dyssynchrony, discordant lead position, and myocardial scar in the segment targeted by the LV lead.[85] CRT optimization has four major goals: (1) achieve biventricular pacing as close to 100% as possible; (2) select the best LV lead position (discussed later); (3) program the AV interval to achieve the maximum contribution of LA contraction to LV filling (i.e., AV resynchronization); and (4) eliminate residual LV dyssynchrony after simultaneous biventricular pacing.[94]

Routine echocardiography-guided CRT optimization has not translated into improvement in outcomes compared with nominal settings. Large, multicenter trials suggest that routine optimization is mostly ineffective, compared with empiric programming of a 100- to 120-ms sensed AV delay.[95] However, optimization of AV delay should be considered for CRT nonresponders, particularly when the mitral inflow pattern by pulsed-wave Doppler demonstrates pseudonormal or restrictive filling. If the post-CRT echocardiogram demonstrates a normal or diastolic stage I inflow pattern at a given, empiric AV delay setting, no further changes to AV delay are warranted.

The role of interventricular optimization is less clear but is also reserved predominantly for nonresponders. Pulsed-wave Doppler interrogation of the LV outflow to estimate stroke volume can be used as a measure of global LV function, and maximizing stroke volume by changes to CRT settings should be considered for nonresponders.[75,76]

TARGETED LV LEAD PLACEMENT

Theoretically, localizing the LV lead to the site of latest mechanical activation should result in optimal resynchronization. However, routine clinical practice entails placing the LV lead through the coronary sinus to target the anatomic posterior or lateral LV region. Researchers have investigated whether CRT response can be improved by targeting the site of the latest LV mechanical activation using speckle-tracking strain. Studies have shown that radial strain–guided LV lead placement based on the latest time-to-peak strain[96] or at the latest site of radial strain thickening of more than 10% to avoid scar[41] may result in an improved CRT response and decrease rates of death or HF-related hospitalization compared with the routine fluoroscopic approach.

HEART FAILURE RISK SCORES

There are numerous risk scores for predicting adverse events in patients with chronic HF.[97–103] Some have attempted to incorporate imaging parameters. Although these models contain a large number of clinical and laboratory variables, in most cases, LVEF is the only echocardiographic parameter that has been included (Table 12.7). The potential additive benefit of other established echocardiographic predictors in HF (e.g., strain) to these existing risk indices bears further evaluation.

TABLE 12.7 Risk Models of Chronic Ambulatory Heart Failure That Include LV Ejection Fraction as a Predictor.

Risk Model	*Variables in Model*
Heart Failure Survival Score (1997)[97]	Mean blood pressure, resting heart rate, intraventricular conduction delay on ECG, peak VO_2, ischemic cause, LVEF, mean pulmonary capillary wedge pressure on invasive measurement, serum sodium level
CHARM model (2006)[108]	21 predictor variables; three strongest predictors were older age, diabetes, and lower LVEF; other predictors that increased risk included higher NYHA class, cardiomegaly, prior HF hospitalization, male gender, lower body mass index, and lower diastolic blood pressure
Seattle Heart Failure Model (2006)[101]	Demographics (age, gender, body mass index, NYHA class, blood pressure), medications, laboratory values (serum sodium level, creatinine, cholesterol, white blood cell count, hemoglobin, % lymphocytes, uric acid), device therapy
MAGGIC Model (2012)[103]	Age, LVEF, NYHA class, serum creatinine, diabetes, lower systolic blood pressure, lower body mass, time since diagnosis, current smoker, chronic obstructive pulmonary disease, male gender, not prescribed a beta-blocker, not prescribed an ACE inhibitor or angiotensin-receptor blocker
GISSI-HF Model (2013)[99]	Age, NYHA class, GFR, LVEF, COPD, SBP, diabetes mellitus, male gender, uricemia, lower BMI, lower hemoglobin concentration, aortic stenosis
MECKI Score (2013)[98]	Hemoglobin level, sodium level, kidney function, LVEF, peak oxygen consumption, VE/VCO_2 slope

ACE, Angiotensin-converting enzyme; *BMI*, body mass index; *COPD*, chronic obstructive pulmonary disease; ECG, electrocardiogram; *GFR*, glomerular filtration rate; *HF*, heart failure; *LVEF*, LV ejection fraction; *LVOT*, LV outflow tract; *NYHA*, New York Heart Association; *SBP*, systolic blood pressure; *VE/VCO_2*, minute ventilation/carbon dioxide production; *VO_2*, oxygen consumption.

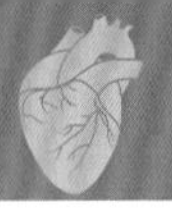

SUMMARY Dilated Cardiomyopathy

Component of Examination	Image Acquisition	Poor Prognostic Markers for Dilated Cardiomyopathy	Comments
LV function	• LVEF by 2D and 3D imaging • Mitral annular displacement • Estimate stroke volume • Rate of LV pressure change during isovolumic contraction *(dP/dt)* • MPI • Global longitudinal strain by speckle tracking • Chapters 2 and 4 detail quantification of LV systolic function	• LVEF < 35%–40% • *dP/dt* < 600 • S_m < 2.8 cm/s • MPI > 0.4 • Abnormal LV global longitudinal strain	• With 2D imaging, foreshortening and poor lateral resolution may be limitations. • Mitral annular displacement is invalid if there are focal wall motion abnormalities. • Stroke volume estimates depend highly on accurate estimation of the LVOT. • Advantages of MPI are that it is independent of heart rate, blood pressure, and ventricular geometry. • TDI is angle dependent. • Speckle-derived strain is not affected by translational motion of the heart and is not angle dependent.
LV size and geometry	• Measure LV size and volumes by conventional 2D echocardiography. • LV mass can be estimated from LV end-diastolic diameter and wall thickness. • Sphericity index can be calculated at end-systole and end-diastole as 2D measurements or by volumes.	• Increased LV end-systolic and diastolic diameters • Increased LV end-systolic and diastolic volumes • Increased LV mass > 298 g • LV sphericity index > 1.5	• Indexed size and volumes are beneficial by adjusting for body size. • Progressive LV remodeling results in an increasing spherical LV shape.
LV diastolic function	• Parameters can be obtained by pulsed-wave Doppler of the mitral inflow and TDI of mitral annulus. • Velocity of flow progression during diastole can be obtained with color Doppler M-mode. • Pulsed-wave Doppler of pulmonary venous flow should be performed. • LA size should be considered. • LA strain can be incremental, but data remain limited. • Chapter 5 details quantification of diastolic dysfunction.	• Pseudonormal filling pattern • Restrictive filling pattern (high E/A ratio, rapid deceleration time < 150 ms, E/e′ > 14, decreased lateral and septal e′) • Increased LA volume • Decreased LA reservoir strain	• Almost all patients with systolic dysfunction have some degree of diastolic dysfunction. • Progressive diastolic dysfunction is associated with worse outcomes, particularly for patients with restrictive filling. • LA size is independently prognostic.

Continued

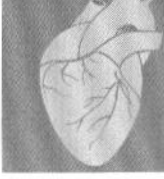

SUMMARY Dilated Cardiomyopathy—cont'd

Component of Examination	Image Acquisition	Poor Prognostic Markers for Dilated Cardiomyopathy	Comments
Right-sided involvement	• Chapter 6 describes RV anatomy, function, and echocardiographic evaluation. • RV free wall strain can be incremental, but data remain limited.	• Decreased fractional area change • Dilated RV • Decreased TAPSE • Abnormal RV global longitudinal strain	• RV function is more difficult to quantitate than LV function due to complex RV anatomy. • RV dysfunction independently predicts death and hospitalization.
Valvular assessment	• Chapter 24 discusses evaluation of MR. • Chapter 28 discusses tricuspid valve evaluation.	Secondary MR • Severe secondary MR (EROA ≥ 20 mm^2, regurgitant volume ≥ 30 mL, regurgitant fraction of ≥ 50%) • Mitral valve tenting area ≥ 3.4 cm^2 Tricuspid assessment • Severe tricuspid regurgitation • Increased pulmonary artery pressures	• Secondary MR occurs from LV remodeling, decreased closing forces from systolic dysfunction, mitral annular dilation and flattening, and displacement of papillary muscles. • Secondary MR orifice is usually elliptical, making accurate assessment challenging. • Quantitative thresholds for severe secondary MR are lower than those for severe primary MR.
Contractile reserve	• Low-dose dobutamine infusion and assessment of stroke volume, cardiac output, wall motion stress index, and/or strain analysis	• Decreased contractile reserve of LV and RV with dobutamine infusion	• Presence of contractile reserve is associated with a better prognosis.

LVEF, Left ventricular ejection fraction; *LVOT*, left ventricular outflow tract; *MPI*, myocardial performance index; *MR*, mitral regurgitation; *EROA*, effective regurgitant orifice area; S_m, longitudinal systolic mitral annular velocity; *TAPSE*, tricuspid annular plane systolic excursion; *TDI*, tissue Doppler imaging.

REFERENCES

1. Richardson P, McKenna W, Bristow M, et al. Report of the 1995 World Health Organization/International Society and Federation of Cardiology Task Force on the Definition and Classification of Cardiomyopathies. *Circulation*. 1996;93:841–842.
2. Maron BJ, Towbin JA, Thiene G, et al. Contemporary definitions and classification of the cardiomyopathies: an American Heart Association Scientific Statement from the Council on Clinical Cardiology, Heart Failure and Transplantation Committee; Quality of Care and Outcomes Research and Functional Genomics and Translational Biology Interdisciplinary Working Groups; and Council on Epidemiology and Prevention. *Circulation*. 2006;113:1807–1816.
3. Elliott P, Andersson B, Arbustini E, et al. Classification of the cardiomyopathies: a position statement from the European society of Cardiology Working group on myocardial and pericardial diseases. *Eur Heart J*. 2008;29:270–276.
4. Arbustini E, Narula N, Tavazzi L, et al. The MOGE(S) classification of cardiomyopathy for clinicians. *J Am Coll Cardiol*. 2014;64:304–318.
5. Manolio TA, Baughman KL, Rodeheffer R, et al. Prevalence and etiology of idiopathic dilated cardiomyopathy (summary of a National Heart, Lung, and Blood Institute workshop. *Am J Cardiol*. 1992;69:1458–1466.
6. Hershberger RE, Hedges DJ, Morales A. Dilated cardiomyopathy: the complexity of a diverse genetic architecture. *Nat Rev Cardiol*. 2013;10:531–547.
7. Hershberger RE, Morales A, Siegfried JD. Clinical and genetic issues in dilated cardiomyopathy: a review for genetics professionals. *Genet Med*. 2010;12:655–667.
8. McNally EM, Golbus JR, Puckelwartz MJ. Genetic mutations and mechanisms in dilated cardiomyopathy. *The Journal of clinical investigation*. 2013;123:19–26.
9. Thomas DE, Wheeler R, Yousef ZR, Masani ND. The role of echocardiography in guiding management in dilated cardiomyopathy. *Eur J Echocardiogr*. 2009;10:iii15–21.
10. Yancy CW, Jessup M, Bozkurt B, et al. ACCF/AHA guideline for the management of heart failure: a report of the American College of Cardiology Foundation/American Heart Association Task Force on practice guidelines. *Circulation*. 2013;128:e240–327. 2013.
11. Baig MK, Goldman JH, Caforio AL, Coonar AS, Keeling PJ, McKenna WJ. Familial dilated cardiomyopathy: cardiac abnormalities are common in asymptomatic relatives and may represent early disease. *J Am Coll Cardiol*. 1998;31:195–201.
12. Hershberger RE, Lindenfeld J, Mestroni L, et al. Genetic evaluation of cardiomyopathy—a Heart Failure Society of America practice guideline. *J Card Fail*. 2009;15:83–97.
13. Douglas PS, Garcia MJ, Haines DE, et al. ACCF/ASE/AHA/ASNC/HFSA/HRS/SCAI/SCCM/SCCT/SCMR 2011 appropriate Use criteria for echocardiography. A report of the American College of Cardiology Foundation Appropriate Use Criteria Task Force, American Society of Echocardiography, American Heart Association, American Society of Nuclear Cardiology, Heart Failure Society of America, Heart Rhythm Society, Society for Cardiovascular Angiography and Interventions, Society of Critical Care Medicine, Society of Cardiovascular Computed Tomography, Society For Cardiovascular Magnetic Reso-

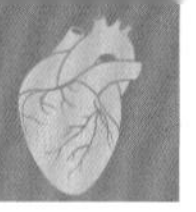

nance American College of Chest Physicians. *J Am Soc Echocardiogr*. 2011;24:229–267.

14. Doherty JU, Kort S, Mehran R, et al. ACC/AATS/AHA/ASE/ASNC/HRS/SCAI/SCCT/SCMR/STS 2019 appropriate use criteria for multimodality imaging in the assessment of cardiac structure and function in nonvalvular heart disease: a report of the American College of Cardiology Appropriate Use Criteria Task Force, American Association for Thoracic Surgery, American Heart Association, American Society of Echocardiography, American Society of Nuclear Cardiology, Heart Rhythm Society, Society for Cardiovascular Angiography and Interventions, Society of Cardiovascular Computed Tomography, Society for Cardiovascular Magnetic Resonance, and the Society of Thoracic Surgeons. *J Am Coll Cardiol*. 2019;73:488–516.
15. Tei C, Ling LH, Hodge DO, et al. New index of combined systolic and diastolic myocardial performance: a simple and reproducible measure of cardiac function—a study in normals and dilated cardiomyopathy. *J Cardiol*. 1995;26:357–366.
16. Dujardin KS, Tei C, Yeo TC, Hodge DO, Rossi A, Seward JB. Prognostic value of a Doppler index combining systolic and diastolic performance in idiopathic-dilated cardiomyopathy. *Am J Cardiol*. 1998;82:1071–1076.
17. Solomon SD, Anavekar N, Skali H, et al. Influence of ejection fraction on cardiovascular outcomes in a broad spectrum of heart failure patients. *Circulation*. 2005;112:3738–3744.
18. Wong M, Staszewsky L, Latini R, et al. Severity of left ventricular remodeling defines outcomes and response to therapy in heart failure: Valsartan heart failure trial (Val-HeFT) echocardiographic data. *J Am Coll Cardiol*. 2004;43:2022–2027.
19. Kolias TJ, Aaronson KD, Armstrong WF. Doppler-derived dP/dt and -dP/dt predict survival in congestive heart failure. *J Am Coll Cardiol*. 2000;36:1594–1599.
20. Bogaard MD, Houthuizen P, Bracke FA, et al. Baseline left ventricular dP/dtmax rather than the acute improvement in dP/dtmax predicts clinical outcome in patients with cardiac resynchronization therapy. *Eur J Heart Fail*. 2011;13:1126–1132.
21. Anavekar NS, Mirza A, Skali H, et al. Survival and ventricular enlargement I. Risk assessment in patients with depressed left ventricular function after myocardial infarction using the myocardial performance index—survival and ventricular enlargement (SAVE) experience. *J Am Soc Echocardiogr*. 2006;19:28–33.
22. Quinones MA, Greenberg BH, Kopelen HA, et al. Echocardiographic predictors of clinical outcome in patients with left ventricular dysfunction enrolled in the SOLVD registry and trials: significance of left ventricular hypertrophy. Studies of left ventricular dysfunction. *J Am Coll Cardiol*. 2000;35:1237–1244.
23. Douglas PS, Morrow R, Ioli A, Reichek N. Left ventricular shape, afterload and survival in idiopathic dilated cardiomyopathy. *J Am Coll Cardiol*. 1989;13:311–315.
24. Grayburn PA, Appleton CP, DeMaria AN, et al. Echocardiographic predictors of morbidity and mortality in patients with advanced heart failure: the Beta-blocker Evaluation of Survival Trial (BEST). *J Am Coll Cardiol*. 2005;45:1064–1071.
25. Verma A, Meris A, Skali H, et al. Prognostic implications of left ventricular mass and geometry following myocardial infarction: the VALIANT (VALsartan in Acute myocardial iNfarcTion) Echocardiographic study. *JACC Cardiovasc Imaging*. 2008;1:582–591.
26. Tischler MD, Niggel J, Borowski DT, LeWinter MM. Relation between left ventricular shape and exercise capacity in patients with left ventricular dysfunction. *J Am Coll Cardiol*. 1993;22:751–757.
27. Gulati VK, Katz WE, Follansbee WP, Gorcsan J 3rd. Mitral annular descent velocity by tissue Doppler echocardiography as an index of global left ventricular function. *Am J Cardiol*. 1996;77:979–984.
28. Nikitin NP, Loh PH, Silva R, et al. Prognostic value of systolic mitral annular velocity measured with Doppler tissue imaging in patients with chronic heart failure caused by left ventricular systolic dysfunction. *Heart*. 2006;92:775–779.
29. Jan MF, Tajik AJ. Modern imaging techniques in cardiomyopathies. *Circ Res*. 2017;121:874–891.
30. Greenberg NL, Firstenberg MS, Castro PL, et al. Doppler-derived myocardial systolic strain rate is a strong index of left ventricular contractility. *Circulation*. 2002;105:99–105.
31. Saito K, Okura H, Watanabe N, et al. Comprehensive evaluation of left ventricular strain using speckle tracking echocardiography in normal adults: comparison of three-dimensional and two-dimensional approaches. *J Am Soc Echocardiogr*. 2009;22:1025–1030.
32. Wen H, Liang Z, Zhao Y, Yang K. Feasibility of detecting early left ventricular systolic dysfunction using global area strain: a novel index derived from three-dimensional speckle-tracking echocardiography. *Eur J Echocardiogr*. 2011;12:910–916.
33. Meluzin J, Spinarova L, Hude P, et al. Left ventricular mechanics in idiopathic dilated cardiomyopathy: systolic-diastolic coupling and torsion. *J Am Soc Echocardiogr*. 2009;22:486–493.
34. Bella JN, Palmieri V, Roman MJ, et al. Mitral ratio of peak early to late diastolic filling velocity as a predictor of mortality in middle-aged and elderly adults: the Strong Heart study. *Circulation*. 2002;105:1928–1933.
35. Hirata K, Hyodo E, Hozumi T, et al. Usefulness of a combination of systolic function by left ventricular ejection fraction and diastolic function by E/E' to predict prognosis in patients with heart failure. *Am J Cardiol*. 2009;103:1275–1279.
36. Pozzoli M, Traversi E, Cioffi G, Stenner R, Sanarico M, Tavazzi L. Loading manipulations improve the prognostic value of Doppler evaluation of mitral flow in patients with chronic heart failure. *Circulation*. 1997;95:1222–1230.
37. Rossi A, Cicoira M, Zanolla L, et al. Determinants and prognostic value of left atrial volume in patients with dilated cardiomyopathy. *J Am Coll Cardiol*. 2002;40:1425.
38. Freed BH, Daruwalla V, Cheng JY, et al. Prognostic utility and clinical significance of cardiac mechanics in heart failure with preserved ejection fraction: importance of left atrial strain. *Circ Cardiovasc Imaging*. 2016;9.
39. Thomas L, Marwick TH, Popescu BA, Donal E, Badano LP. Left atrial structure and function, and left ventricular diastolic dysfunction: JACC state-of-the-art review. *J Am Coll Cardiol*. 2019;73:1961–1977.
40. Singh A, Medvedofsky D, Mediratta A, et al. Peak left atrial strain as a single measure for the non-invasive assessment of left ventricular filling pressures. *Int J Cardiovasc Imaging*. 2019;35:23–32.
41. Khan FZ, Virdee MS, Palmer CR, et al. Targeted left ventricular lead placement to guide cardiac resynchronization therapy: the TARGET study: a randomized, controlled trial. *J Am Coll Cardiol*. 2012;59:1509–1518.
42. Karaca O, Avci A, Guler GB, et al. Tenting area reflects disease severity and prognosis in patients with non-ischaemic dilated cardiomyopathy and functional mitral regurgitation. *Eur J Heart Fail*. 2011;13:284–291.
43. Koelling TM, Aaronson KD, Cody RJ, Bach DS, Armstrong WF. Prognostic significance of mitral regurgitation and tricuspid regurgitation in patients with left ventricular systolic dysfunction. *Am Heart J*. 2002;144:524–529.
44. Zoghbi WA, Adams D, Bonow RO, et al. Recommendations for noninvasive evaluation of native valvular regurgitation: a report from the American Society of Echocardiography developed in collaboration with the Society for Cardiovascular Magnetic Resonance. *J Am Soc Echocardiogr*. 2017;30:303–371.
45. Nishimura RA, Otto CM, Bonow RO, et al. AHA/ACC guideline for the management of patients with valvular heart disease: a report of the American College of Cardiology/American Heart Association Task Force on Practice Guidelines. *J Am Coll Cardiol*. 2014;63:e57–185. 2014.
46. Onishi T, Onishi T, Marek JJ, et al. Mechanistic features associated with improvement in mitral regurgitation after cardiac resynchronization therapy and their relation to long-term patient outcome. *Circ Heart Fail*. 2013;6:685–693.
47. Wu AH, Aaronson KD, Bolling SF, Pagani FD, Welch K, Koelling TM. Impact of mitral valve annuloplasty on mortality risk in patients with mitral regurgitation and left ventricular systolic dysfunction. *J Am Coll Cardiol*. 2005;45:381–387.
48. Nishimura RA, Otto CM, Bonow RO, et al. AHA/ACC focused update of the 2014 AHA/ACC guideline for the management of patients with valvular heart disease: a report of the American College of Cardiology/American Heart Association Task Force on Clinical Practice Guidelines. *J Am Coll Cardiol*. 2017;70:252–289. 2017.
49. Obadia JF, Messika-Zeitoun D, Leurent G, et al. Percutaneous repair or medical treatment for secondary mitral regurgitation. *N Engl J Med*. 2018;379:2297–2306.
50. Stone GW, Lindenfeld J, Abraham WT, et al. Transcatheter mitral-valve repair in patients with heart failure. *N Engl J Med*. 2018;379:2307–2318.
51. Grayburn PA, Sannino A, Packer M. Proportionate and disproportionate functional mitral regurgitation: a new conceptual framework that reconciles the results of the MITRA-FR and COAPT trials. *JACC Cardiovasc Imaging*. 2019;12:353–362.
52. Marmor A, Schneeweiss A. Prognostic value of noninvasively obtained left ventricular contractile reserve in patients with severe heart failure. *J Am Coll Cardiol*. 1997;29:422–428.
53. Otasevic P, Popovic Z, Pratali L, Vlahovic A, Vasiljevic JD, Neskovic AN. Right vs. left ventricular contractile reserve in one-year prognosis of patients with idiopathic dilated cardiomyopathy: assessment by dobutamine stress echocardiography. *Eur J Echocardiogr*. 2005;6:429–434.
54. Gulati A, Ismail TF, Jabbour A, et al. The prevalence and prognostic significance of right ventricular systolic dysfunction in nonischemic

dilated cardiomyopathy. *Circulation*. 2013;128:1623–1633.
55. Lewis JF, Webber JD, Sutton LL, Chesoni S, Curry CL. Discordance in degree of right and left ventricular dilation in patients with dilated cardiomyopathy: recognition and clinical implications. *J Am Coll Cardiol*. 1993;21:649–654.
56. Ghio S, Recusani F, Klersy C, et al. Prognostic usefulness of the tricuspid annular plane systolic excursion in patients with congestive heart failure secondary to idiopathic or ischemic dilated cardiomyopathy. *Am J Cardiol*. 2000;85:837–842.
57. Meluzin J, Spinarova L, Hude P, et al. Prognostic importance of various echocardiographic right ventricular functional parameters in patients with symptomatic heart failure. *J Am Soc Echocardiogr*. 2005;18:435–444.
58. Ghio S, Gavazzi A, Campana C, et al. Independent and additive prognostic value of right ventricular systolic function and pulmonary artery pressure in patients with chronic heart failure. *J Am Coll Cardiol*. 2001;37:183–188.
59. Motoki H, Borowski AG, Shrestha K, et al. Right ventricular global longitudinal strain provides prognostic value incremental to left ventricular ejection fraction in patients with heart failure. *J Am Soc Echocardiogr*. 2014;27:726–732.
60. Park JH, Park JJ, Park JB, Cho GY. Prognostic value of biventricular strain in risk stratifying in patients with acute heart failure. *J Am Heart Assoc*. 2018;7:e009331.
61. Grant AD, Smedira NG, Starling RC, Marwick TH. Independent and incremental role of quantitative right ventricular evaluation for the prediction of right ventricular failure after left ventricular assist device implantation. *J Am Coll Cardiol*. 2012;60:521–528.
62. Lieback E, Hardouin I, Meyer R, Bellach J, Hetzer R. Clinical value of echocardiographic tissue characterization in the diagnosis of myocarditis. *Eur Heart J*. 1996;17:135–142.
63. Afonso L, Hari P, Pidlaoan V, Kondur A, Jacob S, Khetarpal V. Acute myocarditis: can novel echocardiographic techniques assist with diagnosis? *Eur J Echocardiogr*. 2010;11:E5.
64. Friedrich MG, Sechtem U, Schulz-Menger J, et al. Cardiovascular magnetic resonance in myocarditis: a JACC White Paper. *J Am Coll Cardiol*. 2009;53:1475–1487.
65. Ammirati E, Veronese G, Brambatti M, et al. Fulminant versus acute nonfulminant myocarditis in patients with left ventricular systolic dysfunction. *J Am Coll Cardiol*. 2019;74:299–311.
66. Acquatella H, Asch FM, Barbosa MM, et al. Recommendations for multimodality cardiac imaging in patients with Chagas disease: a report from the American Society of Echocardiography in collaboration with the Inter American Association of Echocardiography (ECOSIAC) and the Cardiovascular Imaging Department of the Brazilian Society of Cardiology (DIC-SBC). *J Am Soc Echocardiogr*. 2018;31:3–25.
67. Barros MV, Leren IS, Edvardsen T, et al. Mechanical dispersion assessed by strain echocardiography is associated with malignant arrhythmias in Chagas cardiomyopathy. *J Am Soc Echocardiogr*. 2016;29:368–374.
68. Jenni R, Oechslin E, Schneider J, Attenhofer Jost C, Kaufmann PA. Echocardiographic and pathoanatomical characteristics of isolated left ventricular non-compaction: a step towards classification as a distinct cardiomyopathy. *Heart*. 2001;86:666–671.
69. Bellavia D, Michelena HI, Martinez M, et al. Speckle myocardial imaging modalities for early detection of myocardial impairment in isolated left ventricular non-compaction. *Heart*. 2010;96:440–447.
70. Gianni M, Dentali F, Grandi AM, Sumner G, Hiralal R, Lonn E. Apical ballooning syndrome or takotsubo cardiomyopathy: a systematic review. *Eur Heart J*. 2006;27:1523–1529.
71. Bybee KA, Kara T, Prasad A, et al. Systematic review: transient left ventricular apical ballooning: a syndrome that mimics ST-segment elevation myocardial infarction. *Ann Intern Med*. 2004;141:858–865.
72. Wittstein IS, Thiemann DR, Lima JA, et al. Neurohumoral features of myocardial stunning due to sudden emotional stress. *N Engl J Med*. 2005;352:539–548.
73. Baccouche H, Maunz M, Beck T, Fogarassy P, Beyer M. Echocardiographic assessment and monitoring of the clinical course in a patient with Tako-Tsubo cardiomyopathy by a novel 3D-speckle-tracking-strain analysis. *Eur J Echocardiogr*. 2009;10:729–731.
74. Sharkey SW, Lesser JR, Zenovich AG, et al. Acute and reversible cardiomyopathy provoked by stress in women from the United States. *Circulation*. 2005;111:472–479.
75. Epstein AE, DiMarco JP, Ellenbogen KA, et al. 2012 ACCF/AHA/HRS focused update incorporated into the ACCF/AHA/HRS 2008 guidelines for device-based therapy of cardiac rhythm abnormalities: a report of the American College of Cardiology Foundation/American Heart Association Task Force on Practice Guidelines and the Heart Rhythm Society. *J Am Coll Cardiol*. 2013;61:e6–75.
76. Brignole M, Auricchio A, Baron-Esquivias G, et al. ESC guidelines on cardiac pacing and cardiac resynchronization therapy: the Task Force on Cardiac Pacing and Resynchronization Therapy of the European Society of Cardiology (ESC). Developed in collaboration with the European Heart Rhythm Association (EHRA). *Eur Heart J*. 2013;34:2281–2329. 2013.
77. Yu CM, Sanderson JE, Gorcsan J 3rd. Echocardiography, dyssynchrony, and the response to cardiac resynchronization therapy. *Eur Heart J*. 2010;31:2326–2337.
78. Chung ES, Leon AR, Tavazzi L, et al. Results of the predictors of response to CRT (PROSPECT) trial. *Circulation*. 2008;117:2608–2616.
79. Ruschitzka F, Abraham WT, Singh JP, et al. Cardiac-resynchronization therapy in heart failure with a narrow QRS complex. *N Engl J Med*. 2013;369:1395–1405.
80. European Heart Rhythm Association, European Society of Cardiology, Heart Rhythm Society, et al. EHRA/HRS expert consensus statement on cardiac resynchronization therapy in heart failure: implant and follow-up recommendations and management. *Heart Rhythm*. 2012;9:1524–1576. 2012.
81. Ponikowski P, Voors AA, Anker SD, et al. 2016 ESC guidelines for the diagnosis and treatment of acute and chronic heart failure: the Task Force for the Diagnosis and Treatment of Acute and Chronic Heart Failure of the European Society of Cardiology (ESC). Developed with the special contribution of the Heart Failure Association (HFA) of the ESC. *Eur J Heart Fail*. 2016;18:891–975.
82. Stankovic I, Prinz C, Ciarka A, et al. Relationship of visually assessed apical rocking and septal flash to response and long-term survival following cardiac resynchronization therapy (PREDICT-CRT). *Eur Heart J Cardiovasc Imaging*. 2016;17:262–269.
83. Donal E, Delgado V, Magne J, et al. Rational and design of EuroCRT: an international observational study on multi-modality imaging and cardiac resynchronization therapy. *Eur Heart J Cardiovasc Imaging*. 2017;18:1120–1127.
84. Tanaka H, Nesser HJ, Buck T, et al. Dyssynchrony by speckle-tracking echocardiography and response to cardiac resynchronization therapy: results of the Speckle Tracking and Resynchronization (STAR) study. *Eur Heart J*. 2010;31:1690–1700.
85. Delgado V, van Bommel RJ, Bertini M, et al. Relative merits of left ventricular dyssynchrony, left ventricular lead position, and myocardial scar to predict long-term survival of ischemic heart failure patients undergoing cardiac resynchronization therapy. *Circulation*. 2011;123:70–78.
86. Marechaux S, Guiot A, Castel AL, et al. Relationship between two-dimensional speckle-tracking septal strain and response to cardiac resynchronization therapy in patients with left ventricular dysfunction and left bundle branch block: a prospective pilot study. *J Am Soc Echocardiogr*. 2014;27:501–511.
87. Risum N, Tayal B, Hansen TF, et al. Identification of typical left bundle branch block contraction by strain echocardiography is additive to electrocardiography in prediction of long-term outcome after cardiac resynchronization therapy. *J Am Coll Cardiol*. 2015;66:631–641.
88. Cazeau SJ, Daubert JC, Tavazzi L, Frohlig G, Paul V. Responders to cardiac resynchronization therapy with narrow or intermediate QRS complexes identified by simple echocardiographic indices of dyssynchrony: the DESIRE study. *Eur J Heart Fail*. 2008;10:273–280.
89. Cleland JG, Freemantle N, Erdmann E, et al. Long-term mortality with cardiac resynchronization therapy in the Cardiac Resynchronization-Heart Failure (CARE-HF) trial. *Eur J Heart Fail*. 2012;14:628–634.
90. Sade LE, Ozin B, Atar I, Demir O, Demirtas S, Muderrisoglu H. Right ventricular function is a determinant of long-term survival after cardiac resynchronization therapy. *J Am Soc Echocardiogr*. 2013;26:706–713.
91. St John Sutton M, Ghio S, Plappert T, et al. Cardiac resynchronization induces major structural and functional reverse remodeling in patients with New York Heart Association class I/II heart failure. *Circulation*. 2009;120:1858–1865.
92. Sutton MG, Plappert T, Hilpisch KE, Abraham WT, Hayes DL, Chinchoy E. Sustained reverse left ventricular structural remodeling with cardiac resynchronization at one year is a function of etiology: quantitative Doppler echocardiographic evidence from the Multicenter InSync Randomized Clinical Evaluation (MIRACLE). *Circulation*. 2006;113:266–272.
93. Goldenberg I, Moss AJ, Hall WJ, et al. Predictors of response to cardiac resynchronization therapy in the multicenter automatic defibrillator implantation trial with cardiac resynchronization therapy (MADIT-CRT). *Circulation*. 2011;124:1527–1536.

94. Ponikowski P, Voors AA, Anker SD, et al. ESC guidelines for the diagnosis and treatment of acute and chronic heart failure. *Rev Esp Cardiol.* 2016;69:1167. 2016.
95. Ellenbogen KA, Gold MR, Meyer TE, et al. Primary results from the SmartDelay determined AV optimization: a comparison to other AV delay methods used in cardiac resynchronization therapy (SMART-AV) trial: a randomized trial comparing empirical, echocardiography-guided, and algorithmic atrioventricular delay programming in cardiac resynchronization therapy. *Circulation.* 2010;122:2660–2668.
96. Saba S, Marek J, Schwartzman D, et al. Echocardiography-guided left ventricular lead placement for cardiac resynchronization therapy: results of the Speckle Tracking Assisted Resynchronization Therapy for Electrode Region trial. *Circ Heart Fail.* 2013;6:427–434.
97. Aaronson KD, Schwartz JS, Chen TM, Wong KL, Goin JE, Mancini DM. Development and prospective validation of a clinical index to predict survival in ambulatory patients referred for cardiac transplant evaluation. *Circulation.* 1997;95:2660–2667.
98. Agostoni P, Corra U, Cattadori G, et al. Metabolic exercise test data combined with cardiac and kidney indexes, the MECKI score: a multiparametric approach to heart failure prognosis. *Int J Cardiol.* 2013;167:2710–2718.
99. Barlera S, Tavazzi L, Franzosi MG, et al. Predictors of mortality in 6975 patients with chronic heart failure in the Gruppo Italiano per lo Studio della Streptochinasi nell'Infarto Miocardico-Heart Failure trial: proposal for a nomogram. *Circ Heart Fail.* 2013;6:31–39.
100. Lee DS, Austin PC, Rouleau JL, Liu PP, Naimark D, Tu JV. Predicting mortality among patients hospitalized for heart failure: derivation and validation of a clinical model. *J Am Med Assoc.* 2003;290:2581–2587.
101. Levy WC, Mozaffarian D, Linker DT, et al. The Seattle Heart Failure Model: prediction of survival in heart failure. *Circulation.* 2006;113:1424–1433.
102. Motoki H, Borowski AG, Shrestha K, et al. Incremental prognostic value of assessing left ventricular myocardial mechanics in patients with chronic systolic heart failure. *J Am Coll Cardiol.* 2012;60:2074–2081.
103. Pocock SJ, Ariti CA, McMurray JJ, et al. Predicting survival in heart failure: a risk score based on 39 372 patients from 30 studies. *Eur Heart J.* 2013;34:1404–1413.
104. Zhang KW, French B, May Khan A, et al. Strain improves risk prediction beyond ejection fraction in chronic systolic heart failure. *J Am Heart Assoc.* 2014;3:e000550.
105. Hung J, Capoulade R. Therapy for secondary mitral regurgitation: time to 'cut the chord'? *Heart.* 2015;101:996–997.
106. Sengelov M, Jorgensen PG, Jensen JS, et al. Global longitudinal strain is a superior predictor of all-cause mortality in heart failure with reduced ejection fraction. *JACC Cardiovasc Imaging.* 2015;8:1351–1359.
107. Park JJ, Park JB, Park JH, Cho GY. Global longitudinal strain to predict mortality in patients with acute heart failure. *J Am Coll Cardiol.* 2018;71:1947–1957.
108. Pocock SJ, Wang D, Pfeffer MA, et al. Predictors of mortality and morbidity in patients with chronic heart failure. *Eur Heart J.* 2006;27:65–75.

中文导读

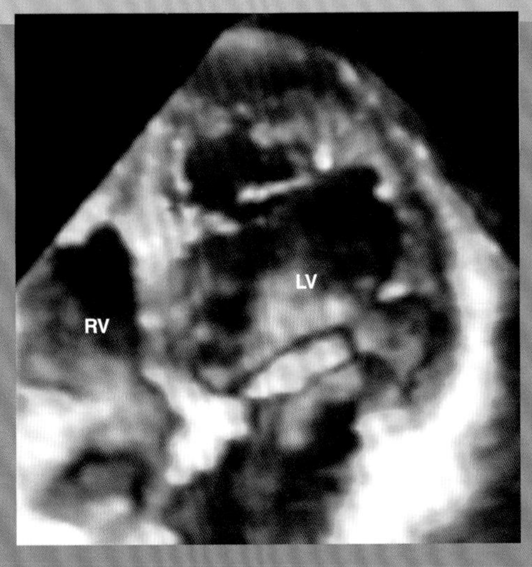

第13章
肥厚型心肌病

肥厚型心肌病是一类显性遗传性以心肌肥厚为特征的心肌病，合并左心室流出道梗阻或无左心室流出道梗阻，其病理特征为：肌纤维肥大、排列紊乱和细胞外基质纤维化。肥厚型心肌病诊断标准是成年人左心室心肌最厚处厚度>15 mm（儿童：室壁最厚处厚度z值>2），前提是排除了诸如主动脉瓣狭窄，主动脉瓣下隔膜，主动脉弓缩窄等引起左心室后负荷增高的疾病，排除代谢性疾病和运动引发的心脏重构等。

目前认为，肥厚型心肌病的病理生理是基于肌动蛋白基因的突变，突变致细胞结构和肌动蛋白功能改变（如收缩和舒张功能）。这些病变包括左心室肥厚、二尖瓣叶病变、二尖瓣下结构病变、纤维化和微血管病变。肥厚型心肌病是一种个体性强的疾病，其病程往往难以预测。临床症状从无症状，运动耐力下降到心力衰竭不一。随着现代医学和治疗手段的进步，肥厚型心肌病呈现一种整体性预后改善的态势。

肥厚型心肌病的治疗手段包括：药物治疗、外科切除术、酒精消融术、心脏复律除颤器植入（针对存在心源性猝死风险的患者）和心脏移植（针对终末期患者）。在对肥厚型心肌病认识逐步提升的过程中，超声心动图发挥着非常重要的作用，尤其是以下几个方面：解剖特征、流行病学调查、诊断和治疗。

肖明虎

13 Hypertrophic Cardiomyopathy

DAVID S. OWENS, MD

Hypertrophic cardiomyopathy (HCM) is an uncommon, inherited form of heart disease whose cardinal feature is unexplained left ventricular hypertrophy (LVH), with or without obstruction of the left ventricular outflow tract (LVOT).[1,2] HCM was first described by British pathologist Donald Teare in 1958, who reported autopsy findings from a series of patients with sudden death and unexplained LVH that was initially and mistakenly described as a cardiac hamartoma.[3] In this report, he defined what is now considered the pathologic triad of HCM: myocyte hypertrophy, myofibrillar disarray, and interstitial fibrosis (Fig. 13.1).

Since that time, enormous advances have been made in understanding HCM, including the epidemiology, pathogenesis, complex pathophysiology, and heterogeneous clinical pictures associated with this disorder.[4] The modern understanding of HCM is that it is a disorder of cardiac hypertrophy and fibrosis caused by a pathogenic variation in one of several sarcomeric genes.[5] These genetic changes alter cellular architecture and sarcomeric function (i.e., contraction and relaxation). Although no single pathway causes the disease, the changes induce LVH, alterations in mitral leaflet and subvalvular anatomy, myocardial and perivascular fibrosis, and microvascular coronary artery disease.

HCM is notable for its heterogeneous and often unpredictable disease course. Clinical manifestations range from asymptomatic disease to exercise intolerance to overt heart failure, and this clinical picture is often punctuated by atrial and ventricular arrhythmias. Initially considered to be a harrowing disease with high morbidity and mortality rates, HCM now has an overall good prognosis with modern therapies, including timely invasive management of LVOT obstruction, cardioverter-defibrillator (ICD) implantation for individuals at high risk for sudden cardiac death (SCD), and advanced heart failure treatments for end-stage disease, including heart transplantation.[4]

Since its inception, echocardiography has played a central role in advancing the understanding of HCM on an anatomic, pathophysiologic, and epidemiologic basis, and it remains the cornerstone of HCM diagnosis and management.

GENETIC BASIS AND EPIDEMIOLOGY

The familial basis of HCM became clear soon after its recognition as a distinct disease entity, but it was not until the 1990s that several groups reported genetic mutations in *MYH7*, a gene that encodes the β heavy-chain subunit of cardiac myosin, as the cause of HCM.[6,7] With advances in genetic sequencing technology, several thousand causal genetic variants have been reported, and HCM is now understood as a genetic condition largely resulting from changes in sarcomeric protein structure and function.[5]

Most cases of HCM are caused by a pathogenic variation in the *MYH7* gene or in the myosin binding protein C (*MYBPC3*) gene, which together account for 70% to 80% of gene-positive HCM. Genes encoding thin-filament sarcomeric proteins, including α-tropomyosin (*TPM1*), troponin T (*TNNT3*), and troponin I (*TNNI2*), individually occur in less than 5% of HCM patients. These genes cause what is occasionally referred to as thin-filament HCM, which may have a slightly different phenotype and course from HCM caused by mutations in *MYH7* or *MYBPC3*.

Data from the Sarcomeric Human Cardiomyopathy Registry (SHaRe) suggest that although there is considerable overlap in cardiac morphology and clinic course, *MYH7* variants are more closely associated with heart failure and atrial fibrillation, whereas the presence of thin-filament disease or two or more sarcomeric variants increases the risk of left ventricular (LV) systolic dysfunction.[8,9] However, there is marked phenotypic diversity and clinical heterogeneity among individuals with the same genetic changes, potentially due to gene-gene or gene-environment interactions or epigenetic modification. Information from specific genetic variants has limited utility for guiding management but can be critical in family screening.

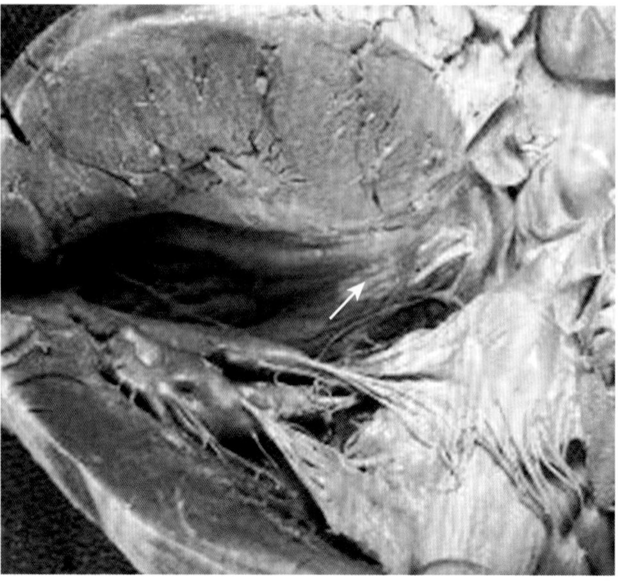

Fig. 13.1 Pathologic findings in hypertrophic cardiomyopathy. Gross pathologic specimen of a heart from a patient with hypertrophic cardiomyopathy and left ventricular outflow tract (LVOT) obstruction. Notable findings include severe asymmetric hypertrophy of the interventricular septum, apical displacement of the papillary muscles, and a narrowed LVOT. Repetitive systolic contact by the mitral leaflets may lead to scarring of the endothelial surface of the basal septum *(arrow)*.

Based on numerous population-based echocardiographic studies involving a wide range of ethnic and racial cohorts, the estimated overall prevalence of HCM is 1 in 500 individuals (0.2%).[10,11] This leads to an estimate of approximately 660,000 HCM patients in the United States and 15 million patients worldwide.[12] Using inferences from population genetic studies, however, the overall lifetime prevalence of HCM is estimated to be 1 in 200 (0.5%).[11] A population-based cardiac magnetic resonance imaging (MRI) study suggested that the prevalence of unexplained LVH (>15 mm wall thickness in two or more adjacent segments) is 1.4%.[13]

DIAGNOSIS

There are no firm diagnostic criteria for HCM.[1,2] A diagnosis of HCM is based on the presence of LVH that is unexplainable by other causes such as pressure overload states or infiltrative conditions. Imaging findings and clinical factors are central to diagnosis; the finding of a causal genetic variant is not required.

Hypertrophy in HCM is usually asymmetric and often involves the septum, but any pattern of hypertrophy can exist (Fig. 13.2). A cut point of 15 mm in maximal wall thickness (or +2 standard deviations in children) is commonly used, but

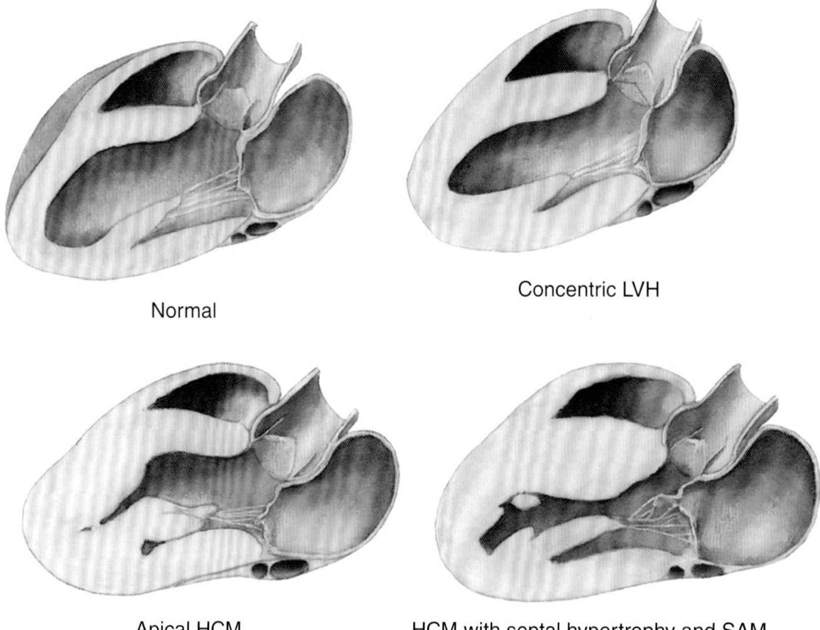

Fig. 13.2 Patterns of septal hypertrophy in hypertrophic cardiomyopathy. Schematic representations of the most common morphologies of left ventricular hypertrophy (LVH), viewed from along the LV long axis. *Upper left*: Normal cardiac anatomy with normal septal wall thickness and normal mitral valve and papillary muscle anatomy. *Upper right*: Concentric LVH with normal mitral valve and papillary muscle anatomy. Although this morphology is compatible with nonobstructive hypertrophic cardiomyopathy (HCM), it is also commonly seen with HCM mimics, including pressure overload conditions and genetic phenocopies. *Lower left*: Hypertrophy of the distal LV cavity and apex with sparing of the basal segments. This morphology is consistent with apical HCM. Notice the apicalized papillary muscle and small distal cavity. *Lower right*: Classic HCM with asymmetric septal hypertrophy and maximal wall thickness in the mid-septum giving a convex (i.e., reverse curve) appearance. Notice the normal posterior wall thickness, elongation of the mitral leaflets, antero-apically displaced papillary muscles and mitral coaptation, and systolic anterior motion of the mitral leaflets with resultant narrowing of the LV outflow tract.

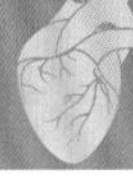

TABLE 13.1 Differential Diagnosis for Hypertrophic Cardiomyopathy.

Pressure Overload Conditions

- Uncontrolled hypertension
- Coarctation of the aorta
- Aortic valve stenosis
- Subaortic membrane
- Supravalvular aortic stenosis

Infiltrative Cardiomyopathies

- Amyloidosis
- Sarcoidosis

Metabolic/Storage Disorders

- Fabry disease
- PRKAG2 syndrome
- Danon disease
- Other glycogen storage disorders

Other Genetic Conditions

- Noonan syndrome
- Noonan syndrome with multiple lentigines
- Friedreich ataxia
- Mitochondrial myopathy

in theory any degree of hypertrophy is compatible with HCM, especially in the setting of a family history of HCM or sarcomeric variant carrier status. A septal-to-posterior wall ratio of 1.3 cm or greater is strongly associated with HCM.[14] The finding of dynamic LVOT obstruction is common in HCM, but it is neither specific to HCM nor required for diagnosis.

DIFFERENTIAL DIAGNOSIS

Because many conditions can result in the phenotype of LVH, HCM is primarily a diagnosis of exclusion. Disorders that can produce sufficient LVH to mimic HCM include pressure overload conditions, metabolic disorders, genetic syndromes, infiltrative conditions, and exercise-induced cardiac remodeling (Table 13.1).

PRESSURE OVERLOAD CONDITIONS

Chronic exposure to high LV systolic pressures induces an adaptive hypertrophic response in the myocardium. Factors that contribute to high LV systolic pressures include uncontrolled hypertension, coarctation of the aorta, and obstruction to LV outflow at the subvalvular, valvular, or supravalvular level. Although pressure overload frequently results in concentric hypertrophy, as many as 15% to 20% of individuals with moderate to severe aortic stenosis develop asymmetric, predominantly septal hypertrophy that can closely mimic HCM.[15] Whether the magnitude of hypertrophy is explainable by the observed degree of pressure overload requires clinical judgment. Subvalvular membranes can be missed on transthoracic echocardiography (TTE) but should be suspected when there is color-flow acceleration within the LVOT in the setting of normal mitral and aortic leaflet motion and an early- to mid-peaking Doppler profile.

GENETIC PHENOCOPIES AND INFILTRATIVE CONDITIONS

Several genetic conditions can result in sufficient LVH to mimic HCM. Fabry disease, caused by a genetic variation in the α-galactosidase (*GLA*) gene, results in intracellular glycosphingolipid accumulation that can manifest as a classic phenotype with multiorgan involvement or as a cardiac-limited phenotype.[16] As with most X-linked conditions, XY males exhibit more severe phenotypes, but disease is twice as common in XX females. Hypertrophy is commonly concentric, but septal- and apical-predominant morphologic subtypes occur.[17] A binary appearance to the endocardium has been proposed as a specific marker of Fabry disease, but it also occurs in many other patients with LVH.[18,19]

Danon disease is another X-linked condition caused by pathogenic variants in the lysosomal-associated membrane protein 2 (*LAMP2*) that results in autophagy dysregulation and subsequent vacuolar glycogen accumulation.[20] This produces a cardiac phenotype of LVH with often extensive fibrosis. Skeletal myopathy and cognitive disability may also occur. Transition from a hypertrophic to a dilated cardiomyopathy can occur, and males with Danon disease often develop end-stage cardiomyopathy by 20 years of age.

PRKAG2 syndrome is an autosomal dominant genetic condition caused by genetic variation in the γ-2 subunit of adenosine monophosphate–activated protein kinase (*PRKAG2*) that plays a crucial role in cardiomyocyte energy metabolism.[20,21] Pathogenic PRKAG2 syndrome variants result in glycogen accumulation and LVH, with presentation occurring at different ages. Atrial fibrillation and conduction system disorders are common, and Danon disease and PRKAG2 syndrome variants have been associated with a Wolff-Parkinson-White preexcitation syndrome.

Transthyretin (TTR) cardiac amyloidosis is caused by deposition of the wild-type or mutated TTR protein, which usually results in concentric LVH and reduced ventricular compliance.[22] It is more insidious than light-chain (AL) amyloidosis, which is caused by plasma cell dyscrasias and often has a rapidly declining clinical course. One TTR polymorphism, Val122Ile, is carried by 3% to 5% of black individuals and is associated with late-life heart failure, although overall disease penetrance is low.[23,24] TTR stabilizers and TTR-interfering RNAs are under clinical investigation, and early recognition of disease is essential.

Echocardiographic features that favor a diagnosis of amyloidosis over HCM include concentric hypertrophy, decreased LV ejection fraction (LVEF), right ventricular (RV) hypertrophy, biatrial enlargement, and interatrial septal thickening. End-stage HCM with reduced EF is characterized by progressive fibrosis with wall thinning, whereas amyloidosis with reduced EF involves wall thickening as disease progresses. Strain maps can be useful in differentiating these disorders because amyloidosis often manifests with apical preservation.[25]

ATHLETE'S HEART

Chronic exercise can induce cardiac remodeling (so-called athlete's heart) that results in eccentric and/or concentric hypertrophy, depending on exercise modality and habits.[26,27] Studies of healthy athletes have shown the upper limit of physiologic hypertrophy to be 11 to 13 mm of wall thickness in women and 14 to 16 mm in men, with black athletes having thicker hearts on average.[28] Echocardiographic features that help to distinguish HCM from athlete's heart include atypical patterns of hypertrophy, wall thickness of 7 mm or greater, nondilated cardiac chambers, impaired LV diastolic relaxation, and reduced longitudinal strain.[29,30] Clinical parameters, family history, response to deconditioning, and the results of cardiopulmonary stress testing can further aid in differentiation.

ECHOCARDIOGRAPHIC ASSESSMENT OF HYPERTROPHY AND FUNCTION

SEVERITY, DISTRIBUTION, AND PATTERNS OF HYPERTROPHY

HCM can be classified into several different morphologic subtypes that often share clinical features. Septal-predominant HCM can manifest as three different morphologies defined by septal shape. In *reverse curvature* septal morphology, LVH often spirals from the basal anterior wall through the septum and extends variably into the mid-inferior and inferolateral walls (Fig. 13.3A–C). The region of greatest septal hypertrophy is commonly in the basal to mid-anterior septum, giving the septum a convex appearance. This morphology is strongly associated with sarcomeric genetic variation.[31]

In *sigmoidal* HCM, LVH is isolated to the most basal portion of the septum, creating a concave appearance (see Fig. 13.3D–F). This has been informally referred to as *septal knuckle*. Sigmoidal HCM is uncommonly caused by sarcomeric variation; it is associated with advanced age, hypertension, and acute ventricular-aortic angulation.[32,33]

With *neutral* septal morphology, the septum is neither convex nor concave and remains similarly hypertrophied throughout (see Fig. 13.3G–I). This morphology has intermediate association with the sarcomeric genetic variation, and it is more common in thin-filament HCM.

There are two additional sub-basilar HCM morphologies. In *mid-ventricular* HCM, hypertrophy occurs circumferentially at the mid-ventricular/papillary level, sparing the basal segments.[34,35] This can lead to mid-ventricular systolic obstruction due to cavity obliteration, resulting in a pressurized LV apex, and development of an apical aneurysm is common with this morphology. In *apical* HCM, hypertrophy occurs predominantly in the LV apex with different degrees of septal involvement and with narrowing of the ventricular cavity to create a spade-like appearance.[36] Apicalized papillary muscles may contribute to the hypertrophy in this region. Sub-basilar HCM is less commonly associated with sarcomeric genetic variation compared with reverse curvature septal morphology.

ECHOCARDIOGRAPHIC ASSESSMENT OF HYPERTROPHY

Proper measurement of septal and maximal LV wall thickness is important in HCM clinical management and SCD risk stratification, and it is important to recognize the role and limitations of echocardiography in this regard.[37,38] For all imaging planes, care must be taken to avoid oblique angulation, which can falsely increase hypertrophy. Basal anterior septal wall thickness is standardly reported but frequently does not represent the region of maximal hypertrophy. When measuring septal wall thickness, care should be taken to differentiate the septum from RV bundles and the *crista interventricularis* (Fig. 13.4).[39] The use of parasternal short-axis (PSAX) views may be helpful in this regard. Acoustic dropout of the inferior septum or lateral wall, particularly of the epicardial surface, may limit wall thickness assessment in these regions. The use of echocardiographic contrast, which improves endocardial but not epicardial definition, does not overcome this issue, and alternative imaging should be considered. The LV apex is prone to suboptimal imaging, and a high index of suspicion is often needed.[38]

HYPERCONTRACTILITY, CAVITY SIZE, AND ADVERSE REMODELING

HCM characteristically has been associated with normal LV cavity size and normal to hyperdynamic systolic function as assessed by LVEF or by the rate of change of ventricular pressures ($+dP/dt$). Hypercontractility, although not fully understood on a molecular basis, is a direct consequence of the genetic variation that alters sarcomeric structure and function.[40] Hypercontractility occurs before the development of hypertrophy and may contribute to disease pathogenesis, including hypertrophy, myocardial ischemia, and fibrosis.[41]

Although HCM is conceived as a disorder of cardiac hypertrophy, it is also marked by various degrees of interstitial fibrosis.[42] The fibrosis is commonly in regions of hypertrophy, and progressive fibrosis may result in thinning and hypokinesis in the affected segments. There is an inverse relationship between fibrosis and LV systolic function such that LVEF declines as fibrosis increases. Approximately 5% of HCM patients progress to end-stage HCM, which is characterized by LV systolic dysfunction with an LVEF of less than 50% with or without LV cavity dilation.[43] These individuals often develop overt heart failure due to combined systolic dysfunction and restrictive physiology.[44] Advanced heart failure therapies such as LV assist devices are often contraindicated because of the lack of LV dilation, and primary transplantation is frequently needed.

MITRAL VALVE ABNORMALITIES

Abnormalities of the mitral valve (MV) leaflets, papillary muscles, and chordal insertions are common in patients with HCM, and these abnormalities contribute greatly to the susceptibility for systolic deformation of the MV leaflets.[45–47] Elongation of one or both mitral leaflets is common, with altered coaptation in the body of one or both leaflets rather than at the tips (Fig. 13.5). The cause of this leaflet elongation is unknown, but it is observed in genotype-positive, LVH-negative individuals and may be related to a hyperdynamic contractile milieu present during organogenesis.[48]

Studies have shown that papillary muscle architecture is often altered in HCM, commonly with anterior and apical displacement of the papillary muscles.[47,49] This produces papillary muscles that are in closer proximity, with a decrease in relative chordal tension. The valve coaptation zone becomes more anteriorly displaced, exposing the posterior undersurface of the leaflet to systolic ejection flow.

Alterations in chordal connections to the mitral leaflets may also occur.[47] Aberrant chordal connections between the leaflet and the septum occur, with the net effect of anterior displacement of the mitral tethering forces; surgical release of these attachments is a key component of obstruction relief. Chordae may be absent, with direct insertion of the papillary muscles in the mitral leaflet (Fig. 13.6).[45] Apical-basal muscle bundles are identified in about 60% of HCM patients (compared with 10% of control subjects); although not unique to HCM, they have been postulated to be remnants of aberrant papillary muscles.[50]

DYNAMIC LV OUTFLOW TRACT OBSTRUCTION

Dynamic LVOT obstruction is a common feature of HCM, and the obstruction is a major cause of symptoms and exercise limitation.[51] LVOT obstruction is defined as a peak LVOT gradient of more than 30 mmHg at rest or more than 50 mmHg

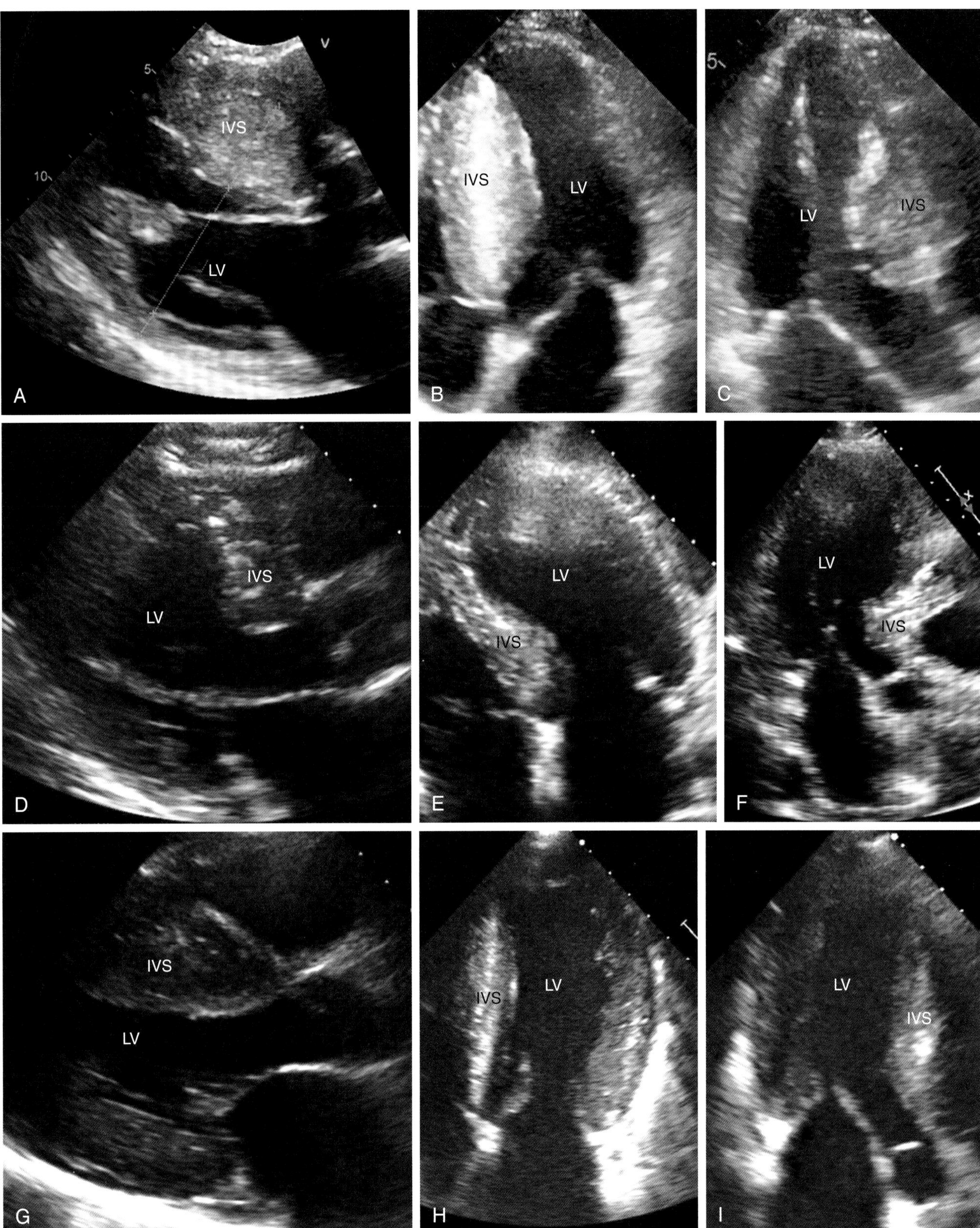

Fig. 13.3 **2D echocardiographic views of reverse curvature and sigmoid septal morphologies in hypertrophic cardiomyopathy (HCM).** *Top row*: Parasternal long-axis (A), apical 4-chamber (B), and apical 3-chamber (C) views of a patient with HCM and reverse curvature septal morphology. Notice the convex septal shape with maximal hypertrophy in the basal to mid-anterior and inferior septum. Genetic testing confirmed a pathogenic *MYPBC3* variant. *Middle row*: Parasternal long-axis (D), apical 4-chamber (E), and apical 3-chamber (F) views of a patient with HCM and sigmoid septum morphology. Notice hypertrophy isolated to the basal septum. Genetic sequencing was normal. *Bottom row*: Parasternal long-axis (G), apical 4-chamber (H), and apical 3-chamber (I) views of a patient with neutral septal morphology. Genetic testing confirmed a pathogenic *TNNI3* variant. *IVS*, Interventricular septum.

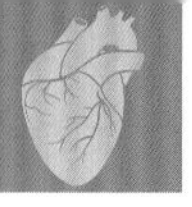

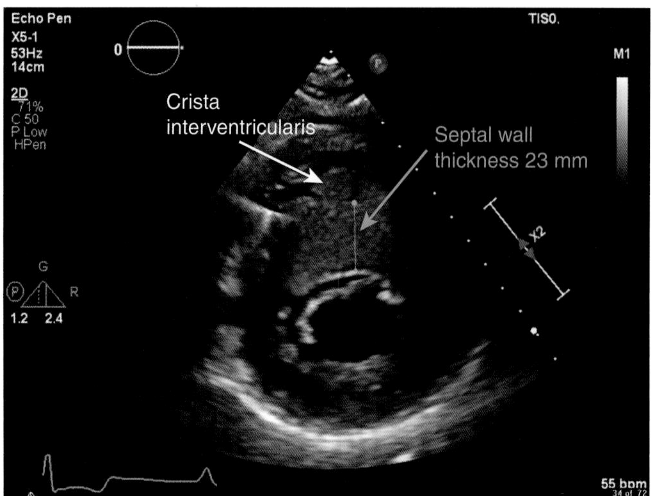

Fig. 13.4 **Parasternal short-axis view of ventricular septum in hypertrophic cardiomyopathy.** Parasternal short-axis (PSAX) view of a patient with reverse curvature HCM demonstrates the method of measuring wall thickness. Notice the prominent crista interventricularis anterior to the septum, which is avoided during wall thickness measurement. Maximal septal wall thickness is 23 mm.

with provocation. It has proved clinically effective to categorize patients into three hemodynamic groups, with about one third of patients having obstruction at rest, one third having obstruction only with provocation, and one third having no obstruction under either condition.[51] Resting and latent LVOT obstruction can be sources of symptoms and exercise intolerance, and medical therapies and interventions directed at the relief of obstruction have often led to marked clinical improvement.

The causes and mechanisms of this dynamic LVOT obstruction are complex and historically have been the source of considerable controversy. Decades of careful hemodynamic and echocardiographic assessments have helped to define the pathophysiologic and anatomic contributors to obstruction (Table 13.2),[52,53] including the role of loading and contractile conditions on obstruction severity. LVOT gradients demonstrate daily and intraday variation related to patient activity, positioning, and fasting status.

SYSTOLIC ANTERIOR MOTION OF THE MITRAL LEAFLETS

Dr. E. Douglas Wigle and others, leveraging advances in echocardiographic technologies, were instrumental in showing that

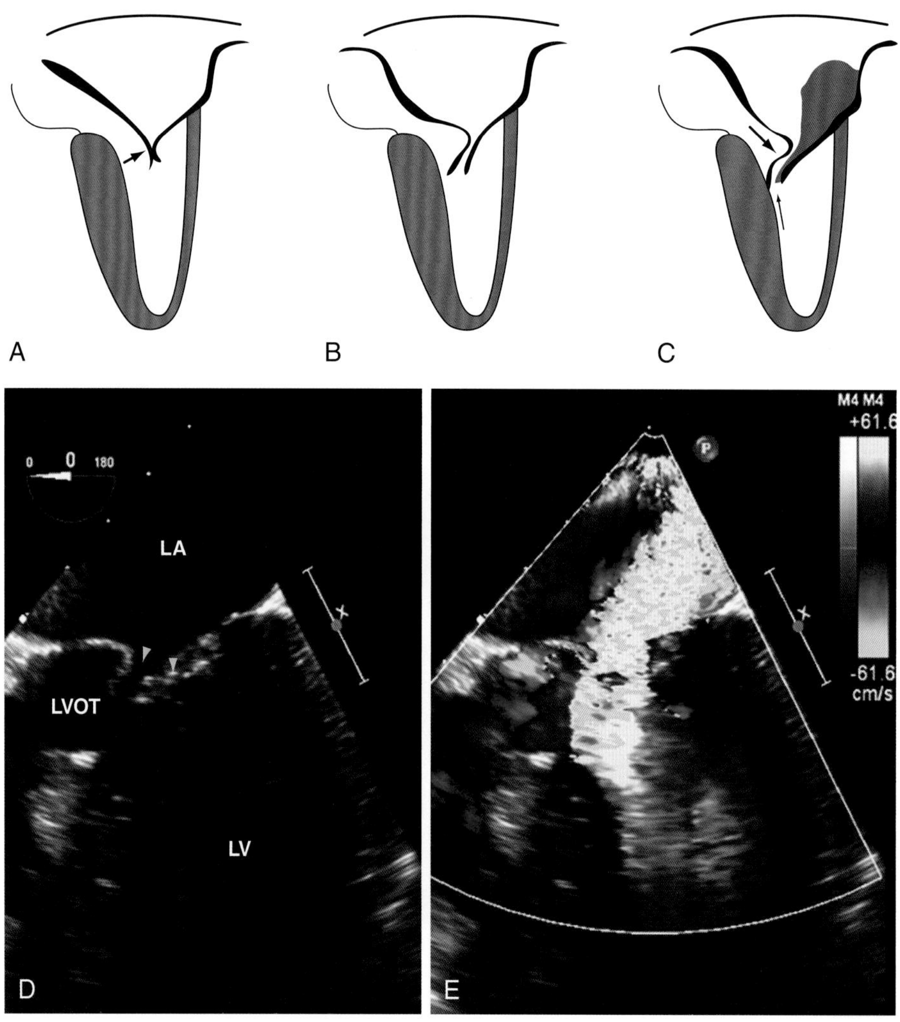

Fig. 13.5 **Systolic mitral leaflet deformation, resulting in dynamic left ventricular outflow tract (LVOT) obstruction and mitral regurgitation.** In patients with obstructive hypertrophic cardiomyopathy (HCM), the mitral leaflets are characteristically elongated and demonstrate anterior displacement of the coaptation line. These anatomic changes result in greater exposure of the undersurface of the leaflet to LV outflow. At the onset of systole (A), leaflet coaptation is at the tips, with minimal leaflet deformation and an open LVOT. During early systole (B), there is anterior bending of the mid-portion of the leaflets, with resultant progressive narrowing of the LVOT. During mid- to late systole (C), there is continued anterior leaflet deformation, resulting in contact with the basal septum and variable loss of coaptation. This characteristically results in a posteriorly directed mitral regurgitation jet. (D) and (E) show 2D and color Doppler echocardiographic correlates to this process. The *orange arrowheads* highlight the loss of leaflet coaptation due to leaflet deformation.

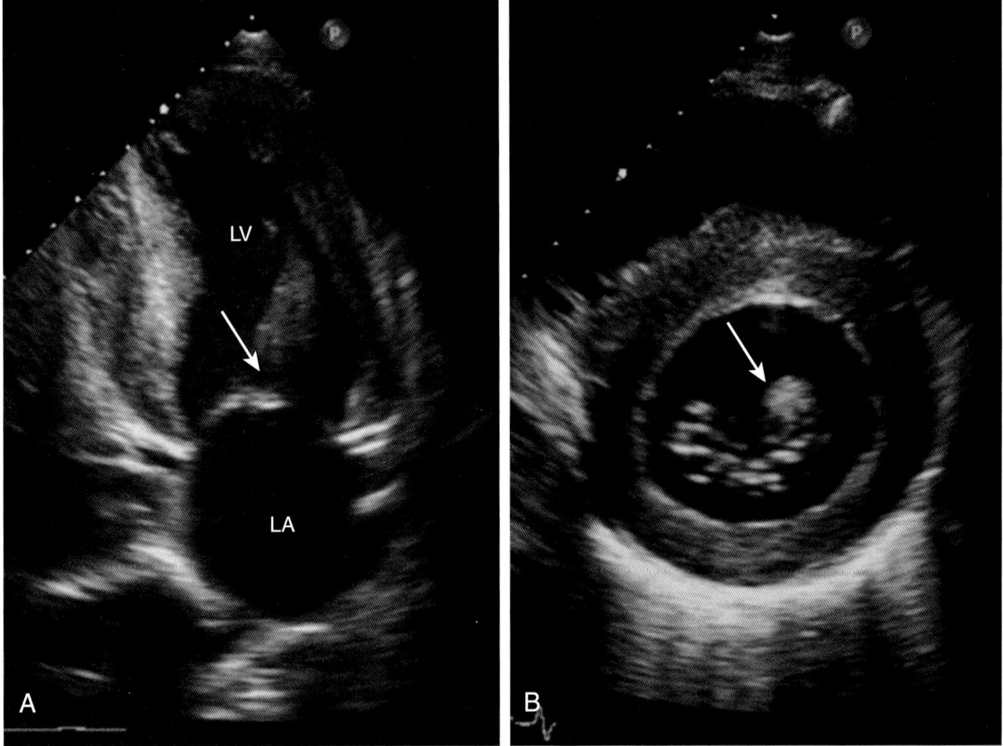

Fig 13.6 Direct insertion of the papillary muscle into the mitral leaflets. Papillary muscle abnormalities are common in hypertrophic cardiomyopathy. Parasternal long-axis (A) and parasternal short-axis (B) views show a papillary muscle directly inserting into the anterior mitral leaflet (*white arrows*).

TABLE 13.2 Factors Contributing to Dynamic LV Outflow Tract Obstruction in Hypertrophic Cardiomyopathy.

Narrowing of LVOT

- Hypertrophy of the basal septum
- Small LV cavity size

Altered Outflow Forces

- Hyperdynamic systolic function
- Rapid LV ejection
- Posterior-to-anterior flow vectors
- Acute ventricular-aortic angulation

Intrinsic Mitral Valve Abnormalities

- Mitral leaflet elongation (anterior or posterior)
- Anterior displacement of mitral apparatus
- Posterior leaflet clefts
- Myxomatous mitral valve degeneration
- Mitral annular calcification

Papillary Muscle Abnormalities

- Antero-apical displacement of the papillary muscle heads
- Bifid papillary muscles
- Hypertrophied papillary muscles
- Aberrant chordal attachment to anterior septum
- Direct insertion into mitral leaflet (absent chordae)

Loading Conditions

- Reduced preload
- Reduced afterload
- Increased contractility

LVOT, Left ventricular outflow tract.

systolic anterior motion (SAM) of the mitral leaflets, along with progressive systolic narrowing of the LVOT due to systolic septal hypertrophy and contraction, is the major cause of dynamic LVOT obstruction.[53,54]

Careful hemodynamic studies have shown that drag forces play a central role in the obstructive process, with lift and Venturi forces likely also contributing.[52,55] In early systole, fluid arising posteriorly flows upward against the posterior surface of the mitral leaflets, creating upward drag forces, akin to a sail in the wind.[56] The total force on the mitral leaflets is a factor of the velocity and acceleration of systolic ejection and of the surface area of the exposed mitral leaflet. These forces are countered by the tethering forces of the papillary muscles, but when these tethering vectors are altered or insufficient, mitral leaflet SAM can occur.

Mitral leaflet SAM is commonly limited to the tips of the leaflets distal to the coaptation zone, resulting in an acute angulation of the leaflets (i.e., typical SAM; Fig. 13.7A and B) and progressive systolic motion leading to SAM-septal contact.[57] Less commonly, the body of the leaflet slides anteriorly without bending (i.e., atypical SAM; see Fig. 13.7B and C). In both cases, there is a direct correlation between the degree of leaflet SAM and the development of an outflow pressure gradient. M-mode, with high temporal resolution, is optimal for observing the degree and duration of SAM (see Fig. 13.7E). This can be often achieved from the parasternal long-axis (PLAX) view, although in some patients, SAM is more medial and best observed from the apical 5-chamber or PSAX view.

Leaflet deformation due to SAM may result in dynamic malcoaptation, leading to mitral regurgitation (MR). This process

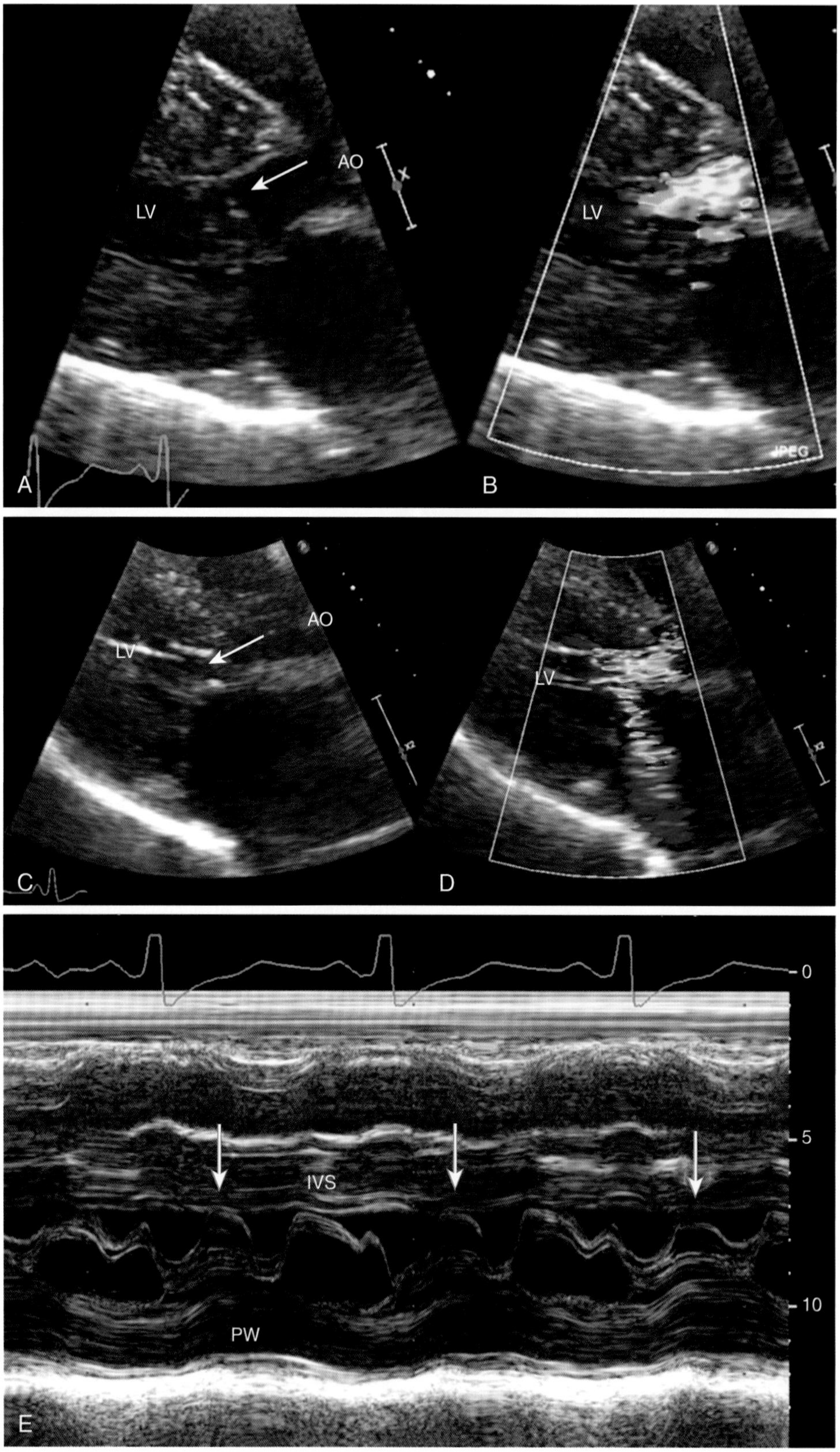

Fig. 13.7 Typical versus atypical systolic anterior motion of the mitral leaflets. Parasternal long-axis views depicting two different mechanisms of systolic anterior motion (SAM) of the mitral leaflets. In typical SAM (A and B), anterior motion is limited to the tips of the leaflets distal to the coaptation zone, resulting in an acute angulation of the leaflets *(arrow)*. Progressive systolic motion leads to SAM-septal contact. In atypical SAM (C and D), the body of the leaflet slides anteriorly without bending *(arrow)*. In both cases, there is a direct relationship between the degree of leaflet SAM and the development of an outflow pressure gradient. (E) M-mode tracing at the level of the mitral tips shows SAM of the mitral leaflets with septal contact *(white arrows)*. *AO*, Aorta; *IVS*, interventricular septum; *PW*, pulsed wave.

depends largely on the relative differences in anterior and posterior leaflet elongation and tethering. When the anterior leaflet is elongated in isolation, it experiences disproportionate drag forces and more SAM, resulting in a progressive loss of leaflet coaptation. MR in this setting is often highly eccentric and posteriorly directed, with late systolic accentuation due to progressive malcoaptation and a progressive increase in LV pressures caused by dynamic LVOT obstruction. Conversely, if posterior leaflet elongation is prominent or the leaflets demonstrate proportionate SAM, leaflet deformation results in less malcoaptation, and MR is absent or less severe.

Classification of SAM severity is based on the presence and duration of SAM-septal contact, which is directly related to the resultant pressure gradient.[58] Mild SAM is defined as a SAM-septal distance of greater than 10 mm, moderate SAM as a distance of less than 10 mm or brief SAM-septal contact, and severe SAM as SAM-septal contact lasting longer than 30% of systole.

There is a direct linear relationship between the time of onset of SAM and the duration of SAM-septal contact and the peak LVOT gradient that ensues. The increasing outflow velocity during systole progressively increases the drag forces on the mitral leaflet and Venturi forces in the LVOT, further narrowing the LVOT. The longer the duration of this feed-forward process, the more severe the peak LVOT obstruction becomes. This physiologic effect is the main target of pharmacologic therapy in the treatment of LVOT obstruction, and short delays in the onset of SAM can result in large effects on peak gradient.

LOADING CONDITIONS AND PROVOCATIVE MANEUVERS

The severity of dynamic LVOT obstruction varies based on inotropic state and loading conditions. A reduction in preload decreases LVOT diameter by approximating the anterior mitral leaflet to the septum, thereby decreasing the effective outflow orifice and worsening LVOT obstruction. Increases in heart rate (HR) or contractility reduce systolic ejection time and increase the force of LV ejection. This creates added drag forces on the mitral leaflets, worsening leaflet SAM and increasing peak LVOT gradients.

Physiologic factors that increase LVOT obstruction include standing or upright position, Valsalva maneuver, postprandial state, and physical exercise. In the echocardiography laboratory, Valsalva maneuvers and upright exercise are the most common forms of assessing LVOT obstruction. When properly performed, the Valsalva maneuver (i.e., forced exhalation against a closed glottis) raises intrathoracic pressure, reduces preload, reduces LV chamber size, and thereby brings mitral leaflets closer to the septum, worsening LVOT obstruction. Amyl nitrite inhalation is used at some centers to unmask LVOT obstruction, but there is only a modest correlation between the severity of the induced gradient and the gradients seen during more physiologic conditions.[59] The American College of Cardiology/American Heart Association (ACC/AHA) and European Society of Cardiology (ESC) guidelines do not recommend use of dobutamine to assess LVOT gradients because the combined increase in inotropy and vasodilation can induce obstruction even in patients without HCM.[1,2]

Exercise stress testing in HCM is safe and improves sensitivity for detecting latent LVOT obstruction compared with Valsalva maneuver. It should be considered for all HCM patients to assess functional capacity, blood pressure (BP) response to exercise, and presence and severity of latent LVOT obstruction and MR.[60,61] Upright exercise methods (i.e., treadmill or bicycle) confer lower preload and higher HR responses compared with supine exercise and therefore have greater sensitivity for detecting obstruction.

Doppler assessment of LVOT gradients can be performed during or immediately after exercise, although systolic BP may decrease early after cessation of muscle contraction, causing a transient increase in LVOT gradients. Doppler assessment may also reveal latent severe MR, which can contribute to a drop in BP at peak exercise.[62] In a small subset of HCM patients, LVOT gradients may paradoxically improve with exercise.[63]

DOPPLER ASSESSMENT OF OBSTRUCTION

Doppler echocardiography is the principal method of monitoring obstruction in patients with HCM. Because obstruction can occur at multiple levels in the LV, color-guided pulsed-wave (PW) Doppler assessment using apical windows (3-chamber or 5-chamber) is ideal for defining the location of obstruction. The PW sample volume can be marched from apex to base to assess the presence of mid-cavitary and LVOT obstruction. The PW Doppler velocity gradually increases as the sample volume becomes closer to the level of obstruction. High pulse repetition frequency (HPRF) or continuous-wave (CW) Doppler imaging of LV outflow may be substituted when Doppler aliasing occurs. Peak LVOT velocity can be converted to pressure gradients using the modified Bernoulli equation ($\Delta P = 4 \bullet [V_{LVOT}]^2$). CW Doppler assessment of MR should also be performed, and if Doppler alignment is adequate, these data can be used to assess or confirm LV pressure estimates.

Dynamic LVOT obstruction arises at the level of the mitral tips and has a characteristic late-peaking Doppler envelope that is often referred to as *dagger shaped* (Fig. 13.8A). This shape is derived from progressive systolic narrowing of the LVOT during systole caused by mitral leaflet SAM, culminating in SAM-septal contact. This late-peaking envelope is distinct from the mid-peaking Doppler profile seen with fixed stenosis at the subvalvular or valvular level (see Fig. 13.8C) and from the asymptotic-appearing Doppler profile of mid-cavitary obstruction (see Fig. 13.8B). Mid-cavitary and LVOT level obstruction can coexist in the same patient, and this may result in merging CW Doppler signals.

For patients with severe LVOT obstruction (>60 mmHg), a PW Doppler signal obtained in the body of the LV just proximal to the mitral tips may demonstrate a mid-systolic drop in velocity that is a consequence of the mechanical effects of the obstruction on LV systolic function.[64] This pattern has been called the *lobster claw* signal because of its appearance (Fig. 13.9). This finding indicates that the progressive decrease in LVOT orifice size due to mitral SAM (and consequent progressive increase in afterload) is reducing LV systolic function and LVOT flow. This effect can similarly be seen in premature closure of the aortic valve on M-mode and in the abrupt termination of LV longitudinal shortening on tissue Doppler. These findings are associated with decreased exercise capacity and increased risk of heart failure.

PITFALLS OF DOPPLER EVALUATION

Advances in ultrasound technology have improved image quality and the ability to obtain discrete LVOT Doppler signals. When discrete PW Doppler signals cannot be obtained due to aliasing, HPRF or CW Doppler signals of LVOT outflow can be used to determine peak outflow gradient.

Mitral leaflet SAM results in leaflet deformation and separation such that the MR jet originates from within the LVOT, which may create challenges in obtaining a distinct Doppler

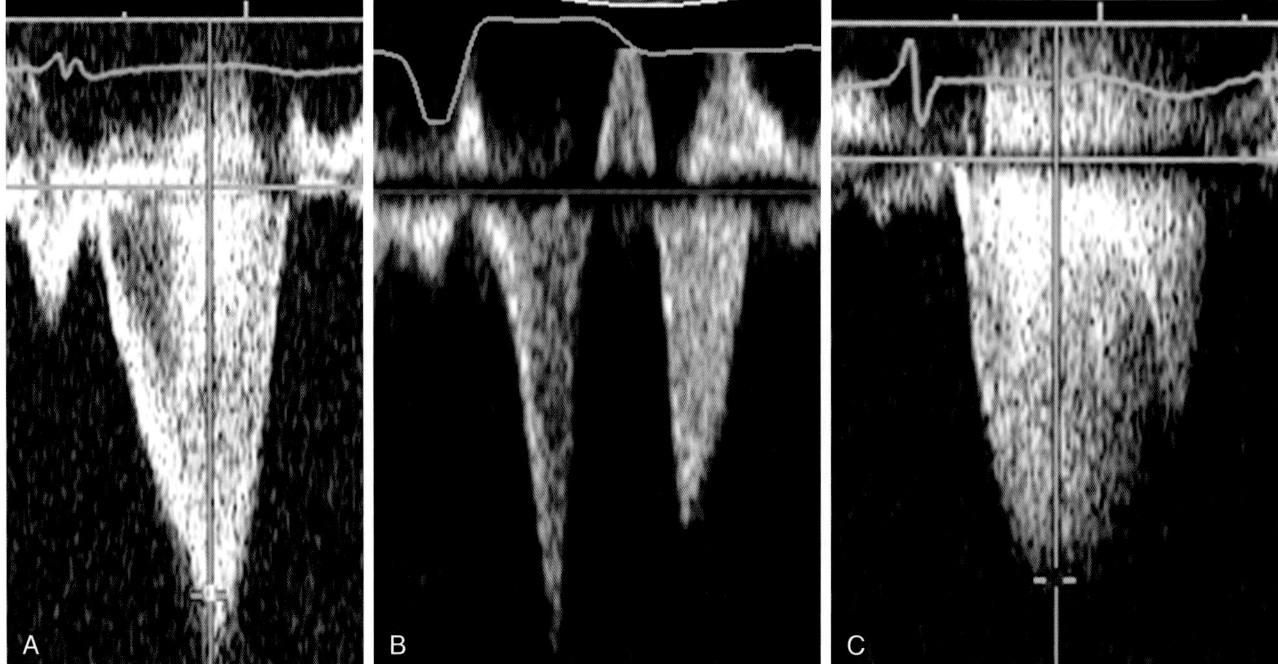

Fig. 13.8 Doppler signal patterns for obstruction in hypertrophic cardiomyopathy. The location of obstruction in HCM can often be deduced by the Doppler pattern. (A) Dynamic obstruction of the left ventricular outflow tract (LVOT) shows a characteristic late peaking signal caused by progressive narrowing of the LVOT due to anterior leaflet deformation. (B) Mid-cavitary obstruction shows a sharp drop in Doppler signal during middle to late systole caused by cavity obliteration. This may be followed by a resumption of basally directed flow during early diastole if the apex remains pressurized while cavity obliteration resolves. (C) Fixed obstruction due to subvalvular or valvular aortic stenosis shows earlier peaking and a rounded Doppler signal.

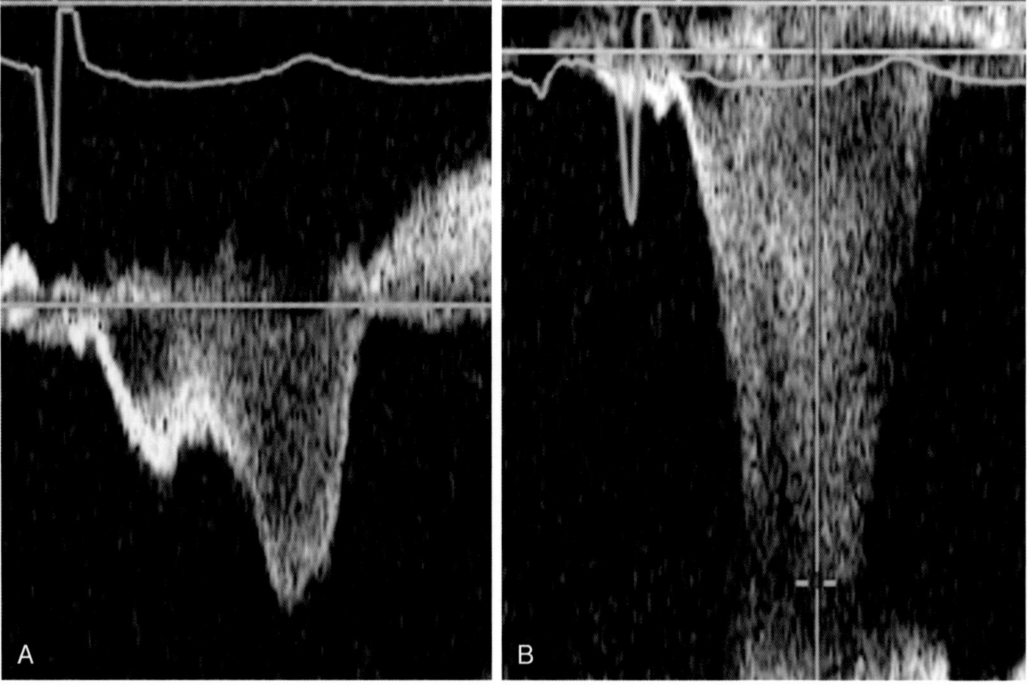

Fig. 13.9 Pulsed-wave Doppler signal from within the LV shows the characteristic lobster claw pattern. A pulsed-wave Doppler sample obtained just apical to the level of dynamic obstruction at the mitral tips (A) shows a mid-systolic drop in outflow velocities. The point at which velocity decreases corresponds to the onset of leaflet-septal contact; the velocity nadir represents the time of peak left ventricular outflow tract (LVOT) gradient, as shown in the CW Doppler signal of LV outflow (B). This lobster claw pattern indicates severe obstruction that is reducing LV contractile function and decreasing LVOT outflow.

outflow signal. If the MR is a result of leaflet SAM, the jet will most often be eccentric and posteriorly directed. Orientation of the transducer beam anteriorly and medially should help isolate the LVOT flow. MR onset occurs earlier, with a more rapid initial increase in velocity, and it often has a rounded, convex appearance (Fig. 13.10). It is uncommon for LV pressures to exceed 300 mmHg at rest, and peak Doppler velocities in excess of 6.0 m/s most likely represent MR.

In some patients with HCM, the LVOT Doppler profile is contaminated by MR and cannot be independently isolated.

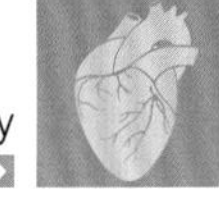

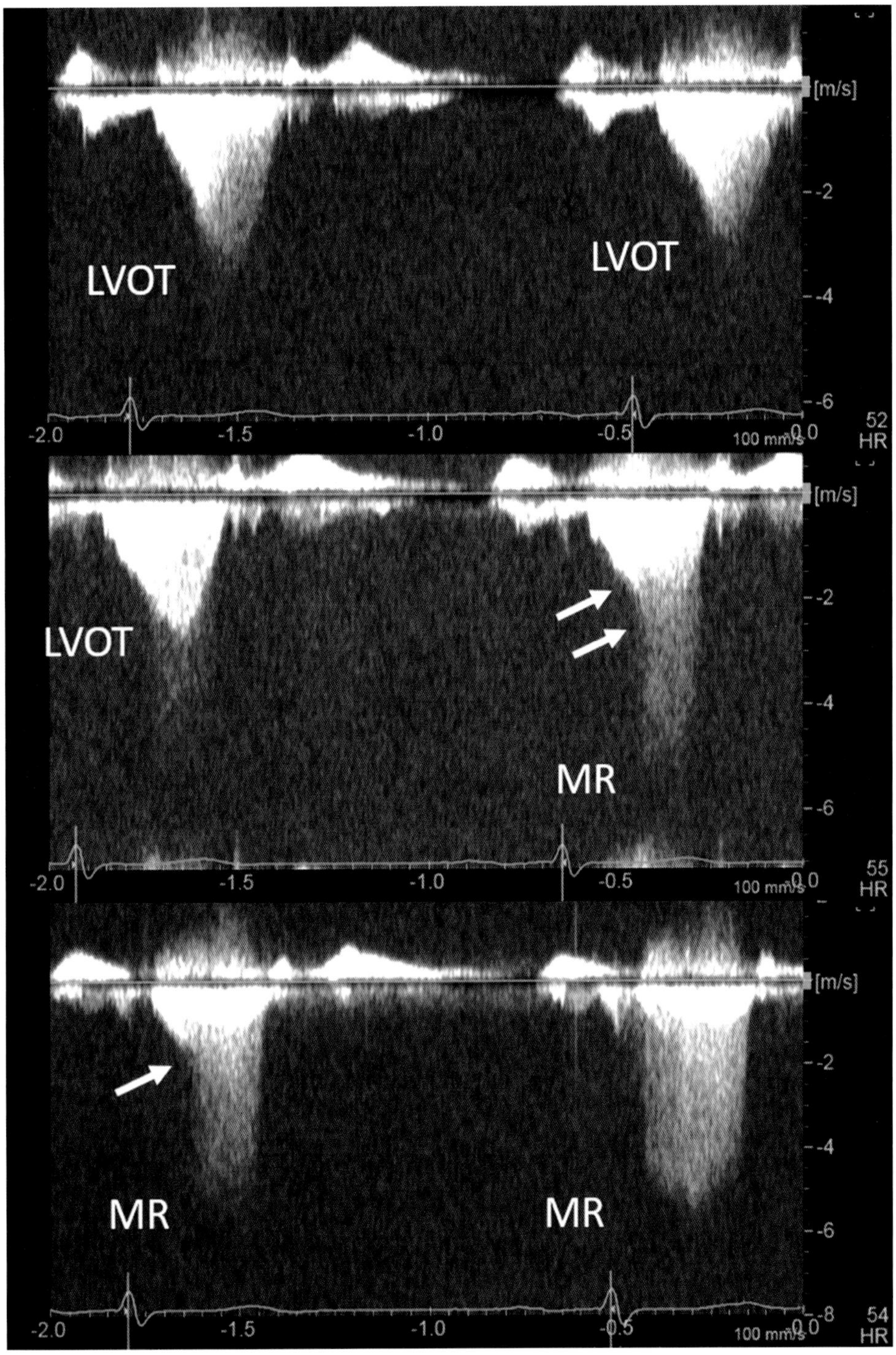

Fig. 13.10 **Comparison of Doppler signals in obstructive hypertrophic cardiomyopathy.** CW Doppler echocardiographic sweep through the left ventricular outflow tract *(LVOT)* shows the transition from LVOT Doppler signal to mitral regurgitation *(MR)* Doppler signal. (A) The CW Doppler signal is obtained from the anterior LVOT and shows a discrete LVOT signal (peak 3.0 m/s) with a characteristic dagger-shaped, late-peaking jet. In the middle panel, the CW Doppler is moved to the posterior LVOT, and the signal begins to be contaminated with MR. The MR signal has a higher velocity, and because of the progressive increase in LV pressure, it takes on a convex appearance *(white arrows)*. (B) The CW Doppler is moved further posteriorly, and the MR envelope (peak ≈ 5.2 m/s) begins to occur earlier in systole. When MR is solely due to leaflet deformation caused by systolic anterior motion (SAM), it begins in early to mid-systole in concert with the increase in LVOT gradient; when MR is present before leaflet deformation, it begins during isovolumetric contraction.

Because of the anterior mitral leaflet deformation, the MR originates from within the LVOT, making contamination more likely. When this occurs, indirect methods for estimating LVOT gradients using peak MR velocity, assumed left atrial (LA) pressure, and measured systolic BP can be employed (Fig. 13.11).

MYOCARDIAL DEFORMATION AND STRAIN

Speckle tracking echocardiography (STE) is a newer echocardiography technique that has provided insights into global and regional myocardial mechanics. HCM often demonstrates

$GRAD_{LVOT} = LVSP - SBP$

$LVSP = GRAD_{LV\text{-}LA} + LAP_{est}$

$GRAD_{LVOT} = GRAD_{LV\text{-}LA} + LAP_{est} - SBP$

$GRAD_{LV\text{-}LA} = (4^*(V_{MR})^2)$

$GRAD_{LVOT} = (4^*(V_{MR})^2) + LAP_{est} - SBP$

Abbreviations
$GRAD_{LVOT}$, LVOT pressure gradient.
LVSP, LV systolic pressure.
SBP, Systolic blood pressure.
$GRAD_{LV\text{-}LA}$, LA-LV pressure gradient
LAP_{est}, estimated LA pressure.
V_{MR}, peak MR velocity.

Example

If V_{MR} = 7.0 m/s, LAP = 15 mmHg, and SBP = 120 mmHg

$GRAD_{LV\text{-}LA} = (4^*(7.0)^2) = 196$
$LVSP = GRAD_{LV\text{-}LA} + LAP_{est} = 196 + 15 = 211$

$GRAD_{LVOT} = LVSP - SBP = 211 - 120 = 91$ mmHg.

Fig. 13.11 **Method for indirectly estimating peak left ventricular outflow tract (LVOT) gradient.** Method for indirectly estimating peak LVOT gradient using peak mitral regurgitation (MR) velocity. This method is useful for confirming LVOT gradients when MR is highly eccentric, or when LVOT Doppler signal is contaminated by MR. LVOT gradient *($GRAD_{LVOT}$)* can be obtained using measured peak MR velocity *(V_{MR})*, measured systolic blood pressure *(SBP)*, and estimated LA pressure *(LA_{est})*.

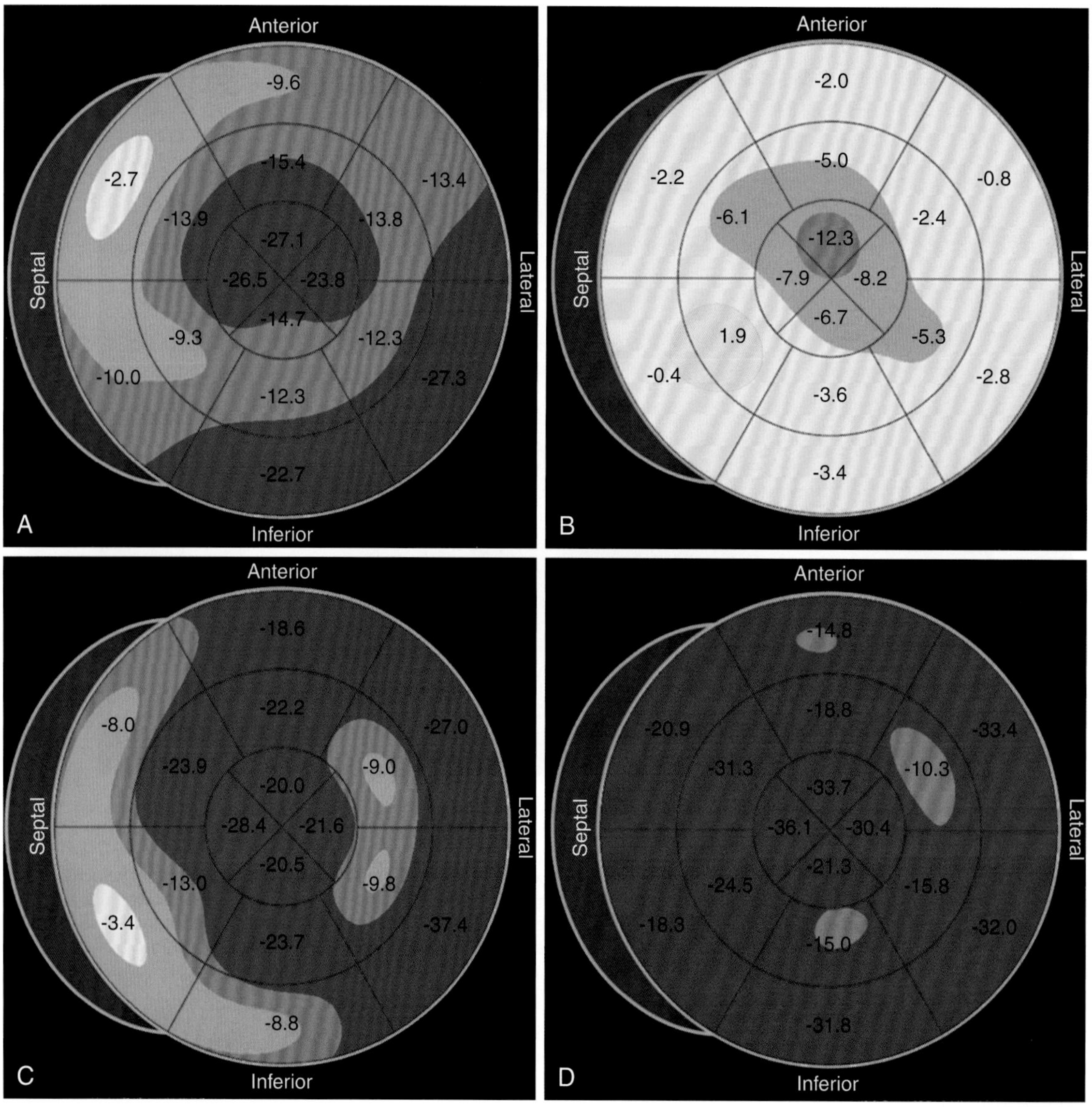

A: Anterior; -9.6; -2.7; -15.4; -13.4; -13.9; -13.8; -27.1; Septal; -26.5; -23.8; Lateral; -14.7; -9.3; -12.3; -10.0; -27.3; -12.3; -22.7; Inferior

B: Anterior; -2.0; -2.2; -5.0; -0.8; -6.1; -2.4; -12.3; Septal; -7.9; -8.2; Lateral; -6.7; 1.9; -5.3; -0.4; -2.8; -3.6; -3.4; Inferior

C: Anterior; -18.6; -22.2; -8.0; -27.0; -23.9; -9.0; -20.0; Septal; -28.4; -21.6; Lateral; -20.5; -13.0; -9.8; -3.4; -37.4; -23.7; -8.8; Inferior

D: Anterior; -14.8; -18.8; -20.9; -33.4; -31.3; -10.3; -33.7; Septal; -36.1; -30.4; Lateral; -21.3; -24.5; -15.8; -18.3; -32.0; -15.0; -31.8; Inferior

Fig. 13.12 **Longitudinal strain patterns in patients with LV hypertrophy.** Longitudinal strain patterns in patients with various forms of LV hypertrophy. (A) Amyloidosis typically demonstrates equally reduced strain in the basal to middle myocardium, with preservation of strain apically. (B) Hypertrophic cardiomyopathy demonstrates reduced strain in the regions of hypertrophy, typically in the basal to middle septum. (C) Fabry disease usually involves reduced strain in the basal inferior and posterior region but can be variable depending on the extent of sphingolipid deposition. (D) Athlete's heart demonstrates globally normal to increased strain without clear regionality.

TABLE 13.3 Factors Contributing to Diastolic Dysfunction in Hypertrophic Cardiomyopathy.

Molecular and Ccellular Function

- Reduced ability of sarcomeres to achieve super-relaxed state
- Myocardium calcium overload
- Myofibrillar disarray

Increased Relaxation Load

- Late systolic loading
- Reduced end-systolic deformation (restoring forces)
- Microvascular ischemia/altered coronary filling
- Dyssynchronous/heterogeneous relaxation

Increased Contraction Load

- Dynamic LVOT obstruction
- Hypertension or other sources of afterload

Decreased Compliance

- Increased LV mass
- LV volume
- Myocardial fibrosis

LVOT, Left ventricular outflow tract.

decreased longitudinal deformation and strain, particularly in regions of hypertrophy and perhaps due to the underlying myofibrillar disarray and fibrosis.[65,66] This is countered by a compensatory increase in circumferential deformation and strain, such that the overall ejection fraction usually remains normal.

STE has revealed important insights into twist mechanics in HCM, which can vary by phenotype.[67,68] Septal hypertrophy results in normal to decreased twisting of the base, a paradoxical clockwise rotation of the mid-ventricle (in the direction of the base rather than the apex), and increased twisting of the apical segments. Overall torsion remains normal to increased. This alteration in the geometry of systolic deformation is reflected in diastolic relaxation, resulting in a delay in the onset of LV untwisting, particularly in patients with LVOT obstruction.[69]

Strain analysis can be a useful diagnostic aid, particularly in differentiating HCM from other causes of LVH such as cardiac amyloidosis, Fabry disease, or exercise-induced cardiac remodeling (Fig. 13.12). The strain map in HCM typically shows a decrease in longitudinal strain in areas of hypertrophy and fibrosis, most commonly the septum. In contrast, the strain map in cardiac amyloidosis shows apical preservation of strain with abnormal longitudinal strain in other segments. Fabry disease demonstrates a reduction in longitudinal and circumferential strain due to the accumulation of glycosphingolipids.[70] Scarring and fibrosis is most commonly seen in the basal to mid-posterior wall, which may be reflected as abnormal strain in this region. LVH due to exercise-induced remodeling (i.e., athlete's heart) is typically associated with normal longitudinal strain and significant increases in circumferential and radial strain.

DIASTOLIC FUNCTION

FACTORS CONTRIBUTING TO IMPAIRED DIASTOLIC FUNCTION

Almost all patients with HCM have some degree of diastolic dysfunction, ranging from impaired relaxation to reduced LV compliance. Diastolic dysfunction that is more severe may contribute to dyspnea on exertion, elevated LA and pulmonary artery (PA) pressures, progressive LA enlargement, and risk of atrial fibrillation. Often, elevated filling pressures are isolated to the left heart, with preserved RV filling pressures.

Innate and acquired factors, along with loading conditions, contribute to diastolic dysfunction in HCM, with specific contributions varying by individual (Table 13.3). Studies suggest that many HCM genetic variants reduce the ability of myosin to achieve a super-relaxed conformation, resulting in an increase in the number of myosin-actin interactions and an increase in metabolic expenditure.[40,71] These factors are postulated to simultaneously increase contractility and reduce relaxation velocities. This may explain the reduction in medial and lateral E′ early relaxation velocities seen in patients with HCM compared with controls, including those with preclinical HCM before the development of LVH.[41]

Several acquired factors contribute to diastolic dysfunction. LVH, increased LV mass, and reduced LV cavity size increase myocardial stiffness, resulting in increased pressure per ventricular volume. Chamber stiffness is directly proportional to myocardial mass and inversely proportional to LV chamber volume. The myocyte hypertrophy and myofibrillar disarray that occurs in HCM creates inefficiencies in energy use, making myocardial ischemia more likely.

The asymmetric hypertrophy seen with HCM may create inhomogeneity of contraction and relaxation. In patients with septal hypertrophy, early relaxation of the LV apex creates a basal-to-apical pressure gradient during isovolumic relaxation. In patients with apical HCM, early relaxation of the basal segments results in apical-to-basal flow during this same period. This may be exacerbated in patients with mid-ventricular obstruction and apical aneurysm, in which flow from the pressurized apex occurs during early diastole after release of the obstruction. Intraventricular and interventricular dyssynchrony occurs in HCM, despite absence of conduction system disease, and its severity correlates with the degree of LVH.

LVOT obstruction, which is common in HCM, places a load on LV contraction, increases oxygen demands, delays the onset of relaxation, and reduces ventricular filling. Surgical myectomy can improve diastolic function and reduce LA and PA pressures. Microvascular coronary artery disease may reduce coronary flow and oxygen supply and thereby contribute to relaxation loads.

Interstitial fibrosis occurs to various degrees in HCM patients and is a major contributor to reduced LV compliance and elevated filling pressures. An important subset of patients has progressive fibrosis that includes a progressive decline in contractility (which may result in loss of obstruction) and reduction in ventricular compliance. These patients may develop a restrictive phenotype with markedly elevated filling pressures.

ECHOCARDIOGRAPHIC ASSESSMENT OF DIASTOLIC FUNCTION

Echocardiographic assessment of diastolic function in patients with HCM is challenging due to disease regionality, myocardial disarray, and alteration of the typical relationship between active relaxation and reduced compliance. There are marked variations among patients in contractility, the location and extent of hypertrophy, the presence and severity of obstruction and MR, and the degree of myocardial disarray and fibrosis.

Annular E′ velocities can be decreased as a result of the underlying genetic change because of the effects of myofibrillar disarray on myocardial deformation or because

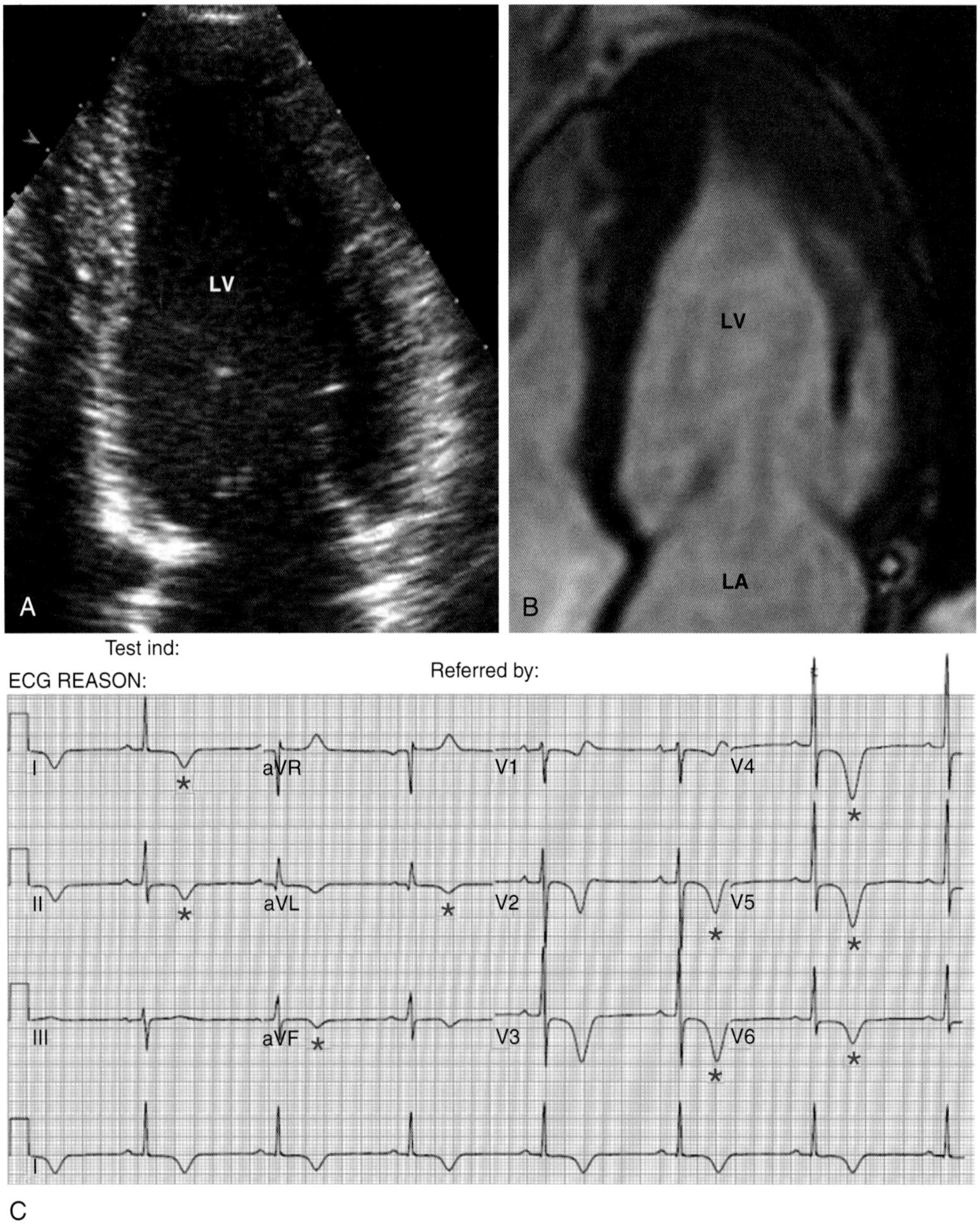

Fig. 13.13 Apical hypertrophic cardiomyopathy with and without echocardiographic contrast. (A) Apical 4-chamber image of a patient with apical variant hypertrophic cardiomyopathy (HCM). (B) A cardiac magnetic resonance imaging (MRI) correlate of the apical 4-chamber view. The extent of hypertrophy can be underappreciated on echocardiography if contrast is not used. Notice the sparing of the basal segments and the overall spade-like configuration of the ventricle caused by the decrease in cavity volume apically. (C) The electrocardiogram (ECG) in patients with apical HCM is often markedly abnormal, showing deep T-wave inversions across the precordial leads *(red asterisks)*.

of septal hypertrophy and fibrosis. They can have varied effects on filling pressures and overall functional capacity. MR is common in HCM and can confound indices of diastolic filling. Although there is a modest correlation between the E:E′ ratio and filling pressures, it is less accurate in patients with HCM compared with other cardiomyopathic conditions.[72]

Because of these factors, a more holistic approach to assessing diastolic function should be undertaken.[73] Conventional indices that correlate with adverse outcomes and/or increased filling pressures include the E:e′ ratio, LA volume index, tricuspid regurgitation (TR) jet velocity, and pulmonary vein A-wave reversal duration ($A_r - A_{dur} > 30$ ms). The latter two indices can be assessed in the setting of moderate or greater MR. LA size in particular negatively correlates with functional capacity, is associated with an increased risk of atrial fibrillation, and is associated with incident heart failure and increased all-cause and HCM-related mortality rates.[74,75]

ASSESSMENT OF HYPERTROPHIC CARDIOMYOPATHY SUBTYPES

Several clinically important HCM subtypes are identified by the location of hypertrophy and/or the genetic basis of disease, and they have unique echocardiographic features.

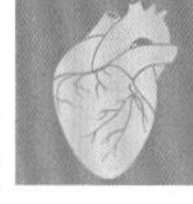

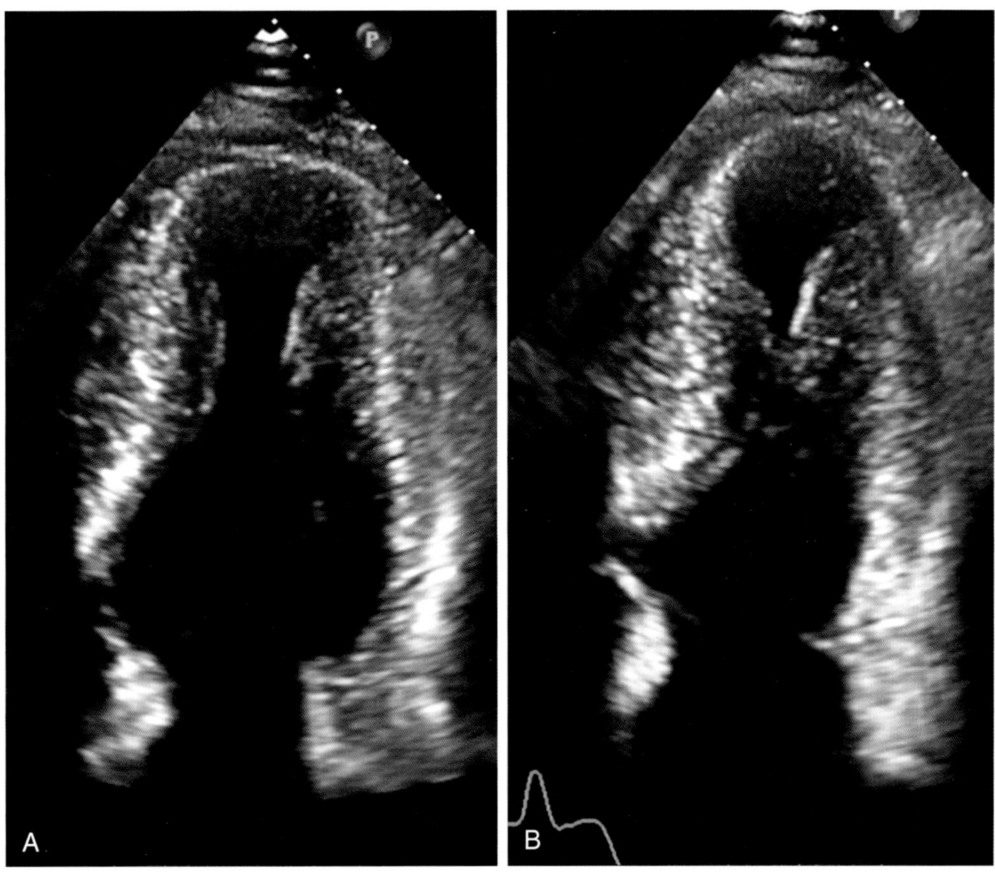

Fig. 13.14 **Mid-ventricular hypertrophic cardiomyopathy with apical aneurysm.** Mid-ventricular hypertrophic cardiomyopathy (HCM) seen on apical 4-chamber views during end-diastole (A) and end-systole (B) shows cavitary obliteration at the mid-ventricular level and an apical aneurysm. Use of contrast imaging can be helpful to exclude apical thrombi.

APICAL VARIANT HYPERTROPHIC CARDIOMYOPATHY

LV wall thickness normally tapers from base to apex. Apical variant HCM (Fig. 13.13) is characterized by hypertrophy that chiefly involves the distal one third of the ventricular chamber circumferentially, although more regional involvement can be seen. This typically results in a spade-like configuration of the distal LV chamber and is commonly associated with a markedly abnormal electrocardiographic (ECG) pattern with deep T-wave inversions across the precordial leads.[36] Apicalized papillary muscles are common in this variant and may contribute to the appearance of apical hypertrophy.[76] The basal and middle septum may be mildly hypertrophied, although this is not the site of maximal wall thickness. Apical HCM has been postulated to be a more benign variant, although it is associated with an increased risk of atrial fibrillation, and SCD can occur.[77]

The LV apex is best seen from apical windows, although it is in the near field from this view. Use of echocardiographic contrast should be considered in all patients with known or suspected apical HCM to better define wall thickness and to exclude an apical outpouching or aneurysm.

MID-VENTRICULAR OBSTRUCTION

Another important subtype of HCM is mid-ventricular HCM (Fig. 13.14), with or without an apical aneurysm.[34] The characteristic feature is circumferential hypertrophy at the mid-ventricular or papillary level, which usually results in late-systolic cavity obliteration, creating an apical-basal pressure. The characteristic asymptotic Doppler profile (see Fig. 13.14) represents the highest detectable gradient, but continued apical contraction may result in higher apical-basal gradients that are undetectable by Doppler due to complete cavity obliteration and absence of flow. Apical-to-basal flow frequently resumes during early diastole, after relief of cavity obliteration.

The thin-walled, high-pressured LV apex is prone to progressive scarring even in the absence of epicardial coronary disease, and development of apical aneurysms is common. Patients with mid-ventricular HCM and apical aneurysms are at increased risk for ventricular tachycardia and cardioembolic strokes, presumably due to thrombus formation within the apical aneurysm.[35,77] Echocardiographic contrast should be considered in all patients with mid-ventricular HCM for detection of aneurysm and thrombus.

THIN-FILAMENT HYPERTROPHIC CARDIOMYOPATHY

Thin-filament HCM is a collective term for the subset of HCM caused by genetic variation in the actin filament and the troponin regulatory complex. Collectively, this group accounts for approximately 20% of all cases of genetically confirmed HCM. Thin-filament HCM more frequently manifests with milder or atypically distributed LVH but with higher degrees of fibrosis (Fig. 13.15). There are higher rates of severe heart failure

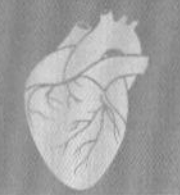

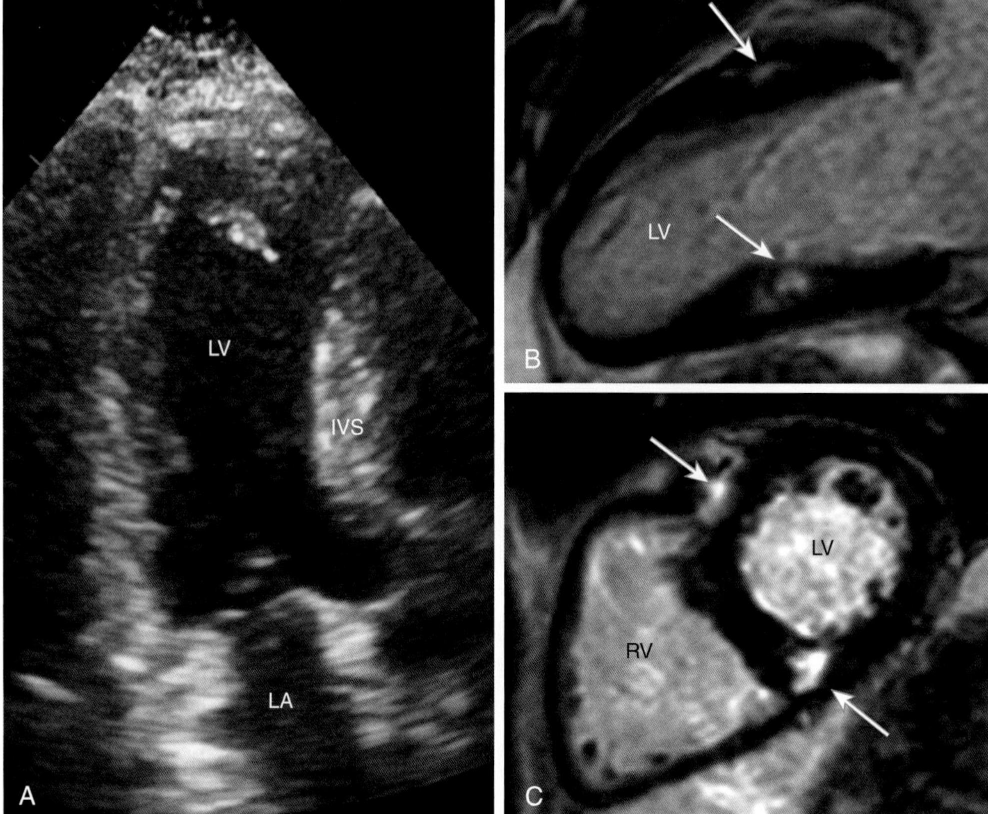

Fig. 13.15 **Thin-filament hypertrophic cardiomyopathy.** Echocardiographic and cardiac magnetic resonance images (MRI) of a patient with thin-filament hypertrophic cardiomyopathy (HCM) demonstrate a combination of mild hypertrophy and significant fibrosis. (A) In a patient with the pathogenic tropomyosin *TPM1* variant, mild hypertrophy (12 mm) of the interventricular septum *(IVS)* is seen on an apical long-axis view. Significant late gadolinium enhancement *(arrows)* is demonstrated on cardiac MRI 2-chamber (B) and short-axis (C) views.

and restrictive and/or triphasic diastolic filling, a marker of advanced LV diastolic dysfunction.[78]

Because of the atypical morphology, patients may be initially mistakenly diagnosed as having hypertensive heart disease or infiltrative conditions. However, the risk of sudden death and/or ventricular arrhythmias is similar between thin-filament and thick-filament HCM, making proper recognition of this disease essential.

NONFAMILIAL HYPERTROPHIC CARDIOMYOPATHY

Not all patients with LVH and LVOT obstruction have a genetic basis for their disease. One group, which has been referred to as *HCM of the elderly*, represents a subset of nonfamilial HCM that is characterized by age-related adverse cardiac remodeling, often in the setting of hypertension or metabolic disease. These patients have unique clinical and echocardiographic features that distinguish them from patients with genetic HCM, although they often require similar management. Patients are older and have milder hypertrophy that is often isolated to the basal septum (i.e., septal knuckle).

Primary abnormalities of mitral leaflets or papillary muscles are less common, and major factors contributing to LVOT obstruction include a small LV cavity, which leads to increased chordal slack; acute ventricular-aortic angulation; and mitral annular calcification, which shifts the mitral apparatus anteriorly and exposes the undersurface of the mitral leaflets. Together, these changes direct LV outflow in a posterior-to-anterior direction, resulting in mitral leaflet SAM similar in effect to that seen with genetic HCM.

MANAGEMENT OF LV OUTFLOW TRACT OBSTRUCTION

Echocardiography remains the primary tool to guide management of HCM, particularly in the assessment of LVOT obstruction. On initial assessment, all patients should undergo thorough echocardiographic assessment for the presence and severity of LVOT obstruction and with the aim of identifying the main contributors to LVOT obstruction in each patient.

The first step in medical management is medication reconciliation. Agents that reduce preload (e.g., diuretics, nitrates) or increase contractility (e.g., digoxin, methylphenidate) can worsen LVOT obstruction and are contraindicated. Medical therapy for LVOT obstruction is directed at reducing the force of cardiac contraction using negative inotropic agents such as β-blockers, non-dihydropyridine calcium channel blockers (e.g., verapamil), and/or disopyramide.[79] A reduction in cardiac contractility delays the onset of mitral leaflet SAM and SAM-septal contact, thereby reducing mitral leaflet deformation, peak LVOT gradients, and MR severity. Response to therapy can be monitored by using onset of SAM-septal contact as defined by M-mode imaging, but peak LVOT gradients are more commonly followed.

β-Blockers and verapamil have chronotropic benefits, decreasing HR, increasing diastolic filling time, and potentially reducing myocardial ischemia.[79] The main benefit of β-blockers is to limit peak HR during exercise, thereby reducing exertional peak LVOT gradients, but verapamil has a modest effect on resting LVOT gradients (30%–50% reduction). Verapamil has induced heart failure and death in patients with severe LVOT obstruction (>100 mmHg) and elevated filling pressures, and it should be avoided or used with caution in this setting.[80]

Disopyramide is the most potent negative inotropic agent available, with an average reduction in LVOT gradients of approximately 50%, although anticholinergic side effects are often dose limiting.[81] Myosin modulators are a novel class of medications with strong negative inotropic effects that have shown promise in the treatment of obstructive HCM.[82]

RV pacing has an alluring theoretical benefit on LVOT obstruction because pacing-induced ventricular dyssynchrony may lead to reduced contractility and lower LVOT gradients. After initial reports suggested hemodynamic benefit, trials randomizing HCM subjects with pacemakers to active pacing versus no pacing showed no significant improvement in gradients or symptoms.[83,84] Placement of a pacemaker for the primary indication of gradient reduction is therefore discouraged (class III recommendation).[1,2] However, for patients who have other pacing indications, forced RV pacing may be considered.

SEPTAL REDUCTION THERAPIES

Patients with resting or provocable LVOT obstruction and severe (New York Heart Association class III–IV) refractory symptoms should be considered for septal reduction therapies.[1,2] The procedural techniques for reducing septal wall thickness include surgical myectomy and alcohol septal ablation (ASA), and echocardiography plays an important intraprocedural role for both techniques.

Proper patient selection for these procedures is critical. Current guidelines prioritize consideration of surgical myectomy over ASA as the procedure of choice because of its low morbidity and mortality rates, excellent postoperative course, and greater predictability and magnitude of gradient reduction.

SURGICAL MYECTOMY

Surgical myectomy was pioneered by Dr. Andrew Morrow in the early 1960s.[85] The surgical technique has evolved into an aortotomy with extended myectomy, referred to as a modified Morrow procedure. This is a technically challenging surgery; the myectomy is performed across the aortic valve to create a trough within the thickened basal septum, thereby improving LV outflow. There is limited visualization of the surgical field, and an experienced surgeon must ensure that the length and depth of myocardial resection is sufficient to eliminate obstruction while avoiding creation of a ventricular septal defect.

Perioperative transesophageal echocardiography (TEE) plays an important role in guiding surgical myectomy, immediately assessing the hemodynamic response to surgery, and in identifying surgical complications.[86] TEE can help to define the length and depth of the required myectomy, thereby guiding the surgical resection. To avoid the conduction system, the surgical myectomy begins to the right of the nadir of the right coronary cusp and is then directed leftward.[87] The length of the myectomy should be determined in this view, with distal resection to at least 1 cm beyond the point of SAM-septal contact (Fig. 13.16). An image showing these measurements can be saved and projected for surgical reference.

Careful preoperative assessment of the MV is essential and should focus on intrinsic MV abnormalities that would require direct MV intervention.[88] Most posteriorly directed MR is related to SAM and does not require valve intervention.[89] It is also important to identify papillary muscle abnormalities, including direct insertion of the papillary muscle into the mitral leaflet, and any aberrant chordal attachments that may be contributing to LVOT obstruction. These should be corrected as a part of the surgical intervention.

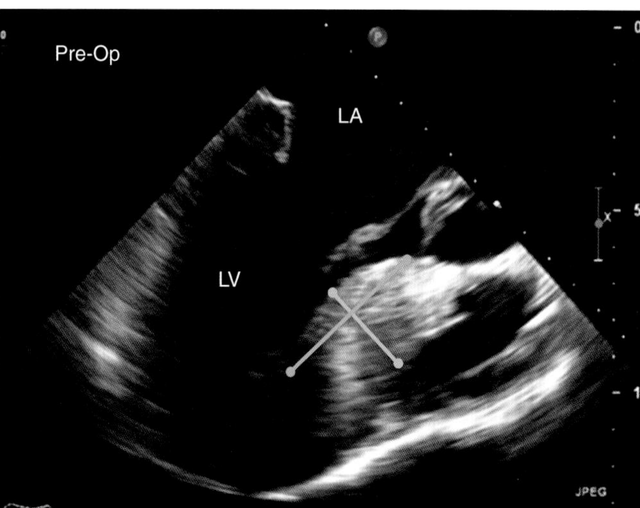

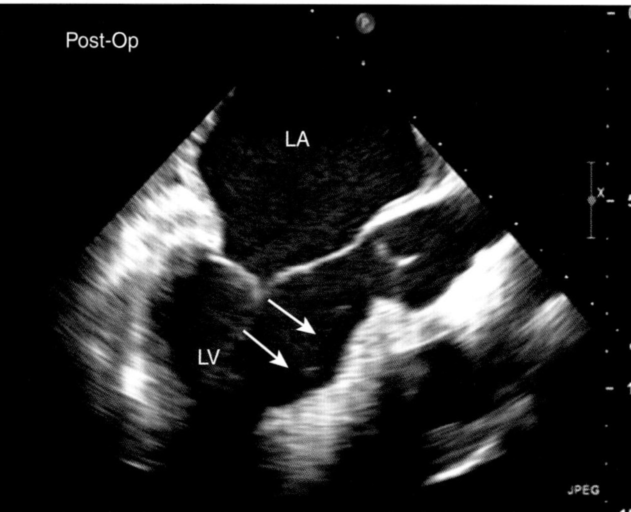

Fig. 13.16 Perioperative TEE for guiding septal ablation. TEE can be used perioperatively to help guide the depth and extent of surgical myectomy. The anterior septum is best visualized on midesophageal long-axis views. (A) Measurement of septal wall thickness *(blue line)* can be performed preoperatively, and the distal extent of the excision *(green line)* can be estimated. The excision should be extended past the region of systolic anterior motion (SAM)-septal contact and ideally to the level of the papillary muscles. (B) Postoperative imaging *(bottom panel)* demonstrates the myectomy trough *(arrows)*.

The presence and severity of LVOT obstruction can be assessed using CW Doppler from deep transgastric long-axis views. General anesthesia reduces cardiac contractility and decreases LVOT gradients. It is standard practice to assess gradients at rest and with isoproterenol or dobutamine provocation.[86,90] Baseline gradients are obtained preoperatively and again after myectomy to determine the effects of surgery. If a residual gradient is detected (>30 mmHg), if there is significant (3+ or greater) MR, or if a ventricular septal defect is detected, the patient can be placed back on cardiopulmonary bypass to extend the myectomy, perform MV intervention, or repair the defect.

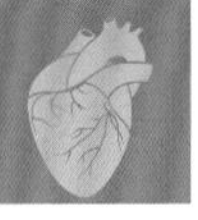

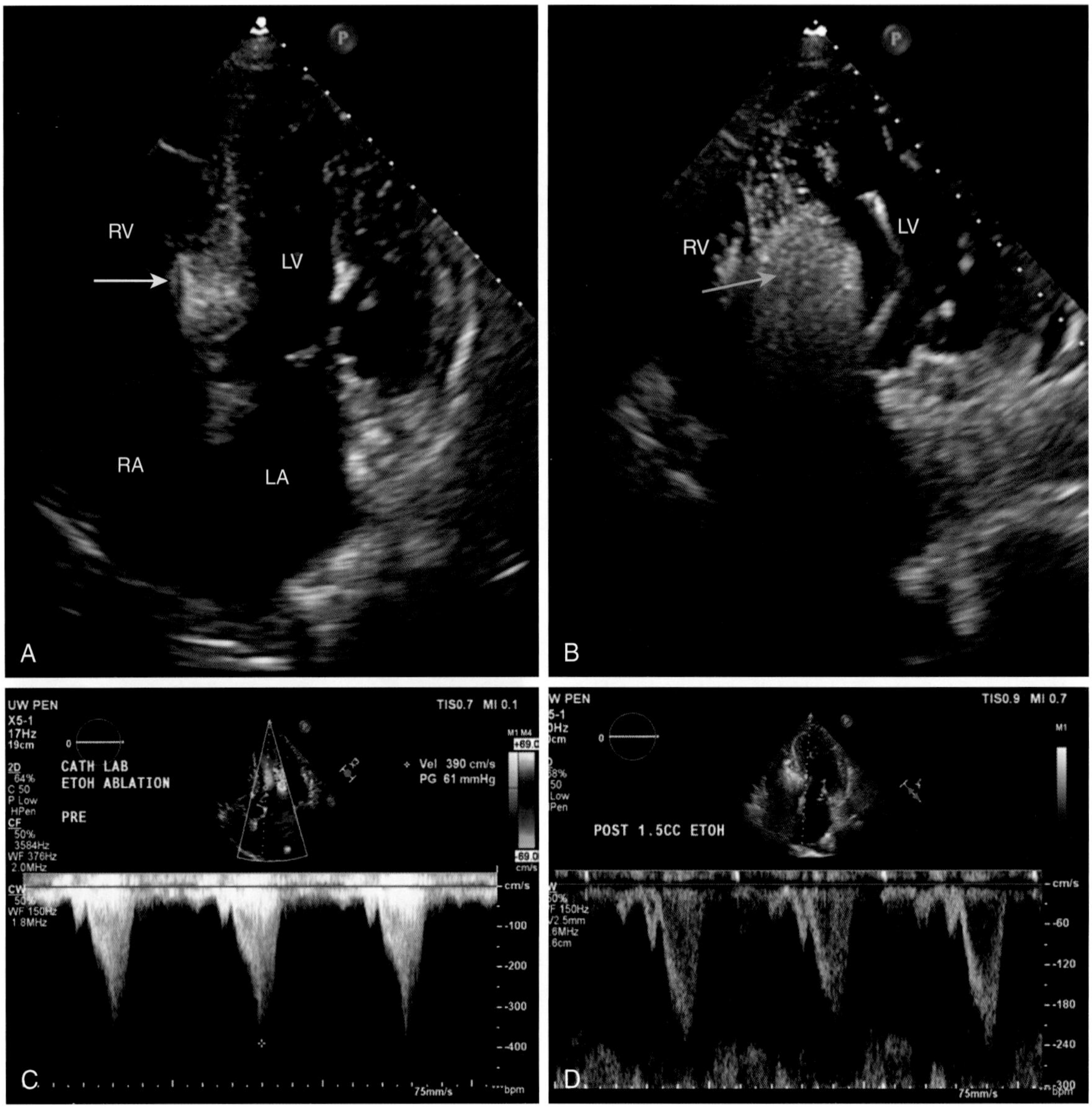

Fig. 13.17 Intraprocedural TTE demonstrating myocardial segments perfused by a candidate septal perforator vessel before ethanol injection. TTE apical 4-chamber views of the LV were performed during alcohol septal ablation. Initial injection of agitated saline contrast into a candidate septal perforator vessel (A) resulted in opacification of the RV side of the basal septum *(yellow arrow)*. A different septal perforator was cannulated, and reinjection of contrast (B) showed opacification of the LV side of the basal septum *(green arrow)*. This region was then injected with 1.5 mL of ethanol. At baseline (C), the peak LV outflow tract (LVOT) gradient was 61 mmHg as measured by CW Doppler. After ethanol injection (D), the peak LVOT gradient was reduced to approximately 16 mmHg.

ALCOHOL SEPTAL ABLATION

ASA involves selective injection of ethanol into the septal perforator branch of the left anterior descending coronary artery, which supplies the hypertrophied basal septum.[91] Occlusion of this artery results in a localized myocardial infarction that has acute hemodynamic benefits and results in septal wall thinning over time due to postinfarct replacement fibrosis. The reduction in LV contractility and widening of the LVOT can result in improved LVOT gradients, although the results vary more than those achieved by myectomy.

Periprocedural echocardiography is essential for localizing the proper site for ethanol injection and for assessment of hemodynamics.[92] Before ethanol injection, agitated saline or echocardiographic contrast can be injected intraarterially into a candidate perforator vessel. This has the same spatial distribution as ethanol, and the segments perfused by the candidate perforator vessel can be visualized (Fig. 13.17).

The target area for ablation is the region of SAM-septal contact or color-flow acceleration, which can best be visualized using the apical long-axis or 5-chamber views. Echocardiographic contrast used in this manner can result in a reflective, echogenic myocardium, and careful attention must be paid to delineating the full spatial extent of contrast. Occasionally, the septal perforator may perfuse distal regions such as the RV, the LV free wall, or papillary muscle, and operators should look for distal opacification, which would be a contraindication to ethanol injection.[93] This use of contrast has improved patient outcomes due to less ethanol use, smaller infarct sizes, and improvement in final LVOT gradients.[92]

Intraprocedural LVOT gradients can be affected by sedation, patient positioning, and a pressure catheter across the region of

SAM-septal contact. LVOT gradients are frequently lower than those obtained preprocedurally under awake conditions, in which case provocation using catheter-induced premature ventricular contractions may be useful in assessing latent obstruction.

The acute improvement in LVOT gradient seen intraprocedurally results primarily from the induction of septal hypokinesis/akinesis, including a reduction in contractility in distal, noninjected segments.[94] As postinfarct remodeling occurs and the septum thins, the LVOT widens, resulting in sustained improvements in LVOT gradients. However, in some cases, the septal myocardium is stunned, and follow-up echocardiography reveals an increase in LVOT gradients. One of the challenges of this procedure is that the final results are not available at the time of the procedure, and a second ablation is occasionally needed.

CLINICAL RESULTS AFTER SEPTAL REDUCTION

Surgical myectomy results in a sustained reduction in LVOT gradients and symptoms, with improvements in diastolic function, PA pressures, and exercise capacity. Surgery allows correction of mitral leaflet, chordal, and papillary muscle abnormalities when needed. Studies have demonstrated a reduction in nonsustained ventricular tachycardia (NSVT) and ICD therapies.[95] Moreover, nonrandomized data from the Mayo Clinic have documented a reduction in mortality rates compared with nonoperative obstruction, with a postoperative life expectancy that is equivalent to age- and gender-matched controls.[96]

Improvement in LVOT gradients using one of these septal reduction techniques is associated with improvement in diastolic function, reduction in LA and PA pressures, and favorable geometric remodeling over time. There is a theoretical concern that a septal ablation scar might induce a proarrhythmic state, but studies have not shown a definitive increased risk of ventricular arrhythmias, ICD shocks, or SCD.[97]

A randomized trial comparing ASA with surgical myectomy is likely not feasible, and retrospective studies are confounded by patient selection, making direct comparison challenging.[98] In general, patients who are younger and at lower operative risk should be considered for surgical myectomy, whereas older individuals, who are more likely to have nonhereditary HCM of the elderly, have tended to undergo ASA. Propensity-adjusted analyses have shown that ASA is associated with a lower likelihood of complete elimination of LVOT obstruction and a higher risk of heart block and the need for a pacemaker.[97] Ultimately, the decision to pursue treatment and the type of septal reduction procedure to perform remain shared decisions between patient and provider after weighing risks and benefits.

ECHOCARDIOGRAPHY IN THE RISK STRATIFICATION FOR SUDDEN DEATH

SCD is one of the most harrowing concerns for HCM patients. The annular risk is approximately 1%, although risk in individual patients can be substantially higher.[1,2] With current treatments and risk stratification measures, including placement of ICDs in at-risk individuals, SCD is a rare event. Echocardiographic factors that have been associated with an increased risk of SCD include maximal wall thickness greater than 30 mm, severe LVOT obstruction, mid-ventricular hypertrophy with an apical aneurysm, and development of end-stage HCM with an EF less than 50%.

All HCM patients should undergo serial assessment of SCD risk using one of two main risk stratification measures. The AHA/ACC HCM guidelines recommend consideration of ICD for individuals with one or more risk markers (i.e., maximal wall thickness > 30 mm, family history of SCD in a first-degree relative, and/or recent unexplained syncope). Clinical factors such as younger age, frequent NSVT, atrial fibrillation, myocardial ischemia, and severe (>15%–20%) late gadolinium enhancement on cardiac MRI are considered modifiers that represent increased risk. Clinical experience is key to identifying higher-risk individuals, although risk prediction is imperfect and shared decision making is needed.

The ESC recommends the use of a validated risk model to estimate a patient's 5-year risk of SCD.[1] The model uses several factors that are not major AHA/ACC risk markers, including LA dimension and degree of LVOT obstruction (at rest or with a Valsalva maneuver). The ESC model has been criticized for its lack of sensitivity, and recommendations should be placed in the context of other findings.

TABLE 13.4 Findings in Preclinical (Genotype Positive, Phenotype Negative) Hypertrophic Cardiomyopathy.

Alterations in Contraction/Relaxation

- Hypercontractility (EF often > 65%)
- Reduced E′ velocities (relative to age)

Myocardial Abnormalities

- Myocardial invaginations/crypts
- Apical hypertrabeculation
- Regional wall thinning (without scarring)

Mitral Valve Abnormalities

- Apical-basal muscle bundles
- Elongation of the mitral leaflets
- Antero-apical displacement of papillary muscles

EF, Ejection fraction.

FAMILY SCREENING AND PRECLINICAL HYPERTROPHIC CARDIOMYOPATHY

HCM due to sarcomeric variants demonstrates an autosomal dominant pattern of inheritance. Offspring of patients with HCM have a 50% chance of inheriting the pathologic genetic variant, and other first-degree relatives (i.e., siblings, parents) are also at high risk. For this reason, current guidelines recommend family screening for HCM using genetic testing or serial echocardiography and ECG for all first-degree relatives.[1,2] If screening is initially normal, serial phenotypic testing should be repeated every 3 to 5 years.

Because of steep reductions in cost, genetic sequencing is increasingly being used as a tool for family screening. Comprehensive sarcomeric genetic sequencing is performed for a family member with definite HCM; if a causal variant is identified, other family members may be tested for this single genetic change.

Increased use of genetic testing has led to increased identification of gene-positive, phenotype-negative individuals—mutation carriers who have not manifested LVH.[99] These patients with so-called preclinical HCM do not have overt HCM, but changes in cardiac anatomy and function can often be identified (Table 13.4). Among first-degree relatives of patients with HCM, the combination of high contractility and impaired relaxation (EF > 68% and E′ velocity < 14 m/s) demonstrated high specificity for gene positivity.[41] Additional morphologic features common in these patients include LV apical hypertrabeculation, elongated mitral leaflets, and clefts or invaginations within the myocardium.[100]

SUMMARY Hypertrophic Cardiomyopathy.

Clinical Facet	Echocardiographic Features
Diagnosis	• HCM is caused by genetic variation in sarcomeric proteins, which alters contractility and relaxation and produces a phenotype of myocardial hypertrophy and fibrosis. • A diagnosis of HCM is based on imaging findings of unexplained LVH, although genetic testing can play a confirmatory role. • Hypertrophy is usually ≥ 15 mm, although any degree of hypertrophy is compatible. • A ratio of septal wall to posterior wall thickness > 1.3 is strongly associated with an HCM diagnosis. • Pressure overload mimics (e.g., severe hypertension, subvalvular or supravalvular aortic stenosis) and genetic phenocopies (e.g., Fabry disease, Danon disease, PRKAG2 syndrome, transthyretin amyloidosis, mitochondrial disorders) often manifest concentric hypertrophy. • Longitudinal strain maps may be helpful if diagnosis is uncertain.
Morphologic subtypes	• HCM involves several common morphologic subtypes. A spiral of hypertrophy extending from the basal anterior wall, through the septum, and into the mid-inferior wall is common. • Reverse curvature septal morphology (thickness in the mid-septum) is strongly associated with gene positivity. • Isolated basal septal hypertrophy is often a variant of cardiac aging. • Mid-ventricular hypertrophy may result in mid-cavitary obstruction and/or apical aneurysm and is associated with ventricular tachycardia and thromboembolism. Echocardiographic contrast should be considered when apical visualization is poor. • Apical variant HCM involves isolated hypertrophy of the distal LV cavity, and apicalized papillary muscles may be present.
Assessment of LV wall thickness	• Hypertrophy most commonly involves the septum, although it can involve any myocardial segment. • Wall thickness is best measured from a stack of PSAX views, although acoustic dropout of the anterior and lateral epicardium can limit reliability. • Wall thickness measurements should exclude the crista interventricularis, which is commonly seen entering the basal septum on the PLAX view. • Consider echocardiographic contrast or cardiac MRI if wall thickness is uncertain.
Assessment of obstruction	• Obstruction can occur at multiple levels, and multilevel obstruction may occur. • To isolate locations of obstruction, the PW Doppler sample volume is marched from apex to base in 1- to 2-cm increments. • In dynamic LVOT obstruction, drag forces on the exposed undersurface of mitral leaflets produce systolic anterior leaflet deformation and progressive LVOT narrowing. • The severity of LVOT obstruction is directly related to the time of onset and duration of SAM-septal contact. • Dynamic LVOT obstruction produces a characteristic late-peaking Doppler profile at the level of the mitral tips. • The magnitude of dynamic LVOT obstruction is affected by contractility and loading conditions. Obstruction is defined as > 30 mmHg at rest and > 50 mmHg with provocation. • LVOT obstruction is preset in approximately one third of HCM patients at rest; one third have LVOT obstruction with provocation only; and one third have no obstruction. • Physiologic provocation methods include squat to stand, Valsalva maneuver, and exercise stress testing. Dobutamine is nonphysiologic and should not be used. • Anterior mitral leaflet deformation can simultaneously induce MR, which is usually posteriorly directed. Medical therapies to reduce LVOT obstruction will reduce MR severity. • SAM-related MR originates from within the LVOT, and the LVOT Doppler signal can be contaminated by MR. • LVOT and MR signals can be differentiated by time of onset, Doppler shape, and peak gradients. A resting LVOT velocity > 6 m/s is uncommon. • LVOT gradients can be estimated using MR velocity and systolic blood pressure, along with an assumed LA pressure (see Fig. 13.11).

Continued

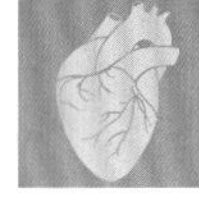

SUMMARY Hypertrophic Cardiomyopathy.—cont'd

Clinical Facet	Echocardiographic Features
Assessment of mitral valve	• Intrinsic MV and subvalvular abnormalities are common in HCM and contribute to LVOT obstruction. • Mitral leaflet elongation can affect one or both of the anterior and posterior leaflets. • Papillary muscle location and anatomy affect tethering forces on the mitral leaflets. Antero-apical displacement commonly contributes to SAM. • Aberrant chordal connections between the mitral leaflets and the anterior wall or septum can occur, tethering the mitral leaflets anteriorly. • MV abnormalities reduce the response rate to negative inotropic therapies and should influence the approach to septal reduction.
Diastology and assessment of filling pressures	• Diastolic function and filling are complex in HCM, and standard measures of diastolic function are less reliable. • Sarcomeric genetic variants alter the contraction-relaxation relationship; relaxation abnormalities can occur before hypertrophy develops. • Regional hypertrophy and fibrosis can lead to heterogeneity in relaxation and compliance. • Twist mechanics and myocardial deformation are altered in HCM, with decreased longitudinal but increased radial and circumferential strain, perhaps due to underlying myofibrillar disarray. • E:e′ ratio is an unreliable measure of filling pressures in HCM. • Conventional indices that correlate with adverse outcomes and/or increased filling pressures include LA volume index, tricuspid regurgitation jet velocity, and pulmonary vein A-wave reversal duration ($A_r - A_{dur} > 30$ ms).
Risk stratification for sudden death	• Maximal wall thickness > 30 mm confers an increased risk of SCD and should prompt consideration of ICD therapy. • LVOT obstruction confers a small increased risk of SCD and is not considered an independent risk marker. • The ESC risk stratification tool includes echocardiographic factors of maximal wall thickness, LA dimension, and degree of LVOT obstruction (at rest or with Valsalva maneuver).
Prognosis	• With contemporary therapies and timely use of septal reduction therapies and ICDs, the overall prognosis for HCM is good. • Severe (>100 mmHg) or symptomatic LVOT obstruction confers an increased risk of heart failure, and retrospective data suggest a possible mortality benefit for septal myectomy. • A subset of HCM patients experience progressive fibrosis, with progressive wall thinning and decreasing contractility, with or without cavity dilation. • About 5% of HCM patients develop end-stage HCM with EF < 50%. These subjects can be considered for advanced heart failure therapies. • The presence of an apical aneurysm, with or without mid-ventricular obstruction, is associated with an increased risk of ventricular tachycardia and thromboembolism. • LA enlargement (LA dimension > 45 mm or LA volume index > 34 mL/m^2) confers an increased risk of atrial fibrillation.
Septal reduction therapies	• Intraprocedural echocardiography plays an important role in guiding septal reduction therapies. • Doppler echocardiography can help to define acute procedural changes in obstructive gradients. • During surgical septal myectomy, TEE imaging can be used intraoperatively to define the extent and depth of surgical resection. • TEE-guided dobutamine or isoproterenol provocative testing can assess the effectiveness of surgical myectomy on LVOT gradients, with repeat myectomy or MV intervention if obstruction remains. • During alcohol septal ablation, 2D imaging after intracoronary injection of contrast aids selection of septal perforators by defining the candidate vessel perfusion territory, resulting in improved patient outcomes.

EF, Ejection fraction; *ESC*, European Society of Cardiology; *HCM*, hypertrophic cardiomyopathy; *ICD*, implantable cardioverter-defibrillator; *LVH*, left ventricular hypertrophy; *LVOT*, left ventricular outflow tract; *MR*, mitral regurgitation; *MRI*, magnetic resonance imaging; *MV*, mitral valve; *PLAX*, parasternal long-axis; *PSAX*, parasternal short-axis; *PW*, pulsed-wave; *SAM*, systolic anterior motion; *SCD*, sudden cardiac death.

REFERENCES

1. Authors/Task Force, Elliott PM, Anastasakis A, et al. 2014 ESC guidelines on diagnosis and management of hypertrophic cardiomyopathy: the Task Force for the Diagnosis and Management of Hypertrophic Cardiomyopathy of the European Society of Cardiology (ESC). *Eur Heart J.* 2014;35(39):2733–2779.
2. Gersh BJ, Maron BJ, Bonow RO, et al. 2011 ACCF/AHA guideline for the diagnosis and treatment of hypertrophic cardiomyopathy: executive summary: a report of the American College of Cardiology Foundation/American Heart Association Task Force on Practice Guidelines. *Circulation.* 2011;124(24):2761–2796.
3. Teare D. Asymmetrical hypertrophy of the heart in young adults. *Br Heart J.* 1958;20(1):1–8.
4. Maron BJ, Rowin EJ, Casey SA, Maron MS. How hypertrophic cardiomyopathy became a contemporary treatable genetic disease with low mortality: shaped by 50 years of clinical research and practice. *JAMA Cardiol.* 2016;1(1):98–105.
5. Marian AJ, Braunwald E. Hypertrophic cardiomyopathy: Genetics, pathogenesis, clinical manifestations, diagnosis, and therapy. *Circ Res.* 2017;121(7):749–770.
6. Geisterfer-Lowrance AA, Kass S, Tanigawa G, et al. A molecular basis for familial hypertrophic cardiomyopathy: a beta cardiac myosin heavy chain gene missense mutation. *Cell.* 1990;62(5):999–1006.
7. Watkins H, Rosenzweig A, Hwang DS, et al. Characteristics and prognostic implications of myosin missense mutations in familial hypertrophic cardiomyopathy. *N Engl J Med.* 1992;326(17):1108–1114.
8. Marstrand P, Han L, Day SM, et al. Hypertrophic cardiomyopathy with left ventricular systolic dysfunction: insights from the SHaRe Registry. *Circulation.* 2020;141(17):1371–1383.
9. Lee SP, Ashley EA, Homburger J, et al. Incident atrial fibrillation is associated with MYH7 sarcomeric gene variation in hypertrophic cardiomyopathy. *Circ Heart Fail.* 2018;11(9). e005191.
10. Maron BJ, Gardin JM, Flack JM, Gidding SS, Kurosaki TT, Bild DE. Prevalence of hypertrophic cardiomyopathy in a general population of young adults. Echocardiographic analysis of 4111 subjects in the CARDIA Study. Coronary Artery Risk Development in (Young) Adults. *Circulation.* 1995;92(4):785–789.
11. Semsarian C, Ingles J, Maron MS, Maron BJ. New perspectives on the prevalence of hypertrophic cardiomyopathy. *J Am Coll Cardiol.* 2015;65(12):1249–1254.
12. Maron BJ, Rowin EJ, Maron MS. Global burden of hypertrophic cardiomyopathy. *JACC Heart Fail.* 2018;6(5):376–378.
13. Massera D, McClelland RL, Ambale-Venkatesh B, et al. Prevalence of unexplained left ventricular hypertrophy by cardiac magnetic resonance imaging in MESA. *J Am Heart Assoc.* 2019;8(8). e012250.
14. Henry WL, Clark CE, Glancy DL, Epstein SE. Echocardiographic measurement of the left ventricular outflow gradient in idiopathic hypertrophic subaortic stenosis. *N Engl J Med.* 1973;288(19):989–993.
15. Dweck MR, Joshi S, Murigu T, et al. Left ventricular remodeling and hypertrophy in patients with aortic stenosis: insights from cardiovascular magnetic resonance. *J Cardiovasc Magn Reson.* 2012;14:50.
16. Serra W, Marziliano N. Role of cardiac imaging in Anderson-Fabry cardiomyopathy. *Cardiovasc Ultrasound.* 2019;17(1):1.
17. Deva DP, Hanneman K, Li Q, et al. Cardiovascular magnetic resonance demonstration of the spectrum of morphological phenotypes and patterns of myocardial scarring in Anderson-Fabry disease. *J Cardiovasc Magn Reson.* 2016;18:14.
18. Pieroni M, Chimenti C, De Cobelli F, et al. Fabry's disease cardiomyopathy: echocardiographic detection of endomyocardial glycosphingolipid compartmentalization. *J Am Coll Cardiol.* 2006;47(8):1663–1671.
19. Kounas S, Demetrescu C, Pantazis AA, et al. The binary endocardial appearance is a poor discriminator of Anderson-Fabry disease from familial hypertrophic cardiomyopathy. *J Am Coll Cardiol.* 2008;51(21):2058–2061.
20. Sweet ME, Mestroni L, Taylor MRG. Genetic infiltrative Cardiomyopathies. *Heart Fail Clin.* 2018;14(2):215–224.
21. Lopez-Sainz A, Dominguez F, Lopes LR, et al. Clinical features and natural history of PRKAG2 variant cardiac glycogenosis. *J Am Coll Cardiol.* 2020;76(2):186–197.
22. Ruberg FL, Grogan M, Hanna M, Kelly JW, Maurer MS. Transthyretin amyloid cardiomyopathy: JACC State-of-the-Art Review. *J Am Coll Cardiol.* 2019;73(22):2872–2891.
23. Jacobson DR, Alexander AA, Tagoe C, et al. The prevalence and distribution of the amyloidogenic transthyretin (TTR) V122I allele in Africa. *Mol Genet Genomic Med.* 2016;4(5):548–556.
24. Quarta CC, Falk RH, Solomon SD. V122I transthyretin variant in elderly black Americans. *N Engl J Med.* 2015;372(18):1769.
25. Phelan D, Collier P, Thavendiranathan P, et al. Relative apical sparing of longitudinal strain using two-dimensional speckle-tracking echocardiography is both sensitive and specific for the diagnosis of cardiac amyloidosis. *Heart.* 2012;98(19):1442–1448.
26. Finocchiaro G, Dhutia H, D'Silva A, et al. Effect of sex and sporting discipline on LV adaptation to exercise. *JACC Cardiovasc Imaging.* 2017;10(9):965–972.
27. Weiner RB, DeLuca JR, Wang F, et al. Exercise-induced left ventricular remodeling among competitive athletes: a phasic phenomenon. *Circ Cardiovasc Imaging.* 2015;8(12) e003651.
28. Whyte GP, George K, Sharma S, et al. The upper limit of physiological cardiac hypertrophy in elite male and female athletes: the British experience. *Eur J Appl Physiol.* 2004;92(4-5):592–597.
29. Weiner RB, Baggish AL. Exercise-induced cardiac remodeling. *Prog Cardiovasc Dis.* 2012;54(5):380–386.
30. Maron BJ, Pelliccia A, Spirito P. Cardiac disease in young trained athletes. Insights into methods for distinguishing athlete's heart from structural heart disease, with particular emphasis on hypertrophic cardiomyopathy. *Circulation.* 1995;91(5):1596–1601.
31. Binder J, Ommen SR, Gersh BJ, et al. Echocardiography-guided genetic testing in hypertrophic cardiomyopathy: septal morphological features predict the presence of myofilament mutations. *Mayo Clin Proc.* 2006;81(4):459–467.
32. Dalldorf FG, Willis PW. Angled aorta ("sigmoid septum") as a cause of hypertrophic subaortic stenosis. *Hum Pathol.* 1985;16(5):457–462.
33. Krasnow N. Subaortic septal bulge simulates hypertrophic cardiomyopathy by angulation of the septum with age, independent of focal hypertrophy. An echocardiographic study. *J Am Soc Echocardiogr.* 1997;10(5):545–555.
34. Falicov RE, Resnekov L, Bharati S, Lev M. Mid-ventricular obstruction: a variant of obstructive cardiomyopathy. *Am J Cardiol.* 1976;37(3):432–437.
35. Maron MS, Finley JJ, Bos JM, et al. Prevalence, clinical significance, and natural history of left ventricular apical aneurysms in hypertrophic cardiomyopathy. *Circulation.* 2008;118(15):1541–1549.
36. Yamaguchi H, Ishimura T, Nishiyama S, et al. Hypertrophic nonobstructive cardiomyopathy with giant negative T waves (apical hypertrophy): ventriculographic and echocardiographic features in 30 patients. *Am J Cardiol.* 1979;44(3):401–412.
37. Maron MS, Rowin EJ, Maron BJ. How to image hypertrophic cardiomyopathy. *Circ Cardiovasc Imaging.* 2017;10(7).
38. Nagueh SF, Bierig SM, Budoff MJ, et al. American Society of Echocardiography clinical recommendations for multimodality cardiovascular imaging of patients with hypertrophic cardiomyopathy: endorsed by the American Society of Nuclear Cardiology, Society for Cardiovascular Magnetic Resonance, and Society of Cardiovascular Computed Tomography. *J Am Soc Echocardiogr.* 2011;24(5):473–498.
39. Maron MS, Hauser TH, Dubrow E, et al. Right ventricular involvement in hypertrophic cardiomyopathy. *Am J Cardiol.* 2007;100(8):1293–1298.
40. Spudich JA. Three perspectives on the molecular basis of hypercontractility caused by hypertrophic cardiomyopathy mutations. *Pflugers Arch.* 2019;471(5):701–717.
41. Ho CY, Sweitzer NK, McDonough B, et al. Assessment of diastolic function with Doppler tissue imaging to predict genotype in preclinical hypertrophic cardiomyopathy. *Circulation.* 2002;105(25):2992–2997.
42. Olivotto I, Maron BJ, Appelbaum E, et al. Spectrum and clinical significance of systolic function and myocardial fibrosis assessed by cardiovascular magnetic resonance in hypertrophic cardiomyopathy. *Am J Cardiol.* 2010;106(2):261–267.
43. Harris KM, Spirito P, Maron MS, et al. Prevalence, clinical profile, and significance of left ventricular remodeling in the end-stage phase of hypertrophic cardiomyopathy. *Circulation.* 2006;114(3):216–225.
44. Maron BJ, Rowin EJ, Udelson JE, Maron MS. Clinical spectrum and management of heart failure in hypertrophic cardiomyopathy. *JACC Heart Fail.* 2018;6(5):353–363.
45. Klues HG, Maron BJ, Dollar AL, Roberts WC. Diversity of structural mitral valve alterations in hypertrophic cardiomyopathy. *Circulation.* 1992;85(5):1651–1660.
46. Kaple RK, Murphy RT, DiPaola LM, et al. Mitral valve abnormalities in hypertrophic cardiomyopathy: echocardiographic features and surgical outcomes. *Ann Thorac Surg.* 2008;85(5):1527–1535. 1535 e1521–1522.

47. Cavalcante JL, Barboza JS, Lever HM. Diversity of mitral valve abnormalities in obstructive hypertrophic cardiomyopathy. *Prog Cardiovasc Dis*. 2012;54(6):517–522.
48. Maron MS, Olivotto I, Harrigan C, et al. Mitral valve abnormalities identified by cardiovascular magnetic resonance represent a primary phenotypic expression of hypertrophic cardiomyopathy. *Circulation*. 2011;124(1):40–47.
49. Kwon DH, Setser RM, Thamilarasan M, et al. Abnormal papillary muscle morphology is independently associated with increased left ventricular outflow tract obstruction in hypertrophic cardiomyopathy. *Heart*. 2008;94(10):1295–1301.
50. Gruner C, Chan RH, Crean A, et al. Significance of left ventricular apical-basal muscle bundle identified by cardiovascular magnetic resonance imaging in patients with hypertrophic cardiomyopathy. *Eur Heart J*. 2014;35(39):2706–2713.
51. Maron MS, Olivotto I, Zenovich AG, et al. Hypertrophic cardiomyopathy is predominantly a disease of left ventricular outflow tract obstruction. *Circulation*. 2006;114(21):2232–2239.
52. Sherrid MV, Wever-Pinzon O, Shah A, Chaudhry FA. Reflections of inflections in hypertrophic cardiomyopathy. *J Am Coll Cardiol*. 2009;54(3):212–219.
53. Pollick C, Morgan CD, Gilbert BW, Rakowski H, Wigle ED. Muscular subaortic stenosis: the temporal relationship between systolic anterior motion of the anterior mitral leaflet and the pressure gradient. *Circulation*. 1982;66(5):1087–1094.
54. Pollick C, Rakowski H, Wigle ED. Muscular subaortic stenosis: the quantitative relationship between systolic anterior motion and the pressure gradient. *Circulation*. 1984;69(1):43–49.
55. Sherrid MV, Chu CK, Delia E, Mogtader A, Dwyer EM Jr, An echocardiographic study of the fluid mechanics of obstruction in hypertrophic cardiomyopathy. *J Am Coll Cardiol*. 1993;22(3):816–825.
56. Sherrid MV, Gunsburg DZ, Moldenhauer S, Pearle G. Systolic anterior motion begins at low left ventricular outflow tract velocity in obstructive hypertrophic cardiomyopathy. *J Am Coll Cardiol*. 2000;36(4):1344–1354.
57. Klues HG, Roberts WC, Maron BJ. Morphological determinants of echocardiographic patterns of mitral valve systolic anterior motion in obstructive hypertrophic cardiomyopathy. *Circulation*. 1993;87(5):1570–1579.
58. Gilbert BW, Pollick C, Adelman AG, Wigle ED. Hypertrophic cardiomyopathy: subclassification by m mode echocardiography. *Am J Cardiol*. 1980;45(4):861–872.
59. Marwick TH, Nakatani S, Haluska B, Thomas JD, Lever HM. Provocation of latent left ventricular outflow tract gradients with amyl nitrite and exercise in hypertrophic cardiomyopathy. *Am J Cardiol*. 1995;75(12):805–809.
60. Drinko JK, Nash PJ, Lever HM, Asher CR. Safety of stress testing in patients with hypertrophic cardiomyopathy. *Am J Cardiol*. 2004;93(11):1443–1444. A1412.
61. Sorensen LL, Liang HY, Pinheiro A, et al. Safety profile and utility of treadmill exercise in patients with high-gradient hypertrophic cardiomyopathy. *Am Heart J*. 2017;184:47–54.
62. Feneon D, Schnell F, Galli E, et al. Impact of exercise-induced mitral regurgitation on hypertrophic cardiomyopathy outcomes. *Eur Heart J Cardiovasc Imaging*. 2016;17(10):1110–1117.
63. Lafitte S, Reant P, Touche C, et al. Paradoxical response to exercise in asymptomatic hypertrophic cardiomyopathy: a new description of outflow tract obstruction dynamics. *J Am Coll Cardiol*. 2013;62(9):842–850.
64. Sherrid MV, Gunsburg DZ, Pearle G. Mid-systolic drop in left ventricular ejection velocity in obstructive hypertrophic cardiomyopathy—the lobster claw abnormality. *J Am Soc Echocardiogr*. 1997;10(7):707–712.
65. Carasso S, Yang H, Woo A, et al. Systolic myocardial mechanics in hypertrophic cardiomyopathy: novel concepts and implications for clinical status. *J Am Soc Echocardiogr*. 2008;21(6):675–683.
66. Popovic ZB, Kwon DH, Mishra M, et al. Association between regional ventricular function and myocardial fibrosis in hypertrophic cardiomyopathy assessed by speckle tracking echocardiography and delayed hyperenhancement magnetic resonance imaging. *J Am Soc Echocardiogr*. 2008;21(12):1299–1305.
67. Takeuchi M, Borden WB, Nakai H, et al. Reduced and delayed untwisting of the left ventricle in patients with hypertension and left ventricular hypertrophy: a study using two-dimensional speckle tracking imaging. *Eur Heart J*. 2007;28(22):2756–2762.
68. Williams LK, Misurka J, Ho CY, et al. Multilayer myocardial mechanics in genotype-positive left ventricular hypertrophy-negative patients with hypertrophic cardiomyopathy. *Am J Cardiol*. 2018;122(10):1754–1760.
69. Wang J, Buergler JM, Veerasamy K, Ashton YP, Nagueh SF. Delayed untwisting: the mechanistic link between dynamic obstruction and exercise tolerance in patients with hypertrophic obstructive cardiomyopathy. *J Am Coll Cardiol*. 2009;54(14):1326–1334.
70. Gruner C, Verocai F, Carasso S, et al. Systolic myocardial mechanics in patients with Anderson-Fabry disease with and without left ventricular hypertrophy and in comparison to nonobstructive hypertrophic cardiomyopathy. *Echocardiography*. 2012;29(7):810–817.
71. Toepfer CN, Garfinkel AC, Venturini G, et al. Myosin sequestration regulates sarcomere function, cardiomyocyte energetics, and metabolism, informing the pathogenesis of hypertrophic cardiomyopathy. *Circulation*. 2020;141(10):828–842.
72. Geske JB, Sorajja P, Nishimura RA, Ommen SR. Evaluation of left ventricular filling pressures by Doppler echocardiography in patients with hypertrophic cardiomyopathy: correlation with direct left atrial pressure measurement at cardiac catheterization. *Circulation*. 2007;116(23):2702–2708.
73. Nagueh SF, Smiseth OA, Appleton CP, et al. Recommendations for the evaluation of left ventricular diastolic function by echocardiography: an update from the American Society of Echocardiography and the European Association of Cardiovascular Imaging. *J Am Soc Echocardiogr*. 2016;29(4):277–314.
74. Nistri S, Olivotto I, Betocchi S, et al. Prognostic significance of left atrial size in patients with hypertrophic cardiomyopathy (from the Italian Registry for Hypertrophic Cardiomyopathy). *Am J Cardiol*. 2006;98(7):960–965.
75. Sachdev V, Shizukuda Y, Brenneman CL, et al. Left atrial volumetric remodeling is predictive of functional capacity in nonobstructive hypertrophic cardiomyopathy. *Am Heart J*. 2005;149(4):730–736.
76. To AC, Lever HM, Desai MY. Hypertrophied papillary muscles as a masquerade of apical hypertrophic cardiomyopathy. *J Am Coll Cardiol*. 2012;59(13):1197.
77. Eriksson MJ, Sonnenberg B, Woo A, et al. Long-term outcome in patients with apical hypertrophic cardiomyopathy. *J Am Coll Cardiol*. 2002;39(4):638–645.
78. Coppini R, Ho CY, Ashley E, et al. Clinical phenotype and outcome of hypertrophic cardiomyopathy associated with thin-filament gene mutations. *J Am Coll Cardiol*. 2014;64(24):2589–2600.
79. Sherrid MV. Pharmacologic therapy of hypertrophic cardiomyopathy. *Curr Cardiol Rev*. 2015.
80. Epstein SE, Rosing DR. Verapamil: its potential for causing serious complications in patients with hypertrophic cardiomyopathy. *Circulation*. 1981;64(3):437–441.
81. Sherrid MV, Barac I, McKenna WJ, et al. Multicenter study of the efficacy and safety of disopyramide in obstructive hypertrophic cardiomyopathy. *J Am Coll Cardiol*. 2005;45(8):1251–1258.
82. Olivotto I, Oreziak A, Barriales-Villa R, et al. Mavacamten for treatment of symptomatic obstructive hypertrophic cardiomyopathy (EXPLORER-HCM): a randomised, double-blind, placebo-controlled, phase 3 trial. *Lancet*. 2020;396(10253):759–769.
83. Kappenberger L, Linde C, Daubert C, et al. Pacing in hypertrophic obstructive cardiomyopathy. A randomized crossover study. PIC Study Group. *Eur Heart J*. 1997;18(8):1249–1256.
84. Nishimura RA, Trusty JM, Hayes DL, et al. Dual-chamber pacing for hypertrophic cardiomyopathy: a randomized, double-blind, crossover trial. *J Am Coll Cardiol*. 1997;29(2):435–441.
85. Morrow AG, Lambrew CT, Braunwald E. Idiopathic hypertrophic subaortic stenosis. Ii. Operative treatment and the results of pre- and postoperative hemodynamic evaluations. *Circulation*. 1964;30(suppl 4):120–151.
86. Thaden JJ, Malouf JF, Rehfeldt KH, et al. Adult intraoperative echocardiography: a comprehensive review of current practice. *J Am Soc Echocardiogr*. 2020;33(6):735–755 e711.
87. Nguyen A, Schaff HV. Surgical myectomy: subaortic, midventricular, and apical. *Cardiol Clin*. 2019;37(1):95–104.
88. Nampiaparampil RG, Swistel DG, Schlame M, Saric M, Sherrid MV. Intraoperative two- and three-dimensional transesophageal echocardiography in combined myectomy-mitral operations for hypertrophic cardiomyopathy. *J Am Soc Echocardiogr*. 2018;31(3):275–288.
89. Hang D, Schaff HV, Nishimura RA, et al. Accuracy of jet direction on Doppler echocardiography in identifying the etiology of mitral regurgitation in obstructive hypertrophic cardiomyopathy. *J Am Soc Echocardiogr*. 2019;32(3):333–340.
90. Bedair Elsayes A, Basura A, Zahedi F, et al. Intraoperative provocative testing in patients with obstructive hypertrophic cardiomyopathy undergoing septal myectomy. *J Am Soc Echocardiogr*. 2020;33(2):182–190.
91. Sigwart U. Non-surgical myocardial reduction for hypertrophic obstructive cardiomyopathy. *Lancet*. 1995;346(8969):211–214.

92. Faber L, Seggewiss H, Welge D, et al. Echo-guided percutaneous septal ablation for symptomatic hypertrophic obstructive cardiomyopathy: 7 years of experience. *Eur J Echocardiogr.* 2004;5(5):347–355.
93. Monakier D, Horlick E, Ross J, et al. Intracoronary myocardial contrast echocardiography in a patient with drug refractory hypertrophic obstructive cardiomyopathy revealing extensive myocardium at risk for infarction with alcohol septal ablation. *J Invasive Cardiol.* 2004;16(9):482–484.
94. Flores-Ramirez R, Lakkis NM, Middleton KJ, Killip D, Spencer WH 3rd, Nagueh SF. Echocardiographic insights into the mechanisms of relief of left ventricular outflow tract obstruction after nonsurgical septal reduction therapy in patients with hypertrophic obstructive cardiomyopathy. *J Am Coll Cardiol.* 2001;37(1):208–214.
95. McLeod CJ, Ommen SR, Ackerman MJ, et al. Surgical septal myectomy decreases the risk for appropriate implantable cardioverter defibrillator discharge in obstructive hypertrophic cardiomyopathy. *Eur Heart J.* 2007;28(21):2583–2588.
96. Schaff HV, Nguyen A. Does septal myectomy reduce risk of sudden cardiac death in patients with hypertrophic cardiomyopathy? *J Thorac Cardiovasc Surg.* 2018;156(2):748–749.
97. Nguyen A, Schaff HV, Hang D, et al. Surgical myectomy versus alcohol septal ablation for obstructive hypertrophic cardiomyopathy: a propensity score-matched cohort. *J Thorac Cardiovasc Surg.* 2019;157(1):306–315 e303.
98. Olivotto I, Ommen SR, Maron MS, Cecchi F, Maron BJ. Surgical myectomy versus alcohol septal ablation for obstructive hypertrophic cardiomyopathy. Will there ever be a randomized trial? *J Am Coll Cardiol.* 2007;50(9):831–834.
99. Maron BJ, Ho CY. Hypertrophic cardiomyopathy without hypertrophy: an emerging pre-clinical subgroup composed of genetically affected family members. *JACC Cardiovasc Imaging.* 2009;2(1):65–68.
100. Captur G, Lopes LR, Mohun TJ, et al. Prediction of sarcomere mutations in subclinical hypertrophic cardiomyopathy. *Circ Cardiovasc Imaging.* 2014;7(6):863–871.

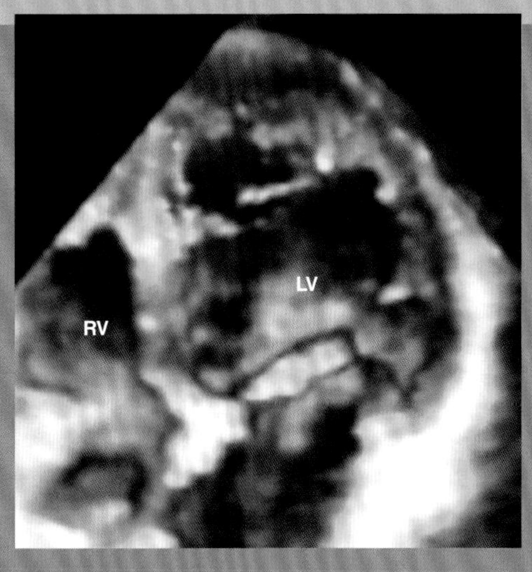

第14章 限制型心肌病

限制型心肌病是一组由不同病因引起的心肌疾病，其晚期的特征性表现是左心室心肌僵硬度的显著增加。临床表现为充血性心力衰竭且左室射血分数正常，以及因左心室顺应性降低所致的血流动力学异常和相关的心脏结构改变。

本章介绍了限制型心肌病的影像学定义、分类和病理生理学改变，包括该病的常规二维超声心动图及多普勒超声特征，以及通过二维斑点追踪成像技术所得的应变成像和其他影像学检查模式对本病诊断的方法。而后介绍了几种特异性限制型心肌病的诊断和治疗，包括：心肌淀粉样变性、特发性限制型心肌病、高嗜酸性粒细胞综合征和心内膜心肌纤维化、蓄积性疾病、结节病、抗肿瘤药物或放射性治疗诱发的心肌病。另外介绍了限制型心肌病和缩窄性心包炎的鉴别诊断。

孙　欣

14 Restrictive Cardiomyopathy

AHMAD MASRI, MD | STEPHEN B. HEITNER, MD

DEFINITION AND PATHOPHYSIOLOGY

Restrictive cardiomyopathies (RCMs) are a heterogeneous group of heart muscle disorders that, in their advanced stages, are characterized by a marked increase in left ventricular (LV) myocardial stiffness. Clinically, this manifests as congestive heart failure, often in the setting of a normal left ventricular ejection fraction (LVEF). The reduction in LV compliance results in hemodynamic abnormalities and associated cardiac structural changes, both of which have characteristics that are detected and characterized by echocardiography. Classically, the increase in left atrial (LA) pressure required to fill a noncompliant LV results in LA enlargement, pulmonary venous congestion, pulmonary edema, and secondary pulmonary hypertension. Reduced LV filling manifests as low cardiac output, which often is very difficult to augment by modulating afterload, preload, or contractility. Later-stage disease is associated with right ventricular (RV) dysfunction, a harbinger of very poor outcome.

The underlying etiopathology of reduced myocardial compliance is varied and includes all aspects of the myocardium, spanning cardiomyocytes, the interstitium, genes, and the proteome. Specifically, increased interstitial or endocardial fibrosis is seen in response to both sarcomeric gene mutations (e.g., MYBPC3, MYH7, troponin, titin) and infiltration or deposition of material from systemic disorders such as amyloidosis, hemochromatosis, and glycogen storage diseases. Table 14.1 shows the classification of the RCMs. The most common type in the developed world is infiltrative cardiomyopathy secondary to amyloidosis.

In almost all RCMs there is a progressive decrease in myocardial compliance over time that is well described and is easily followed using echo-Doppler variables. In the early stages of disease, LV size and LVEF are normal, and only mild abnormalities of diastolic function, such as impaired LV relaxation, are present. With disease progression, LVEF typically remains normal but myocardial compliance decreases, which raises LV and LA filling pressures and leads to atrial enlargement. The increase in LA pressure "normalizes" early diastolic filling at the expense of pulmonary venous congestion, and LA hypertension becomes an important compensatory mechanism to maintain a normal LV end-diastolic volume and cardiac output.

In advanced stages of disease, restrictive physiology is present, with its typical dip-and-plateau hemodynamic waveform seen in invasive hemodynamic assessment. At this stage, very high filling pressures are needed to fill an extremely noncompliant LV, but the rapid rate of early diastolic filling terminates abruptly due to a rapid rise in LV pressure. Filling at atrial contraction becomes greatly reduced because of LA systolic failure. Heart failure symptoms and functional limitation are common because of pulmonary venous congestion and, in many cases, a reduced stroke volume and cardiac output. The stages of progression of diastolic dysfunction resulting in advanced RCM are summarized in Chapter 5.

Fig. 14.1 shows the Doppler echocardiographic characteristics of advanced RCM. At this stage, LV size and LVEF vary depending on the underlying etiology, but in general the diastolic abnormalities tend to be more severe than the systolic dysfunction. Restrictive physiology is characterized by a high spectral early Doppler mitral inflow (E) velocity, together with a high ratio of E to the late-diastolic atrial (A) transmitral velocity (E/A ratio), a rapid mitral deceleration time, a short pulmonary vein diastolic (D) wave deceleration time (<160 ms), a short isovolumic relaxation time (<50 ms), decreased early diastolic mitral septal and lateral E' velocities (3–4 cm/s), and a markedly increased LA volume index (>50 mL/m^2). When present, these features portend a very poor prognosis.

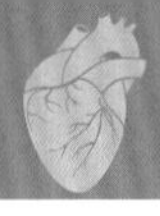

TABLE 14.1 Classification of Restrictive Cardiomyopathy.

Noninfiltrative	Idiopathic
	Scleroderma
Infiltrative	Immunoglobulin amyloidosis
	Hereditary transthyretin amyloidosis (hATTR)
	Wild-type transthyretin amyloidosis (wtATTR)
	Light-chain amyloidosis (AL)
	Sarcoid
Storage disease	Gaucher disease
	Hurler–Hunter syndrome
	Hemochromatosis
	Pompe disease
	Fabry disease
Endomyocardial	Endomyocardial fibrosis
	Hypereosinophilic syndrome
	Carcinoid
	Scleroderma
	Ehlers–Danlos syndrome
	Systemic lupus erythematosus
	Metastatic malignancy
	Radiation
	Anthracycline toxicity
	Drugs causing fibrous endocarditis (serotonin, methysergide, ergotamine, mercury-containing agents, busulfan, chloroquine)

INTRODUCTION TO IMAGING IN RESTRICTIVE CARDIOMYOPATHY

Although it is convenient to envision systole and diastole as separate hemodynamic events, in reality they are intricately intertwined. Good diastolic function depends on good myocardial contraction. This is now evident from recently developed echocardiographic (and other imaging) techniques. Myocardial deformation imaging (strain) using two-dimensional (2D) speckle tracking clearly demonstrates abnormal systolic mechanics in patients traditionally classified as having diastolic heart failure or heart failure with preserved ejection fraction (HFpEF). Currently there is a groundswell of evidence based on the use of this technique to diagnose,[1] prognosticate,[2] and guide treatment of patients with amyloid cardiomyopathy. In particular, incorporation of the evaluation of longitudinal strain analysis into clinical practice is resulting in the earlier diagnosis of amyloid cardiomyopathies. This is a direct result of the unique distribution of segmental strain abnormalities in these disorders (i.e., relative apical sparing with predominant basal segmental involvement)[3] (Fig. 14.2).

Complimentary imaging with cardiac magnetic resonance imaging (MRI), using gadolinium to augment tissue characteristics (late gadolinium enhancement [LGE]), enables evaluation for the presence and distribution of myocardial fibrosis (replacement and interstitial), as well as quantification of myocardial extracellular volume (ECV). Similar to characteristic patterns observed with strain echocardiography, there are clues in the degree, distribution, and nature of abnormalities seen with LGE and ECV that are associated with specific pathologies. Additionally, bone scintigraphy, mainly using technetium pyrophosphate or technetium 99m–labeled

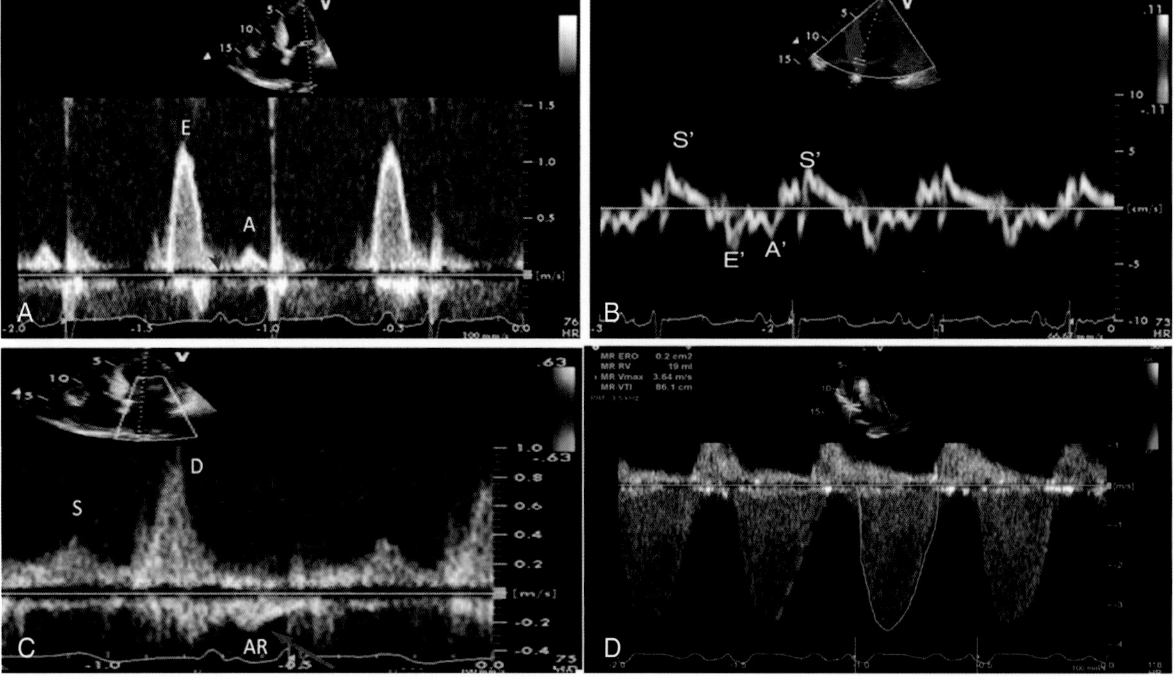

Fig. 14.1 **Doppler characteristics in advanced restrictive cardiomyopathy.** (A) Pulsed Doppler mitral inflow shows a restrictive pattern with a high early diastolic LV filling velocity, a steep deceleration slope *(dotted arrow)*, and low late-diastolic atrial-induced LV filling velocity. (B) Doppler tissue imaging shows low-early *(E')* and late *(A')* diastolic mitral annular velocity and low systolic wave (S'). (C) Pulmonary vein flow demonstrates an increased and prolonged atrial reversal velocity *(AR; red arrow)* consistent with high LV filling pressures, as well as systolic flow *(S)* blunting with diastolic flow *(D)* predominance. (D) The CW Doppler mitral regurgitant jet obtained from the LV apical 3-chamber view is of relatively low velocity with a slow deceleration slope *(dotted red arrow)* due to a high LV end-diastolic pressure and impaired diastolic relaxation.

3,3-diphosphono-1,2-propanodicarboxylicacid (^{99m}Tc-DPD), has re-emerged as a highly sensitive and specific imaging technique for transthyretin amyloidosis (ATTR) deposition in the myocardium, and in combination with targeted genotyping, it has enabled the diagnosis of ATTR cardiomyopathy without the need for myocardial biopsy.

Reducing the technical limitations of three-dimensional (3D) echocardiography for single-beat 3D strain will likely enable better quantification of global LV contractility and compliance and link the benefits of echocardiography for functional assessment with the advantages of 3D structural evaluation (LV geometry). Additionally, strain imaging is proving to be a promising technology for the evaluation of atrial function.[4,5]

2D ECHOCARDIOGRAPHIC AND DOPPLER FEATURES

Echocardiographic assessment for RCM includes a comprehensive evaluation using multiple echocardiographic modalities that evaluate cardiac structure and function. These include M-mode, 2D imaging, color Doppler, spectral Doppler (CW and pulsed wave [PW]), and strain imaging (Tables 14.2 and 14.3).

M-MODE IMAGING

Parasternal views in the long and short axes are used to measure LV chamber dimension and interventricular septum and posterior wall thickness and to calculate LV mass (see Chapter 8). Color M-mode in the apical 4-chamber view is used to assess the velocity of flow propagation (Vp) and to measure isovolumic relaxation time by placing the M-mode cursor in the center of the LV.[2] Vp values are expressed in centimeters per second, and normal values are greater than 50 cm/s.

2D IMAGING

Parasternal views (2D parasternal long- and short-axis views) are now the most commonly used and recommended views to measure LV dimensions, wall thickness, and LV mass. The mid-short-axis view is also used to assess LV radial and circumferential strain and the strain rate of all myocardial segments by speckle tracking and the strain rate of the anterior interventricular septum and inferolateral wall by tissue Doppler imaging (TDI) (see Chapters 4 and 8).

Apical views allow assessment of the biplane LVEF by the Simpson method. Inherent variability in the LVEF measurement (±5%) and lack of endocardial border visualization occur in up to 31% of patients undergoing stress echocardiography.[6] Use of contrast imaging improves the accuracy of LV volume measurements and LVEF. LV volume measurements by contrast-enhanced 2D imaging[3] and by 3D echocardiography[4] have superior reproducibility and closer approximation to results of the cardiac MRI technique than does non-contrast-enhanced 2D echocardiography (see Chapter 3). Longitudinal LV strain and strain rate are assessed in the apical 4-, 3-, and 2-chamber focused LV views, and right ventricular (RV) strain and strain rate are assessed in the RV focused view (see Chapter 2). Calculation of global longitudinal strain (GLS) and segmental strain analysis are possible from high-quality apical views with sufficiently high frame rates (50–80 fps). Additionally, the apical views are used for

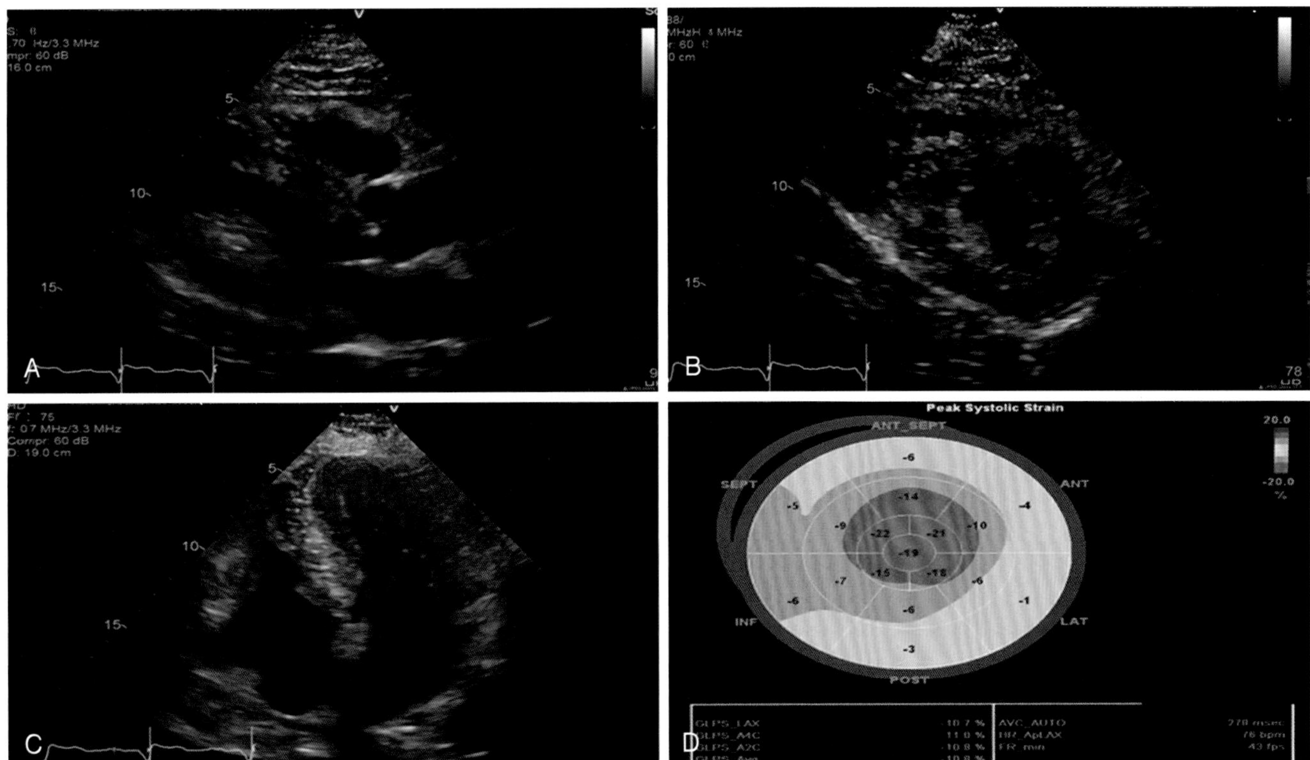

Fig. 14.2 **Echocardiographic findings in ATTR amyloidosis.** The patient was a 70-year-old man with the pV50M mutation (or V30M; valine-to-methionine substitution at position 30). Parasternal long-axis (A), parasternal short-axis (B), and apical 4-chamber (C) views show concentric hypertrophy and decreased longitudinal motion of the LV. (D) Polar map of all myocardial segments shows the reduced global longitudinal strain (GLS) at −10.8% and an apical-sparing pattern: >2:1 apical/basal ratio, >1:1 apical/(mid+basal) ratio, or "cherry-on-top" (Videos 14.2A, 14.2B, and 14.2C).

TABLE 14.2 **Echocardiographic Features of Restrictive Cardiomyopathy.**

M-mode and color M-mode	Square root sign in the interventricular septum and the inferolateral wall motion
	LV hypertrophy
	Small LV dimensions
	Decreased velocity of flow propagation (Vp)
	Prolonged IVRT in early stages, short IVRT in late stages
2D findings	Decreased LV volumes
	Preserved LV systolic function (early stages)
	Biatrial enlargement
	Unexplained myocardial hypertrophy
	Myocardial speckling
	Atrial septal thickening
	Homogenous AV valve thickening
	Small pericardial effusion
	Ventricular thrombi or apical mass despite normal underlying wall motion
Mitral PW Doppler	Large E wave, small A wave; E/A ratio >2
	Short DT <150 ms; short IVRT <60 ms
	No significant change in mitral E wave, deceleration time, or IVRT with Valsalva maneuver
	Abnormal relaxation pattern with E/A ratio <1 and DT in early stages
	Pseudonormal and reversible restrictive patterns in intermediate stages
Tricuspid PW Doppler	Restrictive filling; increased E/A ratio and short DT; with inspiration, further shortening of the DT and minimal change in E/A ratio
Pulmonary veins	Dilated pulmonary veins, diastolic dominant pattern, and S/D ratio <0.5
	Prominent atrial reversal velocity with pulmonary vein atrial A duration > mitral inflow A duration
	Rapid D wave deceleration time in late stages
	No change in D wave with respiration
Mitral regurgitation	Increased *dP/dt* in early stages, reduced *dP/dt* in late stages, and elevated LA filling pressure [SBP − 4(MR velocity)^2]
Tricuspid regurgitation	Pulmonary artery systolic pressure [4 × (tricuspid insufficiency jet^2]
Pulmonary regurgitation	Pulmonary artery diastolic pressure [4 × (pulmonary insufficiency jet^2] plus RA pressure
Color Doppler findings	MR and TR due to leaflet or papillary muscle involvement (as in endomyocardial fibrosis)
	TR secondary to pulmonary hypertension
	Diastolic MR due to increased LV end-diastolic pressure
	Diastolic TR and MR due to first-degree AV block or complete heart block
Mitral annulus TDI	E/E′ ratio to assess LV filling pressure; in RCM, E′ usually <8 cm/s and E/E′ >15 due to elevated filling pressure
Tricuspid annulus TDI	Decreased RV function *s* <1 cm/s
	RA pressure E/E′ >6
Color M-mode examination	Vp <45 cm/s in RCM; E/Vp >1.5 can be used to assess LV filling pressure
Hepatic vein/flow	Dilated hepatic veins, S/D ratio <0.5
	Prominent atrial reversals that increase with inspiration
Inferior vena cava	Dilated (>2.1 cm) with reduced respiratory variation (<50%)

AV, Atrioventricular; *BP,* blood pressure; *DT,* deceleration time; *IVRT,* isovolumic relaxation time; *MR,* mitral regurgitation; *PW,* pulsed-wave; *RCM,* restrictive cardiomyopathy; *S/D ratio,* ratio of pulmonary vein systolic to diastolic flow; *SBP,* systolic blood pressure; *TDI,* tissue Doppler imaging; *TR,* tricuspid regurgitation; *Vp,* propagation velocity.

evaluation of atrial strain, giving insight into LA pump and LA reservoir function.

SPECTRAL DOPPLER IMAGING

Parasternal and apical views allow assessment of LV and RV diastolic function and filling pressures. The technique and specific information for data acquisition using both PW and CW are detailed in Chapter 8. We provide here a summary of spectral Doppler findings that are used to characterize various stages of RCM.

Mitral inflow PW Doppler is used to measure the peak mitral inflow E-wave and A-wave velocities, the E/A ratio, E-wave deceleration time, and mitral A-wave duration.

Pulmonary vein PW Doppler is used to measure peak pulmonary vein systolic (S) and diastolic (D) velocities, D-wave deceleration time, and atrial reversal velocity and duration (see Fig. 14.1). Use of contrast improves the pulmonary vein PW Doppler signal in technically difficult studies.[7]

Mitral annular PW TDI in the apical 4-chamber view is used to measure mitral annular systolic and early and late diastolic velocities (S′, E′, and A′, respectively) from the medial and lateral mitral annuli (see Chapter 5).

FINDINGS

Specific echocardiographic features of various types of RCMs are summarized in Table 14.2. RCMs are characterized by concentric hypertrophy (elevated LV mass) or remodeling (elevated wall thickness with normal LV mass), with marked increase in wall thickness relative to cavity size, and normal or small LV end-diastolic volume. Atrial enlargement is associated with the grade of diastolic dysfunction: mild, moderate, and severe diastolic dysfunction are reflected by progressively

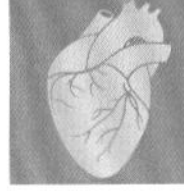

TABLE 14.3 Other Approaches in the Diagnosis of Restrictive Cardiomyopathies.

Diagnostic Modality	*Key Findings*	*Limitations*
2D/Doppler echocardiography	LV hypertrophy	Comorbidities of advanced age and coexisting hypertension renders LVH nonspecific and commonly a late finding with limited impact on guiding treatment or affecting prognosis. Nonreproducible measurements make regression difficult to follow.
	Restrictive filling	Does not provide etiologic information in amyloidosis.
Systemic markers	Light chains, serum amyloid P component, troponin, and pro-BNP in primary amyloidosis	
Biopsy (tongue, subcutaneous fat pads, kidneys, bone marrow, gastric mucosa, rectal mucosa, and EMB)	May reveal specific cause of restrictive cardiomyopathy. Eosinophilic interstitial deposits on H&E, apple-green birefringence on Congo red staining, and fibrillar protein on EM in cardiac amyloid.	Procedural risk and uncertainty about sampling error limits use in monitoring disease.
Cardiac catheterization	Systolic area index	Procedural risk Radiation exposure
	Dip and plateau	
	RV systolic pressure usually >50 mmHg	
	Often, LVEDP > 5 mmHg > RVEDP	
	RVEDP <⅓ of RV systolic pressure.	
CT imaging	Pericardium of normal thickness. No pericardial calcification	Radiation exposure Contrast agent side effects
MRI	Amyloidosis: global subendocardial LGE, increased native T1 relaxation time, and increased extracellular volume	Use in early stages of the disease has not been evaluated.
	Significantly decreased T1 relaxation time in Fabry and hemochromatosis; decreased T2* in hemochromatosis.	
Nuclear scintigraphy with 99Tc pyrophosphate or indium-labeled systemic amyloid protein scan	Tc pyrophosphate scan (semiquantitative visual grade II and III) differentiates between AL and ATTR.	Radiation exposure

AL, Immunoglobulin light-chain amyloidosis; ATTR, transthyretin amyloidosis; *BNP*, brain natriuretic peptide; *EM*, electron microscopy; *EMB*, endoscopic muscle biopsy; *H&E*, hematoxylin and eosin stain; *LGE*, late gadolinium enhancement; *LVEDP*, LV end-diastolic pressure; *LVH*, LV hypertrophy; *MRI*, magnetic resonance imaging; *RVEDP*, RV end-diastolic pressure; *Tc*, technetium.

increasing LV stiffness and resultant filling pressures. Mild, moderate, and severe LA enlargement are defined by the American Society of Echocardiography guidelines[8] as an LA volume index of more than 34 mL/m^2, 40 to 47 mL/m^2, and more than 48 mL/m^2, respectively, as measured by the Simpson method.

Mitral Inflow Pulsed-Wave Doppler Imaging

Diastolic variables in RCM usually progress through a spectrum of increasing severity, beginning with abnormal relaxation, followed by a pseudonormal pattern, and ultimately restrictive filling. In the early stages, the mitral inflow filling pattern shows an E/A ratio lower than 1, a prolonged mitral inflow E-wave deceleration time, and a prolonged isovolumic relaxation time. As the disease progresses and LV stiffness increases, the compensatory increase in LA pressure results in a return to an apparently normal E/A ratio (>1), known as pseudonormalization; however, the increase in E-wave velocity results solely from increased LA pressure. This pattern is recognized by LA enlargement and reduced mitral annular *e′* velocity. Temporary reduction of preload (and LA filling pressure) by Valsalva maneuver, nitroglycerine administration, or diuresis unmasks the underlying disordered relaxation and reveals the abnormal E/A (<1). With severe abnormalities of ventricular compliance, advanced diastolic dysfunction develops, characterized by an increased E velocity and a reduced atrial contribution due to LA systolic failure. The E wave decelerates rapidly as pressure between the LA and LV quickly equilibrates earlier in diastole (see Fig. 14.1). Because of poor LA function and a limited late-diastolic left atrioventricular pressure gradient due to elevated LV diastolic pressure, the atrial amplitude becomes small, and a restrictive pattern develops that is irreversible (unresponsive to preload-reducing maneuvers). Because of a marked increase in LV end-diastolic pressure, diastolic mitral regurgitation may be seen, especially in the presence of first-degree heart block.

Pulmonary Vein Pulsed-Wave Doppler Imaging

In early stages of the disease, pulmonary venous flow may show a systolic-dominant pattern with an S/D ratio greater than 1 and normal atrial reversal. As LA pressures rise, the A-wave velocity and duration progressively increase. This is followed by a blunting of the S-wave velocity[7] and an increased D-wave velocity, with resultant reversal of the normal S/D ratio (see Fig. 14.1). In the presence of atrial fibrillation, there is further absence of the early systolic component (S_1) of pulmonary vein filling, which is related to atrial relaxation after atrial contraction, and resultant marked blunting of the totality of the S wave. The pulmonary vein D wave is a result of the pulmonary vein–LA pressure gradient created during atrioventricular filling in early LV diastole (LA conduit), and it is dependent on the same factors that influence the early mitral velocity and its deceleration time. In advanced stages of the disease, there is a tall D wave with a shortened deceleration time, truncated atrioventricular filling with atrial contraction, and prominent regurgitation into the pulmonary vein (A-wave reversal > mitral E-wave duration). Finally, impairment of LA contraction due to mechanical atrial failure leads to a decrease in the amplitude and duration of the pulmonary vein atrial wave.

Tissue Doppler Imaging of the Mitral Annulus

TDI of the septal and lateral mitral annulus interrogates myocardial tissue motion directly; it is a key modality for the assessment of myocardial relaxation and is less load-dependent than mitral inflow Doppler imaging.[8] As one would expect, progressive decline in LV compliance is mirrored by a decline in early tissue velocities. Relating the early velocities of mitral inflow to the tissue velocities enables one to ascertain whether the myocardium is sufficiently compliant to accept mitral inflow normally, or whether the tissue is too stiff to do so. This ratio (E/*E′*) has been associated with the mean pulmonary capillary wedge pressure.[9] Decreased RV systolic and diastolic velocities reflect a global impairment in myocardial relaxation.

Additionally, this metric (E/*E′* ratio) is critical for the echocardiographic differentiation of restrictive from constrictive cardiomyopathy. Diminished tissue velocities are observed in patients with RCM, whereas patients with constrictive pericarditis have normal or even increased velocities. Furthermore, as opposed to the positive correlation between E/*E′* and pulmonary capillary wedge pressure in patients with myocardial disease, there is an inverse relationship between these values in patients with constrictive pericarditis (annulus paradoxus).[10]

Color M-Mode

Impaired LV relaxation causes a reduction in the Vp of blood from the mitral annulus deep into the LV cavity. Using color M-mode, this can be calculated as the slope of a linear approximation of an isovelocity contour of the color-flow jet; it is obtained from the apical views. Unlike PW TDI, color M-mode provides spatial information along with velocity and time data and is relatively load-independent; however, it is more difficult to perform. A slope greater than 100 cm/s has 74% sensitivity and 91% specificity in identifying constrictive pericardial disease.[11]

Tissue Doppler Imaging and Longitudinal Strain

Longitudinal systolic strain echocardiography is an accurate technique for the detection of systolic dysfunction in amyloidosis. TDI can be used to detect impaired LV systolic function even when no evidence of cardiac involvement exists on standard 2D and Doppler echocardiography. Doppler-based strain imaging is confounded by a relatively low signal-to-noise ratio, is subject to the usual technical limitations of Doppler signals (discussed later), and as such has largely been replaced by speckle tracking strain imaging.

Limitations and Pitfalls of Pulsed-Wave Doppler and Color M-Mode

The effect of the incident angle, the amplitude of the reflected echoes, scattering, sweep speed, Nyquist limit, and low wall filters remain important considerations for Doppler imaging,[12] including TDI. The TDI sample volume should be placed at the junction of the annulus with the base of the myocardium. The sample volume moves in relation to the myocardial wall dynamics in such a way that the selected region of interest of the ventricular myocardium under analysis is not always the same, causing frequent motion artifacts superimposed on the pulsed Doppler images. Because of the physiologic beat-to-beat variability of PW TDI data, an averaged value from a few cardiac cycles should be obtained. Vp cannot be measured when a linear wave front for early filling is not available in patients with poor acoustic windows, when there is a lack of continuity in the blood column, or when apical blood flow is not present due to reduced forward propagation. In these cases, the Nyquist limit should be lowered. In patients with a significantly dilated LV, in which the mitral inflow progresses along the posterolateral wall, alignment of the M-mode cursor parallel to blood flow may be difficult, resulting in a falsely low propagation speed.

2D SPECKLE TRACKING STRAIN IMAGING

Unlike TDI, 2D strain imaging is independent of the angle of insonation and can be used in multiple planes to interrogate longitudinal shortening, circumferential rotation, and radial thickening of the myocardium. Speckle tracking involves placing tissue markers on the myocardium adjacent to any of the cardiac chambers and tracking the complex movement of that chamber throughout the cardiac cycle. Of all the types of strain, speckle tracking LV global longitudinal strain (LV-GLS) is the most studied and is currently being utilized in clinical practice. An array of postprocessing packages can be used to perform tissue tracking and calculate LV-GLS. Although it remains challenging to standardize LV-GLS across all vendors and postprocessing software, patterns for specific cardiac diseases have been identified, adding to the diagnostic and prognostic value of echocardiography in RCMs. Individual strain patterns for specific cardiomyopathies (e.g., amyloidosis, Fabry disease) are described later. LV-GLS is widely used as a marker of subclinical LV systolic dysfunction, especially in patients who are receiving cardiotoxic chemotherapeutic agents.[13] LA strain parameters have been shown to be associated with the development of atrial arrhythmias and ischemic stroke.[14] LA strain provides detailed information on the LA reservoir (peak atrial longitudinal strain) and on contractile functions (peak atrial contraction strain). In patients with cardiac amyloidosis, LA function is impaired and is highly correlated with LV deformation parameters.[5] In one study, LA function was abnormal irrespective of LA cavity size.[15]

OTHER IMAGING MODALITIES

Complimentary imaging using cardiac MRI, cardiac computed tomography, and nuclear scintigraphy are increasingly employed in an attempt to accurately phenotype these cardiomyopathies (see Table 14.3). This is of particular importance in light of the discoveries of disease-specific therapies. Specific applications of each of these modalities are discussed in the following sections.

SPECIFIC RESTRICTIVE CARDIOMYOPATHIES

Many disease processes can result in an RCM (see Table 14.1). Echocardiography plays a central role in establishing the diagnosis of RCM and potentially characterizing the disease process. In most cases, a thorough clinical and multimodality imaging evaluation is needed to establish an accurate diagnosis. Characteristics of the relatively common RCMs are described in the following sections.

AMYLOIDOSIS

Amyloidosis is a common cause of RCM that is increasing in prevalence. The advancement of non-invasive imaging technologies has uncovered a 15% to 20% prevalence of amyloidosis in certain common conditions such as aortic stenosis and HFpEF.[16,17]

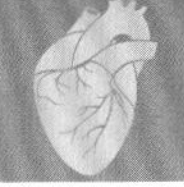

Definition

Numerous types of amyloidosis that affect the human body have been described. From a cardiac standpoint, two major subtypes affect the myocardium.[18,19]

Light-chain amyloidosis (AL) is a plasma cell dyscrasia that results in the uncontrolled production of immunoglobulin light chains (most commonly lambda) that are ordinarily used for antibody formation. These abnormal circulating light chains conglomerate, form amyloid fibrils, and are deposited in a variety of organs. The estimated age- and sex-adjusted incidence of AL is 1.2 cases per 100,000 person-years,[20] with more than 50% of patients demonstrating cardiac deposition. There is an overlap between AL and multiple myeloma: approximately 10% of patients with AL will be diagnosed with overt multiple myeloma. Early recognition of this disease is critical because prognosis is directly related to the degree of cardiac involvement. Historical data show that the median survival time without treatment is only 6 months from the onset of heart failure.[21]

ATTR either results from a point mutation (hereditary of hATTR) or is sporadic (wild-type or wtATTR). The disease process results from deposition of transthyretin fibrils (misfolded and aggregated into the amyloid configuration) in various tissues. The familial variants tend to affect the heart and the peripheral nervous system to varying degrees; more than 80 unique mutations having been described to date. The sporadic type is overall the most common form of cardiac amyloidosis, with increased prevalence in older men in particular.

Clinical Features

Deposition of amyloid fibrils in the myocardium occurs in about 50% of patients with AL and in most patients with wtATTR. Histologically, alterations in cellular metabolism, calcium transport, receptor regulation, and cellular edema occur. Such changes lead to features of RCM, conduction system disorders, and amyloid angiopathy. Clinically, patients predominantly present with symptoms of heart failure, chest pain, atrial and/or ventricular arrhythmias, embolic stroke, autonomic dysfunction, and syncope. A history of carpal tunnel syndrome (especially bilateral), lumbar stenosis, or bicep tendon rupture should raise the suspicion for ATTR.[22,23] Macroglossia and spontaneous periorbital hematoma ("raccoon eyes") are seen more commonly in AL amyloidosis. The electrocardiographic signs (pseudoinfarct pattern and/or low-voltage QRS) provide important clinical clues but generally lack sensitivity and specificity, whereas serum urine free light chains and immunofixation electrophoresis have a high negative predictive value for AL.[24] Serum troponin and N-terminal pro B-type natriuretic peptide (NT-proBNP) are of prognostic value and are used in disease staging.[25]

Imaging

Echocardiography

The following echocardiographic characteristics are suggestive but not diagnostic of cardiac amyloidosis (see Fig 14.2) and do not discriminate between the AL and ATTR types. The hallmark features of the disease are increased LV wall thickness and mass in most cases (ATTR > AL). In a minority of patients, especially those with AL, the LV wall may be normal or only slightly thickened. LV volumes and LVEF tend to remain normal, except in advanced disease, and predict an adverse outcome. The RV is invariably involved, mainly showing a thickened RV wall. The classic finding of a brilliant speckled appearance is neither sensitive nor specific because harmonic imaging has replaced fundamental imaging in the current era.[26] With long-standing elevated LV end-diastolic pressure, bi-atrial dilatation occurs. Infiltration of the valves also gives a typical appearance of thickened valve leaflets and may lead to mitral regurgitation.

Systematic screening of patients presenting for evaluation of aortic stenosis revealed a prevalence of 16% for ATTR cardiac amyloidosis in these patients, but it remains uncertain why this relationship exists.[17] The myocardial contraction fraction (MCF), defined as the ratio of LV stroke volume to myocardial volume, is a simple metric that provides additional prognostic information in patients with amyloid cardiomyopathy. In a cohort of patients with AL, the MCF was an independent predictor of overall survival,[27] and in a follow-up study, the stroke volume index performed similarly to MCF, leading the authors to conclude that stroke volume index should be reported routinely in patients with AL cardiomyopathy.[28]

Echo-Doppler Imaging

PW Doppler of the LV can reveal the entire range of diastolic abnormalities seen in RCMs (Fig. 14.3)[29] with associated elevated pulmonary systolic pressures. The ratio of E to E' as determined by PW TDI is typically more elevated in diastolic dysfunction secondary to amyloidosis than in hypertensive heart disease.[30] Rarely, dynamic LV outflow obstruction can occur in amyloidosis and may masquerade as obstructive hypertrophic cardiomyopathy. A histopathologic study showed that approximately 1% of patients undergoing septal myectomy had evidence of amyloid deposition.[31] In patients with aortic stenosis, an average mitral annular S' wave velocity of less than 6 cm/s had a 100% sensitivity for a positive technetium pyrophosphate scintigraphy study indicating ATTR.[17]

Tissue deformation assessment using strain and strain rate imaging by TDI or speckle tracking significantly improves the ability to screen for and diagnose cardiac amyloidosis and provides prognostic[32] information. Using segmental longitudinal strain analysis, one frequently notes the well-described pattern of relative apical sparing ("cherry-on-top" sign), with an overall reduction in absolute GLS (see Fig. 14.2). Contrary to the common belief, the apical sparing pattern is a result of segmental differences in the distribution of the total amyloid mass rather than the proportion of amyloid deposits.[33] In a cohort of 97 AL patients, those with cardiac involvement and heart failure had the worst basal LV strain compared to those without cardiac involvement or heart failure.[1] GLS in patients with AL undergoing stem cell transplantation provided added prognostic value to the Mayo AL Staging Model.[34] In a cohort of 249 AL patients, strain of the basal RV and tricuspid annular plane systolic excursion by M-mode echocardiography (TAPSE) were associated with cardiac involvement in AL and subsequent death.[35]

The concept of relative apical sparing was quantified and defined using the following equation:

$$(\text{Average apical longitudinal strain}) \div (\text{Average basal longitudinal strain} + \text{Mid-longitudinal strain}) \geq 1.0$$

This equation was tested in 55 patients with amyloidosis compared with normal controls (patients with hypertrophic cardiomyopathy or aortic stenosis) and showed 93% sensitivity and 82% specificity in differentiating cardiac amyloidosis from controls (area under the curve, 0.94).[3] This relative apical sparing pattern was later shown to be associated with the outcome of death or heart transplantation.[36] Subsequent studies, however, showed that although relative apical sparing is specific, it lacks sensitivity; in one study of

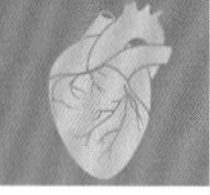

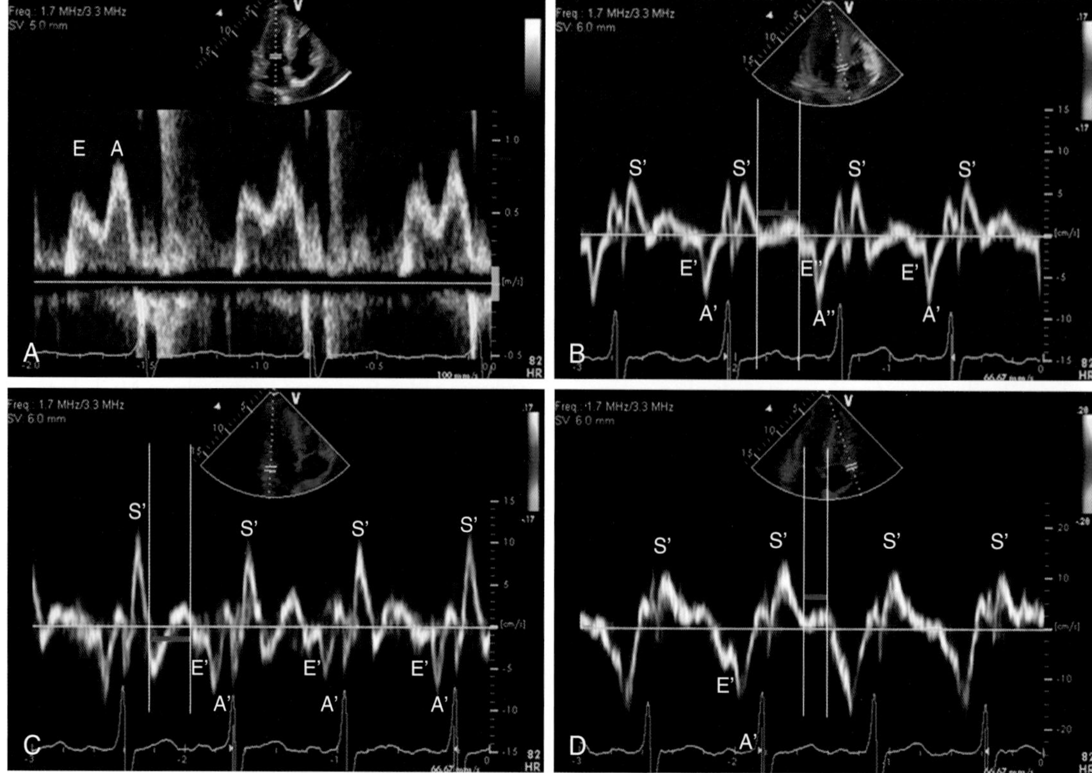

Fig. 14.3 Doppler findings in immunoglobulin light-chain (AL) amyloidosis. (A) Mitral inflow pulsed-wave Doppler image obtained at the level of the mitral valve leaflets from a reverse 2D apical 4-chamber view. (B) Medial annular tissue Doppler image. (C) Lateral annular tissue Doppler image. (D) Tricuspid annular tissue Doppler image. Reversed mitral inflow E/A ratio, as shown in A, can occur in restrictive cardiomyopathy. Marked prolongation of isovolumic relaxation times (*red lines* in B and D) indicate impaired relaxation of the LV (B and C) and RV (D) along with markedly reduced E′ velocities of both the LV (B and C) and RV (D). S′ and A′ velocities are preserved.

79 patients with proven amyloidosis, only 48% demonstrated this pattern.[37] In another study of 40 patients with amyloidosis, 40 with hypertrophic cardiomyopathy, and 20 with hypertensive heart disease, relative apical sparing greater than 1.0 showed a sensitivity of only 37.5% for the diagnosis of cardiac amyloidosis.[38]

Typically, absolute GLS is related to LVEF by a factor of 3 (e.g., absolute GLS 20% ≈ LVEF of 60%). In patients with cardiac amyloidosis, this relationship is decoupled: worsening (less negative) GLS occurs in amyloidosis but LVEF remains the same, leading to deviation of the GLS and LVEF relationship from a factor of 3 to a factor of 4 or 5. This finding has enabled improved diagnostic accuracy (90% sensitivity and 92% specificity).[38] Some challenges remain for the use of GLS in routine practice, including the need for high-quality echocardiographic images, the load dependency of GLS, and the vendor-dependent normative values for strain.[39]

3D strain echocardiography offers the promise of single-beat acquisition for whole-ventricle analysis of cardiac mechanics. The technology remains limited by temporal and spatial resolution, and more work is needed before adoption into routine practice.[40,41]

Magnetic Resonance Imaging

Advanced amyloidosis on cardiac MRI has similar morphologic features to those identified by echocardiography, but cardiac MRI also enables tissue characterization (Fig. 14.4). Deposition of amyloid fibrils leads to diffuse LV subendocardial, and at times transmural, LGE. With increasing amyloid burden, the RV, RA, and LA walls may show LGE. Gadolinium kinetics are affected by the infiltration of amyloid fibrils, leading to difficulty in nulling of the myocardium despite varying inversion times. Amyloid deposits lead to myocardial edema and fibrosis, with subsequent prolongation of myocardial T1 relaxation time.[42] Another measure is the ECV fraction, which is calculated from pre- and postcontrast myocardial and blood T1 values after correcting for a patient's hematocrit. ECV reflects the extent of interstitial expansion, either by myocardial fibrosis or by deposition of foreign materials (amyloid fibrils in the case of cardiac amyloidosis), and it can aid in both diagnosis and prognosis.[43] Thicker left ventricles, LGE of the RV, higher T1, and higher ECV are likely to be associated with ATTR; however, as with echocardiography, cardiac MRI is not able to reliably differentiate ATTR from AL. One study suggested the use of a scoring system to differentiate ATTR from AL on cardiac MRI,[44] but that was only a single study, and the results have not been duplicated.

Nuclear Imaging

Several nuclear techniques are either approved or being investigated for use in the diagnosis and monitoring of amyloidosis.[45] A diagnostic algorithm[46] endorsed by multiple professional societies combines bone scintigraphy (technetium pyrophosphate in the United States[47] [Fig 14.5], ^{99m}Tc-DPD in Europe) and serum biomarkers (serum and urine free light chains and immunofixation electrophoresis). It has resulted in a 100% positive predictive value for the diagnosis of ATTR cardiac amyloidosis and obviates the need for endomyocardial biopsy in most patients. Early data using positron emission tomography and the radionucleotide tracer florbetapir for the diagnosis and quantification of AL amyloidosis are very promising,[48,49] but more research is needed before this technology can be incorporated clinically. Fig. 14.6 provides a practical approach to the diagnosis of cardiac amyloidosis.

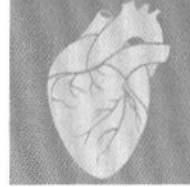

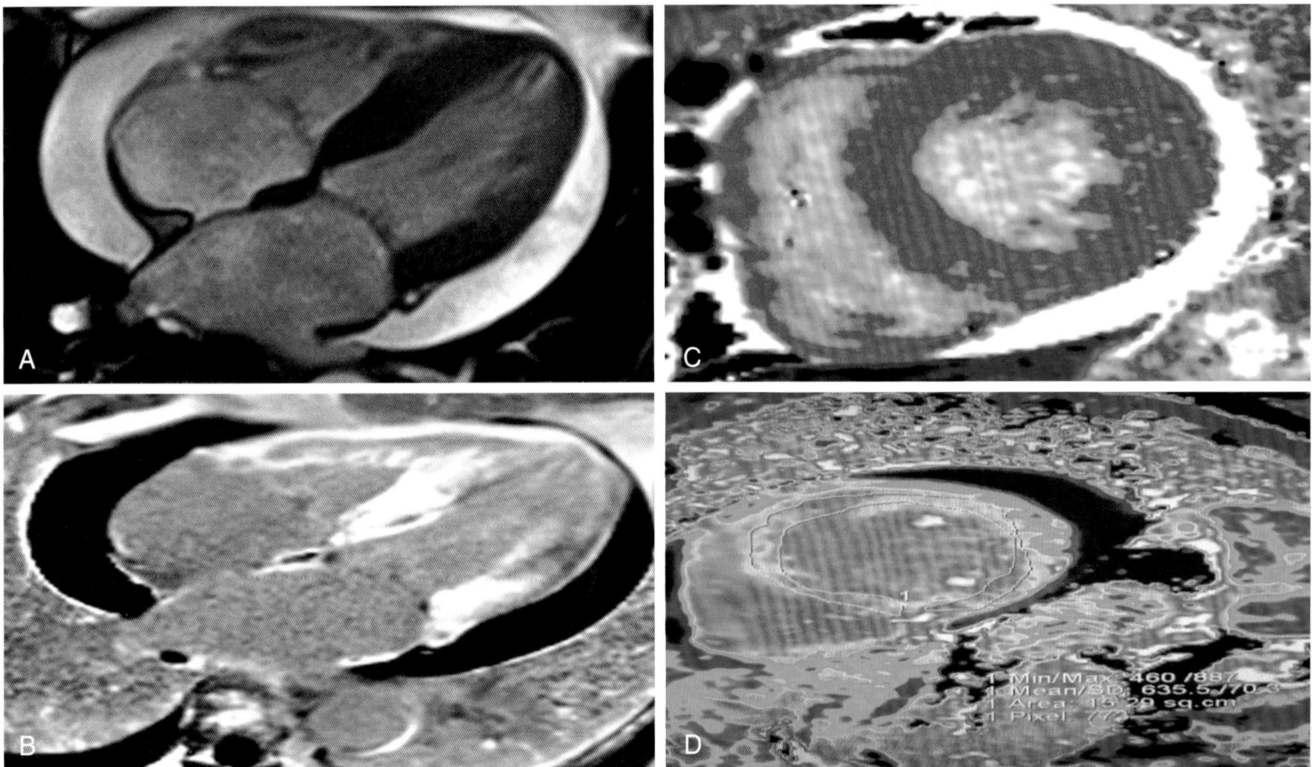

Fig. 14.4 Cardiac MRI findings in ATTR cardiac amyloidosis. (A) A 4-chamber steady-state free precession sequence shows increased LV thickness, dilated atria, and moderate-sized pleural effusion. (B) Four-chamber phase-sensitive inversion recovery image taken 10 minutes after gadolinium bolus shows extensive global late gadolinium enhancement in the LV (transmural at bases, subendocardial toward the apex), the RV, and the LA. (C) Native T1 mapping shows increased T1 relaxation time at the LV base (1200 ms; normal, <1050 ms). (D) Significantly elevated extracellular volume fraction at the LV base (64%; normal, <28%) reflects the expansion of the interstitium by deposition of amyloid fibrils.

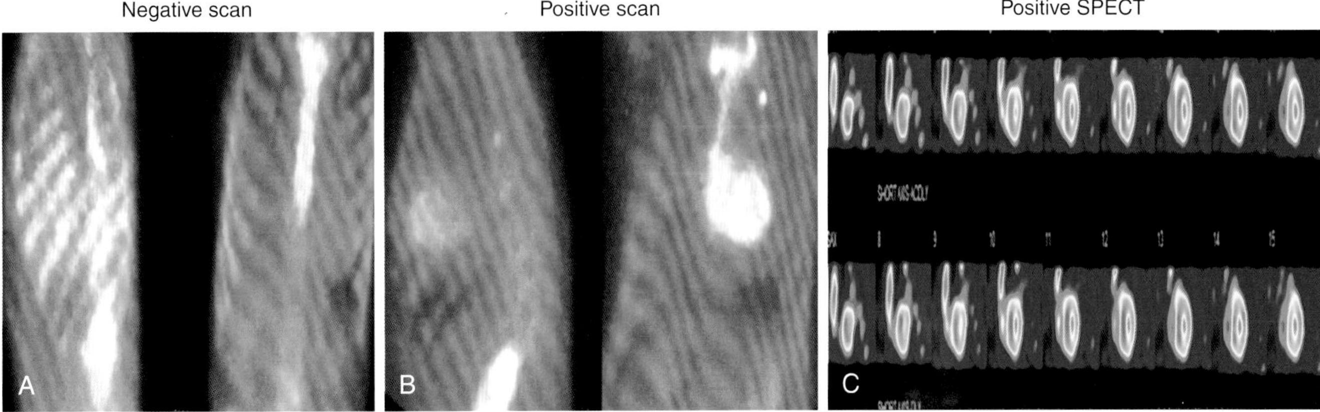

Fig. 14.5 Technetium pyrophosphate scintigraphy. (A) A negative planar scan in a 72-year-old patient with heart failure with preserved ejection fraction (HFpEF). The sternum and ribs show avid uptake of the tracer, whereas the heart does not. (B) A positive scan in a 78-year-old male patient with transthyretin amyloid cardiomyopathy. The tracer is avidly taken up by the myocardium, more intensely than in the adjacent ribs (visual semi-quantitative grade III, heart to contralateral side count ratio of 2.3). (C) A single-photon emission computed tomography (SPECT) study from the same patient as in B shows uptake in the myocardium and not in the blood pool.

Treatment

The treatment of patients with AL (and overlapping multiple myeloma) is rapidly changing. The primary goal of treatment is to abolish the culprit clonal plasma cell population, eliminating the production of amyloidogenic free light chains. Secondarily, cardiologists are key in the supportive care and treatment of congestive heart failure and in deprescribing therapies that are traditionally used in patients with non-amyloid heart failure (i.e., beta blockers, calcium channel blockers, angiotensin-converting enzyme [ACE] inhibitors, angiotensin II receptor blockers [ARBs], and, potentially, digoxin). Given the complexity of this condition, patients benefit from a multidisciplinary team. Details of the various treatment strategies for AL amyloidosis are beyond the scope of this chapter.

Recent advances in the treatment of ATTR amyloid have transformed it from a disease without any available treatment to one with multiple options. For ATTR cardiomyopathy, the Transthyretin Amyloidosis Cardiomyopathy Clinical Trial

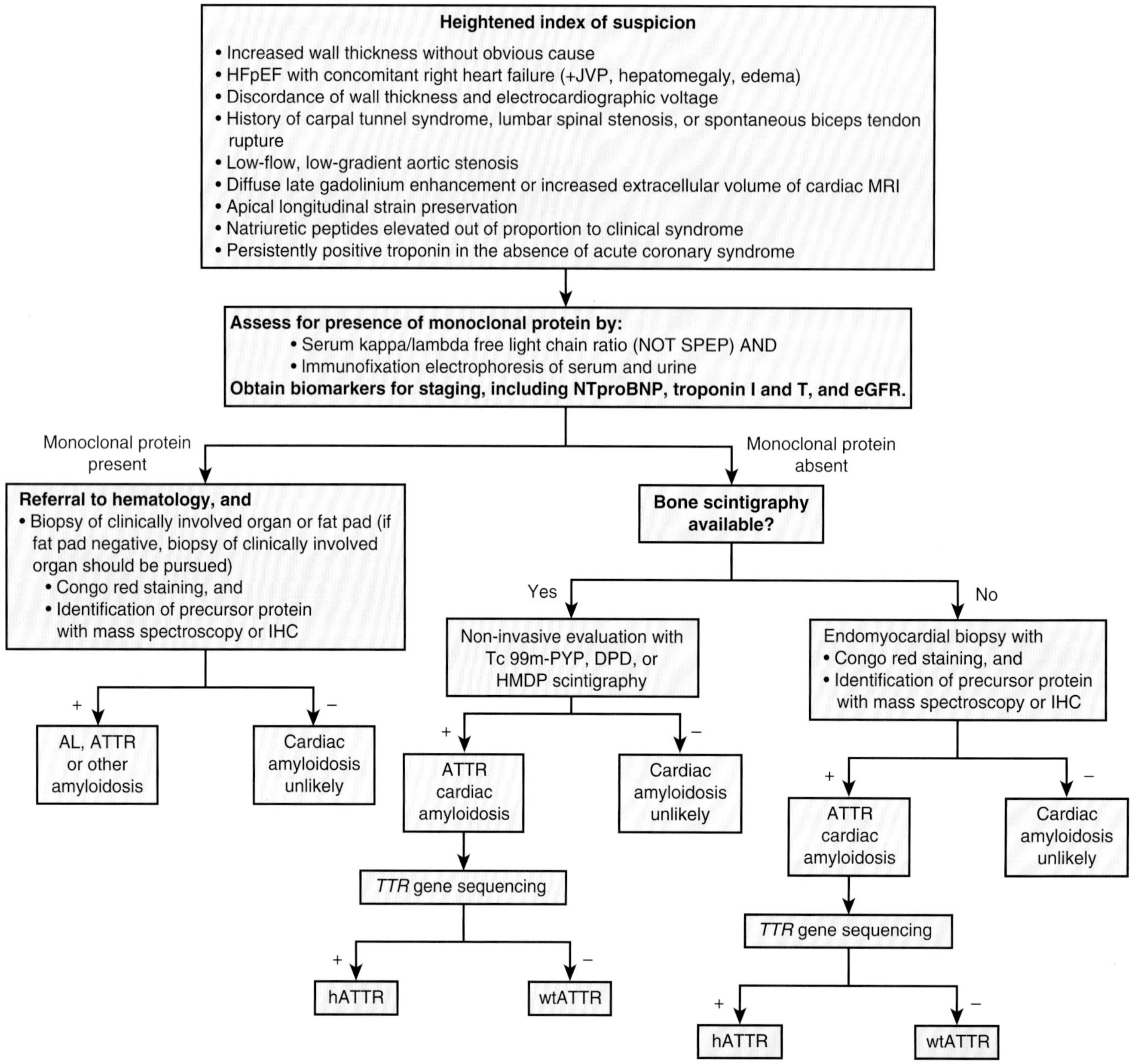

Heightened index of suspicion
- Increased wall thickness without obvious cause
- HFpEF with concomitant right heart failure (+JVP, hepatomegaly, edema)
- Discordance of wall thickness and electrocardiographic voltage
- History of carpal tunnel syndrome, lumbar spinal stenosis, or spontaneous biceps tendon rupture
- Low-flow, low-gradient aortic stenosis
- Diffuse late gadolinium enhancement or increased extracellular volume of cardiac MRI
- Apical longitudinal strain preservation
- Natriuretic peptides elevated out of proportion to clinical syndrome
- Persistently positive troponin in the absence of acute coronary syndrome

Assess for presence of monoclonal protein by:
- Serum kappa/lambda free light chain ratio (NOT SPEP) AND
- Immunofixation electrophoresis of serum and urine

Obtain biomarkers for staging, including NTproBNP, troponin I and T, and eGFR.

Monoclonal protein present

Referral to hematology, and
- Biopsy of clinically involved organ or fat pad (if fat pad negative, biopsy of clinically involved organ should be pursued)
  - Congo red staining, and
  - Identification of precursor protein with mass spectroscopy or IHC

+ AL, ATTR or other amyloidosis

− Cardiac amyloidosis unlikely

Monoclonal protein absent

Bone scintigraphy available?

Yes

Non-invasive evaluation with Tc 99m-PYP, DPD, or HMDP scintigraphy

+ ATTR cardiac amyloidosis

TTR gene sequencing

+ hATTR

− wtATTR

− Cardiac amyloidosis unlikely

No

Endomyocardial biopsy with
- Congo red staining, and
- Identification of precursor protein with mass spectroscopy or IHC

+ ATTR cardiac amyloidosis

TTR gene sequencing

+ hATTR

− wtATTR

− Cardiac amyloidosis unlikely

Fig. 14.6 A practical approach for the workup and diagnosis of patients with suspected amyloidosis. Flow chart details indications and procedures for diagnosing amyloidosis. *AL*, Light-chain amyloidosis; *ATTR*, transthyretin amyloidosis; *DPD*, 3,3-diphosphono-1,2-propanodicarboxylic acid; *eGFR*, estimated glomerular filtration rate; *hATTR*, hereditary transthyretin cardiomyopathy; *HFpEF*, heart failure with preserved ejection fraction; *HMDP*, hydroxymethylene diphosphonate; *IHC*, immunohistochemistry; *JVP*, jugular vein pressure; *MRI*, magnetic resonance imaging; *NT-proBNP*, N-terminal pro B-type natriuretic peptide; *PYP*, pyrophosphate; *SPEP*, serum protein electrophoresis; *wtATTR*, wild-type transthyretin cardiomyopathy. (Adapted from Ruberg FL, Grogan M, Hanna M, Kelly JW, Maurer MS. Transthyretin amyloid cardiomyopathy: JACC state-of-the-art review. *J Am Coll Cardiol.* 2019;73[22]:2872–2891.)

(ATTR-ACT) tested the efficacy of tafamidis (20 mg or 80 mg) in 264 patients against placebo in 177 patients.[50] At 30 months, tafamidis was associated with lower all-cause mortality than placebo (29.5% vs. 42.9%, hazard ratio [HR]: 0.70; 95% confidence interval [CI]: 0.51–0.96) and a lower rate of cardiovascular-related hospitalizations (0.48 vs. 0.7 per year; 95% CI: 0.56–0.81). Tafamidis was also associated with a lower rate of decline in distance for the 6-minute walk test and a lower rate of decline in the Kansas City Cardiomyopathy Questionnaire–Overall Summary score. Tafamidis is a stabilizer for ATTR, so it halts the progression of the disease rather than leading to a regression, and it seems to perform better if started earlier in the disease process (New York Heart Association [NYHA] class I–II vs. NYHA class III).[50]

Other recently approved novel agents include patisiran (a small interfering RNA–based drug) and inotersen (an antisense oligonucleotide); however, both agents were tested in patients with neuropathy and have not undergone dedicated ATTR cardiac amyloidosis trials. Another stabilizer, AG10, is currently undergoing a phase 3 randomized clinical trial after showing promising results in phase 2.[51] Last, limited data have shown utility of diflunisnal for ATTR and doxycycline with tauro-deoxycholic acid for AL.

IDIOPATHIC RESTRICTIVE CARDIOMYOPATHY

When all diagnostic approaches fail to elucidate a cause for the RCM, especially in the young, the disease is termed idiopathic

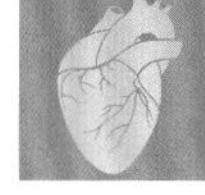

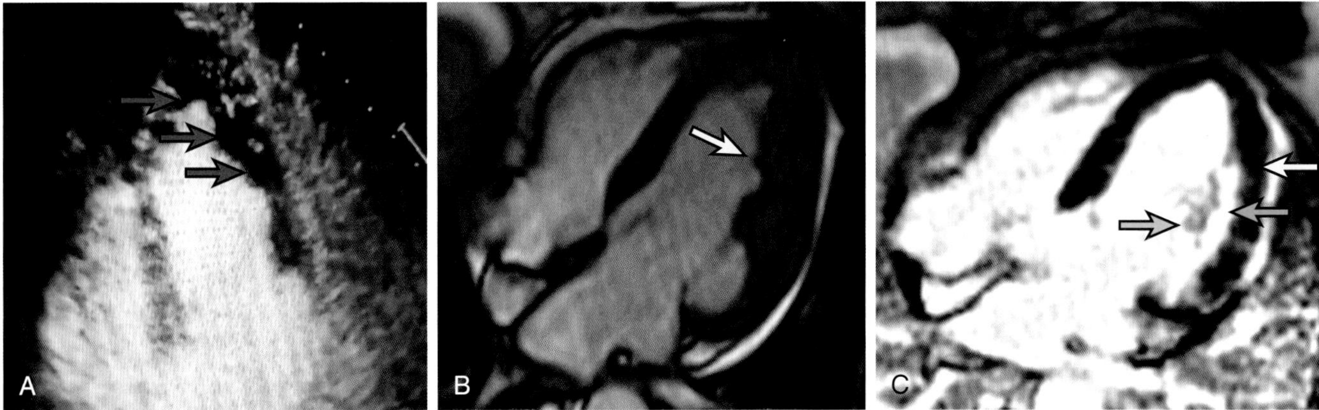

Fig. 14.7 **A 45-year-old woman presenting with a stroke was found to have hypereosinophilic syndrome.** (A) Apical 4-chamber view obtained after microbubble contrast administration shows a layered thrombus extending from the base of the inferolateral wall to the apex *(red arrows)*. (B) A cardiac MRI, 4-chamber steady-state free precession acquisition shows the thickened "myocardium" with rigged appearance representing a thrombus overlying the myocardium *(yellow arrow)*. (C) Cardiac MRI, 4-chamber phase-sensitive inversion recovery images taken 10 minutes after gadolinium bolus show the three-layered appearance: a thrombus *(blue arrow)* overlying the injured myocardium (*green arrow*, late gadolinium enhancement imaging, boundaries mixed with blood pool), with underlying normal "nulled" black myocardium *(yellow arrow)*. *MRI*, Magnetic resonance imaging.

restrictive cardiomyopathy (iRCM). With the improvements in multimodality imaging and genetic testing, many patients previously diagnosed with iRCM are now being given specific phenotypic diagnoses. In one study of 32 patients with iRCM, 84% of whom required heart transplantation, next-generation sequencing and genetic analysis revealed that 60% had disease-causing genetic mutations: *MYH7* (4 patients), *DES* (3), *FLNC* (3), *MYBPC3* (2), *LMNA* (2), *TCAP* (1), *TNNI3* (1), *TNNT2* (1), *TPM1* (1), and *LAMP2* (1).[52] In another cohort of 24 patients, 54% were ultimately found to be gene positive, mainly for a combination of sarcomeric and cytoskeletal gene mutations.[53] It is important to note that symptoms at presentation do not reflect on the poor prognosis of this condition, and timely heart transplantation is associated with better outcomes.[54]

HYPEREOSINOPHILIC SYNDROME AND ENDOMYOCARDIAL FIBROSIS

Hypereosinophilic syndrome (HES) is a leukoproliferative disorder characterized by idiopathic sustained peripheral blood eosinophilia (>1.5 × 10^9/L) noted on two separate tests at least 1 month apart or the finding of tissue hypereosinophilic infiltration (>20% eosinophils on bone marrow section), extensive tissue infiltration by eosinophils validated by a pathologist, or marked deposition of eosinophilic granule proteins in tissue.[55]

Cardiac dysfunction (i.e., endomyocardial fibrosis [EMF]) is the most common cause of morbidity and mortality and is termed Loeffler's endocarditis (although classically Loeffler syndrome refers to eosinophilia associated with parasitic infections). HES is classified as primary, secondary, or idiopathic. There are three defined stages of the disease: an acute necrotic stage, an intermediate phase during which thrombi form along the injured endocardium, and a fibrotic stage characterized by altered cardiac function and RCM.[55] Clinically, patients present with symptoms of biventricular heart failure including dyspnea, ascites, and peripheral edema. Because of the tendency to form intracardiac thrombi, embolic stroke is a potential presentation of the disease.

Echocardiography plays a central role in the diagnosis of cardiac involvement in these diseases. Classically, M-mode shows the Merlon and square root signs, which occur secondary to basal hypercontractility opposing an obliterated LV apex.[56] Depending on the stage of the disease, thrombi in any chamber can be found, typically layered over the injured endocardium (Fig. 14.7). Contrast echocardiography is useful in evaluating the endocardium and in assessing for the presence of biventricular thrombi. Valvular involvement is not uncommon and typically leads to mitral regurgitation due to leaflet or subvalvular restriction without obvious thickening; it is distinct from rheumatic heart disease. Careful evaluation on echocardiography is required so as not to confuse HES with apical variant hypertrophic cardiomyopathy. Cardiac MRI is helpful in the evaluation of HES and eosinophilic myocarditis. Inflammation leads to increased T2 and T1 signal in a distinct continuous subendocardial pattern[57]; with the use of gadolinium agents, thrombi can be carefully evaluated, and the classic V sign (or double V if both ventricles are involved) can be appreciated.[58] The combination of echocardiography and cardiac MRI results in clear differentiation of HES and EMF from other forms of cardiomyopathy.

Endomyocardial biopsy is rarely required, but if done, it typically shows fibrous thickening of the endocardium, made up of collagen fibers without elastic fibers and sometimes organized thrombus.

Treatment requires a multidisciplinary team and rests on defining the underlying etiology of HES. Corticosteroids are often used, in conjunction with targeted therapies, to suppress the eosinophilic inflammation. Patients with the specific myeloproliferative variant, the Fip1-like1–platelet-derived growth factor receptor α (*FIP1L1-PDGFRA*) fusion gene, require a tyrosine kinase inhibitor such as imatinib.[59]

HEMOCHROMATOSIS

The most common form of hereditary hemochromatosis results from the C282Y gene mutation in the *HFE* gene. Both *HFE* and non-*HFE* genes have been implicated in this disease.[60] Less commonly, hemochromatosis occurs secondary to iron overload, mainly from repeated blood transfusions. Deposition of iron in various body tissues leads to toxic damage. Symptoms depend on the affected organ system, with cardiac symptoms mainly deriving from heart failure. Biochemical studies, imaging, and genetic testing can be carried out to confirm diagnosis.[60] Cardiac involvement is evaluated through the use of echocardiography and cardiac MRI. On echocardiography, the main features are consistent with restrictive disease without significant

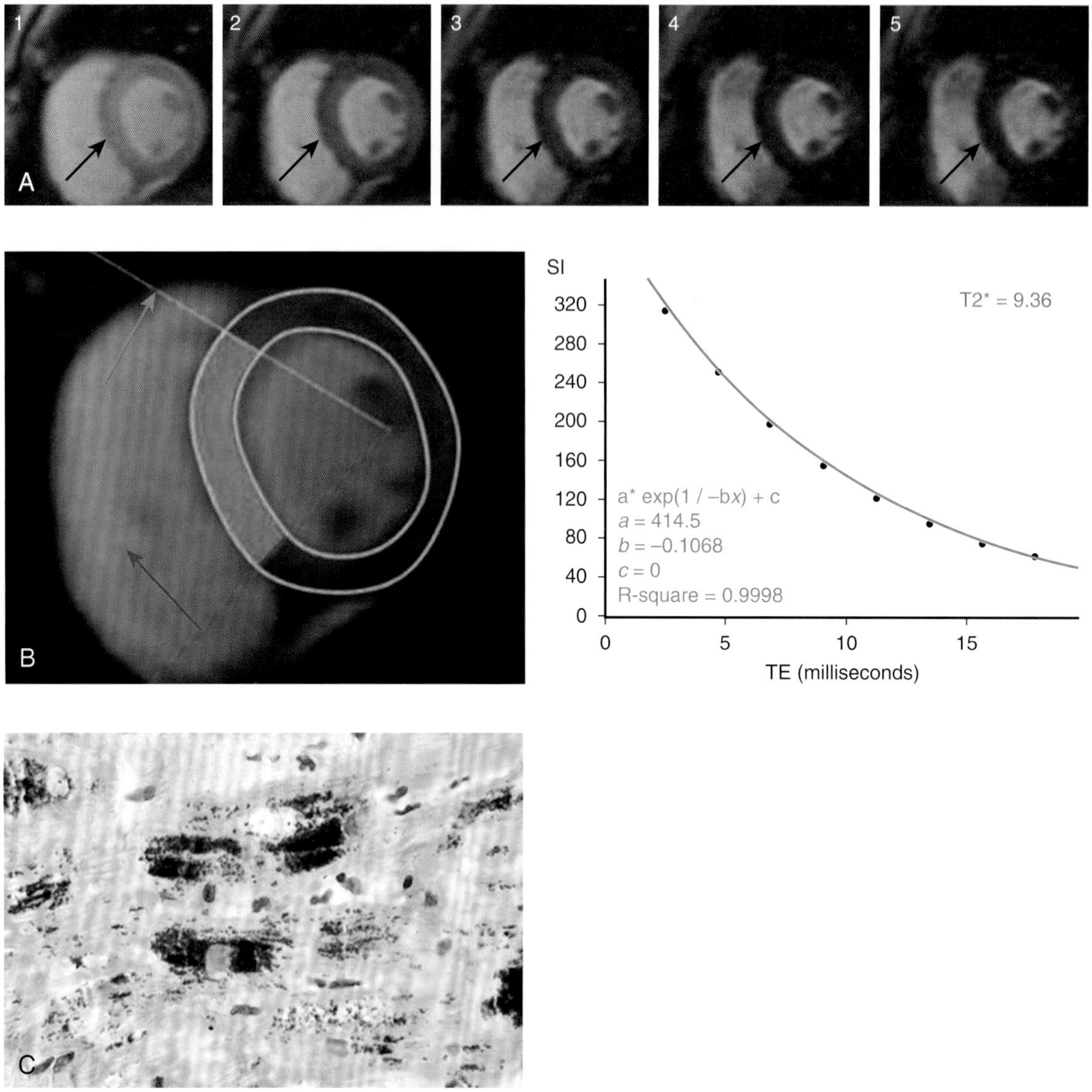

Fig. 14.8 Cardiac magnetic resonance imaging of iron-overload cardiomyopathy. (A) Short-axis imaging demonstrates bright-blood T2* sequence from a transfusion-dependent thalassemia patient. The myocardium *(arrows)* is initially bright, but the signal decays quickly due to the high myocardial iron content. (B) The calculated T2* value is 9.4 ms, which is indicative of severe iron overload. (C) High-power photomicrograph of ventricular myocytes with extensive sarcoplasmic iron accumulation *(blue)* (Prussian blue stain; original magnification ×400). (A and B, Adapted from Gupta A, Gulati GS, Seth S, Sharma S. Cardiac MRI in restrictive cardiomyopathy. *Clin Radiol.* 2012;67:95–105. C, Adapted from Pereira NL, Grogan M, Dec GW. Spectrum of restrictive and infiltrative cardiomyopathies: part 2 of a 2-part series. *J Am Coll Cardiol.* 2018;71:1149–1166.)

hypertrophy.[61] Systolic dysfunction can occur and is related to the degree and duration of iron overload. The cardiac MRI relaxation parameter R2* (assessed clinically via its reciprocal, T2*) has the ability to diagnose, estimate iron load, and monitor therapy in patients with cardiac hemochromatosis[62] (Fig. 14.8).

Treatment consists of maintenance phlebotomy and iron chelation therapy. Myocardial iron overload and resultant heart failure improve with the depletion of iron. Some patients present late in the advanced stages of a dilated cardiomyopathy and may require heart transplantation.[60]

SARCOIDOSIS

Sarcoidosis is a granulomatous disease of unknown etiology with a predilection for certain ethnic groups, particularly African Americans. Pulmonary sarcoid is often the first manifestation of the disease. Endomyocardial biopsy in the presence of noncaseating granulomas has a low sensitivity (19.2%) for diagnosis[56] due to a patchy distribution of the pathology and a predilection of granulomas for the cephalad portion of the septum, which is less accessible to biopsy. The yield of endomyocardial biopsy can be increased by utilizing electroanatomic mapping (electrophysiology study) to identify areas of low voltage that might represent granulomas that can be biopsied.[63] Historically, cardiac involvement was thought to occur in up to 25% of sarcoid cases; however, emerging data from cardiac MRI studies suggest that the prevalence is closer to 5% to 10%.

Clinical presentations vary and can include nonspecific palpitations, atrioventricular block, sudden cardiac death, and heart failure. RCM remains uncommon in sarcoidosis, and a high degree of suspicion is required because cardiac sarcoidosis is often misdiagnosed as genetic arrhythmogenic cardiomyopathy, hypertrophic cardiomyopathy, or dilated cardiomyopathy. Echocardiographic features of cardiac sarcoidosis include diastolic dysfunction with preserved systolic function,[61] wall motion abnormalities, LV aneurysm, systolic dysfunction, dilated cardiac chambers, conduction

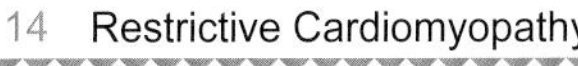

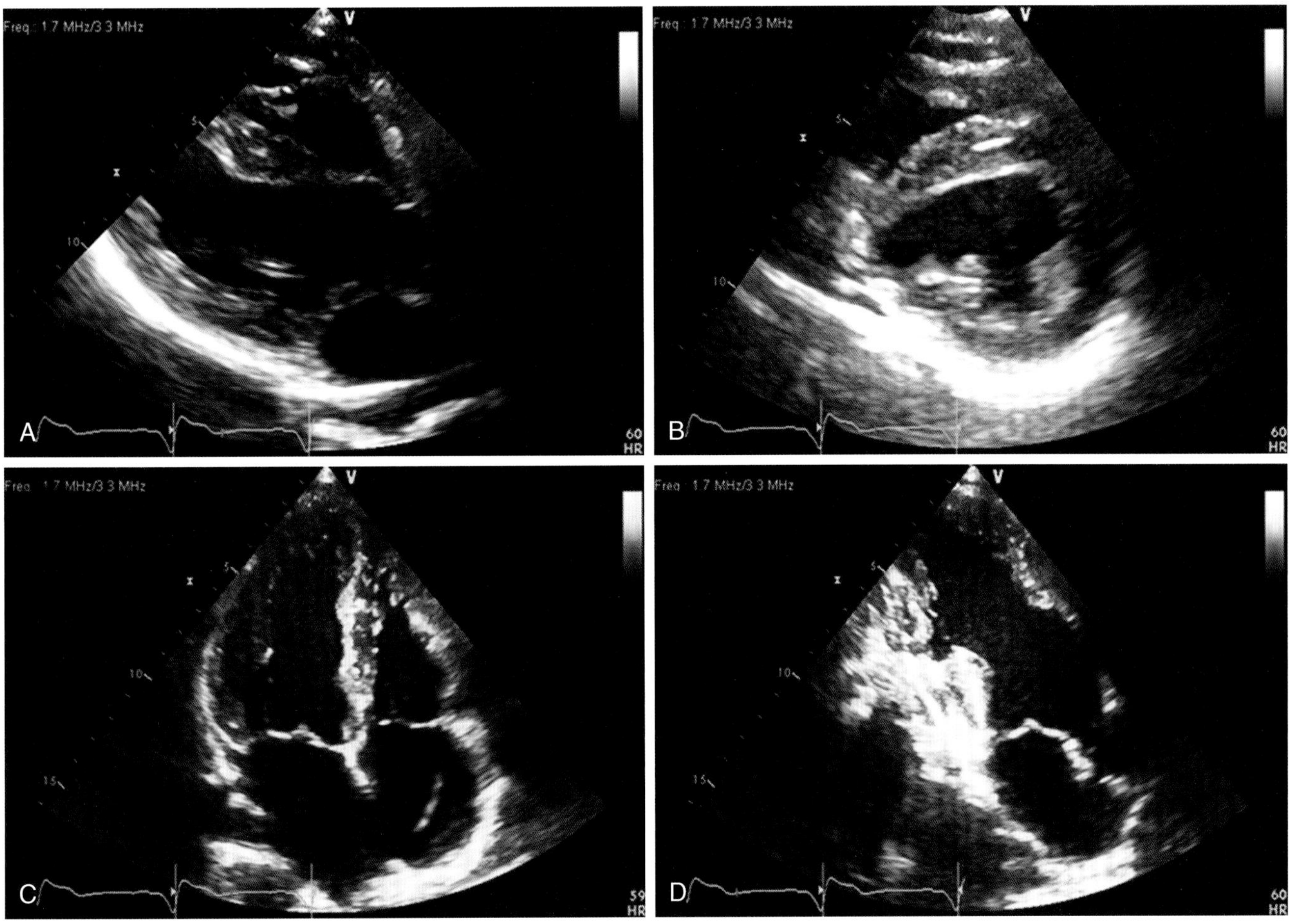

Fig. 14.9 Echocardiographic features of cardiac sarcoidosis. A 52-year-old man was diagnosed with sarcoid cardiomyopathy at age 34 years. He required an implanted cardiac defibrillator and pacemaker at age 35 years for complete heart block and reduced LV ejection fraction. New York Heart Association functional classification improved from class IV at presentation to class II. A parasternal long-axis view (A), a short-axis view at the mid-papillary muscle level (B), an apical 4-chamber view (LV on left side of the image) (C), and an apical 2- and 3-chamber view (D; Video 14.9D) are shown. Features include thinning of the basal septum (in A) and focal aneurysmal segments in the mid-inferior and basal inferolateral and basal lateral walls (in B and D). The ejection fraction was 45%.

abnormalities with diastolic mitral and tricuspid regurgitation, and pericardial effusion (Figs. 14.9 and 14.10). Sarcoid lesions are more prominent in the upper portions of the interventricular septum, where thinning, wall motion abnormalities, and asymmetric septal hypertrophy may be present.[62]

Cardiac MRI is the next step, after an echocardiogram, to evaluate the LV and RV morphology and for tissue characterization. Findings include increased T2 relaxation signals in areas of inflammation and LGE, typically in the basal inferolateral and/or septal walls, in a noncoronary distribution sparing the endocardium. Cardiac MRI is used as a screening test, followed by cardiac fluorodeoxyglucose (^{18}F) positron emission tomography (FDG-PET) as a confirmatory test. FDG-PET can be used to monitor response to therapy.[64] Cardiac involvement portends a worse prognosis, and treatment should be started immediately. Immunosuppression, typically with corticosteroids, is first-line therapy, combined with specific therapy for heart failure and device therapy (i.e., pacemaker, defibrillator) if needed.

STORAGE DISORDERS[63]

Glycogen Storage Disorder: Pompe Disease

Pompe disease is caused by alpha-1,4-glucosidase deficiency and is characterized by progressive deposition of glycogen in all tissues. The disease has an autosomal recessive inheritance with a predicted frequency of 1:40,000.

In 90% to 95% of patients with Pompe disease, there is an elevation of muscle enzymes (creatine phosphokinase, lactate dehydrogenase, alanine aminotransferase, and aspartate aminotransferase), and the diagnosis is confirmed by detection of a deficiency in leukocyte, fibroblast, or muscle alpha-glucosidase enzyme levels. More recently, gene testing has shown excellent diagnostic capability,[64a] and it is now the preferred method of diagnosis.

The classic infantile form of the disease occurs shortly after birth and is characterized by generalized muscular hypotonia and severe thickening of the myocardial walls; the juvenile and adult forms are typically without cardiac manifestations at presentation. Echocardiography reveals a hypertrophied LV, similar to what is seen in sarcomeric hypertrophic cardiomyopathy[65]; however, the underlying histopathology is completely different (see later discussion). Cardiac MRI in the juvenile- or adult-onset disease does not yield specific findings. In a study of 17 patients, LGE in a non-ischemic pattern was seen in 18%, and 21% had an elevated ECV fraction, suggestive of interstitial fibrosis.[66] Treatment with recombinant human alpha-glucosidase (enzyme replacement therapy) may result in regression of some of the phenotypic features of the disease.[67]

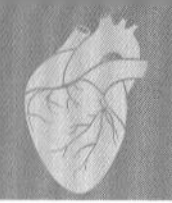

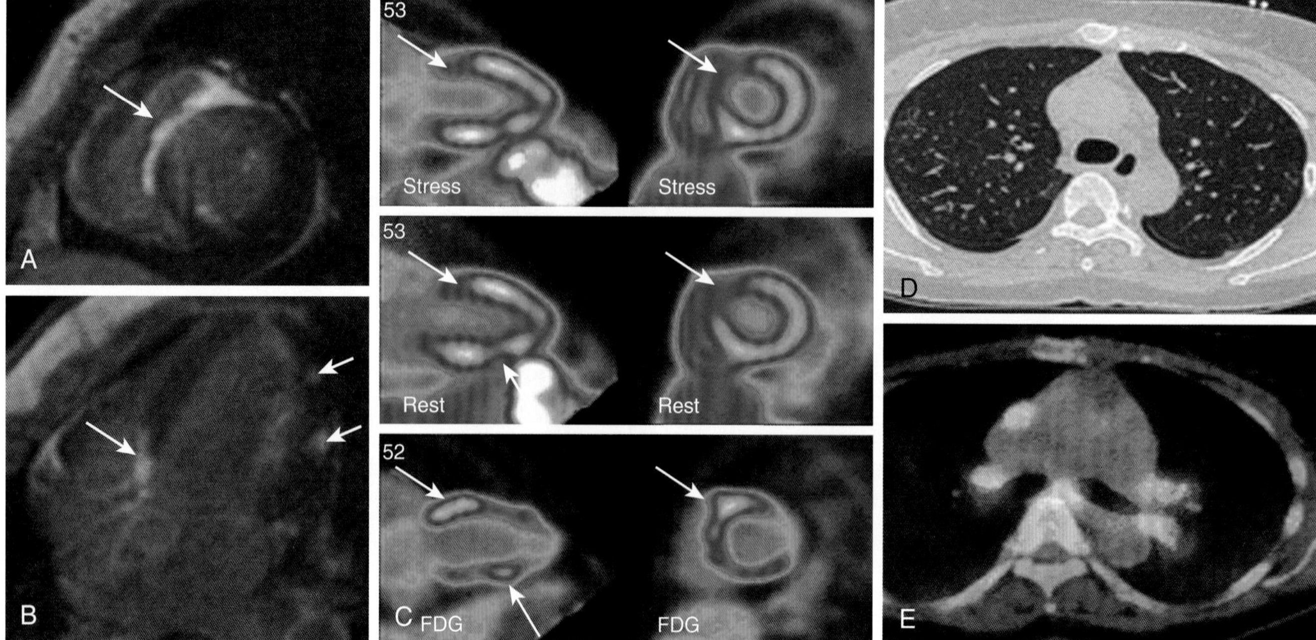

Fig. 14.10 **Multimodality imaging in cardiac sarcoidosis.** (A and B) Cardiac MRI delayed-enhancement images show late gadolinium uptake *(arrows)* in the basal anteroseptum, as well as in the lateral wall in B. (C) Fluorodeoxyglucose (^{18}F) positron emission tomography (FDG-PET) images demonstrate perfusion defects with increased FDG uptake. (D) Computed tomographic (CT) chest image demonstrates perilymphatic micronodules suspicious for pulmonary sarcoidosis. (E) PET/CT image shows multiple enlarged hypermetabolic mediastinal and hilar lymph nodes. (Adapted from Riggs J, Harb S. Cardiac sarcoidosis: a shocking diagnosis. *J Am Coll Cardiol.* 2019;73[9 suppl 1].)

Fabry Disease

Fabry disease is a rare X-linked recessive sphingolipidosis that results from defective activity of the lysosomal enzyme alpha-galactosidase A. Homozygous males have the most severe form of the disease, and heterozygous females usually have a more benign presentation. The enzymatic defect in this lysosomal storage disease leads to the accumulation of globotriaosylceramide (Gb3) in several organs, including skin, kidney, nervous system, cornea, and heart.

Fabry disease is a multisystem disease; cardiac manifestations may occur in conjunction with involvement of other organs or in isolation. Cardiac involvement typically occurs at a later age. Recent work suggests three phases of cardiac involvement: accumulation of Gb3, myocyte hypertrophy, and inflammation (Fig 14.11).[68] Cardiac manifestations are common in males and females, although females tend to have fewer clinical manifestations.[69,70] Notably, Gb3 accumulation within the myocardium does not correlate with the severity of LV hypertrophy.

Echocardiographic findings include concentric LV hypertrophy secondary to the deposition of Gb3 and subsequent cellular hypertrophy. If it is left untreated, systolic dysfunction and dilated cardiomyopathy ensue. The binary sign of the thickened LV myocardium reflects the compartmentalization of the Gb3 deposition in the LV (Fig 14.12). Initially it was thought to be a highly sensitive and specific sign of Fabry disease,[71] but subsequent publications found that it likely lacks the sensitivity for screening.[72,73] Myocardial strain is helpful in patients with LV hypertrophy when there is a suspicion for Fabry disease because the disease classically involves the inferolateral wall, and regional strain abnormalities in that territory may provide a diagnostic clue (Fig 14.13). With cardiac MRI, deposition of Gb3 leads to a decrease in T1 relaxation time,[74] and imaging with LGE tends to show mid-myocardial inferolateral enhancement[75] (see Fig. 14.11).

The diagnostic approach is sex-specific. For males, leukocyte alpha-galactosidase can be used as a screening tool, with decreased enzyme activity (<35%) triggering genetic testing for mutations in the *GLA* gene. In heterozygous females, there is variable expression of alpha-galactosidase A, making the enzyme assay unreliable and requiring genotyping for all females with suspected Fabry disease. Cardiac involvement is suspected on echocardiography and can be further evaluated with cardiac MRI. Endomyocardial biopsy is the gold standard to evaluate cardiac involvement, but it is rarely required today. If a biopsy is obtained, it reveals sarcoplasmic vacuolization (as opposed to myocyte hypertrophy) on light microscopy and concentric lamellar bodies within the sarcoplasm on electron microscopy.

LV systolic function progressively deteriorates in untreated Fabry disease. In a large cross-sectional study of a patient cohort from the Fabry disease clinical and genetic registry, the median cumulative survival time was 50 years, which represents an approximate 20-year reduction of life span.[76] Enzyme replacement therapy has been shown to result in clearing of vascular endothelial deposits of Gb3,[77] with potential improvement of LV mass and systolic function.[78,79] An alternative therapy is oral chaperone therapy with migalastat, which facilitates trafficking of alpha-galactosidase A into lysosomes, but only specific genetic variants are eligible.[80]

DRUG-INDUCED RESTRICTIVE CARDIOMYOPATHY

Although it is a rare consequence of anthracycline chemotherapy, fibrous thickening of the LV endocardium with features of RCM may occur.[81] Hydroxychloroquine has been known to cause an inflammatory RCM; although this complication is rare, it is important to keep it in mind because it resembles cardiac amyloidosis and will provide a false-positive technetium pyrophosphate scan.[82]

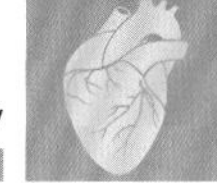

ACCUMULATION PHASE	INFLAMMATION AND MYOCYTE HYPERTROPHY PHASE	FIBROSIS AND IMPAIRMENT PHASE

Women (or men—some mutations)

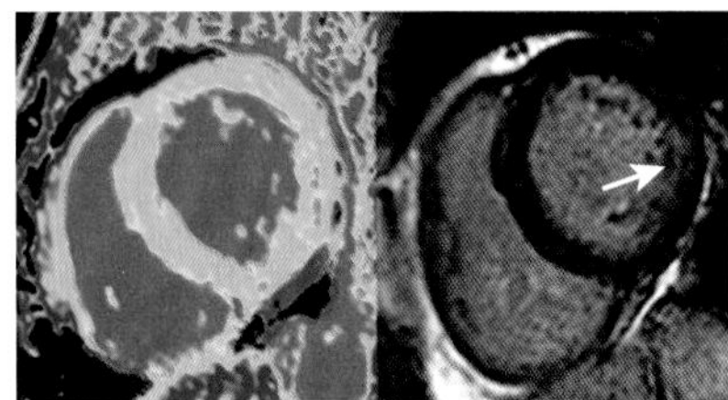

Low T1, LGE +ve
LVH −ve

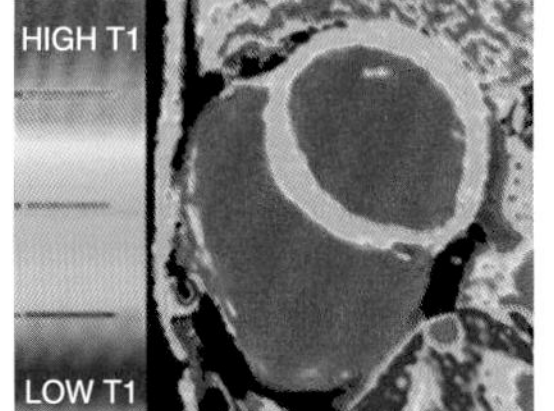

Normal T1,
LVH −ve

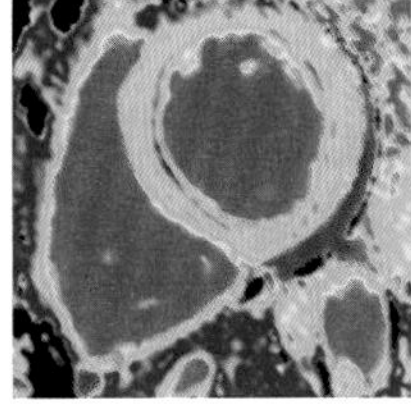

LOW T1,
LVH −ve

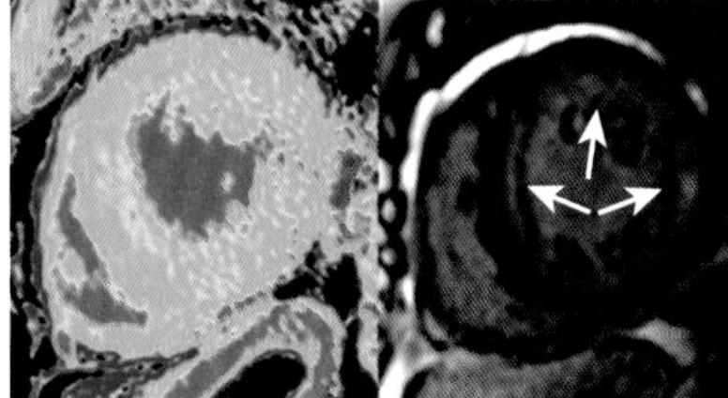

Normalizing T1,
extensive LGE

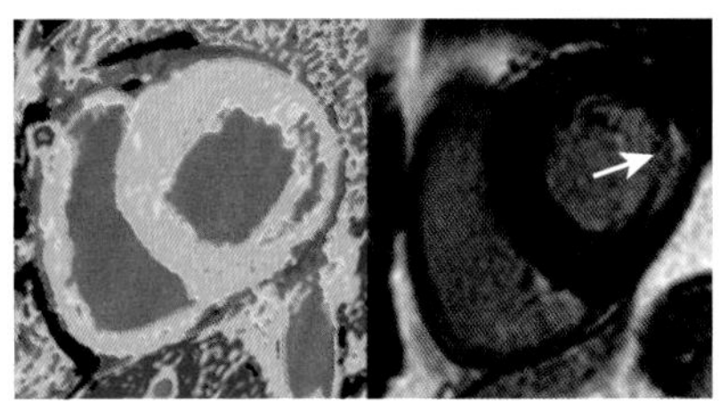

Low T1, LGE +ve
LVH +ve (men >> women)

Abnormal ECG — High troponin — High NT-proBNP

Fig. 14.11 **Proposed stages of Fabry disease based on cardiac magnetic resonance imaging.** The disease developmental model consists of an accumulation phase (silent myocyte storage and greater T1 lowering), an inflammation and myocyte hypertrophy phase, and a fibrosis and impairment (late) phase. *Arrows* indicate areas of late gadolinium enhancement (LGE) on cardiac MRI. *ECG*, Electrocardiogram; *LVH*, LV hypertrophy; *NT-proBNP*, N-terminal pro B-type natriuretic peptide; *-ve*, negative; *+ve*, positive. (Adapted from Nordin S, Kozor R, Medina-Menacho K, et al. Proposed stages of myocardial phenotype development in Fabry disease. *JACC Cardiovasc Imaging.* 2019;12[8 Pt 2]:1673–1683.)

POSTRADIATION CARDIOMYOPATHY

Radiation-induced cardiomyopathy is an uncommon complication of mediastinal radiotherapy. It most commonly occurs in survivors of Hodgkin lymphoma and is typically associated with radiation-induced pericardial and coronary artery diseases. The combination of mediastinal irradiation and anthracycline exposure leads to worse outcomes. Among Hodgkin lymphoma survivors who have received mediastinal radiotherapy with or without anthracyclines, the 40-year cumulative incidence of heart failure or cardiomyopathy was 8.1% for the first cardiac adverse event and 24.8% overall.[83] The risk appears to rise with increasing cumulative dose and sharply rises after a total dose of 21 gray or more, with a variable latent period. These estimates are changing rapidly, mirroring the improvements in radiotherapy technologies designed to target the tumor and decrease the dose to the heart.[84] Patients with prior mediastinal radiotherapy should be followed by cardiology, but management frequently requires a multidisciplinary team given the high incidence of cardiopulmonary disease (Figs. 14.14 and 14.15). Whereas standard supportive therapy is used for complications of irradiation, the damage inflicted by radiotherapy appears to reduce survival in patients undergoing cardiac surgery compared to matched controls with the same disease burden.[85]

OTHER CAUSES OF RESTRICTIVE CARDIOMYOPATHY

Rare causes of RCM include (1) metastatic malignant lymphomas, (2) connective tissue diseases such as scleroderma and systemic lupus erythematosus, (3) carcinoid disease, (4) late stages of hypertrophic obstructive cardiomyopathy, and (5) primary oxaluria; also, calcified endocardial bands may be seen in those with RCM due to pseudoxanthoma elasticum.

DIFFERENTIATING BETWEEN RESTRICTIVE CARDIOMYOPATHY AND CONSTRICTIVE PERICARDITIS

Constrictive pericarditis and RCM should be considered in any patient with a disproportionate degree of right heart failure in the setting of a normal or mildly depressed LV systolic function and normal or mildly abnormal valvular function. Given

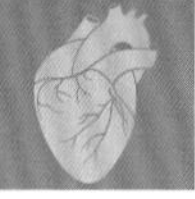

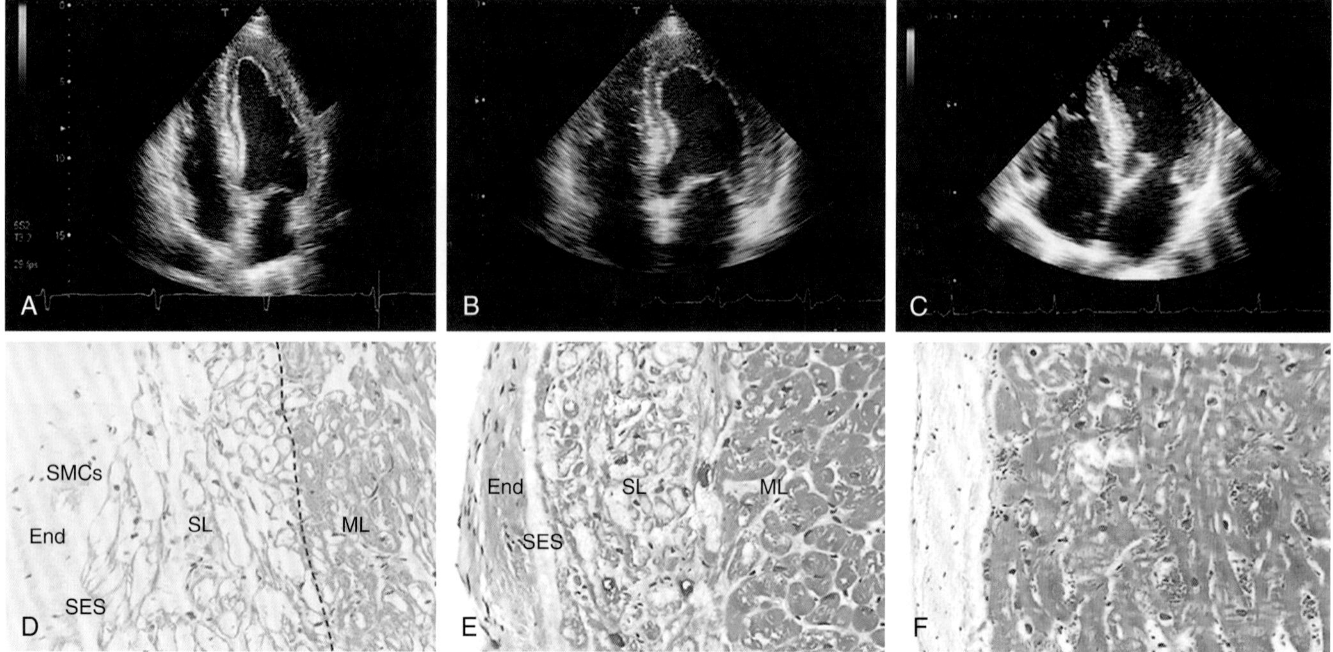

Fig. 14.12 The binary sign on echocardiography. 2D Echocardiograms in 4-chamber apical view (A–C) and LV endomyocardial biopsy specimens (D–F) from two patients with Fabry disease cardiomyopathy (A + D, B + E, respectively) and a patient with hypertrophic cardiomyopathy (C + F). Comparison of the three echocardiographic frames reveals a binary appearance of the LV endocardial border in the two patients with Fabry disease (A, B). This echocardiographic finding reflects the glycosphingolipids compartmentalization involving a thickened endocardium *(End)* with enlarged and engulfed smooth muscle cells *(SMCs)*, a subendocardial empty space *(SES)*, and a prominent involvement of the subendocardial myocardial layer *(SL)*, while the middle layer *(ML)* appears partially spared (D, E). This echocardiographic pattern is absent in hypertrophic cardiomyopathy (C), despite a similar thickening of the endocardium (F). (Adapted from Pieroni M, Chimenti C, De Cobelli F, et al. Fabry's disease cardiomyopathy: echocardiographic detection of endomyocardial glycosphingolipid compartmentalization. *J Am Coll Cardiol*. 2006;47[8]:1663–1671.)

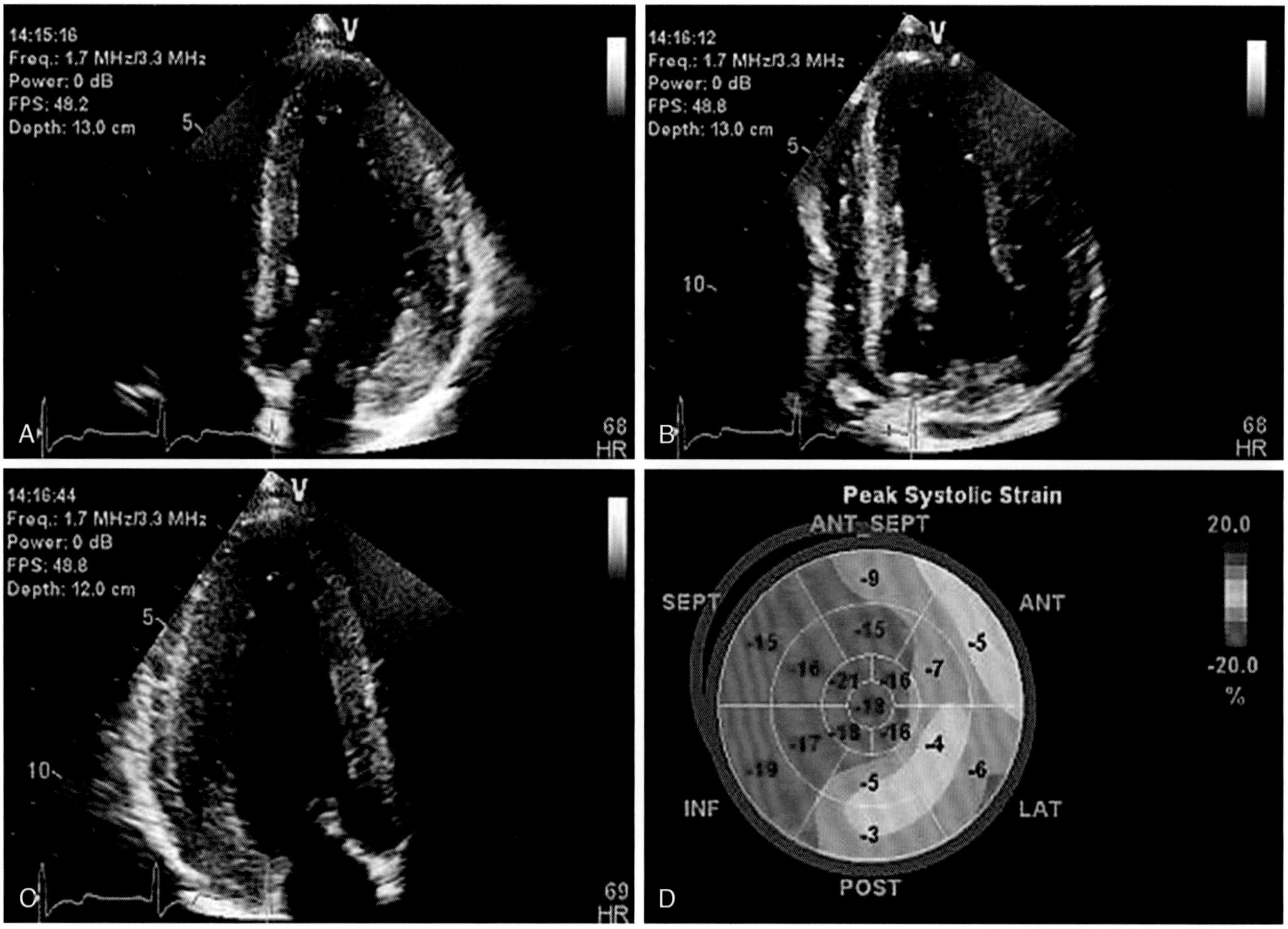

Fig. 14.13 A 37-year-old man with Fabry disease. The apical 4-chamber view (A), apical 2-chamber view (B), apical 3-chamber view (C), and strain pattern on a polar map (D) reveal LV hypertrophy, the binary sign of the LV, and a typical strain pattern with decreased longitudinal strain in the lateral and inferolateral walls.

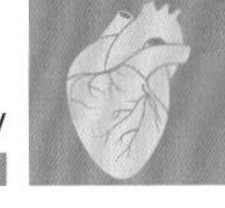

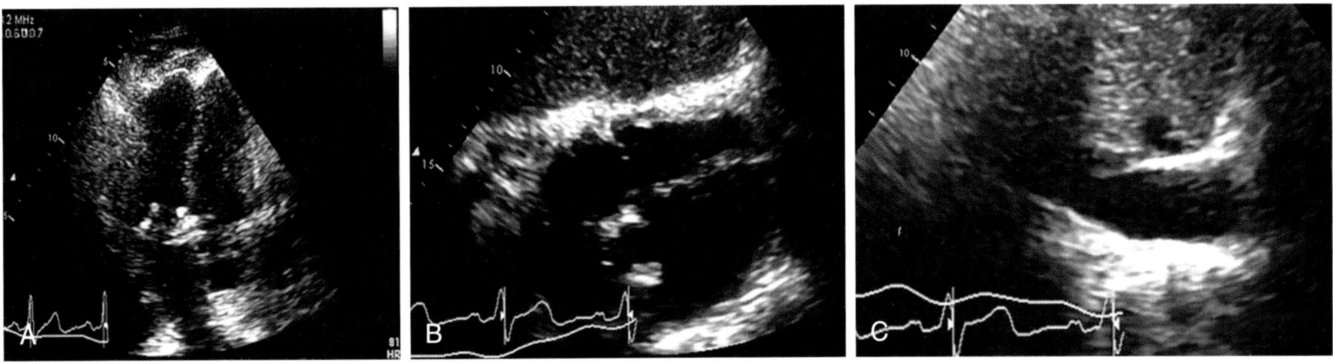

Fig. 14.14 Echocardiographic findings in radiation-induced cardiomyopathy. The patient was a 59-year-old man with chronic dyspnea on exertion and a history of radiation treatment for Hodgkin lymphoma requiring bioprosthetic mitral valve replacement. (A) Apical 4-chamber view shows paradoxical interventricular septal motion and a normal-appearing bioprosthetic mitral valve (the LV and LA are shown on the left side). (B) Subcostal view shows the RV adherent to the diaphragm because of pericardial adhesions. (C) Subcostal view shows a dilated inferior vena cava with reduced inspiratory collapse.

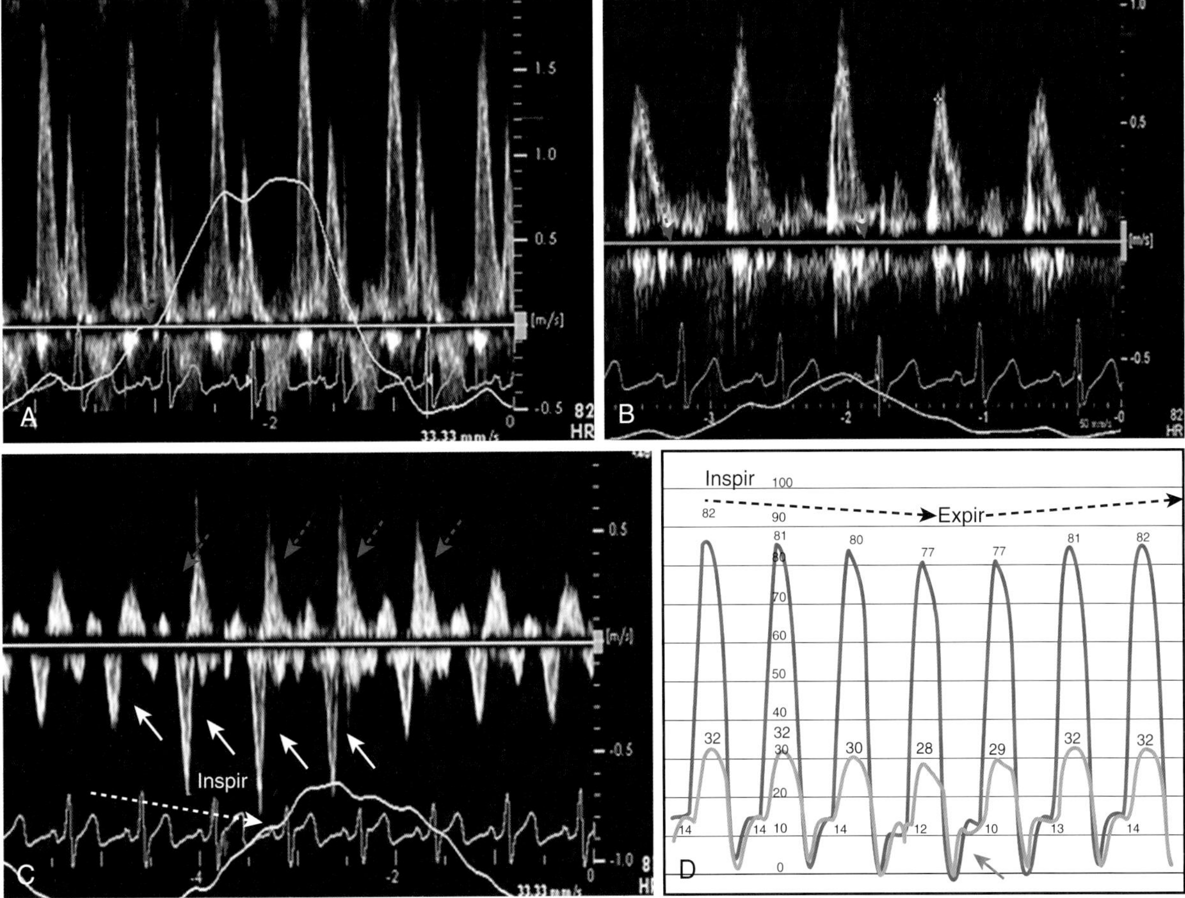

Fig. 14.15 Pulsed-wave Doppler findings in radiation-induced cardiomyopathy. The patient was a 59-year-old man with chronic dyspnea on exertion and a history of radiation therapy for Hodgkin lymphoma requiring bioprosthetic mitral valve replacement. (A) Pulsed-wave (PW) Doppler image of mitral inflow shows no significant respiratory variation and a restrictive filling pattern with a short deceleration time *(red arrow)* despite the presence of a 29-mm bioprosthetic mitral valve, suggesting a stiff LV with high filling pressures. (B) Tricuspid inflow PW Doppler image shows minimal A-wave forward flow with inspiration and prominent backward atrial flow into the hepatic vein, indicating RV noncompliance. The tricuspid deceleration time shortens progressively during inspiration *(red arrows)*. The deceleration times were 210 ms during apnea, 180 ms during the first beat of inspiration, and 160 ms during the second beat of inspiration, indicating RV noncompliance. (C) PW Doppler image of the hepatic vein. Velocities below the baseline reflect venous flow into the heart, and those above the baseline reflect reflux back into the hepatic vein. On inspiration *(white arrows)*, inflow time shortens (shown by the steeper slope of the velocity signal), and increased A-wave reversal *(red arrows)* indicates RV noncompliance due to increased RV volume with inspiration. These changes match the shortening of tricuspid inflow deceleration time in B; they are characteristic of restrictive cardiomyopathy and not of pericardial constriction. (D) LV and RV pressure tracings show equalization of RV and LV end-diastolic pressures. With inspiration the slope of the rise of both RV and LV rapid filling waves *(red arrow)* is increased. Concordance of LV and RV systolic pressures during inspiration and expiration is shown by *dashed black arrows*. These findings are typical of restrictive cardiomyopathy and not of pericardial constriction. These findings were present despite the patient's dehydrated and veno-dilated state at the time of cardiac catheterization, with a drop in systolic blood pressure from 140 mmHg at the start of the procedure to 85 mmHg during catheterization. These changes also match the shortening of tricuspid inflow deceleration time seen on PW Doppler imaging in B.

TABLE 14.4 Echocardiographic Features of Restrictive Cardiomyopathy and Constrictive Pericarditis.

	Restrictive Cardiomyopathy	*Constrictive Pericarditis*
Pericardium	Normal	Thickened
LV	Small	Small
	May show systolic dysfunction	Systolic function is usually normal but may be abnormal, particularly after CABG or radiation
	No septal bounce	Septal bounce and septal shift
Atria	Usually dilated	Usually nondilated but may be dilated in late stages
Mitral and tricuspid inflow	Increased E/A ratio, short DT	Increased E/A ratio, short DT
	No significant respiratory variation of E velocity	>25% expiratory increase in E velocity mitral inflow
		>25%–40% inspiratory increase in tricuspid E velocity
	Diastolic MR	Diastolic MR
Velocities by TDI	Markedly reduced	E/E′ < 15 despite volume overload (annulus paradoxus). Medial E′ > lateral E′ (annulus reversus).
Circumferential strain	Normal	Reduced
Peak radial strain LV base	Normal	Reduced
Net twist	Normal	Reduced
Basal longitudinal strain	Reduced	Normal
Apical untwisting velocities	Normal	Reduced
Pulmonary vein inflow	Decreased S/D ratio (typically <0.5)	S/D ratio = 1
	Prominent atrial reversal	Decrease in S and D wave with inspiration
	No significant respiratory change	
Inferior vena cava	Dilated	Dilated
Hepatic veins	Blunted S/D ratio. Diastolic flow reversal during inspiration.	Inspiration: minimal increase in S and D velocity; diastolic flow reversal during expiration, ratio of expiratory-to-inspiratory flow reversal >0.79, >25% increase in atrial reversal in expiration compared with inspiration.
Peak PA pressure	>40 mmHg	<40 mmHg
Color M-mode	Decreased Vp <45 cm/s	Normal or increased >100 cm/s
Mitral annular Doppler	Low velocity <8 cm/s	High velocity ≥8 cm/s

CABG, Coronary artery bypass grafting surgery; *D*, diastolic; *DT*, deceleration time; *MR*, mitral regurgitation; *PA*, pulmonary artery; *S*, systolic; *TDI*, tissue Doppler imaging; *Vp*, propagation velocity.
Adapted from Kushwaha S, Fallon JT, Fuster V. Restrictive cardiomyopathy. *N Engl J Med*. 1997;336:267–276; Goldstein JA. Cardiac tamponade, constrictive pericarditis, and restrictive cardiomyopathy. *Curr Probl Cardiol*. 2004;29:503–567.

that the treatment approach is completely different for these two entities, differentiation between them is critical. A number of studies have reported specific 2D and Doppler features that help differentiate RCM from constrictive pericarditis.[92] Echocardiographic features differentiating the two conditions are listed in Table 14.4.

A history of prior pericarditis, cardiac surgery, or irradiation makes a diagnosis of constriction more likely. Pericardial calcification on chest radiography and thickened pericardium on computed tomography or cardiac MRI are diagnostic findings of constriction. However, absence of thickened pericardium or calcification does not rule out pericardial constriction. For example, in about 18% of patients with surgically proven constriction, pericardial thickness was not increased on noninvasive imaging because of the patchy nature of pericardial involvement.[86] Cardiac MRI provides morphoanatomic insights, similar to echocardiography, in addition to comprehensive and superior direct imaging of the pericardium. As such, cardiac MRI is a key modality in the diagnostic evaluation of pericardial constriction.[87] The outcome of surgical pericardectomy is best for patients with idiopathic pericarditis followed by postoperative constriction; patients with radiation pericarditis have an overall difficult clinical course and a poor overall prognosis.

Both constrictive pericarditis and RCM are associated with increased intracardiac filling pressures. The most important pathophysiologic feature of constrictive pericarditis is dissociation of intrathoracic and intracardiac pressures with increased ventricular interdependence. Negative chest pressure during inspiration is not transmitted to the cardiac chambers, and this causes a decrease in transmitral gradient during the inspiratory phase, secondary to a more pronounced decrease in pulmonary venous pressure relative to LV diastolic pressure. In constrictive pericarditis, there is an abrupt diastolic shift in the ventricular septum toward the LV during inspiration and toward the RV during expiration. Doppler echocardiography demonstrates exaggerated interventricular interdependence in constrictive pericarditis by showing marked respiratory variations on mitral and tricuspid flow Doppler images. The characteristic respiratory variations in Doppler flow velocities in patients with constriction that are not seen in patients with restriction include the following: more than 25% expiratory increase in mitral E velocity; expiratory decrease in hepatic vein diastolic flow velocity (mnemonic: RICE [restriction inspiratory, constriction expiratory]); more than 25% increase in diastolic hepatic vein flow reversals compared with inspiratory velocity; greater respiratory variation in pulmonary venous flows; and a systolic pulmonary vein flow velocity lower than diastolic velocity throughout respiration.[29,88] Ventricular interdependence is absent in RCM.

Early diastolic mitral annular velocity (E′) by TDI can be used to differentiate constrictive pericarditis from RCM.[9] Patients with constrictive pericarditis have a significantly higher *e′* at the septal annulus than those with primary RCM or cardiac

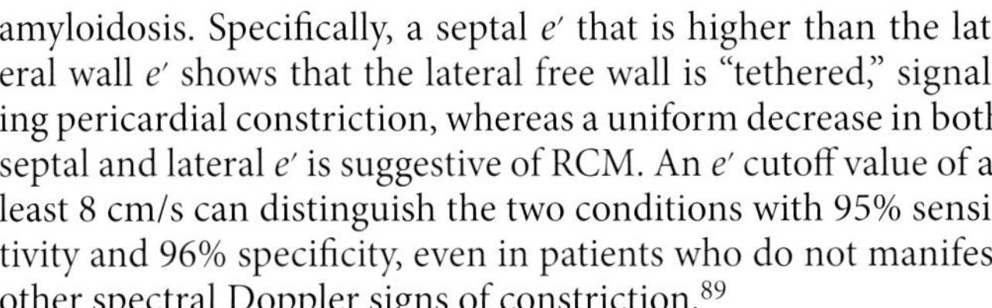

amyloidosis. Specifically, a septal *e′* that is higher than the lateral wall *e′* shows that the lateral free wall is "tethered," signaling pericardial constriction, whereas a uniform decrease in both septal and lateral *e′* is suggestive of RCM. An *e′* cutoff value of at least 8 cm/s can distinguish the two conditions with 95% sensitivity and 96% specificity, even in patients who do not manifest other spectral Doppler signs of constriction.[89]

Along with an increased *e′* mitral annular velocity, patients with constriction and normal diastolic function show a rapid propagation slope on color M-mode images of greater than 100 cm/s. In the constrictive group, the maximal velocity reaches the apex almost instantaneously, compared with a significant delay in the restrictive group. Even if mitral and pulmonary vein inflow are not diagnostic, TDI and color M-mode are able to correctly differentiate patients with constrictive pericarditis from those with RCM. The presence of ventricular septal shift in combination with either a medial *e′* of at least 9 cm/s or a hepatic vein expiratory diastolic reversal ratio of at least 0.79 corresponded to a sensitivity of 87% and a specificity of 91% in diagnosing pericardial constriction and differentiating it from RCM.[89a] In some patients who have undergone aggressive diuresis, volume loading helps to bring out the specific features of constrictive pericarditis.[90] Alternatively, preload reduction helps to bring out the respiratory variation in volume-overloaded patients.[91]

Some patients may have features of mixed RCM and constrictive pericarditis, such as those with active myocarditis, postradiation cardiomyopathy, or concomitant underlying cardiomyopathy with superimposed pericarditis. In patients with clinical and echo-Doppler features of RCM, constriction should still be excluded given the dramatically different treatment strategies.

Recent observations using 2D speckle tracking have shown that deformation of the LV is constrained in the circumferential direction in constrictive pericarditis and in the longitudinal direction in RCM.[92] A longitudinal TDI *e′* velocity of 5 cm/s had 92% sensitivity and 90% specificity; peak untwisting velocity of −50 degrees/s had 57% sensitivity and 95% specificity; and net LV twist of 10 degrees had 83% sensitivity and 84% specificity in differentiating constrictive pericarditis from RCM[92] (see Fig. 14.15).

At times, echocardiographic characteristics are not diagnostic and hemodynamic characterization with invasive catheterization, with the option of endomyocardial biopsy, is indicated. Importantly, most hemodynamic metrics are relatively unreliable in differentiating constrictive pericarditis from RCM. The only sign that has shown good performance is the systolic area index. Using simultaneous LV and RV pressure waveforms, the ratio of RV to LV waveform area on inspiration versus expiration is quantified. A cutoff value of greater than 1.1 has a sensitivity of 97% and a specificity of 100% for constrictive pericarditis. This finding reflects the hallmark of constrictive pericarditis, respirophasic ventricular interdependence.[93]

Patients with atrial fibrillation and irregular RR intervals present another hurdle in diagnostic evaluation for both echocardiographic and hemodynamic assessments. Cardiac MRI offers a wealth of morphoanatomic information; it allows measurement of respirophasic ventricular interdependence (the difference in maximal septal excursion between inspiration and expiration, normalized to biventricular diameter) and aids in making the diagnosis.[94] A practical approach to differentiating constrictive pericarditis from RCM is to start with the history and physical examination, then use echocardiography, followed by cardiac MRI and, for the minority of patients who remain without a diagnosis, move to invasive hemodynamic evaluation.

SUMMARY Restrictive Cardiomyopathy

Element	Modality	Views	Image Acquisition Pearls	Measurement	Key Findings
LV wall thickness	2D, M-mode, 3D	PLAX, PSAX, apical, and SC	Horizontal IVS in parasternal views	IVS, posterior wall, RWT, LV mass (M-mode, 2D, and 3D)	LV hypertrophy
LV size	2D, M-mode	PLAX, PSAX	Perpendicular alignment to IVS	LVEDD, LVESD	Usually small LV dimensions
LV volume	2D, 3D	Apical 4-, 2-, and 3-chamber	Non-foreshortened views, contrast if needed	LVESV, LVEDV, SV	Decreased LV volumes
LV myocardial appearance	2D	PLAX, PSAX			Ventricular thrombi or apical mass despite normal underlying wall motion
IVS motion	2D, M-mode	PLAX, PSAX, apical, SC		Visual	Square root sign in the IVS and in the inferolateral wall motion
LA size	2D	PLAX, apical views	Non-foreshortened atrial views	AP diameter, volume/m^2	Usually marked LA enlargement

SUMMARY Restrictive Cardiomyopathy—Cont'd

Element	Modality	Views	Image Acquisition Pearls	Measurement	Key Findings
RA size	2D	Apical 4-chamber	Non-foreshortened apical views, RV focused	LA AP diameter, volume/m^2	Usually marked RA enlargement
RV size	2D	PLAX, PSAX, RV inflow, apical 4-chamber, SC		RV ED length, RVOT, and basal and mid-RV ED diameter	
Pericardium	2D, M-mode	PLAX, PSAX, RV inflow, apical 4-chamber, SC	Mitral, tricuspid, PV, and hepatic vein flow respiratory variation	Effusion, thickness and brightness	May show small pericardial effusion
Valves	2D, M-mode, color Doppler	PLAX, PSAX, apical views	Focused valve views, use zoom function	Regurgitation severity	Homogenous AV valve thickening, occasional atrial septal thickening
			Quantitation of regurgitation by PISA and continuity equation		MR and TR due to leaflet or papillary muscle involvement (as in endomyocardial fibrosis)
					TR possibly secondary to pulmonary hypertension
					Diastolic MR due to increased LV ED pressure
					Diastolic TR and MR due to first-degree AV block or complete heart block
LV function	2D, M-mode, 3D, speckle tracking	PLAX, PSAX, apical views	Non-foreshortened apical views, contrast if needed, 3D	FS, wall motion, LVEDV, LVESV, LVEF (biplane Simpson), 3D volumes	Normal to increased LVEF in early stages, mildly reduced LV function in later stages
Mitral inflow	PW Doppler	Apical 4-chamber	Parallel alignment to flow	E, A, E/A ratio, E-wave DT, A duration, E/E′	Tall E wave, small A wave; E/A ratio >2
					Short DT <150 ms; short IVRT <60 ms
					No significant change in mitral E wave, DT, or IVRT with Valsalva maneuver
					Abnormal relaxation pattern with E/A ratio <1 and prolonged DT in early stages
					Pseudonormal and reversible restrictive pattern in intermediate stages

Continued

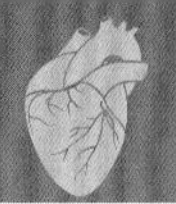

SUMMARY Restrictive Cardiomyopathy—Cont'd

Element	Modality	Views	Image Acquisition Pearls	Measurement	Key Findings
PV inflow	PW Doppler	Apical 4-chamber (2- or 3-chamber may be used)	Parallel alignment, PW sample volume 0.5 cm within the PV	S/D ratio, D DT, A duration	Dilated PVs, diastolic dominant pattern, and S/D ratio <0.5
					Prominent atrial reversal velocity with PV atrial A duration > mitral inflow A duration
					Rapid D wave DT in late stages
					No change in D wave with respiration
Mitral annular TDI	Tissue Doppler	Apical 4-chamber	Appropriate gain, scale, and frame rate	E′, E/E′ (medial and lateral)	E/E′ ratio to assess LVFP; in RCM, E′ usually <8 cm/s and E/E′ >15 due to elevated LVFP
Velocity of propagation	Color M-mode	Apical 4-chamber	Narrow sector, zoom LV, decrease color Doppler scale	Slope of Vp, IVRT, E and A waves	Vp usually <45 cm/s in RCM; E/Vp >1.5 and can be used to assess LVFP
IVRT	CW, PW, M-mode	Apical views	Appropriate frame rate	IVRT	Prolonged IVRT in early stages, short IVRT in late stages
Pulmonary artery pressure	CW Doppler	RV inflow, apical 4-chamber, SC	Use saline contrast if needed	PASP	Usually increased
RA pressure	2D, M-mode	SC	Long loop to show IVC size during respiration	IVC size and respiratory variation	Dilated with reduced respiratory variation; increased in late stages
RV function	2D, TDI	PLAX, PSAX, RV inflow, apical 4-chamber, SC		TAPSE, S′, fractional area change, RV GLS, RV free wall strain	Reduced in later stages; may be reduced by TDI and strain imaging at earlier stages
RV diastolic function	PW, color Doppler, M-mode	SC	Parallel alignment to color Doppler inflow, gain, depth, and scale settings	RV inflow PW Doppler, hepatic vein size, S/D ratio, inspiratory diastolic velocities and diastolic flow reversal	Restrictive filling; increased E/A ratio and short DT; with inspiration, further shortening of the DT and minimal change in E/A ratio, dilated hepatic veins, S/D ratio <0.5, and prominent atrial reversals that increase with inspiration

A, Atrial-induced LV filling velocity; *AP*, anteroposterior; *AV*, atrioventricular; *D*, pulmonary venous diastolic wave; *DT*, deceleration time; *E*, early diastolic LV filling velocity; *E′*, mitral annular early diastolic velocity; *ED*, end-diastolic; *FS*, fractional shortening; *GLS*, global longitudinal strain; *IVS*, interventricular septum; *IVC*, inferior vena cava; *IVRT*, isovolumic relaxation time; *LVEDD*, LV end-diastolic diameter; *LVEDV*, LV end-diastolic volume; *LVEF*, LV ejection fraction; *LVESD*, LV end-systolic diameter; *LVESV*, LV end-systolic volume; *LVFP*, LV filling pressure; *MR*, mitral regurgitation; *PASP*, pulmonary artery systolic pressure; *PISA*, proximal isovelocity surface area; *PLAX*, parasternal long axis; *PSAX*, parasternal short axis; *PV*, pulmonary vein; *RCM*, restrictive cardiomyopathy; *RVOT*, RV outflow tract; *RWT*, relative wall thickness; *S*, PV systolic wave; *S′*, PV systolic wave velocity; *SC*, subcostal; *SV*, stroke volume; *TAPSE*, tricuspid annular plane systolic excursion by M-mode echocardiography; *TDI*, tissue Doppler imaging; *TR*, tricuspid regurgitation; *Vp*, velocity of propagation.

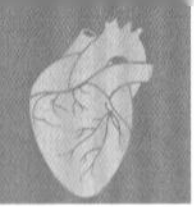

REFERENCES

1. Koyama J, Ray-Sequin PA, Falk RH. Longitudinal myocardial function assessed by tissue velocity, strain, and strain rate tissue Doppler echocardiography in patients with AL (primary) cardiac amyloidosis. *Circulation.* 2003;107(19):2446-2452.
2. Buss SJ, Emami M, Mereles D, et al. Longitudinal left ventricular function for prediction of survival in systemic light-chain amyloidosis: incremental value compared with clinical and biochemical markers. *J Am Coll Cardiol.* 2012;60(12):1067–1076.
3. Phelan D, Collier P, Thavendiranathan P, et al. Relative apical sparing of longitudinal strain using two-dimensional speckle-tracking echocardiography is both sensitive and specific for the diagnosis of cardiac amyloidosis. *Heart (British Cardiac Society).* 2012;98(19):1442–1448.
4. Cameli M, Mandoli GE, Loiacono F, et al. Left atrial strain: a new parameter for assessment of left ventricular filling pressure. *Heart Fail Rev.* 2016;21(1):65–76.
5. Nochioka K, Quarta CC, Claggett B, et al. Left atrial structure and function in cardiac amyloidosis. *Eur Heart J Cardiovasc Imaging.* 2017;18(10):1128–1137.
6. Plana JC, Mikati IA, Dokainish H, et al. A randomized cross-over study for evaluation of the effect of image optimization with contrast on the diagnostic accuracy of dobutamine echocardiography in coronary artery disease the OPTIMIZE Trial. *JACC Cardiovasc Imaging.* 2008;1(2):145–152.
7. Terasawa A, Miyatake K, Nakatani S, et al. Enhancement of Doppler flow signals in the left heart chambers by intravenous injection of sonicated albumin. *J Am Coll Cardiol.* 1993;21(3):737–742.
8. Lang RM, Badano LP, Mor-Avi V, et al. Recommendations for cardiac chamber quantification by echocardiography in adults: an update from the American Society of Echocardiography and the European Association of Cardiovascular Imaging. *J Am Soc Echocardiogr.* 2015;28(1):1–39.e14.
9. Nagueh SF, Mikati I, Kopelen HA, et al. Doppler estimation of left ventricular filling pressure in sinus tachycardia. A new application of tissue Doppler imaging. *Circulation.* 1998;98(16):1644–1650.
10. Ha JW, Oh JK, Ling LH, et al. Annulus paradoxus: transmitral flow velocity to mitral annular velocity ratio is inversely proportional to pulmonary capillary wedge pressure in patients with constrictive pericarditis. *Circulation.* 2001;104(9):976–978.
11. Rajagopalan N, Garcia MJ, Rodriguez L, et al. Comparison of new Doppler echocardiographic methods to differentiate constrictive pericardial heart disease and restrictive cardiomyopathy. *Am J Cardiol.* 2001;87(1):86–94.
12. Nagueh SF, Smiseth OA, Appleton CP, et al. Recommendations for the evaluation of left ventricular diastolic function by echocardiography: an update from the American Society of Echocardiography and the European Association of Cardiovascular Imaging. *J Am Soc Echocardiogr.* 2016;29(4):277–314.
13. Oikonomou EK, Kokkinidis DG, Kampaktsis PN, et al. Assessment of prognostic value of left ventricular global longitudinal strain for early prediction of chemotherapy-induced cardiotoxicity: a systematic review and meta-analysis. *JAMA Cardiol.* 2019.
14. Habibi M, Zareian M, Ambale Venkatesh B, et al. Left atrial mechanical function and incident ischemic cerebrovascular events independent of AF: insights from the MESA study. *JACC Cardiovasc Imaging.* 2019.
15. Henein MY, Suhr OB, Arvidsson S, et al. Reduced left atrial myocardial deformation irrespective of cavity size: a potential cause for atrial arrhythmia in hereditary transthyretin amyloidosis. *Amyloid.* 2018;25(1):46–53.
16. Gonzalez-Lopez E, Gallego-Delgado M, Guzzo-Merello G, et al. Wild-type transthyretin amyloidosis as a cause of heart failure with preserved ejection fraction. *Eur Heart J.* 2015;36(38):2585–2594.
17. Castaño A, Narotsky DL, Hamid N, et al. Unveiling transthyretin cardiac amyloidosis and its predictors among elderly patients with severe aortic stenosis undergoing transcatheter aortic valve replacement. *Eur Heart J.* 2017 38(38):2879–2887.
18. Falk RH, Alexander KM, Liao R, et al. (Light-Chain) cardiac amyloidosis: a review of diagnosis and therapy. *J Am Coll Cardiol.* 2016;68(12):1323–1341.
19. Flodrova P, Flodr P, Pika T, et al. Cardiac amyloidosis: from clinical suspicion to morphological diagnosis. *Pathology.* 2018;50(3): 261–268.
20. Kyle RA, Larson DR, Kurtin PJ, et al. Incidence of AL amyloidosis in Olmsted County, Minnesota, 1990 through 2015. *Mayo Clin Proc.* 2019;94(3):465–471.
21. Kyle RA, Linos A, Beard CM, et al. Incidence and natural history of primary systemic amyloidosis in Olmsted County, Minnesota, 1950 through 1989. *Blood.* 1992;79(7):1817–1822.
22. Sperry BW, Reyes BA, Ikram A, et al. Tenosynovial and cardiac amyloidosis in patients undergoing carpal tunnel Release. *J Am Coll Cardiol.* 2018;72(17):2040–2050.
23. Geller HI, Singh A, Alexander KM, et al. Association between ruptured distal biceps tendon and wild-type transthyretin cardiac amyloidosis. JAMA. 2017;318(10):962–963.
24. Rajkumar SV, Dimopoulos MA, Palumbo A, et al. International Myeloma Working Group updated criteria for the diagnosis of multiple myeloma. *Lancet Oncol.* 2014;15(12):e538–e548.
25. Kumar S, Dispenzieri A, Lacy MQ, et al. Revised prognostic staging system for light chain amyloidosis incorporating cardiac biomarkers and serum free light chain measurements. *J Clin Oncol.* 2012;30(9):989–995.
26. Rahman JE, Helou EF, Gelzer-Bell R, et al. Noninvasive diagnosis of biopsy-proven cardiac amyloidosis. *J Am Coll Cardiol.* 2004;43(3):410–415.
27. Milani P, Dispenzieri A, Gertz MA, et al. In patients with light-chain (AL) amyloidosis myocardial contraction fraction (MCF) is a simple, but powerful prognostic measure that can be calculated from a standard echocardiogram (ECHO). *Blood.* 2015;126(23). 1774–1774.
28. Milani P, Dispenzieri A, Scott CG, et al. Independent prognostic value of stroke volume index in patients with immunoglobulin light chain amyloidosis. *Circ Cardiovasc Imaging.* 2018;11(5). e006588.
29. Klein AL, Hatle LK, Taliercio CP, et al. Prognostic significance of Doppler measures of diastolic function in cardiac amyloidosis. A Doppler echocardiography study. *Circulation.* 1991;83(3):808–816.
30. Schiano-Lomoriello V, Galderisi M, Mele D, et al. Longitudinal strain of left ventricular basal segments and E/e' ratio differentiate primary cardiac amyloidosis at presentation from hypertensive hypertrophy: an automated function imaging study. *Echocardiography (Mount Kisco, NY).* 2016;33(9):1335–1343.
31. Alashi A, Desai RM, Khullar T, et al. Different histopathologic diagnoses in patients with clinically diagnosed hypertrophic cardiomyopathy after surgical myectomy. *Circulation.* 2019;140(4):344–346.
32. Barros-Gomes S, Williams B, Nhola LF, et al. Prognosis of light chain amyloidosis with preserved LVEF: added value of 2D speckle-tracking echocardiography to the current prognostic staging system. *JACC Cardiovasc Imaging.* 2017;10(4):398–407.
33. Bravo PE, Fujikura K, Kijewski MF, et al. Relative apical sparing of myocardial longitudinal strain is explained by regional differences in total amyloid mass rather than the proportion of amyloid deposits. *JACC Cardiovasc Imaging.* 2019;12(7 Pt 1):1165–1173.
34. Pun SC, Landau HJ, Riedel ER, et al. Prognostic and added value of two-dimensional global longitudinal strain for prediction of survival in patients with light chain amyloidosis undergoing Autologous Hematopoietic cell transplantation. *J Am Soc Echocardiogr.* 2018;31(1):64–70.
35. Bellavia D, Pellikka PA, Dispenzieri A, et al. Comparison of right ventricular longitudinal strain imaging, tricuspid annular plane systolic excursion, and cardiac biomarkers for early diagnosis of cardiac involvement and risk stratification in primary systematic (AL) amyloidosis: a 5-year cohort study. *Eur Heart J Cardiovasc Imaging.* 2012;13(8):680–689.
36. Senapati A, Sperry BW, Grodin JL, et al. Prognostic implication of relative regional strain ratio in cardiac amyloidosis. *Heart.* 2016;102(10):748–754.
37. Ternacle J, Bodez D, Guellich A, et al. Causes and consequences of longitudinal LV dysfunction assessed by 2D strain echocardiography in cardiac amyloidosis. *JACC Cardiovascu Imaging.* 2016;9(2):126–138.
38. Pagourelias ED, Mirea O, Duchenne J, et al. Echo parameters for differential diagnosis in cardiac amyloidosis: a head-to-head comparison of deformation and nondeformation parameters. *Circ Cardiovasc Imaging.* 2017;10(3). e005588.
39. Nagata Y, Takeuchi M, Mizukoshi K, et al. Intervendor variability of two-dimensional strain using vendor-specific and vendor-independent software. *J Am Soc Echocardiogr.* 2015;28(6):630–641.
40. Pradel S, Magne J, Jaccard A, et al. Left ventricular assessment in patients with systemic light chain amyloidosis: a 3-dimensional speckle tracking transthoracic echocardiographic study. *Int J Cardiovasc Imag.* 2019;35(5):845–854.
41. Vitarelli A, Lai S, Petrucci MT, et al. Biventricular assessment of light-chain amyloidosis using 3D speckle tracking echocardiography: differentiation from other forms of myocardial hypertrophy. *Int J Cardiol.* 2018;271:371–377.
42. Karamitsos TD, Piechnik SK, Banypersad SM, et al. Noncontrast T1 mapping for the diagnosis of cardiac amyloidosis. *JACC Cardiovasc Imaging.* 2013;6(4):488–497.
43. Martinez-Naharro A, Treibel TA, Abdel-Gadir A, et al. Magnetic resonance in transthyretin

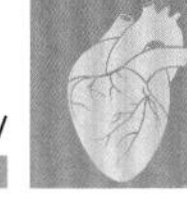

cardiac amyloidosis. *J Am Coll Cardiol.* 2017;70(4):466–477.

44. Dungu JN, Valencia O, Pinney JH, et al. CMR-based differentiation of AL and ATTR cardiac amyloidosis. *JACC Cardiovasc Imaging.* 2014;7(2):133–142.
45. Bravo PE, Dorbala S. Targeted nuclear imaging Probes for cardiac amyloidosis. *Curr Cardiol Rep.* 2017;19(7):59.
46. American Society of Nuclear Cardiology. Available at: https://www.asnc.org/content.asp?contentid=182. m-PIfTCA. Secondary.
47. Bokhari S, Castano A, Pozniakoff T, et al. (99m)Tc-pyrophosphate scintigraphy for differentiating light-chain cardiac amyloidosis from the transthyretin-related familial and senile cardiac amyloidoses. *Circ Cardiovasc Imaging.* 2013;6(2):195–201.
48. Dorbala S, Vangala D, Semer J, et al. Imaging cardiac amyloidosis: a pilot study using (1)(8) F-florbetapir positron emission tomography. *Eur J Nucl Med Mol Imag.* 2014;41(9):1652–1662.
49. Ehman EC, El-Sady MS, Kijewski MF, et al. Early detection of multiorgan light chain (AL) amyloidosis by whole body (18)F-florbetapir PET/CT. *J Nucl Med.* 2019;60(9):1234–1239.
50. Maurer MS, Schwartz JH, Gundapaneni B, et al. Tafamidis treatment for patients with transthyretin amyloid cardiomyopathy. *N Engl J Med.* 2018;379(11):1007–1016.
51. Judge DP, Falk RH, Maurer MS, et al. Transthyretin stabilization by AG10 in symptomatic transthyretin amyloid cardiomyopathy. *J Am Coll Cardiol.* 2019;74(3):285–295.
52. Gallego-Delgado M, Delgado JF, Brossa-Loidi V, et al. Idiopathic restrictive cardiomyopathy is primarily a genetic disease. *J Am Coll Cardiol.* 2016;67(25):3021–3023.
53. Kostareva A, Kiselev A, Gudkova A, et al. Genetic spectrum of idiopathic restrictive cardiomyopathy uncovered by next-generation sequencing. *PLoS One.* 2016;11(9). e0163362.
54. Anderson HN, Cetta F, Driscoll DJ, et al. Idiopathic restrictive cardiomyopathy in children and young adults. *Am J Cardiol.* 2018;121(10):1266–1270.
55. Mankad R, Bonnichsen C, Mankad S. Hypereosinophilic syndrome: cardiac diagnosis and management. *Heart.* 2016;102(2):100–106.
56. Berensztein CS, Pineiro D, Marcotegui M, et al. Usefulness of echocardiography and Doppler echocardiography in endomyocardial fibrosis. *J Am Soc Echocardiogr.* 2000;13(5):385–392.
57. Salemi VM, Rochitte CE, Shiozaki AA, et al. Late gadolinium enhancement magnetic resonance imaging in the diagnosis and prognosis of endomyocardial fibrosis patients. *Circ Cardiovasc Imaging.* 2011;4(3):304–311.
58. Carneiro AC, Mochiduky RI, Zancaner LF, et al. A new typical finding in late gadolinium enhanced images for the diagnosis of endomyocardial fibrosis—the double V sign. *J Cardiovasc Magn Reson.* 2011;13(suppl 1):O40.
59. Cools J, DeAngelo DJ, Gotlib J, et al. A tyrosine kinase created by fusion of the PDGFRA and FIP1L1 genes as a therapeutic target of imatinib in idiopathic hypereosinophilic syndrome. *N Engl J Med.* 2003;348(13):1201–1214.
60. Gulati V, Harikrishnan P, Palaniswamy C, et al. Cardiac involvement in hemochromatosis. *Cardiol Rev.* 2014;22(2):56–68.
61. Palka P, Macdonald G, Lange A, et al. The role of Doppler left ventricular filling indexes and Doppler tissue echocardiography in the assessment of cardiac involvement in hereditary hemochromatosis. *J Am Soc Echocardiogr.* 2002;15(9):884–890.
62. Carpenter JP, He T, Kirk P, et al. On T2* magnetic resonance and cardiac iron. *Circulation.* 2011;123(14):1519–1528.
63. Alizad A, Seward JB. Echocardiographic features of genetic diseases: part 2. Storage disease. *J Am Soc Echocardiogr.* 2000;13:164–170.
64. Chareonthaitawee P, Beanlands RS, Chen W, et al. Joint SNMMI-ASNC expert consensus document on the role of (18)F-FDG PET/CT in cardiac sarcoid detection and therapy monitoring. *J Nucl Cardiol.* 2017;24(5):1741–1758.

64a. Pompe Disease Diagnostic Working Group; Winchester B, Bali D, Bodamer OA, et al. Methods for a prompt and reliable laboratory diagnosis of Pompe disease: report from an international consensus meeting. *Mol Genet Metab.* 2008;93(3):275–281.

65. Limongelli G, Fratta F. S1.4 Cardiovascular involvement in Pompe disease. *Acta Myol.* 2011;30(3):202–203.
66. Boentert M, Florian A, Dräger B, et al. Pattern and prognostic value of cardiac involvement in patients with late-onset pompe disease: a comprehensive cardiovascular magnetic resonance approach. *J Cardiovasc Magn Reson.* 2016;18(1):91.
67. Chen M, Zhang L, Quan S. Enzyme replacement therapy for infantile-onset Pompe disease. *Cochrane Database Syst Rev.* 2017;11:Cd011539.
68. Nordin S, Kozor R, Medina-Menacho K, et al. Proposed stages of myocardial phenotype development in Fabry disease. *JACC Cardiovasc Imaging.* 2018;8 (Part 2):1673–1683.
69. Kampmann C, Baehner F, Whybra C, et al. Cardiac manifestations of Anderson-Fabry disease in heterozygous females. *J Am Coll Cardiol.* 2002;40(9):1668–1674.
70. Linhart A, Kampmann C, Zamorano JL, et al. Cardiac manifestations of Anderson–Fabry disease: results from the international Fabry outcome survey. *Eur Heart J.* 2007;28(10):1228–1235.
71. Pieroni M, Chimenti C, De Cobelli F, et al. Fabry's disease cardiomyopathy: echocardiographic detection of endomyocardial glycosphingolipid compartmentalization. *J Am Coll Cardiol.* 2006;47(8):1663–1671.
72. Kounas S, Demetrescu C, Pantazis AA, et al. The binary endocardial appearance is a poor discriminator of Anderson-Fabry disease from familial hypertrophic cardiomyopathy. *J Am Coll Cardiol.* 2008;51(21):2058–2061.
73. Mundigler G, Gaggl M, Heinze G, et al. The endocardial binary appearance ('binary sign') is an unreliable marker for echocardiographic detection of Fabry disease in patients with left ventricular hypertrophy. *Eur Heart J—Cardiovasc Imaging.* 2011;12(10):744–749.
74. Sado DM, White SK, Piechnik SK, et al. Identification and assessment of Anderson-Fabry disease by cardiovascular magnetic resonance noncontrast myocardial T1 mapping. *Circ Cardiovasc Imaging.* 2013;6(3):392–398.
75. Perry R, Shah R, Saiedi M, et al. The role of cardiac imaging in the diagnosis and management of Anderson-Fabry disease. *JACC Cardiovasc Imaging.* 2019;12(7 Pt 1):1230–1242.
76. MacDermot KD, Holmes A, Miners AH. Anderson-Fabry disease: clinical manifestations and impact of disease in a cohort of 98 hemizygous males. *J Med Genet.* 2001;38(11):750–760.
77. Eng CM, Guffon N, Wilcox WR, et al. Safety and efficacy of recombinant human alpha-galactosidase A replacement therapy in Fabry's disease. *N Engl J Med.* 2001;345(1):9–16.
78. Germain DP, Elliott PM, Falissard B, et al. The effect of enzyme replacement therapy on clinical outcomes in male patients with Fabry disease: a systematic literature review by a European panel of experts. *Mol Genet Metab Rep.* 2019;19:100454.
79. Hughes DA, Elliott PM, Shah J, et al. Effects of enzyme replacement therapy on the cardiomyopathy of Anderson-Fabry disease: a randomised, double-blind, placebo-controlled clinical trial of agalsidase alfa. *Heart.* 2008;94(2):153–158.
80. Germain DP, Nicholls K, Giugliani R, et al. Efficacy of the pharmacologic chaperone migalastat in a subset of male patients with the classic phenotype of Fabry disease and migalastat-amenable variants: data from the phase 3 randomized, multicenter, double-blind clinical trial and extension study. *Genet Med.* 2019.
81. Mortensen SA, Olsen HS, Baandrup U. Chronic anthracycline cardiotoxicity: haemodynamic and histopathological manifestations suggesting a restrictive endomyocardial disease. *Br Heart J.* 1986;55(3):274–282.
82. Chang ICY, Bois JP, Bois MC, et al. Hydroxychloroquine-mediated cardiotoxicity with a false-positive (99m)Technetium-labeled pyrophosphate scan for transthyretin-related cardiac amyloidosis. *Circ Cardiovasc Imaging.* 2018;11(1):e007059.
83. van Nimwegen FA, Schaapveld M, Janus CP, et al. Cardiovascular disease after Hodgkin lymphoma treatment: 40-year disease risk. *JAMA Intern Medicine.* 2015;175(6):1007–1017.
84. van Nimwegen FA, Ntentas G, Darby SC, et al. Risk of heart failure in survivors of Hodgkin lymphoma: effects of cardiac exposure to radiation and anthracyclines. *Blood.* 2017;129(16):2257–2265.
85. Wu W, Masri A, Popovic ZB, et al. Long-term survival of patients with radiation heart disease undergoing cardiac surgery: a cohort study. *Circulation.* 2013;127(14):1476–1485.
86. Talreja DR, Edwards WD, Danielson GK, et al. Constrictive pericarditis in 26 patients with histologically normal pericardial thickness. *Circulation.* 2003;108(15):1852–1857.
87. Miller CA, Dormand H, Clark D, et al. Comprehensive characterization of constrictive pericarditis using multiparametric CMR. *JACC Cardiovasc Imaging.* 2011;4(8):917–920.
88. Hatle LK, Appleton CP, Popp RL. Differentiation of constrictive pericarditis and restrictive cardiomyopathy by Doppler echocardiography. *Circulation.* 1989;79(2):357–370.
89. Ha JW, Oh JK, Ommen SR, et al. Diagnostic value of mitral annular velocity for constrictive pericarditis in the absence of respiratory variation in mitral inflow velocity. *J Am Soc Echocardiogr.* 2002;15(12):1468–1471.

89a. Welch TD, Ling LH, Espinosa RE, et al. Echocardiographic diagnosis of constrictive pericarditis: Mayo Clinic criteria. *Circ Cardiovasc Imaging.* 2014;7:526–553.

90. Abdalla IA, Murray RD, Lee JC, et al. Does rapid volume loading during transesophageal echocardiography differentiate constrictive pericarditis from restrictive cardiomyopathy? *Echocardiography (Mount Kisco, NY).* 2002;19(2):125–134.

91. Oh JK, Tajik AJ, Appleton CP, et al. Preload reduction to unmask the characteristic Doppler features of constrictive pericarditis. A new observation. *Circulation*. 1997;95(4):796–799.
92. Sengupta PP, Krishnamoorthy VK, Abhayaratna WP, et al. Disparate patterns of left ventricular mechanics differentiate constrictive pericarditis from restrictive cardiomyopathy. *JACC Cardiovasc Imaging*. 2008;1(1):29–38.
93. Talreja DR, Nishimura RA, Oh JK, et al. Constrictive pericarditis in the modern era: novel criteria for diagnosis in the cardiac catheterization laboratory. *J Am Coll Cardiol*. 2008;51(3):315–319.
94. Francone M, Dymarkowski S, Kalantzi M, et al. Assessment of ventricular coupling with real-time cine MRI and its value to differentiate constrictive pericarditis from restrictive cardiomyopathy. *Eur Radiol*. 2006;16(4):944–951.

中文导读

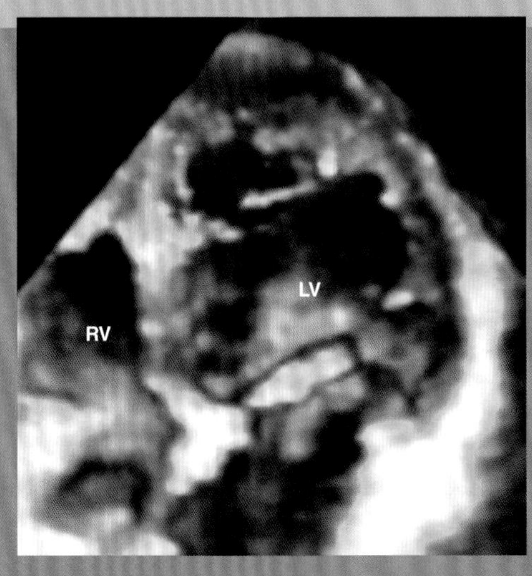

第15章 心脏移植

超声心动图提供的信息，可以协助晚期心力衰竭或移植团队判断预后，指导医疗决策，在心脏移植术前及术后发挥至关重要的作用。本章首先介绍了超声在晚期心力衰竭患者的诊断、移植术前评估中的作用，包括：评估病因、心力衰竭严重程度、疾病进展情况、可逆性肺动脉高压和机械辅助装置。其次介绍了超声评估潜在供体心脏的结构和功能，以及对边缘供体的连续评估。而后又介绍了超声评估移植围术期及术后并发症、超声评估移植后的急性和亚急性期并发症，包括：原发性移植物功能障碍、急性排斥反应、右心衰竭、心包积液或心脏压塞、感染、心内膜心肌活检术后并发症和缩窄性心包炎。另外介绍了超声诊断移植术后慢性期并发症，包括：慢性移植物功能衰竭、慢性排斥反应、移植物血管病和心脏肿瘤。最后，阐述了超声诊断心脏移植并发症所面临的挑战、移植术后超声的预后价值，以及未来的方向。

孙　欣

Cardiac Transplantation

HOLLY GONZALES, MD | KELLY H. SCHLENDORF, MD | DEEPAK K. GUPTA, MD, MSCI

Since the first human heart transplant operation in 1967, the field of advanced heart failure and cardiac transplantation has continued to grow, with more than 5500 heart transplantations performed annually worldwide in each of the past few years.[1] Advancements in surgical technique, histocompatibility testing, and immunosuppression have led to improvements in graft longevity and patient survival. Because of its ready availability, low cost, and safety, echocardiography plays a key role in the assessment of cardiac structure and function in the cardiac transplant donor and the heart recipient.[2] This chapter summarizes the role of echocardiography in the evaluation of patients before and after cardiac transplantation.

EVALUATION BEFORE CARDIAC TRANSPLANTATION

RECIPIENT

All patients under consideration for cardiac transplantation require characterization of cardiac structure and function. Echocardiography has a well-established role in pre-transplantation assessment. It is the most common noninvasive imaging test used in the initial evaluation of the patient with cardiac disease, and it is often the test of choice for serial examination due to its availability, lack of radiation exposure, and compatibility with implanted devices (i.e., pacemakers, defibrillators, and ventricular assist devices).

By the time a patient is being considered for cardiac transplantation, the advanced heart failure/transplantation providers typically have data obtained from one or more prior echocardiograms for their review. The serial studies are used to understand the cause, severity, and progression of cardiac disease, including screening for the presence of irreversible or substantial fixed pulmonary hypertension, which is a contraindication to heart transplantation.[3] Consequently, high-quality comprehensive echocardiography is paramount in the pre-transplantation evaluation of the cardiac patient. The most common underlying conditions in heart transplant operations are shown in Table 15.1.[1] Echocardiographic techniques and analyses for these and other cardiac conditions are detailed elsewhere in this textbook and are applicable to the pre-transplantation patient as well.

Although the underlying cardiomyopathies and indications that lead to cardiac transplantation have not changed drastically through the years, there are two noteworthy temporal changes that pertain to the pre-transplantation echocardiographic assessment. First, the use of temporary and durable mechanical circulatory support as a bridge to transplantation has steadily increased over the past few decades. Mechanical support devices are used before transplantation in approximately 50% of cases.[1] The echocardiographic evaluation of patients with mechanical circulatory support is reviewed in Chapter 16.

Second, the increasing number of patients with complex congenital heart disease surviving into adulthood has led to a greater number of transplantations in this patient group. Echocardiographic evaluation in the adult congenital heart disease population is especially important to help recognize and define unique anatomic features (e.g., pre-Fontan) that may impact the need for reconstructive operations around the time of transplantation.[4,5] The echocardiographic evaluation of congenital heart disease is reviewed in Chapters 42 through 46.

DONOR

Evaluation of potential cardiac allograft donors includes a thorough clinical assessment of comorbidities, cause of brain death, hemodynamic stability (including the need for inotrope or pressor support), cardiac biomarkers, and electrocardiograms.[6] Abnormalities in these clinical parameters are common in the potential donor population, and the evaluation of cardiac structure and function, and therefore suitability for transplantation, is often best assessed by noninvasive imaging, of which echocardiography is the first-line option. Thorough transthoracic echocardiographic (TTE) imaging of cardiac donors may be challenging due to poor acoustic windows as a result of trauma and/or mechanical ventilation. In these circumstances, use of echocardiographic contrast and/or transesophageal

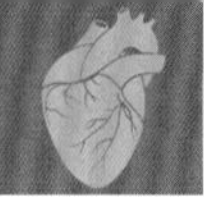

TABLE 15.1 Underlying Conditions in Heart Transplant Operations.[a]

Condition	*Proportion of Heart Transplant Operations (%)*
Non-ischemic cardiomyopathy	49
Ischemic cardiomyopathy	35
Restrictive cardiomyopathy	4
Congenital heart disease	3
Hypertrophic cardiomyopathy	3
Retransplantation	3
Valvular cardiomyopathy	2
Other	1

[a]Primary indications vary slightly by geographic location; shown here are primary diagnoses in North America.

Adapted from Khush KK, Cherikh WS, Chambers DC, et al. The International Thoracic Organ Transplant Registry of the International Society for Heart and Lung Transplantation: thirty-fifth adult heart transplantation report—2018; Focus theme: multiorgan transplantation. *J Heart Lung Transplant*. 2018;37(10):1155–1168.

echocardiography (TEE) may be warranted.[7] The role of alternative cardiac imaging modalities, such as magnetic resonance imaging (MRI) and computed tomography (CT), for donor heart assessment is less certain, in part because of mechanical ventilation, arrhythmias, the need for intravenous contrast, and interference from other life support devices.[8]

The echocardiographic assessment of potential donors includes a comprehensive cardiac study. Features of cardiac structure and function of particular interest to the transplantation team include left ventricular (LV) wall thickness, biventricular systolic function, wall motion, diastolic function, hemodynamics, potentially undiagnosed valvular or congenital heart disease, and cardiac masses. Findings related to these parameters inform the transplantation team's cardiologist and surgeon, who must decide whether to accept the heart for transplantation.

A completely normal donor examination result is not a requisite for organ acceptance.[9] The decision about whether a heart may be acceptable as an allograft is more nuanced because there are no well-established criteria.[10] An LV ejection fraction (LVEF) lower than 45% to 50%, regional wall motion abnormalities, coronary artery disease in more than one vessel, and LV hypertrophy (LVH) are among the strongest factors associated with the decision not to use a potential donor heart.[11,12] However, these criteria are largely based on expert opinion because few studies have systematically examined donor cardiac structure and function in relation to recipient outcomes.

One of the largest studies included data from 22,252 primary orthotopic heart transplantations between 1996 and 2007. In that study, low donor LVEF was the only parameter of cardiac structure and function included in the multivariable analysis found not to be associated with recipient survival at 1 year.[13] In a study of 808 donor hearts that were selected and used for transplantation, LVEF, regional wall motion abnormalities, and LVH were not significantly associated with recipient survival at 1 year.[12] Donor heart LVH was previously thought to be associated with the development of cardiac allograft vasculopathy (CAV); however, later studies with larger sample sizes suggest that some degree of LVH is acceptable in the absence of advanced donor age (>55 years) or prolonged ischemic time (>4 hours).[14–17]

As the discrepancy between organ supply and demand continues to widen, the use of so-called marginal donors or allografts is increasing. This includes the use of donor hearts with mildly depressed LVEF, single-vessel coronary artery disease, hepatitis C, or potentially prolonged ischemic time, with or without the use of ex vivo perfusion systems.[18] Systolic function of potential allografts is assessed using typical quantification methods and strain imaging. Given the potential for transient cardiac stunning or wall motion abnormalities in the setting of trauma and neurologic insults, serial echocardiograms may be needed to assess cardiac recovery with time and/or hormonal resuscitation.[19] Persistent regional wall motion abnormalities may be a manifestation of underlying coronary artery disease. In these cases and in those with persistently reduced LVEF, stress echocardiography may be useful to evaluate for contractile reserve or ischemia that may require further evaluation with coronary angiography.[6,20,21]

Valvular disease in the donor heart is also an important consideration. Because drug overdose is an increasingly common cause of donor death, close attention to valvular structure and function is mandatory, especially when the donor has positive blood cultures and endocarditis must be ruled out.[22] Although systematic evidence is lacking, case reports suggest that mild forms of noninfectious valvular disease, such as regurgitant mitral valves or bicuspid aortic valves, can be surgically addressed in the donor heart with successful subsequent transplantation.[23–26]

POST-TRANSPLANTATION EVALUATION

Echocardiography is an integral part of the management of patients who have undergone heart transplantation. Broadly, it is used to ensure adequate graft function and to monitor for acute and chronic post-transplantation complications in symptomatic and asymptomatic patients. In uncomplicated cases, the follow-up echocardiographic examination is largely similar to that for a normal heart. However, unique physiologic changes and acute and chronic complications can occur. Many of the echocardiographic findings that are seen in the normal transplanted heart can also exist in the setting of early complications, and the echocardiographic examination can serve as a sensitive test for the detection of structural and functional abnormalities that may be markers of complications.

A protocol for a post-transplantation TTE examination is shown in Table 15.2. The post-transplantation echocardiography report should also include the date of cardiac transplantation, the surgical technique, and additional procedures performed that may influence the assessment of cardiac structure and function.

To provide high-quality data that contribute to the care of a patient after transplantation, echocardiographers should understand cardiac transplant surgical techniques and acute and chronic complications (discussed later).[27] Cardiologists who interpret echocardiograms and transplant cardiologists should appreciate the complementary roles of multimodality cardiac imaging, including MRI, CT, nuclear imaging, fluoroscopy, and intravascular ultrasound, to provide robust diagnostic and prognostic information that ultimately informs patient care after transplantation. A full discussion of multimodality imaging after cardiac transplantation is beyond the scope of this chapter and is reviewed elsewhere.[28]

SURGICAL CONSIDERATIONS IN ECHOCARDIOGRAPHIC IMAGING AND INTERPRETATION

Cardiac transplantation has dramatically evolved since its inception in 1967. At first, orthotopic heart transplantation (OHT),

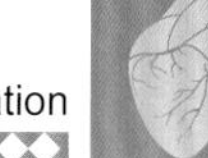

TABLE 15.2 Comprehensive Protocol for Transthoracic Echocardiography After Cardiac Transplantation.

2D View	*M-Mode*	*Doppler*	*Additional or Advanced*
Parasternal Window			
Long-axis	RV, LV, MV, AV, LA	MV and AV (color)	Zoomed LVOT/AV Aortic anastomosis (2D, color, and spectral Doppler) LA anastamosis
RV inflow	—	RV inflow (spectral) TV (color and spectral)	IVC and SVC anastomosis (2D, color, and spectral Doppler) RA anastamosis
Short-axis (base, MV, mid-LV, apex)	AV	AV, TV, PV, MV (color) TV, PV, PA, RVOT (spectral)	PA anastomosis (2D, color, and spectral Doppler)
Apical Window			
4-Chamber	—	MV annulus (TDI) Transmitral LV inflow (spectral) Pulmonary vein (spectral) MV (color and spectral)	Zoomed LA Color M-mode of LV inflow Longitudinal strain 3D LV volume
RV-focused	—	RV inflow (spectral) TV (color and spectral)	IVC and SVC anastomosis (2D, color, and spectral Doppler) RA anastamosis
Short-axis (base, MV, mid-LV, apex)	AV	AV, TV, PV, MV (color) TV, PV, PA, RVOT (spectral)	PA anastomosis (2D, color, and spectral Doppler)
Apical Window			
4-Chamber	—	TV (color and spectral) TV annulus (TDI)	Fractional area change RV longitudinal strain 3D RV volume
2-Chamber	—	MV (color and spectral) MV annulus (TDI)	Zoomed LA Longitudinal strain
Long-axis	—	AV (color and spectral) MV (color and spectral)	Longitudinal strain
Subcostal Window			
5-Chamber	—	LVOT and AV (color and spectral) IVRT	Aortic anastomosis (2D, color, and spectral Doppler)
4-Chamber	—	TV (color and spectral) IAS (color)	—
IVC and hepatic veins	IVC	Hepatic veins (color and spectral)	Sniff IVC anastomosis (2D and color Doppler)
Suprasternal Window			
Aorta	—	Ascending (color and spectral) Descending (spectral)	—

AV, Aortic valve; *IAS*, interatrial septum; *IVC*, inferior vena cava; *IVRT*, isovolumic relaxation time; *LVOT*, left ventricular outflow tract; *MV*, mitral valve; *PA*, pulmonary artery; *PV*, pulmonic valve; *RVOT*, right ventricular outflow tract; *SVC*, superior vena cava; *TDI*, tissue Doppler imaging; *TV*, tricuspid valve; *TAPSE*, tricuspid annular plane systolic excursion.

defined by recipient cardiectomy with donor transplantation, involved biatrial anastomoses in the mid-right and left atria (LA), leading to snowman-shaped atria due to the inclusion of donor and recipient tissue (Figs. 15.1A and 15.2).[27,29] Because of concerns about atrial arrhythmia, mechanical dysfunction, thrombosis, and tricuspid regurgitation from distorted atrial anatomy, this method has largely been supplanted with bicaval anastomosis.[30–32] The bicaval technique involves five anastomoses: superior vena cava, inferior vena cava, LA around all four pulmonary veins, and the ascending aorta and pulmonary artery distal to the semilunar valves (see Fig. 15.1B).

Other heart transplantation methods, including the so-called total technique and the heterotopic technique, were sparingly used in the past. The total technique, similar to the bicaval method but with separate right and left pulmonary vein anastomoses, was mostly abandoned due to issues with bleeding, pulmonary vein stenosis, prolonged procedure times, and an overall higher incidence of postoperative complications.[33] Heterotopic heart transplantation, in which a donor piggyback heart was used to keep the recipient heart in place, was employed for a short period as a means of affording back-up circulatory support in the event of acute rejection or graft failure of the donor heart. Advancements in immunosuppression, postoperative care, and mechanical support have rendered this technique obsolete.[34] Because these surgical approaches are rare in contemporary practice, their post-transplantation echocardiographic assessment is not discussed further here.

In the echocardiographic evaluation of a transplant patient, other relevant surgical aspects include management of the pericardium and the left atrial appendage. Most transplant surgeons do not close the pericardium during OHT, and a partial pericardiectomy with resection of excess anterior pericardial tissue often is performed.[35] Nevertheless, postoperative pericardial effusions may still occur within the residual pericardial space as a result of bleeding and hematoma formation, mediastinitis, and less commonly, acute cellular rejection.[36] The left atrial appendage may also be closed or resected at the time of transplantation, particularly with the biatrial anastomosis technique, due to the greater risk for atrial arrhythmias with this surgical method.[37] For patients with post-transplantation atrial fibrillation/flutter or stroke, knowledge of the left atrial appendage closure method is helpful when performing TEE to assess for thrombus and/or recanalization.

In the contemporary era of adult cardiac transplantation, 1-year survival rates exceed 85%, with a median survival time of 12.4 years.[38] Despite the success of modern cardiac transplantation, complications can still occur (Fig. 15.3).[1] Echocardiography

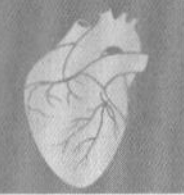

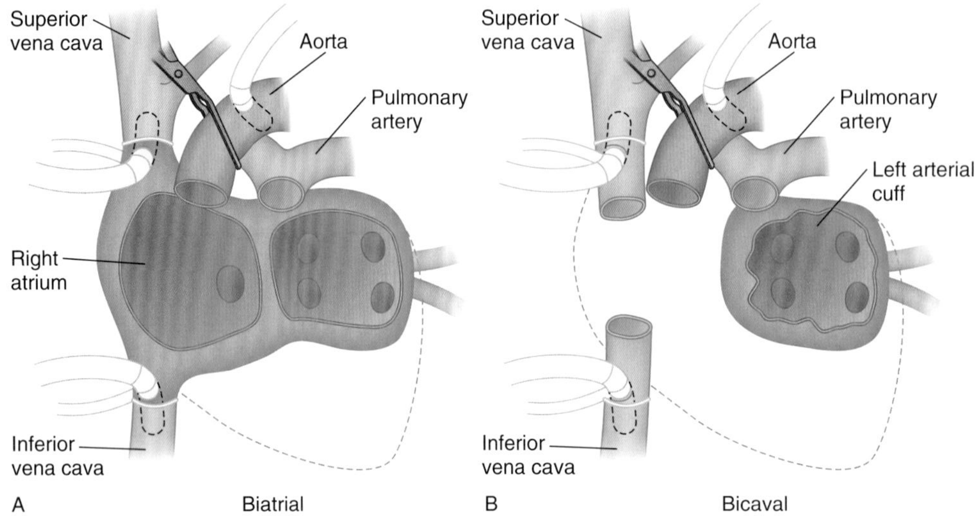

Fig. 15.1 Schematics of the (A) biatrial and (B) bicaval anastomosis surgical techniques for cardiac transplantation. (From Badano LP, Miglioranza MH, Edvardsen T, et al. European Association of Cardiovascular Imaging/Cardiovascular Imaging Department of the Brazilian Society of Cardiology recommendations for the use of cardiac imaging to assess and follow patients after heart transplantation. *Eur Heart J Cardiovasc Imaging.* 2015;16[9]:919–948.)

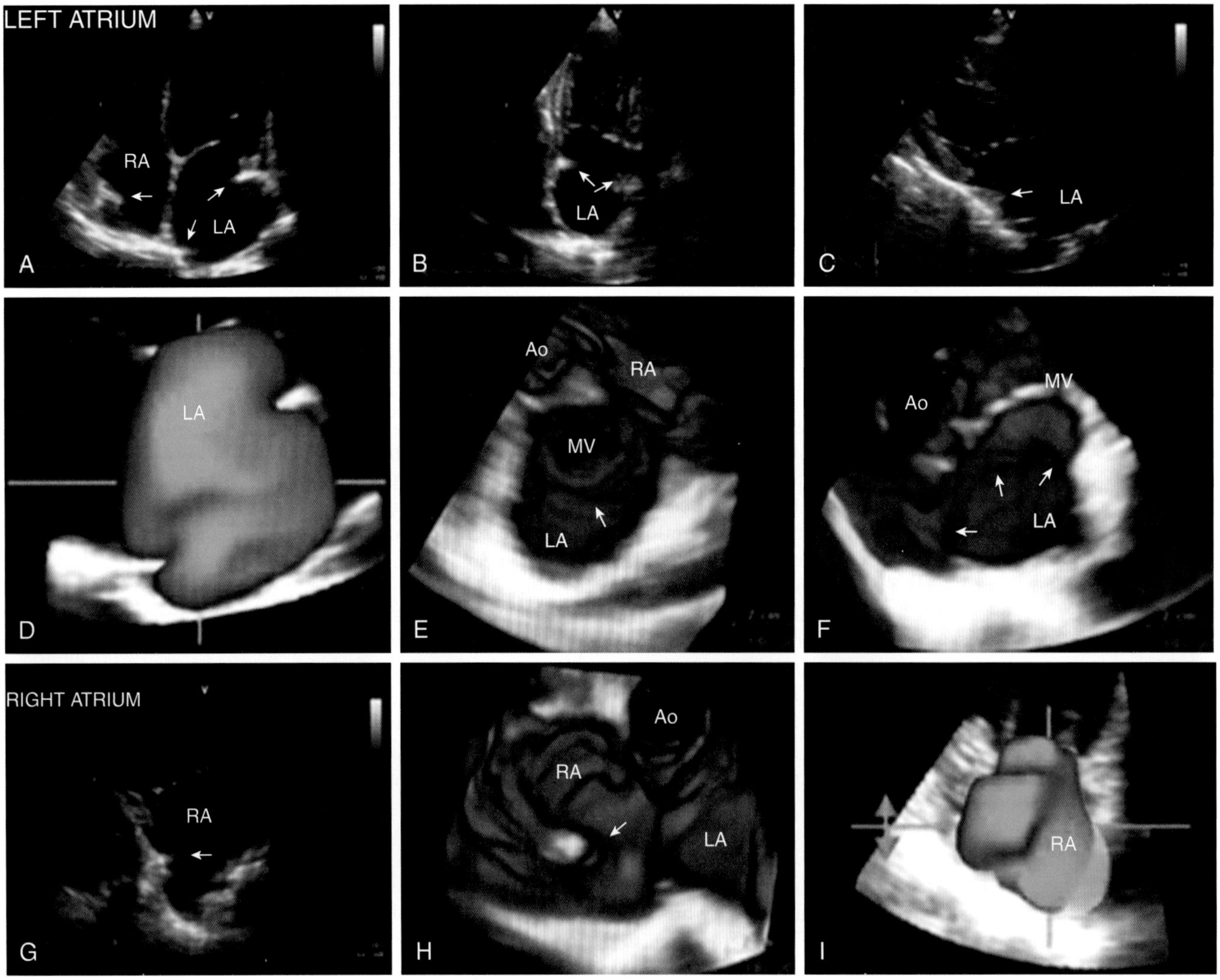

Fig. 15.2 TTE imaging in a cardiac transplant patient with biatrial anastamosis. RA and LA suture lines *(arrows)* are seen on 2D imaging (A–C, G) with the typical atrial snowman appearance and 3D reconstructions (D–F, H, I). *Ao,* Aorta; *MV,* mitral valve. (From Badano LP, Miglioranza MH, Edvardsen T, et al. European Association of Cardiovascular Imaging/Cardiovascular Imaging Department of the Brazilian Society of Cardiology recommendations for the use of cardiac imaging to assess and follow patients after heart transplantation. *Eur Heart J Cardiovasc Imaging.* 2015;16[9]:919–948.)

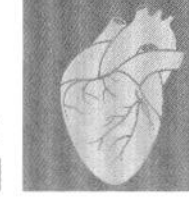

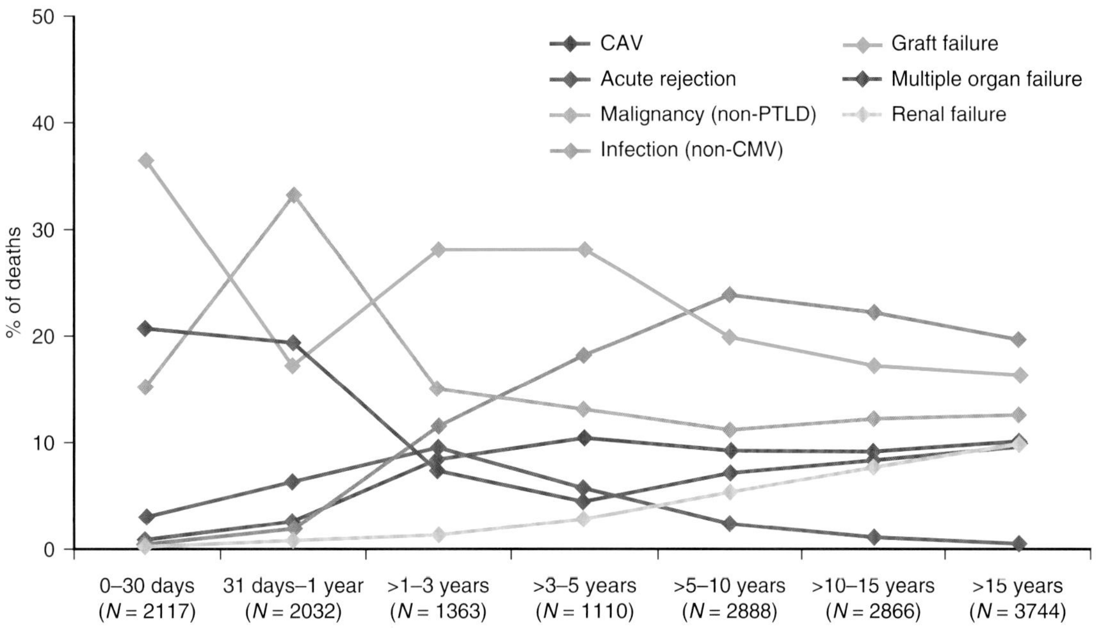

Fig. 15.3 Cause-specific mortality rates for adult heart transplant patients in relation to time from transplantation (January 2009–June 2017). *CAV*, Cardiac allograft vasculopathy; *CMV*, cytomegalovirus; *PTLD*, post-transplantation lymphoproliferative disorder. (From Chambers DC, Cherikh WS, Goldfarb SB, et al. The International Thoracic Organ Transplant Registry of the International Society for Heart and Lung Transplantation: Thirty-fifth adult lung and heart-lung transplant report-2018; Focus theme: Multiorgan Transplantation. *J Heart Lung Transplant.* 2018;37[10]:1169–1183.)

plays an important role in screening for potential complications and assessing response to therapies (Table 15.3).

PERIOPERATIVE POST-TRANSPLANTATION PERIOD

Perioperative complications in OHT are rare but can be devastating. Intraoperative TEE is considered the standard of care during cardiac transplant surgery. After surgery, TEE and TTE can be helpful in evaluating the unstable patient. Diagnostic considerations in this setting include myocardial ischemia or injury, anastomotic strictures or kinks, primary graft dysfunction, hyperacute rejection, bleeding and/or hypovolemia, tricuspid regurgitation, right ventricular (RV) dysfunction, and pericardial effusion. For example, regional wall motion abnormalities may indicate cardiac ischemia due to coronary artery embolism or, rarely, compression from a suture. In contrast, diffuse graft dysfunction with hemodynamic instability may represent primary graft dysfunction or, less commonly, hyperacute rejection. Findings of an underfilled heart and small inferior vena cava may suggest occult bleeding or hypovolemia.

Visualization of anastomotic kinks and strictures by 2D imaging or their inference by high-velocity flow on Doppler imaging may explain abnormal filling pressures or low-output states, especially in the setting of apparently normal biventricular systolic function (Figs. 15.4 and 15.5).[39,40] In one study, mild or worse tricuspid regurgitation and RV dysfunction assessed by TEE at the completion of OHT were associated with almost triple and double the risk of death, respectively.[41]

ACUTE POST-TRANSPLANTATION PERIOD

Following the immediate perioperative period, acute complications (within 1 month) after OHT include ongoing or worsening primary graft dysfunction, acute graft rejection, RV failure, tamponade, infection, and endomyocardial biopsy-related complications (see Table 15.3). Each of these conditions and their corresponding echocardiographic findings are discussed here.

Primary Graft Dysfunction

As the leading cause of early mortality after OHT, primary graft dysfunction (PGD) is defined by LV and/or RV dysfunction manifesting with reduced EF and/or elevated filling pressures and low cardiac output, such that inotropes or mechanical support are required, and for which there is no discernible secondary cause.[42] Echocardiography plays a key diagnostic role in assessing for PGD because it can document ventricular dysfunction, elevated filling pressures, and low output and can facilitate ruling out secondary causes (e.g., anastomotic kinks, pulmonary hypertension). Echocardiography is also critical in serial monitoring for graft recovery over time.

Acute Rejection

Acute cellular and/or antibody-mediated rejection requiring treatment is estimated to occur in approximately 13% of patients within 1 year after OHT.[38] Although endomyocardial biopsy remains the gold standard for the diagnosis of acute rejection, echocardiography plays an important role in alerting providers to the possibility of acute rejection and in monitoring for response to treatment. Findings of normal wall thickness, wall motion, systolic and diastolic function, and filling pressures suggest a low likelihood of acute rejection.[27] In contrast, abnormal echocardiographic findings for one or more of these parameters may be associated with acute rejection due to myocardial edema and inflammation (Table 15.4; see also Table 15.3).

The most sensitive echocardiographic parameters of acute rejection appear to be LV diastolic dysfunction and longitudinal systolic strain (Tables 15.5 and 15.6).[43] Normal diastolic parameters, particularly mitral annular tissue Doppler velocities ($e' >$ 16 cm/s, $a' >$ 9 cm/s), appear to effectively rule out acute rejection. Lateral wall longitudinal systolic strain velocities lower

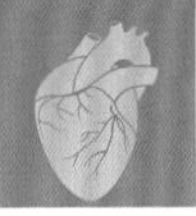

TABLE 15.3 Echocardiographic Correlates of Cardiac Complications in the Transplant Patient.

Complication	*Echocardiographic Correlations*	*Comments*
Perioperative		
Myocardial ischemia/injury	Regional wall motion abnormalities	Coronary artery embolism or compression/ligation by a suture
Anastomotic kinks/strictures	Anastomotic narrowing Turbulence on color Doppler High spectral Doppler velocities	IVC, SVC, PA, pulmonary veins, and/or aorta anastomosis involvement
Primary graft dysfunction	LV or RV systolic dysfunction in the absence of other causes	Hemodynamic instability
Hyperacute rejection	Diffuse graft dysfunction	Hemodynamic instability
Bleeding/hypovolemia	Underfilled heart, small IVC	—
Tricuspid regurgitation	Assess RA, RV size/function, PASP	More than mild at completion of intraoperative TEE associated with increased mortality
RV dysfunction	Dilated RV Low TAPSE, tricuspid S′ velocity, RV FAC High RAP Assess PASP	More than mild at completion of intraoperative TEE associated with increased mortality May be related to irreversible pHTN, rapid changes in hemodynamics, or ischemic time
Pericardial effusion/tamponade	May be located anterior and lateral to RA requiring TEE imaging	Can occur despite pericardium not being closed after transplantation
Acute (<1 mo)		
Primary graft dysfunction	Reduced LVEF or RV systolic dysfunction with low cardiac output and high filling pressures without secondary causes	Leading cause of early mortality
Acute rejection	LV diastolic dysfunction Impaired GLS Reduced LVEF (late finding) Increased LV wall thickness or mass Pericardial effusion	Variable sensitivity and specificity for each parameter Normal echocardiogram has highest NPV
RV failure	Low TAPSE, tricuspid S′ velocity, RV FAC High RAP Assess PASP	3D may be better than 2D assessment of RV function after transplantation
Pericardial effusion/tamponade	May be located anterior and lateral to RA requiring TEE imaging	Can occur despite pericardium not being closed after transplantation
Infections	Can occur with valves and anastomosis sites	Difficult to discern anastamotic infective endocarditis, thrombus, and sutures from TTE
Post-biopsy complications	Tricuspid regurgitation Pericardial effusion Coronary fistulas	Echocardiographic guidance of biopsy has equivocal complication rates compared with fluoroscopic guidance
Subacute (1–12 mo)		
Infection/endocarditis	Can occur with valves and anastomosis sites	Leading cause of death in subacute period
Acute rejection	LV diastolic dysfunction Impaired GLS Reduced LVEF (late finding) Increased LV wall thickness/mass Pericardial effusion	More common in highly allosensitized and noncompliant patients
Constrictive pericarditis	Exaggerated respirophasic variation Tall E waves, short deceleration time Mitral TDI annulus reversus High RAP Usually normal biventricular function	Can occur with parietal or visceral pericardium
Chronic (>12 mo)		
Chronic graft failure	LV diastolic dysfunction Impaired GLS Reduced LVEF Wall motion abnormalities Increased LV wall thickness/mass	Major cause of mortality in chronic period Caused by CAV or repeated acute rejection or infection
Cardiac allograft vasculopathy	Wall motion abnormalities LV or RV dysfunction Impaired GLS Increased LV wall thickness Abnormal DSE	50% of transplant patients at 10 years Often asymptomatic DSE has variable sensitivity and specificity CFR may be most sensitive
Cardiac masses	Differential diagnosis includes malignancy, thrombus, endocarditis	Multimodality imaging may be needed

CAV, Cardiac allograft vasculopathy; *CFR*, coronary flow reserve; *DSE*, dopamine stress echocardiography; *FAC*, fractional area change; *GLS*, global longitudinal strain; *IVC*, inferior vena cava; *LVEF*, left ventricular ejection fraction; *NPV*, negative predictive value; *PA*, pulmonary artery; *PASP*, pulmonary artery systolic pressure; *pHTN*, pulmonary hypertension; *RAP*, right atrial pressure; *SVC*, superior vena cava; *TAPSE*, tricuspid annular plane systolic excursion; *TDI*, tissue Doppler imaging.

than −15.5% also performed well to exclude acute rejection requiring treatment.[44] Although these are sensitive techniques, diastolic dysfunction and global longitudinal strain (GLS) are limited by poor specificity because abnormalities in these parameters can be also be seen in the absence of rejection and in the presence of other conditions, including coronary allograft vasculopathy (CAV).[45] Similarly, whereas reductions in LVEF and increases in wall thickness may be associated with acute rejection, these findings are neither highly sensitive nor specific. Attention to acute increases in LV wall thickness and mass

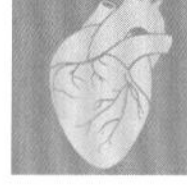

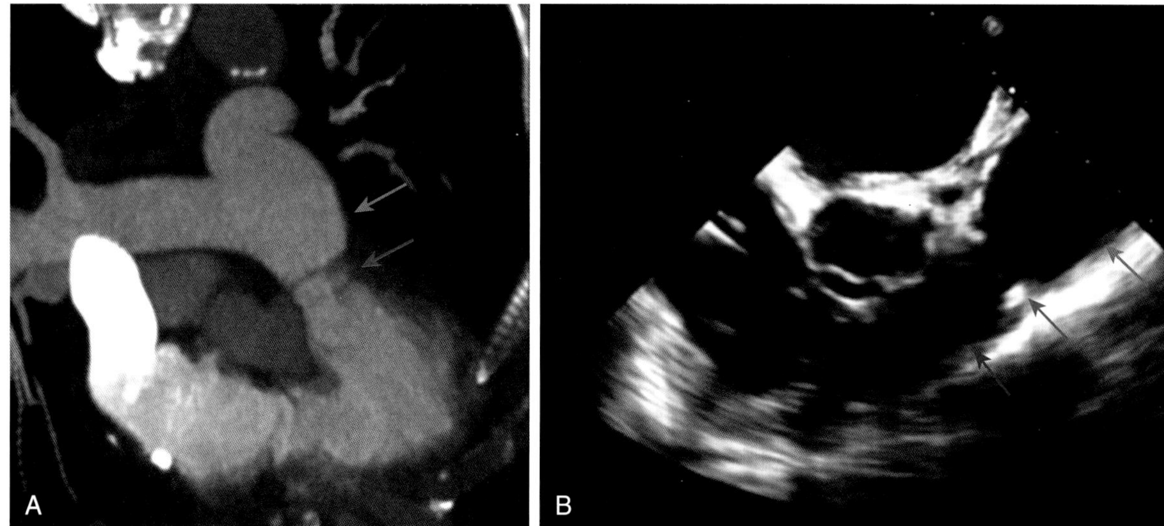

Fig. 15.4 Images obtained after cardiac transplantation show a pulmonary anastamotic stricture. (A) Computed tomography angiogram demonstrates the proximal main pulmonary artery stenosis *(red arrow)* and poststenotic dilatation *(green arrow)*. (B) TEE at the mid-esophageal short-axis view shows the supravalvular anastamotic stenosis *(red arrow)*, pulmonary valve *(blue arrow)*, and poststenotic dilatation *(green arrow)*. (From Lee JZ, Lee KS, Abidov A, Samson RA, Lotun K. Endovascular stenting of suture line supravalvular pulmonic stenosis after orthotopic heart transplantation using rapid pacing stabilization. *JACC Cardiovasc Interv.* 2014;7[8]:e91–e93.)

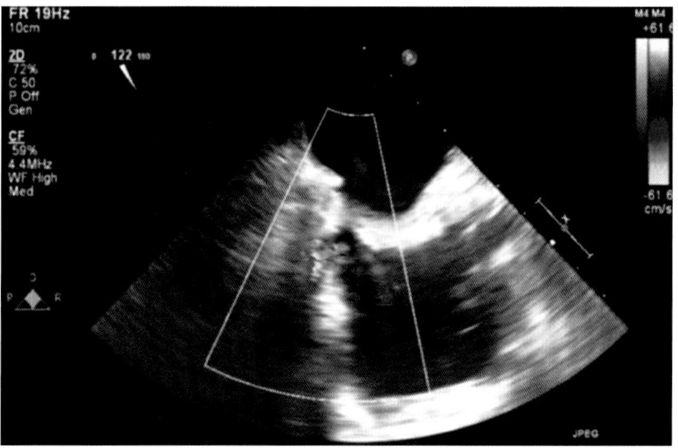

Fig. 15.5 TEE in the mid-esophageal bicaval view shows turbulence by color Doppler at the inferior vena cava anastomosis to the RA, discovered on postoperative day 7 after cardiac transplantation during evaluation for refractory shock. (From Chaney MA, Lowe ME, Minhaj MM, Santise G, Jacobsohn E. Inferior vena cava stenosis after bicaval orthotopic heart transplantation. *J Cardiothorac Vasc Anesth.* 2019;33[9]:2561–2568.)

compared with a prior echocardiogram may enhance specificity for acute rejection.

Fewer data exist on other parameters of cardiac structure and function for diagnosing acute rejection. Examples include the myocardial performance index (MPI), isovolumic contraction and relaxation times, and mitral inflow deceleration time, although these have not been reliably validated or widely used (Fig. 15.6).[27,46] Pericardial effusion may also be a sign of acute rejection, but it is nonspecific.[47]

RV Failure

In the absence of PGD and acute rejection, isolated RV failure is common early after OHT and is associated with poor clinical outcomes.[48] RV failure is thought to be caused by ischemia, postoperative hemodynamic changes, and high pulmonary pressures. The echocardiographic assessment of RV function in the transplanted heart parallels that in the native heart (see Chapters 6 and 36) and includes hemodynamic estimation of RV systolic pressure and right atrial (RA) pressure. However, the geometry of the RV may undergo changes after cardiac transplantation, making 2D-based longitudinal functional assessments (i.e., tricuspid annular plane systolic excursion [TAPSE] and RV tissue Doppler s' velocity) less reliable than the 3D RVEF. Echocardiography can then be used to monitor improvement in RV function over time, which may be seen when hemodynamics normalize postoperatively as pulmonary pressures begin to fall.[27,49]

Pericardial Effusions and Tamponade

Although it is not common practice to close the pericardium after OHT, postoperative pericardial effusions may still develop as a result of residual pericardium and mediastinal space created when a dilated heart is replaced with one that is normal in size (Figs. 15.7, 15.8, and 15.9).[50] Echocardiography plays an important role in characterizing the size and location of effusions and the degree to which they may compromise cardiac function.

In a study of 88 patients after cardiac transplantation, moderate to large pericardial effusions were found in approximately one third, and of those, 9% to 10% of patients had hemodynamic compromise requiring urgent intervention.[51] Because pericardial hematomas after OHT often occur anterior and lateral to the RA, they can be difficult to visualize on transthoracic imaging. In cases of high intrapericardial pressures and low cardiac output, providers should maintain a high index of suspicion and rely on transesophageal imaging when necessary.[52]

Infections

Endocarditis is an uncommon complication after transplantation; it is most likely to occur when underlying valvular heart disease in the donor goes unrecognized or is underappreciated. The echocardiographic evaluation of endocarditis after OHT mirrors that for native heart endocarditis (see Chapter 29), with the additional consideration of interrogating suture lines, particularly at the aorta.

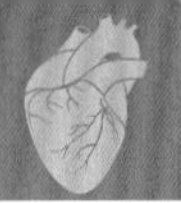

TABLE 15.4 **Common Echocardiographic Parameters and Their Association With Acute Cellular Rejection as Confirmed by RV Biopsy in Heart Transplant Patients.**

Echocardiographic parameter	*No ACR[a] (n = 173)*	*ACR Grade = 1R[a] (n = 50)*	*ACR Grade ≥ 2R[a] (n = 12)*	P[b]	P[c]	P[d]	*Overall P Value[e]*
LVEF (%) (Simpson)	63.6 ± 8.10	63.4 ± 7.5	62.2 ± 9.6	1.00	1.00	1.00	0.88
Septal thickness (mm)	11.3 ± 1.8	12.3 ± 2.2	12.6 ± 1.4	0.01	0.59	0.02	0.001
TAPSE (mm)	14.6 ± 3.9	13.9 ± 3.9	12.6 ± 3.5	0.09	0.83	1.00	0.18
RV wall thickness (mm)	5.3 ± 1.1	5.6 ± 1.2	6.0 ± 1.7	0.11	0.84	0.28	0.13
E/A ratio	2.1 ± 0.7	2.0 ± 1.1	2.5 ± 0.8	0.42	0.35	1.00	0.32
DT (ms)	150.8 ± 40.3	156.5 ± 42.7	126.9 ± 41.4	0.16	0.08	1.00	0.09
IVRT (ms)	93.7 ± 17.6	83.1 ± 20.2	74.2 ± 12.9	0.01	0.38	0.01	<0.001
TDI lateral E (cm/s)	13.0 ± 3.6	12.1 ± 3.3	9.9 ± 3.0	0.01	0.05	0.41	0.04
Lateral E/E′ ratio	6.8 ± 2.8	7.1 ± 3.0	9.6 ± 3.6	0.004	0.02	1.00	0.006
Systolic velocity tricuspid annulus (cm/s)	10.4 ± 2.4	9.9 ± 2.2	9.2 ± 2.3	0.30	1.00	0.36	0.11
LV radial strain (%)	22.5 ± 7.1	20.1 ± 8.0	18.0 ± 6.5	0.56	1.00	0.55	0.20
LV circumferential strain (%) (absolute value)	19.1 ± 3.6	18.5 ± 3.3	17.3 ± 3.9	1.00	1.00	1.00	0.51
LV longitudinal strain (%) (absolute value)	17.8 ± 3.4	15.1 ± 3.7	13.7 ± 2.7	<0.001	0.68	<0.001	<0.001
RV longitudinal strain (%) (absolute value)	19.9 ± 3.8	16.2 ± 3.7	15.2 ± 1.7	<0.001	1.00	<0.001	<0.001
RV free wall longitudinal strain (%) (absolute value)	23.3 ± 5.2	16.9 ± 3.0	16.6 ± 3.6	<0.001	1.00	<0.001	<0.001

[a]Data are expressed as mean ± SD.
[b]No ACR vs. ACR grade ≥ 2R.
[c]ACR grade 1R vs. ACR grade ≥ 2R.
[d]No ACR vs. ACR grade 1R.
[e]Analysis of variance global *P* value between groups.
ACR, Acute cellular rejection; *DT*, deceleration time; *TDI*, tissue Doppler imaging; *IVRT*, isovolumic relaxation time; *LVEF*, left ventricular ejection fraction; *TAPSE*, tricuspid annular plane systolic excursion.
From Mingo-Santos S, Moñivas-Palomero V, Garcia-Lunar I, et al. Usefulness of two-dimensional strain parameters to diagnose acute rejection after heart transplantation. *J Am Soc Echocardiogr*. 2015;28(10):1149–1156.

TABLE 15.5 **Test Characteristics for Tissue Doppler Measures in the Diagnosis of Acute Cellular Rejection After Cardiac Transplantation.**

TDI-Derived Wall Motion Velocity	*Study*	*Patients Evaluated (n)*	*No ACR vs. ACR (P Value)*	*Changes (Cutoff)*	*Sensitivity (%)*	*Specificity (%)*	*PPV (%)*	*NPV (%)*
Peak systolic velocity (S′)	Clemmensen et al.[63] (PW-TDI[a])	64	0.02	—	—	—	—	—
	Dandel et al.[43] (PW-TDI[b])	363	0.001	>10% (↓)	88	94	90	93
	Lunze et al.[87] (PW-TDI[c])	122	<0.001	>15% (↓)	88	93	31	99.5
Peak early diastolic velocity (E′)	Derumeaux et al.[59] (color-coded TDI[d])	34	<0.001	≥10% (↓)	92	—	—	—
	Puleo et al.[88] (PW-TDI[e])	121	<0.001	0.16 cm/s	76	88	—	92
	Dandel et al.[43] (PW-TDI[b])	363	<0.001	>10% (↓)	92	92	87	95
Peak-to-peak mitral annular velocity (S′ + E′)	Mankad et al.[89] (color-coded TDI[f])	78	<0.001	13.5 cm/s	93	71	—	98
Time-to-peak early diastolic velocity (TE′)	Dandel et al.[43] (PW-TDI[b])	363	<0.001	>10% (↓)	92	94	90	95
Peak late diastolic velocity (A′)	Lunze et al.[87] (PW-TDI[c])	122	<0.001	>5% (↓)	95	64	9	99.7

[a]Mitral annular velocity (average of septal, lateral, anterior and posterior) cross-section analysis: no ACR vs. ACR grade 2R.
[b]Basal posterior wall radial wall motion, serial assessment: no ACR vs. biopsy-proven clinically relevant ACR.
[c]Basal longitudinal wall motion, serial assessment in children: ACR < 2R vs. ≥ 2R.
[d]Septum and endocardium of posterior wall serial assessment: no ACR vs. biopsy-proven ACR (including mild ACR).
[e]Inferior wall motion, cross-section analysis: "no" ACR (ISHLT-1990 grades 0, 1A, or 1B) vs. moderate ACR.
[f]Posterior wall and mitral annular velocity analysis: biopsy-proven "no" ACR (ISHLT-1990 Grade < 1B) vs. ≥ 1B.
ACR, Acute cellular rejection; *ISHLT*, International Society for Heart and Lung Transplantation; *NPV*, negative predictive value; *PPV*, positive predictive value; *PW*, pulsed-wave; *TDI*, tissue Doppler imaging; ↓, reduction.
From Dandel M, Hetzer R. Post-transplant surveillance for acute rejection and allograft vasculopathy by echocardiography: usefulness of myocardial velocity and deformation imaging. *J Heart Lung Transplant*. 2017;36(2):117–131.

TABLE 15.6 Test Characteristics for Strain Measures in the Diagnosis of Acute Cellular Rejection After Cardiac Transplantation.

Deformation Imaging Methods	*Studies*	*Evaluated Parameters*	*EMB ACR Grade*[a]	*No ACR vs. ACR (P Value)*	*Changes (Cutoff)*	*Sensitivity (%)*	*Specificity (%)*	*PPV (%)*	*NPV (%)*
TDI-derived strain and strain rate	Kato et al.[90]	LV systolic peak GLS	≥1B[b]	<0.001	−27.4%	82	82	36	97
		LV early diastolic peak LSr	—	<0.001	−2.8/s	76	75	21	96
	Marciniak et al.[91]	LV (SA) systolic peak RS	≥1B	<0.05	≤30%	85	90	80	93
		LV (SA) systolic peak RSr	—	<0.001	≤3.0/s	80	86	72	90
		LV (LW-4CV) systolic peak LS	—	<0.05	—	—	—	—	—
		LV (LW-4CV) systolic peak LSr	—	<0.05	—	—	—	—	—
2D speckle tracking	Sato et al.[92]	% of LV torsion	≥2R	<0.001	25% decrease	74	95	60	97
	Sera et al.[93]	LV systolic peak GLS	≥1B[b]	<0.05	<−14.8%	64	63	24	90
		LV systolic peak GRS	—	>0.05	—	—	—	—	—
		LV systolic peal GCS	—	>0.05	—	—	—	—	—
	Mingo-Santos et al.[44]	LV systolic peak GLS	≥2R	<0.001	<−15.5%	86	81	25	99
		RV free wall peak LS	—	<0.001	<−17%	86	91	43	99
		LV and RV systolic LS	—	<0.001	<−17%; −15.5%	100	77	26	100
		LV systolic peak GRS and GCS	—	>0.05	—	—	—	—	—
	Clemmensen et al.[63]	LV systolic peak GLS	≥2R	<0.001	—	—	—	—	—
	Sehgal et al.[94]	LV systolic peak LS	≥2R	0.05	—	—	—	—	—
		LV systolic peak RS	—	<0.05	—	—	—	—	—
		LV systolic peak CS and CSr	—	<0.01	—	—	—	—	—
	Ambardekar et al.[45] (Velocity Vector Imaging software)	LV systolic peak GLS and GLSr	≥2R[c]	>0.05	—	—	—	—	—
		LV systolic CS and CSr	—	>0.05	—	—	—	—	—
		LV diastolic LSr and CSr	—	>0.05	—	—	—	—	—
	Ruiz Ortiz et al.[95]	LV systolic average RS	2R	0.001	—	100	48	6	100
3D speckle tracking	Du et al.[96]	LV systolic peak GLS	≥1B[d]	<0.05	<25%	87.5	54	—	—
		LV systolic peak RS and CS	—	>0.05	<−9.6%	—	—	—	—

[a]1B grades are based on the ISHLT-1990 system, and 2R grades on the ISHLT-2004 system.
[b]Significant in both univariate and multivariate analyses.
[c]Asymptomatic ACR.
[d]ACR ≥ 1B ($n = 8$).
4CV, 4-Chamber view; *ACR*, acute cellular rejection; *CS*, circumferential strain; *CSr*, circumferential strain rate; *EMB*, endomyocardial biopsy; *GCS*, global circumferential strain; *GLS*, global longitudinal strain; *GLSr*, global longitudinal strain rate; *GRS*, global radial strain; *LS*, longitudinal strain; *LSr*, longitudinal strain rate; *LW*, lateral wall; *NPV*, negative predictive value; *PPV*, positive predictive value; *RS*, radial strain; *SA*, short-axis view; *TDI*, tissue Doppler imaging.
From Dandel M, Hetzer R. Post-transplant surveillance for acute rejection and allograft vasculopathy by echocardiography: usefulness of myocardial velocity and deformation imaging. *J Heart Lung Transplant*. 2017;36(2):117–131.

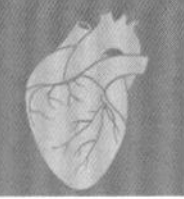

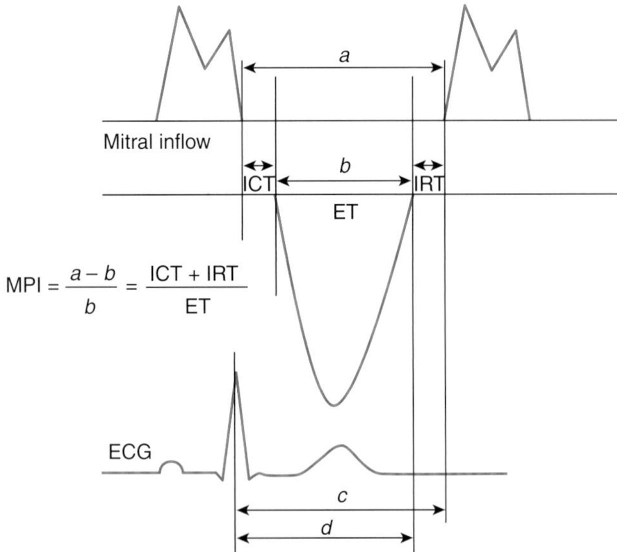

Fig. 15.6 Myocardial performance index schematic. Myocardial performance index *(MPI)* is the sum of the isovolumic contraction time *(ICT)* and isovolumic relaxation time *(IRT)*, divided by the ejection time *(ET)*. (From Toumanidis ST, Papadopoulou ES, Saridakis NS, et al. Evaluation of myocardial performance index to predict mild rejection in cardiac transplantation. *Clin Cardiol.* 2004;27[6]:352–358.)

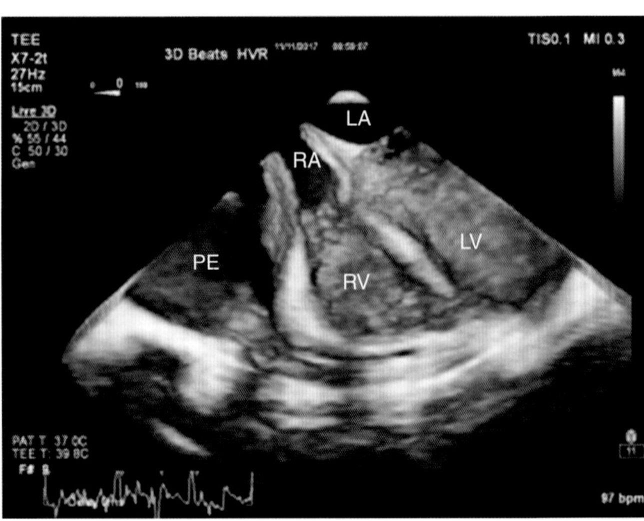

Fig. 15.7 Post-transplantation pericardial effusion (PE) seen on 3D TEE was caused by placement of a normal-size heart within a large pericardial space from a patient with dilated cardiomyopathy with compression of the RA and basal RV. (From Essandoh M. Atypical presentation of a large pericardial effusion after heart transplantation in a patient with dilated cardiomyopathy. *J Cardiothorac Vasc Anesth.* 2018;32[4]:e84.)

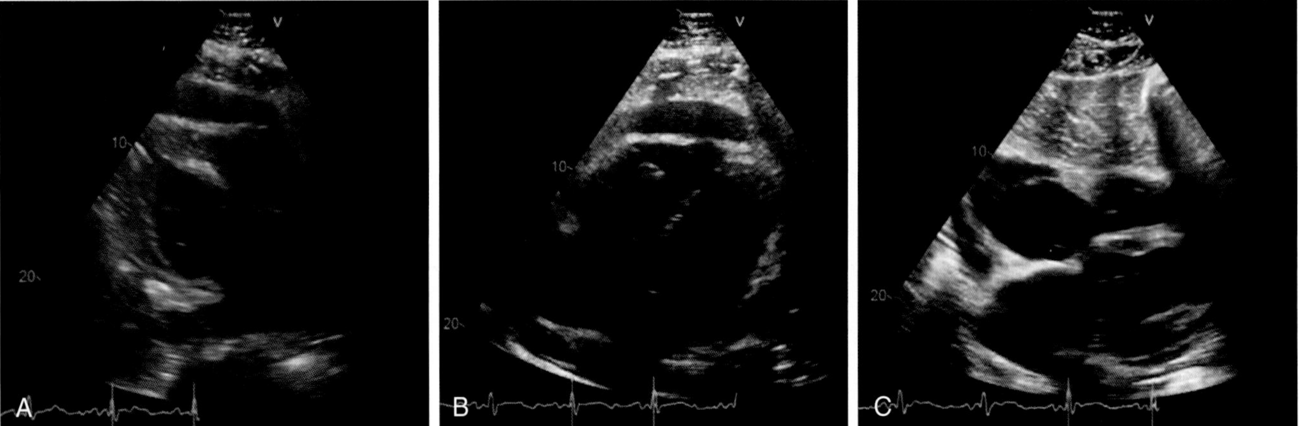

Fig. 15.8 Transthoracic echocardiography of a patient 12 days after cardiac transplantation. A large focal pericardial effusion is shown anterior to the RV, which is seen in the parasternal long-axis (A) and apical 4-chamber (B) views but not in the subcostal view (C), demonstrating the importance of multiple views in the postoperative assessment of transplant patients for possible pericardial effusions (see Video 15.8).

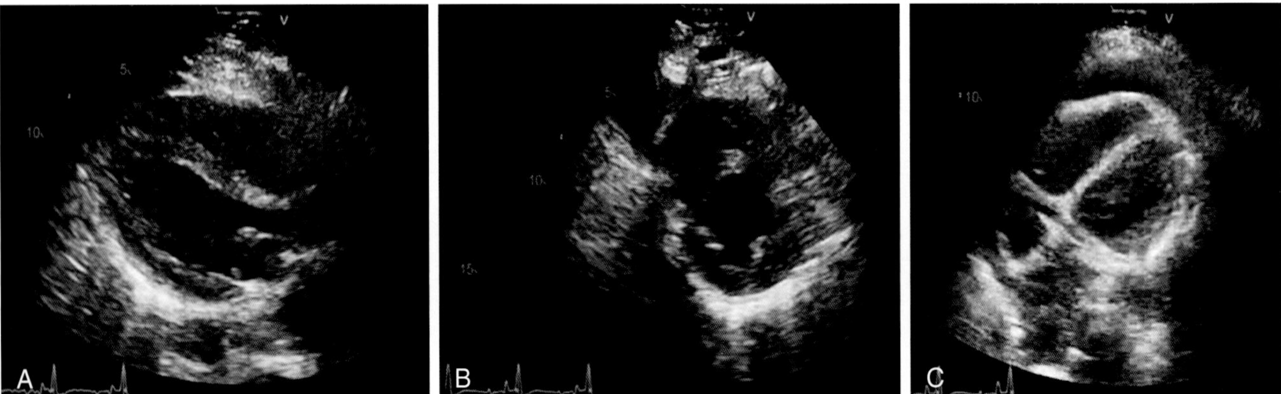

Fig. 15.9 Transthoracic echocardiography of a patient 7 days after cardiac transplantation showing a large focal pericardial effusion anterior to the RV. In this case, the effusion is not seen in parasternal long-axis views (A) but is seen *arrow*) in the parasternal short-axis (B) and apical 4-chamber (C) views (see Video 15.9).

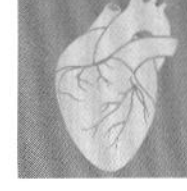

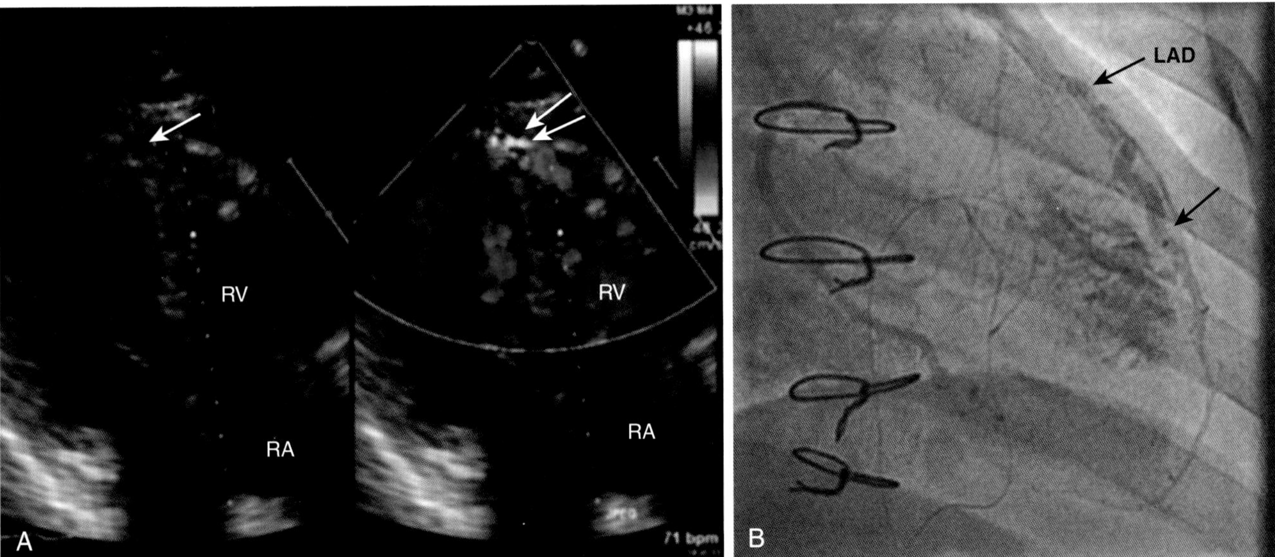

Fig. 15.10 **TTE performed on a cardiac transplant patient presenting with shortness of breath.** Diastolic flow into the RV apex *(arrows)* (A) is shown, which was confirmed to be a coronary artery fistula *(unlabeled arrow)* by coronary angiography (B). *LAD,* Left anterior descending coronary artery. (From Yip AMC, Chong AY, Stadnick E, et al. Treatment of coronary artery fistula post-cardiac transplantation with covered stent: a case study and review of literature. *Int J Transplant Res Med.* 2017;3[2].)

Complications After Endomyocardial Biopsy

Endomyocardial biopsy remains the gold standard for the diagnosis of acute rejection after OHT. Although the overall complication rate associated with any one biopsy is less than 1%, the cumulative risk for transplant patients is higher given the frequent biopsies performed during the first year after OHT. Echocardiography plays an important role in identification and characterization of potential complications, including tricuspid regurgitation due to leaflet injury, pericardial effusion with or without tamponade as a result of myocardial perforation, and less commonly, coronary fistulas (Fig. 15.10).[53,54] Routine echocardiographic assessment after biopsy is typically not warranted in the stable patient, but it should be considered in those patients for whom the biopsy procedure was technically challenging and in those requiring systemic anticoagulation near the time of the biopsy. For patients who become unstable within 24 to 48 hours after biopsy, prompt echocardiographic assessment is mandatory.[55]

In an effort to minimize biopsy complications and radiation exposure, some centers use echocardiographic guidance with or without concomitant fluoroscopy to help steer the bioptome in the direction of the RV septum[56,57] (Fig. 15.11; see https://mmcts.org/tutorial/104). There are no convincing data to suggest that this strategy reduces complication rates.

SUBACUTE POST-TRANSPLANTATION PERIOD

In the subacute period after OHT (1 month to 1 year), complications that may require echocardiographic assessment include infection, acute rejection, and constrictive pericarditis. The leading cause of death among OHT patients in this period is infection. Especially in patients with positive blood cultures, prompt echocardiographic evaluation with TTE or TEE should be performed to rule out endocarditis.

Hemodynamically significant graft rejection during this period, although rare, remains a concern, especially among highly allosensitized patients and those for whom medication adherence is uncertain. Rarely, constrictive pericarditis may occur in this period as a result of postoperative pericarditis, effusions, mediastinitis, or acute rejection. The echocardiogram is well suited to identify features of constrictive pericarditis (see Chapter 17).[35,36]

CHRONIC POST-TRANSPLANTATION PERIOD

The management of cardiac transplant patients in the chronic period (after 1 year) relies heavily on echocardiography to ensure stability of cardiac structure and function over time. This includes follow-up of complications that may have occurred in the acute and subacute periods. This period requires attention to chronic graft failure, the most significant late complication encountered in transplant patients. Chronic graft failure includes chronic graft rejection or CAV. Less frequently, cardiac masses are observed. The echocardiographic assessment of these entities is briefly described in this section.

Chronic Graft Failure

The major limitation to longevity of the cardiac allograft and freedom from death or retransplantation is chronic graft failure. Most often caused by progressive CAV, chronic graft failure may also be attributable to multiple episodes of acute rejection or infectious causes.[27] Echocardiography can be helpful, albeit nonspecific, in the diagnosis of chronic graft failure, with potential findings of diastolic dysfunction, systolic dysfunction with or without wall motion abnormalities, abnormal GLS, and increased wall thickness and mass.

Chronic Rejection

Also known as CAV, chronic rejection affects more than 50% of patients within 10 years after OHT.[58] CAV is thought to be an immune-related phenomenon. It is a fibroproliferative ingrowth of the graft coronary arteries, which leads to microvascular and macrovascular occlusion and ischemia. Like acute rejection, CAV is often asymptomatic in its early stages, and routine surveillance is mandatory.

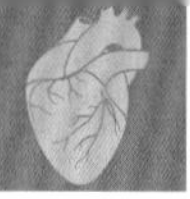

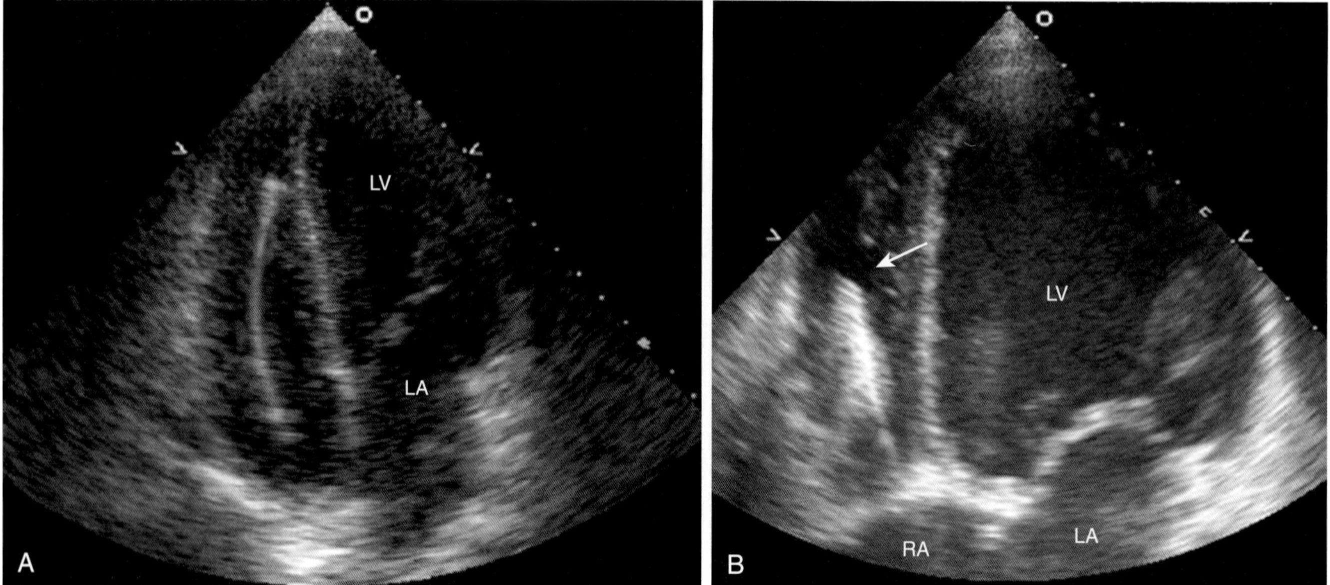

Fig. 15.11 TTE guidance of RV biopsies with (A) optimal bioptome placement at the interventricular septum and (B) suboptimal bioptome placement *(arrow)* with inability to visualize bioptome tip at the septum. (From Silvestry FE, Kerber RE, Brook MM, et al. Echocardiography-guided interventions. *J Am Soc Echocardiogr.* 2009;22[3]:213–231; quiz 316.)

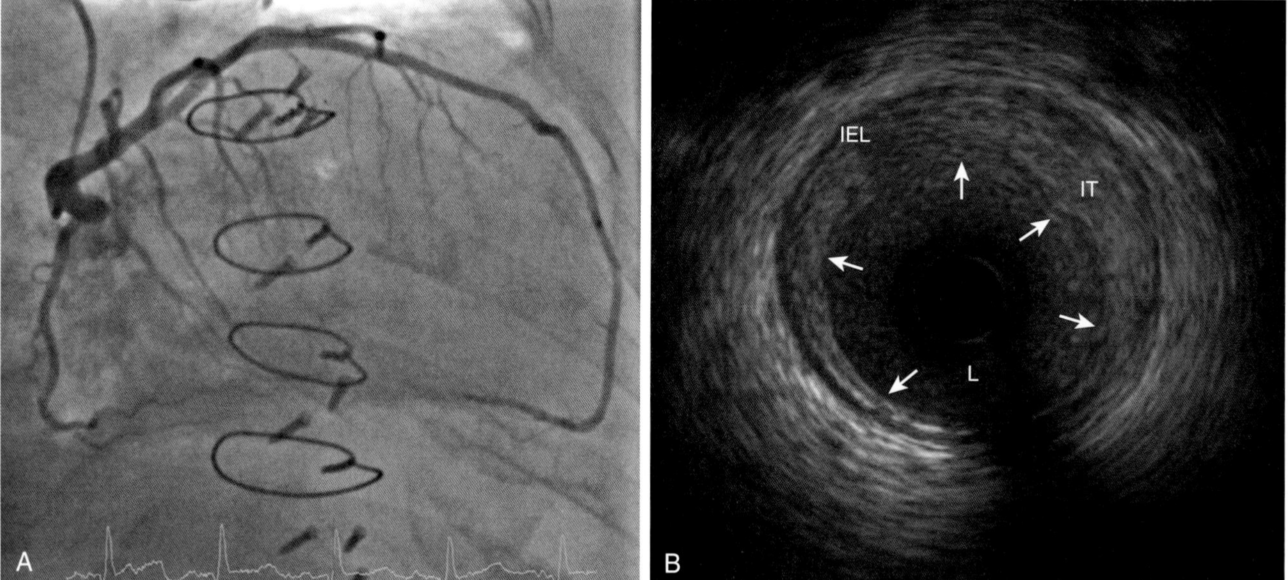

Fig. 15.12 Cardiac allograft vasculopathy (CAV) 1 year after transplantation. (A) The coronary angiogram appears normal. (B) Significant circumferential intimal thickening *(IT)* with reduced lumen area *(arrows)* is visible by intravascular ultrasound. Intravascular ultrasound increases the sensitivity of angiography for the detection of CAV given the diffuse intraluminal narrowing characteristic of this disease process. *IEL*, Internal elastic lamina; *L*, lumen.

Intravascular ultrasound combined with coronary angiography has a high sensitivity for the diagnosis of CAV and has become the gold standard (Fig. 15.12). However, because of the invasiveness of these catheter-based techniques, noninvasive imaging methods have an important role in raising the index of suspicion for CAV. Noninvasive imaging findings that may suggest CAV include new wall motion abnormalities or graft dysfunction, increased LV wall thickness, and changes in GLS. Dobutamine stress echocardiography (DSE), which was heavily relied upon for many years to help diagnose CAV noninvasively, has shown variable sensitivity and specificity for CAV across multiple studies (Table 15.7).[59–62]

Quantification of myocardial deformation with strain has been studied as a potentially more sensitive technique for detection of CAV with varied but promising results.[63] Assessment of coronary flow reserve appears to be the most sensitive noninvasive method of screening for CAV, and therefore alternative imaging modalities, including positron-emission tomography (PET) and cardiac MRI, are increasingly being used, with some evidence for the efficacy of dobutamine stress echocardiography when used with quantitative myocardial contrast echocardiography.[64–66]

Cardiac Masses

Although the incidence of cardiac masses in the transplanted heart is unknown, several case reports have demonstrated that they can occur.[67–69] Because the risk of malignancy increases after transplantation with the use of chronic immunosuppression, echocardiography becomes an important tool for detection and characterization of masses. Contrast echocardiography, along

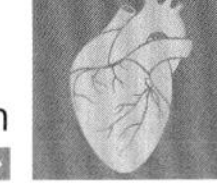

TABLE 15.7 Echocardiography Test Characteristics for the Diagnosis of Cardiac Allograft Vasculopathy.

Echocardiographic Method	*Standard for CAV Diagnosis*	*Studies*	*Sensitivity (%)*	*Specificity (%)*	*PPV (%)*	*NPV (%)*
2D echocardiography at rest	Angiography[a]	Spes et al.[80] Collings et al.[97] Smart et al.[98]	14–58	69–88	44–86	67–87
Exercise stress echocardiography	Angiography[b]	Collings et al.[97] Cohn et al.[99] Chen et al.[100]	33–89	82–92	62–73	86–97
DSE	Angiography[b]	Akosah et al.[60] Derumeaux et al.[59] Bacal et al.[82] Spes et al.[80] Clerkin et al.[101]	0–100	55–99	0–69	82–100
	Angiography[a] plus IVUS	Derumeaux et al.[59] Spes et al.[80] Stork et al.[102] Herregods et al.[103]	50–86	71–95	86	91
	Angiography[a]	Bharat et al.[104]	33	94	67	81
		Sade et al.[64]	78	64	—	—
	IVUS	Spes et al.[80]	79	83	88	71
DSE plus echo-CFR	Angiography[a]	Sade et al.[64]	78	87	—	—
PW-TDI systolic parameters at rest	Angiography[a]	Dandel et al.[43]	77–80	89–90	81–82	88–93
	Angiography[a] plus IVUS	Dandel et al.[43]	89–90	88–94	92–97	83–85
	Angiography[b]	Dandel et al.[43]	51	87–91	63–65	80
2D-STE at rest	Angiography[a] peak systolic GLS[c]	Clemmensen et al.[63]	42	93	78	72
	Angiography[b]	Dandel et al.[43]	—	—	—	—
	Peak GRS/GLS[d]		60/63	84/87	55/58	85/87
	Peak GRSr/GLSr[e]		71/77	97/98	90/95	91/93
	Systolic ASI[f] R/L		71/85	85/87	62/64	91/95
	Systolic DSI[g] R/L		83/89	97/99	90/95	95/97
DSE with 2D-STE analysis	Angiography[a]	Eroglu et al.[105]	88	85	—	—

[a]CAV with and without focal proximal coronary artery stenoses.
[b]CAV with focal proximal stenoses (≥50%) in ≥ 1 coronary vessel.
[c]Cutoff for GLS ≤ −14%.
[d]Cutoff value for GRS < 30% and for GLS ≤ −15%.
[e]Cutoff value for GRSr < 1.4/s and for GLSr < −0.9/s.
[f]Cutoff value for ASI > 20% (for radial and longitudinal strain).
[g]Cutoff for radial strain > 15%, for longitudinal strain > 20%.
ASI, Asynchrony index (standard deviation ÷ mean of regional Q wave to peak global strain time); *CAV*, cardiac allograft vasculopathy; *DSE*, dobutamine stress echocardiography; *DSI*, dyssynergy index (standard deviation / mean [numeric average] of regional strain values at the end of systole); *echo-CFR*, echocardiography-derived coronary flow reserve; *GLS*, global longitudinal strain; *GLSr*, global longitudinal strain rate; *GRS*, global radial strain; *GRSr*, global radial strain rate; *IVUS*, intravascular ultrasound; *NPV*, negative predictive value; *PPV*, positive predictive value; *PW-TDI*, pulsed-wave tissue Doppler imaging; *R/L*, right/left ventricle; *STE*, speckle tracking echocardiography.
From Dandel M, Hetzer R. Post-transplant surveillance for acute rejection and allograft vasculopathy by echocardiography: usefulness of myocardial velocity and deformation imaging. *J Heart Lung Transplant*. 2017;36[2]:117–131.

with multimodality imaging with TEE and cardiac MRI, may be useful after cardiac transplantation to distinguish tumors from other masses, including sutures, thrombus, and endocarditis.[70]

CHALLENGES TO DIAGNOSING COMPLICATIONS BY ECHOCARDIOGRAPHY

Recognition of the complications described previously is important for the care of the cardiac transplant patient, but differentiating echocardiographic abnormalities that are pathologic from those that are within the normal range after transplantation can be challenging. This is in part because of the lack of reference ranges for chamber quantification after heart transplantation. Given the changes that occur immediately postoperatively, it is recommended that a complete echocardiogram be obtained 6 months after transplantation, if the patient is clinically stable, to define the new normal and establish a baseline for serial comparisons.[27]

Parameters of LV structure and function that would be considered abnormal in a native heart may be normal after transplantation.[71,72] For example, increased LV wall thickness and mass are frequently observed in the absence of acute rejection. In some patients, this may be a normal finding in response to perioperative myocardial inflammation, and it generally regresses by 3 months without intervention. Paradoxical septal motion can lead to abnormal longitudinal strain of the septal segments. Abnormal GLS can be observed in the acute post-transplantation period, and it may normalize over time without directed therapy.[73] Persistence of abnormal GLS, however, portends a poor prognosis.

As in all patients, assessment of LV diastolic dysfunction after transplantation typically integrates multiple parameters, including transmitral inflow velocities, mitral annular tissue Doppler velocities, the E/e' ratio, left atrial (LA) size, and estimated pulmonary artery systolic pressure. In the early postoperative period, assessment of diastolic function may be confounded by tachycardia leading to fusion of transmitral E and A waves and by LA enlargement due to surgical technique. A restrictive filling pattern can occur in the acute postoperative phase; it may be related to allograft ischemic time or an undersized heart. Although this phenomenon often improves with time, a restrictive filling pattern can also be the first sign of acute rejection.[74]

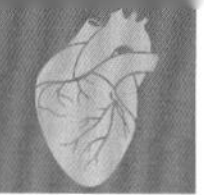

TABLE 15.8 Prognostic Signficance of Selected Echocardiographic Findings in After Cardiac Transplantation.

Parameter	*Studies*	N	*Primary Outcome*	*Risk Estimate*
Systolic Function				
LVEF > 60%	Barbir et al.[75]	91	Event-free survival from acute MI, new onset HF, cardiac mortality, need for coronary revascularization	OR = 0.21 *P* = 0.005
LVEF ≤ 64%	Clemmensen et al.[63]	196	Median time to first MACE	HR = 1.9 95% CI: 1.1–3.6 *P* < 0.05
RV dysfunction	Haddad et al.[48]	548	Death or retransplantation at 1 year	OR = 4.8 *P* = 0.007
RV FAC	Barakat et al.[77]	96	Combined death, moderate-severe CAV, or treated rejection at 1 year after OHT	HR = 0.95 95% CI: 0.91–0.99 *P* = 0.012
Diastolic Function				
E/A	Ambrosi et al.[76]	122	Event-free survival from cardiac death, retransplantation, acute coronary events, hospitalization for HF, treated AR episodes, and coronary revascularization procedures	HR = 2.2 95% CI: 1.1–4.4 *P* = 0.02
E/e′	Ambrosi et al.[76]	122	Event-free survival from cardiac death, retransplantation, acute coronary events, hospitalization for HF, treated AR episodes, and coronary revascularization procedures	HR = 2.3 95% CI: 1.1–4.8 *P* = 0.02
Mitral valve decel time	Barakat et al.[77]	96	Combined death, moderate-severe CAV, or treated rejection at 1 year after OHT	HR = 0.95 95% CI: 0.91–0.99 *P* = 0.012
Strain Imaging				
LV-GLS	Sarvari et al.[79]	176	Mortality at 1 year	HR = 1.42 95% CI: 1.07–1.88 *P* = 0.02
LV-GLS	Barakat et al.[77]	96	Combined death, moderate-severe CAV, or treated rejection at 1 year after OHT	HR = 1.03 95% CI: 0.91–1.16 *P* = 0.662
LV-GLS	Clemmensen et al.[63]	196	Median time to first MACE	HR = 4.9 95% CI: 2.7–8.9 *P* = 0.049
LV-GLS	Eleid et al.[78]	51	Combined risk of death and hospitalization for HF or biopsy-detected rejection	HR = 5.92 95% CI: 1.96–17.91 *P* < 0.0001
RV-FWS	Barakat et al.[77]	96	Combined death, moderate-severe CAV, or treated rejection at 1 year after OHT	HR = 1.11 95% CI: 1.02–1.22 *P* = 0.022
Dobutamine Stress Echocardiography				
Interval worsening on serial DSE	Spes et al.[80]	109	Risk of cardiac events including MI, HF, retrasplantation, cardiac death, new angiographic stenosis ≥ 75% requiring revascularization	RR = 7.26 *P* = 0.0014

AR, Acute rejection; *CAV*, cardiac allograft vasculopathy; *CI*, confidence interval; *DSE*, dobutamine stress echocardiography; *FAC*, fractional area change; *FWS*, free wall strain; *GLS*, global longitudinal strain; *HF*, heart failure; *HR*, hazard ratio; *LVEF*, left ventricular ejection fraction; *MACE*, major adverse cardiac event; *MI*, myocardial infarction; *OHT*, orthotopic heart transplant; *OR*, odds ratio; *RR*, relative risk.

Decreased tissue Doppler *e′* and *s′* velocities can also be seen in the first few weeks after transplantation in the absence of any overt pathology.

Similarly, the RV is commonly dilated after transplantation, with changes in systolic function parameters (i.e., TAPSE, TDI *s′*, and RV FAC), which may improve over time even in the absence of targeted therapies.[73] Because of changes in RV geometry that may occur after transplantation, 3D RV volumes and RV EF may be more reflective of true RV size and systolic function.[27] A size mismatch between donor and recipient pulmonary arteries may cause pseudo-narrowing of the proximal pulmonary artery, seen visually on echocardiography, with no significant gradient.

PROGNOSTIC SIGNIFICANCE OF ECHOCARDIOGRAPHY AFTER TRANSPLANTATION

The preponderance of evidence suggests that abnormal echocardiographic findings are associated with an adverse prognosis. Features of cardiac structure and function that have been examined in association with post-transplantation outcomes are summarized in Table 15.8.[48,63,75–80] However, these abnormalities lack diagnostic sensitivity and specificity, making the therapeutic implications of abnormal findings uncertain. Collectively, the existing evidence suggests that normal findings on resting echocardiography and negative stress testing may be the most informative because they identify transplant patients who are at relatively lower risk of adverse outcomes.[81,82]

FUTURE DIRECTIONS

A major limitation of echocardiography after cardiac transplantation is its uncertain diagnostic value for acute and chronic complications based on any single parameter alone. The reasons for this are complex and include methodological considerations, such as the availability of sensitive, quantitative, and reproducible methods for detection of pathology, and the scientific approach to the evidence base. Conventional measures of cardiac structure and function, such as LV size, wall thickness, wall motion, EF, and diastolic function, provide fundamental information but may be insensitive to detect subtle abnormalities.

Assessment of myocardial mechanics, particularly with strain imaging, has shown promise for early detection of many of the most serious complications after OHT, including acute and chronic graft rejection, but requires further validation. Tissue characterization techniques may provide greater sensitivity and specificity, but they need further study. For example, cardiac MRI T2 mapping with extracellular volume quantification has a high diagnostic accuracy for acute rejection.[83,84] Functional assessments of coronary physiology, such as coronary flow reserve by cardiac MRI, PET, or contrast-enhanced perfusion stress echocardiography may be superior to anatomic or inferential approaches (i.e., DSE, coronary angiography, and intravascular ultrasound).[64] Non–imaging-based approaches are also gaining interest, including identification of novel circulating biomarkers and gene expression profiling to diagnose rejection.[85] Ultimately, the combination of various noninvasive imaging techniques with multimodality imaging and biomarker use may prove more accurate in the detection of transplant-related complications.[86]

Most of the evidence base for the role of echocardiography in cardiac transplantation has been derived from single-center retrospective analyses. Although this evidence is important, it may lead to bias imparted by relatively small sample sizes and local factors. Further, temporal trends in the surgical and medical management of cardiac transplant patients may be influential. Prospective, multicenter studies of adequate sample size using standardized echocardiographic acquisition and interpretation protocols in the era of contemporary surgical and medical management are needed.

CONCLUSIONS

The preoperative and postoperative management of cardiac transplant patients requires robust and accurate quantification of cardiac structure and function to determine the cause, pathophysiology, therapy, and prognosis. Echocardiography can provide additive information to the clinical heart failure/transplantation team to facilitate medical decision making, and it is therefore likely to remain a cornerstone in the evaluation of the cardiac transplant patient.

Normal findings reported from echocardiography before and after cardiac transplantation are reassuring and are associated with low likelihood of acute and chronic complications. In contrast, abnormal findings after transplantation are risk markers for adverse prognoses but have uncertain sensitivity and specificity for the diagnosis of individual acute and chronic complications. The interpretation of echocardiographic findings requires careful integration with a comprehensive clinical assessment to guide medical decision making.

SUMMARY Cardiac Transplantation

Summary: Echocardiography plays a central role in the diagnosis of heart failure patients, their evaluation for cardiac transplantation, and the continued assessment of cardiac graft function to assess for known complications and guide prognosis and clinical management of the patient by the advanced heart failure/transplant team.

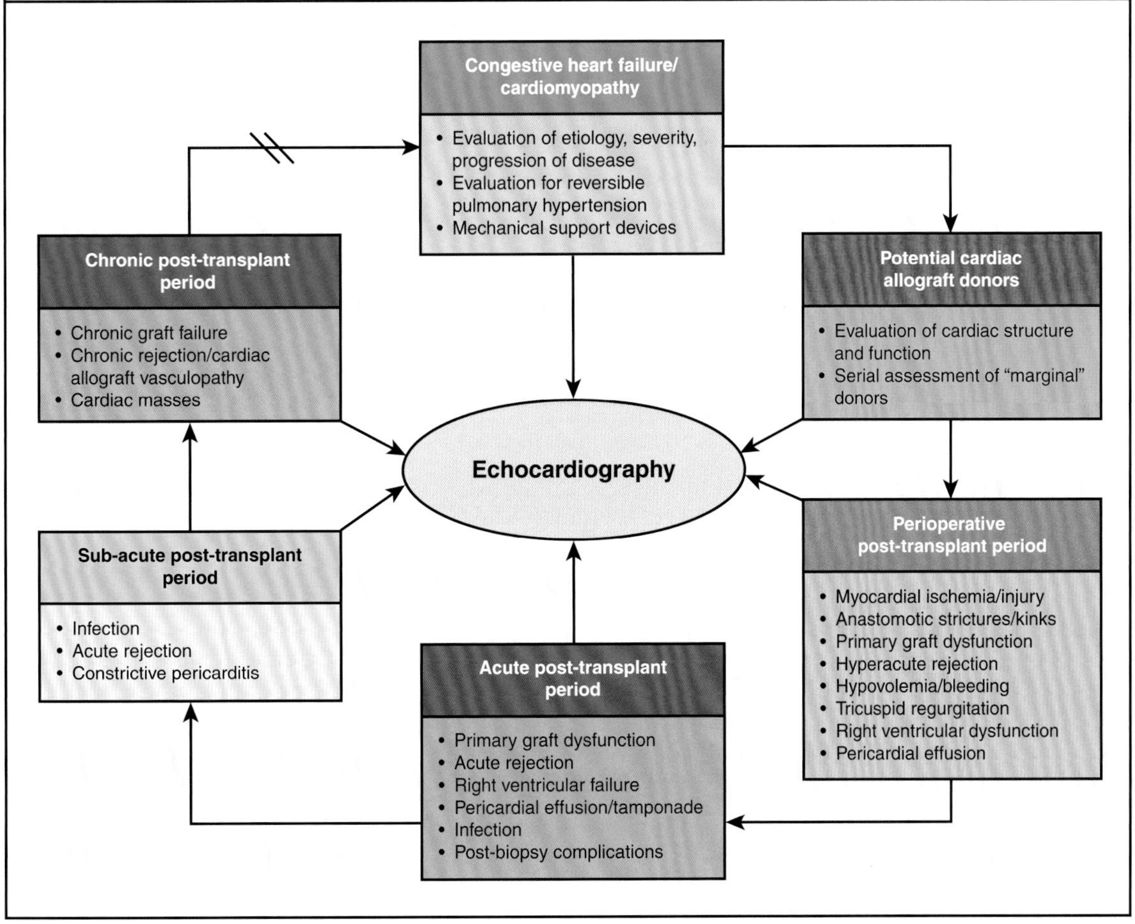

Congestive heart failure/ cardiomyopathy
- Evaluation of etiology, severity, progression of disease
- Evaluation for reversible pulmonary hypertension
- Mechanical support devices

Potential cardiac allograft donors
- Evaluation of cardiac structure and function
- Serial assessment of "marginal" donors

Perioperative post-transplant period
- Myocardial ischemia/injury
- Anastomotic strictures/kinks
- Primary graft dysfunction
- Hyperacute rejection
- Hypovolemia/bleeding
- Tricuspid regurgitation
- Right ventricular dysfunction
- Pericardial effusion

Acute post-transplant period
- Primary graft dysfunction
- Acute rejection
- Right ventricular failure
- Pericardial effusion/tamponade
- Infection
- Post-biopsy complications

Sub-acute post-transplant period
- Infection
- Acute rejection
- Constrictive pericarditis

Chronic post-transplant period
- Chronic graft failure
- Chronic rejection/cardiac allograft vasculopathy
- Cardiac masses

Echocardiography

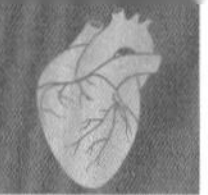

REFERENCES

1. Chambers DC, et al. The International Thoracic Organ Transplant Registry of the International Society for Heart and Lung Transplantation: thirty-fifth adult lung and heart-lung transplant report-2018; Focus theme: multiorgan transplantation. *J Heart Lung Transplant.* 2018;37:1169–1183.
2. Mondillo S, Maccherini M, Galderisi M. Usefulness and limitations of transthoracic echocardiography in heart transplantation recipients. *Cardiovasc Ultrasound.* 2008;6:2.
3. Kuppahally SS, et al. Can echocardiographic evaluation of cardiopulmonary hemodynamics decrease right heart catheterizations in end-stage heart failure patients awaiting transplantation? *Am J Cardiol.* 2010;106:1657–1662.
4. Vouhé PR, et al. Pediatric cardiac transplantation for congenital heart defects: surgical considerations and results. *Ann Thorac Surg.* 1993;56:1239–1247.
5. Lamour JM, et al. The effect of age, diagnosis, and previous surgery in children and adults undergoing heart transplantation for congenital heart disease. *J Am Coll Cardiol.* 2009;54:160–165.
6. Kilic A, Emani S, Sai-Sudhakar CB, Higgins RSD, Whitson BA. Donor selection in heart transplantation. *J Thorac Dis.* 2014;6:1097–1104.
7. Zaroff J. Echocardiographic evaluation of the potential cardiac donor. *J Heart Lung Transplant.* 2004;23:S250–S252.
8. Nair N, Gongora E. Role of cardiovascular imaging in selection of donor hearts. *World J Transplant.* 2015;5:348–353.
9. Venkateswaran RV, et al. Echocardiography in the potential heart donor. *Transplantation.* 2010;89:894–901.
10. Zaroff JG, et al. Consensus conference report: maximizing use of organs recovered from the cadaver donor: cardiac recommendations, March 28–29, 2001, Crystal City, Va. *Circulation.* 2002;106:836–841.
11. Smits JM, et al. Donor scoring system for heart transplantation and the impact on patient survival. *J Heart Lung Transplant.* 2012;31:387–397.
12. Khush KK, Menza R, Nguyen J, Zaroff JG, Goldstein BA. Donor predictors of allograft use and recipient outcomes after heart transplantation. *Circ Heart Fail.* 2013;6:300–309.
13. Weiss ES, et al. Development of a quantitative donor risk index to predict short-term mortality in orthotopic heart transplantation. *J Heart Lung Transplant.* 2012;31:266–273.
14. Kuppahally SS, et al. Outcome in cardiac recipients of donor hearts with increased left ventricular wall thickness. *Am J Transplant.* 2007;7:2388–2395.
15. Pinzon OW, et al. Impact of donor left ventricular hypertrophy on survival after heart transplant. *Am J Transplant.* 2011;11:2755–2761.
16. Marelli D, et al. The use of donor hearts with left ventricular hypertrophy. *J Heart Lung Transplant.* 2000;19:496–503.
17. Goland S, et al. Use of cardiac allografts with mild and moderate left ventricular hypertrophy can be safely used in heart transplantation to expand the donor pool. *J Am Coll Cardiol.* 2008;51:1214–1220.
18. Messer S, et al. Outcome after heart transplantation from donation after circulatory-determined death donors. *J Heart Lung Transplant.* 2017;36:1311–1318.
19. Lazzeri C, Guetti C, Migliaccio ML, Ciapetti M, Peris A. The utility of serial echocardiograms for organ procurement in brain death. *Clin Transplant.* 2017;31. https://doi.org/10.1111/ctr.13094.
20. Powner DJT. Goals during care of adult donors that can influence outcomes of heart transplantation. *Prog. Transpl.* 2005;15:226–232.
21. Bombardini T, et al. Favorable short-term outcome of transplanted hearts selected from marginal donors by pharmacological stress echocardiography. *J Am Soc Echocardiogr.* 2011;24:353–362.
22. Goldberg DS, Blumberg E, McCauley M, Abt P, Levine M. Improving organ utilization to help overcome the tragedies of the opioid epidemic. *Am J Transplant.* 2016;16:2836–2841.
23. Navia JL, et al. Bench repair of donor aortic valve with minimal access orthotopic heart transplantation. *Ann Thorac Surg.* 2005;80:313–315.
24. Larobina ME, Mariani JA, Rowland MA. Aortic valve replacement for aortic stenosis during orthotopic cardiac transplant. *Ann Thorac Surg.* 2008;86:1979–1982.
25. Saito S, et al. Bench replacement of donor aortic valve before orthotopic heart transplantation. *J Heart Lung Transplant.* 2009;28:981–983.
26. Kaczorowski DJ, Woo YJ. Aortic valve repair by sinotubular junctional remodeling to eliminate aortic regurgitation in donor cardiac allograft. *J Thorac Cardiovasc Surg.* 2012;144:722–724.
27. Badano LP, et al. European Association of Cardiovascular Imaging/Cardiovascular Imaging Department of the Brazilian Society of Cardiology recommendations for the use of cardiac imaging to assess and follow patients after heart transplantation. *Eur. Heart J. Cardiovasc. Imaging.* 2015;16:919–948.
28. Estep JD, et al. The role of multimodality cardiac imaging in the transplanted heart. *JACC Cardiovasc. Imaging.* 2009;2:1126–1140.
29. Stehlik J, Kobashigawa J, Hunt SA, Reichenspurner H, Kirklin JK. Honoring 50 years of clinical heart transplantation in circulation: in-depth state-of-the-art review. *Circulation.* 2018;137:71–87.
30. Riberi A, et al. Systemic embolism: a serious complication after cardiac transplantation avoidable by bicaval technique. *Eur J Cardio Thorac Surg.* 2001;19:307–311. discussion 311.
31. Koch A, et al. Influence of different implantation techniques on AV valve competence after orthotopic heart transplantation. *Eur J Cardio Thorac Surg.* 2005;28:717–723.
32. Sun JP, et al. Influence of different implantation techniques on long-term survival after orthotopic heart transplantation: an echocardiographic study. *J Heart Lung Transplant.* 2007;26:1243–1248.
33. Aziz TM, et al. Orthotopic cardiac transplantation technique: a survey of current practice. *Ann Thorac Surg.* 1999;68:1242–1246.
34. Marasco SF, et al. Heterotopic heart transplant: is there an indication in the continuous flow ventricular assist device era? *Eur J Cardio Thorac Surg.* 2014;45:372–376.
35. Bansal R, Perez L, Razzouk A, Wang N, Bailey L. Pericardial constriction after cardiac transplantation. *J Heart Lung Transplant.* 2010;29:371–377.
36. Ueda N, et al. Atypical patterns of constrictive pericarditis after heart transplantation: a case report. *JOT.* 2017;1:32–37.
37. Thajudeen A, et al. Arrhythmias after heart transplantation: mechanisms and management. *J. Am. Heart Assoc.* 2012;1. e001461.
38. Khush KK, et al. The International Thoracic Organ Transplant Registry of the International Society for Heart and Lung Transplantation: thirty-fifth adult heart transplantation report-2018; Focus theme: multiorgan transplantation. *J Heart Lung Transplant.* 2018;37:1155–1168.
39. Chaney MA, Lowe ME, Minhaj MM, Santise G, Jacobsohn E. Inferior vena cava stenosis after bicaval orthotopic heart transplantation. *J Cardiothorac Vasc Anesth.* 2019;33:2561–2568.
40. Lee JZ, Lee KS, Abidov A, Samson RA, Lotun K. Endovascular stenting of suture line supravalvular pulmonic stenosis after orthotopic heart transplantation using rapid pacing stabilization. *JACC Cardiovasc Interv.* 2014;7:e91–e93.
41. Anderson CA, et al. Severity of intraoperative tricuspid regurgitation predicts poor late survival following cardiac transplantation. *Ann Thorac Surg.* 2004;78:1635–1642.
42. Kobashigawa J, et al. Report from a consensus conference on primary graft dysfunction after cardiac transplantation. *J Heart Lung Transplant.* 2014;33:327–340.
43. Dandel M, Hetzer R. Post-transplant surveillance for acute rejection and allograft vasculopathy by echocardiography: usefulness of myocardial velocity and deformation imaging. *J Heart Lung Transplant.* 2017;36:117–131.
44. Mingo-Santos S, et al. Usefulness of two-dimensional strain parameters to diagnose acute rejection after heart transplantation. *J Am Soc Echocardiogr.* 2015;28:1149–1156.
45. Ambardekar AV, Alluri N, Patel AC, Lindenfeld J, Dorosz JL. Myocardial strain and strain rate from speckle-tracking echocardiography are unable to differentiate asymptomatic biopsy-proven cellular rejection in the first year after cardiac transplantation. *J Am Soc Echocardiogr.* 2015;28:478–485.
46. Toumanidis ST, et al. Evaluation of myocardial performance index to predict mild rejection in cardiac transplantation. *Clin Cardiol.* 2004;27:352–358.
47. Ciliberto GR, et al. Significance of pericardial effusion after heart transplantation. *Am J Cardiol.* 1995;76:297–300.
48. Haddad F, et al. Right ventricular dysfunction predicts poor outcome following hemodynamically compromising rejection. *J Heart Lung Transplant.* 2009;28:312–319.
49. Bozbas H, et al. The prevalence and types of cardiovascular disease in patients with end-stage renal disease undergoing renal transplantation. *Transplant Proc.* 2013;45:3478–3480.
50. Essandoh M. Atypical presentation of a large pericardial effusion after heart transplantation in a patient with dilated cardiomyopathy. *J Cardiothorac Vasc Anesth.* 2018;32:e84.
51. Al-Dadah AS, et al. Clinical course and predictors of pericardial effusion following cardiac transplantation. *Transplant Proc.* 2007;39:1589–1592.
52. D'Cruz IA, Overton DH, Pai GM. Pericardial complications of cardiac surgery: emphasis on the diagnostic role of echocardiography. *J Card Surg.* 1992;7:257–268.
53. Amc Y. Treatment of coronary artery fistula post-cardiac transplantation with covered stent: a case study and review of Literature. *Int. J. Transplant. Res. Med.* 2017;3. https://doi.org/10.23937/2572-4045.1510032.
54. Saraiva F, Matos V, Gonçalves L, Antunes M, Providência LA. Complications of endomyocardial biopsy in heart transplant patients: a retrospective study of 2117 consecutive procedures. *Transplant Proc.* 2011;43:1908–1912.

55. Peng DM, et al. Utility of screening echocardiogram after endomyocardial biopsy for identification of cardiac perforation or tricuspid valve injury. *Pediatr Transplant.* 2018;22. e13275.
56. Silvestry FE, et al. Echocardiography-guided interventions. *J Am Soc Echocardiogr.* 2009;22:213–231. quiz 316.
57. Toscano G, et al. Endomyocardial biopsy under echocardiographic monitoring. *Multimed Man Cardiothorac Surg.* 2016 (2016). https://doi.org/10.1093/mmcts/mmw006.
58. Stehlik J, et al. The Registry of the International Society for Heart and Lung Transplantation: twenty-seventh official adult heart transplant report—2010. *J Heart Lung Transplant.* 2010;29:1089–1103.
59. Derumeaux G, et al. Dobutamine stress echocardiography in orthotopic heart transplant recipients. *J Am Coll Cardiol.* 1995;25:1665–1672.
60. Akosah KO, McDaniel S, Hanrahan JS, Mohanty PK. Dobutamine stress echocardiography early after heart transplantation predicts development of allograft coronary artery disease and outcome. *J Am Coll Cardiol.* 1998;31:1607–1614.
61. Spes CH, et al. Dobutamine stress echocardiography for noninvasive diagnosis of cardiac allograft vasculopathy: a comparison with angiography and intravascular ultrasound. *Am J Cardiol.* 1996;78:168–174.
62. Chirakarnjanakorn S, Starling RC, Popović ZB, Griffin BP, Desai MY. Dobutamine stress echocardiography during follow-up surveillance in heart transplant patients: diagnostic accuracy and predictors of outcomes. *J Heart Lung Transplant.* 2015;34:710–717.
63. Clemmensen TS, Eiskjær H, Løgstrup BB et al. Noninvasive detection of cardiac allograft vasculopathy by stress exercise assessment of myocardial deformation. *J Am Soc Echocardiogr.* 2016;29:480–490.
64. Sade LE, et al. Follow-up of heart transplant recipients with serial echocardiographic coronary flow reserve and dobutamine stress echocardiography to detect cardiac allograft vasculopathy. *J Am Soc Echocardiogr.* 2014;27:531–539.
65. Rutz T, et al. Quantitative myocardial contrast echocardiography: a new method for the non-invasive detection of chronic heart transplant rejection. *Eur. Heart J. Cardiovasc. Imaging.* 2013;14:1187–1194.
66. Tona F, et al. Coronary microvascular dysfunction correlates with the new onset of cardiac allograft vasculopathy in heart transplant patients with normal coronary angiography. *Am J Transplant.* 2015;15:1400–1406.
67. Yap WW, Bhattacharya K, Pathi V. Left atrial myxoma in transplanted heart. *Heart.* 2005;91:e49.
68. Yousefzai R, et al. Expecting the unexpected: right atrial mass in a transplant patient. *ESC Heart Fail.* 2015;2:164–167.
69. Neuman Y, et al. Pseudomyxoma originating from the interatrial septum in a heart transplant patient. *J Am Soc Echocardiogr.* 2005;18:e1.
70. Baumwol J, et al. Atrial masses post cardiac transplantation: diagnostic and treatment dilemmas. *Am J Transplant.* 2012;12:2237–2241.
71. Goland S, et al. Changes in left and right ventricular function of donor hearts during the first year after heart transplantation. *Heart.* 2011;97:1681–1686.
72. DeVore AD, et al. Assessment of cardiac allograft systolic function by global longitudinal strain: from donor to recipient. *Clin Transplant.* 2017;31. https://doi.org/10.1111/ctr.12961.
73. Moñivas Palomero V, et al. Two-dimensional speckle tracking echocardiography in heart transplant patients: two-year follow-up of right and left ventricular function. *Echocardiography.* 2016;33:703–713.
74. Valantine HA, et al. A hemodynamic and Doppler echocardiographic study of ventricular function in long-term cardiac allograft recipients. Etiology and prognosis of restrictive-constrictive physiology. *Circulation.* 1989;79:66–75.
75. Barbir M, Lazem F, Banner N, Mitchell A, Yacoub M. The prognostic significance of non-invasive cardiac tests in heart transplant recipients. *Eur Heart J.* 1997;18:692–696.
76. Ambrosi P, Macé L, Habib G. Predictive value of E/A and E/E' Doppler indexes for cardiac events in heart transplant recipients. *Clin Transplant.* 2016;30:959–963.
77. Barakat AF, et al. Prognostic utility of right ventricular free wall strain in low risk patients after orthotopic heart transplantation. *Am J Cardiol.* 2017;119:1890–1896.
78. Eleid MF, et al. Natural history of left ventricular mechanics in transplanted hearts: relationships with clinical variables and genetic expression profiles of allograft rejection. *JACC Cardiovasc. Imaging.* 2010,3.989–1000.
79. Sarvari SI, et al. Early postoperative left ventricular function by echocardiographic strain is a predictor of 1-year mortality in heart transplant recipients. *J Am Soc Echocardiogr.* 2012;25:1007–1014.
80. Spes CH, et al. Diagnostic and prognostic value of serial dobutamine stress echocardiography for noninvasive assessment of cardiac allograft vasculopathy: a comparison with coronary angiography and intravascular ultrasound. *Circulation.* 1999;100:509–515.
81. Ciliberto GR, et al. Resting echocardiography and quantitative dipyridamole technetium-99m sestamibi tomography in the identification of cardiac allograft vasculopathy and the prediction of long-term prognosis after heart transplantation. *Eur Heart J.* 2001;22:964–971.
82. Bacal F, et al. Dobutamine stress echocardiography predicts cardiac events or death in asymptomatic patients long-term after heart transplantation: 4-year prospective evaluation. *J Heart Lung Transplant.* 2004;23:1238–1244.
83. Dedieu N, et al. The importance of qualitative and quantitative regional wall motion abnormality assessment at rest in pediatric coronary allograft vasculopathy. *Pediatr Transplant.* 2018;22. e13208.
84. Vermes E, et al. Cardiovascular magnetic resonance in heart transplant patients: diagnostic value of quantitative tissue markers: T2 mapping and extracellular volume fraction, for acute rejection diagnosis. *J Cardiovasc Magn Reson.* 2018;20:59.
85. Neumann A, et al. MicroRNA 628-5p as a novel biomarker for cardiac allograft vasculopathy. *Transplantation.* 2017;101:e26–e33.
86. Roshanali F, et al. Echo rejection score: new echocardiographic approach to diagnosis of heart transplant rejection. *Eur J Cardio Thorac Surg.* 2010;38:176–180.
87. Lunze FI, Colan SD, Gauvreau K, et al. Tissue Doppler imaging for rejection surveillance in pediatric heart transplant recipients. *J Heart Lung Transplant.* 2013;32(10):1027–1033.
88. Puleo JA, Aranda JM, Weston MW, et al. Noninvasive detection of allograft rejection in heart transplant recipients by use of doppler tissue imaging. *J Heart Lung Transplantat.* 1998;17(2):176–184.
89. Mankad S, Murali S, Kormos RL, et al. Evaluation of the potential role of color-coded tissue Doppler echocardiography in the detection of allograft rejection in heart transplant recipients. *Am Heart J.* 1999;138(4 Pt 1):721–730.
90. Kato TS, Homma S, Mancini D. Novel echocardiographic strategies for rejection diagnosis. *Curr Op Organ Transplant.* 2013;18(5):573–580.
91. Marciniak A, Eroglu E, Marciniak M, et al. The potential clinical role of ultrasonic strain and strain rate imaging in diagnosing acute rejection after heart transplantation. *Eur J Echocardiogr.* 2007;8(3):213–221.
92. Sato T, Kato TS, Komamura K, et al. Utility of left ventricular systolic torsion derived from 2-dimensional speckle-tracking echocardiography in monitoring acute cellular rejection in heart transplant recipients. *J Heart Lung Transplant.* 2011;30(5):536–543.
93. Sera F, Kato TS, Farr M, et al. Left ventricular longitudinal strain by speckle-tracking echocardiography is associated with treatment-requiring cardiac allograft rejection. *J Card Fail.* 2014;20(5):359–364.
94. Sehgal S, Blake JM, Sommerfield J, Aggarwal S. Strain and strain rate imaging using speckle tracking in acute allograft rejection in children with heart transplantation. *Pediatr Transplant.* 2015;19(2):188–195.
95. Ruiz Orti M, Peña ML, Mesa D, et al. Impact of asymptomatic acute cellular rejection on left ventricle myocardial function evaluated by means of two-dimensional speckle tracking echocardiography in heart transplant recipients. *Echocardiography.* 2015;32(2):229–237.
96. Du G-Q, Hsiung M-C, Wu Y, et al. Three-dimensional speckle-tracking echocardiographic monitoring of acute rejection in heart transplant recipients. *J Ultrasound Med.* 2016;35(6):1167–1176.
97. Collings CA, Pinto FJ, Valentine HA. Exercise echocardiography in heart transplant recipients: a comparison with angiography and intracoronary ultrasonography. *J Heart Lung Transplant.* 1994;13:604–613.
98. Smart FW, Balantyne CM, Cocanougher B, et al. Insensitivity of noninvasive tests to detect coronary artery vasculopathy after after heart transplant. *Am J Cardiol.* 1991;67:243–247.
99. Cohn JM, Wilensky RL, O'Donnell JA, et al. Exercise echocardiography, angiography and intra-operative ultrasound after cardiac transplantation. *Am J Cardiol.* 1996;77:1216–1219.
100. Chen HM, Abernathey E, Lunze F, et al. Utility of exercise stress echocardiography in pediatric cardiac transplant recipients: a single-center experience. *J Heart Lung Transplant.* 2012;31:517–523.
101. Clerkin KJ, Farr MA, Restaino SW, et al. Dobutamine stress echocardiography is inadequate to detect early cardiac allograft vasculopathy. *J Heart Lung Transplant.* 2016;35:1040–1041.
102. Stork S, Behr TM, Birk M, et al. Assessment of cardiac vasculopathy late after heart transplantation: when is coronary angiography necessary? *J Heart Lung Transplant.* 2006;25:1103–1108.
103. Herregods MC, Anastasiou I, van Cleemput J, et al. Dobutamine stress echocardiography after heart transplantation. *J Heart Lung Transplant.* 1994;13:1039–1044.
104. Bharat DA, Manlhiot C, Safi M, et al. A prospective study of dobutamine stress echocardiography for assessment of cardiac allograft vasculopathy in pediatric heart transplant recipients. *Pediatr Transplant.* 2008;12:170–176.
105. Eroglu E, D'Hooge J, Sutherland GR, et al. Quantitative dobutamine stress echocardiography for early detection of cardiac allograft vasculopathy in heart transplant recipients. *Heart.* 2008;94(e3):2.

中文导读

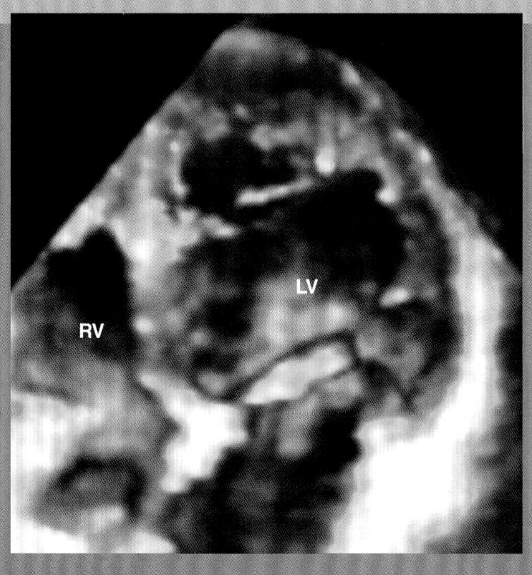

第16章 心脏辅助设备

心力衰竭已成为威胁全球人民健康的一种严重疾病。目前，心脏移植仍然是终末期心力衰竭患者的主要治疗方法，但由于心脏供体数量有限及存在术后排异反应，其应用受到了很大的限制。因此，机械循环支持在治疗晚期心脏疾病方面发挥着越来越重要的作用。超声心动图可以提供心脏辅助设备所支持的心脏的结构、功能和血流动力学方面的信息，已成为机械循环支持植入治疗过程中最重要的影像学检查手段。

本章详细介绍了机械循环支持设备的工作原理和心脏辅助装置的类型，全面阐述了经胸和经食管超声心动图在机械循环支持植入前患者筛选、植入术中监测及植入术后远期随访中的作用、检查时机及检查要点，并客观地说明了超声心动图在评估机械循环支持植入患者时存在的局限性和对未来发展方向的展望。

施怡声

16 Cardiac Assist Devices

JAMES N. KIRKPATRICK, MD

Mechanical circulatory support (MCS) in the form of cardiac assist devices plays an increasingly important role in the treatment of end-stage cardiac disease. Extracorporeal membrane oxygenation (ECMO) devices developed in the middle of the 20th century enabled cardiopulmonary bypass and subsequent advances in cardiac surgery. ECMO began to be used outside of the operating room for temporary support of children with ventricular failure.

A permanent heart replacement device has been under development since the 1950s[1] and spawned the development of the total artificial heart and right (RV) and left (LV) ventricular assist devices (VADs). Early-generation VADs were used as a bridge to recovery to support patients who were expected to recover from reversible cardiac insults.[2,3] Indications soon expanded to include stabilization of patients before organ transplantation (i.e., bridge to transplantation).[4–6]

Technologic improvements reduced VAD size so that the device could be implanted in the abdomen or chest, allowing patients to await transplantation at home. The early devices were the size of small refrigerators; the newest implantable pump fits into the palm of a hand.

Developments in percutaneously placed device technology have expanded the options for temporary cardiac support, although ECMO remains a mainstay in many institutions. In addition to supporting ventricles until recovery, transplantation, or implantation of a long-term VAD platform, temporary devices have been used to stabilize patients with refractory ventricular arrhythmias, to support marginal ventricles through procedures (e.g., high-risk percutaneous coronary or valvular interventions, complex arrhythmia ablations), and to provide a vent to decompress the LV in patients on ECMO.[7]

The success of early VADs,[8] the limited number of donor hearts, and the large number of patients excluded from transplantation candidacy because of age or comorbidities led to the use of VADs as a permanent treatment.[9] This application of VADs as destination therapy set the stage for widespread use.[10,11] A few patients supported on long-term platforms demonstrate sufficient recovery of native heart function to be considered for device explantation, a protracted bridge to recovery.

Echocardiography is the most important imaging modality for all forms of MCS. Echocardiography before implantation identifies pitfalls to MCS device insertion. During implantation, transesophageal echocardiography (TEE) guides surgical placement of the device components and can be used to establish initial device settings. After implantation, echocardiography provides surveillance imaging to detect dysfunction of the device or native heart and to optimize device settings. Echocardiography readily characterizes the causes of device alarms and patient symptoms. Echocardiography also identifies patients with ventricular recovery who are candidates for device explantation.

PRINCIPLES OF MECHANICAL CIRCULATORY SUPPORT AND TYPES OF CARDIAC ASSIST DEVICES

There are three basic types of cardiac assist devices: durable, implanted VADs; percutaneous MCS devices; and total artificial hearts (Table 16.1).

DURABLE, IMPLANTED VENTRICULAR ASSIST DEVICES

Most implanted VADs consist of a pump, an inflow cannula, an outflow cannula, a power supply, and a controller. The controller collects data from the pump and directs its action through a driveline. VADs are classified according to the location of these components. Extracorporeal VADs have pumps and controllers outside the body. Patients with paracorporeal VADs have pumps strapped close to the body but not inside it. Intracorporeal VADs have implanted pumps, with drivelines connecting to a paracorporeal or extracorporeal controller and batteries or another power supply.

Cardiac assist devices can support the LV as an LV assist device (LVAD), the right ventricle (RV) as an RV assist device (RVAD), or both ventricles as a biventricular assist device (BI-VAD). LVAD inflow cannulas are connected to left-sided chambers, most often the LV apex. The outflow graft cannula can be attached to the aorta in multiple places but is usually anastomosed, end to side,

TABLE 16.1 Examples of Commonly Used Ventricular Assist Devices.

Name (Company)[a]	Pump Location[b]	Mechanism	Cannulas	Specifications	Indications
EXCOR Pediatric (Berlin Heart)	Extracorporeal	Pulsatile	Inflow: LV or RV Outflow: Asc Ao or PA	6 different pump sizes: 10–60 mL	BTT
HeartMate II (Abbott)	Anterior abdominal wall	Axial	Inflow: LV apex Outflow: Asc Ao	3–10 L/min 6,000–15,000 rpm	BTT, destination therapy
HeartMate III (Abbott)	Pericardium	Centrifugal	Inflow: LV apex Outflow: Asc Ao	Up to 10 L/min 4800–6500 rpm	BTT, destination therapy
HeartWare[a] HVAD (Medtronic)	Pericardium	Centrifugal	Inflow: LV apex Outflow: Asc Ao	Up to 10 L/min 2000–3000 rpm	BTT, destination therapy
CentriMag (Abbott)	Extracorporeal	Centrifugal	Inflow: LA or LV by RSPV, RA Outflow: Asc Ao, PA	Up to 9.9 L/min	Up to 6 h
PediMag (Abbott)	Extracorporeal	Centrifugal	As above	Up to 1.5 L/min	Acute BTR or bridge to decision
Impella Recover 2.5, 5.0, CP (Abiomed)	Catheter	Axial	Single cannula, femoral artery access, retrograde across aortic valve Inflow: LVOT Outflow: Asc Ao	2.5 L/min or 5 L/min	Up to 4 days for the 2.5, and up to 6 days for others
TandemHeart (LivaNova)	Extracorporeal	Centrifugal	Transseptal LA and femoral artery cannulation	2–5 L/min	Up to 6 h
Impella Recover RP (Abiomed)	Catheter	Axial	Single cannula, femoral vein access, placed antegrade Inflow: IVC Outflow: PA	2–5 L/min	Up to 14 days
ProtekDuo	Extracorporeal	Centrifugal	Internal jugular vein access, placed antegrade Inflow: RA Outflow: PA	2–5 L/min	Up to 6 h
CardioWest (SynCardia)	TAH	—	Pumps replace LV and RV	Up to 9.5 L/min	BTT

[a]Company Headquarters: Abbott (Abbott Park, IL), Berlin Heart (Berlin, Germany), HeartWare (Minneapolis, MN), Abiomed (Danvers, MA), LivaNova (London, UK), SynCardia (Tucson, AZ).
[b]Pumps located in or near inflow cannula create imaging artifacts.
Asc Ao, Ascending aorta; *BTR,* bridge to recovery; *BTT,* bridge to transplant; *IVC,* inferior vena cava; *LVOT,* left ventricular outflow tract; *PA,* pulmonary artery; *RSPV,* right superior pulmonary vein; *TAH,* total artificial heart.

to the ascending aorta. RVADs involve right atrial (RA) or RV inflow and pulmonary artery outflow cannulation.

Devices are also characterized by mechanism. Early-generation cardiac VADs included a pneumatically compressed, distensible chamber or a pusher-plate mechanism to expel blood into the outflow cannula. These early-generation devices simulated cardiac pulsatile action through one-way inlet and outlet valves.[12]

The second-generation VADs produce continuous flow by a rotating propeller and are called *axial-flow pumps.* The HeartMate II (Abbott, Abbott Park, IL) draws blood from the heart through an inflow cannula and propels it into the outflow graft cannula (Fig. 16.1A).

The third-generation continuous-flow VADs, HeartWare HVAD (Medtronic, Minneapolis, MN), and HeartMate 3, use centrifugal force to propel blood. Magnetic or hydrodynamic forces levitate and spin a disklike impeller rather than a propeller (see Fig. 16.1B). The speed of the propeller or impeller (in revolutions per minute [rpm]) and the pressure difference between the inflow and outflow cannulas determine the rate of flow. There is greater flow during systole, when the aortic-LV pressure difference drops (i.e., LV pressure rises with ventricular contraction) than during diastole, when LV pressure falls with ventricular relaxation and the pressure difference increases.

The continuous-flow pumps provide greater flow at lower pressures than pulsatile pumps do. They also tend to be more durable because they lack valves (which wear out over time).[13,14] Centrifugal pumps lack bearings and may reduce the amount of hemolysis, and they appear to be associated with lower rates of reoperation for pump dysfunction.[15] The HeartMate 3 device has an additional feature that rapidly and briefly alters pump speed, asynchronous to heart rate, with the intention of lowering rates of thrombosis.

Continuous-flow devices are called *nonpulsatile* VADs, but residual ventricular function and non-uniform pressure differences between the inflow and outflow cannulas produce some pulsatility. Centrifugal-flow devices, particularly the HeartMate 3, demonstrate greater pulsatility than the axial-flow devices.[16,17]

PERCUTANEOUS MECHANICAL CIRCULATORY SUPPORT DEVICES

Percutaneous MCS devices are inserted through peripheral arteries and veins and can be placed relatively quickly to provide temporary support. The Impella Recover devices (Abiomed, Danvers, MA) consist of an axial-flow (propeller) pump within a catheter that is placed into the femoral artery, through the aorta, and across the aortic valve into the LV (Fig. 16.2A). The inflow port draws blood from the LV outflow tract (LVOT) and ejects it through the outflow port in the aorta. A right-sided Impella is placed into the RV and across the pulmonic valve; it draws blood from the RV outflow tract (RVOT) and pumps it into the proximal pulmonary artery. Several different sizes are available, corresponding to the amount of support in liters per minute. The larger devices have traditionally required surgical cutdown of a large artery for insertion.

The TandemHeart (LivaNova, London, UK) devices consist of a paracorporeal centrifugal-flow pump connected to an inflow catheter, which is placed through the venous system into the RA, and then into the left atrium (LA) across the interatrial septum, and an outflow cannula that is in the distal aorta through the femoral artery (see Fig. 16.2B). The TandemHeart cannulas can also be positioned in the RA (inflow) and the pulmonary artery (outflow) to support the RV and can be

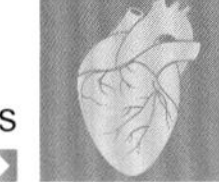

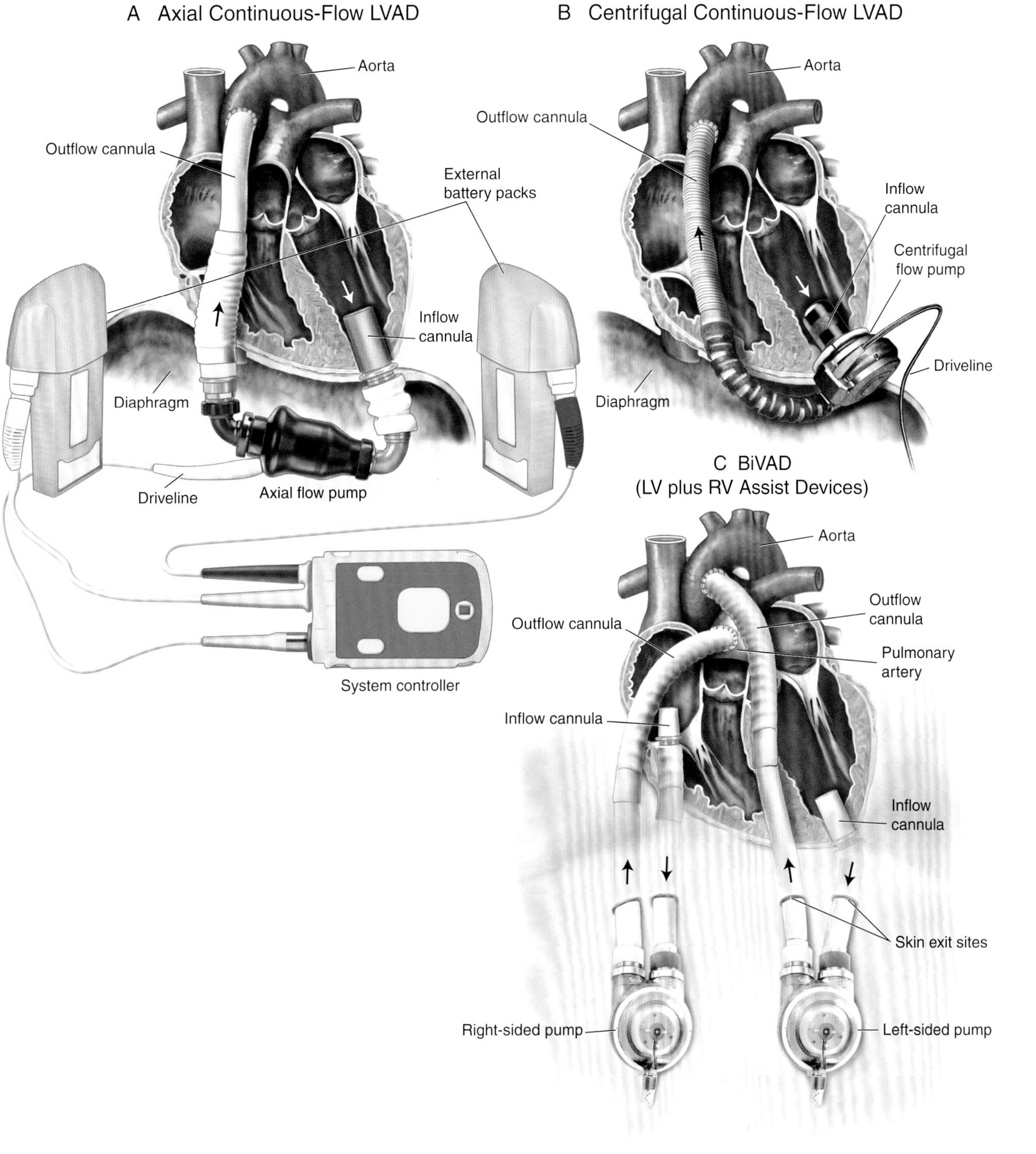

Fig. 16.1 Examples of ventricular assist devices. (A) Axial continuous-flow LV assist device *(LVAD)* (HeartMate II, Abbott, Abbott Park, IL). (B) Centrifugal continuous-flow LVAD (HVAD, Medtronic, Minneapolis, MN). (C) Biventricular assist device *(BiVAD)*.

connected to an oxygenator to provide lung support, similar to venovenous ECMO. The TandemHeart devices improve the cardiac index and pulmonary pressures in patients with decompensated heart failure after myocardial infarction and have been used to stabilize patients with incessant ventricular tachycardia.

The CentriMag (Abbott, Abbott Park, IL) consists of a paracorporeal, centrifugal pump with a magnetically levitated impeller. It can be connected with catheters placed in any of the cardiac chambers to provide left (LA or LV inflow, aortic outflow), right (RA or RV inflow, pulmonary artery outflow), biventricular, or cardiopulmonary support. The CentriMag has been used to provide temporary support of the RV in patients with a durable LVAD.

TOTAL ARTIFICIAL HEART

The current version of the total artificial heart, the temporary Total Artificial Heart (TAH-t; SynCardia Systems, Tucson, AZ)

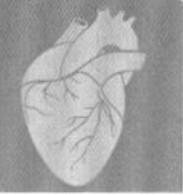

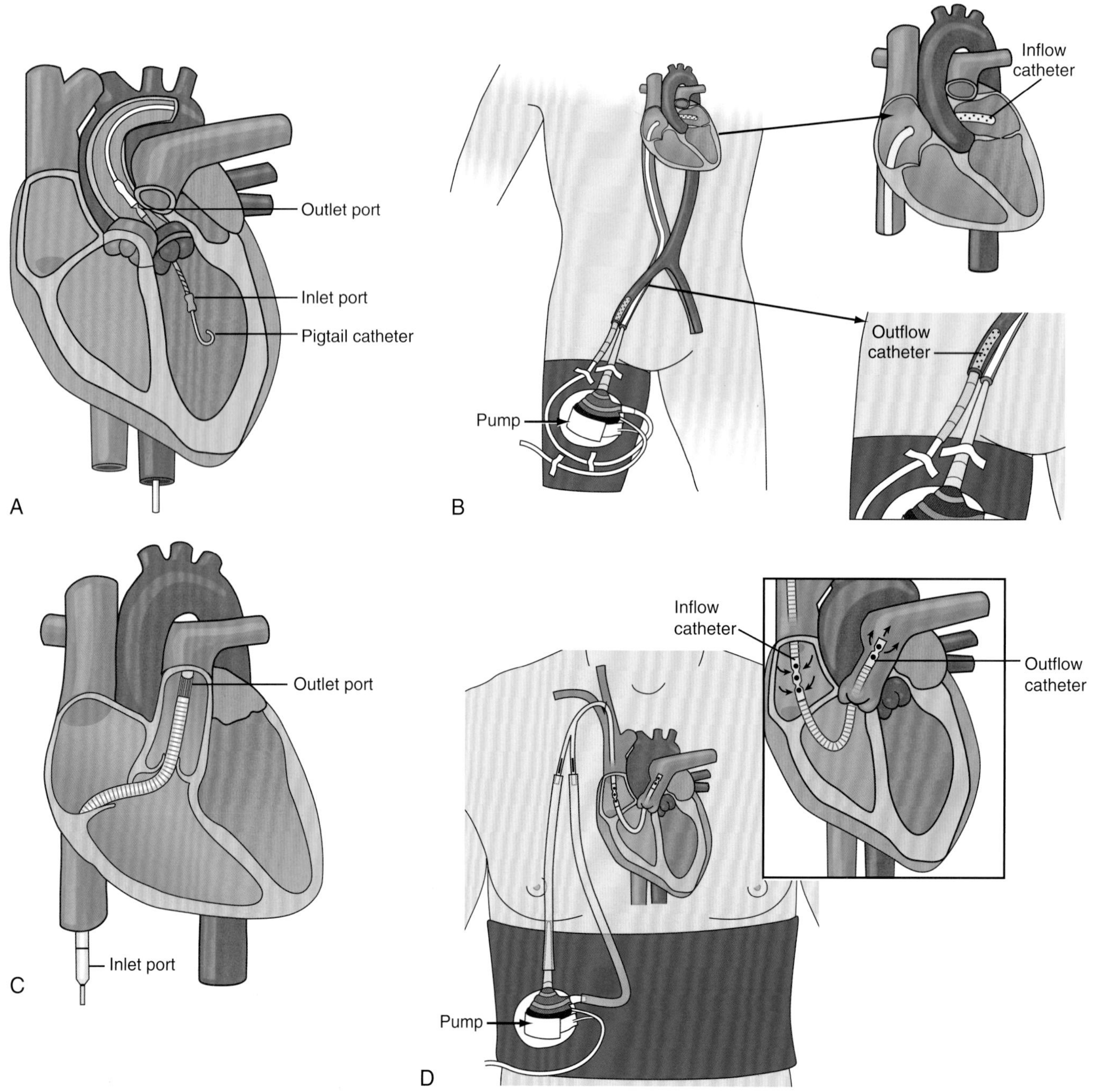

Fig. 16.2 Percutaneous ventricular assist devices. (A) Impella Recover device (Abiomed, Danvers, MA) consists of an axial-flow pump (propeller) inside a catheter that has a distal inflow port and a more proximal outflow port. The catheter is inserted into the femoral artery, through the aorta, and across the aortic valve into the LV. A pigtail catheter is left in the central lumen for stabilization. The inflow port is positioned below the aortic valve to draw blood from the LV outflow tract. The outflow port is located in the ascending aorta. Flow is determined by the propeller speed and the aortic-LV pressure difference. The Impella can also be inserted through the chest into the ascending aorta. (B) The TandemHeart (LivaNova, London, UK) has a paracorporeal centrifugal-flow pump connected to an inflow cannula that is inserted in the femoral vein and advanced into the RA, across an interatrial septotomy, and into the LA. A separate outflow cannula is inserted into one femoral artery and advanced into the distal aorta. Alternatively, an outflow catheter can be inserted into each femoral artery. (C) The Impella RP device supports the right ventricle with an inflow port in the inferior vena cava and the outflow port in the proximal pulmonary artery. (D) The TandemHeart cannula can also be positioned in the RA (inflow) and the pulmonary artery (outflow) to support the RV.

replaces the RV and LV with pulsatile pumps and metallic atrioventricular valves anastomosed to the native atria. The pumping component is attached by drivelines to an extracorporeal controller and battery (Fig. 16.3). The SynCardia device is approved by the U.S. Food and Drug Administration (FDA) as a bridge to transplantation.

ECHOCARDIOGRAPHIC APPROACH TO MECHANICAL CIRCULATORY SUPPORT

PREIMPLANTATION ASSESSMENT

Specific criteria for placement of an LVAD as destination therapy include an LV ejection fraction (LVEF) of less than 25%

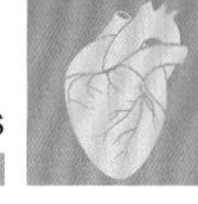

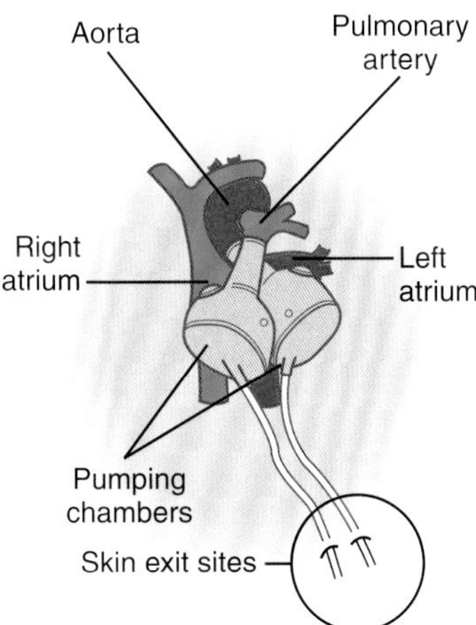

Fig. 16.3 **Total artificial heart.** The SynCardia device (SynCardia Systems, Tucson, AZ) consists of two pumping chambers attached to the native atria and great arteries.

to 30%, most often measured by echocardiography. Although the hemodynamic criteria refer to invasively determined measurements, echocardiography can provide noninvasive assessment of the cardiac index and intracardiac pressures. A small ventricular size (<6.3 cm) portends a worse outcome after LVAD implantation, possibly because patients with smaller cavity sizes and severe LV dysfunction suffer from infiltrative cardiomyopathies.[18]

Echocardiography identifies factors that warrant interventions, complicate cardiac assist device placement, or support the use of one type of device over another (Table 16.2). It is particularly important to detect thrombi that can embolize after an MCS device is placed. Use of an ultrasound enhancing agent (i.e., microbubble contrast) may be necessary to exclude ventricular thrombi in patients with inadequate images, and TEE should be used to examine LA and RA appendages in patients with atrial fibrillation or atrial flutter. Intracardiac shunting produces systemic hypoxemia and/or paradoxical emboli after LVAD placement with left-sided decompression and a potential right-to-left pressure gradient. Intracardiac shunts should be repaired at the time of implantation. High LA pressure may prevent passage of agitated saline contrast across a patent foramen ovale (PFO), even after a Valsalva maneuver, leading to false-negative examination results for shunting at the atrial level.

Moderate or greater aortic regurgitation (AR) complicates the use of MCS devices.[19] Placement of an outflow cannula in the ascending aorta or an Impella Recover device across the aortic valve may worsen baseline AR, leading to circulation of blood from the LV to the pump, to the aorta, and back into the LV. High LV pressure and low diastolic pressure in the aortic root from severe AR can reduce coronary perfusion pressure, which is exacerbated by the fact that the TandemHeart draws blood from the LA and ejects it into the distal aorta (bypassing the coronary ostia).

Preimplantation grading of the degree of AR is complicated in patients with end-stage heart failure, who commonly have low systemic pressure and high LV diastolic pressure. The low aortic-to-LV pressure gradient may artificially decrease the amount of regurgitation through an incompetent aortic valve. In the case of greater than moderate AR, the aortic valve should be replaced, repaired, or (rarely) oversewn.[20] Although significant mitral stenosis must be corrected at the time of implantation of an LVAD or Impella device because it impedes flow into the device, aortic stenosis does not necessarily require intervention because the aortic valve is bypassed. However, severe aortic stenosis, aortic valve oversewing to prevent AR, and aortic valve cusp fusion prevent cardiac output in the setting of LVAD pump failure. Significant mitral regurgitation should be ameliorated

TABLE 16.2 Echocardiographic Findings That Complicate Ventricular Assist Device Implantation.

Finding	*Implications*
Thrombus in cardiac chamber	Thrombectomy at time of implantation
	Placement of cannula in alternate chamber
Intracardiac shunting	Repair of shunt
Aortic aneurysms, tortuosity, atheromas	Graft repair of aneurysm
	Placement of outflow graft cannula away from atheroma
	Caution with Impella Recover
Aortic stenosis (moderate or greater)	Bioprosthetic valve replacement[a]
	Impella Recover contraindicated
Aortic regurgitation (moderate or greater)	Bioprosthetic valve replacement[a]
	Oversew valve cusps, use Park stitch to oppose two commissures
	Cannulation of descending aorta
	Orient ascending aortic graft cannula away from aortic valve
	Caution with TandemHeart
	Impella Recover contraindicated
Mitral stenosis	Valvuloplasty
	Bioprosthetic valve replacement[a]
	Placement of inflow cannula in LA
	Caution with Impella Recover
Mitral regurgitation	Repair or bioprosthetic valve replacement[a]
	Caution with Impella Recover
RV systolic dysfunction	Caution with left-sided MCS devices
	Right-sided MCS device
Ventricular septal defect	Caution with Impella Recover (right-to-left shunting)
	Repair at implantation[a]
Atrial septal defect	Caution with TandemHeart and LA cannulation (right-to-left shunting)
	Repair at implantation[a]
Interatrial septal aneurysm	Caution with TandemHeart and ECMO or CentriMag atrial cannulation (aneurysm can be drawn into and obstruct cannula)
Heavy LV trabeculation, aneurysms/dyskinetic walls, redundant chords, prominent ridges, small inflow chamber	Orient inflow cannula away from potentially obstructing structures
	Excise trabeculation
	Excise aneurysm
Clotting diathesis	Avoid LA cannulation, caution with TandemHeart, ECMO, CentriMag (stasis in bypassed LV)
	Ensure aortic valve opening to "wash" aortic root
	Higher INR target, additional antiplatelet agents
Pericardial effusion (chambers can collapse after decompression with VAD)	Effusion drainage
Peripheral vascular disease	Caution with Impella Recover
	Caution with TandemHeart

[a]Mechanical valves are generally not used in VAD patients because of concerns for thrombus formation despite anticoagulation.
INR, International normalized ratio; *ECMO,* extracorporeal membrane oxygenation; *MCS,* mechanical circulatory support; *VAD,* ventricular assist device.
Adapted from Stainback RF, Estep JD, Agler DA, et al. Echocardiography in the management of patients with left ventricular assist devices: recommendations from the American Society of Echocardiography. *J Am Soc Echocardiogr*. 2015;28:853–909.

by a functioning LVAD and does not represent a pitfall for implantation.

Mechanical prosthetic aortic valves should be replaced with a bioprosthesis at the time of implantation because reduced transaortic flow increases the risk of thrombosis. Transmitral flow, however, is preserved, and a functional mechanical mitral valve need not be replaced.[20,21]

Before implantation, identification and characterization of RV dysfunction is vitally important. RV failure is a significant cause of morbidity and mortality.[22] LVAD placement produces a higher cardiac output and increased venous return to the RV. An RV with preexisting dysfunction may fail in the setting of increased preload.[23] The LVAD influence on septal motion reduces RV function and can worsen baseline tricuspid regurgitation. However, decompression of the LV by a VAD can reduce pulmonary pressures and RV afterload, improving RV function. Identification of RV dysfunction can lead to a decision to delay durable LVAD implantation to optimize RV function through medical therapy or a temporary RVAD; to implant a TAH, a BIVAD, or an RVAD with an LVAD; or to forego durable MCS device implantation entirely. For patients with known RV dysfunction, planned early placement of an RVAD improves survival compared with delayed placement.[24] In light of the potential worsening of RV function with increased tricuspid regurgitation after LVAD implantation, expert consensus documents recommend tricuspid repair if tricuspid regurgitation is greater than moderate.[21]

TEE may be necessary to assess valvular anatomy and function and to exclude vegetations in patients with suspected endocarditis.[21] Imaging of the ascending aorta may reveal aneurysms, dissections, or severe or mobile atheromatous plaques, all of which complicate placement of an outflow graft.

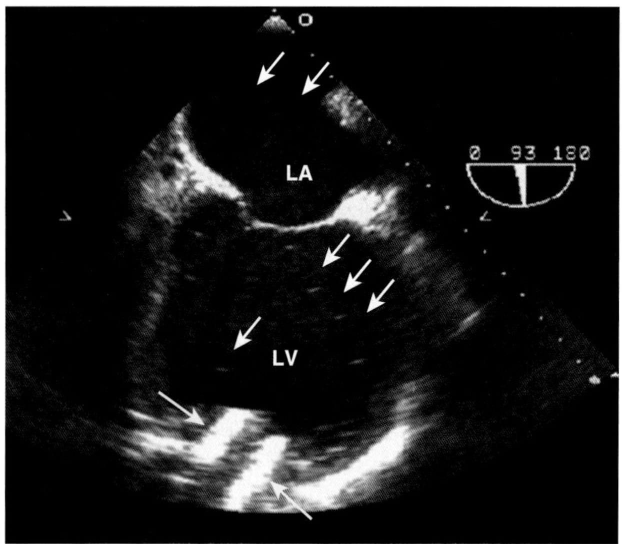

Fig. 16.4 Intracardiac air after LV assist device implantation. This mid-esophageal TEE apex-down 2-chamber view demonstrates air bubbles *(white arrows)* in the LV and LA after placement of an LV apical inflow cannula (sides defined by *yellow arrows*). Echocardiography can detect bubbles arising at anastomotic sites. Ventricular chambers should be deaired before coming off bypass.

PERIPROCEDURAL GUIDANCE

Intracardiac echocardiography and TEE provide real-time visualization to direct cannula placement away from potentially obstructing cardiac structures. The Impella device can be guided to position the inflow port in the LVOT and the outflow port above the aortic valve. Echocardiography can guide transseptal puncture in TandemHeart insertion, preventing inadvertent puncture of the LA or RA wall or the aortic root.

As with other cardiac surgical procedures, TEE is useful in deairing the heart before taking the patient off bypass. Air bubbles arise at cannula anastomosis sites and can embolize if not detected before the aortic cross-clamp is removed. Anterior structures, including the ascending aorta, the RV, and anterior portions of the LV, should be examined for air bubbles[25] (Fig. 16.4).

Periprocedural TEE is useful to reassess the degree of AR, identify a potentially missed PFO, and guide initial speed settings (see Optimization Studies). After chest closure, periprocedural TEE can assess for changes in cannula orientation.

POSTIMPLANTATION SURVEILLANCE AND COMPLICATIONS

When there is no suspicion of MCS device dysfunction, longitudinal surveillance echocardiographic studies are part of protocols for many institutions that follow patients with cardiac assist devices (Table 16.3). The protocols vary in the frequency and timing of echocardiography. The goals of these echocardiograms are to monitor baseline changes in native heart and device performance and to detect dysfunction before clinical manifestations. Examples include worsening AR with LV enlargement

TABLE 16.3 Postimplantation Echocardiographic Imaging Studies for Mechanical Circulatory Support Devices.

Parameter	*Surveillance*	*Problem Focus*	*Recovery*
Purpose	Establish parameters for LVAD and native heart function Early diagnosis of occult pathology/dysfunction Screen for recovery	Determine cause of clinical symptoms Determine cause of LVAD controller alarms	Determine candidacy for explantation
Timing/setting	Before discharge from implantation hospitalization At 1, 3, 6, and 12 mo Every 6–12 mo	Congestive symptoms Lightheadedness or syncope Arrhythmias High flow/power Low flow/power	Ventricular remodeling on surveillance echocardiography or after resolution of insult or clinical improvement Improvement in systolic function on surveillance echocardiography or after resolution of insult or clinical improvement
Speed change	Optimization of parameters: LV filling, AoV opening, AR, RV systolic function	Ramp Position change	Weaning/turndown: at minimal level of support ± after exercise

AR, Aortic regurgitation; *AoV,* aortic valve; *LVAD,* LV assist device.

Adapted from Stainback RF, Estep JD, Agler DA, et al. Echocardiography in the management of patients with left ventricular assist devices: recommendations from the American Society of Echocardiography. *J Am Soc Echocardiogr.* 2015;28:853–909.

and detection of intracardiac thrombi. Surveillance echocardiography may be performed with speed changes to optimize devices with echocardiographic parameters directing the optimal setting (discussed later). In certain cases, improvement in cardiac function detected on surveillance echocardiography may warrant consideration for explantation.

Echocardiography is also performed for symptoms such as dyspnea, edema, and lightheadedness and for MCS device alarms (Table 16.4). Current MCS devices have alarms tied to changes in power consumption and/or flow, although the latter are limited in accuracy. Alarms signal that dysfunction exists, but defining the cause of the dysfunction often requires an imaging study[26] (Table 16.5).

TABLE 16.4 Mechanical Circulatory Support Controller Readings and Alarms.

Power: measurement of average power consumption of the device over time; directly related to speed
- Power spike, high power: increase in power without an increase in speed suggests mechanical obstruction

Flow: given as L/min; directly related to speed and power; calculated for durable LVADs and measured for ECMO
- Low flow:
  - Suction events
  - RV failure
  - Tamponade
  - Underfilling
  - Inflow cannula obstruction
  - Outflow graft kink
  - Hypertension
  - Arrhythmias
- High flow:
  - Pump thrombosis (in reality, high power with low flow)
  - Sepsis/vasodilation
  - Aortic regurgitation
  - Recovery of native ventricular function

ECMO, Extracorporeal membrane oxygenation; *LVAD*, LV assist device.

TABLE 16.5 Echocardiographic Findings in Ventricular Assist Device Dysfunction.

Obstruction or Overfilling

- ↑ LVEDd (especially axial-flow devices)
- Septum → RV (especially for axial-flow devices)
- Spontaneous echocardiographic contrast
- ↑ Aortic valve opening
- ↑ Outflow cannula velocities
  - Pulsatile: >2.3 m/s peak inflow, >2.1 m/s peak outflow[a]
  - Axial flow: >1.5 m/s peak inflow, >2.0 m/s outflow[a]
  - Centrifugal flow: >3.4 m/s peak outflow[b]
- Inflow cannula regurgitation (pulsatile and axial flow)
  - Pulsatile: VAD peak outflow < 1.8 m/s
  - Flow reversal by color, spectral Doppler
  - Thrombus or vegetation obstructing cannula

Underfilling

- ↓ LVEDd
- Septum → LV
- ↓ Aortic valve opening
- Pericardial effusion with chamber collapse
- Suction of cardiac structures into inflow cannula
- ↑ Cannula velocities

[a]Few data exist on normal velocities, but for most continuous-flow devices, patients have peak velocities of <1.5 m/s.
[b]Data from Grinstein J, Kruse E, Sayer G, et al. Screening for outflow cannula malfunction of left ventricular assist devices (LVADs) with the use of Doppler echocardiography: new LVAD-specific reference values for contemporary devices. *J Card Fail.* 2016;22(10):808–814.
LVEDd, LV end-diastolic diameter; *VAD*, ventricular assist device; ↑, increased; ↓, decreased;. →, shifted toward.
From Stainback RF, Estep JD, Agler DA, et al: Echocardiography in the management of patients with left ventricular assist devices: recommendations from the American Society of Echocardiography. *J Am Soc Echocardiogr*. 2015;28:853–909.

Overfilling

Regurgitation, obstruction, and malfunction cause overfilling and pressure increase in the supported ventricle. In pulsatile VADs, failure of the one-way valves leads to regurgitation. Cannula regurgitation can occur in continuous-flow devices when the systemic vascular resistance is elevated. Cannula obstruction can result from kinking, malposition, or thrombosis and can be partial, complete, or intermittent. VAD pumping mechanisms may become partially or completely obstructed, leading to increased shear stress and hemolysis.

There can be primary failure of VAD components: battery, controller, or pump. Pump failure can result from failure of the pumping mechanism but is more likely to result from pump thrombosis. The ensuing ventricular dilation and reduced cardiac output can lead to intracavitary stasis and thrombus formation in the LV or aortic root (Fig. 16.5). Failure of the power supply or of the controller can be catastrophic unless the patient has adequate residual cardiac function and an unobstructed aortic outflow.

Underfilling

Underfilling of the supported ventricle shrinks the cavity size and can cause obstruction of the inflow cannula due to encroachment by normal cardiac structures, which is called a *suction event*. Trabeculations, papillary muscles, chordal structures, ridges, and septa are drawn into the orifice of the inflow cannula as chamber size decreases (Fig. 16.6). Obstruction of the orifice decreases flow, reduces cardiac output, and causes arrhythmias.

Anything that reduces preload can predispose to obstruction of the inflow orifice, including dehydration, overdiuresis, sepsis, and tamponade (Fig. 16.7). RV failure with an inability to fill the left side can lead to LV suction events. Bleeding is a special concern because some form of anticoagulation is advised for most VAD patients to prevent thrombosis. Continuous-flow VADs have been associated with an increased risk of gastrointestinal bleeding.[27]

Valvular Dysfunction

Relatively mild AR before device implantation may worsen after LVAD placement. Development of de novo AR can occur months after implantation and may be related to changes in aortic sinus size and lack of aortic valve opening.[28] AR after LVAD placement can be difficult to quantify because it can be continuous throughout systole and diastole.

Acquired aortic stenosis due to cusp fusion is a rare but recognized complication in native and bioprosthetic valves.[29] Echocardiographic examination of the valve leaflets can reveal a relatively normal structure. When the aortic valve does not open or opens minimally, there is a risk of thrombus formation in the aortic root, especially in continuous-flow VADs, because of the lower, mostly nonpulsatile flows.[30] AR that is refractory to medical and device speed management and cusp fusion in the setting of possible recovery may require transcatheter aortic valve intervention.[30]

Mitral regurgitation usually improves when an LVAD is placed, but the Impella Recover devices may interfere with the chordal apparatus or the anterior mitral valve leaflet, causing an increase in mitral regurgitation. Suction events that tether chordae or papillary muscles may have the same result. Tricuspid regurgitation can increase after LVAD placement because septal shift and annular distortion can lead to tethering on the septal leaflet.

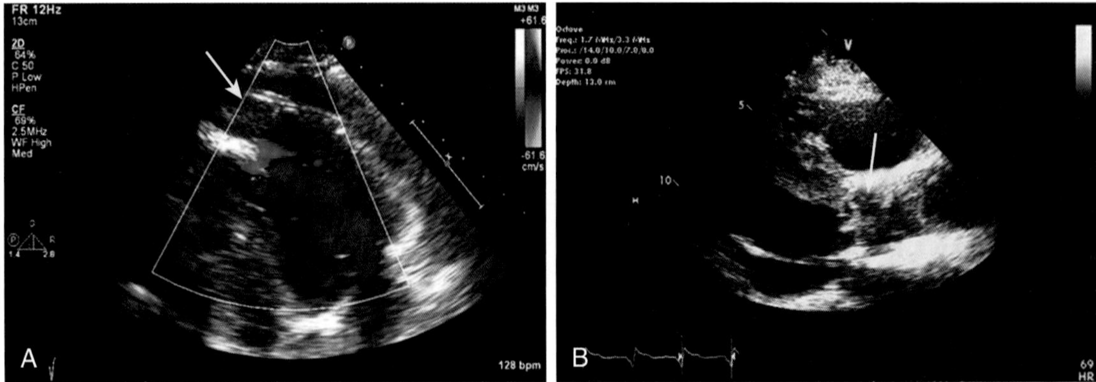

Fig. 16.5 **Intracardiac thrombi after implantation of an LV assist device.** (A) Modified apical 4-chamber view demonstrates thrombus in the LV apex *(arrow)* alongside the LV assist device inflow cannula. (B) Parasternal long-axis view demonstrates thrombus in the aortic root *(arrow)*.

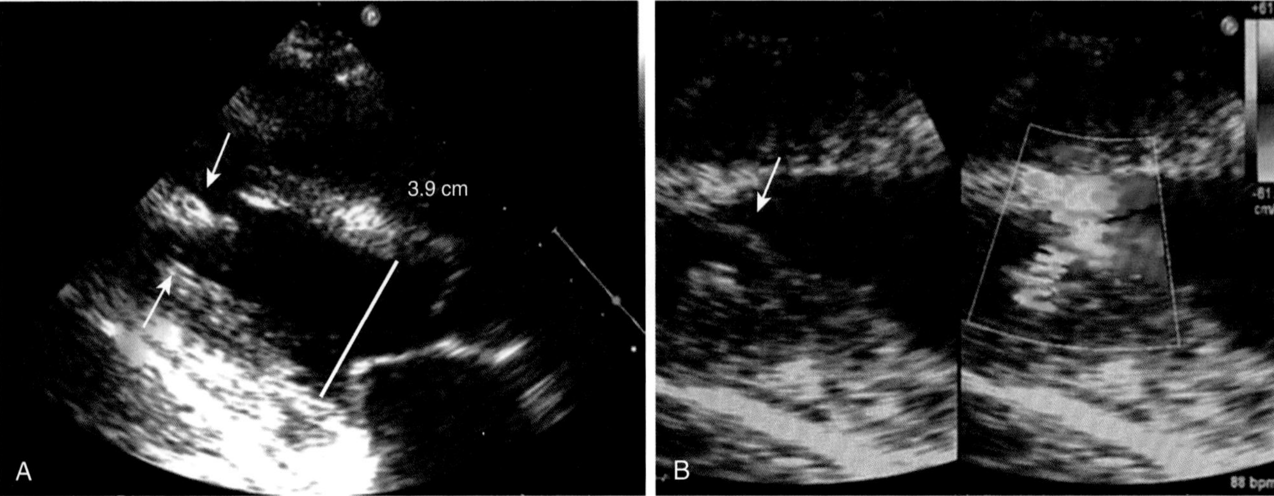

Fig. 16.6 **Inflow cannula obstruction with a small LV.** (A) Parasternal long-axis views of the LV demonstrate an apical HeartMate II LVAD inflow cannula (*large arrows* define sides of cannula). The ventricular cavity is small (LVEDd of 3.9 cm). (B) Zoomed view of the cannula shows a papillary or chordal structure *(arrow)* being drawn into the cannula orifice. Color Doppler imaging shows color aliasing, indicative of high velocities from partial obstruction. *Ao*, Aorta; *LVAD*, LV assist device; *LVEDd*, LV end-diastolic diameter.

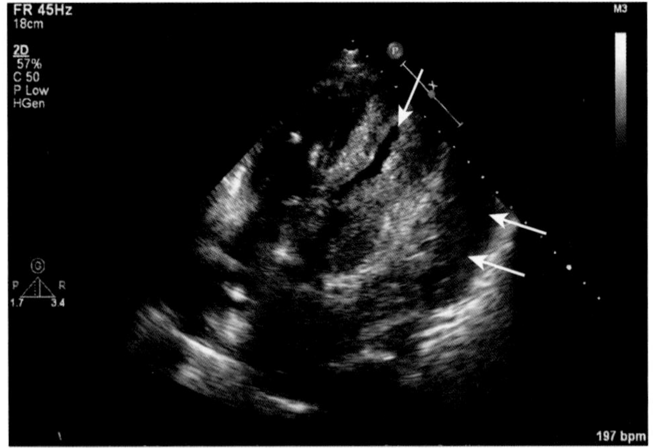

Fig. 16.7 **Pericardial clot compressing the LV.** In a modified apical view, a large thrombus is seen lateral to the LV wall *(double arrows)*. The LV cavity *(single arrow)* is severely compressed (see Video 16.7).

Endocarditis of native valves or MCS device components is another significant concern. Infection is a cause of death in the VAD population and often begins as an infection at the driveline exit site.[31] Vegetations on intracorporeal VAD cannulas or pump components put patients at risk for obstruction and septic embolism. Device explantation is often necessary.

EFFECTS OF SPEED CHANGES

In some cases, MCS device settings must be adjusted to address hemodynamic challenges or to optimize cardiac function. Reducing the pump speed increases preload. A higher preload may improve LV systolic function through Starling mechanisms, increasing ejection through the aortic valve. For continuous-flow devices, some degree of aortic valve opening is considered desirable. Alternatively, reduced LVAD flow may overdistend the LV, leading to a reduction in residual function and to symptoms of congestion. Increasing the pump speed decreases ventricular preload, potentially alleviating distention and congestion. However, LV systolic function may fall, and the aortic valve may cease to open, increasing the risk of root thrombosis. Excessive reduction of the pumping rate produces underfilling and impingement of the inflow cannula.

Pump Thrombosis

Pump thrombosis should be suspected in the setting of increased power consumption and markers of hemolysis such as elevated

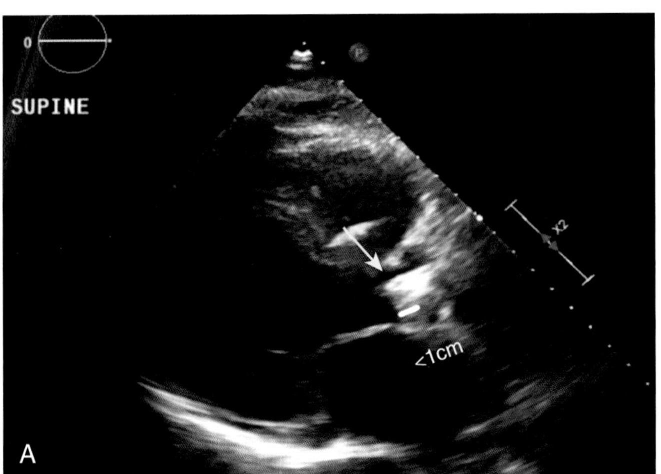

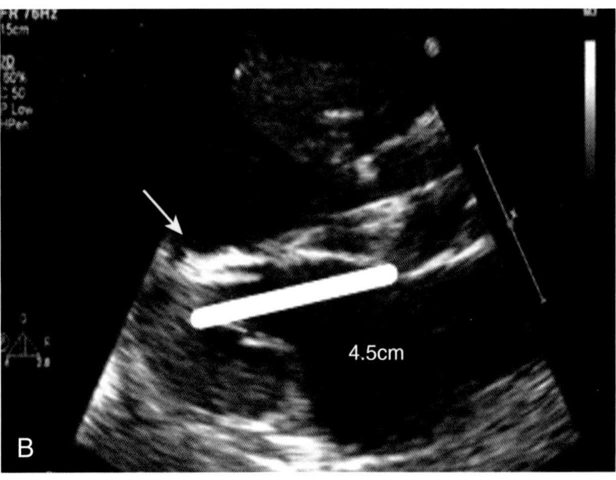

Fig. 16.8 Impella Recover device distance from the aortic annulus. (A) In a parasternal long-axis view, the inflow port of the device (*arrow*, identified as the terminus of the parallel lines of the catheter) is <1 cm below the aortic valve annulus and at significant risk for migrating above the annulus, which would cause the blood to be ineffectually circulated by the device in the aorta. After appropriate initial placement, the device migrated, likely during patient positioning (see Video 16.8A). (B) In contrast, in the parasternal long-axis view, the cannula is placed too far into the LV (4.5 cm) and is at risk for further migration such that both the inflow and outflow ports would be located within the LV (see Video 16.8B).

lactate dehydrogenase, low haptoglobin, and high plasma-free hemoglobin levels. Pump thrombosis can be treated by intensification of anticoagulation, use of thrombolytics, or pump exchange. In the case of pump thrombosis, increasing the speed has little effect on echocardiographic parameters, but in the setting of no pump thrombosis, increases in speed progressively unload the LV, reducing the opening of the aortic valve, the size of an LV supported by the HeartMate II device, and possibly, the degree of mitral regurgitation.

Ventricular Recovery

MCS devices are increasingly used to temporarily support patients with reversible causes of heart failure, both acute (i.e., percutaneous, temporary devices) and chronic (i.e., durable VADs), although recovery after durable VAD implantation remains rare.[32] In patients with chronic heart failure and VADs, ventricular unloading can produce reverse remodeling, including normalization of chamber sizes, regression of LV hypertrophy, recovery of beta receptor responsiveness, and normalization of calcium handling.[33–35]

With decompression, however, reduced preload produces loss of systolic function due to reduced ventricular fiber stretch. Reductions in systolic function on VAD support are therefore not necessarily indicative of progression of myocardial dysfunction. Improvements in systolic function may be a sign of overfilling or may portend resolution of an acute insult and/or reverse remodeling over time.

Turning down VAD flows leads to increases in afterload and preload. In patients with recovered heart function, increasing preload leads to improvement in ventricular function and maintenance of ventricular size. In patients who depend on VAD support, ventricles fail and/or dilate because of an inability to accommodate increased preload and afterload.

Percutaneous Mechanical Circulatory Support Device Position

Percutaneous MCS device positioning may require guided adjustment. When an Impella device outflow port migrates out of the LVOT, the device circulates blood within the aorta in the blind loop (Fig. 16.8A). If the inflow portion migrates into the ventricle, the same thing happens within the LV (see Fig. 16.8B). Pressure sensors at each port can often identify that there is a problem.

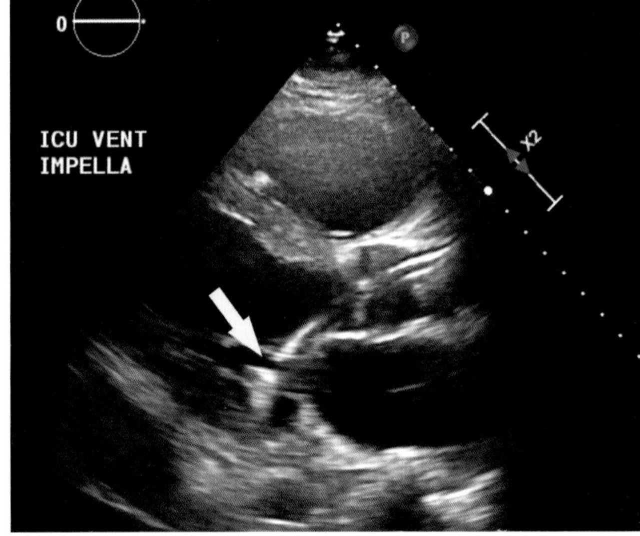

Fig. 16.9 Impella Recover device and mitral regurgitation. The Impella cannula inflow port (*arrows*, identified as the terminus of the parallel lines of the catheter) is located <4 cm from the aortic valve, but it is directed posteriorly into the mitral valve chordal apparatus.

The device may interfere with the mitral apparatus, leading to significant regurgitation (Fig. 16.9). The transseptally placed TandemHeart can move backward into the RA, drawing deoxygenated blood through the inflow cannula and delivering it to the system circulation, or it can migrate forward into the left atrial appendage (Fig. 16.10).

TECHNICAL DETAILS, QUANTITATION, AND DATA ANALYSIS

Standard echocardiographic imaging protocols provide structural, functional, and hemodynamic information about hearts

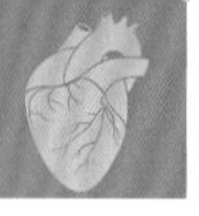

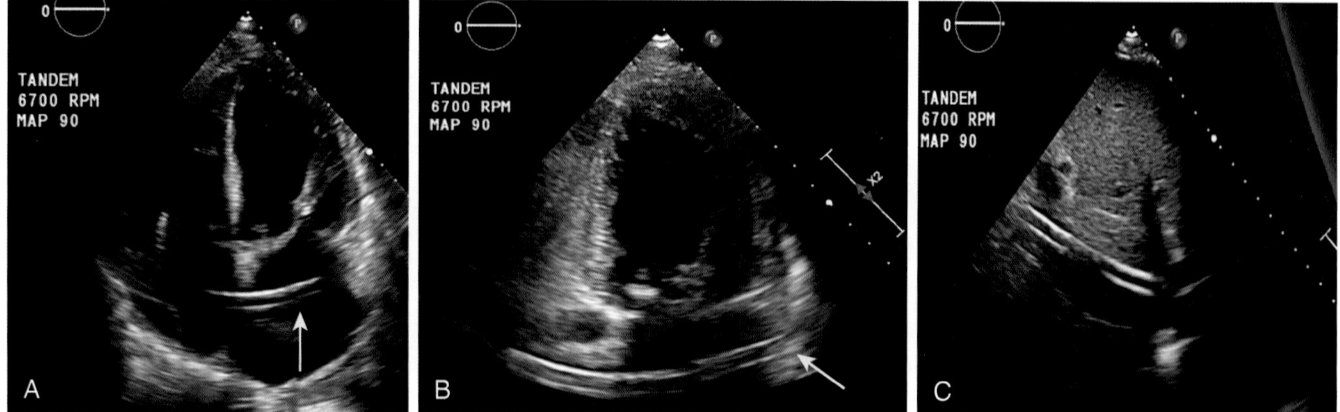

Fig. 16.10 TandemHeart device. (A) The TandemHeart inflow cannula (*arrow*) is seen traversing the interatrial septum in the apical 4-chamber view. (B) In the apical 2-chamber view, the terminus of the TandemHeart inflow catheter (*arrow*) is seen just above the location of the left atrial appendage (LAA). Echocardiography can help to guide the cannula away from any potential LAA thrombus. (C) The TandemHeart inflow cannula is seen in the inferior vena cava in this subcostal view.

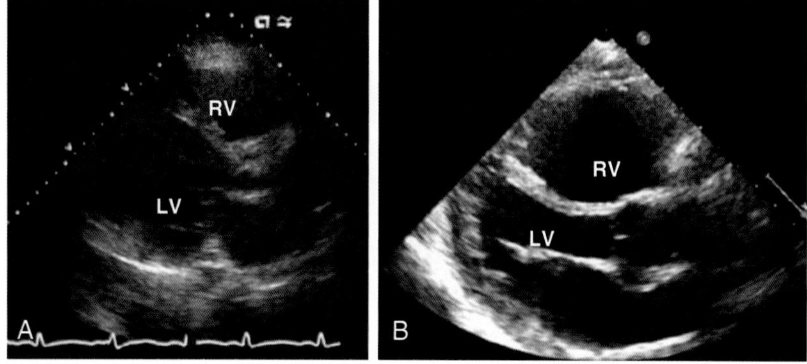

Fig. 16.11 Abnormal septal positions. (A) Distended LV with rightward septal shift toward the RV. The inflow cannula is not seen in this view, but in Video 16.11A, the aortic valve does not open, consistent with an LV assist device. (B) Leftward septal shift. In a parasternal long-axis view, diastolic septal shift into the LV is seen, suggesting LV underfilling or RV enlargement and dysfunction. The inflow cannula is seen in the apex (see Video 16.11B).

supported by cardiac assist devices. Specific indications for the examination, device type, cannulation, mode, and pump settings should be noted on every examination report, as should blood pressure (taken with a Doppler cuff in patients with continuous-flow devices to obtain an approximation of the mean arterial pressure[36]). Certain standard acquisitions deserve special emphasis, and specialized views to assess device components are necessary additions.

Comparison with prior echocardiograms is essential because changes in parameters on surveillance examinations may herald clinical decompensation. Examinations performed to assess for complications may provide the clue to pathologic processes. The same imaging planes should be used in all examinations to ensure validity of measurements.

LV END-DIASTOLIC DIAMETER AND SEPTAL ORIENTATION

LV end-diastolic diameter (LVEDd) from the parasternal long-axis view is traditionally used as a surrogate marker for filling status in patients with axial-flow devices. It also reflects the position of the interventricular septum, which indicates the interaction between the LV and RV. In most VAD patients, the ideal position of the septum is neutral between the ventricles or bowed slightly to the right (relative to the long axis of the LV) (Fig. 16.11). This septal orientation denotes adequate ventricular decompression without underfilling and likely optimizes the septal contribution to RV contraction. In the case of a dysfunctional LVAD and overfilling, the LVEDd increases, in part because of a shift of the septum into the RV.

In axial-flow devices, cannula obstruction related to a small LV and suction events can manifest as a decrease in LVEDd and septal bowing into the LV. However, septal orientation toward the LV can also result from high right-sided pressures (see Fig. 16.11). Dyssynchrony from interventricular conduction delay, ischemic wall motion abnormalities, poststernotomy state, pericardial constriction, and RV pacing can also influence the septal position.

LVEDd measured in the 2-dimensional (2D) parasternal long-axis view at the mitral valve leaflet tips is generally reproducible, allowing detection of differences in size and septal position in serial studies and in response to changes in VAD pump settings during optimization and weaning. Nonetheless, care must be taken to record images in the same plane each time and to measure at the same level. 2D-directed M-mode can be used if the M-mode cursor can achieve a perpendicular axis with respect to the ventricular walls.

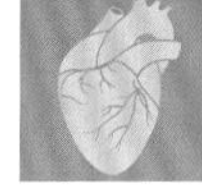

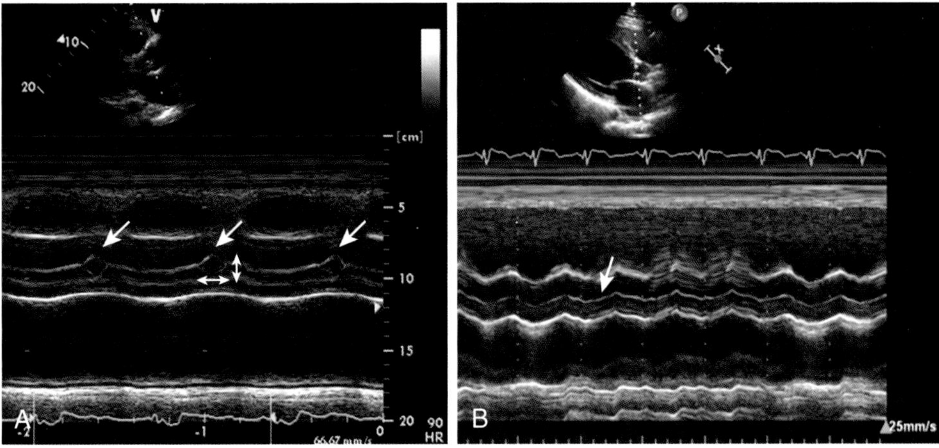

Fig. 16.12 **Aortic valve opening.** (A) M-mode tracing from the parasternal long-axis view demonstrates reduced opening of the aortic valve with each beat *(arrows)*, consistent with normal LV assist device (LVAD) function that prevents thrombus formation in the aortic root. *Double-headed arrows* show duration and extent of opening, which can be measured to allow quantitative comparisons between studies or at different LVAD pump settings. Increased opening can be a sign of overfilling or of ventricular recovery, (B) No aortic valve opening is seen *(arrow)*, consistent with very low residual cardiac output, high LVAD pump flow, oversewn valve to prevent aortic regurgitation, or leaflet fusion.

Unlike with axial-flow devices, changes in LVEDd may not be an accurate marker of filling dynamics with centrifugal-flow devices.[37] Centrifugal-flow devices are placed up against the apex of the heart, whereas axial-flow devices are placed in the abdomen. Placement determines whether the device pushes (centrifugal) or pulls (axial) on the apex of the heart. The pushing effect is probably transmitted to the basal portion of the heart, making it less reflective of changes in ventricular volume. Instead of changes in LVEDd, changes in aortic valve opening, outflow Doppler profile, and possibly, mitral regurgitation may be better markers of filling status in centrifugal-flow devices.

VENTRICULAR FUNCTION

In patients with an LVAD, it is often difficult to quantify LVEF using the biplane apical method because of artifact from the apical inflow cannula. Use of an ultrasound enhancing agent to improve endocardial border definition in MCS can be considered. Calculation of LVEF from linear measurements is confounded by LVAD effects on septal orientation and ventricular dimensions. The Quinones method, which calculates LVEF from measurements of multiple diameters in two views and does not account for motion of the apex (which is akinetic in most VAD patients), is theoretically attractive but has not been well validated.[26]

Comprehensive imaging of RV function requires 2D assessment of size and systolic motion and careful assessment of tricuspid regurgitation and measurement of right-sided hemodynamics. Examination of the tricuspid valve should include assessment of leaflet flattening or prolapse, septal leaflet tethering, and annular dilation. Noninvasive pulmonary vascular resistance can be measured as a marker of LVAD effect on RV afterload.[38]

AORTIC VALVE OPENING

Aortic valve opening is normally reduced in left-sided MCS devices. Relative aortic valve opening can be a marker for LVAD and the ventricular contribution to cardiac output. The aortic valve may open minimally, briefly, intermittently, or not at all when the ventricle is severely dysfunctional. The aortic-LV pressure difference opposes opening because the LV pressure is low as a result of decompression, and the LVAD outflow increases pressure in the proximal aorta. Conversely, the aortic valve may open normally when there is ventricular recovery or LVAD dysfunction leading to high LV pressures. It has been proposed that the degree and frequency of aortic valve opening be assessed as opening with each cardiac cycle, opening intermittently, or remaining closed.[26]

Quantitation of the degree of opening can be obtained by planimetry of the open valve in the short-axis view or by linear measurement of systolic cusp separation in the long-axis view. M-mode imaging at a low sweep speed (25–50 mm/s) gives a quantitative frequency of aortic valve opening as a percentage of recorded cardiac cycles (Fig. 16.12). Duration of opening can be measured by M-mode as time of opening or as a percentage of the RR interval in which the valve is open. Translational motion during systole can move the aortic valve relative to the M-mode probe, leading to the appearance of opening when the valve is actually closed. Opening can be confirmed with a long 2D clip or the use of color M-mode.[26]

PERICARDIAL PATHOLOGY

2D imaging can visualize effusions or thrombus in the pericardial space that are compressing cardiac chambers, leading to underfilling and inflow cannula obstruction (see Fig. 16.7). Exaggerated Doppler flow variation across valves in the supported ventricle may be unhelpful as a marker of intrapericardial pressure because flow is affected by VAD function, which is affected by afterload and preload. The total artificial heart chambers are opaque to ultrasound, but the native atria, the superior and inferior vena cavae, and the pulmonary veins can be assessed for compression or collapse.

CANNULAS

2D imaging, especially with TEE, can determine orientation of the cannulas and whether cardiac structures (e.g., trabeculations, septa, chordal structures) are sucked into the cannulas (see Fig. 16.6). 2D imaging should also assess for thrombi and vegetations on the cannulas. The inflow cannulas should be imaged from all windows. 3D may be helpful to define the

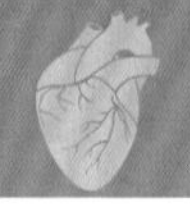

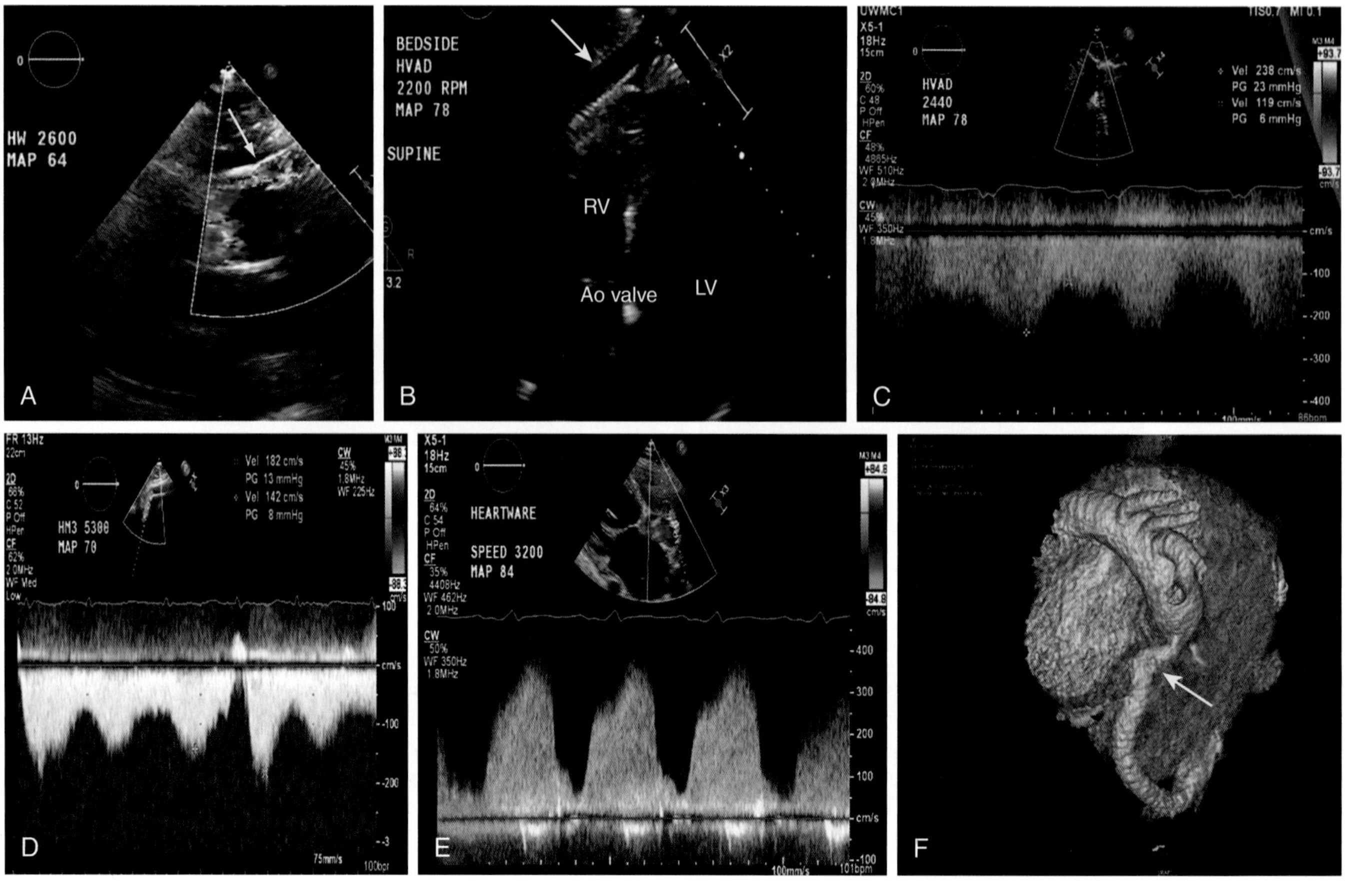

Fig. 16.13 Imaging LV assist device outflow graft cannula. The LV assist device (LVAD) outflow graft cannula can be visualized by TTE in many patients in the right upper sternal border. (A) The outflow graft (*arrow*) is anastomosed, end to side, in a short-axis view of the ascending aorta. The best imaging window depends on the location of the cannula, which can vary (see Video 16.13A). (B) Subcostal views may provide the best visualization of the midportion of the cannula (*arrow*) and the best Doppler angle of insonation (see Video 16.13B). (C) Normal velocity profile for a HeartWare HVAD outflow cannula. (D) Normal velocity profile for a HeartMate 3 outflow cannula. Notice the dip and spike pattern in the velocity profile that reflects the normal speed alterations in this device. (E) A very high systolic peak velocity is seen, and subsequent volume-rendered cardiac computed tomography (F) demonstrates a kink in the outflow cannula (*arrow*). *Ao Valve*, Aortic valve.

cannula orientation and its relation to other structures (e.g., septum). For LVAD inflow cannulas in axial-flow devices, the most parallel Doppler angle of insonation is often found in the apical views. The orientation of LVAD inflow cannulas can vary, however, and the most parallel angle is sometimes found in the parasternal long-axis view or the subcostal view, especially if the cannula was placed by an inferior approach.

MCS device inflow cannulas placed in other cardiac chambers, especially ECMO, CentriMag, and TandemHeart cannulas in the atria, often require TEE for adequate visualization. The LVAD outflow cannula in the ascending aorta can be inconsistently located and oriented. Multiple windows should be employed, including the right parasternal, upper left parasternal, right supraclavicular, suprasternal notch, and subcostal views (Fig. 16.13A and B). It is usually easily seen by TEE.

The Impella Recover percutaneous VAD cannula is normally well seen from the parasternal long-axis view, but it may be necessary to angle the transducer off-axis to ensure that the tip is visualized. The distance from the aortic annulus to the inflow cannula is a marker of correct positioning. Proper location of the inflow port (i.e., near the tip of the cannula) is 3 to 4 cm below the aortic valve. The inflow port may be in the LVOT or at risk for migration above the aortic valve (see Fig. 16.8A), or the outflow port may be in the LVOT rather than in the aorta (see Fig.16.8B), leading to ineffective device function because the inlet and outflow are in the same chamber. The outflow port is not as easily identified; it can sometimes be located by a jet of color Doppler ultrasound, although artifact often obscures its location. It should be 1.5 to 2 cm above the sinuses of Valsalva.[39] Impella cannula orientation, particularly assessment of its relation to the mitral valve apparatus, may require biplane or 3D imaging[40] (see Fig 16.9).

Color Doppler examination of normal cannulas reveals laminar flow with minimal or no regurgitant flow. Aliasing of color flow may be seen in cases of partial obstruction. The intensity of color Doppler inflow jets may be reduced or absent in complete obstruction or pump failure. The color Doppler jet can also help to direct angulation of the transducer to achieve a parallel alignment for spectral Doppler interrogation.

Pulsed-wave (PW) Doppler should be performed inside and immediately outside of the cannula orifice, and continuous-wave (CW) Doppler should be performed, aligned as much as possible with the cannula long axis. Normal and abnormal Doppler profiles through inflow and outflow cannulas are illustrated in Fig. 16.13. Partial obstruction leads to increases in inflow and outflow velocities, depending on the site of obstruction. Complete obstruction (i.e., from thrombotic occlusion or kinking) leads to loss of the Doppler signal or low velocities in the VAD cannulas.[41] Regurgitation, inflow obstruction, and pump failure can lead to low outflow velocities.

Pump thrombosis may manifest as reduced background, nadir, or basal velocities through the inflow cannula. Usually found in diastole, these velocities reflect VAD function, whereas systolic peak velocities represent a combination of VAD function and residual systolic ventricular contraction forcing blood into the cannula. Significant AR may lead to increases in the basal velocities over the course of diastole.[42] Because it is often difficult to obtain a completely aligned angle of insonation through the inflow cannula, background velocities must be considered in relation to prior values and the systolic peak velocities (i.e., peak-to-background or -nadir ratio), rather than relying on a specific value to diagnose obstruction. Interrogation of inflow in a centrifugal-flow device is compromised by artifact in many patients (Fig. 16.14), and the outflow graft peak-to-background or -nadir ratio may need to be used instead. CW Doppler interrogation is necessary to resolve high velocities, but because of range ambiguity, the CW Doppler signal may become contaminated by other flows (e.g., LVAD inflow, AR).

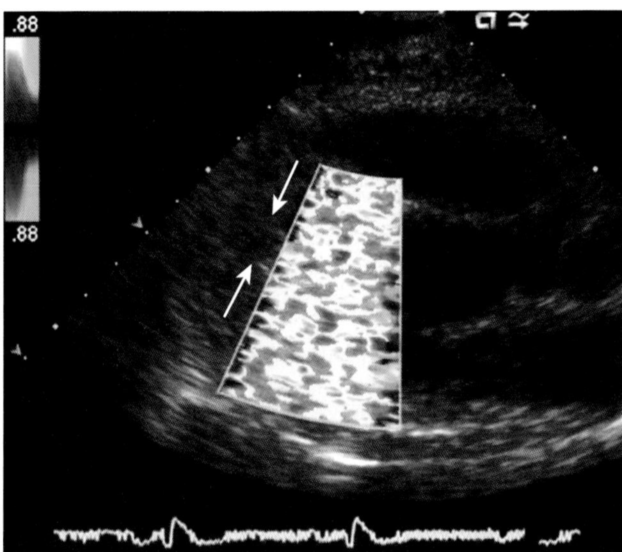

Fig. 16.14 Centrifugal-flow device color Doppler artifact. Ventricular assist devices with continuous-flow pumps located close to the heart create Doppler artifacts, seen here filling the entire Doppler sector in the parasternal long-axis view. The artifact is located in the mid-LV and precludes any assessment of flow into or out of the inflow cannula (sides denoted by *arrows*).

Table 16.6 provides the formulas used to calculate the stroke volume through pulsatile VADs, flow through continuous-flow VADs, and VAD regurgitation using cross-sectional orifice area and PW Doppler velocity–time integral (VTI). Because continuous-flow VADs technically have no discrete stroke volume, VAD flows (in L/min) must be calculated indirectly using the residual output through the aortic valve and the output through the pulmonic valve or RVOT, or they may be calculated directly by measuring the Doppler VTI over 3 seconds (multiplied by 20 seconds to convert to a per-minute flow rate).[42]

OPTIMIZATION STUDIES

Depending on the type of VAD, different parameters can be used as optimization targets. For an axial-flow VAD, the rotor speed is adjusted until the septum is neutrally positioned at a near-normal LVEDd. For both kinds of VADs, the aortic valve optimally opens to a small degree, for a brief period of time, and/or with less than 1:1 cardiac cycle frequency. The optimal opening characteristics to prevent aortic root thrombus and cusp fusion while signaling appropriate ventricular decompression have not been well defined.

Other targets of optimization include mitral regurgitation, AR, pulmonary artery pressures, outflow Doppler profiles, and Doppler-derived cannula flows. Optimization of RVAD and BI-VAD function has not been well described but could apply the same principles to RV size, septal positioning, and pulmonic valve opening.

RAMP STUDIES

Echocardiographic indices examined during ramp protocol echocardiography assess structural and functional changes as speed is increased and define suction events. In the setting of a negative ramp (i.e., no pump thrombosis), the LVEDd should decrease, and/or the aortic valve should exhibit a reduced degree and duration or frequency of opening, eventually remaining closed throughout the cardiac cycle. Spectral Doppler interrogation of the cannulas should demonstrate increases in basal or nadir flow.[43] Mitral deceleration time

TABLE 16.6 Doppler Formulas for Ventricular Assist Device Flow Volumes.

Formulas	*Measurements*
Pulsatile VAD (VAD_p) stroke volume (SV_{VADp}): $SV_{VADp} = \pi(D_{can}/2)^2 \times VTI_{can}$	D_{can} = cannula diameter (usually 12–25 mm) VTI_{can} = VTI of the PW Doppler signal measured just within the cannula orifice
Continuous-flow LVAD (VAD_c): $SV_{VADc} = \left[\pi(D_{RVOT}/2)^2 \times VTI_{RVOT}\right] - \left[\pi(D_{LVOT}/2)^2 \times VTI_{LVOT}\right]$	D_{RVOT} = RV outflow tract diameter VTI_{RVOT} = RV outflow tract VTI D_{LVOT} = LV outflow tract diameter VTI_{LVOT} = LV outflow tract VTI
$SV_{VADc} = VTI_{can3sec} \times 20 \times \pi(D_{can}/2)^2 \times C$	C = correction factor for inflow cannula = 0.67 $VTI_{can3sec}$ = 3-second tracing of VTI continuous flow in the VAD cannula
Pulsatile VAD regurgitant volume (RV_{VADp}): $RV_{VADp} = \left[\pi(D_{IN}/2)^2 \times VTI_{IN}\right] - \left[\pi(D_{out}/2)^2 \times VTI_{OUT}\right]$	VTI_{IN} = inflow cannula VTI VTI_{OUT} = outflow cannula VTI D_{OUT} = outflow cannula diameter D_{IN} = inflow cannula diameter
Continuous-flow VAD regurgitant volume (RV_{VADc}): $RV_{VADc} = \left[\pi(D_{asc}/2)^2 \times VTI_{asc}\right] - \left[\pi(D_{PA}/2)^2 \times VTI_{PA}\right]$	D_{asc} = ascending aorta diameter D_{PA} = pulmonary artery diameter VTI_{asc} = ascending aorta VTI measured above the outflow cannula VTI_{PA} = pulmonary artery VTI

D, Diameter; *LVAD*, LV assist device; *LVOT*, LV outflow tract; *PA*, pulmonary artery; *PW*, pulsed wave; *RVOT*, RV outflow tract; *VAD*, ventricular assist device; *VTI*, velocity–time integral.

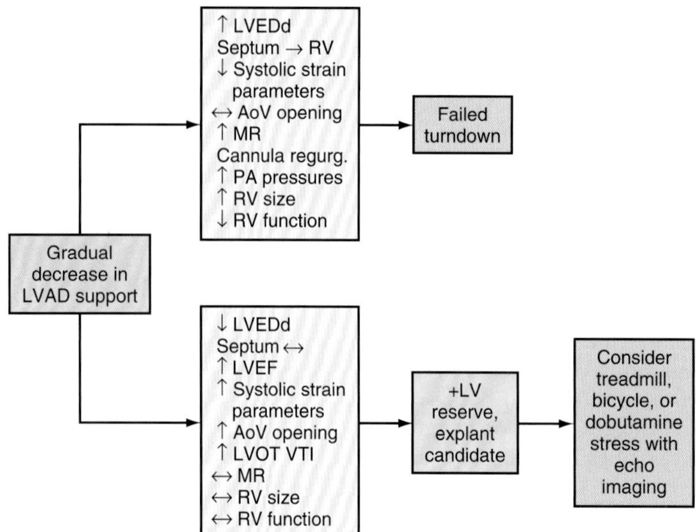

Fig. 16.15 LV assist device weaning. The flow chart outlines echocardiographic parameters that can be used to determine whether a patient has experienced LV recovery and may be a candidate for device explantation. The same parameters used during the turndown phase can be assessed during exercise or dobutamine stress, including LV end-diastolic diameter *(LVEDd)*, septal orientation, LV ejection fraction *(LVEF)*, AV opening, LV outflow tract *(LVOT)*, velocity–time integral *(VTI)*, degree of mitral regurgitation *(MR)*, and RV size and function. Few data exist on the ability of any specific measures to definitively predict recovery. *AoV*, Aortic valve; *echo*, echocardiographic; *LVAD*, LV assist device; *PA*, pulmonary artery.

should lengthen, and the degree of mitral regurgitation may decrease. Because increased left-sided output delivers more blood to the RV, the RVOT VTI, as a marker of cardiac output, should increase. However, the increased RV preload in conjunction with septal shift into the LV can lead to increased tricuspid regurgitation.

AR may worsen, and central aortic pressure can rise with increased outflow in the ascending aorta. Worsening AR or increasing mean arterial pressure during a ramp study can lead to an inability to decompress the LV and a false-positive ramp study result.[44] Echocardiographic ramp studies can predict pump thrombosis, but partial thrombosis may be more difficult to detect by current measures. Investigations have found that a negative ramp study result may be falsely reassuring in the setting of clinical parameters that suggest thrombosis, although clinical parameters can vary.[45] Before initiating a ramp protocol, it is imperative to exclude thrombus in the LV and aortic root because changes in speed may lead to systemic embolization.

TURNDOWN STUDIES FOR VENTRICULAR RECOVERY

Before MCS device explantation, weaning is usually necessary to demonstrate the impact of reduced support on cardiac structure and function. Protocols differ but usually involve echocardiography with or without invasive arterial and venous pressure monitoring. Cardiac assist device support is decreased gradually to prevent acute decompensation. Fig. 16.15 summarizes the echocardiographic parameters used during turndown. If the results are favorable after turndown to minimal levels of support, some protocols call for exercise or dobutamine stress testing. Sometimes, oxygen consumption measurement is added. Echocardiographic imaging at peak exercise is facilitated with supine bicycle stress. There may be adequate cardiac reserve to support the patient after MCS explantation if the LVEF improves, the aortic valve opens more, and stroke volume increases in response to dobutamine.[46]

Echocardiography can also guide weaning protocols for right-sided assist devices and ECMO. As flows are decreased, RV failure or recovery may be predicted by central venous pressure, RV function, LV filling pressures, and tricuspid regurgitation.[47] For weaning from durable VADs and temporary percutaneous MCS devices, a failed turndown study is characterized by marked chamber enlargement and/or increased atrioventricular valve regurgitation and sometimes by a decrement in ventricular systolic function.

CLINICAL UTILITY AND OUTCOME DATA

Echocardiography plays a major role in guiding the care of patients with MCS devices, from establishing an indication for MCS to uncovering the cause of device alarms, but there are few studies demonstrating specific outcome measures tied to echocardiography.

Preimplantation echocardiographic indices of RV structure and function have been reported to predict RV dysfunction after LVAD implantation. Different studies tested different parameters, and most studies represent only single-center experiences. A 2015 study investigated multiple different risk scores for RV failure after implantation and found only modest predictive value, but the study did not incorporate risk scores with quantitative echocardiographic parameters.[47] Later work suggested that RV and RA strain parameters, along with assessment of intra-RV dyssynchrony, may best correlate with need for RVAD support.[48]

Regular echocardiography has been recommended during the postimplantation period and to guide weaning of temporary RVAD support. RV function after implantation and the effects on clinical parameters have been investigated in a number of studies. Maeder et al.[23] showed that reduced mortality rates and improved renal function were associated with improved RV function after LVAD implantation. Lam et al.[52] reported

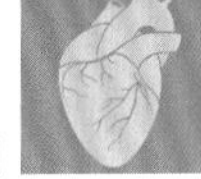

Fig. 16.16 **3D imaging of LV assist device cannulas.** (A) Real-time 3D TEE in the mid-esophageal position demonstrates normal positioning of the inflow cannula *(arrow)* in the LV apex. The 3D data set is rotated to look inferiorly and posteriorly from the anterior perspective. The orifice is unobstructed by any cardiac structures. (B) Real-time 3D TEE in upper mid-esophageal position shows the orifice of the outflow graft cannula *(arrow)* as viewed from inside the proximal ascending aorta. In contrast to the inflow cannula, the outflow graft cannula is anastomosed, end to side, to the aorta.

that a greater than 10% reduction in RV fractional area change after implantation portended worse quality of life and exercise capacity.

The initial studies investigating the use of echocardiographic measures of LV size and systolic function to predict successful LVAD explantation involved pulsatile devices.[53,54] Protocols for imaging continuous-flow pumps have also used standard LV size and LVEF measurements during sequentially decreased LVAD support (i.e., turndown examinations) and have suggested that favorable responses to exercise or dobutamine stress testing may correlate with successful explantation.[55]

A 2019 study employed a protocol using echocardiographic measures made during turndown examination as the first step in determining the safety of explantation. Only patients with favorable measures (LVEF/RVEF > 45%, LVEDd < 55 mm or 3.2 mm/m^2, RVOT < 40 mm, less than mild valvular regurgitation, and aortic valve opening with each beat) at a speed producing zero net flow and at pump stoppage subsequently underwent right heart catheterization with graft occlusion (targeting a pulmonary capillary wedge pressure of <16 mmHg) and eventually explantation.[57]

POTENTIAL LIMITATIONS AND FUTURE DIRECTIONS

Echocardiographic imaging is complicated in the postimplantation state, when bandages, mechanical ventilation, and patient positioning compromise imaging windows. In addition to the attenuation artifacts created by inflow cannulas, significant artifacts are caused by centrifugal-flow devices that have pumps located very close to or in the inflow cannula. Doppler distortion results from the ultrasonic signals produced by the rotating disk (see Fig. 16.14). It is possible to avoid Doppler sampling near the device and to attempt off-axis imaging and thereby interrogate other cardiac structures with color and spectral Doppler.

Cannula orientation, orifice location, and proximity to ventricular structures are not always clear from 2D imaging planes. Real-time 3D echocardiography can play a role in more precisely defining cannula position. 3D TEE images of the LVAD inflow and outflow cannulas are obtained from the mid-esophageal position (Fig. 16.16). 3D TEE also provides the best images of cannulas placed in the RA and LA. Real-time 3D imaging may facilitate visualization of the entire Impella Recover cannula, which tends to traverse 2D imaging planes.

A precise and load-independent measure of intrinsic myocardial reserve may augment traditional assessments of ventricular recovery. Measures of myocardial deformation, including strain and strain rate, may provide a better way to predict recovery.

ALTERNATIVE APPROACHES

Cardiac magnetic resonance imaging (MRI) provides highly accurate measures of ventricular volumes and function. MRI accurately measures RV size and function, potentially improving prediction of RV function after implantation. MRI can also accurately image the aorta and define pitfalls for Impella Recover and outflow cannula placement.[58] However, MRI cannot be used with current-generation MCS devices after implantation.

Computed tomography (CT) can be used after implantation. Studies suggest high sensitivity and specificity for the detection of cannula thrombosis and inflow cannula malposition.[59,60] Most cannulas do not cause significant CT artifact, and direct visualization of the cannula orientation is easily achieved from data sets. The entire length of cannulas can be examined. CT also provides excellent preimplantation imaging of the aorta. The downsides to CT include radiation exposure and the nephrotoxicity of the contrast agent, which is a concern in VAD patients, who often have compromised renal function.

Although preliminary studies suggest that Doppler-based estimation of pulmonary pressures and pulmonary vascular resistance is valid after LVAD implantation, validation in larger numbers of patients is needed. In the meantime, invasive measures of intracardiac hemodynamics may be necessary to establish accurate filling pressures, cardiac output, and pulmonary vascular resistance to guide therapy. Invasive hemodynamic measurements may also be necessary to assess the severity of valvular lesions, especially when echocardiographic images are limited.

SUMMARY Diagnosis-Oriented Practical Imaging Guide.

Evaluation	Parameters	Important Imaging Approaches/Techniques
Preimplantation assessment	LV systolic function	LVEF by biplane method of disks 3D volumetric measurement Contrast enhancement
	LV size	LVEDd at MV leaflet tips (particularly for axial-flow devices) Biplane methods of disks 3D volumetric measurements Contrast enhancement
	Intracardiac thrombus	Careful scanning of LV apex Ultrasound enhancing agent TEE to assess LA appendage (atrial fibrillation, atrial flutter)
	RV size	Standard techniques (e.g., basal, middle, and longitudinal diameters) Consider 3D imaging
	RV systolic function	Standard techniques (e.g., fractional area change, TAPSE, free wall s′, free wall peak systolic longitudinal strain, RVOT VTI) PASP and RAP Consider 3D RV volumes and RVEF
	Tricuspid regurgitation	More than moderate regurgitation is an indication for tricuspid repair at the time of LVAD implantation Integrate assessments of jet size with other parameters (e.g., hepatic vein spectral Doppler, IVC size and collapse, interatrial septal leftward shift, RA size, PASP)
	Mitral regurgitation	Standard techniques (e.g., vena contracta, PISA-derived EROA and regurgitant volume, pulmonary vein flow reversal) Functional MR should improve with LVAD
	Mitral stenosis	Stenotic mitral valve should be replaced at time of LVAD implantation Standard techniques (e.g., pressure half time, peak and mean gradients, area by 3D-directed measurement) Integrate with other parameters (e.g., PASP)
	Aortic regurgitation	May worsen after implantation Standard techniques (e.g., vena contracta)
	Aortic stenosis	Although bypassed by LVAD, may create a problem in the setting of device failure Standard techniques (e.g., peak velocities, mean gradients, AVA)
	Intracardiac shunts	Right-to-left shunt may develop after LVAD implantation Agitated saline contrast with Valsalva maneuver to exclude PFO
	Aorta	Proximal aortic aneurysm Plaque in ascending aorta and aortic arch Consider CT or MRI
Perioperative TEE	Aortic regurgitation	Reassessment (anesthetic loading conditions may unmask significant aortic regurgitation)
	Intracardiac shunts	Reassessment for unmasked interatrial shunt
	Tricuspid regurgitation	Standard techniques to assess for worsening after use of MCS device
	Mitral regurgitation	Standard techniques, compare with baseline to guide speed settings
	Guide device placement	LVAD inflow cannula pointed toward mitral valve CentriMag use in appropriate chambers ECMO inflow cannula in RA
	Deairing	Careful assessment of anterior structures and sites of cannula anastomoses
Postimplantation surveillance	LV systolic function	LVEF by biplane method of disks 3D volumetric measurement Ultrasound enhancing agent

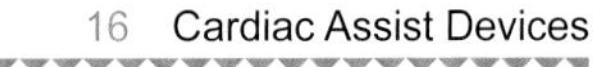

SUMMARY Diagnosis-Oriented Practical Imaging Guide.—cont'd

Evaluation	Parameters	Important Imaging Approaches/Techniques
	LV size	LVEDd at MV leaflet tips (particularly for axial-flow devices) using same imaging plane each time Biplane methods of disks 3D volumetric measurements Ultrasound enhancing agent
	Intracardiac thrombus	Careful scanning of LV apex, LVOT, and aortic root Ultrasound enhancing agent
	RV size	Standard techniques (e.g., basal, middle, and longitudinal diameters) Consider 3D
	RV systolic function	Standard techniques (e.g., fractional area change, TAPSE, free wall s′, free wall peak systolic longitudinal strain, RVOT VTI) PASP and RAP Consider 3D
	Tricuspid regurgitation	Septal shift and septal leaflet tethering can worsen TR after LVAD implant Integrate assessments of jet size with other parameters (e.g., hepatic vein spectral Doppler, IVC size and collapse, interatrial septal leftward shift, RA size, PASP)
	Mitral regurgitation	Worsening/unchanged MR may signal overfilling Standard techniques (e.g., vena contracta, PISA-derived EROA and regurgitant volume, pulmonary vein flow reversal)
	Aortic valve opening	Marker of LV systolic function and filling. M-mode of AoV leaflets in PLAX view Color M-mode
	Aortic regurgitation	May worsen after implantation and become continuous Standard techniques (e.g., vena contracta) but note severity is increased when continuous
	Cannulas/device location and velocities	Often requires off-axis imaging LVAD inflow cannula oriented centrally; inflow peak and basal/nadir spectral Doppler velocities Outflow graft peak and basal/nadir spectral Doppler velocities Impella device inflow port 3–4 cm below aortic valve Consider biplane or 3D to assess proximity to mitral apparatus TandemHeart inflow cannula in LA CentriMag use in appropriate chambers ECMO inflow cannula in RA
Postimplantation problem-focused assessment	LV systolic function	LVEF by biplane method of disks 3D volumetric measurement Ultrasound enhancing agent
	LV size	Marker of overfilling, device dysfunction, suction event, or underfilling (particularly change from baseline) LVEDd at MV leaflet tips (particularly for axial-flow devices); same imaging plane each time Biplane methods of disks 3D volumetric measurements Ultrasound enhancing agent
	Intracardiac thrombus	Key in stroke, device thrombosis Careful scanning of LV apex, LVOT, and aortic root Ultrasound enhancing agent
	RV size	Standard techniques (e.g., basal, middle, and longitudinal diameters) Consider 3D

Continued

SUMMARY Diagnosis-Oriented Practical Imaging Guide.—cont'd

Evaluation	Parameters	Important Imaging Approaches/Techniques
	RV systolic function	Dysfunction may cause low-flow alarms Standard techniques (e.g., fractional area change, TAPSE, free wall s′, free wall peak systolic longitudinal strain, RVOT VTI) PASP and RAP Consider 3D
	Tricuspid regurgitation	Septal shift and septal leaflet tethering can worsen TR after LVAD implantation Integrate assessments of jet size with other parameters (e.g., hepatic vein spectral Doppler, IVC size and collapse, interatrial septal leftward shift, RA size, PASP)
	Mitral regurgitation	Worsening/unchanged MR may accompany device dysfunction or overfilling Standard techniques (e.g., vena contracta, PISA-derived EROA and regurgitant volume, pulmonary vein flow reversal)
	Aortic valve opening	May increase in setting of overfilling and device dysfunction May decrease in underfilling/suction event M-mode of AoV leaflets in PLAX view. Color M-mode
	Aortic regurgitation	May worsen after implant and become continuous Standard techniques (e.g., vena contracta) but note severity increased when continuous
	Cannulas/device location	Often requires off-axis imaging LVAD inflow cannula oriented toward septum, obstructed by trabeculation Color Doppler aliasing, elevated spectral Doppler velocities, regurgitation, elevated peak to basal/nadir spectral Doppler velocities suggest device thrombosis Elevated or low outflow graft spectral Doppler velocities may signal partial or complete obstruction by kinking or thrombus, respectively Consider CT Impella device inflow port < or > 3–4 cm below aortic valve TandemHeart inflow cannula in RA or LA appendage CentriMag migration ECMO inflow cannula migration into caval structure
	Pericardium	Low-flow alarms caused by tamponade Chamber compression may be more reliable than spectral Doppler inflow or outflow variance
Postimplantation optimization	LV size	LVEDd at MV leaflet tips (particularly for axial-flow devices), same imaging plane each time
	RV size	Standard techniques (e.g., basal, middle, and longitudinal diameters)
	RV systolic function	Standard techniques (e.g., fractional area change, TAPSE, free wall s′, free wall peak systolic longitudinal strain, RVOT VTI) PASP and RAP
	Tricuspid regurgitation	Integrate assessments of jet size with other parameters (e.g., hepatic vein spectral Doppler, IVC size and collapse, interatrial septal leftward shift, RA size, PASP)
	Mitral regurgitation	Standard techniques (e.g., vena contracta, PISA-derived EROA and regurgitant volume, pulmonary vein flow reversal)
	Aortic valve opening	M-mode of AoV leaflets in PLAX view Color M-mode
	Aortic regurgitation	May worsen after implant and become continuous Standard techniques (e.g., vena contracta) but note severity increased when continuous

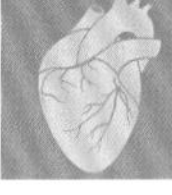

SUMMARY Diagnosis-Oriented Practical Imaging Guide.—cont'd

Evaluation	Parameters	Important Imaging Approaches/Techniques
Postimplantation ramp study	LV size	LVEDd at MV leaflet tips (particularly for axial-flow devices), same imaging plane each time
	Mitral valve inflow	Deceleration time
	Mitral regurgitation	Standard techniques (e.g., vena contracta, PISA-derived EROA and regurgitant volume, pulmonary vein flow reversal)
	Aortic valve opening	M-mode of AoV leaflets in PLAX view Color M-mode
	Aortic regurgitation	May lead to false-positive ramp study Standard techniques (e.g., vena contracta) but note severity is increased when continuous
	Cannulas	LVAD inflow cannula spectral Doppler to assess change in basal/nadir velocities.
Recovery	LV size	LVEDd at MV leaflet tips (particular for axial-flow devices), same imaging plane each time
	LV systolic function	LVEF by biplane method of disks 3D volumetric measurement Ultrasound enhancing agent
	RV systolic function	Standard techniques (e.g., fractional area change, TAPSE, free wall s′, free wall peak systolic longitudinal strain, RVOT VTI) PASP and RAP
	Aortic valve opening	M-mode of AoV leaflets in PLAX view
	Cannulas	Often requires off-axis imaging LVAD inflow cannula color and spectral Doppler to exclude regurgitation during turndown

AoV, Aortic valve; *AVA,* aortic valve area; *CT,* computed tomography; *ECMO,* extracorporeal membrane oxygenation; *EROA,* effective regurgitant orifice area; *IVC,* inferior vena cava; *LVAD,* LV assist device; *LVEDd,* LV end-diastolic diameter; *LVEF,* LV ejection fraction; *LVOT,* LV outflow tract; *MCS,* mechanical circulatory support; *MRI,* magnetic resonance imaging; *MV,* mitral valve; *PASP,* pulmonary artery systolic pressure; *PFO,* patent foramen ovale; *PISA,* proximal isovelocity surface area; *PLAX,* parasternal long axis; *RAP,* right atrial pressure; *RVEF right ventricular ejection fraction; RVOT,* RV outflow tract; *TAPSE,* tricuspid annular plane systolic excursion; *TR,* tricuspid regurgitation; *VTI,* velocity–time integral.

REFERENCES

1. Jauhar S. The artificial heart. *N Engl J Med.* 2004;350:542–544.
2. Hetzer R, Muller JH, Went Y, et al. Bridging-to-recovery. *Ann Thorac Surg.* 2001;71:S109–S113.
3. Boehmer JP, Popjes E. Cardiac failure: mechanical support strategies. *Crit Care Med.* 2006;34(Suppl):S268–S277.
4. Friedel N, Viazis P, Schiessler A, et al. Recovery of end-organ failure during mechanical circulatory support. *Eur J Cardio Thorac Surg.* 1992;6:519–522.
5. Farrar DJ, Hill JD. Recovery of major organ function in patients awaiting heart transplantation with Thoratec ventricular assist devices. *J Heart Lung Transplant.* 1994;13:1125–1132.
6. Frazier OH, Rose EA, Oz MC, et al. Multicenter clinical evaluation of the HeartMate vented electric left ventricular assist system in patients awaiting heart transplantation. *J Thorac Cardiovasc Surg.* 2001;122:1186–1195.
7. Dangas GD, Kini AS, Sharma SK, et al. Impact of hemodynamic support with Impella 2.5 versus intra-aortic balloon pump on prognostically important clinical outcomes in patients undergoing high-risk percutaneous coronary intervention (from the PROTECT II randomized trial). *Am J Cardiol.* 2014;113:222–228.
8. Lietz K, Miller LW. Improved survival of patients with end-stage heart failure listed for heart transplantation. Analysis of organ Procurement and Transplantation network/U.S. United Network of Organ Sharing Data, 1990 to 2005. *J Am Coll Cardiol.* 2007;50:1282–1290.
9. Rose EA, Gelijns AC, Moskowitz AJ, et al. Randomized evaluation of mechanical assistance for the treatment of congestive heart failure (REMATCH) study group. Long-term mechanical left ventricular assistance for end-stage heart failure. *N Engl J Med.* 2001;345:1435–1443.
10. Lietz K, Long JW, Kfoury AG, et al. Outcomes of left ventricular assist device implantation as destination therapy in the post-REMATCH era: implications for patient selection. *Circulation.* 2007;116:497–505.
11. Westaby S, Frazier OH, Banning A. Six years of continuous mechanical circulatory support. *N Engl J Med.* 2006;355:325–327.
12. Iqbal I, Ventura HO, Smart FW, Stapleton DD. Difficult cases in heart failure: left ventricular assist device implantation for the treatment of recurrent ventricular tachycardia in end stage heart failure. *Congest Heart Fail.* 1999;5:129–130.
13. Miller LW, Pagani FD, Russell SD, et al. Use of a continuous-flow device in patients awaiting heart transplantation. *N Engl J Med.* 2007;357:885–896.
14. John R, Kamdar F, Liao K, et al. Improved survival and decreasing incidence of adverse events using the HeartMate II left ventricular assist device as a bridge-to-transplant. *Ann Thorac Surg.* 2008;86:1227–1234.
15. Mehra MR, Naka Y, Uriel N, et al. A fully magnetically levitated circulatory pump for advanced heart failure. *N Engl J Med.* 2017;376:440–450.
16. Slaughter MS, Rogers JG, Milano CA, et al. Advanced heart failure treated with continuous-flow left ventricular assist device. *N Engl J Med.* 2009;361:2241–2251.
17. Farrar DJ, Bourque K, Dague CP, et al. Design features, developmental status, and experimental results with the HeartMate III centrifugal left ventricular assist system with a magnetically levitated rotor. *ASAIO J.* 2007;53:310–315.

18. Topilsky Y, Oh JK, Shah DK, et al. Echocardiographic predictors of adverse outcomes after continuous left ventricular assist device implantation. *JACC Cardiovasc Imaging.* 2011;4:211–222.
19. John R, Mantz K, Eckman P, et al. Aortic valve pathophysiology during left ventricular assist device support. *J Heart Lung Transplant.* 2010;29:1321–1329.
20. Feldman D, Pamboukian SV, Teuteberg JJ, et al. The 2013 International Society for Heart and Lung Transplantation Guidelines for mechanical circulatory support: executive summary. *J Heart Lung Transpl.* 2013;32:157–187.
21. Potapov EV, Antonides C, Crespo-Leiro MG, et al. EACTS Expert Consensus on long-term mechanical circulatory support. *Eur J Cardio Thorac Surg.* 2019;56(2):230–270. 2019.
22. Kormos RL, Teuteberg JJ, Pagani FD, et al. Right ventricular failure in patients with the HeartMate II continuous-flow left ventricular assist device: incidence, risk factors, and effect on outcomes. *J Thorac Cardiovasc Surg.* 2010;139:1316–1324.
23. Maeder MT, Leet A, Ross A, et al. Changes in right ventricular function during continuous-low left ventricular assist device support. *J Heart Lung Transplant.* 2009;28:360–366.
24. Fitzpatrick JR III, Frederick JR, Hiesinger W, et al. Early planned institution of biventricular mechanical circulatory support results in improved outcomes compared with delayed conversion of a left ventricular assist device to a biventricular assist device. *J Thorac Cardiovasc Surg.* 2009;137:971–977.
25. Tingleff J, Joyce FS, Pettersson G. Intraoperative echocardiographic study of air embolism during cardiac operations. *Ann Thorac Surg.* 1995;60:673–677.
26. Stainback RF, Estep JD, Agler DA, et al. Echocardiography in the management of patients with left ventricular assist devices: recommendations from the American Society of Echocardiography. *J Am Soc Echocardiogr.* 2015;28:853–909.
27. Pagani FD, Miller LW, Russell SD, et al. Extended mechanical circulatory support with a continuous-flow rotary left ventricular assist device. *J Am Coll Cardiol.* 2009;54:312–321.
28. Bhagra S, Bhagra C, Özalp F, et al. Development of de novo aortic valve incompetence in patients with the continuous-flow HeartWare ventricular assist device. *J Heart Lung Transplant.* 2016;35(3):312–319.
29. Mudd JO, Cuda JD, Halushka M, et al. Fusion of aortic valve commissures in patients supported by a continuous axial-flow left ventricular assist device. *J Heart Lung Transplant.* 2008;27:1269–1274.
30. Phan K, Haswell JM, Xu J, et al. Percutaneous transcatheter interventions for aortic insufficiency in continuous-flow left ventricular assist device patients: a systematic review and meta-analysis. *ASAIO J.* 2017;3(2):117–122.
31. Topkara VK, Kondareddy S, Malik F, et al. Infectious complications in patients with left ventricular assist device: etiology and outcomes in the continuous flow era. *Ann Thorac Surg.* 2010;90:1270–1277.
32. Kirklin JK, Pagani FD, Kormos RL, et al. Eighth annual INTERMACS report: special focus on framing the impact of adverse events. *J Heart Lung Transplant.* 2017;36(10):1080–1086.
33. Terracciano CM, Harding SE, Adamson D, et al. Changes in sarcolemmal Ca entry and sarcoplasmic reticulum Ca content in ventricular myocytes from patients with end-stage heart failure following myocardial recovery after combined pharmacological and ventricular assist device therapy. *Eur Heart J.* 2003;24:1329–1339.
34. Thohan V, Stetson SJ, Nagueh SF, et al. Cellular and hemodynamics responses of failing myocardium to continuous flow mechanical circulatory support using the DeBakey-Noon left ventricular assist device: a comparative analysis with pulsatile-type devices. *J Heart Lung Transplant.* 2005;24:566–575.
35. Simon MA, Primack BA, Teuteberg J, et al. Left ventricular remodeling and myocardial recovery on mechanical circulatory support. *J Card Fail.* 2010;16:99–105.
36. Li S, Beckman JA, Welch NG, et al. Accuracy of Doppler blood pressure measurement in continuous-flow left ventricular assist device patients. *ESC Heart Fail.* 2019;6(4): 793–798.
37. Addetia K, Uriel N, Maffessanti F, et al. 3D morphological changes in LV and RV during LVAD ramp studies. *JACC Cardiovasc Imaging.* 2018;(2 Pt 1):159–169.
38. Abbas AE, Fortuin FD, Schiller NB, et al. A simple method for noninvasive estimation of pulmonary vascular resistance. *J Am Coll Cardiol.* 2003;41:1021–1027.
39. Meyns B, Dens J, Sergeant P, et al. Initial experiences with the Impella device in patients with cardiogenic shock—Impella support for cardiogenic shock. *Thorac Cardiovasc Surg.* 2003;51:312–317.
40. Nguyen VP, Qin A, Kirkpatrick JN. Three-dimensional echocardiography of mechanical circulatory support devices. *Echocardiography.* 2018;35(12):2071–2078.
41. Estep JD, Vivo RP, Cordero-Reyes AM, et al. A simplified echocardiographic technique for detecting continuous-flow left ventricular assist device malfunction due to pump thrombosis. *J Heart Lung Transplant.* 2014;33:575–586.
42. Schwarz KQ, Parikh SS, Chen X, et al. Non-invasive flow measurement of a rotary pump ventricular assist device using quantitative contrast echocardiography. *J Am Soc Echocardiogr.* 2010;23:324–329.
43. Uriel N, Morrison KA, Garan AR, et al. Development of a novel echocardiography ramp test for speed optimization and diagnosis of device thrombosis in continuous-flow left ventricular assist devices: the Columbia ramp study. *J Am Coll Cardiol.* 2012;60:1764–1775.
44. Adatya S, Holley CT, Roy SS, et al. Echocardiographic ramp test for continuous-flow left ventricular assist devices: do loading conditions matter? *JACC Heart Fail.* 2015;3:291–299.
45. Birati EY, Quiaoit Y, Wald J, et al. Ventricular assist device thrombosis: a wide spectrum of clinical presentation. *J Heart Lung Transplant.* 2015;34:613–615.
46. Khan T, Delgado RM, Radovancevic B, et al. Dobutamine stress echocardiography predicts myocardial improvements in patients supported by left ventricular assist devices (LVADs): hemodynamic and histologic evidence of improvement before LVAD explantation. *J Heart Lung Transplant.* 2003;22:137–146.
47. Kalogeropoulos AP, Kelkar A, Weinberger JF, et al. Validation of clinical scores for right ventricular failure prediction after implantation of continuous-flow left ventricular assist devices. *J Heart Lung Transplant.* 2015;34:1596–1603.
48. Charisopoulou D, Banner NR, Demetrescu C, Simon AR, Rahman Haley S. Right atrial and ventricular echocardiographic strain analysis predicts requirement for right ventricular support after left ventricular assist device implantation. *Eur Heart J Cardiovasc Imaging.* 2019;20(2):199–208.
49. Geisen M, Spray D, Nicholas Fletcher S. Echocardiography-based hemodynamic management in the cardiac surgical intensive care unit. *J Cardiothorac Vasc Anesth.* 2014;28:733–744.
50. Kato TS, Jiang J, Schulze PC, et al. Serial echocardiography using tissue Doppler and speckle tracking imaging to monitor right ventricular failure before and after left ventricular assist device surgery. *JACC Heart Fail.* 2013;1: 216–222.
51. Riebandt J, Haberl T, Wiedemann D, et al. Extracorporeal membrane oxygenation support for right ventricular failure after left ventricular assist device implantation; temporary right ventricular support following left ventricle assist device implantation: a comparison of two techniques. *Eur J Cardio Thorac Surg.* 2017;19: 49–55.
52. Lam KMT, Ennis S, O'Driscoll G, et al. Observations from non-invasive measures of right heart hemodynamics in left ventricular assist device patients. *J Am Soc Echocardiogr.* 2009;22:1055–1062.
53. Dandel M, Weng Y, Siniawski H, et al. Prediction of cardiac stability after weaning from left ventricular assist devices in patients with idiopathic dilated cardiomyopathy. *Circulation.* 2008;118(suppl 1):S94–S105.
54. Dandel M, Weng Y, Siniawski H, et al. Heart failure reversal by ventricular unloading in patients with chronic cardiomyopathy: criteria for weaning from ventricular assist devices. *Eur Heart J.* 2011;32:1148–1160.
55. Birks EJ, George RS, Hedger M, et al. Reversal of severe heart failure with a continuous-flow left ventricular assist device and pharmacological therapy: a prospective study. *Circulation.* 2011;123:381–390.
56. Birks EJ, Tansley PD, Hardy J, et al. Left ventricular assist device and drug therapy for the reversal of heart failure. *N Engl J Med.* 2006;355:1973–1984.
57. Knierim J, Heck R, Pieri M, et al. Outcomes from a recovery protocol for patients with continuous-flow left ventricular assist devices. *J Heart Lung Transplant.* 2019;38(4):440–448.
58. Lohan DG, Krishnam M, Saleh R, et al. MR imaging of the thoracic aorta. *Magn Reson Imaging Clin North Am.* 2008;16:213–234.
59. Raman SV, Sahu A, Merchant AZ, et al. Non-invasive assessment of left ventricular assist devices with cardiovascular computed tomography and impact on management. *J Heart Lung Transplant.* 2010;29:79–85.
60. Acharya D, Singh S, Tallaj JA, et al. Use of gated cardiac computed tomography angiography in the assessment of left ventricular assist device dysfunction. *ASAIO J.* 2011;57:32–37.

中文导读

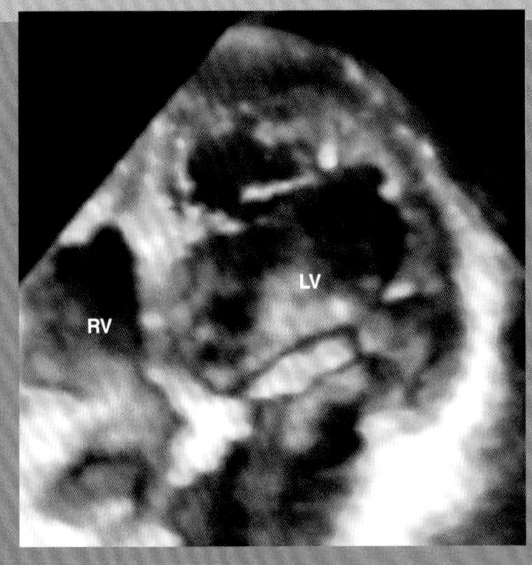

第17章 心包疾病

心包疾病的患病率相对不高，但其病因多样，严重的也可以危及生命。心包疾病不易诊断，经常会被误诊成其他疾病，如果诊断正确的话，通常是可以治疗的。本章将介绍几种最常见的心包疾病：缩窄性心包炎、心包积液、心脏压塞、急性心包炎，以及相对少见的心包缺失和心包囊肿等。

缩窄性心包炎的超声表现主要包括室间隔的异常摆动、肝静脉呼气相的显著逆流、二尖瓣环组织多普勒的异常和二尖瓣血流E峰随呼吸变化率的增加等。心包积液的超声诊断需要关注积液的回声、心包粘连、分析积液是否为血性或肿瘤来源，并对积液进行半定量。心脏压塞的超声诊断需要注意各个腔室的塌陷征象、下腔静脉的扩张及其随呼吸的变化；局限性的心包血肿或积液亦可导致局部的心脏压塞，尤其是在心脏术后。

心脏影像诊断要结合临床病史、体格检查、心电图、胸片和实验室检查等。当怀疑心包疾病时，首先推荐超声心动图来评估心脏解剖和血流动力学异常。超声心动图具有便捷、应用广泛、无放射性和价廉等优点，常作为心包疾病的首选检查方法。除此之外，CT和MRI可以确定诊断或提供其他有用的鉴别诊断信息。

李鸣瑶

17 Pericardial Disease

TERRENCE D. WELCH, MD

Although relatively few in number, pericardial diseases have a multitude of causes (Table 17.1) and may have life-threatening effects. They frequently masquerade as other diseases and may be missed if not considered in the differential diagnosis. Treatments are usually available if the condition is correctly diagnosed. For these reasons, pericardial diseases have long fascinated the medical community.[1] Constrictive pericarditis, pericardial effusion and tamponade, and acute pericarditis remain the most important and frequently encountered clinical entities. Less common problems include congenital absence of the pericardium and pericardial cysts.

Cardiac imaging should be performed in conjunction with a careful history and physical examination, electrocardiography, chest radiography, and appropriate laboratory assessment. Comprehensive echocardiography is recommended for all patients with suspected pericardial disease for the assessment of anatomic and hemodynamic abnormalities.[2,3] Advantages include its wide availability, portability, lack of ionizing radiation, and relative cost-effectiveness. Additional cross-sectional imaging with computed tomography (CT) and magnetic resonance imaging (MRI) may be required to confirm findings or offer additional diagnostic information, but echocardiography remains the first-line imaging test in most cases.[4]

PERICARDIAL ANATOMY AND FUNCTION

ANATOMY OF THE PERICARDIUM

The pericardium surrounds the heart and consists of a fibrous sac and a serous membrane.[5,6] The outer, fibrous sac is a thick structure that attaches to the great vessels superiorly, the sternum anteriorly, the vertebral column posteriorly, and the diaphragm inferiorly. The inner, serous membrane consists of a single layer of mesothelial cells that lines the epicardial fat, where it is called the visceral pericardium. This layer extends to the proximal portions of the aorta, pulmonary artery, vena cavae, and pulmonary veins, and then reflects back along the underside of the fibrous sac. Together, the reflected serous membrane and the fibrous sac form the parietal pericardium.

The space between the visceral and parietal pericardium contains a variable amount of fluid and is limited superiorly by the attachments of the fibrous pericardium to the great vessels and posteriorly by the reflections of the serous membrane around the pulmonary veins and vena cavae (Fig. 17.1). These reflections create two pericardial sinuses. The oblique sinus is posterior to the left atrium (LA), bordered by the pulmonary veins and inferior vena cava (IVC). The transverse sinus is superior to the LA, bordered by the great arteries, the superior vena cava, and the roof of the LA (see Fig. 17.1).

The primary arterial blood supply to the pericardium is from the pericardiophrenic arteries, which are branches of the internal thoracic arteries. Venous drainage occurs through the pericardiophrenic veins, which then drain into the brachiocephalic veins. The pericardium receives sympathetic, parasympathetic, and sensory innervation; the phrenic nerve provides the sensory component.

PERICARDIAL FLUID

The pericardial space normally contains 20 to 60 mL (average, 20–25 mL) of fluid in an average-sized man.[5] This fluid is an ultrafiltrate of plasma and contains proteins, electrolytes, and phospholipids. Pericardial fluid is drained by lymphatic channels along the epicardial surface and in the parietal pericardium.

FUNCTIONS OF THE PERICARDIUM

Although not considered essential for life, the pericardium is proposed to have beneficial ligamentous, membranous, and mechanical functions.[7] Ligamentous function refers to maintenance of the heart in a stable position within the thorax. Membranous functions include reduction of friction between the heart and contiguous structures and provision of a barrier

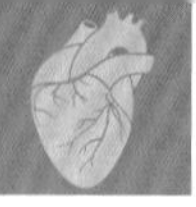

TABLE 17.1 Causes of Pericardial Disease.

Category	*Causes*
Idiopathic	
Infectious diseases	Bacterial, including tuberculosis, *Chlamydia*, borreliosis, *Treponema pallidum*, *Haemophilus*, *Meningococcus*, *Pneumococcus*, *Gonococcus*
	Fungal, including *Candida*, histoplasmosis
	Viral, including coxsackievirus, echovirus, mumps, Epstein-Barr, cytomegalovirus, *Varicella*, rubella, human immunodeficiency virus (HIV), parvovirus B19
	Parasitic, including *Toxoplasma*, *Echinococcus*, *Entamoeba histolytica*
Trauma	Blunt or penetrating trauma
	Cardiac surgery
Cardiac	Myocardial infarction
	Dressler syndrome
	Effusion and tamponade may be caused by myocardial rupture or aortic dissection
Systemic inflammatory disorders	Rheumatoid arthritis, systemic lupus erythematosus, systemic sclerosis, Reiter syndrome
Neoplasia	Primary benign or malignant pericardial tumors
	Secondary, including lung, breast, gastric, or colon cancer; leukemia; and melanoma
Metabolic and endocrine disorders	Renal failure, hypothyroidism, adrenal insufficiency
Miscellaneous	Mediastinal irradiation
	Pulmonary asbestosis

to inflammation or infection. Mechanical functions are more complex and may include limitation of excessive acute chamber dilation, preservation of ventricular diastolic pressure-volume curves, and mediation of cardiac chamber coupling.

PERICARDIAL PRESSURE AND NORMAL RESPIRATORY EFFECTS ON HEMODYNAMICS

The pressure within the pericardial space affects cardiac chamber filling through the *transmural pressure relationship*, defined as the pressure within the cardiac chamber minus pericardial pressure.[7–9] Changes in intrapleural pressure normally lead to equal changes in pericardial pressure. These pressure changes cause a normal, slight respiratory variation in left ventricular (LV) stroke volume and systemic blood pressure.[7,10] With inspiration, negative intrapleural pressure increases the gradient between the systemic venous reservoir and the right heart and increases transmural distention pressure for the right heart chambers. This leads to augmented venous return to the right heart, which expands outward. Total cardiac volume therefore increases.[11] There is a corresponding, slight decrease in left heart filling that is likely multifactorial in origin.[7,10]

In contrast to the right heart, the pressure gradient to fill the left heart should not increase with inspiration because the pulmonary veins and left heart chambers are intrapleural and exposed to the same pressure changes. Increased right ventricular (RV) preload may reduce LV diastolic compliance by lowering the transseptal diastolic pressure gradient. Effective afterload on the LV may be increased by the effect of negative

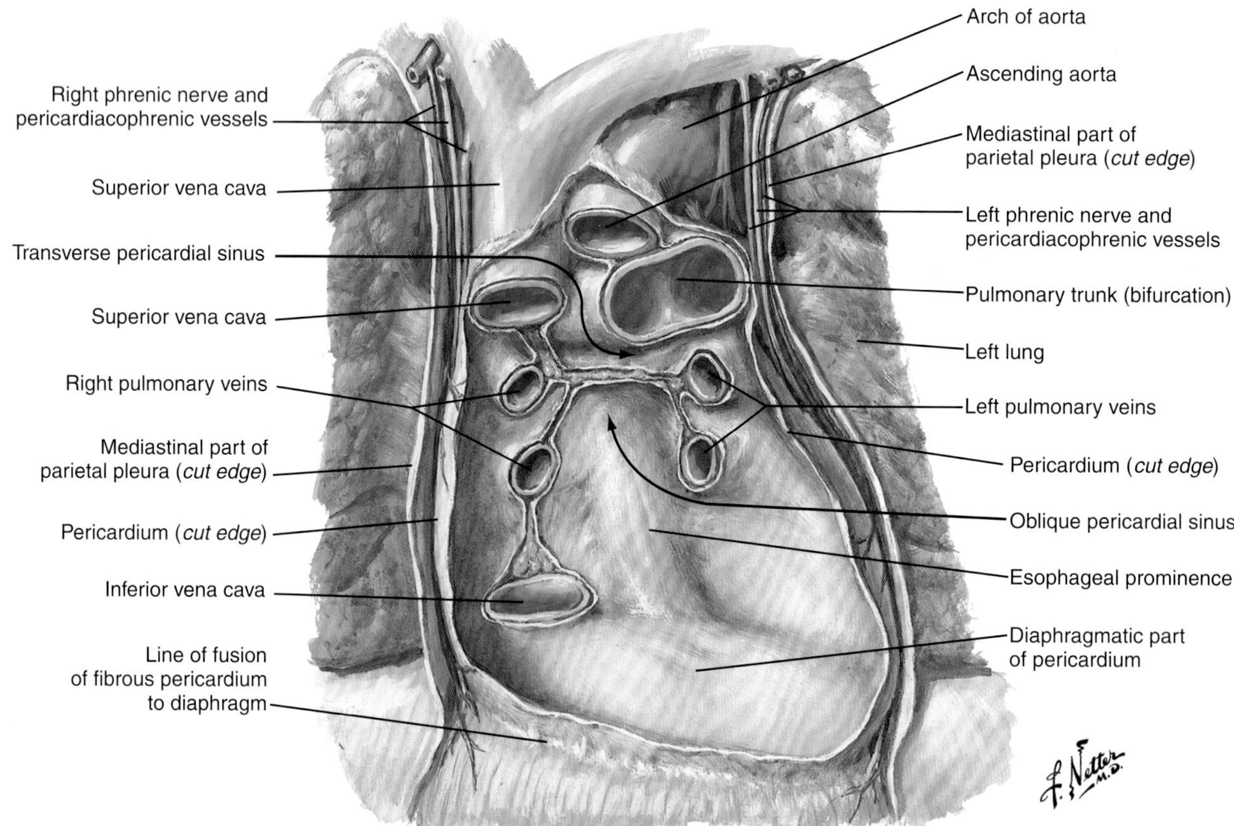

Fig. 17.1 Pericardial anatomy. Anterior view of the pericardial sac with the heart removed. (From Netter FH. *Atlas of Human Anatomy.* 1st ed. Ciba-Geigy Pharmaceutical; 1989.)

intrapleural pressure. The combined effects of decreased preload and increased afterload lead to slight reductions in LV stroke volume and aortic systolic pressure (<10 mmHg) during inspiration. These changes reverse with the rise in intrapleural pressure that occurs with expiration. A diseased pericardium may create spatial constraints or insulate the cardiac chambers from intrapleural pressure changes, either of which may magnify the respiratory changes in right- and left-sided filling and output.

PATHOPHYSIOLOGIC PRINCIPLES IN COMPRESSIVE PERICARDIAL DISEASE

The normal pericardium exhibits some elasticity, and its stretched volume represents the maximal pericardial volume. The difference between maximal pericardial volume and cardiac volume represents the pericardial *reserve volume*, into which the heart intermittently expands with respiration. With normal respiratory effort and in the absence of pericardial disease, the reserve volume is adequate, and *pericardial restraint* does not significantly affect cardiac filling. However, in compressive pericardial disease, the pericardial reserve volume is decreased because the pericardium is relatively inelastic, as in the case of constriction, or because the pericardial space has increased fluid contents under pressure, as in the case of tamponade. A combination of the two may occur in effusive-constrictive disease. In this setting of pericardial restraint, total cardiac volume is limited by the pericardium, and the ventricles must compete with each other for space. Recognition of this phenomenon is critical to echocardiographic diagnosis. RV expansion during inspiration must occur at the expense of the LV. This *enhanced ventricular interaction* manifests by a shift in the ventricular septum toward the left (Fig. 17.2). Increased LV filling during expiration is associated with a shift in the interventricular septum toward the RV and reduced RV filling.[12,13]

Variation in right and left heart filling also occurs because the diseased pericardium insulates the heart, such that the pericardial and intracardiac pressures no longer track intrapleural pressure changes. This phenomenon is called *dissociation of intrapleural and intracardiac pressures.* Inspiration decreases intrapleural and pulmonary venous pressures, but the pericardial and left heart chamber pressures are affected to a lesser extent. The pressure gradient for left heart filling therefore decreases and leads to reduced LV preload and subsequent stroke volume. The onset of expiration increases intrapleural pressure and the pressure gradient for left heart filling. Although dissociation of intrapleural and intracardiac pressures has been described in tamponade (Fig. 17.3), it appears to be a much more prominent mechanism in constriction. The two principles of *enhanced ventricular interaction* and *dissociation of intrapleural and intracardiac pressures* explain the *pulsus paradoxus* (i.e., decrease in systolic blood pressure by more than 10 mmHg with inspiration) that is observed in some patients with constrictive pericarditis and in most patients with tamponade.

With progressive, compressive pericardial disease, the reserve volume is lost completely, and pericardial volume steadily encroaches on cardiac volume throughout the respiratory cycle. This leads to progressive elevation in venous filling pressures, reduction in cardiac output, and worsening clinical heart failure. In tamponade, pericardial pressure may rise above intracardiac pressure, leading to chamber compression, markedly inadequate cardiac filling, and acutely life-threatening hemodynamic collapse.

ECHOCARDIOGRAPHIC EVALUATION OF PERICARDIAL DISEASE

Several components must be added to standard transthoracic echocardiography (TTE) to create an optimal pericardial disease protocol study that can accurately identify compressive pericardial disease. The Summary table reviews these components.

CONSTRICTIVE PERICARDITIS

DEFINITION AND ETIOLOGY

Constrictive pericarditis is a form of heart failure in which the diseased pericardium stiffens and restricts diastolic filling. Many disease states can involve the pericardium and lead to constrictive pericarditis (see Table 17.1). In North America and Europe, constrictive pericarditis is most commonly idiopathic or due to prior cardiac surgery, chest irradiation, or pericarditis.[14–18] Globally, tuberculosis remains a dominant cause.[19–21] Less common causes include rheumatologic disease, other infections, malignancy, trauma, and asbestosis.

PATHOLOGY AND PATHOPHYSIOLOGY

The pathologic changes in constriction typically affect the parietal pericardium but may also affect the visceral pericardium. Most diagnosed cases of constriction are chronic and are caused

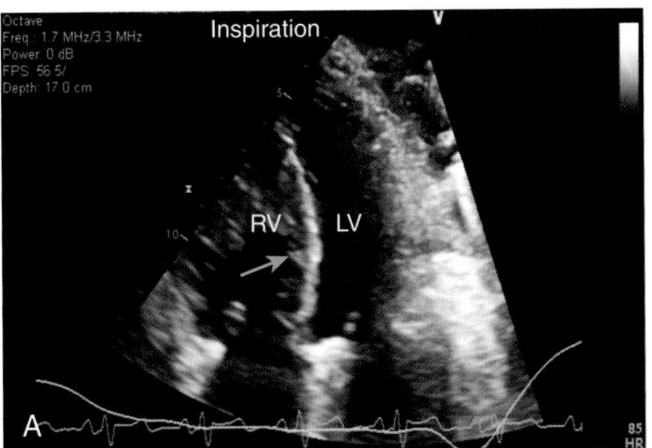

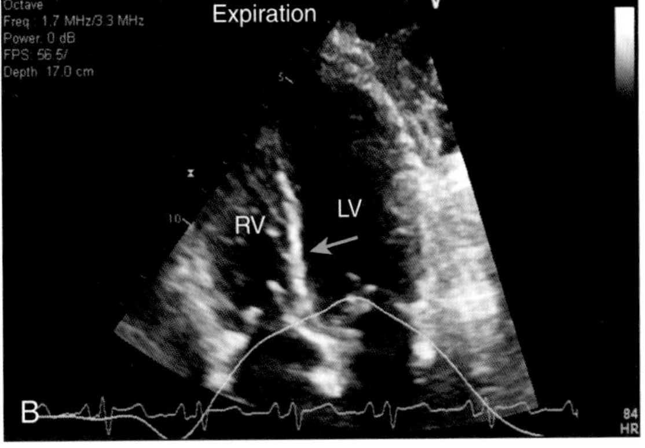

Fig. 17.2 Septal shift. Enhanced ventricular interaction in constriction is shown by the respiratory ventricular septal shift in these apical 4-chamber images. The ventricular septum shifts toward the left *(arrow)* during inspiration (A) and back toward the right *(arrow)* during expiration (B). The same phenomenon may be observed in tamponade (see Video 17.2).

by a scarred, calcified pericardium. The pericardium is usually thickened, but a substantial minority of patients with chronic constriction may have a normal pericardial thickness.[22] In a smaller number of cases, inflammation is the dominant pathologic finding, which suggests a subacute, potentially transient, and medically treatable process.

The diseased, stiffened pericardium loses its reserve volume and progressively limits the ability of the heart to expand and fill, particularly during inspiration, when cardiac volume normally increases.[11] The pathophysiologic principles of *enhanced ventricular interaction* and *dissociation of intrapleural and intracardiac pressures* become operative and serve as the basis for the echocardiographic and invasive hemodynamic diagnosis of constrictive pericarditis.[12,23]

As cardiac volume and ventricular diastolic filling are progressively restricted, filling pressures become elevated and equalized in the cardiac chambers. Increased atrial pressures lead to rapid early diastolic ventricular filling that abruptly terminates when the ventricle reaches the volume limit imposed by the constrictive pericardium. This is marked by a steep, deep *y* descent in the jugular venous pressure waveform. Venous pressure rises, and cardiac output falls, leading to progressive clinical symptoms.

CLINICAL PRESENTATION AND TREATMENT

The clinical presentation is a heart failure syndrome, which is often insidious and is characterized by dyspnea on exertion and signs of venous congestion, including elevated jugular venous pressure, ascites, and edema.[14] Some patients have recurrent pleural effusions or present with cirrhosis due to hepatic congestion.

The clinical features of constriction overlap almost entirely with those of other causes of predominantly right-sided heart failure, often creating a diagnostic dilemma.[24] The differential diagnosis typically includes heart failure with preserved ejection fraction, severe tricuspid regurgitation, severe pulmonary hypertension, and RV infarction, but restrictive cardiomyopathy is the classic and most difficult contending diagnosis.

Treatment of chronic constriction consists of surgical pericardiectomy. In a minority of cases, the constrictive process is subacute, caused by inflammation of the pericardium, and may improve or resolve with anti-inflammatory therapy.[25]

ECHOCARDIOGRAPHIC DIAGNOSIS

The echocardiographic diagnosis of constrictive pericarditis relies on recognition of the unique hemodynamic properties of constriction. In addition to the previously described principles of enhanced ventricular interaction and dissociation of intrapleural and intracardiac pressures, the unique diastolic properties of the myocardium in constriction allow a more confident diagnosis of constriction and differentiation from restrictive cardiomyopathy.[12,26–28] A dedicated pericardial-protocol echocardiogram (see Summary table) provides an important opportunity to use two-dimensional (2D), spectral Doppler, and tissue Doppler imaging to reveal a treatable form of heart failure.

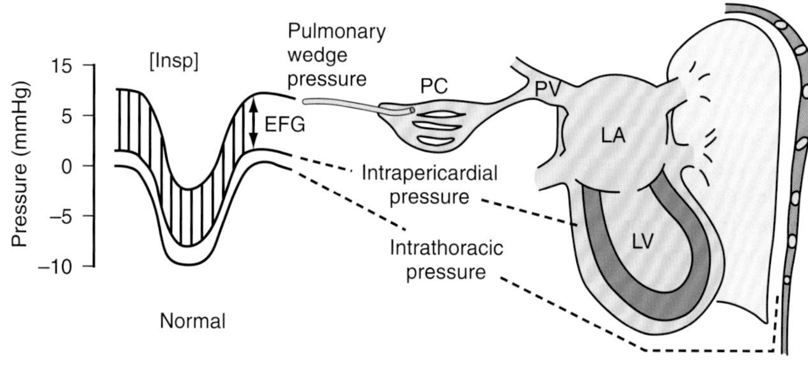

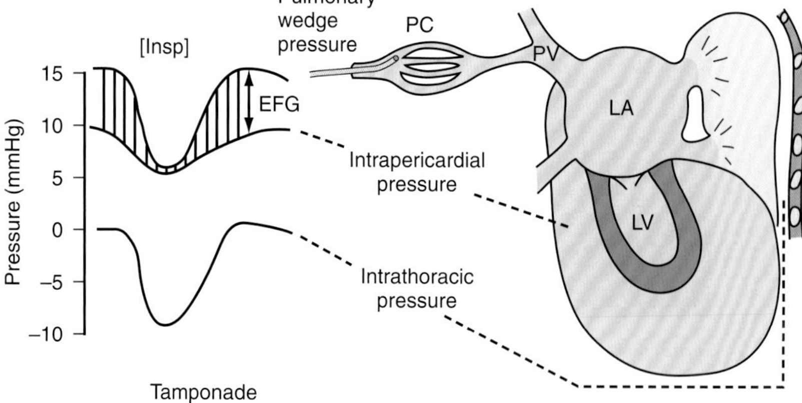

Fig. 17.3 Physiology of constrictive pericardial disease. Dissociation of intrapleural and intracardiac pressures in compressive pericardial disease. *Top*, Normal situation in which changes in intrathoracic pressure are transmitted to the pericardial sac and pulmonary veins (*PV*). The effective filling gradient (*EFG*) changes only slightly during respiration. *Bottom*, In compressive pericardial disease, changes in intrathoracic pressure are transmitted to PVs but not to the pericardial sac. EFG falls during inspiration (*Insp*). Although pictured in tamponade, this phenomenon is more prominent in constriction. *PC*, Pulmonary capillaries. (From Sharp JT, Bunnell IL, Holland JF, et al. Hemodynamics during induced cardiac tamponade in man. *Am J Med*. 1960;29:640–646.)

Assessment should begin with the five principal echocardiographic findings that were evaluated in the largest, blinded comparison of patients with constriction (n = 130) versus patients with restriction or severe tricuspid regurgitation (n = 36) at the Mayo Clinic and subsequently at the Cleveland Clinic (Table 17.2).[29,30] However, there are no universally accepted diagnostic criteria, and all available echocardiographic information should be considered in the diagnostic work-up.

Abnormal Ventricular Septal Motion: Ventricular Septal Shift and Shudder

Assessment of ventricular septal motion and position often provides the first clue to the diagnosis of constrictive pericarditis because wall motion analysis is included in all standard echocardiographic examinations. Unexplained abnormal ventricular septal motion should always prompt consideration of full pericardial-protocol echocardiography for patients with clinical heart failure.

Ventricular Septal Shift

Respiration-related shifting in the position of the ventricular septum is a manifestation of the previously described principles of enhanced ventricular interaction and dissociation of intrapleural and intracardiac pressures. Decreased filling of the left-sided cardiac chambers in inspiration leads to an obligatory shift of the ventricular septum toward the LV (Fig. 17.4; see Fig. 17.2). Increased filling of the left-sided cardiac chambers during expiration causes the ventricular septum to shift back toward the RV. With the highest reported sensitivity (93%) and an independent association with the diagnosis of constriction, this finding may be the most important of the echocardiographic criteria.[29]

TABLE 17.2 Test Performance Characteristics for Five Principal Echocardiographic Findings in Constrictive Pericarditis.

Variable[a]	*Sensitivity (%)*	*Specificity (%)*	*Positive Predictive Value (%)*	*Negative Predictive Value (%)*
Individual Variables				
1. Ventricular septal shift	**93**	**69**	**92**	**74**
2. Change in mitral E velocity ≥ 14.6%[b]	84	73	92	55
3. Medial e′ velocity ≥ 9 cm/s	**83**	**81**	**94**	**57**
4. Medial e′/lateral e′ ≥ 0.91	75	85	95	50
5. Hepatic vein ratio in expiration ≥ 0.79	**76**	**88**	**96**	**49**
Combinations of Variables 1, 3, and 5[c]				
1 (with or without 3 and/or 5)	93	69	92	74
1 and 3 (with or without 5)	80	92	97	56
1 with 3 or 5	87	91	97	65
1 with both 3 and 5	64	97	99	42

[a]Cut points for continuous variables were selected from receiver operating characteristic (ROC) analysis.
[b]Limited to echocardiographic findings (in bold) that were independently associated with the diagnosis of constrictive pericarditis. HV ratio = diastolic reversal velocity/forward velocity.
[c]Based on [(expiratory velocity − inspiratory velocity)/inspiratory velocity × 100]; the value will be slightly lower if the currently recommended formula [(expiratory velocity − inspiratory velocity)/expiratory velocity × 100] is used.
From Welch TD, Ling LH, Espinosa RE, et al. Echocardiographic diagnosis of constrictive pericarditis: Mayo Clinic criteria. *Circ Cardiovasc Imaging*. 2014;7(3):526–534.

Ventricular Septal Shudder

In addition to ventricular septal shift with respiration, there is almost always an abnormality in beat-to-beat (regardless of phase in the respiratory cycle) diastolic septal motion that is called a *shudder* and may be visualized on 2D and M-mode recordings (see Fig. 17.4) and with tissue Doppler imaging.[31] The oscillatory diastolic motion of the septum may be related to enhanced ventricular interaction on a millisecond scale that arises from subtle differences in timing of tricuspid and mitral valve opening and right atrial (RA) and LA contraction.[32–34]

A septal shudder is probably less clinically useful than the respiration-related septal shift because beat-to-beat septal abnormalities are relatively common (e.g., due to conduction abnormalities or to prior cardiac surgery). They also appear to be less specific for constriction (reported in 44% of patients with restrictive cardiomyopathy or severe tricuspid regurgitation).[29]

Respiratory Variation in the Hepatic Vein Doppler Profile: Prominent Diastolic Flow Reversals in Expiration

The hepatic vein Doppler profile is affected by right heart hemodynamics and provides another clue to the dissociation of intrapleural and intracardiac pressures and the enhanced ventricular interaction expected in constrictive pericarditis. Hepatic vein forward flow in constriction is typically biphasic, with a systolic waveform and a more prominent diastolic waveform. This pattern arises because elevated RA pressure inhibits venous return during systole, and tricuspid valve opening allows increased venous return in early diastole. Brief flow reversals are usually seen at the end of systole and diastole.

The diagnosis of constriction can be made based on changes in the flows during the respiratory cycle. Increased left heart filling during expiration shifts the ventricular septum back toward the RV, and right heart filling decreases. There is a reduction in hepatic vein diastolic forward flow velocity and an exaggerated late diastolic reversal (Fig. 17.5).[12,26] Although most often qualitatively assessed, this finding may be quantified with the *hepatic vein expiratory diastolic reversal ratio.*[29] The ratio is the expiratory diastolic reversal velocity divided by the diastolic forward velocity, and it therefore incorporates the expected decrease in diastolic forward flow and the exaggerated diastolic flow reversal.

In restriction and severe tricuspid regurgitation, right-sided filling is not as compromised in expiration. The expiratory diastolic forward velocity is higher, and the diastolic reversal velocity is less prominent (but may be more prominent during inspiration). Higher reversal ratio values are therefore expected in constriction (1.4 ± 0.7) as opposed to restriction or severe tricuspid regurgitation (0.5 ± 0.4).[29] A reversal ratio of ≥0.79 appears to be one of the more specific (88%) findings for constriction and is independently associated with the diagnosis.[29]

Mitral Annular Tissue Velocities

Preserved or Elevated e′ Values

Doppler echocardiography allows identification of unique myocardial relaxation properties in constrictive pericarditis. The early diastolic mitral annular tissue velocity (e′) is a measure of diastolic relaxation and is expected to be reduced in restrictive cardiomyopathy and most other forms of heart failure but not in pure constrictive pericarditis. Preserved or elevated e′ velocities therefore provide an important means of differentiating constriction from restriction.[27,28]

Increased medial e′ velocity is independently associated with the diagnosis of constrictive pericarditis, and a medial e′ velocity of ≥9 cm/s allows differentiation of constriction from restriction or severe tricuspid regurgitation with a sensitivity of 83% and a sensitivity of 81%.[29] The important limitation to the use of this single-point velocity is that it may be affected by other processes such as annular calcification and may not be as reliable when pericardial or myocardial disease processes are not uniform.[35]

Mitral e′ velocity is also expected to vary with the cause of constriction. Constriction due to prior radiation therapy or cardiac surgery is associated with relatively lower e′ velocities compared with constriction that is idiopathic or caused by rheumatologic disease or prior pericarditis.[29] Patients who have received radiation treatment represent an especially challenging group; in many cases, they may have a component of restriction in addition to constriction.

Annulus Reversus

Comparison of the medial and lateral mitral annular e′ velocities may help in evaluating constriction. As opposed to the usual pattern of the lateral e′ being higher than the medial e′, the medial e′ velocity is often equal to or higher than the lateral in constriction (Fig, 17.6). This phenomenon has been called *annulus reversus* and is thought to result from tethering of the lateral myocardium by the diseased pericardium with compensation by the medial annulus.[36] However, the ratio of medial to

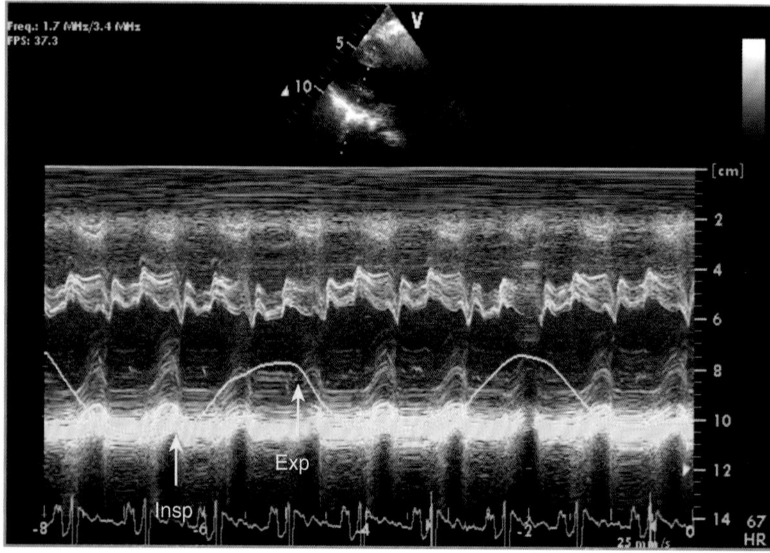

Fig. 17.4 M-mode in constriction. Mid-ventricular septal M-mode recording (parasternal long axis) in a patient with constrictive pericarditis. There is a leftward ventricular septal shift in inspiration *(Insp)* and a beat-to-beat septal diastolic shudder. *Exp*, Expiration. (From Welch TD, Ling LH, Espinosa RE, et al. Echocardiographic diagnosis of constrictive pericarditis: Mayo Clinic criteria. *Circ Cardiovasc Imaging.* 2014;7[3]:526–534.)

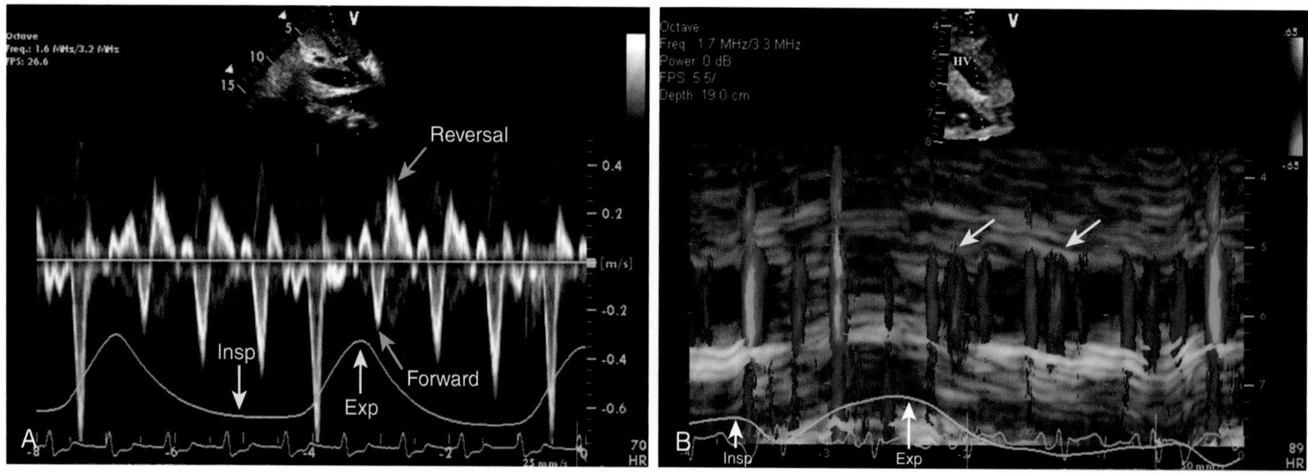

Fig. 17.5 Hepatic vein pulsed Doppler in constriction. (A) Pulsed-wave Doppler recording (subcostal window) within the hepatic vein (HV) in a patient with constrictive pericarditis. Note the prominent diastolic flow reversals in expiration *(Exp)*, with the diastolic reversal ratio defined as reversal velocity divided by forward velocity (≈0.35 m/s reversal velocity divided by ≈ 0.30 cm/s forward flow velocity yields a diastolic reversal ratio of 1.2). (B) Color M-mode recording (subcostal window) within the hepatic vein in a patient with constrictive pericarditis. Prominent diastolic flow reversals *(arrows)* occur during expiration. *Insp*, Inspiration. (From Welch TD, Ling LH, Espinosa RE, et al. Echocardiographic diagnosis of constrictive pericarditis: Mayo Clinic criteria. *Circ Cardiovasc Imaging.* 2014;7[3]:526–534.)

lateral e′ velocities was not found to be independently associated with the diagnosis of constrictive pericarditis in the Mayo Clinic study, making the absolute value of medial e′ the more important echocardiographic finding.

Annulus Paradoxus

The preserved or accentuated e′ velocity in constrictive pericarditis leads to a lower-than-expected early (E)/e′ velocity ratio, despite increased filling pressure. This finding has been called *annulus paradoxus*.[37] Whether there is a true inverse relationship between E/e′ and pulmonary capillary wedge pressure is a matter of debate.[37–39]

Respiratory Variation in Mitral Inflow Velocity

Because filling pressures tend to be elevated in constrictive pericarditis, the ratio of E to late (A) transmitral filling velocities is usually pseudonormal or restrictive and is almost always more than 0.8.[26,40,41] Dissociation of intrapleural and intracardiac pressures is typically evident on Doppler evaluation through an inspiratory decrease in mitral E velocity (Fig. 17.7). With the onset of expiration and increased gradient for left heart filling, the mitral E velocity increases.

The percent change in mitral E velocity during respiration varies with the method of measurement and calculation. The current recommendation is to compare the first beat of expiration with the first beat of inspiration and to calculate the percent change using the following formula: (expiratory velocity − inspiratory velocity)/expiratory velocity × 100.[4] Using this formula, the reported average variation in mitral E velocity ranges from 15% to 35% in constriction.[12,26,29,42] Variation in the range of 10% to 15% has been an optimal cut point for differentiating constriction from restriction, with a reported sensitivity of 84% and specificities ranging from 73% to 91%.[29,42]

There are several reasons why variation in mitral E velocity is helpful but not essential for the diagnosis of constriction. First, modest variation in mitral E velocity may be observed in the absence of constriction, with variation up to 12% in restriction or severe tricuspid regurgitation.[29] Second, up to one-fifth of patients with constriction may lack characteristic changes in mitral E velocity, likely because of hypervolemia and very high LA pressure. Repeating the Doppler study after preload reduction maneuvers, such as head-up tilt or sitting positions, may demonstrate more significant variation in mitral E in these cases.[43] Third, patients with atrial arrhythmias have changes in mitral E velocity that reflect varied diastolic filling periods, such that dissociation between intrapleural and intracardiac pressures cannot be reliably identified. Accordingly, variation in mitral E velocity has not been significantly different between constriction and other disorders in the setting of atrial fibrillation or flutter.[29] Fourth, variation in mitral E velocity has not been independently associated with constriction on multivariable analysis, likely because of the aforementioned issues.[29]

Other Echocardiographic Findings

Other 2D and M-Mode Findings

Plethora of the IVC, as a marker of elevated venous pressure, is expected but not specific for the diagnosis of constriction. Of 130 patients with constriction in the Mayo Clinic series, all but 5 had plethora of the IVC as defined by a diameter of more than 2.1 cm and/or less than 50% collapse with inspiration or sniff.[29]

Pericardial thickening may be suspected in up to 85% of cases. It is not required for the diagnosis and is better assessed with CT or cardiac MRI (CMR).[29]

A *pericardial effusion* is reported for 10% to 24% of cases that required pericardiectomy. It may indicate effusive-constrictive pericarditis.[29,44]

Diastolic checking or flattening of LV free wall expansion in diastole may be appreciated by 2D and M-mode imaging.[45] *Distortion of the ventricular contour* by an obviously constrictive pericardium can occur in up to 34% of cases and is likely to be a highly specific finding.[29]

Apparent *tethering of the RV free wall* at its interface with the diaphragm and liver, as opposed to the normal independent sliding motion during the cardiac cycle, has been reported in 61% of patients with constriction. However, it does not appear to be specific for the diagnosis.[29]

Other Doppler Findings

Although respiratory variation in hepatic and mitral Doppler profiles receives the most attention, characteristic changes in velocity also occur at the aorta, pulmonary artery, tricuspid valve, and pulmonary veins. According to prior reports, inspiration leads to an average 14% decrease in *aortic velocity*, a 16% increase in *pulmonary artery velocity*, and a 48% to 55% increase in *tricuspid inflow E velocity*.[12,26]

Although not commonly performed for constriction, transesophageal echocardiography (TEE) is the best modality for assessing respiration-related variation in the *pulmonary vein Doppler profile*. The following findings appear to be the most helpful: (1) a greater ratio of systolic to diastolic forward velocities compared with restriction and (2) greater augmentation (>18%) of the peak diastolic forward flow velocity during

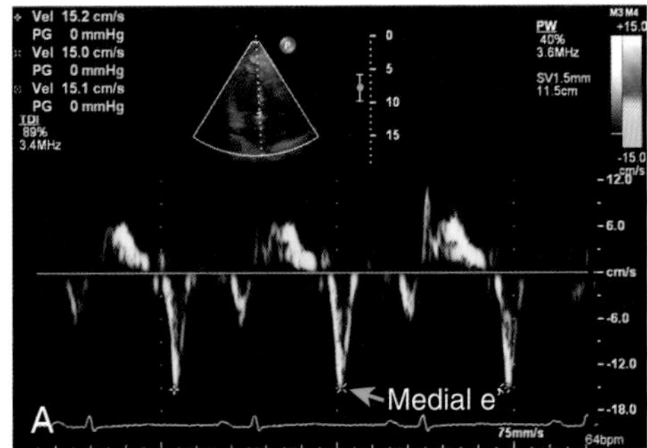

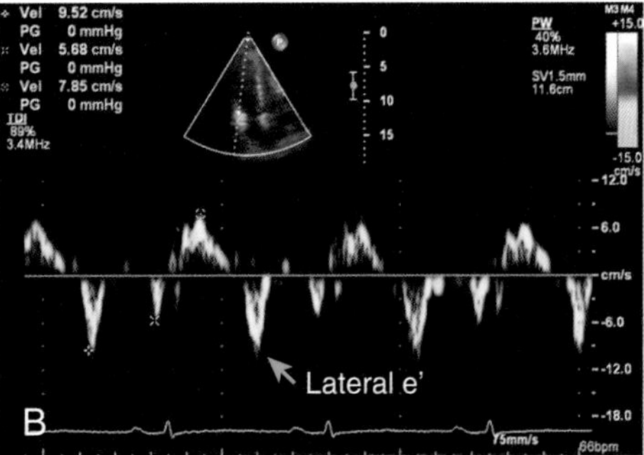

Fig. 17.6 **Tissue Doppler in constriction.** Medial (A) and lateral (B) mitral annular tissue Doppler recording (reversed 4-chamber view) in a patient with constrictive pericarditis. Note the normal to increased early relaxation velocity (*e′*), with a medial velocity greater than the lateral velocity (i.e., annulus reversus). (From Welch TD, Ling LH, Espinosa RE, et al. Echocardiographic diagnosis of constrictive pericarditis: Mayo Clinic criteria. *Circ Cardiovasc Imaging*. 2014;7[3]:526–534.)

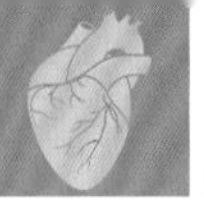

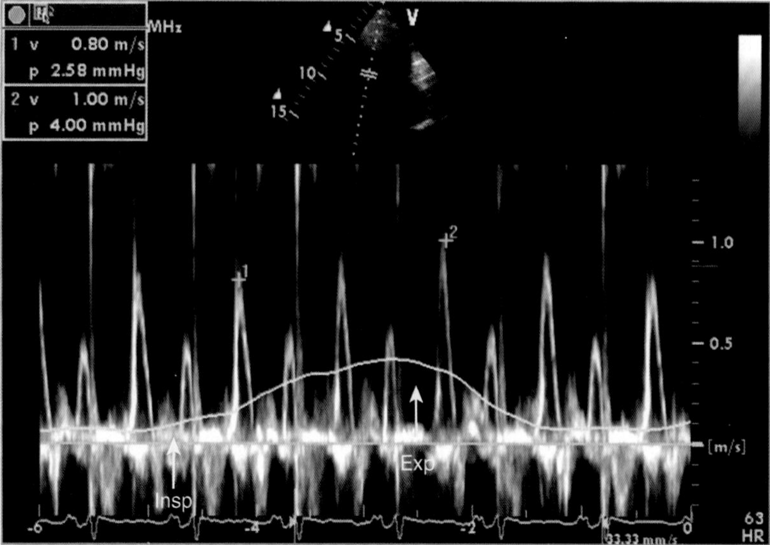

Fig. 17.7 **Transmitral Doppler in constriction.** Pulsed-wave Doppler recording (apical window in Mayo Clinic format) at the level of the open mitral leaflet tips in a patient with constrictive pericarditis. Notice the inspiratory *(Insp)* decrease and expiratory *(Exp)* increase in early (E) inflow velocity. (From Welch TD, Ling LH, Espinosa RE, et al. Echocardiographic diagnosis of constrictive pericarditis: Mayo Clinic criteria. *Circ Cardiovasc Imaging*. 2014;7[3]:526–534.)

expiration in constriction as opposed to restriction.[42,46] The expiratory increase in pulmonary vein diastolic forward velocity mirrors the increase in Doppler velocities found elsewhere in the left heart during expiration.

Other Doppler findings that have been described in the right heart include increased peak velocity and time velocity integral of the tricuspid regurgitation jet and premature termination of the pulmonary regurgitation jet during inspiration.[47,48]

Color M-mode Doppler is more difficult to use, but it may help in differentiating constriction from restriction through assessment of flow propagation slope, which is related to ventricular relaxation properties and tends to be higher (>100 cm/s) in constriction.[42]

Doppler assessment of the superior vena cava is an important component of pericardial-protocol echocardiography because it helps to differentiate constriction from obstructive lung disease and other conditions that may cause false-positive echocardiographic findings in the absence of pericardial disease. In obstructive lung disease, respiratory variation in Doppler velocities is caused by marked swings in intrapleural pressure and is accompanied by significantly increased (≥35%) flow velocity from the superior vena cava to the RA during inspiration.[49] In contrast, inspiratory forward flow velocities in the superior vena cava do not increase significantly and may even decrease during inspiration in constrictive pericarditis (Fig. 17.8). This is the echocardiographic correlate of the Kussmaul sign (i.e., inspiratory increase in jugular venous pressure) that is sometimes seen in constriction.

The flat superior vena cava Doppler profile in constriction contrasts with the inspiratory augmentation of hepatic vein forward flow (see Fig. 17.5). This finding likely is related to competitive flow from the superior vena cava and IVC (and therefore hepatic veins) when RA pressure is high. During inspiration, hepatic vein and IVC flow is driven by increased intraabdominal pressure that arises because of diaphragmatic descent.[50] The increased return from the IVC cava limits inflow from the superior vena cava because cardiac filling is constrained by the diseased pericardium.

Strain Imaging

Speckle-tracking strain imaging can elucidate the uniquely abnormal myocardial mechanics in constriction, and it provides another tool for differentiating constriction from restriction. Global longitudinal systolic strain is typically preserved in constriction and reduced in restriction.[51] Circumferential systolic strain, torsion, and early diastolic untwisting tend to be reduced in constriction and preserved in restriction. This situation is likely related to the fact that subendocardial muscle fibers, which are responsible for longitudinal deformation, are affected in restriction, whereas subepicardial muscle fibers, which are responsible for circumferential deformation, are affected in constriction.

Significant differences in regional longitudinal systolic strain have also been demonstrated for constriction versus restriction. In constriction, regional myocardial strain inversely correlates with the thickness of the adjacent pericardium as measured by MRI.[52] The lateral LV and RV walls have reduced longitudinal systolic strain compared with the septal wall because they are tethered by the diseased pericardium (Fig. 17.9). The same degree of regional heterogeneity is not expected in restriction, and the ratio of lateral LV to septal strain can be used to discriminate between constriction and restriction.[52] The discrepancy between lateral and septal strain appears to resolve after pericardiectomy or resolution of an inflammatory constrictive process.

DIFFERENTIATION FROM RESTRICTIVE CARDIOMYOPATHY

Constrictive pericarditis and restrictive cardiomyopathy may manifest similarly despite having different pathologic mechanisms. The diastolic filling impairment results from a noncompliant myocardium in restriction and an inelastic pericardium in constriction. Treatment therefore differs markedly, and constriction may be curable by removal of the abnormal pericardium or sometimes with antiinflammatory treatment. Comprehensive echocardiography provides vital information

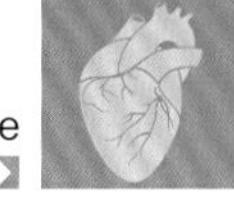

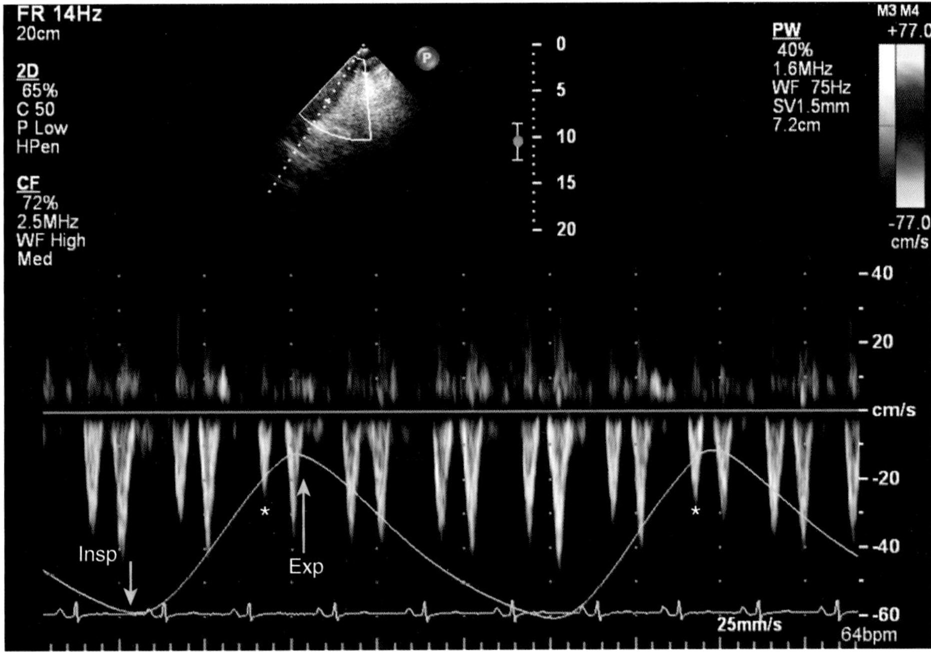

Fig. 17.8 Superior vena cava Doppler in constriction. Pulsed-wave Doppler recording (right supraclavicular window) from the superior vena cava in a patient with constrictive pericarditis. The forward velocities (below the baseline) do not increase with inspiration *(Insp)*; in this case, they actually decrease (*asterisks* mark decreased end-inspiratory systolic velocities). This contrasts with what is found in obstructive lung disease. *Exp*, Expiration.

that can distinguish the two disorders. Table 17.3 summarizes important echocardiographic differences between constriction and restriction.

2D echocardiographic assessment of cardiac morphology typically is not diagnostic. Thickening of the pericardium may be more common in constriction but is difficult to assess accurately by TTE. LA enlargement and increased ventricular wall thickness may be more common in restriction. Plethora of the IVC occurs in both disorders.

The key to the diagnosis of constriction and differentiation from restriction is to recognize the echocardiographic signs of its distinct pathophysiologic properties, including (1) enhanced ventricular interaction, (2) dissociation of intrapleural and intracardiac pressures, and (3) unique myocardial relaxation properties. Although all aspects of the echocardiogram should be considered, three echocardiographic findings have been independently associated with the diagnosis of constrictive pericarditis and are therefore likely to be the most important: (1) ventricular septal shift, (2) preserved or increased medial e′, and (3) exaggerated hepatic vein diastolic flow reversals in expiration.[29] The finding of ventricular septal shift along with either of the other two findings may yield the optimal combination of sensitivity (87%) and specificity (91%).

There is no universally accepted algorithm for the echocardiographic diagnosis of constrictive pericarditis. A proposed algorithm from the Mayo Clinic is presented in Fig. 17.10.[40] A plethoric IVC and mitral E/A ratio of at least 0.8 are expected in both constriction and restriction. Detection of a respiration-related ventricular septal shift provides a highly sensitive starting point for the diagnosis of constriction. Thereafter, finding a preserved medial e′ velocity and/or exaggerated hepatic vein expiratory diastolic flow reversal offers progressively increased specificity for the diagnosis of constriction. In some cases, constriction and restriction may coexist. An unexpectedly low e′ velocity in the setting of other findings that suggest constriction may be the clue. If the diagnosis remains uncertain after meticulous clinical evaluation and a pericardial-protocol echocardiogram, additional investigation is advisable and may include hemodynamic catheterization, CT, and/or CMR.

EFFUSIVE-CONSTRICTIVE PERICARDITIS AND TRANSIENT CONSTRICTIVE PERICARDITIS

There is some overlap among the compressive pericardial syndromes. *Effusive-constrictive pericarditis* is the term used when pericardial fluid accumulates between the layers of a constrictive pericardium, such that constrictive hemodynamics persist even after removal of the pericardial fluid.[53,54] Limited data suggest that this is an uncommon disease entity, identified in 8% of patients referred for pericardiocentesis.[54] Although historically suspected when RA pressure remains elevated after a successful therapeutic pericardiocentesis, there are echocardiographic findings (before and after pericardiocentesis) that can help distinguish effusive-constrictive pericarditis from effusive tamponade and constrictive pericarditis without effusion.[55] Before pericardiocentesis, the medial and lateral e′ velocities and E/A ratios are higher in effusive-constrictive pericarditis than in tamponade. Compared with constrictive pericarditis without effusion, hepatic vein forward diastolic flow during expiration is significantly lower in effusive-constrictive pericarditis and tamponade. After pericardiocentesis, IVC plethora is more common in effusive-constrictive pericarditis than in tamponade, and hepatic vein diastolic reversals in expiration decrease in tamponade but not in effusive-constrictive pericarditis. Effusive-constrictive pericarditis appears to be most commonly caused by idiopathic pericarditis and malignancy, but it is also seen after radiation therapy, after cardiac surgery, and in tuberculous pericarditis.[54] Some cases may require pericardiectomy, which is technically challenging because the visceral pericardium is

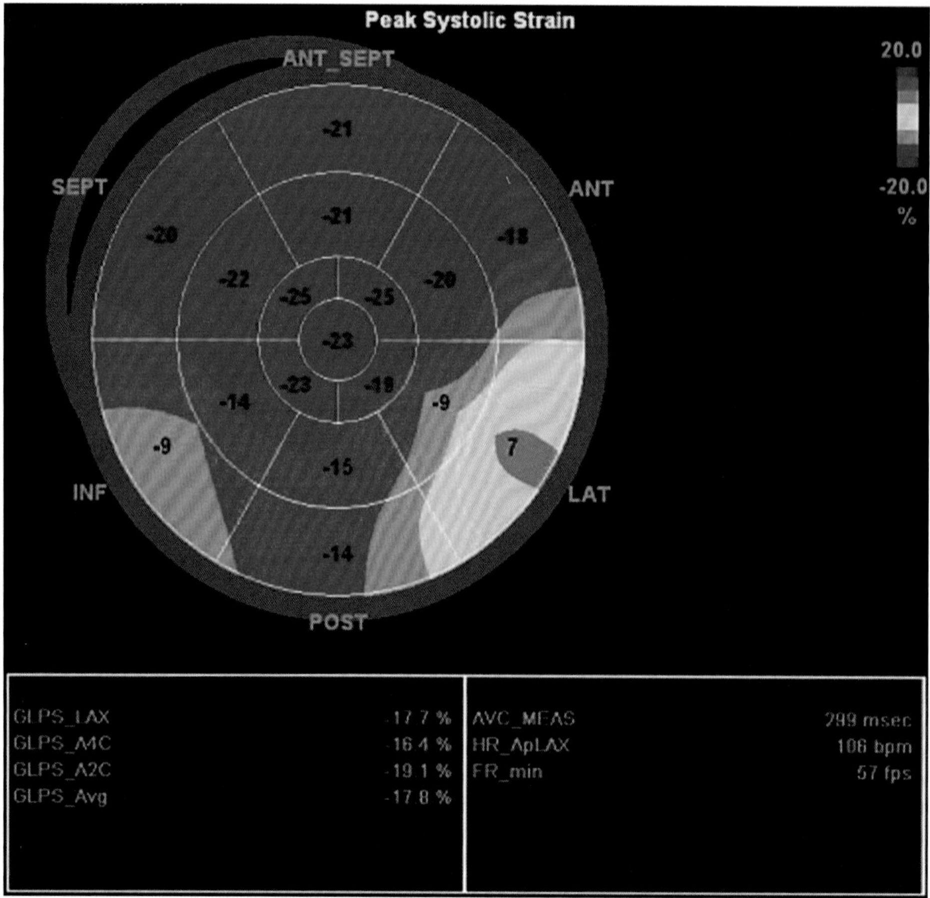

Fig. 17.9 Strain imaging in constriction. Longitudinal systolic strain (speckle-tracking) bull's-eye map in a patient with constrictive pericarditis. Global average longitudinal systolic strain is almost normal (−17.8%). Lateral strain is prominently reduced compared with septal strain because of the tethering effects of the diseased pericardium. *ANT*, Anterior; *INF*, inferior; *LAT*, lateral; *POST*, posterior; *SEPT*, septal.

TABLE 17.3 Constriction Versus Restriction: Typical Echocardiographic Findings.

Assessment	*Constriction*	*Restriction*
Respiratory ventricular septal shift	Present	Absent
Hepatic vein diastolic reversals	Prominent in expiration	Prominent in inspiration
Mitral medial e′ velocity	Preserved or increased	Decreased
Respiratory variation in mitral E velocity	Typically prominent	Minimal
Longitudinal systolic strain	Globally preserved, with reduction in lateral compared with septal	Globally decreased without significant difference between lateral and septal

predominantly involved and must be painstakingly removed through sharp dissection along the surface of the heart. Other cases may improve with antiinflammatory therapy.

A few patients with constriction have an inflammatory *transient constrictive pericarditis*, which resolves over a period of weeks to months with antiinflammatory therapies.[25,56] In a series of 212 patients with constriction, a transient process occurred in 36 (17%), and most of these were effusive-constrictive.[25] Determination of which patients have potentially transient constriction is accomplished with assessment of serum inflammatory markers and CMR (discussed in the next section); echocardiography is not useful for this purpose.

MULTIMODALITY IMAGING OF CONSTRICTIVE PERICARDITIS

Multimodality imaging is often used to supplement echocardiography in clinching the diagnosis of constrictive pericarditis and in guiding treatment. CT reveals pericardial thickening and calcification better than echocardiography, although neither finding is required for the diagnosis.[22] CT also allows careful assessment of any deformation in the contour of the heart (due to the constrictive pericardium) and helps define the relationship between the pericardium and the coronary arteries (for patients who may need surgical intervention).[4]

Like CT, gated CMR offers detailed information about cardiac anatomy. Like echocardiography, CMR allows assessment of enhanced ventricular interaction and respiratory variation in flows across the atrioventricular valves.[4,57] Unlike CT or echocardiography, CMR facilitates tissue characterization of the pericardium and helps identify patients who may benefit from a course of antiinflammatory therapy. Late gadolinium enhancement (LGE) in the pericardium signifies increased fibroblast proliferation and neovascularization along with chronic inflammation and granulation tissue.[58] When LGE of the pericardium occurs, the constrictive process is more likely to be inflammatory and modifiable with medical therapy.[59]

PERICARDIAL EFFUSION

A multitude of conditions may lead to accumulation of excess pericardial fluid; they may be broadly categorized into idiopathic,

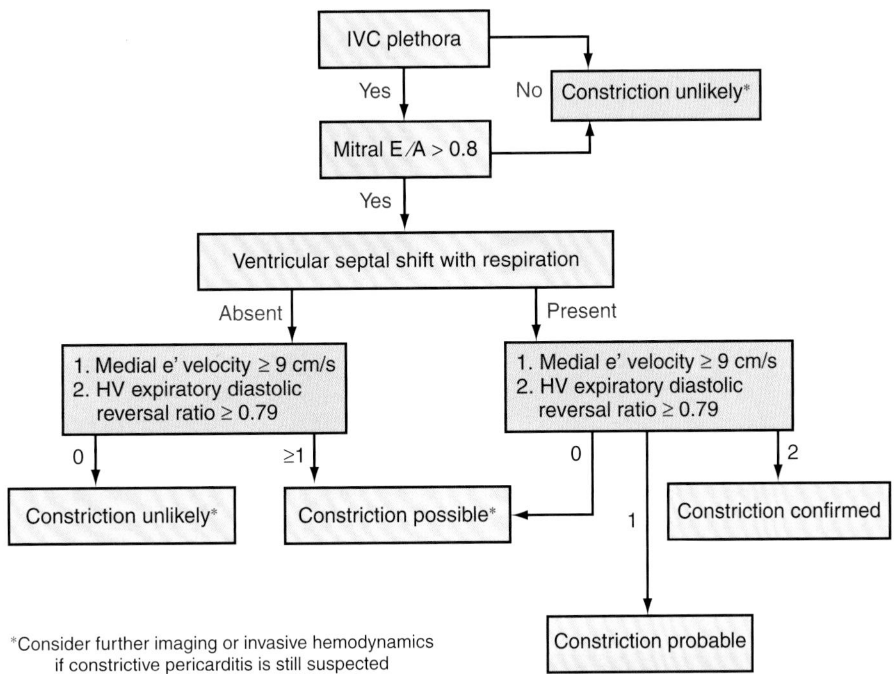

Fig. 17.10 Suggested diagnostic algorithm for the echocardiographic diagnosis of constrictive pericarditis, based on the Mayo Clinic criteria. The numbers indicate how many of the criteria in the green boxes are present. Note, however, an important caveat. Patients with obstructive lung disease or increased respiratory effort may have enhanced ventricular interaction, and the e′ may be normal, particularly in a young patient. This situation may be distinguished from constriction by the marked respiratory variation observed in superior vena cava velocities. The numbers indicate how many of the criteria in the *green boxes* are present. *A*, Late mitral inflow velocity; *E*, early mitral inflow velocity; *e′*, early diastolic mitral annular relaxation velocity. *HV*, Hepatic vein; *IVC*, inferior vena cava. (From Syed FF, Schaff HV, Oh JK. Constrictive pericarditis—a curable diastolic heart failure. *Nat Rev Cardiol.* 2014;11[9]:530–544.)

infectious, traumatic, cardiac, inflammatory, neoplastic, metabolic, and miscellaneous (including radiation) causes (see Table 17.1). Mechanisms underlying the development of a pericardial effusion include obstructed lymphatic flow, increased central venous pressure, and increased pericardial permeability.

Echocardiography should be the first-line imaging test used to identify a pericardial effusion, estimate the size or volume of the effusion, and determine the hemodynamic significance of the effusion.[4]

ECHOCARDIOGRAPHIC DIAGNOSIS

A pericardial effusion appears as an echo-lucent space between the epicardium and parietal pericardium. When evident only in systole, a physiologic or trivial amount of fluid is present. When evident throughout the cardiac cycle, a greater than physiologic (>50 mL) amount of fluid is present.[4] The fluid may be present in a circumferential space around the heart and easily visible or, less commonly, may be loculated and visible only from some imaging windows.

Pericardial effusions need to be distinguished from nonpericardial processes and normal anatomic variants. A left pleural effusion may mimic a posterior pericardial effusion. The key to differentiation is in observing the relationship of the fluid to the descending thoracic aorta from the parasternal imaging window; pericardial fluid tracks anterior to the aorta, whereas pleural fluid does not (Fig. 17.11).[60] An epicardial fat layer may mimic a pericardial effusion, but it may be distinguished from fluid based on its relatively echo-bright appearance and movement in concert with the myocardium (Fig. 17.12). A transudative pericardial effusion typically has an echo-lucent appearance and is motionless.[4]

Echocardiographic lucency may not characterize exudative pericardial effusions, which often contain strands or adhesions. Blood or tumor may also be found in the pericardial space. The presence of echo-bright coagulum (Fig. 17.13) in the pericardial space is an especially ominous sign that may occur with myocardial perforation or ascending aortic dissection. A clot or loculated effusion in the pericardial space can be a dangerously elusive cause of focal chamber compression and hemodynamic collapse, particularly after cardiac surgery (Fig. 17.14); TEE or cross-sectional imaging is frequently required.[4,61–63]

Semiquantitative sizing of pericardial effusions by 2D echocardiography is performed by measuring the rim of fluid between the epicardium and parietal pericardium at end-diastole. A small effusion has a rim less than 10 mm; a moderate effusion has a rim of 10 to 20 mm; and a large effusion has a rim greater than 20 mm.[4] Additional categories of trivial (rim < 5 mm) or very large (rim > 25 mm) are sometimes used. For a significant effusion, the spatial distribution of fluid should be reported to guide decision making about pericardiocentesis (i.e., feasibility and optimal site to access the pericardial space).

PERICARDIAL TAMPONADE

DEFINITION AND ETIOLOGY

Cardiac tamponade is a potentially life-threatening heart failure condition in which cardiac filling is impaired because of excess pericardial fluid under pressure. Tamponade may arise from any condition or event that leads to increased fluid contents within the pericardial space. The diagnosis requires a clinical assessment that is informed by echocardiographic findings. Tamponade is best considered a spectrum of hemodynamic abnormalities rather than an all-or-none phenomenon.

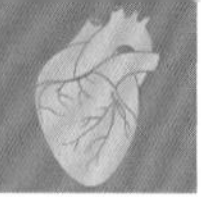

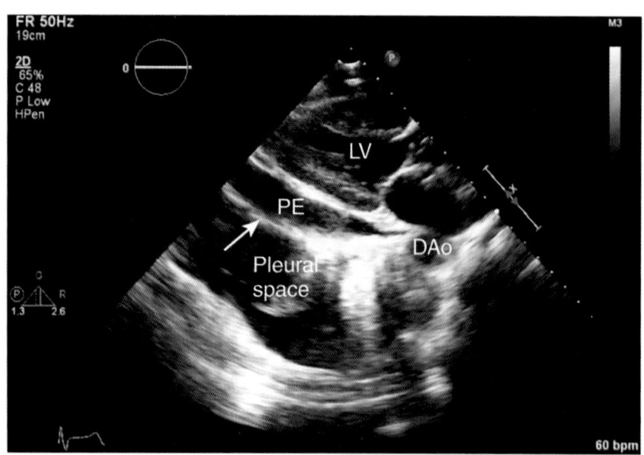

Fig. 17.11 **Pericardial effusion on 2D imaging.** Parasternal long-axis image in a patient with pericardial and pleural effusions. The pericardial effusion *(PE)* tracks anterior to the descending thoracic aorta *(DAo)*. The pleural space, which in this case contains an effusion and collapsed lung, is more posterior. The parietal pericardium *(arrow)* separates the two fluid layers.

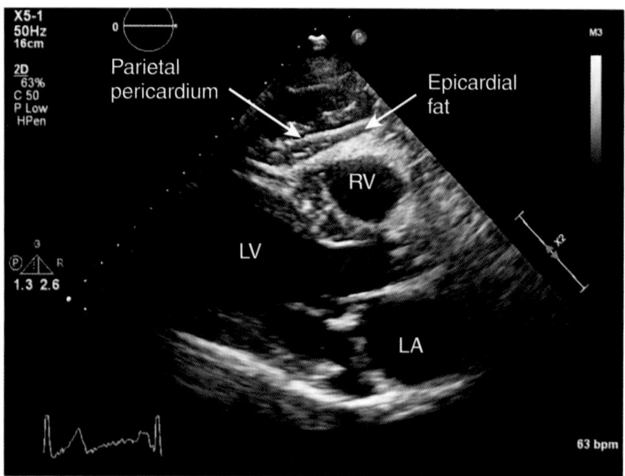

Fig. 17.12 **Pericardial adipose tissue.** Parasternal long-axis image shows a prominent anterior fat layer. There are two layers separated by the parietal pericardium.

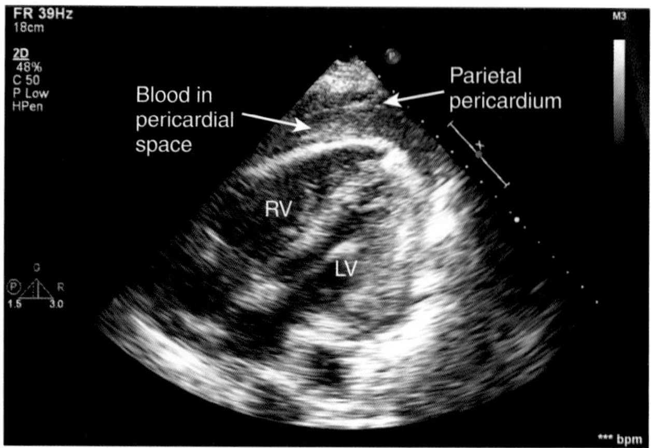

Fig. 17.13 **Pericardial thrombus.** Extensive echo-bright coagulum is seen in the pericardial space after procedure-related myocardial perforation (see Video 17.13).

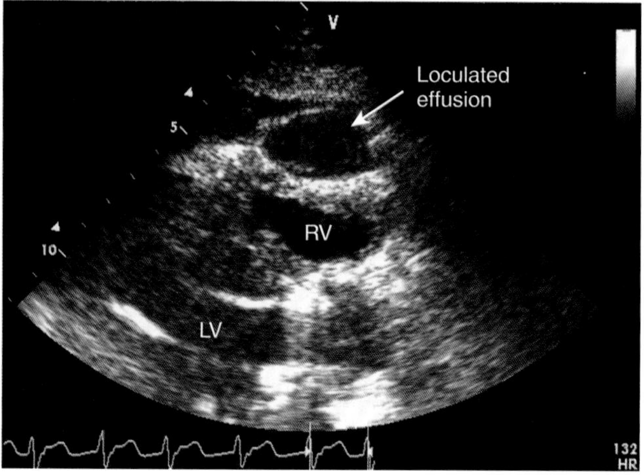

Fig. 17.14 **Loculated, anterior pericardial effusion.** Parasternal long-axis image shows a loculated, anterior fluid collection causing diastolic collapse of the RV (see Video 17.14). (Courtesy Sunil Mankad, MD.)

PATHOPHYSIOLOGY

Although the normal pericardium has some limited capacity to stretch, an acutely accumulating pericardial effusion can quickly fill the reserve volume and exhaust the pericardial stretch capacity such that pericardial pressure begins to rapidly rise (Fig. 17.15). When effusions collect more slowly, the pericardium is able to stretch to a greater degree and accommodate more fluid volume before the pericardial pressure begins to rapidly rise.[64] Rising pericardial pressure reduces the myocardial transmural distending pressure (i.e., pressure within the cardiac chamber minus pericardial pressure) and thereby reduces cardiac filling, first for the right heart but eventually for all the cardiac chambers, which must compete with the pericardial fluid for space within the fixed total pericardial volume. Decreased compliance of the stretched pericardium therefore dictates compliance for all cardiac chambers, which become smaller and have equalized diastolic pressures that are equivalent to pericardial pressure.[9,65]

Because of spatial constraints inside the fixed total pericardial volume in tamponade, the ventricles fill at the expense

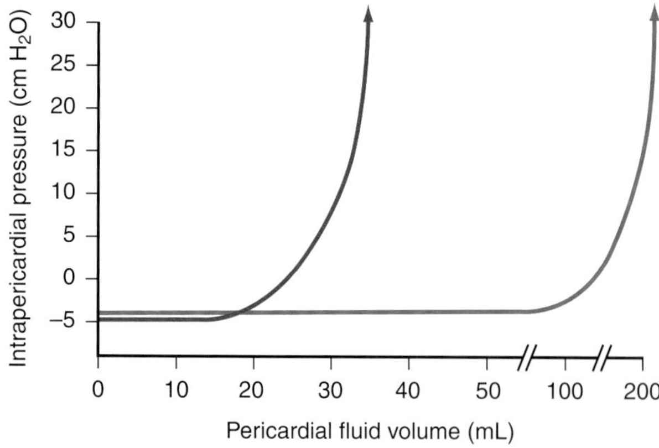

Fig. 17.15 **Normal pericardial pressure-volume relationships.** The relationship between pericardial volume and pressure is diagramed for a patient who has rapidly developed a pericardial effusion *(red line)* and for a patient who has gradually developed a pericardial effusion *(blue line)*. (Adapted from Edmunds HL Jr. *Cardiac Surgery in the Adult.* New York: McGraw-Hill; 1997:1305.)

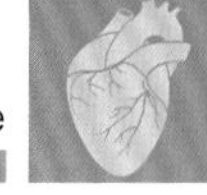

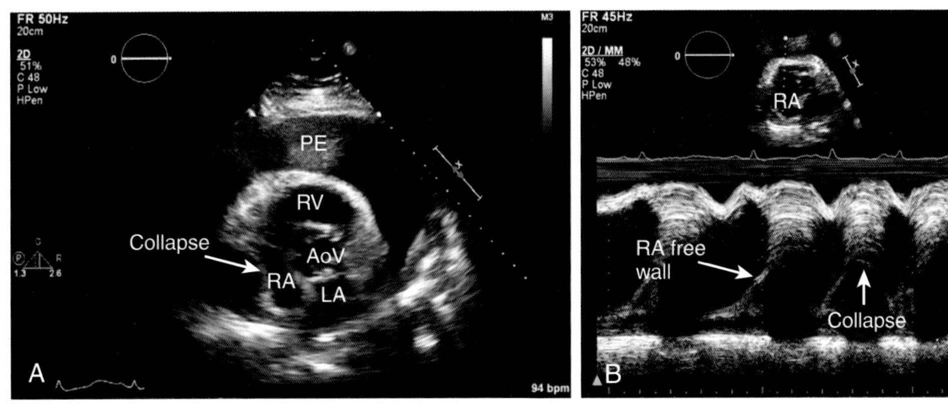

Fig. 17.16 2D and M-mode imaging in pericardial tamponade. Parasternal short-axis imaging in a patient with tamponade shows RA collapse persisting well into ventricular systole by 2D (A) and M-mode (B) assessment (see Video 17.16). *AV,* Aortic valve; *PE,* pericardial effusion.

of each other, which leads to characteristic clinical findings. Increased *ventricular interdependence* or *enhanced ventricular interaction* (Fig. 17.2 shows the analogous phenomenon in constriction) is one of the principle mechanisms for the *pulsus paradoxus* (i.e., decrease in systolic blood pressure by more than 10 mmHg with inspiration) found in most patients with tamponade.[10] There is normal slight respiratory variation in LV stroke volume and systolic blood pressure. In tamponade, this becomes exaggerated (rather than paradoxical, as the name implies). During inspiration, increased venous return to the right heart still occurs in tamponade, but this volume can be accommodated only through a shift in the ventricular septum toward the left because the RV is unable to expand outward. LV filling and output become compromised, leading to a decrease in stroke volume and systolic blood pressure during inspiration.[10,66] The opposite changes occur with expiration.

Although *dissociation of intrapleural and intracardiac pressures,* with an inspiratory decrease in pressure gradient between the pulmonary veins and LA (see Fig. 17.3), has been postulated[65] as an additional contributing mechanism, it has not been consistently shown in experimental studies and is likely to play a only a minor role.[10,66] In other words, the fluid-filled pericardium may have some insulating effect on intracardiac pressure changes, but not as much as the diseased, constrictive pericardium does.

As pericardial pressure continues to increase, systemic and pulmonary venous pressure must also increase to preserve filling. Atrial filling occurs more in systole than diastole because cardiac volume and pericardial pressure transiently decrease only in early systole.[4] Diastolic ventricular filling is progressively compromised, leading to a blunted *y* descent in the jugular venous waveform. In addition to increased venous pressure, other compensatory mechanisms may include tachycardia and arterial vasoconstriction. Ultimately, they are overwhelmed, and hemodynamic collapse will ensue if intervention does not occur.

ECHOCARDIOGRAPHIC DIAGNOSIS

Echocardiography is the pivotal imaging modality in cases of suspected tamponade.[4] A pericardial effusion may cause a spectrum of hemodynamic effects, and the echocardiogram helps define the patient's position in that spectrum. Despite different pathophysiologic mechanisms, the assessment for tamponade bears many similarities to the assessment for constriction.

A dedicated pericardial-protocol echocardiogram (see Summary table) allows characterization of the effusion and identification of chamber collapse, plethora of the IVC, and respiratory variation in right- and left-sided cardiac filling. This information should be considered in conjunction with bedside clinical assessment. Serial echocardiography or invasive hemodynamics may be necessary when the initial echocardiogram is not consistent with tamponade but clinical suspicion remains elevated.

Characterization of the Pericardial Effusion

Echocardiographic assessment begins with identification of the pericardial effusion, which is typically moderate to large. The heart may exhibit a characteristic swinging motion within the fluid, which is responsible for the electrocardiographic finding of *electrical alternans.* However, even a small or focal effusion may cause life-threatening tamponade in the acute setting after trauma, aortic dissection, infarction-association myocardial rupture, or procedure-related perforation.

Cardiac Chamber Collapse

When pericardial pressure exceeds the pressure within a given cardiac chamber, compression or collapse of that chamber will occur. This phenomenon typically is phasic during the cardiac cycle because of the dynamic changes in myocardial transmural pressure that occur. Because the right heart chambers have more compliant walls, they are most commonly affected. This may be clinically described as chamber compression, inversion, or collapse.

RA Compression, Inversion, or Collapse

Because RA pressures tend to be the lowest throughout the cardiac cycle, RA collapse occurs earliest and is considered to be a highly sensitive sign of increased pericardial pressure and tamponade.[67–69] RA collapse typically becomes evident at the end of ventricular diastole (Fig. 17.16) (i.e., near the QRS on the electrocardiogram) and may persist into ventricular systole until filling increases atrial pressure above pericardial pressure. Although brief collapse may occur in the absence of clinical tamponade and therefore lack specificity, collapse that persists for at least one third of the cardiac cycle is a highly sensitive (94%) and specific (100%) finding for tamponade.[69] RA hypertension and ventricular pacing may decrease the reliability of this sign.[69]

RV Compression, Inversion, or Collapse

The RV collapses at a higher pericardial pressure than the RA, making RV collapse a generally less sensitive but more specific

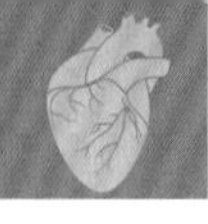

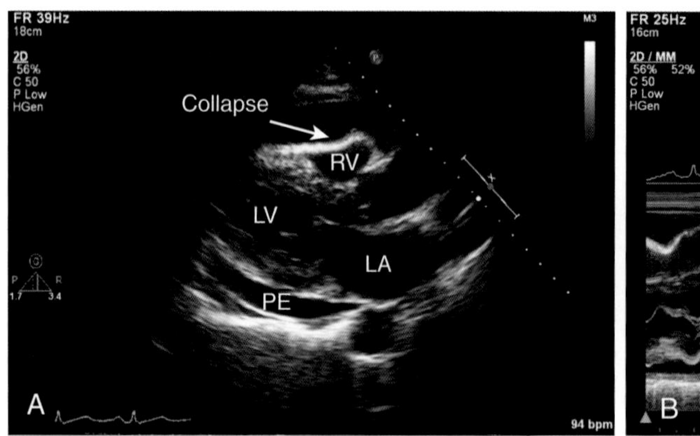

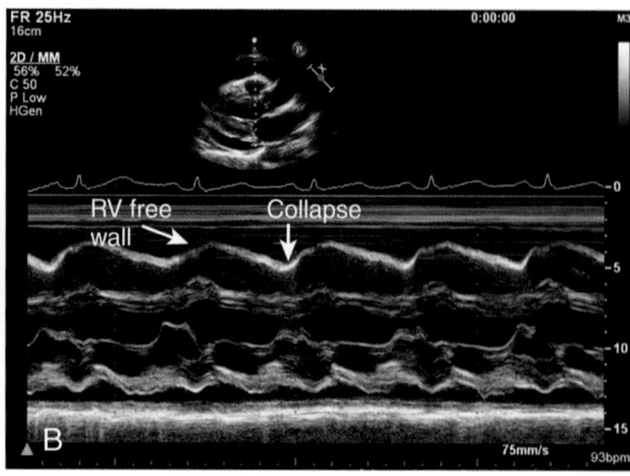

Fig. 17.17 **RV diastolic collapse.** Parasternal long-axis imaging in a patient with tamponade shows RV collapse extending into late diastole by 2D (A) and M-mode (B) assessment (see Video 17.17). *PE*, Pericardial effusion.

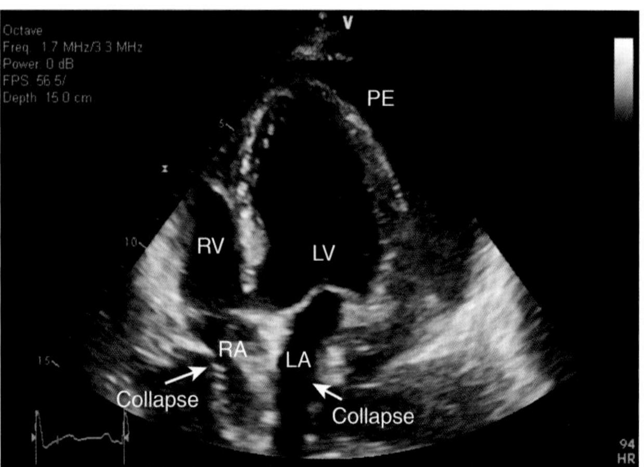

Fig. 17.18 **LA and RA diastolic collapse.** Apical 4-chamber imaging in a patient with tamponade shows LA and RA collapse extending well into ventricular systole (see Video 17.18). *PE*, Pericardial effusion.

finding for tamponade.[67,70–73] RV collapse occurs in early diastole (Fig. 17.17), when ventricular volume and pressure are lowest, and persists until filling increases ventricular pressure above pericardial pressure. Echocardiographic evaluation ideally consists of a combination of 2D and M-mode imaging. Collapse is initially most evident during expiration, but it can be observed throughout the respiratory cycle as tamponade becomes more severe. RV collapse is associated with a hemodynamically important reduction in cardiac output despite preserved systemic arterial pressure.[74] However, if the RV is hypertrophied or has significantly increased diastolic pressure, as may occur with pulmonary hypertension or hypervolemia, RV collapse may not be a reliable indicator of tamponade.[74,75]

Left Heart Chamber Collapse

Because LA pressure is normally higher than RA pressure, LA collapse (Fig. 17.18) is a less common finding in tamponade.[68] Nevertheless, LA collapse is a specific sign of tamponade and may be the only chamber collapse evident in cases of tamponade with pulmonary hypertension or regional tamponade after trauma or cardiac surgery.[76,77] LV chamber collapse is an even less common phenomenon, but it can occur with localized effusion, such as after trauma or surgery.[76,78]

Plethora of the Inferior Vena Cava

Impaired cardiac filling leads to increased venous pressure in most cases of tamponade. Plethora of the IVC (<50% decrease in diameter with deep inspiration or sniff) is one of the echocardiographic correlates for increased venous pressure, and it is highly sensitive (97%) for tamponade.[72] However, plethora of the IVC can occur with any cause of elevated venous pressure, and it is not specific for the diagnosis of tamponade.

Respiratory Variation in Right and Left Heart Filling

Because of enhanced ventricular interaction, the 2D examination typically reveals respiration-related variation in the position of the ventricular septum, with a shift toward the LV in inspiration and toward the RV in expiration (see Fig. 17.2 for analogous finding in constriction).

Cyclic variation in right and left heart filling may also be detected with the use of Doppler echocardiography.[13,79,80] Because of enhanced ventricular interaction, right- and left-sided Doppler velocities vary with respiration and are 180 degrees out of phase with each other. With inspiration, right heart filling increases at the expense of left heart filling, and then this reverses with expiration. Accordingly, the tricuspid inflow E velocity increases with inspiration and decreases with expiration, with a percent change of more than 60%. It is calculated as the (expiratory velocity − inspiratory velocity)/expiratory velocity × 100, using the first beats of expiration and inspiration (Fig. 17.19).[4,13] The pulmonary artery velocity is expected to change concordantly with the tricuspid inflow velocity. However, mitral inflow velocity increases with expiration and decreases with inspiration, with a typical percent change of more than 30% (see Fig. 17.19).[4,13,79] This variation in peak filling velocity should occur even when diastolic filling predominantly results from atrial contraction (recorded as the A wave in the mitral inflow profile), as sometimes occurs in tamponade.[4] The pulmonary vein and aortic velocities are expected to change concordantly with the mitral inflow velocity. Although less commonly used in clinical practice, respiratory changes in LV isovolumic relaxation time (which increases with inspiration) and ejection time (which increases with expiration) have also been reported.[13]

Respiratory variation in the hepatic vein Doppler profile may be clinically helpful in making the diagnosis of tamponade. Hepatic vein systolic forward flow predominates in tamponade, because intrapericardial pressure falls only during ventricular contraction (Fig. 17.20).[55] As tamponade

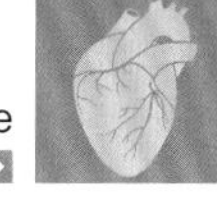

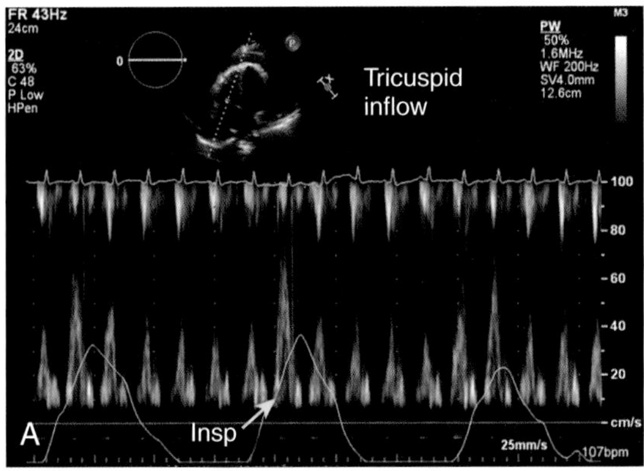

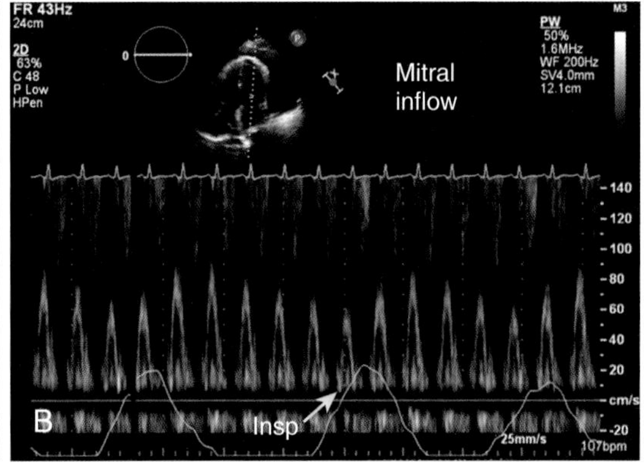

Fig. 17.19 Respiratory variation in ventricular inflow velocities. Tricuspid (A) and mitral (B) inflow Doppler profiles in cardiac tamponade. Inspiration leads to increased tricuspid and decreased mitral E-wave velocities (last beat of inspiration marked by *arrows*). Expiration leads to decreased tricuspid and increased mitral E-wave velocities. *Insp,* Inspiration.

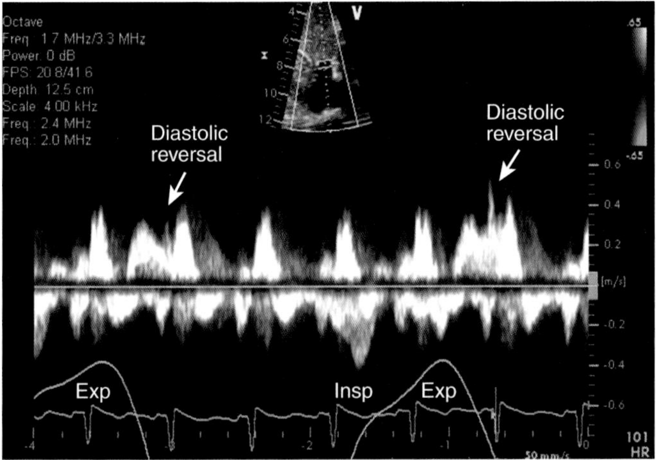

Fig. 17.20 Hepatic venous Doppler profile in tamponade. Inspiration *(Insp)* leads to augmentation of hepatic vein forward velocity. With the onset of expiration *(Exp)*, when left heart filling is favored at the expense of the right, hepatic vein diastolic forward flow reverses as indicated.

progresses, hepatic vein diastolic forward flow diminishes and ultimately becomes undetectable by Doppler. Inspiration leads to augmentation of hepatic vein forward velocities. With the onset of expiration, when left heart filling is favored at the expense of the right, hepatic vein diastolic forward flow markedly decreases or reverses.[13,55,79] Similar findings are seen in the superior vena cava.

Abnormal hepatic vein venous flow (i.e., systolic predominance and expiratory reduction or reversal of the diastolic flow) has high positive and negative predictive values for the diagnosis of tamponade.[70] However, hepatic vein interrogation in tamponade is technically challenging and may not be of diagnostic quality in many cases.

Combining Chamber Collapse With Abnormal Hepatic Venous Flow: Test Performance Characteristics

A prospective study of 110 patients with moderate to large pericardial effusions (38 patients had tamponade, 72 patients did not) assessed the test performance characteristics of chamber collapse, abnormal hepatic or superior vena caval flow, and combinations thereof (Table 17.4).[70] The absence of any chamber collapse correlated well with the absence of tamponade and accordingly had the highest sensitivity (90%). Abnormal venous flow in combination with RA and RV collapse correlated well with the presence of tamponade and had the highest specificity (98%).

TABLE 17.4 Test Performance Characteristics for Echocardiographic Findings in Tamponade.

Characteristic	*Sensitivity (%)*	*Specificity (%)*
Any collapse	90	65
RA collapse	68	66
RV collapse	60	90
RA + RV collapse	45	92
Abnormal venous flow[a]	75	91
Abnormal venous flow + 1 collapse	67	91
Abnormal venous flow + 2 collapses	37	98

[a]Abnormal venous (hepatic vein or superior vena cava) flow defined as marked systolic over diastolic component, expiratory accentuation of this difference, and expiratory reversal of diastolic flow.

From Merce J, Sagrista-Sauleda J, Permanyer-Miralda G, Evangelista A, Soler-Soler J. Correlation between clinical and Doppler echocardiographic findings in patients with moderate and large pericardial effusion: implications for the diagnosis of cardiac tamponade. *Am Heart J.* 1999;138(4 pt 1):759–764.

REGIONAL TAMPONADE

Localized cardiac chamber compression may occur because of a loculated effusion or hematoma (see Fig. 17.14). This may be most likely to occur after cardiac surgery.[77] Diagnosis may be challenging because typical clinical and echocardiographic findings may be absent. A high index of clinical suspicion is essential, and echocardiographic imaging should include a careful search for localized compression of any cardiac chamber, including the LA and LV.[76–78] This may require TEE, particularly when TTE quality is suboptimal.[4,61,62] If there is continued uncertainty about the presence of a loculated effusion or about the hemodynamic effect of an effusion, invasive hemodynamic assessment or surgical exploration may be required for diagnostic and therapeutic purposes.[77]

ECHOCARDIOGRAPHICALLY GUIDED PERICARDIOCENTESIS

After clinical tamponade is confirmed, expeditious removal of the pericardial fluid is the most effective and potentially life-saving treatment. This is most rapidly accomplished with percutaneous pericardiocentesis, which has become the procedure of choice for most cases.[2] When performed blindly, with the subxyphoid approach as the standard, percutaneous pericardiocentesis has been reported to be successful in 86% of cases and is associated with an approximately 4% rate of death and at least 11% risk of hemopericardium due to cardiac puncture.[81]

The use of 2D echocardiography to guide the procedure has improved the success rate and safety of the procedure considerably, and it is therefore recommended whenever possible.[82] Echocardiographic imaging allows identification of the optimal needle entry site and direct visualization of the needle as it enters the pericardial fluid. In the largest published series from the Mayo Clinic, 1127 pericardiocenteses were performed over 21 years with a procedural success rate of 97% and a major complication rate of 1.2%.[83] The reported major complications in this series were death (1 patient), cardiac laceration (5), vessel laceration (1), pneumothorax (5), infection (1), and sustained ventricular tachycardia (1).

Contraindications

Percutaneous pericardiocentesis is relatively contraindicated for tamponade due to aortic dissection, penetrating thoracic trauma, or myocardial rupture.[2,82,84] These cases should be managed with emergent surgery. Severe coagulopathy is also a relative contraindication.[2,82] Although any form of traumatic hemopericardium was traditionally considered an indication for surgery, tamponade due to cardiac perforation at the time of an invasive cardiac diagnostic or therapeutic procedure may in many cases be handled definitively with percutaneous pericardiocentesis alone.[85]

Procedural Steps

The procedural approach to echocardiographically guided percutaneous pericardiocentesis has been well described.[82,86,87] The online video from Fitch et al. is an especially helpful resource.[82] Although some institutional variation is expected, the following is a summary of the basic procedural principles, with an emphasis on the role of echocardiography.

1. Select and mark the optimal site for needle entry. Echocardiographic imaging allows identification of the most direct and safest route to the largest collection of fluid. Peri-xyphoid, parasternal, and apical approaches are possible. The parasternal approach was used most frequently in the largest published series.[83] When this approach is used, care must be taken to avoid the course of the internal mammary artery, which courses lateral to the sternal border, and the intercostal vessels, which course along the inferior borders of the ribs.
2. While imaging the effusion from the optimal access site, carefully note the angulation of the transducer and the distance between skin and fluid. The transducer angulation in three-dimensional (3D) space needs to be replicated with the pericardiocentesis needle.
3. Establish a sterile field, and administer local anesthesia along the anticipated tract of the needle.
4. Perform pericardiocentesis. Ideally, a second operator or sonographer images from a window remote from the puncture site for monitoring during the procedure. Correct needle position may be confirmed with administration of agitated saline, which should be visualized only in the pericardial space.
5. Place a pigtail catheter in the pericardial space. The pericardial fluid is drained as completely as possible. Echocardiographic imaging confirms this. The catheter is typically left in place for 1 to 3 days until intermittent suction yields less than approximately 50 mL of fluid in a 24-hour period. Limited echocardiographic assessment should be repeated to ensure that the effusion has resolved before removing the catheter.

ACUTE PERICARDITIS

Acute pericarditis is an inflammatory pericardial process that may be caused by numerous conditions, including those in Table 17.1. Most cases are idiopathic and presumed to be viral.[88,89] Diagnosis is established by finding two or more of the following: (1) chest pain consistent with pericarditis, (2) pericardial friction rub, (3) typical electrocardiographic changes, and (4) a new or worsening pericardial effusion.[89]

Echocardiography is recommended within 24 hours of presentation in all cases to evaluate for effusion and to exclude tamponade physiology if an effusion is present.[4] In many cases, there is no effusion, and the echocardiogram is essentially normal. Other possible findings on the echocardiogram that suggest a pericardial process include increased pericardial brightness or thickness or constrictive physiology. In some cases, LV regional wall motion abnormalities may occur due to associated myocarditis. The echocardiogram also allows evaluation for other causes of chest pain. For example, LV regional wall motion abnormalities occurring in a coronary artery-specific distribution may indicate that an acute coronary syndrome is more likely than pericarditis.

Cardiac CT and CMR offer incremental information about the pericardium and may be useful when the diagnosis remains uncertain, when antiinflammatory treatment fails, or when the case is otherwise complicated.[4] Key clinical-echocardiographic correlates for acute pericarditis, tamponade, and constriction are summarized in Table 17.5.

CONGENITAL ABSENCE OF THE PERICARDIUM

The pericardium rarely is absent from birth. The defect may be partial, most commonly involving the left side of the pericardium, or complete, in which case the entire pericardium is absent. Up to 30% of patients have associated congenital cardiac defects, including atrial septal defect, bicuspid aortic valve, patent ductus arteriosus, and tetralogy of Fallot.[90] Patients with a congenitally absent pericardium may be asymptomatic or have paroxysmal stabbing chest discomfort or dyspnea. Rarely, a portion of the heart may herniate through a partial pericardial defect, leading to acute complications such as ST-elevation myocardial infarction or sudden death due to cardiac strangulation.[91,92] Surgical treatment may be necessary for those with severe symptoms or for cases of cardiac herniation through a partial defect.

The absent pericardium causes the echocardiographic evaluation to be abnormal in multiple respects (Fig. 17.21). The position of the heart is typically shifted to the left, and the heart acquires a teardrop configuration, characterized by elongation

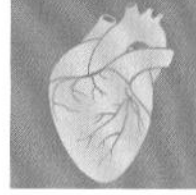

TABLE 17.5 Pericardial Disease: Clinical-Echocardiographic Correlates.

Disease	*Clinical Presentation*	*Echocardiographic Findings*
Constrictive pericarditis	May include dyspnea on exertion and signs of venous congestion (elevated venous pressure, ascites, and edema)	• Ventricular septal shift • Hepatic vein diastolic flow reversals in expiration • Preserved or increased medial e′ velocity, often with medial e′ > lateral e′ velocities • Respiratory variation in mitral E velocities • Plethora of the inferior vena cava • Decreased lateral longitudinal strain compared with medial value
Pericardial effusion	Varies, depends on cause; may be asymptomatic and incidentally discovered	• Pericardial effusion may range from trivial to very large and be circumferential or loculated • Fluid echocardiographic brightness varies with characteristics (transudative, exudative, or frankly bloody)
Tamponade	Varies, often nonspecific; may include hypotension, tachycardia, elevated venous pressure, and pulsus paradoxus	• Chamber collapse • Plethora of the inferior vena cava • Respiratory variation in right- and left-heart filling and venous flow patterns
Acute pericarditis	Characteristic chest pain and electrocardiographic changes; pericardial friction rub may be present	• Effusion may be present and helps secure the diagnosis • Ventricular regional wall motion abnormalities suggest associated myocarditis or an alternative diagnosis • Tamponade or constrictive physiology may be observed

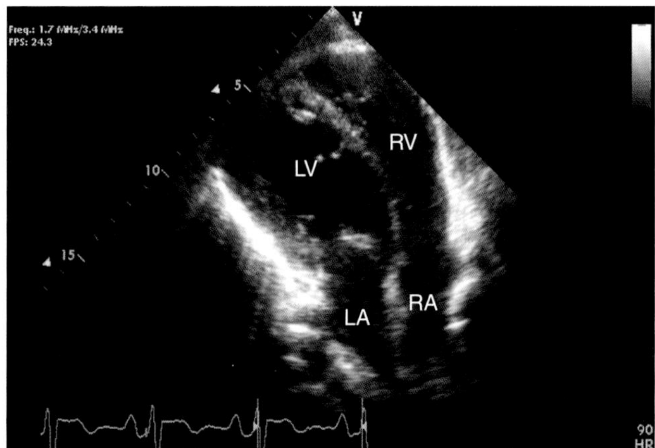

Fig. 17.21 Congenital absence of the pericardium. Apical 4-chamber image (reversed orientation) shows the characteristic echocardiographic appearance of a congenitally absent pericardium. The heart is shifted toward the left and acquires a teardrop configuration (see Video 17.21). (Courtesy Sunil Mankad, MD.)

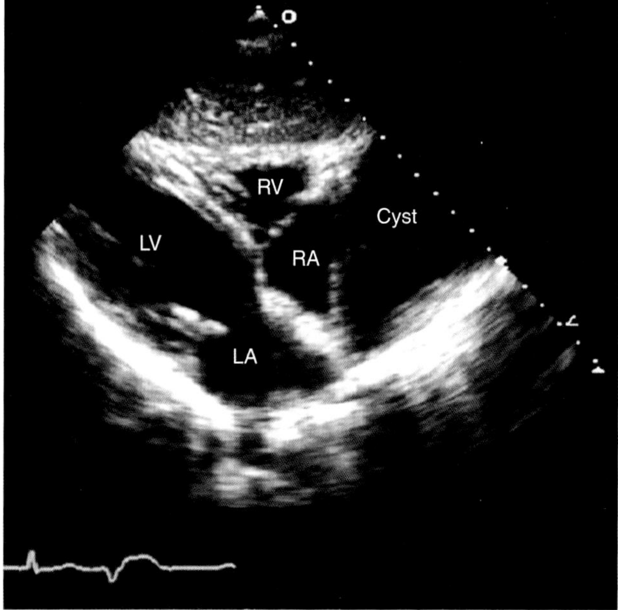

Fig. 17.22 Pericardial cyst. Subcostal 4-chamber image shows a pericardial cyst adjacent to the right heart border (see Video 17.22). (Courtesy Sunil Mankad, MD.)

of the atria and bulbous-appearing ventricles.[90] Other findings include higher and more lateral imaging windows, cardiac hypermobility, paradoxical or flat ventricular septal systolic motion, and abnormal swinging of the heart.[93]

PERICARDIAL CYSTS

Pericardial cysts are rare, benign, and usually incidentally discovered on a chest radiograph or echocardiogram. They are typically located at the right cardiophrenic angle but may also be found at the left cardiophrenic angle or other locations.[94] On echocardiographic evaluation, a pericardial cyst appears as a round or oval, echo-lucent space surrounded by a wall and adjacent to the cardiac border (Fig. 17.22).[95]

Pericardial cysts appear to follow a benign course, and therapy is not required for asymptomatic patients. However, there are isolated reports of complications from cysts, including tamponade and erosion into adjacent structures.[94]

SUMMARY Pericardial Protocol Echocardiogram: Full 2D and Doppler Examination With Simultaneous Recording of Respiration With Emphasis on Certain Parameters.

Parameter	Modality	View	Recording	Assessment	Comment
Ventricular septal motion	2D and M-mode	Parasternal (long- and short-axis) and apical	Extended loops (e.g., 10 cardiac cycles)	Evaluate for shift in septal position during respiration (toward the LV in inspiration, toward the RV in expiration)	Respiratory ventricular septal shift signifies enhanced ventricular interaction, as seen in constriction and tamponade
Mitral inflow	Pulsed-wave Doppler	Apical	Include slow sweep speed with extended recording	Evaluate for respiratory variation in peak E velocity (lower with inspiration, higher with expiration)	Typical change of 15%–35% in constriction and >30% in tamponade; consider also assessing tricuspid inflow, LV outflow, and pulmonary outflow velocities
Mitral annular tissue Doppler	Pulsed-wave Doppler	Apical	Medial and lateral mitral annulus	Assess medial e′ velocity and compare with lateral e′ velocity	Expect preserved (≥9 cm/s) or increased medial e′ in constriction (without concomitant myocardial disease); medial e′ velocity is often higher than lateral e′ velocity
Hepatic vein flow	Pulsed-wave Doppler, possibly color M-mode	Subcostal	Zoom, set sample volume to 3–4 mm, include slow sweep speed with extended recording	Evaluate for prominent diastolic flow reversals in expiration; consider calculating hepatic vein expiratory diastolic reversal ratio	Expect prominent reversals in expiration in constriction (reversal ratio > 0.79) and tamponade
Inferior vena cava	2D, possibly M-mode	Subcostal	Standard	Measure diameter and % collapse with sniff	Expect plethora (diameter > 2.1 cm and/or < 50% collapse with sniff) in constriction and tamponade; not a specific finding

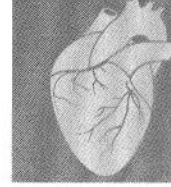

SUMMARY Pericardial Protocol Echocardiogram: Full 2D and Doppler Examination With Simultaneous Recording of Respiration With Emphasis on Certain Parameters.—cont'd

Parameter	Modality	View	Recording	Assessment	Comment
Superior vena cava	Pulsed-wave Doppler	Right supraclavicular	Slow sweep speed	Examine change in forward systolic velocity during respiratory cycle	Expect little change in forward systolic velocity in constriction (compared with COPD); expect expiratory reduction in diastolic forward flow (or even reversal) in tamponade
Chamber collapse (if pericardial effusion is present)	2D, M-mode	All imaging windows	Include extended loops (e.g., 10 cardiac cycles)	Evaluate for inversion or collapse of any cardiac chamber; RA collapses in late diastole (assess duration compared with cardiac cycle); RV collapses in early diastole	Chamber collapse signifies elevated pericardial pressure and possibly tamponade
Strain imaging	Speckle-tracking (systolic, longitudinal)	Apical	Standard	Evaluate global and regional strain pattern; compare lateral wall with septal wall	GLS typically preserved in constriction; lateral wall often reduced compared with septal wall; circumferential strain is typically reduced in constriction

COPD, Chronic obstructive pulmonary disease; *GLS*, global longitudinal strain.

REFERENCES

1. Spodick DH. Medical history of the pericardium. The hairy hearts of hoary heroes. *Am J Cardiol.* 1970;26(5):447–454.
2. Maisch B, Seferovic PM, Ristic AD, et al. Guidelines on the diagnosis and management of pericardial diseases executive summary; the task force on the diagnosis and management of pericardial diseases of the European Society of Cardiology. *Eur Heart J.* 2004;25(7):587–610.
3. Douglas PS, Garcia MJ, Haines DE, et al. ACCF/ASE/AHA/ASNC/HFSA/HRS/SCAI/SCCM/SCCT/SCMR 2011 appropriate use criteria for echocardiography. A report of the American College of Cardiology Foundation Appropriate Use Criteria Task Force, American Society of Echocardiography, American Heart Association, American Society of Nuclear Cardiology, Heart Failure Society of America, Heart Rhythm Society, Society for Cardiovascular Angiography and Interventions, Society of Critical Care Medicine, Society of Cardiovascular Computed Tomography, and Society for Cardiovascular Magnetic Resonance endorsed by the American College of Chest Physicians. *J Am Coll Cardiol.* 2011;57(9):1126–1166.
4. Klein AL, Abbara S, Agler DA, et al. American Society of Echocardiography clinical recommendations for multimodality cardiovascular imaging of patients with pericardial disease: endorsed by the Society for Cardiovascular Magnetic Resonance and Society of Cardiovascular Computed Tomography. *J Am Soc Echocardiogr.* 2013;26(9):965–1012 e1015.
5. Holt JP. The normal pericardium. *Am J Cardiol.* 1970;26(5):455–465.
6. Ishihara T, Ferrans VJ, Jones M, Boyce SW, Kawanami O, Roberts WC. Histologic and ultrastructural features of normal human parietal pericardium. *Am J Cardiol.* 1980;46(5):744–753.
7. Spodick DH. The normal and diseased pericardium: current concepts of pericardial physiology, diagnosis and treatment. *J Am Coll Cardiol.* 1983;1(1):240–251.
8. Boltwood CM Jr. Ventricular performance related to transmural filling pressure in clinical cardiac tamponade. *Circulation.* May 1987;75(5):941–955.
9. Spodick DH. Acute cardiac tamponade. *N Engl J Med.* 2003;349(7):684–690.
10. McGregor M. Current concepts: pulsus paradoxus. *N Engl J Med.* 1979;301(9):480–482.
11. Anavekar NS, Wong BF, Foley TA, et al. Index of biventricular interdependence calculated using cardiac MRI: a proof of concept study in patients with and without constrictive pericarditis. *Int J Cardiovasc Imaging.* 2013;29(2):363–369.
12. Hatle LK, Appleton CP, Popp RL. Differentiation of constrictive pericarditis and restrictive cardiomyopathy by Doppler echocardiography. *Circulation.* 1989;79(2):357–370.
13. Appleton CP, Hatle LK, Popp RL. Cardiac tamponade and pericardial effusion: respiratory variation in transvalvular flow velocities studied by Doppler echocardiography. *J Am Coll Cardiol.* 1988;11(5):1020–1030.
14. Ling LH, Oh JK, Schaff HV, et al. Constrictive pericarditis in the modern era: evolving clinical

spectrum and impact on outcome after pericardiectomy. *Circulation*. 1999;100(13):1380–1386.

15. Bertog SC, Thambidorai SK, Parakh K, et al. Constrictive pericarditis: etiology and cause-specific survival after pericardiectomy. *J Am Coll Cardiol*. 2004;43(8):1445–1452.
16. Szabo G, Schmack B, Bulut C, et al. Constrictive pericarditis: risks, aetiologies and outcomes after total pericardiectomy: 24 years of experience. *Eur J Cardio Thorac Surg* 2013;44(6):1023–1028: discussion 1028.
17. George TJ, Arnaoutakis GJ, Beaty CA, Kilic A, Baumgartner WA, Conte JV. Contemporary etiologies, risk factors, and outcomes after pericardiectomy. *Ann Thorac Surg*. 2012;94(2): 445–451.
18. Avgerinos D, Rabitnokov Y, Worku B, Neragi-Miandoab S, Girardi LN. Fifteen-year experience and outcomes of pericardiectomy for constrictive pericarditis. *J Card Surg*. 2014;29(4): 434–438.
19. Mutyaba AK, Balkaran S, Cloete R, et al. Constrictive pericarditis requiring pericardiectomy at Groote Schuur Hospital, Cape Town, South Africa: causes and perioperative outcomes in the HIV era (1990–2012). *J Thorac Cardiovasc Surg*. 2014;148(6):3058–3065.
20. Lin Y, Zhou M, Xiao J, Wang B, Wang Z. Treating constrictive pericarditis in a Chinese single-center study: a five-year experience. *Ann Thorac Surg*. 2012;94(4):1235–1240.
21. Ghavidel AA, Gholampour M, Kyavar M, Mirmesdagh Y, Tabatabaie MB. Constrictive pericarditis treated by surgery. *Tex Heart Inst J*. 2012;39(2):199–205.
22. Talreja DR, Edwards WD, Danielson GK, et al. Constrictive pericarditis in 26 patients with histologically normal pericardial thickness. *Circulation*. 2003;108(15):1852–1857.
23. Talreja DR, Nishimura RA, Oh JK, Holmes DR. Constrictive pericarditis in the modern era: novel criteria for diagnosis in the cardiac catheterization laboratory. *J Am Coll Cardiol*. 2008;51(3):315–319.
24. Nishimura RA. Constrictive pericarditis in the modern era: a diagnostic dilemma. *Heart. Dec*. 2001;86(6):619–623.
25. Haley JH, Tajik AJ, Danielson GK, Schaff HV, Mulvagh SL, Oh JK. Transient constrictive pericarditis: causes and natural history. *J Am Coll Cardiol*. 2004;43(2):271–275.
26. Oh JK, Hatle LK, Seward JB, et al. Diagnostic role of Doppler echocardiography in constrictive pericarditis. *J Am Coll Cardiol*. 1994;23(1):154–162.
27. Garcia MJ, Rodriguez L, Ares M, Griffin BP, Thomas JD, Klein AL. Differentiation of constrictive pericarditis from restrictive cardiomyopathy: assessment of left ventricular diastolic velocities in longitudinal axis by Doppler tissue imaging. *J Am Coll Cardiol*. 1996;27(1):108–114.
28. Ha JW, Ommen SR, Tajik AJ, et al. Differentiation of constrictive pericarditis from restrictive cardiomyopathy using mitral annular velocity by tissue Doppler echocardiography. *Am J Cardiol*. 2004;94(3):316–319.
29. Welch TD, Ling LH, Espinosa RE, et al. Echocardiographic diagnosis of constrictive pericarditis: Mayo Clinic criteria. *Circ Cardiovasc Imaging*. 2014;7(3):526–534.
30. Qamruddin S, Alkharabsheh SK, Sato K, et al. Differentiating constriction from restriction (from the Mayo Clinic echocardiographic criteria). *Am J Cardiol*. 2019;124(6):932–938.
31. Sengupta PP, Mohan JC, Mehta V, Arora R, Khandheria BK, Pandian NG. Doppler tissue imaging improves assessment of abnormal interventricular septal and posterior wall motion in constrictive pericarditis. *J Am Soc Echocardiog*. 2005;18(3):226–230.
32. Himelman RB, Lee E, Schiller NB. Septal bounce, vena cava plethora, and pericardial adhesion: informative two-dimensional echocardiographic signs in the diagnosis of pericardial constriction. *J Am Soc Echocardiogr*. 1988;1(5):333–340.
33. Coylewright M, Welch TD, Nishimura RA. Mechanism of septal bounce in constrictive pericarditis: A simultaneous cardiac catheterisation and echocardiographic sudy. *Heart*. 2013 http://dx.doi.org/10.1136/heartjnl-2013-304070.
34. Tei C, Child JS, Tanaka H, Shah PM. Atrial systolic notch on the interventricular septal echogram: an echocardiographic sign of constrictive pericarditis. *J Am Coll Cardiol*. 1983;1(3):907–912.
35. Sengupta PP, Mohan JC, Mehta V, Arora R, Pandian NG, Khandheria BK. Accuracy and pitfalls of early diastolic motion of the mitral annulus for diagnosing constrictive pericarditis by tissue Doppler imaging. *Am J Cardiol*. 2004;93(7):886–890.
36. Reuss CS, Wilansky SM, Lester SJ, et al. Using mitral 'annulus reversus' to diagnose constrictive pericarditis. *Eur J Echocardiogr* 2009;10(3):372–375.
37. Ha JW, Oh JK, Ling LH, Nishimura RA, Seward JB, Tajik AJ. Annulus paradoxus: transmitral flow velocity to mitral annular velocity ratio is inversely proportional to pulmonary capillary wedge pressure in patients with constrictive pericarditis. *Circulation*. 2001;104(9):976–978.
38. Alraies MC, Kusunose K, Negishi K, et al. Relation between echocardiographically estimated and invasively measured filling pressures in constrictive pericarditis. *Am J Cardiol*. 2014;113(11):1911–1916.
39. Welch TD, Oh JK. Constrictive pericarditis: the mitral annulus remains paradoxical. *Am J Cardiol*. 2015;115(5). 704–704.
40. Syed FF, Schaff HV, Oh JK. Constrictive pericarditis—a curable diastolic heart failure. *Nature reviews. Cardiology. Sep*. 2014;11(9):530–544.
41. Welch TD, Oh JK. Constrictive pericarditis: old disease, new approaches. *Current Cardiology Reports*. 2015;17(4):20 https://doi.org/10.1007/s11886-015-0576-x.
42. Rajagopalan N, Garcia MJ, Rodriguez L, et al. Comparison of new Doppler echocardiographic methods to differentiate constrictive pericardial heart disease and restrictive cardiomyopathy. *Am J Cardiol*. 2001;87(1):86–94.
43. Oh JK, Tajik AJ, Appleton CP, Hatle LK, Nishimura RA, Seward JB. Preload reduction to unmask the characteristic Doppler features of constrictive pericarditis—a new observation. *Circulation*. 1997;95(4):796–799.
44. Cameron J, Oesterle SN, Baldwin JC, Hancock EW. The etiologic spectrum of constrictive pericarditis. *Am Heart J*. 1987;113(2):354–360.
45. Voelkel AG, Pietro DA, Folland ED, Fisher ML, Parisi AF. Echocardiographic features of constrictive pericarditis. *Circulation*. 1978;58(5):871–875.
46. Klein AL, Cohen GI, Pietrolungo JF, et al. Differentiation of constrictive pericarditis from restrictive cardiomyopathy by Doppler transesophageal echocardiographic measurements of respiratory variations in pulmonary venous flow. *J Am Coll Cardiol*. 1993;22(7): 1935–1943.
47. Klodas E, Nishimura RA, Appleton CP, Redfield MM, Oh JK. Doppler evaluation of patients with constrictive pericarditis: use of tricuspid regurgitation velocity curves to determine enhanced ventricular interaction. *J Am Coll Cardiol*. 1996;28(3):652–657.
48. Gilman G, Ommen SR, Hansen WH, Higano ST. Doppler echocardiographic evaluation of pulmonary regurgitation facilitates the diagnosis of constrictive pericarditis. *J Am Soc Echocardiog*. 2005;18(9):892–895.
49. Boonyaratavej S, Oh JK, Tajik AJ, Appleton CP, Seward JB. Comparison of mitral inflow and superior vena cava Doppler velocities in chronic obstructive pulmonary disease and constrictive pericarditis. *J Am Coll Cardiol*. 1998;32(7):2043–2048.
50. Takata M, Beloucif S, Shimada M, Robotham JL. Superior and inferior vena caval flows during respiration: pathogenesis of Kussmaul's sign. *Am J Physiol*. 1992;262(3 Pt 2):H763–H770.
51. Sengupta PP, Krishnamoorthy VK, Abhayaratna WP, et al. Disparate patterns of left ventricular mechanics differentiate constrictive pericarditis from restrictive cardiomyopathy. *JACC. Cardiovasc Imaging*. 2008;1(1):29–38.
52. Kusunose K, Dahiya A, Popovic ZB, et al. Biventricular mechanics in constrictive pericarditis comparison with restrictive cardiomyopathy and impact of pericardiectomy. *Circ Cardiovasc Imaging*. 2013;6(3):399–406.
53. Hancock EW. Subacute effusive-constrictive pericarditis. *Circulation*. 1971;43(2):183–187.
54. Sagrista-Sauleda J, Angel J, Sanchez A, Permanyer-Miralda G, Soler-Soler J. Effusive-constrictive pericarditis. *New Engl J Med*. 2004;350(5):469–475.
55. Miranda WR, Newman DB, Sinak LJ, et al. Pre- and post-pericardiocentesis echo-Doppler features of effusive-constrictive pericarditis compared with cardiac tamponade and constrictive pericarditis. *Eur Heart J Cardiovasc Imaging*. 2019;20(3):298–306.
56. Sagristasauleda J, Permanyermiralda G, Candellriera J, Angel J, Solersoler J. Transient cardiac constriction—an unrecognized pattern of evolution in effusive acute idiopathic pericarditis. *Am J Cardiol*. 1987;59(9):961–966.
57. Thavendiranathan P, Verhaert D, Walls MC, et al. Simultaneous right and left heart real-time, free-breathing CMR flow quantification identifies constrictive physiology. *JACC. Cardiovasc Imaging*. 2012;5(1):15–24.
58. Zurick AO, Bolen MA, Kwon DH, et al. Pericardial delayed hyperenhancement with CMR imaging in patients with constrictive pericarditis undergoing surgical pericardiectomy: a case series with histopathological correlation. *JACC. Cardiovasc Imaging*. 2011;4(11):1180–1191.
59. Feng D, Glockner J, Kim K, et al. Cardiac magnetic resonance imaging pericardial late gadolinium enhancement and elevated inflammatory markers can predict the reversibility of constrictive pericarditis after antiinflammatory medical therapy: a pilot study. *Circulation*. 2011;124(17):1830–1837.
60. Haaz WS, Mintz GS, Kotler MN, Parry W, Segal BL. 2 dimensional echocardiographic recognition of the descending thoracic aorta—value in differentiating pericardial from pleural effusions. *Am J Cardiol*. 1980;46(5):739–743.
61. Kochar GS, Jacobs LE, Kotler MN. Right atrial compression in postoperative cardiac patients—detection by transesophageal echocardiography. *J Am Coll Cardiol*. 1990;16(2):511–516.
62. Brooker RF, Farah MG. Postoperative left atrial compression diagnosed by transesophageal echocardiography. *J Cardiothor Vasc An*. 1995;9(3):304–307.

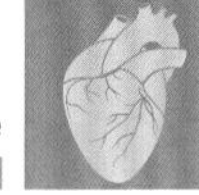

63. Duvernoy O, Larsson SG, Persson K, Thuren J, Wikstrom G. Pericardial-effusion and pericardial compartments after open-heart-surgery—an analysis by computed-tomography and echocardiography. *Acta Radiol.* 1990;31(1):41–46.
64. Spodick DH. Acute cardiac tamponade. *N Engl J Med.* 2003;349(7):684–690.
65. Reddy PS, Curtiss EI, Otoole JD, Shaver JA. Cardiac-tamponade—hemodynamic observations in man. *Circulation.* 1978;58(2):265–272.
66. Shabetai R, Fowler NO, Fenton JC, Masangka M. Pulses paradoxus. *J Clin Invest.* 1965;44(11). 1882-1898.
67. Singh S, Wann LS, Schuchard GH, et al. Right ventricular and right atrial collapse in patients with cardiac-tamponade—a combined echocardiographic and hemodynamic-study. *Circulation.* 1984;70(6):966–971.
68. Kronzon I, Cohen ML, Winer HE. Diastolic atrial compression—a sensitive echocardiographic sign of cardiac-tamponade. *J Am Coll Cardiol.* 1983;2(4):770–775.
69. Gillam LD, Guyer DE, Gibson TC, King ME, Marshall JE, Weyman AE. Hydrodynamic compression of the right atrium: a new echocardiographic sign of cardiac tamponade. *Circulation.* 1983;68(2):294–301.
70. Merce J, Sagrista-Sauleda J, Permanyer-Miralda G, Evangelista A, Soler-Soler J. Correlation between clinical and Doppler echocardiographic findings in patients with moderate and large pericardial effusion: implications for the diagnosis of cardiac tamponade. *Am Heart J.* 1999;138(4 Pt 1):759–764.
71. Armstrong WF, Schilt BF, Helper DJ, Dillon JC, Feigenbaum H. Diastolic collapse of the right ventricle with cardiac-tamponade—an echocardiographic study. *Circulation.* 1982;65(7):1491–1496.
72. Himelman RB, Kircher B, Rockey DC, Schiller NB. Inferior vena cava plethora with blunted respiratory response: a sensitive echocardiographic sign of cardiac tamponade. *J Am Coll Cardiol.* 1988;12(6):1470–1477.
73. Engel PJ, Hon H, Fowler NO, Plummer S. Echocardiographic study of right ventricular wall motion in cardiac-tamponade. *Am J Cardiol.* 1982;50(5):1018–1021.
74. Leimgruber PP, Klopfenstein HS, Wann LS, Brooks HL. The hemodynamic derangement associated with right ventricular diastolic collapse in cardiac-tamponade—an experimental echocardiographic study. *Circulation.* 1983;68(3):612–620.
75. Klopfenstein HS, Cogswell TL, Bernath GA, et al. Alterations in intravascular volume affect the relation between right ventricular diastolic collapse and the hemodynamic severity of cardiac-tamponade. *J Am Coll Cardiol.* 1985;6(5):1057–1063.
76. Fusman B, Schwinger ME, Charney R, Ausubel K, Cohen MV. Isolated collapse of left-sided heart chambers in cardiac tamponade: demonstration by two-dimensional echocardiography. *Am Heart J.* 1991;121(2 Pt 1):613–616.
77. Chuttani K, Tischler MD, Pandian NG, Lee RT, Mohanty PK. Diagnosis of cardiac-tamponade after cardiac-surgery—relative value of clinical, echocardiographic, and hemodynamic signs. *Am Heart J.* 1994;127(4):913–918.
78. Chuttani K, Pandian NG, Mohanty PK, et al. Left-ventricular diastolic collapse—an echocardiographic sign of regional cardiac tamponade. *Circulation. Jun.* 1991;83(6):1999–2006.
79. Burstow DJ, Oh JK, Bailey KR, Seward JB, Tajik AJ. Cardiac tamponade: characteristic Doppler observations. *Mayo Clin Proc.* 1989;64(3):312–324.
80. Leeman DE, Levine MJ, Come PC. Doppler echocardiography in cardiac-tamponade - exaggerated respiratory variation in transvalvular blood-flow velocity integrals. *J Am Coll Cardiol.* 1988;11(3):572–578.
81. Krikorian JG, Hancock EW. Pericardiocentesis. *Am J Med.* 1978;65(5):808–814.
82. Fitch MT, Nicks BA, Pariyadath M, McGinnis HD, Manthey DE. Emergency pericardiocentesis. *New Engl J Med.* 2012;366(12):E17–U19.
83. Tsang TS, Enriquez-Sarano M, Freeman WK, et al. Consecutive 1127 therapeutic echocardiographically guided pericardiocenteses: clinical profile, practice patterns, and outcomes spanning 21 years. *Mayo Clin Proc.* 2002;77(5):429–436.
84. Isselbacher EM, Cigarroa JE, Eagle KA. Cardiac-tamponade complicating proximal aortic dissection—is pericardiocentesis harmful. *Circulation.* 1994;90(5):2375–2378.
85. Tsang TSM, Freeman WK, Barnes ME, Reeder GS, Packer DL, Seward JB. Rescue echocardiographically guided pericardiocentesis for cardiac perforation complicating catheter-based procedures—the Mayo Clinic experience. *J Am Coll Cardiol.* 1998;32(5):1345–1350.
86. Salem K, Mulji A, Lonn E. Echocardiographically guided pericardiocentesis - the gold standard for the management of pericardial effusion and cardiac tamponade. *Can J Cardiol.* 1999;15(11):1251–1255.
87. Tsang TSM, Freeman WK, Sinak LJ, Seward JB. Echocardiographically guided pericardiocentesis: evolution and state-of-the-art technique. *Mayo Clin Proc.* Jul 1998;73(7):647–652.
88. Troughton RW, Asher CR, Klein AL. Pericarditis. *Lancet.* 2004;363(9410):717–727.
89. LeWinter MM. Acute pericarditis. *New Engl J Med.* 2014;371(25):2410–2416.
90. Abbas AE, Appleton CP, Liu PT, Sweeney JP. Congenital absence of the pericardium: case presentation and review of literature. *Int J Cardiol.* 2005;98(1):21–25.
91. Wilson SR, Kronzon I, Machnicki SC, Ruiz CE. A constrained heart: a case of sudden onset unrelenting chest pain. *Circulation.* 2014;130(18):1625–1631.
92. Shah AB, Kronzon I. Congenital defects of the pericardium: a review. *Eur Heart J Cardiovasc Imaging.* 2015;16(8):821–827.
93. Connolly HM, Click RL, Schattenberg TT, Seward JB, Tajik AJ. Congenital absence of the pericardium: echocardiography as a diagnostic tool. *J Am Soc Echocardiogr.* 1995;8(1):87–92.
94. Patel J, Park C, Michaels J, Rosen S, Kort S. Pericardial cyst: case reports and a literature review. *Echocardiogr-J Card.* 2004;21(3):269–272.
95. Pezzano A, Belloni A, Faletra F, Binaghi G, Colli A, Rovelli F. Value of two-dimensional echocardiography in the diagnosis of pericardial cysts. *Eur Heart J.* 1983;4(4):238–246.

中文导读

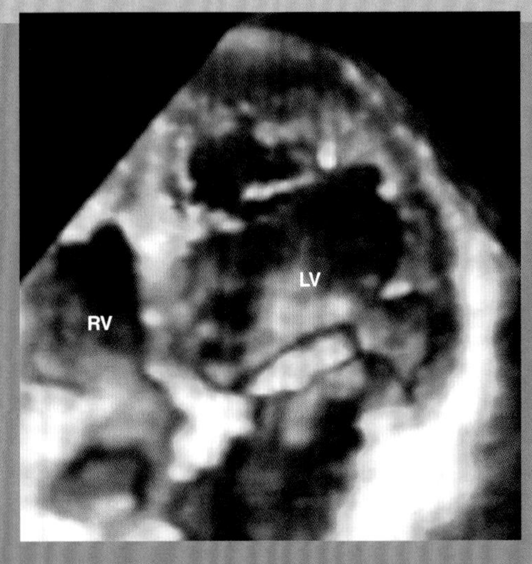

第18章 心脏肿瘤及心脏肿瘤学

心脏肿瘤学是一个快速发展的领域，旨在识别、监测和治疗由癌症和癌症相关治疗导致的心血管并发症。超声心动图在肿瘤患者的基线评估和随访中发挥重要作用。

左室射血分数下降≥5%至最终射血分数<55%伴充血性心力衰竭症状，或无症状性时左室射血分数下降≥10%至最终射血分数<55%定义为心脏毒性。该定义存在争议，但左室射血分数定量在心脏肿瘤学实践中有特殊地位。

左室射血分数的单数字测量在肿瘤学中有着悠久的历史。超声心动图、斑点追踪成像技术也用于评价心脏毒性。辐射诱发的心脏病包括一系列心包疾病、瓣膜疾病、冠状动脉或微血管疾病、功能障碍及限制型心肌病。这些病理过程通常是晚期表现，在放射治疗多年后才具有临床意义。

超声心动图是评价和诊断心脏占位（无论是血栓、赘生物或肿瘤）的首选方法。评价重点包括占位的形态、大小、位置、与相邻结构的关系、肿块植入的位置、肿块进入心脏的途径、血流动力学影响和滋养血管形成情况等。

心脏肿瘤很罕见，分为原发性和继发性。继发性或转移性心脏肿瘤的发病率约是原发性恶性肿瘤的30倍，原发性心脏肿瘤的尸检率仅为0.002%～0.3%，80%以上为良性肿瘤，最常见的是黏液瘤。当遇到可疑心脏占位时，应将整合所有可用信息，进行鉴别诊断，首先需要排除血栓、赘生物、变异的正常结构，再考虑心脏肿瘤的可能性。心脏恶性肿瘤预后差，手术切除结合化疗和放疗可一定程度提高患者生存率。

陶　瑾

18 Cardiac Tumors and Cardio-oncology

JOSE BANCHS, MD

Cardio-oncology is a growing field aimed at recognizing, monitoring, and treating cardiovascular complications resulting from cancer and cancer-related treatments. Echocardiography plays an essential role in the baseline assessment and serial follow-up of oncology patients and remains the test most often used to evaluate cardiac function in patients of all ages who undergo a variety of anti-cancer therapies. Although several echocardiographic variables are capable of evaluating systolic function, the left ventricular ejection fraction (LVEF) continues to be the most widely used.

In the clinical setting and in many research protocols, cardiotoxicity has been defined as a decline in LVEF of 5% or greater to a final ejection fraction (EF) less than 55% with symptoms of congestive heart failure or an asymptomatic decline of 10% or greater to a final ejection fraction less than 55%. Although this definition is controversial and somewhat arbitrary,[1] LVEF quantification has a special place in cardio-oncology practice.

Cardiac tumors have diverse histologies and natural histories. They are divided into primary and secondary tumors. Primary cardiac tumors are rare based on the reported autopsy prevalence.[2,3] Primary cardiac tumors include benign and malignant neoplasms that originate from cardiac tissue. Secondary or metastatic cardiac tumors are approximately 30 times more common than primary malignancies.[4]

CHEMOTHERAPEUTIC CARDIOTOXICITY

QUANTITATIVE ASSESSMENT OF LV EJECTION FRACTION IN CARDIO-ONCOLOGY

Echocardiography is frequently used for sequential measurement of EF in the assessment of potential cardiotoxicity caused by chemotherapy or immune therapy for patients with malignancies (Table 18.1). In most oncology practices, the LVEF is followed closely and given a great deal of clinical importance.

In clinical practice, the most commonly accepted definition of cardiac toxicity comes from a retrospective review by the independent Cardiac Review and Evaluation Committee (CREC) of cardiotoxicity of patients enrolled in a variety of trastuzumab clinical trials.[5]

In practice, given the use of singular measures for any particular cardiotoxicity definition, it has been common for echocardiography clinicians to report single numbers and to avoid reporting EF ranges. Oncologists make critical clinical decisions based on a 5% or 10% EF change or a drop to less than 50% or 55%. When the value reported from one study to the next is 55% to 60% followed by 50% to 55%, confusion, if not inappropriate clinical consequences from decisions to halt anticancer therapy, may ensue.[6]

Single-digit measures of LVEF have a long history in oncology. Cardiac imaging was established in the late 1970s and early 1980s, when a number of publications[7–11] supported the use of different modalities for assessing cardiac toxicity. Measurement of LVEF by nuclear methods (i.e., multigated acquisition [MUGA]) soon became the established practice and was considered the gold standard for LV function assessment during chemotherapy. LVEF by radionuclide imaging proved to be sensitive, specific, and reproducible and was reported as a single measure.

Measurement of LVEF by MUGA as a sole indicator of cardiotoxicity has significant limitations, including image quality and the technical difficulty of the measurement. For instance, MUGA is subject to variations related to the use of a particular cardiac cycle, operator experience, and volume drawing style. The EF is the relative volume ejected in systole, a measurement that does not necessarily reflect intrinsic myocardial systolic function, particularly because it can be load dependent.

The ready availability, ease, and improvements in image quality of transthoracic echocardiography (TTE) have made it a more attractive option for the assessment of LVEF in cancer patients. The most commonly used LVEF measures in routine practice are two-dimensional (2D) methods, and among the 2D options, the most common method for volume calculations is the biplane method of disks summation (i.e., modified Simpson rule). It is the recommended 2D echocardiographic method by consensus and by current published LV quantification guidelines[12] (see Chapter 4).

The literature is clear that the use of microbubble enhancement offers the best results in terms of intraobserver and interobserver variability, and contrast agents are recommended when needed to improve endocardial border delineation, specifically

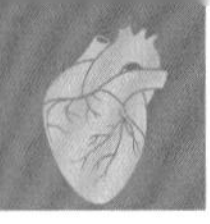

TABLE 18.1 Cancer Therapies Associated With LV Dysfunction.

Therapeutic Agents	*Percentage Reported in Research/Literature*
Anthracyclines	
Doxorubicin (Adriamycin)	3–26
Epirubicin (Ellence)	0.9–3.3
Idarubicin (Idamycin)	5–18
Alkylating Agents	
Cyclophosphamide (Cytoxan)	7–28
Ifosfamide (Ifex)	17
Antimetabolites	
Clofarabine (Clolar)	27
Antimicrotubule Agents	
Docetaxel (Taxotere)	2.3–8
Monoclonal Antibody–Based Tyrosine Kinase Inhibitors	
Bevacizumab (Avastin)	1.7–3
Trastuzumab (Herceptin)	2–28
Proteasome Inhibitors	
Bortezomib (Velcade)	2–5
Small-Molecule Tyrosine Kinase Inhibitors	
Dasatinib (Sprycel)	2–4
Imatinib mesylate (Gleevec)	0.5–1.7
Lapatinib (Tykerb)	1.5–2.2
Sunitinib (Sutent)	2.7–11
Immunotherapies	
Chimeric antigen receptor T-cell therapy, associated with cytokine release syndrome/stress-induced effects	Case reports
Interferon (immune modulator)	Case reports
Interleukins (immune modulators), associated with myocarditis	Case reports
Immune checkpoint inhibitors, associated with myocarditis	Case reports

when two or more contiguous LV endocardial segments are poorly visualized in apical views. Microbubble-enhanced images provide larger volumes than unenhanced images. Volumes obtained in this fashion are closer to those obtained with cardiac magnetic resonance (CMR)[13] (see Chapter 3).

Three-dimensional echocardiography (3DE) is more accurate than 2D methods for ventricular volume and EF measurements compared with CMR imaging, and 3DE should be used when available[14,15] (see Chapter 1). This method, which is still not routine in most centers, has been shown to offer the lowest temporal variability for EF and ventricular volumes, on the basis of multiple echocardiograms done over a period of 1 year in women with breast cancer receiving chemotherapy (Fig. 18.1).[16]

DOPPLER METHODS FOR DETECTION OF CARDIOTOXICITY

Earlier detection of cardiotoxicity allows a time advantage in risk stratification. Measurements of diastolic function by Doppler echocardiography could represent a marker for the early detection of toxicity. One study found that the isovolumetric relaxation time was significantly prolonged (from 66 ± 18 to 84 ± 24 ms; $P < 0.05$) after a cumulative doxorubicin dose of 100 to 120 mg/m^2.[16a] An increase of more than 37% in isovolumetric relaxation time was 78% sensitive (7 of 9 cases) and 88% specific (15 of 17 cases) for predicting the subsequent development of doxorubicin-induced systolic dysfunction.[17] Overall, however, the results regarding the value of diastolic dysfunction as an indicator of the diagnosis of cardiotoxicity have been inconsistent. Because of the influence of hypertension and other risk factors on diastolic function, this signal appears to be nonspecific.

The myocardial performance (Tei) index is another important Doppler-derived tool.[18] This index expresses the ratio of the sum of isovolumetric contraction time and isovolumetric relaxation time divided by the ejection time. This formula combines systolic and diastolic myocardial performance without geometric assumptions, and it correlates well with the results of invasive measurements. It is appealing for use with cancer patients because it appears to be independent of heart rate, mean arterial pressure, and degree of mitral regurgitation. It is sensitive and accurate in detecting subclinical cardiotoxicity associated with anthracycline therapy.[19] Studies have shown that the Tei index is better than EF in detecting anthracycline-induced deterioration in LV function among adults: it detects deterioration earlier in the course of treatment and is more likely to detect statistically significant differences.[20]

SPECKLE TRACKING CHARACTERISTICS OF CARDIAC MECHANICS IN CARDIO-ONCOLOGY

New techniques have aimed at detecting cardiotoxicity before the onset of a measurable decrease in LVEF or symptoms. These methods include echocardiographic assessment for strain using speckle tracking imaging and testing for elevations in cardiac biomarkers, including troponin.

Speckle tracking takes full advantage of the capacity for image acquisition at higher frame rates. Use of this particular technology in the realm of cardiac dysfunction related to cancer therapeutics has yielded important results, particularly the use of longitudinal deformation measures, including global longitudinal strain (GLS).

It was first reported in 2009 that changes in tissue deformation assessed by myocardial strain and strain rate were able to identify LV dysfunction earlier than LVEF in women undergoing treatment with trastuzumab for breast cancer.[21] Two subsequent reports produced comparable findings.[22,23]

A multicenter collaboration[23] investigated the cooperative use of troponin and longitudinal strain measures to predict the development of cardiotoxicity in patients treated with anthracyclines and trastuzumab. Patients who demonstrated decreases in longitudinal strain measures or elevations in hypersensitive troponin had a ninefold increase in risk of cardiotoxicity at 6 months compared with those who had no changes in either of these markers. LVEF alone and diastolic function parameters failed to predict cardiotoxicity.

In a review that included more than 30 studies, although the best GLS cutoff value to predict cardiotoxicity was not clear, an early relative change of between 10% and 15% appeared to have the best specificity.[24] Similar studies, however, found a stronger correlation from ventricular-arterial coupling and circumferential strain than from longitudinal measures.[25] A consensus statement on the evaluation of adult patients during and after cancer therapy that was published by the American Society of Echocardiography and the European Association of Cardiovascular Imaging; based on the current literature, it recommended that a relative reduction in GLS of more than 15% is very likely to be abnormal, whereas a change of less than 8% appears to be of no clinical significance (Fig. 18.2).[26]

The same consensus statement recommended that an abnormal GLS value be confirmed by a repeat study. The repeat study should be performed 2 to 3 weeks after the initial abnormal

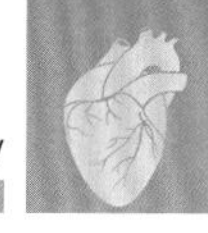

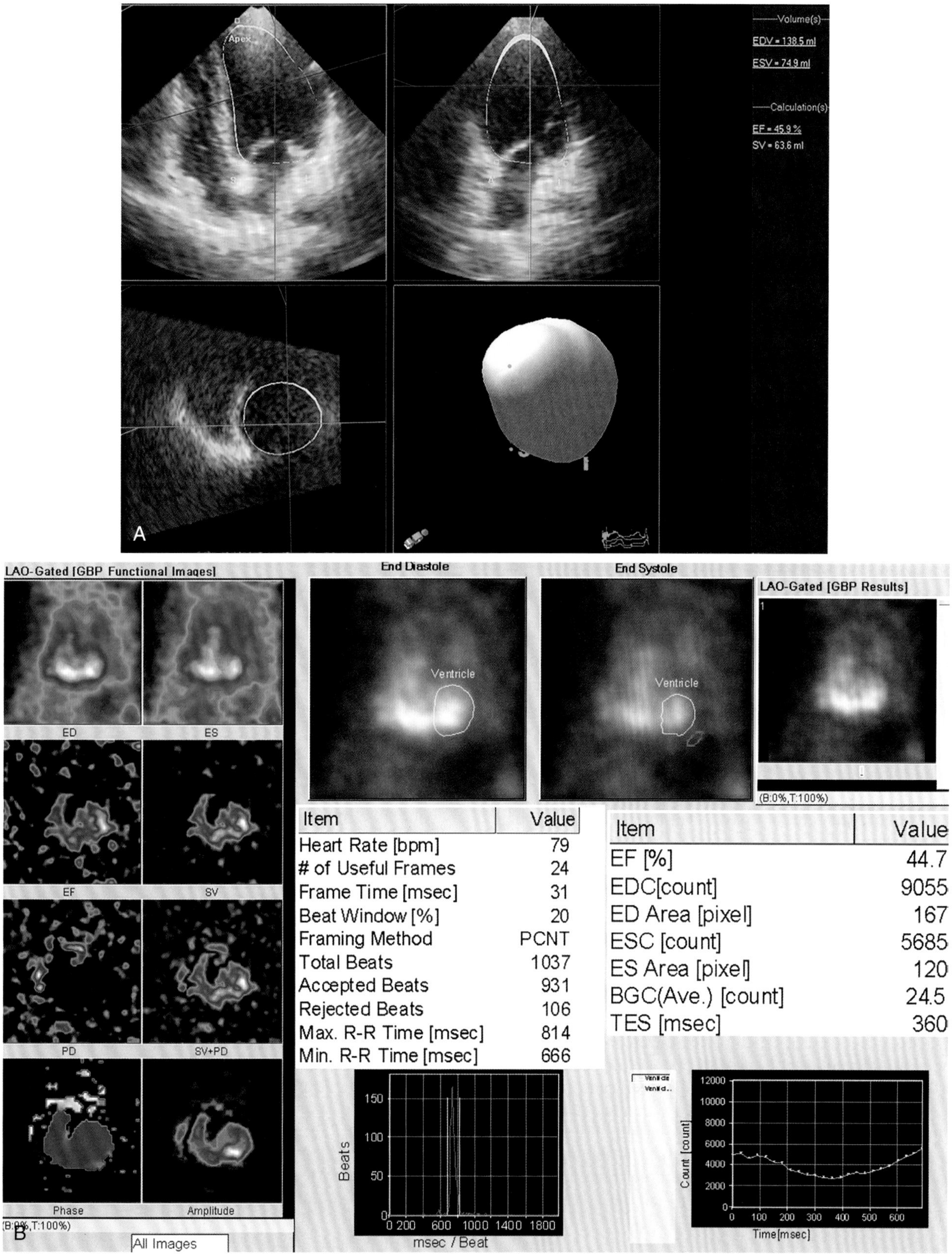

Volume(s)
EDV = 138.5 ml
ESV = 74.9 ml
Calculation(s)
EF = 45.9 %
SV = 63.6 ml
Apex
A
LAO-Gated [GBP Functional Images]
End Diastole
End Systole
LAO-Gated [GBP Results]
Ventricle
Ventricle
ED
ES
EF
SV
PD
SV+PD
Phase
Amplitude
(B:0%,T:100%)
(B:0%,T:100%)
B
All Images
Item | Value
Heart Rate [bpm] 79
# of Useful Frames 24
Frame Time [msec] 31
Beat Window [%] 20
Framing Method PCNT
Total Beats 1037
Accepted Beats 931
Rejected Beats 106
Max. R-R Time [msec] 814
Min. R-R Time [msec] 666
Item | Value
EF [%] 44.7
EDC[count] 9055
ED Area [pixel] 167
ESC [count] 5685
ES Area [pixel] 120
BGC(Ave.) [count] 24.5
TES [msec] 360
Beats
msec / Beat
Count [count]
Time[msec]

Fig. 18.1 **Quantification of LV ejection fraction.** (A) In a 62-year-old woman with breast cancer during therapy with trastuzumab, a new low ejection fraction *(EF)* was reported by 3D echocardiography with LV ejection fraction (LVEF) at 45.9%. (B) Comparison of 3D and multigated acquisition (MUGA). The same patient as in A was evaluated with MUGA because of doubts from the oncology team, and the EF was confirmed to be 44.7%.

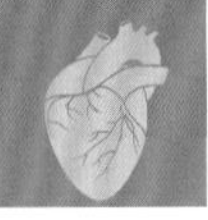

study result. These recommendations have been reported mostly for the breast cancer population, and it remains to be seen whether the same cardiac imaging benefit extends to other malignancies and their treatment regimens (Fig. 18.3).

CHEMOTHERAPEUTIC IMPACT ON THE RV

Right ventricular (RV) function is a prognostic indicator in patients with LV systolic dysfunction and various LV pathologies, but there is limited literature concerning the specific effects of cardiotoxic agents on the RV. For low-dose anthracycline chemotherapy regimens, it has been reported that a differential effect on ventricular function is detected using the myocardial performance index measure; a significant negative impact on LV function is produced, but RV function is spared.[27,28] A later study challenged that notion. Using a comprehensive list of measures, a retrospective analysis showed statistically significant decreases in RV fractional area change and longitudinal deformation in patients exposed to relatively low doses of anthracyclines.[28]

CONSIDERATIONS IN RADIATION-INDUCED HEART DISEASE

Radiation-induced heart disease (RIHD) includes a spectrum of pericardial disease, valvular disease, coronary or microvascular disease or dysfunction, and restrictive cardiomyopathy. These pathologic processes are usually late manifestations, becoming clinically significant years after radiation therapy.

Fibrosis is a common cause of radiation therapy, which leads to fibrotic thickening of the pericardium. Up to 70% to 90% of patients with significant mediastinal radiation exposure may have evidence of pericardial disease. Pericardial disease is one of the most common manifestations of RIHD and occurs if a significant proportion of heart, usually greater than 30%, receives a dose of 5000 rad.

Initial injury to the pericardium is a result of microvascular damage that leads to episodic ischemia.[29,30] Acute and late pericardial types of injury are driven by inflammation and immediate fibrin deposition. Tortuous, immature, and permeable vascularization occurs later in the irradiated pericardium, leading to ischemia and late fibrosis. Additional fibrosis of venous and lymphatic channels in the heart decreases the ability to drain extracellular fluid, leading to accumulation of a fibrin-rich exudate. Early clinical pericardial disease typically manifests as effusions, and almost one fifth of patients who experienced late significant fibrosis of the pericardium may have had effusions initially.

Characteristic echocardiographic findings of constrictive pericarditis include a thickened pericardium, prominent respiratory phasic diastolic motion of the interventricular septum, a restrictive diastolic filling pattern, and significant inspiratory variation of the mitral E-wave velocity. Other secondary findings include inferior vena cava (IVC) dilation and expiratory diastolic flow reversal in the hepatic veins. Typically, tissue Doppler interrogation of the medial mitral annulus reveals a normal or increased velocity that can be higher than the lateral annulus velocity[31] (see Chapter 17).

Another important consideration in RIHD is effusive-constrictive pericarditis. This clinical syndrome is characterized by concurrent pericardial effusion and pericardial constriction, with constrictive hemodynamics that persist after drainage of the pericardial effusion. Effective recognition of this syndrome is important because pericardiectomy is often indicated.

Manifestations of radiation-induced valvular disease include fibrosis and patchy calcification of structures such as the aortic root, annulus, and leaflets; the aortic-mitral intervalvular fibrosa; the mitral annulus; and the base and midportions of the mitral valve (MV) leaflets. This process typically spares the tips and commissures—a key difference from the pattern seen in rheumatic heart disease.[32] However, thickening and fibrosis may manifest in any area that was in the radiation treatment field (Fig. 18.4).

Stenotic lesions more commonly involve the aortic valve. Reported incidences of clinically significant valve disease are 1% at 10 years, 5% at 15 years, and 6% at 20 years after radiation exposure. The incidence of valve disease increases significantly beyond 20 years after chest radiation, with mild aortic regurgitation (AR) in up to 45% of patients, moderate AR in up to 15%, aortic stenosis in up to 16%, mild mitral regurgitation in up to 48%, and mild pulmonic regurgitation in up to 12%.[33,34] Grading of the severity of valvular disease should be based on the published guidelines (see Chapters 22–28). Valve regurgitation is more commonly encountered than stenosis in RIHD.

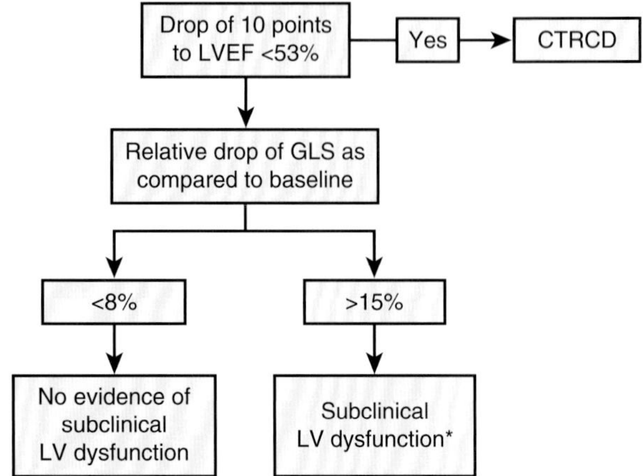

Fig. 18.2 Identification of subclinical LV dysfunction using longitudinal deformation measures. Global longitudinal strain *(GLS)* can be used to identify subclinical LV dysfunction. When baseline strain is available, a relative percentage decrease of greater than 15% compared with baseline is likely to be of clinical significance, but a decrease of less than 8% should be considered not significant. *CTRCD*, Chemotherapy-related cardiac dysfunction; *LVEF*, LV ejection fraction.

CARDIAC MASSES AND TUMORS

Cardiac tumors are rare and are divided into primary and secondary types. Primary cardiac tumors have an autopsy incidence of only 0.002% to 0.3%.[35,36] Primary cardiac tumors include benign and malignant neoplasms that originate from cardiac tissue. Secondary or metastatic cardiac tumors are approximately 30 times more common than primary malignancies, with a reported autopsy incidence of 1.7% to 14% (Table 18.2).[37] A diagnostic approach to cardiac masses is presented in Fig. 18.5.

Other possible categories of tumors could include those from the lower body that reach the cardiac cavities by extension through the IVC and tumors that extend from the mediastinal space, invading directly and usually involving pericardial layers. Infradiaphragmatic tumors of almost any cell type can occur, but most have been attributed to renal cell carcinoma (RCC). Up to 10% of patients with RCC have tumor extension into the IVC.[38] In patients with RCC, involvement of the right atrium

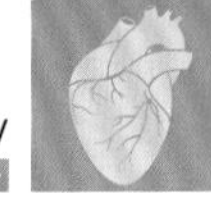

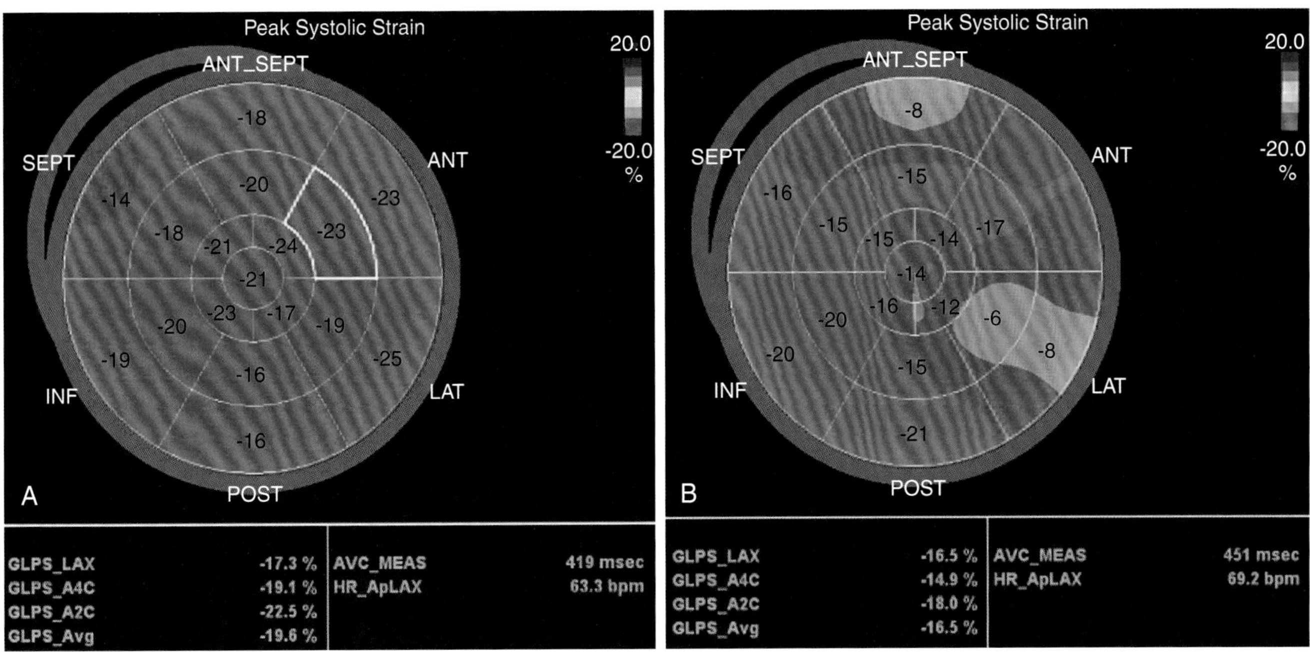

Fig. 18.3 **Example in clinical practice of the use of global longitudinal strain in follow-up.** (A) A 60-year-old woman, before chemotherapy with anthracyclines and trastuzumab, had a normal baseline LV ejection fraction (LVEF) of 59% and a global longitudinal strain (GLS) of −19.6. (B) In a 3-month follow-up study of the same patient as in A, the GLS was -16.5, a relative change of greater than 15%. At this time the LVEF was unchanged, but 3 months later, the LVEF was 42%.

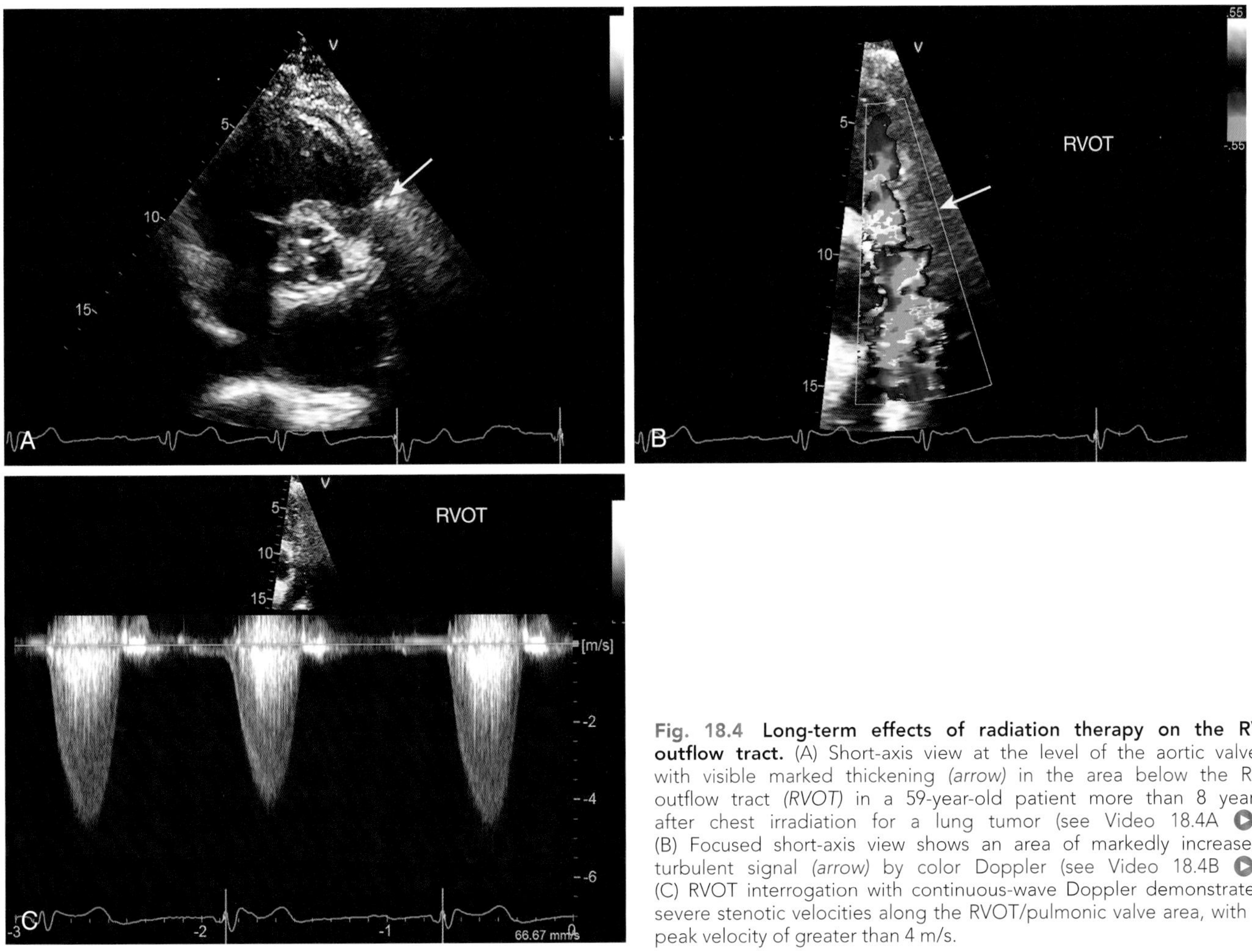

Fig. 18.4 **Long-term effects of radiation therapy on the RV outflow tract.** (A) Short-axis view at the level of the aortic valve, with visible marked thickening *(arrow)* in the area below the RV outflow tract *(RVOT)* in a 59-year-old patient more than 8 years after chest irradiation for a lung tumor (see Video 18.4A). (B) Focused short-axis view shows an area of markedly increased turbulent signal *(arrow)* by color Doppler (see Video 18.4B). (C) RVOT interrogation with continuous-wave Doppler demonstrates severe stenotic velocities along the RVOT/pulmonic valve area, with a peak velocity of greater than 4 m/s.

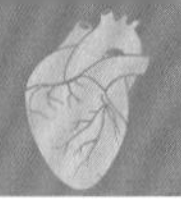

TABLE 18.2 Cardiac Masses.

Neoplastic Masses			
Primary	*Secondary*	*Nonneoplastic Masses*	*Others*
Benign	Direct extension	Hamartomas	Thrombus
Myxoma	Breast cancer	Rhabdomyoma	Vegetation
PFE[a]	Lung cancer	Fibroma	CAT
Lipoma	Esophageal cancer	PFE[a]	Normal structure
Malignant	Mediastinal tumor	Age-related growths	Image artifact
Sarcoma	Hematogenous spread	Lipomatous hypertrophy	
Lymphoma	Melanoma	Reactive proliferation	
	GU cancer	Lambl excrescence	
	GI cancer	PFE[b]	
	Venous extension		
	Renal cancer		
	Adrenal cancer		
	Thyroid cancer		
	Hepatoma		
	Lymphatic extension		
	Lymphoma		
	Leukemia		

[a]PFE arising de novo.
[b]PFE arising in the setting of hypertrophic cardiomyopathy or after endocardial injury.
CAT, Calcified amorphous tumor; *GI,* gastrointestinal; *GU,* genitourinary; *PFE,* papillary fibroelastoma.

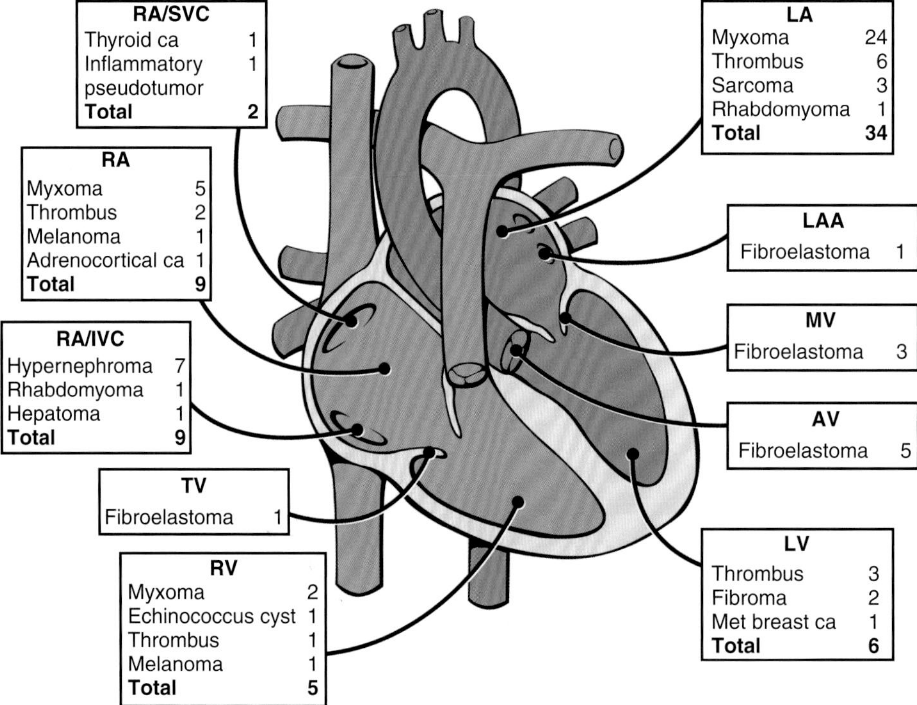

Fig. 18.5 Distribution of cardiac masses according to intracardiac attachment site among 75 patients undergoing surgery. *AV,* Aortic valve; *ca,* carcinoma; *IVC,* inferior vena cava; *LAA,* LA appendage; *Met,* metastatic; *MV,* mitral valve; *SVC,* superior vena cava; *TV,* tricuspid valve. (Reproduced with permission from Dujardin KS, Click RL, Oh JK. The role of intraoperative transesophageal echocardiography in patients undergoing cardiac mass removal. *J Am Soc Echocardiogr.* 2000;13:1080–1083.)

(RA) is encountered in up to 5% of cases, and pulmonary artery tumor emboli are observed but are uncommon.[35,36]

Other sources for this route of invasion include uterine malignancies[37] and hepatocellular carcinoma.[39,40] Tumors with direct extension in the mediastinal space can involve almost any cell type. Thymoma comprises 20% to 25% of all mediastinal tumors and is the most commonly described anterior mediastinal tumor[41]; however, in most case reports, direct mediastinal invasion is not from thymic origin.[42,43]

The clinical manifestations of cardiac tumors vary and depend on location, size, and cause.[44–49] A growing mass inside a contractile and moving cavity eventually compromises blood flow in the affected or receiving chamber and disrupts valve coaptation. In this setting, symptoms of congestive

TABLE 18.3 Features of Benign Primary Cardiac Tumors.

Type of Tumor	*Patient Age at Diagnosis*	*Associated Syndromes*	*Most Common Location*	*Typical Morphologic Features*	*Echocardiographic Features*	*CT Features*	*MRI Features*
Myxoma	30–60 y (younger if associated with Carney complex)	Carney complex	Interatrial septum at fossa ovalis; LA more common than RA	Gelatinous, attached to stalk; calcification common; hemorrhage or necrosis common	Mobile tumor, narrow stalk	Heterogeneous, low attenuation	Heterogeneous, bright on T2WI; heterogeneous enhancement
Papillary fibroelastoma	Middle-aged, elderly	None	Cardiac valves	Small (<1 cm), frondlike, narrow stalk; calcification rare; no hemorrhage or necrosis	Shimmering edges	Usually small pedunculated mass; may have calcifications and frondlike appearance when large	Usually small pedunculated mass; may have frondlike appearance when large
Lipoma	Varies	Multiple fatty lesions in tuberous sclerosis may be lipomas or angiomyolipomas	Pericardial space or any cardiac chamber	Large, broad-based; no calcification, hemorrhage, or necrosis	Usually hypoechoic in the pericardial space, echogenic in a cardiac chamber	Homogeneous fat attenuation (low attenuation)	Homogeneous fat signal intensity (increased T1); no enhancement
Hemangioma	All ages; mean, 4th decade	None	Anywhere; one third in RV, one third in LV; one fourth in RA	Multilobulated, unilocular, cystic, <1–8 cm	Solid echo-dense	Intense central contrast enhancement	Rapid enhancement increased T2WI signal
Rhabdomyoma	Infants, children < 4 y	Tuberous sclerosis	Walls of RV and/or LV; outflow tract on aortic valves	Mural pedunculated multiple, variable size, spontaneous regression	Brighter than surrounding myocardium	Hypodense on contrast CT	Isointense to myocardium T2WI; hyperintense to myocardium T2WI
Fibroma	Infants, children, young adults	Gorlin syndrome	Ventricles	Large, intramural; calcification common; no hemorrhage or necrosis	Intramural, calcified	Low attenuation, calcified	Isointense on T1W1; dark on T2WI; usually little or no enhancement
Paraganglioma	Young adults	Many possible but almost always sporadic	LA, coronary arteries, aortic root	Broad-based, infiltrative or circumscribed; calcification rare; hemorrhage or necrosis common	Echogenic, relatively immobile	Low attenuation; avidly enhancing	Typically isointense or heterogeneous on T1W1, bright on T2WI; marked enhancement

CT, Computed tomography; *MRI*, magnetic resonance imaging; *T1WI*, T1-weighted images; *T2WI*, T2-weighted images.
Adapted from Araoz PA, Mulvagh SL, Tazelaar HD, et al. CT and MR imaging of benign primary cardiac neoplasms with echocardiographic correlation. *Radiographics*. 2000;20:1303–1319.

failure can be identified and are exacerbated by myocardial involvement and secondary limitations of contractility. Even in asymptomatic patients, cardiac tumors may be found on routine surveillance echocardiograms or other chest imaging studies (Table 18.3).

The pediatric population seems to have different clinical manifestations than most adults with cardiac tumors. In one of the few and largest series in children, primary malignant tumors of the heart were rare, and benign tumors showed minimal growth over time, with some even exhibiting spontaneous regression (Table 18.4).[50]

BENIGN TUMORS

Almost 90% of primary cardiac tumors excised surgically are benign. In a report of 323 consecutive patients undergoing surgical resection of primary cardiac tumors between 1957 and 2006 at the Mayo Clinic, 94% of tumors were benign, and 50% of those were myxomas.[51] The remaining benign tumors, in descending order of frequency, included papillary fibroelastomas (26%), fibromas (6%), lipomas (4%), and others, including calcified amorphous tumors, hemangiomas, teratomas, unilocular developmental cysts, and rhabdomyomas (see Table 18.4).

TABLE 18.4 Relative Incidence of Benign Tumors of the Heart in Adults and Children.

Tumor Type	Incidence (%)	
	Adults	*Children*
Myxoma	45	15
Lipoma	20	—
Papillary fibroelastoma	15	—
Angioma	5	5
Fibroma	3	15
Hemangioma	5	5
Rhabdomyoma	1	45
Teratoma	<1	15

Adapted from Shapiro LM. Cardiac tumors: diagnosis and management. *Heart*. 2001;85:218–222.

Myxomas occur in all age groups but most frequently between the third and sixth decades of life. Women are more commonly affected than men. Although myxomas usually occur sporadically as an isolated tumor in the LA, familial myxomas have been reported (accounting for 7% of myxomas). Familial myxomas occur as an inherited autosomal dominant disorder in combination with two or more of the following conditions: skin myxomas (single or multiple), cutaneous lentiginosis, myxoid fibroadenomas of the breast, pituitary adenomas, primary adrenocortical micronodular dysplasia with Cushing syndrome, and testicular tumors (characteristically large-cell calcifying Sertoli cell tumors).

Although multiple acronyms (e.g., LAMB for *l*entigines, *a*trial *m*yxomas, and *b*lue nevi; NAME for *n*evi, *a*trial myxoma, *m*yxoid neurofibromas, and *e*phelides) have been used to describe these associations in the past, these syndromes are now grouped under the broader category of Carney complex, named after the physician who first described the familial nature of the disorder (Fig. 18.6).[52]

The second most common benign tumor, papillary fibroelastoma, usually develops on cardiac valves (75%–90%) but may arise anywhere in the heart, originating from the LV, ostium of the right and left coronary arteries, LA appendage, atrial and ventricular septum, and LV outflow tract. They have also been found in the RA, RA appendage, eustachian valve, Chiari network, and RV outflow tract. Left-sided valves are affected 95% of the time, with aortic valve involvement slightly more common than MV involvement. Almost 50% of papillary fibroelastomas are discovered incidentally during echocardiography for unrelated reasons or during evaluation of a cardiac source of embolism.[51,53]

Like most cardiac tumors, the clinical profile of papillary fibroelastomas depends on many factors, including tumor location, size, growth rate, and tendency to embolize. The most common manifestations include cerebral and systemic embolization and coronary artery occlusion (Fig. 18.7).

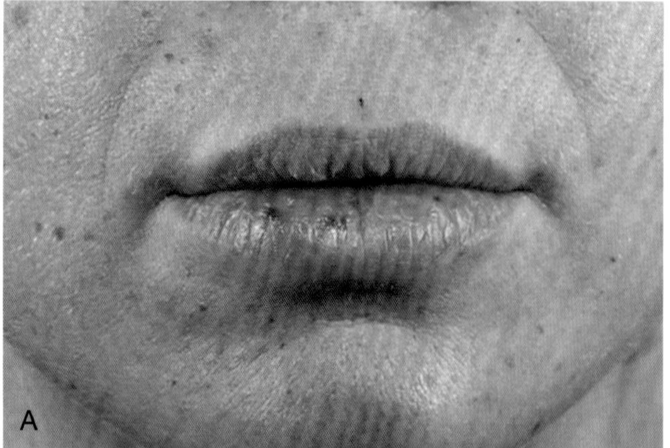

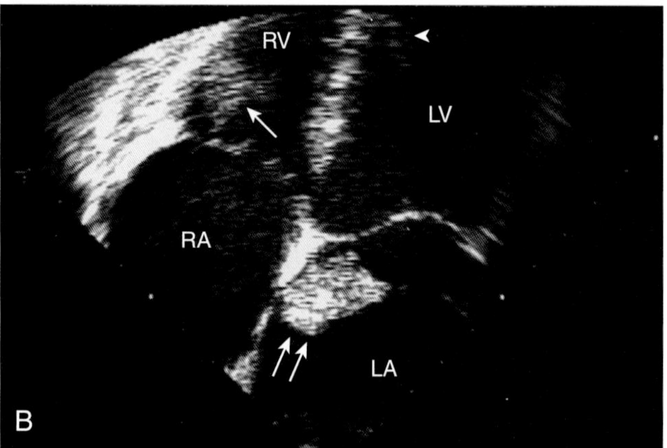

Fig. 18.6 Carney complex. (A) A 19-year-old woman presented with a stroke. Examination revealed cutaneous myxomas and lentigines of the lips. (B) The TEE shows multiple intracardiac myxomas. Tumors are seen in the LA near the fossa ovalis *(double arrows)* and related to the anterior tricuspid valve leaflet *(single arrow)*. An LV myxoma attached to the anterior septum is also present but is poorly seen in this still-frame image *(arrowhead)*. At surgery, an additional small RV apical myxoma was also identified with a thoracoscope that was not appreciated on preoperative or intraoperative echocardiography. This patient was diagnosed with Carney complex. Although there was no evidence of myxoma recurrence after 4 years, 10 years later echocardiography demonstrated recurrent myxomas in the RV that were surgically removed.

OTHER BENIGN CARDIAC TUMORS: LIPOMAS AND LIPOMATOUS HYPERTROPHY

Lipomatous hypertrophy of the atrial septum is a benign condition and not a true tumor. It is discussed here because it is often confused with a lipoma. Lipomatous hypertrophy is "any deposit of fat in the atrial septum at the level of the fossa ovalis that exceeds 2 cm in transverse dimension."[54]

Lipomatous hypertrophy involves the interatrial septum, sparing the fossa ovalis membrane and resulting in a characteristic dumbbell shape. It results from adipose cell hyperplasia and is associated with increasing age and obesity. It is a nonneoplastic condition and may be associated with atrial arrhythmias or may rarely result in superior vena cava obstruction. Echocardiographically, the atrial septum can be up to 3 cm thick and appears hyperechoic.

Unlike lipomatous hypertrophy, lipomas are much less common. Unfortunately, the number of reported cases is not clear from the literature because some series do not differentiate between lipomas and lipomatous hypertrophy. These homogeneous, fatty, encapsulated tumors may arise from epicardial or endocardial surfaces. Subendocardial lipomas are often small and sessile, whereas subepicardial lipomas tend to be larger. Subendocardial lipomas may grow as broad-based, pedunculated masses protruding into the cardiac chambers. Subepicardial lipomas also tend to be broad based and protrude into the pericardial space.

Lipomas are usually asymptomatic but may cause symptoms from local compression (rarely, lipomas become quite large, weighing as much as 4.8 kg), or they may cause arrhythmias. They occasionally arise from the interatrial septum and extend into the LA cavity, mimicking a cardiac myxoma. However, compared with myxomas, lipomas have a broad base of attachment and are not as mobile.

The echocardiographic appearance of lipomas depends on their particular location. In the pericardial space, they may appear echogenic or entirely hypoechoic or have hypoechoic regions. Intracavitary lipomas are homogeneous and hyperechoic. The reason for this difference is not known.

If diagnostic uncertainty exists with respect to identification of lipomatous hypertrophy or lipoma, computed tomography (CT) and magnetic resonance imaging (MRI) are diagnostic because of their high specificity in identifying fat.[55,56] Because the dumbbell appearance is characteristic for lipomatous hypertrophy and noninvasive imaging is specific for fat, a percutaneous tissue biopsy or surgical biopsy is unnecessary (Table 18.5).

ECHOCARDIOGRAPHY AND CARDIAC TUMORS

Because of its noninvasive nature, availability, relative portability, and affordability compared with other modalities,

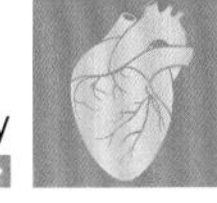

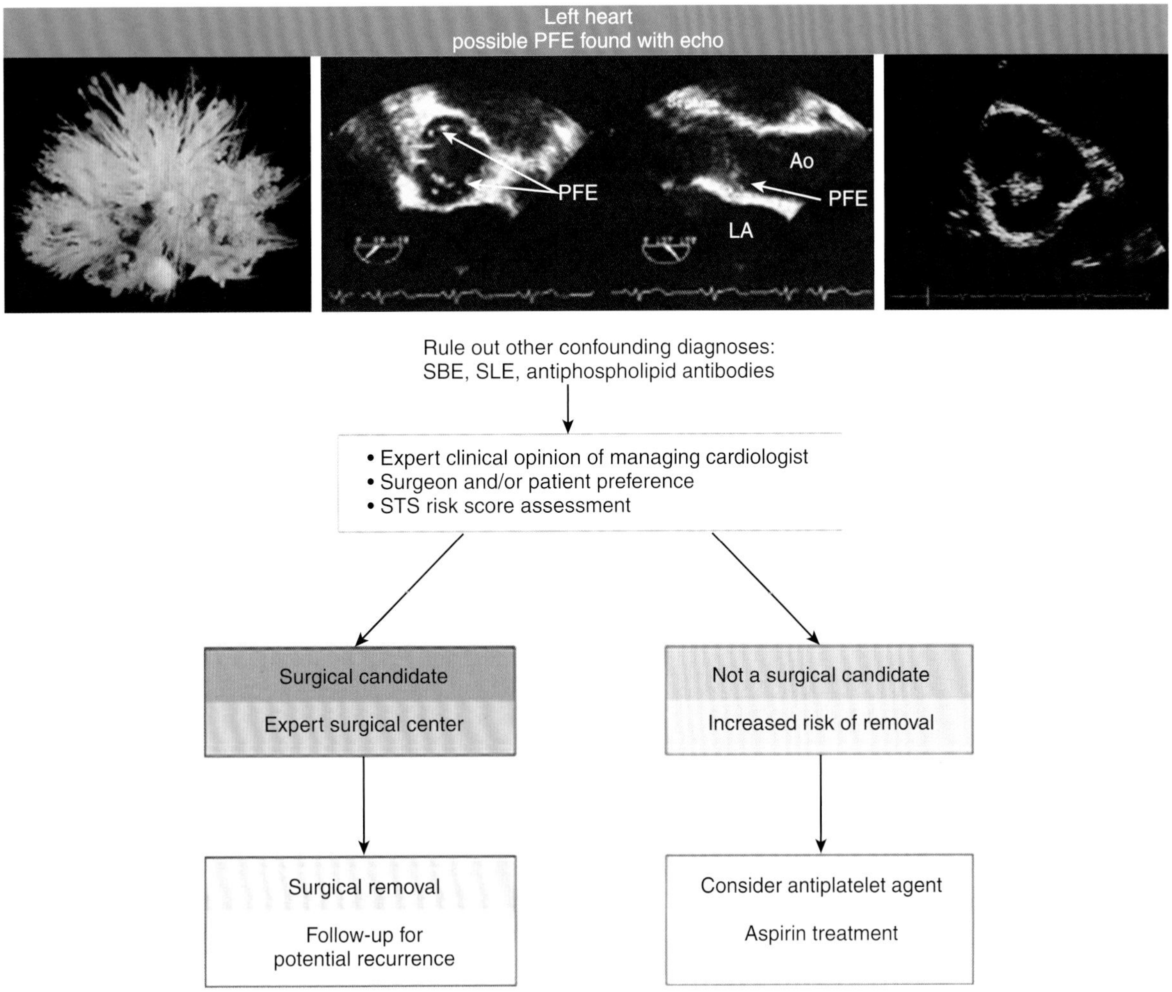

Left heart
possible PFE found with echo

PFE
Ao
PFE
LA

Rule out other confounding diagnoses:
SBE, SLE, antiphospholipid antibodies

- Expert clinical opinion of managing cardiologist
- Surgeon and/or patient preference
- STS risk score assessment

Surgical candidate
Expert surgical center

Not a surgical candidate
Increased risk of removal

Surgical removal
Follow-up for potential recurrence

Consider antiplatelet agent
Aspirin treatment

Fig. 18.7 Proposed management of PFEs based on echocardiography findings. *Ao*, Aorta; *PFE*, papillary fibroelastoma; *SBE*, subacute bacterial endocarditis; *SLE*, systemic lupus erythematous; *STS*, Society of Thoracic Surgeons. (Reproduced with permission from Tamin SS, Maleszewski JJ, Scott CG, et al. Prognostic and bioepidemiologic implications of papillary fibroelastomas. *J Am Coll Cardiol.* 2015;65:2420–2429.)

echocardiography is the most widely used diagnostic modality for the evaluation of cardiac tumors (Table 18.6).

Echocardiography is the method of choice for the diagnosis and evaluation of cardiac masses, whether they are thrombi, vegetation, or tumors. Assessment begins with a detailed description of the location of the mass and its relation to any adjacent structure. Masses can be intracardiac or extracardiac. The description should include the location and mechanism of implantation of the mass (i.e., a pedunculated mass attached to the apical segment of the inferior wall through a long stalk) or the route of access of the mass to the heart (superior vena cava, IVC, or pulmonary veins) if the mass is not primarily attached to the heart. The characterization of the shape, the longest dimensions, and ideally, the volume of the mass are impotant components. Maximum diameter measurements obtained with 2D echocardiography are routinely used to define the size of the mass. However, actual volume calculations are feasible with real-time 3DE. The size of an intracardiac mass has important clinical relevance as a predictor of embolic events, congestive heart failure, and death and as an efficacy assessment after treatment.[57]

A description of the hemodynamic consequences of the mass should be reported. The echocardiographer should then integrate all of the available information to generate a differential diagnosis. After this information has been obtained, a decision can be made about the most appropriate treatment for the patient (i.e., anticoagulation, chemotherapy, or surgery).

Beyond characterization of mass and volume, 3DE is useful for assessing cardiac masses, particularly in demonstrating their relationships with cardiac structures. Evaluation of a cardiac mass by transthoracic 3DE should include full-volume acquisition in the parasternal long-axis and apical views. If the mass in question is located in the RA, full-volume acquisition, live 3D, and subcostal images are obtained from right-sided modified views.

After a 3D data set has been acquired, it can be sliced and cropped or processed and manipulated to provide multiple nonstandard views and planes and to align structures in ways that were previously impossible with 2D imaging. This feature is particularly useful for situations in which the images captured by a sonographer are later interpreted by the physician, and the patient is no longer available to provide additional images (Fig. 18.8).

Echocardiographic technology has advanced to include mechanical function analysis, which may increase the sensitivity to recognize more subtle impacts of cardiac tumors. Repolarization changes in patients with cardiac metastases are thought to occur as a result of myocardial ischemia caused by the tumor's direct invasion and resulting myocardial injury. This presentation has been found for people without obstructive

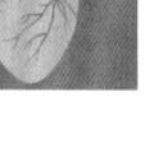

TABLE 18.5 Echocardiographic Findings That May Be Confused With Cardiac Tumors.

Normal or Normal-Variant Cardiac Structures
RA
Crista terminalis
Eustachian valve
Chiari network
LA
Floor of left upper pulmonary vein adjacent to the LA appendage (ligament of Marshall)
RV
Moderator band
LV
Papillary muscles
Nontumor Cardiac Pathology
Intracardiac
Thrombi
Valves
Vegetations (infective and marantic)
Lambl excrescence
Flail or prolapsing leaflet
Severed mitral valve apparatus after mitral valve replacement
Fatty tricuspid valve annulus
Mitral annular calcification
Myocardium
Asymmetric ventricular hypertrophy
Noncompaction of the LV
Hypereosinophilic syndrome
Atrial septum
Lipomatous hypertrophy
Atrial septum aneurysm
Extracardiac
Compression of LA by aorta
Coronary aneurysm or fistula
Potential space of the transverse sinus
Left lower lobe atelectasis
Hematoma
Hiatal hernia
Pericardial fat infiltration
Mediastinal tumor
Intracardiac Hardware
Pacing leads
Pulmonary artery catheter
Central line catheter

coronary lesions by angiography.[58] Careful attention to segmental dysfunction is pertinent because direct occlusive pressure or direct extension of the tumor into the lumens of coronary arteries (including embolization of tumor fragments) has also been described.[59]

Transesophageal echocardiography (TEE) complements TTE, providing a significant upgrade in spatial resolution and overall image clarity. This technique often provides superior 3D images. Echocardiographic images are also used in cardio-oncology to guide procedures.

Guidance from echocardiography is used during endomyocardial biopsy. In some institutions, echocardiographic guidance is frequently used for right-sided cardiac mass biopsy. Echocardiographic guidance helps illustrate bioptome direction, which is particularly helpful in avoiding damage to adjacent normal structures. Echocardiographic guidance also allows monitoring of the pericardial space and prompt identification of pericardial effusions. There is the potential for monitoring any embolization during the procedure. Assistance and details in regard to pericardiocentesis are discussed in detail in Chapter 17 (Fig. 18.9).

The use of echocardiographic contrast provides signifcant advantages in detection of cardiac masses.[60] Many other studies have demonstrated that 2D echocardiography using contrast

TABLE 18.6 Echocardiography in the Evaluation, Diagnosis, and Treatment of Cardiac Tumors.

Evaluation of Cardiac Masses
Normal-variant anatomy
Nontumor masses and disorders that mimic tumors
Thrombi
Vegetation
Infiltrative disorder
Device hardware
Diagnosis of Tumor
Morphology
Location
Attachment site
Mobility
Size
Shape
Hemodynamic impact
Guiding Interventions
Percutaneous biopsy
Pericardiocentesis
Intraoperative assessment before and after cardiopulmonary bypass

agents is an accurate method for definition of the contours and tissue characterization of intracardiac tumors. Contrast echocardiography is a reliable means of differentiating tumor from thrombus (Figs. 18.10 and 18.11).

ALTERNATIVE IMAGING MODALITIES

CMR often provides a more detailed characterization of a malignant lesion infiltrating the myocardium, and cardiac CT can give a more complete view of the mediastinum, particularly illustrating attachments of a mass located outside the cardiac cavities. This is considered critical information for surgeons planning resection. These modalities also offer advantages when it comes to tissue characterization. They do not suffer from the acoustic window limitations that often make echocardiographic examination technically difficult particularly in obese patients, in those with a history of previous chest surgery, and in those with chronic lung disease (Figs. 18.12 and 18.13).

Cardiac interventional procedures used in the diagnosis of cardiac tumors (Table 18.7) include endomyocardial biopsy[61] and pericardiocentesis. The latter has been frequently used to confirm malignant cells in the fluid.

TUMOR TYPES, PHYSIOLOGY, AND TREATMENT CONSIDERATIONS

The history of cardiac tumor detection began in the late 1550s, when a case of primary cardiac neoplasm was first described.[62] The first series of cases was published in 1845[63] and included six arterial tumors consistent with myxoma. The classification system that is still in use today originated 86 years later, when Yater reported nine postmortem cases of cardiac tumors in 1931.[64]

There are few large series describing the characteristics of cardiac tumors in the existing literature. One of the largest reports was published by the MD Anderson Cancer Center. This 12-year experience, based on an echocardiogram database of cardiac tumors, found that roughly one fourth of cardiac tumors were primary and almost three fourths were secondary. Dyspnea was the most common symptom described by patients.[58]

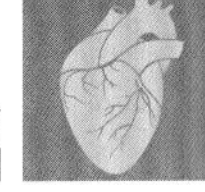

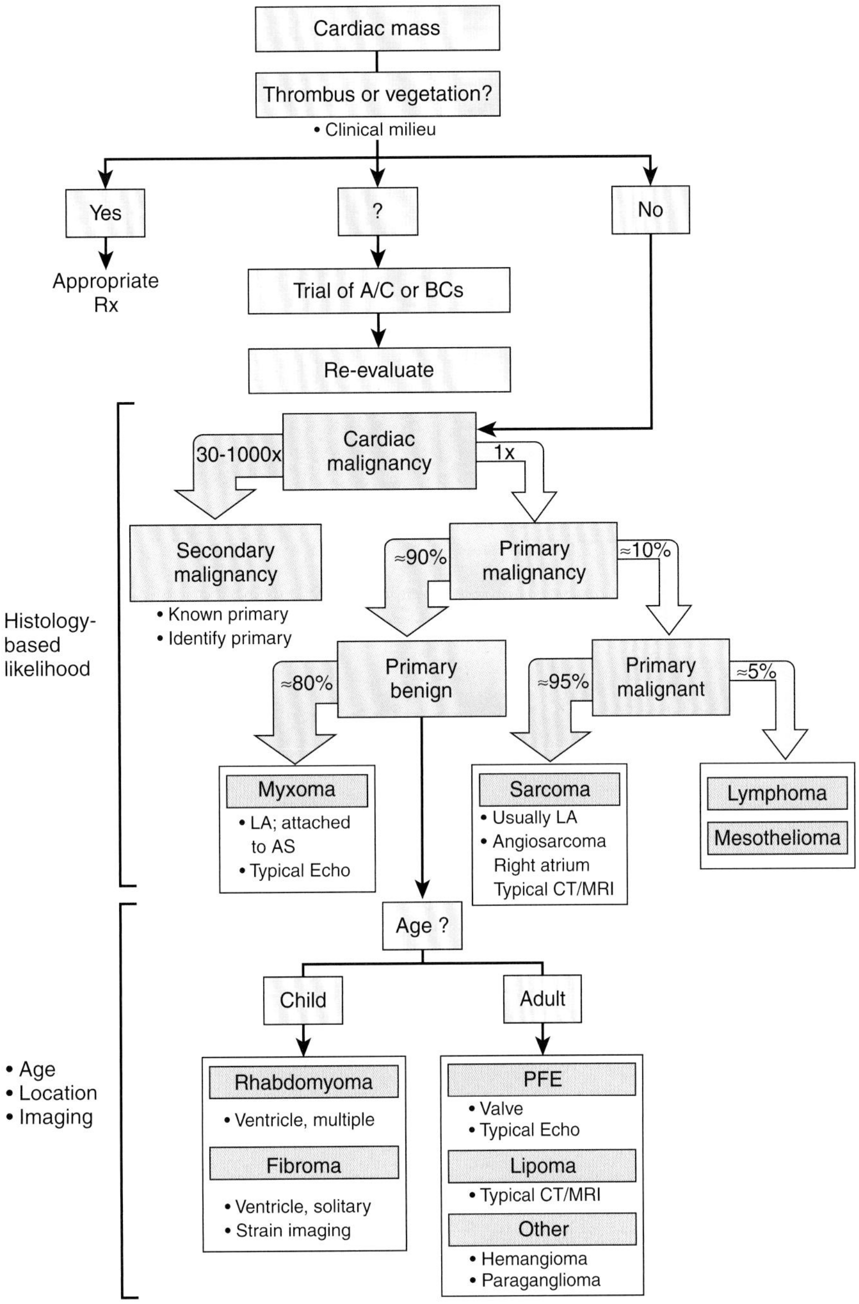

Cardiac mass

Thrombus or vegetation?
• Clinical milieu

Yes → Appropriate Rx

? → Trial of A/C or BCs → Re-evaluate

No → Cardiac malignancy

Histology-based likelihood

Cardiac malignancy: 30-1000x → Secondary malignancy; 1x → Primary malignancy

Secondary malignancy
• Known primary
• Identify primary

Primary malignancy: ≈90% → Primary benign; ≈10% → Primary malignant

Primary benign: ≈80% → Myxoma

Myxoma
• LA; attached to AS
• Typical Echo

Primary malignant: ≈95% → Sarcoma; ≈5% → Lymphoma, Mesothelioma

Sarcoma
• Usually LA
• Angiosarcoma
Right atrium
Typical CT/MRI

Lymphoma

Mesothelioma

• Age
• Location
• Imaging

Age ?

Child:

Rhabdomyoma
• Ventricle, multiple

Fibroma
• Ventricle, solitary
• Strain imaging

Adult:

PFE
• Valve
• Typical Echo

Lipoma
• Typical CT/MRI

Other
• Hemangioma
• Paraganglioma

Fig. 18.8 Diagnostic algorithm for evaluation of a cardiac mass. This approach relies on histology-based likelihood, age, location, and imaging characteristics. *A/C*, Anticoagulation; *AS*, aortic stenosis; *BCs*, blood cultures; *CT*, computed tomography; *IAS*, interatrial septum; *MRI*, magnetic resonance imaging; *PFE*, papillary fibroelastoma; *Rx*, treatment.

More than 80% of primary cardiac tumors are benign; myxoma is the most common.[65,66] The remaining 20% of primary cardiac tumors are malignant. The most common malignant primary tumor type in every large series has been sarcoma. In the MD Anderson series, sarcomas were followed in prevalence by paragangliomas and myxomas.

PRIMARY CARDIAC MALIGNANT TUMORS

Most primary cardiac sarcomas are angiosarcomas in the RA.[67] Osteosarcomas and unclassified sarcomas are predominantly found on the left side of the heart.[68,69] Pericardial angiosarcomas are rare. About 29% of cardiac sarcomas have metastasized by the time of diagnosis.[70] In the pediatric population, rhabdomyosarcoma is the most common form of cardiac sarcoma. Leiomyosarcoma, synovial sarcoma, osteosarcoma, fibrosarcoma, myxoidsarcoma, liposarcoma, mesenchymal sarcoma, neurofibrosarcoma, and malignant fibrous histiocytoma are other cardiac sarcomas observed.[69,70]

SECONDARY (METASTATIC) CARDIAC MALIGNANT TUMORS

Compared with older series, there was a significant increase in the incidence of cardiac metastases in cancer patients after 1970,[66] probably related to improvements in technique and availability of cardiac imaging modalities. The pericardium is most often involved by direct invasion by thoracic malignancies.

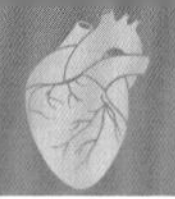

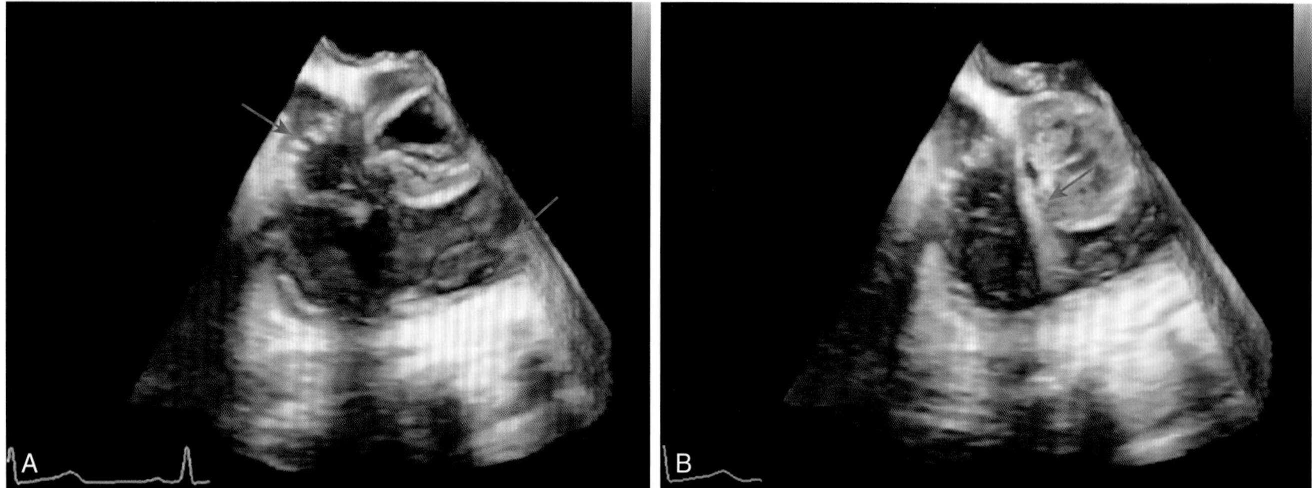

Fig. 18.9 Visualization of RV outflow tract mass with echocardiography-guided myocardial biopsy. 3D TEE images were obtained during an echocardiography-guided myocardial biopsy for a 66-year-old man with colorectal cancer. Biopsy was performed to investigate whether the mass was a metastatic lesion or a new primary tumor. (A) 3D short-axis view at the level of the aortic valve shows a suture line for a tricuspid valve annulolasty ring *(arrow on left)* and a mass in the RV outflow tract *(arrow on right)* (see Video 18.9A). (B) 3D TEE imaging was then used to guide the bioptome *(arrow)* (see Video 18.9B).

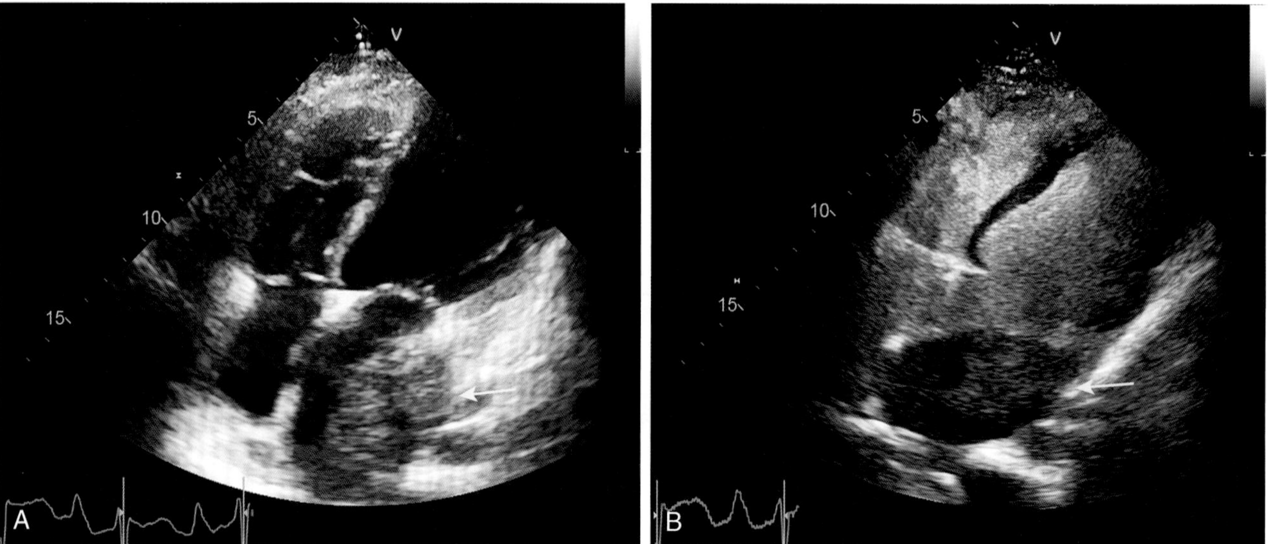

Fig. 18.10 Use of contrast in imaging of an extracardiac mass. A 21-year-old woman with synovial sarcoma in the mediastinum had a tumor pressing on the LA and apparent mass effect causing a convex deformity of the LA wall. (A) A mass outside the LA *(arrow)* compresses the chamber (see Video 18.10A). (B) In the same patient, images with microbubble enhancement improve visualization of the mass *(arrow)* (see Video 18.10B).

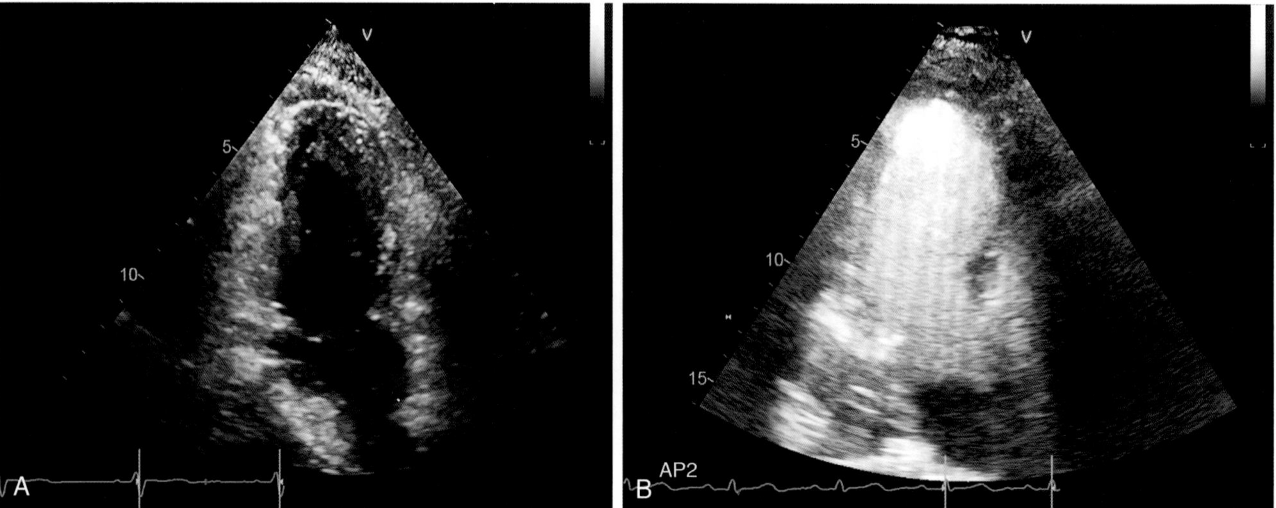

Fig. 18.11 LA mass was identified as a melanoma metastasis. (A) Apical view in a 70-year-old woman with melanoma and a tumor lesion in the LA. (B) In the same patient, the mass is easier to recognize using microbubble enhancement.

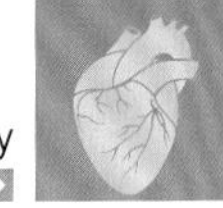

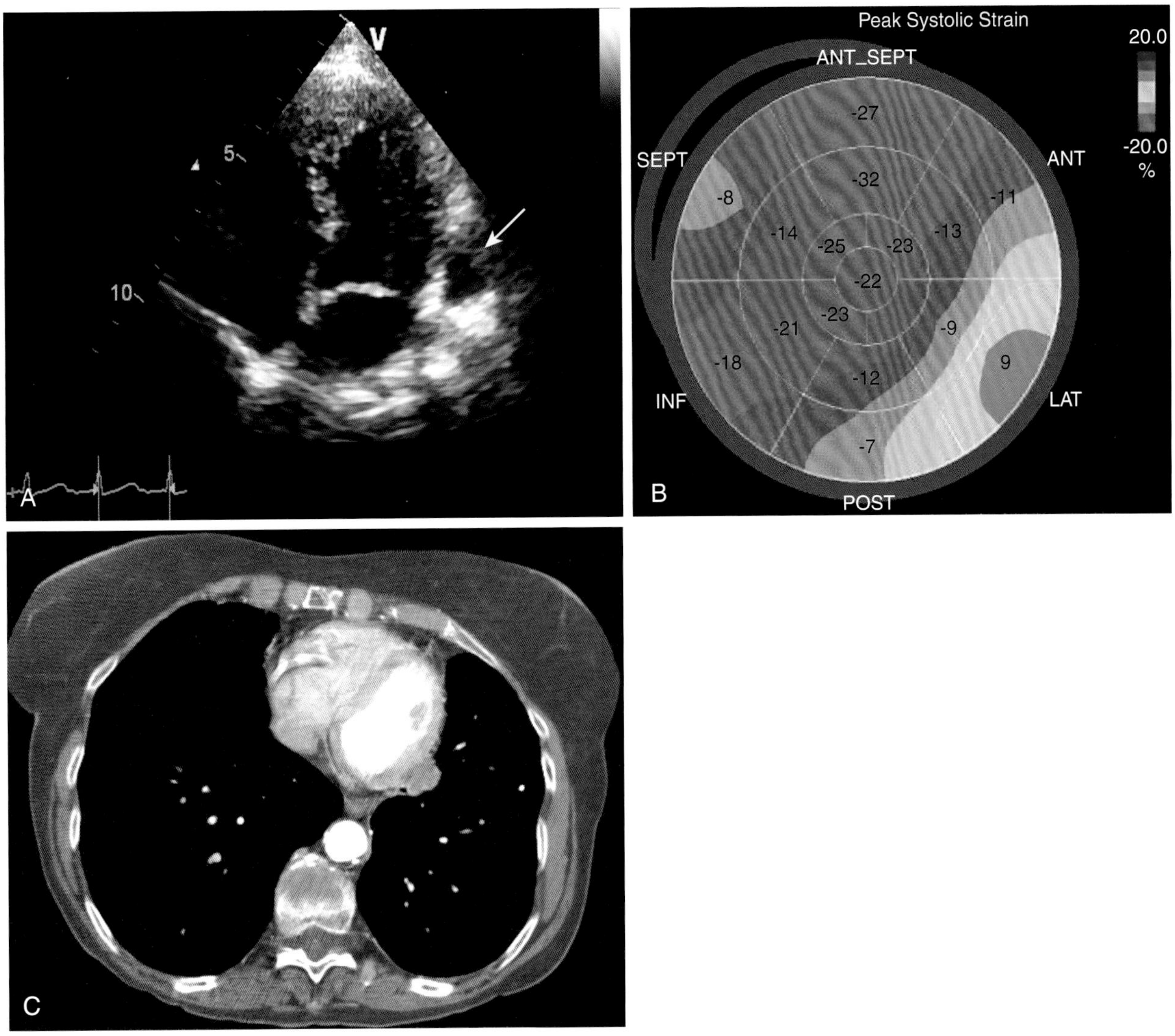

Fig. 18.12 **Mass invading the lateral wall base visualized by multimodality imaging.** (A) Apical 4-chamber view in an 80-year-old woman with a history of left upper lobectomy for adenocarcinoma years earlier who presented with tachycardia, dyspnea, and an echolucency *(arrow)* at the lateral wall base on 2D echocardiography (see Video 18.12A ▶). (B) Longitudinal strain polar map representation suggests a significant systolic abnormality corresponding to the lateral wall base. (C) Chest CT confirms a mass invading the lateral wall base. This was identified as a recurrence of the primary lung tumor.

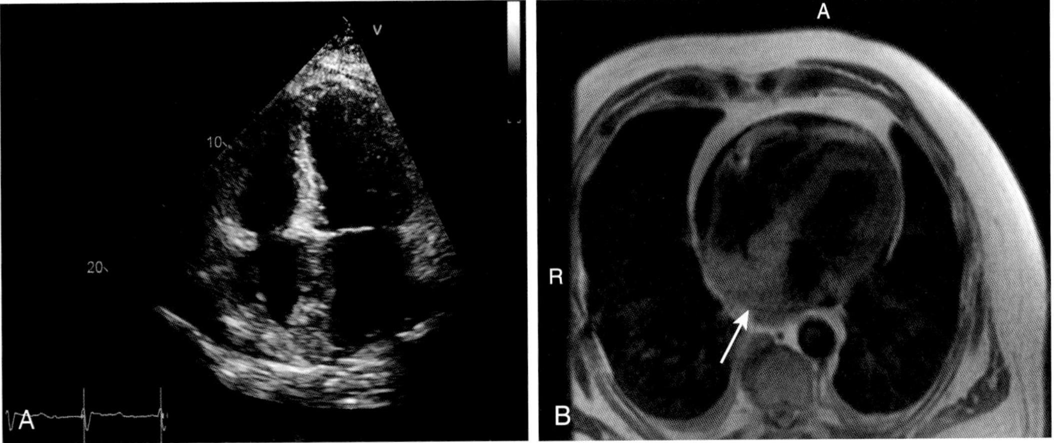

Fig. 18.13 **Lymphoma invading the heart.** (A) In a 70-year-old man with mantle cell lymphoma after multiple courses of chemotherapy and refractory mediastinal disease, the 4-chamber view shows marked thickening of the interatrial septum in a straight pattern, suggesting tumor infiltration; this is different from the lipomatous infiltration for which a bilobed pattern is more common. (B) Cardiac magnetic resonance image shows extensive mass infiltration *(arrow)* extending along the epicardial surface and involving the interatrial septum. There was encasement of the ascending thoracic aorta and partial atrial encasement with associated pericardial effusion.

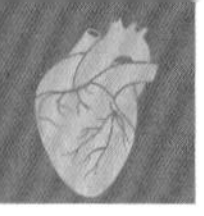

TABLE 18.7 **Techniques for the Diagnosis of Cardiac Tumors.**

Tumor	*Echocardiography*	*CT*	*MRI*
Primary benign myxoma	+++++	+++	+++
Lipoma	+++	+++++	+++++
Fibroelastoma	+++++	++	++
Rhabdomyoma	+++++	+++	+++
Fibroma	++++	++++	+++
Primary malignant sarcomas	+++	++++	+++++
Mesotheliomas	++	+++++	++++
Lymphomas	++	++++	+++++
Secondary tumors direct extension	+++	+++++	+++++
Venous extension	++++	++++	+++++
Metastatic spread	++	+++++	++++

CT, Computed tomography; *MRI*, magnetic resonance imaging; +, of limited use; ++, may be of use; +++, useful; ++++, very useful; +++++, preferred diagnostic tool.

The myocardium or epicardium is most commonly involved through lymphatic spread, and endocardial metastases are the result of hematogenous spread.

Patients with secondary (metastatic) cardiac tumors are, on average, older than those with sarcomas. The RA is the most common location. For secondary tumors, the second most common site in the MD Anderson series[58] was the LA, followed by the RV, the RA and RV combined, the LA, and the MV. There was one instance in which all three left-sided structures were involved (Fig. 18.14).

Most secondary cardiac tumors were metastases from renal cell carcinoma; 14% were from extracardiac sarcomas. The primary solid tumor location varied considerably (i.e., pleura, retroperitoneum, pelvis, endometrium, mediastinum and IVC). Lung cancer is found as frequently as sarcomas, followed by breast and carcinoid tumors. Despite melanoma being described in a few reports as a neoplasm with a propensity to metastasize to the heart, this represented a minority of cases in the MD Anderson series.[71–73]

DIFFERENTIAL DIAGNOSIS

When confronted with a suspicious mass, it is important to integrate all the clinical information (e.g., patient age, history of malignant disease) with all the echocardiographic information. The most likely cause of an intracardiac mass is a thrombus, followed by a vegetation. Often, a cardiac mass is diagnosed when in fact there is only an unusual plane of a normal cardiac structure or a normal anatomic variant. It is important to distinguish these findings from cardiac tumors.

Associated echocardiographic findings provide important clues about the cause of the mass. For example, thrombi and vegetations have characteristic echocardiographic features, but they can often be distinguished from one another and from other cardiac masses by their particular intracardiac location (e.g., LA appendage or ventricular apex versus valve leaflets) and by their associated conditions (e.g., atrial fibrillation, LA enlargement, MV disease, valvular destruction, bacteremia).

Thrombi seldom occur as an isolated finding. Ventricular thrombi usually occur in the setting of coronary artery disease with associated akinetic or dyskinetic myocardial segments, most commonly an aneurysmal LV apex with concomitant LV dysfunction. Atrial thrombi usually occur within the LA appendage in patients with atrial fibrillation, MV disease, amyloidosis, and LA enlargement. Ancillary features of sluggish blood flow, such as spontaneous echocardiographic contrast and reduced LA appendage emptying velocity, may be present.

Another useful clinical strategy for determining whether a mass is a thrombus or a tumor is to perform a serial echocardiographic evaluation after a period of systemic anticoagulation therapy. Thrombi usually resolve after 4 weeks of anticoagulation therapy, whereas tumors increase in size or remain unchanged.

Vegetations may be confused with cardiac tumors. However, apart from papillary fibroelastomas, primary tumors of the cardiac valves are rare. Vegetations appear as mobile echogenic masses attached to valves and are usually diagnosed in the setting of known or suspected valve disease and bacteremia. Valvular vegetations in the setting of infective endocarditis are usually accompanied by features of valvular destruction and consequent regurgitation. Occasionally, when vegetations are seen in the absence of bacteremia, underlying malignant disease may represent nonbacterial thrombotic endocarditis (NBTE) or marantic endocarditis. Libman–Sacks endocarditis, a form of nonbacterial endocarditis, can be seen in association with systemic lupus erythematosus. Nonvalvular vegetations occur at sites of turbulence and may be attached to the ventricular endocardial surface in patients with hypertrophic obstructive cardiomyopathy and in patients with septal defects.

Infiltrative disorders that involve the heart may mimic cardiac tumors. They include cardiac involvement by sarcoidosis, Wegener's granulomatosis,[63] hypereosinophilic syndrome,[64] and tuberculosis. Specific pathologic cardiac disorders that have been confused with cardiac tumors[65] include cardiac varices, coronary artery fistula,[66] coronary artery aneurysm,[66,67] atrial septal aneurysm,[68,69] intramyocardial hematoma[69] after percutaneous intervention, blood cysts, and pericardial cysts.

Normal cardiac structures potentially confused with tumors include a prominent crista terminalis, eustachian valves, Chiari network, lipomatous hypertrophy of the atrial septum, and the ridge of tissue seen between the left superior pulmonary vein and the LA appendage on TEE, also known as the ligament of Marshall. Even a diaphragmatic hernia may be confused with a cardiac tumor. It can be readily identified by having the patient drink a carbonated beverage while being imaged and confirming the presence of gas bubbles in the lumen. Knowledge of these normal cardiac structures and normal variants of cardiac anatomy is important to prevent unnecessary additional evaluation, biopsy, or repeated cardiac imaging tests, which can cause significant anxiety for the patient.

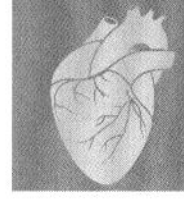

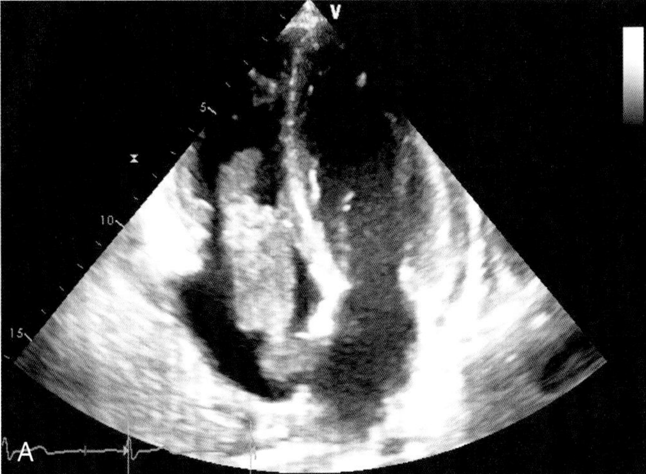

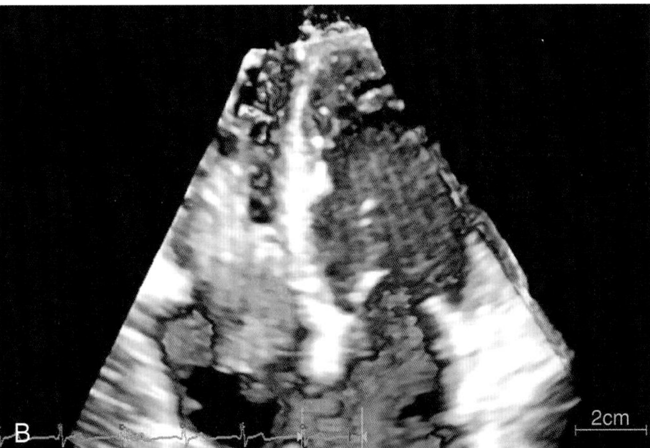

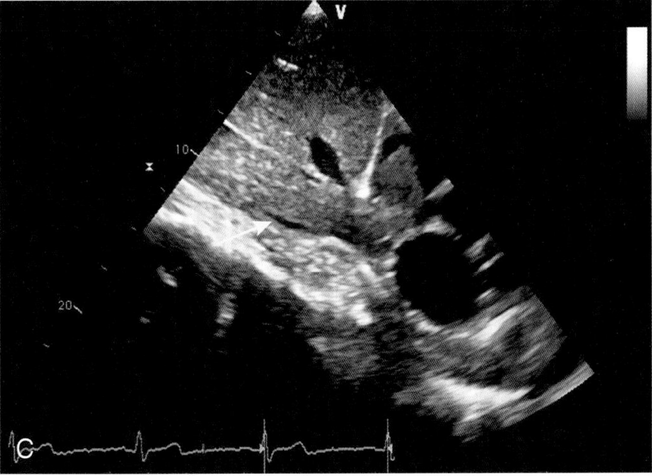

Fig. 18.14 **Large mass in the RA and RV invading from inferior vena cava.** (A) 4-Chamber view in a 59-year-old man with renal cell carcinoma (RCC); a large mass is protruding into the RA and moving deep into the RV in diastole (see Video 18.14A). (B) The same view as a full-volume 3D image shows the mass making contact with the RV moderator band in diastole (see Video 18.14.B). (C) Subcostal view with the mass *(arrow)* in longitudinal view as it comes from the inferior vena cava (see Video 18.14C).

PROGNOSIS

Recognition of cardiac lesions portends a significant change in prognosis. Almost one half (44%) of patients with malignant primary cardiac tumors die within 12 months after diagnosis. Unlike other sarcomas, cardiac sarcomas have a very poor prognosis, with a median survival rate of 6 to 25 months after diagnosis.[68,69] Tumor necrosis and metastases are associated with a poor prognosis.[68,70] A systematic review of the literature revealed a cumulative 30-day mortality rate of 6.7% for primary cardiac sarcomas in children.[74] Sarcomas other than angiosarcomas, sarcomas in the left heart, and completely resected sarcomas have a better prognosis.[68,70] Angiosarcomas grow faster, infiltrate widely, and metastasize early; they therefore have a poor prognosis.

After metastasizing to other organs, melanoma is by definition stage IV and associated with poor survival rates. The reported 5-year survival rate in this case is 15% to 20%.[75] Similarly, sarcomas that metastasize to the myocardium are frequently high-grade tumors that progress quickly. Myocardial infiltration, outflow obstruction, and distant metastasis result in death within a few weeks to 2 years after onset of symptoms, with median survival ranging from 6 to 12 months. Different series document the metastatic rate to be between 26% and 43% at presentation and 75% at the time of death.[68,70,76–83] More than one half of patients with a secondary tumor die within 12 months after diagnosis. Of the patients with secondary cardiac tumors who do not undergo surgery, 65% are dead within 1 year after diagnosis.

TREATMENT

Surgical treatment of cardiac tumors began in the late 1930s, when an intrapericardial cystic teratoma that extended to the patient's RV was removed.[84] The surgical treatment of cardiac tumors radically changed and progressed after the introduction of cardiopulmonary bypass in 1953.[85] This allowed controlled access to the interior chambers of the heart and led to multiple reports of successful cardiac mass excisions, mostly myxomas.[86,87] Cardiac tumor resection has continued despite challenges related to the inherent technical difficulties of any major cardiac resection and the aggressive biology of some tumors. Survival improves with surgical resection.[88] Novel approaches allowing a more complete tumor resection, such as cardiac autotransplantation, have proved succesful.[89,90]

For treatment purposes, cardiac sarcomas are divided into three groups: right heart sarcomas, left heart sarcomas, and pulmonary artery sarcomas.[91] The treatment for right heart and left heart sarcomas is chemotherapy and surgical resection. Direct cardiac radiation therapy is avoided because it can injure the myocardium. Treatment of metastatic cardiac tumors is usually palliative.

Different series have shown that the median survival time is 17 to 24 months for patients who can undergo complete tumor resection and 6 to 10 months for those who are unable to do so.[70,92] One study showed that 14.8% of the resected tumors were low grade, and all of those patients were alive at follow-up.[95] This underlies the importance of early detection and tumor grade in the survival of postoperative patients.

Surgery with postoperative chemotherapy and/or radiation therapy to prevent local recurrence is indicated for patients with a better prognosis and when they have only cardiac metastases without disseminated disease. Orthotopic heart transplantation is an option for selected patients and is associated with improved survival.[93,94]

For patients with disseminated disease, limited life expectancy, and poor performance status, radiation therapy is sometimes offered. Chemotherapy is recommended for tumors that are chemosensitive. End-of-life care should be discussed with all patients, and all efforts should be made to improve the patient's quality of life.

SUMMARY Cardiac Tumors and Cardio-oncology.

Cancer-Related Cardiac Pathology	Clinical Elements	Key Imaging Aspects

Cardiac chemotoxicity	• Anthracyclines
	  • Doxorubicin (Adriamycin) Epirubicin (Ellence)
	  • Idarubicin (Idamycin)
	• Alkylating agents
	  • Cyclophosphamide (Cytoxan)
	  • Ifosfamide (Ifex)
	• Antimetabolites
	  • Clofarabine (Clolar)
	• Antimicrotubule agents
	  • Docetaxel (Taxotere)
	• Monoclonal antibody–based tyrosine kinase inhibitors
	  • Bevacizumab (Avastin)
	  • Trastuzumab (Herceptin)
	• Proteasome inhibitor
	  • Bortezomib (Velcade)
	• Small-molecule tyrosine kinase inhibitors
	  • Dasatinib (Sprycel)
	  • Imatinib mesylate (Gleevec)
	  • Lapatinib (Tykerb)
	  • Sunitinib (Sutent)
	  • Chimeric antigen receptor (CAR) T-cell therapy (CRS/stress induced)
	• Immune modulators
	  • Interferon
	• Immune modulators
	  • Interleukins (myocarditis related)
	• Immune checkpoint inhibitors (myocarditis related)
		• The most commonly clinically used LVEF measure in practice is the biplane method of disks (i.e., modified Simpson rule).
		• Microbubble enhancement offers the best results for 2D echocardiography in terms of intraobserver and interobserver variability, a key factor in serial assessments of LVEF.
		• 3D echocardiography is more accurate than 2D echocardiography for ventricular volume and EF measurements compared with CMR imaging.
		• GLS is an important modality to detect cardiotoxicity before decrements in LVEF occur.
		• A relative percentage reduction in GLS of >15% is very likely to be abnormal, whereas a change of <8% appears to be of no clinical significance.
		• Abnormalities in LVEF and GLS should be confirmed by repeat echocardiography in 2–3 weeks.

Radiation-induced cardiac damage	Pericarditis Pericardial effusion Valvular stenosis Valvular regurgitation Epicardial coronary artery disease Microvascular disease and dysfunction	• Presentation is usually many years after exposure.

Cardiac tumors—general	• Primary
	• Secondary
	• Benign
	• Malignant
		• Key echocardiographic descriptors of cardiac masses
		  • Location
		  • Attachment
		  • Shape
		  • Dimensions/volume
		  • Hemodynamic consequences
		  • Impact on myocardial function
		• TEE advantages
		  • Spatial resolution
		  • Image clarity
		  • 3D images
		• Microbubble contrast can be used to improve definition and characterization of cardiac masses.
		• CMR and cardiac CT can give a more complete view of the mediastinum, particularly illustrating attachments of a mass outside of the cardiac cavities, and have advantages in terms of tissue characterization.

Continued

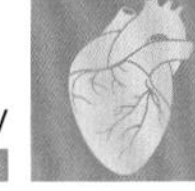

SUMMARY Cardiac Tumors and Cardio-oncology.—cont'd

Cancer-Related Cardiac Pathology	Clinical Elements	Key Imaging Aspects

Cardiac tumors—specific	• Myxoma
	  • 30–60 y
	  • Interatrial septum at fossa ovalis; LA
	  • Calcification common
		• Mobile, narrow stalk
		• Homogeneous or heterogeneous echotexture

	• Papillary fibroelastoma
	  • Middle-aged, elderly
	  • Cardiac valves
		• Small (<1 cm), frondlike, narrow stalk
		• "Shimmering" edges

	• Lipoma (variable)
	  • Multiple fatty lesions in tuberous sclerosis
	  • May be lipomas or angiomyolipomas
	  • Pericardial space or any cardiac chamber
		• Large, broad-based
		• Homogeneous
		• Usually hypoechoic in the pericardial space, echogenic in a cardiac chamber

	• Hemangioma
	  • All ages; mean, 4th decade
	  • One third in RV, one third in LV, one fourth in RA
		• Multilobulated, unilocular, cystic, <1–8 cm
		• "Solid" echo-dense

	• Rhabdomyoma
	  • Infants, children <4 y
	  • Tuberous sclerosis
	  • Spontaneous regression
	  • LV, RV, in walls of aortic valves, outflow tract
		• Mural, pedunculated multiple, variable size
		• Brighter than surrounding myocardium

	• Fibroma
	  • Infants, children, young adults
	  • Gorlin syndrome
	  • Ventricles
		• Large, intramural
		• Calcifications
		• Broad-based, infiltrative or circumscribed

	• Paraganglioma
	  • Young adults
	  • Almost always sporadic
	  • LA, coronary arteries, aortic root
		• Echogenic
		• Relatively immobile

CMR, Cardiac magnetic resonance; *CRS*, cytokine release syndrome; *CT*, computed tomography; *EF*, ejection fraction; *GLS*, global longitudinal strain; *LVEF*, left ventricular ejection fraction.

REFERENCES

1. Lambert JT, Thavendiranathan P. Controversies in the definition of cardiotoxicity: do we care? American College of Cardiology. 2016. Available at: https://www.acc.org/latest-in-cardiology/articles/2016/07/07/14/59/controversies-in-the-definition-of-cardiotoxicity.
2. Al-Mamgani A, Baartman L, Baaijens M, de Pree I, Incrocci L, Levendag PC. Cardiac metastases. *Int J Clin Oncol.* 2008;13:369–372.
3. Virmani RS, Burke A, Farb A. *Atlas of Cardiovascular Pathology*. 1st ed. Philadelphia, PA: Saunders; 1996.
4. Eisenhauer EA, Therasse P, Bogaerts J, et al. New response evaluation criteria in solid tumours: revised RECIST guideline (version 1.1). *Eur J Cancer.* 2009;45:228–247.
5. Seidman A, Hudis C, Pierri MK, et al. Cardiac dysfunction in the trastuzumab clinical trials experience. *J Clin Oncol.* 2002;20:1215–1221.
6. Moja L, Tagliabue L, Balduzzi S, et al. Trastuzumab containing regimens for early breast cancer. *Cochrane Database Syst Rev.* 2012. 2012(4):CD006243.
7. Alcan KE, Robeson W, Graham MC, Palestro C, Oliver FH, Benua RS. Early detection of anthracycline-induced cardiotoxicity by stress radionuclide cineangiography in conjunction with Fourier amplitude and phase analysis. *Clin Nucl Med.* 1985;10:160–166.
8. Lenzhofer R, Dudczak R, Gumhold G, Graninger W, Moser K, Spitzy KH. Noninvasive methods for the early detection of doxorubicin-induced cardiomyopathy. *J Canc Res Clin Oncol.* 1983;106:136–142.
9. McKillop JH, Bristow MR, Goris ML, Billingham ME, Bockemuehl K. Sensitivity and specificity of radionuclide ejection fractions in doxorubicin cardiotoxicity. *Am Heart J.* 1983;106:1048–1056.
10. Pauwels EK, Horning SJ, Goris ML. Sequential equilibrium gated radionuclide angiocardiography for the detection of doxorubicin cardiotoxicity. *Radiother Oncol.* 1983;1:83–87.
11. Ramos A, Meyer RA, Korfhagen J, Wong KY, Kaplan S. Echocardiographic evaluation of adriamycin cardiotoxicity in children. *Canc Treat Rep.* 1976;60:1281–1284.
12. Lang RM, Badano LP, Mor-Avi V, et al. Recommendations for cardiac chamber quantification by echocardiography in adults: an update from the American Society of Echocardiography and the European Association of Cardiovascular Imaging. *J Am Soc Echocardiogr.* 2015;28:1–39. e14.
13. Hoffmann R, von Bardeleben S, Kasprzak JD, et al. Analysis of regional left ventricular function by cineventriculography, cardiac magnetic resonance imaging, and unenhanced and contrast-enhanced echocardiography: a multicenter comparison of methods. *J Am Coll Cardiol.* 2006;47:121–128.
14. Jenkins C, Chan J, Hanekom L, Marwick TH. Accuracy and feasibility of online 3-dimensional echocardiography for measurement of left ventricular parameters. *J Am Soc Echocardiogr.* 2006;19:1119–1128.
15. Jenkins C, Moir S, Chan J, Rakhit D, Haluska B, Marwick TH. Left ventricular volume measurement with echocardiography: a comparison of left ventricular opacification, three-dimensional echocardiography, or both with magnetic resonance imaging. *Eur Heart J.* 2009;30:98–106.
16. Thavendiranathan P, Grant AD, Negishi T, Plana JC, Popovic ZB, Marwick TH. Reproducibility of echocardiographic techniques for sequential assessment of left ventricular ejection fraction and volumes: application to patients undergoing cancer chemotherapy. *J Am Coll Cardiol.* 2013;61:77–84.

16a. Stoddard MF, Seeger J, Liddell NE, Hadley TJ, Sullivan DM, Kupersmith J. Prolongation of isovolumetric relaxation time as assessed by Doppler echocardiography predicts doxorubicin-induced systolic dysfunction in humans. *J Am Coll Cardiol.* 1992;20(1):62–69.

17. McCall R, Stoodley PW, Richards DA, Thomas L. Restrictive cardiomyopathy versus constrictive pericarditis: making the distinction using tissue Doppler imaging. *Eur J Echocardiogr.* 2008;9:591–594.
18. Tei C, Ling LH, Hodge DO, et al. New index of combined systolic and diastolic myocardial performance: a simple and reproducible measure of cardiac function—a study in normals and dilated cardiomyopathy. *J Cardiol.* 1995;26:357–366.

19. Ishii M, Tsutsumi T, Himeno W, et al. Sequential evaluation of left ventricular myocardial performance in children after anthracycline therapy. *Am J Cardiol.* 2000;86:1279–1281, a9.
20. Belham M, Kruger A, Mepham S, Faganello G, Pritchard C. Monitoring left ventricular function in adults receiving anthracycline-containing chemotherapy. *Eur J Heart Fail.* 2007;9:409–414.
21. Hare JL, Brown JK, Leano R, Jenkins C, Woodward N, Marwick TH. Use of myocardial deformation imaging to detect preclinical myocardial dysfunction before conventional measures in patients undergoing breast cancer treatment with trastuzumab. *Am Heart J.* 2009;158:294–301.
22. Fallah-Rad N, Walker JR, Wassef A, et al. The utility of cardiac biomarkers, tissue velocity and strain imaging, and cardiac magnetic resonance imaging in predicting early left ventricular dysfunction in patients with human epidermal growth factor receptor II-positive breast cancer treated with adjuvant trastuzumab therapy. *J Am Coll Cardiol.* 2011;57:2263–2270.
23. Sawaya H, Sebag IA, Plana JC, et al. Early detection and prediction of cardiotoxicity in chemotherapy-treated patients. *Am J Cardiol.* 2011;107:1375–1380.
24. Thavendiranathan P, Poulin F, Lim KD, Plana JC, Woo A, Marwick TH. Use of myocardial strain imaging by echocardiography for the early detection of cardiotoxicity in patients during and after cancer chemotherapy: a systematic review. *J Am Coll Cardiol.* 2014;63:2751–2768.
25. Narayan HK, French B, Khan AM, et al. Noninvasive measures of ventricular-arterial coupling and circumferential strain predict cancer therapeutics-related cardiac dysfunction. *JACC Cardiovasc Imaging.* 2016;9:1131–1141.
26. Plana JC, Galderisi M, Barac A, et al. Expert consensus for multimodality imaging evaluation of adult patients during and after cancer therapy: a report from the American Society of Echocardiography and the European Association of Cardiovascular Imaging. *J Am Soc Echocardiogr.* 2014;27:911–939.
27. Belham M, Kruger A, Pritchard C. The Tei index identifies a differential effect on left and right ventricular function with low-dose anthracycline chemotherapy. *J Am Soc Echocardiogr.* 2006;19:206–210.
28. Boczar KE, Aseyev O, Sulpher J, et al. Right heart function deteriorates in breast cancer patients undergoing anthracycline-based chemotherapy. *Echo Res Pract.* 2016;3:79–84.
29. Brosius 3rd FC, Waller BF, Roberts WC. Radiation heart disease. Analysis of 16 young (aged 15 to 33 years) necropsy patients who received over 3,500 rads to the heart. *Am J Med.* 1981;70:519–530.
30. Veinot JP, Edwards WD. Pathology of radiation-induced heart disease: a surgical and autopsy study of 27 cases. *Hum Pathol.* 1996;27:766–773.
31. Reuss CS, Wilansky SM, Lester SJ, et al. Using mitral 'annulus reversus' to diagnose constrictive pericarditis. *Eur J Echocardiogr.* 2009;10:372–375.
32. Hering D, Faber L, Horstkotte D. Echocardiographic features of radiation-associated valvular disease. *Am J Cardiol.* 2003;92:226–230.
33. Heidenreich PA, Hancock SL, Lee BK, Mariscal CS, Schnittger I. Asymptomatic cardiac disease following mediastinal irradiation. *J Am Coll Cardiol.* 2003;42:743–749.
34. Lund MB, Ihlen H, Voss BM, et al. Increased risk of heart valve regurgitation after mediastinal radiation for Hodgkin's disease: an echocardiographic study. *Heart.* 1996;75:591–595.
35. Columbo MR. *De Re Anatomica Libri XV.* Venice: Nicolò Bevilacqua; 1559.
36. Hanfling SM. Metastatic cancer to the heart. Review of the literature and report of 127 cases. *Circulation.* 1960;22:474–483.
37. Xu ZF, Yong F, Chen YY, Pan AZ. Uterine intravenous leiomyomatosis with cardiac extension: imaging characteristics and literature review. *World J Clin Oncol.* 2013;4:25–28.
38. Marshall VF, Middleton RG, Holswade GR, Goldsmith EI. Surgery for renal cell carcinoma in the vena cava. *J Urol.* 1970;103:414–420.
39. Jun CH, Sim da W, Kim SH, et al. Risk factors for patients with stage IVB hepatocellular carcinoma and extension into the heart: prognostic and therapeutic implications. *Yonsei Med J.* 2014;55:379–386.
40. Steinberg C, Boudreau S, Leveille F, Lamothe M, Chagnon P, Boulais I. Advanced hepatocellular carcinoma with subtotal occlusion of the inferior vena cava and a right atrial mass. *Case Rep Vasc Med.* 2013;2013:489373.
41. Detterbeck FC, Parsons AM. Thymic tumors. *Ann Thorac Surg.* 2004;77:1860–1869.
42. Ban-Hoefen M, Zeglin MA, Bisognano JD. Diffuse large B cell lymphoma presenting as a cardiac mass and odynophagia. *Cardiol J.* 2008;15:471–474.
43. El Banna M, Geraldes L, Grapsa J, et al. Large mediastinal neoplasm penetrating the myocardium. *Perfusion.* 2019;34:170–172.
44. Aoyagi S, Tayama E, Yokokura Y, Yokokura H. Right atrial myxoma in a patient presenting with syncope. *Kurume Med J.* 2004;51:91–93.
45. Kubota H, Takamoto S, Kotsuka Y, et al. Surgical treatment of malignant tumors of the right heart. *Jpn Heart J.* 2002;43:263–271.
46. Alzeerah MA, Singh R, Jarrous A. Large B-cell lymphoma of the atria. *Tex Heart Inst J.* 2003;30:74–75.
47. Rettmar K, Stierle U, Sheikhzadeh A, Diederich KW. Primary angiosarcoma of the heart. Report of a case and review of the literature. *Jpn Heart J.* 1993;34:667–683.
48. Marti G, Galve E, Huguet J, Soler Soler J. [Cardiac metastases of malignant melanoma mimicking sick sinus syndrome]. *Revista espanola de cardiologia.* 2004;57:589–591.
49. Schrepfer S, Deuse T, Detter C, et al. Successful resection of a symptomatic right ventricular lipoma. *Ann Thorac Surg.* 2003;76:1305–1307.
50. Uzun O, Wilson DG, Vujanic GM, Parsons JM, De Giovanni JV. Cardiac tumours in children. *Orphanet J Rare Dis.* 2007;2:11.
51. Elbardissi AW, Dearani JA, Daly RC, et al. Survival after resection of primary cardiac tumors: a 48-year experience. *Circulation.* 2008;118:S7–S15.
52. Carney JA, Gordon H, Carpenter PC, Shenoy BV, Go VL. The complex of myxomas, spotty pigmentation, and endocrine overactivity. *Medicine (Baltim).* 1985;64:270–283.
53. Elbardissi AW, Dearani JA, Daly RC, et al. Embolic potential of cardiac tumors and outcome after resection: a case-control study. *Stroke.* 2009;40:156–162.
54. Pugliatti P, Patane S, De Gregorio C, Recupero A, Carerj S, Coglitore S. Lipomatous hypertrophy of the interatrial septum. *Int J Cardiol.* 2008;130:294–295.
55. Araoz PA, Mulvagh SL, Tazelaar HD, Julsrud PR, Breen JF. CT and MR imaging of benign primary cardiac neoplasms with echocardiographic correlation. *Radiographics.* 2000;20:1303–1319.
56. Restrepo CS, Largoza A, Lemos DF, et al. CT and MR imaging findings of benign cardiac tumors. *Curr Prob Diag Radiol.* 2005;34:12–21.
57. Asch FM, Bieganski SP, Panza JA, Weissman NJ. Real-time 3-dimensional echocardiography evaluation of intracardiac masses. *Echocardiography.* 2006;23:218–224.
58. Yusuf SW, Bathina JD, Qureshi S, et al. Cardiac tumors in a tertiary care cancer hospital: clinical features, echocardiographic findings, treatment and outcomes. *Heart Int.* 2012;7:e4.
59. Reddy G, Ahmed MI, Lloyd SG, Brott BC, Bittner V. Left anterior descending coronary artery occlusion secondary to metastatic squamous cell carcinoma presenting as ST-segment-elevation myocardial infarction. *Circulation.* 2014;129:e652–e653.
60. Kirkpatrick JN, Wong T, Bednarz JE, et al. Differential diagnosis of cardiac masses using contrast echocardiographic perfusion imaging. *J Am Coll Cardiol.* 2004;43:1412–1419.
61. Cooper LT, Baughman KL, Feldman AM, et al. The role of endomyocardial biopsy in the management of cardiovascular disease: a scientific statement from the American Heart Association, the American College of Cardiology, and the European Society of Cardiology. *Circulation.* 2007;116:2216–2233.
62. Burns A. Observations on some of the most frequent and important diseases of the heart, etc.; oon the aneurism of the thoracic aorta; Illustrated by cases. *Edinburgh: Printed by James Muirhead, for Thomas Bryce and Co., Etc.* 1809.
63. Yater WM. Tumors of the heart and pericardium: pathology, symptomatology, and report of nine cases. *Arch Intern Med.* 1931;48(4):627–666.
64. Barnes AR, Beaver DC, Snell AM. Primary sarcoma of the heart: report of a case with electrocardiographic and pathological studies. *Am Heart J.* 1934;9(4):480–491.
65. Centofanti P, Di Rosa E, Deorsola L, et al. Primary cardiac tumors: early and late results of surgical treatment in 91 patients. *Ann Thorac Surg.* 1999;68:1236–1241.
66. Perchinsky MJ, Lichtenstein SV, Tyers GF. Primary cardiac tumors: forty years' experience with 71 patients. *Cancer.* 1997;79:1809–1815.
67. Bear PA, Moodie DS. Malignant primary cardiac tumors. The Cleveland Clinic experience, 1956 to 1986. *Chest.* 1987;92:860–862.
68. Burke AP, Cowan D, Virmani R. Primary sarcomas of the heart. *Cancer.* 1992;69:387–395.
69. Kim CH, Dancer JY, Coffey D, et al. Clinicopathologic study of 24 patients with primary cardiac sarcomas: a 10-year single institution experience. *Hum Pathol.* 2008;39:933–938.
70. Simpson L, Kumar SK, Okuno SH, et al. Malignant primary cardiac tumors: review of a single institution experience. *Cancer.* 2008;112:2440–2446.
71. Allen BC, Mohammed TL, Tan CD, Miller DV, Williamson EE, Kirsch JS. Metastatic melanoma to the heart. *Current problems in diagnostic radiology.* 2012;41:159–164.
72. Ambrosio GB. [Frequency of cardiac metastasis: review of 2222 autopsies and critical assessment]. *Arch Sci Med.* 1980;137:29–32.
73. Glancy DL, Roberts WC. The heart in malignant melanoma. A study of 70 autopsy cases. *Am J Cardiol.* 1968;21:555–571.
74. Tzani A, Doulamis IP, Mylonas KS, Avgerinos DV, Nasioudis D. Cardiac tumors in pediatric patients: a systematic review. *World J Pediatr Congenit Heart Surg.* 2017;8:624–632.

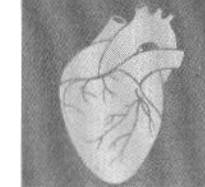

75. Aerts BR, Kock MC, Kofflard MJ, Plaisier PW. Cardiac metastasis of malignant melanoma: a case report. *Neth Heart J*. 2014;22:39–41.
76. Burke APTH, Butany J, et al. *Cardiac Sarcoma*. Lyon, France: IARC Press; 2004.
77. Mayer F, Aebert H, Rudert M, et al. Primary malignant sarcomas of the heart and great vessels in adult patients—a single-center experience. *Oncol*. 2007;12:1134–1142.
78. Llombart-Cussac A, Pivot X, Contesso G, et al. Adjuvant chemotherapy for primary cardiac sarcomas: the IGR experience. *Br J Cancer*. 1998;78:1624–1628.
79. Burgert SJ, Strickman NE, Carrol CL, Falcone M. *Catheter Cardiovasc Interv*. 2000;49:208–212.
80. Raaf HN, Raaf JH. Sarcomas related to the heart and vasculature. *Semin Surg Oncol*. 1994;10:374–382.
81. Knobel B, Rosman P, Kishon Y, Husar M. Intracardiac primary fibrosarcoma. Case report and literature review. *Thorac Cardiovasc Surg*. 1992;40:227–230.
82. Laya MB, Mailliard JA, Bewtra C, Levin HS. Malignant fibrous histiocytoma of the heart. A case report and review of the literature. *Cancer*. 1987;59:1026–1031.
83. Donsbeck AV, Ranchere D, Coindre JM, Le Gall F, Cordier JF, Loire R. Primary cardiac sarcomas: an immunohistochemical and grading study with long-term follow-up of 24 cases. *Histopathology*. 1999;34:295–304.
84. Mauer E. Successful removal of tumor of the heart. *J Thorac Surg*. 1952;3:479.
85. Craaford C. Panel discussion of late results of mitral commissurotomy. In: Lam CR, ed. *Henry Ford Hospital International Symposium on Cardiovascular Surgery*. 1955:202–203.
86. Kay JH, Anderson RM, Meihaus J, et al. Surgical removal of an intracavitary left ventricular myxoma. *Circulation*. 1959;20:881–886.
87. Gerbode F, Kerth WJ, Hill JD. Surgical management of tumors of the heart. *Surgery*. 1967;61:94–101.
88. Cooley DA, Reardon MJ, Frazier OH, Angelini P. Human cardiac explantation and autotransplantation: application in a patient with a large cardiac pheochromocytoma. *Tex Heart Inst J*. 1985;12:171–176.
89. Hoffmeier A, Scheld HH, Tjan TD, et al. Ex situ resection of primary cardiac tumors. *Thorac Cardiovasc Surg*. 2003;51:99–101.
90. Ewer MS, Benjamin RS. *Doxorubicin Cardiotoxicity: Clinical Apect, Recognition, Monitoring, Treatment, and Prevention*. In *Cancer and the Heart*. Hamilton: BC Decker, Ontario, 9–32. 2006.
91. Reardon MJ, Walkes JC, Benjamin R. Therapy insight: malignant primary cardiac tumors. *Nat Clin Pract Cardiovasc Med*. 2006;3:548–553.
92. Gross BH, Glazer GM, Francis IR. CT of intracardiac and intrapericardial masses. *AJR Am J Roentgenol*. 1983;140:903–907.
93. Winther C, Timmermans-Wielenga V, Daugaard S, Mortensen SA, Sander K, Andersen CB. Primary cardiac tumors: a clinicopathologic evaluation of four cases. *Cardiovasc Pathol*. 2011;20:63–67.
94. Putnam JB Jr, Sweeney MS, Colon R, Lanza LA, Frazier OH, Cooley DA. Primary cardiac sarcomas. *Ann Thorac Surg*. 1991;51:906–910.
95. Zhang PJ, Brooks JS, Goldblum JR, et al. Primary cardiac sarcomas: a clinicopathologic analysis of a series with follow-up information in 17 patients and emphasis on long-term survival. *Hum Pathol*. 2008;39:1385–1395.

PART Ⅳ
第四部分

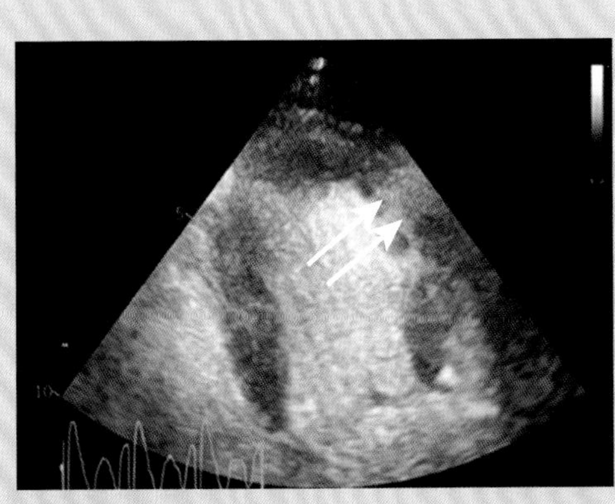

Ischemic Heart Disease
缺血性心肌病

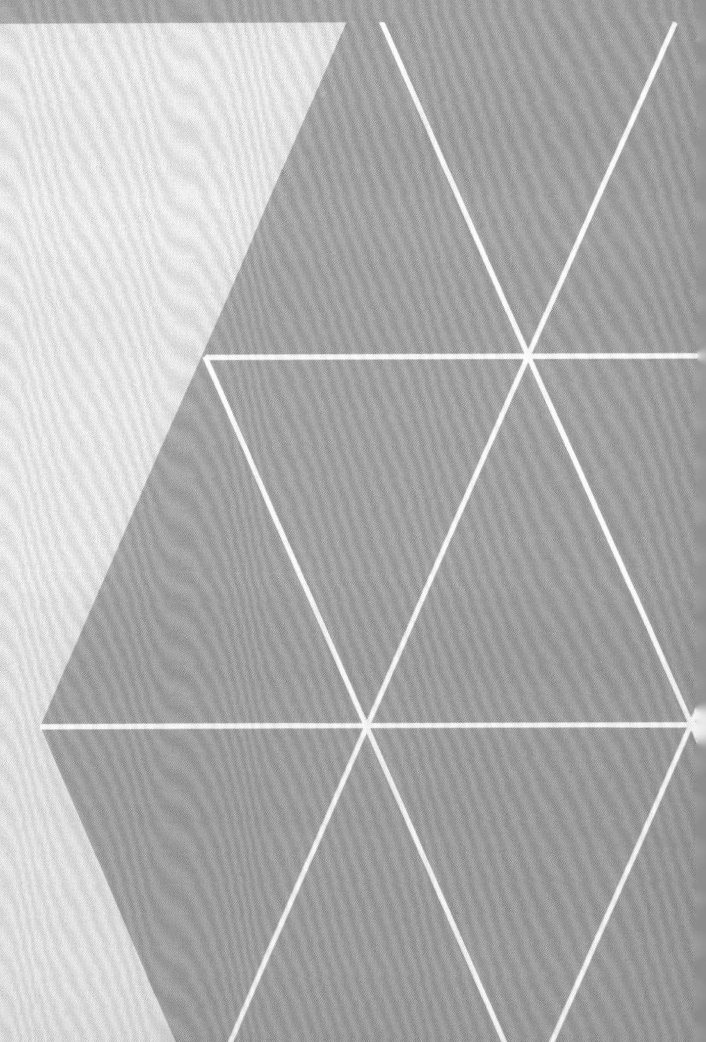

中文导读

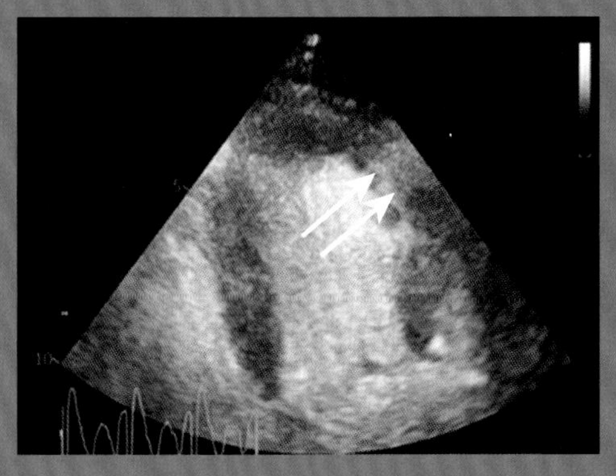

第19章
负荷超声心动图评价冠状动脉缺血

负荷超声心动图是指通过运动或使用药物等方法，增加心肌耗氧量，诱发心肌缺血，同时使用超声心动图对比观察静息状态和负荷状态下室壁运动的变化，并同步记录心电图变化，是无创识别冠心病所致心肌缺血最特异、最敏感的方法。

运动负荷、多巴酚丁胺和血管扩张剂等药物负荷，均会诱发冠状动脉明显狭窄患者的室壁运动异常。运动负荷超声心动图还可以诱发隐匿性心肌缺血，评价心功能储备、运动耐量、运动过程中心率和血压的变化。由于负荷超声心动图的最终影响是诱发心肌缺血，因此要严格把握检查的适应证与禁忌证，规范检查流程，检查者要熟练掌握操作并对检查结果进行判读。负荷超声心动图和超声造影、三维超声、超声应变、CT等其他影像技术联合应用，在评价冠状动脉缺血方面具有更强的优势和更广阔的应用前景。

陶　瑾

19 Stress Echocardiography for Detecting Coronary Ischemia

FLORIAN RADER, MD | ROBERT J. SIEGEL, MD

EXERCISE ECHOCARDIOGRAPHY FOR THE DIAGNOSIS OF CORONARY DISEASE

Stress echocardiography—exercise or pharmacologic stress electrocardiography (ECG) coupled with echocardiography—is the most specific and sensitive method to noninvasively identify patients with inducible myocardial ischemia due to coronary artery disease (CAD) without the use of ionizing radiation. As early as 1935, Tennant and Wiggers[1] demonstrated that coronary occlusion impairs myocardial contraction. In the 1970s, studies[2–4] showed that regional wall motion abnormalities could be identified using M-mode echocardiography in canine models of coronary artery occlusion and reduced myocardial perfusion. These pivotal studies provided the basis for the development of clinical stress echocardiography.

Segmental wall motion abnormalities are more sensitive and specific for the detection of myocardial ischemia than symptoms or ECG changes. The advent of two-dimensional (2D) echocardiography improved the feasibility of stress echocardiography. In 1979, segmental wall motion abnormalities due to exercise induced by ischemia was first reported in a patient performing supine bicycle exercise.[5] The development of digital acquisition of echocardiographic images in the 1980s enabled side-by-side comparison of resting ventricular wall motion and left ventricular (LV) wall motion at peak stress or immediately after exercise.

Digitization greatly facilitated the ability to accurately interpret stress echocardiography because it allows direct comparison of the motions of individual LV myocardial segments before and during or immediately after exercise, enhancing the sensitivity and specificity of stress echocardiography. Harmonic imaging and echocardiographic contrast further improved image resolution and identification of the LV endocardial border and the detection of segmental ventricular wall motion abnormalities.

Stress echocardiography has an excellent safety profile. The use of pharmacologic stress echocardiography is detailed in Chapter 14. Exercise, dobutamine, and vasodilators at appropriate doses are equally effective for inducing wall motion abnormalities in the setting of a significant coronary arterial stenosis. However, exercise stress echocardiography has the added diagnostic value of providing information on inducible myocardial ischemia, functional capacity, exercise tolerance, appropriateness of heart rate response to exercise, heart rate recovery after exercise, and exercise-induced hypertension or hypotension. These data provide important prognostic information that is not evaluated with pharmacologic or pacing stress testing.

The method for stress echocardiography has evolved with improvements in imaging quality, new indications, and new ultrasound techniques, including LV echocardiographic contrast for chamber opacification and LV endocardial border definition, as well as myocardial perfusion, LV strain, three-dimensional (3D) LV volumes, and wall motion analysis. Concerns about radiation exposure with nuclear perfusion imaging[6] and coronary computed tomography (CT) angiography have prompted a renewed interest in stress echocardiography.[7]

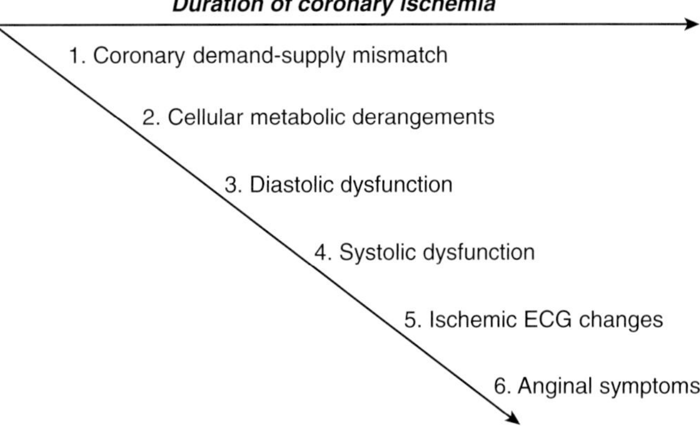

Fig. 19.1 The ischemic cascade. The ischemic cascade is a sequence of events that occurs after the onset of myocardial ischemia. The cardinal symptom of myocardial ischemia, angina pectoris, is the last step in a series of cellular and macroscopic responses to the supply–demand imbalance.

PHYSIOLOGIC AND PATHOPHYSIOLOGIC PRINCIPLES OF STRESS ECHOCARDIOGRAPHY IN ISCHEMIC HEART DISEASE

THE ISCHEMIC CASCADE

The primary goal of stress echocardiography is to safely induce and detect an imbalance between myocardial oxygen consumption and oxygen delivery (i.e., myocardial ischemia). The ischemic cascade is a sequence of events that occurs after the onset of myocardial ischemia. The cardinal symptom of myocardial ischemia, angina pectoris, is the last step in a series of cellular and macroscopic responses to this demand–supply imbalance.

As shown in Fig. 19.1, the first step consists of cellular metabolic derangements, such as lactate accumulation and electrolyte disturbances within the myocytes. These cellular changes precede clinical manifestations of ischemia, lack of myocardial wall thickening, hypokinetic wall motion, ECG changes, and chest pain. Diastolic dysfunction is usually the first manifestation of myocardial ischemia. Although it is not routinely assessed, abnormal diastolic function during stress echocardiography is useful for the detection of myocardial ischemia and has incremental prognostic value.[8]

With continuing ischemia during stress, the main echocardiographic sign of stress-induced myocardial ischemia becomes evident by a lack of myocardial segmental wall thickening and focal or global systolic dysfunction (i.e., myocardial hypokinesia, akinesia, or dyskinesia). ECG signs of ischemia occur after wall motion abnormalities can be detected, sometimes even after cessation of exercise, during the recovery period.[9] Symptomatic angina pectoris is the last indicator of myocardial ischemia and probably the least reliable because of subjectivity in perception and variations in reporting the symptoms.

Stress-induced increases in LV filling pressures from diastolic or systolic dysfunction often cause chest pressure and dyspnea during stress testing and may be difficult to distinguish from typical angina. It is desirable to detect myocardial ischemia as early as possible to reduce the ischemic burden and the risk of complications during stress testing. The risk profile of stress echocardiography is more favorable than that of stress ECG, although it still is recommended for many patients as the first-line test for inducible ischemia.[10,11] Stress echocardiography increases test sensitivity and specificity compared with stress ECG, especially in patients with LV hypertrophy, in those with hypertension, and in women (for whom the positive predictive value of ST abnormalities is lower than for men)[12–15]; however, the cost of stress echocardiography is greater.

DETERMINANTS OF MYOCARDIAL OXYGEN DEMAND AND SUPPLY

Major determinants of myocardial oxygen demand are (1) LV wall tension, (2) heart rate, and (3) systolic blood pressure (BP). LV wall tension is influenced by myocardial wall thickness, ventricular size, and intraventricular pressure.[16,17] Examples of situations in which these three respective determinants are altered are LV and right ventricular (RV) hypertrophy, eccentric LV remodeling, and LV pressure overload from hypertension or aortic stenosis. During stress testing, the so-called double product of heart rate times systolic BP yields the external work of the heart—which is increased and reflects myocardial oxygen demand. Increased LV contractility also augments myocardial oxygen consumption ($M\dot{V}O_2$).[18] Other determinants of metabolic demand, including calcium handling (i.e., calcium-adenosine triphosphatase [Ca^{2+}-ATPase] activity) and excitation-contraction coupling,[19,20] are harder to quantify and less well understood. Adaptation to increased oxygen demand is limited by myocardial blood flow and by oxygen extraction.[21]

A decrease in oxygen delivery to the myocardium may also induce myocardial ischemia. Several mechanisms can lead to a diminished oxygen supply: (1) decreased oxygen carrying capacity (e.g., anemia); (2) decreased epicardial or microvascular coronary blood flow from a fixed stenosis such as atherosclerotic plaque; (3) abnormal epicardial or microvascular coronary blood flow from dynamic obstruction such as impaired vasodilatory capacity (e.g., endothelial dysfunction, endothelium-independent smooth muscle cell dysfunction) or vasospasm; (4) external systolic compression of intramural coronary arteries from myocardial bridging or increased extracellular matrix in infiltrative or hypertrophic cardiomyopathies; (5) decreased microvascular subendocardial blood flow in situations of ventricular pressure overload (e.g., hypertension, aortic stenosis, pulmonary hypertension, pulmonary embolism); (6) decreased diastolic time (e.g., tachycardia) because most[22] coronary perfusion occurs during diastole; and (7) reduced diastolic flow gradient for myocardial perfusion, as is seen with acute severe aortic regurgitation with low diastolic aortic pressure and an elevated LV end-diastolic pressure (LVEDP). Reduction in the myocardial perfusion gradient can occur in any setting in which the LVEDP is high and aortic diastolic pressure is low (e.g., cardiogenic shock, hypotension in the setting of severe LV hypertrophy). We have even seen this occur during stress testing in a patient with pericardial constriction.

During stress echocardiography, myocardial oxygen demand increases with exercise, adrenergic stimulation with dobutamine, or incremental intracardiac or external (transesophageal) electrical pacing. The common goal of these stress modalities is to increase the myocardial work and O_2 consumption by increasing heart rate, contractility, and systolic BP during exercise to unmask coronary artery stenoses that may not be severe enough to cause symptoms or cardiac dysfunction at rest. Coronary stenoses with a reduction of the cross-sectional luminal diameter to 75% or a diameter of less than 50% can be detected with usual stress testing modalities. However, all the factors that influence supply and demand of coronary blood flow also influence the detection of significant coronary stenoses during stress echocardiography.

INDICATIONS AND CONTRAINDICATIONS FOR STRESS ECHOCARDIOGRAPHY

Table 19.1 lists general advantages, limitations, and developing areas of stress echocardiography. The most common and effective exercise stress modalities are treadmill, upright bicycle, and supine bicycle ergometers. If the patient is unable to exercise, pharmacologic stress or pacing protocols can be applied.

TABLE 19.1 Advantages, Limitations, and Developing Areas of Exercise Stress Echocardiography.

Advantages

Exercise or pharmacologic stress can be used
Assessment of cardiac structure
Assessment of global LV and RV function
Assessment of segmental wall motion at rest and with stress for location of coronary ischemia territory
Prognostication for future cardiac events

Limitations

Image quality varies, depending on patient characteristics and position, equipment, and sonographer's experience
Limited time for image acquisition with treadmill exercise stress testing
Inability to reach ischemic threshold with bicycle exercise

Developing Areas

Strain exercise echocardiography (tissue Doppler, speckle tracking)
3D stress echocardiography
Myocardial contrast echocardiography

Treadmill stress echocardiography is hampered by time constraints for imaging after exercise. Optimally, ultrasound images should be obtained as soon as the patient stops exercising. However, it takes time to get the patient off the treadmill and safely onto a gurney or bed so that the echocardiographic images can be obtained. The longer the delay, the lower the sensitivity of the test if the myocardial ischemia resolves. This issue is not applicable to supine bicycle stress testing, in which imaging can readily be performed during peak exercise. Bicycle testing is the preferred method at our stress laboratory.

INDICATIONS

Indications for stress echocardiography for CAD include symptoms of myocardial ischemia, chest pain in the absence of an acute coronary syndrome (ACS) or myocardial infarction, recent ACS without coronary angiography, stable CAD or a change in clinical status, and suspected risk of CAD before noncardiac surgery.

The appropriateness of stress echocardiography in various patient subsets was defined in the 2013 multimodality appropriate use criteria[23] for detection and risk assessment of stable CAD (Tables 19.2, 19.3, and 19.4). The previous appropriateness categories of testing modalities were changed from those of prior guidelines to *Appropriate, May be appropriate,* and *Rarely appropriate* by an expert panel for each of the modalities.

The 2020 American Society of Echocardiography guidelines on stress echocardiography[24] list indications for stress testing together with recommendation class (I, IIa, IIb, or III) and level of supporting evidence (A–C) (Table 19.5). In symptomatic patients, these indications include a low or intermediate likelihood of CAD in those who can exercise but have an

TABLE 19.2 Appropriateness of Noninvasive and Invasive Testing Modalities in Symptomatic Patients.[a]

	Indication Text	*Exercise ECG*	*Stress RNI*	*Stress Echocardiography*	*Stress CMR*	*Calcium Scoring*	*CCTA*	*Invasive Coronary Angiography*
1	Low pretest probability of CAD ECG interpretable *and* able to exercise	A	R	M	R	R	R	R
2	Low pretest probability of CAD ECG uninterpretable *or* unable to exercise	—	A	A	M	R	M	R
3	Intermediate pretest probability of CAD ECG interpretable *and* able to exercise	A	A	A	M	R	M	R
4	Intermediate pretest probability of CAD ECG uninterpretable *or* unable to exercise	—	A	A	A	R	A	M
5	High pretest probability of CAD ECG interpretable *and* able to exercise	M	A	A	A	R	M	A
6	High pretest probability of CAD ECG uninterpretable *or* unable to exercise	—	A	A	A	R	M	A

[a]Appropriate use categories: A, appropriate; M, may be appropriate; R, rarely appropriate.
CAD, Coronary artery disease; *CCTA*, coronary computed tomography angiography; *CHD*, coronary heart disease; *CMR*, cardiac magnetic resonance; *ECG*, electrocardiogram; *RNI*, radionuclide imaging.
From Wolk MJ, Bailey SR, Doherty JU, et al. ACCF/AHA/ASE/ASNC/HFSA/HRS/SCAI/SCCT/SCMR/STS 2013 Multimodality appropriate use criteria for the detection and risk assessment of stable ischemic heart disease. *J Am Coll Cardiol.* 2014;4:380–406.

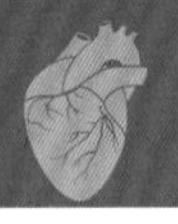

TABLE 19.3 Appropriateness of Noninvasive and Invasive Testing Modalities in Asymptomatic Patients.[a]

	Indication Text	Exercise ECG	Stress RNI	Stress Echo-cardiography	Stress CMR	Calcium Scoring	CCTA	Invasive Coronary Angiography
7	Low global CHD risk Regardless of ECG interpretability and ability to exercise	R	R	R	R	R	R	R
8	Intermediate global CHD risk ECG interpretable *and* able to exercise	M	R	R	R	M	R	R
9	Intermediate global CHD risk ECG uninterpretable *or* unable to exercise	—	M	M	R	M	R	R
10	High global CAD risk ECG interpretable *and* able to exercise	A	M	M	M	M	M	R
11	High global CAD risk ECG uninterpretable *or* unable to exercise	—	M	M	M	M	M	R

[a]Appropriate use categories: A, appropriate; M, may be appropriate; R, rarely appropriate.
CAD, Coronary artery disease; *CCTA*, coronary computed tomography angiography; *CHD*, coronary heart disease; *CMR*, cardiac magnetic resonance; *ECG*, electrocardiogram; *RNI*, radionuclide imaging.
From Wolk MJ, Bailey SR, Doherty JU, et al. ACCF/AHA/ASE/ASNC/HFSA/HRS/SCAI/SCCT/SCMR/STS 2013 Multimodality appropriate use criteria for the detection and risk assessment of stable ischemic heart disease. *J Am Coll Cardiol.* 2014;4:380–406.

TABLE 19.4 Appropriateness of Noninvasive and Invasive Testing Modalities in Various Cardiac Conditions.[a]

	Indication Text	Exercise ECG	Stress RNI	Stress Echo-cardiography	Stress CMR	Calcium Scoring	CCTA	Invasive Coronary Angiography
Newly Diagnosed Heart Failure (Resting LV Function Previously Assessed but No Prior CAD Evaluation)								
12	Newly diagnosed systolic heart failure	M	A	A	A	R	A	A
13	Newly diagnosed diastolic heart failure	M	A	A	A	R	M	M
Evaluation of Arrhythmias Without Ischemic Equivalent (No Prior Cardiac Evaluation)								
14	Sustained VT	A	A	A	A	R	M	A
15	Ventricular fibrillation	M	A	A	A	R	M	A
16	Exercise-induced VT or nonsustained VT	A	A	A	A	R	M	A
17	Frequent PVCs	A	A	A	M	R	M	M
18	Infrequent PVCs	M	M	M	R	R	R	R
19	New-onset atrial fibrillation	M	M	M	R	R	R	R
20	Before initiation of antiarrhythmia therapy in patients with high global CAD risk	A	A	A	A	R	M	R
Syncope Without Ischemic Equivalent								
21	Low global CAD risk	M	M	M	R	R	R	R
22	Intermediate or high global CAD risk	A	A	A	M	R	M	R

[a]Appropriate use categories: A, appropriate; M, may be appropriate; R, rarely appropriate.
CAD, Coronary artery disease; *CCTA*, coronary computed tomography angiography; *CMR*, cardiac magnetic resonance; *ECG*, electrocardiogram; *PVCs*, premature ventricular contractions; *RNI*, radionuclide imaging; *VT*, ventricular tachycardia.
From Wolk MJ, Bailey SR, Doherty JU, et al. ACCF/AHA/ASE/ASNC/HFSA/HRS/SCAI/SCCT/SCMR/STS 2013 Multimodality appropriate use criteria for the detection and risk assessment of stable ischemic heart disease. *J Am Coll Cardiol.* 2014;4:380–406.

uninterpretable ECG, and a high pretest likelihood of CAD even with an interpretable ECG. In asymptomatic patients, stress echocardiography was deemed useful only in selected cases when CAD risk is intermediate or high and the ECG uninterpretable.

Indications for stress echocardiography by prior guidelines[25] included possible ACS without ischemic ECG changes or left bundle branch block (LBBB) and normal or minimally elevated troponin levels (which is a contraindication for some practitioners). The 2013 guidelines listed stress echocardiography in patients without chest pain but with new-onset congestive heart failure or LV dysfunction, certain arrhythmias, and syncope.

Exercise Stress Echocardiography for Preoperative Risk Assessment in Noncardiac Surgery

Preoperative risk is heightened in patients with known peripheral arterial disease, ischemic heart disease, diabetes, or

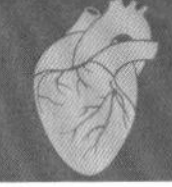

TABLE 19.5 Recommendations for Stress Echocardiography in Patients With Symptoms or Suspected Stable Coronary Artery Disease.

Recommendations	*Class of Recommendation*	*Level of Evidence*
Recommendations for Noninvasive Testing for IHD		
In patients with suspected stable CAD, intermediate pretest probability and preserved ejection fraction, stress imaging, such as stress echocardiography, is preferred as the initial test option.	I	B
In patients without typical angina, an imaging stress test, such as stress echocardiography, is recommended as the initial test for diagnosing stable CAD if the pretest probability is high or if LVEF is reduced.	I	B
In patients with suspected CAD and with resting ECG abnormalities that prevent accurate interpretation of ECG changes during stress, an imaging stress test, such as stress echocardiography, is recommended.	I	B
In patients with LBBB and symptoms consistent with IHD, stress echocardiography (ESE or DSE) is preferred over SPECT imaging because of its greater specificity and its versatility for detecting other cardiac conditions associated with LBBB.	I	B
Stress echocardiography is the preferred test for women with an indication for a noninvasive imaging test for known or suspected CAD because of its safety (absence of radiation to the breasts) and greater specificity (absence of breast attenuation artifact).	I	B
ESE is the preferred imaging stress test for children with suspected IHD because of the absence of radiation to developing tissues, absence of need for an intravenous line, and provision of the prognostically important assessment of exercise capacity.	I	B
A pharmacologic stress test, such as DSE, is recommended for patients with the above indications for a stress imaging test who are unable to exercise.	I	B
Stress echocardiography is the preferred test in patients with exertional dyspnea of uncertain etiology. For these patients, in addition to assessment of regional wall motion, tricuspid regurgitation velocity and diastolic function should be assessed at rest and with stress.	I	B
An imaging stress test, such as stress echocardiography, should be considered in patients with prior coronary artery revascularization (PCI or CABG) and new cardiac symptoms.	IIa	B
An imaging stress test, such as stress echocardiography, should be considered to assess the functional severity of intermediate lesions on coronary arteriography.	IIa	B
Recommendations for Risk Stratification Using Ischemia Testing		
A stress imaging test such as stress echocardiography for risk stratification is recommended in patients with an inconclusive exercise ECG.	I	B
A stress imaging test, such as stress echocardiography, is recommended for risk stratification in patients with known stable CAD and a deterioration in symptoms if the site and extent of ischemia would influence clinical decision making.	I	B
In asymptomatic adults with diabetes, peripheral vascular disease, or a strong family history of CAD, or when previous risk assessment testing suggests a high risk of CAD (e.g., coronary artery calcium score ≥ 400), a stress imaging test, such as stress echocardiography, may be considered for advanced cardiovascular risk assessment.	IIb	B
Recommendation for Reassessment in Patients With Stable CAD		
An exercise ECG or stress imaging test, such as stress echocardiography, is recommended in the presence of recurrent or new symptoms after instability has been ruled out.	I	C
In symptomatic patients with revascularized stable CAD, a stress imaging test, such as stress echocardiography, is indicated rather than stress ECG.	I	C
Reassessment of prognosis using a stress test, such as stress echocardiography, may be considered in asymptomatic patients after the expiration of the period for which the previous test was thought to be valid.	2b	B
Recommendations for Noninvasive Stress Testing of IHD		
A pharmacologic stress imaging test such as DSE is recommended before high-risk surgery in patients with more than two clinical risk factors and poor functional capacity (<4 METs).	I	B
A pharmacologic stress imaging test such as DSE may be considered before high- or intermediate-risk surgery in patients with suspected cardiac symptoms and poor functional capacity (<4 METs).	I	B

CABG, Coronary artery bypass grafting; *CAD*, coronary artery disease; *DSE*, dobutamine stress echocardiography; *ECG*, electrocardiographic; *ESE*, exercise stress echocardiography; *IHD*, ischemic heart disease; *LBBB*, left bundle branch block; *LVEF*, LV ejection fraction; *METs*, metabolic equivalents; *PCI*, percutaneous coronary intervention; *SPECT*, single-photon emission computed tomography.
From Pellikka PA, Arruda-Olson A, Chaudhry FA, et al. Guidelines for performance, interpretation, and application of stress echocardiography in ischemic heart disease: from the American Society of Echocardiography. *J Am Soc Echocardiol*. 2020;33(1):1–41 e48.

congestive heart failure, especially in the setting of poor functional capacity (Table 19.6). It is recommended that high-risk patients with a previous history of CAD undergo stress echocardiography before noncardiac surgery.[23]

Although exercise testing is the preferred modality, pharmacologic stress testing can be used for those patients who are unable to exercise. Compared with myocardial perfusion scintigraphy, dobutamine stress echocardiography has been shown to be as sensitive and more specific with a better accuracy of predicting cardiac events.[26–28] Table 19.7 lists advantages and disadvantages of various testing modalities for the evaluation of CAD.

CONTRAINDICATIONS

There are no side effects associated with exercise echocardiography other than those associated with physical exercise. Absolute contraindications for exercise echocardiography are acute myocardial infarction, unstable angina, serious cardiac arrhythmias, acute pulmonary embolism, aortic dissection, a significant aortic aneurysm, active myocarditis or pericarditis, decompensated heart failure, and symptomatic severe aortic stenosis. Other contraindications include known left main coronary stenosis, severe systemic hypertension (e.g., 200/100 mmHg), severe pulmonary hypertension (e.g., 60 mmHg), and inability to adequately exercise.

TABLE 19.6 **Stress Echocardiography: Predictors of Risk.**

Very Low Risk[a]: Myocardial Infarction, Cardiac Events < 1%/y	*Factors Increasing Risk[b]*	*High Risk[c]: RR > Fourfold Low Risk*
Normal exercise echocardiogram result with good exercise capacity >7 METs men >5 METs women	Increasing age Male sex Diabetes High pretest probability History of dyspnea or CHF History of myocardial infarction Limited exercise capacity Inability to exercise Stress ECG with ischemia Rest WMA LV hypertrophy Stress echocardiography with ischemia Reduced baseline EF No change or increased ESV with stress[d] No change or decreased EF with stress[d] Increasing wall motion score with stress	Extensive WMA at rest (4–5 segments of LV) Baseline EF < 40% Extensive ischemia (4–5 segments of LV) Multivessel ischemia Rest WMA and remote ischemia Low ischemic threshold Ischemic WMA, no change or decrease in exercise EF[d]

[a]High pretest probability of CAD, poor exercise capacity or low rate-pressure product, increased age, angina during stress, LV hypertrophy, history of infarction, history of CHF, and anti-ischemic therapy are factors known to increase risk in patients with normal stress echocardiogram results.

[b]The degree to which each factor increases risk varies.

[c]Cutoff values for high-risk group are approximate values derived from available studies. Studies have shown that increased rest and low- and peak-dose wall motion scores can identify individuals at high risk, especially those with reduced global LV function, but threshold values used to define patients at high risk have varied (e.g., peak exercise scores ranging from 1.4 to >1.7).

[d]For treadmill and dobutamine stress.

CAD, Coronary artery disease; *CHF*, congestive heart failure; *ECG*, electrocardiogram; *EF*, ejection fraction; *ESV*, end-systolic volume; *HR*, heart rate; *METs*, metabolic equivalents; *WMA*, wall motion abnormalities.

Adapted from Pellikka PA, Arruda-Olson A, Chaudhry FA, et al. Guidelines for performance, interpretation, and application of stress echocardiography in ischemic heart disease: from the American Society of Echocardiography. *J Am Soc Echocardiol.* 2020;33(1):1–41 e48.

TABLE 19.7 **Advantages and Disadvantages of Cardiac Imaging Modalities.**

Cardiac Imaging Modality	*Advantages*	*Disadvantages*
Stress echocardiography	Portable, inexpensive Both exercise and pharmacologic stress No radiation Concurrent structural information Future use of echocardiographic perfusion imaging	Operator dependent Quality affected by patient body habitus, poor acoustic windows (but improved with appropriate use of contrast)
CT angiography	High diagnostic accuracy (particularly high sensitivity and NPV) Early detection of nonobstructive CAD (coronary calcification, non-calcified atherosclerotic plaque Future use of CT MPI may provide both anatomic and functional assessment	Accuracy affected by high coronary calcification Involves radiation Anatomic, so unable to predict functional significance of stenotic lesion (will improve in future with CTA MPI) Use of iodinated contrast
MPI SPECT	Both exercise and pharmacologic stress Both perfusion and LV functional assessment with gated SPECT Robust data validating Less operator-dependent than echocardiography	Radiation Soft tissue attenuation artifacts
MPI PET	Superior diagnostic accuracy compared with SPECT Absolute blood flow quantification Accurate attenuation correction	Radiation Expensive Mainly employs only pharmacologic stress
Stress CMR	No radiation No soft tissue attenuation artifacts Excellent concurrent structural information	Expensive, time consuming Contraindicated in patients with CRMD, claustrophobia, severe renal impairment
MR coronary angiography	No radiation No soft tissue attenuation artifacts	Inferior spatial resolution compared with CTA
Exercise ECG	Added prognostic value of exercise (Duke treadmill score) Inexpensive No radiation	Inferior diagnostic accuracy Requires ability to exercise Uninterpretable with baseline ECG abnormalities (e.g., LBBB, significant resting ST depression)

CAD, Coronary artery disease; *CMR*, cardiac magnetic resonance imaging; *CRMD*, cardiac rhythm management device; *CT*, computed tomography; *CTA*, computed tomography angiography; *ECG*, electrocardiogram; *LBBB*, left bundle branch block; *MPI*, myocardial perfusion imaging; *MR*, magnetic resonance; *NPV*, negative predictive value; *PET*, positron emission tomography; *SPECT*, single-photon emission computed tomography.

Adapted from Dowsley T, Al-Mallah M, Ananthasubramaniam K, et al. The role of noninvasive imaging in coronary artery disease detection, prognosis, and clinical decision making. *Can J Cardiol.* 2013;29:285–296.

Additional relative contraindications, such as hypertrophic cardiomyopathy or asymptomatic critical aortic stenosis, are readily identified from the baseline echocardiogram; therefore, a built-in safeguard exists against the inappropriate stressing of patients with these entities. Nonserious arrhythmias that may preclude adequate wall motion interpretation and poor acoustic windows that are not resolved with echocardiographic contrast can prevent accurate interpretation of segmental wall motion abnormalities and therefore are relative contraindications for exercise echocardiography. Tables 19.2, 19.3, and 19.4 list the appropriate indications for stress echocardiography in symptomatic and asymptomatic patients.

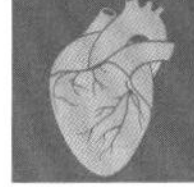

COST-EFFECTIVENESS OF EXERCISE STRESS ECHOCARDIOGRAPHY

The cost-effectiveness of stress echocardiography relates to the pretest likelihood of CAD. If there is a very low or very high pretest probability of CAD, the value of stress testing is limited. The greatest value of stress echocardiography is for patients with an intermediate probability of CAD of 20% to 80%.[29] However, when considering stress test costs and further downstream testing from equivocal results, adding echocardiography to stress testing is cost-effective, especially if stress ECG has a high likelihood of being nondiagnostic.

Stress echocardiography has an equal or higher specificity than alternative imaging modalities.[30] This makes it a more cost-effective method than nuclear perfusion studies, which cost more than twice as much.[31]

STRESS PROTOCOLS

GENERAL CONSIDERATIONS

The goal of stress echocardiography is to safely reach a workload high enough to increase myocardial oxygen demand to a level at which coronary artery stenosis can be detected with an optimal sensitivity and specificity. The exercise target at which CAD can be detected with a high level of confidence may be different for each patient, but by convention, it is 85% of the age-dependent maximal predicted heart rate.

Other exercise targets, such as a rate times pressure value (i.e., double product) of at least 20,000 or the development of symptoms, may be reasonable depending on the clinical context. For safety monitoring and for the detection of signs of myocardial ischemia or cardiac decompensation, continuous monitoring of the ECG, heart rate, BP, pulse oximetry, and symptom status, in addition to the echocardiogram, is required before, during, and after the exercise protocol.

Clinical context is particularly relevant in athletes, for whom a higher double product and greater duration and degree of exercise are often warranted to ensure that the individual will be safe during sports activities. The timing of echocardiographic imaging depends on the stress modality. However, imaging during bicycle stress testing is more sensitive and equally specific compared with treadmill protocols.[32] Table 19.8 shows some of the advantages and disadvantages of bicycle versus treadmill exercise stress modalities.[30]

TABLE 19.8 Advantages and Disadvantages of Bicycle Versus Treadmill Ergometry.

Bicycle Ergometry	*Treadmill Ergometry*
Advantages	
Easier monitoring of blood pressure and pulse oximetry	Standard exercise modality in the United States
Less artifact on electrocardiogram	Greater percentage of patients achieve target heart rate
Continuous/intermittent imaging	More validated data on exercise duration, workload, heart rate recovery
Ability to maintain target heart rate for a prolonged period for comprehensive echocardiographic evaluation (e.g., diastology, valvular function)	
May increase sensitivity for the detection of ischemic wall motion abnormalities	
Disadvantages	
Some patients are not familiar with bicycle exercise	Noncontinuous imaging
Smaller percentage of patients achieve target heart rate	Delay between peak exercise and image acquisition
Less validated data on exercise duration and prognosis	Limited time to obtain imaging
Higher risk of pulmonary congestion (supine position)	Greater risk of fall/injury
	More difficult monitoring of blood pressure and pulse oximetry
	More artifact on electrocardiogram

EQUIPMENT AND PERSONNEL

Fig. 19.2 shows the setup for supine bicycle and treadmill stress echocardiographic testing in our laboratory. Whereas certain standard equipment and personnel are necessary to maximize safety and efficiency, requirements for different stress testing modalities vary. The motorized treadmill or bicycle ergometer; a lateral-tilting echocardiography table with a left lateral cutout for optimal apical imaging; stress testing equipment that can integrate workload, ECG, and vital signs for monitoring and reporting; and the echocardiography machine should be set up so that they can be controlled and inspected by the laboratory staff at any time during the test. With treadmill exercise testing, the echocardiography bed should be in immediate proximity to the treadmill so that patients can be quickly transferred for postpeak exercise imaging, which must occur within seconds of exercise cessation.

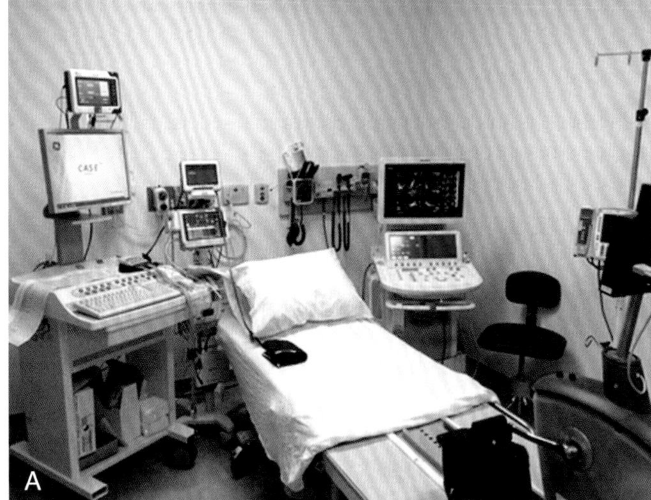

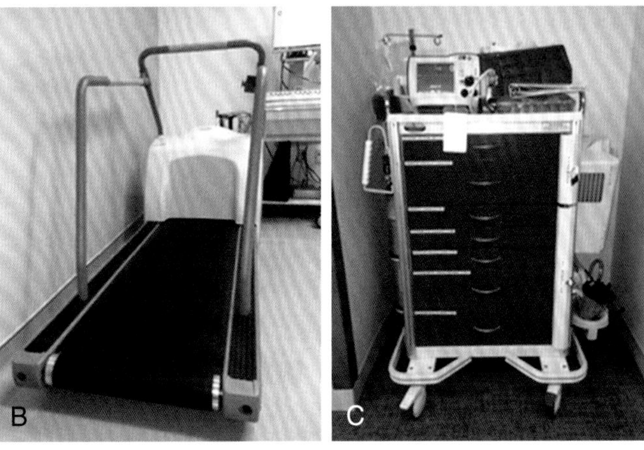

Fig. 19.2 Equipment and setup of a stress echocardiography room. (A) Typical arrangement *(left to right)* of stress ECG machine, vital sign monitor, echocardiography bed with built-in supine bicycle ergometer, echocardiogram machine, and infusion pump for administration of intravenous medication. (B) Motorized treadmill. (C) Crash cart with defibrillator.

TABLE 19.9 Recommended Steps for Patient Preparation and Evaluation Before Stress Echocardiography.

Assess brief medical history, physical examination, and indication for the stress test.
Review allergies.
Confirm fasting state.
Obtain written informed consent.
Place blood pressure cuff.
Place ECG leads (allowing adequate imaging windows).
Obtain baseline ECG.
Obtain baseline echocardiogram.
Recommended: Place intravenous access line.
Review above data.
Perform a time-out to verify patient identity, review indications for the test, review medication allergies and contraindications to frequently used medications (e.g., atropine).

ECG, Electrocardiogram.

Other necessary equipment consists of a crash cart with a defibrillator and medications used during stress testing, including those to reverse or treat the adverse effects of pharmacologic stress agents. In a hospital setting, a code blue alert system should be in every stress room. It is controversial and depends on hospital or facility policy about whether a nurse or physician assistant or only a physician can directly supervise a stress test.[33] At a minimum, a physician needs to be available without delay in case a complication occurs during or immediately after the stress test.

PATIENT PREPARATION

Table 19.9 lists necessary and recommended steps before starting the stress protocol.

EXERCISE STRESS TESTING

In the United States, the most common form of stress testing employs a motorized treadmill. It is used for stress ECG and nuclear exercise stress tests and for stress echocardiography. Although treadmill ergometry has advantages in terms of maximizing body workload (e.g., increasing speed and incline), and therefore more frequently achieves target heart rate, it has significant disadvantages, particularly for stress echocardiography.

Supine and, to a lesser degree, upright bicycle ergometry allows continuous or intermittent echocardiographic surveillance during exercise. With leg bicycle machines the upper body motion is minimized, which decreases ECG artifacts and allows much easier BP assessment by oscillometric rather than manual methods. Exclusive arm bicycle ergometry often does not provide an adequate workload to achieve target end points. Ideally, both treadmill and bicycle ergometry should be available in a stress echocardiography laboratory to allow tests to be individualized for patients' needs and limitations. Table 19.8 provides a more comprehensive list of advantages and disadvantages of bicycle versus treadmill exercise ergometry.

EXERCISE STRESS PROTOCOLS

All exercise stress protocols are designed to gradually increase workload, depending on the estimated functional capacity of the exercising patient. The ideal stress protocol allows the patient to reach maximal workload after 6 to 12 minutes. If the maximal workload is reached too quickly, respiratory rather than cardiac limitations set in; if the stress protocol exercises patients too long, musculoskeletal rather than cardiac limitations may determine the exercise duration. If the target heart rate is not reached, handgrip exercise or intravenous atropine can be added to any of the stress modalities.[34]

Treadmill Protocols

The most commonly used treadmill protocol is the Bruce protocol, which prescribes consecutive 3-minute stages. The modified Bruce protocol, used for more sedentary patients, includes two additional lower-intensity stages at the beginning of the test, followed by a regular Bruce protocol.

The Naughton protocol is appropriate for more sedentary patients and uses 2-minute stages. The Balke and Cornell protocols have shorter stages and therefore provide more data points. The Costill protocol is intended for highly trained individuals and is typically used for cardiopulmonary exercise testing. The detailed stages and metabolic equivalents of the Bruce, modified Bruce, and Naughton protocols are listed in Fig. 19.3.[35]

Bicycle Protocols

Bicycle protocols usually have 1- or 2-minute stages, increasing the workload by 15 to 25 watts per stage until test end points are reached. Approximately 20% of patients undergoing supine bicycle exercise in our laboratory do not achieve their target heart rate (i.e., at least 85% of predicted maximal heart rate).

Among patients with a nondiagnostic supine bicycle stress test result, 80% of those receiving 0.5 to 2.0 mg of atropine achieved a diagnostic test with a target heart rate of 85% of maximal predicted or greater. There were no major adverse effects from the administration of atropine. The use of atropine to augment the heart rate or rate–pressure product during supine bicycle exercise stress echocardiography is safe, enables the assessment of ischemia at peak effort, and allows assessment of exercise hemodynamics in patients with submaximal exercise capacity or chronotropic incompetence.[36]

Handgrip

Handgrip exercise alone typically is not sufficient as a cardiac stressor, but it is a useful adjunct to bicycle stress protocols and pharmacologic stress protocols to further raise cardiac workload.

EFFECTS OF MEDICAL THERAPY

Antianginal therapy decreases the sensitivity of stress echocardiography by decreasing myocardial oxygen demand. A positive test result while on medical therapy indicates that these patients are at higher risk for ischemic cardiovascular events. However, the ability of anti-ischemic therapy to prevent an ischemic response to stress testing is an effective way to assess the adequacy of medical therapy.

Exercise echocardiography for patients with known ischemic heart disease while on anti-ischemic therapy is useful to assess the adequacy of treatment. Observational data suggest that for patients on beta-blocker therapy, a lower predicted maximal heart rate threshold (65%) has a prognostic power similar to that of the usual 85% threshold for patients not treated with beta-blockers.[37] However, this finding needs to be reproduced in a controlled trial. In general, if the goal of the test is

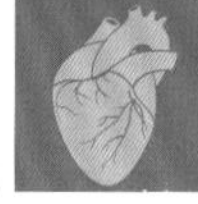

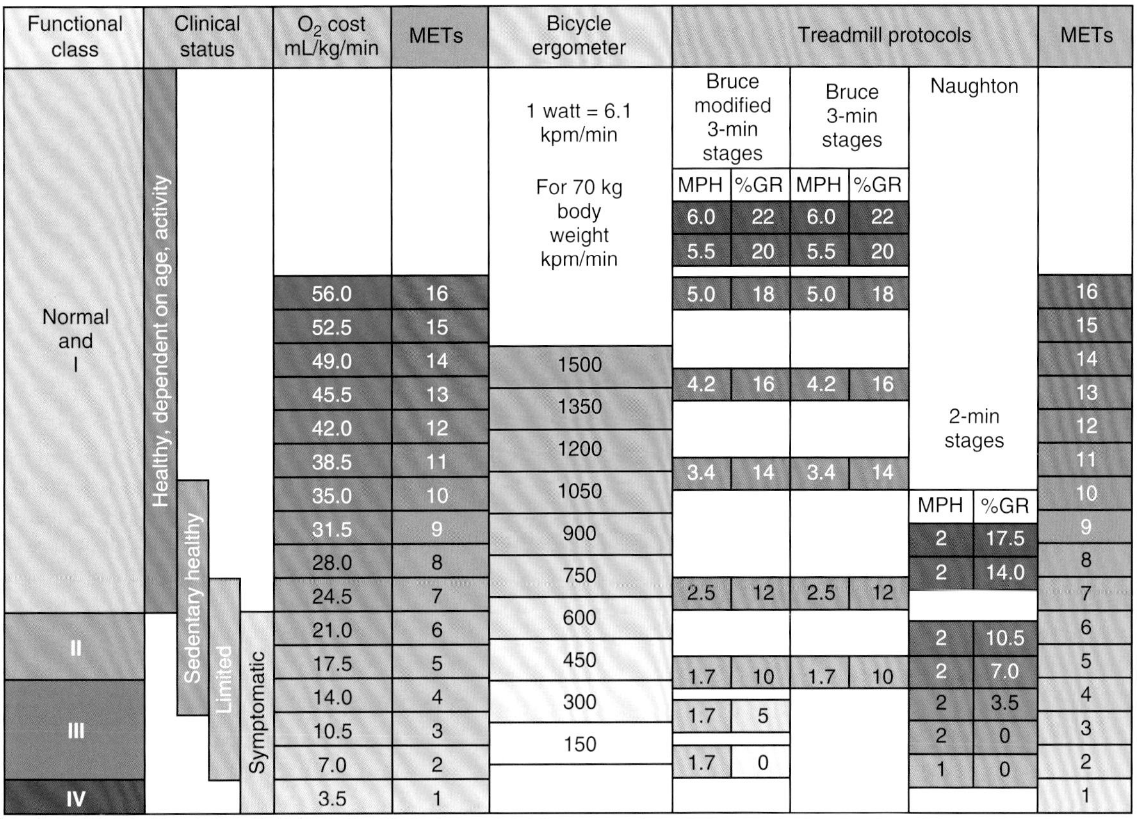

Functional class	Clinical status	O_2 cost mL/kg/min	METs	Bicycle ergometer (1 watt = 6.1 kpm/min; For 70 kg body weight kpm/min)	Bruce modified 3-min stages MPH	Bruce modified 3-min stages %GR	Bruce 3-min stages MPH	Bruce 3-min stages %GR	Naughton 2-min stages MPH	Naughton 2-min stages %GR	METs
					6.0	22	6.0	22			
					5.5	20	5.5	20			
Normal and I	Healthy, dependent on age, activity	56.0	16		5.0	18	5.0	18			16
Normal and I	Healthy, dependent on age, activity	52.5	15								15
Normal and I	Healthy, dependent on age, activity	49.0	14	1500							14
Normal and I	Healthy, dependent on age, activity	45.5	13		4.2	16	4.2	16			13
Normal and I	Healthy, dependent on age, activity	42.0	12	1350							12
Normal and I	Healthy, dependent on age, activity	38.5	11	1200							11
Normal and I	Healthy, dependent on age, activity; Sedentary healthy	35.0	10	1050	3.4	14	3.4	14			10
Normal and I	Healthy, dependent on age, activity; Sedentary healthy	31.5	9	900					2	17.5	9
Normal and I	Healthy, dependent on age, activity; Sedentary healthy	28.0	8						2	14.0	8
Normal and I	Healthy, dependent on age, activity; Sedentary healthy; Limited	24.5	7	750	2.5	12	2.5	12			7
II	Sedentary healthy; Limited; Symptomatic	21.0	6	600					2	10.5	6
II	Sedentary healthy; Limited; Symptomatic	17.5	5	450	1.7	10	1.7	10	2	7.0	5
III	Sedentary healthy; Limited; Symptomatic	14.0	4	300					2	3.5	4
III	Limited; Symptomatic	10.5	3		1.7	5			2	0	3
III	Limited; Symptomatic	7.0	2	150	1.7	0			1	0	2
IV	Symptomatic	3.5	1								1

Fig. 19.3 Correlation of metabolic workload and functional class in commonly used exercise stress protocols. Listed examples are the Bruce, the modified Bruce, and the Naughton treadmill exercise protocols. *GR*, Grade; *kpm/min*, kilopond meters per minute; *METs*, metabolic equivalents; *MPH*, miles per hour. (From Fletcher GF, Balady GJ, Amsterdam EA, et al. Exercise standards for testing and training: a statement for healthcare professionals from the American Heart Association. *Circulation*. 2001;104:1694–1740.)

to identify the existence of CAD, antianginal therapy should be withheld 24 to 48 hours before the test.[31]

OUTCOME ASSESSMENT OF STRESS ECHOCARDIOGRAPHY

SYMPTOMS, ANGINA, AND PERCEIVED EFFORT

Although symptoms are classically the last step of the ischemic cascade, they do not necessarily indicate myocardial ischemia. Dyspnea, fatigue, chest pressure, lightheadedness, and syncope can be signs of ischemia, but more frequently, they are the result of limited functional capacity, increased LA pressure (e.g., diastolic dysfunction, hypertensive exercise response), pulmonary causes, dynamic obstruction (specifically, during dobutamine stress testing or in hypertrophic obstructive cardiomyopathy), or dehydration.

There is no standardized way to assess these symptoms, but patients should be instructed to report any exertional symptom to the medical staff. A scale ranging from 0 to 10 may be useful to describe the severity of chest pain or other symptoms and follow their evolution during and after the stress test. The scale most commonly used for perceived exercise effort is the Borg scale of perceived exertion, which by convention is a 15- or 10-grade scale.[38]

HEART RATE

During stress echocardiography, the unifying goal is to reach a certain external cardiac workload. Heart rate is the most important exercise target during stress testing. By convention, reaching a target heart rate equal to 85% of the age-adjusted maximal heart rate is desirable because it has been validated as a reasonable cutoff for the prediction of cardiac events.[39] Chronotropic incompetence, atrioventricular nodal blocker therapy, and submaximal effort are possible causes for an inability to reach this goal. Addition of handgrip exercise or intravenous atropine to the stress test protocol has been effective in augmenting heart rate during exercise, enabling patients to achieve target heart rate and thereby increasing the detection rate of ischemia.[40]

A submaximal normal stress echocardiography test result requires further workup if patients are at high risk (e.g., after coronary artery bypass surgery, prior myocardial infarction, resting wall motion abnormalities); if functional capacity during the test was limited (<7 METs in men, <5 METs in women); or if significant BP or ECG abnormalities or chest pain occurred during testing. Conversely, in low-risk patients with good exercise capacity and a slightly submaximal test, further workup may not be necessary.[41]

HEART RATE RECOVERY

A normal heart rate recovery after exercise stress testing is 12 or more beats per minute with stress ECG (when a cool-down period is performed after exercise). During exercise echocardiography with no cool-down period, a heart rate recovery of at least 18 beats/min within the first minute is considered normal. Among patients who do not achieve this cutoff, mortality risk doubles even after adjustment for other stress-dependent cardiovascular risk factors (hazard ratio = 2.13; 95% confidence interval [CI] 1.63–2.78; $P < 0.001$).[39,42]

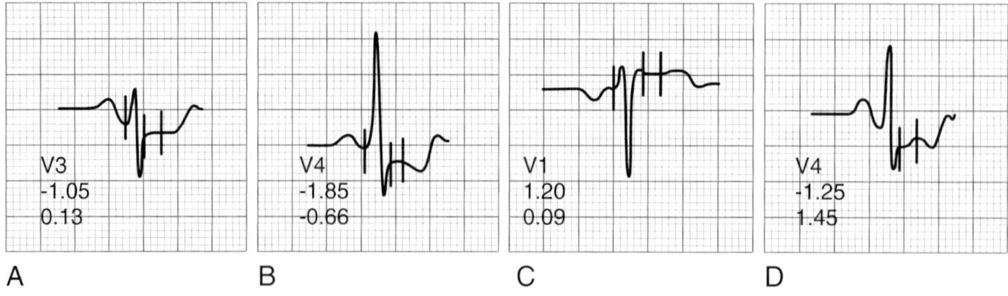

Fig. 19.4 Abnormal ST changes indicate myocardial ischemia. (A) Horizontal ST depression. (B) Down-sloping ST depression. (C) ST elevation of greater than 1 mm magnitude, indicative of myocardial ischemia. (D) Up-sloping ST depression of less than 1.5 mm, which does not meet criteria for ischemia.

BLOOD PRESSURE

BP rises significantly during exercise stress testing. It is the second major determinant of external cardiac work during stress testing, and the combination of heart rate and BP (rate–pressure product or double product) during stress testing is often reported. The assessment of BP during stress testing predicts risk and is useful to determine adequate control of exertional hypertension in treated hypertensives.[43,44] A normal systolic BP response at peak exercise is considered to be 190 mmHg or less in women and 210 mmHg or less in men.[45]

There is observational evidence that exercise-induced hypertension increases the odds of a cardiovascular event 3.6-fold and new-onset resting hypertension by 2.4-fold.[46] Other studies confirmed the predictive value of a hypertensive response to exercise for the presence of hypertension even at a lower peak systolic BP threshold of 181 mmHg.[47,48] Although initiation of antihypertensive medications based on exercise-induced hypertension cannot be uniformly recommended, vigilant monitoring of BP in the clinic and in daily life—ideally with ambulatory BP monitoring—is indicated in patients with an excessive pressor response to exercise.

FUNCTIONAL CAPACITY

Functional capacity is the exercise limit at which a person can perform aerobic work defined by the maximal oxygen uptake ($\dot{V}O_2max$). Mathematically, $\dot{V}O_2max$ is the product of cardiac output and the arteriovenous oxygen difference ($a - \dot{V}O_2$) at physical exhaustion. It is thought that $\dot{V}O_2max$ is limited by cardiac output.

Unless directly measured (as is done in cardiopulmonary exercise testing), the amount of performed exercise (i.e., functional capacity) is usually expressed in metabolic equivalents (METs), with 1 MET representing the resting energy expenditure ($\approx$3.5 mL $O_2 \cdot kg^{-1} \cdot min^{-1}$). By convention, patients who achieve less than 5, 5 to 8, 9 to 11, and 12 or more METs are considered to have poor, fair, good, and excellent functional capacity, respectively (see Fig. 19.3).[35] Exercise duration also has prognostic value; a maximal exercise duration of less than 6 minutes carries an increased mortality risk, especially for patients with systolic heart failure.[49]

ELECTROCARDIOGRAPHIC CHANGES

One major indicator for myocardial ischemia during or after stress testing is a deviation of the ST segment (Fig. 19.4). Both depression and elevation of the ST segment can be evidence of myocardial ischemia. Guideline-recommended thresholds for an ischemic ECG response during stress testing (measured at 80 ms after the J-point) are an upsloping ST-segment depression of 1.5 mm or more and a horizontal or downsloping ST-segment depression of 1 mm or more. Furthermore, 12-lead ECG monitoring during stress echocardiography provides information on exercise-induced arrhythmias (which sometimes can result from myocardial ischemia) or exertional heart rate control (e.g., in patients with atrial fibrillation).[31]

ECHOCARDIOGRAPHIC IMAGING

Imaging protocols vary by stress modality. For instance, with treadmill exercise stress, the echocardiogram is performed before and immediately after exercise (with some delay to transfer the patient from the treadmill to the imaging bed), whereas supine bicycle stress or supine/left lateral dobutamine stress testing allows intermittent or continuous imaging. A list of required steps for image acquisition is shown in Table 19.10. For the detection of stress-induced wall motion abnormalities, parasternal short-axis and apical 4-chamber, 2-chamber, and 3-chamber (apical long-axis) views are obtained at baseline and after (or during) exercise.

Baseline images identify noncoronary causes of cardiac chest pain, some of which are shown in Fig. 19.5, that may merit cancellation of the stress test or initiation of additional diagnostic evaluations. They also can identify baseline wall motion abnormalities, which if previously unknown, may indicate a need for an invasive angiogram or a coronary CT angiogram for a more definitive diagnosis of CAD. Some laboratories use a parasternal long-axis view, but we prefer the apical 3-chamber view because it allows more rapid imaging, more complete visualization of the apical segments, and better imaging with echocardiographic contrast; contrast opacification of the RV may limit visualization of the LV in parasternal views.

Baseline wall motion abnormalities and abnormal thickening should be identified and compared with stress images. When the endocardial border zone is difficult to visualize, specifically if two or more segments are not well seen, echocardiographic contrast should be given unless contraindicated. Imaging software allows side-by-side comparisons to detect differences in systolic motion.

A normal response is hyperdynamic LV function and normal myocardial thickening. Hypokinetic, akinetic, dyskinetic, or aneurysmal wall motion can be a sign of subendocardial, or transmural ischemia. Subjective assessment of LV wall motion and thickening is the standard for assessment of stress echocardiograms, and among trained and experienced echocardiologists, interobserver variability is very good.[31]

As shown in Fig. 19.6, localization of wall motion abnormalities is performed according to a standardized 17-segment

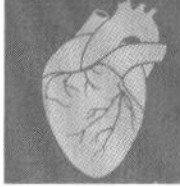

TABLE 19.10 Image Acquisition in Echocardiographic Stress Testing and Implications of Significant Findings During Baseline Imaging.

Baseline and Pretest Imaging	*Imaging During Peak Exercise and Early Recovery*
Full baseline study, including valvular function in most patients, except those recently tested and without change in clinical status since then. Patient is in left lateral supine position	The sequence of imaging can be tailored to the priority of echocardiographic assessment (e.g., ischemia, diastology, valvular assessment)
Parasternal views, including long- and short-axis views Stack of short-axis views to capture basal, middle, and apical segments; RV assessment	Parasternal views, including long- and short-axis views Stack of short-axis views to capture basal, middle, and apical segments
Apical views, including 4-chamber, 2-chamber, long-axis views for LV and RV assessment	Apical views, including 4-chamber, 2-chamber, long-axis views Assessment of diastology, including pulsed-wave Doppler mitral inflow, tissue Doppler, pulmonary vein flow, and when E-A wave separation occurs during recovery
Valvular assessment, including color and spectral Doppler measurements	Valvular assessment if indicated, including color and spectral Doppler measurements
Assessment of diastology, including pulsed-wave Doppler mitral inflow, tissue Doppler, pulmonary vein flow	
RV assessment and pulmonary artery pressure measurement	RV assessment and pulmonary artery pressure measurement
Assessment of RA pressure from inferior vena cava imaging in subcostal views	Assessment of RA pressure from inferior vena cava imaging in subcostal views
For supine bicycle stress, evaluate image quality in supine position, administer echocardiographic contrast if necessary, and repeat parasternal and apical views for wall motion assessment	For supine bicycle stress, administer echocardiographic contrast for wall motion assessment after any planned valvular assessment. Diastology assessment usually can be done with echocardiographic contrast
Baseline Imaging Findings	***Implications***
Baseline wall motion abnormalities	Reassess appropriateness of test; if new wall motion abnormalities, anatomic imaging of coronary arteries recommended (invasive or CT coronary angiogram)
Baseline diastolic dysfunction	Compare with exertional diastolic function
Severe aortic stenosis	Reassess appropriateness of test (symptomatic severe aortic stenosis is a contraindication to stress testing; test may be appropriate for asymptomatic patients)
Severe pulmonary hypertension	For most cases, abort test

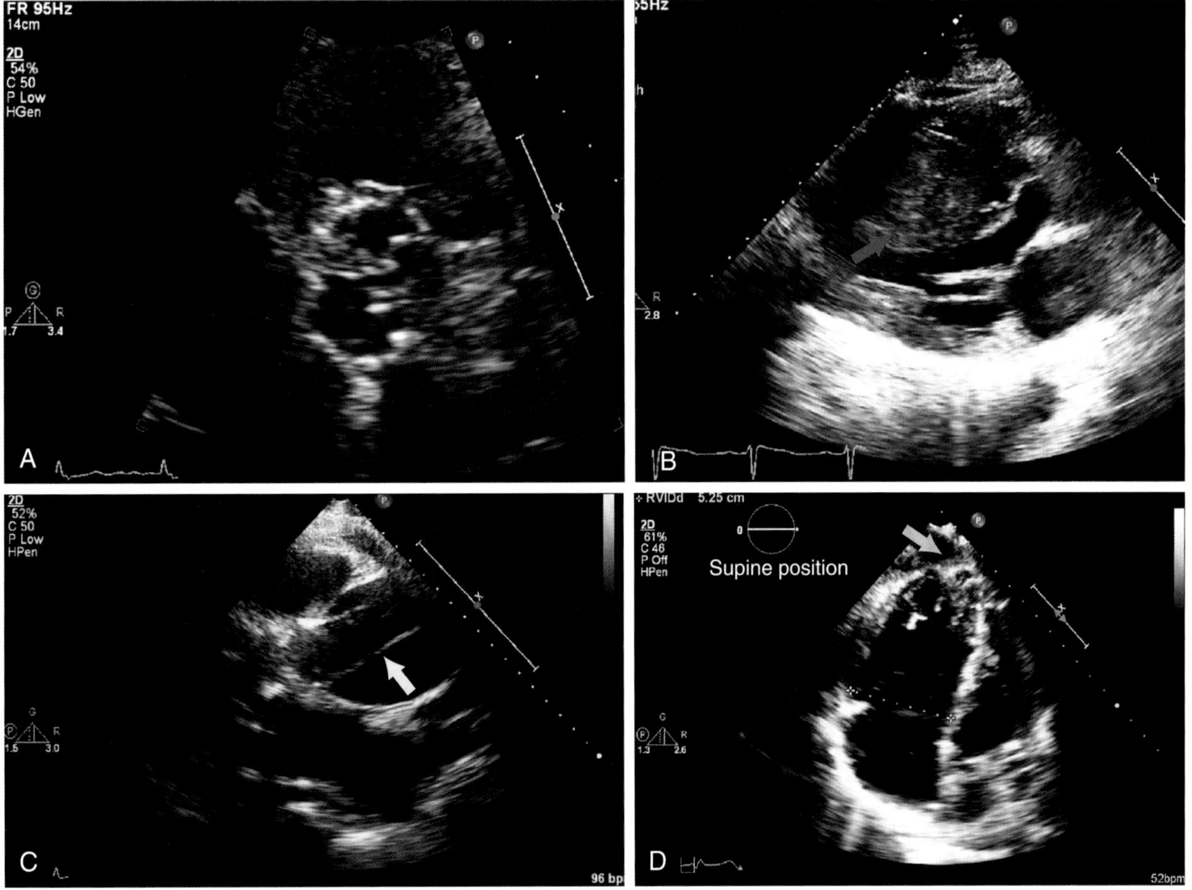

Fig. 19.5 Nonischemic causes of chest pain detected from baseline echocardiograms. (A) Parasternal short-axis view of a severely stenosed aortic valve (see Video 19.5A). (B) Parasternal long-axis view in a patient with hypertrophic cardiomyopathy *(red arrow)* (see Video 19.5B). (C) Parasternal long-axis view of the ascending aorta with a clear aortic dissection flap *(yellow arrow)* (see Video 19.5C). (D) Dilated and dysfunctional RV with relatively preserved apical contraction in systole (i.e., McConnell's sign) *(blue arrow)* in a patient with subacute pulmonary embolism (see Video 19.5D).

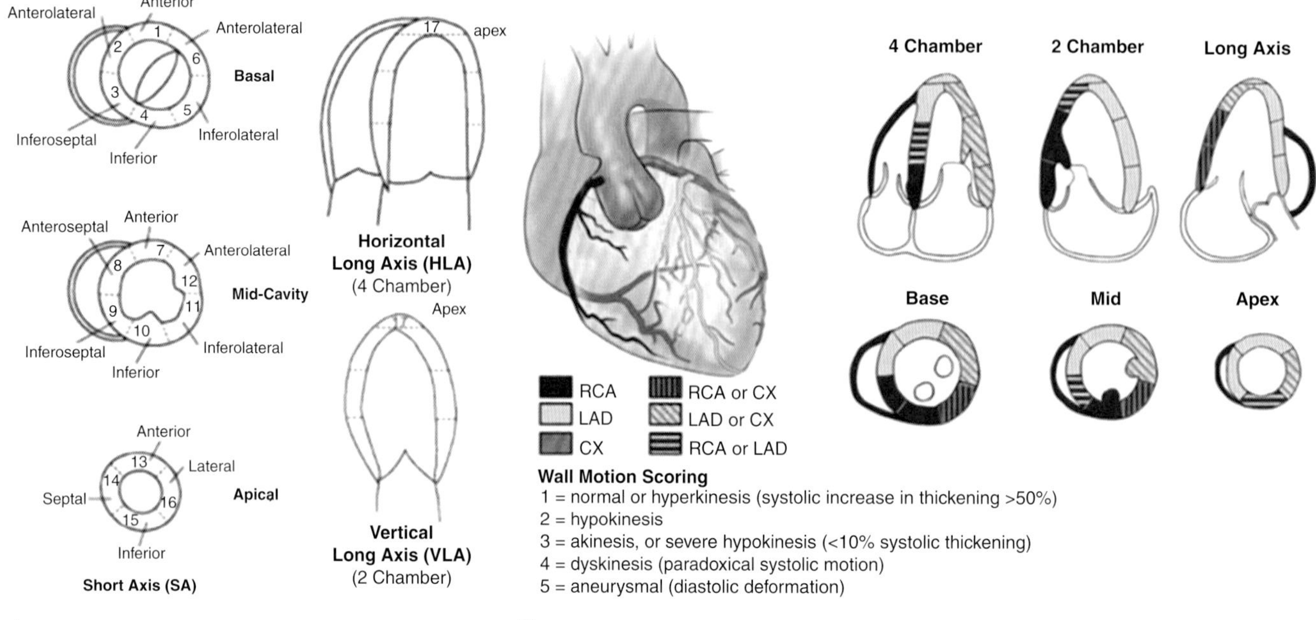

Fig. 19.6 Seventeen-segment model for the description of wall motion abnormalities in stress echocardiography. (A) Notice that the basal short-axis view should include the tips of the mitral valve leaflets, the mid-short-axis view at the level of the papillary muscles, and the apical short-axis view beyond the papillary muscles. Descriptions of the apical segments seen in the 4- and 2-chamber views separate this recommended model from the older 16-segment model. (B) Coronary artery distribution supplying the myocardial segments at the base, in mid-cavity, and at the apex and wall motion scoring chart. *CX*, Circumflex artery; *LAD*, left anterior descending coronary artery; *RCA*, right coronary artery. (Adapted from Cerqueira MD, Weissman NJ, Dilsizian V, et al. Standardized myocardial segmentation and nomenclature for tomographic imaging of the heart: a statement for healthcare professionals from the Cardiac Imaging Committee of the Council on Clinical Cardiology of the American Heart Association. *Circulation.* 2002;105:539–542; Pellikka PA, Arruda-Olson A, Chaudhry FA, et al. Guidelines for performance, interpretation, and application of stress echocardiography in ischemic heart disease: from the American Society of Echocardiography. *J Am Soc Echocardiogr.* 2020;33:1–41.)

model. Localization of segmental wall motion abnormalities to a given coronary territory provides reliable information about whether the coronary arteries and their branches supplying the anterior and anteroseptal segments (i.e., left anterior descending [LAD] coronary artery) or those supplying the inferior or inferolateral segments (i.e., right coronary artery [RCA] or left circumflex coronary artery [LCx]) are likely the source of myocardial ischemia.[50] Wall motion scores provide a quantitative estimation of myocardial ischemia and must be compared with baseline scores.

Other quantitative methods, such as myocardial strain assessment, have not become standard (discussed later). Left (or right) ventricular dilation at peak stress can be an indication of severe, proximal three-vessel CAD or balanced ischemia and has been confirmed to be an important prognosticator.[51] Figs. 19.7A through E show examples of abnormal stress echocardiography test findings with corresponding wall motion abnormalities on echocardiography, ST deviations on ECG, and the responsible coronary lesion. Fig. 19.7C demonstrates transient ischemic dilation during contrast-enhanced stress echocardiography in a patient with apical wall motion abnormalities at baseline.

Table 19.11 lists potential causes for false-negative and false-positive stress echocardiography test results.[52] It is important for the physician interpreting a stress echocardiogram to be aware of these limitations. Patients with false-positive stress echocardiograms had a mortality rate similar to those with true-positive stress echocardiograms.[53] The presence of microvascular ischemia among false-positive stress tests with open epicardial coronary arteries may explain this phenomenon.

DUKE TREADMILL SCORE

The Duke treadmill score[54] integrates functional capacity, exertional angina, and ischemic changes on ECG. It provides useful information in combination with stress echocardiography.[55] It is calculated as

$$\text{Exercise time} - (5 \times \text{ST deviation}) - (4 \times \text{exercise angina})$$

Angina is graded as follows: 0 = none, 1 = non-limiting angina, and 2 = exercise-limiting angina. The ST segment deviation is measured in millimeters, and maximum exercise time is measured in minutes. Scores range from −25 to +15, and more negative scores indicate higher risk.[54] Although scores such as the Duke treadmill score are helpful, the cardiologist should consider each component of the score individually.

OTHER IMPORTANT STRESS ECHOCARDIOGRAPHIC OUTCOMES

Exertional diastolic function can be evaluated with exercise stress echocardiography, particularly to work up causes of exertional dyspnea.[24,56,57] Several studies have described the association between exercise capacity and diastolic function[8,58,59] and the correlation with ischemia detection.[8] This concept is also useful in evaluating whether exercise-induced dyspnea is caused by diastolic dysfunction (cardiac origin) or has a pulmonary cause.

Fig. 19.8 shows normal and abnormal diastology findings in response to exercise. Normally, the E wave and e' increase with exercise because of increased cardiac output and systolic function. In exercise-induced diastolic dysfunction, the E/e' ratio increases rather than staying constant. Evaluation of mitral inflow may be limited to fusion of the early and atrial contraction mitral inflow streams (E wave and A wave) and must be evaluated during recovery with a high sweep speed to separate the E from the A wave.

Evaluation of *RV systolic function*, either as a sign for RV ischemia or as a risk indicator for RV arrhythmias,[60] and *pulmonary artery systolic pressure* are important parts of the diagnostic evaluation.[61,62] Assessment of pulmonary pressure during exercise is important in the assessment of exertional dyspnea, diastolic dysfunction, primary pulmonary hypertension, and valvular heart disease.[61,62] It is also useful for identifying calcifications of the aortic root, the aortic valve, and the mitral annulus, conditions that are associated with a greater risk of CAD.[63]

TERMINATION OF STRESS ECHOCARDIOGRAPHY

Table 19.12 outlines the absolute and relative indications for terminating a stress echocardiographic study, such as definitive ischemic ECG changes (see Fig. 19.4) and wall motion abnormalities or hemodynamic instability and intolerable symptoms.

REPORTING OF STRESS ECHOCARDIOGRAPHY FINDINGS

Table 19.13 lists stress echocardiographic findings that should be reported in addition to standard echocardiographic findings.

ACCURACY OF EXERCISE STRESS ECHOCARDIOGRAPHY

As shown in Table 19.14, the reported sensitivity and specificity of stress echocardiography is about 80% and just below 90%, respectively. One study showed a relatively high rate of false-positive test results. However, the prognosis of patients with false-positive test results was similar to that of patients with true-positive tests.[53]

Wide ranges in diagnostic accuracy likely reflect differences in laboratory procedures, the types of patients being studied (e.g., poor echocardiographic imaging windows due to obesity, chronic obstructive pulmonary disease, prior surgery, chest wall deformity), the experience and expertise of the sonographers

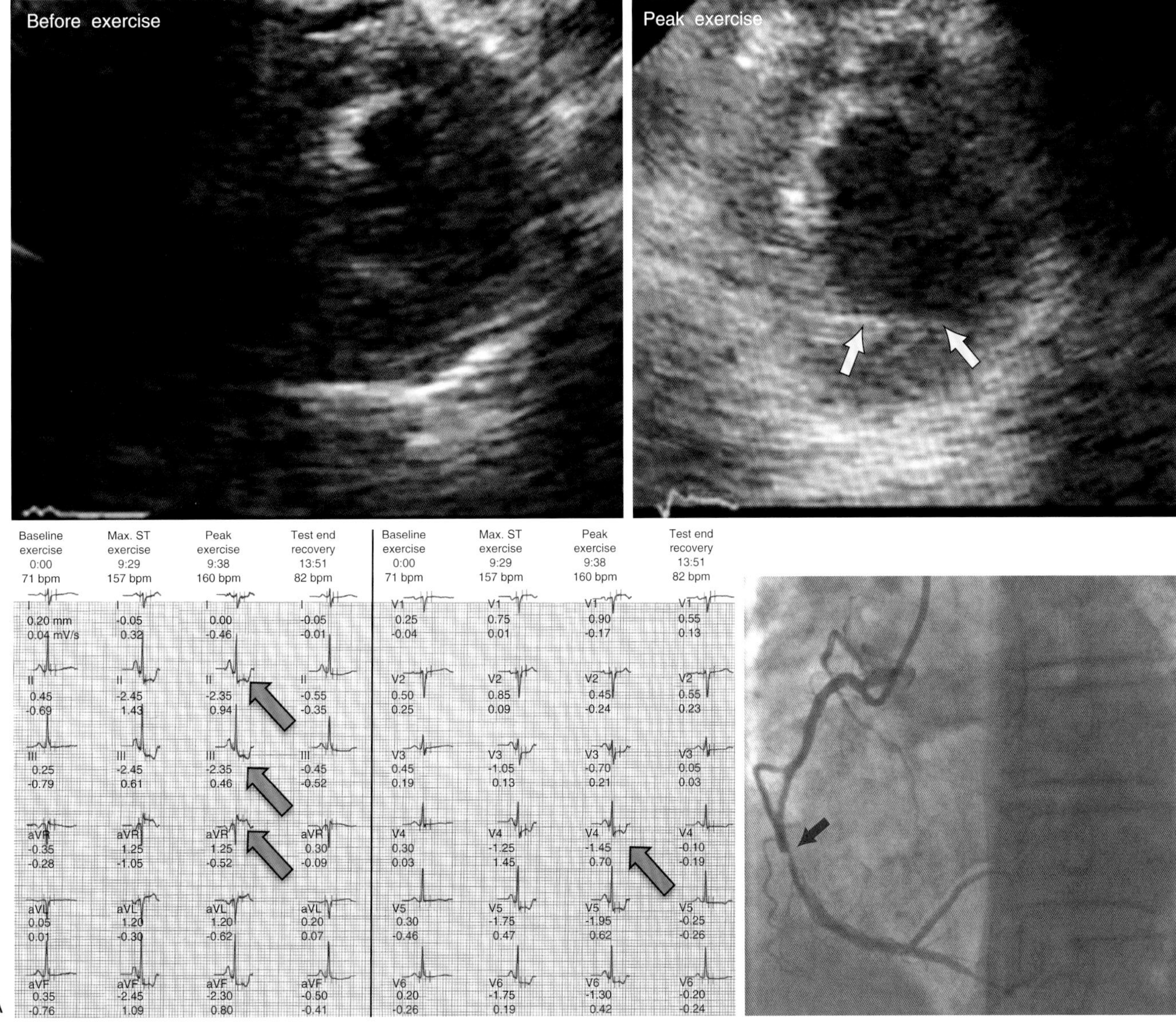

Fig. 19.7 Examples of abnormal stress echocardiography test findings. (A) Ischemic response to exercise stress: inferior and inferolateral stress-induced hypokinesis *(white arrows)* on echocardiography with diffuse ST depressions on ECG *(green arrows)*. Subsequent coronary angiography demonstrated a focal critical right coronary artery stenosis *(red arrow)* (see Video 19.7A).

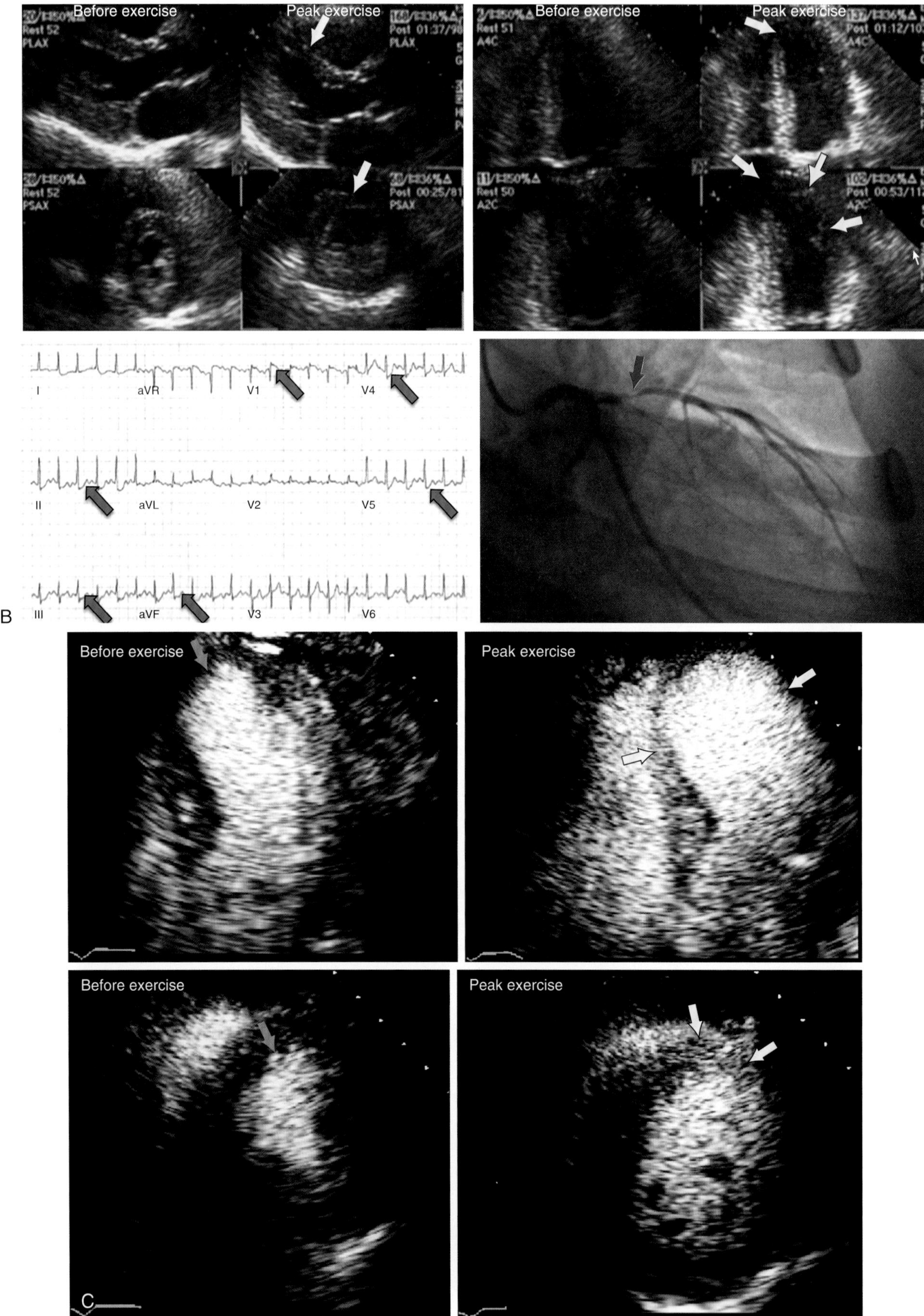

Fig. 19.7—cont'd (B) Ischemic response to exercise stress: anteroseptal, anterior, and lateral stress-induced hypokinesis *(white arrows)* on echocardiography with diffuse ST depressions and ST elevation in the aVR lead on ECG *(green arrows)*. Subsequent coronary angiography demonstrated a focal critical LAD artery stenosis *(red arrow)*. (C) Ischemic response to exercise stress: a patient with apical baseline hypokinesis *(brown arrows)* during contrast-enhanced echocardiography developed extensive apical and lateral stress-induced hypokinesis *(white arrows)* with transient ischemic dilation of the LV. Subsequent coronary angiography demonstrated significant three-vessel coronary artery disease (angiogram not shown) (see Video 19.7C).

Continued

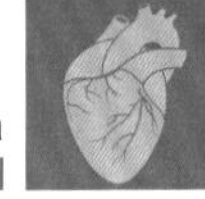

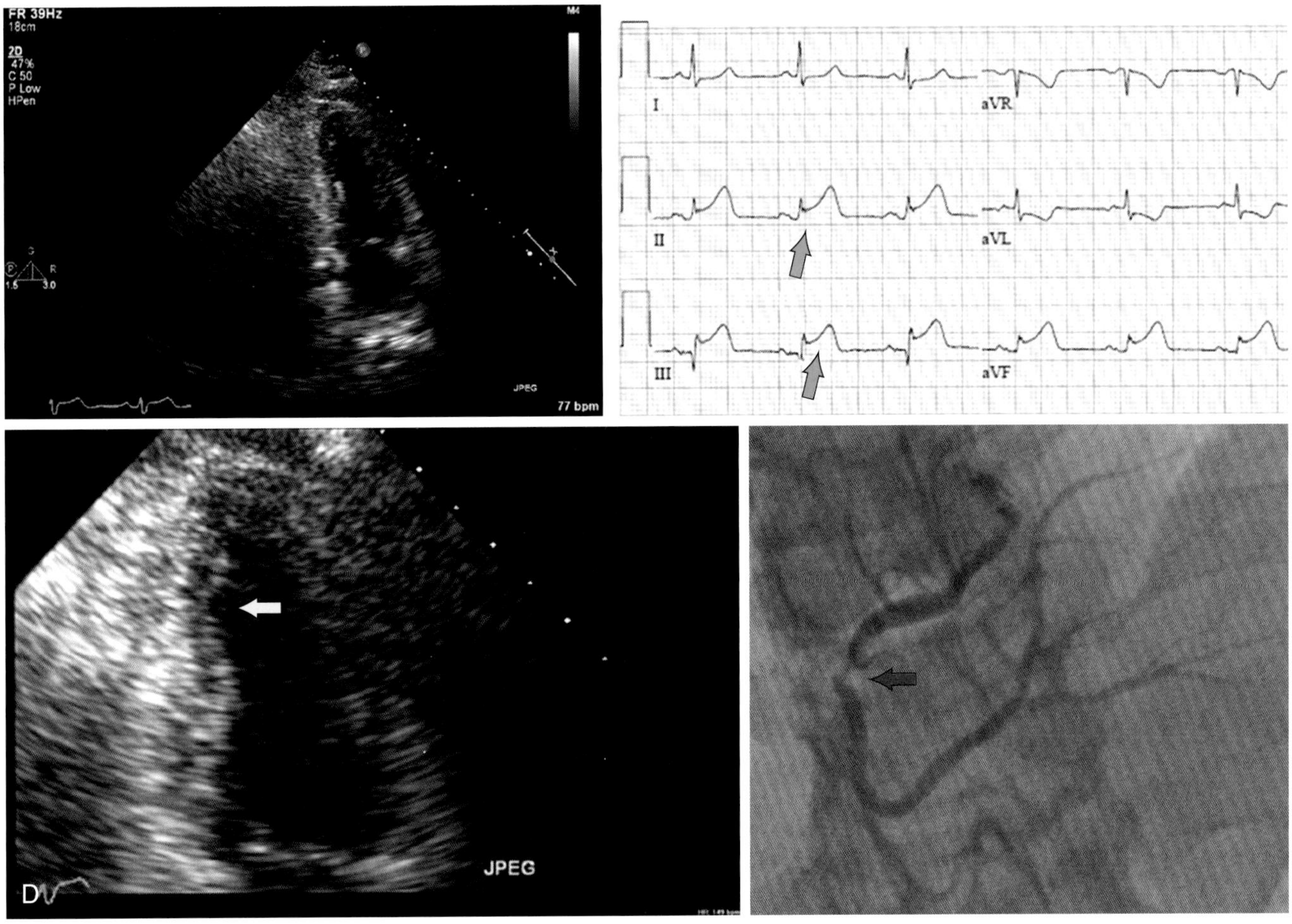

Fig. 19.7—cont'd (D) Possible plaque rupture during exercise stress. At baseline, there was no definitive echocardiographic evidence of wall motion abnormalities. During stress, the patient developed chest pain and inferior wall hypokinesis of the basal and mid-cavitary segments *(yellow arrow at hinge point)*. Inferior ST segment elevation developed on stress ECG *(blue arrows)*, and persisted during recovery. The patient was emergently brought to the catheterization laboratory, where a hazy, possibly acute high-grade stenosis of the mid-right coronary artery was detected and repaired *(red arrow)* (see Video 19.7D).

and the interpreting echocardiographer, and the quality of echocardiographic instrumentation.

Factors that influence sensitivity include poor image quality, delay in post-exercise imaging, studying patients with a low pretest probability, inability to achieve target heart rate and/or double product, and coronary factors such as lack of critical coronary stenosis, single-vessel disease, balanced ischemia in multivessel disease, and lateral wall abnormalities. Specificity can be lowered by lack of contractile reserve associated with valvular heart disease and cardiomyopathy, segmental wall motion abnormalities of the basal inferior wall, and tethering of myocardial segments. Interventricular conduction delays paced rhythms, and a hypertensive response to stress also reduces specificity.

As shown in Fig. 19.9, for identifying and localizing coronary artery obstruction, stress echocardiography was 75% sensitive for LAD stenosis, 33% for LCx stenosis, 78% for RCA lesions, and 65% when assessing all coronary vessels. These findings were comparable to those obtained with single-photon emission computed tomography (SPECT), with the exception of LCx disease, for which stress echocardiography was less sensitive.[64]

Stress echocardiography is more sensitive for identifying patients who have greater myocardial ischemia due to multivessel CAD. Supine bicycle exercise is superior to treadmill exercise for identifying the extent of myocardial ischemia (i.e., number of ischemic segments), but the severity of the wall motion abnormality is similar with both methods.[65] Stress echocardiography is feasible and prognostic for cardiovascular events in high-risk populations, including octogenerians[66] and morbidly obese patients,[67] in whom the use of echocardiographic contrast is strongly encouraged.

SENSITIVITY, SPECIFICITY, AND PROGNOSTIC VALUE OF STRESS ECHOCARDIOGRAPHY

Meta-analyses[30,68,69] have shown that stress echocardiography and nuclear perfusion studies (i.e., SPECT, positron emission tomography [PET]) have similar sensitivity, specificity, and predictive accuracy. In a comprehensive literature review, Dowsley et al.[30] compared stress echocardiography with cardiac CT, PET, cardiac magnetic resonance imaging (CMR)–stress wall motion, CMR–stress perfusion, SPECT, and exercise ECG. The highest sensitivities were with CT, PET, and CMR–stress perfusion, all being greater than 90%. The sensitivities for stress echocardiography, CMR–stress wall motion, and SPECT were similar (79%–85%). Although the specificity of stress echocardiography was the highest of all the modalities studied (87%), overall specificities of the other imaging methods were similar, ranging from 82% to 86%.

A meta-analysis by Metz et al.[69] compared the prognostic value of a normal result on stress radionuclide myocardial

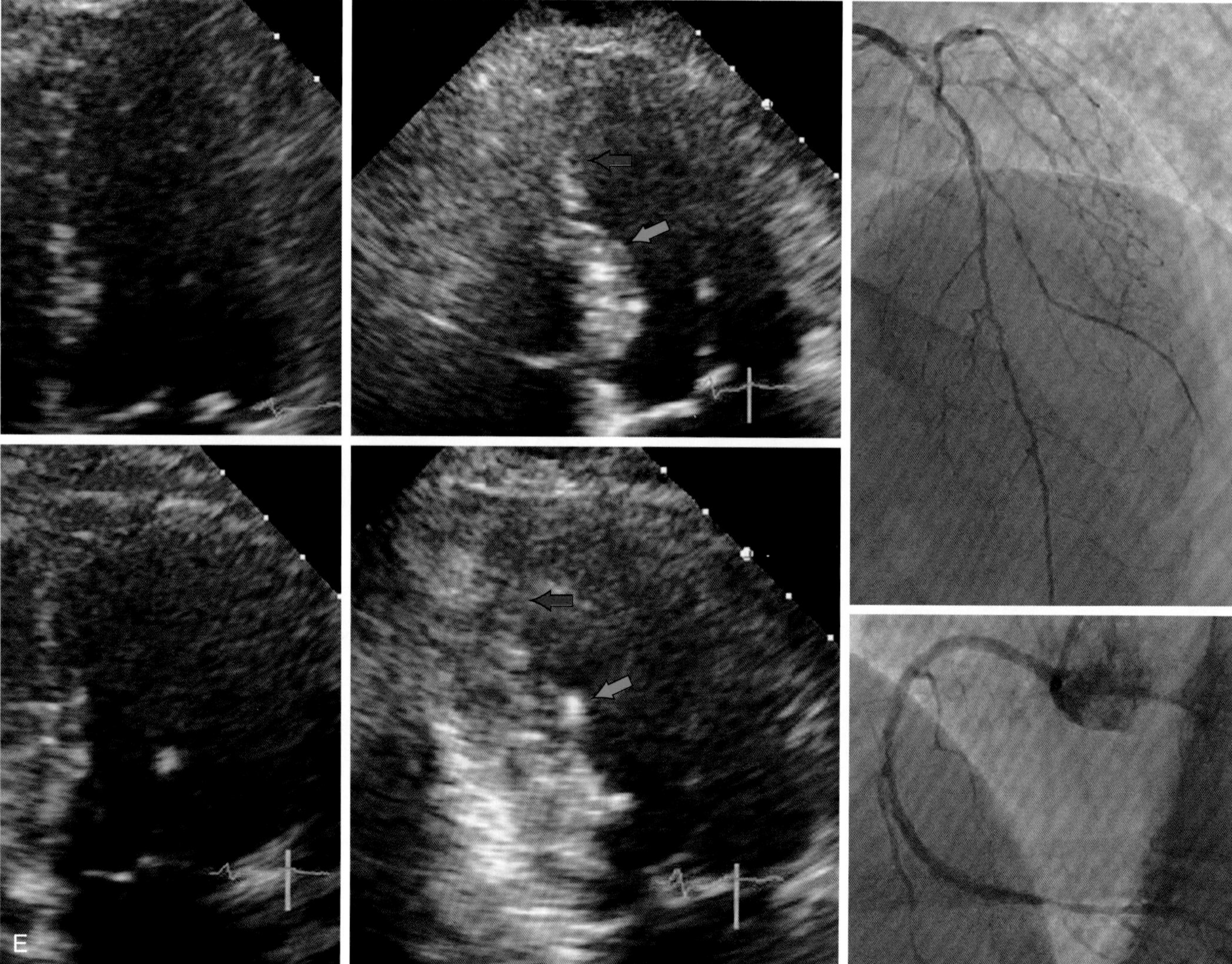

Fig. 19.7—Cont'd (E) LAD ischemia in a setting of three-vessel coronary disease. At baseline there was normal LV function without wall motion abnormalities. At peak stress, the patient reported significant dyspnea and chest pressure and had marked ST depressions. Stress echocardiography detected a middle to distal septal and distal inferior hypokinesis *(red arrows)* with a clear hinge point *(blue arrows)*. Coronary angiography demonstrated multivessel coronary artery disease, and the patient underwent coronary bypass surgery (see Video 19.7E). *ECG*, Echocardiography; *LAD*, left anterior descending coronary artery.

perfusion imaging (rMPI) using thallium, sestamibi, or both with that of a normal stress echocardiogram. The prognosis after a normal test with either imaging modality was excellent. The negative predictive value (NPV) of each test was similarly high. For rMPI, the NPV at 36 months for myocardial infarction and cardiac death was 98.8% (95% CI: 98.5%–99.0%). The follow-up data for stress echocardiography at 33 months indicated a similarly high NPV (98.4%; 95% CI: 97.9%–98.9%); event rates were similar for men and women. Given the high and comparable NPV of either imaging modality for up to almost 3 years, they are both clinically useful.

LBBB on ECG is associated with an increased risk of CAD and death and poses a challenge for stress testing. Bouzas-Mosquera et al.[70] evaluated the prognostic value of stress echocardiography in the setting of LBBB. Of 8050 patients undergoing stress echocardiography, 618 (7.7%) had LBBB. Ischemia was defined as a new or worsening wall motion abnormality with exertion, excluding the septal wall segments.

After 4.6 years of follow-up, patients who developed ischemia (n = 177) had a greater 5-year mortality rate than those with a nonischemic test result (24.6% vs. 12.6%, $P = 0.001$) and almost twice as many major cardiac events (18.1% vs. 9.7%, $P = 0.003$). A multivariate analysis demonstrated that a new wall motion abnormality was a major independent predictor of mortality (hazard ratio = 2.42; 95% CI: 1.30 to 8.82, $P = 0.013$).[70] The investigators also found that stress echocardiography in

TABLE 19.11 Potential Causes of False-Positive and False-Negative Stress Echocardiography Test Results.

False Positives	*False Negatives*
Isolated basal inferior wall motion abnormality	Submaximal exercise
Bundle branch block	Treatment with antianginal medications
Ventricular pacing	Coronary artery stenosis < 50%
After open heart surgery	Poor visualization of the endocardial border zone
Significant hypertension during stress	Changes in imaging plane between pretest and posttest images (i.e., foreshortening)
Interpretation bias (i.e., high pretest probability)	Balanced ischemia
Cardiomyopathies, particularly hypertrophic cardiomyopathy	LV hypertrophy
Changes in imaging plane between pretest and posttest images	

Adapted from Marwick TH. Stress echocardiography. *Heart*. 2003;89(1):113–118.

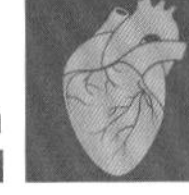

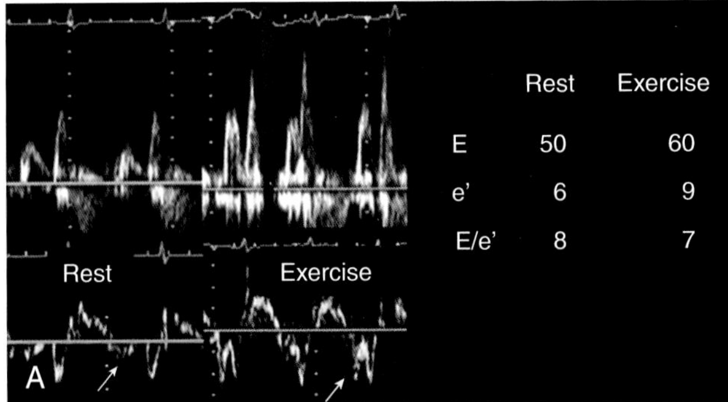

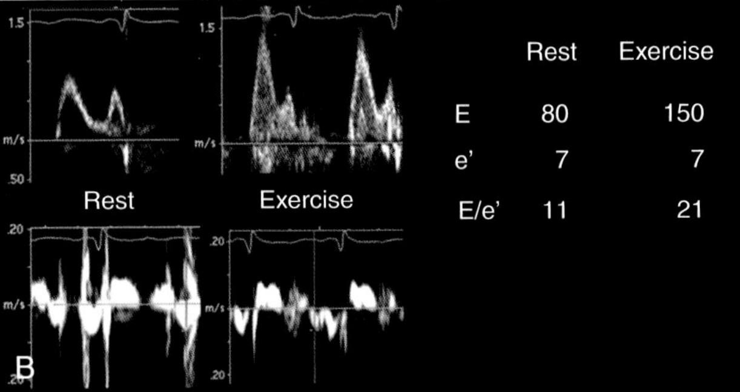

Fig. 19.8 Diastolic stress echocardiography. Stress echocardiographic Doppler data before and after a symptom-limited exercise stress echocardiography test. (A) Data from a patient with a normal response. The rises in E and *e′* velocity are similar, so the E/*e′* ratio stays essentially unchanged. The rises in E and e′ *(yellow arrows)* velocity are similar, so the E/e′ ratio stays essentially unchanged. (B) Data from a patient with a normal vs. pseudonormal filling pattern at rest and a marked increase of both E-wave velocity and E/*e′* ratio, indicating exercise-induced diastolic dysfunction.

TABLE 19.13 Stress Echocardiographic Findings to Report in Addition to Standard Echocardiographic Findings.

Relevant history
- Coronary artery disease
- Exertional angina
- Dyspnea
- Symptom status
- Preoperative evaluation findings
- Other relevant information

Exercise stress testing
- Exercise modality (e.g., treadmill, supine bike, handgrip)
- Exercise protocol (e.g., Bruce, Naughton)
- Exercise duration
- Workload achieved (e.g., watts, METs)
- Adjunct medications used (e.g., atropine 0.4 mg)

Pharmacologic stress testing
- Drugs used, including dose administered (i.e., dobutamine 30 μg, atropine 0.8 mg, metoprolol 5 mg)
- Stress duration

Pacing stress testing
- Pacing modality (e.g., permanent pacemaker, transesophageal pacing)
- Pacing ramp protocol (e.g., 10 beats/min increase at 1 minute intervals)
- Maximum pacing rate

Vital signs
- Baseline and peak heart rate, blood pressure, oxygen saturation
- Peak rate–pressure product
- Qualitative description of hemodynamic response: hypotensive, hypertensive, exaggerated hypertensive

Stress-related symptoms

Reason for stress test termination (e.g., predicted heart rate achieved, significant chest pain)

Stress-induced arrhythmias

Baseline and stress ECG findings

Stress echocardiogram findings
- Stress-induced wall motion abnormalities
- Stress-induced valvular dysfunction
- Stress-induced LV outflow gradient
- Increase of LV outflow gradient
- Peak stress pulmonary artery systolic pressure

ECG, Electrocardiogram; *METs*, metabolic equivalents.

TABLE 19.12 Indications for Terminating a Stress Echocardiography Test.

Absolute Indications
- Moderate or severe angina
- Development of severe shortness of breath
- Drop in O_2 saturation to < 90% or drop of ≥ 10% from baseline
- Drop in systolic blood pressure of ≥ 10 mmHg during stress with ischemia
- Evidence of hypoperfusion
- Sustained ventricular tachycardia (VT)
- ST-segment elevation ≥1 mm (not in leads V_1 or aVR)
- Development of multiple segmental wall motion abnormalities or global LV hypokinesis during exercise
- Development of severe pulmonary hypertension (pulmonary artery pressure [PAP] ≥ 60 mmHg)

Relative Indications
- Drop in systolic blood pressure from baseline but no ischemia
- ST depression horizontal or downsloping by ≥ 2 mm
- Supraventricular tachycardia, heart block, bradyarrhythmias, VT not sustained
- Systolic blood pressure ≥ 250 mmHg or diastolic blood pressure ≥ 150 mmHg
- Bundle branch block or intraventricular conduction defect that cannot be distinguished from VT

Routine Indications
- Target heart rate or double product achieved
- Fatigue
- Shortness of breath
- Patient's inability to continue to exercise

TABLE 19.14 Comparison of Stress and Imaging Modalities for Sensitivity and Specificity in Detecting Coronary Artery Disease.

Cardiac Imaging Modality	*Sensitivity (%)*	*Specificity (%)*
CTA	98	82
Stress echocardiography	79	87
PET	92	85
Stress CMR wall motion	83	86
Stress CMR perfusion	91	81
SPECT	85	85
Exercise ECG	68	77

CMR, Cardiac magnetic resonance imaging; *CTA*, computed tomography angiography; *ECG*, electrocardiogram; *SPECT*, single-photon emission computer tomography; *PET*, positron emission tomography.

Adapted from Dowsley T, Al-Mallah M, Ananthasubramaniam K, et al. The role of non-invasive imaging in coronary artery disease detection, prognosis, and clinical decision making. *Can J Cardiol*. 2013;29:285–296.

patients with LBBB was superior to clinical assessment, resting echocardiogram, and stress ECG without echocardiography.

Other high-risk features include stress-induced wall motion abnormalities in multiple segments, particularly when baseline and stress-induced wall motion abnormalities coexist. Ischemia in the distribution of the LAD, multiple inducible wall motion abnormalities, ischemia at a low threshold, lack of an increase in ejection fraction and absence of a reduction in LV end-systolic volume in response to exercise, and presence of LV hypertrophy at baseline are associated with a high risk. Patients with resting wall motion abnormalities and no inducible ischemia are at intermediate risk.[31]

Selecting the appropriate test for the patient depends on echocardiographic image quality and local expertise of the cardiovascular imaging center in stress echocardiography, radionuclide imaging, cardiac CT, or CMR. Additional factors that should be considered include cost and radiation exposure, both of which favor stress echocardiography.

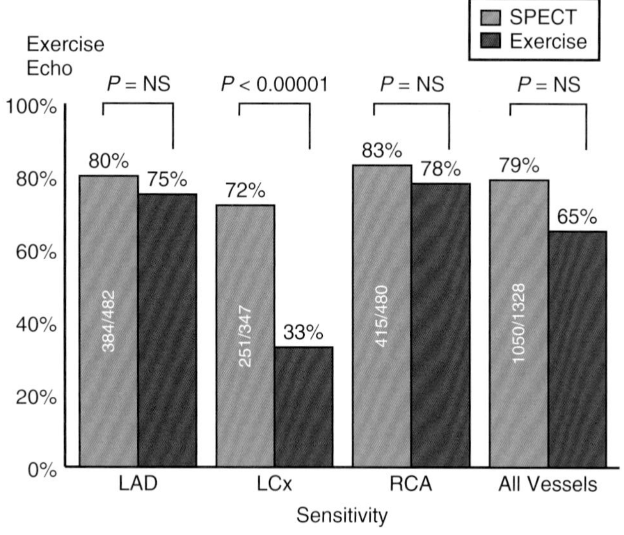

Fig. 19.9 Differential sensitivities for detecting significant stenoses based on coronary distribution. Whereas the sensitivities of SPECT and stress echocardiography were similar in the LAD and RCA distributions, sensitivity was significant lower for stress echocardiography in the LCx distribution. *Echo*, Echocardiography; *LAD*, left anterior descending coronary artery; *LCx*, left circumflex coronary artery; *NS*, nonsignificant; *RCA*, right coronary artery; *SPECT*, single-photon emission computed tomography. (From O'Keefe JH Jr, Barnhart CS, Bateman TM. Comparison of stress echocardiography and stress myocardial perfusion scintigraphy for diagnosing coronary artery disease and assessing its severity. *Am J Cardiol*. 1995;75:25D–34D.)

FUTURE DEVELOPMENTS IN STRESS ECHOCARDIOGRAPHY

STRAIN ECHOCARDIOGRAPHY

Interpretation of stress-induced wall motion abnormalities is largely qualitative, and although the sensitivity and specificity of standard exercise stress echocardiography protocols are excellent,[30] a more quantitative approach may be desirable to reduce interobserver variability. Strain techniques measure deformation of the myocardium by either tissue Doppler imaging or speckle tracking. A major advantage of speckle tracking techniques is a global assessment of myocardial function (global strain), which is useful in the longitudinal surveillance of valvular heart disease or cardio-oncology but less useful in stress echocardiography, for which the goal usually is to detect regional myocardial dysfunction.

As reviewed by Argyle et al.,[71] strain initially increases with heart rate and then plateaus and may even decrease in response to the tachycardia-induced decrease in LV filling and decreased stroke volume. However, strain rate (i.e., changes of strain over time) increases in a linear fashion with increasing heart rate and therefore may be better suited as an indicator of myocardial function during stress echocardiography. Abnormalities in post-systolic strain (i.e., strain occurring after closure of the aortic valve) constitute another determinant of myocardial ischemia.[72]

Strain imaging during stress for the detection of CAD has been evaluated with exercise[73] and dobutamine stress methods.[74–76] Preliminary data show that strain imaging can be useful in the assessment of viability in conjunction with dobutamine stress testing after myocardial infarction.[77] Major limitations of this technique are (1) the assessment of apical segments, particularly with the tissue Doppler method[74]; (2) dependence on excellent image quality, particularly with speckle tracking; (3) differences in tissue Doppler angle, which affect strain measurements; (4) need for manual placement of the detection zone; (5) manual confirmation of tracking with automated software; (6) additional time required for postprocessing and interpretation; and (7) variation in strain imaging quality and normal values among vendors. Much of the available data on stress echocardiography strain measurement are limited to relatively few studies with relatively few patients.[77]

Because of these limitations, current guidelines do not recommend routine use of strain imaging during stress echocardiography. However, newer echocardiographic technologies and improved tracking algorithms may lead to the clinical use of strain technologies for detection of CAD. Recent data showed that four-dimensional echocardiography area strain imaging may be able to detect even mild coronary stenoses (<50%).[78] Fig. 19.10 depicts examples of physiologic and pathologic (i.e., ischemic) strain curves and their evaluation during stress testing.[79]

3D ECHOCARDIOGRAPHY

Real-time 3D echocardiography allows rapid full-volume image acquisition during stress testing. Fig. 19.11 shows an example of how a full-volume data set can be used to evaluate stacks of short-axis images at any level of the LV. Major advantages of this technique are (1) unlimited tomographic images such that multiple planes of any ventricular segment can be imaged; (2) ability to choose pre-exercise and post-exercise cuts of the 3D data to best match corresponding myocardial segments, allowing precise comparison of prestress and poststress segmental wall motion; (3) rapid image acquisition, which reduces image acquisition time and can potentially prevent post-exercise imaging during submaximal heart rate; (4) less difficulty with apical foreshortening; (5) less reliance on the operator for optimal image acquisition; (6) more accurate measurements of LV volumes and ejection fraction; and (7) improved interobserver variability.[80,81] To summarize, the major advantage of 3D echocardiography for stress testing is the ability to quickly and completely acquire the segmental wall motion of the entire LV.

Studies by Peteiro et al.[82] and Jenkins et al.[83] using treadmill stress and 3D stress echocardiography showed that 3D echocardiography had a better sensitivity and specificity for detection of CAD (verified by coronary angiography) than 2D stress echocardiography. However, the disadvantages of 3D imaging include (1) prolonged postprocessing of images; (2) larger imaging transducer footprint, which sometimes makes it more difficult to obtain optimal images; (3) learning curves for sonographers and echocardiologists; and (4) reduction in temporal and spatial resolution compared with 2D techniques.

Despite its limitations, 3D imaging during stress testing will play an increasingly important role in the future as new equipment and imaging software develop. Another potential use of 3D imaging is the assessment of parametric 3D maps with corresponding time–volume curves to assess stress-induced ischemic wall changes (Fig. 19.12).[84]

MYOCARDIAL CONTRAST PERFUSION STRESS ECHOCARDIOGRAPHY

Although assessment of stress-induced wall motion abnormalities during exercise or pharmacologic stress echocardiography has excellent sensitivity and specificity,[30] use of echocardiographic contrast (i.e., lipid-laden microspheres [microbubbles] that pass through the lung circulation) improve assessment by enhancing the endocardial border zones of the LV. The microspheres can enter the myocardial microvasculature and enhance

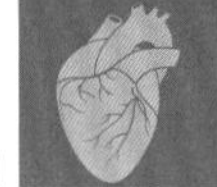

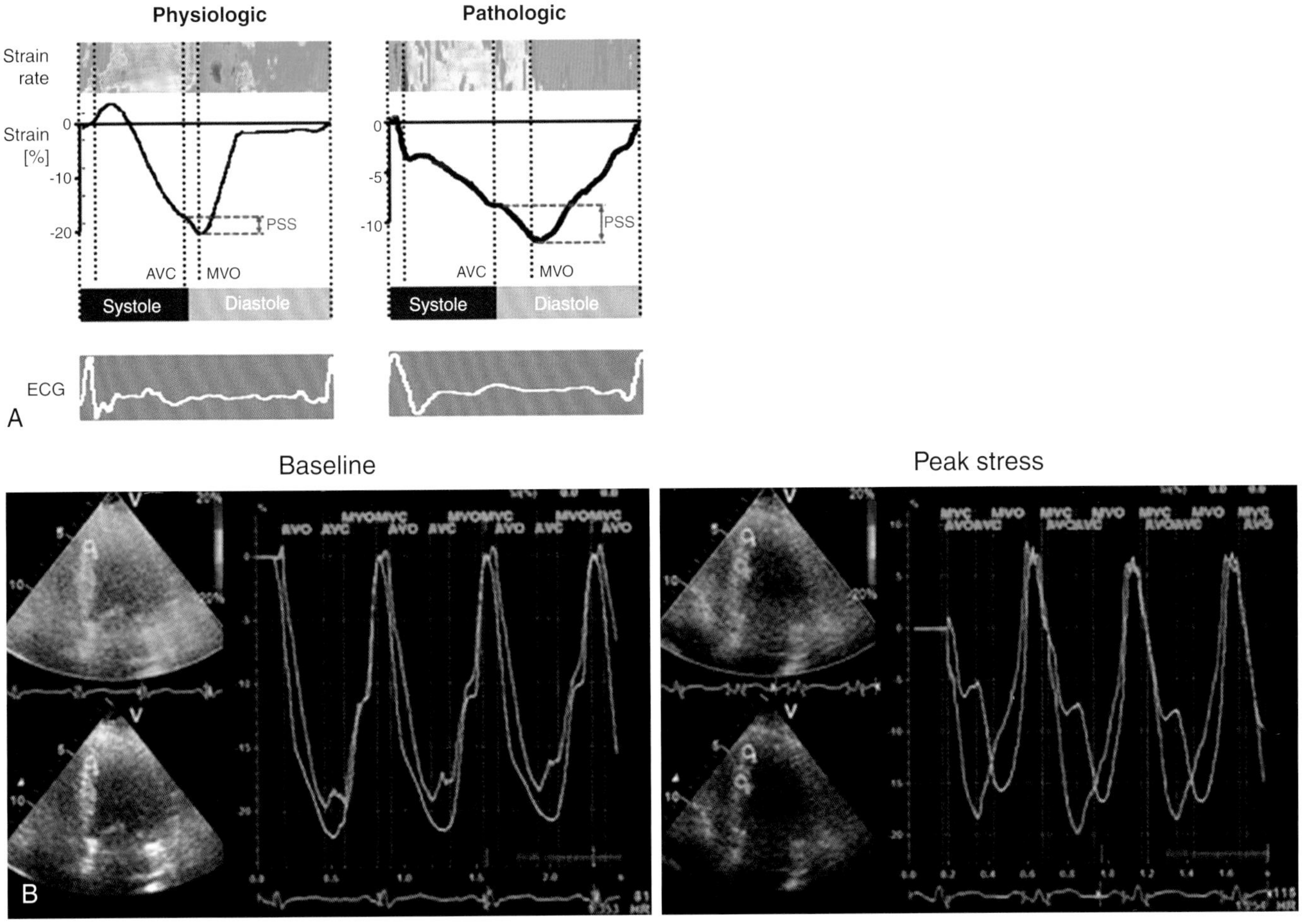

Fig. 19.10 **Strain imaging for the detection of coronary ischemia.** (A) Physiologic *(left)* and pathologic *(right)* strain curves in two myocardial segments, both showing accentuated PSS. (B) Baseline *(left)* and peak stress *(right)* strain curves of an ischemic apical septal segment (left anterior descending artery territory). The *yellow* curve clearly demonstrates reduced systolic strain and marked PSS at peak stress, suggesting inducible ischemia. *AVC*, Aortic valve closure; *AVO*, aortic valve opening; *ECG*, electrocardiogram; *MVC*, mitral valve closure; *MVO*, mitral valve opening; *PSS*, postsystolic shortening. (From Mada RO, Duchenne J, Voight J-U. Tissue Doppler, strain and strain rate in ischemic heart disease "how I do it." *Cardiovasc Ultrasound.* 2014;12:38.)

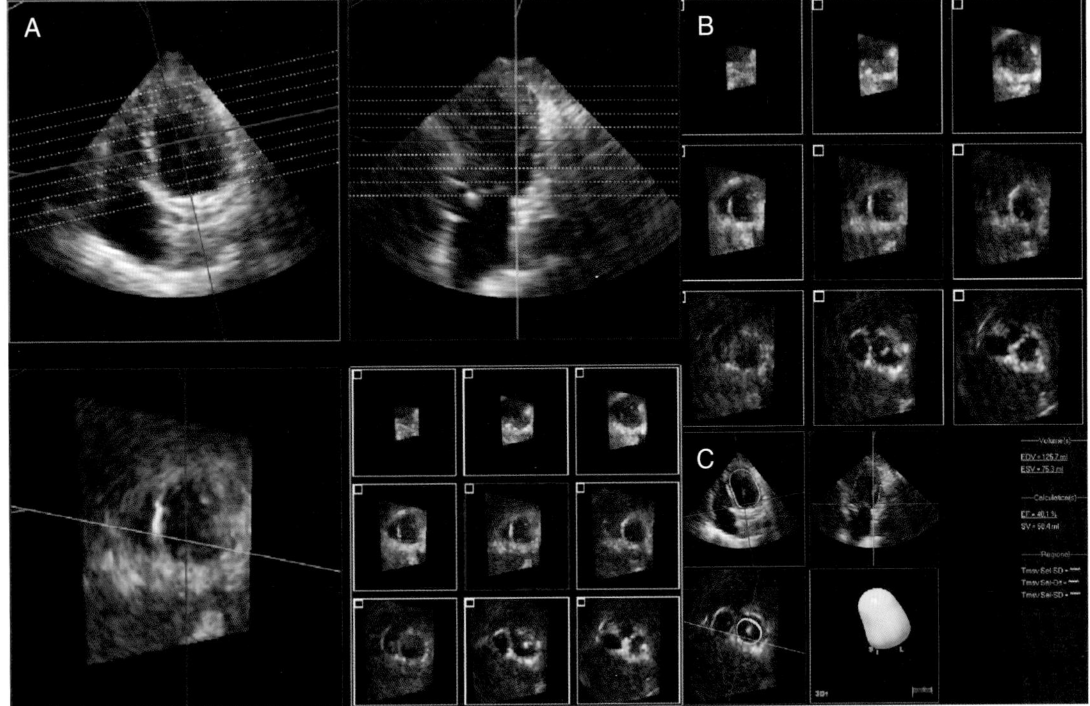

Fig. 19.11 **3D echocardiography.** 3D full-volume image acquisition is used to create short-axis stacks (A and B) and assess wall motion abnormalities and full volumetric measurement of the LV ejection fraction (C).

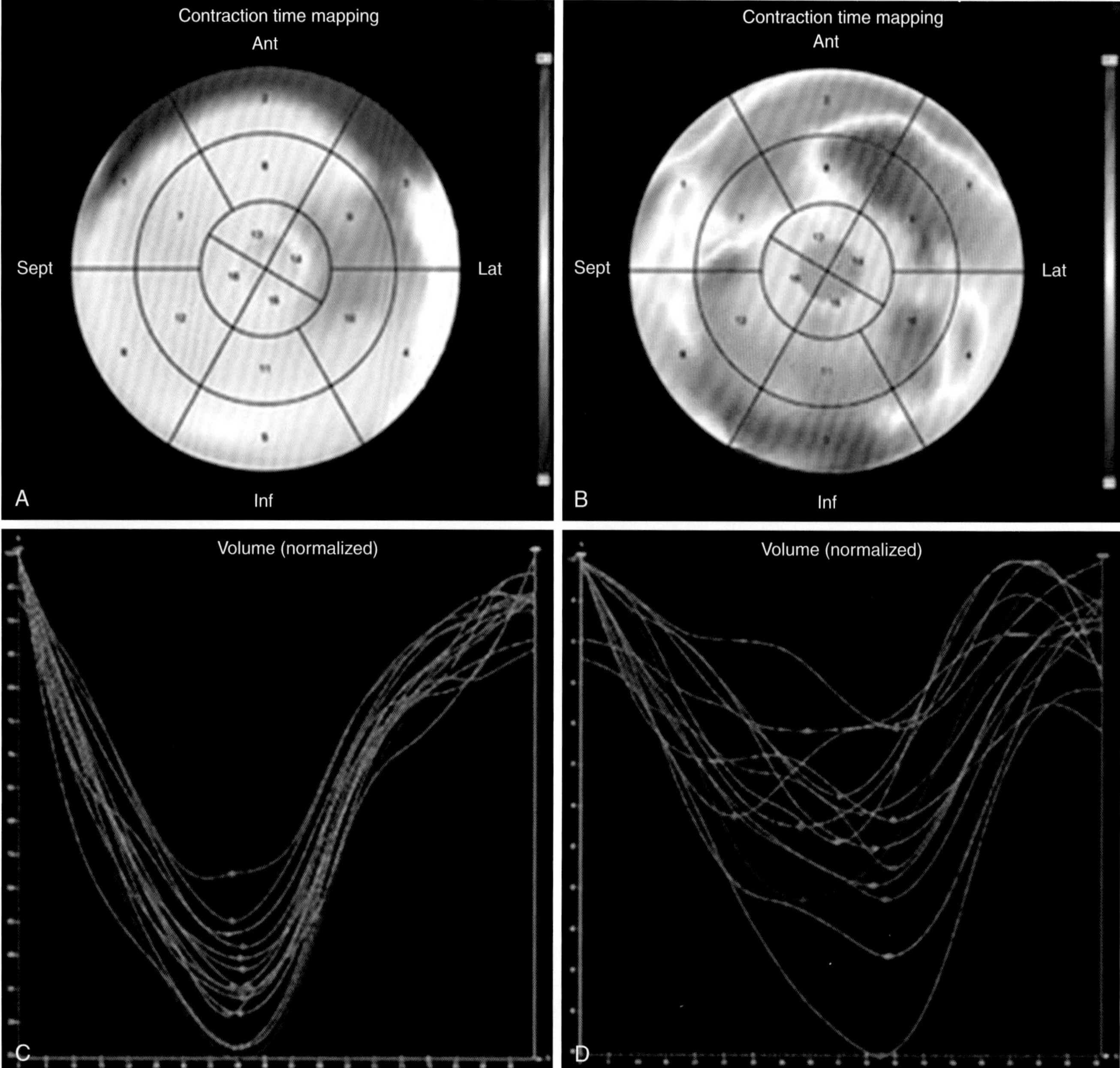

Fig. 19.12 3D imaging to assess stress-induced ischemic wall changes. 3D parametric maps of the LV in the 16-segment model *(top panels)* with corresponding time–volume curves *(bottom panels)*. (A and C) Normal LV contraction at baseline. (B and D) Asynchronous systolic contraction at peak stress, indicating stress-induced wall motion abnormalities. (From Berbarie RF, Dib E, Ahmad M. Stress echocardiography using real-time three-dimensional imaging. *Echocardiography.* 2018;35:1196–1203.)

the myocardial echocardiographic signal, allowing direct assessment of myocardial blood flow.[85,86]

Given the need for optimal imaging conditions and to fully take advantage of myocardial perfusion imaging, most studies have used dobutamine,[87] dipyridamole, or a combination of them with atropine as stressor.[88] However, successful contrast perfusion imaging has also been performed using bicycle ergometry.[89]

Evaluation of myocardial contrast perfusion can be qualitative (i.e., present or absent myocardial contrast), semiquantitative (i.e., normal, reduced, or absent perfusion), or quantitative. Ideally, echocardiographic contrast is infused over several minutes to achieve a steady state, followed by a high-mechanical-index ultrasound flash, which destroys contrast bubbles in the viewing field. Reaccumulation of contrast within the myocardium is observed during the first few beats after the flash to detect segmental perfusion abnormalities (Fig. 19.13).

The video intensity of contrast reaccumulation in a specific myocardial segment can be quantified off-line with specialized software. However, this step is time-consuming and is rarely done for clinical purposes. Typically, the video intensity is measured in ECG-triggered end-systolic imaging frames.[88]

Although quantitative evaluation of myocardial perfusion has many challenges, most of which are related to breathing-induced motion artifact, overall image quality, and reproducibility, qualitative or semiquantitative assessment of contrast perfusion can easily be added to regular stress protocols.[90] There is no expert consensus for the performance of myocardial contrast echocardiography, and current guidelines do not recommend this technique. However, abnormal perfusion has been a useful prognosticator, and this assessment may play an increasingly important role in the future.[85]

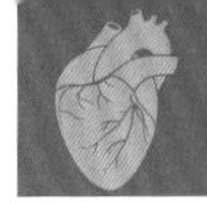

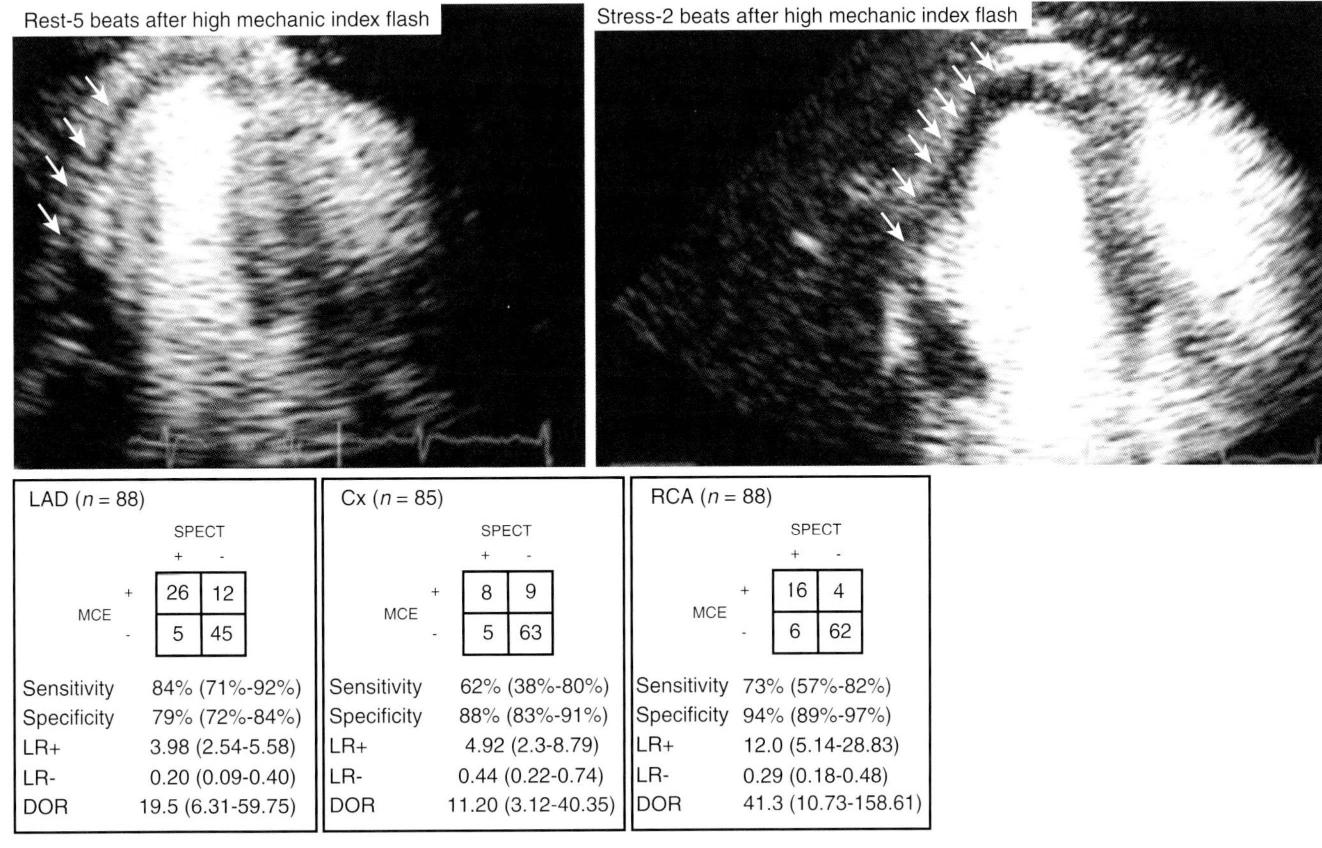

Rest-5 beats after high mechanic index flash
Stress-2 beats after high mechanic index flash
LAD (n = 88)
SPECT
+ -
MCE
+ 26 12
- 5 45
Sensitivity 84% (71%-92%)
Specificity 79% (72%-84%)
LR+ 3.98 (2.54-5.58)
LR- 0.20 (0.09-0.40)
DOR 19.5 (6.31-59.75)
Cx (n = 85)
SPECT
+ -
MCE
+ 8 9
- 5 63
Sensitivity 62% (38%-80%)
Specificity 88% (83%-91%)
LR+ 4.92 (2.3-8.79)
LR- 0.44 (0.22-0.74)
DOR 11.20 (3.12-40.35)
RCA (n = 88)
SPECT
+ -
MCE
+ 16 4
- 6 62
Sensitivity 73% (57%-82%)
Specificity 94% (89%-97%)
LR+ 12.0 (5.14-28.83)
LR- 0.29 (0.18-0.48)
DOR 41.3 (10.73-158.61)

Fig. 19.13 **Myocardial contrast echocardiography.** A fixed perfusion defect in the distribution of the left circumflex coronary artery is seen at rest *(top left)*, with worsening of the defect after stress, in this case, adenosine induced *(top right)*. *Bottom panels*: Sensitivity for MCE compared with SPECT was best for LAD defects and lowest for LCx defects, whereas specificity was best for RCA defects. *DOR*, Diagnostic odds ratio; *LAD*, left anterior descending artery; *LR+*, positive likelihood ratio; *LR−*, negative likelihood ratio; *Cx*, left circumflex artery; *MCE*, myocardial contrast echocardiography; *SPECT*, single-photon emission computed tomography; *RCA*, right coronary artery. (From Abdelmoneim SS, Bernier M, Dhoble A, et al. Diagnostic accuracy of contrast echocardiography during adenosine stress for detection of abnormal myocardial perfusion: a prospective comparison with technetium-99 m sestamibi single-photon emission computed tomography. *Heart Vessels*. 2010;25:121–130.)

SUMMARY Exercise Echocardiography.

Test Stage	Technical Details	Findings	Interpretation
Baseline imaging	Assessment of LV and RV function and wall motion 1. Parasternal long-axis view 2. Parasternal short-axis view 3. Parasternal RV inflow view 4. Apical 4-chamber view 5. Apical 2-chamber view 6. Apical long-axis view (may replace parasternal long-axis view)	Baseline wall motion abnormality	Reassess appropriateness of exercise echocardiogram as diagnostic test.
	7. Assess resting diastolic function (pulsed wave Doppler E-wave velocity, tissue Doppler e′ at high sweep speed)	Normal, grades I to III diastolic dysfunction	Use as baseline for comparison with exercise data.
	Assessment of valvular function	Severe aortic stenosis	Abort test, unless goal of test is to evaluate functional capacity in an asymptomatic patient.
	Assessment of pulmonary artery systolic pressure 1. Peak tricuspid regurgitation velocity 2. IVC size/collapse	Severe pulmonary hypertension (≥60 mmHg)	Reassess appropriateness of test.

SUMMARY Exercise Echocardiography.—cont'd

Test Stage	Technical Details	Findings	Interpretation
Exercise	Treadmill ergometry Upright bicycle ergometry Supine bicycle ergometry Add-on interventions: 1. Handgrip exercise 2. A tropine 0.4 to maximal 2.0 mg	1. Functional capacity (Watts/METs achieved, Borg scale of perceived exertion) 2. External workload achieved (Watts/METs, % of predicted heart rate achieved, heart rate pressure-double product)	<5 METs: poor 5–8 METs: fair 9–11 METs: good ≥12 METs: excellent ≥85% of age-adjusted heart rate considered appropriate workload
Evaluation of ischemia	**Treadmill**: immediately after exercise **Upright/supine bicycle**: during each stage plus at peak exercise		
ECG	1. Continuous ECG monitoring	Arrhythmias	Possible sign of ischemia or exercise-induced diastolic dysfunction
	2. 12-lead ECG at each exercise stage	ST segment deviation (80 ms after the J-point) 1. Upsloping ST segment depression of ≥1.5 mm 2. Horizontal or downsloping ST segment depression ≥1 mm 3. ST segment elevation	Ischemia
Echocardiography	Assessment of LV and RV function and wall motion 1. Parasternal long-axis view 2. Parasternal short-axis view 3. Apical 4-chamber view 4. Apical 2-chamber view 5. Apical long-axis view (may replace parasternal long-axis view) Optional:	1. Hyperdynamic 2. Focal hypokinesis 3. Focal akinesis 4. Global hypokinesis or transient LV dilation	Normal Subendocardial ischemia Transmural ischemia Multivessel (i.e., balanced) ischemia
	6. Parasternal RV inflow view	Hypokinesis or dilation	RV ischemia, exercise-induced pulmonary hypertension
	7. Assess exertional diastolic function (pulsed wave Doppler E-wave velocity, tissue Doppler *e′* at high sweep speed)	1. Parallel increase in E and e′ velocity 2. Increase of E > *e′*	Normal Exercise-induced diastolic dysfunction
Heart rate recovery	No cool down during stress echocardiography compared with stress ECG	≥18 beats/min within the first minute <18 beats/min	Normal Increased cardiovascular risk

ECG, Electrocardiogram; *IVC*, inferior vena cava; *METs*, metabolic equivalents.

REFERENCES

1. Armstrong WF. Acute myocardial ischemia: from Tennant and Wiggers to contrast echocardiography. *J Am Coll Cardiol*. 1986;7(2):393–394.
2. Theroux P, Franklin D, Ross Jr J, Kemper WS. Regional myocardial function during acute coronary artery occlusion and its modification by pharmacologic agents in the dog. *Circ Res*. 1974;35(6):896–908.
3. Theroux P, Ross Jr J, Franklin D, Kemper WS, Sasyama S. Regional myocardial function in the conscious dog during acute coronary occlusion and responses to morphine, propranolol, nitroglycerin, and lidocaine. *Circulation*. 1976;53(2):302–314.
4. Kerber RE, Marcus ML, Ehrhardt J, Wilson R, Abboud FM. Correlation between echocardiographically demonstrated segmental dyskinesis and regional myocardial perfusion. *Circulation*. 1975;52(6):1097–1104.
5. Wann LS, Faris JV, Childress RH, Dillon JC, Weyman AE, Feigenbaum H. Exercise cross-sectional echocardiography in ischemic heart disease. *Circulation*. 1979;60(6):1300–1308.
6. Chatal JF, Rouzet F, Haddad F, Bourdeau C, Mathieu C, Le Guludec D. Story of Rubidium-82 and advantages for myocardial perfusion PET imaging. *Front Med*. 2015;2:65.
7. Fazel R, Shaw LJ. Radiation exposure from radionuclide myocardial perfusion imaging: concerns and solutions. *J Nucl Cardiol*. 2011;18(4):562–565.
8. Holland DJ, Prasad SB, Marwick TH. Prognostic implications of left ventricular filling pressure with exercise. *Circ Cardiovasc Imaging*. 2010;3(2):149–156.

9. Michaelides AP, Fourlas CA, Giannopoulos N, et al. Significance of QRS duration changes in the evaluation of ST-segment depression presenting exclusively during the postexercise recovery period. *Ann Noninvasive Electrocardiol.* 2006;11(3):241–246.
10. Fihn SD, Blankenship JC, Alexander KP, et al. ACC/AHA/AATS/PCNA/SCAI/STS focused update of the guideline for the diagnosis and management of patients with stable ischemic heart disease: a report of the American College of Cardiology/American Heart Association Task Force on Practice Guidelines, and the American Association for Thoracic Surgery, Preventive Cardiovascular Nurses Association, Society for Cardiovascular Angiography and Interventions, and Society of Thoracic Surgeons. *J Am Coll Cardiol.* 2014;64(18):1929–1949.
11. Qaseem A, Fihn SD, Dallas P, et al. Management of stable ischemic heart disease: summary of a clinical practice guideline from the American College of Physicians/American College of Cardiology Foundation/American Heart Association/American Association for Thoracic Surgery/Preventive Cardiovascular Nurses Association/Society of Thoracic Surgeons. *Ann Intern Med.* 2012;157(10):735–743.
12. Morise AP, Diamond GA, Detrano R, Bobbio M. Incremental value of exercise electrocardiography and thallium-201 testing in men and women for the presence and extent of coronary artery disease. *Am Heart J.* 1995;130(2):267–276.
13. Banerjee A, Newman DR, Van den Bruel A, Heneghan C. Diagnostic accuracy of exercise stress testing for coronary artery disease: a systematic review and meta-analysis of prospective studies. *Int J Clin Pract.* 2012;66(5):477–492.
14. Morise AP, Diamond GA. Comparison of the sensitivity and specificity of exercise electrocardiography in biased and unbiased populations of men and women. *Am Heart J.* 1995;130(4):741–747.
15. Akil S, Heden B, Pahlm O, Carlsson M, Arheden H, Engblom H. Gender aspects on exercise-induced ECG changes in relation to scintigraphic evidence of myocardial ischaemia. *Clin Physiol Funct Imaging.* 2018;38(5):798–807.
16. Sarnoff SJ, Braunwald E, Welch Jr GH, Case RB, Stainsby WN, Macruz R. Hemodynamic determinants of oxygen consumption of the heart with special reference to the tension-time index. *Am J Physiol.* 1958;192(1):148–156.
17. Graham Jr TP, Covell JW, Sonnenblick EH, Ross Jr J, Braunwald E. Control of myocardial oxygen consumption: relative influence of contractile state and tension development. *J Clin Invest.* 1968;47(2):375–385.
18. Schwid HA, Buffington CW, Strum DP. Computer simulation of the hemodynamic determinants of myocardial oxygen supply and demand. *J Cardiothorac Anesth.* 1990;4(1):5–18.
19. Suga H, Yamada O, Goto Y, Igarashi Y. Oxygen consumption and pressure-volume area of abnormal contractions in canine heart. *Am J Physiol.* 1984;246(2 Pt 2):H154–H160.
20. Suga H, Yamada O, Goto Y, Igarashi Y, Ishiguri H. Constant mechanical efficiency of contractile machinery of canine left ventricle under different loading and inotropic conditions. *Jpn J Physiol.* 1984;34(4):679–698.
21. Crystal GJ, Silver JM, Salem MR. Mechanisms of increased right and left ventricular oxygen uptake during inotropic stimulation. *Life Sci.* 2013;93(2-3):59–63.
22. Motwani M, Kidambi A, Uddin A, Sourbron S, Greenwood JP, Plein S. Quantification of myocardial blood flow with cardiovascular magnetic resonance throughout the cardiac cycle. *J Cardiovasc Magn Reson.* 2015;17(1):4.
23. Wolk MJ, Bailey SR, Doherty JU, et al. ACCF/AHA/ASE/ASNC/HFSA/HRS/SCAI/SCCT/SCMR/STS 2013 multimodality appropriate use criteria for the detection and risk assessment of stable ischemic heart disease: a report of the American College of Cardiology Foundation Appropriate Use Criteria Task Force, American Heart Association, American Society of Echocardiography, American Society of Nuclear Cardiology, Heart Failure Society of America, Heart Rhythm Society, Society for Cardiovascular Angiography and Interventions, Society of Cardiovascular Computed Tomography, Society for Cardiovascular Magnetic Resonance, and Society of Thoracic Surgeons. *J Am Coll Cardiol.* 2014;63(4):380–406.
24. Pellikka PA, Arruda-Olson A, Chaudhry FA, et al. Guidelines for performance, interpretation, and application of stress echocardiography in ischemic heart disease: from the American Society of Echocardiography. *J Am Soc Echocardiogr.* 2020;33(1):1–41 e48.
25. Fihn SD, Gardin JM, Abrams J, et al. 2012 ACCF/AHA/ACP/AATS/PCNA/SCAI/STS guideline for the diagnosis and management of patients with stable ischemic Heart Disease: Executive Summary: a Report of the American College of Cardiology Foundation/American Heart Association Task Force on Practice Guidelines, and the American College of Physicians, American Association for Thoracic Surgery, Preventive Cardiovascular Nurses Association, Society for Cardiovascular Angiography and Interventions, and Society of Thoracic Surgeons. *Circulation.* 2012;126(25):3097–3137.
26. Shaw LJ, Eagle KA, Gersh BJ, Miller DD. Meta-analysis of intravenous dipyridamole-thallium-201 imaging (1985 to 1994) and dobutamine echocardiography (1991 to 1994) for risk stratification before vascular surgery. *J Am Coll Cardiol.* 1996;27(4):787–798.
27. Poldermans D, Arnese M, Fioretti PM, et al. Sustained prognostic value of dobutamine stress echocardiography for late cardiac events after major noncardiac vascular surgery. *Circulation.* 1997;95(1):53–58.
28. Beattie WS, Abdelnaem E, Wijeysundera DN, Buckley DN. A meta-analytic comparison of preoperative stress echocardiography and nuclear scintigraphy imaging. *Anesth Analg.* 2006;102(1):8–16.
29. Gurunathan S, Zacharias K, Akhtar M, et al. Cost-effectiveness of a management strategy based on exercise echocardiography versus exercise electrocardiography in patients presenting with suspected angina during long term follow up: a randomized study. *Int J Cardiol.* 2018;259:1–7.
30. Dowsley T, Al-Mallah M, Ananthasubramaniam K, Dwivedi G, McArdle B, Chow BJ. The role of noninvasive imaging in coronary artery disease detection, prognosis, and clinical decision making. *Can J Cardiol.* 2013;29(3):285–296.
31. Pellikka PA, Nagueh SF, Elhendy AA, Kuehl CA, Sawada SG, American Society of E. American Society of Echocardiography recommendations for performance, interpretation, and application of stress echocardiography. *J Am Soc Echocardiogr.* 2007;20(9):1021–1041.
32. Caiati C, Lepera ME, Carretta D, Santoro D, Favale S. Head-to-head comparison of peak upright bicycle and post-treadmill echocardiography in detecting coronary artery disease: a randomized, single-blind crossover study. *J Am Soc Echocardiogr.* 2013;26(12):1434–1443.
33. Kane GC, Hepinstall MJ, Kidd GM, et al. Safety of stress echocardiography supervised by registered nurses: results of a 2-year audit of 15,404 patients. *J Am Soc Echocardiogr.* 2008;21(4):337–341.
34. Yao SS, Moldenhauer S, Sherrid MV. Isometric handgrip exercise during dobutamine-atropine stress echocardiography increases heart rate acceleration and decreases study duration and dobutamine and atropine dosage. *Clin Cardiol.* 2003;26(5):238–242.
35. Fletcher GF, Balady GJ, Amsterdam EA, et al. Exercise standards for testing and training: a statement for healthcare professionals from the American Heart Association. *Circulation.* 2001;104(14):1694–1740.
36. Nalawadi SS, Tolstrup K, Cuk O, et al. Atropine as an adjunct to supine bicycle stress echocardiography: an alternative strategy to achieve target heart rate or rate pressure product. *Eur Heart J Cardiovasc Imaging.* 2012;13(7):612–616.
37. Hung RK, Al-Mallah MH, Whelton SP, et al. Effect of beta-blocker therapy, maximal heart rate, and exercise capacity during stress testing on long-term Survival (from the Henry Ford Exercise Testing Project). *Am J Cardiol.* 2016;118(11):1751–1757.
38. Borg GA. Psychophysical bases of perceived exertion. *Med Sci Sports Exerc.* 1982;14(5):377–381.
39. Lauer MS, Francis GS, Okin PM, Pashkow FJ, Snader CE, Marwick TH. Impaired chronotropic response to exercise stress testing as a predictor of mortality. *Jama.* 1999;281(6):524–529.
40. Manganelli F, Spadafora M, Varrella P, et al. Addition of atropine to submaximal exercise stress testing in patients evaluated for suspected ischaemia with SPECT imaging: a randomized, placebo-controlled trial. *Eur J Nucl Med Mol Imag.* 2011;38(2):245–251.
41. Makani H, Bangalore S, Halpern D, Makwana HG, Chaudhry FA. Cardiac outcomes with submaximal normal stress echocardiography: a meta-analysis. *J Am Coll Cardiol.* 2012;60(15):1393–1401.
42. Nishime EO, Cole CR, Blackstone EH, Pashkow FJ, Lauer MS. Heart rate recovery and treadmill exercise score as predictors of mortality in patients referred for exercise ECG. *Jama.* 2000;284(11):1392–1398.
43. Singh JP, Larson MG, Manolio TA, et al. Blood pressure response during treadmill testing as a risk factor for new-onset hypertension. The Framingham Heart Study. *Circulation.* 1999;99(14):1831–1836.
44. Lauer MS, Pashkow FJ, Harvey SA, Marwick TH, Thomas JD. Angiographic and prognostic implications of an exaggerated exercise systolic blood pressure response and rest systolic blood pressure in adults undergoing evaluation for suspected coronary artery disease. *J Am Coll Cardiol.* 1995;26(7):1630–1636.
45. Lauer MS, Levy D, Anderson KM, Plehn JF. Is there a relationship between exercise systolic blood pressure response and left ventricular mass? The Framingham Heart Study. *Ann Intern Med.* 1992;116(3):203–210.
46. Allison TG, Cordeiro MA, Miller TD, Daida H, Squires RW, Gau GT. Prognostic significance of exercise-induced systemic hypertension in healthy subjects. *Am J Cardiol.* 1999;83(3):371–375.

47. Schultz MG, Picone DS, Nikolic SB, Williams AD, Sharman JE. Exaggerated blood pressure response to early stages of exercise stress testing and presence of hypertension. *J Sci Med Sport*. 2016;19(12):1039–1042.
48. Jae SY, Franklin BA, Choo J, Choi YH, Fernhall B. Exaggerated exercise blood pressure response during treadmill testing as a predictor of future hypertension in men: a longitudinal study. *Am J Hypertens*. 2015;28(11):1362–1367.
49. Keteyian SJ, Patel M, Kraus WE, et al. Variables measured during cardiopulmonary exercise testing as predictors of mortality in chronic systolic heart failure. *J Am Coll Cardiol*. 2016;67(7):780–789.
50. Cerqueira MD, Weissman NJ, Dilsizian V, et al. Standardized myocardial segmentation and nomenclature for tomographic imaging of the heart. A statement for healthcare professionals from the Cardiac Imaging Committee of the Council on Clinical Cardiology of the American Heart Association. *Circulation*. 2002;105(4):539–542.
51. Turakhia MP, McManus DD, Whooley MA, Schiller NB. Increase in end-systolic volume after exercise independently predicts mortality in patients with coronary heart disease: data from the Heart and Soul Study. *Eur Heart J*. 2009;30(20):2478–2484.
52. Marwick TH. Stress echocardiography. *Heart (British Cardiac Society)*. 2003;89(1):113–118.
53. From AM, Kane G, Bruce C, Pellikka PA, Scott C, McCully RB. Characteristics and outcomes of patients with abnormal stress echocardiograms and angiographically mild coronary artery disease (<50% stenoses) or normal coronary arteries. *J Am Soc Echocardiogr*. 2010;23(2):207–214.
54. Mark DB, Shaw L, Harrell Jr FE, et al. Prognostic value of a treadmill exercise score in outpatients with suspected coronary artery disease. *N Engl J Med*. 1991;325(12):849–853.
55. Marwick TH, Case C, Vasey C, Allen S, Short L, Thomas JD. Prediction of mortality by exercise echocardiography: a strategy for combination with the duke treadmill score. *Circulation*. 2001;103(21):2566–2571.
56. Kane GC, Oh JK. Diastolic stress test for the evaluation of exertional dyspnea. *Curr Cardiol Rep*. 2012;14(3):359–365.
57. Prasad SB, Holland DJ, Atherton JJ. Diastolic stress echocardiography: from basic principles to clinical applications. *Heart*. 2018;104(21):1739–1748.
58. Grewal J, McCully RB, Kane GC, Lam C, Pellikka PA. Left ventricular function and exercise capacity. *Jama*. 2009;301(3):286–294.
59. Otto ME, Pereira MM, Beck AL, Milani M. Correlation between diastolic function and maximal exercise capacity on exercise test. *Arq Bras Cardiol*. 2011;96(2):107–113.
60. La Gerche A, Claessen G, Dymarkowski S, et al. Exercise-induced right ventricular dysfunction is associated with ventricular arrhythmias in endurance athletes. *Eur Heart J*. 2015;36(30):1998–2010.
61. Ha JW, Choi D, Park S, et al. Determinants of exercise-induced pulmonary hypertension in patients with normal left ventricular ejection fraction. *Heart (British Cardiac Society)*. 2009;95(6):490–494.
62. Shim CY, Kim SA, Choi D, et al. Clinical outcomes of exercise-induced pulmonary hypertension in subjects with preserved left ventricular ejection fraction: implication of an increase in left ventricular filling pressure during exercise. *Heart (British Cardiac Society)*. 2011;97(17):1417–1424.
63. Jeon DS, Atar S, Brasch AV, et al. Association of mitral annulus calcification, aortic valve sclerosis and aortic root calcification with abnormal myocardial perfusion single photon emission tomography in subjects age < or =65 years old. *J Am Coll Cardiol*. 2001;38(7):1988–1993.
64. O'Keefe Jr JH, Barnhart CS, Bateman TM. Comparison of stress echocardiography and stress myocardial perfusion scintigraphy for diagnosing coronary artery disease and assessing its severity. *Am J Cardiol*. 1995;75(11):25D–34D.
65. Badruddin SM, Ahmad A, Mickelson J, et al. Supine bicycle versus post-treadmill exercise echocardiography in the detection of myocardial ischemia: a randomized single-blind crossover trial. *J Am Coll Cardiol*. 1999;33(6):1485–1490.
66. Gurunathan S, Ahmed A, Pabla J, et al. The clinical efficacy and long-term prognostic value of stress echocardiography in octogenarians. *Heart*. 2017;103(7):517–523.
67. Shah BN, Zacharias K, Pabla JS, et al. The clinical impact of contemporary stress echocardiography in morbid obesity for the assessment of coronary artery disease. *Heart*. 2016;102(5):370–375.
68. Ashley EA, Myers J, Froelicher V. Exercise testing in clinical medicine. *Lancet (London, England)*. 2000;356(9241):1592–1597.
69. Metz LD, Beattie M, Hom R, Redberg RF, Grady D, Fleischmann KE. The prognostic value of normal exercise myocardial perfusion imaging and exercise echocardiography: a meta-analysis. *J Am Coll Cardiol*. 2007;49(2):227–237.
70. Bouzas-Mosquera A, Peteiro J, Alvarez-Garcia N, et al. Prognostic value of exercise echocardiography in patients with left bundle branch block. *JACC Cardiovascul Imag*. 2009;2(3):251–259.
71. Argyle RA, Ray SG. Stress and strain: double trouble or useful tool? *Eur J Echocardiogr*. 2009;10(6):716–722.
72. Voigt JU, Exner B, Schmiedehausen K, et al. Strain-rate imaging during dobutamine stress echocardiography provides objective evidence of inducible ischemia. *Circulation*. 2003;107(16):2120–2126.
73. Ishii K, Miwa K, Sakurai T, et al. Detection of postischemic regional left ventricular delayed outward wall motion or diastolic stunning after exercise-induced ischemia in patients with stable effort angina by using color kinesis. *J Am Soc Echocardiogr*. 2008;21(4):309–314.
74. Davidavicius G, Kowalski M, Williams RI, et al. Can regional strain and strain rate measurement be performed during both dobutamine and exercise echocardiography, and do regional deformation responses differ with different forms of stress testing? *J Am Soc Echocardiogr*. 2003;16(4):299–308.
75. Goebel B, Arnold R, Koletzki E, et al. Exercise tissue Doppler echocardiography with strain rate imaging in healthy young individuals: feasibility, normal values and reproducibility. *Int J Cardiovasc Imag*. 2007;23(2):149–155.
76. Kowalski M, Herregods MC, Herbots L, et al. The feasibility of ultrasonic regional strain and strain rate imaging in quantifying dobutamine stress echocardiography. *Eur J Echocardiogr*. 2003;4(2):81–91.
77. Hanekom L, Jenkins C, Jeffries L, et al. Incremental value of strain rate analysis as an adjunct to wall-motion scoring for assessment of myocardial viability by dobutamine echocardiography: a follow-up study after revascularization. *Circulation*. 2005;112(25):3892–3900.
78. Deng Y, Peng L, Liu YY, et al. Four-dimensional echocardiography area strain combined with exercise stress echocardiography to evaluate left ventricular regional systolic function in patients with mild single vessel coronary artery stenosis. *Echocardiography*. 2017;34(9):1332–1338.
79. Mada RO, Duchenne J, Voigt JU. Tissue Doppler, strain and strain rate in ischemic heart disease "how I do it." *Cardiovasc Ultrasound*. 2014;12:38.
80. Caiani EG, Corsi C, Zamorano J, et al. Improved semiautomated quantification of left ventricular volumes and ejection fraction using 3-dimensional echocardiography with a full matrix-array transducer: comparison with magnetic resonance imaging. *J Am Soc Echocardiogr*. 2005;18(8):779–788.
81. Hoffmann R, Barletta G, von Bardeleben S, et al. Analysis of left ventricular volumes and function: a multicenter comparison of cardiac magnetic resonance imaging, cine ventriculography, and unenhanced and contrast-enhanced two-dimensional and three-dimensional echocardiography. *J Am Soc Echocardiogr*. 2014;27(3):292–301.
82. Peteiro J, Pinon P, Perez R, Monserrat L, Perez D, Castro-Beiras A. Comparison of 2- and 3-dimensional exercise echocardiography for the detection of coronary artery disease. *J Am Soc Echocardiogr*. 2007;20(8):959–967.
83. Jenkins C, Haluska B, Marwick TH. Assessment of temporal heterogeneity and regional motion to identify wall motion abnormalities using treadmill exercise stress three-dimensional echocardiography. *J Am Soc Echocardiogr*. 2009;22(3):268–275.
84. Berbarie RF, Dib E, Ahmad M. Stress echocardiography using real-time three-dimensional imaging. *Echocardiography*. 2018;35(8):1196–1203.
85. Xiu J, Cui K, Wang Y, et al. Prognostic value of myocardial perfusion analysis in patients with coronary artery disease: a meta-analysis. *J Am Soc Echocardiogr*. 2017;30(3):270–281.
86. Senior R, Monaghan M, Main ML, et al. Detection of coronary artery disease with perfusion stress echocardiography using a novel ultrasound imaging agent: two Phase 3 international trials in comparison with radionuclide perfusion imaging. *Eur J Echocardiogr*. 2009;10(1):26–35.
87. Shah BN, Gonzalez-Gonzalez AM, Drakopoulou M, et al. The incremental prognostic value of the incorporation of myocardial perfusion assessment into clinical testing with stress echocardiography study. *J Am Soc Echocardiogr*. 2015;28(11):1358–1365.
88. Gaibazzi N, Rigo F, Lorenzoni V, et al. Comparative prediction of cardiac events by wall motion, wall motion plus coronary flow reserve, or myocardial perfusion analysis: a multicenter study of contrast stress echocardiography. *JACC Cardiovasc Imaging*. 2013;6(1):1–12.
89. Miszalski-Jamka T, Kuntz-Hehner S, Schmidt H, et al. Myocardial contrast echocardiography enhances long-term prognostic value of supine bicycle stress two-dimensional echocardiography. *J Am Soc Echocardiogr*. 2009;22(11):1220–1227.
90. Abdelmoneim SS, Bernier M, Dhoble A, et al. Diagnostic accuracy of contrast echocardiography during adenosine stress for detection of abnormal myocardial perfusion: a prospective comparison with technetium-99 m sestamibi single-photon emission computed tomography. *Heart Ves*. 2010;25(2):121–130.

中文导读

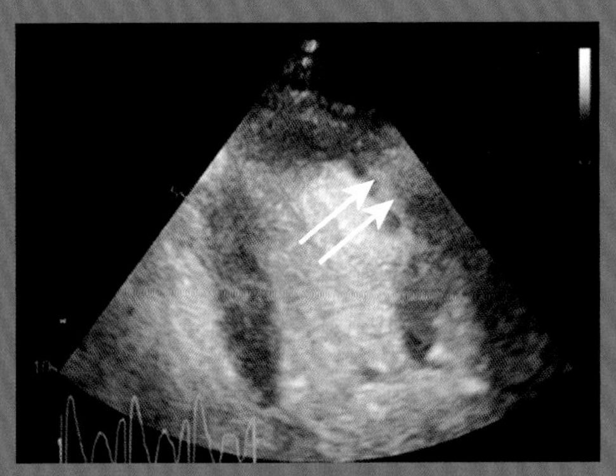

第20章 非运动负荷超声心动图诊断冠心病

负荷超声心动图是缺血性心脏病诊断和风险分级的主要方法。缺血诱导从冠脉灌注和代谢变化受损发展为心室局部收缩功能障碍，表现为室壁运动异常、心电图变化和其他临床症状。检查缺血性左心室收缩功能障碍患者的心肌存活能力是负荷超声心动图的另一个指征。在心率加快的情况下由于显著狭窄而导致心肌缺血时，在较高的应激水平下可观察到双相反应，其特征为室壁局部功能的最初改善，随后恶化。负荷超声心动图的准确性取决于左心室心内膜边界的清晰显示，可通过造影剂增强，从而提高负荷超声心动图诊断的准确性和评估预后价值。30%～40%的患者无法进行负荷运动或运动不耐受。在运动应激峰值时采集图像亦极具挑战性。这时，非运动负荷超声心动图可以作为一种实用的替代方法。

本章重点介绍了非运动负荷超声心动图技术，并提供了药理学和非药理学应激源的概述，以及这些技术的诊断准确性和预后价值。最后讨论了新兴技术（如三维成像、组织多普勒成像和应变成像）在非运动负荷超声心动图中的作用。

非运动负荷超声心动图在当前临床实践中具有无可争议的诊断和预后价值，可用于诊断冠状动脉粥样硬化性心脏病、鉴定心肌存活能力及对不同心脏人群进行风险分层。其安全、经济有效且可重复，并提供了有关心脏结构大小和心功能的测量数据。

施怡声

20 Nonexercise Stress Echocardiography for Diagnosis of Coronary Disease

PIETER VAN DER BIJL, MD, PhD | JEROEN J. BAX, MD, PhD | VICTORIA DELGADO, MD, PhD

Stress echocardiography (SE) is a mainstay of ischemic heart disease diagnosis and risk stratification. For diagnosis of coronary artery disease (CAD), various stressors (e.g., exercise, pharmacologic agents, pacing) are used to create an imbalance between oxygen supply and demand, resulting in myocardial ischemia. The induction of ischemia progresses from impaired perfusion and metabolic changes to regional systolic dysfunction (manifesting as wall motion abnormalities [WMAs]), electrocardiographic changes, and symptoms. This sequence of events is known as the *ischemic cascade*, and regional WMAs are therefore an early, sensitive indicator of ischemia.[1]

Accurate diagnosis of CAD with SE requires a high level of cardiovascular stress. Although exercise is the most physiologic stressor, it is unfeasible or inconclusive in 30% to 40% of patients due to physical limitations (e.g., peripheral vascular disease), deconditioning (i.e., submaximal effort), or an uninterpretable electrocardiogram (ECG).[2] Acquisition of images at peak exercise stress is challenging and requires a high level of expertise to compensate for the image degradation caused by hyperventilation and excessive chest wall motion. Pharmacologic SE is a practical alternative that is widely used for diagnosis and risk stratification of CAD.[2,3]

Detection of myocardial viability in patients with ischemic left ventricular (LV) systolic dysfunction is another indication for SE. Dysfunctional myocardium at rest that has the potential to recover with revascularization usually responds to a low-stress challenge with improvement in regional wall motion (i.e., contractile reserve). In contrast, myocardial segments that remain dysfunctional throughout low-dose stress typically indicate nonviable scar tissue. A biphasic response, characterized by initial improvement of regional function followed by deterioration, can be observed at higher levels of stress when ischemia develops as a consequence of significant stenosis in the setting of an elevated heart rate.

The accuracy of SE relies on adequate visualization of the LV endocardial border, which can be enhanced with contrast media, thereby improving the diagnostic accuracy and prognostic value of SE.[4] This chapter focuses on nonexercise SE techniques, providing an overview of pharmacologic and nonpharmacologic stressors, and the diagnostic accuracy and prognostic value of these techniques. The role of emerging techniques (e.g., three-dimensional [3D] imaging, tissue Doppler imaging [TDI], and strain imaging) in nonexercise SE is discussed.

STRESS ECHOCARDIOGRAPHY SUITE, PHARMACOLOGIC STRESSORS, AND PROTOCOLS

Before performing nonexercise SE, informed patient consent should be obtained and contraindications reviewed (Table 20.1 and Fig. 20.1).[5,6] The quality of echocardiographic windows should be checked beforehand, and use of intravenous contrast is recommended if two or more endocardial segments cannot be visualized. Nonexercise SE should be performed with ECG (remote from echocardiography windows) and blood pressure monitoring; in a dedicated suite comprising a private room with a height-adjustable bed (with a cutout for apical probe placement), appropriate monitoring facilities (e.g., ECG, blood pressure, pulse oximetry), and resuscitation equipment, including drugs and a defibrillator.

Stressors (e.g., dobutamine, dipyridamole) are administered through an intravenous cannula into an antecubital vein. If possible, a medial antecubital vein is preferred because it drains directly through the basilic vein into the axillary vein, whereas use of a lateral antecubital vein may cause a delay in effect (and unpredictable pharmacokinetics) of infused drugs at the entry of the cephalic vein into the axillary vein, where a valve is often found. A three-way stopcock is advisable for administering

TABLE 20.1 Contraindications to the Use of Pharmacologic Stressors.

	Rationale	*Comments*
General Contraindications		
Anti-ischemic therapy (nitrates, β-blockers, calcium channel antagonists)	Influences the diagnostic and prognostic value of the test	If a stress test is conducted, there is a risk of not achieving the target heart rate (i.e., an inadequate test result may be achieved).
Acute coronary syndrome ≤1 week earlier	Risk of cardiac rupture	Stress testing cannot proceed under any circumstances.
LV thrombus	Increased cardiac deformation during stress may dislodge the thrombus	Stress testing cannot proceed under any circumstances.
Recent pulmonary embolism	Cardiac decompensation due to stress	Stress testing cannot proceed under any circumstances.
Recent aortic dissection	Progression due to increased blood pressure during stress	Stress testing cannot proceed under any circumstances.
Decompensated LV failure	Further decompensation due to stress	Stress testing cannot proceed under any circumstances.
Active endocarditis, myocarditis, or pericarditis	Progression of disease	—
Contraindications to Dobutamine		
Uncontrolled or poorly controlled systemic hypertension	Increase of blood pressure with dobutamine stress	Vasodilator (dipyridamole) stress testing can be considered—no significant hypertensive response.
History of (serious) arrhythmias	Precipitation of arrhythmias with dobutamine stress	Vasodilator (dipyridamole) stress testing can be considered—no significant arrhythmic risk.
LV outflow tract obstruction or hypertrophic cardiomyopathy	Peripheral vasodilatation, with increased outflow tract gradient	—
Severe aortic stenosis	Peripheral vasodilatation, with increased outflow tract gradient	Dobutamine stress echocardiography has a role in low-flow, low-gradient aortic stenosis.
Hypokalemia	Potentiates risk of ventricular arrhythmias	Investigate the cause before administration of dobutamine.
Contraindications to Atropine		
Closed-angle glaucoma	Precipitation of acute angle closure glaucoma by mydriasis	—
Benign prostatic hyperplasia	Precipitation of acute urinary retention by parasympatholytic effect on detrusor muscle	—
Contraindications to Vasodilators		
Reactive airways disease	Acute reactivity of airways could be precipitated or worsened by vasodilators	Regadenoson is an alternative. Dobutamine is another option.
Recent xanthine use (<12 h earlier) or caffeine ingestion	Methylxanthines antagonize the effects of vasodilators	Can continue with dobutamine as stressor.
Advanced atrioventricular block (second or third degree)	Potentiation of atrioventricular block by vasodilators	Dobutamine is an alternative.
Sinus node dysfunction	Decrease in spontaneous depolarization of sinoatrial node with vasodilators, leading to potentially severe bradycardia	—
Wolff-Parkinson-White syndrome	Atrioventricular block with vasodilators, allowing conduction through an accessory pathway	—
Carotid artery stenosis	Cerebral ischemia or infarction due to hypoperfusion	—

adjunctive atropine or intravenous contrast medium. A 12-lead ECG is recorded at baseline and at 1-minute intervals (while being continuously displayed on the echocardiography monitor throughout the examination) to detect ischemic changes or arrhythmias. Sphygmomanometric blood pressure readings are obtained at baseline and during each protocol stage.

With the patient in a left lateral decubitus position, echocardiographic data are optimized and acquired at baseline and at each stage (i.e., baseline, low dose, peak dose, and recovery) of the protocol, typically including parasternal long- and short-axis views, apical 4- and 2-chamber views, and a long-axis view.[7] A minimum of three RR intervals should be saved for every view in every stage of the protocol to allow meaningful interpretation.

The definition of low-dose and peak-dose stages and image sets depends on the clinical question, the stressor used, and the patient's response. If viability testing is performed with dobutamine, low-dose images are acquired at an infusion rate of 5 μg/kg per minute, in contrast to ischemia testing, in which the low-dose stage reflects the myocardial response at 10 μg/kg per minute. Dipyridamole low-dose images are obtained after a dose of 0.56 mg/kg has been administered. Peak-dose images are acquired when 85% of the target heart rate is achieved by dobutamine (with or without atropine) stress or after the total dipyridamole dose of 0.84 mg/kg has been administered. Recovery images are taken after administration of the stressor has been terminated (i.e., after 3 minutes or when the peak heart rate has decreased by 10–20 beats/min).

The echocardiography machine reproduces baseline settings for each stage and view of the protocol, simplifying acquisition but also mandating attention to the baseline settings, which are reproduced automatically for every stage. To allow comparative analysis of a single view in various stages, a *quad-screen format* is required.

Segmental wall motion is reported according to the terminology in Table 20.2. A distinction is made between active inward motion and tethering, the latter referring to passive motion of a segment due to forces exerted on it by adjacent myocardium.

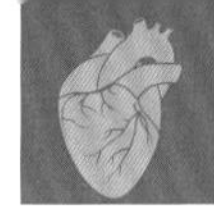

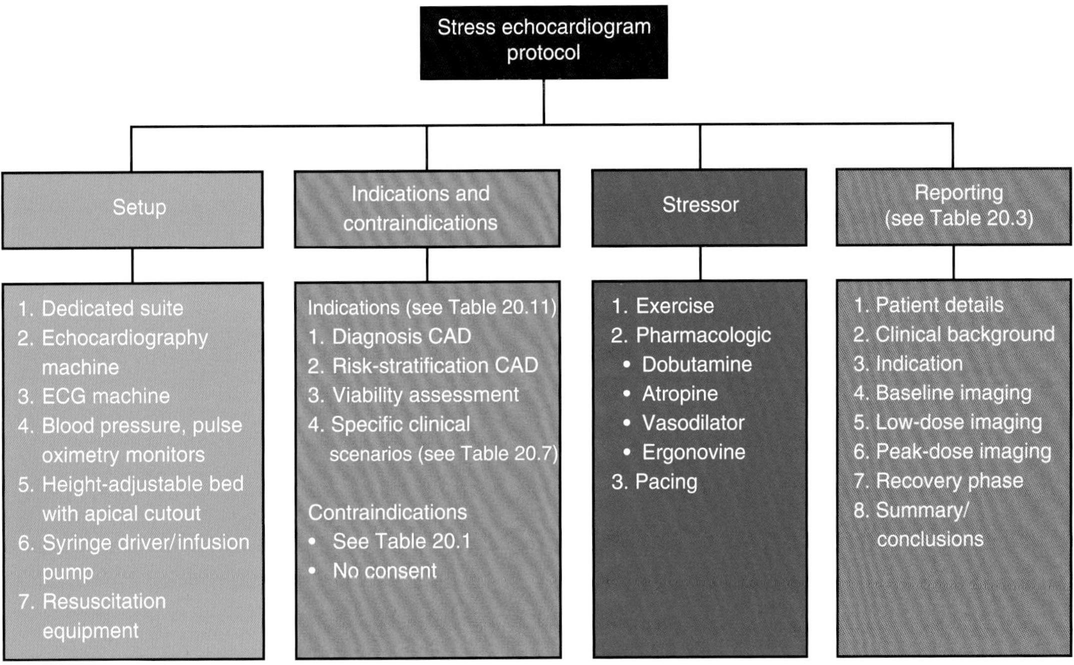

Fig. 20.1 Proposed algorithm for a (pharmacologic) stress echocardiogram. Color coding denotes the following: *green*, setup (including suite and equipment); *orange*, indications and contraindications; *blue*, choice of stressors; *brown*, central components of stress echocardiogram report. *CAD*, Coronary artery disease; *ECG*, electrocardiogram.

TABLE 20.2 Wall Motion Terminology and Qualitative Analysis of Wall Motion at Rest and Peak Stress, Correlated With Underlying Pathophysiology.

Wall Motion Terminology

Term	*Definition*
Normokinesia	Normal inward motion/thickening
Hypokinesia	Reduced inward motion/thickening Hypokinesia is sometimes defined in more detail as (1) reduced amplitude of endocardial motion, (2) reduced velocity of endocardial motion, (3) reduced systolic wall thickening, or (4) delay in onset of segmental motion (tardokinesia)
Akinesia	Absent inward motion/thickening
Dyskinesia	Systolic outward motion

Qualitative Analysis of Wall Motion Correlated With Underlying Pathophysiology

Pathophysiology	*Rest*	*Stress*
Normal	Normokinesia	Normokinesia, hyperkinesia
Ischemia	Normokinesia	Hypokinesia, akinesia, dyskinesia
Viable	Hypokinesia, akinesia	Hypokinesia, normokinesia
Nonviable scar	Akinesia, dyskinesia	Akinesia, dyskinesia

Tethering can be difficult to distinguish visually from active motion. However, decreased myocardial thickening reflects true contractility, and it is therefore a more specific sign of abnormal myocardial wall motion. Ventricular dyssynchrony (e.g., due to an RV pacemaker, bundle branch block, or post-surgical status) can mimic abnormal wall motion, but careful assessment of wall thickening can distinguish it from true WMAs.

Localization of WMAs is performed using a 16- or 17-segment model of the LV, according to the coronary artery territory (Fig. 20.2 and Video 20.2).[7] The anatomic variation among individuals in the myocardial territories supplied by the various coronary arteries should be considered.[8]

Diagnostic end points of pharmacologic SE include (1) administration of the maximum dose of stressor, (2) achievement of the target heart rate ([220 − age in years] × 0.85), (3) new WMAs in at least two contiguous LV segments, and (4) angina and ECG changes indicative of ischemia (>2 mm changes in the ST segment of two contiguous leads (Fig. 20.3).[2] Nondiagnostic end points include intolerable symptoms, hypertension (systolic blood pressure >220 mmHg or diastolic blood pressure >120 mmHg), hypotension (>40 mmHg drop), supraventricular and ventricular arrhythmias, and polymorphic ventricular beats.[2]

If cardiac arrest or life-threatening arrhythmias occur, resuscitation should proceed according to published guidelines such as those proposed by the European Resuscitation Council.[9] The test is concluded when (1) the heart rate has decreased to within 20 beats/min of baseline, and (2) all new WMAs have resolved. The patient is transferred to a recovery area, and the intravenous cannula is left in situ in case of a delayed contrast reaction. The report is subsequently written, including all relevant clinical information (Table 20.3).

DOBUTAMINE AND ATROPINE STRESS ECHOCARDIOGRAPHY

Dobutamine is a racemic mixture of the levo-isomer (α_1-agonist) and the dextro-isomer (α_1-antagonist) and has only weak α-effects as a result. Both isomers are β-receptor agonists, having higher affinity for β_1- than β_2-receptors. Myocardial demand ischemia is provoked by an increase in myocardial contractility due to inotropy (β_1-receptors) at lower doses and by an increase in heart rate due to reflex tachycardia from peripheral vasodilation (β_2-receptors) at higher doses and, to a lesser extent, chronotropy (β_1-receptors) at lower doses (Fig. 20.4). Secondary mechanisms of ischemia include greater oxygen demand due

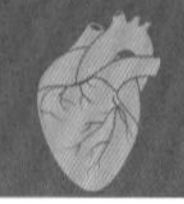

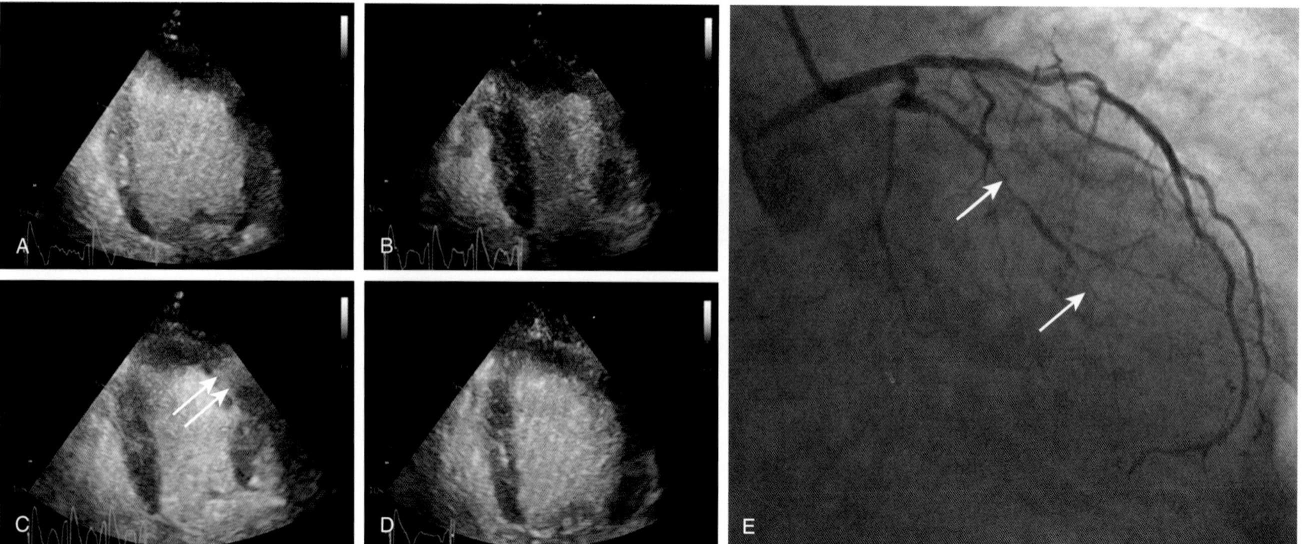

Fig. 20.2 Dobutamine stress echocardiography. The apical 4-chamber view is compared for baseline (A), low-dose (B), peak-dose (C), and recovery (D) phases in a quad-view format. Intravenous contrast is used to enhance endocardial border detection. At peak dose, akinesia in the apical lateral segment *(arrows)* demonstrates inducible ischemia in the territory of the distal left circumflex coronary artery. (E) Invasive coronary angiography demonstrates two sequential, chronic total occlusions *(arrows)* of the left circumflex coronary artery. The cine loop of the apical 4-chamber quad-view is shown in Video 20.2.

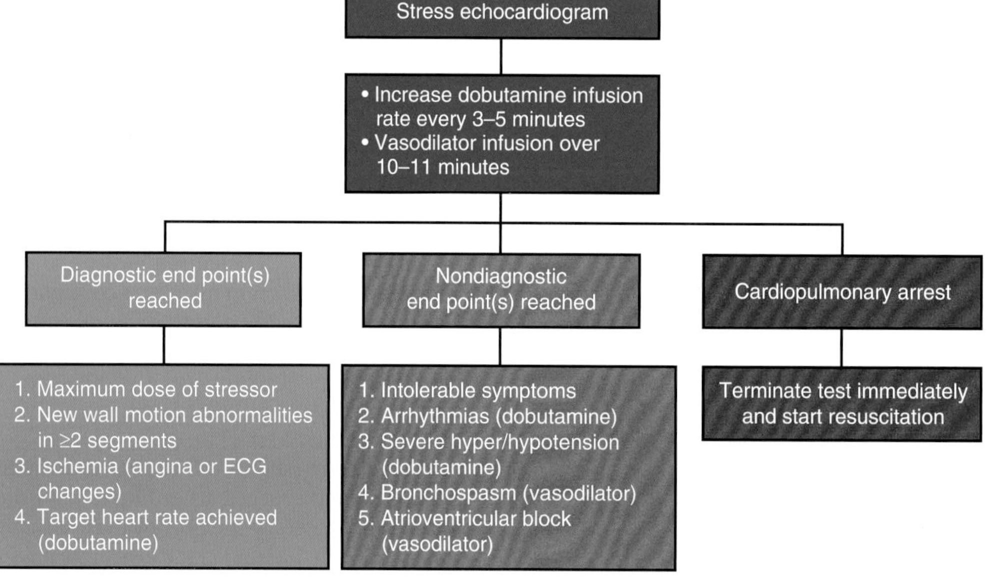

Fig. 20.3 Proposed algorithm for determining the end points of a stress echocardiogram. Color coding denotes the following: *blue*, initiation and performance of the test; *green*, diagnostic end points, which indicate that the test can be stopped; *orange*, nondiagnostic end points, each of which should prompt consideration of terminating the test; *red*, cardiopulmonary arrest, which is an indication for immediate termination of the test and the start of cardiopulmonary resuscitation. *ECG*, Electrocardiogram.

to cellular effects (e.g., inefficient excitation-contraction coupling); this is referred to as an *oxygen-wasting effect.*

For myocardial ischemia detection, dobutamine SE is performed with a continuous intravenous infusion (half-life [$t_{1/2}$] of <2 min), starting at 5 μg/kg per minute and increasing every 3 to 5 minutes by 10 μg/kg per minute until a dose of 40 μg/kg per minute or a diagnostic end point is reached (see Summary table). If the target heart rate is not achieved with a maximal dobutamine dose (e.g., due to a reflex bradycardia in response to hypertension), the maximal rate (40 μg/kg per minute) is maintained while intravenous atropine sulfate is administered, starting with a 0.25-mg atropine bolus and increasing to a maximum of 2 mg.

Atropine is an anticholinergic agent that binds to vagal muscarinic acetylcholine receptors. Its parasympatholytic effect is mediated by inhibition of the sinoatrial and atrioventricular (AV) nodes, which causes a chronotropic and enhanced dromotropic effect and subsequent tachycardia (Fig. 20.5). For myocardial viability assessment, a low-dose dobutamine protocol (maximum dose, 10 μg/kg per minute) is used.

The pharmacodynamic effects of dobutamine and atropine can be counteracted by an intravenous β-blocker (e.g., esmolol 0.5 mg/kg bolus followed by 0.2 mg/kg boluses titrated to heart rate). This may be used to ameliorate unwanted effects (e.g., ischemia) or to shorten the recovery phase (especially when atropine has been administered because its $t_{1/2}$ is longer than that of dobutamine).

Serious unwanted effects of dobutamine include myocardial ischemia, severe hypertension (which also decreases

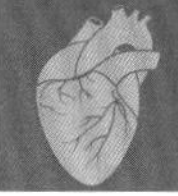

TABLE 20.3 Recommendations for Components of a Standard Stress Echocardiography Report.

Component	*Text*				
Patient details	Name, surname, age, gender, date, hospital number, referring clinician, operator(s)				
Clinical background	Known coronary artery disease? Previous myocardial revascularization? Inability to complete exercise?				
Indication for test	Evaluation of inducible ischemia or viability				
	HR (beats/min)	*BP (mmHg)*	*Heart Rhythm*	*New WMA*	*Symptoms*
Baseline	...	.../...	SR/AF/VT	Yes/No	Yes/No
Low dose	...	.../...	SR/AF/VT	Yes/No	Yes/No
Peak dose	...	.../...	SR/AF/VT	Yes/No	Yes/No
Recovery	...	.../...	SR/AF/VT	Yes/No	Yes/No
Baseline imaging	LV systolic function and wall motion analysis at rest.				
Low-dose imaging	Dose of dobutamine infusion rate (5 or 10 μg/kg per minute). Describe changes in LV wall motion analysis.				
Peak-dose imaging	Dose of dobutamine infusion rate (maximum 40 μg/kg per minute) and dose of atropine if added. Describe changes in LV wall motion analysis.				
Recovery phase	Indicate whether β-blockers were used. Describe changes in LV wall motion analysis.				
Summary/conclusions	The test is positive/negative for ischemia/viability.				

AF, Atrial fibrillation; *BP*, blood pressure; *HR*, heart rate; *SR*, sinus rhythm; *VT*, ventricular tachycardia; *WMA*, wall motion abnormality.

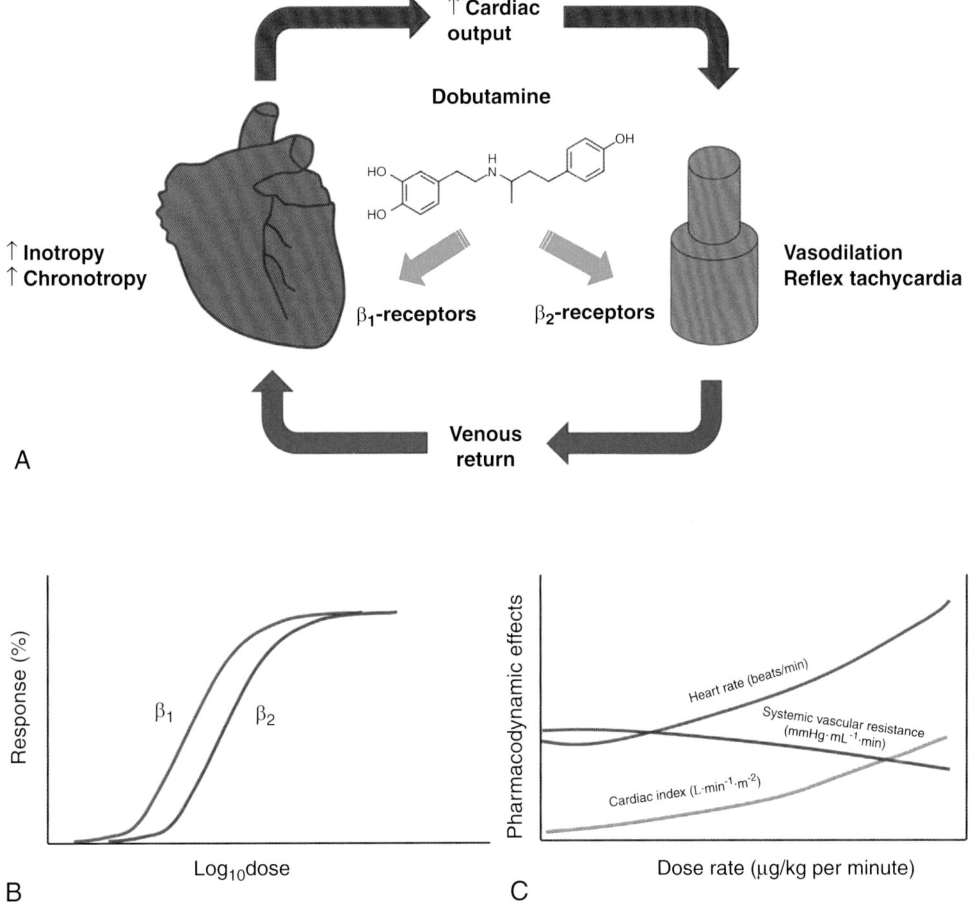

Fig. 20.4 Pharmacodynamics of dobutamine. Dobutamine enhances inotropy and chronotropy by stimulation of cellular cardiac β_1-receptors, leading to an increase in cardiac output. (A) Stimulation of β_2-receptors in the systemic vasculature causes vasodilation and a reflex tachycardia. (B) Schematic dose-response curve for dobutamine demonstrates its higher affinity for β_1-receptors than for β_2-receptors. (C) Schematic representation of the pharmacodynamic effects of dobutamine with increasing dose rate. As the dose rate (infusion rate) increases, heart rate and cardiac index (reflecting the product of heart rate and contractility) increase while systemic vascular resistance decreases. The decrease in systemic vascular resistance becomes more prominent at higher dose rates (β_2-receptor effect).

specificity because regional WMAs may reflect the increased afterload rather than ischemia), life-threatening arrhythmias, and death (3 per 1000 patients).[10] Less severe effects include palpitations, atrial tachyarrhythmias, premature ventricular complexes, urinary urgency, anxiety (potentiated by atropine), nausea, and hypotension. Hypotension is primarily a consequence of the vasodilator effect of high-dose dobutamine, although loss of synchronized AV contraction (due to atrial arrhythmias), LV outflow tract obstruction, and ischemia can also contribute.

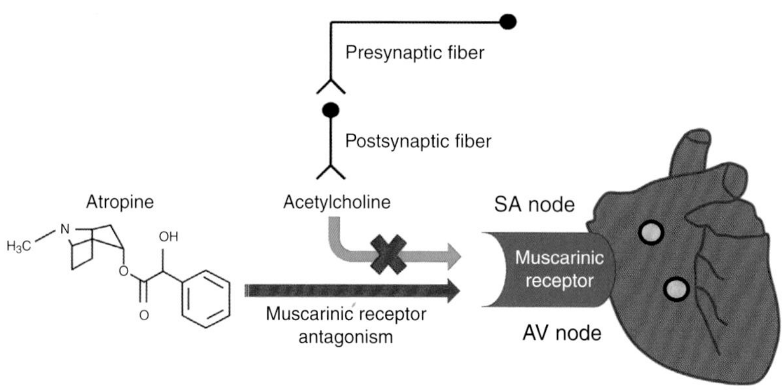

Fig. 20.5 Pharmacodynamics of atropine. Atropine is a competitive antagonist of acetylcholine at vagal muscarinic receptors supplying the sinoatrial *(SA)* and atrioventricular *(AV)* nodes. These receptors are physiologically innervated by postsynaptic vagal fibers close to the SA and AV nodes. The parasympatholytic effect is mediated by inhibition of the SA and AV nodes, which causes a dromotropic (conduction velocity) and enhanced chronotropic (heart rate) effect and subsequent tachycardia.

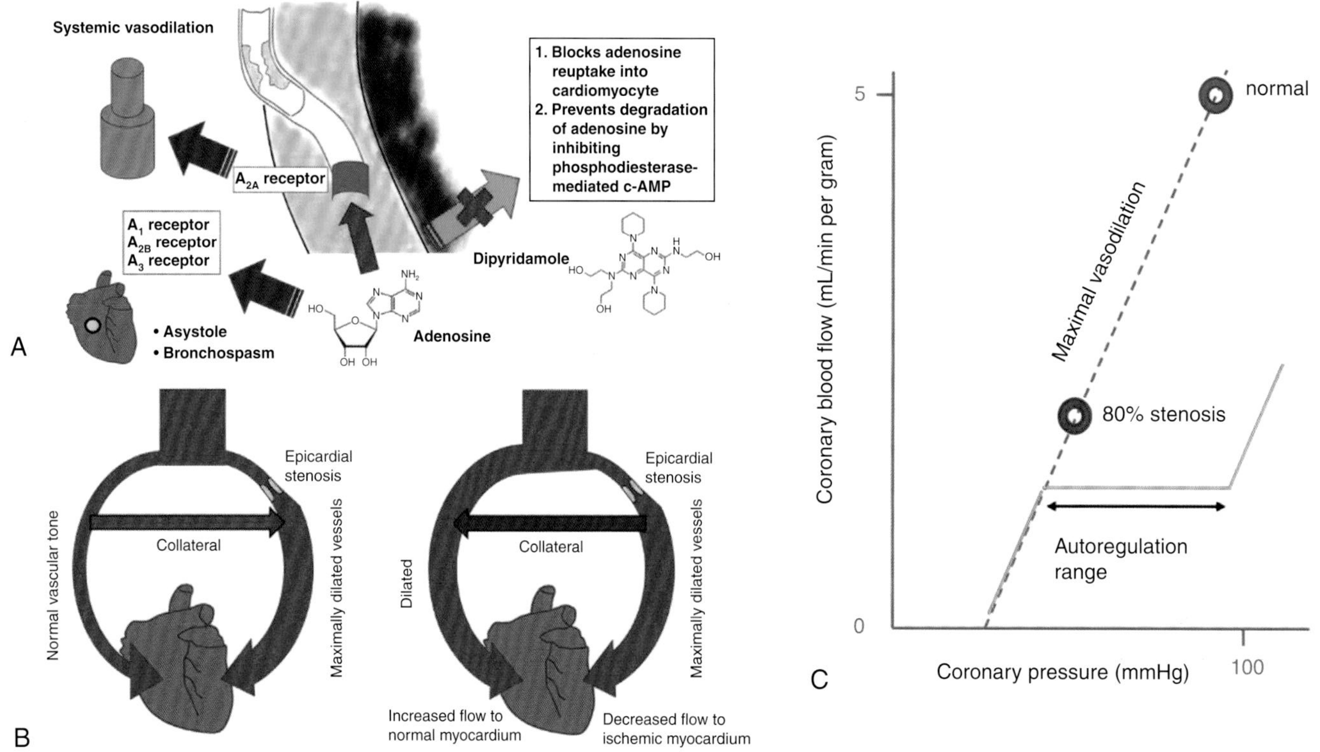

Fig. 20.6 Pharmacodynamics of vasodilators (i.e., adenosine and dipyridamole). (A) Dipyridamole exerts its vasodilatory effects indirectly by inhibition of (1) adenosine degradation (by adenosine deaminase) and (2) adenosine reuptake by cardiomyocytes. Increased concentrations of adenosine stimulate A_{2A} (coronary and systemic vasodilation), A_1, A_{2B}, and A_3 (atrioventricular block and bronchoconstriction) receptors. (B) Preferential vasodilation in myocardial territories supplied by nonobstructed coronary arteries results in a redistribution of blood flow toward nonischemic areas, away from ischemic zones. The flow redistribution effect is enhanced by collaterals and is known as *horizontal steal.* (C) *Vertical steal* refers to a decrease in perfusion across a significant epicardial coronary stenosis when the distal pressure is decreased beyond the point at which distal flow can be increased. *c-AMP,* Cyclic adenosine monophosphate.

DIPYRIDAMOLE, ADENOSINE, AND REGADENOSON STRESS ECHOCARDIOGRAPHY

Dipyridamole is a vasodilator that acts indirectly by inhibition of (1) adenosine degradation (by adenosine deaminase) and (2) adenosine reuptake by cardiomyocytes.[11] Increased adenosine concentrations act on adenosine A_1, A_{2A}, A_{2B}, and A_3 receptors. Coronary vasodilation is mediated by A_{2A} receptors on smooth muscle cells of coronary resistance vessels (<400 μm), whereas stimulation of A_1, A_{2B}, and A_3 receptors cause AV conduction block and bronchoconstriction (Fig. 20.6).[11]

Myocardial ischemia detection using dipyridamole relies on the induction of a steal phenomenon. Preferential vasodilation occurs in myocardial territories subtended by nonobstructed coronary arteries, resulting in a redistribution of blood flow toward nonischemic areas and away from ischemic zones. Collaterals also play a role in the redistribution of blood flow. This is known as *horizontal steal* (see Fig. 20.6). *Vertical steal* also occurs with vasodilator stress; it refers to a decrease in perfusion across a significant epicardial coronary stenosis when the distal pressure is decreased beyond the point at which distal flow can be increased (see Fig. 20.6). Secondary mechanisms are a reflex tachycardia that occurs in response to systemic hypotension and increasing oxygen consumption. Patients should refrain from ingesting methylxanthines (e.g., prescription drugs, food, beverages) for at least 12 hours before dipyridamole (or adenosine) stress testing because they are competitive antagonists of adenosine receptors.

Dipyridamole SE consists of an intravenous infusion of 0.84 mg/kg over 10 minutes in two stages: 0.56 mg/kg administered over 4 minutes and, after 4 additional minutes, 0.28 mg/kg over 2 minutes (see Summary table). A protocol administering the total dose of 0.84 mg/kg over 6 minutes increases the sensitivity of the test. If no end point is reached, atropine (0.25-mg boluses, up to a maximum of 2 mg) can be added. The protocol for use of adenosine is to administer 100 μg/kg per minute for 3 minutes, followed by 140 μg/kg per minute for another 4 minutes, and then increased to a maximum of 200 μg/kg per minute for 4 minutes (see Summary table).[12]

Vasodilator-related side effects include flushing, headache, bronchospasm, complete AV block, cerebral hypoperfusion (in the setting of carotid artery stenosis), nonischemic chest pain from direct stimulation of nociceptors, and ischemic chest pain. Because of the indirect mechanism of action of dipyridamole, its onset of action is slower than that of adenosine, and its unwanted effects are less severe but of longer duration.

Vasodilators are contraindicated in the setting of reactive airways disease or preexisting AV block. Regadenoson is a selective A_{2A} adenosine receptor agonist with a rapid onset of action ($t_{1/2}$ = 3 minutes) (see Summary table).[11,13] It can be used safely in patients with mild or moderate reactive airways disease, and 400 μg is administered over 10 seconds.[11] The effects of dipyridamole, adenosine, and regadenoson can be antagonized with slow intravenous administration of aminophylline (50 mg boluses titrated up to a maximum dose of 250 mg). In the case of adenosine, because of its very short $t_{1/2}$, cessation of the infusion usually suffices to treat unwanted effects.

ERGONOVINE STRESS ECHOCARDIOGRAPHY

Ergonovine is an ergot alkaloid that precipitates coronary vasospasm by stimulation of serotonergic (5-HT2) receptors on vascular smooth muscle.[14] It can be used to diagnose vasospastic angina (i.e., Prinzmetal angina) noninvasively with echocardiography.[15] A sensitivity of 91% and a specificity of 88% have been reported with the following protocol: a 50-μg intravenous bolus of ergonovine maleate every 5 minutes until myocardial ischemia (i.e., WMA) is detected or until the maximum dose of 0.35 mg is reached.[15,16] The action of ergonovine can be antagonized by intravenous nitroglycerin (0.25 mg), sublingual nitroglycerin (0.6 mg), or sublingual nifedipine (10 mg).[15–17]

PACING STRESS ECHOCARDIOGRAPHY

If the target heart rate cannot be achieved with pharmacologic stress alone, the pacing rate can be increased by external programming. If pacing SE is used without a pharmacologic stressor, a suggested protocol is to increase the pacing rate, commencing at 110 beats/min, by 10 beats/min every 2 minutes until the target heart rate is reached or an alternative end point has been achieved.[18] Because RV pacing causes dyssynchronous ventricular contractions, which may simulate regional WMAs, atrial or biventricular pacing is preferred. Regional wall thickening can be still evaluated.

DIAGNOSTIC ACCURACY AND PROGNOSTIC VALUE OF NONEXERCISE STRESS ECHOCARDIOGRAPHY FOR SIGNIFICANT CORONARY ARTERY DISEASE

The echocardiographic diagnosis of CAD relies on WMAs at rest, during, or after stress (i.e., in the recovery phase). Resting WMAs (i.e., hypokinesia, akinesia, or dyskinesia) indicate a previous myocardial infarction or significant obstructive coronary artery lesions that cause ischemia at rest with subsequent LV dysfunction. During stress, a new or worsening WMA or no increase of wall motion from baseline indicates obstructive CAD.

Ischemic WMAs may be delayed, with a normal stress response, manifesting later, during recovery. New WMAs that appear during the recovery phase carry the same diagnostic implications as those appearing during stress. Qualitative description of wall motion permits normal, ischemic, viable, and nonviable myocardium to be distinguished (see Table 20.2). Quantification with the wall motion score index yields prognostic data.[19]

Several meta-analyses have investigated the diagnostic accuracy of nonexercise SE.[20–23] In a meta-analysis of 35,268 patients, SE (i.e., dobutamine and dipyridamole) had a lower sensitivity but a higher specificity for the diagnosis of CAD compared with single-photon emission computed tomography (SPECT) (Fig. 20.7).[21,23] Dipyridamole SE had lower sensitivity and higher specificity compared with dipyridamole SPECT, whereas dobutamine SE has a similar sensitivity but higher specificity compared with dobutamine SPECT.[22] Picano et al.[23] showed that dobutamine and dipyridamole had comparable accuracy to diagnose coronary artery lesions of greater than 50% stenosis in a meta-analysis that included 435 patients (see Fig. 20.7).[23–28] Dipyridamole SE has fewer false-positive results than dobutamine SE.[29]

The relative performance of the various agents used in SE for the diagnosis of CAD was evaluated in two meta-analyses (Fig. 20.8).[23,30] In a meta-analysis of 818 patients, the sensitivity of dobutamine was higher (74%) for single-vessel disease compared with dipyridamole (68%; $P < 0.05$).[6] The sensitivities of these two agents were similar (80%) for multivessel disease, whereas dipyridamole was more specific than dobutamine (93% vs. 87%, respectively; $P < 0.05$).[6]

The prognostic value of SE for death and nonfatal myocardial infarction has been extensively documented in different populations of patients with suspected or known CAD and was found to be similar whether dobutamine or dipyridamole was used.[3,19,31–35] The extent and the severity of WMAs are independent predictors of outcome in patients with suspected or known CAD.[36,37] Even though a greater WMA extent portends a worse prognosis, nonexercise SE still has prognostic value in single-vessel CAD.[38] RV WMAs (at rest or during stress) can sometimes be appreciated and are independently associated with outcome when LV WMAs are taken into account.[39] The RV has not been studied as extensively in the SE context as the LV.

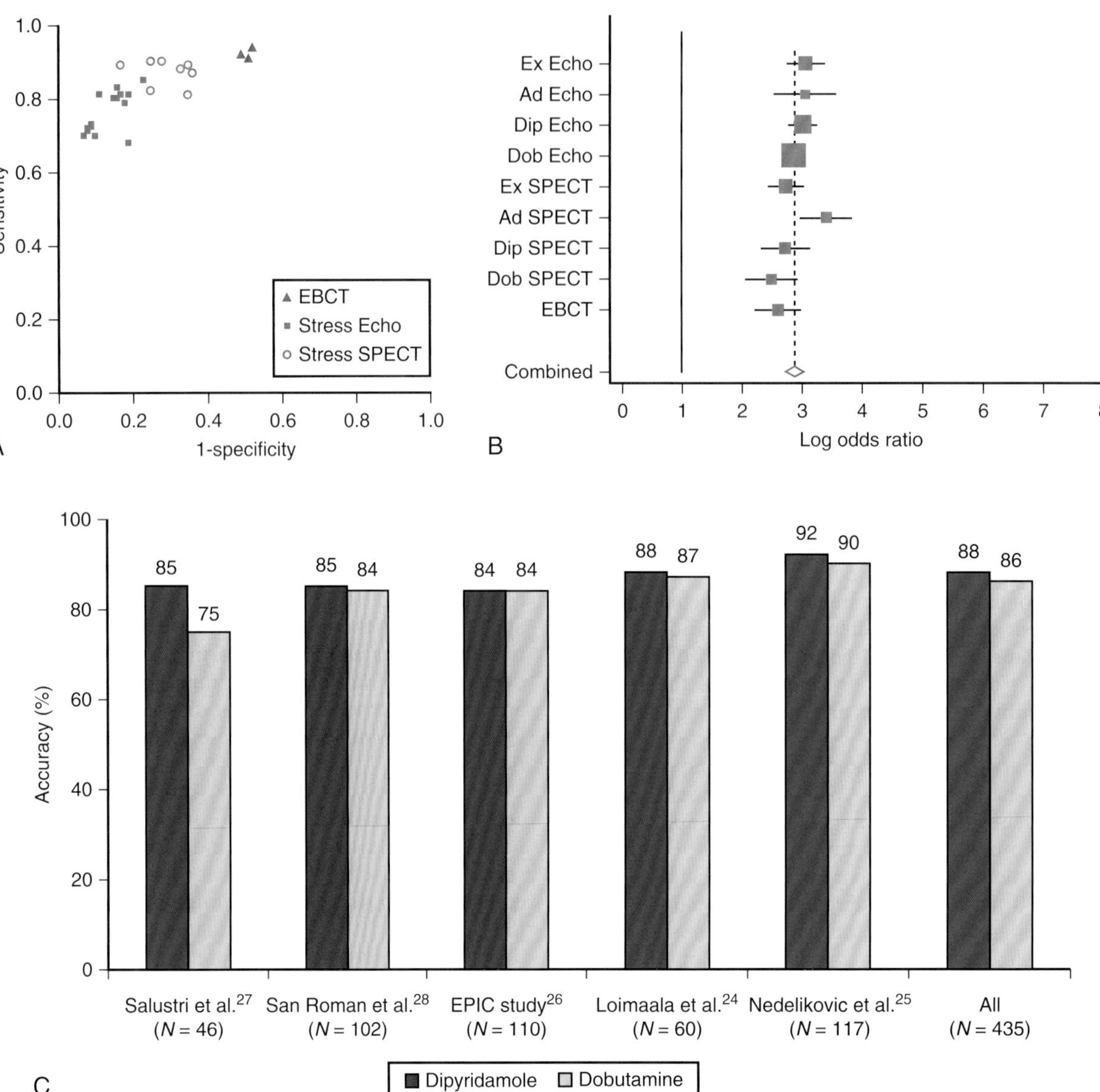

Fig. 20.7 Accuracy of pharmacologic stress echocardiography. (A) Pooled estimates of the sensitivity and specificity of stress echocardiography (SE) for the diagnosis of coronary artery disease (CAD) compared with electron beam computed tomography (EBCT) and stress single-photon emission computed tomography (SPECT). (B) Summary of the diagnostic logarithmic odds ratios and 95% confidence intervals for pharmacologic SE compared with other functional tests (e.g., detection of ischemia by echocardiography) and anatomic tests (e.g., EBCT). Compared with other modalities, there are no significant differences in overall performance of pharmacologic SE for the diagnosis of significant CAD. (C) Diagnostic accuracy of pharmacologic SE for the detection of greater than 50% coronary artery stenosis in various studies. *Vertical bars* represent the accuracy of dobutamine SE *(yellow)* compared with dipyridamole SE *(blue)*. *Ad*, Adenosine; *Dip*, dipyridamole; *Dob*, dobutamine; *EBCT*, electron beam computed tomography; *Echo*, echocardiography; *Ex*, exercise; SPECT, single-photon emission computed tomography. (A and B from Heijenbrok-Kal MH, Fleischmann KE, Hunink MG. Stress echocardiography, stress single-photon-emission computed tomography and electron beam computed tomography for the assessment of coronary artery disease: a meta-analysis of diagnostic performance. *Am Heart J.* 2007;154:415–423; C from Picano E, Molinaro S, Pasanisi E. The diagnostic accuracy of pharmacological stress echocardiography for the assessment of coronary artery disease: a meta-analysis. *Cardiovasc Ultrasound.* 2008;6:30.)

ASSESSMENT OF MYOCARDIAL VIABILITY

Detection of dysfunctional myocardium that may recover after revascularization is the aim of myocardial viability assessment in patients with CAD and chronic LV dysfunction. Myocardium responds to transient ischemia with a reduction in contractile function that may persist for several hours to weeks after restoration of coronary flow; this is known as *stunning* (Table 20.4). Repetitive episodes of stunning may lead to hibernation, with reduction in contractile function but preserved (although down-regulated) metabolism. The chronic reduction in resting perfusion that is seen with hibernation appears to be a consequence rather than a cause of the contractile dysfunction.[40] Severe reduction in coronary perfusion leads to myocyte death and scarring, both of which do not recover with revascularization.

The assessment of viable myocardium and the prediction of recovery of segmental and global LV function (with subsequent improvement in symptoms and prognosis) after revascularization have been the focus of a large body of research.[41] Table 20.5 summarizes the markers of myocardial viability according to imaging technique. Pooled analysis of 158 studies revealed that fluorodeoxyglucose positron emission tomography had the highest sensitivity for predicting recovery of regional and global LV function, followed by SPECT and SE, whereas dobutamine SE had the highest specificity.[41] In a pooled analysis of studies

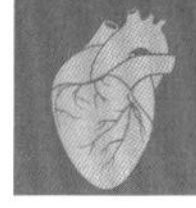

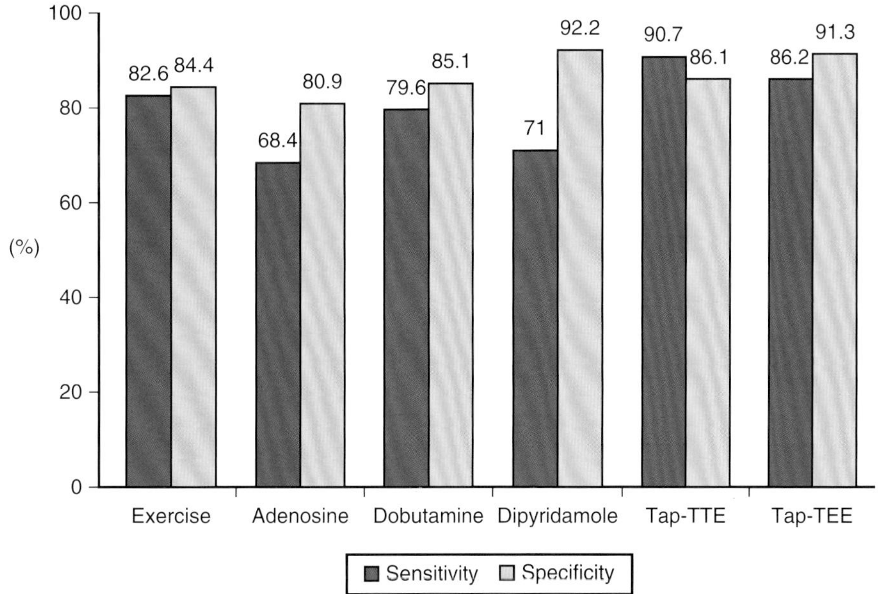

Fig. 20.8 Weighted means of diagnostic sensitivity and specificity for different echocardiographic stressors. Transatrial pacing combined with transesophageal echocardiography *(Tap-TEE)* demonstrated the highest sensitivity and specificity, followed by transatrial pacing and transthoracic echocardiography *(Tap-TTE)*, exercise stress echocardiography, dipyridamole, dobutamine, and adenosine stress echocardiography. (From Noguchi Y, Nagata-Kobayashi S, Stahl JE, et al. A meta-analytic comparison of echocardiographic stressors. *Int J Cardiovasc Imaging.* 2005;21:189–207.)

TABLE 20.4 Assessment of Myocardial Dysfunction in Ischemic Heart Disease: Evaluation of Pathophysiologic Mechanisms.

Substrate	*Coronary Flow Reserve*	*Contractile Reserve*	*Perfusion*	*Metabolism*	*Scar Tissue*
Normal myocardium	Normal	Normal	Normal	Normal	Absent
Stunned myocardium	Reduced	Normal	Normal	Normal	Absent
Hibernating myocardium	Severely reduced	Abnormal	Abnormal	Normal	Absent
Myocardial scar tissue	Severely reduced	Absent	Absent	Absent	Present

TABLE 20.5 Imaging Modalities to Assess Myocardial Viability.

Imaging Modality	*Viability Marker*
SPECT	
201-Thallium	Perfusion, cell membrane integrity
99m-Technetium	Perfusion, cell membrane integrity, intact mitochondria
FDG-PET	Glucose metabolism
Echocardiography	
Low-dose dobutamine infusion	Contractile reserve
Low-dose dipyridamole infusion	Contractile reserve
Magnetic resonance imaging	
Low-dose dobutamine infusion	Contractile reserve
Gadolinium contrast	Scar tissue

FDG-PET, Fluorodeoxyglucose positron emission tomography; *SPECT*, single-photon emission computed tomography.

published before 1998, the sensitivity and specificity of low-dose dobutamine SE for the detection of viability were 84% and 81%, respectively.[42] Similar sensitivities (80%) and specificities (78%) were found in a pooled analysis of later studies (2001–2007).[41]

Large retrospective studies have firmly linked myocardial viability to long-term survival.[41,43,44] In the Surgical Treatment for Ischemic Heart Failure (STICH) trial, 1212 patients with ischemic heart failure (LV ejection fraction ≤35%) and coronary anatomy amenable to surgical revascularization were randomized to receive optimal medical treatment (n = 602) or optimal medical therapy and coronary artery bypass grafting (n = 610).[45] Patients undergoing coronary revascularization demonstrated significantly lower rates of death or hospitalization for cardiovascular events compared with medically treated patients (58% vs. 68%; P <0.001).[46] In a subanalysis, patients with viable myocardium had lower mortality rates than those without myocardial viability (37% vs. 51%; P = 0.003).[46]

After adjustments for LV ejection fraction, LV volume, heart failure symptoms, and comorbidities, viability was not, however, an independent predictor of outcome. This result can be attributed to (1) methodologic issues in the trial design, (2) the fact that surgical revascularization was offset by surgical risk, or (3) understanding that surgical revascularization improves survival regardless of the presence of ischemic or viable tissue by bypassing diseased coronary segments, which are the sites of acute coronary syndromes (the main driver of mortality for patients with CAD).[47] The role of viability testing in ischemic cardiomyopathy is being re-evaluated in the Study of Efficacy and Safety of Percutaneous Coronary Intervention to Improve Survival in Heart Failure (REVIVED-BCIS2; NCT01920048).[48]

Measurement of myocardial thickness in dysfunctional segments is standard practice before low-dose dobutamine SE is performed for viability assessment. An end-diastolic thickness of greater than 6 mm has a sensitivity of 94% for viability but a specificity of only 48%.[49] An even higher sensitivity (but lower specificity) was reported by La Canna et al.[50] This result has been challenged by data from cardiac magnetic resonance imaging, which demonstrated that 18% of segments with a

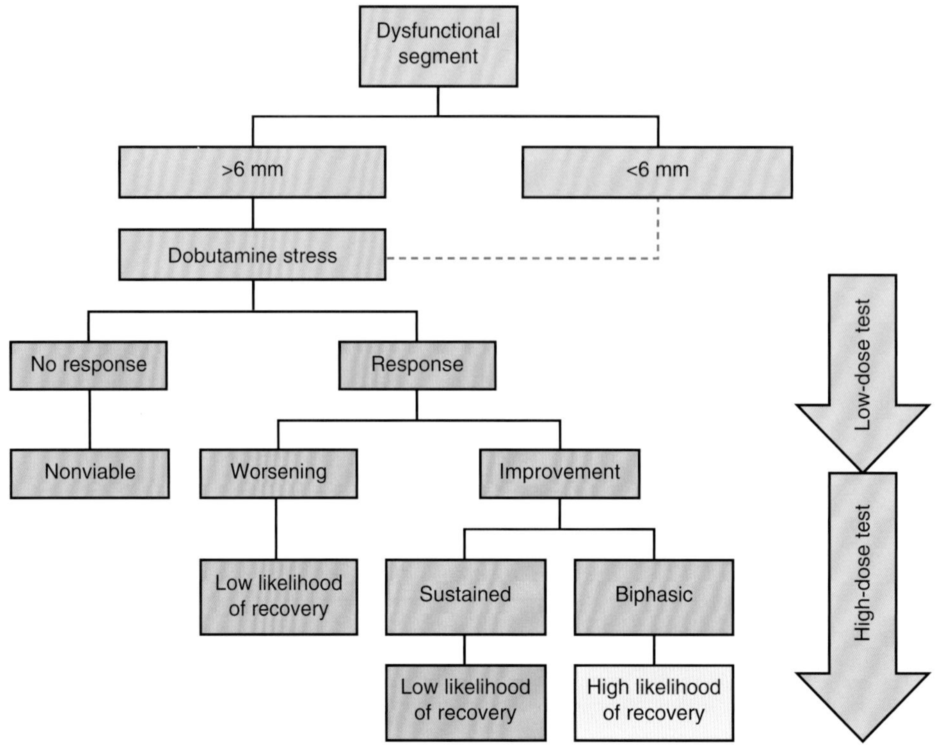

Fig. 20.9 Proposed algorithm for evaluation of myocardial viability with dobutamine stress echocardiography. Dysfunctional segments may be thin (<6 mm), but this does not necessarily indicate nonviability. Various responses to low-dose dobutamine stress echocardiography can be elicited; absence of a response indicates nonviability of a myocardial segment, whereas a response suggests viability. The addition of high-dose dobutamine stress further refines the classification of a segment in which a response is identified: worsening response and sustained improvement predict a low likelihood of recovery after revascularization, whereas a biphasic response indicates a high likelihood of recovery. An example of a biphasic response is shown in Video 20.9.

wall thickness of 5.5 mm or less had only a limited scar burden (on delayed gadolinium enhancement imaging) and improved function after revascularization.[51] Segments with a thickness of 5.5 to 6 mm or less cannot therefore automatically be assumed to be nonviable.

During low-dose dobutamine SE (5–10 μg/kg/min), viable myocardial segments that are dysfunctional at rest show a response, whereas nonviable segments do not. A response is characterized by a change in contraction (i.e., thickening). An akinetic segment that becomes dyskinetic (merely the result of increased intraventricular pressure during stress[52]) is classified as "no response." A worsening function is also considered a response, although these segments have a low likelihood of recovery after revascularization and probably represent a mixture of scar tissue and normal myocardium that becomes ischemic during stress (Fig. 20.9).[53,54]

Improvement in function can be further characterized by increasing the infusion rate of dobutamine beyond 20 μg/kg per minute to induce a chronotropic response. If the viable segments (stunned or hibernating) are subtended by a coronary artery with significant stenosis, the increase in heart rate will cause ischemia and a biphasic response: an initial improvement (at low dose) and subsequent deterioration (at peak dose) in contractile function when ischemia supervenes (see Fig. 20.9 and Video 20.9).[53]

A sustained improvement (i.e., improved at low dose and further improved at high dose) has a poor predictive value for functional improvement after revascularization and probably represents stunned or hibernating myocardium.[54] It is unclear why the identification of stunned or hibernating myocardium does not translate into a better response rate, but it is hypothesized that some of these patients also harbor a mix of stunned or hibernating and infarcted myocardium. A biphasic response to dobutamine is the most specific predictor of functional recovery after coronary revascularization (better than worsening function or sustained improvement).[53]

The different response patterns that resting dysfunctional myocardial segments may show in reaction to dobutamine SE and their pathophysiologic mechanisms are summarized in Table 20.6.[53,54] Dipyridamole has also been used for viability assessment; dipyridamole has a slightly higher specificity than dobutamine, whereas dobutamine has a somewhat better sensitivity.[6]

NONEXERCISE STRESS ECHOCARDIOGRAPHY IN SPECIFIC CLINICAL SCENARIOS

The clinical role of nonexercise SE in specific patient subsets is summarized in Table 20.7.[55–60]

USE OF CONTRAST DURING NONEXERCISE STRESS ECHOCARDIOGRAPHY

Nonexercise SE relies on adequate visualization of the endocardial border, which is not always feasible. The use of contrast media that can traverse the pulmonary vascular bed and provide opacification of the LV greatly enhances endocardial border detection (Fig. 20.10 and Video 20.10).[4,61] Commercially available contrast microbubbles consist of a shell (e.g., phospholipid) containing an insoluble gas with a high molecular mass

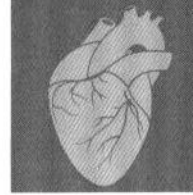

TABLE 20.6 Assessment of Myocardial Viability With Dobutamine Stress Echocardiography: Wall Motion Changes and Pathologic Substrates.

Pathologic Substrate	*Wall Motion Pattern*	*Rest*	*Low-Dose Response*	*Peak-Dose Response*	*Functional Recovery (%)*
Viable myocardium					
Stunned/hibernating + ischemia	Biphasic	Hypokinesia, akinesia	Improvement	Worsening	72–75
Mixture scar and normal	Worsening	Hypokinesia, akinesia	Worsening	Worsening	9–35
Stunned or hibernating ± possible scar tissue	Sustained improvement	Hypokinesia, akinesia	Improvement	Improvement	15–22
Scar tissue	No response	Hypokinesia, akinesia	Hypokinesia, akinesia	Hypokinesia, akinesia	4–13

TABLE 20.7 Clinical Role of Nonexercise Stress Echocardiography in Specific Clinical Scenarios.

Patient Subset	*Clinical Role*	*Evidence*	*Comments*
After acute MI	Requirement for further revascularization vs. medical therapy, especially if complete revascularization was not performed initially	Presence and extent of myocardial ischemia independently associated with cardiac mortality and nonfatal MI, increased risk of recurrent angina, and need for revascularization	Role of viability testing with low-dose dobutamine more controversial
Diabetes mellitus	Commonly accompanied by complications that make exercise SE unfeasible (i.e., obesity, peripheral vascular disease, and neuropathy)	Diagnostic accuracy of nonexercise SE similar to that in nondiabetics Prognostic implications of SE proven for diabetics	Screening of asymptomatic diabetics with SPECT or coronary CT has not decreased death or nonfatal MI when risk factors are well controlled, and is not recommended
Before noncardiac surgery	Coronary artery stenosis may cause supply-demand mismatch during hemodynamic fluctuations induced by anesthesia and surgery. Perisurgical stress can cause plaque rupture. SE is of value for higher-risk procedures and patients, as is nonexercise SE in high-risk vascular surgery patients who are unable to exercise	Nonexercise SE has a high negative predictive value	Also applicable to high-risk surgery in patients with >2 clinical risk factors and poor functional capacity (<4 METs) (class IC) and in high- or intermediate-risk surgery with 1or 2 clinical risk factors and poor functional capacity (<4 METs) (class IIb, C)
LBBB	Dyssynchrony simulates RWMAs, but regional thickening can still be evaluated	Less sensitive than in non-LBBB patients, but more specific than SPECT	—

CT, Computed tomography; *LBBB*, left bundle branch block; *METs*, metabolic equivalents; *MI*, myocardial infarction; *RWMA*, regional wall motion abnormality; *SE*, stress echocardiography; *SPECT*, single-photon emission computed tomography.

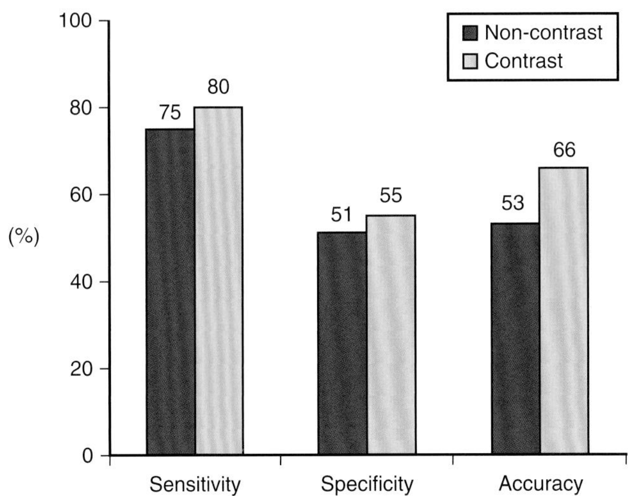

Fig. 20.10 Effect of contrast agent use on the sensitivity, specificity, and diagnostic accuracy of dobutamine stress echocardiography. The addition of contrast media improved the sensitivity, specificity (nonsignificant change), and diagnostic accuracy ($P = 0.002$) of dobutamine stress echocardiography. An example of the use of contrast for improving endocardial border detection is shown in Video 20.10. (From Plana JC, Mikati IA, Dokainish H, et al. A randomized cross-over study for evaluation of the effect of image optimization with contrast on the diagnostic accuracy of dobutamine echocardiography in coronary artery disease The OPTIMIZE Trial. *JACC Cardiovasc Imaging*. 2008;1:145–152.)

(e.g., sulfur hexafluoride). Microbubbles can generate nonlinear backscatter of ultrasound, which can be used to selectively enhance the signal emanating from the contrast. Contrast is injected intravenously in boluses (although a continuous infusion may be used) about 30 seconds before image acquisition; effective opacification lasts for 60 seconds or longer.

The specific storage requirements, indications, and doses published by the manufacturer should be adhered to. Hypersensitivity reactions to echocardiographic contrast are rare (1 in 10,000 patients) and may be delayed, but drugs should be readily available to manage this complication, such as chlorpheniramine (10 mg intravenous bolus), hydrocortisone (200 mg intravenous bolus), and adrenaline (diluted 1:1000 with saline; 1-mL intramuscular injection).

Because intravenous contrast passes from the RV through the pulmonary circulation to the LV, it is interposed between the transducer and the LV in parasternal views, causing shadowing. Apical acquisitions should be performed first or parasternal views eliminated from the protocol altogether when contrast is used.

EMERGING TECHNIQUES IN STRESS ECHOCARDIOGRAPHY

Pharmacologic SE relies on 2-dimensional (2D) assessment of LV wall motion, including wall thickening and excursion. It is subject to a variety of limitations: (1) foreshortening of the LV,

(2) potential misalignment of views acquired at different stages of the protocol, (3) a time-consuming acquisition in which all views have to be recorded for every stage of the protocol, and (4) reliance on subjective, visual analysis for distinguishing active deformation (i.e., true motion) from passive tethering (i.e., translational motion) of myocardial segments. 3D echocardiography and speckle tracking strain echocardiography can potentially overcome these limitations by avoiding off-axis images and foreshortening of the LV apex and allowing quantification of abnormal motion, thereby reducing interobserver variability.

Though SE has traditionally been predicated on the inducibility of WMAs, direct assessment of coronary flow reserve and myocardial perfusion can be assessed echocardiographically. Measurement of the coronary flow velocity reserve at rest and at peak pharmacologic stress in the left anterior descending (LAD) coronary artery increases the diagnostic sensitivity of SE. In the following sections, evidence for the clinical use of these emerging techniques (3D SE, speckle tracking strain echocardiography, coronary flow reserve, and myocardial perfusion) is summarized.

THREE-DIMENSIONAL STRESS ECHOCARDIOGRAPHY

Three-dimensional (3D) SE, in which echocardiographic data are obtained from the apical window using ECG-gating, allows rapid acquisition of a nonforeshortened image. The 3D full volume of the LV is usually constructed from four to seven conical subvolumes obtained during multiple cardiac cycles to maximize volume rate (Fig. 20.11); however, it can be acquired in a single beat. The data are analyzed off-line, allowing tomographic assessment of regional thickening during each stage of the stress study. The diagnostic sensitivity, specificity, and accuracy of 2D and 3D dobutamine SE are similar to those of SPECT (86%, 83%, 84% and 86%, 80%, 82%, respectively).[62] No significant differences in sensitivity or specificity were found with respect to different coronary artery territories.[62] Data acquisition is more rapid with dobutamine 3D SE than with 2D SE (29 ± 4 s vs. 68 ± 6 s, respectively; $P < 0.0001$).[62] Similar results in terms of test performance and speed were reported by Eroglu et al.[63]

When performed with contrast, the sensitivity, specificity, and accuracy of 3D SE were similar to those of 2D SE with contrast (78%, 89%, 85% and 73%, 93%, 86%, respectively).[64] However, what is gained in acquisition time might be lost as a result of the more complex postprocessing involved for 3D image analysis. Multislice analysis of 3D SE demonstrated a higher specificity (95%) than 2D SE when compared with coronary angiography but at the cost of a lower sensitivity (72%).[65] 3D SE outperformed 2D SE for ischemia detection in the right coronary artery territory when using multislice analysis.[65] 3D SE has been used for viability assessment, but not comprehensively in comparison with 2D SE for this indication.[66]

3D SE remains limited by its temporal and spatial resolution and by stitching artifacts (misalignment of subvolumes when images are stitched together), particularly when arrhythmias occur. The role of contrast media in 3D nonexercise SE is still being defined: although they improve endocardial definition, dedicated contrast pulse techniques reduce volume rate (in addition to the already reduced volume rate of 3D compared with the frame rate of 2D acquisitions).[67]

TWO-DIMENSIONAL TISSUE DOPPLER AND SPECKLE TRACKING STRAIN ECHOCARDIOGRAPHY

Measurement of systolic and diastolic myocardial velocities with TDI provides quantitative assessment of regional longitudinal function and has been associated with significant coronary artery stenosis.[68] Myocardial velocity, however, is influenced by tethering from adjacent segments and by angle dependency, limiting its clinical usefulness. In contrast, speckle tracking strain echocardiography, in which myocardial features (i.e., speckles) are tracked throughout the cardiac cycle, permits quantification of regional active shortening or thickening and is less influenced by translational motion (i.e., tethering). Strain represents the magnitude of change in length or thickness of a myocardial segment

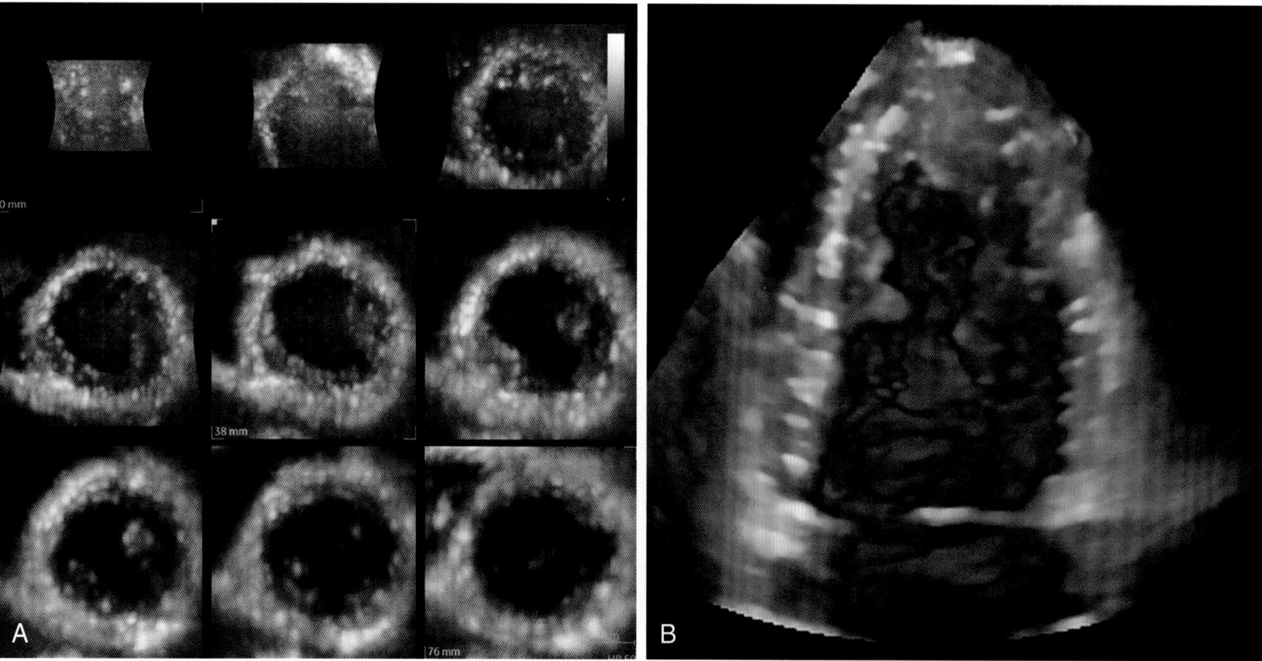

Fig. 20.11 Three-dimensional stress echocardiography. (A) Parallel, slice-rendered views from a full-volume acquisition of the LV. (B) Full-volume rendered view of the LV. Wall motion analysis is more readily performed on the cine loops of A than on those of B.

relative to its original dimension, whereas strain rate quantifies the speed at which the deformation occurs. 2D speckle tracking echocardiography also allows assessment of multidirectional strain (i.e., longitudinal, radial, and circumferential).

The subendocardial layer is located adjacent to the LV cavity, exposing it to high intracavitary pressures. This leads to higher wall stress and a higher rate of oxidative metabolism (i.e., increased oxygen demand) compared with the subepicardial layer. High LV pressure is transmitted to coronary vessels, decreasing oxygen supply in the subendocardial layer. The subendocardium is consequently more susceptible to ischemia than the subepicardium. Because longitudinal function is largely determined by the subendocardial fibers, impairment of longitudinal deformation parameters is detected earlier than impairment in radial function (influenced by all layers) during ischemia (Fig. 20.12).

Ischemia slows the onset of deformation, causing postsystolic shortening. Postsystolic shortening is an early marker of myocardial ischemia and is associated with a reduction in subendocardial blood flow.[69] Regional strain is preload dependent, and a decrease in filling time at a high heart rate during SE may lead to reduced strain as a consequence of the elevated heart rate rather than a decrease in contractile function.[70] The different responses of longitudinal strain, strain rate, and postsystolic shortening during dobutamine SE are summarized in Table 20.8.

The diagnostic value of global and regional TDI-derived strain and strain rate and of 2D speckle tracking strain echocardiography has been demonstrated in various clinical scenarios (Table 20.9) and may be superior to visual assessment of WMAs.[71–78] Most studies have comprised study populations with predominantly single-vessel disease.[72,74,75,77,78] Strain imaging is also useful in the evaluation of viability (Table 20.10)[79–84] and may be of incremental value to wall motion assessment in identifying viable myocardium.

CORONARY FLOW VELOCITY RESERVE

Coronary flow reserve is the capacity of coronary artery blood flow to increase in response to increased myocardial metabolic demand (i.e., the ratio of hyperemic flow in a coronary artery to

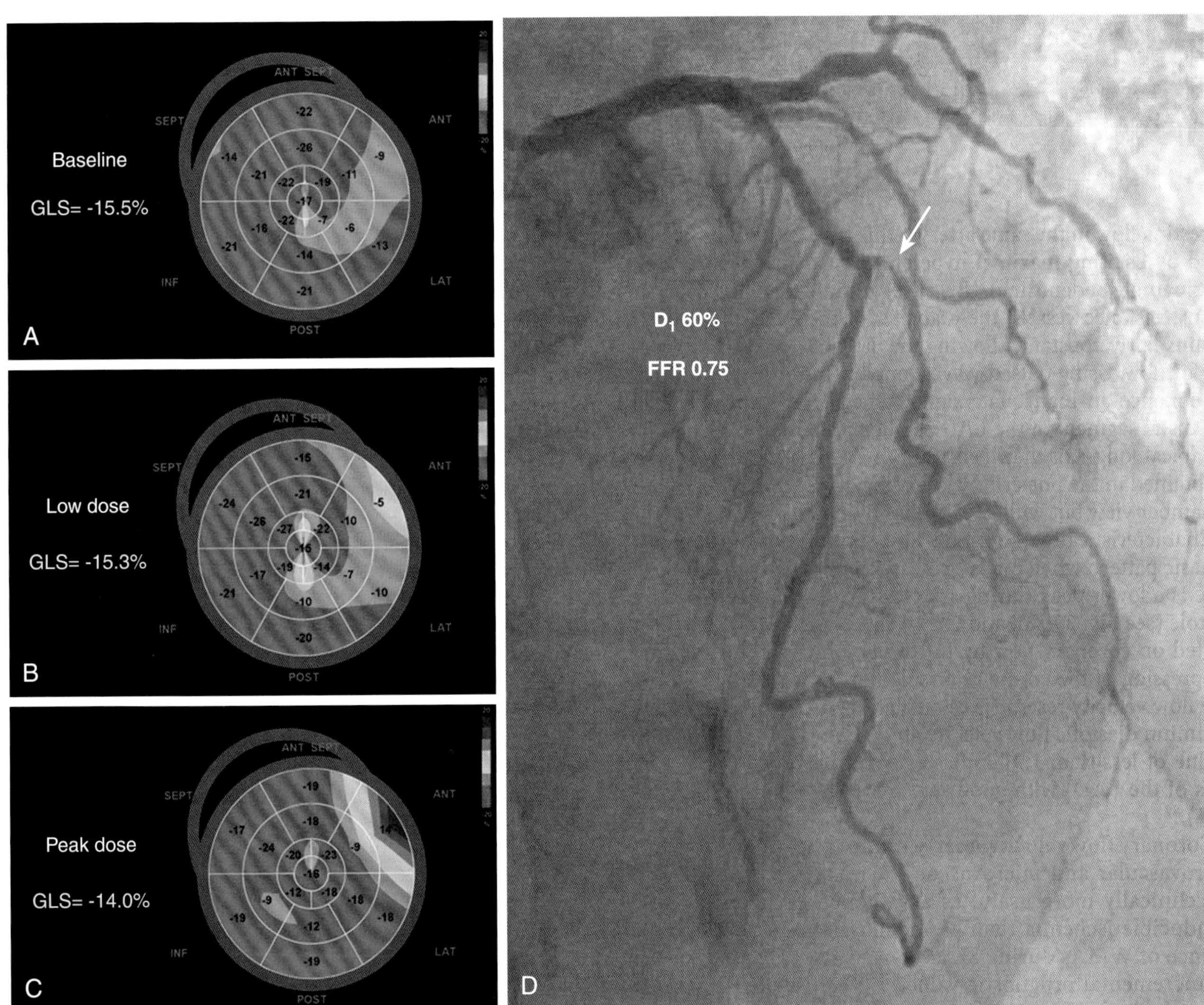

Fig. 20.12 Speckle tracking strain imaging for dobutamine stress echocardiography. (A) At baseline, longitudinal strain was impaired in the anterolateral segments, as displayed on a parametric map. (B) During low-dose dobutamine infusion, longitudinal strain deteriorated further in the anterolateral segments. (C) At peak dose, dyskinesia developed in the affected segments (*blue color* of a segment denotes elongation during systole; *red color* indicates systolic shortening). (D) Invasive coronary angiogram demonstrates a 60% stenosis in the first diagonal branch (D_1) of the left anterior descending coronary artery, which proved to be physiologically flow-limiting with an invasively measured fractional flow reserve *(FFR)* of 0.75. *ANT*, Anterior; *ANT SEPT*, anterior septum; *GLS*, global longitudinal strain; *INF*, inferior; *LAT*, lateral; *POST*, posterior; *SEPT*, septal.

TABLE 20.8 Longitudinal Strain Patterns at Rest and During Dobutamine Stress Echocardiography According to the Ischemic Substrate.

Condition	*Rest*	*Low Dose*	*Peak Dose*
Normal			
Peak systolic strain rate	Normal	Improved	Further improved
Systolic strain	Normal	Improved	Further improved
Postsystolic shortening	Absent	Absent	Absent
Acute ischemia			
Peak systolic strain rate	Reduced	Further reduced	Further reduced
Systolic strain	Reduced	Further reduced	Further reduced
Postsystolic shortening	Present	Pronounced	Further pronounced
Stunning			
Peak systolic strain rate	Reduced	Improved	Further improved
Systolic strain	Reduced	Improved	Improved - reduced
Postsystolic shortening	Present	Reduced	Absent
Hibernation			
Peak systolic strain rate	Reduced	Improved	Reduced
Systolic strain	Reduced	Improved	Reduced
Postsystolic shortening	Present	Pronounced	Further pronounced
Non-transmural infarction			
Peak systolic strain rate	Very reduced	Reduced	Further reduced
Systolic strain	Very reduced	Reduced	Further reduced
Postsystolic shortening	Present	Pronounced	Further pronounced
Transmural infarction			
Peak systolic strain rate	No deformation	Unchanged	Unchanged
Systolic strain	No deformation	Unchanged	Unchanged
Postsystolic shortening	Absent	Unchanged	Unchanged

the resting flow in the same artery). This reserve capacity can be tested by eliciting maximal hyperemia with vasodilators (e.g., dipyridamole, adenosine). Because vasodilators act primarily on resistance vessels, the diameter of the epicardial vessels remains fairly constant, allowing the use of velocity as a surrogate for flow. Using pulsed-wave Doppler (intravenous contrast can enhance an inadequate signal), the blood velocity of the mid-distal segment of the LAD can be measured from a modified apical long-axis view (Fig. 20.13A). Flow velocity can also be obtained in the posterior descending artery from a modified 2-chamber view but with a lower feasibility (58%).[85]

Characteristically, the blood flow velocity profile shows a biphasic pattern when interrogated with pulsed-wave Doppler: there is a lower peak during systole and a higher peak during diastole (see Fig. 20.13B and C).[86] This is caused by the suction exerted on coronary flow by LV relaxation in diastole and by compression of the coronary circulation during systole. Coronary flow velocity reserve is calculated as the ratio between the maximum diastolic flow velocity at peak stress and at baseline; a value of less than 1.91 indicates significant CAD (75% stenosis of the LAD) with good sensitivity (89%) and specificity (80%).[87]

Coronary flow velocity reserve cannot distinguish between macrovascular and microvascular disease.[88] As a corollary, it is clinically more useful as an adjunct to the evaluation of inducible ischemia than as a stand-alone test.[88,89] In the absence of WMAs during SE, coronary flow velocity reserve has incremental prognostic value.[85,87,88,90] Normal coronary flow velocity reserve in patients without WMAs during SE identifies a low-risk group (0.6% annual rate of death and nonfatal myocardial infarction).[85] This technique has potential applications in specific patient subsets when analysis of WMAs is less useful, such as in screening for cardiac allograft vasculopathy.[86]

MYOCARDIAL CONTRAST PERFUSION AND MYOCARDIAL CONTRAST BLOOD FLOW RESERVE

Because abnormal myocardial perfusion is an earlier manifestation of ischemia than regional WMAs (ischemic cascade; discussed earlier), it is an attractive imaging target for CAD diagnosis. Myocardial perfusion defects can be visually identified with contrast echocardiography. Dedicated pulse sequences with high mechanical indices (i.e., flash) are used to disrupt contrast microbubbles, after which inflow (i.e., replenishment) of intact microbubbles is visualized at a lower mechanical index. Myocardial blood flow can be derived from a flash-replenishment protocol by multiplying microbubble velocity (i.e., blood velocity) with peak signal density (representing myocardial blood volume). The physical principles of myocardial blood flow quantification are discussed in more detail in Chapter 3.

In a pooled analysis of 20 studies (1683 patients), myocardial contrast echocardiography was compared with invasive coronary angiography and was found to have a sensitivity of 80% and a specificity of 83% for the diagnosis of CAD.[91] A meta-analysis of eight studies demonstrated a higher diagnostic sensitivity (85%) for myocardial contrast perfusion compared with SPECT/dobutamine SE (71%), with comparable specificity (74% and 71%, respectively).[92]

A later prospective trial found a higher sensitivity for the diagnosis of CAD with 70% or greater stenosis (75%) when compared with SPECT (49%; P <0.0001) but the specificity was lower (52% and 81%, respectively; P <0.0001).[93] In a large study (6075 patients with long-term follow-up), myocardial contrast perfusion was an independent predictor (odds ratio = 2.4; 95% confidence interval: 1.0–5.9) of all-cause mortality and nonfatal myocardial infarction when corrected for WMAs.[94] A study of 1252 patients undergoing myocardial contrast perfusion testing confirmed its incremental prognostic value over WMAs alone.[95]

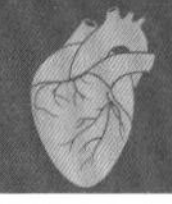

TABLE 20.9 Diagnostic Strain Imaging During Dobutamine Stress Echocardiography for Significant Coronary Artery Disease (After 2010).

Study	*No. of Patients*	*Deformation Imaging Mode*	*Patient Characteristics*	*Comparator*	*Parameters (Global and/or Segmental)*	*Predictive Value*
Yu et al.[71]	76	STE dobutamine	*n* = 34 with severe 3-vessel CAD and preserved LVEF; *n* = 42 controls	CAG (≥70% stenosis)	Global and segmental longitudinal strain, peak systolic strain rate, circumferential strain and strain rate	Peak systolic strain rate at intermediate dose (10 μg/kg per minute) was an independent predictor of multivessel CAD (odds ratio = 1.63; 95% CI: 1.12 to 2.82)
Aggeli et al.[72]	100	STE dobutamine	Known or suspected CAD, without history of transmural infarction (46% single-vessel disease)	CAG (>70% stenosis)	Global longitudinal strain	Change in global longitudinal strain from rest to peak stress had a higher sensitivity (81%) than WMSI (78%) for detecting CAD, although the area under the curve was higher for WMSI
Joyce et al.[73]	105	STE dobutamine	Post-STEMI patients at 3 months' follow-up (56% multivessel disease)	CAG (>70% stenosis)	Global and segmental peak systolic, longitudinal strain	Optimal change in global, peak systolic longitudinal strain from rest to peak stress for detection of CAD was ≥1.9%, and was independently associated with CAD, whereas WMSI was not
Nagy et al.[74]	60	TDI/STE dobutamine	Suspected CAD (28% single-vessel disease; 28% multivessel disease)	Quantitative CAG (≥50% stenosis)	Peak longitudinal systolic strain and strain rate, postsystolic strain	No clear benefit of strain-derived parameters compared with WMA analysis, but study might have been underpowered
Cusmà-Piccione et al.[75]	52	STE dipyridamole	Scheduled for CAG (single-vessel CAD)	CAG (>50% stenosis)	Peak global and coronary artery territory, longitudinal strain	Change between resting and peak stress global longitudinal strain provided higher sensitivity (61%) and specificity (90%) than visual WMAs (44% and 55%, respectively). Change between low dose and peak dose, peak global longitudinal strain, had the highest sensitivity (84%) and specificity (92%) for CAD diagnosis
Dattilo et al.[76]	65	TDI dipyridamole	Previous, nondiagnostic dipyridamole SE	CT coronary angiography (15%–50% stenosis = mild coronary stenosis)	Global systolic strain in longitudinal and circumferential directions	Change ≤0% in global longitudinal strain from rest to peak stress, identified mild coronary artery stenosis with a sensitivity of 95% and a specificity of 93%
Uusitalo et al.[77]	50	STE dobutamine	Intermediate probability of CAD (24% single-vessel disease)	CAG (>75% stenosis) or FFR <0.8 or quantitative $H_2{}^{15}O$-PET adenosine stress perfusion (myocardial blood flow <2.5 mL/g per minute)	Global and regional peak systolic longitudinal strain and strain rate, postsystolic index	Decreased peak systolic strain (<18.4%) and increased post-strain index (>6.2%) during recovery, had the highest areas under the curve for CAD diagnosis
Rumbinaite et al.[78]	127	STE dobutamine	Moderate and high probability of CAD and preserved LVEF (≥55%) (48% single-vessel disease)	CAG (≥70% stenosis) and adenosine stress perfusion CMR (visual perfusion defect)	Global peak systolic, early diastolic, late diastolic strain and strain rate in longitudinal, radial, and circumferential directions	Global longitudinal strain at peak stress had the highest area under the curve (0.96), sensitivity (94%), and specificity (92%) for CAD diagnosis

CAD, Coronary artery disease; *CAG*, coronary angiography; *CI*, confidence interval; *CMR*, cardiac magnetic resonance; *CT*, computed tomography; *FFR*, fractional flow reserve; *LVEF*, left ventricular ejection fraction; *PET*, positron emission tomography; *SE*, stress echocardiography; *STE*, speckle tracking echocardiography; *STEMI*, ST-segment elevation myocardial infarction; *TDI*, tissue Doppler imaging; *WMA*, wall motion abnormality; *WMSI*, wall motion score index.

After a vasodilator (i.e., dipyridamole or adenosine) infusion, contrast is administered as a continuous infusion until steady state is achieved. Microbubbles are cleared by applying a flash pulse with a high mechanical index (0.9–1.0). Replenishment is then assessed in real time with low-power imaging (mechanical index of 0.1–0.2) for 8 to 10 beats (Fig. 20.14).[93] Dobutamine elicits a coronary hyperemic response due to increased cardiac workload and is an alternative agent.

Myocardial perfusion is normal if no perfusion defects are observed during replenishment (within five cardiac cycles at rest or within two cardiac cycles during stress) after a flash. Myocardial ischemia is defined by the presence of (1) a newly

TABLE 20.10 **Strain Imaging During Dobutamine Stress Echocardiography for Assessment of Myocardial Viability (After 2010).**

Study	*No. of Patients*	*Strain Imaging*	*Patient Characteristics*	*Definition of Viability*	*Parameters (Segmental)*	*Predictive Value*
Fujimoto et al.[79]	48	TDI dobutamine	Previous myocardial infarction	Sustained improvement in WMSI at peak stress (uniphasic response) or improvement at low dose followed by worsening at peak dose (biphasic response)	Postsystolic shortening index, ratio of systolic lengthening to the sum of late systolic and postsystolic shortening (L/TS ratio)	The area under the curve of L/TS ratio to predict functional recovery was 0.89, compared with 0.78 for WMSI.
Bansal et al.[80]	55	TDI/STE dobutamine	Known CAD and LVEF <45%	Improvement in resting WMS by ≥1 after CABG	Peak systolic and end-systolic strain and strain rate in longitudinal, radial, and circumferential directions	Longitudinal strain and strain rate, circumferential strain and strain rate at low dose were independent predictors of LV functional recovery.
Rösner et al.[81]	72	TDI dobutamine	Patients undergoing CABG with preoperative MRI	Difference in ejection time strain ≥ 4.4% between pre-CABG and post-CABG	Peak systolic strain and strain rate, postsystolic strain	Increase in systolic strain during dobutamine SE had an area under the curve to predict functional recovery of 0.79.
Gong et al.[82]	42	STE dobutamine	Previous myocardial infarction with LVEF < 50%	Improvement in resting WMS by ≥1 after PCI	End-systolic and peak systolic strain and strain rate in longitudinal, radial, and circumferential directions	Peak longitudinal strain and strain rate at peak stress were independent predictors of viability.
Ismail et al.[83]	60	TDI dobutamine	Previous STEMI, treated with thrombolysis	Viability on ^{99m}Tc-sestamibi scintigraphy	Peak systolic strain and strain rate	Peak systolic strain and strain rate during peak stress differed significantly between viable and nonviable segments.
Li et al.[84]	33	STE dobutamine	Previous myocardial infarction with LVEF < 50%	Improvement in resting WMS by ≥1 after PCI	Peak systolic strain and strain rate in longitudinal, radial, and circumferential directions	Peak longitudinal strain and strain rate at peak stress were independent predictors of viability.

CABG, Coronary artery bypass grafting; *CAD*, coronary artery disease; *LVEF*, left ventricular ejection fraction; *MRI*, magnetic resonance imaging; *PCI*, percutaneous coronary intervention; *SE*, stress echocardiography; *STE*, speckle tracking echocardiography; *STEMI*, ST-segment elevation myocardial infarction; *TDI*, tissue Doppler imaging; *WMS*, wall motion score; *WMSI*, wall motion score index.

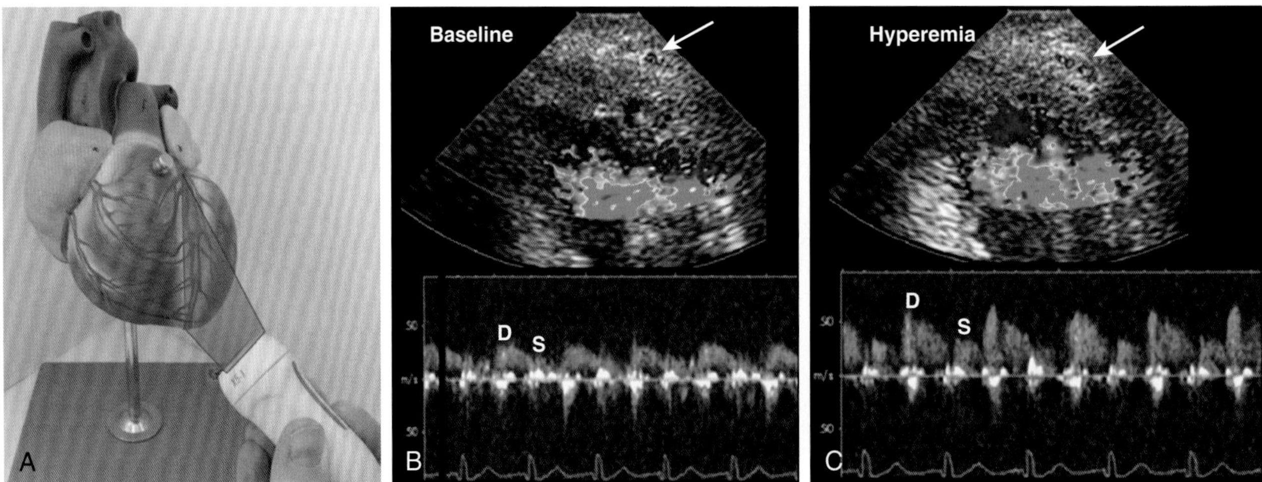

Fig. 20.13 Assessment of coronary flow reserve during stress echocardiography. Using pulsed-wave Doppler imaging, the blood velocity can be measured in the mid-distal segment of the left anterior descending (LAD) coronary artery from a modified apical long-axis view (A). Recordings of the systolic *(S)* and diastolic *(D)* peak blood velocities in the LAD *(arrow)* during rest (B) and at peak stress (C). A ratio of peak diastolic velocity during stress to peak diastolic velocity during rest of 2.5 or more indicates nonsignificant coronary artery disease, whereas a ratio of 2 to 2.5 reflects moderate stenosis (40%–70%), a ratio of <2 indicates severe stenosis (70%–90%), and a ratio of <1 indicates subtotal occlusion (>90% stenosis). (B and C from Sade LE, Eroglu S, Yuce D, et al. Follow-up of heart transplant recipients with serial echocardiographic coronary flow reserve and dobutamine stress echocardiography to detect cardiac allograft vasculopathy. *J Am Soc Echocardiogr.* 2014;27:531–539.)

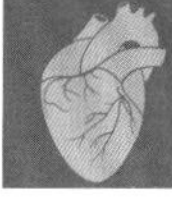

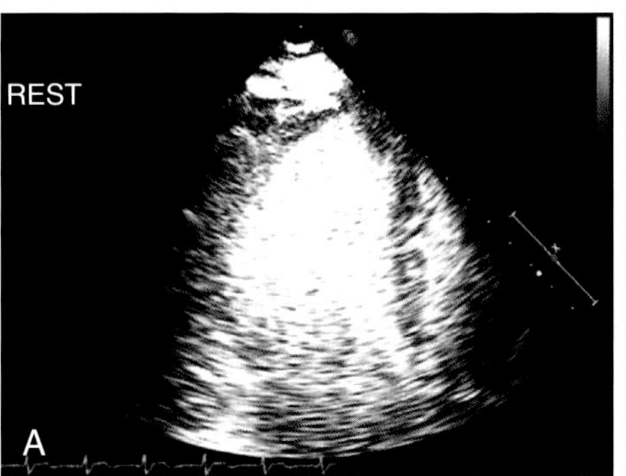

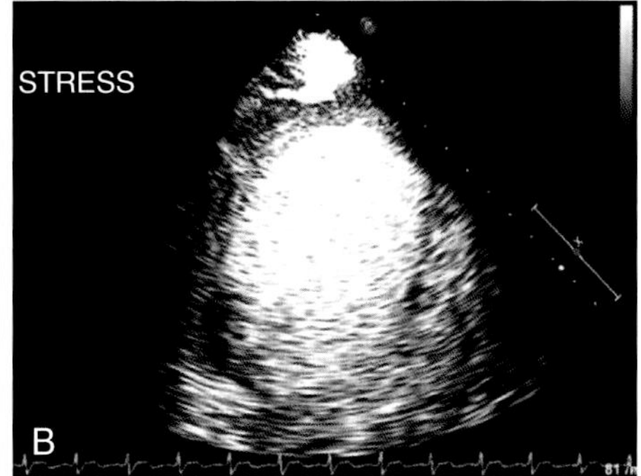

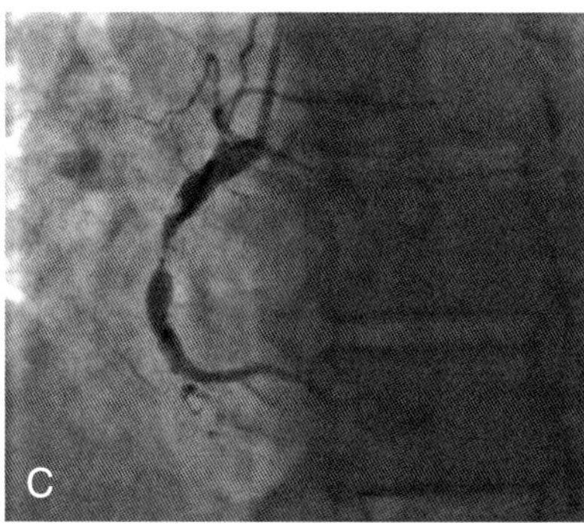

Fig. 20.14 Myocardial contrast echocardiography for detection of coronary artery disease. A reversible myocardial perfusion defect is demonstrated in the inferior wall: (A) at rest; (B) at peak stress. (C) This corresponded to an 80% stenosis of the right coronary artery seen on invasive angiography. (From Senior R, Moreo A, Gaibazzi N, et al. Comparison of sulfur hexafluoride microbubble (SonoVue)–enhanced myocardial contrast echocardiography with gated single-photon emission computed tomography for detection of significant coronary artery disease: a large European multicenter study. *J Am Coll Cardiol.* 2013;62:1353–1361.)

visible patchy or subendocardial defect or (2) a delay in replenishment on at least three cardiac cycles in at least two contiguous segments. Myocardial contrast echocardiography has also been successfully applied to viability assessment.[96]

Although the sensitivity of this test for detection of viable myocardium (90%) has been reported to be similar to that of SPECT (92%) or dobutamine SE (80%), the specificity of myocardial contrast echocardiography (63%) was higher than for either SPECT (45%) or dobutamine SE (54%) ($P < 0.05$).[96] 3D myocardial contrast echocardiography has been performed successfully, but its advantage over 2D acquisition remains to be proven.[66] Myocardial blood flow reserve can be calculated from myocardial blood flow values at rest and during stress[97] but may be discordant with coronary flow velocity reserve (see earlier discussion), depending on the contribution of collateral flow. The clinical role of myocardial blood flow reserve measurement remains to be accurately defined.

NONEXERCISE STRESS ECHOCARDIOGRAPHY: ROLE IN CURRENT CLINICAL PRACTICE

Nonexercise SE has an established role in current clinical practice and has undisputed diagnostic and prognostic value. Noninvasive CAD diagnosis is the primary referral indication for exercise ECG, SE, nuclear imaging, cardiac magnetic resonance, or computed tomography coronary angiography. Invasive coronary angiography is inappropriate as a first-line investigation because of cost, radiation exposure, and risk of procedural complications. Exercise ECG remains the initial test in most patients. If it is unfeasible (e.g., deconditioning), uninterpretable (e.g., resting ST-segment abnormality), incompletely performed (e.g., submaximal effort), or inconclusive, an alternative test has to be used. The choice depends on indications and contraindications (e.g., renal impairment disallowing intravenous contrast administration), local facilities and expertise, and the pretest likelihood of CAD. Similar considerations are applicable to viability testing and risk stratification of special populations (e.g., patients with diabetes mellitus).

TABLE 20.11 Indications for Nonexercise Stress Echocardiography for Patients With Suspected or Known Coronary Artery Disease.

Indications	*Class of Recommendation*	*Level of Evidence*
An imaging stress test is recommended as the initial test for diagnosing SCAD if the PTP is 66%–85% or the LVEF is <50% in patients without typical angina.	I	B
An imaging stress test is recommended for patients with resting ECG abnormalities that prevent accurate interpretation of ECG changes during stress.	I	B
Exercise stress testing is recommended rather than pharmacologic stress testing whenever possible.	I	C
An imaging stress test should be considered for symptomatic patients with prior revascularization (PCI or CABG).	IIa	B
An imaging stress test should be considered to assess the functional severity of intermediate lesions on coronary angiography.	IIa	B

CABG, Coronary artery bypass grafting; *ECG*, electrocardiogram; *LVEF*, left ventricular ejection fraction; *PCI*, percutaneous coronary intervention; *PTP*, pretest probability; *SCAD*, stable coronary artery disease.

Nonexercise SE is a sensitive and specific test for the diagnosis of CAD, identification of myocardial viability, and risk stratification of various cardiac populations. It is safe (i.e., no ionizing radiation or intravenous contrast), cost-effective, and reproducible, and it provides additional data on cardiac structure and function. It has received a class I indication from the European Society of Cardiology for patients with an uninterpretable ECG, inability to exercise, or submaximal or uncertain exercise ECG test results. Table 20.11 summarizes the indications for nonexercise SE in patients with suspected or known CAD.[2,98,99]

FUTURE DIRECTIONS

Although 3D SE is theoretically very attractive, its routine implementation will require compatibility with intravenous contrast and speckle tracking strain, both of which demand improved volume rates. 3D SE image postprocessing will probably become more automated and more standardized in the future, thereby improving workflow. Fusion imaging takes advantage of the strengths of the different imaging modalities and combines functional (e.g., 3D SE) and anatomic (e.g., computed tomography) imaging (Fig. 20.15).[100]

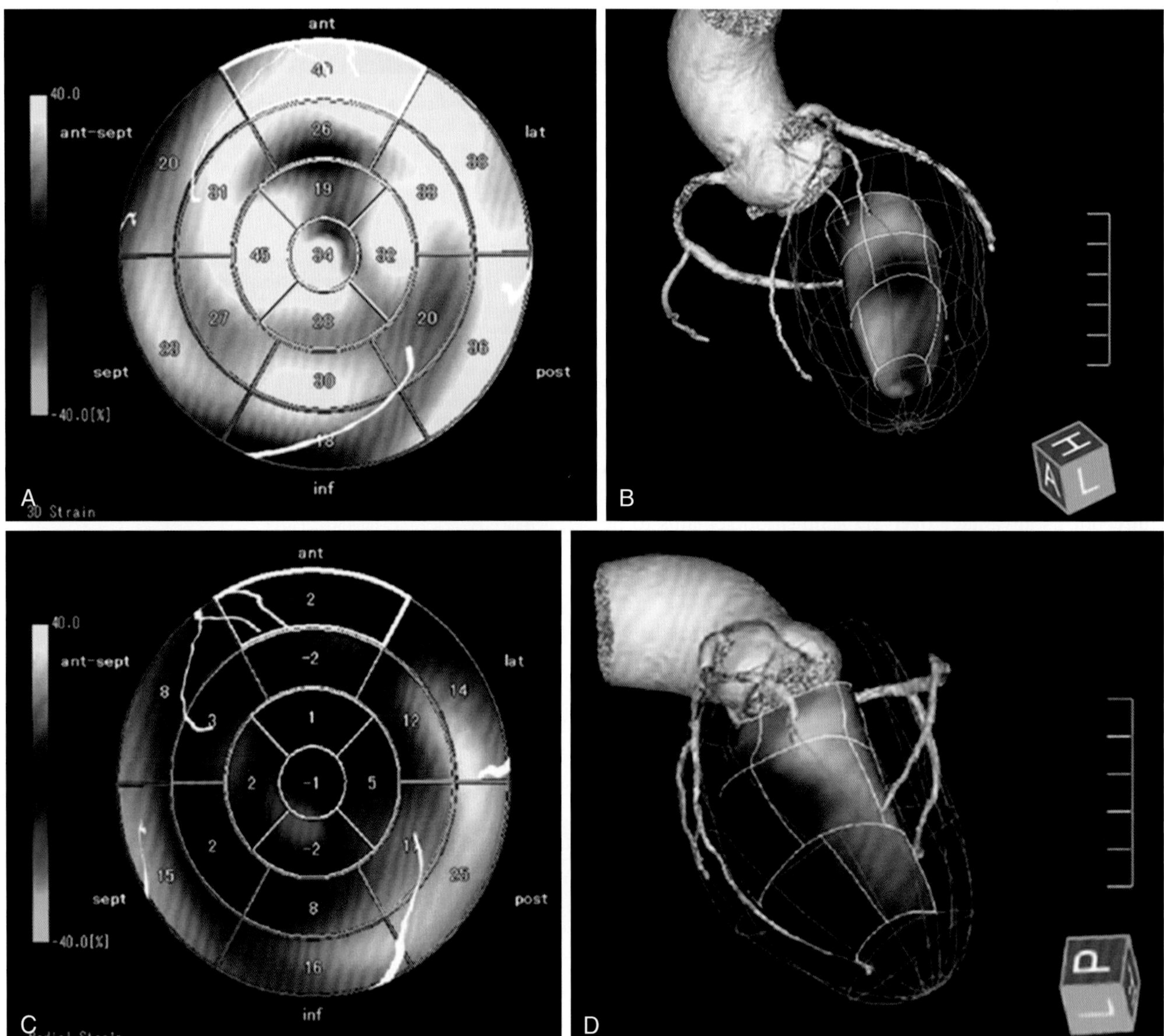

Fig. 20.15 Fusion imaging, combining data from functional (3D) echocardiography and anatomic (computed tomography [CT]) modalities. (A) Parametric map of resting 3D speckle tracking strain echocardiography of the LV segments, with overlying CT-matched coronary arteries. (B) Surface-rendered model of LV strain at rest demonstrates the 3D relation to the coronary arteries. (C) Parametric map of 3D speckle tracking strain at peak stress, with overlying coronary arteries. Ischemia can be discerned as low strain values (darker colors). (D) Surface-rendering at peak stress demonstrates inducible ischemia in the territory of the left anterior descending coronary artery. *ANT,* Anterior; *ANT SEPT,* anterior septum; *INF,* inferior; *LAT,* lateral; *POST,* posterior; *SEPT,* septal. (From Casas Rojo E, Fernandez-Golfin C, Zamorano J. Hybrid imaging with coronary tomography and 3D speckle-tracking stress echocardiography fusion. *Eur Heart J Cardiovasc Imaging.* 2014;15:555.)

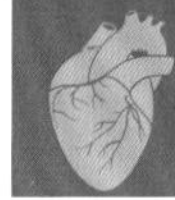

SUMMARY Pharmacologic Stress Echocardiography: Protocols and Clinical Indications.

Stressor	Intravenous Administration (Protocol)	Clinical Indications
Dobutamine	Ischemia detection: 5, 10, 20, 30, 40 μg/kg per minute with 0.25–2 mg atropine	Ischemia detection • New WMA • Strain (rate) imaging • Myocardial contrast perfusion
	Viability assessment: 5, 10, 20 μg/kg per minute	Viability assessment • WMAs • Strain (rate) imaging • Myocardial contrast perfusion
Dipyridamole[a]	0.56 mg/kg for 4 min + 0.28 mg/kg for 2 min or 0.84 mg/kg for 6 min	Ischemia detection • New WMA
Adenosine[a]	100 μg/kg per minute for 3 min + 140 μg/kg per minute for 4 min + 200 μg/kg per minute for 4 min	• Coronary flow velocity reserve • Myocardial contrast perfusion
Regadenoson[a]	400 μg for 10 s	• Strain (rate) imaging Viability assessment • WMAs • Coronary flow reserve

[a]Vasodilator.
WMA, Wall motion abnormality.

REFERENCES

1. Nesto RW, Kowalchuk GJ. The ischemic cascade: temporal sequence of hemodynamic, electrocardiographic and symptomatic expressions of ischemia. *Am J Cardiol.* 1987;59:23C–30C.
2. Sicari R, Nihoyannopoulos P, Evangelista A, et al. Stress echocardiography expert consensus statement - executive summary: European Association of Echocardiography (EAE) (a registered branch of the ESC). *Eur Heart J.* 2009;30:278–289.
3. Biagini E, Elhendy A, Bax JJ, et al. The use of stress echocardiography for prognostication in coronary artery disease: an overview. *Curr Opin Cardiol.* 2005;20:386–394.
4. Plana JC, Mikati IA, Dokainish H, et al. A randomized cross-over study for evaluation of the effect of image optimization with contrast on the diagnostic accuracy of dobutamine echocardiography in coronary artery disease The OPTIMIZE Trial. *JACC Cardiovasc Imaging.* 2008;1:145–152.
5. Sicari R, Cortigiani L, Bigi R, et al. Prognostic value of pharmacological stress echocardiography is affected by concomitant antiischemic therapy at the time of testing. *Circulation.* 2004;109:2428–2431.
6. Picano E, Bedetti G, Varga A, et al. The comparable diagnostic accuracies of dobutamine-stress and dipyridamole-stress echocardiographies: a meta-analysis. *Coron Artery Dis.* 2000;11:151–159.
7. Lang RM, Badano LP, Mor-Avi V, et al. Recommendations for cardiac chamber quantification by echocardiography in adults: an update from the American Society of Echocardiography and the European Association of Cardiovascular Imaging. *Eur Heart J Cardiovasc Imaging.* 2015;16:233–270.
8. Ortiz-Perez JT, Rodriguez J, Meyers SN, et al. Correspondence between the 17-segment model and coronary arterial anatomy using contrast-enhanced cardiac magnetic resonance imaging. *JACC Cardiovasc Imaging.* 2008;1:282–293.
9. Monsieurs KG, Nolan JP, Bossaert LL, et al. European Resuscitation Council guidelines for resuscitation 2015: Section 1. Executive summary. *Resuscitation.* 2015;95:1–80.
10. Secknus MA, Marwick TH. Evolution of dobutamine echocardiography protocols and indications: safety and side effects in 3,011 studies over 5 years. *J Am Coll Cardiol.* 1997;29:1234–1240.
11. Nguyen KL, Bandettini WP, Shanbhag S, et al. Safety and tolerability of regadenoson CMR. *Eur Heart J Cardiovasc Imaging.* 2014;15:753–760.
12. Djordjevic-Dikic AD, Ostojic MC, Beleslin BD, et al. High dose adenosine stress echocardiography for noninvasive detection of coronary artery disease. *J Am Coll Cardiol.* 1996;28:1689–1695.
13. Al Jaroudi W, Iskandrian AE. Regadenoson: a new myocardial stress agent. *J Am Coll Cardiol.* 2009;54:1123–1130.
14. Zaya M, Mehta PK, Merz CN. Provocative testing for coronary reactivity and spasm. *J Am Coll Cardiol.* 2014;63:103–109.
15. Kim MH, Park EH, Yang DK, et al. Role of vasospasm in acute coronary syndrome: insights from ergonovine stress echocardiography. *Circ J.* 2005;69:39–43.
16. Song JK, Lee SJ, Kang DH, et al. Ergonovine echocardiography as a screening test for diagnosis of vasospastic angina before coronary angiography. *J Am Coll Cardiol.* 1996;27:1156–1161.
17. Song JK, Park SW, Kang DH, et al. Safety and clinical impact of ergonovine stress echocardiography for diagnosis of coronary vasospasm. *J Am Coll Cardiol.* 2000;35:1850–1856.
18. Gligorova S, Agrusta M. Pacing stress echocardiography. *Cardiovasc Ultrasound.* 2005;3:36.
19. Yao SS, Qureshi E, Sherrid MV, et al. Practical applications in stress echocardiography: risk stratification and prognosis in patients with known or suspected ischemic heart disease. *J Am Coll Cardiol.* 2003;42:1084–1090.
20. Geleijnse ML, Krenning BJ, van Dalen BM, et al. Factors affecting sensitivity and specificity of diagnostic testing: dobutamine stress echocardiography. *J Am Soc Echocardiogr.* 2009;22:1199–1208.
21. Heijenbrok-Kal MH, Fleischmann KE, Hunink MG. Stress echocardiography, stress single-photon-emission computed tomography and electron beam computed tomography for the assessment of coronary artery disease: a meta-analysis of diagnostic performance. *Am Heart J.* 2007;154:415–423.
22. Kim C, Kwok YS, Heagerty P, et al. Pharmacologic stress testing for coronary disease diagnosis: a meta-analysis. *Am Heart J.* 2001;142:934–944.
23. Picano E, Molinaro S, Pasanisi E. The diagnostic accuracy of pharmacological stress echocardiography for the assessment of coronary artery disease: a meta-analysis. *Cardiovasc Ultrasound.* 2008;6:30.
24. Loimaala A, Groundstroem K, Pasanen M, et al. Comparison of bicycle, heavy isometric, dipyridamole-atropine and dobutamine stress echocardiography for diagnosis of myocardial ischemia. *Am J Cardiol.* 1999;84:1396–1400.
25. Nedeljkovic I, Ostojic M, Beleslin B, et al. Comparison of exercise, dobutamine-atropine and dipyridamole-atropine stress echocardiography in detecting coronary artery disease. *Cardiovasc Ultrasound.* 2006;4:22.
26. Pingitore A, Picano E, Colosso MQ, et al. The atropine factor in pharmacologic stress echocardiography. Echo Persantine (EPIC) and Echo Dobutamine International Cooperative (EDIC) Study Groups. *J Am Coll Cardiol.* 1996;27:1164–1170.
27. Salustri A, Fioretti PM, McNeill AJ, et al. Pharmacological stress echocardiography in the diagnosis of coronary artery disease and

myocardial ischaemia: a comparison between dobutamine and dipyridamole. *Eur Heart J.* 1992;13:1356–1362.
28. San Roman JA, Vilacosta I, Castillo JA, et al. Selection of the optimal stress test for the diagnosis of coronary artery disease. *Heart.* 1998;80:370–376.
29. Beleslin BD, Ostojic M, Djordjevic-Dikic A, et al. Integrated evaluation of relation between coronary lesion features and stress echocardiography results: the importance of coronary lesion morphology. *J Am Coll Cardiol.* 1999;33:717–726.
30. Noguchi Y, Nagata-Kobayashi S, Stahl JE, et al. A meta-analytic comparison of echocardiographic stressors. *Int J Cardiovasc Imaging.* 2005;21:189–207.
31. Bangalore S, Yao SS, Chaudhry FA. Prediction of myocardial infarction versus cardiac death by stress echocardiography. *J Am Soc Echocardiogr.* 2009;22:261–267.
32. Sicari R, Pasanisi E, Venneri L, et al. Stress echo results predict mortality: a large-scale multicenter prospective international study. *J Am Coll Cardiol.* 2003;41:589–595.
33. Shaw LJ, Vasey C, Sawada S, et al. Impact of gender on risk stratification by exercise and dobutamine stress echocardiography: long-term mortality in 4234 women and 6898 men. *Eur Heart J.* 2005;26:447–456.
34. Cortigiani L, Bigi R, Landi P, et al. Prognostic implication of stress echocardiography in 6214 hypertensive and 5328 normotensive patients. *Eur Heart J.* 2011;32:1509–1518.
35. Pingitore A, Picano E, Varga A, et al. Prognostic value of pharmacological stress echocardiography in patients with known or suspected coronary artery disease: a prospective, large-scale, multicenter, head-to-head comparison between dipyridamole and dobutamine test. Echo-Persantine International Cooperative (EPIC) and Echo-Dobutamine International Cooperative (EDIC) Study Groups. *J Am Coll Cardiol.* 1999;34:1769–1777.
36. Yao SS, Qureshi E, Syed A, et al. Novel stress echocardiographic model incorporating the extent and severity of wall motion abnormality for risk stratification and prognosis. *Am J Cardiol.* 2004;94:715–719.
37. Shaw LJ, Berman DS, Picard MH, et al. Comparative definitions for moderate-severe ischemia in stress nuclear, echocardiography, and magnetic resonance imaging. *JACC Cardiovasc Imaging.* 2014;7:593–604.
38. Cortigiani L, Picano E, Landi P, et al. Value of pharmacologic stress echocardiography in risk stratification of patients with single-vessel disease: a report from the Echo-Persantine and Echo-Dobutamine International Cooperative Studies. *J Am Coll Cardiol.* 1998;32:69–74.
39. Bangalore S, Yao SS, Chaudhry FA. Role of right ventricular wall motion abnormalities in risk stratification and prognosis of patients referred for stress echocardiography. *J Am Coll Cardiol.* 2007;50:1981–1989.
40. Canty Jr JM, Suzuki G. Myocardial perfusion and contraction in acute ischemia and chronic ischemic heart disease. *J Mol Cell Cardiol.* 2012;52:822–831.
41. Schinkel AF, Bax JJ, Poldermans D, et al. Hibernating myocardium: diagnosis and patient outcomes. *Curr Probl Cardiol.* 2007;32:375–410.
42. Bax JJ, Wijns W, Cornel JH, et al. Accuracy of currently available techniques for prediction of functional recovery after revascularization in patients with left ventricular dysfunction due to chronic coronary artery disease: comparison of pooled data. *J Am Coll Cardiol.* 1997;30:1451–1460.
43. Allman KC, Shaw LJ, Hachamovitch R, et al. Myocardial viability testing and impact of revascularization on prognosis in patients with coronary artery disease and left ventricular dysfunction: a meta-analysis. *J Am Coll Cardiol.* 2002;39:1151–1158.
44. Inaba Y, Chen JA, Bergmann SR. Quantity of viable myocardium required to improve survival with revascularization in patients with ischemic cardiomyopathy: a meta-analysis. *J Nucl Cardiol.* 2010;17:646–654.
45. Velazquez EJ, Lee KL, Deja MA, et al. Coronary-artery bypass surgery in patients with left ventricular dysfunction. *N Engl J Med.* 2011;364:1607–1616.
46. Bonow RO, Maurer G, Lee KL, et al. Myocardial viability and survival in ischemic left ventricular dysfunction. *N Engl J Med.* 2011;364:1617–1625.
47. Doenst T, Haverich A, Serruys P, et al. PCI and CABG for treating stable coronary artery disease: JACC review topic of the week. *J Am Coll Cardiol.* 2019;73:964–976.
48. Perera D, Clayton T, Petrie MC, et al. Percutaneous revascularization for ischemic ventricular dysfunction: rationale and design of the REVIVED-BCIS2 trial: percutaneous coronary intervention for ischemic cardiomyopathy. *JACC Heart Fail.* 2018;6:517–526.
49. Cwajg JM, Cwajg E, Nagueh SF, et al. End-diastolic wall thickness as a predictor of recovery of function in myocardial hibernation: relation to rest-redistribution T1-201 tomography and dobutamine stress echocardiography. *J Am Coll Cardiol.* 2000;35:1152–1161.
50. La Canna G, Rahimtoola SH, Visioli O, et al. Sensitivity, specificity, and predictive accuracies of non-invasive tests, singly and in combination, for diagnosis of hibernating myocardium. *Eur Heart J.* 2000;21:1358–1367.
51. Shah DJ, Kim HW, James O, et al. Prevalence of regional myocardial thinning and relationship with myocardial scarring in patients with coronary artery disease. *J Am Med Assoc.* 2013;309:909–918.
52. Arnese M, Fioretti PM, Cornel JH, et al. Akinesis becoming dyskinesis during high-dose dobutamine stress echocardiography: a marker of myocardial ischemia or a mechanical phenomenon? *Am J Cardiol.* 1994;73:896–899.
53. Afridi I, Kleiman NS, Raizner AE, et al. Dobutamine echocardiography in myocardial hibernation. Optimal dose and accuracy in predicting recovery of ventricular function after coronary angioplasty. *Circulation.* 1995;91:663–670.
54. Cornel JH, Bax JJ, Elhendy A, et al. Biphasic response to dobutamine predicts improvement of global left ventricular function after surgical revascularization in patients with stable coronary artery disease: implications of time course of recovery on diagnostic accuracy. *J Am Coll Cardiol.* 1998;31:1002–1010.
55. Salustri A, Ciavatti M, Seccareccia F, et al. Prediction of cardiac events after uncomplicated acute myocardial infarction by clinical variables and dobutamine stress test. *J Am Coll Cardiol.* 1999;34:435–440.
56. Elhendy A, van Domburg RT, Poldermans D, et al. Safety and feasibility of dobutamine-atropine stress echocardiography for the diagnosis of coronary artery disease in diabetic patients unable to perform an exercise stress test. *Diabetes Care.* 1998;21:1797–1802.
57. Cortigiani L, Borelli L, Raciti M, et al. Prediction of mortality by stress echocardiography in 2835 diabetic and 11305 nondiabetic patients. *Circ Cardiovasc Imaging.* 2015;8.
58. Muhlestein JB, Lappe DL, Lima JA, et al. Effect of screening for coronary artery disease using CT angiography on mortality and cardiac events in high-risk patients with diabetes: the FACTOR-64 randomized clinical trial. *J Am Med Assoc.* 2014;312:2234–2243.
59. Sicari R, Ripoli A, Picano E, et al. Long-term prognostic value of dipyridamole echocardiography in vascular surgery: a large-scale multicenter study. *Coron Artery Dis.* 2002;13:49–55.
60. Mairesse GH, Marwick TH, Arnese M, et al. Improved identification of coronary artery disease in patients with left bundle branch block by use of dobutamine stress echocardiography and comparison with myocardial perfusion tomography. *Am J Cardiol.* 1995;76:321–325.
61. Moir S, Shaw L, Haluska B, et al. Left ventricular opacification for the diagnosis of coronary artery disease with stress echocardiography: an angiographic study of incremental benefit and cost-effectiveness. *Am Heart J.* 2007;154:510–518.
62. Matsumura Y, Hozumi T, Arai K, et al. Non-invasive assessment of myocardial ischaemia using new real-time three-dimensional dobutamine stress echocardiography: comparison with conventional two-dimensional methods. *Eur Heart J.* 2005;26:1625–1632.
63. Eroglu E, D'Hooge J, Herbots L, et al. Comparison of real-time tri-plane and conventional 2D dobutamine stress echocardiography for the assessment of coronary artery disease. *Eur Heart J.* 2006;27:1719–1724.
64. Aggeli C, Giannopoulos G, Misovoulos P, et al. Real-time three-dimensional dobutamine stress echocardiography for coronary artery disease diagnosis: validation with coronary angiography. *Heart.* 2007;93:672–675.
65. Yoshitani H, Takeuchi M, Mor-Avi V, et al. Comparative diagnostic accuracy of multiplane and multislice three-dimensional dobutamine stress echocardiography in the diagnosis of coronary artery disease. *J Am Soc Echocardiogr.* 2009;22:437–442.
66. Scislo P, Kochanowski J, Koltowski L, et al. Utility and safety of three-dimensional contrast low-dose dobutamine echocardiography in the evaluation of myocardial viability early after an acute myocardial infarction. *Arch Med Sci.* 2018;14:488–492.
67. Krenning BJ, Nemes A, Soliman OI, et al. Contrast-enhanced three-dimensional dobutamine stress echocardiography: between Scylla and Charybdis? *Eur J Echocardiogr.* 2008;9:757–760.
68. Joyce E, Delgado V, Bax JJ, et al. Advanced techniques in dobutamine stress echocardiography: focus on myocardial deformation analysis. *Heart.* 2015;101:72–81.
69. Blessberger H, Binder T. Two dimensional speckle tracking echocardiography: clinical applications. *Heart.* 2010;96:2032–2040.
70. Weidemann F, Jamal F, Sutherland GR, et al. Myocardial function defined by strain rate and strain during alterations in inotropic states and heart rate. *Am J Physiol Heart Circ Physiol.* 2002;283:H792–H799.
71. Yu Y, Villarraga HR, Saleh HK, et al. Can ischemia and dyssynchrony be detected during early stages of dobutamine stress echocardi-

ography by 2-dimensional speckle tracking echocardiography? *Int J Cardiovasc Imaging.* 2013;29:95–102.

72. Aggeli C, Lagoudakou S, Felekos I, et al. Two-dimensional speckle tracking for the assessment of coronary artery disease during dobutamine stress echo: clinical tool or merely research method. *Cardiovasc Ultrasound.* 2015;13:43.
73. Joyce E, Hoogslag GE, Al Amri I, et al. Quantitative dobutamine stress echocardiography using speckle-tracking analysis versus conventional visual analysis for detection of significant coronary artery disease after ST-segment elevation myocardial infarction. *J Am Soc Echocardiogr.* 2015;28:1379–1389 e1371.
74. Nagy AI, Sahlen A, Manouras A, et al. Combination of contrast-enhanced wall motion analysis and myocardial deformation imaging during dobutamine stress echocardiography. *Eur Heart J Cardiovasc Imaging.* 2015;16:88–95.
75. Cusma-Piccione M, Zito C, Oreto L, et al. Longitudinal strain by automated function imaging detects single-vessel coronary artery disease in patients undergoing dipyridamole stress echocardiography. *J Am Soc Echocardiogr.* 2015;28:1214–1221.
76. Dattilo G, Imbalzano E, Lamari A, et al. Ischemic heart disease and early diagnosis. Study on the predictive value of 2D strain. *Int J Cardiol.* 2016;215:150–156.
77. Uusitalo V, Luotolahti M, Pietila M, et al. Two-dimensional speckle-tracking during dobutamine stress echocardiography in the detection of myocardial ischemia in patients with suspected coronary artery disease. *J Am Soc Echocardiogr.* 2016;29:470–479 e473.
78. Rumbinaite E, Zaliaduonyte-Peksiene D, Lapinskas T, et al. Early and late diastolic strain rate vs global longitudinal strain at rest and during dobutamine stress for the assessment of significant coronary artery stenosis in patients with a moderate and high probability of coronary artery disease. *Echocardiography.* 2016;33:1512–1522.
79. Fujimoto H, Honma H, Ohno T, et al. Longitudinal Doppler strain measurement for assessment of damaged and/or hibernating myocardium by dobutamine stress echocardiography in patients with old myocardial infarction. *J Cardiol.* 2010;55:309–316.
80. Bansal M, Jeffriess L, Leano R, et al. Assessment of myocardial viability at dobutamine echocardiography by deformation analysis using tissue velocity and speckle-tracking. *JACC Cardiovasc Imaging.* 2010;3:121–131.
81. Rosner A, Avenarius D, Malm S, et al. Persistent dysfunction of viable myocardium after revascularization in chronic ischaemic heart disease: implications for dobutamine stress echocardiography with longitudinal systolic strain and strain rate measurements. *Eur Heart J Cardiovasc Imaging.* 2012;13:745–755.
82. Gong L, Li D, Chen J, et al. Assessment of myocardial viability in patients with acute myocardial infarction by two-dimensional speckle tracking echocardiography combined with low-dose dobutamine stress echocardiography. *Int J Cardiovasc Imaging.* 2013;29:1017–1028.
83. Ismail M, Nammas W. Dobutamine-induced strain and strain rate predict viability following fibrinolytic therapy in patients with ST-elevation myocardial infarction. *Front Cardiovasc Med.* 2015;2:12.
84. Li L, Wang F, Xu T, et al. The detection of viable myocardium by low-dose dobutamine stress speckle tracking echocardiography in patients with old myocardial infarction. *J Clin Ultrasound.* 2016;44:545–554.
85. Cortigiani L, Rigo F, Bovenzi F, et al. The prognostic value of coronary flow velocity reserve in two coronary arteries during vasodilator stress echocardiography. *J Am Soc Echocardiogr.* 2019;32:81–91.
86. Sade LE, Eroglu S, Yuce D, et al. Follow-up of heart transplant recipients with serial echocardiographic coronary flow reserve and dobutamine stress echocardiography to detect cardiac allograft vasculopathy. *J Am Soc Echocardiogr.* 2014;27:531–539.
87. Cortigiani L, Rigo F, Galderisi M, et al. Diagnostic and prognostic value of Doppler echocardiographic coronary flow reserve in the left anterior descending artery in hypertensive and normotensive patients. *Heart.* 2011;97:1758–1765.
88. Rigo F. Coronary flow reserve in stress-echo lab. From pathophysiologic toy to diagnostic tool. *Cardiovasc Ultrasound.* 2005;3:8.
89. Cortigiani L, Rigo F, Gherardi S, et al. Coronary flow reserve during dipyridamole stress echocardiography predicts mortality. *JACC Cardiovasc Imaging.* 2012;5:1079–1085.
90. Ciampi Q, Zagatina A, Cortigiani L, et al. Functional, anatomical, and prognostic correlates of coronary flow velocity reserve during stress echocardiography. *J Am Coll Cardiol.* 2019;74:2278–2291.
91. Bhatia VK, Senior R. Contrast echocardiography: evidence for clinical use. *J Am Soc Echocardiogr.* 2008;21:409–416.
92. Dijkmans PA, Senior R, Becher H, et al. Myocardial contrast echocardiography evolving as a clinically feasible technique for accurate, rapid, and safe assessment of myocardial perfusion: the evidence so far. *J Am Coll Cardiol.* 2006;48:2168–2177.
93. Senior R, Moreo A, Gaibazzi N, et al. Comparison of sulfur hexafluoride microbubble (SonoVue)-enhanced myocardial contrast echocardiography with gated single-photon emission computed tomography for detection of significant coronary artery disease: a large European multicenter study. *J Am Coll Cardiol.* 2013;62:1353–1361.
94. Dolan MS, Gala SS, Dodla S, et al. Safety and efficacy of commercially available ultrasound contrast agents for rest and stress echocardiography a multicenter experience. *J Am Coll Cardiol.* 2009;53:32–38.
95. Gaibazzi N, Reverberi C, Lorenzoni V, et al. Prognostic value of high-dose dipyridamole stress myocardial contrast perfusion echocardiography. *Circulation.* 2012;126:1217–1224.
96. Shimoni S, Frangogiannis NG, Aggeli CJ, et al. Identification of hibernating myocardium with quantitative intravenous myocardial contrast echocardiography: comparison with dobutamine echocardiography and thallium-201 scintigraphy. *Circulation.* 2003;107:538–544.
97. Moir S, Haluska BA, Jenkins C, et al. Myocardial blood volume and perfusion reserve responses to combined dipyridamole and exercise stress: a quantitative approach to contrast stress echocardiography. *J Am Soc Echocardiogr.* 2005;18:1187–1193.
98. Task Force Members, Montalescot G, Sechtem U, et al. 2013. ESC guidelines on the management of stable coronary artery disease: the Task Force on the management of stable coronary artery disease of the European Society of Cardiology. *Eur Heart J.* 2013;34:2949–3003.
99. Pellikka PA, Arruda-Olson A, Chaudhry FA, et al. Guidelines for performance, interpretation, and application of stress echocardiography in ischemic heart disease: from the American Society of Echocardiography. *J Am Soc Echocardiogr.* 2020;33:1–41 e48.
100. Casas Rojo E, Fernandez-Golfin C, Zamorano J. Hybrid imaging with coronary tomography and 3D speckle-tracking stress echocardiography fusion. *Eur Heart J Cardiovasc Imaging.* 2014;15:555.

中文导读

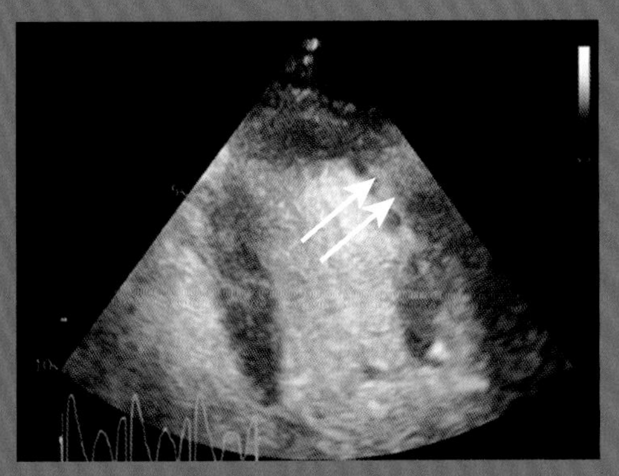

第21章 超声心动图在急性冠状动脉综合征中的作用

急性冠状动脉综合征是用于描述与心肌缺血相关的一系列疾病的总称。超声心动图对急性冠状动脉综合征的辅助诊断起到至关重要的作用，特别是在冠心病监护病房中的使用。本章着重从以下几个方面描述了超声心动图的诊断价值：①如何使用超声心动图诊断心肌梗死及对梗死区域的探查；②急性心肌梗死导致的并发症诊断；③心肌梗死后的风险分层评估。

超声心动图以其高性价比和对血流动力学精确评估等诸多优势成为了冠心病监护病房的常规检查，在评估左心室收缩功能、节段性室壁运动异常、左心室舒张功能、右心室功能和二尖瓣反流均有较高的敏感性和特异性。

本章对于心室壁节段划分和室壁运动评分做了详尽的描述，多项研究表明室壁运动评分与心肌梗死后的并发症有关联。对于血流动力学不稳定的患者来说，合理利用超声心动图诊断及排除早期心脏机械并发症有助于减少患者终末期事件的发生。

利用超声心动图对心肌梗死后的风险分层评估应主要从多个方面入手，例如评价左心室的收缩舒张功能、室壁运动评分、左心房容积、左心室重构等，利用负荷超声可以评估存活心肌以及诊断心肌缺血而引起的二尖瓣反流。以上定量或半定量的分析均可为急性冠状动脉综合征患者提供合理的住院期管理依据。

李羽加

21 Role of Echocardiography in Patients With Acute Coronary Syndrome

IVOR L. GERBER, MD, MBChB | SALLY CAROLINE GREAVES, MMedSci, MBChB

APPLICABLE MODES OF ECHOCARDIOGRAPHY IN THE CORONARY CARE UNIT

Transthoracic echocardiography (TTE) is ideally suited for cardiac imaging in the coronary care unit. It offers major advantages compared with other imaging modalities, including its portability, its relative low cost, and the wealth of anatomic, hemodynamic, and functional information that can be obtained rapidly at the bedside. With further technologic advances, it continues to play a major role in the diagnostic assessment and risk stratification of patients in the coronary care unit[1] (Table 21.1).

For patients with an established myocardial infarction (MI), early echocardiographic evaluation using routine measures of left ventricular (LV) systolic function, regional wall motion, LV diastolic function, right ventricular (RV) function, and mitral regurgitation (MR) greatly assists with management. The use of left-sided contrast agents for LV opacification improves interobserver agreement and is superior to routine evaluation for the measurement of LV ejection fraction (LVEF) and regional wall motion. Real-time three-dimensional (3D) echocardiography allows fast, semiautomated, dynamic measurement of LV volume and LVEF, automated detection of regional wall motion abnormalities (WMAs),[2] and perfusion imaging.[3]

Quantification with myocardial strain techniques is a further significant step to reduce interobserver variability in the assessment of regional WMAs.[4] It may facilitate the exclusion of significant coronary artery stenosis among patients with suspected non–ST-segment elevation acute coronary syndromes (ACSs) who have inconclusive electrocardiographic (ECG) findings and normal cardiac biomarkers.[5]

Because perfusion abnormalities precede WMAs in the ischemic cascade, myocardial contrast echocardiography has a higher sensitivity for the detection of coronary artery disease (CAD).[6] Myocardial contrast echocardiography also has a significant role in the evaluation of myocardial viability.[7] Progressive improvements and miniaturization of handheld echocardiographic instruments have led to its increasing use as an adjunct to physical examination. Several studies have shown the utility of these modalities, but they are not comparable to full-service systems, and care should be exercised to ensure that clinicians using and reporting studies with these instruments are appropriately trained.[8]

With careful sedation and close monitoring, transesophageal echocardiography (TEE) can be performed safely in patients early after acute MI. If there is a concern about the patient's hemodynamic state or respiration, intubation and ventilation by an anesthetist before TEE imaging should be strongly considered. The cause of hemodynamic instability in patients with MI often can be established by bedside TTE. However, TTE may be limited by mechanical ventilation, recent cardiac surgery, and an inability to adequately position the patient, and in such cases, TEE may be invaluable. Other potential uses of TEE in the coronary care unit include exclusion of other diagnoses, particularly aortic dissection (especially in patients with impaired renal function that limits the use of contrast computed tomography [CT]) and evaluation of left atrial appendage thrombus before cardioversion. Two-dimensional (2D) and three-dimensional (3D) TEE are commonly used to guide intracardiac catheter-based interventions, such as closure of a post-MI ventricular septal defect.

ECHOCARDIOGRAPHY IN THE DIAGNOSIS AND LOCALIZATION OF ACUTE MYOCARDIAL INFARCTION

DIAGNOSTIC ROLE OF ECHOCARDIOGRAPHY

The accuracy of echocardiographic diagnosis of an MI depends on its ability to detect WMAs in the involved segment. The severity of the WMA depends on the transmural extent of the infarction, and the circumferential limits depend on the arterial distribution and collateral blood supply. Most patients with ST-elevation

TABLE 21.1 Appropriate Use[a] of TTE for Cardiovascular Evaluation in Acute Settings.

Finding	*Score*
Hypotension or Hemodynamic Instability	
Hypotension or hemodynamic instability of uncertain or suspected cardiac origin	A-9
Assessment of volume status in a critically ill patient	U-5
Myocardial Ischemia/Infarction	
Acute chest pain with suspected MI and nondiagnostic ECG when a resting TTE can be performed during pain	A-9
Evaluation of a patient without chest pain but with other features of an ischemic equivalent or laboratory markers indicative of ongoing myocardial ischemia	A-8
Suspected complication of myocardial ischemia or MI, including but not limited to acute mitral regurgitation, ventricular septal defect, free wall rupture/tamponade, shock, RV involvement, heart failure, or thrombus	A-9
Evaluation of Ventricular Function After Acute Coronary Syndrome	
Initial evaluation of ventricular function after acute coronary syndrome	A-9
Re-evaluation of ventricular function after acute coronary syndrome during recovery phase when result will guide therapy	A-9

[a]Appropriateness is scored 1 to 9: *A*, appropriate indication (7–9); *U*, uncertain indication (4–6).
ECG, Electrocardiogram; *MI*, myocardial infarction.
Adapted from Douglas PS, Garcia MJ, Haines DE, et al. ACCF/ASE/AHA/ASNC/HFSA/HRS/SCAI/SCCM/SCCT/SCMR 2011 appropriate use criteria for echocardiography. A report of the American College of Cardiology Foundation Appropriate Use Criteria Task Force, American Society of Echocardiography, American Heart Association, American Society of Nuclear Cardiology, Heart Failure Society of America, Heart Rhythm Society, Society for Cardiovascular Angiography and Interventions, Society of Critical Care Medicine, Society of Cardiovascular Computed Tomography, Society for Cardiovascular Magnetic Resonance American College of Chest Physicians. *J Am Soc Echocardiogr*. 2011;24:229–267.

TABLE 21.2 Scoring System for Grading Wall Motion.

Score	*Wall Motion*	*Endocardial Motion[a]*	*Wall Thickening[a]*
1	Normal	Normal	Normal (>30%)
2	Hypokinesis	Reduced	Reduced (<30%)
3	Akinesis	Absent	Absent
4	Dyskinesis	Outward	Thinning
5	Aneurysmal	Diastolic deformity	Absent or thinning

[a]In systole.
Modified from Lang RM, Badano LP, Mor-Avi V, et al. Recommendations for cardiac chamber quantification by echocardiography in adults: an update from the American Society of Echocardiography and the European Association of Cardiovascular Imaging. *J Am Soc Echocardiogr*. 2015;28(1):1–39.e14.

TABLE 21.3 Regional Wall Motion Abnormalities Unrelated to Coronary Artery Disease.

Condition	*Comment*
Left bundle branch block	May be an ECG manifestation of acute MI or an incidental and unrelated finding
Wolff-Parkinson-White syndrome	May mimic inferior or posterior MI
Pacemaker	May result in abnormal septal or apical motion depending on the site of attachment of the RV pacemaker lead
Previous cardiac surgery	Septum may be hypokinetic
RV volume overload	Ventricular septal flattening in diastole
RV pressure overload	Ventricular septal flattening in systole
Constrictive pericarditis	Diastolic wobble of the septum
Apical ballooning syndrome (takotsubo cardiomyopathy)	Classically, akinesis or ballooning of the middle and apical LV segments and hyperkinetic basal LV segments
Myocarditis	May result in global or regional LV systolic impairment
Dilated cardiomyopathy	Usually global LV systolic impairment, but there may be regional variation in contractility and wall thickness
Sarcoidosis	May cause areas of hypokinesis and/or thinning

ECG, Electrocardiogram; *MI*, myocardial infarction.

myocardial infarction (STEMI) have some hypokinetic LV segments unless there is very early reperfusion, but it is not unusual for patients who have non-STEMI with a small troponin rise to have no appreciable WMA. The most widely used scoring system for grading the severity of a WMA is shown in Table 21.2.[9]

Other causes of segmental LV dysfunction must be recognized (Table 21.3). An increasingly recognized mimic of acute MI is apical ballooning syndrome, also known as takotsubo cardiomyopathy. It is estimated that approximately 2% of all patients with suspected ACS are ultimately diagnosed with takotsubo cardiomyopathy.[10] In the International Takotsubo Registry,[11] 90% of registrants were women older than 50 years of age. Women are most commonly affected by an emotional trigger, men by a physical trigger, and no trigger is evident in an estimated 28% of cases.

Earlier criteria for the diagnosis of takotsubo cardiomyopathy excluded CAD, but it is now recognized that this syndrome may occur in patients with CAD. The prevalence of CAD

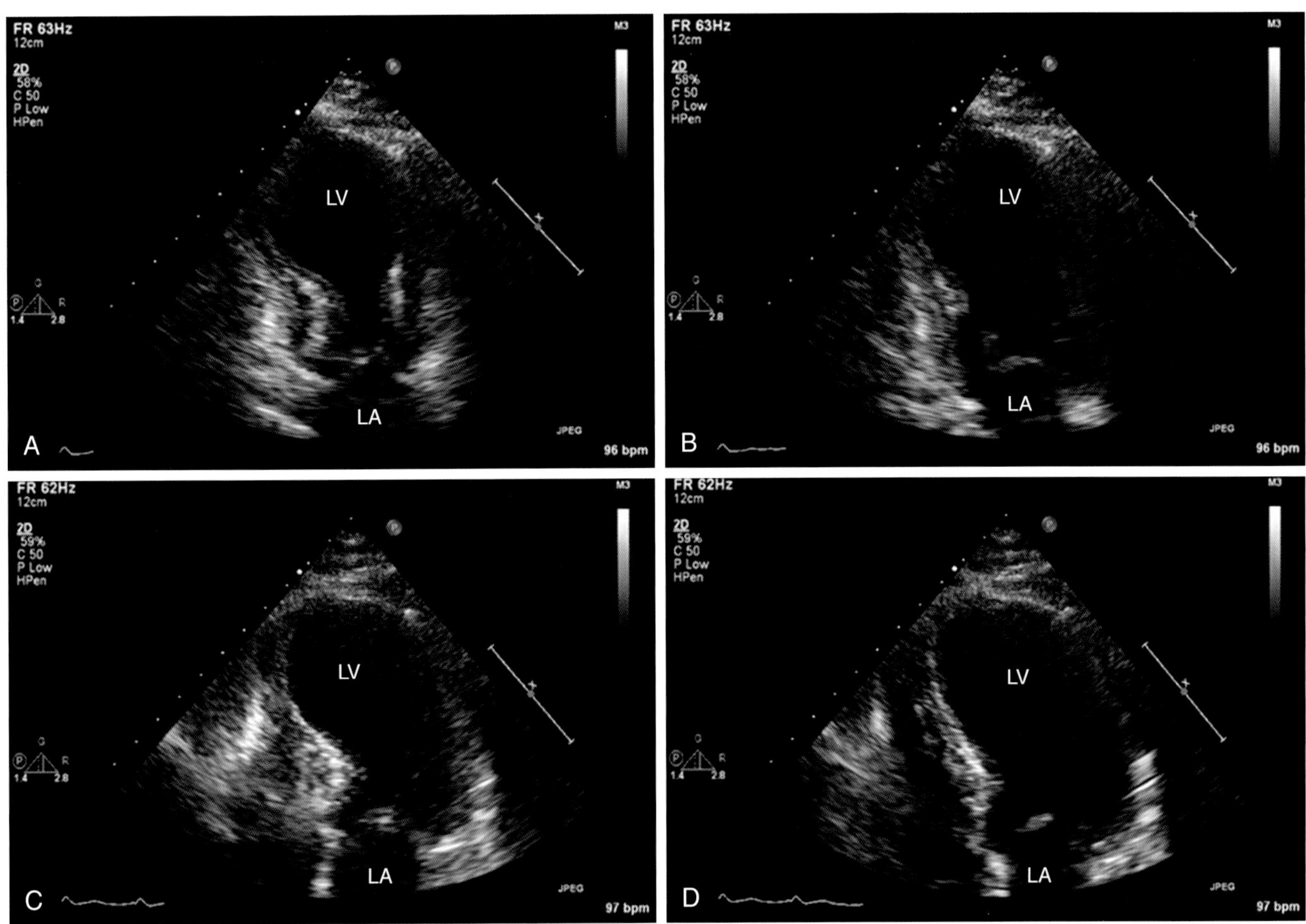

Fig. 21.1 **Takotsubo cardiomyopathy (apical ballooning syndrome).** TTE shows the classic appearance of hypokinesis or akinesis of the midwall and apical LV segments and hyperkinesis of the basal LV segments in apical 2-chamber views (A and B) (see Videos 21.1A and 21.1B) and in 4-chamber views (C and D). Images were taken at end-systole (A and C) and at end-diastole (B and D).

ranges from 10% to 61%, with a 15% prevalence in the International Takotsubo Registry.[11] Specific criteria were proposed by Frangieh et al.[12] to help differentiate takotsubo cardiomyopathy from STEMI and non-STEMI.

TTE is invaluable in the diagnosis of takotsubo cardiomyopathy and reveals characteristic features of LV impairment in a noncoronary distribution and early improvement of LV function consistent with myocardial stunning rather than MI.[13] Although the classic presentation is with midwall and apical LV ballooning and hypercontractile basal LV segments (Fig. 21.1), variant forms such as mid-ventricular ballooning[14] and basal ballooning[15] have also been described.

In a cardiac magnetic resonance (CMR) imaging series of 256 patients with takotsubo cardiomyopathy, 82% were of the apical variety, 17% were mid-ventricular, 1% were basal, and 34% had RV involvement.[16] Up to one third of patients experience early complications, including dynamic LV outflow tract obstruction, acute MR, heart failure, cardiogenic shock, and arrhythmias.[17] Mortality rates vary from 2% to 5%, similar to those for STEMI, and death occurs mainly from cardiogenic shock and ventricular arrhythmias.[18] Natural history studies suggest improvement in LV function in most cases within weeks or months with reported recurrence rates of 5% to 22% at 6 months to 10 years after the index event.[19]

Myocarditis is an important mimic of ACS. Patients typically present with chest pain, a rise in troponin levels, and nonspecific ECG changes. Regional WMAs may exist but with a normal or near-normal coronary angiogram. Shirani et al[20] showed a predominance of subepithelial inflammation in the LV free wall. The posterolateral LV segments are most commonly involved,[21] but other LV segments may be involved, or the LV may be globally dilated and/or impaired. In a study by Mahrholdt et al.,[21] patients with biopsy-proven myocarditis due to parvovirus PVB19, the lateral wall of the LV was predominantly affected, whereas in patients affected with herpesvirus HHV6, the anterior septum was predominantly affected.

Clues to the diagnosis of myocarditis rather than an ACS include clinical features such as a viral prodrome, pleuritic chest pain, a more persistent rise in troponin levels (rather than the typical rise and fall of troponin levels in an ACS), and a pericardial effusion. Magnetic resonance imaging (MRI) with gadolinium is a very accurate modality to confirm myocarditis.

LOCALIZATION OF INFARCTION

In an attempt to establish segmentation standards applicable to all types of imaging, including echocardiography, nuclear perfusion imaging, cardiovascular MRI, and cardiac CT, a 17-segment model of LV segmentation has been proposed.[9] This model includes the apical cap, which is the segment beyond the end of the LV cavity that usually is seen only with some contrast and myocardial perfusion studies. With routine echocardiographic studies, the 16-segment model can be used

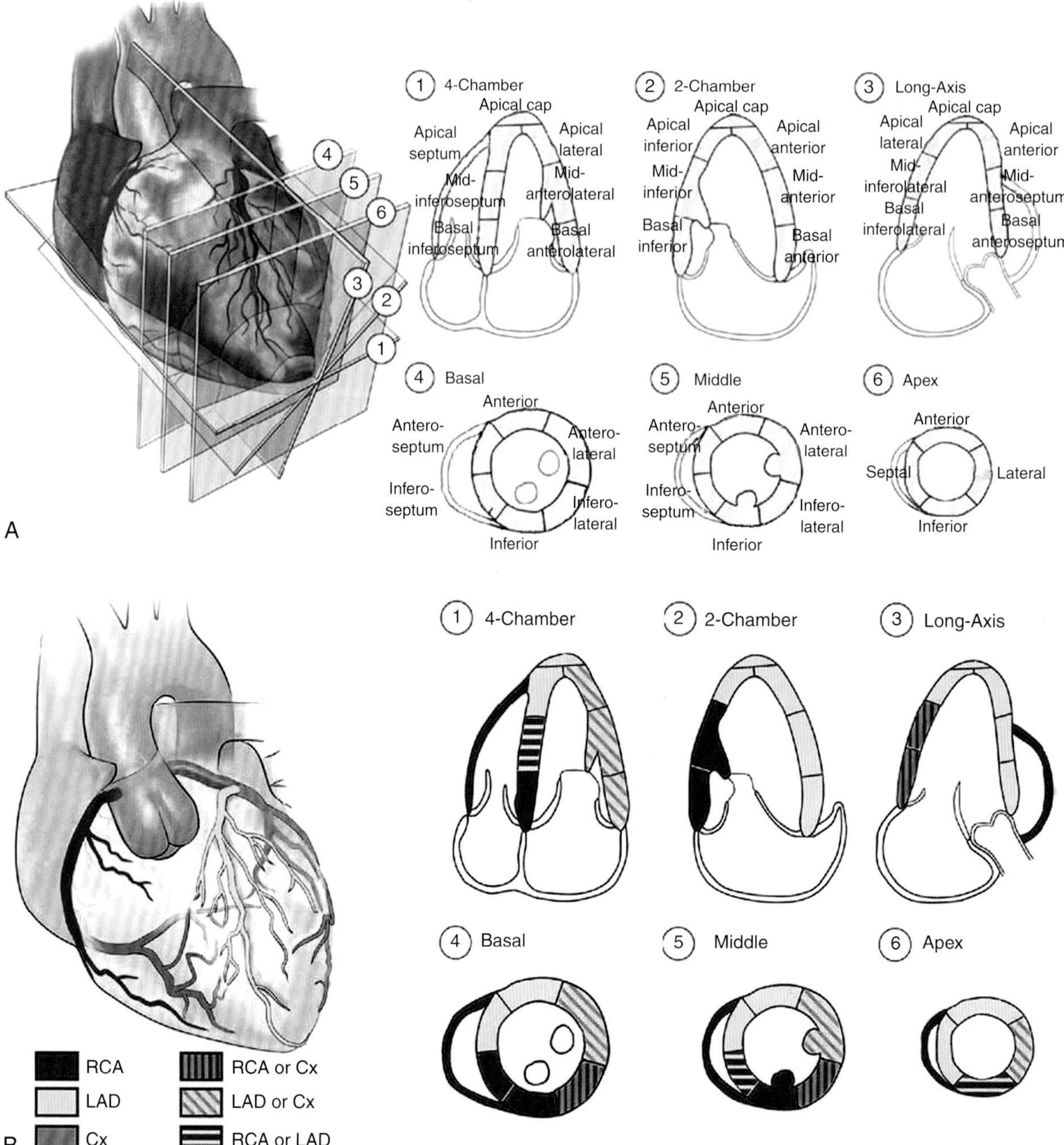

Fig. 21.2 Typical coronary artery distribution of blood flow is shown in apical and parasternal short-axis views. (A) The LV segments. (B) The approximate and most common coronary arterial distributions related to these segments. *Cx*, Circumflex; *LAD*, left anterior descending coronary artery; *RCA*, right coronary artery. (From Lang RM, Badano LP, Mor-Avi V, et al. Recommendations for cardiac chamber quantification by echocardiography in adults: an update from the American Society of Echocardiography and the European Association of Cardiovascular Imaging. *J Am Soc Echocardiogr.* 2015;28:1–39.e14.)

without the apical cap. The LV segments and the approximate and most common coronary arterial distributions in relation to these segments are depicted in Fig. 21.2. The extent of the segmental wall motion is related to the exact coronary anatomy in an individual patient but may vary among patients. The presence of collaterals and previous bypass surgery alters the distribution of ischemia and infarction relative to the involved arterial supply.

Direct visualization of the ostia of the left main coronary artery and right coronary artery (RCA) and the proximal left anterior descending coronary artery (LAD) in adults may be achieved with the use of TTE (Fig. 21.3). This may be helpful to exclude anomalous coronary artery origin, especially in younger patients.

RV INFARCTION

Although RV infarction was first described in the 1930s, it was only after the hemodynamic consequences were recognized in the 1970s that RV infarction was considered a clinical entity.[22]

RV infarction occurs in up to 50% of inferior MIs, but hemodynamic compromise develops in fewer than half of such

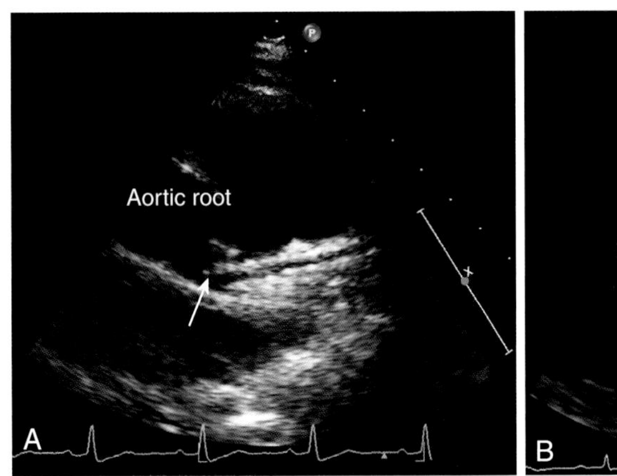

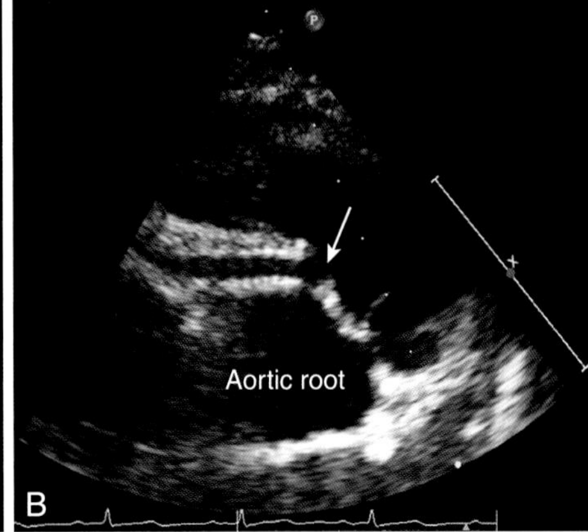

Fig. 21.3 Ostia and proximal courses of the major epicardial coronary arteries. TTE images in the high parasternal short-axis view demonstrate the ostium of the left main coronary artery and proximal left anterior descending coronary artery (A, *arrow*) and the ostium and proximal course of the right coronary artery (B, *arrow*).

cases.[23] The RV is predominantly supplied by acute marginal branches of the RCA, and occlusion of the RCA proximal to the origin of these branches results in ischemic dysfunction of the RV. When the occlusion is distal to the right atrial (RA) branches, augmented RA contractility enhances RV function and cardiac output. Conversely, more proximal occlusions result in ischemic depression of RA contractility, which impairs RV filling and function, resulting in more severe hemodynamic compromise.

Less commonly, RV infarction is associated with acute anteroseptal MI.[24] Isolated RV MI is reported to occur in less than 3% of all acute MIs.[25] The clinical importance of RV infarction is emphasized by higher rates of hemodynamic compromise, arrhythmias, and in-hospital mortality compared with MI involving only the LV.[26]

Echocardiography plays a vital role in the evaluation of patients with suspected RV infarction[27] (Table 21.4). In many cases, the LV inferior WMA may be relatively small with preserved LVEF. Assessment of RV systolic function is complex, and commonly used echocardiographic measures, including RV fractional area change and visual assessment, are associated with significant interobserver variability.

Tricuspid annular plane systolic excursion of less than 10 mm is a useful objective measure of RV dysfunction and should be measured in patients with suspected RV infarction. In a study of 60 patients with a first acute inferior MI, a tricuspid valve annulus peak systolic velocity of less than 12 cm/s had a sensitivity of 81%, a specificity of 82%, and a negative predictive value of 92% for RV infarction.[28]

Global longitudinal strain of the RV can provide greater sensitivity and specificity than RV fractional area change or tricuspid annular plane systolic excursion for major adverse cardiovascular events after RV infarction.[29] Reduced RV compliance can be detected by an increased A-wave velocity on the hepatic vein flow signal and by a short pressure half-time of the pulmonary regurgitant jet (<150 ms).[30]

Characteristic echocardiographic features of RV failure with high RA pressures include bowing of the interatrial septum into the left atrium (LA) and dilation of the inferior vena cava with lack of inspiratory collapse. These indicators of RV function correlate with clinical status and prognosis.[31] Hypoxemia resulting from right-to-left shunting across a patent foramen ovale may occur with a large RV infarction associated with elevated RA pressures.

TABLE 21.4 Echocardiographic Signs of RV Infarction.

Primary Signs
RV dilation
Segmental wall motion abnormality of the RV free wall
Reduced TAPSE
Tricuspid valve annulus peak systolic velocity < 12 cm/s
Reduced RV global longitudinal strain
Reduced RV fractional area change
Secondary Signs
Paradoxical septal motion
Tricuspid regurgitation
Tricuspid papillary muscle rupture
Pulmonary regurgitant jet pressure half-time < 150 ms
Dilated inferior vena cava
Right-to-left interatrial septal bowing
Right-to-left shunting across patent foramen ovale

TAPSE, Tricuspid annular plane systolic excursion.

In most cases of RV infarction, RV function improves and returns to near normal within 3 to 12 months,[32] although the improvement may not be complete. Because the acutely ischemic dysfunctional RV represents predominantly viable myocardium, which may spontaneously recover or respond favorably to successful reperfusion even late after the onset of occlusion, it has been suggested that the term *RV infarction* is largely a misnomer and that the term *RV ischemic dysfunction* should be used.[33] However, it is important to recognize that RV infarction is associated with relatively high in-hospital mortality rates, and early reperfusion enhances recovery of RV function with an improved clinical course and improved survival.[34] The use of RV speckle tracking–derived longitudinal strain has prognostic value for patients with heart failure[35] and may have a role after MI with RV involvement.

DETECTING COMPLICATIONS OF ACUTE MYOCARDIAL INFARCTION

In the acutely hemodynamically unstable patient, it is critical to exclude mechanical complications of MI before concluding that cardiogenic shock is the result of pump failure (Table 21.5). In most cases, TTE (supplemented when necessary by TEE) is sufficient to exclude the major mechanical complications of papillary muscle rupture (PMR), ventricular free wall rupture (VFWR), and ventricular septal rupture (VSR).

A single-center study of 2508 patients admitted with STEMI reported an overall mechanical complication rate of 1.1% (26 patients), including VSR in 17, VFWR in 2, a combination of VSR and VFWR in 2, and PMR in 5 patients. Older age, female sex, no history of angina or revascularization, multivessel CAD, and longer time between symptom onset and coronary angiography were more common factors for patients who developed a mechanical complication.[36]

The prognosis of acute MI has markedly improved with the implementation of strategies for early restoration of culprit coronary artery flow and a reduction in the incidence of mechanical complications. However, the mortality rate remains very high when acute MI is complicated by cardiac rupture.[37]

PAPILLARY MUSCLE RUPTURE

Acute severe mitral valve regurgitation in the setting of MI is usually a result of necrosis and rupture of papillary muscle tissue. It is a life-threatening complication that almost always requires urgent surgical intervention. MR due to LV remodeling and distortion of ventricular architecture may also occur (discussed later).

2D imaging may detect abnormalities in the mitral valve apparatus, including flail leaflets and PMR. Even if not clearly visualized, PMR should be suspected when there is an eccentric jet of MR with a relatively normal-sized LA. Although color-flow parameters are those most often used, accurate grading of MR severity should also encompass other Doppler-echocardiographic signs. For patients with pulmonary edema, the unexpected findings of a small infarction, a hyperdynamic LV, or increased early mitral inflow velocity should prompt a careful search for MR even when color-flow Doppler is unrevealing.

In a review of PMR, 15 of 17 cases occurred in patients with inferior infarction and rupture of the posteromedial papillary muscle.[38] The more common involvement of the posteromedial papillary muscle occurs because its blood supply is from a single coronary artery (i.e., the posterior descending artery) rather than a dual coronary artery supply, as in the anterolateral papillary muscle, which is supplied by the LAD and the left circumflex coronary artery (LCx) (Fig. 21.4).

Chordae to both leaflets arise from each of the papillary muscles, and in cases of *complete* rupture of the entire trunk of a papillary muscle, both leaflets are affected. In less severe cases, the rupture is *incomplete,* and only a single head is torn. The 2D echocardiographic findings may include prolapse of one or both leaflets, a flail leaflet, or liberation of a portion of the papillary muscle. In some patients, the ruptured muscle remains tethered to the chordae, and chaotic motion is present. If only a single head of the papillary muscle is affected (i.e., incomplete rupture), medical stabilization often is possible. When rupture is complete, involving the main trunk of the papillary muscle, the complication is fatal without immediate recognition and prompt surgical repair.

TABLE 21.5 Echocardiography for Complications of Myocardial Infarction.

Hemodynamic States
Hypovolemia
RV infarction
Globally reduced LV contractility
Mechanical Complications
Papillary muscle rupture and severe mitral regurgitation
Ventricular septal rupture
Free wall rupture and tamponade
Other
LV aneurysm
Mural thrombus
Pericardial effusion

VENTRICULAR SEPTAL RUPTURE

Unlike PMR, VSR occurs with similar frequency among patients with anterior (LAD) and inferior (RCA) infarctions but rarely in those with lateral (LCx) infarctions. The incidence of VSR has declined in the modern era of reperfusion, but mortality

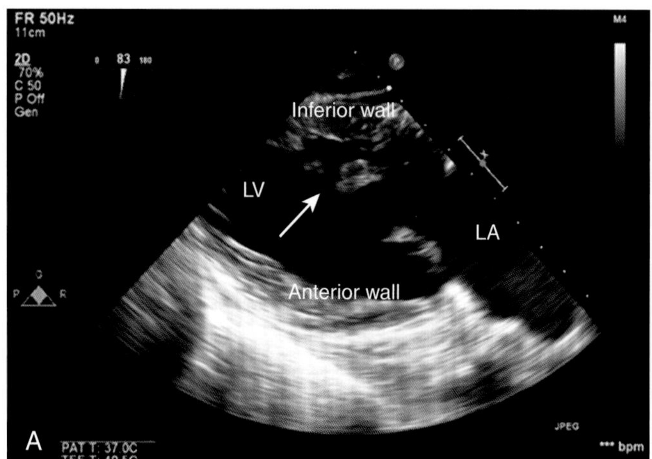

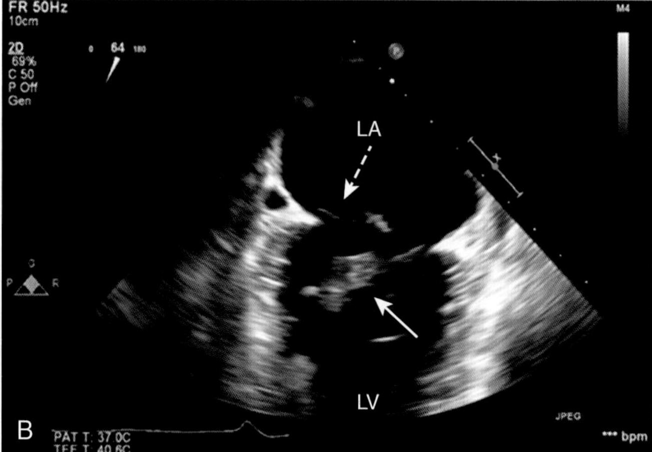

Fig. 21.4 Papillary muscle rupture. (A) TEE (transgastric view) shows posteromedial papillary muscle rupture *(arrow).* Rupture of this muscle is more common, because of its single blood supply, than rupture of the anterolateral papillary muscle, which has a dual blood supply (see Video 21.4A). (B) TEE (mid-esophageal view) shows posteromedial papillary muscle rupture *(solid arrow)* and flail anterior mitral valve leaflet *(dashed arrow)* (see Video 21.4B).

rates remain high. In a series of 408 patients with VSR complicating acute MI between 1990 and 2007, overall in-hospital, 30-day, and 1-year mortality rates were 50%, 54%, and 65%, respectively.[39]

Most VSRs occur within 24 hours after treatment. Bedside echocardiography is highly sensitive and specific for the diagnosis of VSR. The defect may be *discrete*, with ventricular entry and exit sites located at a similar horizontal level, or *complex*, with entry and exit sites at different levels along the ventricular septum. VSR may occur in more than one region, and there may be an associated VFWR or PMR.

VSR due to occlusion of the RCA usually occurs in the basal inferior septum (Fig. 21.5), and VSR after acute anterior MI most often occurs in the distal one third of the septum (Fig. 21.6). When VSR is clinically suspected, it is often necessary to use nonconventional imaging planes, first with color Doppler to locate the defect and then with 2D imaging. The width of the jet by color-flow Doppler correlates with the size of the defect as measured at surgery. Although the peak gradient across the VSR measured with continuous-wave Doppler allows an estimate of RV systolic pressure, this measurement should be used with caution for patients with complex defects involving indirect tracts through the myocardium.

Associated echocardiographic findings of elevated RV pressure include RV dilation, decreased RV systolic function, and paradoxical septal motion. Signs of increased RA pressure include RA dilation, bowing of the interatrial septum toward the left throughout the cardiac cycle, and a plethora of the inferior vena cava.

Although VSR carries a very high mortality rate, echocardiography may allow risk stratification of patients. Complex septal ruptures and RV involvement are significant determinants of adverse clinical outcome.[40] Rupture of the posterior septum after inferior MI is associated with a higher mortality rate, which is related to the degree of associated RV dysfunction. Posterior VSRs tend to be more complex and associated with remote myocardial involvement. In contrast, anterior septal defects more often involve a discrete myocardial region.

The largest study of patients with VSR after MI, from the Society of Thoracic Surgeons database of 2876 patients, showed an operative mortality rate of 54% if repair was performed within 7 days and 18% if repair was delayed more than 7 days after MI.[41] This difference was most likely the result of selection bias; patients operated on later usually had small and less complex ventricular septal defects and were hemodynamically stable. The influence of concomitant coronary bypass grafting on survival is uncertain.[42]

Without surgical intervention, survival to 1 month is very low, estimated at 5% to 10%,[43] but if the patient is hemodynamically stable, surgery can potentially be delayed and the patient managed with medical optimization.[44] In selected patients, a conservative approach may be associated with a good outcome in the mid-term. Sivadasan et al.[40] described 7 patients, of 27 with post-MI VSR, who did not undergo surgery and were followed for a mean of approximately 3 years; all 7 patients had single-vessel disease, small defect size (on average 9.8 mm), minimal left-to-right shunt, and preserved RV function. Spontaneous closure by thrombus of a small post-MI ventricular septal defect (VSD) has been reported.[45]

Percutaneous device closure should be considered in certain cases: to close a residual leak after VSR surgical repair, which occurs in approximately 25% of cases[46]; to stabilize high-risk patients and allow myocardial fibrosis, facilitating delayed surgical correction[47]; and as a primary intervention for selected cases, usually for simple defects that are smaller than 15 mm.[48] The use of two devices for more complex VSRs has been reported.[49] The largest published series of percutaneous device closure of post-MI VSD, in 53 patients, demonstrated a high procedural success rate. The in-hospital mortality rate was

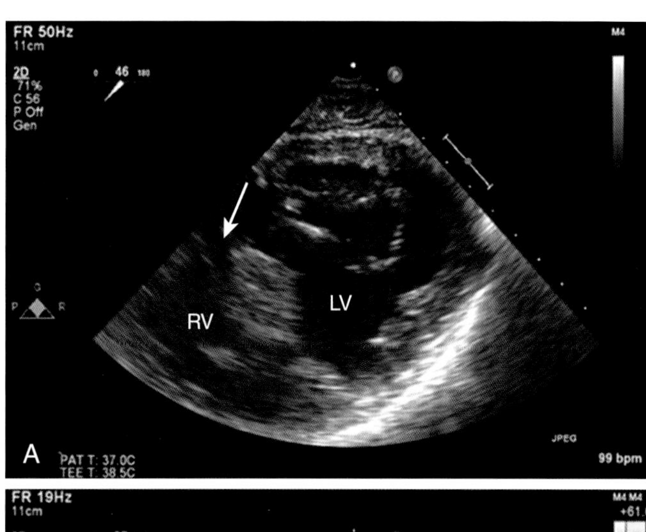

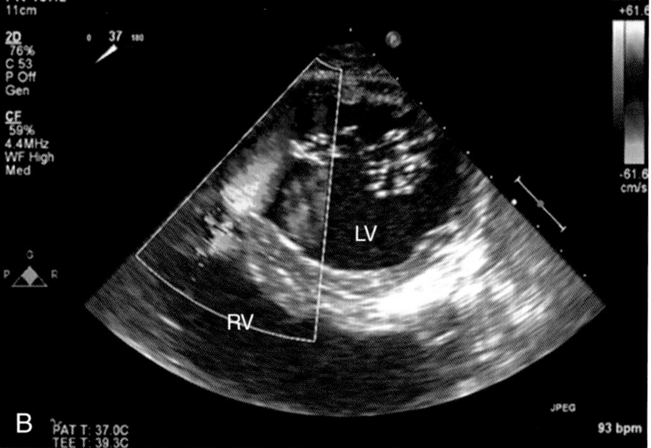

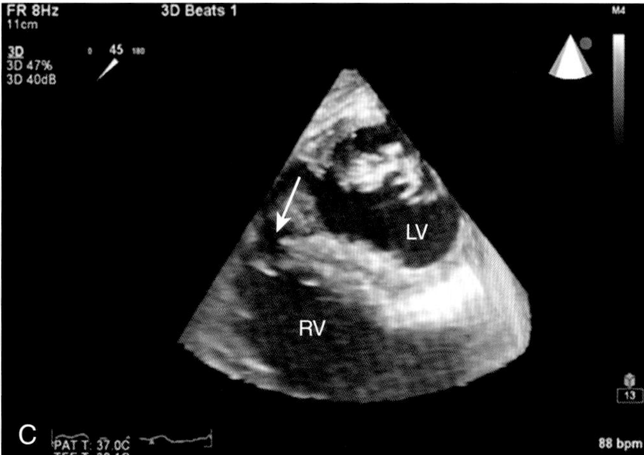

Fig. 21.5 Ventricular septal defect after inferior myocardial infarction. (A) TEE (transgastric view) shows a large ventricular septal defect resulting from rupture in a patient with a large inferior myocardial infarction. (B) Same view with color Doppler technique. (C) Same view with 3D TEE. The area of discontinuity can be visualized as a large, irregularly shaped area of myocardial dropout *(arrow)* in parts A and C. (See Videos 21.5A and 21.5B.)

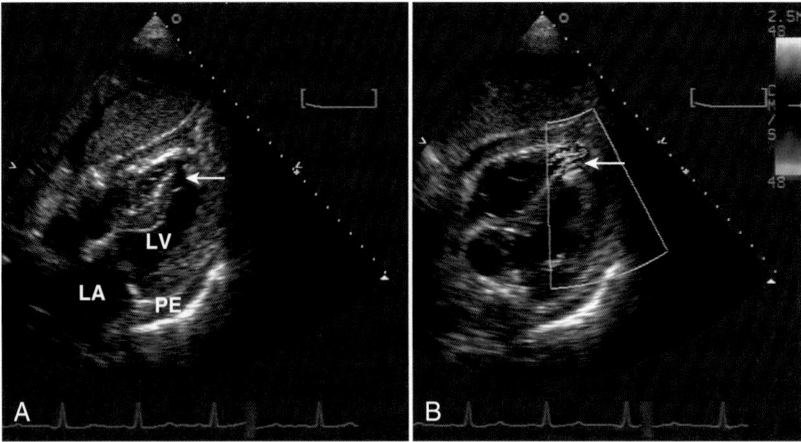

Fig. 21.6 Ventricular septal defect after anterior myocardial infarction. (A) TTE (subcostal view) shows a ventricular septal defect *(arrow)* resulting from rupture involving the apical septum. (B) Color-flow Doppler demonstrates left-to-right shunting across the septal defect *(arrow)*. Also notice the small circumferential pericardial effusion *(PE)* in A.

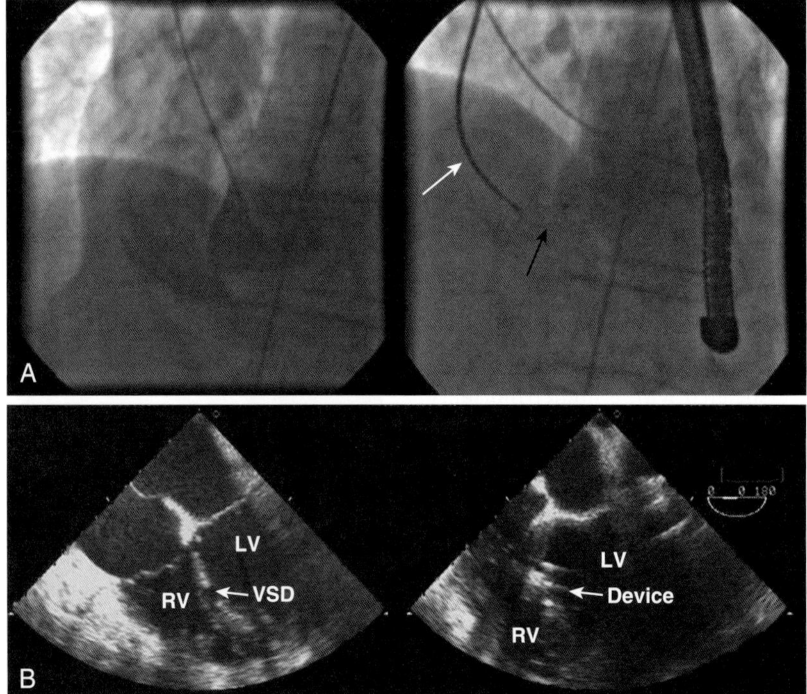

Fig. 21.7 Device closure of postinfarction ventricular septal defect. (A) Left ventriculography before closure of postinfarction ventricular septal defect *(VSD)* shows a left-to-right shunt *(left)*; angiographic image *(right)* shows the Amplatzer device in position *(black arrow)* before release from delivery cable *(white arrow)*. (B) TEE images at 0 degrees show a postinfarction VSD located in the mid-inferior septum *(left)* before the procedure and device placement in the mid-inferior septum *(right)* afterward. (From Ahmed A, Ruygrok P, Wilson N, et al. Percutaneous closure of postmyocardial infarction ventricular septal defects: a single centre experience. *Heart Lung Circ.* 2008;17:119–123.)

high, but patients who survived to discharge did relatively well in the longer term.[50]

TEE is helpful in guiding closure of these defects (Fig. 21.7).[51] Intracardiac echocardiography may be a suitable alternative. For closure of apical defects, TTE guidance may be feasible. The major role of TEE guidance for VSD closure is to evaluate the defective anatomy from multiple views—esophageal and transgastric views are usually needed—including defect size, location, and proximity to the mitral, tricuspid, and aortic valves (for inferior VSD). TEE guidance also assists with catheter manipulation, sizing of the defect, and deployment of the device. Accurate sizing of the defect is critical; this is performed with 2D or 3D TEE, and a device up to 50% bigger than the defect is used to reduce the incidence of device embolization or residual shunts. TEE is also essential to assess any residual defect and to detect complications of the procedure, including device migration, residual shunts, or valvular damage caused by catheter entrapment.

RUPTURE OF THE VENTRICULAR FREE WALL

Rupture of the free wall of the LV is the second most common mechanical cause of death of patients with acute STEMI after cardiogenic shock due to pump failure.[52] This complication is more likely to occur in patients with a transmural MI involving the inferolateral wall associated with a LCx occlusion

(Fig. 21.8) or with an LAD occlusion.[53] Early successful reperfusion appears to decrease the risk of rupture.[54]

VFWR is usually an acute catastrophic event. However, some cases take a subacute or chronic course when a small rupture is temporarily sealed by fibrinous pericardial adhesions or thrombus. Patients diagnosed during this subacute phase and taken promptly to surgery have a greater chance of survival.[55]

An echocardiographic feature of risk for rupture is infarct expansion with significant wall thinning. A small pericardial effusion is a common finding after an uncomplicated transmural MI, but increasing size of a pericardial effusion and the presence of intrapericardial thrombus suggest the diagnosis of rupture; the absence of pericardial effusion virtually excludes rupture. Intrapericardial thrombus significantly increases the diagnostic specificity. It appears as an echo-dense mass that may be *mobile*, undulating within the pericardial space, or *immobile*, impinging on the cardiac chambers.[55] Direct visualization of the myocardial tear with TTE is relatively uncommon. When the diagnosis is uncertain, imaging with left heart contrast may delineate the tear.[56]

The mortality rate for VFWR in the absence of surgical intervention has been very high, although recent series have documented survival rates as high as 50% for patients who underwent pericardiocentesis and conservative medical management.[57] The in-hospital mortality rate for patients who undergo surgical repair is in the range of 40%; those who survive until hospital discharge appear to have a good long-term prognosis.[52] Early echocardiographic diagnosis with prompt management is critical.[58]

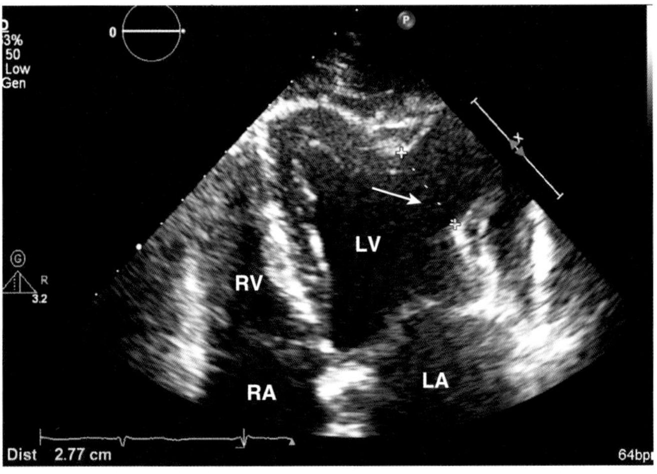

Fig. 21.8 Contained myocardial rupture. Apical 4-chamber view shows contained rupture of the mid-lateral wall of the LV *(arrow)* associated with a small pericardial effusion (see Videos 21.8A and 21.8B).

POSTINFARCTION PERICARDIAL EFFUSION

TTE is sensitive for the detection of pericardial effusion, but compared with cardiac MRI, TTE is not sensitive for the detection of pericardial inflammation without effusion, which is a common cause of chest pain after MI.[59] In a study of 908 patients from 25 French hospitals,[60] a pericardial effusion was identified in 6.6% of patients when assessed by TTE at admission and at discharge.

Infarct-associated pericardial effusion usually occurs within the first 5 days but may occur at any time during the first 3 weeks after MI. The effusion is usually small, and circumferential effusions are rare. Spontaneous resolution of the effusion is usually slow, between 6 and 18 months. Cardiac rupture is the most common cause of a moderate to large pericardial effusion early after acute MI and may be associated with thrombus in the pericardial space (Fig. 21.9).

The differential diagnosis of pericardial effusion in the acute setting must include aortic dissection and perimyocarditis. Iatrogenic pericardial effusion may also occur after interventional procedures, including coronary stenting with vessel rupture, implantation of a temporary pacemaker with perforation of the RV, cardiac biopsy, and transseptal puncture. Localized thrombus around the RA may cause hemodynamic compromise without an associated pericardial effusion and should always be considered in the unstable patient after invasive cardiac procedures and early after cardiac surgery (Fig. 21.10).

PSEUDOANEURYSM

A pseudoaneurysm is a contained rupture of the LV free wall (Fig. 21.11). It usually represents a complication of acute MI, but it may also occur after cardiac surgery, chest trauma, or endocarditis. An LV pseudoaneurysm is often diagnosed incidentally (e.g., in 25 of 52 patients in a series from the Mayo Clinic).[61] Most pseudoaneurysms are located in the inferoposterior or inferolateral regions (associated with RCA or LCx occlusion).

It is important to differentiate a pseudoaneurysm, which has a high likelihood of spontaneous rupture, from a true aneurysm,

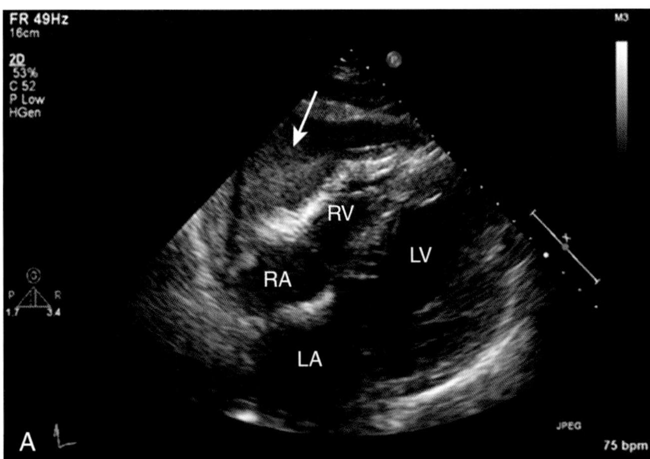

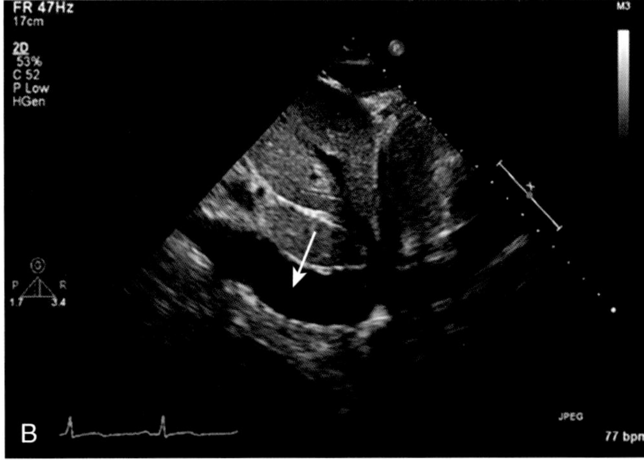

Fig. 21.9 Hemorrhagic pericardial effusion. (A) TTE (subcostal view) shows hemorrhagic pericardial effusion and thrombus within the pericardial space *(arrow)* causing compression of the RV. (B) Notice the dilated inferior vena cava *(arrow)* caused by increased RA pressure.

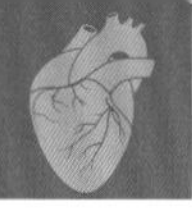

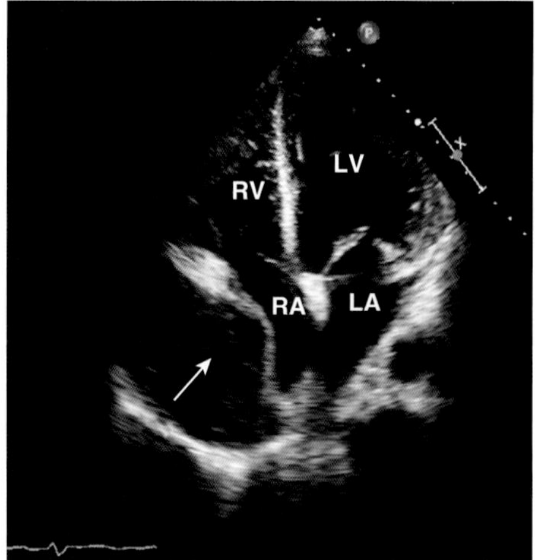

Fig. 21.10 Thrombus around the RA. Large thrombus *(arrow)* around the RA is causing extrinsic compression (see Video 21.10).

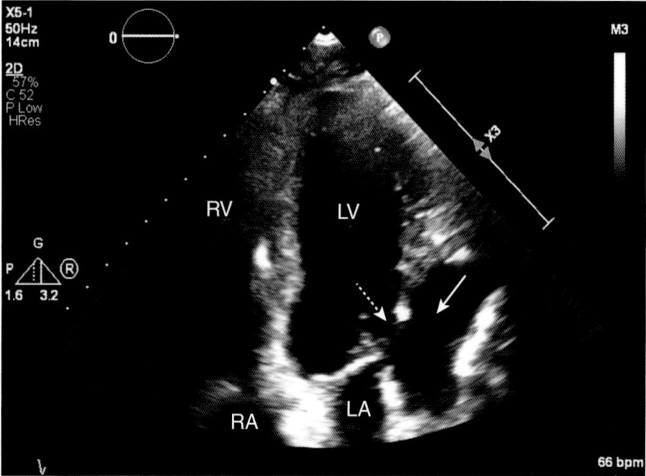

Fig. 21.11 LV pseudoaneurysm. TTE in the apical 4-chamber view demonstrates large pseudoaneurysm of the basal lateral wall *(solid arrow). Dashed arrow* indicates the site of the free wall rupture (see Video 21.11).

which seldom ruptures. The walls of the pseudoaneurysm are composed of organizing thrombus from hemorrhage into the pericardial space after cardiac rupture and various amounts of epicardium and parietal pericardium. In contrast, the wall of a true aneurysm consists of dense fibrous tissue.

A common distinguishing echocardiographic feature of a pseudoaneurysm is the narrow neck; the ratio of neck diameter to maximum aneurysm diameter is less than 0.5, whereas a true aneurysm has a broader opening to the body. However, this sign is only 60% sensitive for differentiating a pseudoaneurysm from a true aneurysm.[61] This is particularly the case with aneurysms at the base of the heart, most commonly after inferior MI. Spectral imaging and color Doppler imaging demonstrate characteristic flow in and out of the pericardial cavity at the site of the tear and show abnormal flow within the pseudoaneurysm.

Surgical repair is the preferred treatment, although conservative medical treatment for certain high-risk patients may be associated with a good outcome.[62] Percutaneous closure of a pseudoaneurysm is a potential approach in carefully selected patients and is performed with TEE guidance (Fig. 21.12).

INFARCT EXPANSION AND TRUE ANEURYSM FORMATION

Infarct expansion represents acute remodeling caused by stretching and thinning of the infarcted zone. This process typically occurs 24 to 72 hours after acute transmural MI. Although any region of the LV may be affected, it is more common after anteroapical MI. Echocardiographic features of infarct expansion include an aneurysmal bulge of the myocardium with reduced local wall thickness. This thin necrotic wall has low tensile strength, and infarct expansion therefore typically precedes mechanical complications, including VSR, VFWR, and PMR.

In the absence of rupture, the final expression of infarct expansion is aneurysm formation, which occurs only with transmural infarction and a full-thickness scar. A true aneurysm is defined as a deformity of the thinned infarct segment that is apparent during diastole and systole. There may be dyskinesis (i.e., outward movement during systole). The involved myocardial segment is scarred and has thin walls (<7 mm) and increased echogenicity due to the increased collagen content. The wall of the aneurysm may eventually calcify.

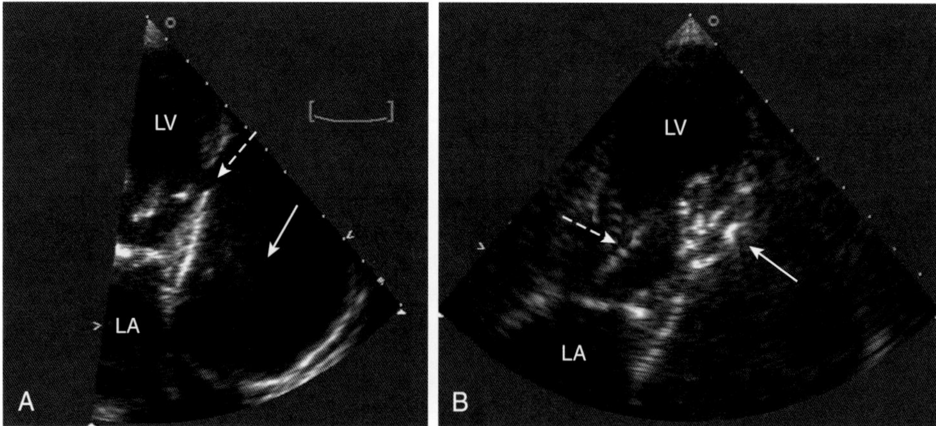

Fig. 21.12 LV pseudoaneurysm. (A) TTE in the apical 4-chamber view demonstrates a large pseudoaneurysm of the mid-inferolateral wall *(solid arrow). Dashed arrow* indicates the site of the free wall rupture. (B) Appearance after transcatheter closure. *Solid arrow,* Amplatzer device; *dashed arrow,* catheter.

Most aneurysms occur in the LV apex and anterior wall (Fig. 21.13); less commonly, they may occur in the inferior wall. Aneurysms of the lateral wall are uncommon. Serial 2D echocardiographic studies indicate that aneurysmal dilation may occur as early as 5 days after MI; new aneurysms after 3 months are unlikely. Spontaneous rupture of an acute aneurysm is rare, and late rupture almost never occurs.

Aneurysms vary in size, and very small aneurysms can be difficult to visualize by echocardiography. Technically, the detection of an apical aneurysm depends on the skill of the operator. Routine employment of high-frequency transducers with a shallow focal point enhances near-field resolution and aids examination of the LV apex. 3D echocardiography and left-sided contrast agents may enable detection of small apical aneurysms or aneurysms in unusual areas (e.g., lateral wall).

Echocardiographic recognition of an LV aneurysm is clinically relevant for several reasons. First, the early formation of an aneurysm adversely affects early (in-hospital) and late (1-year) mortality rates and is associated with an increased incidence of cardiac failure.[63] Second, thrombi are commonly found within aneurysms and are associated with systemic embolization. Third, aneurysms may cause life-threatening ventricular arrhythmias. For patients with heart failure or ventricular arrhythmia, aneurysmectomy may be recommended. When considering aneurysmectomy, it is important to ensure that the basal portions of the LV have vigorous function, and echocardiography plays a key role in patient selection.

LV THROMBUS

LV thrombus is an important complication of acute STEMI because of the risk of systemic embolization, especially stroke. LV thrombus tends to develop on the endocardium of akinetic, nonviable apical LV segments in patients with anterior STEMI due to LAD occlusion. High-risk patients include those with an anterior STEMI, LVEF less than 30%, or LV aneurysm. LV thrombus may occur within a few hours after MI in large areas of apical akinesis or weeks later.

The reported incidence of LV thrombus after STEMI in the modern era varies according to the modality used. TTE with contrast is more sensitive for detection of LV thrombus than standard TTE, especially when image quality is suboptimal (Fig. 21.14). Cardiac MRI with delayed enhancement is the most sensitive imaging modality for detection of LV thrombus. Although

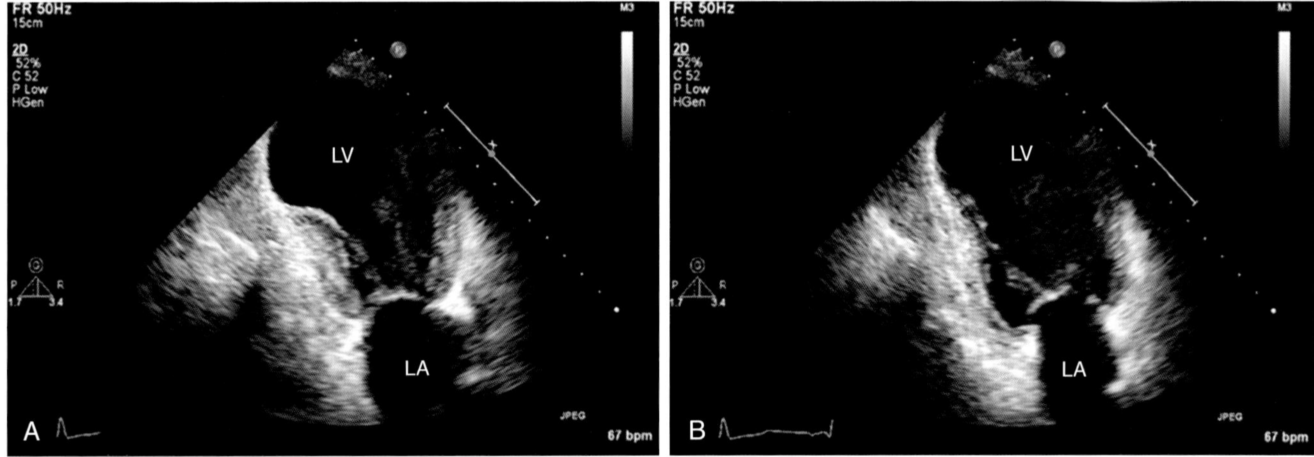

Fig. 21.13 LV true aneurysm. Apical 2-chamber views show a large apical wall aneurysm at end-systole (A) and at end-diastole (B) (see Video 21.13).

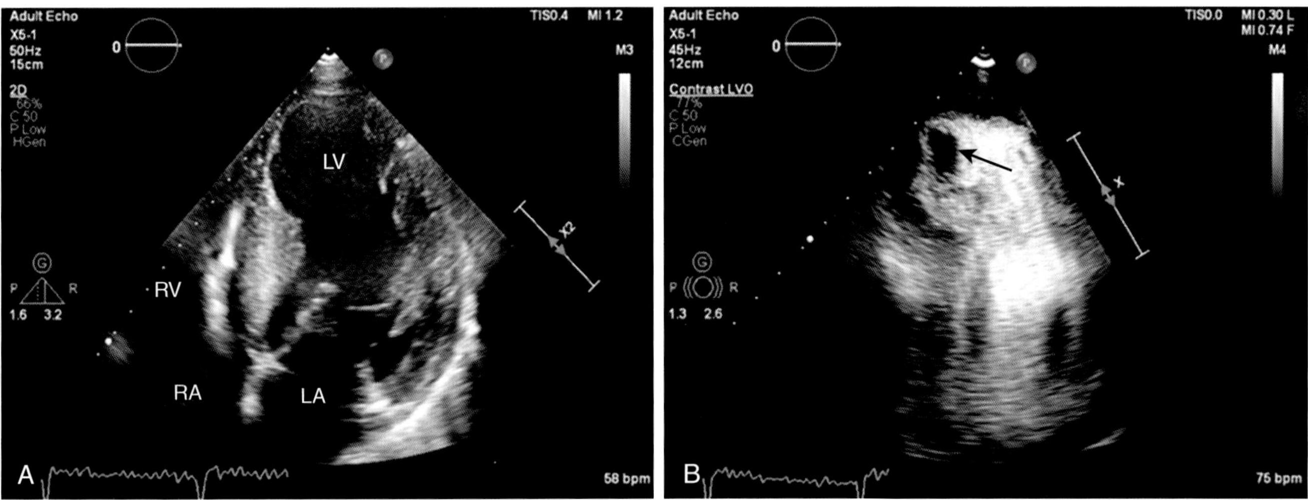

Fig. 21.14 LV thrombus with myocardial contrast. (A) Apical 4-chamber view of LV shows no obvious thrombus (see Video 21.14A). (B) With the use of myocardial contrast, apical thrombus *(black arrow)* is obviously visible as a filling defect (see Video 21.14B).

cardiac MRI is not as widely available as echocardiography, it should be considered in selected cases after MI to evaluate LV thrombus.[64] Cardiac computed tomography is an alternative imaging modality used to detect LV thrombus and may be useful in selected cases.

In a study of 100 consecutive patients with acute anterior STEMI (excluding patients with cardiogenic shock) who were treated with stenting of the LAD within 2 to 12 hours after symptom onset, LV thrombus was diagnosed by echocardiography in 13 patients and by cardiac MRI in 2 patients. All patients underwent echocardiography within the first 1 to 3 days after MI, 4.5 ± 1.1 days after MI, and 3 months after MI.[65] All patients were treated with aspirin 75 mg/day and clopidogrel 75 mg/day, and 50% were treated with a glycoprotein IIb/IIIa inhibitor. Of the 15 patients (15%) diagnosed with LV thrombus, 10 were diagnosed within the first week, 4 between weeks 1 and 4, and 1 between weeks 4 and 12.

Weinsaft et al.[66] studied 201 patients with acute STEMI and found 17 cases of LV thrombus (an overall incidence of 8%) and an incidence of 15% for LAD infarcts. Compared with delayed-enhancement cardiac MRI (which was performed in all patients within 24 hours of the TTE), the sensitivity for LV thrombus detection by TTE was 35% and improved to 65% with the use of ultrasound contrast (used in all cases). Specificity was greater than 98%. Only 12% of patients had an LVEF of less than 30%, and only 18% had LV aneurysm. This study highlighted the surprisingly low sensitivity of non-contrast echocardiography and, to a lesser extent, echocardiography with contrast for the detection of LV thrombus. The impact of these data on clinical management needs to be further studied.

The echocardiographic appearance of a mural thrombus is that of a mass distinct from the endocardium and protruding to some extent into the LV cavity (Fig. 21.15). The tissue characteristics of an acute thrombus are usually similar to those of the myocardium. A chronic thrombus may have increased reflectivity, demonstrate a layered appearance, or contain areas of calcification. The base of attachment to the wall may be broad (i.e., sessile thrombus) or narrow (i.e., pedunculated thrombus). Occasionally, thrombi have areas of relative echolucency. False-positive echocardiographic diagnoses are usually a result of pseudotendons (i.e., false chordae) spanning the LV apex, coarse trabeculations associated with LV hypertrophy, or near-field artifacts (which are common with low-frequency transducers). High-frequency transducers with a short focal point can sometimes differentiate true thrombus from these other phenomena.

The likelihood of an embolic event is highest during the first 2 weeks after an acute MI and decreases over the next 6 weeks. After that time, there is endothelialization of the thrombus associated with reduced embolic potential. Among the characteristics of the thrombus, mobility is most closely associated with embolic events (positive predictive value of 85%), and when mobility and protrusion of the thrombus into the LV cavity occur, embolic rates of up to 40% have been reported.

Anticoagulation with warfarin or a novel oral anticoagulant (NOAC) is recommended for at least 3 months after the diagnosis of LV thrombus. In any patient on anticoagulation, the morphology may change.[67] This emphasizes the need to follow patients with LV thrombus with serial echocardiography.

RISK STRATIFICATION AFTER MYOCARDIAL INFARCTION

LV SYSTOLIC FUNCTION

LVEF is a long-standing echocardiographic measure of global LV systolic function and a well-established predictor of prognosis after acute MI (Table 21.6). Although LVEF is a powerful predictor of outcome, it may be normal, particularly early after acute MI, as a result of compensatory hyperkinesis in the noninfarcted segments despite extensive myocardial damage.[68] LVEF is load dependent and does not provide a true measure of intrinsic LV contractility.

Other measures of LV systolic function have been shown to be better predictors of outcome after MI. In an early study of 605 patients with acute MI, White et al.[69] showed that LV end-systolic volume was superior to LVEF as a prognostic indicator for survival in patients with LVEF less than 50%. Measurement of LV global myocardial strain correlates well with myocardial infarct size and has higher diagnostic value than LVEF for myocardial infarct size measured by single-photon emission tomographic imaging.[70]

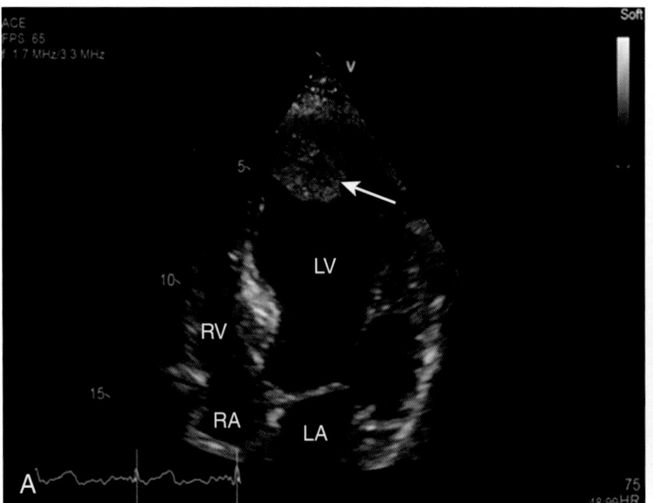

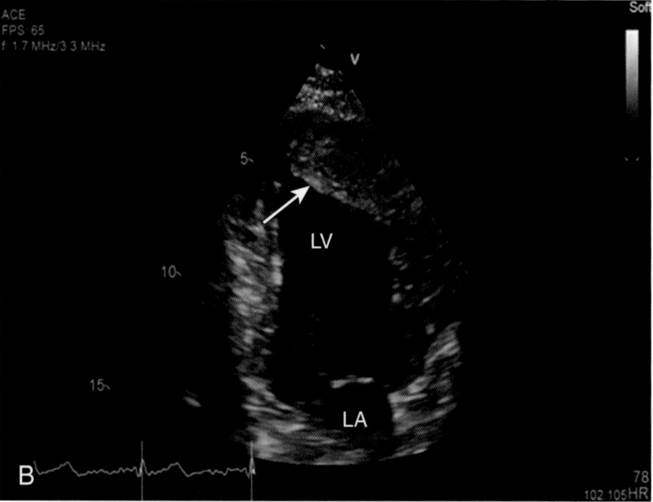

Fig. 21.15 LV thrombus. (A) Apical 4-chamber view of LV shows large thrombus *(arrow)* in the LV apex (see Video 21.15A). (B) Apical 2-chamber view of LV in the same patient shows the large thrombus *(arrow)* adherent to the endocardium of the LV apex and the distal anterior wall (see Video 21.15B).

REGIONAL WALL MOTION SCORE

Semiquantitative assessment of regional systolic function using the wall motion score index can provide an assessment of the extent of WMA.[71] The total score is derived by assigning a grade of 1 through 5 to each myocardial segment that is adequately visualized (see Table 21.2). For a segment to be scored, most of the endocardium within that segment must be apparent. The scores for each segment are added, and then the sum is divided by the number of segments graded. Several studies have demonstrated that a higher wall motion score index (12–24 hours after admission) is associated with a higher rate of in-hospital complications, including malignant arrhythmias, pump failure, cardiac rupture, and death.[72]

WMAs remote from the infarction site may occur early in the course of the infarction, or they may develop in the setting of postinfarction angina. This is strong evidence of multivessel disease. Abnormal wall motion in territories remote from the area of infarction may be a result of (1) previous infarction, (2) increased myocardial oxygen demand in the noninfarcted segment caused by increased wall stress, or (3) reduction in collateral blood supply that originated from the newly occluded vessel.

LV DIASTOLIC FUNCTION

Assessment of LV diastolic function provides prognostic information in the early phase after acute MI[73–79] (Table 21.7). The ratio of early (E-wave) to late (A-wave) transmitral peak velocity and a shortened deceleration time of early transmitral flow were among the earliest measures of LV diastolic function shown to be powerful predictors of outcome, and these results were validated in a 2014 cohort.[80] In a study of 125 consecutive patients with acute MI, Moller et al.[77] demonstrated that the 1-year survival rate was 100% for patients with normal filling, 89% for those with impaired relaxation, 50% for those with a pseudonormal pattern, and 35% for those with a restrictive pattern.

TABLE 21.6 Risk Stratification After Acute Myocardial Infarction.

Echocardiographic Parameter	*Comment*
LV ejection fraction	A well-established predictor of prognosis after acute MI; however, may be normal as a result of compensatory regional hyperkinesis in the noninfarcted segments despite extensive myocardial damage
LV end-systolic volume	Superior to LVEF as a prognostic indicator for survival in patients with LVEF < 50%
Global LV strain	Correlates well with myocardial infarct size and has a higher diagnostic value than LVEF for myocardial infarct size
LV regional wall motion score index	A higher index in acute MI is associated with a higher rate of in-hospital complications, including malignant arrhythmias, pump failure, cardiac rupture, and death
LV diastolic function	Numerous LV diastolic function parameters provide strong and independent prediction for clinical outcomes after MI (see Table 21.7)
LA volume index	An independent predictor of death after MI
Mitral regurgitation	Increased severity of ischemic mitral regurgitation in acute MI correlates with reduced survival
Coronary flow reserve	Noninvasive assessment (especially of the LAD) provides prognostic information early after acute MI
Stress echocardiography	Exercise stressor to detect inducible ischemia; dobutamine stressor to detect inducible ischemia and viability
Myocardial contrast echocardiography	Accurate measure of reperfusion at a microvascular level; predicts LV function and functional recovery after acute MI
Mechanical dispersion	Predicts ventricular arrhythmic events independently of LVEF
LV twist	Peak subepicardial twist strongly reflects infarct transmurality and is independently associated with LV remodeling after MI

LAD, Left anterior descending coronary artery; *LVEF*, LV ejection fraction; *MI*, myocardial infarction.

TABLE 21.7 Role of Diastolic Functional Parameters in Prognosis After Myocardial Infarction.

Study	*N*	*Comment*
MeRGE AMI et al. (2008)[74]	3396	Restrictive filling is an independent predictor of death after acute MI, regardless of LVEF, LV end-systolic volume index, and Killip class.
Kruszewski et al. (2010)[73]	400	Ratio of mitral E wave to early mitral annulus diastolic velocity (E/e′) > 15 when measured on day 1 after acute MI is associated with increased risk of adverse events within 1 year and medium-term mortality.
Whalley et al. (2006)[76]	3855	Mortality rates are four times higher for patients with a restrictive filling pattern than in those with nonrestrictive filling patterns after acute MI.
Moller et al. (2003)[75]	110	Patients with persistently abnormal or deteriorating LV filling pattern, as opposed to improved or normal filling, are at increased risk for cardiac death and readmission as a result of heart failure.
Moller et al. (2000)[77]	125	Restrictive filling and pseudonormal filling independently predicted death.
Hillis et al. (2004)[78]	250	Ratio of mitral E wave to early mitral annulus diastolic velocity (E/e′) > 15 was the most powerful independent predictor of survival.
Moller et al. (2001)[79]	67	Ratio of mitral E wave velocity to color M-mode flow propagation velocity ≥ 1.5 was a significant predictor of the composite of cardiac death and readmission for heart failure.
Fontes-Carvalho et al. (2015)[81]	225	Septal E/e′ was best echocardiographic predictor of reduced functional capacity 1 month after acute MI.
Dokainish et al. (2014)[80]	528	Restrictive LV diastolic filling was a strong and independent predictor of major adverse cardiac events after STEMI across a broad range of LVEF.

LVEF, LV ejection fraction; *MI*, myocardial infarction; *STEMI*, ST elevation myocardial infarction.

The Meta-Analysis Research Group in Echocardiography (MeRGE)[74] showed that a restrictive filling pattern is associated with an almost threefold increase in the mortality rate. This relationship is independent of age, LV size, LVEF, and Killip class. The value of serial echocardiography after MI is emphasized by the finding that patients with a persistently abnormal or deteriorating LV filling pattern (as opposed to improved or normal filling) are at increased risk for cardiac death and readmission as a result of heart failure after acute MI.[79] In addition to providing prognostic information, E/e′ measured 1 month after acute STEMI has been the best echocardiographic predictor of reduced functional capacity.[81]

LA VOLUME AND FUNCTION

The mechanisms influencing LA remodeling are similar to those affecting LV diastolic function. However, in contrast to Doppler indices of LV diastolic function, LA volume is a more stable parameter integrating the effects of elevated left filling pressures from preexisting cardiovascular conditions and acute disease.

Beinart et al.[82] demonstrated that LA volume index measured within 48 hours after an acute MI was an independent predictor of 5-year mortality and a more powerful predictor than LV volumes or MR. Similarly, in the study by Moller et al.,[83] LA volume index was a powerful predictor of mortality and remained an independent predictor after adjustment for clinical factors, LV systolic function, and Doppler-derived parameters of diastolic function. Like measurement of LA size, measurement of LA function with peak systolic strain in acute MI correlates inversely with levels of B-type natriuretic peptide and decreases with deteriorating LV systolic and diastolic function.[84]

LV REMODELING

After transmural MI, alterations in LV structure and function occur; this is commonly referred to as *LV remodeling*.[85] The early phase of LV remodeling is confined to the infarct zone and consists primarily of infarct expansion, whereas the late phase involves changes in the entire myocardium and may continue for months.

The major factors that determine the magnitude and duration of the remodeling process include the size and location of the initial infarct (usually a complication of a larger anterior infarction), the patency and time to restoration of flow in the infarct-related artery, neurohormonal activation, and the ability of the extracellular matrix to form a stable, mature collagen scar. The major clinical significance of remodeling is the resultant ventricular dilation with reduced contractility, which is associated with an increased incidence of cardiac failure, arrhythmias, and death. Remodeling may cause MR as a result of apical and lateral displacement of the papillary muscles, a process that is associated with increased mortality and risk of cardiac failure. Echocardiography plays a major role in predicting ventricular remodeling and functional recovery.

Although percutaneous coronary artery interventions restore patency of the infarct-related artery, myocardial perfusion may be absent, and this is associated with adverse outcomes. Myocardial contrast echocardiography is an accurate measure of reperfusion at a microvascular level; it has been shown in multiple studies to predict LV function after MI,[86] and it may predict functional recovery after acute MI.[87]

LV twist, which is systolic wringing motion derived from rotatory movement of the LV apex and base, has emerged as an accurate index of LV systolic performance. Peak subepicardial twist strongly reflects infarct transmurality and is independently associated with LV remodeling after MI.[88]

LV strain and strain rate, quantified using tissue Doppler or speckle tracking imaging, can differentiate transmural from nontransmural MI and therefore reflect the extent of nonviable myocardium.[89] There is a close correlation between global and regional longitudinal strain and the degree of diminished microcirculation after MI. These strain measures are significantly better tools for assessing coronary flow reserve after a recent MI than conventional echocardiographic measurements.[90] LV strain parameters also can independently predict death or the development of heart failure during follow-up after acute MI.[91] Circumferential strain (but not longitudinal strain) can predict late remodeling, suggesting that preserved circumferential function may serve to restrain ventricular enlargement after MI.[92]

In studies using color tissue Doppler imaging and speckle tracking radial strain analysis for the assessment of LV dyssynchrony after acute MI, the finding of LV dyssynchrony at baseline was significantly related to LV dilation at 6 months' follow-up.[93] LV dyssynchrony is also independently associated with the occurrence of ventricular tachycardia after MI.[94]

LVEF of less than 35% is the main measure of LV function that determines whether an implanted cardiac defibrillator is indicated as primary prophylaxis to prevent sudden cardiac death. However, it is increasingly recognized that LVEF has limited accuracy to risk-stratify patients for sudden cardiac death after MI. It has been suggested that measurement of mechanical dispersion and global longitudinal strain may improve patient selection.[92] Mechanical dispersion by strain echocardiography, a parameter of inhomogeneous ventricular contraction, predicted ventricular arrhythmic events independently of LVEF in a study of 569 patients more than 40 days after acute MI (STEMI and non-STEMI).[95]

STRESS ECHOCARDIOGRAPHY

Stress echocardiography has an important role in the postinfarction period for assessment of myocardial viability and inducible myocardial ischemia.[96] After acute MI, improvement of wall motion during low-dose dobutamine infusion (i.e., contractile reserve) indicates the presence of viable (stunned) myocardium that improves spontaneously in function and is associated with an improved outcome. Higher doses of dobutamine and exercise echocardiography can detect residual ischemia and provide better prognostic value than exercise ECG.

A normal stress echocardiogram provides favorable prognostic information for patients with preserved LVEF after MI, with a reported 5-year survival rate of 94%. A 95% 1-year survival rate after acute MI was reported for patients with a negative stress echocardiogram compared with 85% and 75% for those with high- and low-dose ischemia, respectively.[97]

Caution should be exercised during the first week after a transmural infarction because cases of myocardial rupture during high-dose dobutamine infusion have been reported. A physician should ideally supervise a dynamic stress echocardiogram after an acute coronary syndrome if ventricular function is significantly impaired, there is known severe CAD not revascularized, or there is a concern because of the high risk of arrhythmias.

MITRAL REGURGITATION

MR is common among patients presenting with acute MI, and the prevalence increases twofold for patients with heart failure.

MR diagnosed in acute MI may be a result of preexisting MR caused by structural leaflet disease, which needs to be differentiated from ischemic causes such as PMR or LV remodeling.

Ischemic MR can be defined as valvular incompetence associated with myocardial ischemia or infarction in the absence of primary leaflet or chordal pathology. Papillary muscle dysfunction represents malfunction of the scarred papillary muscle and of the underlying ventricular wall. This results in retraction of the anterior or posterior leaflet and malcoaptation. The LV remodeling process that occurs after a transmural MI may also result in apical and posterior displacement of the LV wall supporting the papillary muscle and of the papillary muscle itself, with abnormal mitral leaflet coaptation and MR.

Dilation of the mitral annulus to various degrees usually contributes to the regurgitation. Depending on the site of the infarction and the degree of remodeling, one mitral leaflet (more commonly the posterior leaflet) may be more involved than the other, and the regurgitation jet may therefore be eccentric, which is a common cause for underestimating the severity of MR.

Ischemic MR is a dynamic condition that may be transient, may worsen in severity with episodes of myocardial ischemia, and may improve with medical therapy. Exercise stress echocardiography is indicated when there is a discrepancy between resting MR severity and the patient's symptoms.[98] Even when mild, ischemic MR in acute MI is associated with an adverse prognosis and increased mortality rates; increased severity correlates with reduced survival.[99]

For patients requiring surgical myocardial revascularization, it is generally accepted that mitral valve surgery is necessary for severe ischemic regurgitation but not for mild regurgitation. However, how to treat moderate ischemic MR is controversial.[100]

SUMMARY The Role of Echocardiography in Patients With an Acute Coronary Syndrome.

Condition	Echocardiographic Findings	Imaging Approach
Diagnosis of MI		
Localization of ischemia/infarction	Regional LV WMA (hypokinesis or akinesis) reflects coronary artery territory	All views required Avoid apical foreshortening LV strain
RV infarction	Dilated, hypokinetic, or akinetic RV Global or regional Severe TR may be present. Inferior LV WMA may be relatively minor.	Standard RV views Additional measures of RV function: TAPSE, DTI S-velocity, FAC, strain
Complications of MI		
Pericardial effusion	Typically small Larger and/or hemorrhagic effusion suggests cardiac rupture or aortic dissection	Standard views for evaluation of effusion Subcostal view to assess inferior vena cava
Ischemic MR	Tethering of posterior mitral valve leaflet with posteriorly directed MR Apical tenting of mitral valve leaflets with dilated LV and/or LV systolic impairment PMR with papillary muscle attached to flail leaflet. Small LA with severe MR suggests acute MR. MR may be intermittently severe during an ischemic episode	Evaluate mitral valve anatomy in standard views, including 3D. Quantitate MR severity. TEE, including 3D imaging, may be needed to determine cause of MR.
Ventricular septal defect	Small or large septal defect in areas of akinesis Inferior septal defect usually associated with RV dilation and impairment Left-to-right flow on color and CW Doppler	May be small and difficult to visualize. Use nonstandard views if needed. Use color Doppler in region of akinesis or apparent septal discontinuity.
Free wall rupture and tamponade	Site of rupture may not be obvious by 2D or 3D imaging; usually associated with large pericardial effusion (hemorrhagic) and tamponade and may be fatal unless sealed by fibrinous pericardial adhesions.	Suspect if hemorrhagic pericardial effusion or pericardial thrombus seen Color Doppler to locate LV-to-pericardial communication

Continued

SUMMARY The Role of Echocardiography in Patients With an Acute Coronary Syndrome.—cont'd

Condition	Echocardiographic Findings	Imaging Approach
LV pseudoaneurysm	Abrupt transition from normal myocardium to aneurysm; narrow neck, with ratio of neck diameter to aneurysm <0.5 Possibly lined with thrombus Often associated with pericardial effusion	Most often at base of inferior wall or mid-lateral wall of LV TEE may be needed.
LV aneurysm	Thin, bright, dyskinetic LV segment with a diastolic contour abnormality Apical and basal inferior LV aneurysm most common; lateral wall aneurysm uncommon Thrombus may be present, especially at LV apex.	Apical aneurysm is best seen in apical views. Avoid foreshortening with TTE. Scan parasternal short axis from base to apex. Apical aneurysm may be missed with TEE.
LV thrombus	Echogenic mass, distinct from myocardium, often protrudes into the chamber. Underlying akinetic LV segment(s), typically at the LV apex May be single or multiple	Use high-frequency transducer and zoom mode; adjust gain and instrument settings. Avoid foreshortening. Contrast to opacify the LV may be needed, especially if LV thrombus not seen when associated with suboptimal image quality and high-risk features (akinetic/aneurysmal LV apex).
Risk Stratification After MI		
LV systolic dysfunction	Location and size of the regional WMAs correspond to infarct size. All measures of LV systolic function are a major determinant of clinical outcome.	Measures include LVEF, LV end-systolic volume index, LV global longitudinal strain, and LV wall motion score index. 3D LV volume and LVEF should be performed when possible.
LV diastolic dysfunction	Pseudonormal pattern and restrictive filling are associated with adverse outcomes.	Transmitral Doppler, pulmonary venous Doppler, DTI LA volume index and PASP
LA volume index	Provides independent prognostic information	Should be measured routinely

DTI, Doppler tissue imaging; *FAC,* fractional area change; *LVEF,* LV ejection fraction; *MI,* myocardial infarction; *MR,* mitral regurgitation; *PASP,* pulmonary artery systolic pressure; *PMR,* papillary muscle rupture; *S,* systolic; *TAPSE,* tricuspid annular plane systolic excursion; *TR,* tricuspid regurgitation; *WMA,* wall motion abnormality.

REFERENCES

1. Prastaro M, Pirozzi E, Gaibazzi N, et al. Expert review on the prognostic role of echocardiography after acute myocardial infarction. *J Am Soc Echocardiogr*. 2017;30:431–443.e2.
2. Corsi C, Lang RM, Veronesi F, et al. Volumetric quantification of global and regional left ventricular function from real-time three-dimensional echocardiographic images. *Circulation*. 2005;112:1161–1170.
3. Toledo E, Lang RM, Collins KA, et al. Imaging and quantification of myocardial perfusion using real-time three-dimensional echocardiography. *J Am Coll Cardiol*. 2006;47:146–154.
4. Pellerin D, Sharma R, Elliott P, et al. Tissue Doppler, strain, and strain rate echocardiography for the assessment of left and right systolic ventricular function. *Heart*. 2003;89(suppl 3):iii9–iii17.
5. Dahlsett T, Karlsen S, Grenne B, et al. Early assessment of strain echocardiography can accurately exclude significant coronary artery stenosis in non-ST-segment elevation acute coronary syndrome. *J Am Soc Echocardiogr*. 2014;27:51209.
6. Lepper W, Belcik T, Wei K, et al. Myocardial contrast echocardiography. *Circulation*. 2004;109:3132–3135.
7. Khumri TM, Nayar S, Idupulapati M, et al. Usefulness of myocardial contrast echocardiography in predicting late mortality in patients with anterior acute myocardial infarction. *Am J Cardiol*. 2006;98:1150–1155.
8. Chamsi-Pasha MA, Sengupta PP, Zoghbi WA. Handheld echocardiography: current state and future perspectives. *Circulation*. 2017;136:2178–2188.
9. Lang RM, Badano LP, Mor-Avi V, et al. Recommendations for cardiac chamber quantification by echocardiography in adults: an update from the American Society of Echocardiography and the European Association of Cardiovascular Imaging. *J Am Soc Echocardiogr*. 2015;28(1):1–39.e14.
10. Rodríguez M, Rzechorzek W, Herzog E, et al. Misconceptions and facts about takotsubo syndrome. *Am J Med*. 2019;132:25–31.
11. Templin C, Ghadri J, Diekmman J, et al. Clinical features and outcomes of takotsubo (stress) cardiomyopathy. *N Engl J Med*. 2015;373:929–938.
12. Frangieh AH, Obeid S, Ghadri JR, et al. ECG criteria to differentiate between takotsubo (stress) cardiomyopathy and myocardial infarction. *J Am Heart Assoc*. 2016;5:e003418.

13. Medina de Chazal H, Del Buono MG, Keyser-Marcus L, et al. Stress cardiomyopathy diagnosis and treatment: JACC state-of-the-art review. *J Am Coll Cardiol*. 2018;72:1955–1971.
14. Siddiqui M, Desiderio M, Ricculli N, et al. Stress related cardiomyopathy with midventricular ballooning: a rare variant. *Case Rep Med*. 2015;2015:154678.
15. Mehta N, Aurigemma G, Rafeq Z, et al. Reverse takotsubo cardiomyopathy after an episode of serotonin syndrome. *Tex Heart Inst J*. 2011;38:568–572.
16. Eitel I, von Knobelsdorff-Brenkenhoff F, Bernhardt P, et al. Clinical characteristics and cardiovascular magnetic resonance findings in stress (Takotsubo) cardiomyopathy. *J Am Med Assoc*. 2011;306:277–286.
17. Citro R, Piscione F, Parodi G, et al. Role of echocardiography in takotsubo cardiomyopathy. *Heart Failure Clin*. 2013;9:153–166.
18. Redfors B, Vedad R, Angeras O, et al. Mortality in takotsubo syndrome is similar to mortality in myocardial infarction—a report from the SWEDEHEART1 registry. *Int J Cardiol*. 2015;185:282–289.
19. Elesber A, Prasad A, Lennon R, et al. Four-year recurrence rate and prognosis of the apical ballooning syndrome. *J Am Coll Cardiol*. 2007;50:448–452.
20. Shirani J, Freant LJ, Roberts WC. Gross and semiquantitative histologic findings in mononuclear cell myocarditis causing sudden death, and implications for endomyocardial biopsy. *Am J Cardiol*. 1993;15:952–957.
21. Mahrholdt H, Wagner A, Deluigi CC, et al. Presentation, patterns of myocardial damage, and clinical course of viral myocarditis. *Circulation*. 2006;114:1581–1590.
22. Cohn JN, Guiha NH, Broder MI et al. Right ventricular infarction. Clinical and hemodynamic features. *Am J Cardiol*. 1974;33:209–214.
23. Goldstein JA. Pathophysiology and management of right heart ischemia. *J Am Coll Cardiol*. 2002;40:841–853.
24. Tahirkheli NK, Edwards WD, Nishimura RA, et al. Right ventricular infarction associated with anteroseptal myocardial infarction: a clinicopathologic study of nine cases. *Cardiovasc Pathol*. 2000;9:175–179.
25. Rallidis LS, Makavos G, Nihoyannopoulos P. Right ventricular involvement in coronary artery disease: role of echocardiography for diagnosis and prognosis. *J Am Soc Echocardiogr*. 2014;27:223–229.
26. Hamon M, Agostini D, Le Page O, et al. Prognostic impact of right ventricular involvement in patients with acute myocardial infarction: meta-analysis. *Crit Care Med*. 2008;36:2023–2033.
27. Kozakova M, Palombo C, Distante A. Right ventricular infarction: the role of echocardiography. *Echocardiography*. 2001;18:701–707.
28. Ozdemir K, Altunkeser BB, Icli A, et al. New parameters in identification of right ventricular myocardial infarction and proximal right coronary artery lesion. *Chest*. 2003;124:219–226.
29. Park S, Park J, Lee H, et al. Impaired RV global longitudinal strain is associated with poor long-term clinical outcomes in patients with acute inferior STEMI. *J Am Coll Cardiol Imaging*. 2015;8:161–169.
30. Cohen A, Logeart D, Costagliola D, et al. Usefulness of pulmonary regurgitation Doppler tracings in predicting in-hospital and long-term outcome in patients with inferior wall acute myocardial infarction. *Am J Cardiol*. 1998;81:276–281.
31. Ketikoglou DG, Karvounis HI, Papadopoulos CE, et al. Echocardiographic evaluation of spontaneous recovery of right ventricular systolic and diastolic function in patients with acute right ventricular infarction associated with posterior wall left ventricular infarction. *Am J Cardiol*. 2004;93:911–913.
32. Hoogslag G, Haeck M, Velders M, et al. Determinants of right ventricular remodeling following ST-segment elevation myocardial infarction. *Am J Cardiol*. 2014;114:1490–1496.
33. Goldstein JA. Right versus left ventricular shock: a tale of two ventricles. *J Am Coll Cardiol*. 2003;41:1280–1282.
34. Kakouros N, Cokkinos D. Right ventricular myocardial infarction: pathophysiology, diagnosis, and management. *Postgrad Med J*. 2010;86:719–728.
35. Houard L, Benaets MB, de Meester de Ravenstein C, et al. Additional prognostic value of 2D right ventricular speckle-tracking strain for prediction of survival in heart failure and reduced ejection fraction: a comparative study with cardiac magnetic resonance. *JACC Cardiovasc Imaging*. 2019;12(12):2373–2385.
36. Lanz J, Wyss D, Räber L, et al. Mechanical complications in patients with ST-segment elevation myocardial infarction: a single centre experience. *PLoS One*. 2019;14:e0209502.
37. Pouleur AC, Barkoudah E, Uno H, et al. Pathogenesis of sudden unexpected death in a clinical trial of patients with myocardial infarction and left ventricular dysfunction, heart failure, or both. *Circulation*. 2010;122:597–602.
38. Nishimura RA, Schaff HV, Shub C, et al. Papillary muscle rupture complicating acute myocardial infarction: analysis of 17 patients. *Am J Cardiol*. 1983;51:373–377.
39. Vargaras-Barron J, Molina-Carrion M, Romero-Cardenas A, et al. Risk factors, angiographic patterns, and outcomes in patients with acute ventricular septal rupture during myocardial infarction. *Am J Cardiol*. 2005;95:1153–1158.
40. Sivadasan Pillai H, Tharakan J, Titus T, et al. Ventricular septal rupture following myocardial infarction. Long-term survival of patients who did not undergo surgery. Single-centre experience. *Acta Cardiol*. 2005;60:403–407.
41. Arnaoutakis G, Zhao Y, George T, et al. Surgical repair of ventricular septal defect after myocardial infarction: outcomes from the society of thoracic surgeons national database. *Ann Thorac Surg*. 2012;94:436–444.
42. Pang P, Sin Y, Lim C, et al. Outcome and survival analysis of surgical repair of post-infarction ventricular septal rupture. *J Cardiothorac Surg*. 2013;8:44.
43. Crenshaw B, Granger C, Birnbaum Y, et al. GUSTO-1 (Global Utilization of Streptokinase and TPA for Occluded Coronary Arteries Trial Investigators. Risk factors, angiographic patterns, and outcomes in patients with ventricular septal defect complicating acute myocardial infarction. *Circulation*. 2000;101:27–32.
44. Papalexopoulou N, Young C, Attia R. What is the best timing of surgery in patients with post-infarct ventricular septal rupture? *Interact Cardiovasc Thorac Surg*. 2013;16:193–197.
45. Mittal C, Aslam N, Mohan B, et al. Spontaneous closure of post-myocardial infarction ventricular septal rupture. *Tex Heart Inst J*. 2011;38:596–597.
46. Baldasare M, Polyakov M, Laub G, et al. Percutaneous repair of post-myocardial infarction ventricular septal defect: current approaches and future perspectives. *Tex Heart Inst J*. 2014;41:613–619.
47. Maltais S, Ibrahim R, Basmadijan A, et al. Postinfarction ventricular septal defects: towards a new treatment algorithm? *Ann Thorac Surg*. 2009;87:687–692.
48. Attia R, Blauth C. Which patients might be suitable for a septal occluder device closure of postinfarction ventricular septal rupture rather than immediate surgery? *Interact Cardiovasc Thorac Surg*. 2010;11:626–629.
49. Capasso F, Caruso A, Valva G, et al. Device closure of 'complex' postinfarction ventricular septal defect. *J Cardiovasc Med*. 2015;16(suppl 1):S15–S17.
50. Calvert P, Cockburn J, Wynne D, et al. Percutaneous closure of postinfarction ventricular septal defect. In-hospital outcomes and long-term follow-up of UK experience. *Circulation*. 2014;129:2395–2402.
51. Kronzon I, Ruize C, Perk G. Guidance of post myocardial infarction ventricular septal defect and pseudoaneurysm closure. *Curr Cardiol Rep*. 2014;16:456.
52. Haddadin S, Milano A, Faggian G, et al. Surgical treatment of postinfarction left ventricular free wall rupture. *J Card Surg*. 2009;24:624–631.
53. Lopez-Sendon J, Gurfinkel E, Lopez de Sa E, et al. Factors related to heart rupture in acute coronary syndromes in the Global Registry of Acute Coronary Events. *Eur Heart J*. 2010;31:1449–1456.
54. Bueno H, Martinez-Selles M, Perez-David E, et al. Effect of thrombolytic therapy on the risk of cardiac rupture and mortality in older patients with first acute myocardial infarction. *Eur Heart J*. 2005;26:1705–1711.
55. Purcaro A, Costantini C, Ciampani N, et al. Diagnostic criteria and management of subacute ventricular free wall rupture complicating acute myocardial infarction. *Am J Cardiol*. 1997;80:397–405.
56. Wilkenshoff UM, Ale Abaei A, Kuersten B, et al. Contrast echocardiography for detection of incomplete rupture of the left ventricle after acute myocardial infarction. *Z Kardiol*. 2004;93:624–629.
57. Figueras J, Cortadellas J, Evangelista A, et al. Medical management of selected patients with left ventricular free wall rupture during acute myocardial infarction. *J Am Coll Cardiol*. 1997;29:512–518.
58. Matteucci M, Fina D, Jiritano F, et al. Treatment strategies for post-infarction left ventricular free-wall rupture. *Eur Heart J Acute Cardiovasc Care*. 2019;8:379–387.
59. Doulaptsis C, Goetschalckx K, Masci P, et al. Assessment of early post-infarction pericardial injury by CMR. *JACC Cardiovasc Imaging*. 2013;6:411–413.
60. Guereta P, Khalifeb K, Jobicc Y, et al. Echocardiographic assessment of the incidence of mechanical complications during the early phase of myocardial infarction in the reperfusion era: a French multicenter prospective registry. *Arch Cardiovasc Dis*. 2008;101:41–47.
61. Yeo TC, Malouf JF, Oh JK, et al. Clinical profile and outcome in 52 patients with cardiac pseudoaneurysm. *Ann Intern Med*. 1998;128:299–305.
62. Tuan J, Kaivani F, Fewins H. Left ventricular pseudoaneurysm. *Eur J Echocardiogr*. 2008;9:107–109.

63. Visser CA, Kan G, Meltzer RS, et al. Incidence, timing and prognostic value of left ventricular aneurysm formation after myocardial infarction: a prospective, serial echocardiographic study of 158 patients. *Am J Cardiol.* 1986;57:729–732.
64. Roifman I, Connelly K, Wright G, et al. Echocardiography vs. cardiac magnetic resonance imaging for the diagnosis of left ventricular thrombus: a systematic review. *Can J Cardiol.* 2015;31:785–791.
65. Solheim S, Seljeflot I, Lunde K, et al. Frequency of left ventricular thrombus in patients with anterior wall acute myocardial infarction treated with percutaneous coronary intervention and dual antiplatelet therapy. *Am J Cardiol.* 2010;106:1197–1200.
66. Weinsaft JW, Kim J, Medicherla CB, et al. Echocardiographic algorithm for post-myocardial infarction LV thrombus: a gatekeeper for thrombus evaluation by delayed enhancement CMR. *JACC Cardiovasc Imaging.* 2016;9:505–515.
67. McCarthy CP, Vaduganathan M, McCarthy KJ, et al. Left ventricular thrombus after acute myocardial infarction: screening, prevention, and treatment. *JAMA Cardiol.* 2018;3:642–649.
68. Mollema S, Nucifora G, Bax J. Prognostic value of echocardiography after acute myocardial infarction. *Heart.* 2009;95:1732–1745.
69. White HD, Norris RM, Brown MA, et al. Left ventricular end-systolic volume as the major determinant of survival after recovery from myocardial infarction. *Circulation.* 1987;76:44–51.
70. Wang Q, Huang D, Zhang L, et al. Assessment of myocardial infarct size by three-dimensional and two-dimensional speckle tracking echocardiography: a comparative study to single photon emission computed tomography. *Echocardiography.* 2015;32:1539–1542.
71. Baron T, Flachskampf F, Johansson K, et al. Usefulness of traditional echocardiographic parameters in assessment of left ventricular function in patients with normal ejection fraction after acute myocardial infarction: results from a large consecutive cohort. *Eur Heart J Cardiovasc Imaging.* 2016;17:413–420.
72. Moller JE, Hillis GS, Oh JK, et al. Wall motion score index and ejection fraction for risk stratification after acute myocardial infarction. *Am Heart J.* 2006;151:419–425.
73. Kruszewski K, Scott A, Barclay J, et al. Noninvasive assessment of left ventricular filling pressure after acute myocardial infarction: a prospective study of the relative prognostic utility of clinical assessment, echocardiography, and B-type natriuretic peptide. *Am Heart J.* 2010;159:47–54.
74. Meta-Analysis Research Group in Echocardiography (MeRGE) AMI Collaborators Independent prognostic importance of a restrictive left ventricular filling pattern after myocardial infarction. *Circulation.* 2008;117:2591–2598.
75. Moller J, Poulsen S, Sondergaard E, et al. Impact of early changes in left ventricular filling pattern on long-term outcome after acute myocardial infarction. *Int J Cardiol.* 2003;89:207–215.
76. Whalley G, Gamble G, Doughty R. Restrictive diastolic filling predicts death after acute myocardial infarction: systematic review and meta-analysis of prospective studies. *Heart.* 2006;92:1588–1594.
77. Moller JE, Sondergaard E, Poulsen SH. Pseudonormal and restrictive filling patterns predict left ventricular dilation and cardiac death after a first myocardial infarction: a serial color M-mode Doppler echocardiographic study. *J Am Coll Cardiol.* 2000;36:1841–1846.
78. Hillis G, Moller J, Pellika P, et al. Noninvasive estimation of left ventricular filling pressure by E/e′is a powerful predictor of survival after acute myocardial infarction. *J Am Coll Cardiol.* 2004;43:360–367.
79. Moller JE, Sondergaard E, Poulsen SH. Color M-mode and pulsed wave tissue Doppler echocardiography: powerful predictors of cardiac events after first myocardial infarction. *J Am Soc Echocardiogr.* 2001;14:757–763.
80. Dokainish H, Rajaram M, Prabhakaran D, et al. Incremental value of left ventricular systolic and diastolic function to determine outcome in patients with acute ST-segment elevation myocardial infarction: the echocardiographic substudy of the OASIS-6 trial. *Echocardiography.* 2014;31:569–578.
81. Fontes-Carvalho R, Sampaio F, Teixeira M, et al. Left ventricular diastolic dysfunction and E/E′ ratio as the strongest echocardiographic predictors of reduced exercise capacity after acute myocardial infarction. *Clin Cardiol.* 2015;38:222–229.
82. Beinart R, Bovko V, Schwamm E, et al. Long-term prognostic significance of left atrial volume in acute myocardial infarction. *J Am Coll Cardiol.* 2004;44:327–334.
83. Moller JE, Hillis GS, Oh JK, et al. Left atrial volume: a powerful predictor of survival after acute myocardial infarction. *Circulation.* 2003;107:2207–2212.
84. Facchini E, Degiovanni A, Marino P. Left atrium function in patients with coronary artery disease. *Curr Opin Cardiol.* 2014;29:423–429.
85. Giannuzzi P, Temporelli P, Bosimi E, et al. Heterogeneity of left ventricular remodeling after acute myocardial infarction: results of the Gruppo Italiano per lo Studio della Sopravvivenza nell'Infarto Miocardico-3 Echo substudy. *Am Heart J.* 2001;141:131–138.
86. Balcells E, Powers ER, Lepper W, et al. Detection of myocardial viability by contrast echocardiography in acute infarction predicts recovery of resting function and contractile reserve. *J Am Coll Cardiol.* 2003;41:827–833.
87. Jeetley P, Swinburn J, Hickman M, et al. Myocardial contrast echocardiography predicts left ventricular remodelling after acute myocardial infarction. *J Am Soc Echocardiogr.* 2004;17:1030–1036.
88. Abate E, Hoogslag G, Leong D, et al. Association between multilayer left ventricular rotational mechanics and the development of left ventricular remodelling after acute myocardial infarction. *J Am Soc Echocardiogr.* 2014;27:239–248.
89. Vartdal T, Brunvand H, Pettersen E, et al. Early prediction of infarct size by strain Doppler echocardiography after coronary reperfusion. *J Am Coll Cardiol.* 2007;49:1715–1721.
90. Logstrup B, Hofsten D, Christophersen T, et al. Correlation between left ventricular global and regional longitudinal systolic strain and impaired microcirculation in patients with acute myocardial infarction. *Echocardiography.* 2012;29:1181–1190.
91. Ersboll M, Valeur N, Andersen M, et al. Early echocardiographic deformation analysis for the prediction of sudden cardiac death and life-threatening arrhythmias after myocardial infarction. *J Am Coll Cardiol Img.* 2013;6:851–860.
92. Hung C, Verma A, Uno H, et al. Longitudinal and circumferential strain rate, left ventricular remodeling, and prognosis after myocardial infarction. *J Am Coll Cardiol.* 2010;56:1812–1822.
93. Mollema S, Liem S, Suffoletto M, et al. Left ventricular dyssynchrony immediately after acute myocardial infarction predicts left ventricular remodelling. *J Am Coll Cardiol.* 2007;50:1532–1540.
94. Leong D, Hoogslag G, Piers S, et al. The relationship between time from myocardial infarction, left ventricular dyssynchrony, and the risk for ventricular arrhythmia: speckle-tracking echocardiographic analysis. *J Am Soc Echocardiogr.* 2015;28:470–477.
95. Haugaa K, Grenne B, Eek C, et al. Strain echocardiography improves risk prediction of ventricular arrhythmias after myocardial infarction. *J Am Coll Cardiol Img.* 2013;6:841–850.
96. Pellikka PA, Arruda-Olson A, Chaudhry FA, et al. Guidelines for the performance, interpretation, and application of stress echocardiography in ischemic heart disease: from the American Society of Echocardiography. *J Am Soc Echocardiogr.* 2020;33:1–41.
97. Sicari R, Landi P, Picano E, et al. Exercise-electrocardiography and/or pharmacological stress echocardiography for non-invasive risk stratification early after uncomplicated myocardial infarction. A prospective international large scale multicentre study. *Eur Heart J.* 2002;23:1030–1037.
98. Varma PK, Krishna N, Jose RL, et al. Ischemic mitral regurgitation. *Ann Card Anaesth.* 2017;20:432–439.
99. Levine RA, Schwammenthal E. Ischemic mitral regurgitation on the threshold of a solution: from paradoxes to unifying concepts. *Circulation.* 2005;112:745–758.
100. Smith P, Puskas J, Ascheim D, et al. Surgical treatment of moderate ischemic mitral regurgitation. *N Engl J Med.* 2014;371:2178–2188.

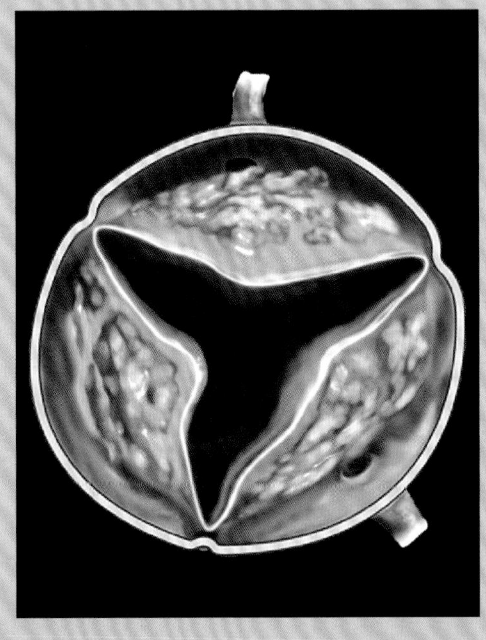

PART V
第五部分

Valvular Heart Disease
瓣膜性心脏病

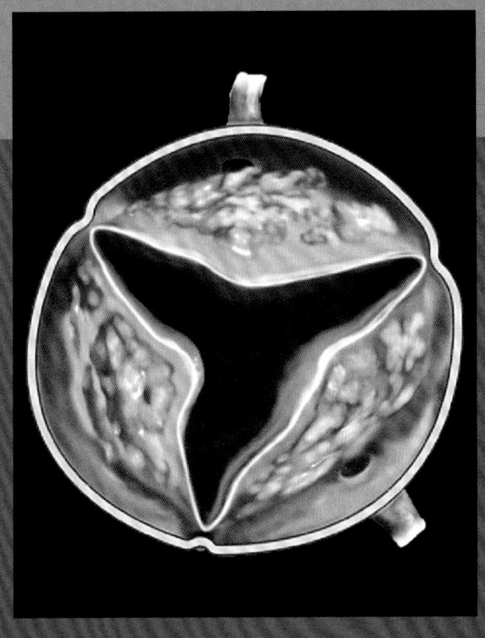

中文导读

第22章 主动脉瓣狭窄（包括经导管主动脉瓣置换术的评估）

主动脉瓣狭窄是发达国家最常见的瓣膜性心脏病。主动脉硬化是主动脉瓣狭窄的前期阶段，年龄大于65岁的老年人中约有超过25%的存在主动脉硬化，主动脉瓣狭窄的患病率随着年龄的增长而增加。本章主要从超声心动图在主动脉瓣狭窄的疾病分期、严重程度及伴发情况、瓣膜形态、血流动力学严重程度、评估的临床挑战、主动脉瓣狭窄的左心室结构和功能改变、主动脉瓣的置换时机、主动脉瓣换瓣类型的选择等多个方面的应用进行了详细介绍。

牛丽莉

22

Aortic Stenosis (Including Evaluation for Transcatheter Aortic Valve Replacement)

NIKOLAUS JANDER, MD | JAN MINNERS, MD, PhD

DISEASE STAGES

Aortic stenosis (AS) is the most common valvular heart disease in developed countries. Aortic sclerosis, the precursor of AS, occurs in more than 25% of patients older than 65 years of age. The prevalence of AS increases with age and is about 3% among patients older than 75 years of age. With an aging population, the widespread use of echocardiography, and percutaneous treatment options, referrals of patients with AS are increasing. The echocardiographic diagnosis of aortic sclerosis alone is associated with an increase of approximately 50% in the risk of death from cardiovascular causes, even in the absence of hemodynamically significant obstruction.[1]

AS in a tricuspid aortic valve is more common among elderly patients. It begins with an active disease process characterized by inflammation, lipid infiltration, and consecutive calcification; mechanisms resembling bone formation are seen in end-stage disease. A congenitally bicuspid valve morphology is a frequent cause of AS in younger patients. Irradiation of the mid-mediastinum may cause valvular dysfunction late after exposure; in such cases, AS is the most common lesion.[2] Rheumatic heart disease is rare in Europe and North America but is the most common cause of valve disease worldwide.

Patients with AS remain asymptomatic for a long period during the development from sclerosis to severe stenosis. Angina pectoris, dyspnea, and dizziness or even syncope with physical exercise are typical symptoms of severe AS and have important clinical implications independent of measures of stenosis severity.

Current guidelines recommend classification of AS by disease stage based on integration of patient symptoms, valve morphology, stenosis severity, and left ventricular (LV) function (Table 22.1).[3]

VALVE MORPHOLOGY

A normal aortic valve consists of three equally sized cusps (Fig. 22.1). Congenitally stenotic aortic valves can be unicuspid, bicuspid, or quadricuspid. Bicuspid valves, which account for most cases, are characterized by two cusps that are typically of different size; the larger cusp often contains a raphe (along the nonseparated cusps). It may be difficult to differentiate from a tricuspid aortic valve because of a prominent raphe, and assessment in the opened position is required.

The aortic valve orifice of tricuspid valves resembles a triangle or star, whereas bicuspid valves open in a lens- or slit-like shape with two edges. Systolic doming is common in a long-axis view because of the nonseparated cusps. The basal part of these cusps may demonstrate preserved mobility, potentially leading to underestimation of AS severity.

Typical rheumatic AS includes symmetric fibrosis, retraction and partial fusion of the edges of the cusps, and possibly doming during opening. Associated aortic regurgitation and mitral valve involvement are common in rheumatic disease.

A certain degree of calcification usually exists in any form of AS, although cases of congenital AS without calcification have been described. The degree of calcification can be classified as

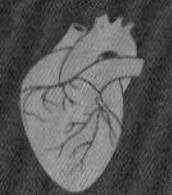

TABLE 22.1 Stages of Valvular Aortic Stenosis.

Stage	*Definition*	*Valve Anatomy*	*Valve Hemodynamics*	*Hemodynamic Consequences*
A	At risk of AS	• Bicuspid aortic valve (or congenital valve anomaly) • Aortic valve sclerosis	• Aortic V_{max} < 2 m/s	• None
B	Progressive AS	• Mild-to-moderate leaflet calcification of a bicuspid or trileaflet valve with some reduction in systolic motion **or** • Rheumatic valve changes with commissural fusion	• Mild AS V_{max} 2.0–2.9 m/s, or mean ΔP < 20 mmHg • Moderate AS V_{max} 3.0–4.0 m/s, or mean ΔP 20–40 mmHg	• Early LV diastolic may exist • Normal LVEF
C	Asymptomatic severe AS			
C1	Asymptomatic severe AS	• Severe leaflet calcification or congenital stenosis with severely reduced leaflet opening	• V_{max} > 4 m/s or mean ΔP > 40 mmHg • AVA typically < 1.0 cm^2 (or indexed AVA < 0.6 cm^2/m^2)	• LV diastolic dysfunction • Mild LV hypertrophy • Normal LVEF
C2	Asymptomatic severe AS with LV dysfunction	• Severe leaflet calcification or congenital stenosis with severely reduced leaflet opening	• V_{max} > 4 m/s or mean ΔP > 40 mmHg • AVA typically < 1.0 cm^2 (or indexed AVA < 0.6 cm^2/m^2)	• LVEF < 50%
D	Symptomatic severe AS			
D1	Symptomatic severe high-gradient AS	• Severe leaflet calcification or congenital stenosis with severely reduced leaflet opening	• V_{max} > 4 m/s or mean ΔP > 40 mmHg • AVA typically < 1.0 cm^2 (or indexed AVA < 0.6 cm^2/m^2) but may be larger with mixed AS/AR	• LV diastolic dysfunction • Mild LV hypertrophy • Pulmonary hypertension may be present
D2	Symptomatic severe low-flow/low-gradient AS with reduced LVEF	• Severe leaflet calcification with severely reduced leaflet opening	• AVA < 1.0 cm^2 with resting V_{max} ≤ 4 m/s or mean ΔP ≤ 40 mmHg • Dobutamine stress echocardiography shows AVA < 1.0 cm^2 with V_{max} > 4 m/s or mean ΔP > 40 mmHg at any flow rate	• LV diastolic dysfunction • LV hypertrophy • LVEF < 50%
D3	Symptomatic severe low-flow/low-gradient AS with normal LVEF	• Severe leaflet calcification with severely reduced leaflet opening	• AVA < 1.0 cm^2 with resting V_{max} ≤ 4 m/s or mean ΔP ≤ 40 mmHg • Indexed AVA < 0.6 cm^2/m^2 **and** • Stroke volume index < 35 mL/m^2 measured when patient is normotensive	• Increased LV relative wall thickness • Small LV chamber with low stroke volume • Restrictive diastolic filling • LVEF ≥ 50%

AR, Aortic regurgitation; *AS*, aortic stenosis; *AVA*, aortic valve area; *indexed AVA*, aortic valve area normalized to body surface area; *LVEF*, left ventricular ejection fraction; *ΔP*, pressure gradient; V_{max}, aortic maximum velocity.

Modified from Nishimura RA, Otto CM, Bonow RO, et al. 2014 AHA/ACC guideline for the management of patients with valvular heart disease: executive summary: a report of the American College of Cardiology/American Heart Association Task Force on Practice Guidelines. *J Am Coll Cardiol*. 2014;63(22):2438–2488.

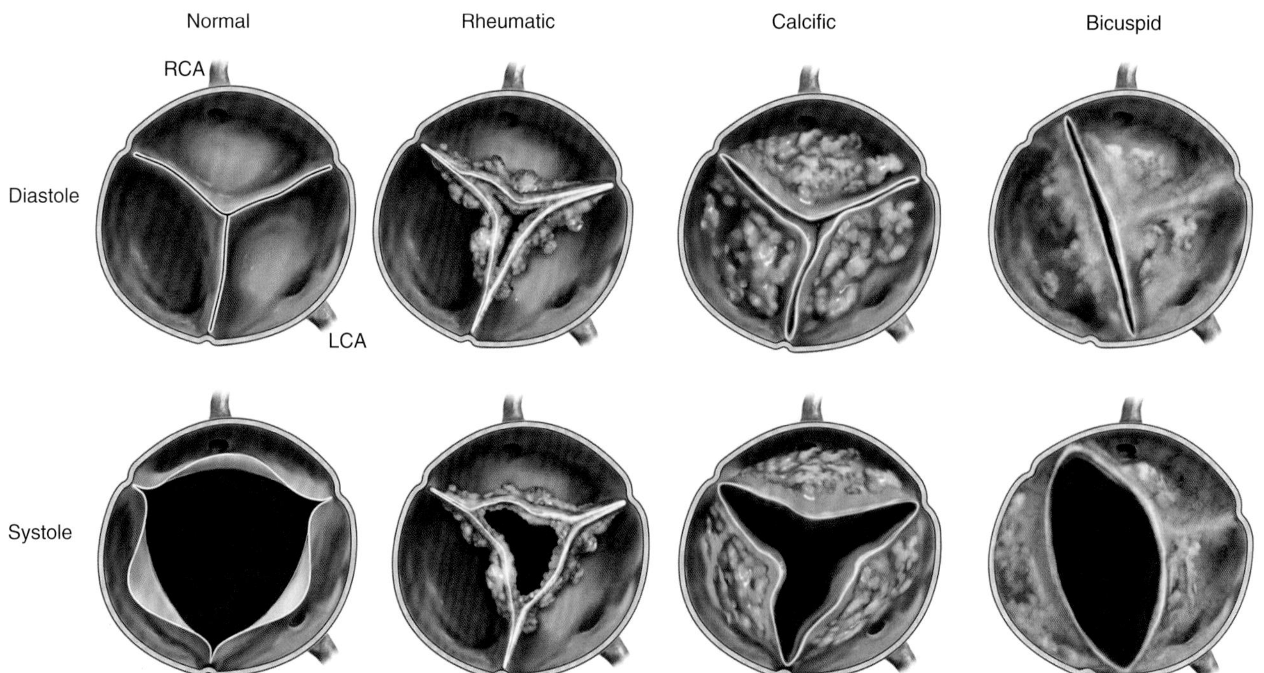

Fig. 22.1 Aortic stenosis morphology. Morphology of normal tricuspid valve; rheumatic and calcific (tricuspid) aortic stenosis; and congenital (bicuspid) aortic stenosis in diastole *(upper row)* and in systole *(lower row)*. *LCA*, Left coronary artery; *RCA*, right coronary artery.

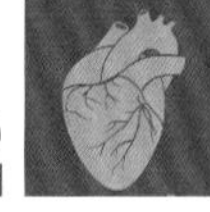

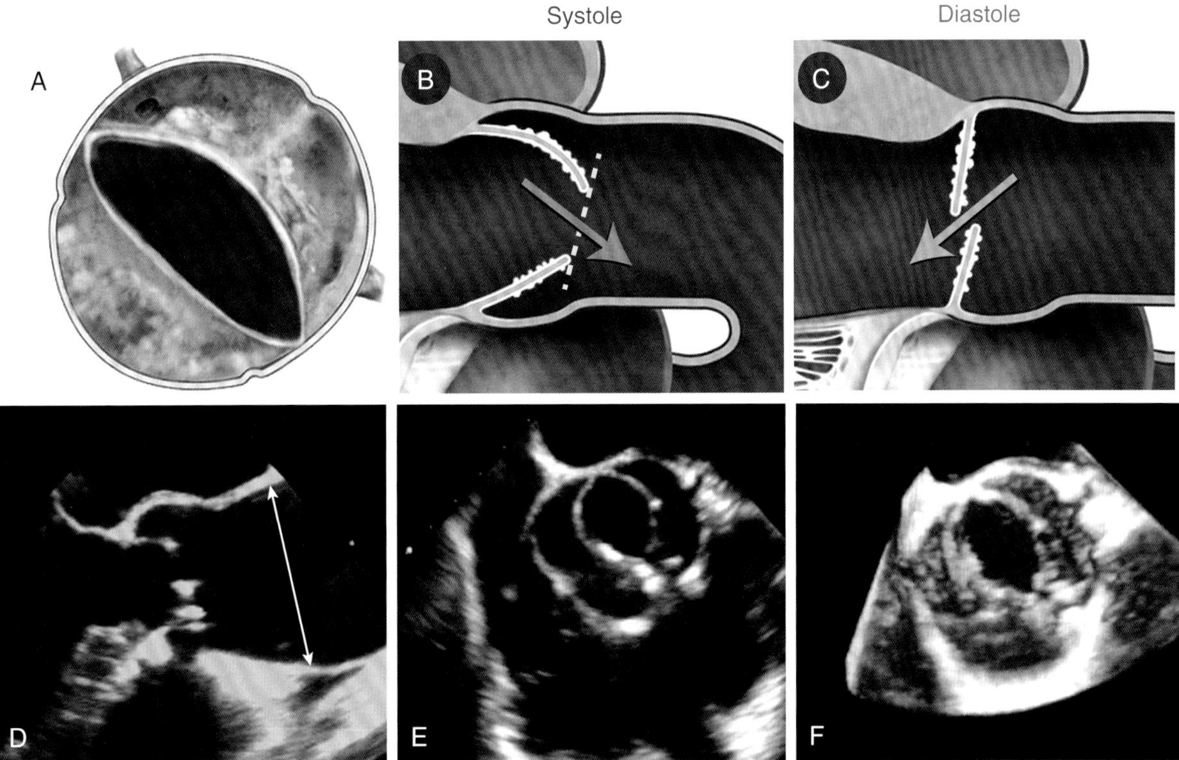

Fig. 22.2 Special features in bicuspid aortic stenosis. (A) Opening of the bicuspid valve often has a slit- or lens-like appearance. (B and C) Two cusps with different sizes account for eccentric stenotic and regurgitant jets, requiring derivation of the Doppler signal from multiple acoustic windows. (D) Because of aortic tissue abnormalities, the aortic root and/or ascending aorta are usually dilated *(arrow)*. Nonseparated cusps account for preserved basal mobility of cusps, possibly leading to underestimation of aortic stenosis severity (see Video 22.2D). Systolic doming requires meticulous inspection of the smallest orifice at the tips of cusps (E) (see Video 22.2E) and may be better appreciated with 3D technology (F) (see Video 22.2F).

mild (isolated, small spots), moderate (multiple bigger spots), or severe (extensive thickening and/or calcification of all cusps).[4] The amount of calcification predicts future cardiac events in asymptomatic patients.[4,5] In the setting of severe calcification, an exact etiologic characterization of AS may be difficult.

Aortic valve morphology is evaluated from parasternal long- and short-axis views in zoom mode. The size of the left ventricular outflow tract (LVOT) and the opening movement of the stenotic valve are best visualized in long-axis views, whereas cuspidity and degree of calcification may best be assessed in short-axis views. The transducer must sometimes be moved away from the sternum along the intercostal space and angulated to the tips of the cusps for optimal display of the stenotic orifice.

Valve morphology gives a first impression of AS severity, but direct planimetry (tracing) of the anatomic valve area is usually not possible and not recommended with a transthoracic approach. In contrast, multiplane transesophageal echocardiography (TEE) allows detailed visualization of valve morphology, differentiation of various forms of congenital AS, and assessment of the degree and distribution of calcifications.

In addition to visualization of valve anatomy on two-dimensional (2D) echocardiography, the combination of imaging and Doppler evaluation allows differentiation of valvular from subvalvular or supravalvular obstruction. Structural abnormalities of the aortic valve confirm the site of obstruction of the LVOT; however, subvalvular or midcavity obstruction is sometimes observed in combination with AS. Turbulent flow shown with color-flow Doppler in a 3- or 5-chamber view usually exhibits the site of relevant stenosis; however, a step-by-step scan along the interventricular septum from the mid-ventricle to the aortic valve with pulsed-wave (PW) Doppler may be necessary to detect consecutive sites of obstruction.

Dilation of the aortic root and ascending aorta is common in patients with AS. Measurements in several long-axis views following the ascending aorta are required (Fig. 22.2).

HEMODYNAMIC SEVERITY

Aortic maximum velocity (V_{max}), mean pressure gradient, and aortic valve area (AVA) are the most important parameters used to assess AS severity, and they should be assessed in all patients with AS.[3,6,7] Three measurements are required to obtain these parameters: aortic velocity within the stenotic valve, prestenotic velocity (i.e., flow velocity in the LVOT just below the aortic valve), and LVOT diameter. The same measurements are used to calculate stroke volume and the velocity ratio, which become important parameters for assessing hemodynamic severity in special circumstances (Figs. 22.3 and 22.4).

AORTIC VELOCITY AND MEAN PRESSURE GRADIENT

The antegrade systolic velocity across the stenotic valve is measured with the use of continuous-wave (CW) Doppler imaging. To obtain the maximum velocity signal, parallel alignment of the Doppler beam with the stenotic jet is mandatory, and multiple acoustic windows must be used. Color flow may help to

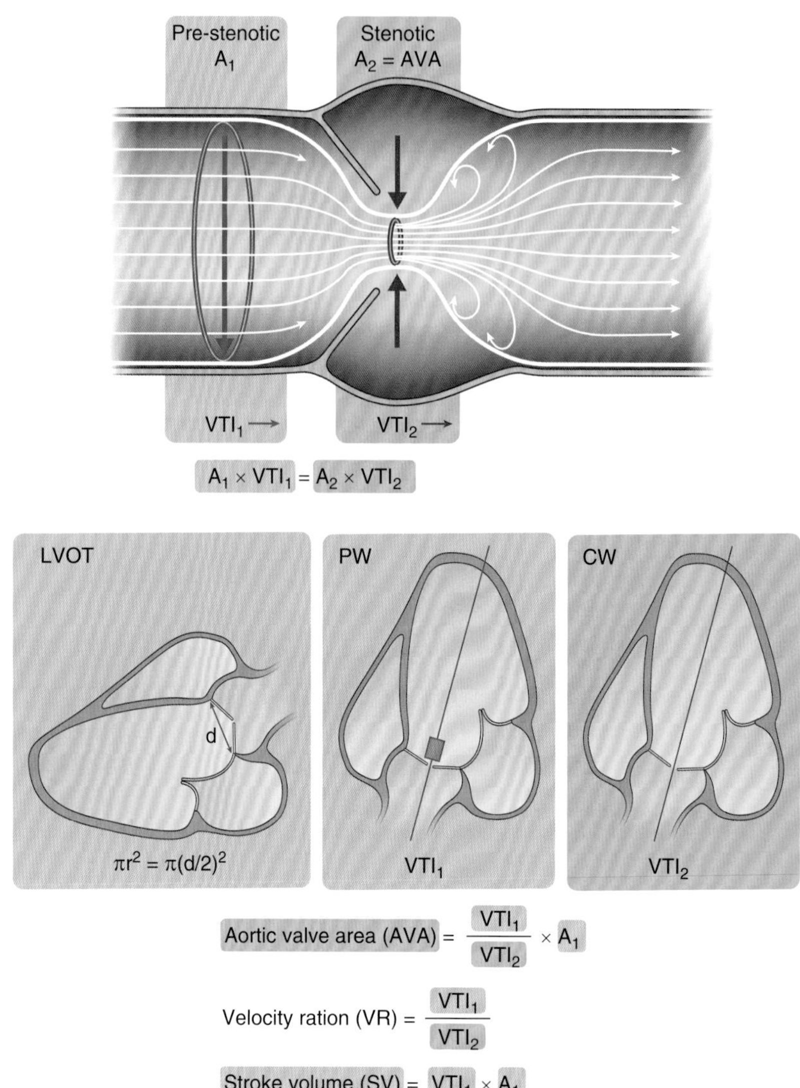

Fig. 22.3 Continuity equation and relationship between aortic valve area, velocity ratio, and stroke volume. The continuity equation states that the flow across the left ventricular outflow tract *(LVOT)* is equal to that across the stenotic aortic valve. Pre-stenotic velocity-time-integral *(VTI)* in the LVOT is measured by pulsed-wave Doppler and stenotic VTI in the aortic valve by CW Doppler. Stroke volume (in mL), as a surrogate marker of flow, in both locations is determined by the product of the area and the VTI of the systolic signal. LVOT area *(A_1)* is derived from the diameter *(d)* using the formula for the area of a circle. The final term, aortic valve area (*A_2 or AVA*), is calculated from A_1, VTI_1, and VTI_2. Velocity ratio and stroke volume are derived from the same measurements. AVA always comprises information about stroke volume; accordingly, measurement error (typically underestimation of LVOT size) results in a double error underestimating the AVA and stroke volume. Likewise, because velocity ratio provides information about the ratio of AVA to LVOT area, it ideally may be used as an individual parameter of aortic stenosis severity in follow-up examinations when LVOT size can be considered constant.

identify jet direction, but the three-dimensional (3D) orientation of the jet may be unpredictable.

Starting with an apical 5-chamber view, the transducer position is modified in such a way that the Doppler beam is truly parallel to the orientation of the LVOT, including positions somewhat dorsal and lateral to the apex. Gain is decreased, wall filter is high, sweep velocity is maximal, and baseline and scale are optimized to display a clear, smooth signal filling the vertical dimension of the monitor. Frayed signals with blurred borders or peak should be neglected.

Next, multiple right parasternal windows are located with the patient lying on the right side (Fig. 22.5). Color flow is helpful for orientation of the Doppler beam parallel to the jet. Sometimes, a dedicated stand-alone CW Doppler transducer is required to allow unusual positioning and angulation. Rarely, additional acoustic windows (i.e., suprasternal, left parasternal, or subcostal) are necessary.

A meticulous search for the maximum velocity is extremely important to avoid underestimation of AS severity, particularly when morphologic changes or clinical symptoms do not match the recorded velocity. The transducer position in which the highest velocity was recorded should be documented in the report for future studies. Aortic maximum velocity (peak velocity) is measured at the peak of the recorded signal. Post-extrasystolic beats should be neglected, and averaging of at least five beats is mandatory in patients with atrial fibrillation (Fig. 22.6).

Aortic maximum velocity may be directly transformed into maximum gradient by the simplified Bernoulli equation:

$$\Delta P = 4V_2^2$$

where ΔP = pressure gradient, and V_2 = peak velocity of the stenotic jet. The original Bernoulli equation is a complex formula describing the general relation between velocity and gradient in stenotic lesions, taking into account (among other parameters)

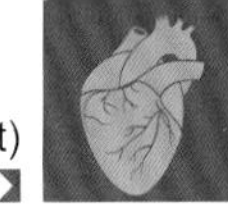

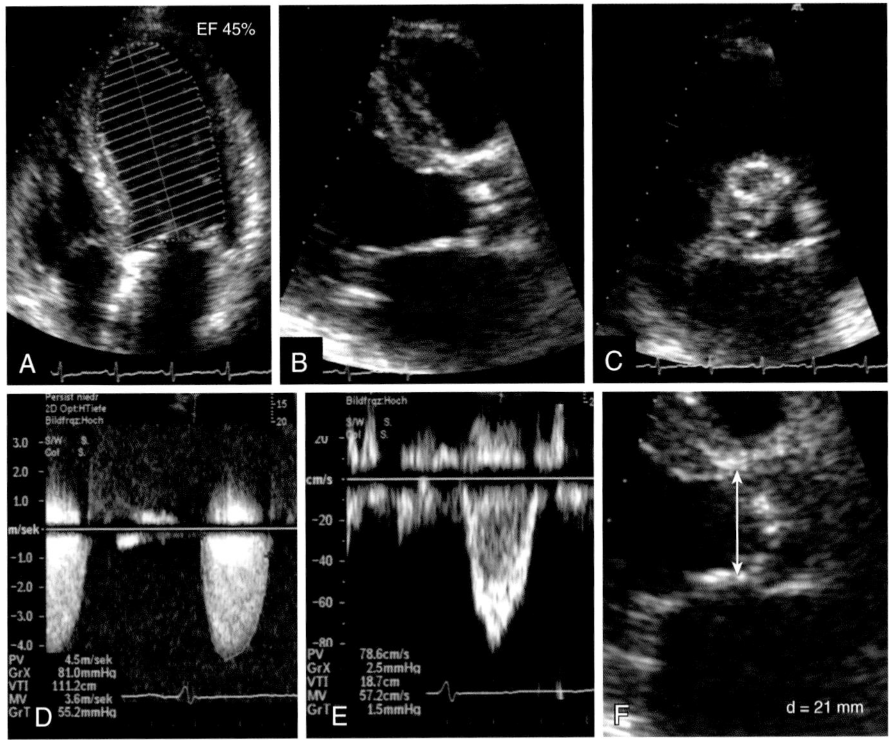

Fig. 22.4 Assessment of aortic stenosis severity. (A) The Simpson method is used to assess LV function by ejection fraction *(EF)*. (B) The long-axis view is used to assess the morphology, degree of calcification, and opening movement (see Video 22.4B ▶). (C) The short-axis view further assesses morphology and the number of cusps (see Video 22.4C ▶). (D) CW Doppler measures peak velocity, mean gradient, and the aortic velocity–time integral (VTI). (E) Pulsed-wave Doppler is used to measure pre-stenotic velocity and the VTI in the LV outflow tract (LVOT). (F) LVOT diameter *(d, double-headed arrow)* in zoom mode is used to calculate LVOT area. Images show a severely stenosed calcified tricuspid aortic valve with a mean gradient of 55 mmHg, a calculated aortic valve area of 0.6 cm^2, and a reduced ejection fraction of 45%.

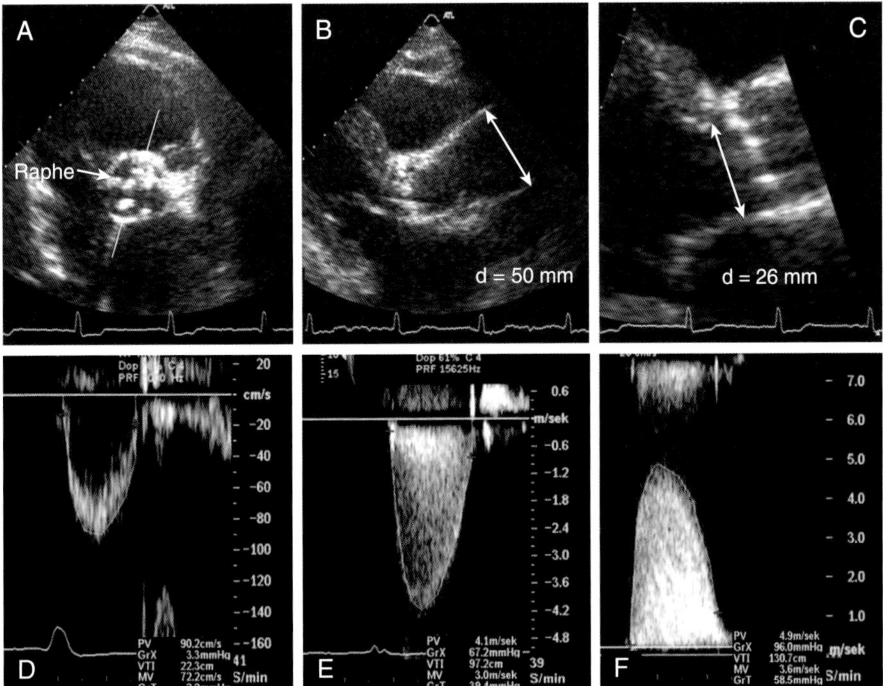

Fig. 22.5 Severe bicuspid aortic stenosis. (A) Short-axis view of the aortic valve shows severe calcification with a slit-like systolic orifice and a raphe *(fusion line)* between the right and noncoronary cusps (see Video 22.5A ▶). (B) Dilated ascending aorta *(double-headed arrow)*. (C) Long-axis view in zoom mode measures LV outflow tract (LVOT) diameter *(d, double-headed arrow)*. (D) Pulsed-wave Doppler image of LVOT near the aortic valve. (E) CW Doppler of the aortic valve from an apical window (mean gradient, 39 mmHg). (F) CW Doppler of the aortic valve from a right parasternal window shows higher velocities (mean gradient, 59 mmHg). Aortic valve area is calculated at 0.9 cm^2.

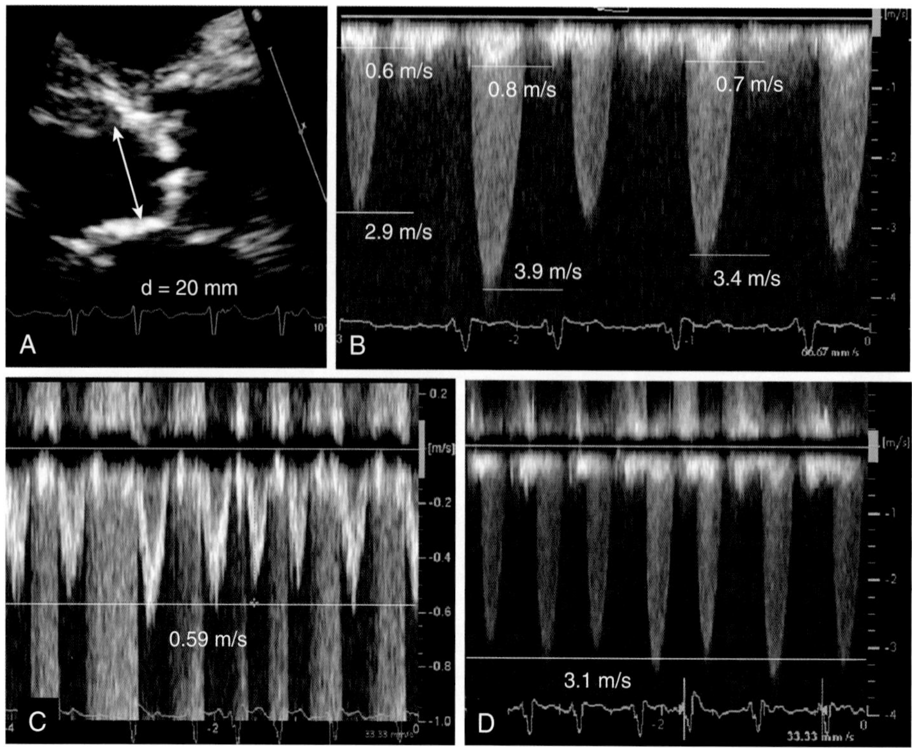

Fig. 22.6 Assessment of aortic stenosis severity in atrial fibrillation. (A) LV outflow tract is measured in zoom mode at mid-systole. (B) Instant peak velocities of pre-stenotic and stenotic velocity may be estimated from CW Doppler. (C and D) Maximum velocity of pre-stenotic and stenotic velocity may be also estimated from the mean of 5 to 10 consecutive beats. Velocity ratio (i.e., the ratio of pre-stenotic and stenotic velocities) is used to calculate aortic valve area (0.6 cm^2 in this case). *d*, Diameter of outflow tract.

flow acceleration and viscous losses that can be neglected in clinical practice. However, the more accurate formula considering pre-stenotic velocity may be sometimes more appropriate:

$$\Delta P = 4\left(V_2^2 - V_1^2\right)$$

where ΔP = pressure gradient, V_2 = peak velocity of the stenotic jet, and V_1 = pre-stenotic velocity. This equation should be used when V_1 is greater than 1.2 m/s.

Mean velocity and velocity–time integral (VTI) are obtained by tracing the outer envelope of the signal. The mean of multiple instant velocities (i.e., mean velocity) is calculated and then integrated over time (VTI). The VTI is used for calculation of AVA by the *continuity equation*. Mean gradient is calculated by averaging the instantaneous gradients over the systolic ejection period derived from the simplified Bernoulli equation, neglecting pre-stenotic velocities.

Aortic maximum velocity and mean pressure gradient are directly derived from the same CW Doppler signal and are closely correlated (Fig. 22.7). The information derived from the two parameters may be considered equivalent, with an aortic maximum velocity of greater than 4 m/s and a mean gradient greater than 40 mmHg indicating severe AS.

Aortic maximum velocity (i.e., peak velocity) is the best validated parameter related to outcomes of patients with AS. A gradual increase of clinical events has been demonstrated with increasing aortic maximum velocity in asymptomatic patients (Fig. 22.8 and Tables 22.2 and 22.3).[8,9] With peak velocities greater than 4 m/s, 1-year event rates rise substantially, providing a clinical rationale for the currently accepted partition value for severe stenosis. Rapid progression of peak velocity (>0.3 m/s per year) has been identified as a marker for future adverse events. A more rapid progression is seen in patients with higher degrees of calcification and valve obstruction and in patients with coronary heart disease.[10]

CONTINUITY EQUATION AORTIC VALVE AREA

If LV function and output are reduced, additional, less flow-dependent parameters to define AS severity are required.[11] To this end, AVA is calculated from the continuity equation, which is based on the consideration that the same stroke volume passes through the LVOT and the aortic valve (see Figs. 22.3 and 22.4). Stroke volume in echocardiography is measured as the product of the VTI of flow and the cross-sectional area; therefore, the equation is

$$A_1 \times VTI_1 = A_2 \times VTI_2$$

where A_1 = LVOT area; VTI_1 = pre-stenotic VTI of flow within the LVOT; A_2 = AVA; and VTI_2 = VTI of the stenotic jet through the aortic valve. Measurement of A_1 and VTI_1 is described later. Three of the four components of the continuity equation can be measured directly, and AVA can be calculated as follows:

$$AVA = A_2 = A_1 \times VTI_1 / VTI_2$$

Because the ejection times of flow within the LVOT and through the aortic valve are considered equal, the maximum (or mean) velocities may be used instead of VTIs, further simplifying the equation:

$$AVA = A_2 = A_1 \times V_1 / V_2$$

Use of maximum velocities results in a slightly higher AVA than when mean velocities are used because the former reflect the largest possible AVA at maximum flow, whereas mean velocities yield an average AVA over the whole systolic period.

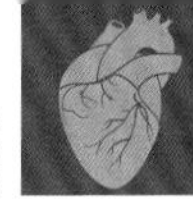

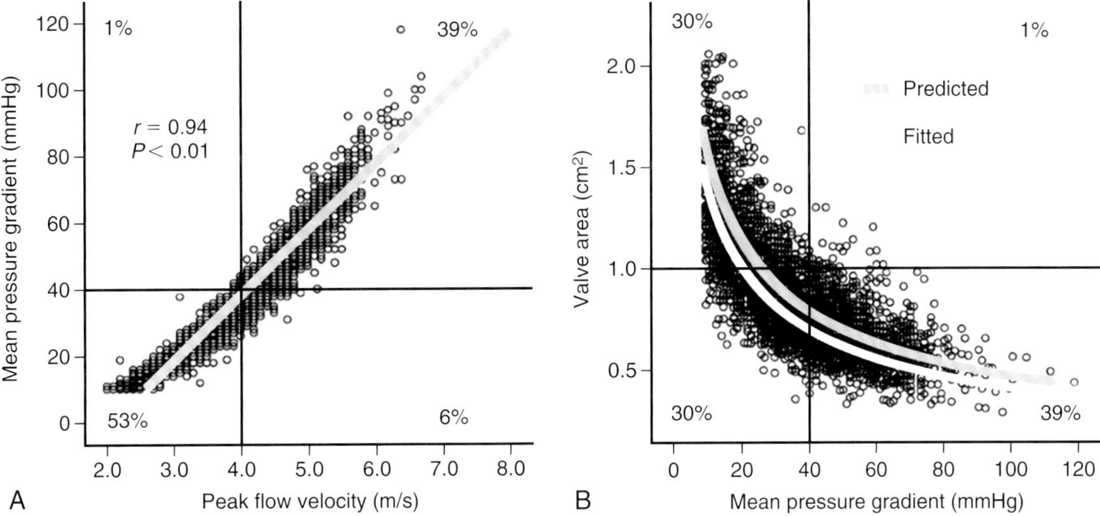

Fig. 22.7 Correlation of parameters for aortic stenosis severity in patients with a normal ejection fraction. (A) Strong correlation between aortic maximum velocity (peak flow velocity) and mean pressure gradient almost exactly crosses the point of both partition values for defining severe aortic stenosis (4 m/s for aortic maximum velocity and 40 mmHg for mean pressure gradient). (B) Relationship between aortic valve area (AVA) and mean pressure gradient (*Fitted* curve) shows that 30% of patients have discordant estimation of aortic stenosis severity (AVA < 1.0 cm^2 and mean pressure gradient ≤ 40 mmHg). For comparison, the related curve derived from the Gorlin formula *(Predicted)*, which presumes normal cardiac output (6 L/min, heart rate 75 beats/min) is shown. (From Minners J, Allgeier M, Gohlke-Baerwolf C, et al. Inconsistencies of echocardiographic criteria for the grading of aortic valve stenosis. *Eur Heart J.* 2008;29;1043–1048.)

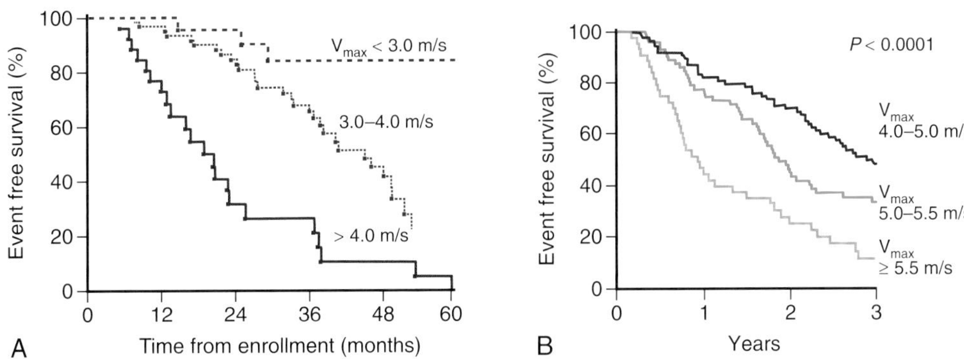

Fig. 22.8 Outcome in asymptomatic patients with aortic stenosis according to velocity. Two landmark studies by Otto et al.[8] (A) and Rosenhek et al.[9] (B) showed a gradual increase of future clinical events with increasing peak velocity. (Modified from Otto CM, et al. Prospective study of asymptomatic valvular aortic stenosis. Clinical, echocardiographic, and exercise predictors of outcome. *Circulation.* 1997;95:2262–2270; and Rosenhek R, et al. Natural history of very severe aortic stenosis. *Circulation.* 2010;121:151–156.)

To account for differences in body surface area (BSA), an indexed AVA (AVAi) may be calculated:

$$\text{AVAi} = \text{AVA/BSA}$$

Severe AS is indicated by an AVA smaller than 1.0 cm^2 or an AVAi smaller than 0.6 cm^2/m^2.

LV Outflow Tract Velocity

The pre-stenotic velocity V_1 is measured within the LVOT using PW Doppler in an apical 5-chamber or 3-chamber view. The transducer position should be optimized in such a way that the Doppler beam is truly parallel to the orientation of the LVOT and includes positions somewhat dorsal and lateral to the apex. Gain is decreased, wall filter is low, sweep velocity is maximal, and baseline and scale are optimized to display a clear, smooth, and laminar flow signal filling the vertical dimension of the monitor. An optimal laminar flow signal shows no spectral dispersion, with a sharp rim and a black center.

The sample volume should be placed as close to the aortic valve as possible. The correct position of the sample volume can be reached by moving it slowly from the aortic valve into the LVOT while the flow signal is changing from turbulent to laminar; the first position with laminar flow is used for measurements.

Mean velocity and VTI are obtained by tracing the outer envelope of the signal. As with aortic velocity, the mean of multiple instant velocities is calculated (mean velocity) and integrated over time (VTI). The VTI_1 is used for the calculation of AVA. It is also required for the calculation of stroke volume (see Fig. 22.3). The correctness of LVOT velocity may be checked by identifying its maximal velocity within the CW signal or with color Doppler (Fig. 22.9).

LV Outflow Tract Diameter

The LVOT diameter is measured in a zoomed parasternal long-axis view at mid-systole (the time of its maximal size). Several attempts may be necessary to obtain the maximal anterior-posterior diameter. Measurements should be performed as close to the aortic valve as possible (reflecting the position of the sample volume used for recording pre-stenotic LVOT velocity), from inner edge to inner edge of the septal wall to the fibrous

TABLE 22.2 Comparison of Guideline Recommendations for Aortic Valve Replacement in Patients With Aortic Stenosis (AS)[a]

AHA/ACC (2020)[3]	*ESC/EACTS (2017)*[6,7]
Cut-Off Values to Define Severe AS	
V_{max} ≥ 4 m/s	V_{max} ≥ 4 m/s
Mean pressure gradient ≥40 mmHg	Mean pressure gradient ≥40 mmHg
AVA ≤1.0 cm²	AVA < 1.0 cm²
Indexed AVA ≤0.6 cm²/m²	Indexed AVA <0.6 cm²/m²
Velocity ratio ≤ 0.25	Velocity ratio <0.25
LV dysfunction: Ejection fraction <50%	LV dysfunction: Ejection fraction <50%
"Low-flow": Stroke volume index <35 mL/m²	"Low-flow": Stroke volume index <35 mL/m²
Symptomatic Patients	
Severe high-gradient AS and AS related symptoms (1,A)	Severe high-gradient AS and AS related symptoms (I,B)
Severe high-gradient AS and symptoms on exercise (1,A)	Severe AS and AS related symptoms on exercise (I,C)
Low-flow/low-gradient severe AS with reduced EF (1,B)	Low-flow/low-gradient AS with reduced EF and evidence of flow reserve excluding pseudosevere AS (I,C)
Dobutamine testing and/or CT calcium score for diagnosis is reasonable in low-flow/low-gradient AS with reduced EF (2a,B)	Low-flow/low-gradient AS with reduced EF without evidence of flow reserve when CT calcium scoring confirms severe AS (IIa,C)
Low-flow/low-gradient severe AS with normal EF, if AS is the most likely cause of symptoms (1,B)	Low-flow/low-gradient AS with normal EF after careful confirmation of severe AS (IIa,C)
Asymptomatic Patients	
Severe AS and EF <50% (1,B)	Severe AS and EF <50% not due to another cause (I,C)
Severe AS and decreased exercise tolerance or blood pressure fall (≥10 mmHg from baseline) on exercise (2a,B)	Severe AS and blood pressure decrease below baseline (IIa,C)
V_{max} ≥5.0 m/s and low surgical risk (2a,B)	V_{max} >5.5 m/s and low surgical risk (IIa,C)
High gradient, severe AS with rapid progression (≥0.3 m/s per year) and low surgical risk (2a,B)	Severe AS, severe calcification with rapid progression (≥0.3 m/s per year) and low surgical risk (IIa,C)
Severe AS, markedly elevated BNP (> 3 times normal) and low surgical risk (2a,B)	Severe AS, markedly elevated BNP (> 3 times normal) and low surgical risk (IIa,C)
Severe AS and progressive decrease of ejection fraction <60% on at least three serial measurements (2b,B)	Severe AS with systolic pulmonary artery pressure >60 mmHg confirmed by invasive measurement (IIa,C)
Patients Undergoing Other Cardiac Surgery	
Severe AS and other cardiac surgery (1,B)	Severe AS and other cardiac surgery (I,C)
Moderate AS and other cardiac surgery (2b,C)	Moderate AS and other cardiac surgery after Heart Team decision (IIa,C)

[a]Recommendation class: *I or 1*, Is indicated; *IIa or 2a*, is reasonable; *IIb or 2b*, may be reasonable. Level of evidence: *A*, High-quality evidence; *B*, moderate quality of evidence; *C*, observational studies or expert opinion.

ACC, American College of Cardiology; *AHA*, American Heart Association; *AS*, aortic stenosis; *AVA*, aortic valve area; *BNP*, B-type natriuretic peptide; *EACTS*, European Association for Cardio-Thoracic Surgery; *EF*, ejection fraction; *ESC*, European Society of Cardiology; *CT*, computed tomography; *indexed AVA*, aortic valve area normalized to body surface area; V_{max}, aortic maximum velocity.

TABLE 22.3 Selected Studies Investigating Hemodynamic Progression of Valvular Aortic Stenosis.

Study	*Year*	*Type of Study*	*Clinical Status at Entry*	N	*Mean Follow-up (y)*	*Increase in Mean ΔP (mmHg/y)*[a]	*Increase in V_{max} (m/s per year)*[a]	*Decrease in AVA (cm²/y)*[a]
Otto et al.[91]	1989	Prospective	Asymptomatic	42	1.7	8 (−7 to 23)	0.36 ± 0.31	0.1 (0–0.5)
Otto et al.[8]	1997	Prospective	Asymptomatic	123	2.5	7 ± 7	0.32 ± 0.34	0.12 ± 0.19
Rosenhek et al.[4]	2000	Prospective	V_{max} > 4.0 m/s	128	1.8	Slow Rapid	0.14 ± 0.18 0.45 ± 0.38	— —
Rosenhek et al.[10]	2004	Retrospective	V_{max} 2.5–3.9 m/s	176	3.8	—	0.24 ± 0.30	—
Rossebø et al.[92,a]	2008	Prospective	V_{max} 2.5–4.0 m/s	1873	5.4	Statin 2.7 ± 0.1 No statin 2.8 ± 0.1	0.15 ± 0.01 0.16 ± 0.01	0.03 ± 0.01 0.03 ± 0.01
Tastet et al.[93]	2017	Prospective	AS on echo	323	2.3	3 (median)	—	—

[a]Data expressed as mean ± standard error.

AS, Aortic stenosis; *AVA*, aortic valve area; *ΔP*, pressure gradient; *echo*, echocardiography; V_{max}, peak aortic jet velocity.

aortic-mitral continuity parallel to the aortic valve. Optimal image quality is necessary to correctly identify tissue–blood interfaces. Localized calcification protruding to the LVOT should be excluded from the measurement (Fig. 22.10). LVOT area is calculated as follows:

$$A_1 = \pi r^2$$

where A_1 = area of LVOT, and r = radius (= diameter/2). LVOT area is required for the calculation of AVA and stroke volume. The AVA has been linked to outcomes for patients with AS, but its gradual impact on prognosis is less strong than with peak velocity in asymptomatic patients (see Table 22.3). However, the assessment of AVA is mandatory to estimate AS severity in any situation when flow is out of the normal range.

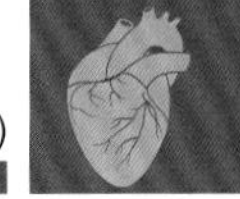

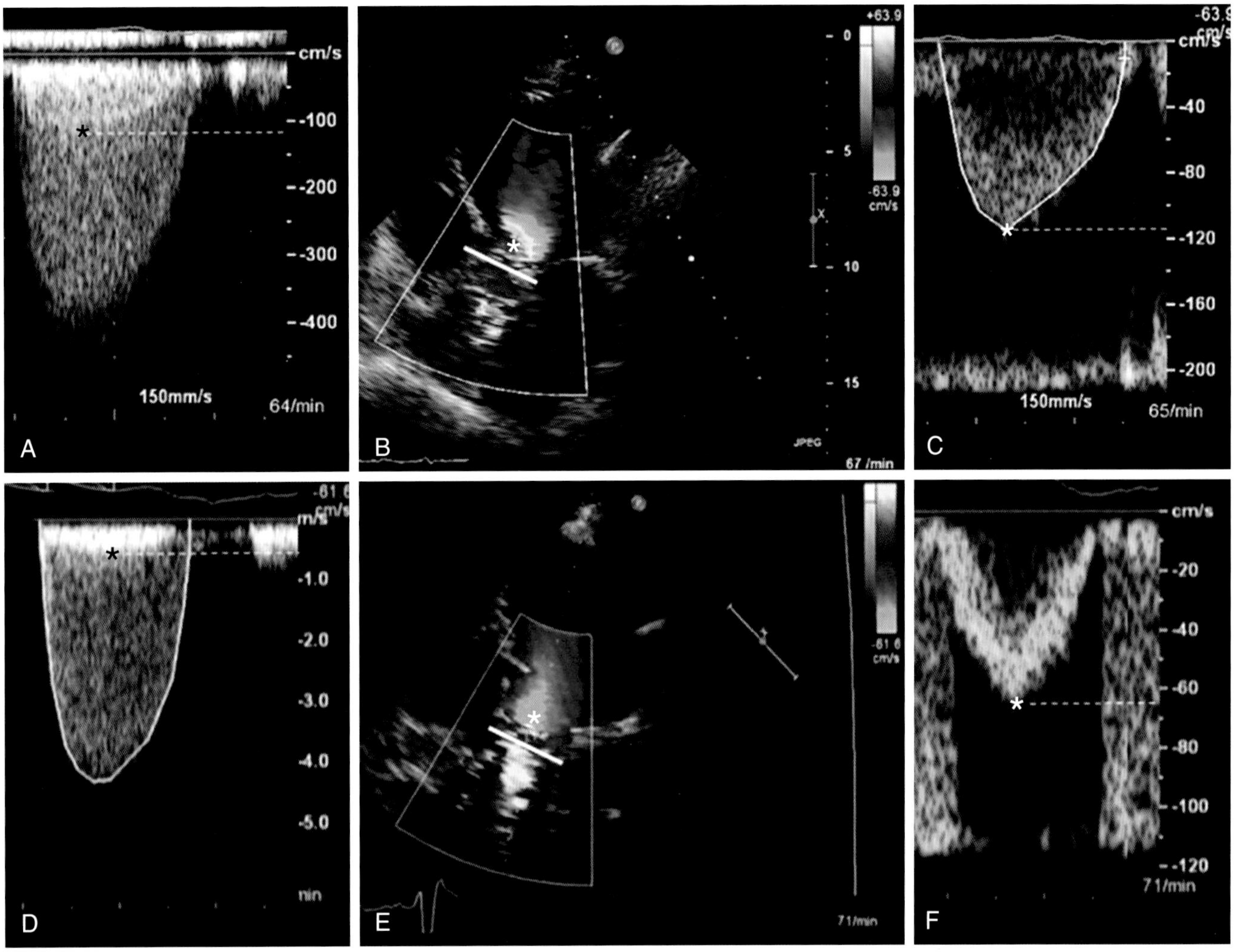

Fig. 22.9 **Possibilities to check correctness of pre-stenotic velocity.** Maximum left ventricular outflow tract (LVOT) velocity of about 1.1 cm/s, estimated by the bright signal within the CW signal *(black asterisk)* (A) and augmented pre-stenotic flow with color *(white asterisk)* (B) (see Video 22.9B), is confirmed by pulsed-wave (PW) Doppler *(white asterisk)* (C). In another patient, maximum LVOT velocity of about 0.6 cm/s is estimated by the bright signal within the CW signal *(black asterisk)* (D) (see Video 22.9E) and by low pre-stenotic flow (no aliasing) with color *(white asterisk)* (E) and confirmed by PW Doppler *(white asterisk)* (F).

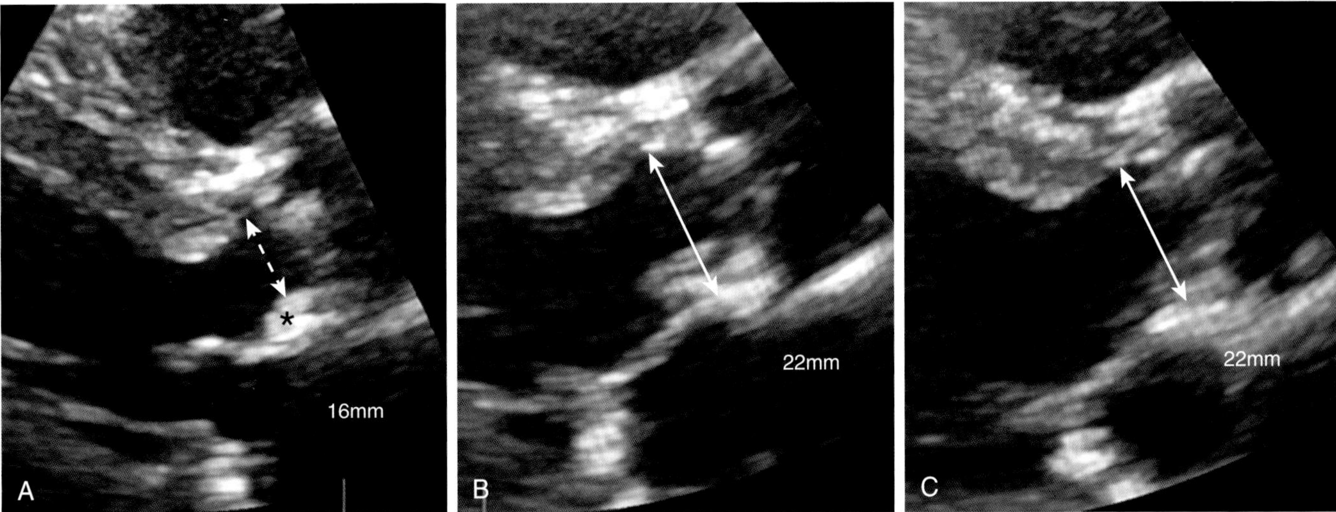

Fig. 22.10 **Correct measurement of LV outflow tract diameter.** (A) A localized calcification *(black asterisk)* protrudes into the LV outflow tract (LVOT) (see Video 22.10A). Measurement of LVOT diameter *(double-headed arrow)* should avoid the calcification because it is not representative of the circumferential LVOT size. (B and C) Possibilities for measurement of a more correct LVOT *(double-headed arrow)* very close to the calcification (see Video 22.10B).

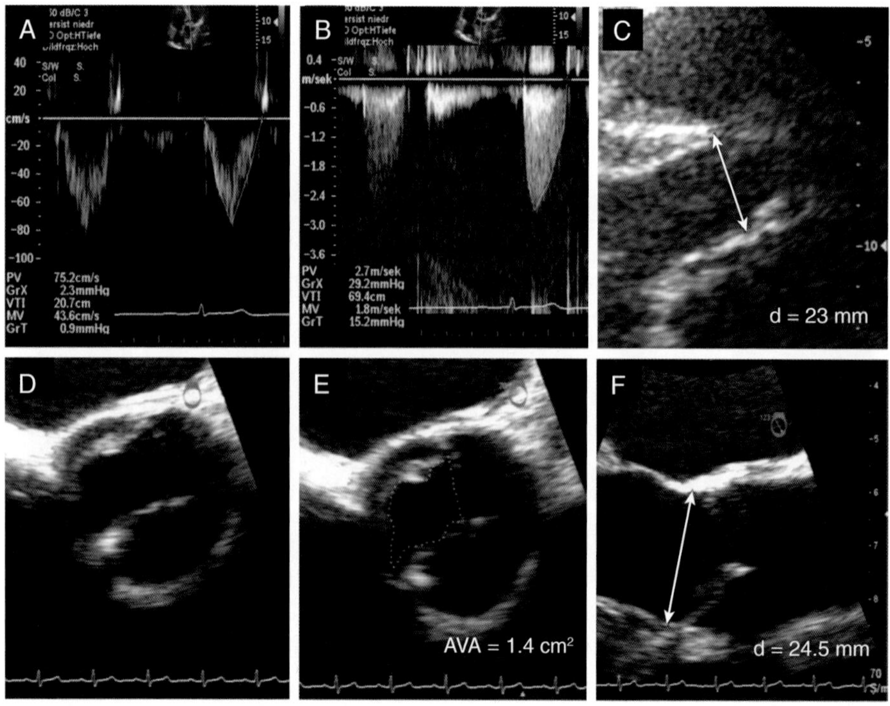

Fig. 22.11 Rheumatic aortic stenosis. A 55-year-old patient with severe rheumatic mitral stenosis and concomitant aortic stenosis. (A) Pulsed-wave Doppler image of the left ventricular outflow tract (LVOT). (B) Continuous-wave Doppler image of the aortic valve. (C) LVOT diameter *(d)* in zoom mode *(double-headed arrow)*. The calculated aortic valve area *(AVA)* is 1.2 cm^2. (D) TEE (see Videos 22.11D1 and 22.11D2) shows fusion of left and right coronary cusps. (E) AVA on TEE. (F) TEE long-axis view to remeasure LVOT diameter *(d)*. The calculated AVA with remeasured LVOT diameter is 1.4 cm^2.

STROKE VOLUME INDEX

Reduced transvalvular flow may occur in patients with apparently normal systolic LV function, and stroke volume index (SVI) has become an important parameter in evaluating AS severity. Low-flow/low-gradient severe AS with preserved ejection fraction (EF) is considered a distinct presentation of severe AS (stage D3) with a unique pathway of concentric LV remodeling.[12,13]

Stroke volume is calculated from the product of the pre-stenotic VTI and the LVOT area and is usually indexed to BSA. An SVI at rest of at least 35 mL/m^2 is considered normal, whereas an SVI of less than 35 mL/m^2 implies low flow.

AVA and stroke volume are calculated using the measurements of pre-stenotic VTI and LVOT diameter volume (see Fig. 22.3). The AVA always contains information on stroke volume. For this reason, measurement error, typically underestimation of the LVOT diameter, results in underestimation of the AVA and stroke volume. Stroke volume should be checked using 2D or 3D ventricular volumes. Concordance of Doppler and anatomic stroke volume may provide more robust evidence of a low-flow state. Indirect signs, including atrial fibrillation, severe hypertrophy, and mitral or tricuspid regurgitation, may help to confirm reduced transvalvular flow.

VELOCITY RATIO

Calculation of LVOT area is a problem for AVA assessment because interobserver reproducibility of the LVOT diameter measurement is low and because the LVOT anatomy is oval rather than circular. The velocity ratio (VR), based on maximal pre-stenotic and stenotic velocities or VTIs, has been used as a simplified measure of AS severity that is less flow dependent than aortic maximum velocity or mean pressure gradient:

$$VR = V_1/V_2 = VTI_1/VTI_2$$

Neglecting LVOT size is a limitation for small and very large LVOTs.[14] However, VR is a helpful parameter in the longitudinal follow-up of patients because the LVOT size in an individual can be expected to remain constant over time. A velocity ratio smaller than 0.25 indicates severe stenosis.

VR based on maximal velocities can frequently be estimated directly from the CW Doppler signal because the pre-stenotic velocity is apparent as a bright area at its base. The VR may be used as a control for the measurement of pre-stenotic velocity in general, but it becomes essential in patients with atrial fibrillation, when subsequent beats vary widely and VR is otherwise difficult to assess (see Fig. 22.6). In that case, at least five simultaneous VR values are calculated from different CW Doppler signals. VR, as part of the continuity equation, may then be used to calculate the AVA in atrial fibrillation.

VR can be used to predict clinical outcomes in asymptomatic patients and to address discrepancies between echocardiographic parameters of AS severity. However, it does not outperform peak velocity or mean gradient as a prognostic marker.[15,16]

TEE PLANIMETRY VALVE AREA

Multiplane TEE allows detailed visualization of valve morphology. Planimetry (i.e., tracing of the anatomic AVA) can be performed in most cases and may be very useful in the context of discrepancies between hemodynamic parameters of stenosis severity in patients with moderate to severe stenosis on transthoracic evaluation. Even without direct measurement of the anatomic AVA, valve morphology provides some information on AS severity.

For planimetry, the aortic valve is displayed in the center of an exact long-axis view, which is the basis for a zoomed short-axis view perpendicular to it. Image parameters are adjusted carefully. Exact recognition of tissue–blood borders in moving loops is a prerequisite for adequate tracing in frozen images (Fig. 22.11).

The anatomic AVA is traced in mid-systole, and several measurements may be required, particularly when there is severe calcification. In bicuspid valves with domed morphology, the maximum flow restriction occurs at the tip of the cusps, and meticulous inspection of the smallest orifice in short-axis views at the highest point in direction of flow is mandatory to avoid overestimation of anatomic AVA. Synchronous display of two perpendicular planes may help to define the appropriate short-axis view for planimetry.

TEE enables a clear delineation of LVOT morphology, which can be difficult to assess in transthoracic echocardiographic (TTE) views. The LVOT is displayed, and its diameter is measured as described for the transthoracic approach. This may be helpful in the setting of additional LVOT obstruction due to a fibrous membrane or a systolic anterior movement (SAM) of parts of the mitral valve. Most importantly, it allows remeasurement of the LVOT diameter in excellent image quality and may therefore serve as a control for TTE assessment and recalculation of the AVA by combining the TTE Doppler parameters with the LVOT diameter from TEE if necessary (see Fig. 22.11).

Modern matrix-array transducers capture real-time volume-rendering images and allow off-line volumetric quantification from a 3D data set. This may help to define anatomic AVA with TEE in difficult cases (e.g., bicuspid valves; see Fig. 22.2). Despite remaining limitations due to severe calcifications, the overall feasibility of this approach was shown to be good.[17]

CLINICAL CHALLENGES IN ASSESSMENT OF AORTIC STENOSIS SEVERITY

MEASUREMENT VARIABILITY AND ERRORS

Aortic maximum velocity and mean pressure gradient are robust measures of AS severity when the maximal jet velocity has been successfully identified from multiple acoustic windows (see Fig. 22.5). Intraobserver and interobserver variability in the assessment of Doppler recordings and measurements are high (coefficient of correlation = 0.9, coefficient of variation, 3.7%–7.7%).[18] The continuity equation yields reliable values for AVA (provided all its components have been assessed correctly) and represents the second most important measure of AS severity, with higher variability due to more complex measurements.

Pre-stenotic flow tends to be overestimated because Doppler echocardiography measures flow velocity at the center of the LVOT, erroneously assuming a homogeneous and flat velocity profile. However, the LVOT area is commonly underestimated because of its oval shape, with the shorter anterior-posterior diameter measured in 2D echocardiography. It has been suggested that slight overestimation of pre-stenotic flow may be compensated by slight underestimation of LVOT area.[19,20]

The most important measurement errors are Doppler misalignment with aortic flow, caused by not using multiple windows (see Fig. 22.5), and underestimation of LVOT diameter, caused by not carefully searching for the widest anterior-posterior distance (see Fig. 22.10). LVOT velocity should always be checked for correctness (see Fig. 22.9).

EFFECT OF TRANSAORTIC FLOW

Aortic maximum velocity and mean pressure gradient are extremely flow dependent. Low-flow and high-flow states have to be considered when interpreting these measures with respect to AS severity because they can result in a gradient that is lower or higher, respectively, than that expected from the calculated AVA. Up to 30% of patients with AS present with low-flow states and reduced or normal EF. Recent guidelines[3,6,7] recommend the assessment of SVI to identify these patients, with a cutoff value of 35 mL/m^2 or less. High flow may be seen in up to 15% of patients, including those with aortic regurgitation, end-stage renal failure, arteriovenous fistula, fever, or anemia, but occasionally the reason may be unidentifiable.[21] A maximum LVOT velocity greater than 1 m/s may suggest an SVI of 58 mL/m^2 or higher, which may be the clue to identifying a high-flow state. However, a cutoff value analogous to the one used to identify low flow has not been validated.

AVA is used as a less flow-dependent measure of AS severity. However, opening of stiff, calcified cusps depends to a certain degree on opening forces and may be incomplete with low flow. This is particularly important if a small AVA is observed in combination with a low mean gradient due to impaired LV function. Stimulation of LV contractility with dobutamine is used to increase transvalvular flow and assess AS severity under normalized flow conditions; this discriminates fixed AS from pseudosevere AS by demonstrating opening reserve with increasing opening forces.[22] Flow rate (FR), measured in milliliters per second, also accounts for the time of flow through the stenotic valve. It therefore mirrors opening forces more accurately than stroke volume does:

$$FR = SV/ET$$

or, alternatively,

$$FR = V_{1mean} \times A_1$$

where SV is stroke volume, ET is ejection time, A_1 is the LVOT area, and V_{1mean} is the mean velocity within the LVOT. The AVA reflects true AS severity down to an FR of 200 mL/s, and dobutamine stimulation may be required only if FR at rest is below this value.[23]

ADJUSTMENT FOR BODY SIZE

Aortic maximum velocity and mean pressure gradient are body size–independent measures of AS severity. In contrast, AVA exhibits a strong correlation to body size. AVAi successfully eliminates this correlation and improves comparability among patients with different body sizes.[24] Small patients have lower oxygen needs, smaller heart chambers, and lower stroke volumes than larger individuals, producing lower mean pressure gradients.

An AVA of 0.9 cm^2 has different hemodynamic implications in small compared with larger individuals, representing moderate stenosis in the former and severe stenosis in the latter. However, the general use of the recommended partition value for AVAi (0.6 cm^2/m^2 for severe stenosis) overestimates stenosis severity in patients with higher BSA,[25] partially due to obesity, and it is useful only in small patients (BSA < 1.6 cm^2).[26] Normalization to height may be an appropriate alterative for obese patients.[27] The velocity ratio may be used as an alternative measure of AS severity, independent of body size and flow and not requiring measurement of LVOT with its potential limitations.[15,16]

CONCURRENT HYPERTENSION

Uncontrolled hypertension may lead to reduced stroke volume, reduced mean gradient, and a smaller AVA compared with blood pressure in the normal range.[28] Blood pressure should be below 140/90 mmHg when AS severity is assessed. Blood pressure at the time of echocardiography should be reported.

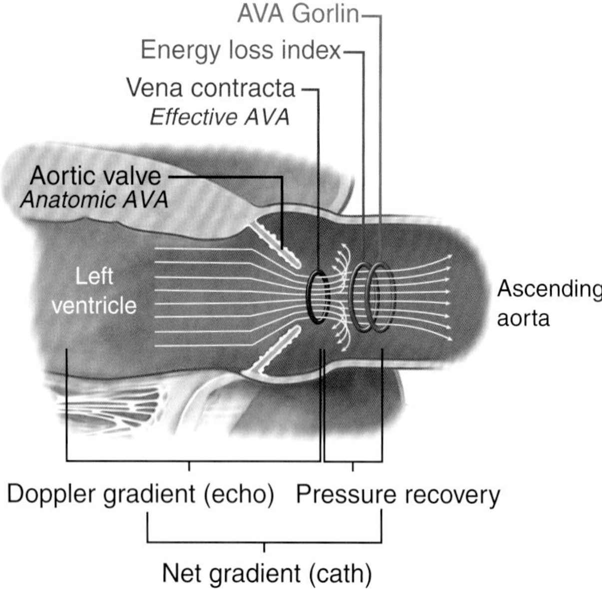

Fig. 22.12 Anatomic and effective aortic valve areas and pressure recovery. The bloodstream passing through the stenotic valve (anatomic AVA) further converges behind the anatomic orifice (vena contracta), forming the effective AVA before turbulent flow appears in the ascending aorta. Doppler imaging measures the maximum pressure drop and calculates the effective AVA. However, some energy loss can be reconverted to pressure energy (pressure recovery) afterward, diminishing the net gradient that is effective for the system. A virtual AVA (indexed to body surface area, called energy loss index) can be calculated, taking into account the net gradient instead of the maximum pressure drop. The AVA is calculated from the catheter-measured net gradient by the Gorlin formula; however, because a constant is introduced, the result is not identical with the energy loss index (see text). *AVA*, Aortic valve area; *BSA*, body surface area; *cath*, catheter; *echo*, echocardiography.

ANATOMIC VERSUS EFFECTIVE AORTIC VALVE AREA AND PRESSURE RECOVERY

The continuity equation calculates an effective AVA, which is slightly smaller than the anatomic AVA because flow further converges downstream of the anatomic orifice (vena contracta) before turbulent flow appears in the ascending aorta (Fig. 22.12). The magnitude of disparity between the effective and the anatomic AVA depends on orifice size and shape, showing increasing differences in small valve areas, flat geometry, and eccentric jets. Significant differences between anatomic and effective AVA are typically observed in patients with bicuspid valves and eccentric jets.[29]

Some of the energy loss in the stenotic jet is reconverted to pressure energy in the ascending aorta. This phenomenon, called *pressure recovery*, leads to a lower net gradient between the LV and aorta than that measured in the immediate vicinity of the aortic valve (see Fig. 22.12). This may explain some differences in mean pressure gradient between catheter and Doppler measurements: Doppler imaging does not account for pressure recovery, whereas catheter pressures are usually recorded in the aorta, after pressure recovery has occurred.

The extent of this phenomenon depends on the difference between the stenotic orifice and the cross-sectional area of the ascending aorta. The smaller the valve orifice relative to the size of the aorta, the more turbulence will occur and the less energy will be available to be recovered as pressure.[30] Significant amounts of pressure recovery are observed in the setting of mild to moderate AS when the ascending aorta is relatively small (<30 mm).

To account for pressure recovery, the energy loss index (ELI) has been proposed. It represents a virtual AVA (adjusted for BSA), assuming that the net gradient was the consequence of a stenosis without the existence of pressure recovery (see Fig. 22.12). ELI is calculated as follows:

$$ELI = AVAi \times A_a/(A_a - AVA)$$

where A_a = the cross-sectional area of the ascending aorta at the sinotubular junction and AVAi = AVA indexed by BSA.

Besides its theoretical advantages, ELI can provide prognostic information. However, it does not outperform other measures of AS severity in patients with mild to moderate AS.[31]

DISCORDANCE BETWEEN MEASURES OF AORTIC STENOSIS SEVERITY

Severe AS is defined as a V_{max} greater 4 m/s and a mean gradient greater than 40 mmHg. The corresponding value for AVA is less than 1 cm^2 (see Table 22.1). Frequently, discordance between mean pressure gradient and AVA is observed, resulting in uncertainty about AS severity (see Fig. 22.7). Any discordance should prompt meticulous review of all measurements involved. However, discordance may persist despite correct assessment of all required components (Table 22.4).

In most discrepant cases, an AVA of less than 1.0 cm^2 indicates severe AS, whereas a mean pressure gradient of less than 40 mmHg points to a nonsevere stenosis. This discordance may be related to low-flow states causing a relatively low mean gradient despite a severely stenotic aortic valve, a combination that may occur with reduced or with normal EF (stages D2 and D3, respectively). First, it may be recognized by direct signs (SVI ≤ 35 mL/m^2) or indirect signs of a reduced flow, which have to be carefully searched for or ruled out. Second, it may be the consequence of small body size, making the use of AVAi necessary for small patients. Third, having excluded the aforementioned reasons for discordance, an inherent inconsistency between AVA and mean pressure gradient partition values for severe stenosis as outlined in the current guidelines[3,7] should be considered. A mean gradient of 40 mmHg correlates with an AVA of 0.8 to 0.9 cm^2 (rather than 1.0 cm^2) in normal flow conditions (i.e., normal EF and normal SVI). Conversely, an AVA of 1.0 cm^2 correlates with a mean gradient close to 30 mmHg (not 40 mmHg), meaning that an AVA of less than 1.0 cm^2 indicates severe AS at an earlier stage of disease than a mean pressure gradient of greater than 40 mmHg.[32,33]

Discordance of AVA and mean gradient in normal flow states is called *normal-flow/low-gradient severe AS*; it shares many characteristics with moderate AS and does not require aortic valve replacement (AVR).[12,34,35] The complex overlay and interactions of various phenomena in low-gradient AS often demand additional diagnostic modalities to confirm AS severity. TEE and calcium scoring by computed tomography (CT) (discussed later) seem to be most helpful in this condition.

In some cases, a reverse discordance is observed, with a mean pressure gradient greater than 40 mmHg, indicating severe AS, but an AVA greater than 1.0 cm^2, pointing to a nonsevere stenosis. It can be explained by high flow, including cardiac and noncardiac causes, as discussed earlier. It is also seen in congenital AS cases, which often exhibit eccentric jets. These jets immediately strike the aortic wall, leading to less pressure recovery and higher gradients than in a comparable AVA, and the Doppler

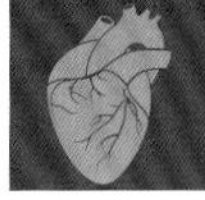

TABLE 22.4 Practical Approach for Assessing Aortic Stenosis Severity in Settings Requiring Increased Attentiveness.

Constellation	*Potential Mechanism*	*Problem Solving*
Small valve area (AVA < 1.0 cm^2) and low gradient (MPG ≤ 40 mmHg)	Measurement error	Underestimation of LVOT size: remeasure LVOT diameter. Underestimation of aortic velocity: use additional acoustic windows. Check LVOT velocity with color and within the CW signal. Consider TEE to display LVOT and valve morphology.
	Small body size (BSA < 1.6 m^2)	Calculate AVAi.
	Reduced ejection fraction (<50%)	Perform dobutamine echocardiography.
	Reduced output despite normal ejection fraction (≥50%)	Calculate SVI, search for indirect signs of reduced SVI. Consider CT (calcium score) and TEE (morphology).
	Mitral insufficiency	Consider low flow and calculate SVI.
	No other explanation	Consider inconsistency of cutoff values for AVA and MPG according to AS severity (normal-flow/low-gradient AS).
High gradient (MPG > 40 mmHg) with large valve area (AVA ≥ 1.0 cm^2)	Measurement error	Remeasure parameters of AS severity.
	High flow as a consequence of aortic regurgitation, bradycardia, anemia, fever, arteriovenous shunts (hemodialysis)	Calculate SVI to detect high flow. Remeasure in case of reversible causes. Overall valve lesion may still be considered severe.
	Eccentric jets	Absence of pressure recovery leading to higher gradients than expected; Doppler gradients mirror true AS severity
	Large body size (BSA > 2.0 cm^2)	Calculate AVAi, but consider overestimation of AS severity by AVAi, especially in obese patients.
Discrepancy between hemodynamic measures of AS and valve morphology	Measurement error	Remeasure parameters of AS severity. Use additional acoustic windows. Consider TEE for better display LVOT and valve morphology.
	Bicuspid valve: doming may give the impression of preserved valve opening	Use additional acoustic windows (eccentric jets). Consider 3D TEE for better display of valve morphology.
	Eccentric jet: underestimation of stenotic velocity V_2	Use additional acoustic windows.
	LVOT obstruction: estimation of AS severity with usual measures problematic	Assess valve morphology (TEE).
	Ascending aorta < 30 mm: Pressure recovery	Calculate ELI.
	Large differences between anatomic and effective AVA	Consider methodical discrepancies between anatomic and effective AVA. Commonly seen in congenital AS.
Symptoms despite moderate AS	Underestimation of stenotic velocity V_2.	Use additional acoustic windows.
	AS is not origin of symptoms.	Consider other symptomatic disease.
	Moderate AS may be symptomatic especially in young and active patients.	Consider valve replacement if AS is the most likely cause of symptoms.

AVA, Aortic valve area; *AVAi*, AVA indexed to BSA; *BSA*, body surface area; *CT*, computed tomography; *ELI*, energy loss index; *LVOT*, left ventricular outflow tract; *MPG*, mean pressure gradient; *SVI*, stroke volume indexed to BSA.

gradient seems to represent the true AS severity.[29] The velocity ratio may also be used because it represents a measure of AS severity independent of body size and flow.[15,16]

LV CHANGES IN AORTIC STENOSIS

LV REMODELING

Almost all patients with significant AS exhibit some kind of LV hypertrophy and/or remodeling. Development of LV hypertrophy depends on genetic factors, gender, body mass index, and coexistent hypertension, and it therefore correlates only weakly with AS severity. The type of hypertrophic remodeling is described by the relative wall thickness (RWT), which is equal to two times the thickness of the posterior wall/end-diastolic dimension, and by the LV mass index. It is characterized as *normal* (i.e., both parameters within the normal range), *concentric remodeling* (RWT > 0.42; LV mass index normal), *concentric hypertrophy* (RWT > 0.42, LV mass index > 95 g/m^2 in women or > 115 g/m^2 in men), or *eccentric hypertrophy* (increased LV mass index, RWT ≤ 0.42). A high LV mass and concentric hypertrophy adversely affect the outcomes of patients with AS.[36]

Hypertrophy, primarily seen as a normal compensatory mechanism in response to pressure overload, is closely related to the development of progressive myocardial fibrosis leading to increased LV stiffness, diminished longitudinal contraction, and diastolic dysfunction. More advanced stages may lead to low-flow/low-gradient AS with preserved EF.[37] Only a part of these changes may resolve after successful AVR, and the outcome of patients may be impaired in terms of symptoms and mortality rates.[38] The detection of myocardial fibrosis may influence decision making for patients in the future.

ASSESSMENT OF LV FUNCTION

Diastolic Function

LV remodeling leads to predominant diastolic dysfunction starting early in the course of the disease; it is related to patients' symptoms and parallels the development of hypertrophy and fibrosis. It is assessed and reported as described in Chapter 5.

Ejection Fraction

Overt systolic dysfunction is a sign of an advanced AS or a coexistent myocardial disease. Regional wall motion abnormalities should always raise the suspicion of concomitant coronary artery disease (CAD). Global systolic function is assessed by visual estimation, and EF is calculated by the Simpson method or by 3D echocardiography (see Chapter 4).

An EF of 50% or greater is considered normal or *preserved.* However, a much higher EF (60%–70%) may be necessary to maintain a normal stroke volume in most patients with relevant AS because the LV is often small due to concentric remodeling. Preoperative EF correlates strongly with overall survival of patients undergoing valve replacement. The worst outcome was reported for patients with an EF lower than 50%; there was gradual improvement in survival with an EF between 50% and 59%, and the lowest risk of death was patients with an EF of 60% or greater, a correlation that appears to be independent of symptom status.[39,40]

Stroke Volume Index

SVI has become the most important parameter of LV function in patients with AS. It may have some advantages over EF because it integrates information on the impact of longitudinal and radial LV function and size, as well as that of concomitant aortic or mitral regurgitation, on forward flow. Reduced stroke volume is linked to increased mortality rates despite a preserved EF (≥50%) for patients with AS; the highest mortality rate correlates with an SVI of 35 mL/m^2 or less.[41]

Longitudinal Function

EF predominantly measures radial contraction, whereas concentric remodeling and myocardial fibrosis may mainly lead to an impaired longitudinal function not adequately represented by EF. Global longitudinal strain (GLS) has become an important marker of myocardial function, with strong predictive value beyond EF (see Chapter 4). A GLS greater than −15% predicted worse outcomes for symptomatic patients,[42] as did a GLS greater than −18% for asymptomatic patients with AS.[43] Despite its unquestionable predictive value and its correlation with the amount of myocardial fibrosis,[44] the role of GLS in clinical decision making, particularly in stage D3 disease, has not been clearly established.

ASSOCIATED FINDINGS

Aortic regurgitation, subvalvular stenosis, and mitral annular calcification may be associated with AS. Potential consequences of AS and subsequent LV changes include mitral regurgitation (MR), left atrial enlargement, pulmonary hypertension, right ventricular (RV) impairment, tricuspid regurgitation, congestion of the inferior vena cava, and pleural effusions, underscoring the need for a comprehensive echocardiographic workup of all patients with AS.

AORTIC REGURGITATION

Aortic regurgitation is common in AS of any cause. A central jet is common in rheumatic and degenerative tricuspid AS, and assessment of severity is usually straightforward. In congenital disease, particularly with bicuspid valves, prolapse of the larger, nonseparated cusp often results in an eccentric jet that requires careful assessment to avoid underestimation (see Figs. 22.2 and 22.5).

Significant aortic regurgitation increases stroke volume through the aortic valve, leading to an elevated gradient compared with solitary AS in a given orifice area. As a result, peak velocity and mean gradient do not reflect the stenotic component but instead mirror the combined hemodynamic burden of the disease, and these parameters are useful in clinical decision making.[45] Severity of the stenotic lesion may be accurately assessed by measurement of the AVA, which is not affected by augmented stroke volume. LV remodeling becomes more eccentric with increasing aortic regurgitation (Fig. 22.13). Preserved EF and SVI may erroneously suggest normal LV function because both measures fail to account for regurgitant volume and therefore do not mirror effective output.

CONCOMITANT SUBVALVULAR OBSTRUCTION

Concomitant subvalvular obstruction may be present, as is seen with fixed membranous subaortic stenosis or dynamic obstruction of the LVOT with advanced hypertrophy or hypertrophic cardiomyopathy. Use of aortic maximum velocity and mean pressure gradient leads to increasingly relevant overestimation of AS severity with increasing pre-stenotic velocities when the simplified Bernoulli equation is applied. A considerably increased maximum pre-stenotic velocity (e.g., >1.2 m/s) should always prompt use of the more complete Bernoulli equation:

$$\Delta P = 4\left(V_2^2 - V_1^2\right)$$

and calculation of the AVA. However, estimation of AS severity may become almost impossible if AS is combined with a relevant subvalvular obstruction; in such cases, CW Doppler may give some idea about the overall pressure burden (Fig. 22.14).

In this complex situation, morphologic information becomes particularly important and is best obtained by TEE, which demonstrates the location and origin of subvalvular obstruction and the morphologic criteria for AS severity. Any reduction of afterload (e.g., with AVR) may aggravate dynamic subvalvular obstruction, and this should be anticipated on the basis of a comprehensive preinterventional echocardiographic assessment.

MITRAL ANNULAR CALCIFICATION AND MITRAL REGURGITATION

Mitral annular calcification is found in about 50% of patients undergoing isolated AVR and is associated with older age, noncongenital tricuspid AS, and renal failure.[46] Significant stenosis occurs in less than 3% of patients.[47] MR frequently coexists in patients with AS and is associated with impaired outcome.[48] Significant hemodynamic interactions have to be considered when estimating the severity of both valve lesions. MR may reduce forward stroke volume and, consequently, the gradient, leading to a low-flow/low-gradient severe AS despite normal EF. Calculation of stroke volume is required. However, elevated LV pressure due to AS may lead to an augmented regurgitant volume in a given effective regurgitant orifice, and direct measurement of regurgitant volume is preferred. Assessment of the cause of MR is mandatory because a decrease of MR after AVR is more likely with secondary than primary causes.[49]

AMYLOIDOSIS

Senile amyloidosis is expected in 6% to 16% of elderly patients with AS.[50,51] It is associated with increased wall thickness, advanced diastolic dysfunction, and the phenotype of low-flow low-gradient AS with mildly reduced EF. Severely impaired longitudinal myocardial function may be an important clue, and

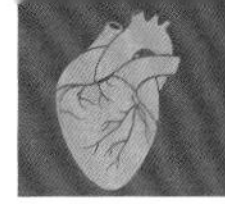

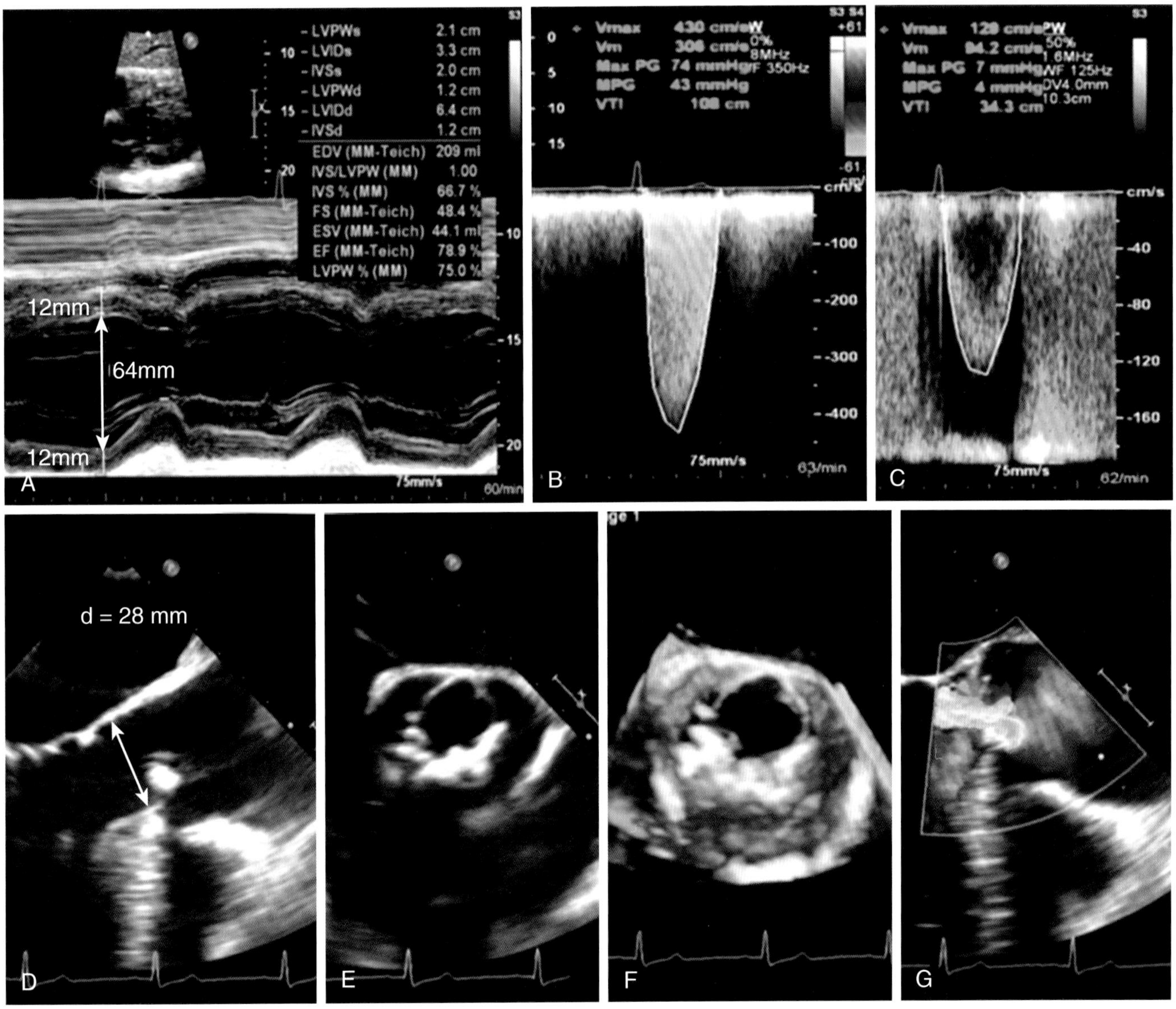

Fig. 22.13 Combined stenotic and regurgitant aortic valve disease. A 56-year-old patient with bicuspid aortic valve, mild aortic stenosis, and severe aortic regurgitation. (A) M-mode imaging shows eccentric remodeling with enlarged LV end-diastolic diameter and hypertrophic walls. (B) CW Doppler indicates a maximum velocity of 4.3 m/s. (C) Increased pre-stenotic maximum velocity is 1.3 m/s. (D) The LV outflow tract *(double-headed arrow)* is large (28 mm); the aortic valve area is 1.7 cm^2, and the stroke volume index is 111 mL/m^2. 2D (E) and 3D (F) TEE images display the aortic valve orifice, indicating nonsevere aortic stenosis. (G) Color Doppler image demonstrates severe aortic regurgitation (see Video 22.13G).

the diagnosis is confirmed by technetium 99m pyrophosphate scintigraphy and/or biopsy.[50] Even after successful AVR, outcome is poor.[51]

CORONARY ARTERY DISEASE

CAD affects about 50% of patients with AS and has a major impact on prognosis.[10] Evidence for CAD, such as regional wall motion abnormalities, should always be sought. Because clinical symptoms of AS and CAD show significant overlap and functional testing has major limitations or may be even contraindicated in symptomatic patients, coronary angiography is required in most cases.

PULMONARY HYPERTENSION

Pulmonary systolic pressure is assessed from the systolic maximum velocity of tricuspid regurgitation and estimated pressure in the inferior vena cava (see Chapter 36). Pulmonary hypertension in patients with AS is independently associated with impaired longitudinal contraction, diastolic dysfunction, and impaired outcome.[52] Pulmonary hypertension may be only partially relieved by AVR and remains a marker of impaired late outcome.[53]

COMPLEMENTARY DIAGNOSTIC MODALITIES

EXERCISE STRESS TESTING

Exercise stress testing is recommended for any asymptomatic patient with severe AS because symptoms may be underreported and unmasked by the test. Inadequate blood pressure response to exercise is a marker of future adverse events.[54] An increase in mean pressure gradient of greater than 20 mmHg and exercise-induced pulmonary hypertension greater than 60 mmHg measured during stress echocardiography have been

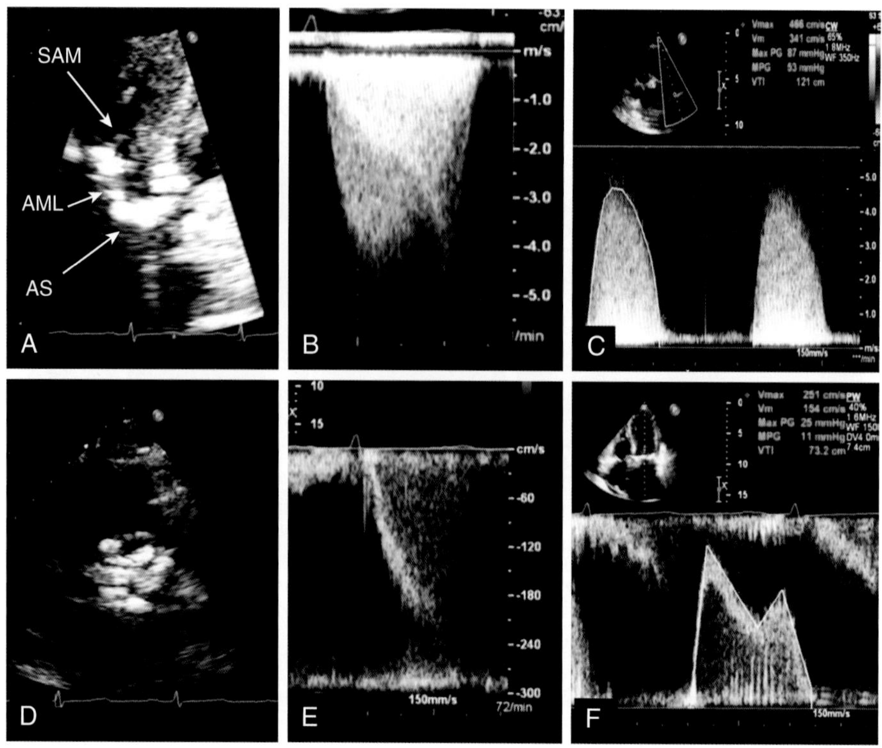

Fig. 22.14 Aortic stenosis in combination with subvalvular obstruction. Complex morphology precluding a reliable calculation of aortic stenosis severity. (A) Severely calcified aortic stenosis *(AS)*, a small LV outflow tract with calcified mitral ring and anterior mitral leaflet *(AML)*, and systolic anterior movement *(SAM)* of the tip of the AML (see Videos 22.14A1 and 22.14A2) are demonstrated in a zoomed 3-chamber view. (B) CW Doppler shows two separated signals, the first with a mid-systolic peak originating from the aortic valve, and the second with a late-systolic peak originating from the obstruction within the LV outflow tract. (C) CW Doppler imaging of the aortic valve from a right parasternal window. (D) Short-axis view of the aortic valve (see Video 22.14D). (E) Pulsed-wave Doppler image of the LV outflow tract near the aortic valve. (F) Pulsed-wave Doppler image of concomitant mitral stenosis. *MPG*, Mean pressure gradient; *VTI*, velocity–time integral.

related to future adverse events in asymptomatic patients with severe AS in small studies.[55,56]

COMPUTED TOMOGRAPHY

Aortic Valve Area Planimetry

Contrast-enhanced CT allows assessment of anatomic AVA with high image quality. Anatomic AVA by CT planimetry shows good correlation with the AVA measured by TEE[57] and may be used as an alternative in selected cases and to confirm echocardiographic assessment of AS severity when indicated anyway in the evaluation process for transcatheter aortic valve implantation (TAVI).[21]

Fusion Approach

Exact delineation of 3D LVOT size by CT has been used for calculation of the effective AVA, together with TTE Doppler, avoiding the most delicate echocardiographic measurement for assessing AS severity. The AVA derived from CT measurement of LVOT is larger than the AVA derived from the diameter as measured by TTE. However, this fusion approach yields an AVA that is even larger than the anatomic AVA measured by planimetry, and it improves neither the concordance of AS severity parameters nor outcome prediction compared with TTE alone.[20,58]

Calcium Scoring

CT enables the exact quantification of aortic valve calcification represented by a calcium score in arbitrary units (AU), similar to the one used in coronary arteries. Different values for women (>1200 AU) and for men (>2000 AU) have been validated to correlate with severe AS, providing information beyond and independent of echocardiographic indices of AS severity (Fig. 22.15).[59–61] Current guidelines endorse the use of a calcium score when doubts about AS severity persist after comprehensive echocardiographic assessment of low-gradient AS.[7]

Preparation for Transcatheter Aortic Valve Implantation

CT is the preferred imaging tool used in preparation for TAVI. It allows exact assessment of the aortic valve annulus size, the distribution of calcifications, the origin of coronary arteries, and the access route within a single acquisition protocol (see Type of Valve Replacement).[7]

CARDIAC MAGNETIC RESONANCE IMAGING

Similar to CT, cardiac magnetic resonance (CMR) imaging has emerged as an alternative method for the assessment of anatomic AVA and LVOT area, and the results are comparable to those of TTE. CMR has the potential to measure four-dimensional flow within the LVOT and the stenotic valve, LV volumes, EF, and LV mass. As a unique feature, it can also quantify and differentiate myocardial fibrosis, which is a strong predictor of adverse events in patients with AS.[19,38,62–64]

CARDIAC CATHETERIZATION

Heart catheterization for the assessment of AS severity is rarely indicated for clinical reasons, but hemodynamic evaluation is often routinely performed before an interventional AVR. Some fundamental differences between echocardiography and catheter measurements should be considered.[30]

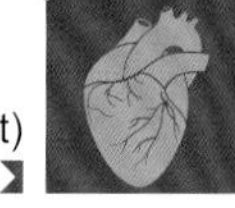

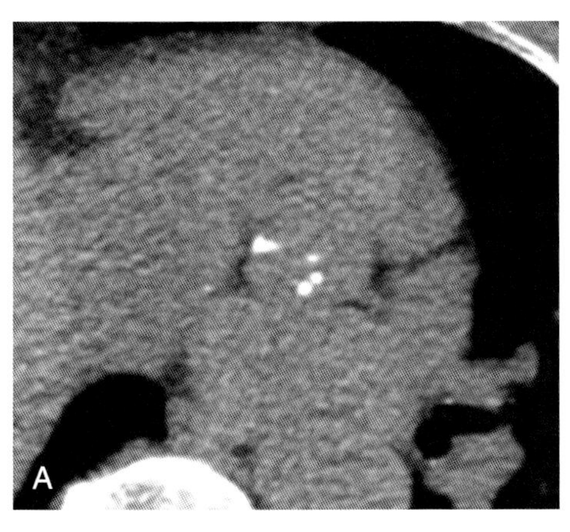

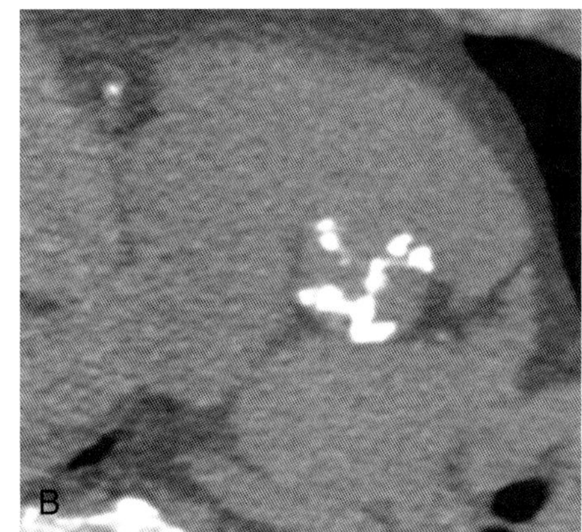

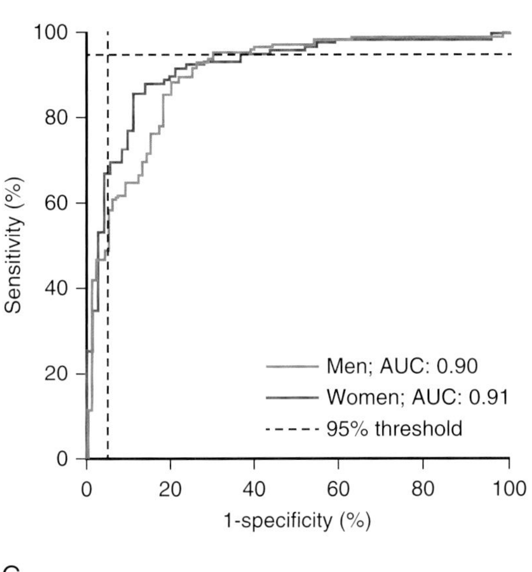

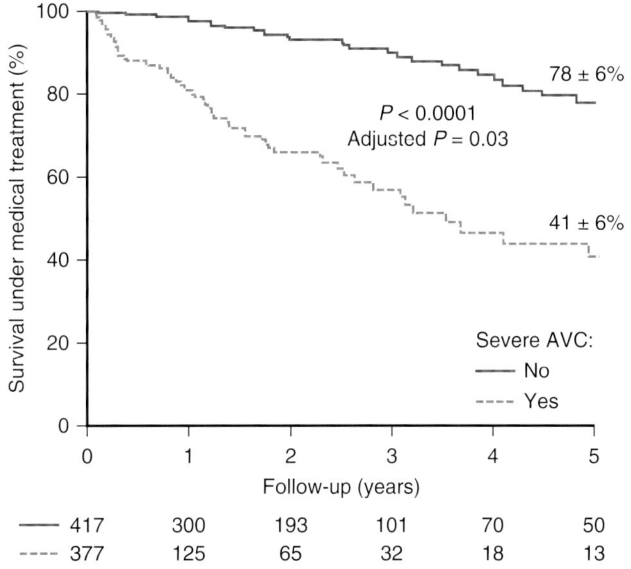

Fig. 22.15 Calcium scoring with computed tomography. Two patients with mild (A) and severe (B) calcification demonstrated by computed tomography (CT).[100] (C) The receiver operating curve of calcium scoring by CT indicates severe or nonsevere aortic stenosis (AS) in 451 patients as assessed by echocardiography with concordant results for AS severity and normal flow (area under the curve [AUC] = 0.90 in men and 0.91 in women).[59] (D) Impact of calcium score (aortic valve calcification [AVC]) on survival under medical treatment in 794 patients. (A and B, From Doris MK, Everett RJ, Shun-Shin M, Clavel M-A, Dweck MR. The role of imaging in measuring disease progression and assessing novel therapies in aortic stenosis. *J Am Coll Cardiol.* 2019;12:185–197. C and D, From Clavel M-A, et al. The complex nature of discordant severe calcified aortic valve disease grading. *J Am Coll Cardiol.* 2013;62:2329– 2338.)

Gradients

Peak-to-peak gradient obtained by catheter measurement indicates the drop in maximal pressure during systole from the LV to the ascending aorta, irrespective of the time point of each maximum; the maximum Doppler gradient is the maximum of instant gradients during systole (Fig. 22.16). In contrast, mean pressure gradients from the two modalities are calculated based on the same principles.

Discrepancies may result from pressure recovery. Whereas Doppler measures the maximal pressure drop from the LV to the vena contracta (effective AVA) and does not account for pressure recovery (discussed earlier), catheter pressure is usually recorded in the aorta after pressure recovery has occurred and therefore reports the net gradient.

Aortic Valve Area

Catheter AVA is calculated from the Gorlin formula:

$$AVA = CO/C \times \Delta P_{mean}$$

where CO = cardiac output, C is a constant, and ΔP_{mean} = mean gradient. Originally, the Gorlin formula calculated an effective AVA similar to Doppler echocardiography, but an empirical constant C was later introduced to convert effective into anatomic AVA (and to account for different units).[30] In general, catheter measurements result in slightly lower mean pressure gradients and slightly higher AVA than echocardiography. Despite these methodological inequalities, neither modality shows a major bias in assessing AS severity.

CLINICAL APPROACH

Symptoms, echocardiographic parameters, and the results of additional diagnostic studies have to be integrated with the clinical context. Fig. 22.17 provides an overview of echocardiographic parameters and diagnostic steps required for the quantification of AS severity and differentiation of AS stages. Table 22.4 summarizes the practical approach and considers specific constellations that may require increased attentiveness.

TIMING OF AORTIC VALVE REPLACEMENT

Timing of intervention is discussed extensively in current guidelines[3,7] (Table 22.5), which are summarized in this section and illustrated in Fig. 22.18.

PROGRESSION OF AORTIC STENOSIS (STAGE B)

In cases of calcific AS, further calcification and hemodynamic alteration are inevitable because there is currently no strategy to mitigate or halt progression. In mild to moderate AS (stage B), the increase in mean gradient is 2.8 mmHg, and the mean reduction in AVA is 0.03 cm^2 per year.[65] However, a more rapid progression has been described associated with advanced age, cardiovascular risk factors, CAD, impaired renal function, and increased aortic valve calcification (see Table 22.2).

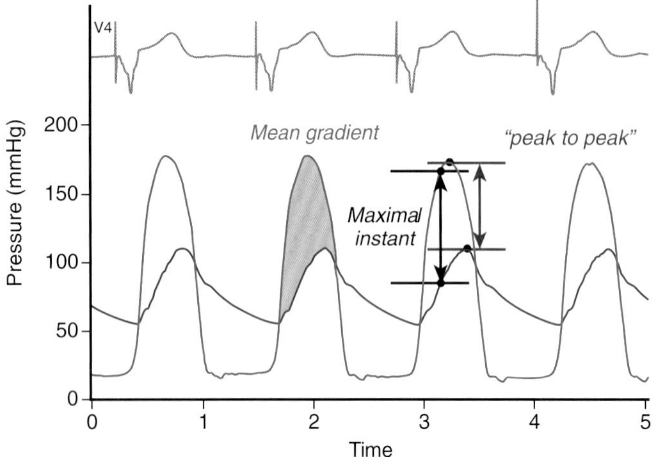

Fig. 22.16 Definitions of gradients. Simultaneous measurement of LV and aortic pressures in a patient with aortic stenosis reveals the difference between peak-to-peak and maximal instant gradients. Peak-to-peak gradient, which is used in catheter evaluations, indicates the drop in maximal pressure during systole from LV to ascending aorta irrespective of the time point of each maximum, whereas maximum Doppler gradient is the maximum of instant gradients during systole. Mean gradient indicates the mean of instant gradients during systole and is similarly calculated from Doppler and from catheter measurements.

ASYMPTOMATIC PATIENTS (STAGE C)

Routine echocardiographic follow-up in asymptomatic patients is recommended every 3 to 5 years for mild AS (maximum velocity < 3 m/s), 1 to 2 years for moderate AS (maximum velocity < 4 m/s), and 6 to 12 months for severe AS.[3] AVR is recommended for asymptomatic patients with severe AS (stage C2) and EF less than 50%, decreased exercise tolerance, or an exercise-induced fall in blood pressure, and likewise for those with very severe AS (stage C1, aortic velocity ≥ 5.0 m/s) and low surgical risk.[66] An AVA of 0.6 cm^2 or less has been identified as an additional marker of high risk for asymptomatic patients and may therefore provide a reason for an early AVR strategy.[67] AVR also may be considered for asymptomatic patients with severe AS, rapid disease progression (maximum velocity progression ≥ 0.3 m/s per year), and low surgical risk

It appears safe to postpone intervention in asymptomatic patients with normal LV function because the risks of sudden death and severe spontaneous complications seem to be lower than the risks of death and severe complications associated with intervention, which is in the range of 1% to 3% for isolated surgical AVR and up to 5% for combined AVR and bypass surgery

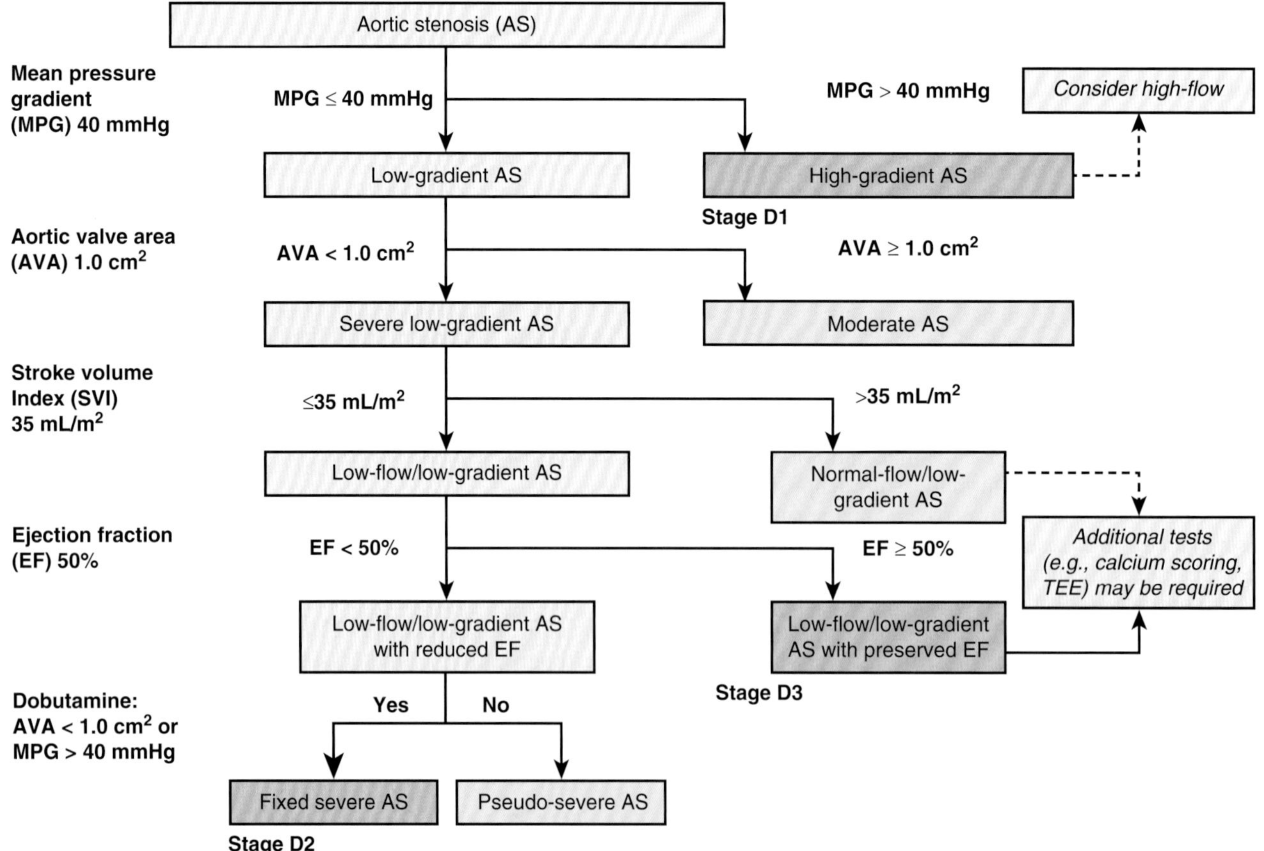

Fig. 22.17 Echocardiographic differentiation of aortic stenosis. Echocardiographic parameters and their respective cutoff values *(left)* are used to differentiate stages of aortic stenosis *(AS)*. *Yellow boxes* signify the need for further evaluation; *red boxes* favor aortic valve replacement; *green boxes* suggest further conservative management. Differentiation between normal-flow/low-gradient AS and low-flow/low-gradient AS requires additional testing beyond TTE in equivocal cases.

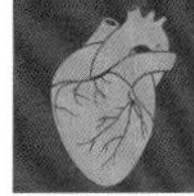

TABLE 22.5 Selected Studies Investigating Incidence of Sudden Death in Patients With Aortic Stenosis.

Study	*Year*	*N*	*Follow-Up (mo)*	*AS Severity at Entry (V_{max} in m/s)*	*AS Severity (AVA in cm²)*	*Sudden Deaths (n)*	*Sudden Deaths (%/y)*
Otto et al.[8]	1997	114	30	3.6 ± 0.6	—	0	0
Rosenhek et al.[4]	2000	128	22	≥4.0	—	1	0.4
Das[54]	2005	125	12		≤1.4	0	0
Pellikka et al.[94]	2005	270	65	≥4.0		11	0.75
Monin et al.[97]	2009	211	22	≥3.0	≤1	2	0.5
Lancellotti et al.[98]	2010	163	20		≤0.6 cm²/m²	3	1.1
Marechaux et al.[56]	2010	135	20		≤1.5	1	0.4
Rosenhek et al.[9]	2010	116	41	≥5.0		1	0.3
Taniguchi et al.[99]	2018	2005[a]	44	V_{max} > 4.0 m/s, or ΔP > 40 mmHg, or AVA < 1.0 cm²	0.67 ± 0.19 cm²	93	1.8
		1808[b]	44	—	0.77 ± 0.17	82	1.4
Kang et al.[100]	2020	145	73	5.1 ± 0.5	0.63 ± 0.09	3[c]	1.0

[a]Symptomatic patients.
[b]Asymptomatic patients.
[c]Within 4 years, conservatively treated patients only.
AS, Aortic stenosis; *AVA*, aortic valve area; V_{max}, peak aortic jet velocity.

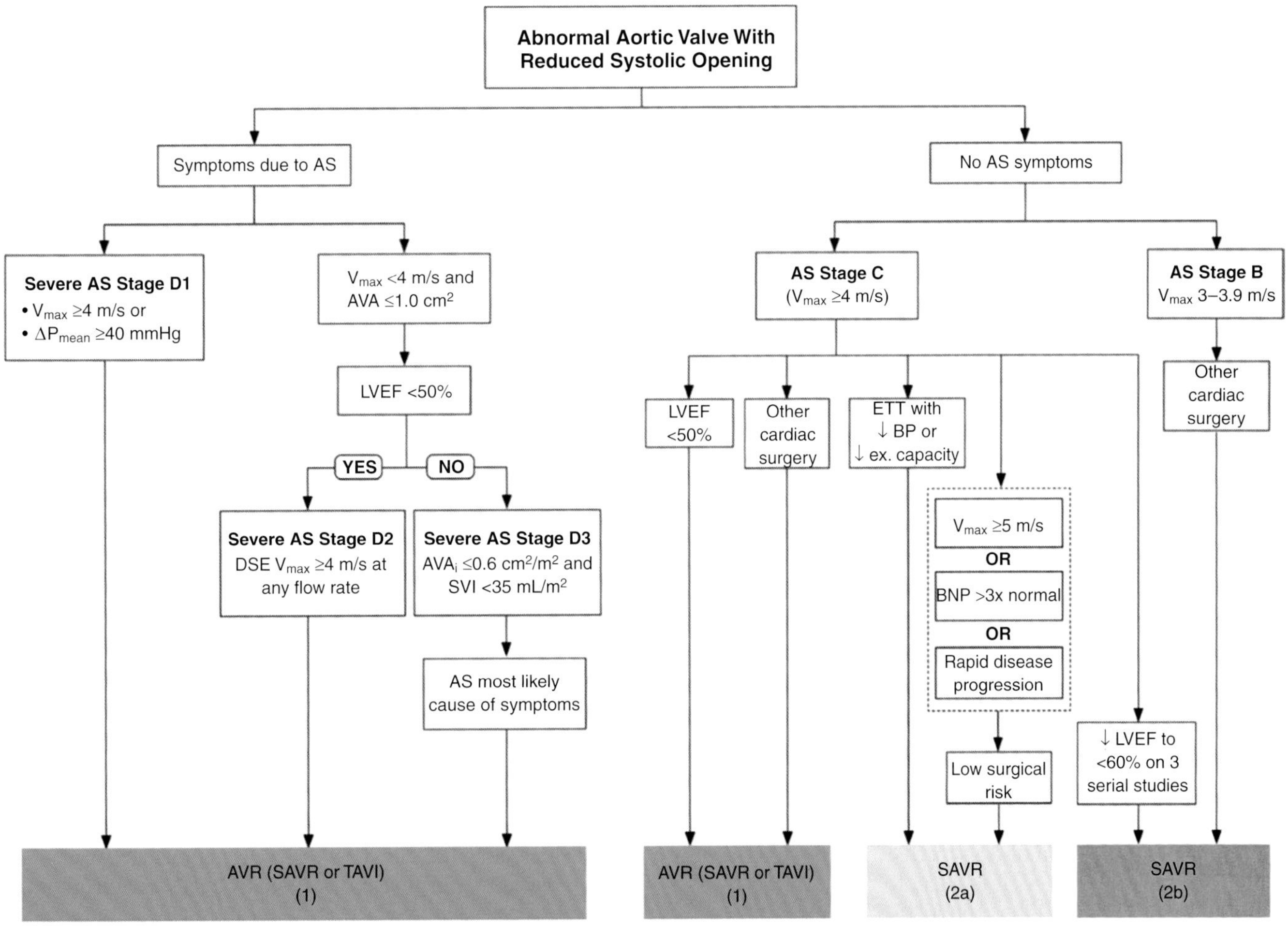

Abnormal Aortic Valve With Reduced Systolic Opening

Symptoms due to AS

No AS symptoms

Severe AS Stage D1
• V_{max} ≥4 m/s or
• ΔP_{mean} ≥40 mmHg

V_{max} <4 m/s and AVA ≤1.0 cm²

LVEF <50%

YES

NO

Severe AS Stage D2
DSE V_{max} ≥4 m/s at any flow rate

Severe AS Stage D3
AVA_i ≤0.6 cm²/m² and SVI <35 mL/m²

AS most likely cause of symptoms

AS Stage C
(V_{max} ≥4 m/s)

AS Stage B
V_{max} 3–3.9 m/s

LVEF <50%

Other cardiac surgery

ETT with ↓ BP or ↓ ex. capacity

V_{max} ≥5 m/s
OR
BNP >3x normal
OR
Rapid disease progression

Low surgical risk

↓ LVEF to <60% on 3 serial studies

Other cardiac surgery

AVR (SAVR or TAVI) (1)

AVR (SAVR or TAVI) (1)

SAVR (2a)

SAVR (2b)

Fig. 22.18 Timing of intervention for AS. *Arrows* show the decision pathways that result in a recommendation for AVR. Periodic monitoring is indicated for all patients in whom AVR is not yet indicated, including those with asymptomatic (stage C) and symptomatic (stage D) AS and those with low-gradient AS (stage D2 or D3) who do not meet the criteria for intervention. *AS*, Aortic stenosis; *AVA*, aortic valve area; *AVAi*, aortic valve area index; *AVR*, aortic valve replacement; *BNP*, B-type natriuretic peptide; *BP*, blood pressure; *DSE*, dobutamine stress echocardiography; *ETT*, exercise treadmill test; *LVEF*, left ventricular ejection fraction; ΔP_{mean} mean systolic pressure gradient between LV and aorta; *SAVR*, surgical aortic valve replacement; *SVI*, stroke volume index; *TAVI*, transcatheter aortic valve implantation; *TAVR*, transcatheter aortic valve replacement; V_{max} maximum velocity. (From Otto CM, Nishimura RA, Bonow RO, et al. 2020 ACC/AHA guideline for the management of patients with valvular heart disease: a report of the American College of Cardiology/American Heart Association Joint Committee on Clinical Practice Guidelines. *Circulation*. 2021;143:e00–e00. DOI: 10.1161/CIR.0000000000000923.

TABLE 22.6 Selected Studies Investigating Event-Free Survival of Asymptomatic Patients With Aortic Stenosis.

Study	Year	Entry Criteria	N	Age (y)	Follow-Up (mo)	AS Severity	Event-Free Survival
Otto et al.[8]	1997	Abnormal valve with V_{max} > 2.6 m/s	123	63 ± 16	30	V_{max} < 3.0 m/s V_{max} 3–4 m/s V_{max} > 4 m/s	84% at 2 y 66% at 2 y 21% at 2 y
Rosenhek et al.[4]	2000	V_{max} ≥ 4.0	128	60 ± 18	22 ± 18	V_{max} 5.0 ± 0.7 m/s	67% at 1 y 56% at 2 y 33% at 4 y
Rosenhek et al.[10]	2004	Abnormal valve with V_{max} 2.5–3.9 m/s	176	58 ± 19	48 ± 19	V_{max} 3.1 ± 0.4 m/s	95% at 1 y 75% at 2 y 60% at 5 y
Pellikka et al.[94]	2005	V_{max} ≥ 4.0	622	72 ± 11	65 ± 48	V_{max} 4.4 ± 0.4 m/s	82% at 1 y 67% at 2 y 33% at 5 y
Rossebø et al.[92]	2008	V_{max} 2.5–4.0	1873	68 ± 9	52 (median)	V_{max} 3.1 ± 0.55	Approx. 65% at 5 y
Rosenhek et al.[9]	2010	V_{max} ≥ 5.0	116	67 ± 15	41 (median)	V_{max} 5.0–5.5 m/s V_{max} ≥ 5.5 m/s	43% at 2 y 25% at 2 y
Kearney et al.[95]	2013	AS on echo	239	74 ± 6	60	Mild Moderate Severe	66% ± 5% 23% ± 7% 20% ± 10%
Maes et al.[82]	2014	AVAi ≤ 0.6 cm²/m²	220	76 ± 13 78 ± 11	28	High gradient (> 40 mmHg) Low gradient (≤ 40 mmHg)	35% ± 7% 59% ± 5%
Taniguchi et al.[96]	2015	V_{max} > 4.0 m/s, or ΔP > 40 mmHg, or AVA < 1.0 cm²	1517	78 ± 9	44	AVA 0.79 ± 0.16 cm²	82% at 1 y 48% at 3 y 17% at 5 y
Lancellotti et al.[66]	2018	AVA < 1.5 cm²	1375	71 ± 13	27	V_{max} 3.8 ± 0.8 AVA 0.94 ± 0.3	93% at 2 y, 86% at 4 y, 75% at 8 y

AS, Aortic stenosis; *AVA*, aortic valve area; *AVAi*, indexed aortic valve area; *echo*, echocardiography; *ΔP*, pressure gradient; V_{max}, peak aortic jet velocity.

(see Table 22.3).[68] AVR as a first-line therapy strategy for asymptomatic patients did not reduce cardiovascular mortality rates in observational studies.[69] The probability of sudden cardiac death without preceding symptoms (reported in a wide range between 0.2% and 3.1% per year) in patients with severe AS does not appear to be closely related to the severity of AS and may be partially attributed to comorbidities such as CAD (Table 22.6).

SYMPTOMATIC PATIENTS (STAGE D1)

After symptoms develop, outcome is dismal unless AVR is performed. AVR is therefore recommended for all symptomatic patients with severe high-gradient AS (stage D1). Similarly, patients initially reporting no symptoms should undergo AVR if they develop symptoms during an exercise test.

The classic triad of symptoms of AS—angina, dyspnea, and exercise-induced dizziness or syncope—occurs late in the disease process, and many patients present with unspecific symptoms such as decreased exercise tolerance and exertional dyspnea, which may in part result from comorbidities such as hypertension, obesity, or chronic lung disease. Echocardiographic quantification of AS severity may provide the only evidence about whether AVR is likely to resolve the patient's symptoms or is indicated for prognostic reasons.

LOW-FLOW, LOW-GRADIENT SEVERE AORTIC STENOSIS WITH REDUCED EJECTION FRACTION (STAGE D2)

Patients with AS and reduced EF frequently require additional diagnostic testing for clinical decision making. Reduced flow in patients with impaired LV function (EF < 50%) precludes an adequate increase in pressure gradient despite a severely reduced valve orifice (AVA < 1.0 cm²). However, low flow may inhibit complete valve opening as a result of diminished opening forces,[70] leading to uncertainty about AS severity if only pressure gradient and AVA at rest are considered. Opening forces may be most adequately mirrored by FR, with an FR < 200 mL/s indicating reduced flow.[23]

With the aim of restoring normal or near-normal flow in these patients, low-dose dobutamine is given intravenously at an increasing dose (5, 10, and 20 µg/kg per minute). In the case of a fixed severe stenosis, restoration of normal flow will increase the mean pressure gradient to above 40 mmHg, leaving AVA unaffected (<1.0 cm²). However, if AVA increases with only minimal changes in mean pressure gradient, the diagnosis of pseudosevere stenosis is made (Fig. 22.19). Pseudostenosis may be treated medically with outcomes similar to those of patients with heart failure without AS,[71] whereas patients with truly severe AS benefit from AVR.

A subset of patients do not exhibit contractile reserve during dobutamine stimulation (i.e., their increase in stroke volume is < 20%). Pseudosevere stenosis may be then excluded by CT calcium scoring. If severe AS is confirmed, increases in EF and long-term survival rates are observed with AVR, but the operative mortality rate is high, and TAVI may be the preferred method.[72,73] Patients with reduced LV function and only moderate AS are at high risk for clinical events[74] and may benefit from early afterload reduction by TAVI, an approach being studied in a randomized trial.[75]

LOW-FLOW, LOW-GRADIENT SEVERE AORTIC STENOSIS WITH PRESERVED EJECTION FRACTION (STAGE D3)

The constellation of a severely reduced AVA (<1.0 cm²) and a low mean pressure gradient (<40 mmHg) despite preserved EF (≥50%) is observed in up to 30% of patients evaluated for AS

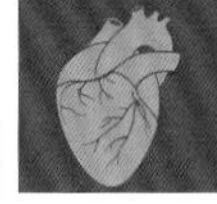

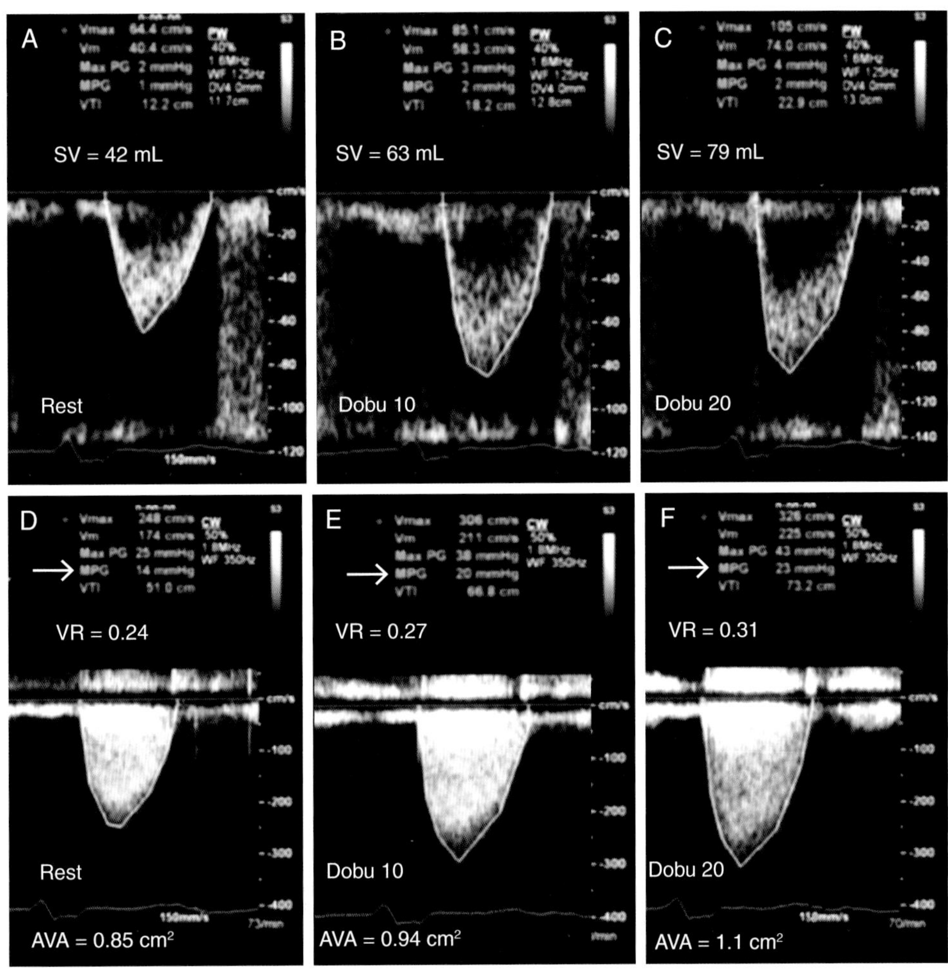

Fig. 22.19 **Dobutamine echocardiography in low-gradient aortic stenosis with reduced ejection fraction.** With increasing doses of dobutamine (*Dobu*), stroke volume (*SV*) increases from 42 to 79 mL (A–C), mean pressure gradient (*MPG, arrows*) from 14 to 23 mmHg, and velocity ratio (*VR*) from 0.24 to 0.31 (D–F). With an LV outflow tract diameter of 21 mm, aortic valve area (*AVA*) is calculated as 0.85 cm^2 at rest and as 1.1 cm^2 with the highest dobutamine dose. Augmentation of SV detects the opening reserve of the aortic valve, and the diagnosis of a pseudosevere aortic stenosis is made. *VTI*, Velocity-time integral.

(see Fig. 22.6). It denotes an inhomogeneous group of individuals with various degrees of AS severity, as discussed earlier (see Discordance Between Measures of Aortic Stenosis Severity).

Patients with definite low-flow/low-gradient AS with preserved EF (stage D3) exhibit reduced flow (Fig. 22.20); this is detected by a reduced SVI (<35 mL/m^2) caused by small ventricular size and reduced longitudinal function[37,76] associated with LV hypertrophy and fibrosis[77] not adequately mirrored by EF. This entity seems to be more likely a distinct presentation of severe AS rather than an advanced stage of high-gradient AS.[13] Patients with this entity had an impaired prognosis in retrospective studies[78,79] and likely can benefit from AVR[35]; however, outcome remains impaired after intervention compared with patients with high-gradient AS.[80,81] AVR is reasonable in symptomatic patients who have low-flow/low-gradient severe AS with preserved EF (stage D3).

Most patients with low-gradient AS and preserved EF exhibit normal flow, as indicated by a normal SVI (≥35 mL/m^2) and by characteristics and outcomes similar to those of patients with moderate AS (normal flow/low gradient severe AS).[12,34,82] These patients do not require AVR.

The differentiation between low-flow and normal-flow low-gradient AS with normal EF (see Fig. 22.17) requires meticulous re-evaluation of echocardiographic measurements and integration of clinical and echocardiographic data for decision making. Age greater than 70 years, mean gradient near 40 mmHg, AVA of 0.8 cm^2 or less, confirmation of low flow by techniques other than Doppler, and reduced longitudinal function may increase the likelihood of severe AS.[6]

Additional diagnostic tools such as TEE may help in estimating AS severity, providing detailed aortic valve morphology, offering the possibility of measuring anatomic AVA by planimetry, and reappraising LVOT size in high-quality images, thereby verifying the calculation of AVA by the continuity equation. Quantification of valvular calcium by CT provides prognostic information beyond echocardiographic measures and is recommended to differentiate patients with low-gradient AS.[59–61]

No randomized studies have been performed in this field, and current recommendations may be questioned by recent findings. For instance, patients with low-flow/low-gradient AS and preserved EF (stage D3) may exhibit reduced valve opening forces, similar to patients with reduced EF (stage D2), and dobutamine echocardiography has been claimed to further elucidate AS severity, with about one third of cases classified as pseudosevere stenosis.[83] Improvement in functional status and

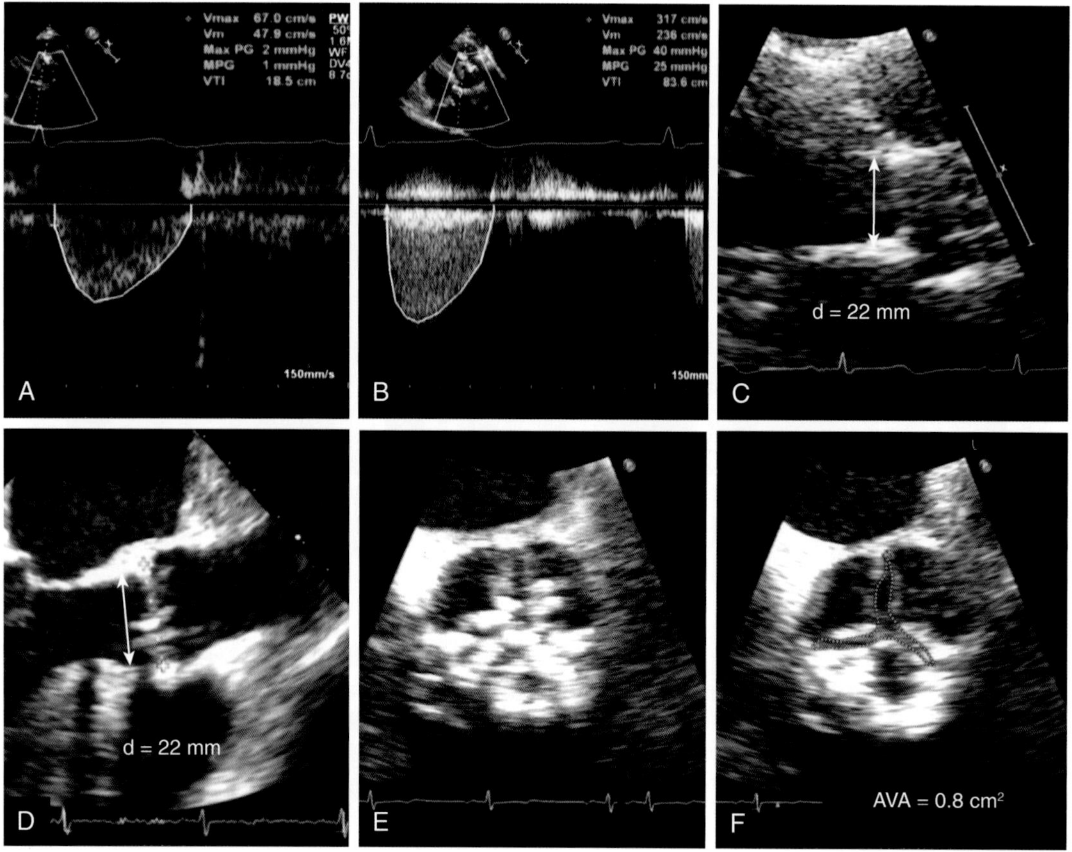

Fig. 22.20 Severe low-flow/low-gradient aortic stenosis with preserved ejection fraction. An 82-year-old patient with a small and hypertrophied LV and an ejection fraction of 52%. (A) Pulsed-wave Doppler image of the LV outflow tract (LVOT) near the aortic valve. (B) CW Doppler of the aortic valve. (C) Long-axis view in zoom mode to measure the diameter *(d)* of the LVOT *(double-headed arrow)*. The calculated aortic valve area *(AVA)* is 0.8 cm^2. (D) Transesophageal long-axis view to remeasure LVOT diameter. (E) Transesophageal short-axis view shows severely calcified tricuspid aortic valve. (F) Planimetry of anatomic AVA.

survival after AVR has been reported for patients with normal-flow/low-gradient AS.[84,85]

PATIENTS UNDERGOING CARDIAC SURGERY FOR OTHER INDICATIONS

AVR is indicated for patients with severe AS, and it is reasonable for those with moderate AS (stage B) who have an aortic velocity of 3.0 to 4.0 m/s or a mean pressure gradient of 20 to 40 mmHg and are undergoing cardiac surgery for other indications.

TYPE OF VALVE REPLACEMENT

TAVI has become the treatment of choice for symptomatic patients with prohibitive surgical risk, and it is an established alternative for surgical aortic valve replacement (SAVR) for patients in the high- and moderate-risk range. Trials enrolling low-risk patients have overall demonstrated excellent results and improved survival with TAVI compared with SAVR.[3,7,86,87]

The role of echocardiography in pre-TAVI evaluation has diminished considerably over the years, and CT angiography is now preferentially used to assess valvular anatomy, particularly annular dimensions for sizing of the prosthetic valve and the position of the coronary ostia in relation to the annular plane. Nonetheless, echocardiography provides important information in the context of pre-TAVI evaluation beyond the correct assessment of stenosis severity, including assessment of additional pathology relevant for risk stratification, evaluation of associated findings potentially amenable to surgical (or interventional) treatment, and delineation of valvular anatomy in case of contraindications to CT angiography.

RISK ASSESSMENT

The contemporary choice regarding type of valve replacement, as outlined in current guidelines, should be made by a heart team and should incorporate a number of clinical, anatomic, and technical characteristics and other cardiac conditions that may require intervention (Table 22.7).[7,88] The current choice between TAVI and SAVR for the individual patient highly depends on perceived surgical risk as estimated by the Society of Thoracic Surgeons' (STS) score or, less frequently, by the EuroSCORE II.

Echocardiographic parameters included in the STS score are EF and concomitant valve pathologies (i.e., aortic regurgitation, mitral stenosis, and/or regurgitation, tricuspid regurgitation). Additional factors, such as RV dimensions and function and pulmonary pressures, also have prognostic importance.[52,53] These factors influence overall (surgical) risk and should be included in the echocardiographic report to allow a well-founded heart team decision. However, as demonstrated in recent trials[86,87] demonstrating favorable outcomes with TAVI also in low-risk

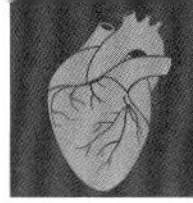

TABLE 22.7 Factors Considered by the Heart Team in Choosing SAVR or TAVI.

Factors Affecting Choice of Procedure	*Favors TAVI*	*Favors SAVR*
Clinical Characteristics		
STS/EuroSCORE II < 4% (logistic EuroSCORE I < 10%)		+
STS/EuroSCORE II ≥ 4% (logistic EuroSCORE I ≥ 10%)	+	
Presence of severe comorbidity (not adequately reflected by scores)	+	
Age < 75 y		+
Age ≥ 75 y	+	
Previous cardiac surgery	+	
Frailty	+	
Restricted mobility and conditions that may affect the rehabilitation process after the procedure	+	
Suspicion of endocarditis		+
Anatomic and Technical Aspects		
Favorable access for transfemoral TAVI	+	
Unfavorable access (any) for TAVI		+
Sequelae of chest irradiation	+	
Porcelain aorta	+	
Intact coronary bypass grafts at risk when sternotomy is performed	+	
Expected patient–prosthesis mismatch	+	
Severe chest deformation or scoliosis	+	
Short distance between coronary ostia and aortic valve annulus		+
Size of aortic valve annulus out of range for TAVI		+
Aortic root morphology unfavorable for TAVI		+
Valve morphology (bicuspid, degree of calcification, calcification pattern) unfavorable for TAVI		+
Presence of thrombi in aorta or LV		+
Cardiac Conditions[a]		
Severe CAD requiring revascularization by CABG		+
Severe primary mitral valve disease that could be treated surgically		+
Severe tricuspid valve disease		+
Aneurysm of the ascending aorta		+
Septal hypertrophy requiring myectomy		+

[a]Conditions in addition to aortic stenosis that require consideration for concomitant intervention.
CABG, Coronary artery bypass grafting; *CAD*, coronary artery disease; *SAVR*, surgical aortic valve replacement; *STS/EuroSCORE*, Society of Thoracic Surgeons/European System for Cardiac Operative Risk Evaluation risk score model; *TAVI*, transcatheter aortic valve implantation.

patients, risk assessment may in the future become less important in deciding on treatment strategy.

ASSOCIATED FINDINGS

Significantly, concomitant MR is frequently seen in patients assessed for AVR, and its severity and mechanism need to be evaluated meticulously. Whereas secondary MR may improve after valve replacement due to decreased ventricular pressures regardless of the type of procedure, primary MR is unlikely to respond, potentially favoring a surgical approach. An aneurysm of the ascending aorta requiring intervention supports a surgical approach. Similarly, in patients with a small, hypertrophied LV showing signs of LVOT obstruction, the possibility to perform a myectomy may have to be considered to avoid postinterventional aggravation of dynamic subvalvular obstruction.

VALVE ANATOMY

A bicuspid aortic valve was initially considered a contraindication to valve replacement in randomized trials comparing TAVI with SAVR because of concerns about prosthesis malpositioning and an increased rate of significant paravalvular leakage. However, cuspidity may be difficult to assess in heavily calcified valves, and a substantial percentage of patients undergoing TAVI present with a bicuspid valve as suggested by CT angiography. Two large propensity score–matched analyses that included patients with bicuspid or tricuspid valves undergoing TAVI showed comparable all-cause mortality rates for up to 2 years.[89]

SUMMARY Measured and Calculated Parameters.

Parameter	Modality/View	Technical Aspects	Caveats/Comments
Measured Parameters			
Aortic velocity	• CW Doppler • Multiple acoustic windows	• Alignment of Doppler parallel to stenotic jet • High wall filter • High sweep velocity • Optimized baseline and scale	• Meticulous search for maximal velocity in multiple acoustic windows
Pre-stenotic velocity	• Pulsed-wave Doppler • Apical 5-chamber view	• Sample volume near the aortic valve • Decreased gain • Low wall filter • High sweep velocity	• Meticulous search for the last laminar flow signal within the LVOT in the direction of flow before turbulence occurs • Check of maximum velocity with Doppler and within the aortic velocity CW signal
LVOT diameter	• 2D echocardiography • Parasternal long-axis view	• Optimized image quality • Zoom • Mid-systole • Near and parallel to the aortic valve • Inner edge	• Multiple attempts to identify maximal anterior-posterior diameter • Can also be measured by TEE in high image quality • Exclusion of localized calcifications from the measurement
TEE planimetry	• 2D or 3D echocardiography • Short-axis view of the aortic valve	• Optimized image quality • Zoom • Mid-systole • Recognition of tissue–blood borders in moving loop before tracing in frozen images	• Requires experienced echocardiographer • Multiple measurements recommended • Domed morphology in bicuspid valves may require 3D imaging • May be helpful if TTE is inconclusive • TEE may be also helpful to re-assess LVOT diameter
Parameter	**Calculation**	**Cutoff Value for Severe AS**	**Strength/Limitation**
Calculated Parameters			
Aortic maximum velocity (V_{max})	Maximum of stenotic spectral CW Doppler signal	>4 m/s	• Best-investigated parameter of AS severity • Gradual increase of adverse events with increasing V_{max} • Flow dependent
Mean pressure gradient (ΔP_{mean})	Derived from CW Doppler instant stenotic velocities: $\Delta P_{mean} = \Sigma(v_1^2 + v_2^2 + \ldots + v_n^2) \times 4/n$	>40 mmHg	• Correlates perfectly with and provides almost identical information as V_{max}
AVA by continuity equation	AVA = VTI_1/VTI_2 × LVOT area	<1.0 cm^2	• Less flow dependent than V_{max} or ΔP_{mean} • Required when flow is reduced • Necessitates calculation of LVOT area (prone to measurement error)
Indexed AVA (AVAi)	AVAi = AVA/BSA	<0.6 cm^2/m^2	• Required in patients with small body size (BSA < 1.6 m^2) • May overestimates AS severity in large and obese patients
Stroke volume index (SVI)	SVI = (VTI_1 × LVOT area)/BSA	Low flow: ≤ 35 mL/m^2	• Important parameter to assess low flow and unmask severe AS with low ΔP_{mean} and normal ejection fraction • Prone to measurement error; should be strengthened by LV volumes and/or indirect signs of reduced flow

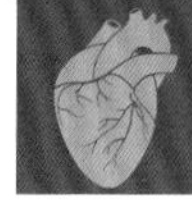

SUMMARY Measured and Calculated Parameters.—cont'd

Parameter	Modality/View	Technical Aspects	Caveats/Comments
Flow rate (FR)	FR = SV/ET	Low flow: FR < 200 mL/s	• More precise parameter to estimate opening forces • Dobutamine stimulation to exclude pseudostenosis may be indicated only with FR < 200 mL/s at rest
Velocity ratio (VR)	$VR = VTI_1/VTI_2$	<0.25	• Ideal parameter for individual follow-up when LVOT size may be considered constant
Energy loss index (ELI)	ELI = AVAi × Aa/ (Aa − AVA)	<0.6 cm^2/m^2	• Useful if pressure recovery is assumed (patients with a diameter of the ascending aorta <30 mm)

Aa, Area of ascending aorta at the sinotubular junction; *AS*, aortic stenosis; *AVA*, aortic valve area; *indexed AVA*, aortic valve area normalized to body surface area; *BSA*, body surface area; *ET*, ejection time; *LVOT*, left ventricular outflow tract; *SV*, stroke volume; VTI_1, velocity–time integral of pre-stenotic velocity; VTI_2, velocity–time integral of stenotic velocity.

REFERENCES

1. Otto CM, Lind BK, Kitzman DW, Gersh BJ, Siscovick DS. Association of aortic-valve sclerosis with cardiovascular mortality and morbidity in the elderly. *N Engl J Med.* 1999;341:142–147.
2. Hull MC, Morris CG, Pepine CJ, Mendenhall N. Valvular dysfunction and carotid, subclavian, and coronary artery disease in survivors of hodgkin lymphoma treated with radiation therapy. *J Am Med Assoc.* 2003;290:2831–2837.
3. Nishimura RA, et al. 2014. AHA/ACC guideline for the management of patients with valvular heart disease: executive summary: a report of the American College of Cardiology/American Heart Association Task force on Practice Guidelines. *J Am Coll Cardiol.* 2014;63(22):e57-185. https://doi.org/10.1016/j.jacc.2014.02.537.
4. Rosenhek R, et al. Predictors of outcome in severe, asymptomatic aortic stenosis. *N Engl J Med.* 2000;343:611–617.
5. Wu VC-C, et al. Prognostic value of area of calcified aortic valve by 2-dimensional echocardiography in asymptomatic severe aortic stenosis patients with preserved left ventricular ejection fraction. *Medicine (Baltim).* 2018;97. e0246.
6. Baumgartner H, et al. Recommendations on the echocardiographic assessment of aortic valve stenosis: a Focused Update from the European Association of Cardiovascular Imaging and the American Society of Echocardiography. *J Am Soc Echocardiogr.* 2017;30:372–392.
7. Baumgartner H, et al. 2017 ESC/EACTS Guidelines for the Management of Valvular Heart Disease. *Eur Heart J.* 2017;38(36):2739-2791. https://doi.org/10.1093/eurheartj/ehx391.
8. Otto CM, et al. Prospective study of asymptomatic valvular aortic stenosis. Clinical, echocardiographic, and exercise predictors of outcome. *Circulation.* 1997;95:2262–2270.
9. Rosenhek R, et al. Natural history of very severe aortic stenosis. *Circulation.* 2010;121:151–156.
10. Rosenhek R. Mild and moderate aortic stenosis natural history and risk stratification by echocardiography. *Eur Heart J.* 2004;25:199–205.
11. Otto CM, et al. Determination of the stenotic aortic valve area in adults using Doppler echocardiography. *J Am Coll Cardiol.* 1986;7:509–517.
12. Eleid MF, et al. Flow-gradient patterns in severe aortic stenosis with preserved ejection fraction: clinical characteristics and predictors of survival. *Circulation.* 2013;128:1781–1789.
13. Dahl JS, et al. Development of paradoxical low-flow, low-gradient severe aortic stenosis. *Heart.* 2015;101(13):1015-23. https://doi.org/10.1136/heartjnl-2014-306838.
14. Michelena HI, et al. Inconsistent echocardiographic grading of aortic stenosis: is the left ventricular outflow tract important? *Heart.* 2013;99:921–931.
15. Jander N, et al. Velocity ratio predicts outcomes in patients with low gradient severe aortic stenosis and preserved EF. *Heart Br Card Soc.* 2014;100:1946–1953.
16. Bradley SM, et al. Use of routinely captured echocardiographic data in the diagnosis of severe aortic stenosis. *Heart.* 2019;105:112–116.
17. Saura D, et al. Aortic valve stenosis planimetry by means of three-dimensional transesophageal echocardiography in the real clinical setting: feasibility, reliability and systematic deviations. *Echocardiogr. Mt. Kisco N.* 2014. https://doi.org/10.1111/echo.12675.
18. Geibel A, Görnandt L, Kasper W, Bubenheimer P. Reproducibility of Doppler echocardiographic quantification of aortic and mitral valve stenoses: comparison between two echocardiography centers. *Am J Cardiol.* 1991;67:1013–1021.
19. Garcia J, Kadem L, Larose E, Clavel M-A, Pibarot P. Comparison between cardiovascular magnetic resonance and transthoracic Doppler echocardiography for the estimation of effective orifice area in aortic stenosis. *J Cardiovasc Magn Reson.* 2011;13:25.
20. Jander N, et al. Anatomic estimation of aortic stenosis severity vs "fusion" of data from computed tomography and Doppler echocardiography. *Echocardiography.* 2018;35:777–784.
21. Mittal TK, et al. Inconsistency in aortic stenosis severity between CT and echocardiography: prevalence and insights into mechanistic differences using computational fluid dynamics. *Open Heart.* 2019;6: e001044.
22. Clavel M-A, et al. Predictors of outcomes in low-flow, low-gradient aortic stenosis results of the Multicenter TOPAS study. *Circulation.* 2008;118:S234–S242.
23. Chahal NS, et al. Resting aortic valve area at normal transaortic flow rate reflects true valve area in suspected low-gradient severe aortic stenosis. *JACC Cardiovasc Imaging.* 2015;8:1133–1139.
24. Minners J, et al. Adjusting parameters of aortic valve stenosis severity by body size. *Heart Br Card Soc.* 2014;100:1024–1030.
25. Jander N, et al. Indexing aortic valve area by body surface area increases the prevalence of severe aortic stenosis. *Heart.* 2014;100:28–33.
26. Saito T, et al. Prognostic value of aortic valve area index in asymptomatic patients with severe aortic stenosis. *Am J Cardiol.* 2012;110:93–97.
27. Tribouilloy C, et al. Outcome implication of aortic valve area normalized to body size in asymptomatic aortic stenosis. *Circ Cardiovasc Imaging.* 2016;9: e005121.
28. Eleid MF, Nishimura RA, Sorajja P, Borlaug BA. Systemic hypertension in low-gradient severe aortic stenosis with preserved ejection fraction. *Circulation.* 2013;128:1349–1353.
29. Abbas AE, et al. The role of jet Eccentricity in generating disproportionately elevated transaortic pressure gradients in patients with aortic stenosis. *Echocardiography.* 2015;32:372–382.
30. Weyman AE, Scherrer-Crosbie M. Aortic stenosis: physics and physiology—what do the numbers really mean? *Rev Cardiovasc Med.* 2005;6:23–32.
31. Bahlmann E, et al. Prognostic value of energy loss index in asymptomatic aortic stenosis. *Circulation.* 2013;127:1149–1156.
32. Minners J, et al. Inconsistencies of echocardiographic criteria for the grading of aortic valve stenosis. *Eur Heart J.* 2008;29:1043–1048.
33. Minners J, et al. Inconsistent grading of aortic valve stenosis by current guidelines: haemodynamic studies in patients with apparently normal left ventricular function. *Heart Br. Card. Soc.* 2010;96:1463–1468.
34. Jander N, et al. Outcome of patients with low-gradient 'severe' aortic stenosis and preserved

ejection fraction. *Circulation*. 2011;123:887–895.

35. Zheng Q, et al. Effects of aortic valve replacement on severe aortic stenosis and preserved systolic function: systematic review and network meta-analysis. *Sci Rep*. 2017;7 (1):5092.
36. Cioffi G, et al. Prognostic effect of inappropriately high left ventricular mass in asymptomatic severe aortic stenosis. *Heart*. 2011;97:301–307.
37. Adda J, et al. Low-flow, low-gradient severe aortic stenosis despite normal ejection fraction is associated with severe left ventricular dysfunction as assessed by speckle-tracking echocardiography: a multicenter study. *Circ Cardiovasc Imaging*. 2012;5:27–35.
38. Treibel TA, et al. Reverse myocardial remodeling following valve replacement in patients with aortic stenosis. *J Am Coll Cardiol*. 2018;71:860–871.
39. Dahl JS, et al. Effect of left ventricular ejection fraction on postoperative outcome in patients with severe aortic stenosis undergoing aortic valve replacement. *Circ Cardiovasc Imaging*. 2015;8(4): e002917.
40. Bohbot Y, et al. Relationship between left ventricular ejection fraction and mortality in asymptomatic and minimally symptomatic patients with severe aortic stenosis. *JACC Cardiovasc Imaging*. 2019;12:38–48.
41. Eleid MF, et al. Survival by stroke volume index in patients with low-gradient normal EF severe aortic stenosis. *Heart*. 2015;101:23–29.
42. Kearney LG, et al. Global longitudinal strain is a strong independent predictor of all-cause mortality in patients with aortic stenosis. *Eur Heart J Cardiovasc Imaging*. 2012;13:827–833.
43. Vollema EM, et al. Association of left ventricular global longitudinal strain with asymptomatic severe aortic stenosis: Natural course and prognostic value. *JAMA Cardiol*. 2018;3:839–847.
44. Fabiani I, et al. Micro-RNA-21 (biomarker) and global longitudinal strain (functional marker) in detection of myocardial fibrotic burden in severe aortic valve stenosis: a pilot study. *J Transl Med*. 2016;14:248.
45. Zilberszac R, et al. Outcome of combined stenotic and regurgitant aortic valve disease. *J Am Coll Cardiol*. 2013;61:1489–1495.
46. Takami Y, Tajima K. Mitral annular calcification in patients undergoing aortic valve replacement for aortic valve stenosis. Heart Vessels. 2016;31(2):183-188. https://doi.org/10.1007/s00380-014-0585-5.
47. Asami M, et al. Transcatheter aortic valve replacement in patients with concomitant mitral stenosis. *Eur Heart J*. 2019;40:1342–1351.
48. Nombela-Franco L, et al. Timing, predictive factors, and prognostic value of cerebrovascular events in a large cohort of patients undergoing transcatheter aortic valve implantation. *Circulation*. 2012;126:3041–3053.
49. Unger P, et al. Mitral regurgitation in patients with aortic stenosis undergoing valve replacement. *Heart*. 2010;96:9–14.
50. Castaño A, et al. Unveiling transthyretin cardiac amyloidosis and its predictors among elderly patients with severe aortic stenosis undergoing transcatheter aortic valve replacement. *Eur Heart J*. 2017;38:2879–2887.
51. Treibel TA, et al. Occult transthyretin cardiac amyloid in severe calcific aortic stenosis prevalence and prognosis in patients undergoing surgical aortic valve replacement. *Circ Cardiovasc Imaging*. 2016;9(8): e005066.
52. Levy F, et al. Impact of pulmonary hypertension on long-term outcome in patients with severe aortic stenosis. *Eur Heart J Cardiovasc Imaging*. 2018;19:553–561.
53. Alushi B, et al. Pulmonary hypertension in patients with severe aortic stenosis: prognostic impact after transcatheter aortic valve replacement. *JACC Cardiovasc Imaging*. 2019;12:591–601.
54. Das P. Exercise testing to stratify risk in aortic stenosis. *Eur Heart J*. 2005;26:1309–1313.
55. Lancellotti P, et al. Determinants and prognostic significance of exercise pulmonary hypertension in asymptomatic severe aortic stenosis. *Circulation*. 2012;126:851–859.
56. Marechaux S, et al. Usefulness of exercise-stress echocardiography for risk stratification of true asymptomatic patients with aortic valve stenosis. *Eur Heart J*. 2010;31:1390–1397.
57. Abdulla J, et al. Evaluation of aortic valve stenosis by cardiac multislice computed tomography compared with echocardiography: a systematic review and meta-analysis. *J Heart Valve Dis*. 2009;18:634–643.
58. Clavel M-A, et al. Aortic valve area calculation in aortic stenosis by CT and Doppler echocardiography. *JACC Cardiovasc Imaging*. 2015;8:248–257.
59. Clavel M-A, et al. The complex nature of discordant severe calcified aortic valve disease grading. *J Am Coll Cardiol*. 2013;62:2329–2338.
60. Clavel M-A, et al. Impact of aortic valve calcification, as measured by MDCT, on survival in patients with aortic stenosis. *J Am Coll Cardiol*. 2014;64:1202–1213.
61. Pawade T, et al. Computed tomography aortic valve calcium scoring in patients with aortic stenosis. *Circ Cardiovasc Imaging*. 2018;11.
62. Bull S, et al. Human non-contrast T1 values and correlation with histology in diffuse fibrosis. *Heart*. 2013;99:932–937.
63. Chin CWL, et al. Myocardial fibrosis and cardiac decompensation in aortic stenosis. *JACC Cardiovasc Imaging*. 2017;10:1320–1333.
64. Ruile P, et al. Pre-procedural assessment of aortic annulus dimensions for transcatheter aortic valve replacement: comparison of a non-contrast 3D MRA protocol with contrast-enhanced cardiac dual-source CT angiography. *Eur Heart J Cardiovasc Imaging*. 2016;17:458–466.
65. Gohlke-Bärwolf C, et al. Natural history of mild and of moderate aortic stenosis-new insights from a large prospective European study. *Curr Probl Cardiol*. 2013;38:365–409.
66. Lancellotti P, et al. Outcomes of patients with asymptomatic aortic stenosis followed up in heart valve clinics. *JAMA Cardiol*. 2018;3:1060–1068.
67. Kanamori N, et al. Prognostic impact of aortic valve area in conservatively managed patients with asymptomatic severe aortic stenosis with preserved ejection fraction. *J Am Heart Assoc*. 2019;8 (3):e010198.
68. Agarwal S, et al. In-hospital mortality and stroke after surgical aortic valve replacement: a nationwide perspective. *J Thorac Cardiovasc Surg*. 2015 150(3):571-8.e8. https://doi.org/10.1016/j.jtcvs.2015.05.068.
69. Lim WY, Ramasamy A, Lloyd G, Bhattacharyya S. Meta-analysis of the impact of intervention versus symptom-driven management in asymptomatic severe aortic stenosis. *Heart*. 2017;103:268–272.
70. Burwash IG, et al. Flow dependence of measures of aortic stenosis severity during exercise. *J Am Coll Cardiol*. 1994;24:1342–1350.
71. Fougeres E, et al. Outcomes of pseudo-severe aortic stenosis under conservative treatment. *Eur Heart J*. 2012;33:2426–2433.
72. Ribeiro HB, et al. Transcatheter aortic valve replacement in patients with low-flow, low-gradient aortic stenosis: the TOPAS-TAVI Registry. *J Am Coll Cardiol*. 2018;71:1297–1308.
73. Maes F, et al. Outcomes from transcatheter aortic valve replacement in patients with low-flow, low-gradient aortic stenosis and left ventricular ejection fraction less than 30%: a substudy from the TOPAS-TAVI Registry. *JAMA Cardiol*. 2019;4:64–70.
74. van Gils L, et al. Prognostic implications of moderate aortic stenosis in patients with left ventricular systolic dysfunction. *J Am Coll Cardiol*. 2017;69:2383–2392.
75. Spitzer E, et al. Rationale and design of the Transcatheter Aortic Valve Replacement to UNload the Left ventricle in patients with ADvanced heart failure (TAVR UNLOAD) trial. *Am Heart J*. 2016;182:80–88.
76. Mehrotra P, et al. Differential left ventricular remodelling and longitudinal function distinguishes low flow from normal-flow preserved ejection fraction low-gradient severe aortic stenosis. *Eur Heart J*. 2013;34:1906–1914.
77. Herrmann S, et al. Low-gradient aortic valve stenosis. *J Am Coll Cardiol*. 2011;58:402–412.
78. Hachicha Z, Dumesnil JG, Bogaty P, Pibarot P. Paradoxical low-flow, low-gradient severe aortic stenosis despite preserved ejection fraction is associated with higher afterload and reduced survival. *Circulation*. 2007;115:2856–2864.
79. Clavel M-A, et al. Outcome of patients with aortic stenosis, small valve area, and low-flow, low-gradient despite preserved left ventricular ejection fraction. *J Am Coll Cardiol*. 2012;60:1259–1267.
80. Eleid MF, et al. Causes of death and predictors of survival after aortic valve replacement in low flow vs. normal flow severe aortic stenosis with preserved ejection fraction. *Eur. Heart J Cardiovasc Imaging*. 2015. https://doi.org/10.1093/ehjci/jev091.
81. Rodriguez-Gabella T, et al. Transcatheter aortic valve implantation in patients with paradoxical low-flow, low-gradient aortic stenosis. *Am J Cardiol*. 2018;122:625–632.
82. Maes F, et al. Natural history of paradoxical low gradient 'severe' aortic stenosis. *Circ Cardiovasc Imaging*. 2014;113. 001695. https://doi.org/10.1161/CIRCIMAGING.113.001695.
83. Clavel M-A, et al. Stress echocardiography to assess stenosis severity and predict outcome in patients with paradoxical low-flow, low-gradient aortic stenosis and preserved LVEF. *JACC Cardiovasc Imaging*. 2013;6:175–183.
84. Saeed S, et al. The impact of aortic valve replacement on survival in patients with normal flow low gradient severe aortic stenosis: a propensity-matched comparison. *Eur Heart J Cardiovasc Imaging*. 2019. https://doi.org/10.1093/ehjci/jez191.
85. Carter-Storch Rasmus, et al. Postoperative reverse remodeling and symptomatic improvement in normal-flow low-gradient aortic stenosis after aortic valve replacement. *Circ Cardiovasc Imaging*. 2017;10(12): e006580.
86. Mack MJ, et al. Transcatheter aortic-valve replacement with a balloon-expandable valve in low-risk patients. *N Engl J Med*. 2019;380:1695-705.
87. Popma JJ, et al. Transcatheter aortic-valve replacement with a self-expanding valve in low-

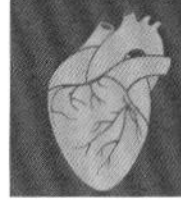

risk patients. *N Engl J Med.* 2019;380:1706–1715.

88. Otto CM, et al. ACC expert consensus decision pathway for transcatheter aortic valve replacement in the management of adults with aortic stenosis: a report of the American College of Cardiology Task Force on Clinical Expert Consensus Documents. *J Am Coll Cardiol.* 2017;69:1313–1346.
89. Makkar RR, et al. Association between transcatheter aortic valve replacement for bicuspid vs tricuspid aortic stenosis and mortality or stroke. *J Am Med Assoc.* 2019;321:2193–2202.
90. Nishimura RA, et al. AHA/ACC Focused Update of the 2014 AHA/ACC guideline for the management of patients with valvular heart disease: a report of the American College of Cardiology/American Heart Association Task Force on Clinical Practice Guidelines. *Circulation.* 2017;135. 2017.
91. Otto CM, Pearlman AS, Gardner CL. Hemodynamic progression of aortic stenosis in adults assessed by Doppler echocardiography. *J Am Coll Cardiol.* 1989;13:545–550.
92. Rossebø AB, et al. Intensive lipid lowering with simvastatin and ezetimibe in aortic stenosis. *N Engl J Med.* 2008;359:1343–1356.
93. Tastet L, et al. Impact of aortic valve calcification and sex on hemodynamic progression and clinical outcomes in AS. *J Am Coll Cardiol.* 2017;69:2096–2098.
94. Pellikka PA, et al. Outcome of 622 adults with asymptomatic, hemodynamically significant aortic stenosis during prolonged follow-up. *Circulation.* 2005;111:3290–3295.
95. Kearney LG, et al. Progression of aortic stenosis in elderly patients over long-term follow up. *Int J Cardiol.* 2013;167:1226–1231.
96. Taniguchi T, et al. Initial surgical versus conservative strategies in patients with asymptomatic severe aortic stenosis. *J Am Coll Cardiol.* 2015;66(25):2827–2838. https://doi.org/10.1016/j.jacc.2015.10.001.
97. Monin J-L, et al. Risk score for predicting outcome in patients with asymptomatic aortic stenosis. *Circulation.* 2009;120:69–75.
98. Lancellotti P, et al. Risk stratification in asymptomatic moderate to severe aortic stenosis: the importance of the valvular, arterial and ventricular interplay. *Heart.* 2010;96:1364–1371.
99. Taniguchi T, et al. Sudden death in patients with severe aortic stenosis: observations from the CURRENT AS Registry. *J Am Heart Assoc Cardiovasc Cerebrovasc Dis.* 2018;7.
100. Kang D-K, Park S-J, Lee S-A, et al. Early surgery or conservative care for asymptomatic aortic stenosis. *N Engl J Med.* 2020;382:111–119.

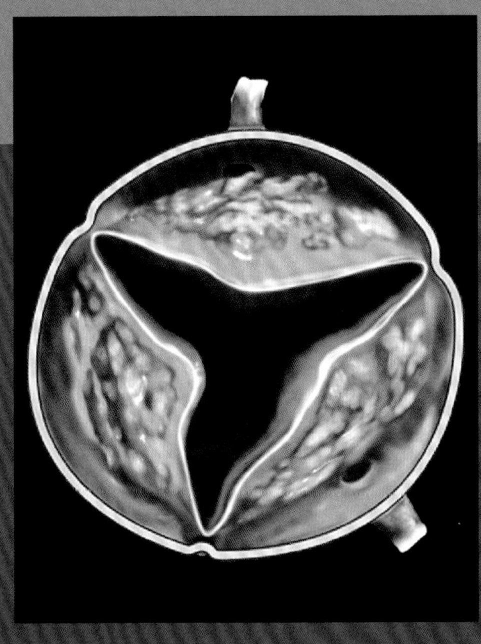

第23章
主动脉瓣反流

主动脉瓣反流是指舒张期血液从升主动脉反流入左心室。其临床表现各异，受多种因素影响，包括发病的缓急、主动脉和左心室的顺应性、血液动力学状况和病变的严重程度。慢性主动脉瓣反流的总患病率为5%～10%，其中大多数患者为轻度反流。中度或重度主动脉瓣反流更少，总发病率为0.5%～2.7%。超声心动图已成为评估主动脉瓣反流最常用的非侵入性方法，包括确定主动脉瓣反流原因（评估升主动脉扩张）、严重程度及对心室功能的影响。推荐采用多个定性和定量参数综合判断主动脉瓣反流的严重程度。

本章主要从主动脉瓣反流的背景、病因、反流严重程度、左心室大小和收缩功能、主动脉根部和升主动脉评估、慢性主动脉瓣反流的自然病史和系列检查、手术的管理和时机、选择和指导手术治疗、急性主动脉瓣反流的手术和随访结果等多个方面进行了详细的介绍。

牛丽莉

23 Aortic Regurgitation

ARTURO EVANGELISTA, MD, PhD | LAURA GALIAN GAY, MD, PhD

BACKGROUND

Aortic regurgitation (AR) is characterized by diastolic reflux of blood from the ascending aorta into the left ventricle (LV). The clinical presentation varies and depends on several factors, including acuity of onset, aortic and LV compliance, hemodynamic conditions, and severity of the lesion.

The overall prevalence of chronic AR is 5% to 10%, with most cases classified as trace or mild. Moderate or severe AR is less common (0.5%–2.7%).[1] In the Euro Heart Survey on Valvular Disease, AR accounted for 13.3% of patients with single native left-sided diseases.[2]

Echocardiography has become the most frequently used noninvasive method for AR assessment, including determination of the cause (with evaluation of ascending aortic dilation), severity of regurgitation, and its effect on ventricular function. Quantitative and qualitative measures are used, and an integrated approach incorporating several parameters is recommended.

ETIOLOGY

AR results from multiple causes involving abnormalities of the aortic valve leaflets or the supporting structures, such as the aortic root and annulus, or both (Table 23.1). Primary leaflet problems include congenital and acquired abnormalities. Although rheumatic heart disease remains the most common cause in developing countries, bicuspid aortic valve (BAV) in younger populations and ascending aortic diseases in older populations are becoming more common causes of AR in developed countries.[3,4]

Transthoracic echocardiography (TTE) evaluation of the anatomy of aortic leaflets, annulus, and aortic root is important for defining the cause and prognosis and for the management of AR. The parasternal long-axis view is classically used to measure the LV outflow tract (LVOT), the aortic annulus, and the dimensions of the aortic sinuses. Leaflet thickness and morphology can be visualized from this window and from the parasternal short-axis view. If the acoustic window is optimal, three-dimensional (3D) echocardiography could provide better delineation of the aortic valve morphology.[5]

In 20% of cases in some series, TTE did not find the cause of AR, probably because of small fenestrations or cusp prolapse. In these cases, transesophageal echocardiography (TEE) can help to assess the mechanisms of AR and aortic root dimensions.

LEAFLET ABNORMALITIES

Several diseases result in AR due to leaflet abnormalities:

Congenital abnormalities include bicuspid and, rarely, unicuspid or quadricuspid valves. The long-axis view reveals an asymmetric closure line and systolic doming or diastolic prolapse of the leaflets. The short-axis view is more specific. The diagnosis is confirmed when only two leaflets are seen in systole with two commissures framing an elliptical systolic orifice[6] (Fig. 23.1). 3D echocardiography may better define morphologic details of the BAV.[7]

The most frequent abnormality (>70%) is fusion of the right and left coronary cusps. The valve orientation of a BAV may be related to the location of aortic enlargement as a consequence of the eccentric direction of the jet and abnormal helical systolic flow in the ascending aorta.[8] BAV with right and left coronary cusp fusion may be related to a larger sinus diameter than BAV with right and noncoronary cusp fusion. The morphology frequently includes a tubular ascending aorta and arch dilation[5] (see Fig. 23.1).

About 50% of patients younger than 30 years of age have aortic dilation, and the 25-year risk of developing an aneurysm (>45 mm) is 26% for this population.[9] Other congenital disorders, such as ventricular septal defect or subvalvular aortic stenosis, may induce AR due to jet lesions.

TABLE 23.1 Causes of Chronic Aortic Regurgitation.

Abnormalities of Aortic Leaflets	*Description or Findings*	*Diseases of the Aortic Root*	*Description or Findings*
Bicuspid aortic valve and other congenital abnormalities	Two leaflets seen in systole with two commissures framing an elliptical orifice; right-left commissural fusion is typical (70%)	Idiopathic aortic root dilation	Dilation occurring at the sinuses of Valsalva level
Aortic valve sclerosis	Calcification appears in the central part of the cusp	Aortoannular ectasia	Dilation of the aortic annulus and aortic root
Rheumatic heart disease	Commissural fusion, thickening and retraction of leaflets; calcification occurs in advanced stages	Marfan syndrome	Aortic dilation mainly in the aortic root; aortic dissection typically occurs in ascending aorta
Myxomatous valve disease	Thickening and redundancy of leaflets; prolapse into the outflow tract in diastole	Ehlers-Danlos syndrome	Dilation of the aortic annulus and aortic root
Infective endocarditis	Infective vegetations can alter diastolic leaflet closure; leaflet perforation can occur	Osteogenesis imperfecta	Aortic root dilation Aortic dissection occurs infrequently
Systemic inflammatory disorders	Leaflet thickening or nodules/vegetations appearing in the free edge of the leaflet	Aortic dissection	Dilation or rupture of the aortic annulus, asymmetric displacement of sigmoid coaptation level, or intima prolapse through the aortic valve
Antiphospholipid syndrome	Leaflet thickening and nodules/vegetations	Syphilitic aortitis	Ascending aorta dilation or aneurysm
Anorectic drugs	Thickening and leaflet retraction	—	—
Subaortic stenosis	Abnormalities due to high-velocity systolic jet that collides with the leaflet	—	—
Leaflet fenestration	Malformation from the early embryonic phase located in the free edge of the cusp near the commissural attachment	—	—

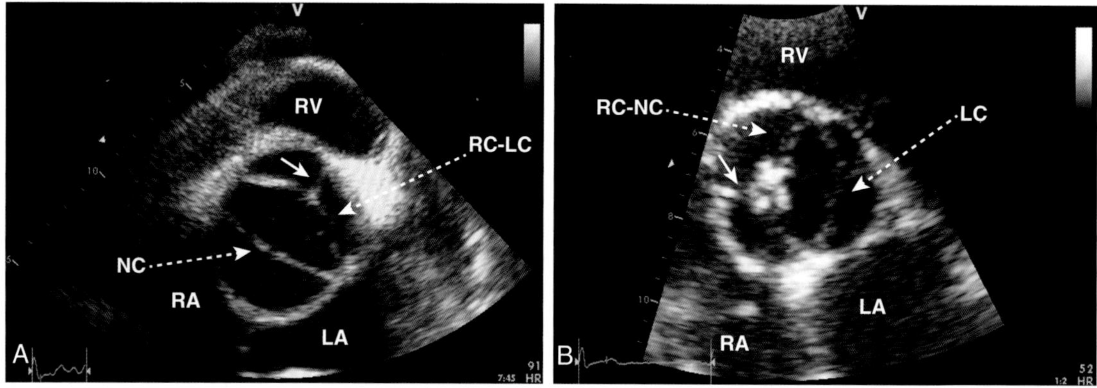

Fig. 23.1 Bicuspid aortic valve. Parasternal short-axis view of a bicuspid aortic valve (BAV). (A) Fusion of the right and left coronary cusps (i.e., anterior-posterior BAV) (see Video 23.1A). (B) Fusion of the right coronary and noncoronary cusps (i.e., right-left BAV). *Small arrows* show the raphe (see Video 23.1B). *LC,* Left coronary cusp; *NC,* noncoronary cusp; *RC,* right coronary cusp.

Aortic valve sclerosis results in AR due to calcifications of the central part of the cusps, a condition that is more prevalent among the elderly.

Rheumatic disease is characterized by commissural fusion, thickening, and retraction of the aortic leaflets, which usually induces a central regurgitation jet (Fig. 23.2).

Endocarditis results in acute AR through leaflet perforation due to the infectious process (see Fig. 23.2) (see Chapter 29) or diastolic leaflet closure deformity caused by a valvular vegetation.[10]

Myxomatous valve disease can affect the aortic and mitral valves. The leaflets are thickened and redundant, with slight sagging into the LVOT during diastole[11] (see Fig. 23.2).

Fenestration of the aortic valve is not a rare malformation. The congenital anomalies can be aggravated by dilation of the ring and increased intravascular pressure with age, but in most cases they do not have functional significance. Fenestrations are located mainly in the free edge of the cusp, near the commissural attachment, Large fenestrations can produce chronic regurgitation, and rupture of the fenestrated fibrous cords can lead to severe regurgitation.[12] Although fenestrations can sometimes be visualized with high-resolution TTE imaging, TEE may be more useful for detecting them.

Less common causes include leaflet thickening induced by drugs or radiation, nonbacterial thrombotic endocarditis, lupus erythematosus, other inflammatory diseases, and complications after transcatheter aortic valve implantation.[13]

AORTIC ROOT ABNORMALITIES

AR may be caused by alterations in the geometry of the structures supporting the leaflets. These conditions may be more common than primary leaflet disease in patients undergoing surgical treatment of isolated AR in developed countries.[4]

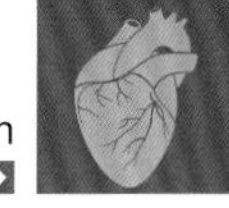

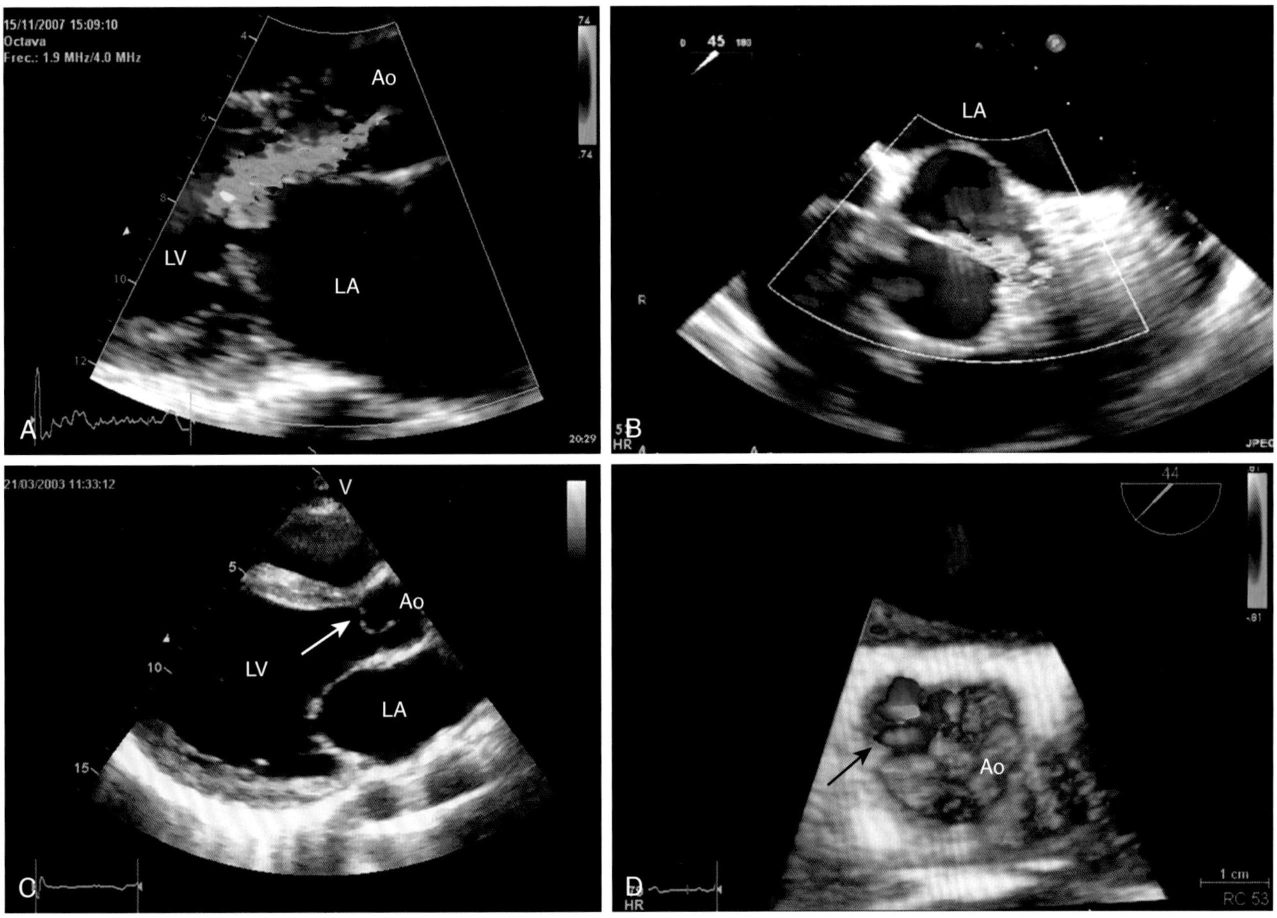

Fig. 23.2 **Causes of aortic regurgitation due to aortic valve leaflet abnormalities.** (A) Rheumatic disease affects the aortic valve and mitral valve (see Video 23.2A). (B) Type I bicuspid aortic valve (see Video 23.2B). (C) Myxomatous aortic valve with right coronary cusp prolapse *(arrow)* (see Video 23.2C). (D) Noncoronary cusp perforation *(arrow)* caused by infective endocarditis (see Video 23.2D). *Ao,* Aorta.

The aortic annulus is a complex, crown-shaped structure located where the leaflets attach to the aortic valve, with the three points of the crown at the commissures and the three lowest points at the midsection of each leaflet. Dilation of this area at the base of the aortic root results in AR due to inadequate coaptation of the stretched leaflets.[14] Aortic root dilation can result from many causes.

Hypertension seems to be associated with modest increases in aortic root size[15] but not AR when age is included in the model. Roberts et al.[4] analyzed the causes of pure AR in 268 patients undergoing isolated aortic valve replacement and showed that the cause was unclear in more than 30% of cases. The group with unclear causes of AR was the oldest; 91% had hypertension, and 29% showed small calcific deposits in the valve cusp.

AORTIC REGURGITATION SEVERITY

COLOR DOPPLER ECHOCARDIOGRAPHY

Color Doppler echocardiography is the key method for the diagnosis and quantification of AR in clinical practice.[16] The regurgitant color Doppler flow pattern has three components: the proximal flow convergence or proximal isovelocity surface area (PISA), the vena contracta, and the distal jet.[16] *Color jet area* correlates only weakly with the degree of AR, mainly in cases of acute or subacute AR that are particularly affected by the aortic-to-LV diastolic pressure gradient and LV compliance.[17]

Despite the limitations, the difference between mild and significant chronic AR may be estimated whenever the same instrument settings are employed and complete visualization of the jet extension using different apical projections is used[23] (Fig. 23.3). In our experience,[18] in cases of chronic AR, a jet area of less than 4 cm^2 or more than 7 cm^2 was specific for mild or significant regurgitation, respectively. However, because of high intermachine variations,[18,19] the use of color flow area of the regurgitant jet is not recommended and should be used only for a visual assessment of AR.

Semiquantitative Methods

Vena contracta width is one of the best methods for grading AR severity.[16] The vena contracta represents the smallest flow diameter at the aortic valve level, immediately below the flow convergence region. The vena contracta is measured in the parasternal long-axis view (Fig. 23.4). A narrow color sector scan and zoom mode are recommended to optimize this measurement. Using a Nyquist limit of 50 to 60 cm/s, a vena contracta width of less than 3 mm correlates with mild AR, whereas a width greater than 6 mm indicates severe AR.[20]

The vena contracta method is limited when the regurgitant orifice is elliptical or irregular. 3D echocardiography permits better vision and analysis of the real vena contracta (Fig. 23.5). With 3D echocardiography, vena contracta areas smaller than 20 cm^2 and larger than 60 cm^2 have been proposed to define mild and severe AR, respectively.[21]

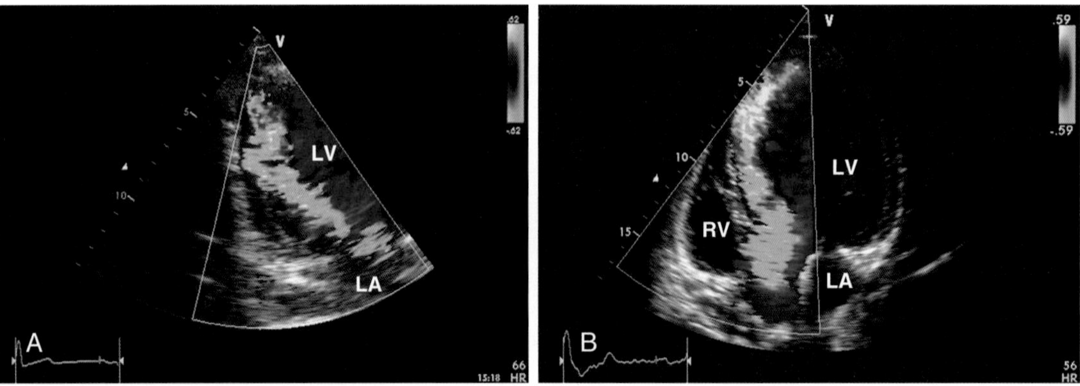

Fig. 23.3 **Aortic regurgitation jet by color Doppler.** (A) The eccentric jet of aortic regurgitation is directed toward the mitral valve. It is better visualized by an apical 3-chamber view in most cases (see Video 23.3A). (B) A very eccentric jet of aortic regurgitation is visualized parallel to the interventricular septum by an apical 5-chamber view (see Video 23.3B).

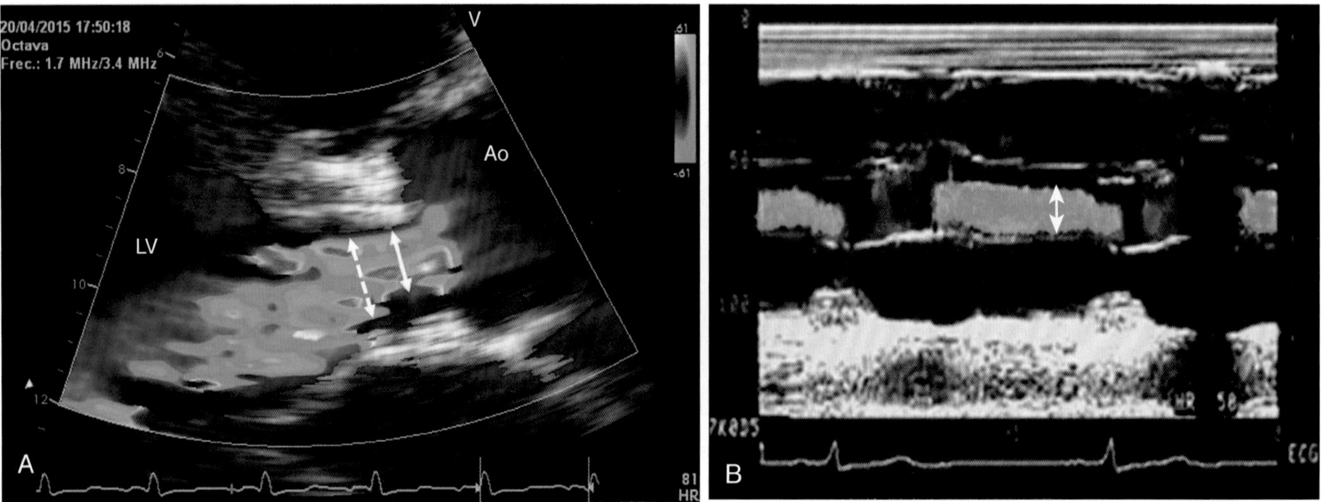

Fig. 23.4 **Parasternal long-axis view of a proximal regurgitant jet width and its vena contracta in severe aortic regurgitation.** (A) Color Doppler signal of aortic regurgitation (AR) occupies more than 65% of the LV outflow tract diameter *(dotted line)*. The vena contracta is the narrowest (waist) diameter of the jet just downstream from the aortic orifice. (B) Color-coded M-mode imaging shows the AR signal during diastole *(double-headed arrow)*. *Ao*, Aorta.

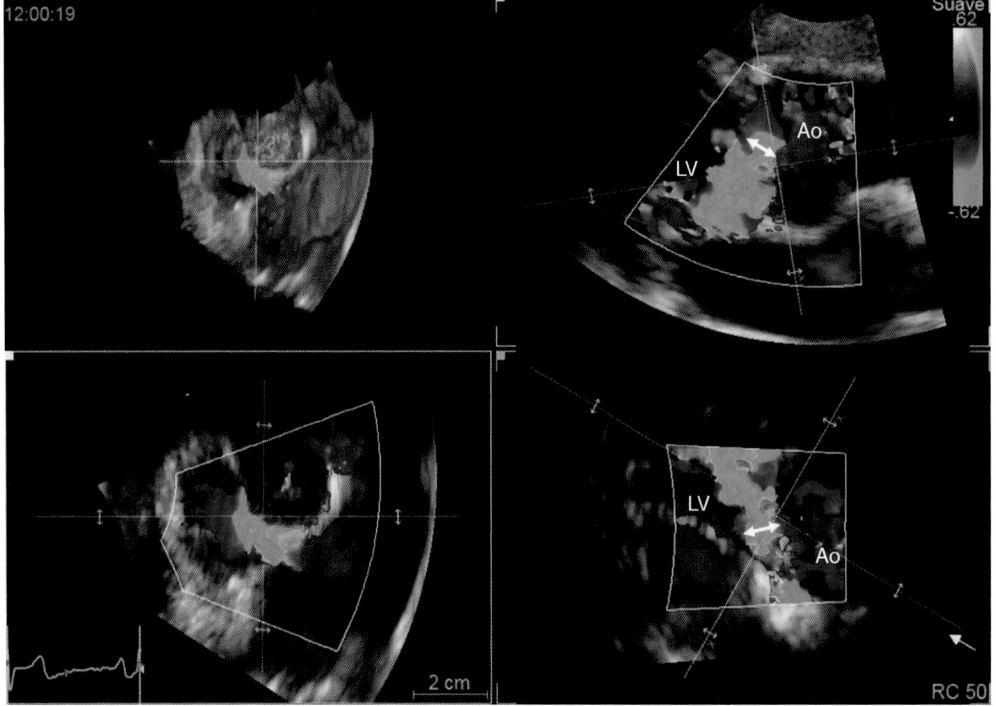

Fig. 23.5 **Multiplanar reconstruction of the aortic regurgitation jet.** From 3D echocardiography *(upper left)*, multiplanar analysis allows the assessment of the direction of the jet and vena contracta size *(double-headed arrows)* of the aortic regurgitant flow (see Video 23.5). *Ao*, Aorta.

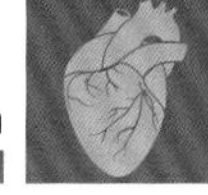

Proximal regurgitant jet width and its ratio to LVOT diameter are obtained from the long-axis views measured immediately below the aortic valve (at the junction of the LVOT and the aortic annulus). A ratio of less than 25% is consistent with mild AR, whereas a ratio greater than 65% indicates severe AR.[22] However, the absolute value of the jet width has similar accuracy and better reproducibility than this ratio, indicating that jet width alone may be sufficient and more practical for follow-up of patients. A jet width greater than 10 mm indicates severe AR, and one less than 7 mm indicates nonsignificant AR[18] (see Fig. 23.4).

This method has some limitations. Jet width should be measured perpendicular to the direction of the jet. However, eccentric jets directed predominantly toward the anterior leaflet of the mitral valve or the septum tend to occupy a small portion of the proximal outflow tract and may appear narrow, leading to underestimation of regurgitation severity.[18] Conversely, central jets tend to expand fully in the outflow tract (i.e., the spray effect) and may be overestimated.

Cross-sectional area of the jet from the parasternal short-axis view and its ratio to the LVOT area are indicators of AR severity.[16] In our experience, an area greater than 1 cm^2 indicates severe AR.[18] The short-axis jet area has limitations because small changes in the LVOT level result in significant differences in jet area, particularly in the setting of eccentric jets, diffuse jets (Fig. 23.6), or jets originating along the coaptation lines.

Quantitative Methods

The *flow convergence method* is less commonly used in AR than in mitral regurgitation to identify a clear proximal flow convergence. When feasible, the PISA method is less sensitive to loading conditions,[23,24] although this method is more technically demanding (Fig. 23.7). The effective regurgitant orifice area (EROA) is obtained by dividing the peak AR flow rate by the peak instantaneous AR velocity (V_{AR}), which is obtained by continuous-wave (CW) Doppler:

$$\text{EROA} = 6.28 \times r^2 \times V_{\text{aliasing}}/\text{peak } V_{AR}$$

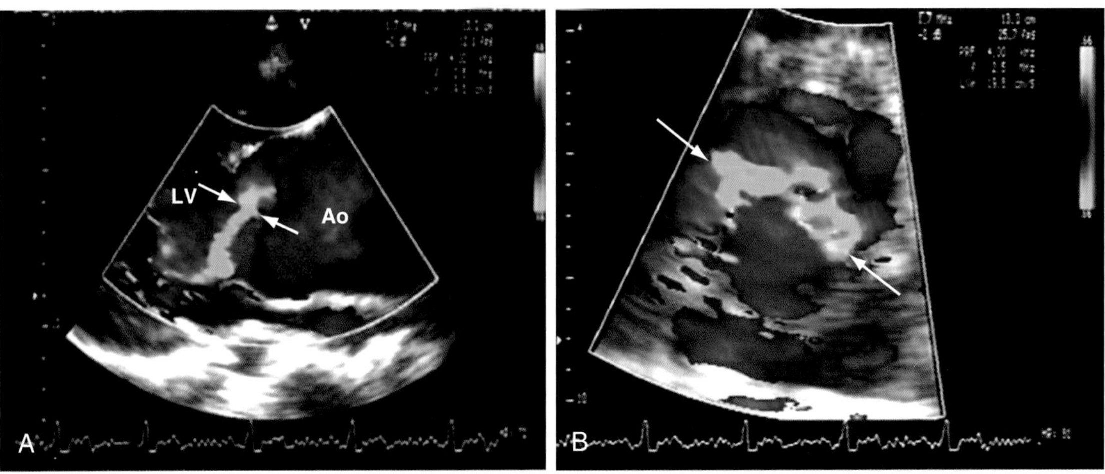

Fig. 23.6 Severe aortic regurgitation due to a bicuspid aortic valve. Although the vena contracta (A, *arrows*) of the eccentric jet directed toward the mitral valve is 5 mm, the short-axis view (B) shows the elliptical shape *(arrows)* of the regurgitant orifice, suggesting greater severity of aortic regurgitation (AR). *Ao*, Aorta.

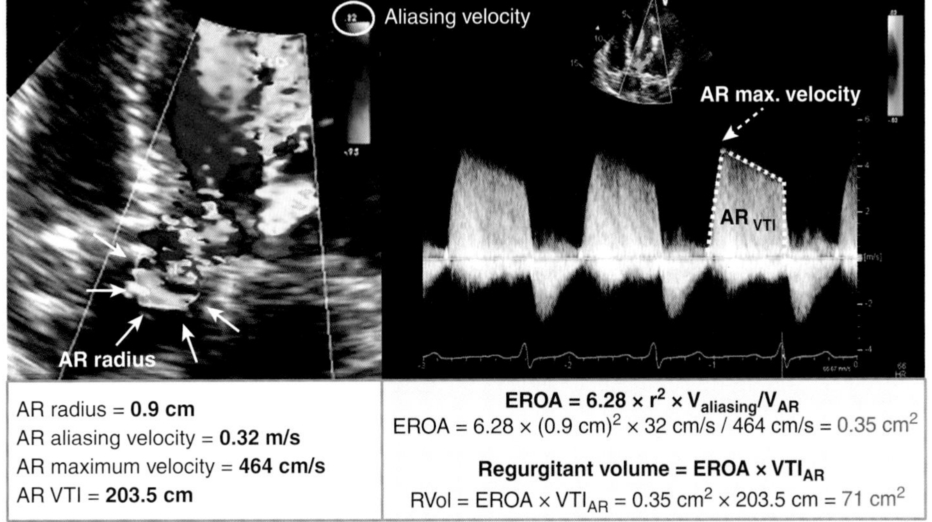

Fig. 23.7 PISA method. *Left,* The proximal isovelocity surface area (PISA) region is imaged ideally in apical or right parasternal views. The area of interest is expanded using the zoom mode, and the sector size is reduced as narrowly as possible to maximize the frame rate. The Nyquist limit should then be shifted in the direction of the aortic regurgitation *(AR)* jet to optimize measurements of the PISA radius. A clearly visible, hemispheric PISA is required for calculation (*arrows* show PISA EROA). Peak flow is calculated as $2\pi r^2$ multiplied by the aliasing velocity ($V_{aliasing}$). Quantitative assessment using the PISA method shows severe AR (EROA ≥ 0.3 cm^2 and RVol ≥ 60 mL/beat). The Nyquist limit is shifted in the direction of the AR jet to obtain hemispheric PISA. *Right,* AR signal to obtain AR maximum velocity and AR VTI. *EROA*, Effective regurgitant orifice area; *r*, radius; V_{AR}, peak instantaneous AR velocity; *VTI*, velocity–time integral.

The regurgitant volume (RVol) is calculated from the EROA by multiplying by the velocity–time integral (VTI) of the AR jet. Possible accumulated errors of each variable in the equation for calculation of the regurgitant orifice render this method unadvisable for groups with limited experience in its routine use. Grading of AR severity classifies an EROA less than 10 mm^2 or an AR RVol less than 30 mL/beat as mild AR and an EROA greater than 30 mm^2, an RVol greater than 60 mL/beat as severe AR, or a regurgitant fraction greater than or equal to 50%.[24]

When imaged from the apical window, the PISA method significantly underestimates AR severity in the setting of noncircular orifices[25] or eccentric AR jets.[23,26] In this situation, imaging the flow convergence zone from the parasternal long axis improves the accuracy of the PISA method.[16]

PULSED-WAVE DOPPLER

To assess *diastolic flow reversal in the descending thoracic aorta*, a pulsed-wave (PW) Doppler sample volume should be placed just distal to the origin of the subclavian artery, aligning it as far as possible along the major axis of the aorta. Diastolic flow reversal should occur throughout most of diastole because there can be brief early diastolic flow in the ascending and descending aorta resulting from elastic recoil in a normal aortic Doppler pattern, particularly in young children and adults. As the degree of regurgitation increases, so do the duration and velocity of reversal flow.[27] In our experience, holodiastolic flow reversal with a diastolic VTI of 15 cm or greater is a reliable qualitative sign of severe AR (Fig. 23.8). However, these methods are influenced by diastolic period duration and aortic distensibility.

Diastolic flow reversal in the abdominal aorta can be evaluated with pulsed-wave Doppler. Significant holodiastolic reversal flow in the abdominal aorta is a very specific sign of severe AR,[16] and assessment is recommended when possible (Fig. 23.9).

CONTINUOUS-WAVE DOPPLER

CW Doppler of the AR jet provides an indirect assessment of AR severity. The deceleration slope of the AR jet reflects the pressure difference between the aorta and the LV during diastole. It is classically best obtained from the apical 5-chamber view (Fig. 23.10). The method is limited in the setting of eccentric jets because an adequate spectral envelope is not easy to obtain. Significant overlap exists between moderate and severe regurgitation.[18]

The deceleration rate of the diastolic regurgitation jet and the derived pressure half-time (PHT) reflect the degree of regurgitation and ventricular end-diastolic pressures. As the degree of AR increases, aortic diastolic pressure decreases and the LV end-diastolic pressure increases. The late diastolic jet velocity is reduced, and the PHT is shortened (see Fig. 23.10). A PHT of less than 200 ms is consistent with severe AR, whereas a value greater than 500 ms suggests mild AR.[28]

This method is influenced by chamber compliance, chamber pressure, peripheral resistance, and aortic compliance.[29] PHT may be more useful in acute AR, before changes in LV compliance occur with chronic volume load.

INTEGRATING DOPPLER INDEXES OF SEVERITY

The best way to evaluate AR severity is to integrate several Doppler methods.[30,31] Based on the literature, a scheme of Doppler parameters for AR severity quantification has been proposed (see Summary table).

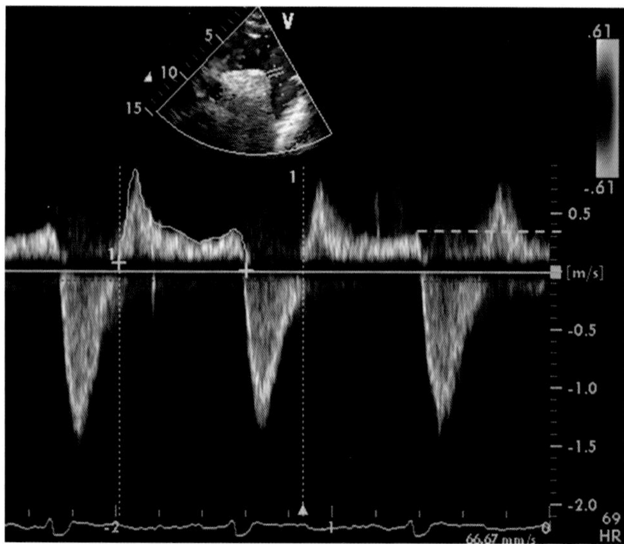

Fig. 23.8 Holodiastolic flow reversal by Doppler echocardiography in the descending thoracic aorta with severe regurgitation. Aortic regurgitation (AR) determined at the aortic isthmus level using the suprasternal view by pulsed Doppler is an easy method for identifying significant AR. End-diastolic velocity exceeding 20 cm/s indicates severe AR. The end-diastolic velocity is 35 cm/s.

AR severity is easy to grade when results from the different parameters are congruent, particularly vena contracta width and holodiastolic flow reversal in the proximal descending aorta and abdominal aorta (Fig. 23.11).[18] When different parameters are contradictory, the clinician must carefully seek technical and physiologic reasons for the discrepancies and rely on the components that have the best quality in the primary data.

Quantitative parameters can overcome certain limitations of some semiquantitative methods. Measures of regurgitant volume and effective regurgitant orifice (ERO) area[1] are better predictors of clinical outcome.[2,3] However, quantitative methods are more technically demanding, require adequate experience, and are vulnerable to the accumulated errors of each variable when image quality is not perfect.[16]

ALTERNATIVE APPROACHES

TEE

TEE is the reference examination for AR quantification in nonechogenic patients (Fig. 23.12). Vena contracta imaging by TEE color flow mapping in the long axis (130 degrees) is an accurate marker of AR severity.[32] In the absence of significant aortic valvular calcification, TEE permits planimetry of the regurgitant jet using color Doppler.[33,34] A regurgitant vena contracta width greater than 6 mm and an area greater than 7.5 mm^2 favor severe AR. Diastolic flow reversal at multiple sites in the descending aorta with biplane TEE may be useful to confirm severe AR.[34]

3D Echocardiography

Studies have demonstrated the feasibility and accuracy of *3D echocardiography* in quantifying AR (Fig. 23.13). Systematic cropping of the acquired 3D TTE data set is used to measure the vena contracta. The first step is to obtain the best AR jet in the long-axis view or from the apical view and, if the parasternal window is poor, by posterior-to-anterior cropping of the 3D TTE data set. The 3D TTE color Doppler data set is cropped from the aortic side to the level of the vena contracta, just below the aortic leaflets, in a plane that is exactly perpendicular to the

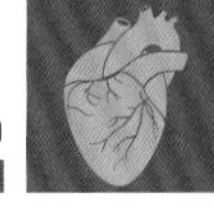

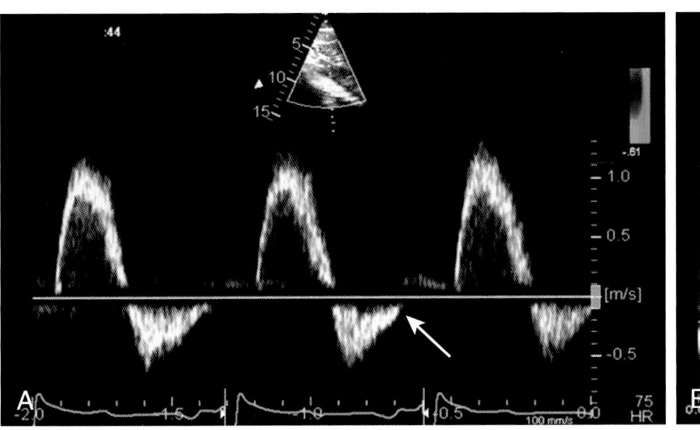

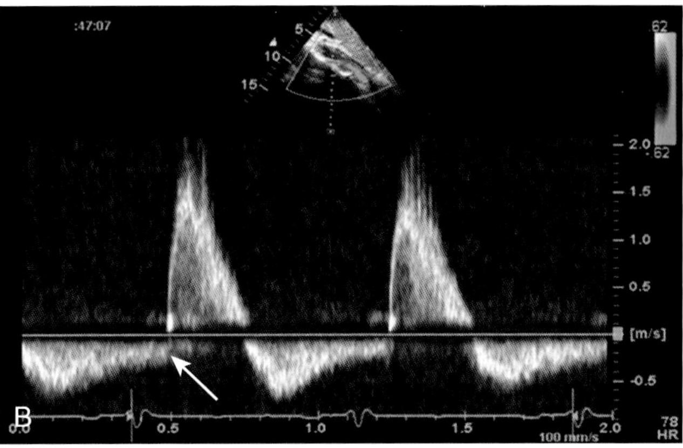

Fig. 23.9 Abdominal aortic flow. (A) Brief diastolic flow in nonsevere aortic regurgitation (AR). (B) Holodiastolic flow reversal in severe AR. *Arrows* indicate the end of the diastolic pulsed-wave Doppler signal.

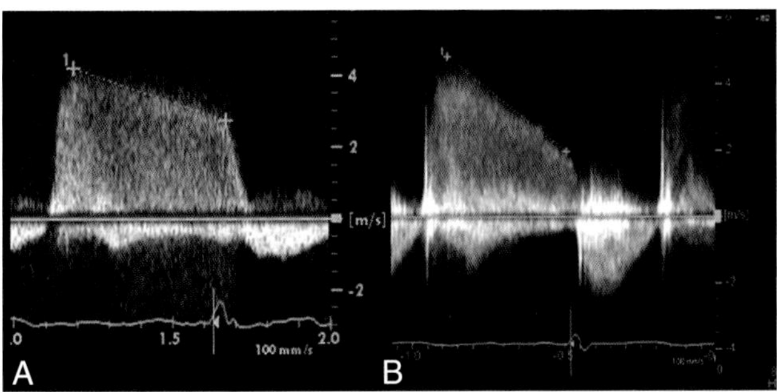

Fig. 23.10 CW Doppler signal of aortic regurgitation with different diastolic deceleration slopes. (A) Moderate aortic regurgitation (AR), (B) Severe acute AR. Notice that the pressure half-time is significantly shorter in B than in A.

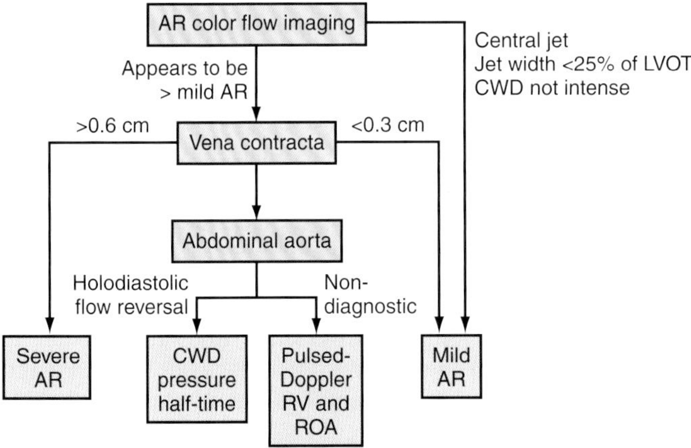

Fig. 23.11 Clinical approach to evaluate aortic regurgitation severity. Flow chart illustrates the clinical approach to evaluating AR severity by echocardiography. *AR*, Aortic regurgitation; *CWD*, continuous-wave Doppler; *LVOT*, left ventricular outflow tract; *ROA*, regurgitant orifice area; *RV*, regurgitant volume. (From Otto CM. *Textbook of Clinical Echocardiography*. 4th ed. Philadelphia: Elsevier; 2009.)

AR jet.[22,26] The image is tilted en face, and the cropped portion of the data set is added back to obtain the maximum area of vena contracta viewed in a short-axis view in systole. The vena contracta area can be multiplied by the VTI to accurately estimate instantaneous RVol.[26]

The 3D TEE approach has proved to be superior to 2D TEE to obtain measurements that are useful for surgeons. An advantage of 3D echocardiography is that it shows the surgeon's view, which aids structure identification. It is also the unique method for quantifying aortic valve measurements (e.g., effective height, coaptation length) for each of the three cusps using the multiplanar reconstruction tool.[35]

Magnetic Resonance Imaging

Current recommendations consider cardiac *magnetic resonance imaging* (MRI) for the noninvasive evaluation of AR when echocardiography is not diagnostic (Fig. 23.14). RVol can be calculated from the difference between antegrade and retrograde flow volume rates in the ascending aorta by phase-contrast sequences.[36] A regurgitant fraction greater than 33% is a good predictor for timing of surgical treatment after 3 years of follow-up.[37]

The good reproducibility of velocity cine MRI for quantitative assessment of RVol and regurgitant fraction indicates the potential of this technique for follow-up and monitoring of response to therapy.[38] Like echocardiography, MRI can also evaluate holodiastolic flow reversal in the descending aorta.

LV SIZE AND SYSTOLIC FUNCTION

LV DIMENSIONS AND CONTRACTILE FUNCTION

Echocardiography is the diagnostic tool most widely used to assess LV diameters, volumes, and ejection fraction (EF). End-diastolic and end-systolic dimensions are measured using the LV minor axis from the parasternal long-axis view, and 2D or 3D imaging is used to optimize alignment. However, higher reproducibility is achieved using guided M-mode because of the clear identification of endocardial borders[38] and excellent temporal resolution. Even with 2D guidance, it may not be possible to align the M-mode cursor perpendicular to the long axis of the LV, which is mandatory for obtaining a true minor axis. Alternatively, chamber dimension and wall thickness can be acquired from the parasternal short-axis view at the level of the mitral chordae (Fig. 23.15).

End-diastolic and end-systolic volumes are obtained according to the Simpson biplane rule using the apical biplane approach. However, 2D echocardiographic methods have limitations, and apical images may foreshorten the true LV length.[39] On serial studies, a review of previous images minimizes measurement variability resulting from changes in the echocardiographic image plane, the measurement site, or foreshortening of the apical view. Decision making is based on consistent

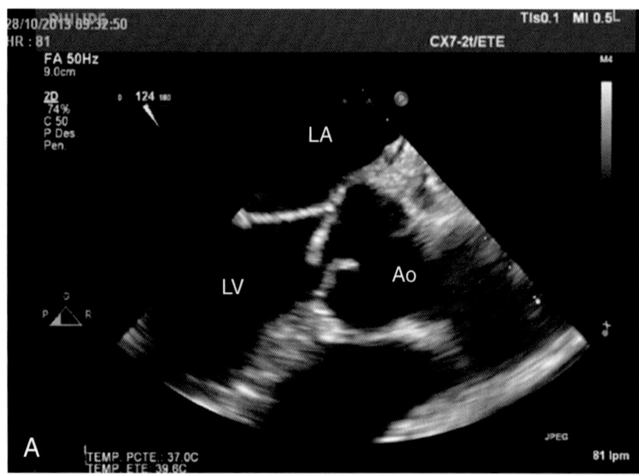

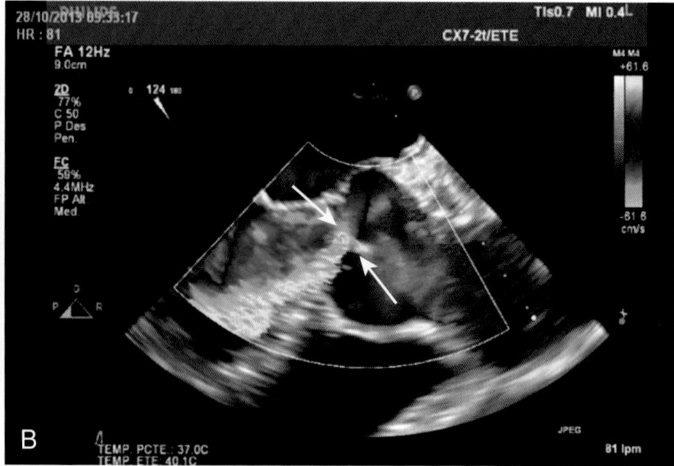

Fig. 23.12 Aortic valve prolapse. TEE shows aortic leaflet prolapse (A), which leads to significant aortic regurgitation (B). *Arrows* indicate the 7-mm vena contracta of an aortic regurgitant jet (see Videos 23.12A and 23.12B). *Ao*, Aorta.

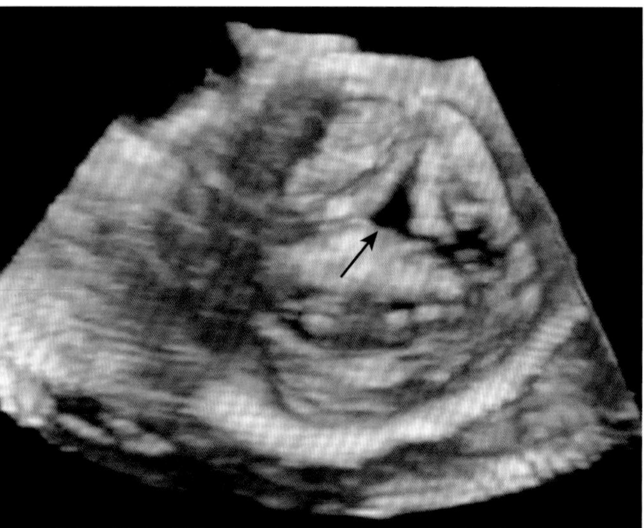

Fig. 23.13 3D TTE utilities in aortic regurgitation. 3D TTE shows the regurgitant orifice *(arrow)* in diastole (see Video 23.13).

directional changes on serial studies.[17] If measurements are approaching a value that would indicate surgical intervention, a repeat evaluation at a shorter time interval or confirmation by an alternative imaging technique is appropriate.

Although LV ejection fraction (LVEF) is the fundamental parameter for evaluating LV contractility, other parameters obtained by tissue Doppler and myocardial deformation imaging may be useful in cases of borderline LVEF values. Two studies showed that a peak systolic wave velocity of less than 9 cm/s at the mitral annulus was a predictor of complications and was related to LV contractile reserve.[40,41] Other studies suggested that 2D strain imaging might be useful for estimating subclinical myocardial dysfunction[41] with preserved EF[42] and for predicting postoperative LV systolic dysfunction.[41]

Global longitudinal strain (GLS) has proved to be an independent predictor of LVEF decrease in patients with severe AR, and a GLS value of less than 18.5% is associated with a worse outcome. In a study of 865 patients with asymptomatic significant AR, Alashi et al. determined that patients with a basal GLS value of less than 19% had higher mortality rates.[43] Persistently impaired GLS values were associated with a lower survival rate.[43] Resting LV and right ventricular (RV) strain and exercise tricuspid annular plane systolic excursion (TAPSE) values were independently associated with the need for earlier surgical treatment of asymptomatic patients with AR.[44]

In cases with suboptimal echocardiographic images or unclear results, MRI may be indicated. MRI has become the gold standard for EF quantification. However, MRI techniques need to be standardized and appropriate thresholds developed because severity thresholds are likely different for MRI and for echocardiography.[45] In cases with discrepancies between AR severity and LV function, imaging techniques such as computed tomography (CT) or MRI can help diagnose coronary artery disease or dilated cardiomyopathy.[46–48]

As procedures continue to improve, real-time acquisitions will shorten scan time and overcome some of the challenges in diagnosing patients with arrhythmia. Four-dimensional (4D) flow sequences acquire flow data in the three MRI dimensions and enable analysis of wall stress and aortic compliance.

MRI permits assessment of reactive fibrosis with the use of T1 mapping techniques and replacement fibrosis with the use of gadolinium contrast enhancement. T1 mapping sequences show different relaxation times for hearts with AR and normal hearts, suggesting the existence of a diffuse myocardial fibrotic process.[49] Later studies confirmed that the extravascular volume fraction obtained by this method correlated well with histologically determined diffuse interstitial fibrosis.[50] The correlation between myocardial replacement fibrosis assessed by late gadolinium enhancement (LGE) MRI and histopathology was also good.[51] However, data on the value of assessing myocardial fibrosis in patients who may benefit from surgery in terms of LV function and clinical symptom improvement remain scant.

CONTRACTILE RESERVE EVALUATION

Exercise testing may be useful when the relationship between symptoms and LV systolic function is uncertain. In this subset of patients, exercise testing can be very useful in eliciting symptoms or determining functional capacity.[48] Assessment of contractile reserve may be helpful for patients with severe AR and equivocal symptoms or borderline values in terms of LVEF (approximately 55%) or an end-systolic diameter (ESD) close to 50 mm or ESD indexed to body surface area (BSA) (ESD/BSA) close to 25 mm/m^2.

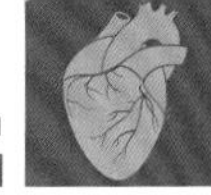

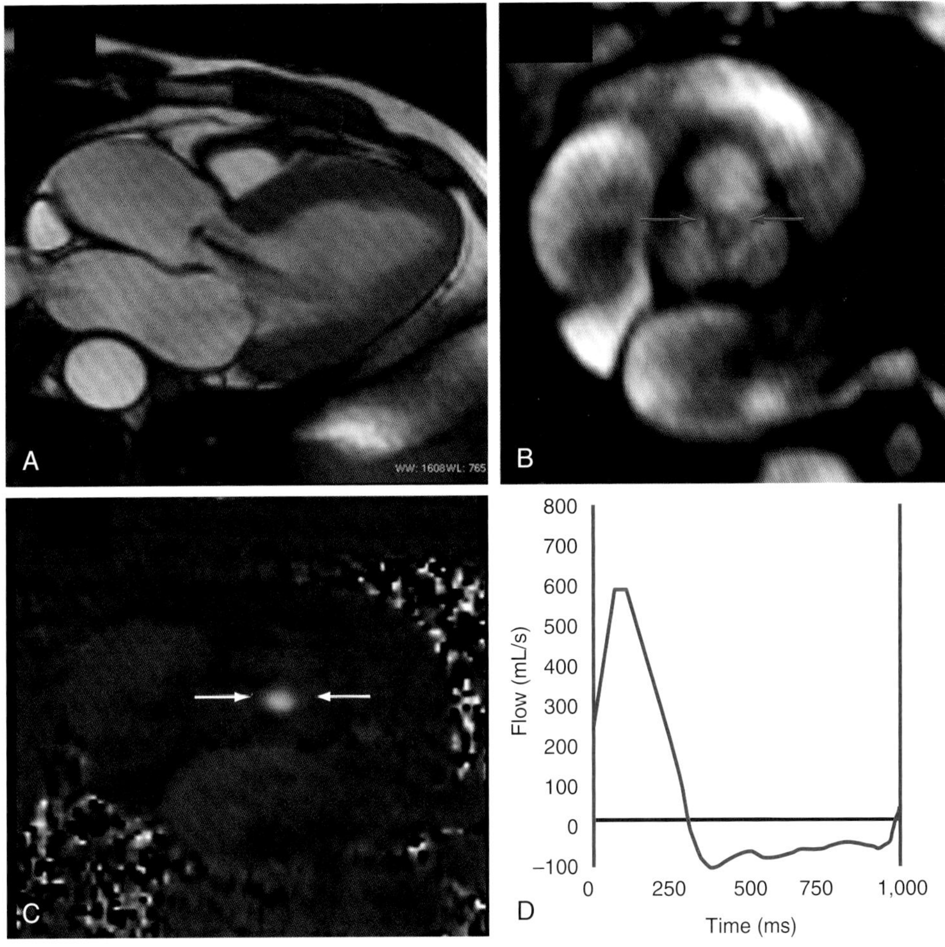

Fig. 23.14 Cardiac magnetic resonance imaging in a patient with aortic regurgitation. (A) Balanced steady-state free precession image. Oblique axial LV inflow/outflow view shows moderate aortic regurgitation (AR). (B) Oblique axial plane in the aortic root, just above the aortic valve at the level of the coronary artery change (opening for ostia) (*arrows*). (C) Phase-contrast velocity mapping. The central jet of AR is seen in white (*arrows*). (D) Flow versus time plot for the ascending aorta. Antegrade flow was 121 mL/s, retrograde flow was 43 mL/s, and the aortic regurgitant fraction was 36% (see Video 23.14).

The absence of contractile reserve seems to be predictive of LV function after surgery.[52] The main limitation is the measurement variability for EF at exercise by echocardiography.

AORTIC ROOT AND ASCENDING AORTA EVALUATION

Assessment of the aortic root and ascending aorta dilation is an important part of the evaluation of patients with AR. Echocardiography is accurate in assessment and follow-up of aortic root size. MRI or CT is recommended for ascending aorta evaluation in patients with an enlarged aorta detected by echocardiography, particularly when enlargement may indicate need for surgery.

AORTIC VALVE AND ROOT FUNCTION

The aortic root is the portion of the aorta that supports the leaflets of the aortic valve. It is delineated superiorly by the sinotubular junction and inferiorly by the aortoventricular junction. It is made up of the sinuses, leaflets, commissures, and interleaflet triangles. The sinotubular ridge is circular, composed primarily of elastic tissue, and supports the peripheral attachments of the valve leaflets.

The valve leaflets are inserted into the aortic wall in semilunar fashion, and their closure determines a complete central coaptation. The level of coaptation is midway between the nadir of their insertion and the commissural areas. The aortoventricular junction or base of the aortic root is defined by the nadirs of attachment of these leaflets and the interleaflet triangles.

Approximately 45% of the circumference of the aortic root is attached to the muscular interventricular septum and 55% to fibrous tissue. This fibrous tissue comprises the membranous interventricular septum and the fibrous body that connect the anterior leaflet of the mitral valve to the aortic root.[53]

Echocardiography can offer dynamic evaluation of the AR mechanism.[14] Accurate aortic root measurement is important for understanding functional AR mechanisms and targeting the optimal time and strategy for aortic valve–sparing surgery. The following parameters should be measured:

- Aortic annulus: distance between the insertions of two basal valve cusps into the aortic root[a]
- Sinuses of Valsalva: maximum diameter of the sinuses
- Sinotubular junction: dimension of the aortic root at the level of commissural cusp-tip insertion into the aortic wall

[a]The annulus is measured in mesosystole; the rest of parameters are measured in protodiastole.

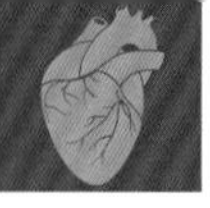

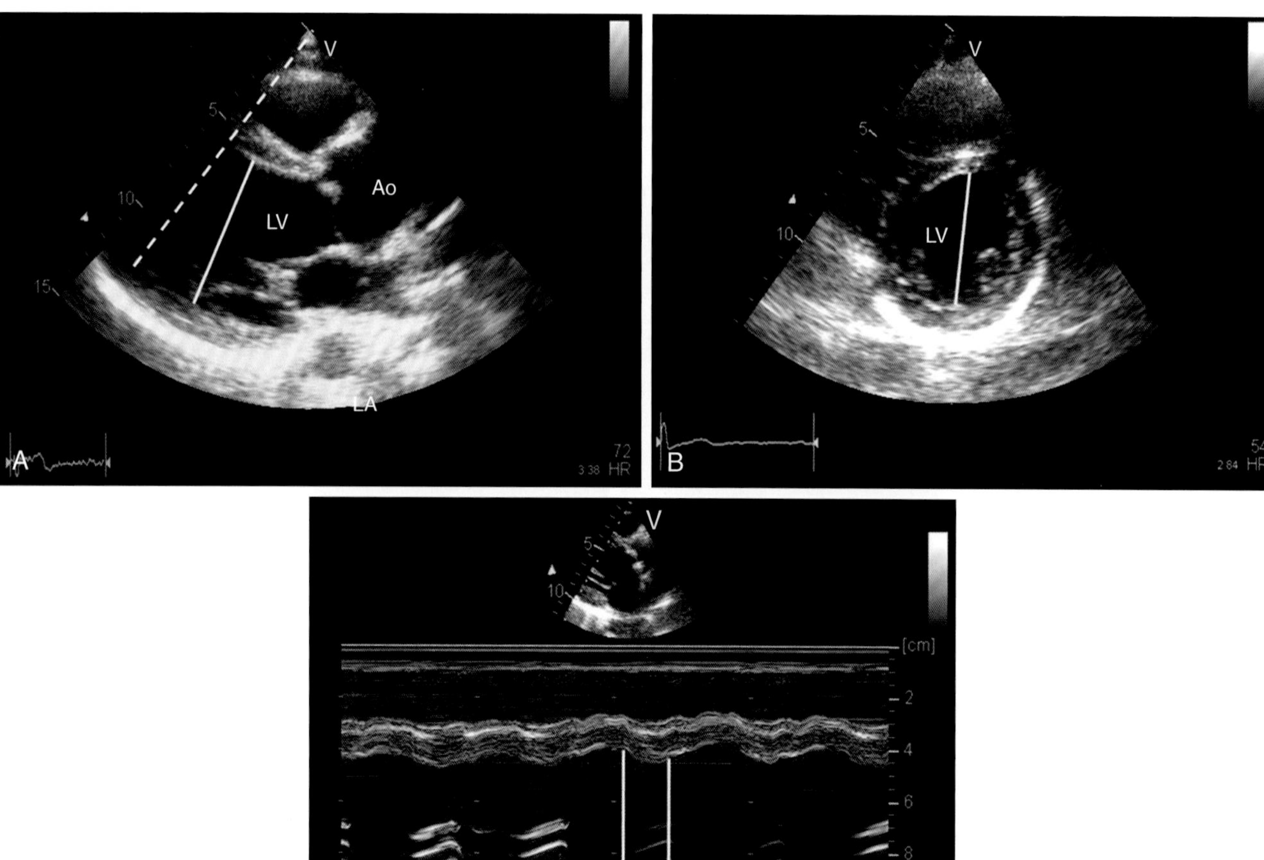

Fig. 23.15 Measurement of LV dimensions in aortic regurgitation. (A and B) LV dimensions in aortic regurgitation can be measured using the LV minor axis with the parasternal long-axis view *(solid line)*, ensuring an optimized alignment. (C) The most accurate measurements are obtained with the guided M-mode method *(dotted line)*. *Ao*, Aorta.

- Tubular tract: maximum diameter of the ascending aorta distal to the sinotubular junction
- Coaptation height: maximum distance between the first point of protodiastolic coaptation of the leaflet tips and the annulus plane corresponding to the basal insertion of the leaflets[54] (Fig. 23.16)
- Coaptation length: maximum distance of coaptation between sigmoides in protodiastole (see Fig. 23.16)
- Tented area: the maximum area subtending the ventricular surface of the leaflets as far as the annular plane

The variable most strongly associated with functional AR severity is diastolic leaflet tenting, which is measured as coaptation height (see Fig. 23.16). Sensitivity and specificity are greater than 95% using a cutoff value of 11 mm. When coaptation length is less than 4 mm, the risk of having significant AR is very high.

Tethering of the leaflets depends on the mismatch of sinotubular junction/annulus diameters rather than the absolute dimension of the proximal aorta. A cutoff value greater than 1.6 strongly identifies diastolic leaflet tenting and is significantly associated with AR severity.[55,56]

NATURAL HISTORY AND SERIAL TESTING IN CHRONIC AORTIC REGURGITATION

Progression of AR involves a complicated interaction of several variables, including AR severity, aortic root disease, and the adaptive response of the LV. Patients with chronic AR typically have slow LV dilation and a prolonged asymptomatic phase. The LV adapts to the volume overload of chronic AR with a series of compensatory mechanisms, including an increase in end-diastolic volume and compliance and eccentric hypertrophy that accommodates the increased volume and maintains cardiac output without raising filling pressures. The compensated phase may last for decades. Eventually, preload reserve is exhausted and/or hypertrophy becomes inadequate; further increases in afterload reduce EF.

The transition may be insidious, and some patients remain asymptomatic until severe LV dysfunction has developed. The decompensated stage is characterized by substantial and progressive LV enlargement, a more spherical geometry, elevated LV diastolic pressures, increased systolic wall stress (i.e., afterload excess), and a decline in the EF.[57]

Natural history information is derived from 12 published series involving 1173 patients and a mean follow-up period of 6.5 years[3,53–66] (Table 23.2). The rate of progression to symptoms and/or LV systolic dysfunction averaged 4.3% per year, development of asymptomatic LV dysfunction was 1.2% per year, and sudden death was 0.2% per year.[48] More than one fourth of patients who died or developed systolic dysfunction did so before the onset of symptoms.[60,61,65]

LV size measured by echocardiography had a major predictive value. Patients with an initial ESD greater than 50 mm had a likelihood of death, symptoms, and/or LV dysfunction

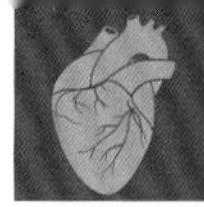

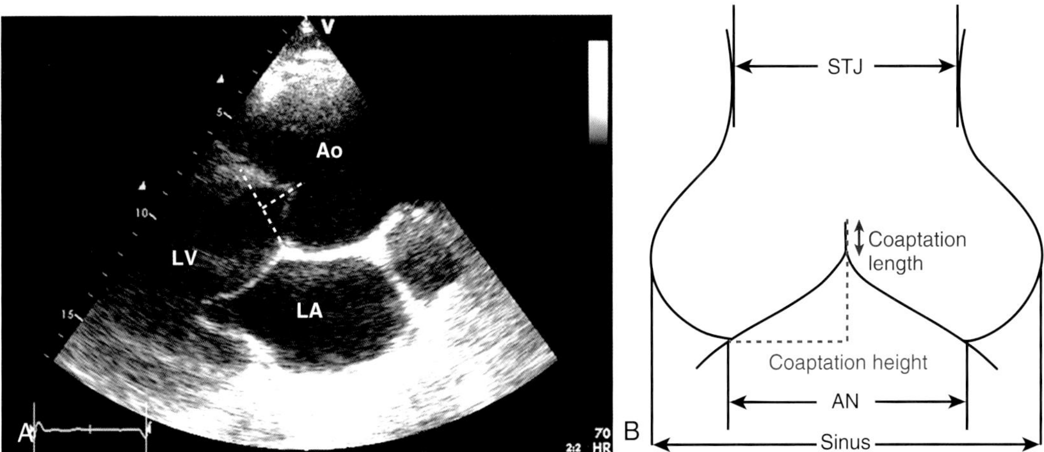

Fig. 23.16 Functional aortic regurgitation. (A) Parasternal long-axis view shows the aortic valve and aortic root in a patient with diastolic cusp tenting and a coaptation height of 14 mm. *Dotted lines* show the annulus level to obtain coaptation height. (B) Schematic drawing of the aortic root with graphic description of coaptation height (see Video 23.16). *AN*, Aortoventricular junction; *Ao*, aorta; *STJ*, sinotubular junction; *Sinus*, maximal sinus diameter. (From Schäfers HJ, Schmied W, Psych D, et al. Cusp height in aortic valves. *J Thorac Cardiovasc Surg.* 2013;146:269–274.)

TABLE 23.2 Studies of the Natural History of Asymptomatic Patients With Aortic Regurgitation.

Study	*No. of Patients*	*Mean Follow-Up (y)*	*Progression to Symptoms, Death, or LV Dysfunction (%/y)*	*Progression to Asymptomatic LV Dysfunction (%/y)*	*No. of Deaths*
Bonow et al.[59,60]	104	8.0	3.8	0.5	2
Scognamiglio et al.[101]	30	4.7	2.1	2.1	0
Siemienczuk et al.[61]	50	3.7	4.0	0.5	0
Scognamiglio et al.[62]	74	6.0	5.7	3.4	0
Tornos et al.[63]	101	4.6	3.0	1.3	0
Ishii et al.[64]	27	14.2	3.6	—	0
Borer et al.[65]	104	7.3	6.2	0.9	4
Tarasoutchi et al.[3]	72	10.0	4.7	0.1	0
Evangelista et al.[66]	31	7.0	3.6	—	1
Detaint et al.[24]	251	8.0	5.0	—	33
Pizarro et al.[102]	294	3.5	10.0	2.8	5
Olsen et al.[42]	35	1.6	14.3	—	0

of 19% per year. For those with an ESD of 40 to 50 mm, the rate was 6% per year, and when the dimension was less than 40 mm, it was zero.[60] However, 25% of asymptomatic patients with depressed systolic function developed symptoms each year.[3,59–69] For symptomatic patients undergoing medical treatment, a mortality rate of 10% to 20% per year has been reported.[64,68,69]

Recent guidelines[70] stratified chronic AR in different stages. Table 23.3 shows the stages ranging from patients at risk of AR (stage A) or with progressive mild to moderate AR (stage B) to severe asymptomatic (stage C) and symptomatic (stage D) AR. Each of these stages is defined by valve anatomy, valve hemodynamics, severity of LV dilation, and LV systolic function, as well as by patient symptoms. Although qualitative measures of AR severity are adequate in many situations, when AR is significant (stages B and C), quantitative measures of regurgitant volume and effective regurgitant orifice (ERO) area[1] are better predictors of clinical outcome.[24,71] Measures of LV systolic function (LVEF or fractional shortening) and LV end-systolic dimension (LVESD) or LV end-systolic volume are predictive of the development of HF symptoms or death in initially asymptomatic patients (Stages B and C1) and are significant determinants of survival and functional results after surgery in asymptomatic and symptomatic patients (stages C2 and D).[3,24,38,59–65,71–77] Symptomatic patients (stage D) with normal LVEF have a significantly better long-term postoperative survival rate than those with depressed systolic function.[78,78a]

For asymptomatic patients with preserved systolic function, initial measurements of LV dimensions and function represent the baseline information with which future serial measurements can be compared. Patients with mild to moderate AR can be seen on a yearly basis, and echocardiography can be performed every 3 years.[79] All patients with severe AR and normal LV function should be seen for follow-up at 6 months after their initial examination. If the LV diameter or EF shows significant changes or becomes close to the threshold for intervention, follow-up should be continued at 6-month intervals.[48,58] Patients with stable parameters can be followed annually.

For patients with a dilated aorta, and especially for those with Marfan syndrome or BAV, echocardiography should be performed on a yearly basis. CT or MRI is advisable when the ascending aorta is not well visualized at the upper part of the sinotubular junction or when surgical indication may be based on aortic enlargement rather than LV size or function.[10]

TABLE 23.3 Stages of Chronic Aortic Regurgitation.

Stage	Definition	Valve Anatomy	Valve Hemodynamics	Hemodynamic Consequences	Symptoms
A	At risk of AR	BAV (or other congenital valve anomaly) Aortic valve sclerosis Diseases of the aortic sinuses or ascending aorta History of rheumatic fever or known rheumatic heart disease IE	AR severity: none or trace	None	None
B	Progressive AR	Mild to moderate calcification of a trileaflet valve BAV (or other congenital valve anomaly) Dilated aortic sinuses Rheumatic valve changes Previous IE	Mild AR: Jet width <25% of LVOT Vena contracta <0.3 cm Regurgitant volume <30 mL/beat Regurgitant fraction <30% ERO <0.10 cm2 Angiography grade 1 Moderate AR: Jet width 25%–64% of LVOT Vena contracta 0.3–0.6 cm Regurgitant volume 30–59 mL/beat Regurgitant fraction 30% to 49% ERO 0.10–0.29 cm^2 Angiography grade 2	Normal LV systolic function Normal LV volume or mild LV dilation	None
C	Asymptomatic severe AR	Calcific aortic valve disease Bicuspid valve (or other congenital abnormality) Dilated aortic sinuses or ascending aorta Rheumatic valve changes IE with abnormal leaflet closure or perforation	Severe AR: Jet width ≥65% of LVOT Vena contracta >0.6 cm Holodiastolic flow reversal in the proximal abdominal aorta Regurgitant volume ≥60 mL/beat Regurgitant fraction ≥50% ERO ≥0.3 cm^2 Angiography grade 3 to 4 In addition, diagnosis of chronic severe AR requires evidence of LV dilation	C1: Normal LVEF (>55%) and mild to moderate LV dilation (LVESD <50 mm) C2: Abnormal LV systolic function with depressed LVEF (≤55%) or severe LV dilation (LVESD >50 mm or indexed LVESD >25 mm/m^2)	None; exercise testing is reasonable to confirm symptom status
D	Symptomatic severe AR	Calcific valve disease Bicuspid valve (or other congenital abnormality) Dilated aortic sinuses or ascending aorta Rheumatic valve changes Previous IE with abnormal leaflet closure or perforation	Severe AR: Doppler jet width ≥65% of LVOT Vena contracta >0.6 cm Holodiastolic flow reversal in the proximal abdominal aorta Regurgitant volume ≥60 mL/beat Regurgitant fraction ≥50% ERO ≥0.3 cm^2 Angiography grade 3 to 4 In addition, diagnosis of chronic severe AR requires evidence of LV dilation	Symptomatic severe AR may occur with normal systolic function (LVEF >55%), mild to moderate LV dysfunction (LVEF 40% to 55%), or severe LV dysfunction (LVEF <40%) Moderate to severe LV dilation is present	Exertional dyspnea or angina or more severe HF symptoms

AR, Aortic regurgitation; *BAV*, bicuspid aortic valve; *ERO*, effective regurgitant orifice; *HF*, heart failure; *IE*, infective endocarditis; *LV*, left ventricular; *LVEF*, left ventricular ejection fraction; *LVESD*, left ventricular end-systolic dimension; *LVOT*, left ventricular outflow tract.

From Otto CM, Nishimura RA, Bonow RO, et al. 2020 ACC/AHA guideline for the management of patients with valvular heart disease: a report of the American College of Cardiology/American Heart Association Joint Committee on Clinical Practice Guidelines. *Circulation.* 2021;143. DOI: 10.1161/CIR.0000000000000923.

MANAGEMENT AND TIMING OF SURGERY

MEDICAL TREATMENT

Medical therapy cannot significantly reduce RVol in normotensive chronic severe AR because the regurgitant orifice area is relatively fixed and diastolic blood pressure is already low. Only two randomized, controlled studies demonstrated significant reductions in LV end-diastolic diameters and an increase in the EF with hydralazine or nifedipine.[62,80] However, a later randomized trial showed no therapeutic benefit of therapy with enalapril or nifedipine compared with placebo.[66]

The use of enalapril or nifedipine is not advised except in the setting of systemic hypertension (i.e., systolic blood pressure greater than 140 mmHg) or overt heart failure en route to surgery.[48,58] Beta-blockers are contraindicated in AR because cardiac output is maintained through an increase in heart rate, and lowering the heart rate may increase diastolic time and regurgitation volume.[48]

INDICATIONS FOR SURGERY

The indication for surgery in patients with severe AR is based on symptoms, LV function and size, and aortic dilation. Determining LV function and dimensions is paramount for the correct management of AR. A curvilinear relationship exists between the preoperative degree of LV dilation and postoperative EF.[81] End-systolic ventricular size is less load dependent and is a more robust predictor of outcome than end-diastolic measurements. Indexing for BSA is recommended, particularly in patients with a small body size and in women (Fig. 23.17).[69,82,83]

Symptomatic Patients With LV Dysfunction

Surgery should not be denied in symptomatic patients with severe LV dysfunction (EF < 30%) or marked LV dilation after carefully ruling out other possible causes. The postoperative outcome is worse for these patients,[84,85] and the likelihood of recovery of systolic function is lower than for patients operated on at an earlier stage.

Patients with a markedly low EF have a higher long-term likelihood of postoperative heart failure; however, at 10 years, only 25% of patients had this complication. Even for patients with New York Heart Association (NYHA) functional class IV symptoms, improvement in LV function and clinical symptoms can be achieved, although the mortality rate associated with aortic valve replacement approaches 10%.[84–86]

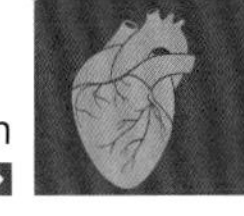

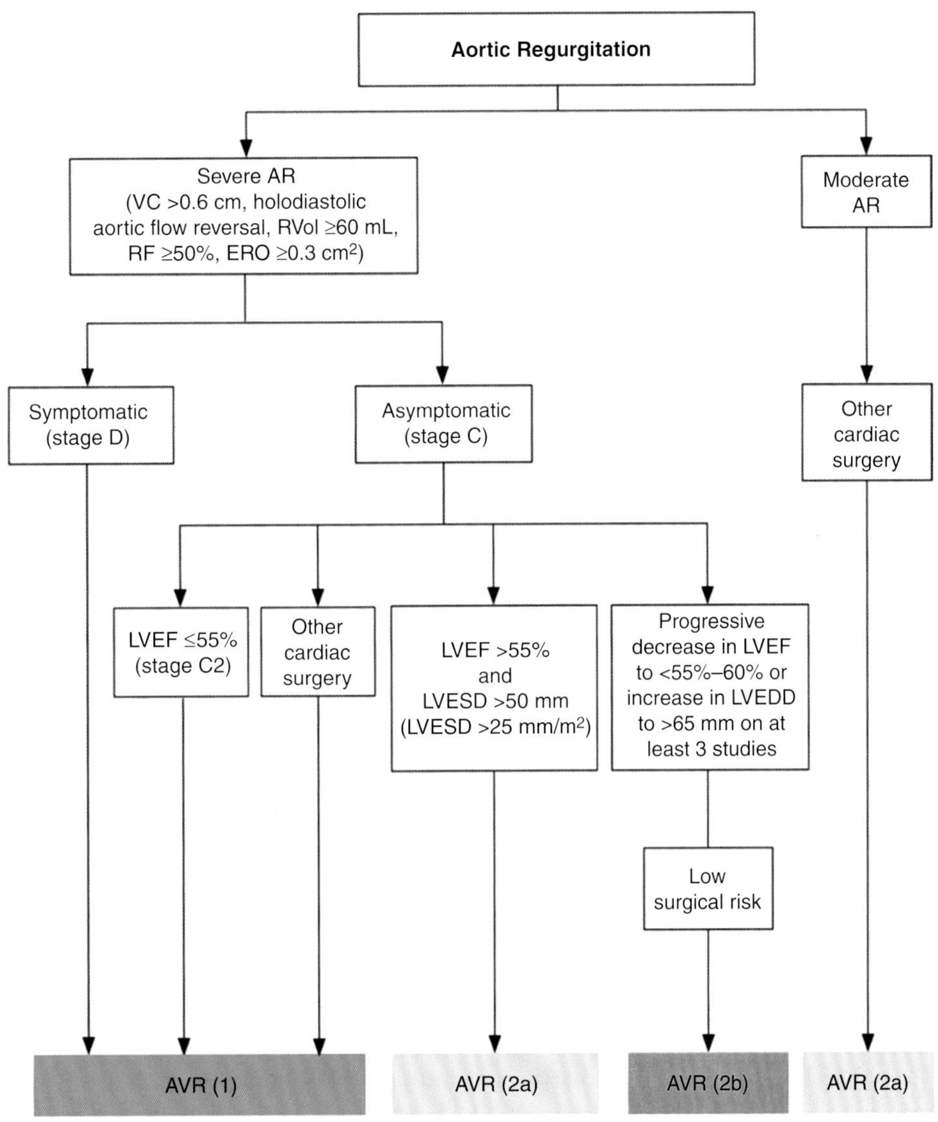

Fig. 23.17 Timing of intervention for AR. *AR,* Aortic regurgitation; *AVR,* aortic valve replacement; *EDD,* end-diastolic dimension; *ERO,* effective regurgitant orifice; *LVEF,* left ventricular ejection fraction; *LVESD,* left ventricular end-systolic dimension; *RF,* regurgitant fraction; *RVol,* regurgitant volume; *VC,* vena contracta. (From Otto CM, Nishimura RA, Bonow RO, et al. 2020 ACC/AHA guideline for the management of patients with valvular heart disease: a report of the American College of Cardiology/American Heart Association Joint Committee on Clinical Practice Guidelines. Circulation. 2021;143. DOI: 10.1161/CIR.0000000000000923.)

Symptomatic Patients With Normal LV Systolic Function

Surgical treatment is indicated for patients with normal LV systolic function (i.e., EF > 55% at rest) and NYHA functional class III or IV symptoms. In patients with NYHA functional class II dyspnea, the cause of symptoms is often unclear. Although a period of observation may be reasonable, an exercise imaging test can help identify the causes of symptoms. Evaluation of other parameters obtained by tissue Doppler and strain rate imaging may be useful in deciphering borderline LVEF values.

Asymptomatic Patients With Reduced Ejection Fraction

Surgical treatment of asymptomatic patients is indicated for those with LV dysfunction (LVEF ≤55%; stage C2); aortic valve surgery is indicated if no other cause for systolic dysfunction is identified.[3,5,8–12] However, it is important to consider the variability of echocardiographic measurements, and exercise tests or other imaging techniques should be performed to confirm LV systolic dysfunction.

Asymptomatic Patients With Normal Ejection Fraction

Surgical treatment is recommended for patients with a normal EF and severe LV dilation (end-diastolic dimension > 65 mm, or ESD > 50 mm or ESD/BSA > 25 mm/m^2).[48,58] Despite a preserved EF, a higher LV end-systolic volume index (≥45 mL/m^2) predicts more cardiac events within each AR grade.[14] Most patients with severe LV dilation and preserved EF are at high risk for complications and reduced exercise tolerance. Class IIb indicators (e.g., enlarged end-diastolic diameter) were not associated with a higher risk of death and hospitalization.[87]

Poorer postoperative outcomes should be anticipated as soon as the EF falls below 55% and the LV ESD/BSA exceeds 22 mm/m^2 in strictly asymptomatic patients. Similar thresholds were reported for a subgroup of patients who never underwent surgery.[76]

Controversy exists about the best approach. Early surgical intervention rather than watchful waiting for asymptomatic patients who fail to meet current surgical criteria was favored by some investigators. However, others observed no benefit with an aggressive approach and considered waiting to be the best option until surgical thresholds are met.[88] Current guidelines[70] have considered an indication type 2b in asymptomatic patients with severe AR and normal LV systolic function at rest (LVEF >55%; stage C1) and low surgical risk. Aortic valve surgery may be considered when there is a progressive decline in LVEF on at least three serial studies to the low-normal range (LVEF 55% to 60%) or a progressive increase in LV dilation into the severe range (LV end diastolic dimension [LVEDD] >65 mm).[38,61,76,77]

Concomitant Aortic Root Disease

Dilation of the ascending aorta is a common cause of isolated AR. In these cases, AR is not severe, and surgical indications should be based more on aortic enlargement than on other parameters.

When valve replacement is required on the basis of AR severity, replacement of the ascending aorta should be considered if the aortic diameter is greater than 45 to 50 mm, depending on age, BSA, the cause of valvular disease, an existing BAV, and the intraoperative shape and thickness of the ascending aorta.[89] Lower thresholds may be used for root replacement if aortic valve repair is planned in surgical centers with established expertise in repair of the aortic root and ascending aorta.

SELECTING AND GUIDING SURGICAL TREATMENT

Treatment of isolated AR has traditionally consisted of valve replacement with a mechanical or biologic prosthesis. Replacement with a pulmonary autograft has been an operation reserved for special instances, primarily in children or very young adults.[90] Repair strategies for the regurgitant aortic valve have been developed in the past 20 years for different morphologies.[91]

Potential advantages of aortic valve repair over replacement include a lower incidence of subsequent thromboembolic events, avoidance of long-term anticoagulation, and reduced risk of endocarditis. Aortic valve repair is increasingly favored over replacement with a prosthetic valve for a variety of lesions causing significant AR.[92,93] Despite the potential benefits, the durability of aortic repair procedures has been a matter of concern.[91,92] Aortic valve repair may show good results in patients undergoing repair of aneurysms of the aorta or aortic root and in other selected patients, such as those with BAV with prolapsing leaflets and minimal sclerosis.

Dilation of the aortic root, regardless of its cause, has been treated by composite replacement of the valve and root or ascending aorta with a mechanical or biologic valve conduit. Valve-sparing aortic replacement is increasingly being employed as an alternative. Supracoronary replacement of the ascending aorta can be used to treat aortic aneurysm when the sinuses of Valsalva are preserved.

Reconstructive leaflet techniques have been applied more frequently in recent years, and a wide range of surgical techniques, such as leaflet plication, nodular unfolding, and leaflet extension with pericardial or artificial patching, has been proposed. Although initial results may be promising, the experience of the surgical team and surgically related aspects (e.g., complex leaflet repair, leaflet extension with patch) may affect long-term outcome.[94–96]

The decision as to the type of surgical treatment should take patient age into consideration.[93] If valve repair or a valve-sparing intervention is considered, TEE may be performed preoperatively to define the anatomy of the cusps and ascending aorta.[14]

ROLE OF ECHOCARDIOGRAPHY

The main roles of echocardiography are to evaluate regurgitation mechanisms, describe valve anatomy, and determine the feasibility of valve repair.[14] 2D TTE does not always show the lesion responsible for leaflet malcoaptation. Analysis of the mechanism of AR influences patient management, particularly when the ascending aorta is dilated or conservative surgery is considered. Several functional classifications have been proposed. The adapted Carpentier classification for AR is the most widely used[97] (Fig. 23.18).

AR Class	Type I Normal cusp motion with FAA dilation or cusp perforation				Type II	Type III
	Ia	Ib	Ic	Id	Cusp prolapse	Type II restriction
Mechanism	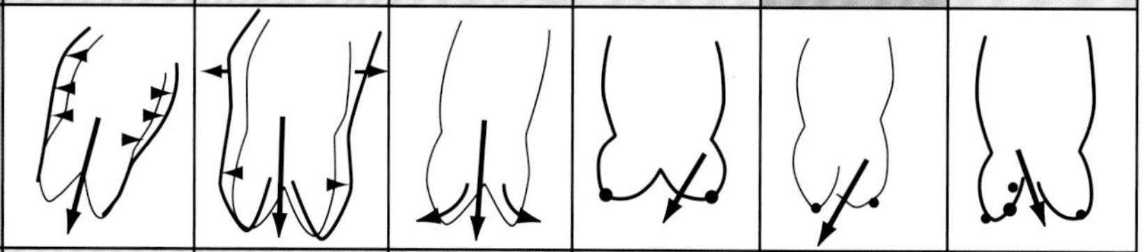					
Repair techniques (Primary)	STJ remodeling *Ascending aortic graft*	Aortic valve sparing: *Reimplantation or Remodeling with SCA*	SCA	Patch repair *Autologous or bovine pericardium*	Prolapse repair *Plication Triangular resection Free margin Resuspension patch*	Leaflet repair *Shaving Decalcification patch*
(Secondary)	SCA		STJ annuloplasty	SCA	SCA	SCA

Fig. 23.18 Classification of aortic regurgitation. Repair-oriented functional classification of aortic regurgitation *(AR)* with descriptions of disease mechanisms and repair techniques used. *FAA*, Functional aortic annulus; *SCA*, subcommissural annuloplasty; *STJ*, sinotubular junction. (Modified from Boodhwani M, de Kaerchove L, Glineur D, et al. Repair-oriented classification of aortic insufficiency: impact on surgical techniques and clinical outcomes. *J Thorac Cardiovasc Surg.* 2009;137:286–294.)

Intraoperative TEE should be mandatory after repair to assess the functional result and identify patients at risk for early AR recurrence.[98] The accuracy of TEE compared with surgical observation is high, even for identification of the various subtypes of aortic cusp prolapse. This identification is necessary for the success of valve-sparing surgery because failure to identify and correct a preexisting cusp prolapse is a frequent cause of failure in valve-sparing operations.[99]

SURGICAL IMPLICATIONS

For Carpentier type I lesions, whenever the AR jet is central and perpendicular to the LVOT, absence of an associated type II lesion is assumed, and surgical correction is based on replacement of the ascending aorta and subcommissural annuloplasty. If the AR jet is not perpendicular to the LVOT, a type II lesion must be suspected and treated. Direction of the jet toward the mitral valve or septum determines the responsible prolapsing cusp; in this case, concomitant surgical valve repair is mandatory.[97]

For type Ib dysfunction due to an aortic root aneurysm, the indication for surgery is often diameter rather than AR severity. Even in patients with severe AR, one or more cusps remain almost normal due to the asymmetric nature of aortic root dilation. After tissue-sparing surgery is achieved by remodeling or reimplantation procedures,[53] a missed prolapse may exist, and it necessitates repair to avoid an immediate valve repair failure.

Patients with type III dysfunction undergoing AR repair are more likely to suffer significant recurrent AR. The primary cause of failure is the persistence or induction of some degree of cusp prolapse at the time of the initial operation.

Repair techniques for BAV have improved. Although some series still consider the presence of BAV to be a predictor of repair failure and reoperation,[95] other series have reported optimistic long-term results.[100,101] A postrepair effective coaptation height of less than 9 mm or coaptation length of less than 4 mm, an aortoventricular diameter greater than 28 mm, and a commissural orientation of less than 160 degrees in patients with BAV have been considered echocardiographic predictors for reoperation.[100] 3D echocardiography and gated high-resolution CT are promising technologies for improving aortic valve imaging.

RESULTS OF SURGERY AND FOLLOW-UP

With the advent of conservative aortic valve surgery, including valve-sparing operations and aortic cusp repair, the management of severe AR has changed significantly. These operations have low operative mortality rates and good long-term durability. Data on reconstructive surgery from expert centers show a hospital mortality rate of less than 2% for isolated valve repair and valve-sparing aortic replacement.[91,92] The mortality rate after pulmonary autograft is approximately 2% and is apparently not increased by the complexity of the operation.[102]

After aortic valve replacement, close follow-up is recommended during the early and mid-term postoperative course to evaluate prosthetic valve and LV function. After isolated surgery for a BAV, patients should have serial CT or MRI evaluations every 2 years. Patients who have an ascending aorta replacement with or without aortic valve surgery should be evaluated annually with echocardiography to assess the size of the retained aortic root, and they should undergo CT or MRI studies of the remaining thoracic and abdominal aorta every 3 to 5 years.

Surgical aortic valve replacement (AVR) has been the preferred therapeutic option for patients with severe AR; however, only 31.5% of those with severe AR and an EF between 30% and 50% were referred for surgery, and only 3.3% with an EF less than 30% underwent aortic valve replacement.[2] Only 2.2% of patients with severe AR received a transcatheter aortic valve.

Several challenges exist in using transcatheter aortic valve replacement (TAVR) for severe AR. Most severe cases of AR coexist with a dilated aortic root, and most devices are not approved for a severely dilated aortic annulus. Moreover, the usual absence of aortic valve calcification in this population renders anchoring of the prosthesis challenging. Despite these limitations and the low implementation rate of TAVR, a meta-analysis of 911 patients undergoing TAVR for AR yielded a device success rate of 80.4%, a moderate or severe paravalvular regurgitation rate of 7.4%, and a 30-day all-cause mortality rate of 9.5%.[103]

ACUTE AORTIC REGURGITATION

In acute severe AR, the sudden large RVol is imposed on a normal-sized LV that has not had time to adapt to the volume overload. The acute increase in diastolic flow into a nondilated LV leads to a marked rise in end-diastolic pressure, and forward cardiac output is decreased. In severe cases, the increased ventricular filling pressures in conjunction with the decrease in aortic diastolic pressure lead to a rapid equalization of aortic and LV pressures at end-diastole.[104] Pulmonary edema results from elevated LV end-diastolic pressure. Coronary flow reserve is impaired, and subendocardial myocardial ischemia may result. The causes of acute AR are shown in Table 23.4.

TABLE 23.4 Randomized, Controlled Trials of Vasodilator Therapy in Asymptomatic Patients With Chronic Severe Aortic Regurgitation.

Study	*Aim*	*Size* (N)	*Follow-Up (y)*	*Intervention vs. Comparator* (n)	*Patient Population*	*Results*
Evangelista et al.[66]	Effects of vasodilator therapy on LV function and time to AVR	95	7	Open-label nifedipine (32 pts) or open-label enalapril (32 pts) vs. no treatment (31 pts)	Asymptomatic, chronic, severe AR and normal LV function	No significant differences in rate of AVR No significant differences in AR severity, LV size, or LVEF
Scognomiglio et al.[62]	Assess whether vasodilator therapy reduces or delays the need for AVR	143	6	Nifedipine (69 pts) vs. digoxin (74 pts)	Asymptomatic, chronic, severe AR and normal LV function	Rate of AVR significantly lower in nifedipine group

AR, Aortic regurgitation; *AVR*, aortic valve replacement; *LVEF*, LV ejection fraction; *pts*, patients.

TABLE 23.5 Echocardiographic Findings in Acute Severe Aortic Regurgitation.

Causes	• Aortic dissection • Native valve infective endocarditis • Prosthetic valve infective endocarditis • Trauma • Spontaneous rupture or prolapse of an aortic cusp with bioprosthetic valve degeneration • Leaflet perforation in the setting of connective tissue disorders • Rupture of a fenestrated cusp • Spontaneous dehiscence of valve commissures • After surgical or catheter valvuloplasty
Specific signs	• Vena contracta > 6 mm • Premature mitral valve closure
Supportive signs	• Pressure half-time < 200 ms • Holodiastolic flow reversal in abdominal aorta • Normal LV size and function
Quantitative parameters	• EROA ≥ 0.30 cm^2 • RVol ≥ 60 mL/beat

EROA, Effective regurgitant orifice area; *RVol*, regurgitant volume.

Many of the physical signs of chronic AR are absent in the acute setting. The diagnosis of acute severe AR can be difficult or underestimated. Physical signs include tachycardia, a sometimes difficult-to-hear diastolic murmur, and heart failure signs; however, pulse pressure is normal and peripheral signs of AR are absent. The lack of physical signs of chronic severe AR renders acute AR difficult to identify, and the diagnosis is usually made by echocardiography.

Echocardiographic findings of acute severe AR are shown in Table 23.5. In acute AR, premature mitral valve closure (before ventricular systole) results from the rapid rise in LV diastolic pressures from the aortic RVol and is indicative of acute severe AR. Premature mitral valve closure is best demonstrated by M-mode imaging because its greater temporal resolution compared with 2D imaging permits delineation of the early closure of the valve.

Quantitative measures of regurgitant severity that are useful for chronic AR are less useful for acute regurgitation. Hemodynamic data have demonstrated the variability in regurgitant orifice area and RVol, depending on afterload and loading conditions.[24] TEE is indicated in most cases of acute AR to define the causes, mainly when acute dissection, endocarditis, or trauma are suspected or when the cause is uncertain.

Patients with acute AR require emergent or urgent surgery to correct the underlying lesion and relieve the acute volume overload of the LV. The type of surgery depends on the underlying cause.

ACUTE TYPE A AORTIC DISSECTION

AR frequently complicates acute type A aortic dissection, occurring in 41% to 76% of patients.[28] Although the need for early aortic surgery is well established, the optimal management of associated AR is controversial.

TEE can define the mechanisms and severity of AR that complicate acute type A aortic dissection. These findings may help the surgeon to differentiate valve and geometry distortions amenable to repair from fixed abnormalities that require replacement. Five mechanisms of AR are identified by TEE, the first three of which are considered reparable without the need for valve replacement:

1. Incomplete closure of intrinsically normal leaflets due to leaflet tethering by a dilated sinotubular junction
2. Leaflet prolapse due to disruption of leaflet attachment by a dissection flap that extends below the sinotubular junction and into the aortic root
3. Prolapse of the dissection flap through intrinsically normal leaflets that disrupts leaflet coaptation
4. BAV with associated leaflet prolapse unrelated to the dissection process
5. Degenerative leaflet thickening resulting in abnormal leaflet coaptation

Some patients have more than one mechanism of AR. TEE can play an important role in determining the optimal management of type A aortic dissection and significant AR.[97]

INFECTIVE ENDOCARDITIS

Heart failure caused by severe aortic or mitral regurgitation is the most common complication of infective endocarditis and represents the most frequent indication for surgery (see Chapters 23–25). Heart failure more often occurs when infective endocarditis affects the aortic rather than the mitral valve.[105] Acute AR in the setting of infective endocarditis may occur as a result of leaflet rupture, leaflet perforation, or, rarely, interference of the vegetation mass with leaflet closure. In addition to the clinical signs of heart failure, TTE and TEE are of crucial importance for the diagnosis and evaluation of AR and for determining the presence of vegetations and perivalvular complications.

In acute severe AR due to infective endocarditis, patients need immediate antibiotics and aggressive medical management. If the hemodynamic situation does not immediately improve, emergency aortic valve replacement may be lifesaving. If the clinical situation stabilizes, patients may benefit from several days of antibiotic treatment before surgery under strict clinical and echocardiographic surveillance.[106] The beneficial impact of surgery for patients with endocarditis and heart failure is clearly established.[107]

SUMMARY Useful Echocardiographic Parameters for Grading Aortic Regurgitation Severity.

Parameters	Mild	Moderate		Severe	Measurements	Planes	Strengths and Limitations
Color Doppler Parameters							
Semiquantitative Parameters							
VC width (cm)[a]	<0.3	0.3–0.6		>0.6	Narrowest flow diameter at the aortic valve level, below the flow convergence region	Parasternal long-axis view	Not circular or irregular regurgitant orifices of very calcified valves
Jet width in LVOT (cm)	Small in central jets (<0.4)	Intermediate (0.4–0.7, 0.7–1)		Large (>1) in central jets; varies in eccentric jets	Measurement just below the aortic valve	Parasternal long-axis view	Eccentric or not circular jets, and central jets with spray effect
Jet width/LVOT width (%)[c]	<25	Mild to moderate 25–45	Moderate to severe 46–64	≥65	Measurement just below the aortic valve	Parasternal long-axis view	Similar to jet width
Jet CSA/LVOT CSA (%)[c]	<5	5–20	21–59	≥60	Measurement of the jet area	Short-axis view	Small changes at LVOT level can cause significant differences in jet area Suboptimal image quality in this view in 20% of cases
Quantitative Parameters							
EROA (cm^2)	<0.10	Mild to moderate 0.10–0.19	Moderate to severe 0.20–0.29	≥0.30	PISA method; Nyquist limit should be shifted in direction of the AR jet Hemispheric PISA is required to obtain PISA radius $EROA = 6.28 \times r^2 \times V_{aliasing}/VAR$	Apical 5-chamber view or parasternal view	Technically demanding Accumulation of errors of each variable can affect final result. EROA can underestimate eccentric jets

Continued

SUMMARY **SUMMARYUseful Echocardiographic Parameters for Grading Aortic Regurgitation Severity—cont'd**

Parameters	Mild	Moderate		Severe	Measurements	Planes	Strengths and Limitations
RVol, mL/beat	<30	30–44	45–59	≥60	Calculated from the EROA by multiplying with the VTI of the AR jet: RVol = EROA × VTI_{AR}	—	—
Pulsed-Wave Doppler Parameters							
Diastolic flow reversal in proximal descending thoracic aorta	Brief, non-holodiastolic reversal flow	Intermediate		End-diastolic velocity > 20 cm/s or VTI > 15 mm	Holodiastolic reversal of flow and VTI measurement	Suprasternal view placed just distal to origin of the subclavian artery	Influenced by heart rate, diastolic time duration, and aortic distensibility
Diastolic flow reversal in abdominal aorta	Brief, early diastolic reversal	Intermediate		Prominent holodiastolic reversal	Holodiastolic reversal of flow	Visualization of abdominal aorta	Similar to proximal descending aorta
Continuous-Wave Doppler Parameters							
Jet deceleration rate (PHT, ms)[b]	Slow > 500	Medium 500–200		Steep < 200	Measurement of half-time from the slope of the regurgitant signal edge	—	Influenced by chamber compliance and pressure, peripheral resistance, and aortic compliance Less reliable in chronic AR, in which the LV is adapted to the chronic volume overload

[a]At Nyquist limit of 50 to 60 cm/s.
[b]PHT is shortened with increasing LV diastolic pressure and vasodilator therapy and may be lengthened in chronic adaptation to severe AR.
AR, Aortic regurgitation; *CSA*, cross-sectional area; *EF*, ejection fraction; *EROA*, effective regurgitant orifice area; *LV*, left ventricle; *LVOT*, left ventricular outflow tract; *PISA*, proximal isovelocity surface area; *PHT*, pressure half-time; *PW*, pulsed-wave Doppler; *RVol*, regurgitant volume; *VC*, vena contracta, *VTI*, velocity time integral.

REFERENCES

1. Singh JP, Evans JC, Levy D, et al. Prevalence and clinical determinants of mitral, tricuspid, and aortic regurgitation (the Framingham Heart Study). *Am J Cardiol.* 1999;83(2):897–902.
2. Iung B, Delgado V, Rosenhek, et al. Contemporary presentation and management of valvular heart diseases: the EURObservational Research Programme valvular heart disease II survey. *Circulation.* 2019;140(14):1156–1169.
3. Tarasoutchi F, Grinberg M, Spina GS, et al. Ten-year clinical laboratory follow-up after application of a symptom-based therapeutic strategy to patients with severe chronic aortic regurgitation of predominant rheumatic etiology. *J Am Coll Cardiol.* 2003;41(8):1316–1324.
4. Roberts WC, Ko JM, Moore TR, et al. Causes of pure aortic regurgitation in patients having isolated aortic valve replacement at a single US tertiary hospital (1993–2005). *Circulation.* 2006;114(5):422–429.
5. Muraru D, Badano LP, Vannan M, et al. Assessment of aortic valve complex by three-dimensional echocardiography: a framework for its effective application in clinical practice. *Eur Heart J Cardiovasc Imaging.* 2012;13(7):541–555.
6. Schaefer BM, Lewin MB, Stout KK, et al. The bicuspid aortic valve: an integrated phenotypic classification of leaflet morphology and aortic root shape. *Heart.* 2008;94(12):1634–1638.
7. Espinola-Zavaleta N, Muñoz-Castellanos L, Attié F, et al. Anatomic three-dimensional echocardiographic correlation of bicuspid aortic valve. *J Am Soc Echocardiogr.* 2003;16(1):46–53.
8. Tadros TM, Klein MD, Shapira OM. Ascending aortic dilatation associated with bicuspid aortic valve. Pathophysiology, molecular biology, and clinical implications. *Circulation.* 2009;119(6):880–890.
9. Michelena HI, Khanna AD, Mahoney D, et al. Incidence of aortic complications in patients with bicuspid aortic valves. *J Am Med Assoc.* 2011;306(10):1104–1112.
10. Evangelista A, González-Alujas MT. Echocardiography in infective endocarditis. *Heart.* 2004;90(6):614–617.
11. Iung B, Baron G, Butchart EG, et al. A prospective survey of patients with valvular heart disease. *Eur Heart J.* 2003;24(13):1231–1243.
12. Schäfers HJ, Langer F, Glombitza P, et al. Aortic valve reconstruction in myxomatous degeneration of aortic valves: are fenestrations a risk factor for repair failure? *J Thorac Cardiovasc Surg.* 2010;139(3):660–664.
13. Lerakis S, Hayekk SS, Douglas PS. Paravalvularaortic leak after transcatheter aortic valve replacement: current knowledge. *Circulation.* 2013;127(3):397–407.
14. Le Polain de Waroux JB, Pouleur AC, et al. Functional anatomy of aortic regurgitation. Accuracy, prediction of surgical repairability and outcome implications of transesophageal echocardiography. *Circulation.* 2007;116(Suppl):I264–I269.
15. Teixido-Tura G, Almeida AL, Choi EY, et al. Determinants of aortic root dilatation and reference values among young adults over a 20-year period: coronary artery risk development in young adults study. *Hypertension.* 2015;66:23–29.
16. Lancelloti P, Tribouilloy C, Hagendorff A, et al. European Association of Echocardiography recommendations for the assessment of valvular regurgitation. Part 1: aortic and pulmonary regurgitation (native valve disease). *Eur J Echocardiogr.* 2010;11(3):223–244.
17. Taylor AL, Eichhorn EJ, Brickner ME, et al. Aortic valve morphology: an important in vitro determinant of proximal regurgitant jet width by Doppler color flow mapping. *J Am Coll Cardiol.* 1990;16(2):405–412.
18. Evangelista A, García del Castillo H, Calvo F, et al. Strategy for optimal aortic regurgitation quantification by Doppler echocardiography: agreement among different methods. *Am Heart J.* 2000;139(5):773–781.
19. Smith MD, Grayburn PA, Michael D, et al. Observer variability in the quantitation of Doppler color flow jet areas for mitral and aortic regurgitation. *J Am Coll Cardiol.* 1988;11(3):579–584.
20. Tribouilloy CM, Enriquez-Serrano M, Bailey KR, et al. Assessment of severity of aortic regurgitation using the width of the vena contracta: a clinical color Doppler imaging study. *Circulation.* 2000;102(5):558–564.
21. Eren M, Eksik A, Gorgulu S, et al. Determination of vena contracta and its value in evaluating severity of aortic regurgitation. *J Heart Valve Dis.* 2002;11(4):567–575.
22. Perez de Isla L, Zamorano J, Fernandez-Golfin C, et al. 3D color-Doppler echocardiography and chronic aortic regurgitation: a novel approach for severity assessment. *Int J Cardiol.* 2013;166(3):640–645.
23. Pouleur AC, de Waroux JB, Goffinet C, et al. Accuracy of the flow convergence method for quantification of aortic regurgitation in patients with central versus eccentric jets. *Am J Cardiol.* 2008;102(4):475–480.
24. Detaint D, Messika-Zeitoun D, Maalouf J, et al. Quantitative echocardiographic determinants of clinical outcome in asymptomatic patients with aortic regurgitation: a prospective study. *JACC Cardiovasc Imaging.* 2008;1(1):1–11.
25. Pirat B, Little SH, Igo SR, et al. Direct measurement of proximal isovelocity surface area by real-time three-dimensional color Doppler for quantitation of aortic regurgitant volume: an in vitro validation. *J Am Soc Echocardiogr.* 2009;22(3):306–313.
26. Ewe SH, Delgado V, van der Geest R, et al. Accuracy of three-dimensional versus two-dimensional echocardiography for quantification of aortic regurgitation and validation by three-dimensional three-directional velocity-encoded magnetic resonance imaging. *Am J Cardiol.* 2013;112(4):560–566.
27. Tribouilloy C, Avinée P, Shen WF, et al. End diastolic flow velocity just beneath the aortic isthmus assessed by pulsed Doppler echocardiography: a new predictor of the aortic regurgitant fraction. *Br Heart J.* 1991;65(1):37–40.
28. Griffin BP, Flachskampf FA, Siu S, et al. The effects of regurgitant orifice size, chamber compliance, and systemic vascular resistance on aortic regurgitant velocity slope and pressure half-time. *Am Heart J.* 1991;122(4 Pt 1):1049–1056.
29. Griffin BP, Flachskampf FA, Reimold SC, et al. Relationship of aortic regurgitant velocity slope and pressure half-time to severity of aortic regurgitation under changing haemo-dynamic conditions. *Eur Heart J.* 1994;15(5):681–685.
30. Gottdiener JS, Panza JA, John Sutton M, et al. Testing the test: the reliability of echocardiography in the sequential assessment of valvular regurgitation. *Am Heart J.* 2002;144(1):115–121.
31. Zarauza J, Ares M, González Vilchez F, et al. An integrated approach to the quantification of aortic regurgitation by Doppler echocardiography. *Am Heart J.* 1998;136(6):1030–1041.
32. Willett DL, Hall SA, Jessen ME, et al. Assessment of aortic regurgitation by transesophageal color Doppler imaging of the vena contracta: validation against an intraoperative aortic flow probe. *J Am Coll Cardiol.* 2001;37(5):1450–1455.
33. Sato Y, Kawazoe K, Kamata J, et al. Clinical usefulness of the effective regurgitant orifice area determined by transesophageal echo-cardiography in patients with eccentric aortic regurgitation. *J Heart Valve Dis.* 1997;6(6):580–586.
34. Sutton DC, Kluger R, Ahmed SU, et al. Flow reversal in the descending aorta: a guide to intraoperative assessment of aortic regurgitation with transesophageal echocardiography. *J Thorac Cardiovasc Surg.* 1994;108(3):576–582.
35. Hagendorff A, Evangelista A, Fehske W, et al. Improvement in the assessment of aortic valve and aortic aneurysm repair by 3-dimensional echocardiography. *JACC Cardiovasc Imaging.* 2019;Mar;(8) doi: 10.1016/j.jcmg.2018.06.032.
36. Gabriel RS, Renapurkar R, Bolen MA, et al. Comparison of severity of aortic regurgitation by cardiovascular magnetic resonance versus transthoracic echocardiography. *Am J Cardiol.* 2011;108(7):1014–1020.
37. Myerson SG, d'Arcy J, Mohiaddin R, et al. Aortic regurgitation quantification using cardiovascular magnetic resonance: association with clinical outcome. *Circulation.* 2012;126(12):1452–1460.
38. Cawley PJ, Hamilton-Craig C, Owens DS, et al. Prospective comparison of valve regurgitation quantitation by cardiac magnetic resonance imaging and transthoracic echocardiography. *Circ Cardiovasc Imaging.* 2013;6(1):48–57.
39. Lang RM, Badano LP, Mor-AVi V, et al. Recommendations for cardiac chamber quantification by echocardiography in adults: an update from the American Society of Echocardiography and the European Association of Cardiovascular Imaging. *J Am Soc Echocardiogr.* 2015;28(1):1–39.
40. Vinereanu D, Ionescu AA, Fraser G. Assessment of left ventricular long axis contraction can detect early myocardial dysfunction in asymptomatic patients with severe aortic regurgitation. *Heart.* 2001;85(1):30–36.
41. Paraskevaidis IA, Kyrzopoulos S, Farmakis D, et al. Ventricular long-axis contraction as an earlier predictor of outcome in asymptomatic aortic regurgitation. *Am J Cardiol.* 2007;100(11):1677–1682.
42. Olsen NT, Sogaard P, Larsson HB, et al. Speckle-tracking echocardiography for predicting outcome in chronic aortic regurgitation during conservative management and after surgery. *JACC Cardiovasc Imaging.* 2011;4(3):223–230.
43. Alashi A, Khullar T, Mentias A, et al. Long-term outcomes after aortic valve surgery in patients with asymptomatic chronic aortic regurgitation and preserved LVEF: impact of baseline and follow-up global longitudinal strain. *JACC Cardiovasc Imaging.* 2019;13(1 Pt 1):12–21. https://doi.org/10.1016/j.jcmg.2018.12.021.

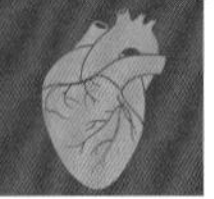

44. Ewe SH, Haeck ML, Ng AC, et al. Detection of subtle left ventricular systolic dysfunction in patients with significant aortic regurgitation and preserved left ventricular ejection fraction: speckle tracking echocardiographic analysis. *Eur Heart J Cardiovasc Imaging.* 2015;16(9):992–999.
45. Gabriel RS, Renapurkar R, Bolen MA, et al. Comparison of severity of aortic regurgitation by cardiovascular magnetic resonance versus transthoracic echocardiography. *Am J Cardiol.* 2011;108:1014–1020.
46. Kusunose K, Agarwal S, Marwick TH, et al. Decision making in asymptomatic aortic regurgitation in the era of guidelines: incremental values of resting and exercise cardiac dysfunction. *Circ Cardiovasc Imaging.* 2014;7(2):352–362.
47. Le Polain de Waroux JB, Pouleur AC, Goffinet C, et al. Combined coronary and late-enhanced multidetector-computed tomography for delineation of the etiology of left ventricular dysfunction: comparison with coronary angiography and contrast-enhanced cardiac magnetic resonance imaging. *Eur Heart J.* 2008;29(20):2544–2551.
48. Otto CM, Nishimura RA, Bonow RO, et al. 2020 ACC/AHA guideline for the management of patients with valvular heart disease: a report of the American College of Cardiology/American Heart Association Joint Committee on Clinical Practice Guidelines. *J Am Coll Cardiol.* 2021;77(4):e25–e197.
49. Sparrow P, Messroghli DR, Reid S, et al. Myocardial T1 mapping for detection of left ventricular myocardial fibrosis in chronic aortic regurgitation: pilot study. *AJR Am J Roentgenol.* 2006;187(6):W630–W635.
50. De Meester de Ravenstein C, Bouzin C, Lazam S, et al. Histological validation of measurement of diffuse interstitial myocardial fibrosis by myocardial extravascular volume fraction from Modified Look-Locker Imaging (MOLLI) T1 mapping at 3 T. *J Cardiovasc Magn Reson.* 2015;11:17–48.
51. Azevedo CF, Nigri M, Higuchi ML, et al. Prognostic significance of myocardial fibrosis quantification by histopathology and magnetic resonance imaging in patients with severe aortic valve disease. *J Am Coll Cardiol.* 2010;56:278–287.
52. Wahi S, Haluska B, Pasquet A, et al. Exercise echocardiography predicts development of left ventricular dysfunction in medically and surgically treated patients with asymptomatic severe aortic regurgitation. *Heart.* 2000;84(6):606–614.
53. Fazel SS, David TE. Aortic valve-sparing operations for aortic root and ascending aortic aneurysms. *Curr Opin Cardiol.* 2007;22(6):497–503.
54. Schäfers HJ, Schmied W, Marom G, et al. Cusp height in aortic valves. *J Thorac Cardiovasc Surg.* 2013;146(2):269–274.
55. La Canna G, Maisano F, De Michele L, et al. Determinants of the degree of functional aortic regurgitation in patients with anatomically normal aortic valve and ascending thoracic aorta aneurysm. Transoesophageal Doppler Echocardiography study. *Heart.* 2009;95(2):130–136.
56. Evangelista A, Flachskampf, Erbel R, et al. Echocardiography in aortic diseases: EAE recommendations for clinical practice. *Eur J Echocardiogr.* 2010;11(8):645–658.
57. Gaasch WH, Sundaram M, Meyer TH. Managing asymptomatic patients with chronic aortic regurgitation. Chest 111:1702-1709, 1997.
58. Baumgartner H, Falk V, Bax JJ, et al. 2017 ESC/EACTS guidelines for the management of valvular heart disease. *Eur Heart J.* 2017;38(36):2739–2791.
59. Bonow RO, Rosing DR, McIntosh CL, et al. The natural history of asymptomatic patients with aortic regurgitation and normal left ventricular function. *Circulation.* 1983;68(3):509–517.
60. Bonow RO, Lakatos E, Maron BJ, et al. Serial long-term assessment of the natural history of asymptomatic patients with chronic aortic regurgitation and normal left ventricular systolic function. *Circulation.* 1991;84(4):1625–1635.
61. Siemienczuk D, Greenberg B, Morris C, et al. Chronic aortic insufficiency: factors associated with progression to aortic valve replacement. *Ann Intern Med.* 1989;110(8):587–592.
62. Scognamiglio R, Rahimtoola SH, Fasoli G, et al. Nifedipine in asymptomatic patients with severe aortic regurgitation and normal left ventricular function. *N Engl J Med.* 1994;331(11):689–694.
63. Tornos MP, Olona M, Permanyer-Miralda G, et al. Clinical outcome of severe asymptomatic chronic aortic regurgitation: a long-term prospective follow-up study. *Am Heart J.* 1995;130(2):333–339.
64. Ishii K, Hirota Y, Suwa M, et al. Natural history and left ventricular response in chronic aortic regurgitation. *Am J Cardiol.* 1996;78(3):357–361.
65. Borer JS, Hochreiter C, Herrold EM, et al. Prediction of indications for valve replacement among asymptomatic or minimally symptomatic patients with chronic aortic regurgitation and normal left ventricular performance. *Circulation.* 1998;97(6):525–534.
66. Evangelista A, Tornos P, Sambola A, et al. Long-term vasodilator therapy in patients with severe aortic regurgitation. *N Engl J Med.* 2005;353(13):1342–1349.
67. Reference deleted in review.
68. Aronow WS, Ahn C, Kronzon I, et al. Prognosis of patients with heart failure and unoperated severe aortic valvular regurgitation and relation to ejection fraction. *Am J Cardiol.* 1994;74(3):286–288.
69. Dujardin KS, Enriquez-Sarano M, Schaff HV, et al. Mortality and morbidity of aortic regurgitation in clinical practice: a long-term follow-up study. *Circulation.* 1999;99(14):1851–1857.
70. Otto CM, Nishimura RA, Bonow RO. 2020 ACC/AHA guideline for the management of patients with valvular heart disease: a report of the American College of Cardiology/American Heart Association Joint Committee on Clinical Practice Guidelines. *Circulation.* 2021;143. DOI: 10.1161/CIR.0000000000000923.
71. Pizarro R, Bazzino OO, Oberti PF, et al. Prospective validation of the prognostic usefulness of B-type natriuretic peptide in asymptomatic patients with chronic severe aortic regurgitation. *J Am Coll Cardiol.* 2011;58(16):1705–1714.
72. Bonow RO, Picone AL, McIntosh CL. et al. Survival and functional results after valve replacement for aortic regurgitation from 1976 to 1983: impact of preoperative left ventricular function. *Circulation.* 1985;72:1244–1256.
73. Cunha CL, Giuliani ER, Fuster V, et al. Preoperative M-mode echocardiography as a predictor of surgical results in chronic aortic insufficiency. *J Thorac Cardiovasc Surg.* 1980;79:256–265.
74. Scognamiglio R, Fasoli G, Dalla Volta S. Progression of myocardial dysfunction in asymptomatic patients with severe aortic insufficiency. *Clin Cardiol.* 1986;9(4):151–156.
75. Saisho H, Arinaga K, Kikusaki S, et al. Long term results and predictors of left ventricular function recovery after aortic valve replacement for chronic aortic regurgitation. *Ann Thorac Cardiovasc Surg.* 2015;21:388–395.
76. Mentias A, Feng K, Alashi A, et al. Long-term outcomes in patients with aortic regurgitation and preserved left ventricular ejection fraction. *J Am Coll Cardiol.* 2016;68(20):2144–2153.
77. Yang L-T, Michelena HL, Scott CG, et al. Outcomes in chronic hemodynamically significant aortic regurgitation and limitations of current guidelines. *J Am Coll Cardiol.* 2019;73:1741–1752.
78. Bonow RO. Chronic mitral regurgitation and aortic regurgitation have indications for surgery changed? *J Am Coll Cardiol.* 2013;61:693-701.
78a. Borer JS, Supino PG, Herrold EM, et al. Survival after aortic valve replacement for aortic regurgitation: prediction from preoperative contractility measurement. *Cardiology.* 2018;140(4): 204–212.
79. Kusunose K, Cremer PC, Tsutsui RS, et al. Regurgitant volume informs rate of progressive cardiac dysfunction in asymptomatic patients with chronic aortic or mitral regurgitation. *JACC Cardiovasc Imaging.* 2015;8(1):14–23.
80. Greenberg BH, DeMots H, Murphy E, et al. Beneficial effects of hydralazine on rest and exercise hemodynamics in patients with chronic severe aortic insufficiency. *Circulation.* 1980;62(1):49–55.
81. Tornos P, Olona M, Permanyer-Miralda G, et al. Heart failure after aortic valve replacement for aortic regurgitation: prospective 20-year study. *Am Heart J.* 1998;136(4):681–687.
82. Enriquez-Sarano M, Tajik AJ. Clinical-practice: aorticregurgitation. *N Engl J Med.* 2004;351(15):1539–1546.
83. Sambola A, Tornos P, Ferreira-Gonzalez I, Evangelista A. Prognostic value of preoperative indexed end-systolic left ventricle diameter in the outcome after surgery in patients with chronic aortic regurgitation. *Am Heart J.* 2008;155(6):1114–1120.
84. Chaliki HP, Mohty D, Avierinos J-F, et al. Outcomes after aortic valve replacement in patients with severe aortic regurgitation and markedly reduced left ventricular function. *Circulation.* 2002;106(21):2687–2693.
85. Tornos P, Sambola A, Permanyer-Miralda G, et al. Long-term outcome of surgically treated aortic regurgitation: influence of guidelines adherence toward early surgery. *J Am Coll Cardiol.* 2006;47(5):1012–1017.
86. Bonow RO, Dodd JT, Maron BJ, et al. Long-term serial changes in left ventricular function and reversal of ventricular dilatation after valve replacement for chronic aortic regurgitation. *Circulation.* 1988;78(5):1108–1120.
87. De Meester C, Gerber BL, Vancraeynest D, et al. Do guideline-based indications result in an outcome penalty for patients with severe aortic regurgitation?. *JACC Cardiovasc Imaging.* 2019;12(11 Pt 1):2126–2138.
88. De Meester, Gerber BL, Vancraeynest D, et al. Early surgical intervention versus watchful waiting and outcomes for asymptomatic severe aortic regurgitation. *J Thorac Cardiovasc Surg.* 2015;150:1100–1108.

89. Borger MA, Preston M, Ivanov J, et al. Should the ascending aorta be replaced more frequently in patients with bicuspid aortic valve disease? *J Thorac Cardiovasc Surg.* 2004;128(5):677–683.
90. Chiappini B, Absil B, Rubay J, et al. The Ross procedure: clinical and echocardiographic follow-up in 219 consecutive patients. *Ann Thorac Surg.* 2007;83(4):1285–1289.
91. Kari FA, Siepe M, Sievers HH, et al. Repair of the regurgitant bicuspid or tricuspid aortic valve: background, principles, and outcomes. *Circulation.* 2013;128(8):854–863.
92. Pacini D, Ranocchi F, Angeli E, et al. Aortic root replacement with composite valve graft. *Ann Thorac Surg.* 2003;76(1):90–98.
93. Hiratzka LF, Bakris GL, Beckman JA, et al. ACCF/AHA/AATS/ACR/ASA/SCA/SCAI/SIR/STS/SVM guidelines for the diagnosis and management of patients with thoracic aortic disease. *Circulation.* 2010;122(4):e410.
94. Mazzitelli D, Stamm C, Rankin JS, et al. Leaflet reconstructive techniques for aortic valve repair. *Ann Thorac Surg.* 2014;98(6):2053–2060.
95. Jasinsky MJ, Gocol R, Malinowski M, et al. Predictors of early and medium-term outcome of 200 consecutive aortic valve and root repairs. *J Thorac Cardiovasc Surg.* 2015;149(1):123–129.
96. Charitos EI, Stierle U, Tietze C, et al. Clinical outcomes and lessons learned with aortic valve repair in 508 patients. *J Heart Valve Dis.* 2014;23(5):550–557.
97. Khoury E, Glineur D, Rubay J, et al. Functional classification of aortic root/valve abnormalities and their correlation with etiologies and surgical procedures. *Curr Opin Cardiol.* 2005;20(2):115–121.
98. Petterson GB, Crucean AC, Savage R, et al. Towards predictable repair of regurgitant aortic valve. A systematic morphology-directed approach to bicomissural repair. *J Am Coll Cardiol.* 2008;52(1):40–49.
99. David TE, Armstrong S, Maganti M, et al. Long-term results of aortic valve-sparing operations in patients with Marfan syndrome. *J Thorac Surg.* 2009;138(4):859–864.
100. Aicher D, Kunihara T, AbouIssa O, et al. Valve configuration determines long-term results after repair of the bicuspid aortic valve. *Circulation.* 2011;123(2):178–185.
101. Svensson LG, Al Kindi AH, Vivacqua A, et al. Long-term durability of bicuspid aortic valve repair. *Ann Thorac Surg.* 2014;97(5):1539–1547.
102. Takkenberg JJ, Klieverik LM, Schoof PH, et al. The Ross procedure: a systematic review and meta-analysis. *Circulation.* 2009;119(2):222–228.
103. Takagi H, Hari Y, Kawai N, Ando T. Meta-analysis and meta-regression of transcatheter aortic valve implantation for pure native aortic regurgitation. *Heart Lung Circ.* 2020;29(5):729–774.
104. Movsowitz HD, Levine RA, Higenberg AD, et al. Transesophageal echocardiography description of the mechanisms of aortic regurgitation in acute type A aortic dissection: implications for aortic valve repair. *J Am Coll Cardiol.* 2000;36(3):884–890.
105. Tornos P, Iung B, Permanyer-Miralda G, et al. Infective endocarditis in Europe: lessons from the Euro Heart Survey. *Heart.* 2005;91(5):571–575.
106. Habib G, Lancellotti P, Antunes MJ, et al. ESC guidelines for the management of infective endocarditis: the Task Force for the Management of Infective Endocarditis of the European Society of Cardiology (ESC). *Eur Heart J.* 2015;36(44):3075–3128.
107. Vikram HR, Buenconsejo J, Hasbun R, Quagliarello VJ. Impact of valve surgery on 6-month mortality in adults with complicated, left-sided native valve endocarditis: a propensity analysis. *J Am Med Assoc.* 2003;290(24):3207–3214.

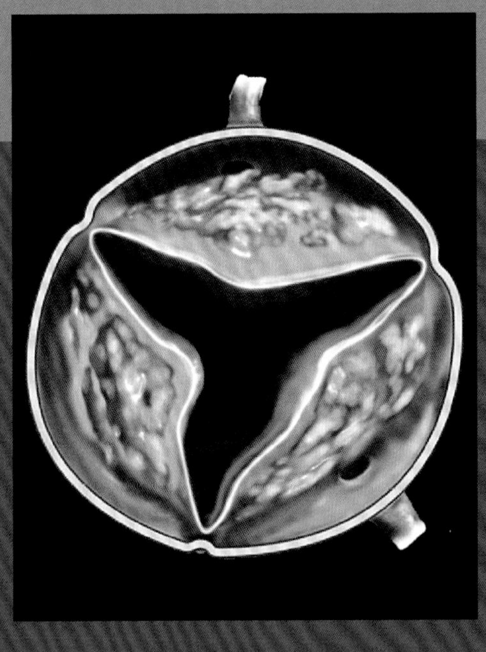

中文导读

第24章 二尖瓣反流：瓣膜解剖、反流严重程度和干预时机

二尖瓣反流是一种常见的心脏瓣膜疾病，是心血管疾病发病率及死亡率增加的重要原因。二尖瓣反流可分为原发性瓣膜病变（瓣膜本身病变）和继发性瓣膜病变（缺血性或功能性）。原发性二尖瓣反流常见的病因是二尖瓣叶、瓣下腱索脱垂或断裂、感染性心内膜炎。继发性二尖瓣反流常见的病因是心肌缺血或心肌重构导致二尖瓣下支持结构乳头肌功能异常。原发性或继发性二尖瓣反流病因的鉴别、准确评估和量化对于临床治疗管理至关重要。超声心动图多普勒成像技术是二尖瓣反流定量研究的准确、无创的方法。本章主要讲述了二尖瓣的解剖基础、二尖瓣反流的病因分类、运用多普勒技术定量评估二尖瓣反流的常用指标及诊断要点、二尖瓣反流定量评估规范化流程，并对指南推荐的原发性和继发性二尖瓣反流临床干预方式和时机进行了详细的说明。

李　慧

24

Mitral Regurgitation: Valve Anatomy, Regurgitant Severity, and Timing of Intervention

JUDY HUNG, MD | JACQUELINE DANIK, MD, DrPH

Mitral regurgitation (MR) is a common valvular disorder that is a significant cause of morbidity and mortality in cardiovascular disease.[1–5] Population studies have estimated the prevalence of mild or greater MR to be 20%.[6–8] More than 30,000 patients undergo mitral valve (MV) surgery annually for significant (moderate or severe) MR in the United States.[9]

MR can be categorized as primary (valvular) or secondary (ischemic or functional). Primary MR results from abnormalities of the mitral leaflets and chordal structures, such as prolapse, flail, or endocarditis. Secondary MR results from abnormalities of the left ventricle (LV) from ischemic or myopathic remodeling of the ventricular myocardium underlying the papillary muscles (PMs) that support the MV apparatus. It is important to distinguish the mechanism of MR because therapy is based on whether MR is primary or secondary.

Accurate quantification of MR plays an important role in clinical practice. Doppler techniques in echocardiography in the early 1980s transformed the diagnosis and management of MV disease, providing accurate, noninvasive quantification of MR. Management of MR relies on accurate assessment of cause and quantification of MR. This chapter reviews the mechanistic basis and quantification of MR and how these factors guide clinical decision making.

MITRAL VALVE ANATOMY AND MECHANISMS OF MITRAL REGURGITATION

MITRAL VALVE ANATOMY

Embryology and Components of the Mitral Valve

The MV apparatus forms from delamination of the ventricular myocardium after formation of the atrioventricular valves from the endocardial cushions. The MV apparatus includes the mitral annulus, mitral leaflets, chordae tendineae, and PMs. Knowledge of the anatomy of the MV apparatus is important for understanding MV function and the mechanisms of primary and secondary MR.

Mitral Annulus

The mitral annulus is part of the fibrous skeleton of the heart. It is composed of a fibromuscular ring situated between the left atrium (LA) and LV, and it anchors the leaflets. The normal mitral annulus is elliptical and has an area between 5 and 11 cm^2 (mean, 7 cm^2). It also has a bimodal or saddle shape, with the anterior and posterior points superiorly oriented (toward the LA) and the medial and lateral points inferiorly oriented (toward the LV).[10] In vitro testing and computer modeling studies have demonstrated that the bimodal shape is optimal for minimizing stress on the mitral leaflets during opening and closing.[11–13]

The anteromedial portion of the mitral annulus, which forms the straight edge of the D-shaped aspect, shares a common wall with the aortic annulus at the attachment of noncoronary and left coronary cusps. This shared wall, which is called the *intervalvular fibrosa* (i.e., aortomitral curtain), is more rigid than the posterior annulus due to fibrous attachments.

The posterior portion of the annulus accounts for a greater circumferential length than the anterior portion. Because the anterior annulus is relatively fixed compared with the posterior annulus, dilation of the mitral annulus predominantly occurs posteriorly.[14] The mitral annular area is dynamic throughout the cardiac cycle and is influenced by LA contraction and filling mechanics.

Mitral Leaflets

The two leaflets of the MV are referred to as anterior and posterior based on their anatomic locations. The broad anterior leaflet has a greater surface area and thickness than the posterior leaflet and accounts for most of the closing surface area of the MV (Fig. 24.1).

The anterior leaflet is attached to the anterior mitral annulus through fibrous continuity with the noncoronary and left aortic cusps. The posterior leaflet is crescent shaped and has overall less surface area than the anterior leaflet, despite having a greater circumferential attachment length to the mitral

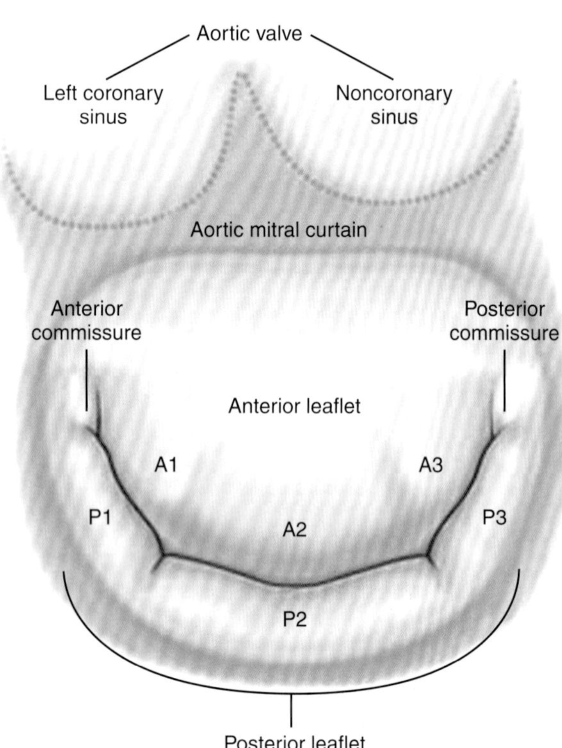

Fig. 24.1 Mitral valve leaflets. The schematic drawing of the mitral valve from the LA aspect is oriented similar to a 3D TEE view of the valve. The anterior leaflet is semicircular and provides two thirds of the leaflet's closing surface area. The posterior leaflet is crescent shaped with three distinct segments that are separated by two small clefts between the segments. Each leaflet can be divided into three segments, numbered from lateral to medial: *A1*, *A2*, and *A3* on the anterior leaflet; *P1*, *P2*, and *P3* on the posterior leaflet. This allows precise description of the location of valve dysfunction with close correlation between echocardiographic and surgical anatomy.

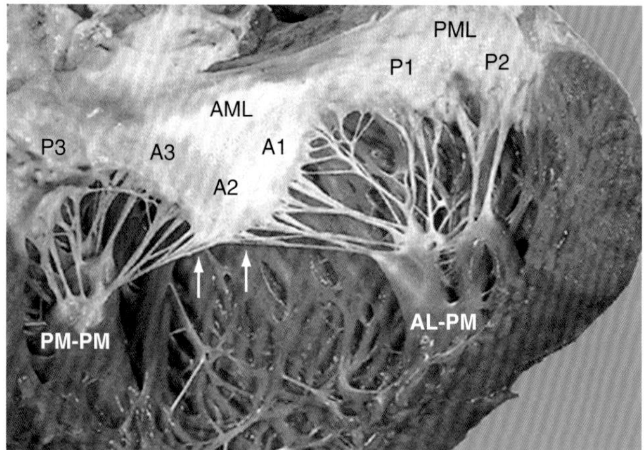

Fig. 24.2 Mitral valve chordae. Chordae originating from the posteromedial papillary muscle *(PM-PM)* attach to the medial half of each leaflet (*A3* and one half of *A2*; *P3* and one half of *P2*). Chordae from the anterolateral papillary muscle *(AL-PM)* attach to the lateral one half of each leaflet (*A1* and one half of *A2*; *P1* and one half of *P2*). Primary chordae *(arrows)* have a branching pattern and insert at the edge of the leaflets. *AML*, Anterior mitral leaflet; *PML*, posterior mitral leaflet. (Adapted from Mills SE, ed. *Histology for Pathologists*. 3rd ed. Baltimore: Lippincott Williams & Wilkins; 2007.)

annulus. The shape of the posterior leaflet forms three scalloped segments separated by thin clefts between each segment.

Both leaflets are attached at the posterior and anterior commissures. The common nomenclature divides each leaflet into three segments or scallops, labeled 1 through 3, indicating the anterolateral, middle, and posteromedial segments, respectively. The anterior leaflet segments are labeled A and the posterior ones B (see Fig. 24.1).

Compensatory Leaflet Growth

Cardiac valves were once seen as static structures, but the data suggest that compensatory leaflet growth may result from altered cardiac dimensions.[15] An increase in leaflet area and thickness occurred in response to subvalvular leaflet tethering in sheep.[16] These changes were attributed to endothelial cells coexpressing smooth muscle α-actin more in tethered leaflets, which indicated endothelial-mesenchymal transdifferentiation.

Chordae Tendineae and Papillary Muscles

The mitral chordae tendineae, which typically number 25, are thin, fibrous structures composed of collagen interwoven with elastin fibers that extend from the PMs to attach to the mitral leaflets. The chordae anchor the mitral leaflets during systole, allowing symmetric coaptation and preventing prolapse of the leaflets into the LA.

The chordae are attached to the LV by the PMs. During systole, the PMs contract to facilitate closure of the leaflets by the chordae. The PMs arise from the area between the apical and middle thirds of the LV free wall and are divided into anterolateral and posteromedial PMs. The anterolateral PM is the larger of the two, has a single body but two heads (i.e., anterior and posterior), and is supplied by the first obtuse marginal branch of the circumflex artery and the first diagonal branch of the anterior descending artery. The posteromedial PM is smaller, has two bodies and three heads (i.e., anterior, intermediate, and posterior), and is supplied by the posterior descending artery, a branch of the right coronary artery in 90% of cases and by the circumflex artery in the other 10%, making it much more vulnerable to ischemic episodes.[17]

Equal numbers of chordae come from each PM to insert into each of the leaflets. Chordae originating from the posteromedial PM attach to the medial one half of each leaflet, and chordae from the anterolateral PM attach to the lateral one half of each leaflet.

Primary, secondary, and tertiary chordae exist. The primary chordae (i.e., marginal chordae) extend from the PMs in a branching pattern to attach along the coaptation line (i.e., margin) of the leaflets (Fig. 24.2). The main role of these primary chordae is to maintain coaptation of the leaflets.[18] Rupture or elongation of the primary chordae results in loss of coaptation and development of prolapse or flail leaflet and, invariably, MR.

The secondary chordae (i.e., intermediate or strut chordae) attach at the midbody of the leaflets in the transition area between the rough and smooth zones of the leaflets. Their main function is to provide the basic support from the PM to the leaflet.[18] They prevent the valve leaflet from developing excess tension by distributing tension across the ventricular surface of the leaflets, preventing leaflet billowing and potentially maintaining dynamic ventricular shape and function.[19] Secondary chordae are thicker and longer than primary chordae and do not have a branching pattern. Secondary chordae may rupture without compromising leaflet coaptation.

Basal or tertiary chordae are associated only with the posterior leaflet. They connect the base of the leaflet and the posterior mitral annulus to the PMs.[15]

MECHANISMS OF MITRAL REGURGITATION

Mechanisms of MR are broadly categorized as primary or secondary. Primary MR is caused by abnormalities of the valvular

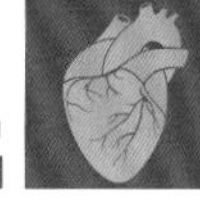

TABLE 24.1 Causes of Primary and Secondary Mitral Regurgitation.

Causes of Regurgitation	*Lesions or Diseases*
Primary MR (Leaflet Abnormality)	
Mitral valve prolapse and myxomatous changes	Prolapse, flail, ruptured or elongated chordae
Degenerative changes	Calcification, thickening of leaflets
Infectious endocarditis	Vegetations, perforations, aneurysm
Noninfectious endocarditis	Collagen vascular disease (Libman-Sacks lesions); malignancy-associated (marantic endocarditis)
Inflammatory disease	Rheumatic or collagen vascular disease, radiation, drugs
Rheumatic disease	Leaflet thickening, often with restriction of the posterior leaflet; mixed mitral valve disease (MS and MR)
Radiation	Diffuse leaflet thickening and calcification; often mixed mitral disease (MS and MR)
Drug-induced (e.g., anorexigen, ergotamine)	Diffuse leaflet thickening
Congenital disorder	Cleft leaflet, parachute mitral valve
Secondary MR (Ventricular Remodeling)	
Ischemia	Ventricular distortion of the mitral apparatus from coronary disease (regional variation or cardiomyopathy)
Cardiomyopathy	Ventricular distortion of the mitral apparatus
Mitral annular dilation	Atrial fibrillation, restrictive cardiomyopathy
MR due to systolic anterior motion of the mitral valve	Hypertrophic cardiomyopathy

MR, Mitral regurgitation; *MS*, mitral stenosis.
From Zoghbi WA, Adams D, Bonow RO, et al. Recommendations for noninvasive evaluation of native valvular regurgitation: a report from the American Society of Echocardiography developed in collaboration with the Society for Cardiovascular Magnetic Resonance. *J Am Soc Echocardiogr.* 2017;30(4):303–371.

leaflets or chordae, whereas secondary MR is caused by chamber (LV or LA) dilation from ischemic, myopathic, or arrhythmic processes. Chamber dilation leads to distortion of the normal geometric relationships of the MV apparatus and the LV. In the latter case, the leaflets are morphologically normal.

Table 24.1 summarizes the causes of MR based on mechanism. Therapeutic options depend on the mechanism of MR. MR can also result from mixed mechanisms, in which both primary and secondary factors contribute.

Primary Mitral Regurgitation

Degenerative MV disease is a common mechanism for primary MR. It includes the mitral valve prolapse (MVP) spectrum and nonspecific calcification and thickening of the leaflets associated with age and comorbidities such as chronic kidney disease, diabetes, and hypertension. *Organic MV disease* is another commonly used term for primary valvular disease that includes the MVP spectrum.

MVP is a common cause of primary MR. MVP is defined as displacement of the mitral leaflets during systole of at least 2 mm from the annular plane (Fig. 24.3).[10] It can occur with or without MR or leaflet thickening. Leaflet thickening on echocardiography is often associated with myxomatous changes. Some patients have mitral annular disjunction (MAD), which is abnormal atrial displacement of the MV leaflet hinge point. In MAD, the posterior leaflet is often involved. MAD has been associated with MVP and ventricular arrhythmias.[20]

The reported prevalence of MVP is approximately 2.4%, and MR due to MVP accounts for most of the more than 10,000 isolated MV operations performed annually in the United States.[9]

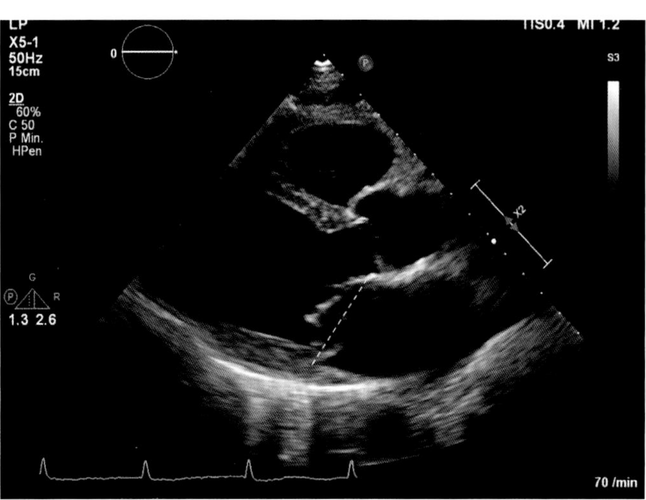

Fig. 24.3 Mitral valve prolapse. (A) The parasternal long-axis view demonstrates prolapse of the posterior mitral leaflet, defined as 2 mm or greater displacement into the LA from the annular plane *(dashed line)* in systole in a long-axis view (see Video 24.3A). (B) The resulting eccentric jet of mitral regurgitation (see Video 24.3B).

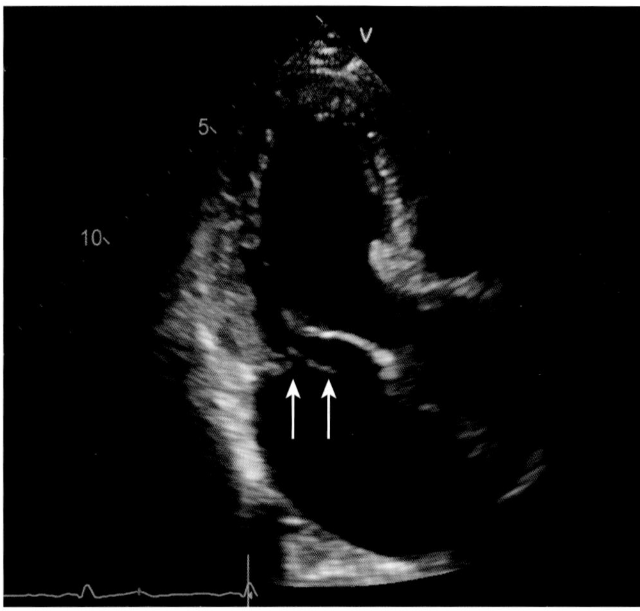

Fig. 24.4 Mitral flail leaflet. The enlarged apical long-axis view shows a flail mitral leaflet *(arrows)*, which occurs when there is chordal disruption (rupture or elongation) resulting in eversion of the leaflet.

MVP has a familial basis, with an autosomal dominant mode of inheritance and variable penetrance influenced by age and sex.[21–23]

Echocardiographically, MVP encompasses a spectrum from minimal prolapse to flail leaflet. Flail leaflet is an eversion of the leaflet segment with loss of its normal concave shape (Fig. 24.4); as a result, the tip of the leaflet is located in the LA. Flail is almost always associated with severe MR, which results from rupture of the primary chordae. Rarely, elongation of the chordae without frank rupture can also result in flail leaflet (Fig. 24.5).

The MVP spectrum includes two distinct clinical entities: fibroelastic deficiency (FD) and Barlow disease (BD).[24] FD is the more common of the two, and in this entity, the abnormalities of the connective tissue structure or function are localized to a single segmental prolapse or flail leaflet (see Fig. 24.5). It is typically diagnosed in patients in their sixth decade with a

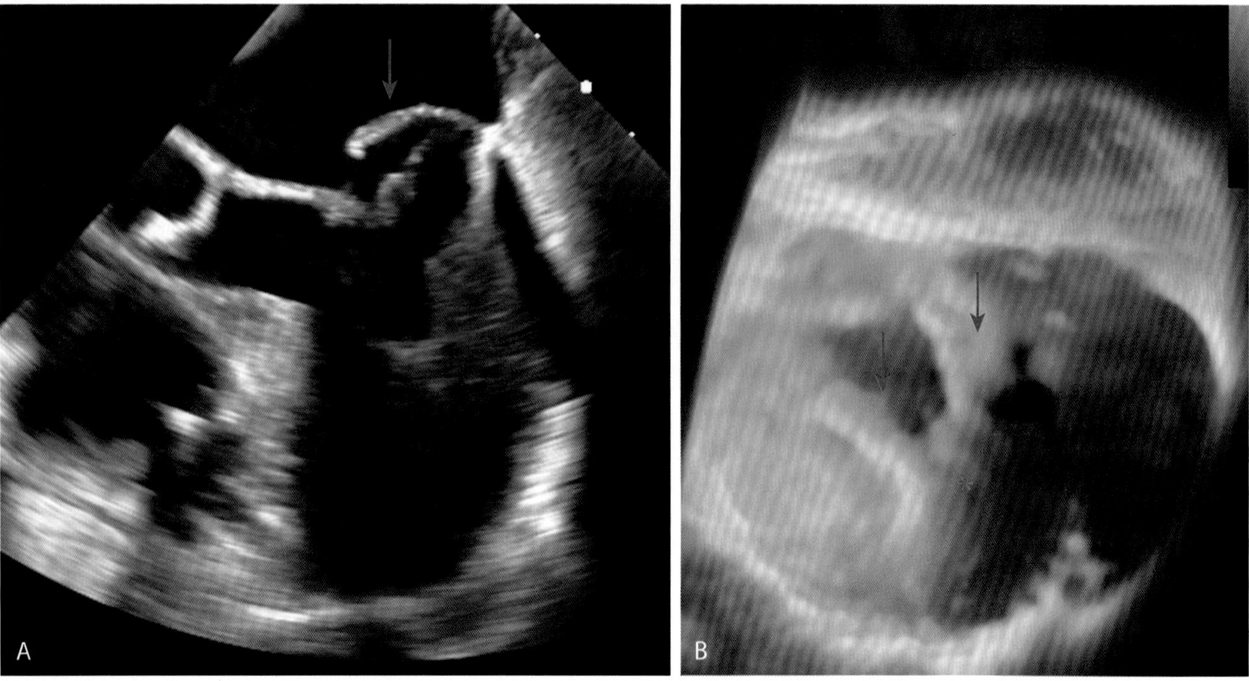

Fig. 24.5 P2 flail leaflet. (A) In the 2D TEE image, the *red arrow* indicates the prolapsed and flail P2 segment (see Video 24.5A). (B) 3D TEE image shows the prolapsed and flail P2 segment *(red asterisk)* with associated ruptured chords *(red arrows)* (see Video 24.5B).

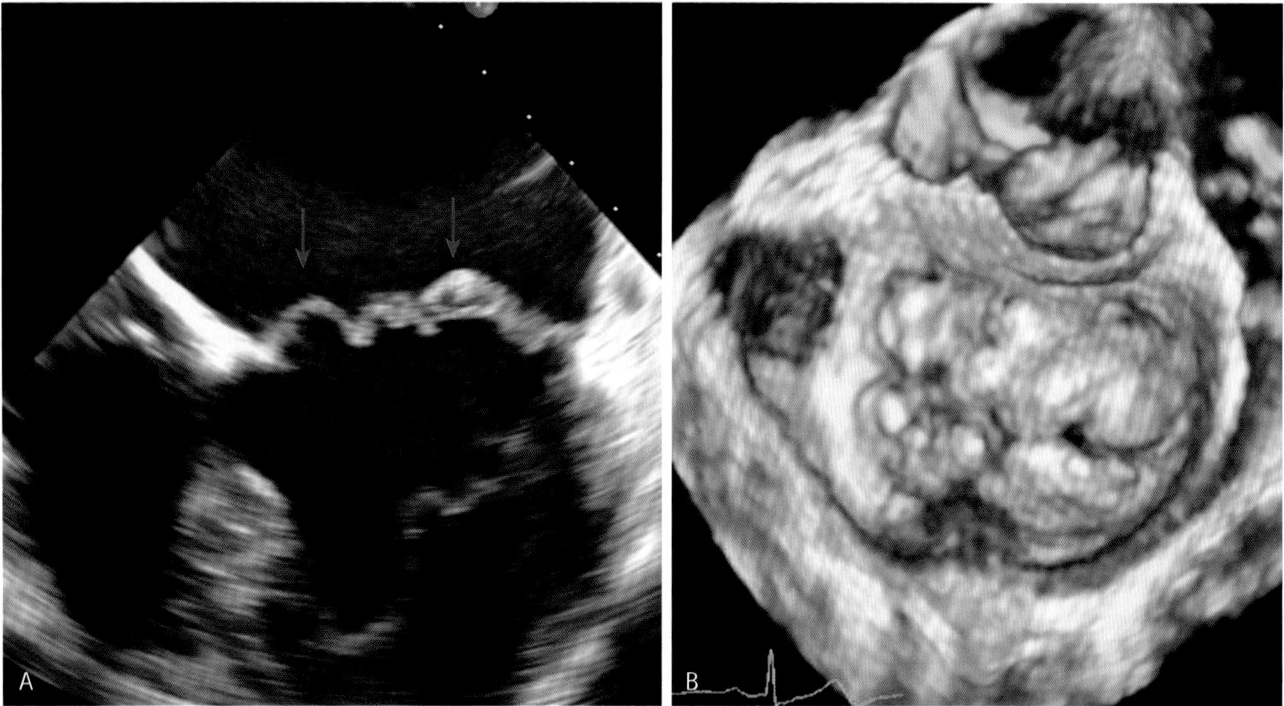

Fig. 24.6 Bileaflet prolapse. (A) 2D TEE image shows bileaflet prolapse with diffuse involvement of both leaflets *(arrows)* (see Video 24.6A). (B) 3D TEE of the mitral valve in an en face or surgeon's view indicates diffuse bileaflet prolapse (see Video 24.6B).

short, acute history of MR that is likely caused by rupture of a single mitral chord. Patients with FD typically have chordal rupture due to progressive weakening and elongation of the chordae tendineae, usually involving the middle segment of the posterior leaflet. The leaflets and the segments are often normal, with no change in height, size, or tissue properties.

BD is caused by an abnormal accumulation of mucopolysaccharides in the leaflets and chordae, which results in thick, bulky, redundant, billowing leaflets and elongated chordae, leading to prolapse of the leaflets (Fig. 24.6). This condition is typical in younger females and usually remains relatively stable until the fourth decade.[25] In BD, the leaflets have diffuse and complex lesions, with prolapse and myxomatous degeneration of many segments in one or both leaflets caused by excessive leaflet tissue, leaflet thickening, and/or rupture of many chordae tendineae. Patients with BD frequently have a dilated annulus and various degrees of annular and subvalvular apparatus calcification, which often affects the posterior face of the annulus and the anteromedial PM.

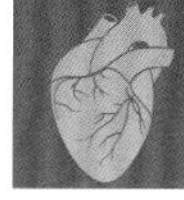

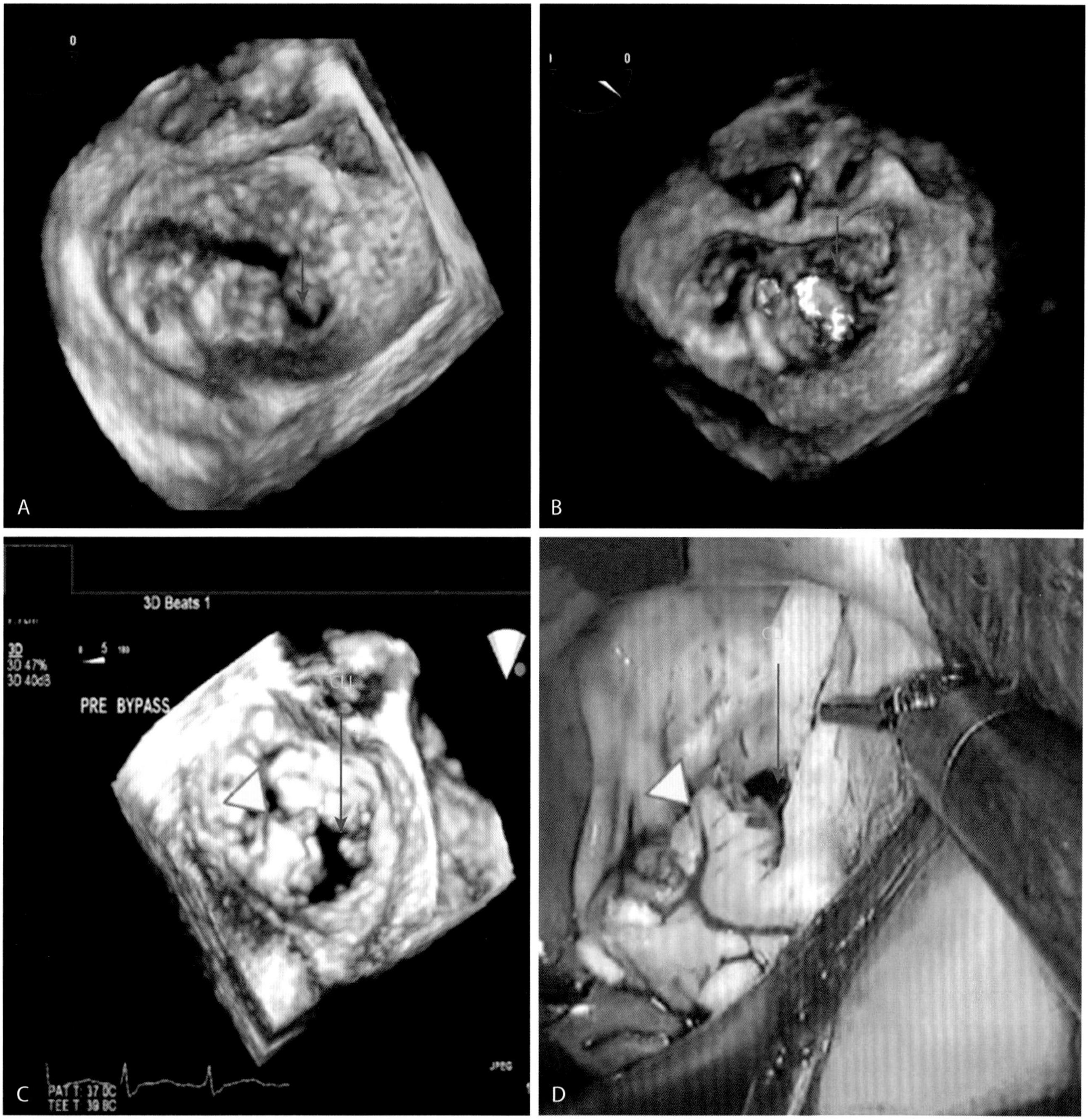

Fig, 24.7 Patient with myxomatous mitral valve disease and a cleft-like indentation. (A) 3D TEE view of the mitral valve from the LA position. There is a cleft-like indentation *(arrow)* between P2 and P3 (see Video 24.7A). (B) The MR jet originates through a gap *(arrow)* (see Video 24.7B). (C and D) A cleft was visualized with a direct mitral valve view during surgical inspection. The cleft-like indentation *(red arrow)* of the posterior mitral valve leaflet is seen near the prolapsing middle scallop *(yellow arrowhead)* of the posterior leaflet. The deep indentation between P2 and P3 is identified by 3D imaging and direct visualization of the mitral valve. (C and D from Mantovani F, Clavel MA, Vatury O, et al. Cleft-like indentations in myxomatous mitral valves by three-dimensional echocardiographic imaging. *Heart*. 2015;101[14]:1111–1117.)

Cleft-like indentations are abnormal exaggerations of the normal small indentations that occur between the lateral and middle segments and the medial and middle segments of the posterior leaflet (Fig. 24.7). They are associated with mitral flail leaflet and can be a source of significant MR. In a single-center study, cleft-like indentations occurred in up to one third of patients with degenerative MV disease who underwent surgical repair.

Cleft-like indentations are visualized with three-dimensional (3D) imaging, but they are difficult to diagnose directly by two-dimensional (2D) imaging. Clues to their presence include a central MR jet or MR jet originating at the base of the leaflet rather than at the coaptation line. 3D transesophageal echocardiography (TEE) can improve the diagnosis of cleft-like indentations (see Fig. 24.7A–C). Features of cleft-like indentations on 3D TEE are the presence of a gap located where normal indentations occur with demonstration of the MR jet originating through this gap. Corroboration of the location of the MR jet through the CLI with color Doppler is important as there can be "drop out" of the acoustic signal, which can be mistaken for a cleft-like indentation. A cleft-like indentation of the posterior mitral leaflet should be distinguished from a congenital cleft of the anterior

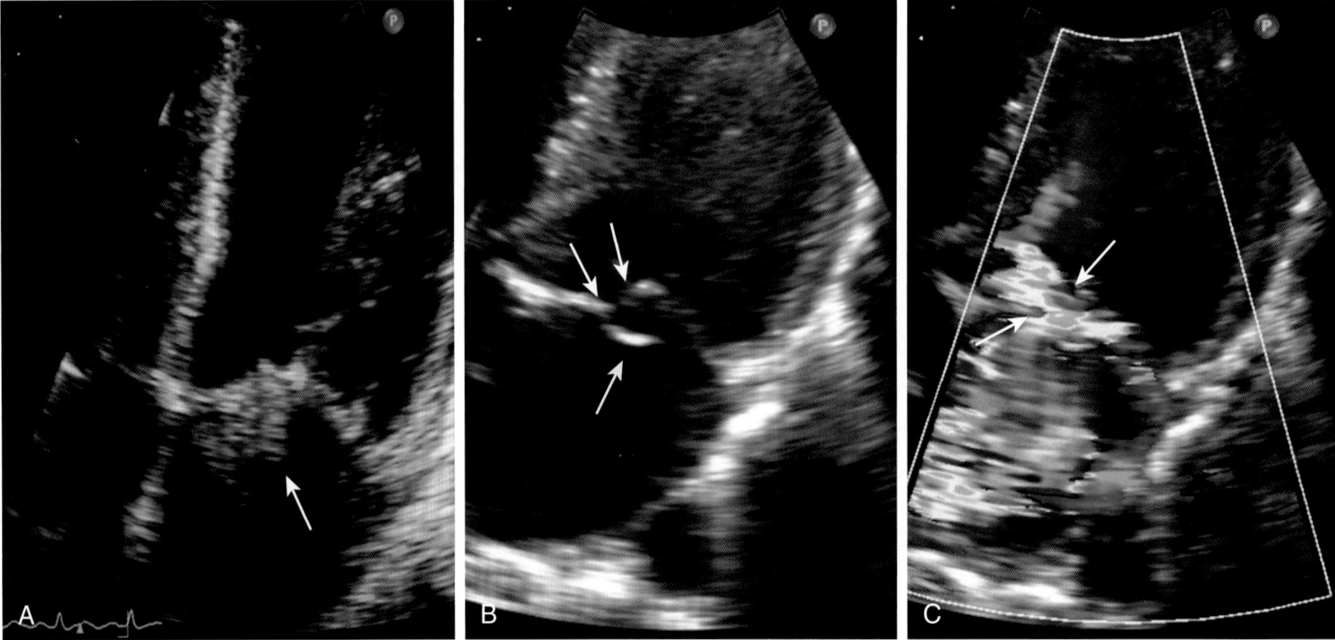

Fig. 24.8 Mitral valve endocarditis. (A) Large mitral valve vegetation *(arrow)*. (B) A mitral leaflet fenestration (dropout space between the *white arrows*) and vegetation *(yellow arrow)*. (C) Color jet of the mitral regurgitation originates through the fenestration *(arrows)*.

mitral leaflet and from an abnormal pathologic exaggeration of a normal posterior leaflet indentation.[26]

Other valvular causes of MR include endocarditis manifesting as valvulitis with leaflet thickening, vegetation with leaflet destruction, and leaflet perforation (Fig. 24.8). In developed countries, rheumatic MR is relatively uncommon, and MR usually occurs in conjunction with rheumatic mitral stenosis. Rheumatic MR remains a common cause of MR in developing countries.[27]

In rheumatic MR, leaflet thickening and scarring and/or restricted posterior leaflet motion prevent complete coaptation (Fig. 24.9). This pattern is also seen with MR induced by anorexigens or other drugs. A less common cause of MR is nonbacterial thrombotic endocarditis (NBTE), which encompasses a spectrum of sterile MV vegetations associated with malignancy and collagen vascular disease, radiation exposure, and drug-induced MV disease. Calcific mitral annular disease, in which annular calcification extends onto the leaflet bodies, often results in mixed MV disease with mitral stenosis and MR.

Congenital abnormalities of the MV account for a small percentage of adult patients with MR. The most common congenital abnormality in the pediatric population that causes MR is MVP.[28] Cleft of the anterior mitral leaflet is a congenital abnormality that occurs most commonly as part of an endocardial cushion defect complex and less commonly as an isolated cleft of the MV caused by failure of the common anterior leaflet to fuse.[29] Other congenital MV abnormalities include double-orifice MV and parachute MV, which can often result in mixed mitral disease with stenosis and regurgitation.[30]

Secondary Mitral Regurgitation

Secondary MR results from nonvalvular pathology, typically in the setting of chamber dilation due to coronary artery disease, non-ischemic cardiomyopathy, or congestive heart failure. It has also been referred to as *functional MR*, indicating MR that occurs in the absence of any structural abnormality of the MV leaflets or chordal apparatus. Secondary MR is the most common mechanism of MR because ischemic heart disease is more prevalent than primary mitral valvular disorders. Secondary MR is associated with an adverse prognosis.

Geometric changes and remodeling of the LV and/or LA occur, distorting the normal spatial relationship of the valve apparatus and tethering the leaflets. Leaflet morphology is initially normal in secondary MR, but structural changes in leaflet architecture can occur over time, worsening coaptation. The mechanism of secondary MR in most cases is dilation or ischemic distortion of the myocardium underlying the PMs. The resulting lateral displacement of the PMs leads to tethering of the mitral leaflets and incomplete leaflet coaptation. Closing forces from LV contraction work to counteract the tethering forces. In secondary MR, the tethering forces overcome the closing forces and prevent the leaflets from closing properly (Fig. 24.10).

The estimated prevalence of mild or greater MR after myocardial infarction (MI) is as much as 50%, and the MR is associated with a worse prognosis.[4,5,31] Patients who present with congestive heart failure due to systolic dysfunction have an approximately 50% incidence of moderate or greater MR.[32]

Ischemic MR and functional MR are types of secondary MR. Ischemic MR is related to MR that results from coronary artery disease. PM rupture is an uncommon but dramatic type of ischemic MR. Up to 1% of patients with MI can develop PM rupture.[33] Ischemic MR can also develop from acute myocardial ischemia. This type of MR is usually transient, resolving after the acute ischemia subsides.

A more common type of ischemic MR results from chronic LV remodeling after MI that causes geometric distortion of the MV apparatus.[34] Development of akinesis, scar, or aneurysm of the infarcted or ischemic myocardium underlying the PMs results in lateral displacement of the affected PMs, which leads to tethering of the mitral leaflets and incomplete closure (Fig. 24.11).

Echocardiographic features include apical tenting of the mitral leaflets, which are best imaged in the apical 4-chamber view in mid-systole. Often, the anterior mitral leaflet has a bend caused by tethering of the midportion of the anterior leaflet

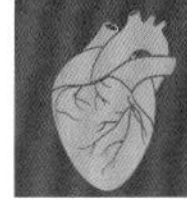

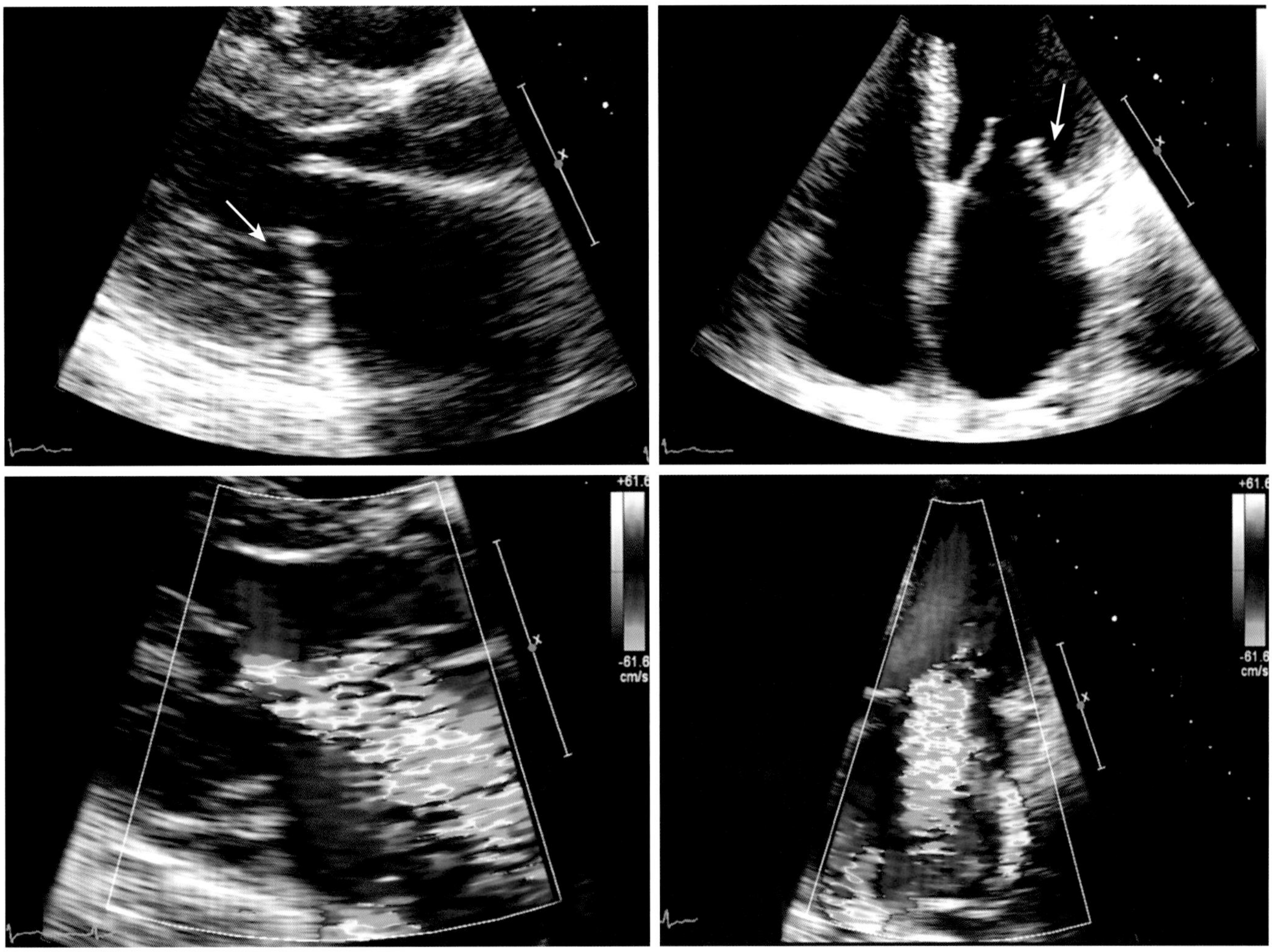

Fig. 24.9 Rheumatic mitral regurgitation. With rheumatic mitral valve disease, the posterior leaflet becomes rigid *(arrows in top panels)* (see Video 24.9A). Rigidity results in poor coaptation and mitral regurgitation (see Video 24.9B) *(bottom panels)*.

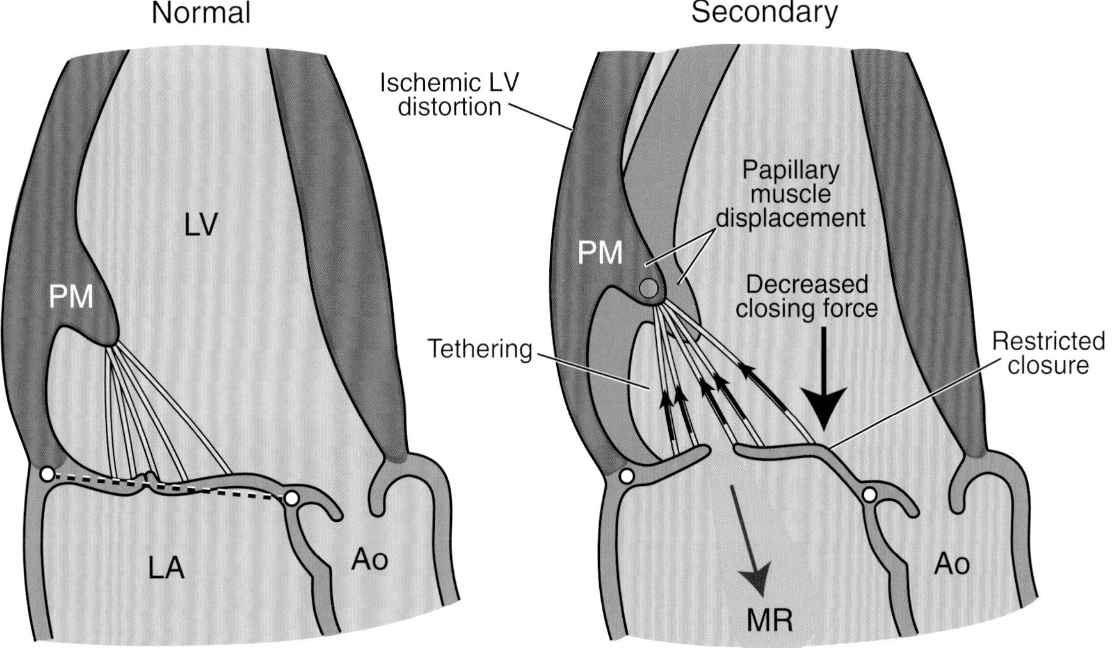

Fig. 24.10 Mechanisms of secondary mitral regurgitation. The normal forces that contribute to a competent mitral valve *(left panel)* and the changes that result in secondary mitral regurgitation *(MR) (right panel)*. The normal angle between the papillary muscle *(PM)* and the mitral annular plane *(dashed line in left panel)* determines the tethering effect of the mitral chords. Diseases that displace the PM or distort the LV shape (e.g., ischemic disease) adversely affect the normal tethering mechanism, resulting in decreased closing force and restricted closure *(right panel)*. Dilation of the mitral annulus may further contribute to inadequate leaflet closure.

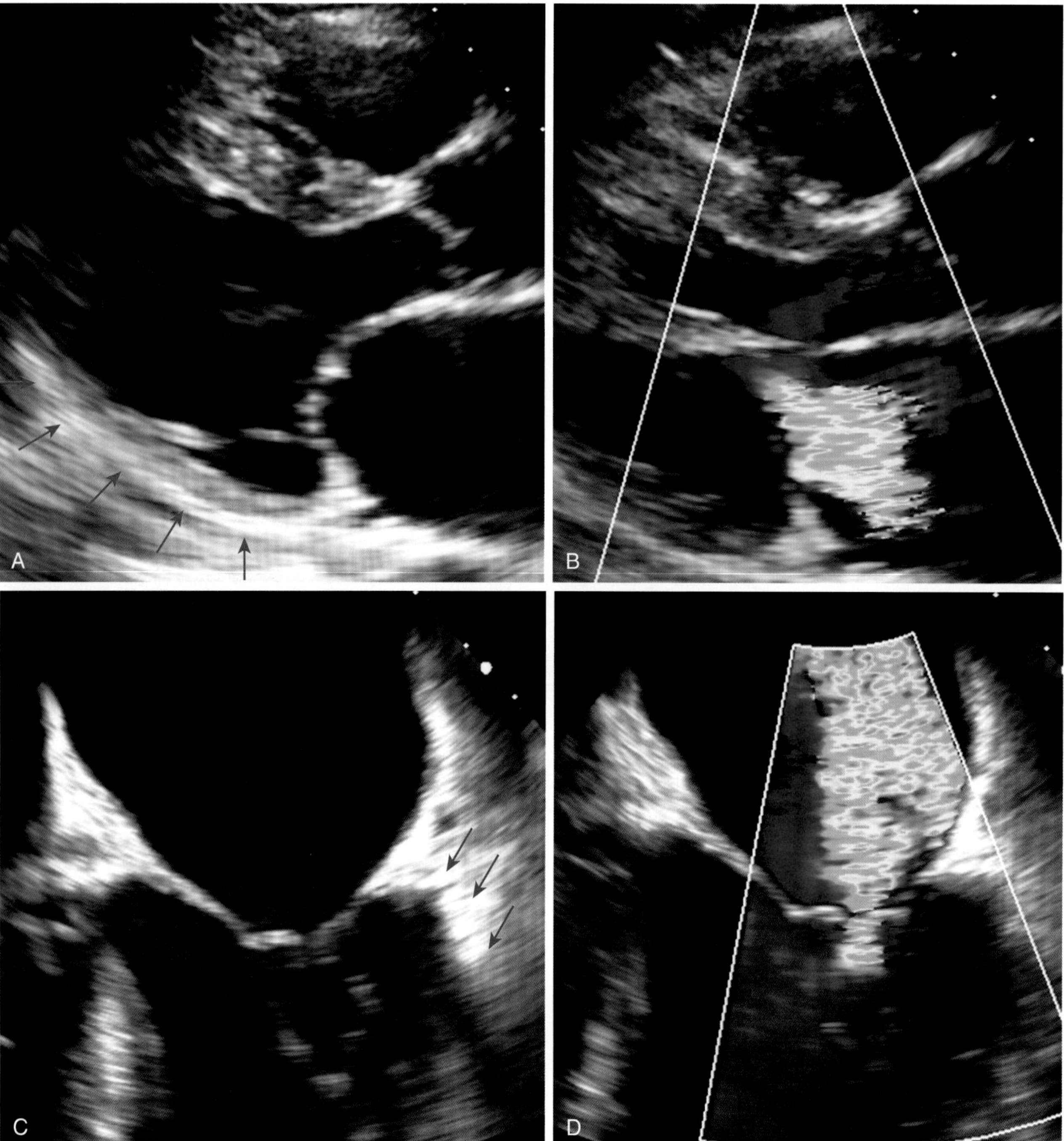

Fig. 24.11 **Inferior basal aneurysm.** Secondary mitral regurgitation (MR) from a basal aneurysm is a type of ischemic MR. (A) Aneurysm of the basal inferolateral wall caused by infarction *(red arrows)* results in distortion of the LV wall (see Video 24.11A). (B) The changes lead to mitral leaflet tethering and restricted closure with development of MR (see Video 24.11B). (C and D) TEE images of the same patient. *Red arrows* in C show the area of the aneurysm (see Videos 24.11C and 24.11D).

from a secondary (strut) chord (Fig. 24.12). Secondary MR can result in a centrally directed jet, which typically occurs in diffusely dilated LVs and results in symmetric tethering, or a posteriorly directed MR jet due to asymmetric tethering, in which the posterior mitral leaflet is more tethered than the anterior leaflet (see Fig. 24.12C and D).

Because the PMs are located along the inferior posterolateral walls, the incidence of ischemic MR is greater for inferior MIs than for anterior MIs.[35] However, inferior MR can develop with any large MI that results in significant LV dilation and remodeling and affects MV geometry.

An uncommon but often catastrophic form of secondary MR due to MI is PM rupture. MI can cause tissue necrosis of the PM head, which can result in a flail leaflet. Compared with the lateral PM with its dual coronary artery blood supply (i.e., left anterior descending and/or left circumflex artery), the medial PM is more susceptible to rupture due to its single coronary artery supply (i.e., right coronary artery).[36] This results in acute and severe MR into the LA, which has not had time to adapt to the sudden increase in LA pressure, leading to pulmonary edema. The absence of prior LV remodeling and dilation underlies the inability to maintain forward stroke volume and possible cardiogenic shock.

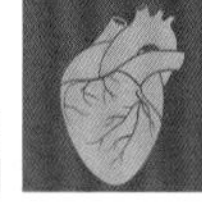

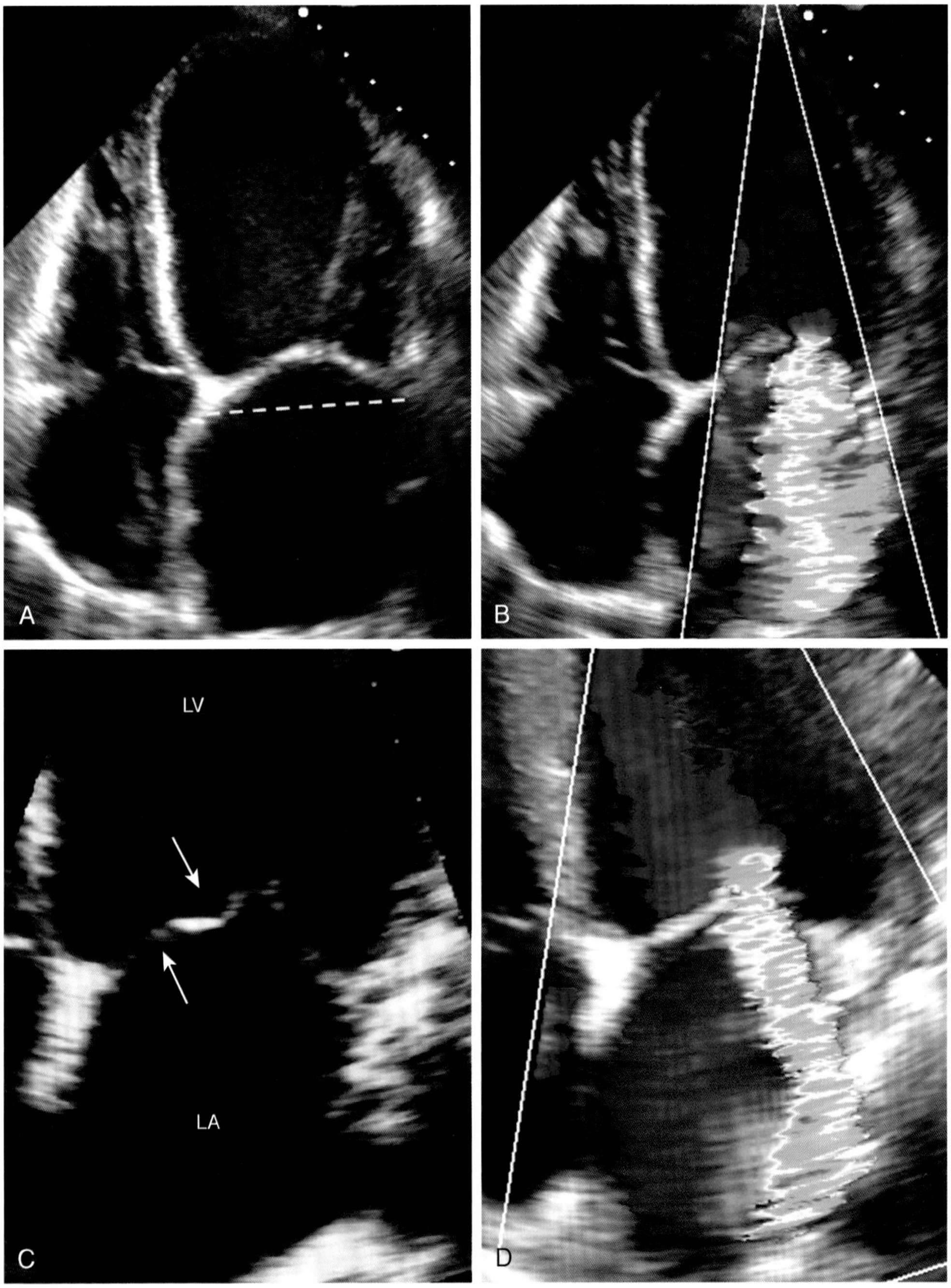

Fig. 24.12 Secondary mitral regurgitation with symmetric versus asymmetric tethering. (A) Echocardiographic features of ischemic mitral regurgitation include apical tenting of the mitral leaflets, which is best imaged in the apical 4-chamber view in mid-systole (see Video 24.12A). The mitral leaflets coapt apically instead of at the annular plane *(dashed line)*. (B) Symmetric MR (see Video 24.12B). (C and D) Secondary MR can result in a posteriorly directed MR jet due to asymmetric tethering. There can be loss of the normal convex shape, which can become concave or bend *(arrow)*, as occurs in the anterior mitral leaflet due to tethering from secondary strut chords (C). Symmetric and asymmetric tethering can be caused by ischemic MR (see Videos 24.12C and 24.12D). *MR,* Mitral regurgitation.

Atrial Functional Mitral Regurgitation

Atrial functional MR is a type of secondary MR that can occur in the setting of atrial fibrillation and a rate control strategy. It is often marked by heart failure with a preserved ejection fraction and a dilated mitral annulus.[37] Structurally, there is minimal to no apical tethering of the leaflets. Instead, there is incomplete closure of structurally normal MV leaflets in the setting of mitral annular dilation relative to leaflet length, annular flattening (i.e., loss of the nonplanar saddle shape), and insufficient atrial or annular dynamics to enhance leaflet coaptation (Fig. 24.13). Posterior leaflet tethering can sometimes be observed in atrial functional MR. It has been hypothesized that this is related to outward displacement of the posterior mitral annulus, leading to iatrogenic leaflet tethering.[38]

Restoration of sinus rhythm decreases the severity of MR.[39] The data suggest that compensatory mitral leaflet area adaptation may occur in patients with persistent atrial fibrillation.[40] The valve may grow, but adaptation may be limited by atrial fibrillation and a concomitant increase in annular area.

Management aims to optimize heart failure therapy because atrial functional MR is frequently associated with heart failure with a preserved ejection fraction and diastolic dysfunction.

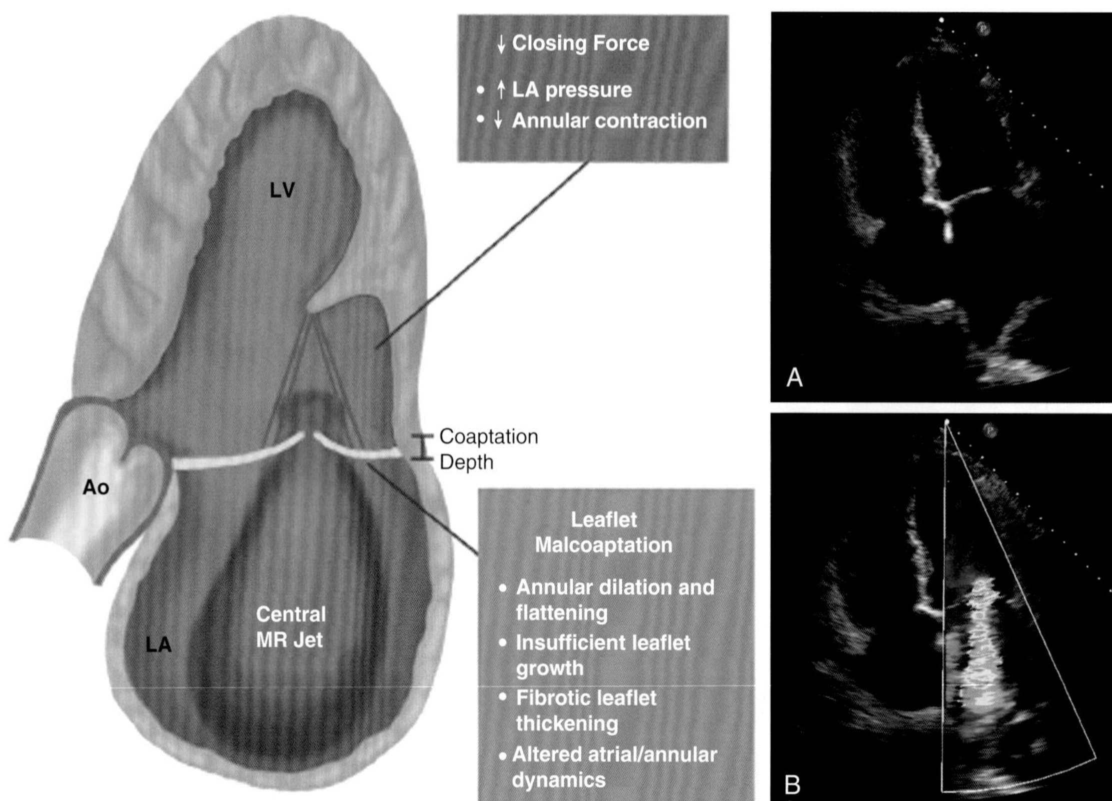

Fig. 24.13 Atrial functional mitral regurgitation. The schematic diagram *(left)* shows mechanisms of MR related to atrial function, such as in atrial fibrillation. (A and B) Atrial annular dilation leads to leaflet malcoaptation and mitral regurgitation (see Videos 24.13A and 24.13B). (From Deferm S, Bertrand PB, Verbrugge FH, et al. Atrial functional mitral regurgitation: JACC review topic of the week. *J Am Coll Cardiol*. 2019;73[19]:2465–2476.)

A rhythm control strategy for atrial fibrillation in patients with significant atrial functional MR may be preferred over rate control. MV intervention can be pursued if medical management and rhythm control strategies are not successful.

Carpentier Classification

An MR classification used predominantly by the cardiac surgery community is one proposed by Alain Carpentier, based on motion of the mitral leaflets[41] (Fig. 24.14). In type I, mitral leaflet motion is normal, and MR results from annular dilation. Type II MR results from excessive leaflet motion such as prolapse or flail leaflet. Type III is caused by restricted leaflet motion and is subdivided into types IIIa and IIIb MR. In type IIIa, leaflets have restricted motion in systole and diastole; rheumatic MR is an example. Ischemic MR and functional MR are grouped as type IIIb MR, for which there is restricted motion during systole. Atrial functional MR is type 1.

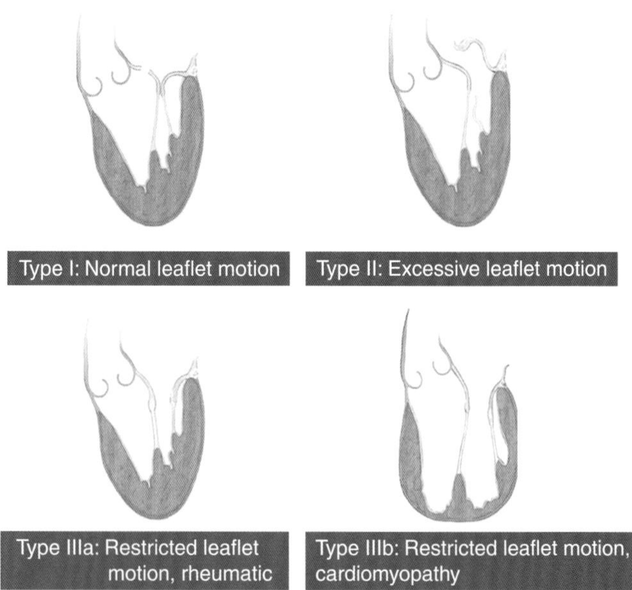

Fig. 24.14 Carpentier classification of mitral regurgitation. In type I, mitral leaflet motion is normal and mitral regurgitation (MR) results from annular dilation. Type II MR is caused by excessive leaflet motion, such as a prolapsed or flail leaflet. Type III is caused by restricted leaflet motion and is subdivided into types IIIa and IIIb. In type IIIa MR, leaflets have restricted motion in systole and diastole. Rheumatic MR falls into this category. Type IIIb refers to restriction of leaflet motion during systole due to secondary MR such as ischemic or other functional MR.

QUANTIFICATION OF MITRAL REGURGITATION

Echocardiography is valuable as a noninvasive tool for identifying the structure of the MV and for assessing cardiac hemodynamics. Advances in ultrasound technology, such as 3D echocardiography, have broadened the application of this imaging modality to include guidance for interventional approaches to management of this disease.

Color Doppler techniques are the most commonly used method for quantification of valvular regurgitation in clinical

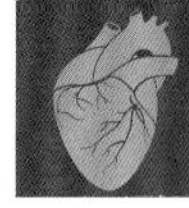

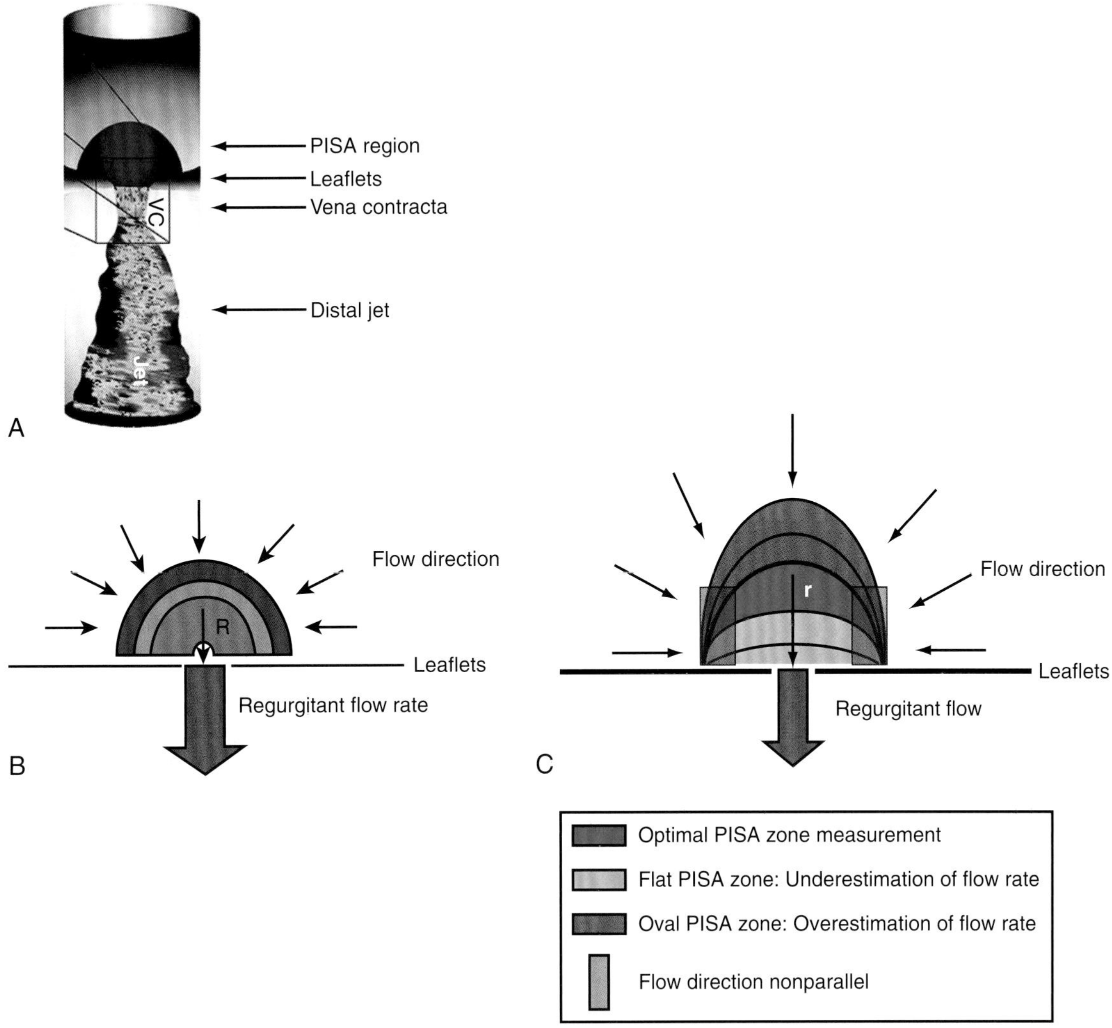

Fig. 24.15 Fluid dynamics of a regurgitant jet. (A) Components of a regurgitant jet: proximal isovelocity surface area *(PISA)* region (i.e., proximal flow convergence region), vena contracta *(VC)*, and distal jet. The effective regurgitant orifice area is defined by the narrowest regurgitant flow stream and typically occurs distal to the anatomic orifice, which is defined by the valve leaflets. (B) Fluid dynamic theory predicts that as flow approaches a circular, finite orifice, it forms a series of concentric, hemispherical shells with gradually decreasing area and increasing velocity. *Arrows* indicate the direction of flow as it approaches the PISA region. *R* is the radius of a hemispherical shell. According to the principle of conservation of mass, Flow through the regurgitant orifice = Flow through the isovelocity surface = $2\pi r^2$ × Aliasing velocity. (C) The PISA region is optimally measured where the region is hemispherical *(r)*. Flows farthest away from the orifice assume an elongated or oval contour, overestimating flows, whereas flows closest to the orifice assume a flat contour, underestimating flows. Measurement of the radius should be avoided along the sides of the PISA region, because flow here is perpendicular to the ultrasound beam, resulting in underestimation of the velocity component with drop-out of flow display at angles perpendicular to flow. (A from Roberts BJ, Grayburn PA. Color flow imaging of the vena contracta in mitral regurgitation: technical considerations. *J Am Soc Echocardiogr.* 2003;16[9]:1002–1006.)

practice and are based on assessment of the components of the regurgitant MR jet. The regurgitant jet has three components: the proximal flow convergence or proximal isovelocity surface area (PISA), the vena contracta. and the distal jet (Fig. 24.15). The proximal flow convergence region occurs proximal to the regurgitant orifice (i.e., proximal to the leaflets).

The vena contracta is the narrowest point at the level of or just distal to the leaflets. The vena contracta is the effective orifice area, not the anatomic orifice area. The latter is defined as an orifice at the level of the leaflets, whereas the effective orifice area is defined by the narrowest point of the flow steam, which typically occurs just distal to the leaflets as flow continues to converge for a short distance beyond the anatomic orifice (see Fig. 24.15A).[42]

The final component is the distal regurgitant jet. It is the regurgitant flow that has passed the leaflets and moved into the receiving chamber.

COLOR DOPPLER METHODS

Distal Jet Area Method

The *distal jet* is defined as the turbulent mosaic color flow within the LA during systole that emanates from the mitral leaflets.[43,44] The maximal jet area (JA) is traced in multiple views, and an average of the areas is calculated. The distal MR JA is normalized relative to the LA area (LAA),[45,46] and the MR JA and LAA are measured in the same systolic frame to obtain a JA/LAA ratio (see Summary table).[46,47] MR JA/LAA ratios of less than 20% correspond to mild MR, whereas ratios greater than 40% correspond to severe MR (Table 24.2).[48] Because the MR flow is entering a constrained chamber (i.e., the LA), the behavior of the MR jet is influenced by factors such as physical containment by the LA wall, entrainment of a blood pool in the LA into the MR flow, and the influence of flow from the pulmonary veins.

Accuracy is affected when the JA/LAA ratio method assumes a relatively linear relationship between JA size and the LAA.

TABLE 24.2 **Grading of Chronic Mitral Regurgitation With Echocardiography.**

Parameter	Mitral Regurgitation Severity			
	Mild	*Moderate*		*Severe*
Structural				
MV morphology	None or mild leaflet abnormality	Moderate leaflet abnormality or moderate tenting		Severe valve lesions (primary: flail leaflet, ruptured papillary muscle, severe retraction, large perforation; secondary: severe tenting, poor leaflet coaptation)
LV and LA size (mostly for primary MR)	Usually normal	Normal or mildly dilated		Dilated
Qualitative Doppler				
Color flow jet area	Small, central, narrow, often brief	Varies		Large central jet (>50% of LA) or eccentric wall-impinging jet of variable size
Flow convergence	Not visible, transient or small (usually <0.3 cm at Nyquist limit of 20–30 cm/s)	Intermediate in size and duration		Large throughout systole (usually ≥1 cm at Nyquist limit of 20–30 cm/s)
CW Doppler	Faint, partial, parabolic	Dense but partial or parabolic		Holosystolic, dense, can be triangular
Semiquantitative				
VCW (cm)	<0.3	Intermediate		≥0.7 (>0.8 for biplane)
Pulmonary vein flow	Systolic dominance (may be blunted in LV dysfunction or AF)	Normal or systolic blunting		Minimal to no systolic flow/systolic flow reversal
Mitral inflow	A-wave dominant	Varies		E-wave dominant (>1.2 m/s)
Quantitative				
EROA, 2D PISA (cm^2)	<0.20	0.20–0.29	0.30–0.39	≥0.40 (may be lower in secondary MR with elliptical ROA)
RVol (mL)	<30	30–44	45–59	≥60 (may be lower in low flow conditions)
RF (%)	<30	30–39	40–49	≥50

AF, Atrial fibrillation; *EROA*, effective regurgitant orifice area; *MR*, mitral regurgitation; *MV*, mitral valve; *PISA*, proximal isovelocity surface area; *RF*, regurgitant fraction; *ROA*, regurgitant orifice area; *RVol*, regurgitant volume; *VCW*, vena contracta width.

From Zoghbi WA, Adams D, Bonow RO, et al. Recommendations for noninvasive evaluation of native valvular regurgitation: a report from the American Society of Echocardiography developed in collaboration with the Society for Cardiovascular Magnetic Resonance. *J Am Soc Echocardiogr*. 2017;30(4):303–371.

However, this is not always the case, and the actual MR volume is sometimes greater than suggested by the JA/LAA ratio, as in cases of chronic MR in which there has been extensive LA remodeling.

Eccentric MR jets are subject to impingement from the LA wall, which can result in a decreased size of the mitral regurgitant jet. Wall jets also are subject to the Coanda effect, which is the tendency of flow to follow along a wall. This effect influences the direction and ultimately the display of the MR jet.[45,49] Eccentric jets in which the MR jet courses out of the plane of the ultrasound beam can be missed or underestimated. Due to limitations of eccentric jets, the JA method is probably best applied to centrally directed jets.[45,50]

Machine settings can also influence the distal MR jet. Too much gain can overestimate the size of the jet. In contrast, too little gain underestimates the jet size. Low Nyquist settings can also overestimate the true MR jet because lower-velocity blood flows in the LA are merged with the true MR jet. Nyquist limits should be at least 50 cm/s for color flow mapping of MR jets. The distal JA is influenced by hemodynamic conditions such as blood pressure and volume status.[51–53]

The distal JA method is a relatively simple and commonly applied technique for the qualitative assessment of MR. However, several technical and physiologic factors can limit its reliability in grading MR. Despite these limitations, distal jets can be used as a useful screen, especially for centrally directed jets, to exclude moderate or greater MR because small distal jets (<20% JA/LAA ratio) with a narrow vena contracta and/or without visible PISA can be considered to be mild.

Vena Contracta Width Method

The vena contracta width (VCW) is the narrowest portion of the MR jet, and it provides a simple linear measurement of the proximal MR jet.[47,54–56] The vena contracta is measured in a parasternal long-axis view, if it is available; if not, it can be measured in the apical long-axis view because reference ranges for VCW were established along the anterior-posterior dimension (see Summary table).

The VCW has a narrow range, so small differences in measurement can have a large impact on the MR value. Care must be taken to optimize the vena contracta region for measurement by magnifying and by adjusting depth and sector settings for optimal color Doppler resolution. It can be difficult to define the narrowest portion of the MR jet because in some cases, the neck of the proximal MR jet is not easily seen or is obscured by the leaflets. The vena contracta is thought to be less influenced by physiologic loading conditions, and it may therefore be more reproducible than JA methods.[47]

VCW measurements of less than 3 mm correspond to mild MR; values of 0.3 to 0.69 mm correspond to moderate MR, and values of 0.7 mm or greater correspond to severe MR (see Table 24.2). The broad range of values for which the vena contracta is considered to be in the moderate range limits the VCW as a quantitative measure. Despite this, VCW remains a clinically useful semiquantitative and simple measure of MR.

Proximal Isovelocity Surface Area Method

The PISA method is based on the fluid dynamic principle that as flow approaches a circular finite orifice, it forms concentric hemispherical shells with gradually decreasing surface area and increasing velocity (see Fig. 24.15B and C).[57] This principle can be applied to mitral regurgitant flow, for which the PISA region is the hemispherical shell that forms proximal to the mitral leaflets on the LV side and the finite orifice is the effective regurgitant orifice area (EROA) at the level of the leaflets.[52,57,58]

By the conservation of mass principle, the flow rate of each of the isovelocity shells equals the flow rate at the regurgitant orifice. Assuming a hemispherical shape for the isovelocity shells,

$$\text{Flow rate} = \text{Surface area of a hemisphere} = 2\pi r^2 \times \text{Aliasing velocity}$$

where r is the radius of the hemispherical shell. The flow rate of the hemispherical shell equals the MR rate at the orifice by the conservation of mass principle.

After the flow rate is calculated, the EROA and the MR regurgitant volume (RVol) can be derived using the following formula:

$$\text{EROA} = \text{MR flow rate/Peak MR velocity determined by CW Doppler}$$

where *CW* is continuous wave (see Fig. 24.15). Because the EROA is calculated from an instantaneous peak flow rate, EROA obtained using the PISA method represents a maximal instantaneous regurgitation orifice area.

To calculate RVol, the EROA is divided by the velocity–time integral (VTI) of the MR jet:

$$\text{RVol} = \text{EROA} \times \text{VTI}_{\text{MR}}$$

The regurgitant fraction is calculated as RVol divided by the stroke volume. Stroke volume can be calculated with the following formula:

$$\text{(End-diastolic volume} - \text{End systolic volume)/End-diastolic volume}$$

To optimize measurement of the radius (r), baseline shifting of the Nyquist limit toward the direction of flow is recommended. In general, a range of 30 to 45 cm/s in Nyquist limit provides an optimal balance of maximal radius resolution and integrity of the PISA shape. Very low Nyquist limits overestimate the size of the PISA region, in which case there will be elongation in the axial dimension; conversely, high Nyquist limits minimize the PISA region, making accurate measurements difficult.[59–61] This is an important consideration when deciding at what time point during systole to measure the PISA radius. For example, with functional MR, there is typically a bimodal pattern, with peak MR flow rates in early and late systole and the least MR flow rate during mid-systole.

In patients with MVP, peak MR flow occurs in middle to late systole. For rheumatic MR, the MR flow rate is constant during systole. The PISA radius measurement should be avoided very early or very late in systole because these are times when the mitral leaflets are just closing or about to open and the flow rate may not be at equilibrium. In general, the PISA radius measurement should occur at the same time as the peak MR velocity (as measured by CW Doppler).

Accuracy and reproducibility of the PISA method depends on careful attention to technique of acquisition and measurements. The PISA region should be magnified with the sector and depth optimized for color Doppler resolution and with the PISA region and mitral leaflets encompassing most of the sector. Measurement of the PISA should be aligned parallel to flow direction because this optimizes Doppler resolution.

Geometric Factors Influencing the PISA Method

In theory, the PISA method provides an accurate quantitative measure of MR. However, there are technical and practical aspects of the PISA method that should be considered. The PISA region is influenced by the surrounding geometry of the orifice.[57] This principle is important when examining eccentrically directed PISA regions, such as occur with a flail mitral leaflet. This typically results in overestimation of the PISA radius due to distortion of the PISA region caused by constraint from the LA wall and a falsely increased radius.[58]

To overcome this problem, an angle correction factor can be applied to the surface area calculation.[57] Angle correction is performed by multiplying the surface area calculation by $\alpha/180$, where α is the angle between the mitral leaflet and the end of the PISA region confined by the LA wall.[62] Angle correction for eccentric PISA regions adds complexity to the MR flow rate calculation, creating additional opportunities for measurement error. Because of LV wall confinement, it is not always possible to accurately measure the α angle. The practical difficulties in applying angle correction have limited its clinical use.

Technical Factors

The operator should measure the radius of the PISA region at Nyquist velocities, which are reliably displayed by color Doppler flow mapping. A major limitation of the PISA method has been that the calculated results vary widely when the radius is measured at different distances from the orifice because of different 3D shapes of the isovelocity surface. The contour of the PISA region changes depending on where the flow rate is measured relative to the regurgitant orifice.[57,60] The contour flattens close to the orifice, whereas the contour assumes an elongated or more oval shape farthest from the orifice (see Fig. 24.15C). These variations in PISA contour result in systematic overestimation of flow rates farthest from the orifice and underestimation closest to the orifice.

Measurement of the radius should be avoided along the sides of the PISA region because the flow there is perpendicular to the ultrasound beam, resulting in underestimation of the velocity component and frank dropout of flow display at angles perpendicular to flow. Dropout of color display where the flow is perpendicular gives the PISA region a rounded appearance at its base. Fig. 24.15B and C show an ideal zone for PISA radius measurement as well as zones in which to avoid measurement.

A hemispherical assumption is used for surface area calculation, but the regurgitant orifice may not be circular, particularly in view of the elliptical coaptation zone of the mitral leaflets. This may be especially important in secondary MR, in which there is symmetric tethering of the mitral leaflets that results in an elliptical regurgitant orifice. A hemispherical assumption of the PISA region has underestimated the regurgitant flow rate, especially with rectangular regurgitant orifices.[63–65]

The hemi-elliptical surface area formula is complex, requiring measurement of three radii that are orthogonally oriented and integrated for surface area calculation. This adds considerable complexity to the PISA method and has limited clinical application. The PISA region appears to be less influenced by changes in machine settings such as gain, wall filter, frame rate, or packet size compared with distal JA methods.[66]

EROA in Primary and Secondary Mitral Regurgitation

US and European guidelines in 2012 and 2014[67,68] proposed different cutoff values for EROA and RVol for severity of MR depending on its cause. For primary MR, the cutoff values for EROA and RVol for severe MR remained ≥ 0.4 cm^2 and ≥ 60 mL, respectively, in 2014,[67] whereas for secondary MR, cutoff values of EROA ≥ 0.2 cm^2 and RVol > 30 mL were suggested for severe MR. The differential cutoff values were predicated on worse prognostic data for mild or greater secondary MR compared with primary MR.[5,67–69] However, limitations of applying a lower EROA standard for secondary MR became apparent. EROA and RVol values depend on LV volumes, which can account for lower EROA values in secondary MR.

Compared with primary MR, adverse outcomes are associated with a smaller calculated EROA in secondary MR, possibly because a smaller RVol may still represent a large regurgitant fraction in the setting of compromised LV systolic function (and low total stroke volume) added to the effects of elevated filling pressures. A hemispherical assumption inherently underestimates the EROA and RVol, and the underestimation in EROA is likely to be magnified to a greater degree in secondary MR than in primary MR due to the more elliptical shape of the PISA region in secondary MR.

Given the limitations and on the basis of the criteria used for determination of severe MR in randomized controlled trials of surgical interventions for secondary MR,[70–72] the recommended definition of severe secondary MR has become the same as for primary MR (EROA ≥ 0.4 cm^2 and RVol ≥ 60 mL), with the understanding that the EROA cutoff of greater than 0.2 cm^2 is more sensitive and greater than 0.4 cm^2 is more specific for severe MR (see Table 24.2). Criteria for severe MR are listed in Fig. 24.16.

3D-Guided Vena Contracta Area

3D echocardiography allows direct planimetry of the vena contracta area (VCA), which is a measure of the regurgitant orifice area (ROA). This technique does not rely on geometric assumptions to calculate the ROA. To perform planimetry of the VCA, a full-volume 3D color Doppler acquisition is obtained. Sector size is narrowed to maximize frame rate. Using multiplanar reconstruction software available on commercial 3D analysis systems, two orthogonal image planes parallel to the regurgitant jet direction are cropped across the regurgitant jet. A third cropping plane oriented perpendicular to the jet direction can be aligned until the cross-sectional area at the level of the vena contracta is visualized. The frame with the largest VCA in systole is measured by direct planimetry of the color Doppler flow signal[73] (see Summary table).

Validation studies have demonstrated that 3D-guided direct planimetry of the VCA correlates well with the ROA derived by the volumetric Doppler approach.[74,75] A limitation is the relatively low 3D spatial resolution, particularly in the nonaxial planes. Optimization of spatial and color resolution is therefore important. 3D color-guided planimetry of the VCA is best applied for moderate or greater MR because of the limitations of 3D spatial resolution. This determination of EROA can provide a complementary or alternative method to 2D imaging.

PULSED-WAVE AND CW DOPPLER METHODS

Pulmonary Venous Inflow Pattern: Systolic Flow Reversal

The pulmonary venous inflow pattern provides confirmatory data for assessing MR severity. Systolic flow reversal in the pulmonary vein inflow pattern, as detected by transthoracic imaging, had a sensitivity of 61% and a specificity of 92% for severe MR as measured by the PISA method.[76] Studies using TEE have demonstrated sensitivities of 82% to 90% and specificity

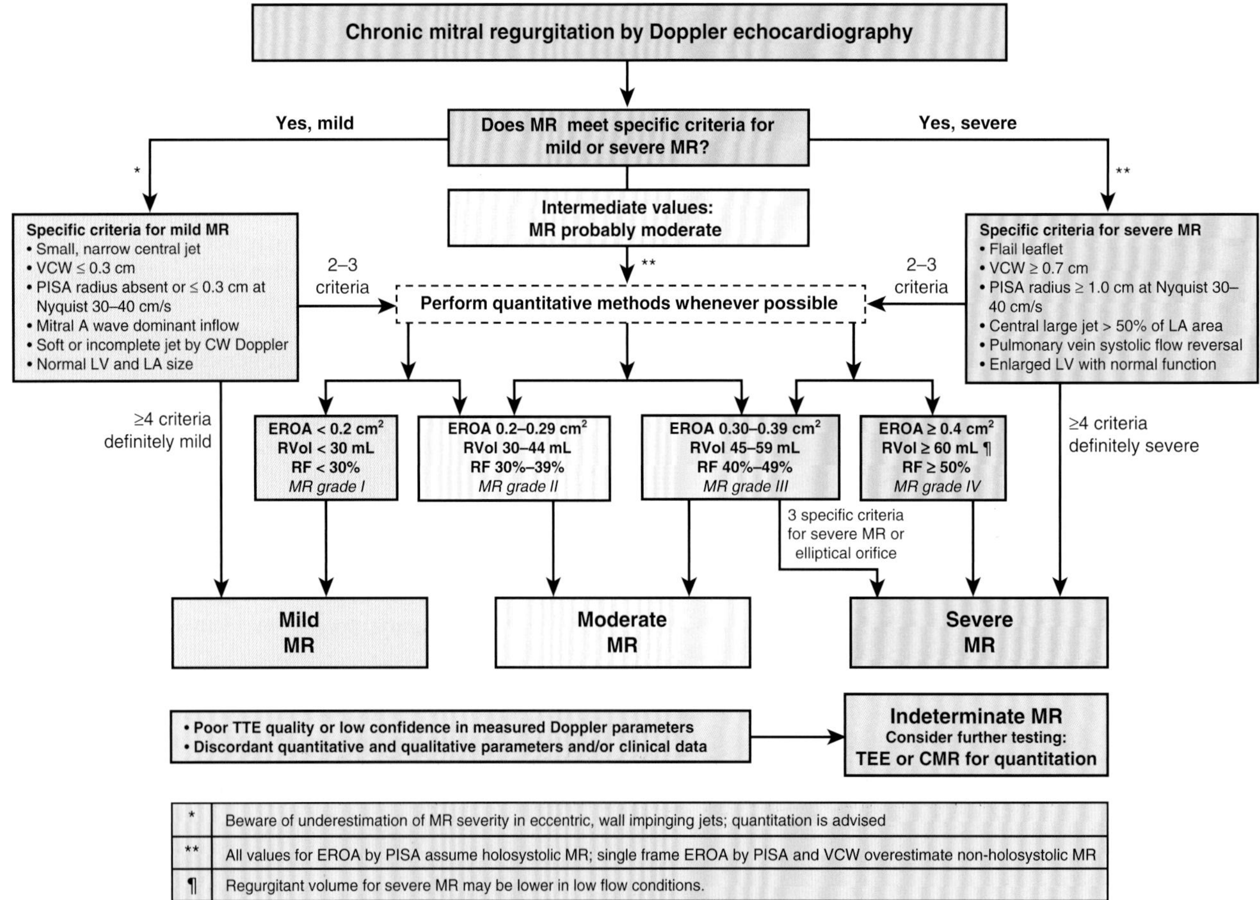

Fig 24.16 Algorithm for the integration of multiple parameters of mitral regurgitation *(MR)* severity. *CMR*, Cardiac magnetic resonance imaging; *CW*, continuous-wave Doppler; *EROA*, effective regurgitant orifice area; *PISA*, proximal isovelocity surface area; *RF*, regurgitant flow rate; *RVol*, regurgitant volume; *VCW*, vena contracta width. (From Zoghbi WA, Adams D, Bonow RO, et al. Recommendations for noninvasive evaluation of native valvular regurgitation: a report from the American Society of Echocardiography developed in collaboration with the Society for Cardiovascular Magnetic Resonance. *J Am Soc Echocardiogr.* 2017;30[4]:303–371.)

of 100% for systolic flow reversal as indicative of severe MR.[77,78] An elevated RV systolic pressure also suggests clinically important MR due to the effect of RVol on the pulmonary vasculature.

Peak E-Wave Velocity

Severe MR results in an increased volume load in the LA, which often translates to an elevated peak E-wave velocity. However, LA volume load is common in other disorders, and an elevated peak E-wave velocity is a nonspecific sign for severe MR. The E-wave velocity is also influenced by LA compliance, and when there is a significant amount of MR volume but a very compliant LA, the E-wave velocity may not be elevated. Nevertheless, a peak E-wave velocity of more than 1.5 m/s is consistent with severe MR.[48]

CW Doppler Pattern

CW Doppler imaging of the MR jet provides an indirect assessment of MR severity. The more intense the CW signal of the MR, the greater the number of red blood cell reflectors and therefore RVol. The more complete the MR CW signal, the greater the likelihood that the MR is significant.

Studies have demonstrated that the signal intensity of the MR CW tracing correlates with MR severity compared against an angiographic standard.[79,80] Rapid equilibration of the LV–LA gradient occurring with severe MR can result in a V-shaped pattern compared with the normal parabolic CW MR jet. CW intensity and pattern should be assessed as supportive evidence for MR severity because signal intensity and shape can vary greatly with machine settings and with alignment of the CW beam along the regurgitant jet.

Volumetric Methods Using Pulsed-Wave Doppler

Volumetric methods use PW Doppler techniques to calculate flow rates and stroke volumes. The stroke volume across a valve annulus is equal to the VTI across the valve annulus multiplied by the cross-sectional area of the annulus. The RVol can be calculated from the flow across cardiac valves.[81,82] Although many combinations can be employed, this is a common way to derive RVol (Fig. 24.17):

$$\text{MR volume} = \text{Mitral inflow} - \text{Aortic outflow}$$

Mitral inflow volume is calculated as follows: VTI of mitral inflow × Cross-sectional area of the mitral annulus. The VTI of mitral inflow should be measured at the level of the mitral annular plane because that is where the cross-sectional area is measured. The cross-sectional area of the mitral annulus is assumed to be circular and is calculated as πr^2, where r is the diameter measured in the in apical 4-chamber view divided by 2.

Anatomically, the mitral annulus has a D shape and is shaped more like an ellipse rather than a circle. However, using a circular assumption for the annulus is reasonable in patients who have developed at least moderate MR because of the annular dilation that occurs with development of moderate or greater MR. Alternatively, the mitral annulus can be calculated as an ellipse in which the area is πab, with a and b being the diameters measured in the apical 4- and 2-chamber views divided by 2.

Aortic outflow is the VTI of aortic outflow multiplied by the cross-sectional area of the left ventricular outflow tract (LVOT). This method assumes that there is no aortic regurgitation; otherwise, pulmonary artery outflow can be used, assuming no significant pulmonary regurgitation. The mitral RVol can also be obtained by calculating LV stroke volume and subtracting aortic outflow volume, assuming there is no aortic insufficiency.

Although volumetric methods are straightforward in concept, they are subject to increased variation related to the number of measurements necessary to calculate cardiac flows from PW Doppler imaging and annular areas. Because the radius is squared in the area term, small errors in measurement are amplified, and accurate resolution of the annulus is important in minimizing measurement errors.

VALVE MORPHOLOGY AND LEFT-SIDED CHAMBER SIZE

Valve morphology provides important clues in the assessment of MR. Apical tenting of the mitral leaflets is associated with functional MR that develops in the setting of LV cardiomyopathy.[17,83,84] Flail leaflet, valvular vegetations, and PM rupture are associated with severe MR. Increased left-sided chamber size is associated with significant MR due to a volume effect in increasing chamber size, and LV dilation is a specific criterion for severe primary MR. However, in secondary MR, left-sided chamber enlargement can develop with intrinsic cardiomyopathy, and it is not a reliable criterion for severe secondary MR.

HOLOSYSTOLIC VERSUS NON-HOLOSYSTOLIC JETS

Non-holosystolic jets are almost never associated with severe MR. The severity of MR is based on total RVol during systole. However, it is important to consider that the quantitative and semiquantitative color Doppler parameters are calculated using an instantaneous value during systole, and it is assumed that this is constant throughout systole.[59] For MR jets that are not holosystolic, this assumption is not applicable, and total RVol in non-holosystolic jets is rarely in the severe range.[85]

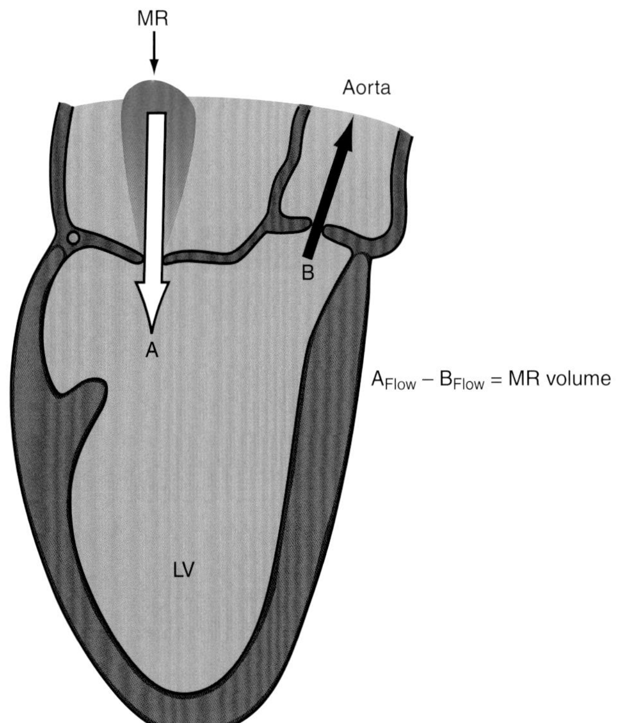

Fig 24.17 Volumetric flow method for mitral regurgitation. Schematic demonstrates the volumetric method for calculating mitral regurgitant volume (RVol). $A_{Flow} - B_{Flow}$ = MR volume, provided there is no significant aortic regurgitation. *A*, Mitral inflow; *B*, aortic outflow.

Non-holosystolic jets are frequently detected in cases of MVP without flail leaflet, in which the MR occurs during middle to late systole. Holosystolic MR almost always is present in severe MR. When flail leaflet develops in MVP due to ruptured marginal chordae, the MR becomes holosystolic, and flail leaflet is therefore typically associated with severe MR. Color M-mode of holosystolic MR is compared with late systolic MR in the Summary table.

DYNAMIC NATURE OF MITRAL REGURGITATION

Hemodynamic and Physiologic Factors

The degree of MR is influenced by hemodynamic factors, including volume status, afterload (blood pressure), and use of inotropic agents in intraoperative and intensive care unit settings. Increased volume or afterload worsens MR.[86] When symptoms are related to exertion, stress echocardiography can be performed to determine whether significant MR develops.[87] Inotropic agents such as dobutamine decrease MR due to afterload-reducing effect and increased inotropy, which decreases cavity size and may mask MR in normal physiologic conditions. Acute myocardial ischemia may worsen MR because of PM function or the effect on global LV function, reducing closing forces on the MV. Ideally, MR grade should be assessed in an optimized loading state and without inotropic agents.

MR also varies temporally across systole, depending on the cause and on hemodynamic and physiologic conditions. For MVP, the peak MR flow occurs during middle to late systole. For secondary MR, the temporal pattern is bimodal, with peaks in early and late systole and a decrease in mid-systole.[88]

Grading Mitral Regurgitation With an Integrative Method

Because a single reference standard for MR grading does not exist and because each method has inherent limitations (see Summary table), the guidelines of the American Society of Echocardiography (ASE), European Society of Cardiology (ESC, 2012), American College of Cardiology/American Heart Association (ACC/AHA, 2014), and American Society of Echocardiography (ASE, 2017) have recommended an integrated approach to grading MR. Multiple parameters, including morphologic features, Doppler techniques, and hemodynamic data, are considered when grading MR, rather than depending on a single measurement (Fig. 24.18). When data are discordant or echocardiographic imaging is poor, 3D Doppler echocardiography–guided direct planimetry of the VCA and/or cardiac MR should be considered.

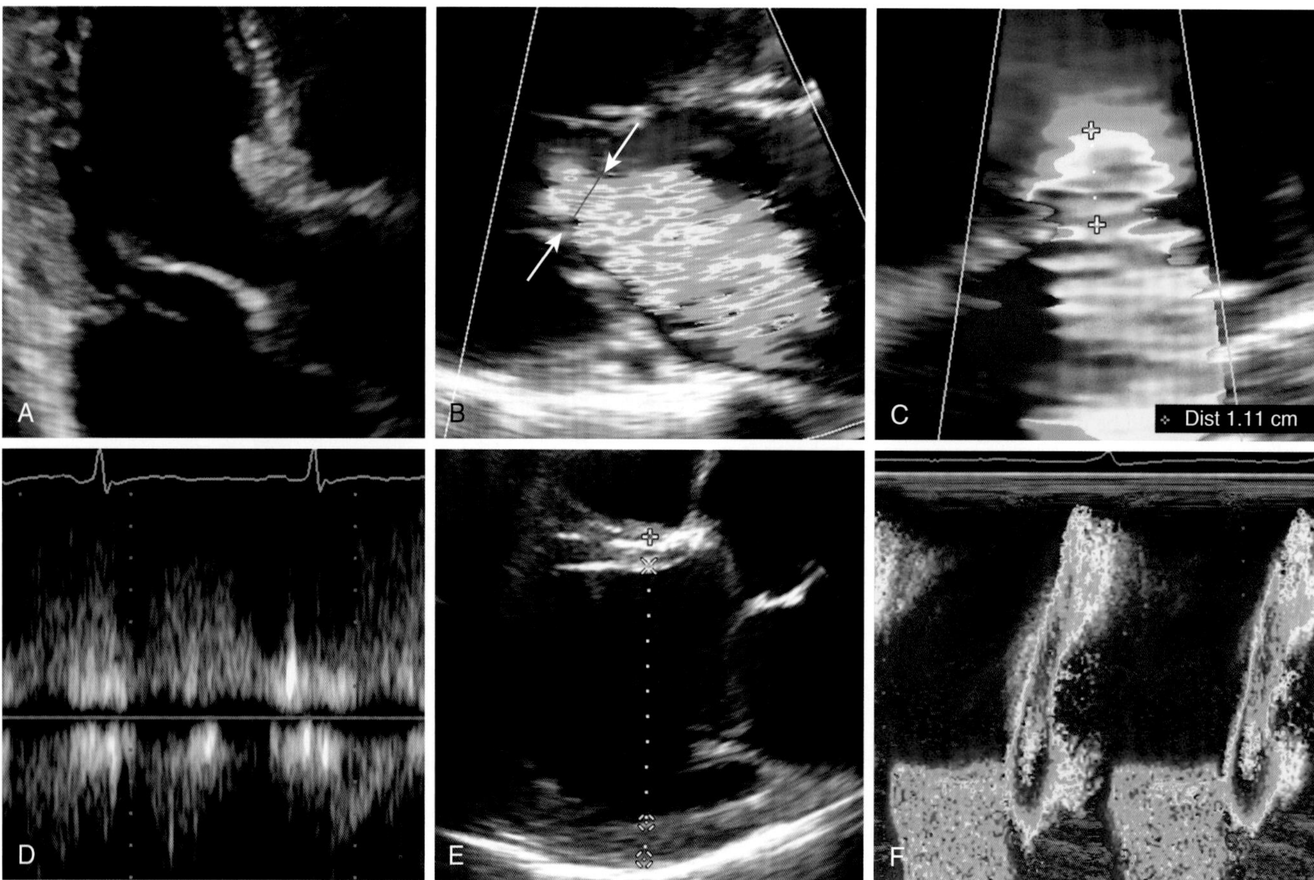

Fig 24.18 Characteristics of severe mitral regurgitation. (A) Flail leaflet. (B) Vena contracta width ≥ 0.7 cm; central large jet > 50% of LA area. (C) PISA radius ≥ 1.0 cm at Nyquist 30–40 cm/s. (D) Pulmonary vein systolic flow reversal. (E) Enlarged LV with normal function; four or more criteria define severe disease. (F) Holosystolic mitral regurgitation seen in color M-mode. *PISA,* Proximal isovelocity surface area. (From Zoghbi WA, Adams D, Bonow RO, et al. Recommendations for noninvasive evaluation of native valvular regurgitation: a report from the American Society of Echocardiography developed in collaboration with the Society for Cardiovascular Magnetic Resonance. *J Am Soc Echocardiogr.* 2017;30[4]:303–371.)

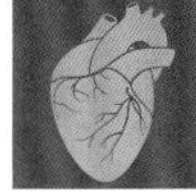

SURGICAL INTERVENTION FOR MITRAL REGURGITATION

PATHOPHYSIOLOGY

MR results in a significant fraction of the LV ejection volume returning to the LA. To maintain the same forward stroke volume, the LV compensates by increasing the dilation and the ejection fraction, resulting in hyperdynamic LV function. Eventually, the LV becomes unable to compensate for the increased volume workload, and the left ventricular ejection faction (LVEF) begins to decrease while the LV end-systolic volume increases. The development of MR can be acute, such as in acute MV endocarditis, or it can be chronic, such as frequently occurs with MVP.

Acute MR can occur in the setting of chronic MR, such as with the development of flail leaflet from a ruptured chord in a patient with chronic MR due to MVP. The presentation and pathophysiology of acute and chronic MR are different. In acute MR, the LA cannot accommodate the sudden volume load because it has not had time to adapt. This results in acute pulmonary edema, elevated right-sided pressures, and severe dyspnea. The LV function becomes hyperdynamic to compensate but may not be able to dilate adequately to maintain forward stroke volume, resulting in decreased cardiac output and hypotension.

Treatment for acute MR focuses on acute unloading with afterload agents, if blood pressure allows, or insertion of an intraaortic balloon pump. These are often temporary measures because surgical correction is ultimately needed.

In chronic MR, the LV has time to remodel. The additional volume load on the LV leads to eccentric hypertrophy as part of the remodeling process. Histologic examination of the myocardium reveals myocyte hypertrophy, predominantly through the addition of sarcomeres in series, resulting in elongation of the myofibers. This remodeling process causes LV dilation and augmented contraction, resulting in hyperdynamic LV function that provides a larger total ejection volume to maintain forward stroke volume.

The LA similarly remodels by dilating to increase compliance and accommodate the MR volume. This lessens the transmitted pressure from backward flow of blood directly into the pulmonary circulation and results in less elevation of right-sided pressures and dyspnea.

Eventually, the LV is unable to compensate; myocyte mass is gradually replaced by interstitial fibrosis as the remodeling process progresses.[2,89,90] LV volumes increase further but cannot fully compensate, resulting in a decrease in LVEF, predominantly by a relatively greater increase in end-systolic volume. The forward stroke volume falls, and without intervention, heart failure occurs.

Patients with chronic severe MR can be asymptomatic for a long period. Studies have reported an average of 5 to 10 years from the time of diagnosis to the appearance of signs and symptoms or other indications for surgical intervention.[89,90] Treatment with afterload-unloading agents for chronic severe primary MR has not shown benefit.[91] Because the pathophysiology of MR does not include increased afterload, use of these agents cannot address the mechanistic derangement and may mask the development of LV dysfunction by unloading the ventricle.

TIMING OF INTERVENTION

Guidelines have characterized four stages of MR for determining prognosis and guiding therapy. Patients classified as stage A do not have MR but are at risk for MR. Those with stage B disease have progressive MR. Patients with stage C disease have asymptomatic severe MR, and those with stage D disease have symptomatic severe MR.[67,92]

Therapy primarily targets stages C and D. It is critical to determine the mechanism of MR because that dictates the therapeutic course, especially because treatments for primary versus secondary MR are different.

Therapy for Primary Mitral Regurgitation

Consensus guidelines supporting class I indications for surgical intervention with MV repair or replacement for primary severe MR are summarized in Tables 24.3 and 24.4. Symptomatic

TABLE 24.3 AHA/ACC 2020 Recommendations for Intervention for Chronic Primary Mitral Regurgitation.

COR	*LOE*	*Recommendations*
1	B-NR	1. In symptomatic patients with severe primary MR (stage D), mitral valve intervention is recommended irrespective of LV systolic function.
1	B-NR	2. In asymptomatic patients with severe primary MR and LV systolic dysfunction (LVEF ≤60%, LVESD ≥40 mm) (stage C2), mitral valve surgery is recommended.
1	B-NR	3. In patients with severe primary MR for whom surgery is indicated, mitral valve repair is recommended in preference to mitral valve replacement when the anatomic cause of MR is degenerative disease, if a successful and durable repair is possible.
2a	B-NR	4. In asymptomatic patients with severe primary MR and normal LV systolic function (LVEF ≥60% and LVESD ≤40 mm) (stage C1), mitral valve repair is reasonable when the likelihood of a successful and durable repair without residual MR is >95% with an expected mortality rate of <1%, when it can be performed at a primary or comprehensive valve center.
2b	C-LD	5. In asymptomatic patients with severe primary MR and normal LV systolic function (LVEF >60% and LVESD <40 mm) (stage C1) but with a progressive increase in LV size or decrease in EF on ≥3 serial imaging studies, mitral valve surgery may be considered irrespective of the probability of a successful and durable repair.
2a	B-NR	6. In severely symptomatic patients (NYHA class III or IV) with primary severe MR and high or prohibitive surgical risk, TEER is reasonable if mitral valve anatomy is favorable for the repair procedure and patient life expectancy is at least 1 year.
2b	B-NR	7. In symptomatic patients with severe primary MR attributable to rheumatic valve disease, mitral valve repair may be considered at a comprehensive valve center by an experienced team when surgical treatment is indicated, if a durable and successful repair is likely.
3: Harm	B-NR	8. In patients with severe primary MR where leaflet pathology is limited to less than one-half the posterior leaflet, mitral valve replacement should not be performed unless mitral valve repair has been attempted at a primary or comprehensive valve center and was unsuccessful.

COR, Class of recommendation; *LOE*, level of evidence; *LVEF*, left ventricular ejection fraction; *LVESD*, left ventricular end-systolic diameter; *MR*, mitral regurgitation; *NYHA*, New York Heart Association; *TEER*, transcatheter edge-to-edge repair.

From Otto CM, Nishimura RA, Bonow RO, et al. 2020 ACC/AHA guideline for the management of patients with valvular heart disease: a report of the American College of Cardiology/American Heart Association Joint Committee on Clinical Practice Guidelines. *Circulation*. 2021; ;77(4):450–500. https://doi.org/10.1016/j.jacc.2020.11.035.

TABLE 24.4 ESC 2017 Guidelines for Chronic Primary Mitral Regurgitation Intervention.

Recommendation	*COR*	*LOE*
Mitral valve repair should be the preferred technique when the results are expected to be durable.	I	C
Surgery is indicated in symptomatic patients with LVEF > 30%.	I	B
Surgery is indicated in asymptomatic patients with LV dysfunction (LVESD ≥ 45 mm[a] and/or LVEF ≤ 60%).	I	B
Surgery should be considered in asymptomatic patients with preserved LV function (LVESD < 45 mm and LVEF > 60%) and atrial fibrillation due to mitral regurgitation or pulmonary hypertension[b] (systolic pulmonary pressure at rest > 50 mmHg).	IIa	B
Surgery should be considered in asymptomatic patients with preserved LVEF (>60%) and LVESD 40–44 mm[a] when a durable repair is likely, surgical risk is low, the repair is performed in a heart valve center, and at least one of the following findings exists: • Flail leaflet • Significant LA dilation (volume index ≥ 60 mL/m² BSA) in sinus rhythm.	IIa	C
Mitral valve repair should be considered in symptomatic patients with severe LV dysfunction (LVEF < 30% and/or LVESD > 55 mm) refractory to medical therapy when the likelihood of successful repair is high and comorbidity is low.	IIa	C
Mitral valve replacement may be considered in symptomatic patients with severe LV dysfunction (LVEF < 30% and/or LVESD > 55 mm) refractory to medical therapy when the likelihood of successful repair is low and comorbidity is low.	IIb	C
Percutaneous edge-to-edge procedure may be considered in patients with symptomatic severe primary mitral regurgitation who fulfill the echocardiographic criteria of eligibility and are judged inoperable or at high surgical risk by the heart team, avoiding futility.	IIb	C

[a]Cutoffs refer to average-size adults and may require adaptations in patients with unusually small or large stature.
[b]If an elevated SPAP is the only indication for surgery, the value should be confirmed by invasive measurement.
BSA, Body surface area; *COR*, class of recommendation; *LOE*, level of evidence; *LVEF*, left ventricular ejection fraction; *LVESD*, left ventricular end-systolic diameter; *SPAP*, systolic pulmonary artery pressure.
From Baumgartner H, Falk V, Bax JJ, et al. 2017. ESC/EACTS guidelines for the management of valvular heart disease. *Eur Heart J*. 2017;38(36):2739–2791.

patients with an LVEF greater than 30% or asymptomatic patients with LV dilation or an LVEF of less than 60% should undergo surgical intervention.

Asymptomatic patients with severe MR with preserved LV function are an important but challenging group to treat. Early mitral repair in asymptomatic patients with chronic severe MR and preserved LV function is a class IIa indication in selected cases for which there is a high likelihood of MV repair (>95%), and the operative mortality rate is low (≤1%). Tables 24.3 and 24.4 summarize the class II and III indications for MV surgery in cases of severe primary MR. MV repair is associated with improved survival of patients compared with MV replacement. If MV repair is not possible, MV replacement should be performed with chordal preservation.

One difficulty is determining whether patients are truly asymptomatic because decreased functional capacity may be attributed to deconditioning and age or may manifest as nonspecific symptoms. Some patients subtly reduce their activity in response and may not be aware or recognize a reduction in functional capacity. In these cases, exercise testing echocardiography can provide objective evidence of functional capacity, and if performed with echocardiography, it can also provide hemodynamic data such as right-sided pressure changes and valvular and ventricular function in response to exercise.[87]

Therapy for Secondary Mitral Regurgitation

Optimal therapy for chronic secondary MR remains an area of active investigation. Class I indications for medical management include heart failure optimization and cardiac resynchronization therapy.[67] Until recently, studies have not demonstrated a survival advantage for patients who underwent MV repair or replacement for moderate or greater ischemic MR at the time of bypass graft surgery.[70,72,93] This may reflect the fact that it is unclear whether secondary MR is a bystander of the cardiomyopathic process or the MR may directly impact comorbidity and mortality rates due to its detrimental effect on LV remodeling and function by increasing volume load.

Reflecting the lack of a consensus for benefit, there are no class I recommendations for performing MV surgery in patients with severe secondary MR. Surgical MV repair or replacement for ischemic MR is most often performed at the time of coronary artery bypass grafting (CABG) in patients with moderate or severe ischemic MR. Valve guidelines[92] and ESC valvular guidelines[94] suggest MV surgery for severe secondary MR at the time of CABG or aortic valve replacement as a class IIa recommendation (Tables 24.5 and 24.6). In trials by the National Institutes of Health (NIH), National Heart, Lung, and Blood Institute (NHLBI), and Cardiothoracic Surgical Network (CTSN), patients with severe ischemic MR were randomized to MV repair with restrictive ring annuloplasty or MV replacement. Results showed no difference in the primary end point (LV end-systolic volume [LVESV] index) between the two groups at 1 year, suggesting that MV repair and replacement for severe ischemic MR were comparable.[70,72]

For patients with moderate ischemic MR, performing MV repair is a class IIb recommendation. Two randomized trials examined the benefit of MV repair for moderate ischemic MR at the time of CABG surgery. The RIME trial enrolled 75 patients who were randomized to CABG alone or CABG plus MV repair. The trial showed improved functional status with an improvement in myocardial oxygen consumption ($M\dot{V}O_2$) for the CABG plus MV repair group.[95] The CTSN conducted a much larger trial that enrolled patients with moderate ischemic MR. The randomized groups were similar, but LVESV index was used as a primary end point. The CTSN trial showed no difference in the LVESV index between the CABG alone and CABG plus MV repair groups.[72]

The advent of transcatheter MV repair has increased options for patients with secondary MR. The French Percutaneous Repair with the MitraClip Device for Severe Functional/Secondary Mitral Regurgitation (Mitra-FR) trial was a study of patients with chronic heart failure and reduced LVEF. The study used European guidelines for severe secondary MR (detected as an EROA > 20 mm²) and randomized patients with severe MR to percutaneous MV repair or medical therapy. At 12 months,

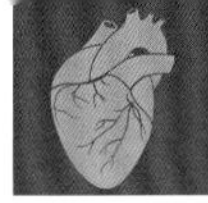

TABLE 24.5 AHA/ACC 2020 Recommendations for Intervention for Secondary Mitral Regurgitation.

COR	*LOE*	*Recommendation*
2a	B-R	1. In patients with chronic severe secondary MR related to LV systolic dysfunction (LVEF <50%) who have persistent symptoms (NYHA class II, III, or IV) while on optimal GDMT for HF (stage D), TEER is reasonable in patients with appropriate anatomy as defined on TEE and with LVEF between 20% and 50%, LVESD ≤70 mm, and pulmonary artery systolic pressure ≤70 mmHg.
2a	B-NR	2. In patients with severe secondary MR (stages C and D), mitral valve surgery is reasonable when CABG is undertaken for the treatment of myocardial ischemia.
2b	B-NR	3. In patients with chronic severe secondary MR from atrial annular dilation with preserved LV systolic function (LVEF ≥50%) who have severe persistent symptoms (NYHA class III or IV) despite therapy for HF and therapy for associated AF or other comorbidities (stage D), mitral valve surgery may be considered.
2b	B-NR	4. In patients with chronic severe secondary MR related to LV systolic dysfunction (LVEF <50%) who have persistent severe symptoms (NYHA class III or IV) while on optimal GDMT for HF (stage D), mitral valve surgery may be considered.
2b	B-R	5. In patients with CAD and chronic severe secondary MR related to LV systolic dysfunction (LVEF <50%) (stage D) who are undergoing mitral valve surgery because of severe symptoms (NYHA class III or IV) that persist despite GDMT for HF, chordal-sparing mitral valve replacement may be reasonable to choose over downsized annuloplasty repair.

CAD, Coronary artery disease; *COR*, class of recommendation; *GDMT*, guideline-directed medical therapy; *HF*, heart failure; *LOE*, level of evidence; *LVEF*, left ventricular ejection fraction; *LVESD*, left ventricular end-systolic diameter; *MR*, mitral regurgitation; *NYHA*, New York Heart Association; *TEER*, transcatheter edge-to-edge repair.
From Otto CM, Nishimura RA, Bonow RO, et al. 2020 ACC/AHA guideline for the management of patients with valvular heart disease: a report of the American College of Cardiology/American Heart Association Joint Committee on Clinical Practice Guidelines. *Circulation*. 2021; ;77(4):450–500. doi: 10.1016/j.jacc.2020.11.035.

TABLE 24.6 European Guidelines for Secondary Mitral Regurgitation Intervention.

Recommendation	*COR*	*LOE*
Surgery is indicated in patients with severe secondary mitral regurgitation undergoing CABG and with an LVEF > 30%.	I	C
Surgery should be considered in symptomatic patients with severe secondary mitral regurgitation, an LVEF < 30% but with an option for revascularization and evidence of myocardial viability.	IIa	C
When revascularization is not indicated, surgery may be considered in patients with severe secondary mitral regurgitation and LVEF > 30% who remain symptomatic despite optimal medical management (including CRT if indicated) and have a low surgical risk.	IIb	C
When revascularization is not indicated and surgical risk is not low, a percutaneous edge-to-edge procedure may be considered in patients with severe secondary mitral regurgitation and an LVEF > 30% who remain symptomatic despite optimal medical management (including CRT if indicated) and who have a suitable valve morphology by echocardiography, avoiding futility.	IIb	C
For patients with severe secondary mitral regurgitation and an LVEF < 30% who remain symptomatic despite optimal medical management (including CRT if indicated) and who have no option for revascularization, the heart team may consider a percutaneous edge-to-edge procedure or valve surgery after careful evaluation for a ventricular assist device or heart transplant according to individual patient characteristics.	IIb	C

CABG, Coronary artery bypass grafting; *COR*, class of recommendation; *CRT*, cardiac resynchronization therapy; *LOE*, level of evidence; *LVEF*, left ventricular ejection fraction.
From Baumgartner H, Falk V, Bax JJ, et al. 2017. ESC/EACTS guidelines for the management of valvular heart disease. *Eur Heart J*. 2017;38(36):2739–2791.

the rate of death or unplanned hospitalization for heart failure was not significantly different for patients who underwent percutaneous MV repair in addition to receiving medical therapy and those who received medical therapy alone.[96]

In contrast, in the Cardiovascular Outcomes Assessment of the MitraClip Percutaneous Therapy for Heart Failure Patients with Functional Mitral Regurgitation (COAPT) study followed patients from 78 US and Canadian sites who had heart failure and moderate to severe or severe secondary MR and who remained symptomatic despite the use of maximal doses of guideline-directed medical therapy. Patients were assigned to transcatheter MV repair plus medical therapy or medical therapy alone. Among patients with heart failure and moderate to severe or severe secondary MR who remained symptomatic despite the use of maximal doses of guideline-directed medical therapy, transcatheter MV repair resulted in a lower rate of hospitalization for heart failure and a lower all-cause mortality rate during 24 months of follow-up compared with medical therapy alone.[97]

The concept of proportionate and disproportionate MR was offered by Grayburn et al.[98] as a framework for reconciling the results of the Mitra-FR and COAPT trials. The investigators suggested that the Mitra-FR trial might have had more patients with proportionate MR (i.e., MR that is proportional to the degree of LV dilation and can respond to drugs and devices that reduce LV end-diastolic volume [LVEDV]) compared with COAPT, which might have had more patients with disproportionate MR (i.e., MR with disproportionate LVEDV) and therefore could benefit from correction of a structural MV defect with further reduction in LVEDV.[98]

Analyses of the discordant data highlighted the importance of optimizing medical therapy before consideration of transcatheter MV repair (i.e., COAPT). Many patients in the COAPT were found to have insufficient MR after medical optimization, and the need for strict application of echocardiographic and clinical criteria to identify persistence of symptomatic and severe MR after optimization of medical therapy may help identify a subset of patients with severe secondary MR who can benefit from transcatheter MV repair.[99] Therapeutic options for secondary MR are likely to expand, and perhaps there will be increasing options for more targeted approaches to individual pathologic anatomy.

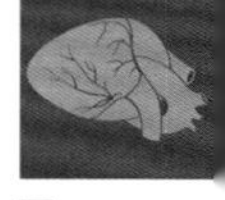

SUMMARY Echocardiographic Parameters in the Evaluation of Mitral Regurgitation Severity.

Parameter	Method of Measurement	Advantages	Disadvantages	Clinical Reference Values
JA or JA/LAA ratio	Turbulent mosaic color flow within the LA during systole emanating from the mitral leaflets that can be normalized relative to the LA area Trace maximal JA to LAA ratio (same frame) in apical views Nyquist set ≥ 50 cm/s Assessed in apical views	Simple, technically less demanding	Subject to machine settings and physiologic conditions, such as LV systolic pressure Eccentric jets may underestimate Overestimation when MR not holosystolic	Mild or less: <20% of LAA Moderate: 20%–39% of LAA (best if central jets) Severe: ≥40% of LAA 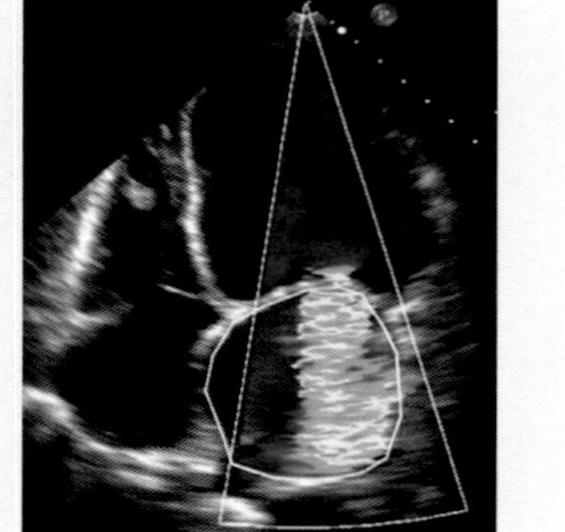
Vena contracta width	Width of narrowest portion of the MR jet, typically at level of or just distal to level of leaflets No need to change scale or Nyquist levels Should be performed in PLAX zoomed view; avoid measurement in 2-chamber view because reference values are established in long-axis views Scan across MV orifice by using medial to lateral tilt of transducer to ensure that VC is being captured fully Best measured when proximal flow convergence, VC, and MR jet are aligned in the same plane	Simple linear measurement Less subject to physiologic loading conditions than JA Surrogate for regurgitant orifice size Can be used in eccentric jets	Narrow reference range, so small differences in measurement can mean a change in MR grade Can be difficult to image due to narrow range Difficult to use for multiple jets Convergence zone needs visualization Overestimation when MR is not holosystolic	Mild or less: <0.3 cm Moderate: 0.3–0.69 cm Severe: ≥ 0.7 cm 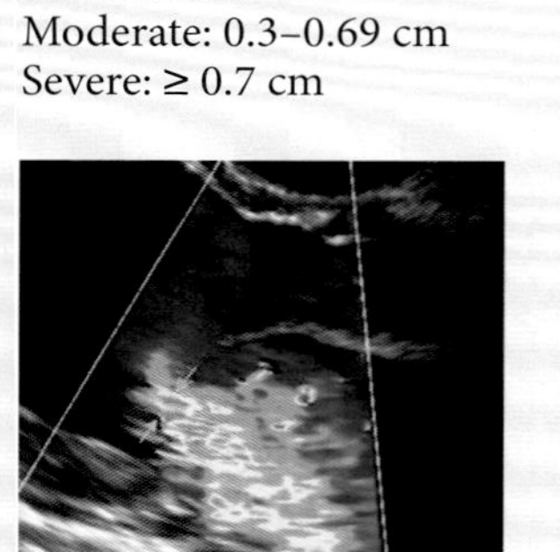

Continued

SUMMARY Echocardiographic Parameters in the Evaluation of Mitral Regurgitation Severity.—cont'd

Parameter	Method of Measurement	Advantages	Disadvantages	Clinical Reference Values
EROA by 2D PISA, quantitative Doppler, RVol, R fraction	The hemispherical shell that forms proximal to the mitral leaflets on the LV side Zoom on PISA region in Apical 4-, 2-, or 3-chamber views; choose view that resources PISA region the best Baseline shift toward direction of MR flow; if TTE apical view: baseline shift down to a lower Nyquist of 30–40 cm/s (depending on level where hemisphere outline is optimal). Acquire digital clip of 2–3 beats Choose PISA region with well-formed hemispherical shape at or near mid-systole or beginning of a T wave on ECG Measure the radius from the point of color aliasing to the VC Measure peak CW MR jet velocity and VTI	Provides a quantitative measure of MR Absence of proximal flow convergence is usually a sign of mild MR EROA predicts outcomes in cases of degenerative and functional MR	Technically challenging High variability Geometric assumptions may underestimate true EROA Eccentric PISA regions subject to wall or leaflet constraint May not be accurate in multiple jets, eccentric jets or very crescent-shaped orifices, or other non-hemispherical shapes, as in functional MR Overestimation when MR not holosystolic	*Reference ranges for EROA:* Mild: <0.20 cm^2 Moderate: <0.4 cm^2 Severe: ≥0.4 cm^2 Flow convergence method (PISA): Va PISA radius (r) Reg Flow = $2\pi r^2 \times Va$ EROA = Reg Flow/PKV_{Reg}
3D VC area	Optimize 3D settings for frame rate and spatial resolution Capture 3D color Doppler digital clip Using multiplanar reconstruction mode (MPR) on 3D software, align orthogonal views of vena contracta to localize the level of the narrowest portion (neck) of the MR jet Crop in from the transverse plane to the level of the narrowest jet Color flow sector should be narrow to improve volume rates and line density Planimeter the high-velocity aliased signal of VC, avoiding low velocity (dark color) signals	Provides a direct planimetry measure of EROA without need of geometric or physiologic assumptions Multiple jets of different directions may be measured Can identify severe functional MR in some cases when PISA underestimates EROA	Subject to poor lateral resolution, often overestimates true EROA Technically challenging to obtain adequate 3D color Doppler data set of VC region for measurement Multiple jets may be in different planes, which must be analyzed separately and then added	None established; reference ranges similar to EROA by 2D PISA Moderate or less: <0.4 cm^2 Severe: ≥0.4 cm^2 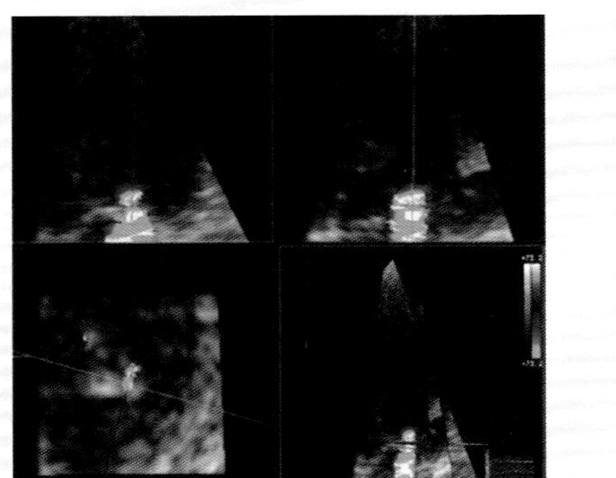

Volumetric Doppler measure of MR RVol 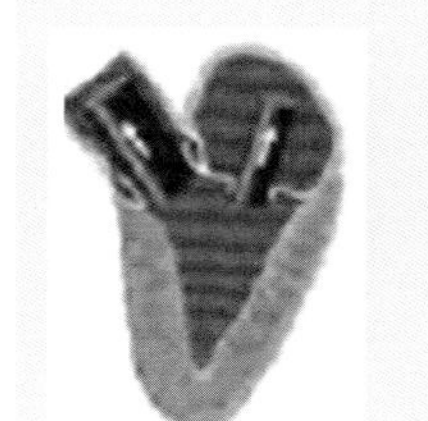 RVol = $SV_{MV} - SV_{LVOT}$	Measure VTI of mitral inflow at level of mitral annulus Measure mitral annulus diameter at mid diastole Measure LVOT diameter and VTI of LVOT outflow in systole Total LV SV can be measured at mitral annulus or by the difference between LV end-diastolic volume and end-systolic volume	Provides a quantitative measure of MR RVol Can be used if color Doppler resolution of jet is poor or jet is complex (eccentric, multiple); valid with multiple jets and eccentric jets Provides lesion severity (EROA, RF) and volume overload (RVol)	Technically challenging, multiple measures required increases variability of technique Cannot be performed if significant (moderate or greater) aortic regurgitation present unless pulmonic site is used	*Reference ranges*[a] Mild: Regurgitant volume < 30 mL Regurgitant fraction < 30% Moderate: Regurgitant volume 30–59 mL Regurgitant fraction 30%–49% Severe: Regurgitant volume ≥ 60 mL Regurgitant fraction ≥ 50% 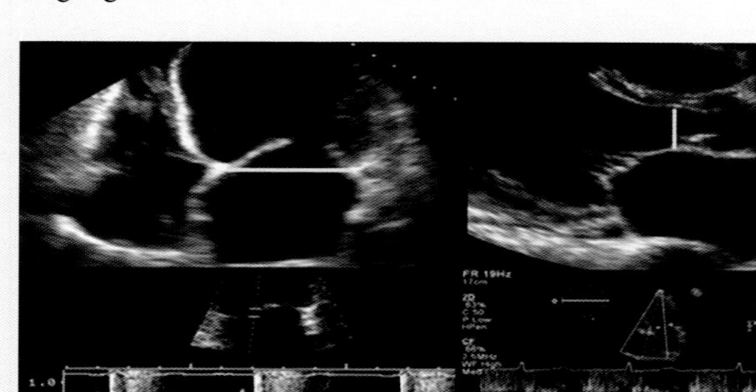
Pulmonary vein flow reversal	Measured in apical views Use small sample volume (3–5 mm) placed 1 cm into pulmonary vein For eccentric MR jet, best assessed in pulmonary vein in which MR jet is directed	A relatively specific but not sensitive parameter of severe MR Systolic flow reversal in more than one pulmonary vein is specific for severe MR Normal pulmonary vein pattern suggests low LA pressure and therefore nonsevere MR	Technically challenging due to depth of sample volume Best assessed with TEE Eccentric MR of mild or moderate severity directed into a pulmonary vein alters flow pattern Systolic blunting is not specific for significant MR (common in secondary MR and present in elevated LA pressure, atrial fibrillation)	Pulmonary vein flow reversal supports severe MR 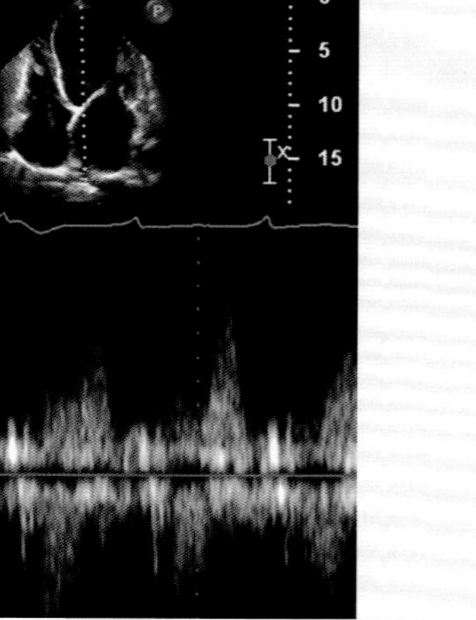 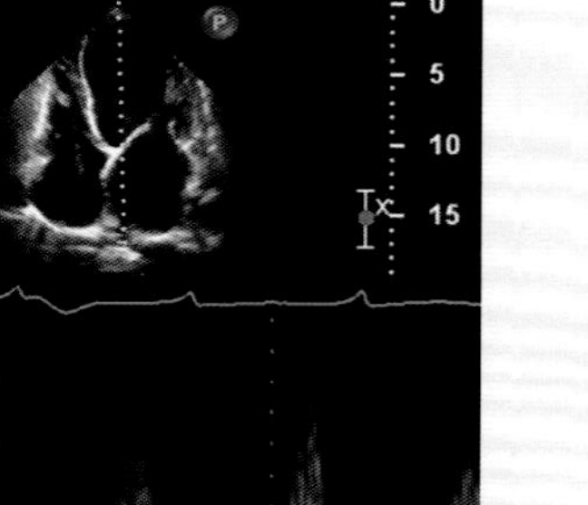

Continued

SUMMARY Echocardiographic Parameters in the Evaluation of Mitral Regurgitation Severity.—cont'd

Parameter	Method of Measurement	Advantages	Disadvantages	Clinical Reference Values
Chamber dilation (LA and LV)	Measured as single dimensions or volumes (area-length method or method of disks for LA; method of disks for LV volumes)	Widely measured with extensive longitudinal and outcome data	Nonspecific parameter because several factors other than MR volume affect chamber size	LA volume index abnormal[a] > 34 mL/m^2 *LV volumes*[b] EDV (mL) normal range Male: 62–150 Female: 46–106 ESV (mL) normal range Male: 21–61 Female: 14–42
E-wave velocity (mitral inflow velocity)	Performed in apical views (apical 4-chamber view). Align beam with flow across the MV at leaflet tips in apical 4-chamber view	Simple reproducible measurement Depends on LV relaxation and filling pressures High E velocity not specific for severe MR in secondary MR, atrial fibrillation, and mitral inflow stenosis Dominant A-wave inflow pattern virtually excludes severe MR	Nonspecific parameter because several factors other than MR volume affect E-wave velocity (loading conditions, LV compliance, mitral stenosis)	E velocity > 1.2 m/s is a simple supportive sign of severe MR (volume overload)
CW Doppler profile of MR jet	Performed in view parallel to MR jet flow (apical views) Important to angle transducer to obtain complete profile especially with eccentric MR jets	Simple measurement Sensitive Doppler measure Density is proportional to the number of red blood cells reflecting the signal Faint or incomplete jet compatible with mild MR A triangular contour (early MR peak velocity denotes a large regurgitant pressure wave and hemodynamic significance)	Can be difficult to obtain complete Doppler profile with eccentric jets Nonspecific measure of MR severity Perfectly central jets may appear denser than eccentric jets of higher severity Density is gain dependent A contour with an early peak velocity is not sensitive for severe MR	Intense CW Doppler signal supports severe MR V-shaped CW Doppler profile supports severe MR

Holosystolic vs. non-holosystolic MR jets	Can measure duration of MR jet throughout systole using color Doppler or color M-mode imaging	Parameter that takes into account duration of MR flow to quantitate MR volume	Technical factors (e.g., eccentric jets, frame rate) can make assessment of whether MR jet is holosystolic difficult	Holosystolic MR jets are almost always associated with severe MR Non-holosystolic MR jets are consistent with moderate or less MR (bottom two panels) *Top panels:* Color M-mode imaging of a patient with secondary MR shows holosystolic regurgitation with early and late flow peaks *Bottom panels:* Color M-mode imaging of a patient with MV prolapse and mostly late-systolic MR 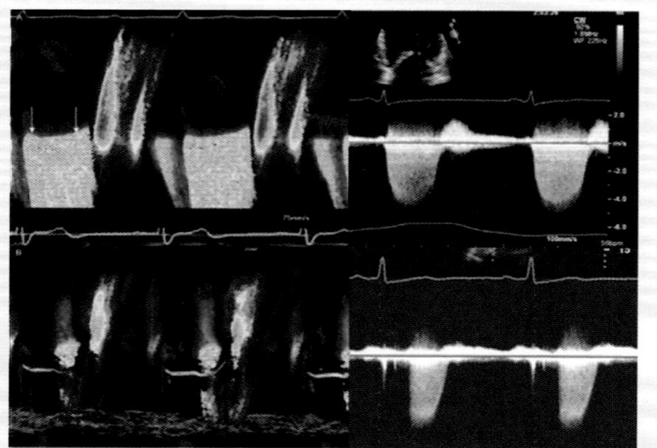

CW, Continuous wave; *ECG,* electrocardiogram; *EDV,* end-diastolic volume; *EROA,* effective regurgitant orifice area; *ESV,* end-systolic volume; *JA,* jet area; *LAA,* left atrial area; *LVOT,* LV outflow tract; *MR,* mitral regurgitation; *MV,* mitral valve; *PISA,* proximal isovelocity surface area; *PLAX,* parasternal long axis; *RF,* regurgitant fraction; *RVol,* regurgitant volume; *SV,* stroke volume; *TTE,* transthoracic echocardiography; *VC,* vena contracta; *VTI,* velocity-time integral.

From [a]Nishimura RA, Otto CM, Bonow RO, et al. 2017 AHA/ACC focused update of the 2014 AHA/ACC guideline for the management of patients with valvular heart disease: a report of the American College of Cardiology/American Heart Association Task Force on Clinical Practice Guidelines. *J Am Coll Cardiol.* 2017;70(2):252–289; [b]reference values from Lang RM, Badano LP, Mor-Avi V, et al. Recommendations for cardiac chamber quantification by echocardiography in adults: an update from the American Society of Echocardiography and the European Association of Cardiovascular Imaging. *J Am Soc Echocardiogr*. 2015;28:1–39; additional data from Zoghbi WA, Adams D, Bonow RO, et al. Recommendations for noninvasive evaluation of native valvular regurgitation: a report from the American Society of Echocardiography developed in collaboration with the Society for Cardiovascular Magnetic Resonance. *J Am Soc Echocardiogr*. 2017;30(4):303–371.

REFERENCES

1. Ling LH, Enriquez-Sarano M, Seward JB, et al. Clinical outcome of mitral regurgitation due to flail leaflet. *N Engl J Med.* 1996;335(19):1417–1423.
2. Rosen SE, Borer JS, Hochreiter C, et al. Natural history of the asymptomatic/minimally symptomatic patient with severe mitral regurgitation secondary to mitral valve prolapse and normal right and left ventricular performance. *Am J Cardiol.* 1994;74(4):374–380.
3. Nishimura RA, McGoon MD, Shub C, Miller FA Jr,, Ilstrup DM, Tajik AJ. Echocardiographically documented mitral-valve prolapse. Long-term follow-up of 237 patients. *N Engl J Med.* 1985;313(21):1305–1309.
4. Lamas GA, Mitchell GF, Flaker GC, et al. Clinical significance of mitral regurgitation after acute myocardial infarction. Survival and Ventricular Enlargement Investigators. *Circulation.* 1997;96(3):827–833.
5. Grigioni F, Enriquez-Sarano M, Zehr KJ, Bailey KR, Tajik AJ. Ischemic mitral regurgitation: long-term outcome and prognostic implications with quantitative Doppler assessment. *Circulation.* 2001;103(13):1759–1764.
6. Nkomo VT, Gardin JM, Skelton TN, Gottdiener JS, Scott CG, Enriquez-Sarano M. Burden of valvular heart diseases: a population-based study. *Lancet.* 2006;368(9540):1005–1011.
7. Jones EC, Devereux RB, Roman MJ, et al. Prevalence and correlates of mitral regurgitation in a population-based sample (the Strong Heart Study). *Am J Cardiol.* 2001;87(3):298–304.
8. Singh JP, Evans JC, Levy D, et al. Prevalence and clinical determinants of mitral, tricuspid, and aortic regurgitation (the Framingham Heart Study). *Am J Cardiol.* 1999;83(6):897–902.
9. Gammie JS, Sheng S, Griffith BP, et al. Trends in mitral valve surgery in the United States: results from the Society of Thoracic Surgeons Adult Cardiac Surgery Database. *Ann Thorac Surg.* 2009;87(5):1431–1437; discussion 7–9.
10. Levine RA, Triulzi MO, Harrigan P, Weyman AE. The relationship of mitral annular shape to the diagnosis of mitral valve prolapse. *Circulation.* 1987;75(4):756–767.
11. Jimenez JH, Liou SW, Padala M, et al. A saddle-shaped annulus reduces systolic strain on the central region of the mitral valve anterior leaflet. *J Thorac Cardiovasc Surg.* 2007;134(6):1562–1568.
12. Padala M, Hutchison RA, Croft LR, et al. Saddle shape of the mitral annulus reduces systolic strains on the P2 segment of the posterior mitral leaflet. *Ann Thorac Surg.* 2009;88(5):1499–1504.
13. Kunzelman KS, Reimink MS, Cochran RP. Annular dilatation increases stress in the mitral valve and delays coaptation: a finite element computer model. *Cardiovasc Surg.* 1997;5(4):427–434.
14. Mihalatos DG, Joseph S, Gopal A, et al. Mitral annular remodeling with varying degrees and mechanisms of chronic mitral regurgitation. *J Am Soc Echocardiogr.* 2007;20(4):397–404.
15. Levine RA, Hagége AA, Judge DP, et al. Mitral valve disease—morphology and mechanisms. *Nat Rev Cardiol.* 2015;12(12):689–710.
16. Dal-Bianco JP, Aikawa E, Bischoff J, et al. Active adaptation of the tethered mitral valve: insights into a compensatory mechanism for functional mitral regurgitation. *Circulation.* 2009;120(4):334–342.
17. Godley RW, Wann LS, Rogers EW, Feigenbaum H, Weyman AE. Incomplete mitral leaflet closure in patients with papillary muscle dysfunction. *Circulation.* 1981;63(3):565–571.
18. He S, Weston MW, Lemmon J, Jensen M, Levine RA, Yoganathan AP. Geometric distribution of chordae tendineae: an important anatomic feature in mitral valve function. *J Heart Valve Dis.* 2000;9(4):495–501; discussion 2–3.
19. Rodriguez F, Langer F, Harrington KB, et al. Importance of mitral valve second-order chordae for left ventricular geometry, wall thickening mechanics, and global systolic function. *Circulation.* 2004;110(11 suppl 1):II115–I122.
20. Dejgaard LA, Skjolsvik ET, Lie OH, et al. The mitral annulus disjunction arrhythmic syndrome. *J Am Coll Cardiol.* 2018;72(14):1600–1609.
21. Disse S, Abergel E, Berrebi A, et al. Mapping of a first locus for autosomal dominant myxomatous mitral-valve prolapse to chromosome 16p11.2-p12.1. *Am J Hum Genet.* 1999;65(5):1242–1251.
22. Freed LA, Acierno JS Jr, Dai D, et al. A locus for autosomal dominant mitral valve prolapse on chromosome 11p15.4. *Am J Hum Genet.* 2003;72(6):1551–1559.
23. Nesta F, Leyne M, Yosefy C, et al. New locus for autosomal dominant mitral valve prolapse on chromosome 13: clinical insights from genetic studies. *Circulation.* 2005;112(13):2022–2030.
24. Fornes P, Heudes D, Fuzellier JF, Tixier D, Bruneval P, Carpentier A. Correlation between clinical and histologic patterns of degenerative mitral valve insufficiency: a histomorphometric study of 130 excised segments. *Cardiovasc Pathol.* 1999;8(2):81–92.
25. Anyanwu AC, Adams DH. Etiologic classification of degenerative mitral valve disease: Barlow's disease and fibroelastic deficiency. *Semin Thorac Cardiovasc Surg.* 2007;19(2):90–96.
26. Mantovani F, Clavel MA, Vatury O, et al. Cleft-like indentations in myxomatous mitral valves by three-dimensional echocardiographic imaging. *Heart.* 2015;101(14):1111–1117.
27. Rothenbuhler M, O'Sullivan CJ, Stortecky S, et al. Active surveillance for rheumatic heart disease in endemic regions: a systematic review and meta-analysis of prevalence among children and adolescents. *Lancet Glob Health.* 2014;2(12):e717–e726.
28. Sattur S, Bates S, Movahed MR. Prevalence of mitral valve prolapse and associated valvular regurgitations in healthy teenagers undergoing screening echocardiography. *Exp Clin Cardiol.* 2010;15(1):e13–e15.
29. Kohl T, Silverman NH. Comparison of cleft and papillary muscle position in cleft mitral valve and atrioventricular septal defect. *Am J Cardiol.* 1996;77(2):164–169.
30. Bano-Rodrigo A, Van Praagh S, Trowitzsch E, Van Praagh R. Double-orifice mitral valve: a study of 27 postmortem cases with developmental, diagnostic and surgical considerations. *Am J Cardiol.* 1988;61(1):152–160.
31. Bursi F, Enriquez-Sarano M, Nkomo VT, et al. Heart failure and death after myocardial infarction in the community: the emerging role of mitral regurgitation. *Circulation.* 2005;111(3):295–301.
32. Koelling TM, Aaronson KD, Cody RJ, Bach DS, Armstrong WF. Prognostic significance of mitral regurgitation and tricuspid regurgitation in patients with left ventricular systolic dysfunction. *Am Heart J.* 2002;144(3):524–529.
33. Clements SD Jr, Story WE, Hurst JW, Craver JM, Jones EL. Ruptured papillary muscle, a complication of myocardial infarction: clinical presentation, diagnosis, and treatment. *Clin Cardiol.* 1985;8(2):93–103.
34. Levine RA, Schwammenthal E. Ischemic mitral regurgitation on the threshold of a solution: from paradoxes to unifying concepts. *Circulation.* 2005;112(5):745–758.
35. Kumanohoso T, Otsuji Y, Yoshifuku S, et al. Mechanism of higher incidence of ischemic mitral regurgitation in patients with inferior myocardial infarction: quantitative analysis of left ventricular and mitral valve geometry in 103 patients with prior myocardial infarction. *J Thorac Cardiovasc Surg.* 2003;125(1):135–143.
36. Harari R, Bansal P, Yatskar L, Rubinstein D, Silbiger JJ. Papillary muscle rupture following acute myocardial infarction: anatomic, echocardiographic, and surgical insights. *Echocardiography.* 2017;34(11):1702–1707.
37. Deferm S, Bertrand PB, Verbrugge FH, et al. Atrial functional mitral regurgitation: JACC review topic of the week. *J Am Coll Cardiol.* 2019;73(19):2465–2476.
38. Silbiger JJ. Does left atrial enlargement contribute to mitral leaflet tethering in patients with functional mitral regurgitation? Proposed role of atriogenic leaflet tethering. *Echocardiography.* 2014;31(10):1310–1311.
39. Gertz ZM, Raina A, Saghy L, et al. Evidence of atrial functional mitral regurgitation due to atrial fibrillation: reversal with arrhythmia control. *J Am Coll Cardiol.* 2011;58(14):1474–1481.
40. Kim DH, Heo R, Handschumacher MD, et al. Mitral valve adaptation to isolated annular dilation: insights into the mechanism of atrial functional mitral regurgitation. *JACC Cardiovasc Imaging.* 2019;12(4):665–677.
41. Carpentier A. Cardiac valve surgery—the "French correction". *J Thorac Cardiovasc Surg.* 1983;86(3):323–337.
42. Roberts BJ, Grayburn PA. Color flow imaging of the vena contracta in mitral regurgitation: technical considerations. *J Am Soc Echocardiogr.* 2003;16(9):1002–1006.
43. Miyatake K, Izumi S, Okamoto M, et al. Semiquantitative grading of severity of mitral regurgitation by real-time two-dimensional Doppler flow imaging technique. *J Am Coll Cardiol.* 1986;7(1):82–88.
44. Omoto R, Yokote Y, Takamoto S, et al. The development of real-time two-dimensional Doppler echocardiography and its clinical significance in acquired valvular diseases. With special reference to the evaluation of valvular regurgitation. *Jpn Heart J.* 1984;25(3):325–340.
45. Enriquez-Sarano M, Tajik AJ, Bailey KR, Seward JB. Color flow imaging compared with quantitative Doppler assessment of severity of mitral regurgitation: influence of eccentricity of jet and mechanism of regurgitation. *J Am Coll Cardiol.* 1993;21(5):1211–1219.

46. Spain MG, Smith MD, Grayburn PA, Harlamert EA, DeMaria AN. Quantitative assessment of mitral regurgitation by Doppler color flow imaging: angiographic and hemodynamic correlations. *J Am Coll Cardiol.* 1989;13(3):585–590.
47. Fehske W, Omran H, Manz M, Kohler J, Hagendorff A, Luderitz B. Color-coded Doppler imaging of the vena contracta as a basis for quantification of pure mitral regurgitation. *Am J Cardiol.* 1994;73(4):268–274.
48. Zoghbi WA, Adams D, Bonow RO, et al. Recommendations for noninvasive evaluation of native valvular regurgitation: a report from the American Society of Echocardiography developed in collaboration with the Society for Cardiovascular Magnetic Resonance. *J Am Soc Echocardiogr.* 2017;30(4):303–371.
49. Chen CG, Thomas JD, Anconina J, et al. Impact of impinging wall jet on color Doppler quantification of mitral regurgitation. *Circulation.* 1991;84(2):712–720.
50. Zoghbi WA, Enriquez-Sarano M, Foster E, et al. Recommendations for evaluation of the severity of native valvular regurgitation with two-dimensional and Doppler echocardiography. *J Am Soc Echocardiogr.* 2003;16(7):777–802.
51. Maciel BC, Moises VA, Shandas R, et al. Effects of pressure and volume of the receiving chamber on the spatial distribution of regurgitant jets as imaged by color Doppler flow mapping. An in vitro study. *Circulation.* 1991;83(2):605–613.
52. Rivera JM, Mele D, Vandervoort PM, Morris E, Weyman A, Thomas JD. Physical factors determining mitral regurgitation jet area. *Am J Cardiol.* 1994;74(5):515–516.
53. Simpson IA, Valdes-Cruz LM, Sahn DJ, Murillo A, Tamura T, Chung KJ. Doppler color flow mapping of simulated in vitro regurgitant jets: evaluation of the effects of orifice size and hemodynamic variables. *J Am Coll Cardiol.* 1989;13(5):1195–1207.
54. Lesniak-Sobelga A, Olszowska M, Pienazek P, Podolec P, Tracz W. Vena contracta width as a simple method of assessing mitral valve regurgitation. Comparison with Doppler quantitative methods. *J Heart Valve Dis.* 2004;13(4):608–614.
55. Hall SA, Brickner ME, Willett DL, Irani WN, Afridi I, Grayburn PA. Assessment of mitral regurgitation severity by Doppler color flow mapping of the vena contracta. *Circulation.* 1997;95(3):636–642.
56. Heinle SK, Hall SA, Brickner ME, Willett DL, Grayburn PA. Comparison of vena contracta width by multiplane transesophageal echocardiography with quantitative Doppler assessment of mitral regurgitation. *Am J Cardiol.* 1998;81(2):175–179.
57. Vandervoort PM, Thoreau DH, Rivera JM, Levine RA, Weyman AE, Thomas JD. Automated flow rate calculations based on digital analysis of flow convergence proximal to regurgitant orifices. *J Am Coll Cardiol.* 1993;22(2):535–541.
58. Rodriguez L, Anconina J, Flachskampf FA, Weyman AE, Levine RA, Thomas JD. Impact of finite orifice size on proximal flow convergence. Implications for Doppler quantification of valvular regurgitation. *Circ Res.* 1992;70(5):923–930.
59. Enriquez-Sarano M, Miller FA Jr, Hayes SN, Bailey KR, Tajik AJ, Seward JB. Effective mitral regurgitant orifice area: clinical use and pitfalls of the proximal isovelocity surface area method. *J Am Coll Cardiol.* 1995;25(3):703–709.
60. Schwammenthal E, Chen C, Giesler M, et al. New method for accurate calculation of regurgitant flow rate based on analysis of Doppler color flow maps of the proximal flow field. Validation in a canine model of mitral regurgitation with initial application in patients. *J Am Coll Cardiol.* 1996;27(1):161–172.
61. Utsunomiya T, Ogawa T, Doshi R, et al. Doppler color flow "proximal isovelocity surface area" method for estimating volume flow rate: effects of orifice shape and machine factors. *J Am Coll Cardiol.* 1991;17(5):1103–1111.
62. Pu M, Vandervoort PM, Griffin BP, et al. Quantification of mitral regurgitation by the proximal convergence method using transesophageal echocardiography. Clinical validation of a geometric correction for proximal flow constraint. *Circulation.* 1995;92(8):2169–2177.
63. Hopmeyer J, He S, Thorvig KM, et al. Estimation of mitral regurgitation with a hemielliptic curve-fitting algorithm: in vitro experiments with native mitral valves. *J Am Soc Echocardiogr.* 1998;11(4):322–331.
64. Rivera JM, Vandervoort PM, Thoreau DH, Levine RA, Weyman AE, Thomas JD. Quantification of mitral regurgitation with the proximal flow convergence method: a clinical study. *Am Heart J.* 1992;124(5):1289–1296.
65. Yosefy C, Levine RA, Solis J, Vaturi M, Handschumacher MD, Hung J. Proximal flow convergence region as assessed by real-time 3-dimensional echocardiography: challenging the hemispheric assumption. *J Am Soc Echocardiogr.* 2007;20(4):389–396.
66. Utsunomiya T, Ogawa T, Tang HA, et al. Doppler color flow mapping of the proximal isovelocity surface area: a new method for measuring volume flow rate across a narrowed orifice. *J Am Soc Echocardiogr.* 1991;4(4):338–348.
67. Nishimura RA, Otto CM, Bonow RO, et al. AHA/ACC guideline for the management of patients with valvular heart disease: a report of the American College of Cardiology/American Heart Association Task Force on Practice Guidelines. *J Am Coll Cardiol.* 2014;63(22):e57–185.
68. Vahanian A, Alfieri O, Andreotti F, et al. Guidelines on the management of valvular heart disease (version 2012): the Joint Task Force on the Management of Valvular Heart Disease of the European Society of Cardiology (ESC) and the European Association for Cardio-Thoracic Surgery (EACTS). *Eur J Cardio Thorac Surg.* 2012;42(4):S1–S44.
69. Lancellotti P, Moura L, Pierard LA, et al. European Association of Echocardiography recommendations for the assessment of valvular regurgitation. Part 2: mitral and tricuspid regurgitation (native valve disease). *Eur J Echocardiogr.* 2010;11(4):307–332.
70. Acker MA, Parides MK, Perrault LP, et al. Mitral-valve repair versus replacement for severe ischemic mitral regurgitation. *N Engl J Med.* 2014;370(1):23–32.
71. Michler RE, Smith PK, Parides MK, et al. Two-year outcomes of surgical treatment of moderate ischemic mitral regurgitation. *N Engl J Med.* 2016;374(20):1932–1941.
72. Smith PK, Puskas JD, Ascheim DD, et al. Surgical treatment of moderate ischemic mitral regurgitation. *N Engl J Med.* 2014;371(23):2178–2188.
73. Kahlert P, Plicht B, Schenk IM, Janosi RA, Erbel R, Buck T. Direct assessment of size and shape of noncircular vena contracta area in functional versus organic mitral regurgitation using real-time three-dimensional echocardiography. *J Am Soc Echocardiogr.* 2008;21(8):912–921.
74. Marsan NA, Westenberg JJ, Ypenburg C, et al. Quantification of functional mitral regurgitation by real-time 3D echocardiography: comparison with 3D velocity-encoded cardiac magnetic resonance. *JACC Cardiovasc Imaging.* 2009;2(11):1245–1252.
75. Yosefy C, Hung J, Chua S, et al. Direct measurement of vena contracta area by real-time 3-dimensional echocardiography for assessing severity of mitral regurgitation. *Am J Cardiol.* 2009;104(7):978–983.
76. Enriquez-Sarano M, Dujardin KS, Tribouilloy CM, et al. Determinants of pulmonary venous flow reversal in mitral regurgitation and its usefulness in determining the severity of regurgitation. *Am J Cardiol.* 1999;83(4):535–541.
77. Castello R, Pearson AC, Lenzen P, Labovitz AJ. Effect of mitral regurgitation on pulmonary venous velocities derived from transesophageal echocardiography color-guided pulsed Doppler imaging. *J Am Coll Cardiol.* 1991;17(7):1499–1506.
78. Kamp O, Huitink H, van Eenige MJ, Visser CA, Roos JP. Value of pulmonary venous flow characteristics in the assessment of severity of native mitral valve regurgitation: an angiographic correlated study. *J Am Soc Echocardiogr.* 1992;5(3):239–246.
79. Utsunomiya T, Patel D, Doshi R, Quan M, Gardin JM. Can signal intensity of the continuous wave Doppler regurgitant jet estimate severity of mitral regurgitation? *Am Heart J.* 1992;123(1):166–171.
80. Jenni R, Ritter M, Eberli F, Grimm J, Krayenbuehl HP. Quantification of mitral regurgitation with amplitude-weighted mean velocity from continuous wave Doppler spectra. *Circulation.* 1989;79(6):1294–1299.
81. Dujardin KS, Enriquez-Sarano M, Bailey KR, Nishimura RA, Seward JB, Tajik AJ. Grading of mitral regurgitation by quantitative Doppler echocardiography: calibration by left ventricular angiography in routine clinical practice. *Circulation.* 1997;96(10):3409–3415.
82. Tribouilloy C, Shen WF, Slama MA, et al. Non-invasive measurement of the regurgitant fraction by pulsed Doppler echocardiography in isolated pure mitral regurgitation. *Br Heart J.* 1991;66(4):290–294.
83. Otsuji Y, Gilon D, Jiang L, et al. Restricted diastolic opening of the mitral leaflets in patients with left ventricular dysfunction: evidence for increased valve tethering. *J Am Coll Cardiol.* 1998;32(2):398–404.
84. Yiu SF, Enriquez-Sarano M, Tribouilloy C, Seward JB, Tajik AJ. Determinants of the degree of functional mitral regurgitation in patients with systolic left ventricular dysfunction: a quantitative clinical study. *Circulation.* 2000;102(12):1400–1406.
85. Topilsky Y, Michelena H, Bichara V, Maalouf J, Mahoney DW, Enriquez-Sarano M. Mitral valve prolapse with mid-late systolic mitral regurgitation: pitfalls of evaluation and clinical outcome compared with holosystolic regurgitation. *Circulation.* 2012;125(13):1643–1651.
86. Stevenson LW, Bellil D, Grover-McKay M, et al. Effects of afterload reduction (diuretics

and vasodilators) on left ventricular volume and mitral regurgitation in severe congestive heart failure secondary to ischemic or idiopathic dilated cardiomyopathy. *Am J Cardiol.* 1987;60(8):654–658.

87. Lancellotti P, Pellikka PA, Budts W, et al. The clinical use of stress echocardiography in non-ischaemic heart disease: recommendations from the European Association of Cardiovascular Imaging and the American Society of Echocardiography. *J Am Soc Echocardiogr.* 2017;30(2):101–138.
88. Schwammenthal E, Chen C, Benning F, Block M, Breithardt G, Levine RA. Dynamics of mitral regurgitant flow and orifice area. Physiologic application of the proximal flow convergence method: clinical data and experimental testing. *Circulation.* 1994;90(1):307–322.
89. Enriquez-Sarano M, Avierinos JF, Messika-Zeitoun D, et al. Quantitative determinants of the outcome of asymptomatic mitral regurgitation. *N Engl J Med.* 2005;352(9):875–883.
90. Rosenhek R, Rader F, Klaar U, et al. Outcome of watchful waiting in asymptomatic severe mitral regurgitation. *Circulation.* 2006;113(18):2238–2244.
91. Tischler MD, Rowan M, LeWinter MM. Effect of enalapril therapy on left ventricular mass and volumes in asymptomatic chronic, severe mitral regurgitation secondary to mitral valve prolapse. *Am J Cardiol.* 1998;82(2):242–245.
92. Nishimura RA, Otto CM, Bonow RO, et al. AHA/ACC focused update of the 2014 AHA/ACC guideline for the management of patients with valvular heart disease: a report of the American College of Cardiology/American Heart Association Task Force on Clinical Practice Guidelines. *J Am Coll Cardiol.* 2017;70(2):252–289.
93. Smith PK, Hung JW, Michler RE. Surgical treatment of moderate ischemic mitral regurgitation. *N Engl J Med.* 2015;372(18):1773–1774.
94. Baumgartner H, Falk V, Bax JJ, et al. ESC/EACTS guidelines for the management of valvular heart disease. *Eur Heart J.* 2017;38(36):2739–2791. 2017.
95. Chan KM, Punjabi PP, Flather M, et al. Coronary artery bypass surgery with or without mitral valve annuloplasty in moderate functional ischemic mitral regurgitation: final results of the Randomized Ischemic Mitral Evaluation (RIME) trial. *Circulation.* 2012;126(21):2502–2510.
96. Obadia JF, Messika-Zeitoun D, Leurent G, et al. Percutaneous repair or medical treatment for secondary mitral regurgitation. *N Engl J Med.* 2018;379(24):2297–2306.
97. Stone GW, Lindenfeld J, Abraham WT, et al. Transcatheter mitral-valve repair in patients with heart failure. *N Engl J Med.* 2018;379(24):2307–2318.
98. Grayburn PA, Sannino A, Packer M. Proportionate and disproportionate functional mitral regurgitation: a new conceptual framework that reconciles the results of the MITRA-FR and COAPT trials. *JACC Cardiovasc Imaging.* 2019;12(2):353–362.
99. Asch FM, Grayburn PA, Siegel RJ, et al. Echocardiographic outcomes after transcatheter leaflet approximation in patients with secondary mitral regurgitation: the COAPT trial. *J Am Coll Cardiol.* 2019;74(24):2969–2979.
100. Lang RM, Badano LP, Mor-Avi V, et al. Recommendations for cardiac chamber quantification by echocardiography in adults: an update from the American Society of Echocardiography and the European Association of Cardiovascular Imaging. *J Am Soc Echocardiogr.* 2015;28(1):1–39.e14.

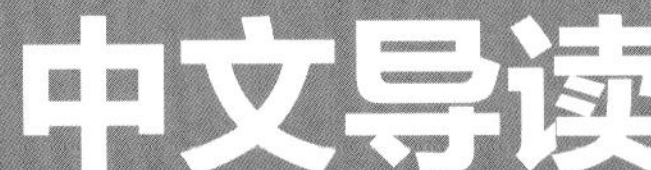

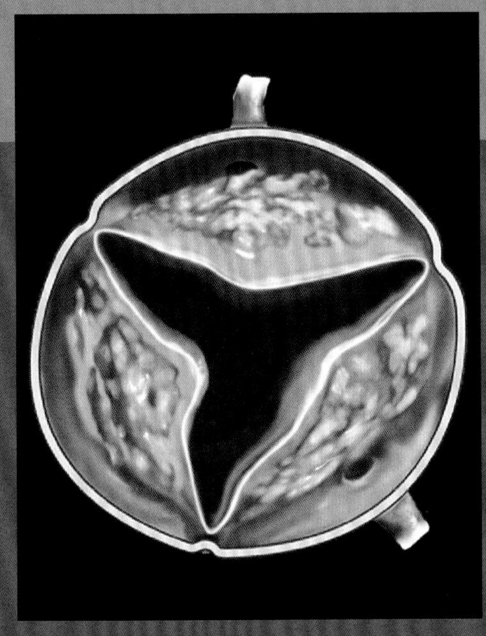

第25章 经食管超声心动图在指导二尖瓣关闭不全手术中的作用

传统二尖瓣病变的手术方式是二尖瓣置换术和二尖瓣修复术，对于原发性二尖瓣反流及瓣膜条件适合的原发性二尖瓣反流患者，二尖瓣修复术是理想的手术方式。经食管超声心动图在筛选可修复二尖瓣病变并指导二尖瓣手术中发挥着重要的作用。

本章重点介绍了常见原发性二尖瓣病变（退行性或黏液样变、感染性心内膜炎、风湿性、放射引起的瓣膜功能障碍、瓣叶钙化）和继发性二尖瓣病变的解剖及病理生理，经食管超声心动图评估二尖瓣病变的标准切面，常见原发性二尖瓣病变和继发性二尖瓣病变的术前、术中及术后经食管超声心动图评估要点，包括左心室结构及功能、残存二尖瓣反流，新发二尖瓣狭窄、室壁运动异常、二尖瓣前叶收缩期前向运动等。此外，还简要介绍了经食管三维超声心动图在上述方面的应用。

李 慧

25

Transesophageal Echocardiography for Surgical Repair of Mitral Regurgitation

DANIEL H. DRAKE, MD | KAREN G. ZIMMERMAN, BS, ACS, RVT | DAVID A. SIDEBOTHAM, MBChB

The superiority of mitral repair over replacement for treating primary mitral regurgitation (MR) is well established.[1,2] In appropriately selected patients, mitral repair is also optimal for treating secondary MR.[3–6] Transesophageal echocardiography (TEE) is ideal for identifying reparable mitral valve disease and guiding surgical repair.[3,7] This chapter focuses on the use of TEE to guide surgical repair and to identify complications after repair. The indications for surgical intervention and the echocardiographic quantification of MR are covered in Chapter 24.

THE TEAM APPROACH TO ECHOCARDIOGRAPHY-GUIDED MITRAL REPAIR

The concept of echocardiography-guided mitral repair stems from two observations: first, that surgical repair is the preferred treatment option for most patients with severe MR,[1] and second, that echocardiographic imaging provides valuable insights into mitral pathoanatomy that help guide surgical decision making and can potentially improve outcome.

Achieving optimal outcomes for patients undergoing mitral repair requires a team approach with input from appropriately trained surgeons, cardiologists, anesthesiologists, and cardiac sonographers. A joint report from the American Association for Thoracic Surgery (AATS), American College of Cardiology (ACC), American Society of Echocardiography (ASE), Society for Cardiovascular Angiography and Interventions (SCAI), and Society of Thoracic Surgeons (STS) recommended that patients with complex valve disease be managed by a multidisciplinary team.[8] The minimum requirements for this team are presented in Table 25.1.

There are several elements to the team approach to echocardiography-guided repair. First, suitable patients must be referred to a skilled mitral valve surgeon. Surgeon volume is an important determinant of outcome, with higher rates of successful repair and fewer complications reported for high-volume than low-volume surgeons.[8–10]

Second, appropriate imaging of the mitral valve is essential. Transthoracic echocardiography (TTE) is suitable for the initial evaluation and ongoing surveillance of patients with MR.[11] However, to assess the likelihood of a successful repair procedure and to determine the appropriate surgical technique, it is necessary to quantify the mitral pathoanatomy. Three-dimensional (3D) TEE offers unprecedented insight into the anatomic location and mechanism of MR compared with TTE or conventional multiplane TEE.[12,13] Quantitative 3D analysis using multiplanar reconstruction allows reproducible measurements of valvular dimensions and leaflet distortion to be obtained, which further aids surgical decision making.[3] Ideally, TEE should be performed in advance of surgery to facilitate operative planning and allow the patient to make an informed decision about his or her treatment.[14]

Third, TEE should be performed by imaging specialists with appropriate training and experience. Recommendations for physician training and credentialing in TEE are summarized in the guideline for performing a comprehensive TEE examination published by the ASE and the Society of Cardiovascular Anesthesiologists.[15] In addition to the physician-echocardiographer, the assistance of an advanced cardiovascular sonographer is invaluable, particularly for the quantitative analysis of 3D data sets.[16] In addition to general training and credentialing in TEE, it is essential that practitioners have specific knowledge of the anatomy, pathology, and imaging techniques of the mitral valve.

Fourth, a standardized approach to TEE imaging should be used to ensure that findings are accurate and reproducible. Measurements should be performed in appropriate views. Uniform approaches to image display and quantitative analysis should be used.

Communications among team members should use standard terminology. For instance, the Carpentier nomenclature (described later) should be used to refer to leaflet segments, rather than using potentially confusing terms such as *medial scallop.* Terms such as *flail* and *prolapse* should be used to convey specific meanings. Ambiguous phrases such as *billowing* or *mild plus regurgitation* should be avoided.

ESSENTIAL ANATOMY

Accurate evaluation of the anatomic and pathophysiologic basis of mitral valve dysfunction requires an understanding of normal valvular anatomy. The mitral valve is best thought of as a valve complex consisting of an annulus, leaflets, chordae, papillary muscles, and associated left ventricular (LV) muscle. The mitral valve and associated cardiac structures are demonstrated in Fig. 25.1. The annulus is a fibrous ring with a 3D shape that resembles a riding saddle.[17,18] The annulus has two axes: a shorter, more basal, anteroposterior axis and a longer, more apical, commissural axis. During systole, the annulus shortens along its anteroposterior axis and folds along its commissural axis, deepening the saddle.[19–21] Systolic shortening and folding help appose the leaflets, particularly during early systole when ventricular pressure is too low to close the valve.[19,22]

The mitral valve has two leaflets: anterior and posterior. The leaflets have approximately the same surface area; however, the posterior leaflet has a longer annular attachment and a shorter base-to-tip length. The posterior leaflet usually has three distinct scallops, which are not present on the anterior leaflet. As the circumferential attachment of the posterior leaflet shortens during systole, pleating between the scallops facilitates valve closure and coaptation. The anterior leaflet does not substantially alter its circumferential attachment during systole, and there is no pleating mechanism. The posterior scallops and corresponding segments of the anterior leaflet are named using the system proposed by Carpentier.[23] The leaflets join at the anterolateral and posteromedial commissures. Leaflet coaptation occurs at or just below the annular plane, and there is normally 8 to 10 mm of leaflet overlap (i.e., coaptation) at end-systole.

There are two papillary muscles, the anterolateral and the posteromedial, located below the commissures of the same names. Each papillary muscle supports both anterior and posterior leaflets symmetrically. The blood supply to the anterolateral muscle is from branches of the left anterior descending and circumflex coronary arteries; the right coronary artery (RCA) provides the sole blood supply to the posteromedial muscle. The

TABLE 25.1 The Multidisciplinary Team: Minimum Requirements.

Interventional cardiologist
Cardiac surgeon
Echocardiographic and radiologic image specialist[a]
Clinical cardiology valve expertise[a]
Heart failure specialist[b]
Cardiovascular anesthesiologist
Nurse practitioner/physician assistant for preprocedural and periprocedural care and MDT consultations
Valve coordinator/program navigator
Institutionally supported data manager for STS/ACC TVT Registry
Hospital administration representative, as necessary

[a]A single individual may provide clinical and imaging expertise.
[b]For patients with heart failure due to LV systolic dysfunction and secondary mitral regurgitation.
ACC, American College of Cardiology; *MDT*, multidisciplinary team; *STS*, Society of Thoracic Surgeons; *TAVR*, transcatheter aortic valve replacement; *TVT*, transcatheter valve therapy.
Reproduced with permission from Nishimura RA, O'Gara PT, Bavaria JE, et al. 2019 AATS/ACC/ASE/SCAI/STS expert consensus systems of care document: a proposal to optimize care for patients with valvular heart disease: a joint report of the American Association for Thoracic Surgery, American College of Cardiology, American Society of Echocardiography, Society for Cardiovascular Angiography and Interventions, and Society of Thoracic Surgeons. *J Am Coll Cardiol.* 2019;73:2609–2635.

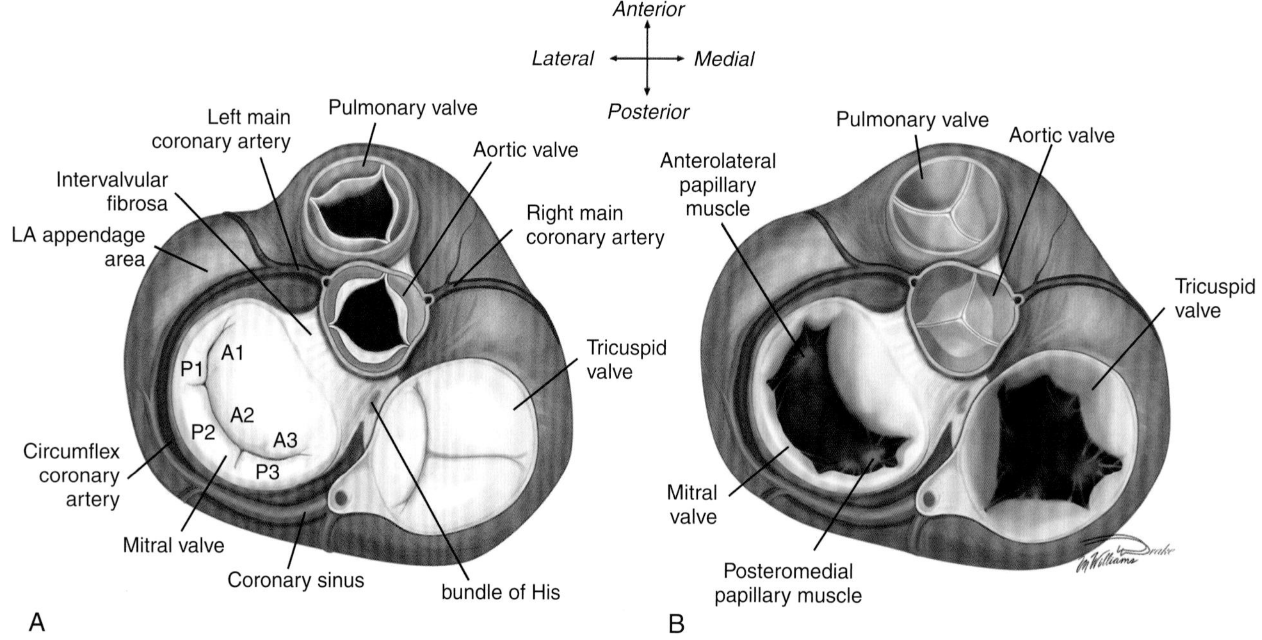

Fig. 25.1 Anatomic relationships of the mitral valve. The base of the heart is shown in an anatomic orientation from the LA aspect to demonstrate the relationship of the mitral valve to adjacent cardiac structures. (A) Systole. The posterior leaflet of the mitral valve normally has two natural clefts. These clefts divide the posterior leaflet into three segments; using the Carpentier nomenclature, they are called P1, P2, and P3. Although there are no natural clefts in the anterior leaflet, its corresponding segments are called A1, A2, and A3. For purposes of echocardiographic orientation, it is useful to note that P1 is adjacent to the LA appendage and P3 is adjacent to the tricuspid valve. (B) Diastole. The anterolateral and posteromedial papillary muscles support the anterior and posterior leaflets symmetrically. The anterolateral muscle supports A1/P1 and the anterolateral one half of A2/P2; the posteromedial muscle supports A3/P3 and the posteromedial one half of A2/P2.

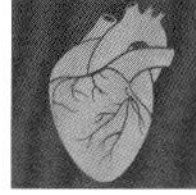

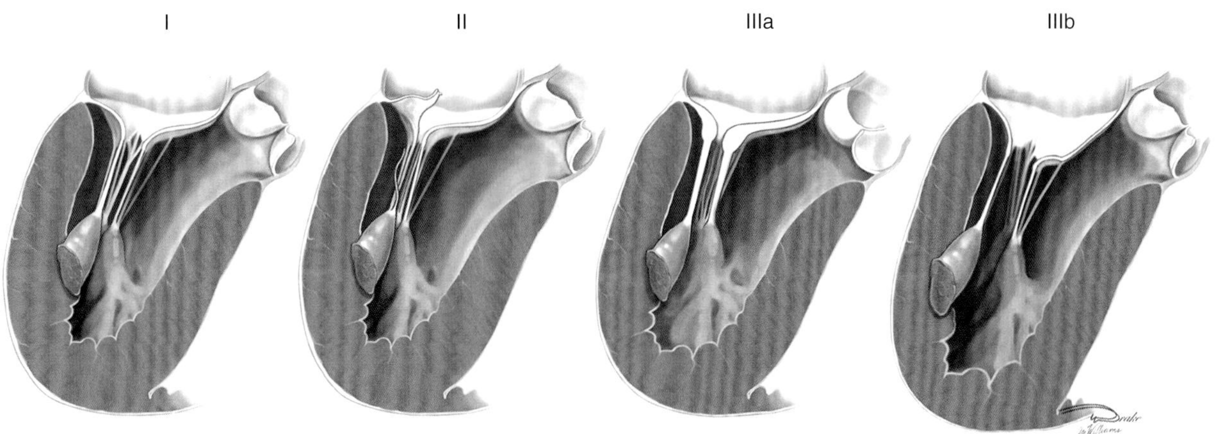

Fig. 25.2 Carpentier classification for leaflet dysfunction. *Type I dysfunction* is defined as mitral regurgitation in the setting of normal leaflet motion. Examples include annular dilation, leaflet perforation, and leaflet cleft. Type I dysfunction can also result from a combination of degenerative and secondary disease. *Type II dysfunction* refers to excessive leaflet motion. Examples include leaflet prolapse and flail caused by degenerative disease. *Type III dysfunction* is characterized by restricted leaflet motion. In *type IIIa* (e.g., rheumatic disease, radiation-induced valvulopathy, dystrophic calcification), leaflet restriction occurs predominantly in diastole. *Type IIIb* dysfunction, in which leaflet restriction occurs predominantly in systole, may be symmetric (e.g., dilated cardiomyopathy) or asymmetric (e.g., myocardial infarction) (see Video 25.2).

leaflets are attached to the papillary muscles by chordae tendineae. Primary (marginal) chordae attach to the free edges of the leaflets, and secondary chordae attach to the ventricular surfaces of the leaflets between the margin and the annulus.

MITRAL VALVE DISEASE

Mitral valve disease is broadly categorized as primary or secondary. Primary disease results from lesions that directly alter the anatomy of the valve complex. It includes conditions such as myxomatous degeneration, endocarditis, rheumatic disease, and papillary muscle rupture. Secondary disease results from lesions that distort LV geometry, primarily as a consequence of LV dilation.

Regardless of the cause, MR results from leaflet dysfunction. The Carpentier classification of leaflet dysfunction is shown in Fig. 25.2.[23] The relationship between lesions of the valve complex and leaflet dysfunction is usefully characterized using the concept of the mitral trapezoid (Fig. 25.3).

DEGENERATIVE (MYXOMATOUS) DISEASE

Degenerative disease is the most common form of mitral valve disease in developed countries and encompasses a spectrum of pathology from fibroelastic deficiency to Barlow disease.[24,25] Fibroelastic deficiency is characterized by thin, delicate leaflet tissue that is relatively deficient in mucopolysaccharides, collagen, and elastic fibers. There is little excess leaflet tissue, and the disease process is usually localized to a single leaflet segment. MR results from leaflet flail due to chordal rupture. The posterior leaflet is affected more commonly than the anterior leaflet, and P2 is affected more commonly than P1 or P3. Noninvolved segments are morphologically normal, and the mitral annulus is typically only mildly dilated.[26]

Barlow disease is a generalized process characterized by an excess of thickened, redundant leaflet tissue and elongated primary chordae. Typically, there is marked annular dilation, which is maximal along the commissural axis.[27] Annular dynamics are blunted, with diminished systolic shortening and folding compared with normal function.[26] Histologically, there is an accumulation of glycosaminoglycans in the extracellular matrix, a process called *myxomatous degeneration*.[28] MR primarily results from leaflet prolapse, which may involve multiple segments. Leaflet flail can also occur after rupture of primary chordae. Mitral clefts or deep posterior scallops are associated with Barlow disease, and they can contribute to MR.

Barlow disease may occur in isolation or in association with genetically mediated systemic diseases such as Marfan syndrome.[28] Barlow disease is also associated with hypertrophic cardiomyopathy, bicuspid aortic valve, and dystrophic calcification.[29,30] Myxomatous degeneration of the tricuspid valve occurs in 40% to 50% of patients with Barlow disease.[31] Advanced Barlow disease is commonly associated with mitral annular disjunction, in which there is a wide separation between the LV shoulder and the posterior annulus.[32] Mitral annular disjunction is associated with ventricular arrhythmias and sudden death.[33,34]

The terminology used to describe degenerative disease is somewhat confusing and reflects the overlapping spectrum of pathology. The terms *fibroelastic deficiency* and *Barlow disease* are widely used in the surgical community. The term *myxomatous mitral valve disease* is often used synonymously with *degenerative disease*. The two features of degenerative disease that are important in terms of surgical repair are the distribution of disease (e.g., single segment, multiple segments, bileaflet involvement) and the amount of redundant leaflet tissue. The terms *Barlow disease* and *fibroelastic deficiency* capture these distinctions and are used throughout this chapter.

Successful repair of degenerative disease is possible in most patients. Rates of successful repair approach 100% for isolated posterior leaflet flail.[11] Repair rates are lower in cases of complex anterior leaflet or bileaflet disease, although successful repair rates in excess of 90% have been reported from high-volume centers.[3,8,10]

INFECTIVE ENDOCARDITIS

Endocarditis of native heart valves usually occurs in the context of underlying valve disease, which for the mitral valve is typically rheumatic or degenerative. Endocarditis is also associated with diabetes, renal failure, immunosuppression, and prosthetic devices such as pacing wires. Vegetations, the characteristic lesion of endocarditis, arise from the deposition of fibrin and platelets at a site of endocardial injury, which subsequently becomes infected

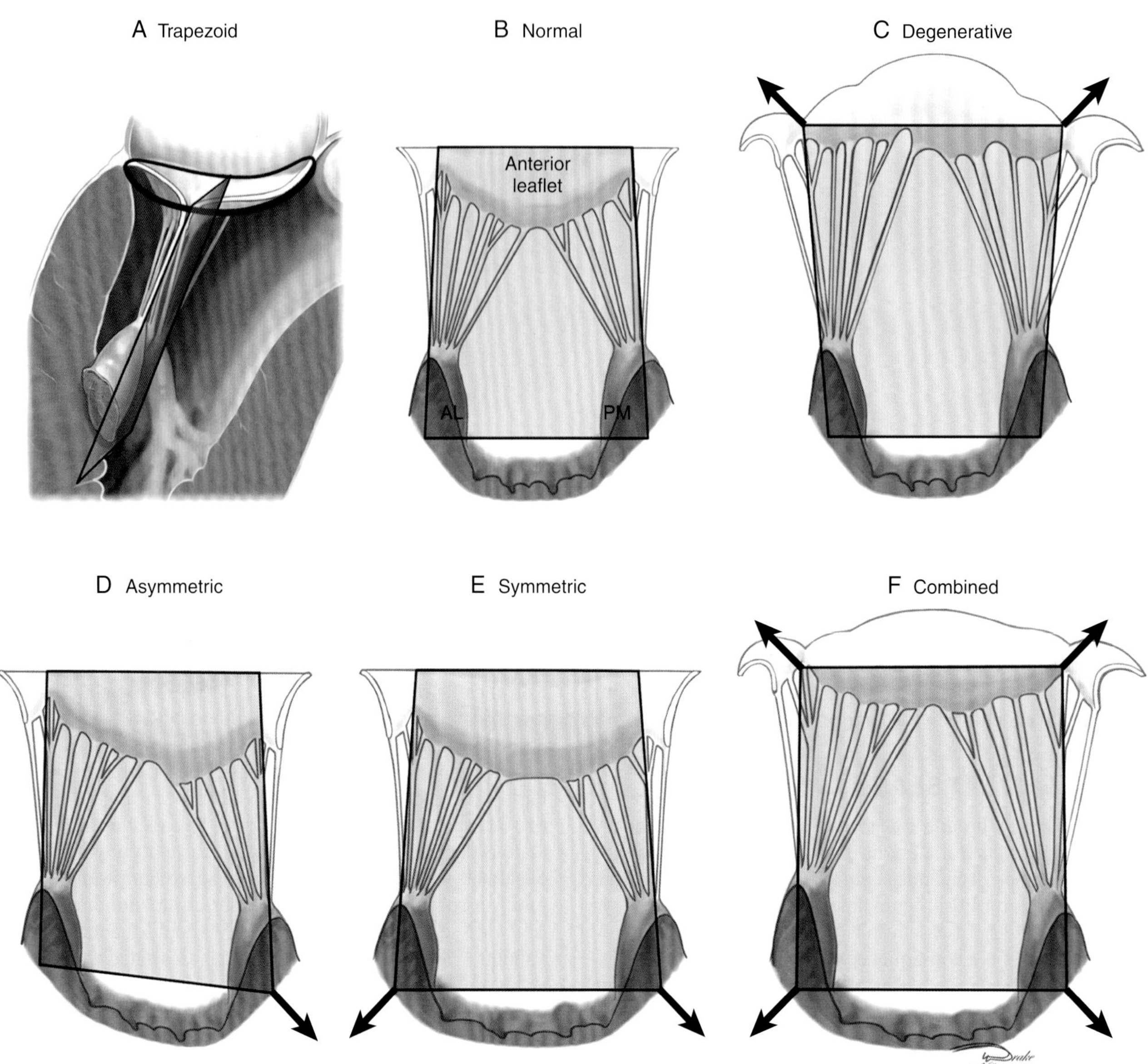

Fig. 25.3 The mitral trapezoid. The relationship between valvular and subvalvular lesions and subsequent leaflet dysfunction can be characterized by the concept of the mitral trapezoid. Distortion of the trapezoid exemplifies disease-specific lesions that result in leaflet dysfunction. The concept of the subvalvular trapezoid is helpful for understanding mitral pathoanatomy and planning surgical intervention. (A and B) The normal trapezoid. The mitral trapezoid is defined by four points in a single plane: (1) the anterolateral commissure, (2) the posteromedial commissure, (3) the base of the anterolateral papillary muscle *(AL)*, and (4) the base of the posteromedial papillary muscle *(PM)*. The vertical sides of the trapezoid extend from the bases of the papillary muscles to the commissures. Superiorly, the horizontal side of the trapezoid is defined as a line that traverses the annulus between the two commissures (the mid-commissural annular width). Inferiorly, the horizontal line of the trapezoid extends between the bases of the papillary muscles (the interpapillary distance). (C) Degenerative disease (Barlow type) results in annular enlargement and elongation of the subvalvular apparatus. The interpapillary distance is usually normal, but the mid-commissural width is typically markedly increased. Mitral regurgitation results from excessive leaflet motion (Carpentier type II dysfunction). (D) Asymmetric secondary disease. Lateral and apical displacement of the posteromedial papillary muscle results in an increased interpapillary muscle distance with little or no elongation of the subvalvular apparatus. Annular enlargement is modest, and the mid-commissural width is not significantly increased. Leaflet motion is restricted asymmetrically in systole (Carpentier type IIIb dysfunction). (E) Symmetric secondary disease. Lateral and apical displacement of both papillary muscles results in a greatly increased interpapillary distance and reduced shortening of the interpapillary distance during systole. There is little or no elongation of the subvalvular apparatus. The mid-commissural width is often substantially increased. Leaflet motion is restricted symmetrically in systole (Carpentier type IIIb dysfunction). (F) Combined degenerative and secondary disease. Degenerative disease results in annular enlargement and elongation of the subvalvular apparatus that initially displaces the leaflets substantially above the plane of the annulus (Carpentier type II dysfunction). Subsequent ventricular dilation causes lateral and apical displacement of the papillary muscles and restricts leaflet motion (Carpentier type IIIb dysfunction). The net effect is to return the leaflets back to the plane of the annulus (Carpentier type I dysfunction). Typically, this combination results in enlargement of the mid-commissural width and the interpapillary distance.

with microorganisms circulating in the blood. Staphylococci and streptococci are the most common causative agents, accounting for 80% of cases.[35] MR results from leaflet perforation or chordal rupture, which often occurs at the site of attachment of vegetations. Abscesses and fistulas to surrounding structures can develop.

Valve repair is possible for most patients with mitral valve endocarditis and is associated with low mortality rates and high rates of freedom from reoperation.[36,37] Valve replacement is required when leaflet destruction is extensive or in the setting of abscesses or fistulas.

RHEUMATIC DISEASE

Rheumatic heart disease remains the most common cause of valvular heart disease in developing nations; it is less common in developed nations but is still responsible for about 20% of valvular heart disease cases.[38] In Europe, rheumatic heart disease is responsible for approximately 85% of cases of mitral stenosis and 15% of cases of MR.[39] Rheumatic disease leads to thickening, fibrosis, and calcification of the leaflets and subvalvular structures. Mitral stenosis typically results from commissural fusion, whereas MR results from leaflet and chordal retraction.

Surgical repair of rheumatic MR is challenging and is not possible in many patients, and valve replacement is commonly indicated. However, in selected patients, repair results in 80% to 90% long-term freedom from reoperation.[40]

RADIATION NECROSIS

Radiation-induced valvular dysfunction typically manifests 10 to 20 years after mediastinal irradiation.[41] Mitral valve dysfunction results from thickening, retraction, and calcification of leaflets and subvalvular apparatus. Associated abnormalities include restrictive cardiomyopathy, calcification of the great vessels, coronary stenosis, pericardial constriction, conduction abnormalities, and pulmonary fibrosis. If surgery is indicated, valve replacement is usually required.

DYSTROPHIC CALCIFICATION

Dystrophic calcification, also known as mitral annular calcification, is common in elderly patients; its risk factors are similar to those of atherosclerosis.[42] Calcification primarily involves the annulus but can extend into the bodies of the leaflets. Dystrophic calcification does not usually cause hemodynamically significant mitral valve dysfunction, but it does complicate surgery for other indications, notably degenerative disease.[43]

PAPILLARY MUSCLE RUPTURE

Papillary muscle rupture arises as a consequence of myocardial infarction. Rupture usually involves the posteromedial muscle because of its sole blood supply from the RCA. Complete rupture of a papillary muscle causes torrential bileaflet regurgitation. Urgent surgery, usually involving mitral valve replacement, is mandatory.[1] Partial rupture, which involves a single papillary muscle head, typically causes severe (but not torrential) unileaflet regurgitation. For cases of partial rupture, surgery can often be delayed, and valve repair is usually possible.

SECONDARY REGURGITATION

Secondary MR can arise from atrial fibrillation, decreased LV systolic function, and increased LV systolic function. All three are ventricular cardiomyopathies.

MR resulting from atrial fibrillation is known as atrial functional MR. Patients with chronic atrial fibrillation develop enlarged atria. Atrial enlargement or loss of atrial contraction is not sufficient to cause MR. Systolic annular contraction is linked to ventricular contraction.[44] Atrial functional MR results from subtle impairment of ventricular dynamics adjacent to the mitral annulus.[45] Echocardiographically, atrial functional MR appears as isolated annular enlargement. Compensatory leaflet area adaptation eventually becomes insufficient.[46] Systolic LV dimensions and function are preserved, and there is no leaflet tethering. Atrial functional MR is classified as Carpentier type I dysfunction (i.e., normal leaflet motion).

The mechanism of secondary MR associated with decreased LV function is LV dilation. LV dilation causes lateral and apical displacement of the papillary muscles, which results in leaflet tethering in systole.[47,48] This leads to Carpentier type IIIb dysfunction (i.e., leaflet motion restricted in systole).

The relationship between LV dilation and MR is complex. MR is more common after inferior and posterior infarction than after anterior infarction, despite greater ventricular dilation with the latter.[49,50] This apparent anomaly may be explained by regional differences in myocardial function affecting the orientation of the papillary muscles to each other and to the valve leaflets. In particular, an increased interpapillary distance and reduced systolic shortening of the interpapillary distance have been implicated as mechanisms of secondary MR that are independent of the severity of LV dilation.[48] Annular dilation is a consistent finding.[51,52] Adaptive remodeling of the leaflet area and chordae tendineae eventually becomes insufficient, leading to MR.[53]

Two patterns of leaflet tethering are recognized: asymmetric and symmetric. Asymmetric tethering is the most common form and typically results from localized remodeling of the basal inferior or inferolateral LV wall after inferior or posterior infarction, with resultant lateral displacement of the posteromedial papillary muscle. Posterior leaflet tethering is more marked than anterior leaflet tethering, and P3 is more severely affected than P1 or P2.[13,54] Distortion of the anterior leaflet also occurs, mainly caused by increased tension due to secondary chordae originating from the posteromedial papillary muscle. Annular dilation is asymmetric and is most marked along the anteroposterior axis. Ventricular dimensions and LV ejection fraction (LVEF) may be relatively normal.[54,55]

In contrast, symmetric tethering results from global LV dilation, most commonly caused by dilated cardiomyopathy or global remodeling after a large (usually anterior) myocardial infarction.[53,54] Apical and lateral displacement of both papillary muscles occurs with symmetric annular dilation.[56] The LV typically demonstrates marked spherical enlargement, and LVEF is usually severely reduced.[57] Symmetric leaflet tethering can also occur in patients with degenerative disease when spherical LV enlargement arises as a consequence of chronic severe MR.

There are seemingly conflicting data on the role of surgical repair for treating secondary MR. In a small randomized trial of patients with severe ischemic regurgitation, repair with a simple reductive ring annuloplasty was associated with increased recurrence of moderate or severe regurgitation compared with valve replacement (32% vs. 2.3%, $P < 0.001$).[58] Image guidance was not used in this study. Nonetheless, the investigators were able to demonstrate that for durable repairs, reverse remodeling was superior to replacement.[59]

Challenging data were offered from the Surgical Treatment for Ischemic Heart Failure trial, which compared coronary revascularization, coronary revascularization plus ventricular reconstruction, and medical therapy in patients with a low LVEF.[60] Among the 1460 patients randomized to coronary revascularization, 234 also underwent mitral valve surgery, which involved mitral valve repair in 94% of cases. Mitral valve surgery performed at the time of coronary revascularization was associated with significantly improved short- and long-term survival. Part of the difficulty with these data is that reductive annuloplasty, the only widely accepted repair technique at the time, is associated with early failure when leaflet tethering is severe.[55,61,62]

The Cardiovascular Assessment of MitraClip Percutaneous Therapy for Heart Failure Patients with Functional Mitral Regurgitation (COAPT) trial[62a] used detailed TEE imaging before enrollment to limit patient selection to those with valve anatomy suitable for durable percutaneous edge-to-edge repair. Using image guidance, they achieved a 95% rate of freedom from recurrent MR at 12 months and improved survival at 24 months.

These three trials demonstrate that durable repair in suitable patients improves ventricular remodeling and prolongs survival in patients with severe secondary MR. The trials also demonstrate that detailed image guidance is mandatory. Echocardiography-guided patient selection and more complex repair techniques can overcome the high failure rate for repair of secondary regurgitation.[3–5]

Secondary MR can arise from dynamic LV outflow tract (LVOT) obstruction in patients with hypertrophic cardiomyopathy or isolated asymmetric septal hypertrophy.[63–65] The main mechanism of regurgitation is septal hypertrophy causing systolic anterior motion (SAM), in which the anterior mitral leaflet is entrained into the LVOT (see Chapter 13). However, some patients with hypertrophic cardiomyopathy develop LVOT obstruction and severe MR in the absence of septal hypertrophy. Mechanisms of MR in this circumstance include an elongated anterior mitral leaflet, abnormal chordal attachments, and a bifid papillary muscle.[66] Mitral valve repair with or without myectomy is typically indicated.

Distinct from hypertrophic cardiomyopathy, *asymmetric septal hypertrophy* refers to isolated hypertrophy of the basal anterior septum. The condition is associated with increased age, hypertension, diabetes, aortic stenosis, and dystrophic calcification.[65] Asymmetric septal hypertrophy typically requires no surgical intervention but predisposes to postoperative SAM in patients undergoing repair for degenerative disease.

TRANSESOPHAGEAL IMAGING OF THE MITRAL VALVE

STANDARD MULTIPLANE IMAGING

For two-dimensional (2D) imaging, knowledge of the expected anatomic-echocardiographic relationships helps identify the correct leaflet segments. Expected segmental relationships for standard multiplane TEE views are demonstrated in Fig. 25.4.

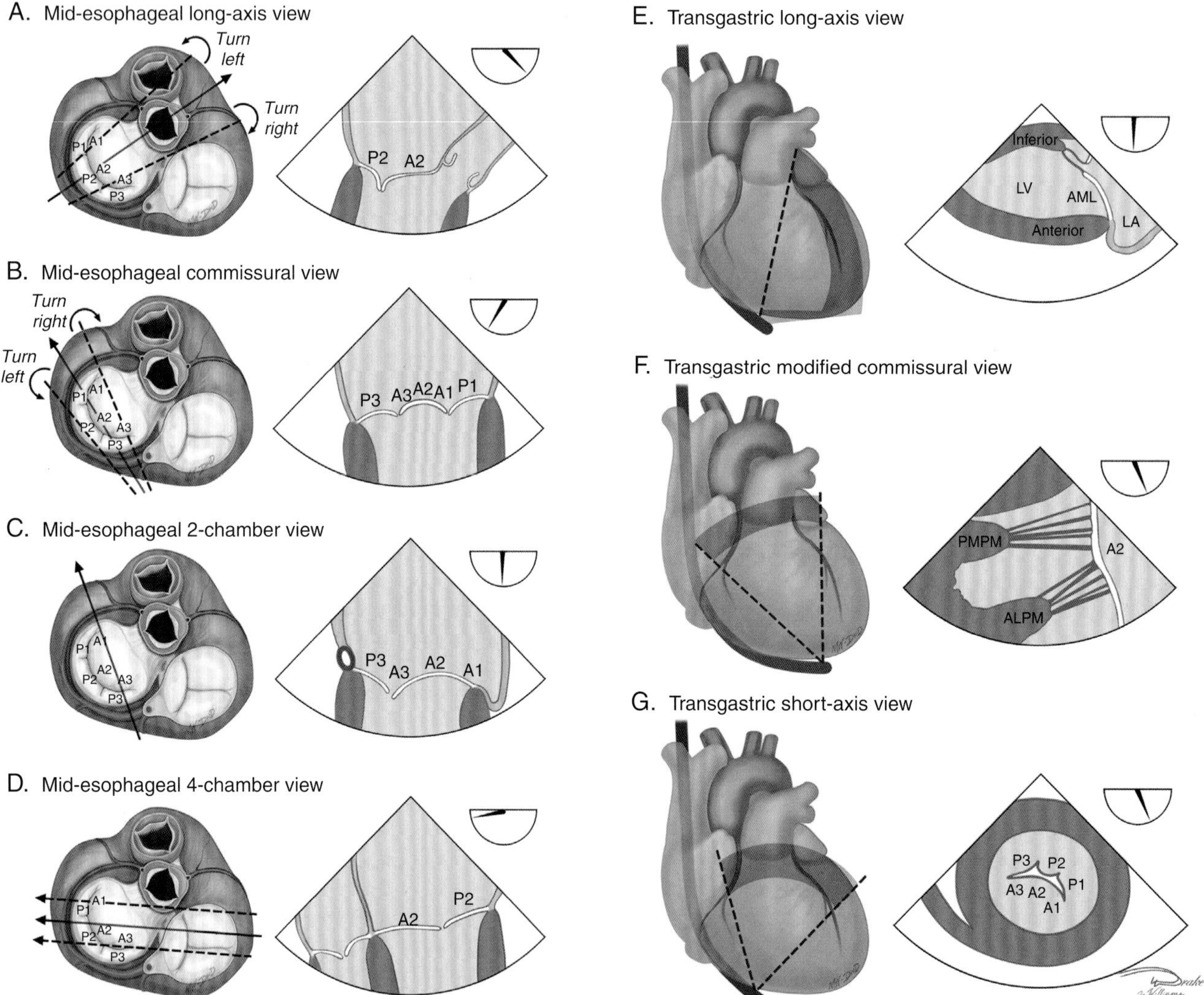

Fig. 25.4 Standard 2D TEE views for assessing the mitral valve. *Solid lines* indicate the expected positions of the scan planes in different views. (A and B) In the mid-esophageal long-axis and commissural positions, *dashed lines* indicate the effect of turning the probe left (counterclockwise) or right (clockwise) from the standard positions. Use of the landmarks described in Fig. 25.8 ensures that the long-axis view reliably visualizes the A2/P2 coaptive surface and the commissural view visualizes the A1/P1 and A3/P3 coaptive surfaces. (C and D) The mid-esophageal 2- and 4-chamber views are demonstrated. In the 2-chamber view, the coronary sinus can be seen adjacent to the base of the posterior leaflet and the left atrial appendage can be seen near the base of the anterior leaflet. In the 4-chamber view, *dashed lines* indicate the effect of withdrawing/anteflexing or advancing/retroflexing the probe from the standard position. As seen in Figure 25.5, the 2- and 4- chamber views are not aligned with the axes of the valve. This makes correct identification of the mitral leaflet segments less reliable. (E and F) The transgastric long-axis and commissural views identify the same segments as their corresponding mid-esophageal views. Note that the posterior papillary muscle is closest to the probe in the transgastric commissural view. (G) All six segments can be identified in the transgastric short-axis view. *ALPM*, Anterolateral papillary muscle; *AML*, anterior mitral leaflet; *LAA*, LA appendage; *PMPM*, posteromedial papillary muscle. (Courtesy David Sidebotham, Auckland City Hospital, Auckland, NZ.)

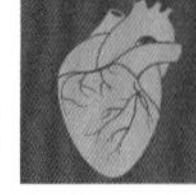

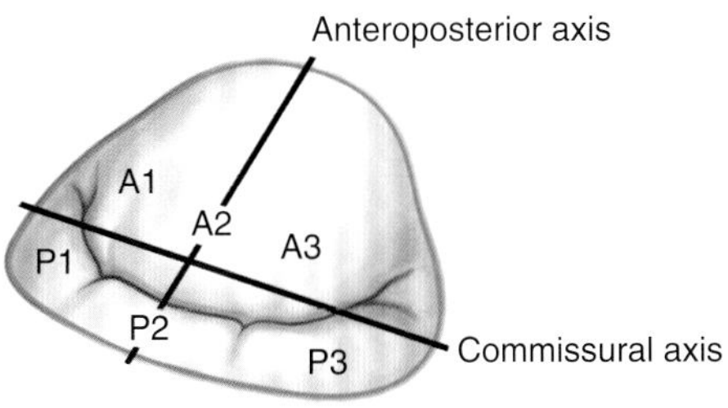

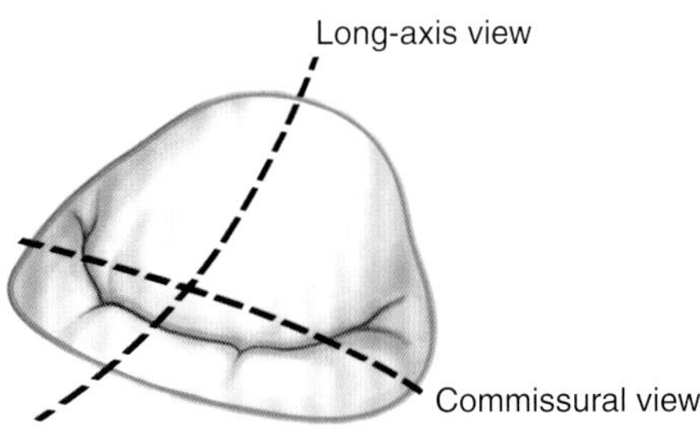

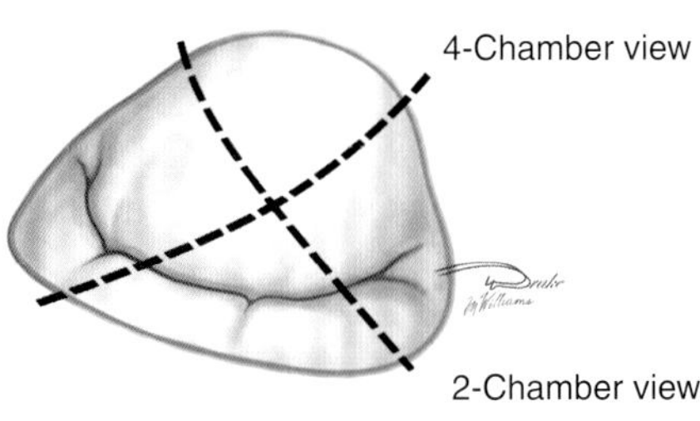

Fig. 25.5 Cross-sectional imaging of the mitral valve. The image planes of the mid-esophageal long-axis, commissural, 4-chamber, and 2-chamber views are indicated. When correctly positioned, the long-axis and commissural views are perpendicular to each other and are aligned, respectively, with the anteroposterior and commissural axes of the valve. By contrast, the 4- and 2-chamber views are oblique to the axes of the valve. Consequently, measurements of annular dimensions and leaflet distortion obtained in the 4- and 2-chamber views are less useful than those obtained in long-axis and commissural views.

The mid-esophageal long-axis and commissural views run parallel to the axes of the valve and are therefore the most important imaging planes for quantifying segmental mitral pathology (Fig. 25.5). The long-axis view is parallel to the anteroposterior axis, and when the image plane passes through the center of the valve, it visualizes the P2/A2 coaptive surface. Turning the probe counterclockwise (left) moves the sector scan toward the anterolateral commissure, visualizing P1/A1. Turning the probe clockwise (right) moves the sector scan toward the posteromedial commissure, visualizing P3/A3. The commissural view is perpendicular to the long-axis view and runs parallel to the commissural axis, traversing the curved coaptation line twice. When the commissural view runs through the center of the valve, the P3/A3 coaptive surface is visualized on the left, and the A1/P1 coaptive surface is visualized on the right.

In the mid-esophageal 4- and 2-chamber views, imaging is oblique to the axes of the valve. Consequently, these views are less useful for quantifying segmental pathology.

Even with careful 2D multiplane imaging, it can be difficult to be confident about which leaflet segments are visualized in a particular view. In one study in which a sequence of standard mid-esophageal views were shown to experienced anesthesiologists, overall accuracy of leaflet segment identification was only 30%.[68] In the mid-esophageal long-axis view, the A2/P2 segments were correctly identified 70% of the time, whereas the A1/P1 and A3/P3 segments were identified 14% and 6% of the time, respectively. Correct identification of leaflet segments occurred 92% of the time in the commissural view. The main reason for low accuracy in the long-axis view is lack of obvious anatomic landmarks (Fig. 25.6). The technique of axial imaging has been introduced to overcome these limitations.[3]

PRINCIPLES OF AXIAL IMAGING

Mathematically, the mitral annulus approximates a hyperbolic paraboloid[17] with three orthogonal axes: anteroposterior (x-axis), commissural (y-axis), and vertical (z-axis). The mitral–LV apex axis is defined as a line running from the LV apex to the center of the valve, approximately parallel to the z-axis (Fig. 25.7).[3] When the commissural and long-axis views are perpendicular to each other and intersect at the mitral–LV apex axis, the image planes reliably visualize the expected leaflet segments shown in Fig. 25.4A and B. Imaging parallel to the mitral–LV apex axis ensures that the resultant image planes are perpendicular to the annulus and that subsequent measurements are not distorted by oblique orientation. The landmarks for 2D and 3D axial acquisition and the appearance of common mitral valve diseases seen in these views are shown in Fig. 25.8.

3D IMAGING

For 3D imaging, wide-sector (full-volume) and focused wide-sector (zoom) modes should be used.[15,67] Axial 2D long-axis and commissural views should be used as the regions of interest for 3D acquisition. The sector dimensions should be adjusted to include the entire annulus, leaflets, and part of the aortic valve throughout the cardiac cycle. Single-beat acquisition is appropriate for standard 3D imaging. To prevent an unacceptably low frame rate, multibeat acquisition should be used with 3D color Doppler imaging. The valve should be displayed from the atrial aspect in the so-called surgical orientation (i.e., with the aortic valve positioned directly above the mitral valve in the 12-o'clock position).[3,15,67,68] This orientation displays all mitral segments simultaneously and facilities unambiguous communication between the echocardiographer and the surgeon. Additional information may be obtained by displaying the valve from the LV aspect. The mitral valve should be oriented so that the aortic valve is displayed in the 12-o'clock position.

Quantitative analysis of 3D data sets using multiplanar reconstruction allows indices of leaflet distortion (e.g., prolapse height, tenting height, closing angles) to be measured accurately and reproducibly in the long-axis and commissural views. The technique of post-acquisition analysis of 3D data sets and the elimination of parallax are described in Figs. 25.9 and 25.10, respectively. Volumetric analysis of the LV using full-volume data sets is also useful for confirming the cause and severity of mitral valve disease, particularly for patients with secondary disease.

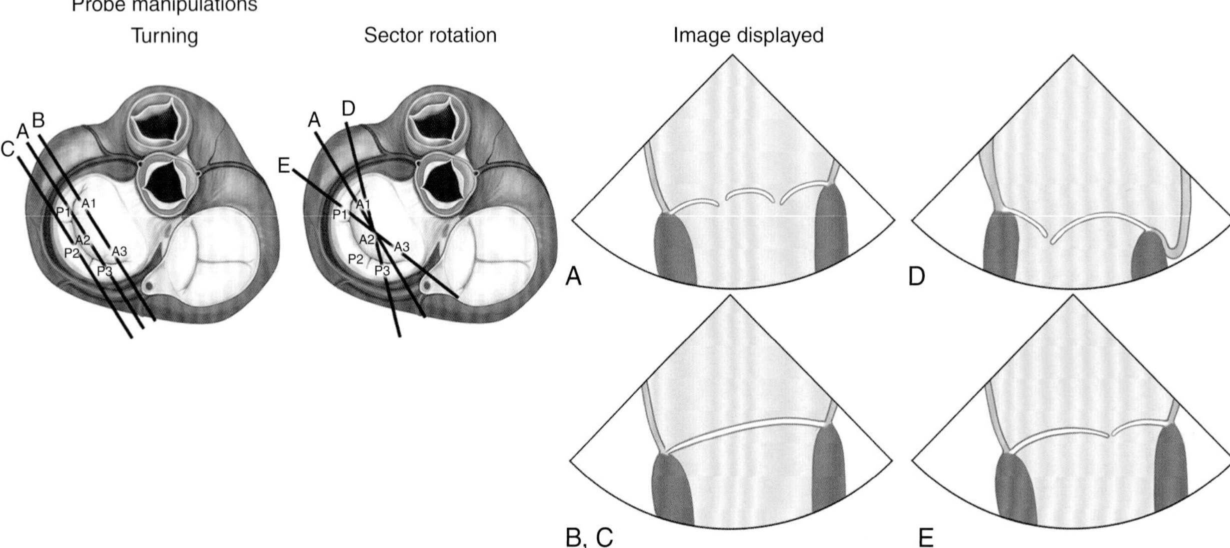

Fig. 25.6 Landmarks for imaging in the mid-esophageal long-axis view. Mid-esophageal long-axis and commissural views are demonstrated. For the long-axis view, turning the probe or adjusting sector rotation from the standard positions results in minimal change in the displayed image but important changes in which mitral segments are being interrogated. For the commissural view, turning the probe or adjusting the sector rotation from the standard positions results in changes to the displayed images coincident with changes in the displayed mitral segments. The technique of axial imaging helps overcome ambiguity in the long-axis view. The scan plane labels (A through E) correspond to the displayed images on the right. (Modified from Sidebotham DA, Allen SJ, Gerber IL, Fayers T. Intraoperative transesophageal echocardiography for surgical repair of mitral regurgitation. *J Am Soc Echocardiogr.* 2014;27:345–366.)

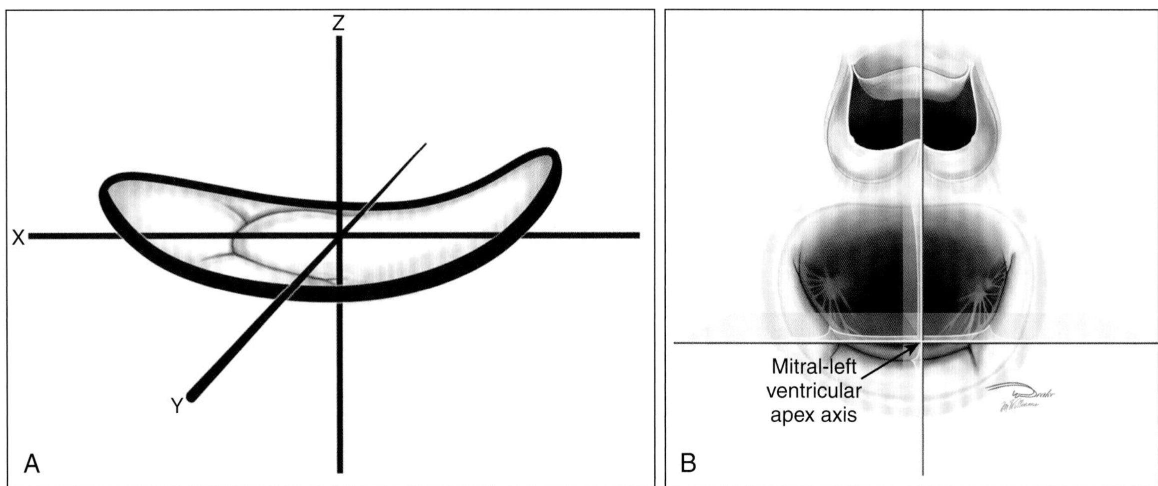

Fig. 25.7 Axes of the mitral valve. (A) Three axes of the annulus. The mitral annulus resembles a hyperbolic paraboloid (riding saddle), with three orthogonal axes; anteroposterior (x-axis), commissural (y-axis), and vertical (z-axis). (B) The mitral–LV apex axis. The mitral–LV axis is the line passing from the LV apex to the center of the valve at the point of intersection between the anteroposterior (x-z) and commissural (y-z) planes. Imaging parallel or perpendicular to the mitral–LV apex axis minimizes geometric distortion from oblique orientation. Imaging along the anteroposterior plane visualizes the A2/P2 coaptive surface; imaging along the commissural plane visualizes the A1/P1 and A3/P3 coaptive surfaces. Using the axial imaging technique described in Fig. 25.8, the mid-esophageal long-axis view is aligned with the anteroposterior plane, and the mid-esophageal commissural view is aligned with the commissural plane. (B, From Drake DH, Zimmerman KG, Hepner AM, Nichols CD. Echo-guided mitral repair. *Circ Cardiovasc Imaging.* 2014;7:132–141.)

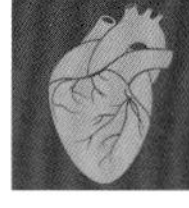

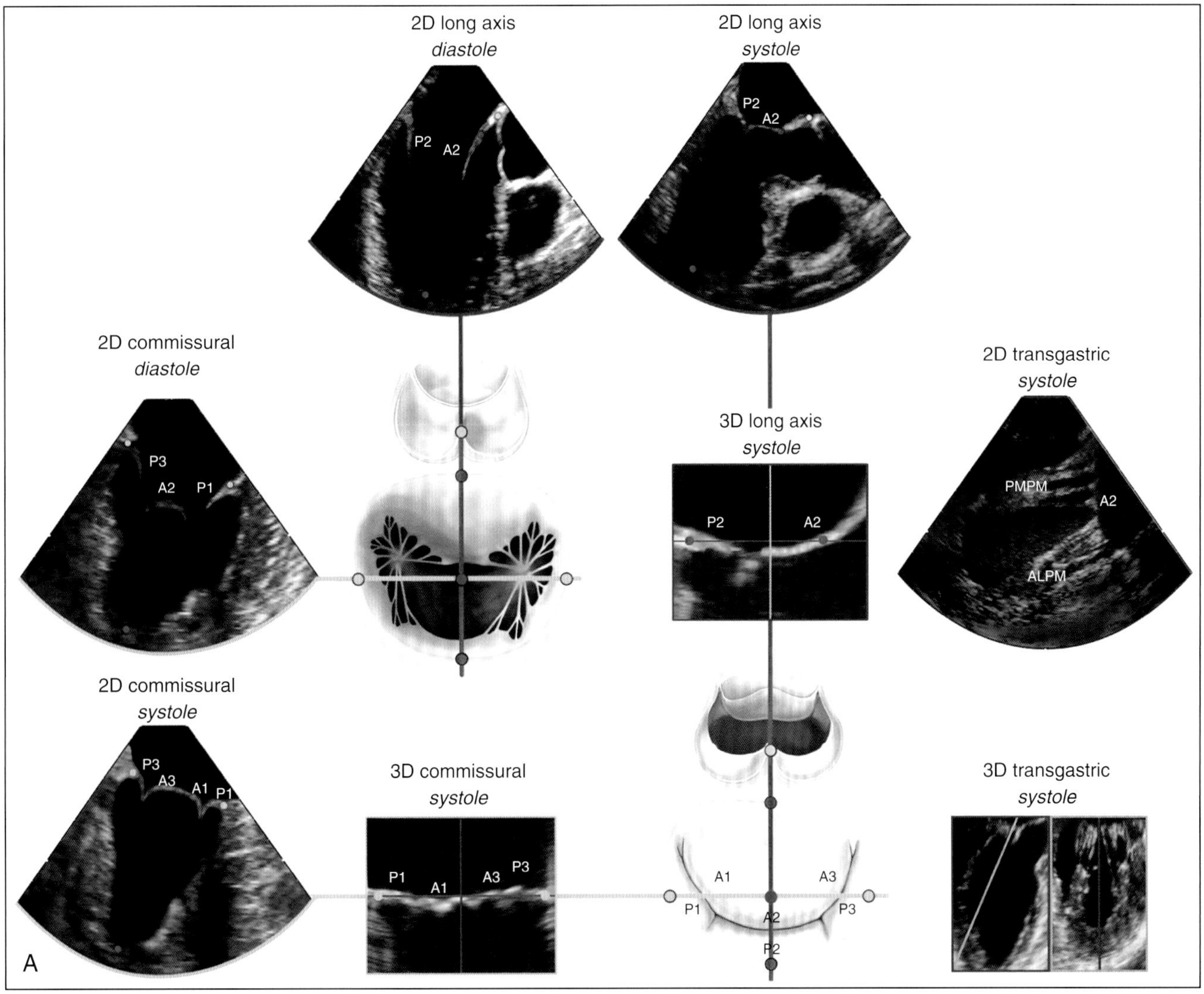

Fig. 25.8 Image acquisition for axial imaging of the mitral valve and examples of common mitral pathologies. (A) Image acquisition for 2D and 3D axial imaging. The 2D multiplane images are shown as gray-scale pyramidal sectors. Landmarks for axial imaging are obtained from diastolic frames. The diastolic landmarks ensure that the long-axis and commissural views are parallel to the mitral–LV apex and perpendicular to each other in systole, which is when measurements are made. Diastolic landmarks for the long-axis view are (1) the commissure between the left and noncoronary leaflets of the aortic valve *(yellow dot)*, (2) the maximum anteroposterior annular width *(red dots)*, and (3) the apex of the LV *(blue dot)*. Diastolic landmarks for the commissural view are (1) the free-floating central A2 segment, (2) the maximum annular width *(green dots)*, and (3) the apex of the LV *(blue dot)*. Measurements of annular dimensions and leaflet distortion are then made from systolic frames. In systole, the long-axis view demonstrates the anteroposterior axis, the A2 and P2 segments, and the A2/P2 coaptive surface. In systole, the commissural view demonstrates the commissural axis, the A1, P1, A3, and P3 segments, and the A1/P1 and A3/P3 coaptive surface surfaces. It is important that all landmarks remain within view throughout the cardiac cycle. Each gray-scale acquisition is followed by an acquisition using color flow Doppler of approximately the same cycle length. Without moving the probe, the zoom function is used to acquire axial 2D and color images focusing on the mitral apparatus. The landmarks for 3D acquisition are the same as for standard multiplane imaging. The initial 3D data sets are acquired using full-volume mode with and without color Doppler imaging. Without moving the probe, additional 3D data sets are acquired using zoom mode, again with and without color Doppler imaging. 3D data sets are then analyzed using multiplanar reconstruction to obtain 2D axial long-axis and commissural images, as described in Fig. 25.9. Systolic frames obtained using multiplanar reconstruction from 3D data sets are shown as rectangular boxes in the figure.

Continued

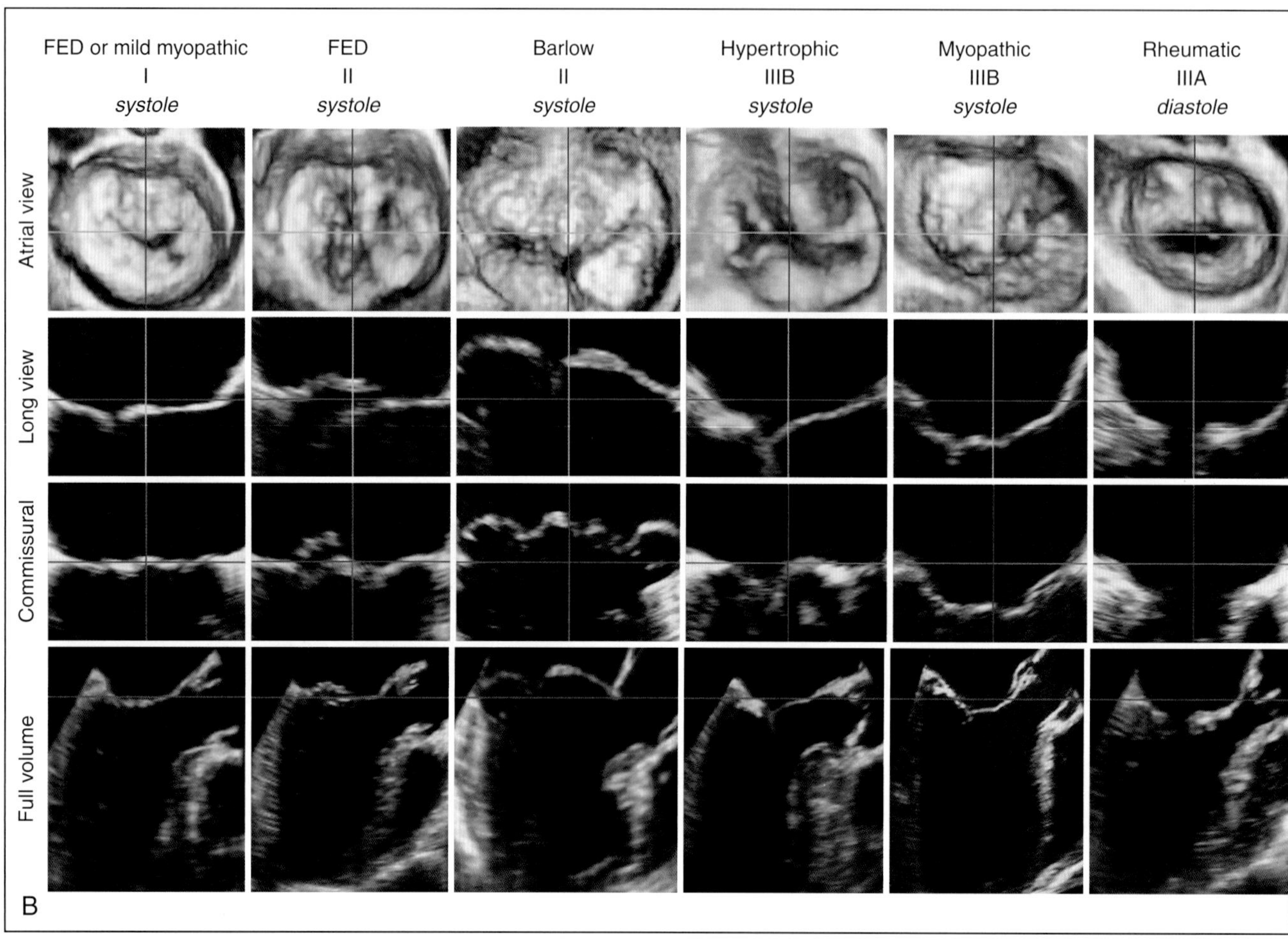

Fig. 25.8, cont'd (B) Axial imaging of common diseases. The images were obtained using quantitative analysis of 3D data sets. Volume-rendered atrial views of the mitral valve are shown in the top row. The middle two rows are mid-esophageal long-axis and commissural views, which were obtained from zoomed 3D data sets using multiplanar reconstruction. The bottom row is a long-axis view that includes the LV apex, obtained from a full-volume 3D data set using multiplanar reconstruction. All frames are obtained in late systole except those demonstrating rheumatic disease, which are late diastolic frames. Column 1 demonstrates normal leaflet motion (Carpentier type I dysfunction) in a patient with atrial function MR or another mild myopathy. There is mild annular dilation and poor central coaptation, best appreciated in the long-axis view. Column 2 demonstrates leaflet flail (Carpentier type II dysfunction) involving the P2 segment in a patient with fibroelastic deficiency (FED). The remaining leaflet tissue, annulus, and LV appear normal. Column 3 demonstrates multisegment prolapse (Carpentier type II dysfunction) in a patient with Barlow disease. Excessive leaflet tissue is evident in all views. The commissural view shows a dramatically enlarged annulus that appears to migrate into the atrium. Concomitant hypertrophy of the basal septum is apparent in the full-volume view. Column 4 is from a patient with hypertrophic cardiomyopathy and systolic anterior motion (SAM) (Carpentier type IIIB dysfunction). SAM and septal hypertrophy are evident in the long-axis view. Column 5 is from a patient with secondary (myopathic) disease resulting in leaflet tethering in systole (Carpentier type IIIB dysfunction). The long-axis and commissural views demonstrate severe bileaflet tethering. The full-volume view shows marked LV dilation. Column 6 is from a patient with rheumatic disease. Leaflet motion is restricted in systole (not shown) and in diastole, consistent with Carpentier type IIIA dysfunction. Leaflet thickening and reduced diastolic leaflet excursion are seen in all views but are most apparent in the long-axis view (see Video 25.8). ALPM, Anterolateral papillary muscle; PMPM, posteromedial papillary muscle. (Modified from Drake DH, Zimmerman KG, Hepner AM, Nichols CD. Echo-guided mitral repair. *Circ Cardiovasc Imaging*. 2014;7:132–141.)

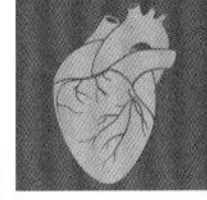

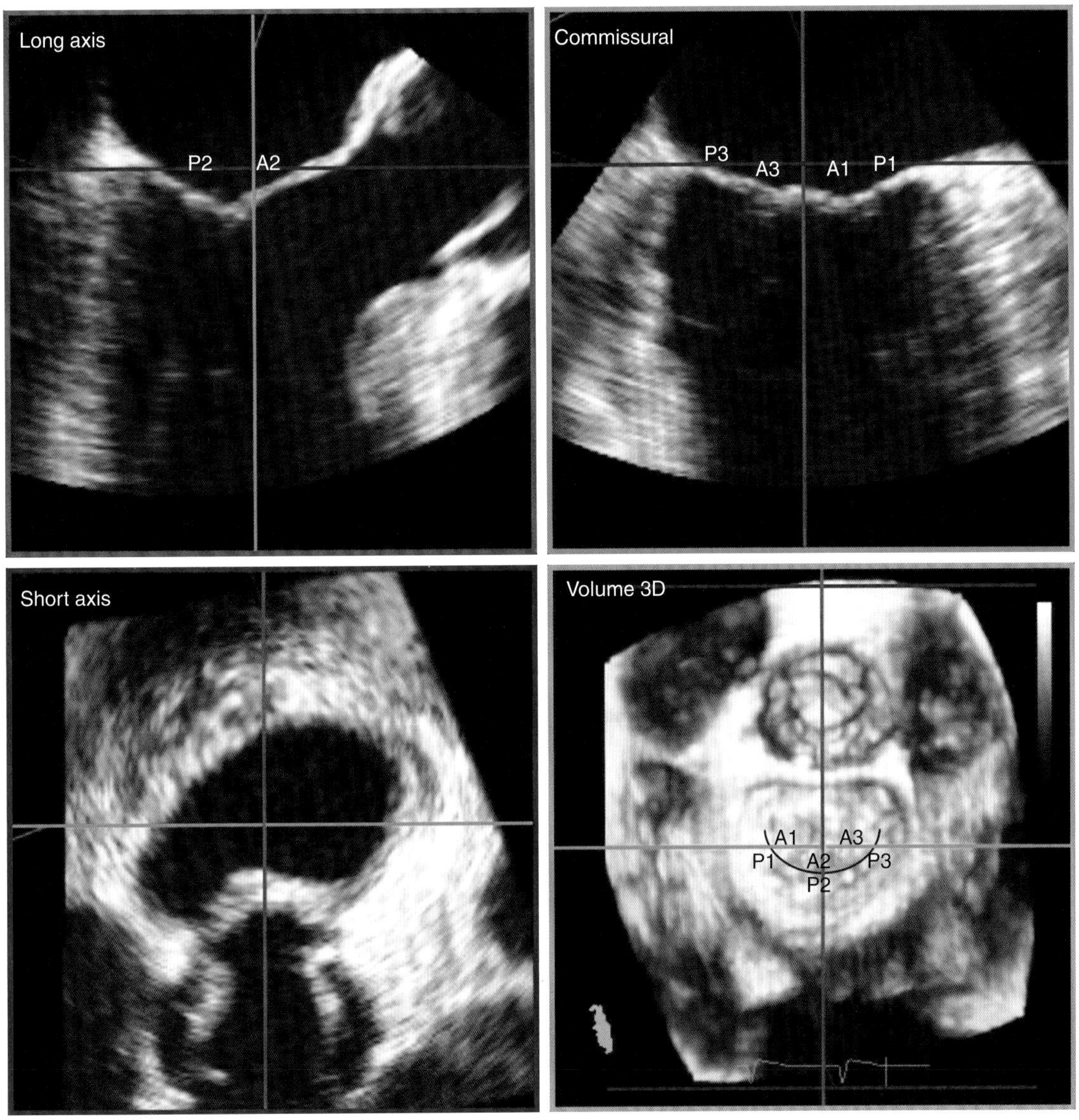

Fig. 25.9 Post-acquisition analysis of axial 3D data sets using multiplanar reconstruction. Full-volume and zoomed 3D data sets should be obtained from axial mid-esophageal long-axis and commissural views, as described in Fig. 25.8. The 3D data sets should then be opened in an analysis package (e.g., 3DQ, Philips Healthcare, Andover, MA), and a late systolic frame should be chosen for analysis. In the zoomed data set shown, three orthogonal 2D slices are demonstrated: the long-axis plane in the top left quadrant *(red box)*, the commissural plane in the top right quadrant *(green box)*, and a short-axis view in the bottom left quadrant *(blue box)*. A volume-rendered view showing all the mitral valve leaflets is presented in the bottom right quadrant. Video 25.9 is a step-by-step guide to analyzing a zoomed 3D data set to obtain long-axis and commissural 2D images. (Courtesy Daniel Drake, Traverse City, MI.)

PRE-REPAIR TEE

Although the timing of surgical intervention for MR is based on the pathophysiology (i.e., regurgitation severity and LV function), the repair procedure is based on the pathoanatomy. The main goals of the pre-repair TEE examination are to determine the mechanisms of MR to identify the anatomic location of the lesions and to quantify leaflet distortion.

The concepts of echocardiography-based pathoanatomic staging of mitral valve disease are presented in Fig. 25.11. Staging facilitates selection of the appropriate repair technique. Quantification of regurgitation is usually less important. The exception is in patients with secondary MR who are scheduled for coronary revascularization. In this situation, MR may not have been accurately quantified or may have changed since earlier assessment.

A comprehensive TEE examination should be performed for all patients according to published guidelines.[15] However, the focus of the examination should be the mitral valve and associated structures, notably the LV and tricuspid valve. The mitral valve should be imaged in all standard views using 2D and color Doppler. 3D imaging from the atrial surface, with and without color Doppler, should also be performed routinely. Annular dimensions and indices of leaflet distortion should be evaluated in axially acquired long-axis and commissural views. Specific findings should be sought according to the underlying disease process.

DEGENERATIVE DISEASE

Leaflet flail or prolapse should be assessed at the three coaptive surfaces (A1/P1, A2/P2, A3/P3) (Table 25.2). With flail, the tip

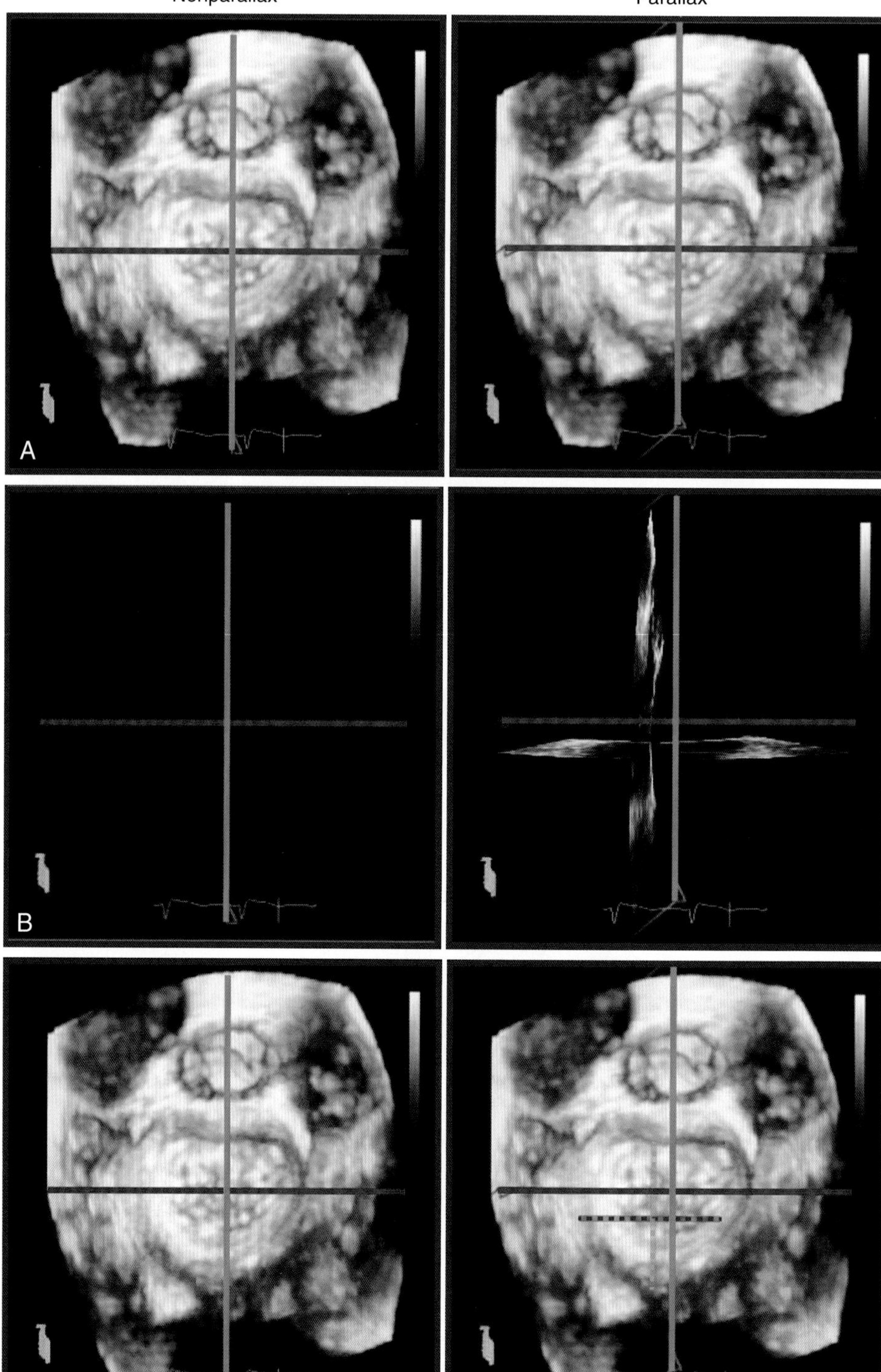

Fig. 25.10 Technique for eliminating parallax. (A) A volume-rendered 3D data set of the mitral valve in the surgical orientation. The pairs of colored reference lines suggest that the long-axis *(green)* and commissural *(red)* planes cross the center of the mitral valve in the correct position; however, the slight perception of depth on the *red* and *green lines* on the right-hand image indicate parallax. (B) The mitral valve using slice mode. The left-hand image is perpendicular to the observer, and there is no parallax. In this circumstance, the 2D planes appear as colored lines with no echo data or depth perception evident. The right-hand image is not perpendicular to the observer, meaning that there is parallax. In this circumstance, the 2D planes demonstrate echo data and a perception of depth. When there is parallax, it is impossible to know where the 2D planes cross the 3D image. (C) The mitral valve in volume mode. *Dashed red and green lines* on the right-hand image indicate the position at which the 2D image planes cross the mitral valve. To eliminate parallax, the position of the long-axis and commissural image planes are adjusted in slice mode so that the echo data disappear and only the *red and green lines* remain (left-hand image) (see Video 25.10). (Courtesy Daniel Drake, Traverse City, MI.)

of the affected leaflet is directed into the left atrium (LA) in systole. Ruptured chordae may be seen extending in the LA in late systole. Prolapse is defined as doming of the body of the leaflet above the annular plane by more than 2 mm.[25] In contrast to flail, the leaflet tip is directed toward the LV, and no ruptured chordae are seen. In practice, a prolapse height of less than 5 mm rarely is associated with significant MR and typically does not require surgical correction. With prolapse and flail, the jet of MR is eccentric and is directed *away* from the affected segment.

It is important to confirm the functional significance of leaflet prolapse because not all prolapsing segments are regurgitant. Close cropping onto the atrial surface of the leaflets with color 3D imaging is useful to confirm the functional significance of prolapsing segments. Associated clefts are most easily

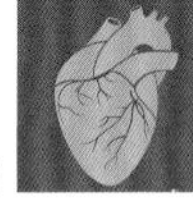

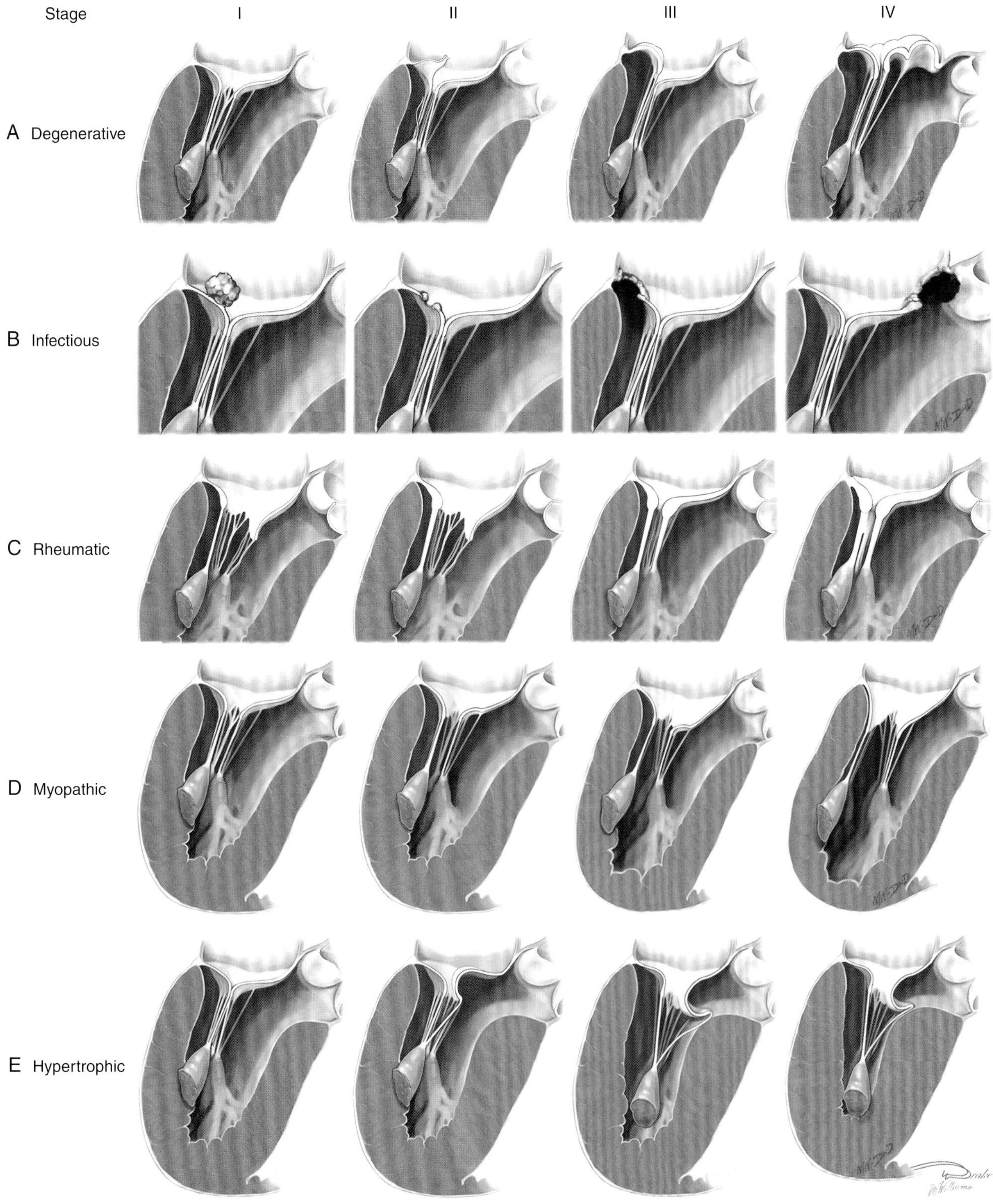

Stage I II III IV

A Degenerative

B Infectious

C Rheumatic

D Myopathic

E Hypertrophic

Fig. 25.11 Staging of mitral valve disease. (A) Degenerative disease. Stages include simple annular dilation (stage I), isolated segmental prolapse/flail (stage II), extensive posterior leaflet prolapse/flail (stage III), and advanced bileaflet disease (stage IV). (B) Infective endocarditis. Stages include simple vegetation without perforation (stage I), isolated leaflet perforation (stage II), annular destruction (stage III), and extensive destruction involving the annulus and fibrous skeleton (stage IV). (C) Rheumatic disease. Stages include isolated posterior leaflet scarring and calcification with minimal chordal and commissural involvement (stage I), extensive leaflet and subvalvular destruction limited to the posterior leaflet (stage II), bileaflet or subvalvular involvement (stage III), and severe commissural fusion and extensive calcification of the leaflets and subvalvular apparatus (stage IV). (D) Secondary (myopathic) disease. Stage I is simple annular dilation, typically from atrial functional MR or another mild myopathy. Stages II to IV represent mild to severe leaflet tethering with progressive distortion of the leaflets and subvalvular apparatus. Indices of leaflet tethering are demonstrated in Fig. 25.14. (E) Hypertrophic cardiomyopathy. Stage I is septal hypertrophy without LV outflow tract obstruction or systolic anterior motion (SAM). Stage II is hypertrophic cardiomyopathy with LV outflow tract obstruction and mitral regurgitation from SAM. Stage III is hypertrophic cardiomyopathy and SAM with significant abnormalities of the mitral leaflets or papillary muscles. Stage IV is hypertrophic cardiomyopathy and SAM with extensive LV hypertrophy extending beyond the LV outflow tract into the LV cavity and apex.

TABLE 25.2 Transesophageal Echocardiographic Assessment for Degenerative Mitral Valve Disease.

Parameter	*Views*	*Implication*
Annular dimensions	2D: ME LAX and commissural views 3D: MPR, LAX, and commissural planes	Severe dilation along commissural axis is highly suggestive of Barlow disease Helps size annuloplasty ring, quantify severity, and confirm cause
Location and severity of prolapse/flail	2D: all standard ME views (see Fig. 25.6); LAX and commissural views are the most useful 3D: en face LA view; MPR, LAX, and commissural planes	Single-segment involvement suggests FED; P2 is the most commonly affected segment Multisegment involvement suggests Barlow disease. Anterior and bileaflet disease are most difficult to successfully repair; required repair guided by TEE findings (see Fig. 25.18A)
Prolapse height in nonflail segment	2D: ME LAX and commissural views 3D: MPR, LAX, and commissural planes	Prolapse < 5 mm above annular plane in late systole rarely requires intervention Correlate with origins of regurgitant jets
Presence of mitral clefts	2D: ME LAX view 3D: en face LA view, including color Doppler with close cropping onto atrial surface; MPR with adjustment of 2D planes to display the defect (see Fig. 25.12)	May need to be repaired as part of surgical procedure
Presence of ventriculo-annular disjunction	2D: ME LAX and commissural views 3D: MPR, LAX, and commissural planes	May need to be repaired as part of surgical procedure
Risk factors for systolic anterior motion	2D: ME LAX view (see Fig. 25.13) 3D: MPR, LAX plane	Increased risk with Barlow disease; minimal risk with FED Increased risk may indicate the need for modification of surgical procedure
Presence and location of valvular calcification	2D: all standard ME views (see Fig. 25.6); specifically include TG two-chamber view for evaluation of subvalvular apparatus	Causes acoustic shadowing Complicates surgical intervention May require surgical debridement
Location, direction, and severity of regurgitant jets	2D + color: ME LAX and commissural views Jet direction away from prolapsing/flail segment(s) Severity quantified by vena contracta width and PISA method (ME LAX view) 3D + color Doppler: en face LA view with close cropping onto LA surface. Severity quantified by vena contracta area using MPR	Jets displaced from coaptation line suggest cleft Complex or multiple jets suggest Barlow disease or clefts Not all prolapsing segments are associated with a regurgitant jet
LV size and function	2D: LVEF from standard ME views 3D: volumetric (parametric) analysis of full volume data sets Can derive volumes, LVEF, and segmental analysis	Severe LV dysfunction indicates increased perioperative risk Likely to deteriorate postoperatively, and preoperative measurements are useful for comparison
Presence and severity of TR	2D: ME 4-chamber view. Severity assessed by vena contracta width	May need concomitant TV surgery (consider if TR > mild or annulus > 4 cm)
Pulmonary artery pressure	2D + CW Doppler: velocity of TR jet (several ME views)	Severe pulmonary hypertension indicates increased perioperative risk Useful when comparing with postoperative function
RV size and function	2D: ME 4-chamber view	Useful when comparing with postoperative function

FED, Fibroelastic deficiency; *LAX*, long-axis; *LVEF*, LV ejection fraction; *ME*, mid-esophageal; *MPR*, multiplanar reconstruction; *PISA*, proximal isovelocity surface area; *TG*, transgastric; *TR*, tricuspid regurgitation; *TV*, tricuspid valve.

recognized in early diastole with 3D imaging from the atrial surface (Fig. 25.12). Close cropping onto the atrial surface with color 3D imaging can confirm the existence of clefts or deep scallops by demonstrating regurgitant jets that are displaced from the coaptation line.

Mitral annular disjunction is most easily recognized in the long-axis and commissural views. Severe mitral annular disjunction (>10 mm) should be discussed with the surgeon because it may require surgical correction. Patients with Barlow disease are at increased risk for postoperative SAM. Risk factors for SAM are demonstrated in Fig. 25.13.[69]

ENDOCARDITIS

The location and size of vegetations should be noted and the mechanism of regurgitation determined (Table 25.3). Vegetations most commonly form on the upstream side (i.e., atrial surface) of the valve. The existence of perforations or significant leaflet destruction should be noted. 3D imaging from the *ventricular* aspect is useful for directly visualizing perforations that are obscured by vegetations when imaging from the atrial aspect. However, 3D imaging from the *atrial* aspect with color Doppler may demonstrate regurgitant jets associated with perforations. A careful search should be made for abscess cavities or fistulous connections. Imaging from nonstandard views, with and without color Doppler, may be necessary to identify fistulas.

RHEUMATIC DISEASE

With rheumatic MR, the likelihood of successful repair is influenced by the amount of freely mobile leaflet tissue and the degree of subvalvular involvement (Table 25.4). A careful assessment of leaflet mobility, leaflet retraction, and valvular calcification is mandatory. Rheumatic MR is often associated with a characteristic rolled-edge appearance to the leaflet tips. Leaflet motion is best assessed in the mid-esophageal long-axis view, whereas the subvalvular apparatus is best seen in the transgastric 2-chamber and mid-esophageal commissural views.

PAPILLARY MUSCLE RUPTURE

With papillary muscle rupture, it is important to identify which papillary muscle is involved, the site of rupture (i.e., base or head of the muscle), and whether rupture is partial or complete. The transgastric 2-chamber and mid-esophageal commissural views are usually best for determining the site and extent of muscle detachment.

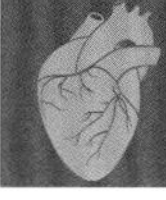

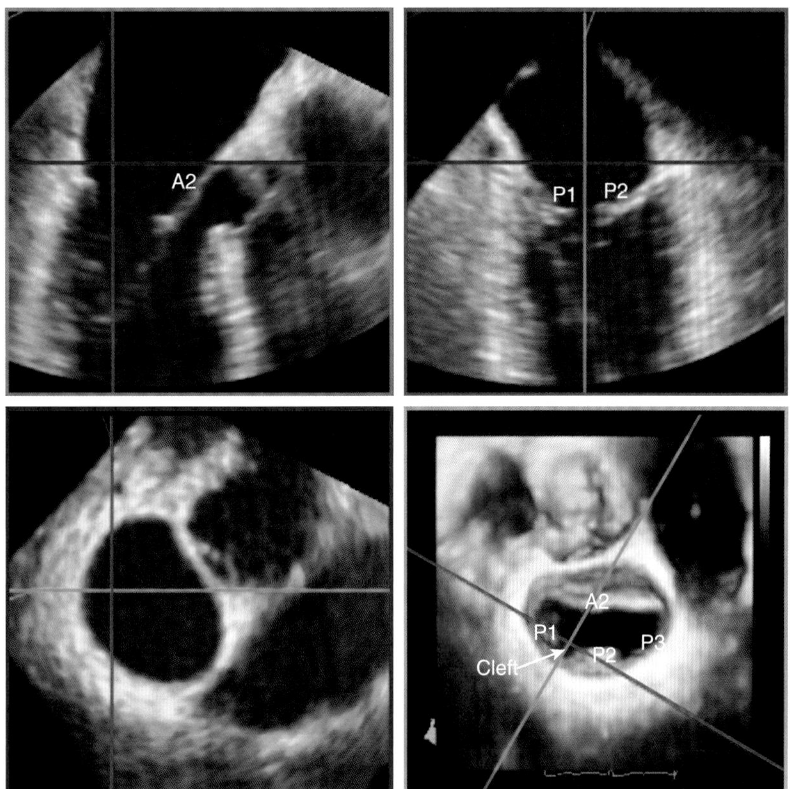

Fig. 25.12 Mitral cleft. Multiplanar reconstruction of an axial 3D data set with elimination of parallax. The 2D cross-sectional views *(green and red boxes)* have been adjusted from the standard long-axis and commissural planes to demonstrate the cleft; their positions can be seen in the volume-rendered view *(bottom right panel)*. Notice that the *green* and *red image planes* are still parallel to the mitral–LV apex axis. A cleft between P1 and P2 can be seen extending to the annulus. Notice the gap between P1 and P2 in the *red box* and the absence of posterior leaflet tissue in the *green box*. The short-axis plane (*blue box*) is located at the level of the commissure between the left and non-coronary leaflets of the aortic valve. In this case, marked regurgitation was seen in this region of the valve with color 3D imaging (not shown). The defect was repaired with simple suture closure.

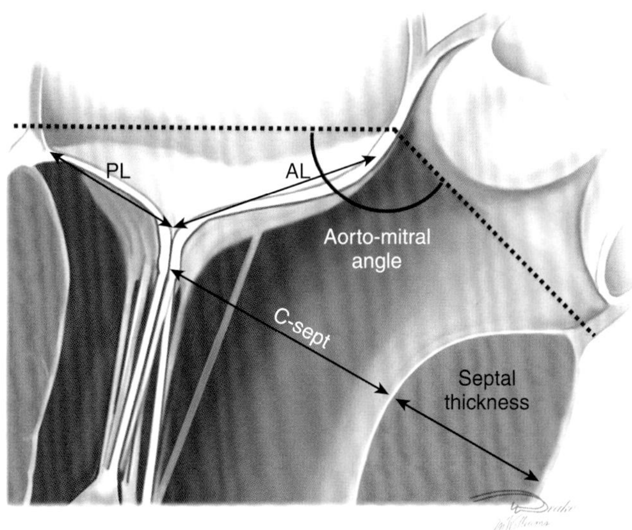

Fig. 25.13 Echocardiographic predictors of systolic anterior motion. The predictors of postoperative systolic anterior motion (SAM) from the pre-repair echocardiogram. An increased risk of postoperative SAM is indicated by (1) posterior leaflet length greater than 1.5 cm; (2) anterior leaflet length greater than 2.0 cm; (3) ratio of posterior leaflet *(PL)* to anterior leaflet *(AL)* length (AL/PL) less than 1.3; (4) C-sept distance less than 2.5 cm; (5) aortomitral angle less than 120 degrees; (6) septal thickness greater than 1.5 cm; and (7) LV end-diastolic diameter (LVEDD) less than 45 mm.[69] *C-sept* is the shortest distance between the coaptation point and the anterior septal wall. Other than LVEDD, all measurements should be obtained in late systole in the mid-esophageal long-axis view.

SECONDARY REGURGITATION

Secondary MR is highly dynamic. Regurgitation severity must be assessed under loading conditions that equate to the awake state (Table 25.5). Recommended techniques for assessing severity are vena contracta width and the flow convergence method.[1,70]

The *pattern* (i.e., asymmetric or symmetric) and *severity* of leaflet tethering should be assessed in the mid-esophageal long-axis view. Leaflet tethering may be quantified by measuring tenting height, tenting area, A2 and P2 closing angles, and anterior leaflet inversion (Fig. 25.14). With asymmetric tethering, regurgitation is usually eccentric and directed *toward* the affected side (i.e., posteriorly). With symmetric tethering, regurgitation tends to be more central. With asymmetric tethering, annular dilation is typically maximal in the anteroposterior dimension, whereas with symmetric tethering, annular dilation tends to affect the anteroposterior and commissural axes. Measurements of LV dimensions, LVEF, and the distribution of segmental wall motion abnormalities also help differentiate symmetric from asymmetric tethering.

DISEASE COMBINATIONS

Mitral dysfunction commonly involves more than one pathologic process. Three scenarios warrant mentioning. First, endocarditis commonly complicates underlying rheumatic or degenerative disease (Fig. 25.15). Distinguishing between vegetations and myxomatous change can be difficult.

TABLE 25.3 Transesophageal Echocardiographic Assessment of Endocarditis.

Parameter	Views	Implication
Underlying mitral valve pathology (degenerative, rheumatic)	2D: all standard ME views (see Fig. 25.6); LAX and commissural views are the most useful 3D: en face LA view; MPR, LAX, and commissural planes	May need repair targeted at underlying degenerative or rheumatic disease
Annular dimensions	As for degenerative disease (see Table 25.1)	Helps size annuloplasty ring, quantify severity, and confirm underlying cause
Presence, size, and location of vegetations	2D: all standard ME views (see Fig. 25.6) 3D: en face LA view	Communicate embolic risk Require debridement or excision at the time of surgery
Presence and location of perforations	2D: all standard ME views (see Fig. 25.6) 3D + color Doppler: en face LA view and LV view (to visualize perforations hidden by vegetations); MPR with adjustment of 2D planes to display defect	Require repair at the time of surgery
Presence and location of fistulas or abscesses	2D + color Doppler: all standard ME views (see Fig. 25.6); may need atypical views focusing on a suspected lesion 3D + color Doppler: MPR with adjustment of 2D planes for atypical views	Require repair at the time of surgery Increased likelihood of requiring valve replacement
Location, direction, and severity of regurgitant jets	As for degenerative disease (see Table 25.1)	Jets displaced from coaptation line suggest perforation Complex or multiple jets suggest perforation and significant leaflet destruction
Involvement of other valves or structures	Comprehensive assessment using standard views Careful assessment of pacing wires	May require concomitant valve surgery or the debridement or removal of pacing wires

LAX, Long axis; *ME*, mid-esophageal; *MPR*, multiplanar reconstruction.

TABLE 25.4 Transesophageal Echocardiographic Assessment of Rheumatic Disease.

Parameter	Views	Implication
Annular dimensions	As for degenerative disease (see Table 25.1)	Helps size annuloplasty ring, quantify severity, and confirm cause
Mobility, thickening, and retraction of the leaflets or subvalvular structures	2D: all standard ME views (see Fig. 25.6); specifically include TG 2-chamber view for evaluation of the subvalvular apparatus	Indicates the need for specific surgical intervention (e.g., debridement, patch augmentation)
Calcification of annulus, valve, and subvalvular apparatus	2D: all standard ME views (see Fig. 25.6); specifically includes TG 2-chamber view for evaluation of the subvalvular apparatus	May require surgical decalcification/debridement
Location, direction, and severity of regurgitant jets	As for degenerative disease (see Table 25.1)	Indicates likelihood of successful valve repair
Presence and severity of concomitant mitral stenosis (i.e., mixed mitral disease)	2D + CW Doppler: diastolic pressure gradient and pressure half-time 3D: MV area assessed using MPR	May require commissural release as part of the repair procedure
Presence of thrombus in LA or LA appendage	2D: all standard ME views (see Fig. 25.6)	Only if concomitant mitral stenosis exists
Involvement of other valves	As for endocarditis (see Table 25.2)	As for endocarditis (see Table 25.2)

ME, Mid-esophageal; *MPR*, multiplanar reconstruction; *MV*, mitral valve; *TG*, transgastric.

TABLE 25.5 Transesophageal Echocardiographic Assessment of Secondary Disease.

Parameter	Views	Implication
Annular dimensions	As for degenerative disease (see Table 25.1)	Helps size annuloplasty ring, quantify severity, and confirm cause Predicts risk of failure of simple reductive annuloplasty band when dilation is severe (see Table 25.6)
Severity of leaflet tethering (tenting area, tenting height, anterior closing angle, posterior closing angle, anterior leaflet inversion, interpapillary distance, and shortening)	2D: ME LAX view (see Fig. 25.14) 3D: MPR, LAX plane	Predicts risk of failure of simple reductive annuloplasty band when dilation is severe (see Table 25.6)
Pattern of leaflet tethering	2D: ME LAX and commissural views. 3D: MPR, LAX, and commissural planes, with adjustment of LAX scan lines to scroll along the coaptation line	Helps guide the surgical procedure (see Fig. 25.18)
LV volumes, ejection fraction, and regional wall motion abnormalities	As for degenerative disease (see Table 25.1)	Indicates perioperative risk
Severity of mitral regurgitation	As for degenerative disease (see Table 25.1) Note reduced cutoff for defining severe regurgitation compared with primary MR Regurgitation severity highly depends on loading conditions	Indicates the need for surgical intervention in patients undergoing primary coronary revascularization
Presence and severity of tricuspid regurgitation	As for degenerative disease (see Table 25.1)	As for degenerative disease (see Table 25.1)
Pulmonary artery pressure	As for degenerative disease (see Table 25.1)	As for degenerative disease (see Table 25.1)
RV size and function	As for degenerative disease (see Table 25.1)	As for degenerative disease (see Table 25.1)

LAX, Long axis; *ME*, mid-esophageal; *MPR*, multiplanar reconstruction; *MR*, mitral regurgitation.

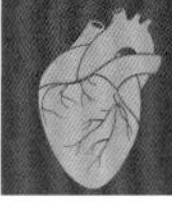

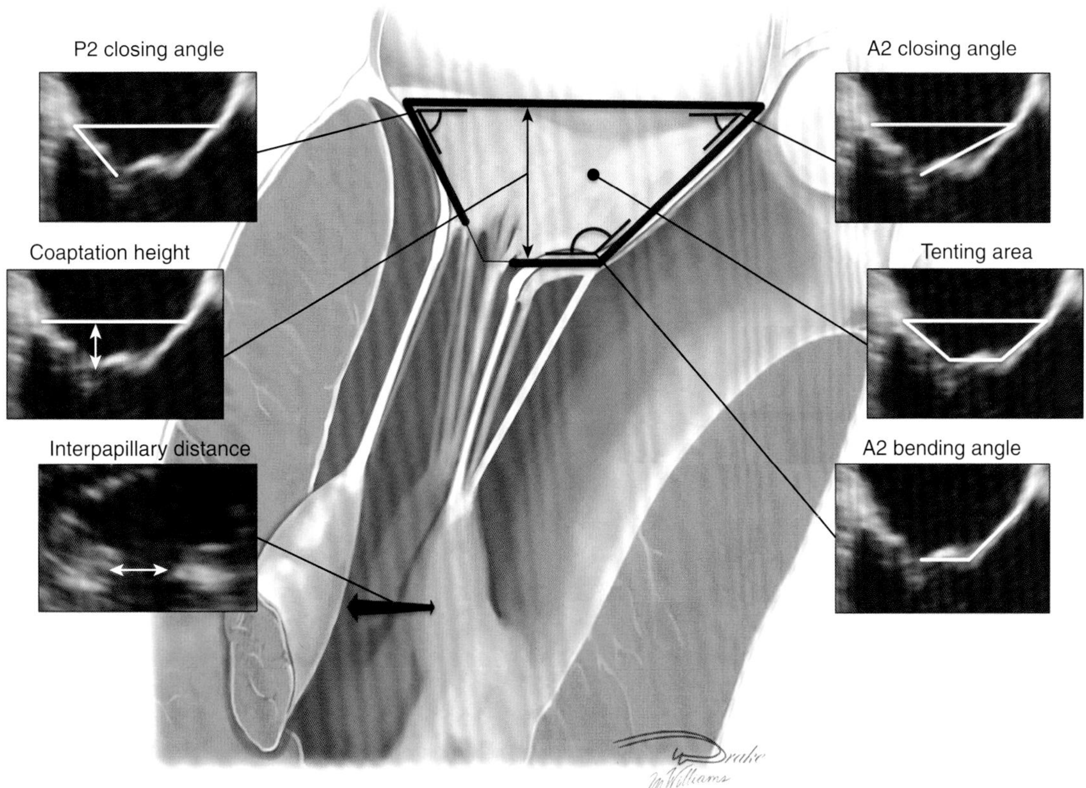

Fig. 25.14 Indices of leaflet distortion with secondary mitral regurgitation. The A2 closing angle is normally less than 25 to 30 degrees, and the P2 closing angle is normally less than 30 to 35 degrees. Values greater than 40 to 45 degrees indicate severe leaflet tethering.[77] Normally, there is no anterior leaflet inversion (i.e., bending angle is 180 degrees). For the interpapillary distance, mid-systolic values greater than 2.0 cm are common in patients with ischemic mitral regurgitation.[87] Reduced systolic shortening of the interpapillary distance (<0.9 cm) is associated with moderate-to-severe ischemic regurgitation.[48] Measurement of these indices can help predict failure of a simple reductive annuloplasty ring for treating myopathic mitral regurgitation (see Video 25.14 ▶). (Courtesy David Sidebotham, Auckland City Hospital, Auckland, New Zealand, and Daniel Drake, Webber Heart Center, Munson Healthcare, Traverse City, MI.)

Second, degenerative disease can coexist with secondary disease. It is important to identify leaflet tethering due to LV dilation in patients with underlying degenerative disease because it influences the surgical technique. In this circumstance, leaflet tethering is most apparent in morphologically normal segments. Prolapsing segments may be less obvious than normal because prolapse height is reduced as a consequence of altered LV geometry and annular dilation. However, signs of myxomatous change (e.g., leaflet thickening, redundant tissue) are typical. The LV is typically markedly enlarged, and LVEF is often reduced. Annular dilation is usually severe. Quantitative 3D analysis of the mitral leaflets and LV function is particularly helpful to elucidate the mechanisms of the regurgitation (Fig. 25.16).

Third, subclinical hypertrophic cardiomyopathy may be complicated by ischemic cardiomyopathy (Fig. 25.17). It is important to determine whether the dominant lesion resulting in regurgitation is leaflet tethering or an LVOT obstruction and SAM. Quantitative 3D analysis of LV function is useful. Features that suggest hypertrophic cardiomyopathy include a normal LVEF, septal hypertrophy, and a narrowed LVOT. Features suggesting ischemic cardiomyopathy include leaflet tethering, increased ventricular volumes, and remodeling involving the basal inferior and inferolateral LV walls.

SURGICAL TECHNIQUES OF IMAGE-GUIDED MITRAL REPAIR

The goals of any repair procedure are to reestablish anatomically normal mitral geometry, dimensions, and function. Achieving these goals requires sufficient, but not excessive, freely mobile leaflet tissue with an adequate coaptive surface located at or just below the annular plane.[3] An annuloplasty ring should be placed in all patients to correct annular dilation, increase coaptation, and prevent further annular remodeling.[23] The techniques of image-guided mitral repair based on pathoanatomy are illustrated in Fig. 25.18.

DEGENERATIVE DISEASE

The classic approach to treating posterior leaflet prolapse is leaflet resection, a technique popularized by Carpentier. Localized posterior leaflet flail, which is typical of fibroelastic deficiency, requires nothing more than narrow triangular resection (see Figs. 25.11A, stage II, and 25.18A). More extensive posterior leaflet prolapse or flail, which is typical of Barlow disease, may be corrected with segmental resection and sliding posterioplasty (see Figs. 25.11A, stage III, and 25.18A).

Height reduction of the nonprolapsing segments may be required to ensure that excess posterior leaflet tissue does not result in postoperative SAM. If segmental involvement is limited, anterior

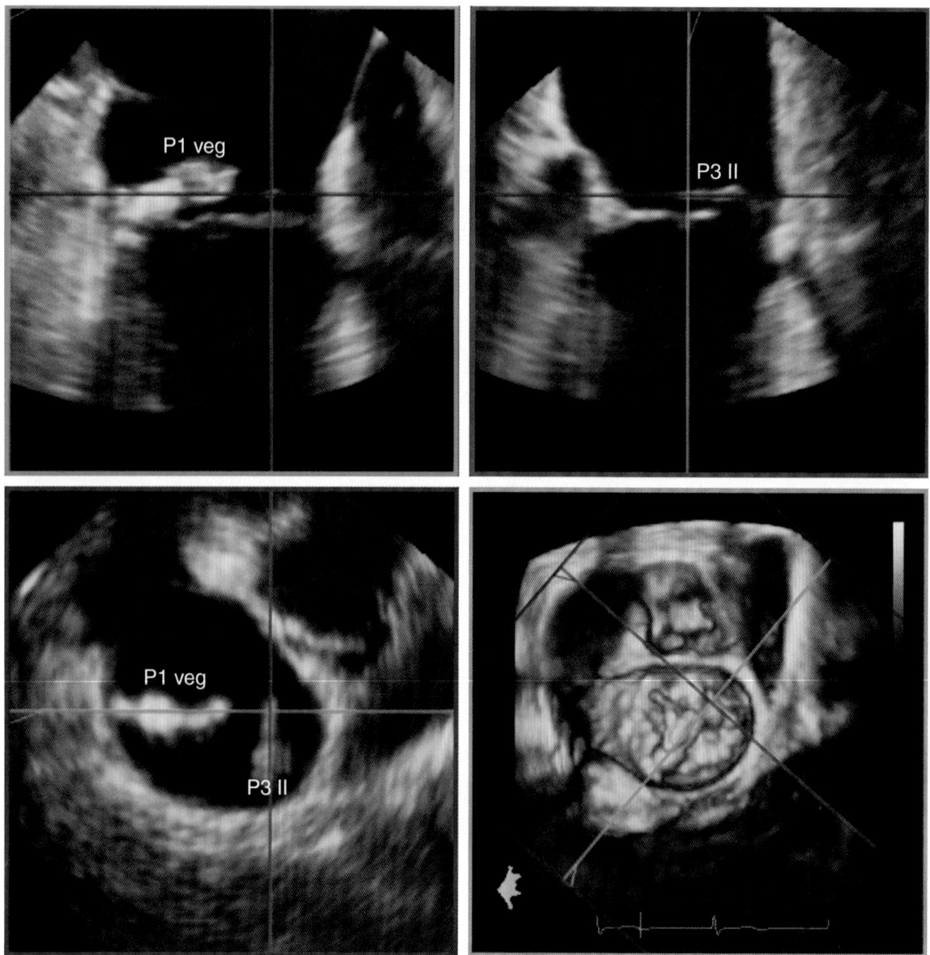

Fig. 25.15 **Combined degenerative disease and endocarditis.** These images were obtained using multiplanar reconstruction of an axial 3D data set. The 2D cross-sectional views *(green and red boxes)* have been adjusted from the standard long-axis and commissural planes to demonstrate the pathology; their positions are demonstrated in the volume-rendered view *(bottom right panel)*. Parallax has been eliminated so that the locations of the *red* and *green planes* as they traverse the volume-rendered LA view are accurate. A large vegetation can be seen arising from the base of P1 *(P1 veg)* in the *green and blue boxes.* A flail segment involving P3 can be seen in the *red and blue boxes (P3 II).* Surgical repair involved excision of the P1 vegetation, annular reconstruction adjacent to P1, narrow P3 parabolic resection, and ring annuloplasty.

leaflet prolapse may be treated with narrow resection or chordal transfer. More extensive anterior leaflet prolapse may require papillary muscle shortening (see Figs. 25.11A, stage IV, and 25.18A).

Leaflet resection, particularly when there is minimal excess leaflet tissue, may result in a small coaptive surface and increased leaflet tension, predisposing to failure of the repair. However, excellent long-term results have been obtained with resection techniques.[71,72]

Replacement of ruptured or elongated chordae with polytetrafluoroethylene neochordae has gained acceptance as an alternative to leaflet resection.[72,73] Potential advantages are a larger coaptation surface, preserved leaflet mobility, reduced leaflet tension, and use of a larger annuloplasty ring. Conversely, neochordal length, even if premeasured, introduces an additional variable that may result in failure of the repair. Similar long-term durability has been achieved with both repair techniques.[71,72]

Several issues particular to Barlow disease must be considered. Repair of associated clefts or annular disjunction may be required. Severe dystrophic calcification may require excision of calcified tissue and reconstruction of the annulus and associated leaflet tissue.[74] Modifications of the surgical technique may be required for patients who are at increased risk for postoperative SAM (see Figs. 25.11A, stage IV; 25.11E, stage I; and 25.13). It is important to avoid undersized annuloplasty rings in this situation.

For excess posterior leaflet tissue, extensive leaflet resection or displacement of bulky posterior leaflet tissue into the LV with shortened neochordae is acceptable. Ideally, the atrial surface of the posterior leaflet should be less than 1.5 cm, and it should never exceed 2.0 cm. For excess anterior leaflet tissue, horizontal elliptical leaflet excision, papillary muscle shortening, secondary chord lysis, or oversized ring annuloplasty placement can be performed. When neochordae are used for anterior leaflet prolapse, it is important that the chordae are not too short because this displaces coaptation closer to the LVOT.

ENDOCARDITIS

Surgery for endocarditis involves excision of vegetations, leaflet debridement, and suture or pericardial patch closure of perforations. Chordal replacement is occasionally required.

RHEUMATIC DISEASE

Repair of rheumatic regurgitation typically requires debriding the leaflets and subvalvular apparatus. Anterior leaflet augmentation and subvalvular reconstruction may be required.

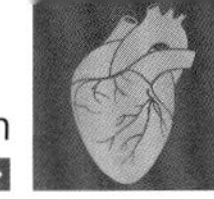

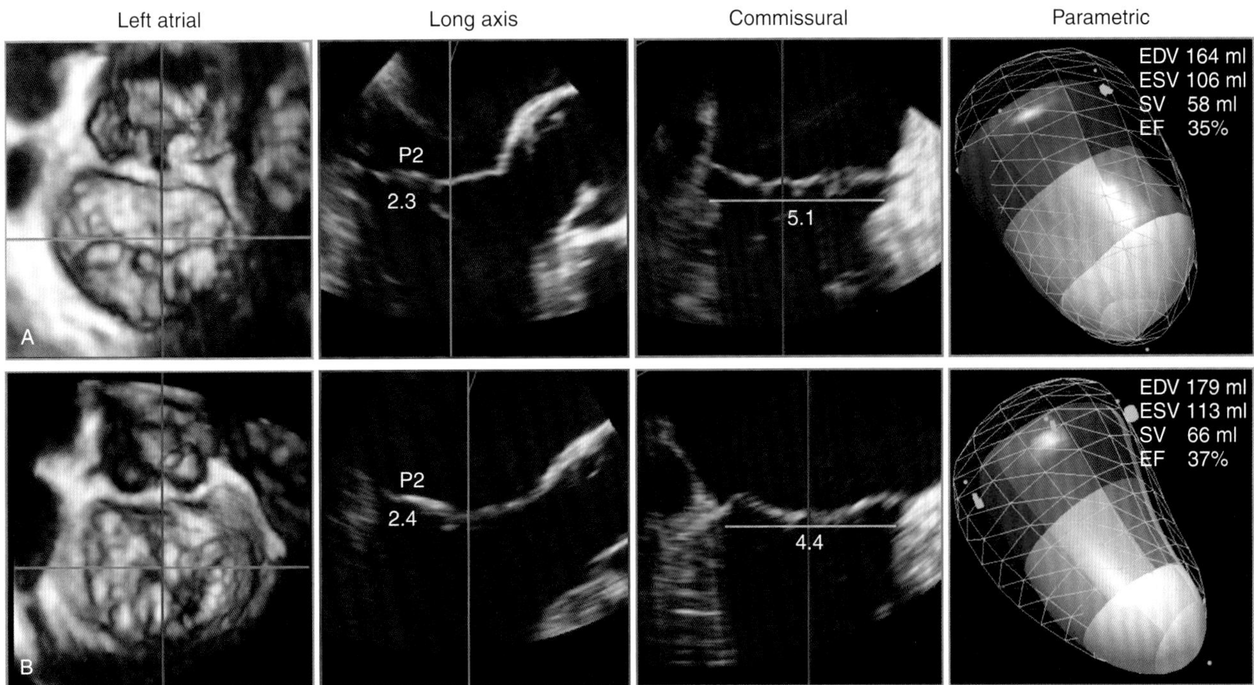

Fig. 25.16 Combined degenerative and secondary (myopathic) disease. 3D views of the mitral valve and LV from two patients who had combined degenerative and secondary mitral valve disease. Volume-rendered 3D views from the atrial aspect are shown in the left-hand column. 2D long-axis and commissural views obtained from zoomed 3D data sets are shown in the middle two columns. Late systolic frames have been chosen for analysis. Volumetric (parametric) 3D views of the LV are shown in the right-hand column. (A) A patient with long-standing Barlow disease that caused severe mitral regurgitation (MR). The atrial view shows redundant tissue typical of Barlow disease. In the long-axis plane, several risk factors for postoperative systolic anterior motion (SAM) are apparent: P2 is elongated (>2 cm), there is mild chordal SAM, the aortomitral angle is reduced, and the basal septum is prominent. The commissural width is increased (5.1 cm; normal < 3.5 cm), which is typical of Barlow disease. However, in the long-axis and commissural views, there is minimal leaflet prolapse. Unlike atrial functional MR, the volumetric (parametric) analysis demonstrates LV enlargement and reduced LV ejection fraction (EF). Despite normal leaflet motion, simple reductive ring annuloplasty is contraindicated due to the increased risk of postoperative SAM. (B) A patient with a recent myocardial infarction and moderate MR presented for coronary revascularization. Initially, regurgitation was assumed to be ischemic in origin. In the atrial view, mild prolapse of the posterior leaflet is apparent, suggesting degenerative disease. In the long-axis and commissural planes, there is no evidence of segmental prolapse; however, the posterior leaflet is elongated (2.4 cm) and the commissural dimension is increased, both of which suggest degenerative disease. There is minimal leaflet tethering, which is atypical for pure secondary MR. Volumetric analysis demonstrates LV dilation and reduced LV EF. The patient initially underwent coronary revascularization; however, he presented later with severe MR due to bileaflet prolapse. *EDV*, End-diastolic volume; *ESV*, end-systolic volume; *MR*, mitral regurgitation; *SV*, stroke volume.

PAPILLARY MUSCLE RUPTURE

Ideally, surgery to repair papillary muscle rupture should be delayed to allow myocardial recovery and infarct demarcation; however, this is not possible for complete rupture because patients are typically critically ill. Partial rupture of a single head of the papillary muscle may be treated by direct suture repair. Complete rupture of the papillary muscle head may be repaired by suture reattachment of the fibrous cap and, if necessary, chordal transfer or placement of neochordae to provide additional leaflet support.[75,76]

SECONDARY REGURGITATION

The surgical approach to repair of secondary MR continues to evolve. Historically, reductive ring annuloplasty was used for the full spectrum of ischemic distortion.[23] However, this approach results in unacceptably high rates of recurrent MR in patients with severe leaflet tethering (Table 25.6).[77] More complex repair techniques (described later) may be used to achieve a durable repair in patients with advanced leaflet tethering.[3–5] We and others have proposed an integrated approach to image-guided repair for secondary MR (see Fig. 25.18B).[3,78]

As an isolated technique, simple reductive ring annuloplasty is appropriate only when leaflet tethering is minimal (see Figs. 25.11D, stage I, and 25.18B). The dominant cause should be atrial functional MR or another mild myopathy affecting the basilar segments of the LV.

Several adjuvants have been developed to reduce the high failure rate associated with simple reductive ring annuloplasty for advanced tethering (see Fig. 25.11D, stages II–IV). They include cutting (lysis) of secondary chordae, chordal translocation, patch extension of the anterior leaflet, papillary muscle approximation, and ventricular aneurysmectomy (see Fig. 25.18B). We have reported encouraging results using a graduated protocol based on the severity of leaflet tethering, progressing from simple reductive ring annuloplasty to secondary chord cutting and patch augmentation of the anterior leaflet.[3] However, for the most advanced secondary disease, ring annuloplasty and chordal cutting may be insufficient, in which case papillary approximation or patch augmentation of the entire anterior leaflet should be considered.[4,79,80] Currently, many surgeons elect to perform mitral valve replacement when tethering is severe.

Patients with Barlow disease and leaflet tethering due to LV dilation are at risk for postoperative SAM if a simple ring

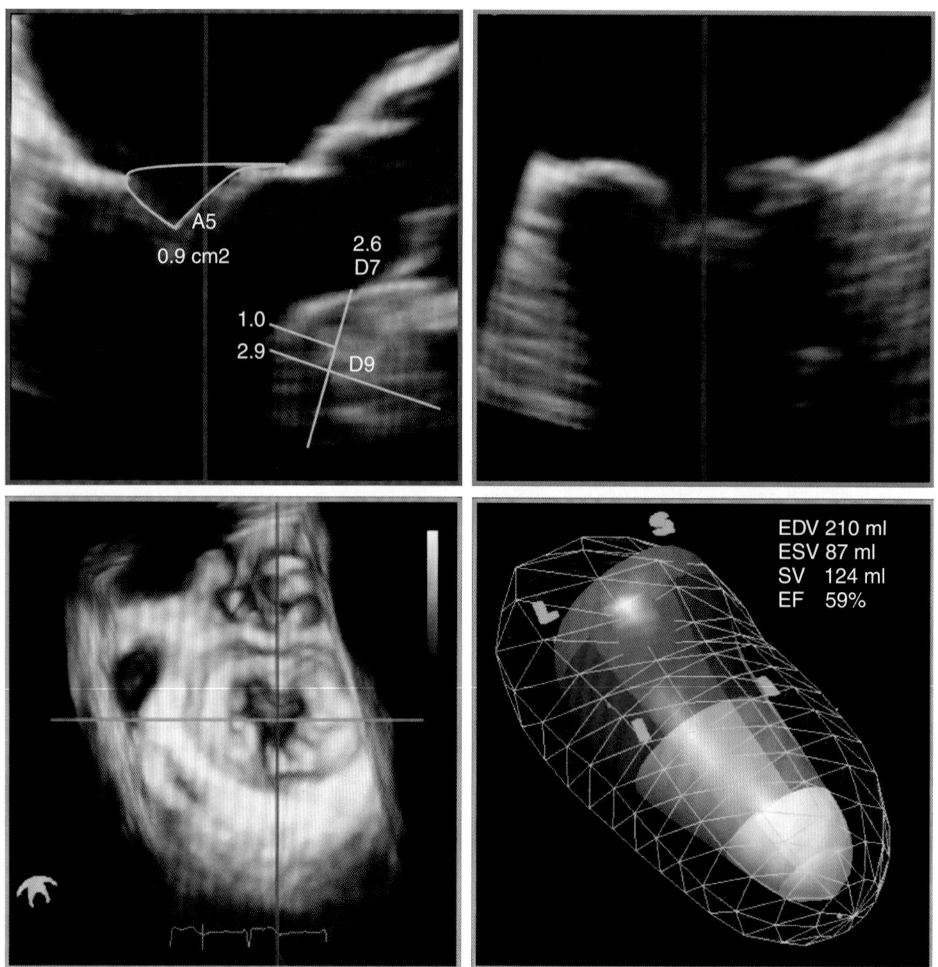

Fig. 25.17 Combined ischemic and hypertrophic disease. Quantitative analysis of a zoomed 3D data set of the mitral valve *(top panels, bottom left panel)* and a full-volume 3D data set of the LV *(bottom right panel)* from a patient with hypertrophic cardiomyopathy and concomitant leaflet tethering due to LV dilation due to ischemic heart disease. Images of the mitral valve were taken in late systole. Parallax has been eliminated so that the long-axis plane *(green box, top left)* and the commissural plane *(green box, top right)* can be accurately located in the volume-rendered atrial view *(bottom left)*. In the long-axis view, there is marked hypertrophy of the basal anterior septum (2.9 cm) over a distance of 2.6 cm. There is moderate leaflet tenting (tenting area, 0.9 cm^2), and the coaptation point is approximately 1 cm below the annular plane. Leaflet tethering, predominantly involving A2, is apparent in the commissural view. Systolic anterior motion (SAM) is not seen in the long-axis or the commissural view. Leaflet restriction is also apparent in the atrial view. Volumetric analysis of the LV demonstrates marked LV dilation with relatively preserved ejection fraction (EF). The findings are consistent with mitral regurgitation (MR), primarily due to LV dilation (i.e., ischemic cardiomyopathy) with subclinical hypertrophic cardiomyopathy. Surgical intervention with coronary revascularization and septal myectomy alone in this circumstance would predispose to recurrent MR from uncorrected leaflet tethering. Surgical intervention with coronary revascularization and reductive annuloplasty alone would predispose to postoperative SAM. In this case, combined revascularization, septal myectomy, secondary chord lysis, anterior leaflet augmentation, and reductive ring annuloplasty produced a successful and durable repair. *EDV,* End-diastolic volume; *ESV,* end-systolic volume; *SV,* stroke volume.

annuloplasty is used for repair (see Figs. 25.3F and 25.16). Despite minimal prolapse, posterior leaflet height reduction is required. This can be accomplished with posterior leaflet elliptical excision, segmentectomy and sliding posterioplasty, or short neochordae.

POST-REPAIR TEE

After repair, the focus of the TEE examination should be to (1) assess leaflet morphology and function; (2) determine the presence and severity of any residual MR; and (3) exclude complications such as mitral stenosis, ventricular dysfunction, and SAM. Routine 2D and 3D imaging with and without color Doppler is usually sufficient to exclude residual regurgitation. However, if there is significant residual MR, quantitative 3D imaging is useful to help elucidate the mechanism and location of the jets.

LEAFLET STRUCTURE AND FUNCTION

The leaflets should open widely in diastole and close fully in systole. Coaptation should be at least 5 mm and ideally more than 8 mm; it should occur at or just below the annular plane and should not intrude into the LVOT. The annuloplasty ring should be correctly seated.

The normal postoperative appearance of the valve depends on the underlying disease and the repair technique used. After posterior leaflet resection, the coaptation point may lie in the acoustic shadow of the annuloplasty ring, making coaptation height difficult to assess and giving the appearance of a unileaflet valve. Repair with neochordae typically results in more extensive, easily visualized coaptation. If shortened neochordae have been used to displace bulky posterior leaflet tissue into the LV, coaptation occurs below the annular plane and is displaced posteriorly. Conversely, if neochordae have been used to treat posterior flail

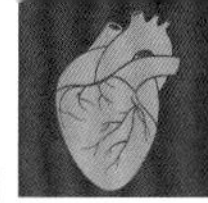

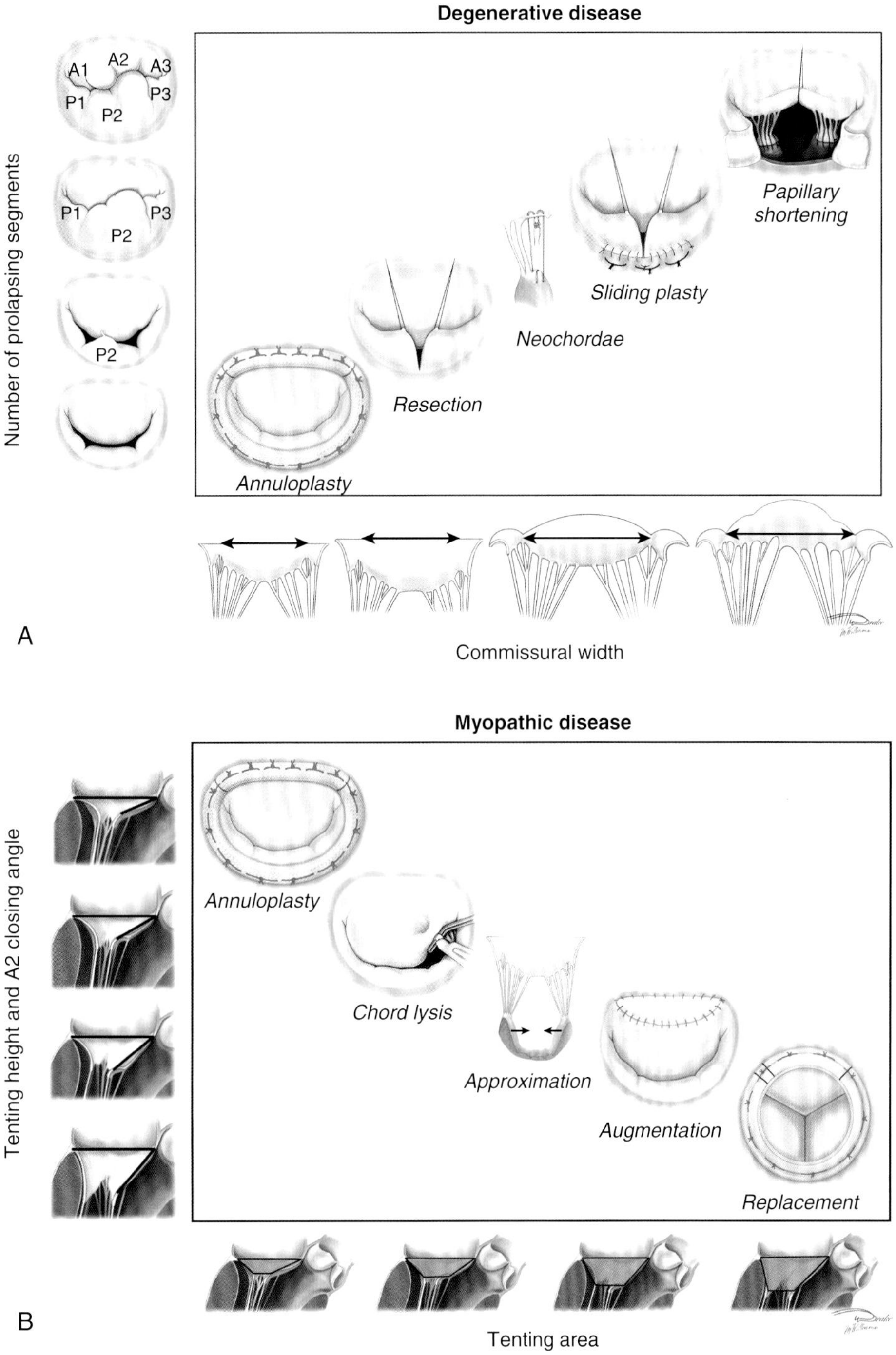

Fig. 25.18 Anatomically based surgical treatment of mitral valve disease. Intervention is based on echocardiography-derived anatomic measurements. (A) Degenerative disease. Echocardiographic indices guiding treatment of degenerative disease include commissural width and the number prolapsing segments. From the left, the procedures illustrated are simple ring annuloplasty, simple triangular resection, neochordae implantation, sliding posterioplasty, and papillary muscle shortening combined with sliding posterioplasty. (B) Secondary (myopathic) disease. Echocardiographic indices guiding treatment of secondary disease include tenting height, tenting area, and A2 closing angle. From the left, the procedures illustrated are simple reductive ring annuloplasty, secondary chord lysis, papillary muscle approximation, partial anterior leaflet augmentation (D-plasty), and complete anterior leaflet augmentation or valve replacement. Ring annuloplasty is used to complete all repairs (see Video 25.18). (Modified from Drake D, Zimmerman K, Sidebotham D. Comment on surgical treatment of moderate ischemic mitral regurgitation. *N Engl J Med.* 2015;372:1771–1773.)

TABLE 25.6 Predictors of Recurrence of Mitral Regurgitation After Simple Reductive Annuloplasty for Treatment of Ischemic Mitral Regurgitation.

Parameter	*TTE or TEE*	*Cutoff Value*	*Sensitivity/ Specificity (%)*
Mitral annular diameter	TEE	≥37 mm	84/76
Tenting area	TEE TTE	≥1.6 cm^2 ≥2.5 cm^2	80/54 64/95
Tenting height	TEE TTE	>1 cm >1 cm	— 64/90
Posterior leaflet closing angle	TTE	≥45 degrees	100/95
LV end-systolic volume	TTE	≥145 mL	90/90
Interpapillary muscle distance	TTE	>20 mm	96/97
Systolic sphericity index[a]	TTE	≥0.7	100/100
Diastolic function	TTE	Restrictive	—

[a]Sphericity index is the ratio of the long axis of the LV/short axis; other parameters are explained in the text.
From Magne J, Senechal M, Dumesnil JG, Pibarot P. Ischemic mitral regurgitation: a complex multifaceted disease. *Cardiology*. 2009;112:244–259.

TABLE 25.7 Mechanisms of Residual Mitral Regurgitation After Repair.

Persistent prolapse (degenerative disease)
Persistent tethering (secondary disease)
Uncorrected clefts (degenerative disease)
Inadequate leaflet coaptation
Leaflet tension causing separation of posterior scallops (degenerative disease with leaflet resection technique)
Leaflet perforation (e.g., from the annuloplasty ring or misplaced suture)
Systolic anterior motion (Barlow disease, hypertrophic cardiomyopathy)

caused by fibroelastic deficiency, coaptation should be at or just below the annular plane and positioned more centrally.

After mitral repair for secondary disease, the anterior leaflet should appear normal, with minimal tethering and satisfactory coaptation occurring just below the annular plane. Anterior leaflet inversion should be completely eliminated. However, residual posterior tethering is common, especially with more advanced disease.

RESIDUAL MITRAL REGURGITATION

Assessment of residual regurgitation should be performed after cardiac function has recovered from the effects of cardiopulmonary bypass (CPB) and under loading conditions that mimic the awake hemodynamic state. This is particularly important after repair for secondary disease because LV function is commonly impaired and alterations in contractility, preload, and afterload greatly affect regurgitation severity.

More than mild residual regurgitation is an indication to revise the repair or replace the valve because this finding increases the probability of needing reoperation.[81,82] There are few data on the long-term implications of mild residual MR. However, the goal should be to achieve no residual regurgitation. Factors to consider when deciding to revise the repair for mild residual regurgitation are the likelihood of improving the repair, the risks of returning to CPB, and the risks of late reoperation.

The severity of residual regurgitation should be quantified by measuring the vena contracta width or vena contracta area (see Chapter 24). The flow convergence technique is not appropriate

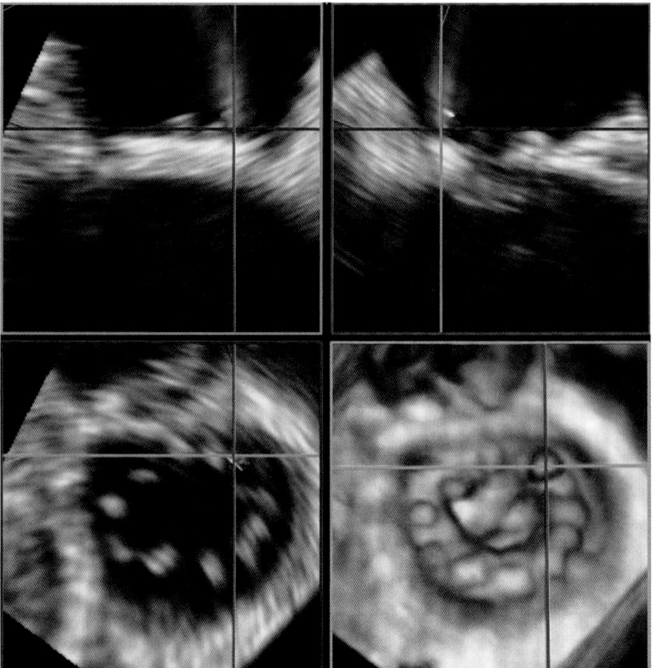

Fig. 25.19 Residual regurgitation after mitral repair. Multiplanar reconstruction of an axial 3D data set with color Doppler imaging. The 2D cross-sectional views *(green and red boxes)* have been adjusted from the standard long-axis and commissural positions to demonstrate the residual leak; their positions are demonstrated in the volume-rendered atrial view *(bottom right panel)*. The short-axis 2D view *(blue box, bottom left)* has been located on the atrial surface of the valve close to the annuloplasty ring. The residual jet is displayed in all four views. The findings are consistent with mild residual regurgitation arising from a suture tear in the anterior annulus located at approximately 1 o'clock on the prosthetic ring. Return to cardiopulmonary bypass and reexploration of the valve revealed no anatomically identifiable leak. However, sutures placed empirically based on the echocardiographic findings eliminated the leak (see Video 25.19).

for quantitating milder degrees of regurgitation because the flow convergence zone is too small to measure accurately. Vena contracta width should be measured in the mid-esophageal long-axis view, turning the probe left and right to scan along the line of coaptation. The narrowest part of the widest jet should be chosen for analysis, and the average of several measurements should be reported. Vena contracta area is measured by quantitative planimetry of color 3D data sets. Brief jets that are seen for only one or two frames in early systole usually diminish over time and should be ignored.

Residual regurgitation may significantly improve with recovery of ventricular function. In difficult cases, it may be appropriate to wait for up to 30 minutes after discontinuation of CPB before making a final decision on the success of the repair.

If there is unacceptable residual regurgitation, it is important to identify the mechanisms (Table 25.7) and location of the regurgitation. Scanning along the coaptation line in the mid-esophageal long-axis view is useful for identifying uncorrected leaflet prolapse or tethering. If leaflet distortion is seen on 2D imaging, it may be quantified with 3D imaging. Color 3D imaging from the atrial aspect, with close cropping onto the valve, is extremely useful to identify the anatomic location of the residual regurgitation (Fig. 25.19). Uncorrected clefts and separation of the posterior scallops can also be identified with this technique.

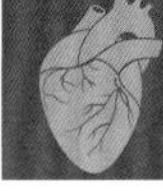

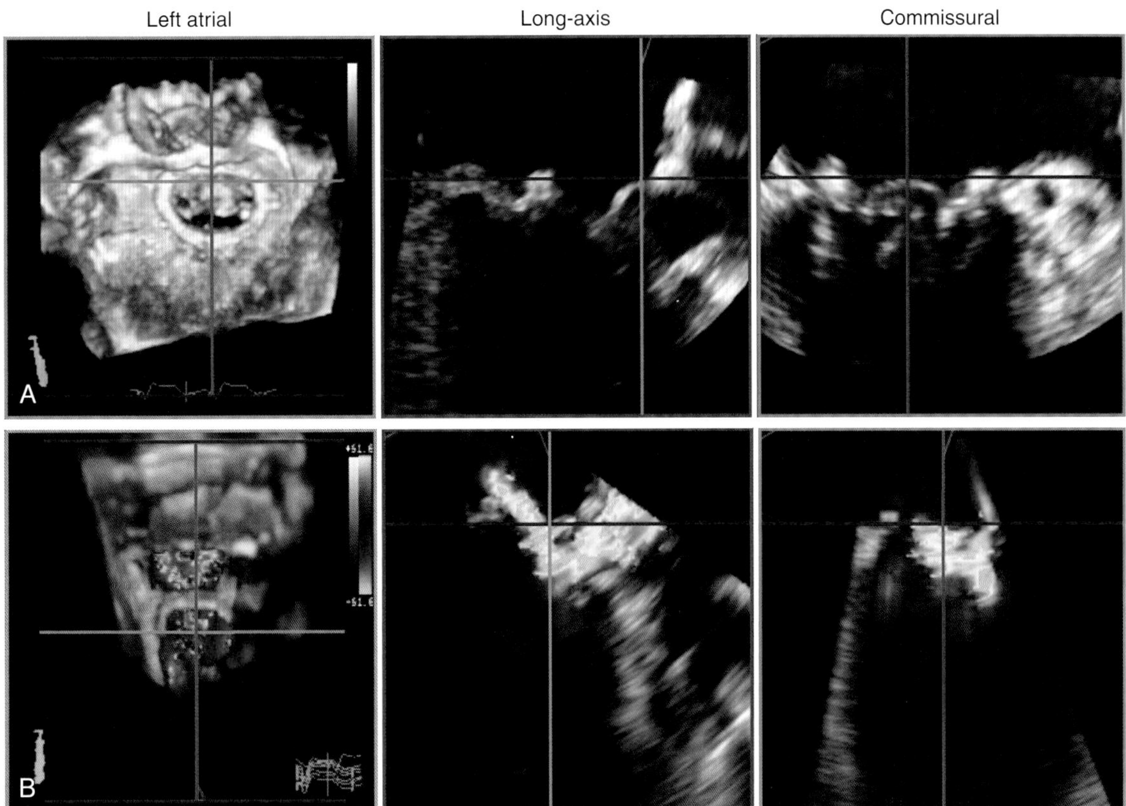

Fig. 25.20 Post-repair systolic anterior motion. Multiplanar reconstruction of axial 3D data sets without color (A) and with color Doppler imaging (B) after mitral repair. All frames were obtained in late systole. Volume-rendered atrial views are shown in the left column. 2D long-axis and commissural views are shown in the middle and right columns. Notice that the position of the commissural view has been moved slightly anteriorly from the standard position (*green line* in the *top left panel*) to demonstrate the pathology. (A) The volume-rendered atrial view demonstrates retraction of A2. In the long-axis view, the anterior mitral leaflet can be seen bending into the LV outflow tract, indicating systolic anterior motion (SAM). In the commissural view, the anterior leaflet can be seen folding back on itself adjacent to the anterior aspect of the prosthetic ring. (B) The volume-rendered atrial view demonstrates the regurgitant jet extending posteriorly into the LA. There is marked systolic turbulence in the region of the aortic valve. The long-axis view confirms a posteriorly directed regurgitant jet and LV outflow tract turbulence. The commissural view also confirms turbulence within the prosthetic annulus, consistent with severe mitral regurgitation.

NEW MITRAL STENOSIS

Clinically significant mitral stenosis is rare but can result from residual rheumatic dysfunction, small annuloplasty rings, or extensive commissural plication. Evaluation of mitral stenosis is complicated by elevated diastolic flow resulting from tachycardia, hyperdynamic contractility, and reduced ventricular compliance, which are common during the post-CPB period. Diastolic mean gradients up to 5 mm Hg are not uncommon in the early period after repair. Although data are limited, a retrospective analysis of 557 patients found that a mean diastolic pressure gradient of 7 mmHg or greater was associated with the need for reoperation.[83]

VENTRICULAR DYSFUNCTION

Ventricular dysfunction is common after mitral valve surgery. Correction of MR increases LV afterload, which exacerbates preexisting LV dysfunction. Injury to the circumflex coronary artery can occur and is suggested by new wall motion abnormality involving the inferolateral LV wall. Transient right ventricular dysfunction may occur due to poor myocardial protection, gas embolus to the RCA, or exacerbation of preexisting pulmonary hypertension.

SYSTOLIC ANTERIOR MOTION

Postoperative SAM occurs almost exclusively in patients with Barlow disease or underlying hypertrophic cardiomyopathy. SAM is best diagnosed in the mid-esophageal long-axis view. Characteristic features are displacement of the anterior mitral leaflet into the LVOT; turbulent, high-velocity flow in the LVOT; and a posteriorly directed jet of MR (Fig. 25.20). LVOT velocity should be measured with continuous-wave (CW) Doppler in a transgastric view. Velocity is typically maximal in late systole and results in a characteristic sharply peaked waveform.

A peak velocity in the LVOT of less than 2 m/s that is associated with mild MR can be safely ignored. More severe SAM should be treated with fluid loading, vasoconstrictors, and cessation of inotropic support. Medical therapy is usually effective, and only rarely is surgical revision necessary.[84] Failure of medical therapy to achieve an LVOT velocity less than 3.5 m/s with mild or less MR is an indication for surgical revision.[85] Options for further repair include placement of a larger annuloplasty ring, maneuvers that displace the coaptation point posteriorly, and limited myectomy.[86]

SUMMARY Surgical Mitral Valve Repair.

Imaging Modality	Views	Utility	Comments
2D imaging of valvular anatomy (+ color Doppler)	ME LAX	Anteroposterior dimension A2/P2 segments and coaptive surface Prolapse vs. flail; prolapse height Mitral-annular disjunction Risk factors for SAM (see Fig. 25.13) Quantification of leaflet tethering (see Fig. 25.15) Regurgitant jet direction Vena contracta width PISA radius	Difficult to be sure of exact position of scan plane (see Fig. 25.6); use axial imaging to overcome this problem Axial imaging ensures that the image plane passes through the anteroposterior axis and traverses the A2/P2 coaptive surfaces
	ME commissural	Commissural dimension A1/P1 and A3/P3 segments and coaptive surfaces Regurgitant jet direction	Axial imaging ensures that the image plane passes through the anteroposterior axis and traverses the A1/P1 and A3/P3 coaptive surfaces
	ME 4-chamber	Mitral leaflet morphology and MR jet direction RV function, TV annular size, and TR severity	Imaging is oblique to axes of valve Avoid measuring mitral leaflet and annular dimensions in this view
	ME 2-chamber	Mitral leaflet morphology and MR jet direction	As for ME 4-chamber view
	TG 2-chamber	Assessing subvalvular apparatus	—
	TG 5-chamber and TG LAX views	Assessing dynamic LVOT obstruction after repair with CW Doppler	Important to ensure close alignment between Doppler beam and blood flow in LVOT
3D imaging of valvular anatomy (+ color Doppler)	En face LA aspect	Identification of anatomic sites of valvular lesions (prolapse, flail, vegetation, perforation, cleft, calcification) and regurgitant jets Vena contracta area	Use axially acquired ME LAX and commissural views as starting images (see Fig. 25.8) Include LA appendage and AoV to facilitate orientation of image Display with AoV in 12-o'clock position Close cropping onto the atrial surface with color Doppler is useful to determine origin of regurgitant jets
	En face LV aspect	Identification of perforations obscured by vegetations on LA view	Display with AoV in 12-o'clock position
Quantitative 3D imaging (MPR)	ME LAX (axial)	As for ME LAX (above)	Axial imaging ensures that the image plane passes through the anteroposterior axis and traverses the A2/P2 coaptation surface Data acquisition and analysis described in Figs. 25.8–25.10
	ME commissural (axial)	As for ME commissural view (above)	Axial imaging ensures that the image plane passes through the commissural axis and traverses the A1/P1 and A3/P3 coaptation surfaces Data acquisition and analysis described in Figs. 25.8–25.10
LV size and function	2D: Modified Simpson (ME 4- and 2-chamber views)		Provides information on LV volumes and LVEF
	3D: Quantitative analysis of full volume data sets		Provides information on LV volumes, LVEF, and wall motion abnormalities Useful for assessing tethering pattern in secondary MR and for assessing secondary MR in setting of degenerative disease
Regurgitation severity (see Chapter 24)	Vena contracta width, EROA: PISA, vena contracta area		Severe organic MR: VCW ≥0.7 cm, EROA ≥ 0.4 cm^2 Severe secondary MR: ≥0.2 cm^2

AoV, Aortic valve; *EROA*, effective regurgitant orifice area; *LAX*, long-axis; *LVEF*, LV ejection fraction; *LVOT*, LV outflow tract; *ME*, mid-esophageal; *MPR*, multiplanar reconstruction; *MR*, mitral regurgitation; *PISA*, proximal isovelocity surface area; *TG*, transgastric; *TR*, tricuspid regurgitation; *TV*, tricuspid valve; *VCW*, vena contracta width.

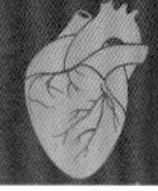

REFERENCES

1. Otto CM, Nishimura RA, Bonow RO, et al. 2020. AHA/ACC guideline for the management of patients with valvular heart disease: a report of the American College of Cardiology/American Heart Association Joint Committee on Clinical Practice Guidelines. *Circulation.* 2021;143(5):e72-e227. doi: 10.1161/CIR.0000000000000923.
2. Badhwar V, Peterson ED, Jacobs JP, et al. Longitudinal outcome of isolated mitral repair in older patients: results from 14,604 procedures performed from 1991 to 2007. *Ann Thorac Surg.* 2012;94:1870–1877; discussion 1877–1879.
3. Drake DH, Zimmerman KG, Hepner AM, Nichols CD. Echo-guided mitral repair. *Circ Cardiovasc Imaging.* 2014;7:132–141.
4. Harmel EK, Reichenspurner H, Girdauskas E. Subannular reconstruction in secondary mitral regurgitation: a meta-analysis. *Heart.* 2018;104:1783–1790.
5. Calafiore AM, Refaie R, Iaco AL, et al. Chordal cutting in ischemic mitral regurgitation: a propensity-matched study. *J Thorac Cardiovasc Surg.* 2014;148:41–46.
6. Vassileva CM, Boley T, Markwell S, Hazelrigg S. Meta-analysis of short-term and long-term survival following repair versus replacement for ischemic mitral regurgitation. *Eur J Cardio Thorac Surg.* 2011;39:295–303.
7. Sidebotham DA, Allen SJ, Gerber IL, Fayers T. Intraoperative transesophageal echocardiography for surgical repair of mitral regurgitation. *J Am Soc Echocardiogr.* 2014;27:345–366.
8. Nishimura RA, O'Gara PT, Bavaria JE, et al. 2019. AATS/ACC/ASE/SCAI/STS expert consensus systems of care document: a proposal to optimize care for patients with valvular heart disease: a joint report of the American Association for Thoracic Surgery, American College of Cardiology, American Society of Echocardiography, Society for Cardiovascular Angiography and Interventions, and Society of Thoracic Surgeons. *J Am Coll Cardiol.* 2019;73:2609–2635.
9. Kilic A, Shah AS, Conte JV, Baumgartner WA, Yuh DD. Operative outcomes in mitral valve surgery: combined effect of surgeon and hospital volume in a population-based analysis. *J Thorac Cardiovasc Surg.* 2013;146:638–646.
10. Chikwe J, Toyoda N, Anyanwu AC, et al. Relation of mitral valve surgery volume to repair rate, durability, and survival. *J Am Coll Cardiol.* 2017. https://doi.org/10.1016/j.jacc.2017.02.026
11. O'Gara PT, Grayburn PA, Badhwar V, et al. 2017. ACC expert consensus decision pathway on the management of mitral regurgitation: a report of the American College of Cardiology Task Force on Expert Consensus Decision Pathways. *J Am Coll Cardiol.* 2017;70:2421–2449.
12. Ben Zekry S, Nagueh SF, Little SH, et al. Comparative accuracy of two- and three-dimensional transthoracic and transesophageal echocardiography in identifying mitral valve pathology in patients undergoing mitral valve repair: initial observations. *J Am Soc Echocardiogr.* 2011;24:1079–1085.
13. Wijdh-den Hamer IJ, Bouma W, Lai EK, et al. The value of preoperative 3-dimensional over 2-dimensional valve analysis in predicting recurrent ischemic mitral regurgitation after mitral annuloplasty. *J Thorac Cardiovasc Surg.* 2016;152:847–859.
14. Biaggi P, Jedrzkiewicz S, Gruner C, et al. Quantification of mitral valve anatomy by three-dimensional transesophageal echocardiography in mitral valve prolapse predicts surgical anatomy and the complexity of mitral valve repair. *J Am Soc Echocardiogr.* 2012;25:758–765.
15. Hahn RT, Abraham T, Adams MS, et al. Guidelines for performing a comprehensive transesophageal echocardiographic examination: recommendations from the American Society of Echocardiography and the Society of Cardiovascular Anesthesiologists. *J Am Soc Echocardiogr.* 2013;26:921–964.
16. Umland M. Advanced cardiac sonographer: a reality at last. *J Am Soc Echocardiogr.* 2015;28:A15.
17. Levine RA, Triulzi MO, Harrigan P, Weyman AE. The relationship of mitral annular shape to the diagnosis of mitral valve prolapse. *Circulation.* 1987;75:756–767.
18. Muraru D, Cattarina M, Boccalini F, et al. Mitral valve anatomy and function: new insights from three-dimensional echocardiography. *J Cardiovasc Med.* 2013;14:91–99.
19. Grewal J, Suri R, Mankad S, et al. Mitral annular dynamics in myxomatous valve disease: new insights with real-time 3-dimensional echocardiography. *Circulation.* 2010;121:1423–1431.
20. Silbiger JJ, Bazaz R. Contemporary insights into the functional anatomy of the mitral valve. *Am Heart J.* 2009;158:887–895.
21. Levack MM, Jassar AS, Shang EK, et al. Three-dimensional echocardiographic analysis of mitral annular dynamics: implication for annuloplasty selection. *Circulation.* 2012;126:S183–S188.
22. Salgo IS, Gorman JH 3rd, Gorman RC, et al. Effect of annular shape on leaflet curvature in reducing mitral leaflet stress. *Circulation.* 2002;106:711–717.
23. Carpentier AAD, Filsoufi F. In: *Carpentier's Reconstructive Valve Surgery.* 1st ed. Philadelphia, PA: Elsevier; 2010.
24. Anyanwu AC, Adams DH. Etiologic classification of degenerative mitral valve disease: Barlow's disease and fibroelastic deficiency. *Semin Thorac Cardiovasc Surg.* 2007;19:90–96.
25. Foster E. Clinical practice. Mitral regurgitation due to degenerative mitral-valve disease. *N Engl J Med.* 2010;363:156–165.
26. Clavel MA, Mantovani F, Malouf J, et al. Dynamic phenotypes of degenerative myxomatous mitral valve disease: quantitative 3-dimensional echocardiographic study. *Circ Cardiovasc Imaging.* 2015;8.
27. Obase K, Weinert L, Hollatz A, et al. Leaflet-chordal relations in patients with primary and secondary mitral regurgitation. *J Am Soc Echocardiogr.* 2015;28:1302–1308.
28. Delling FN, Vasan RS. Epidemiology and pathophysiology of mitral valve prolapse: new insights into disease progression, genetics, and molecular basis. *Circulation.* 2014;129:2158–2170.
29. Maron MS, Olivotto I, Harrigan C, et al. Mitral valve abnormalities identified by cardiovascular magnetic resonance represent a primary phenotypic expression of hypertrophic cardiomyopathy. *Circulation.* 2011;124:40–47.
30. Charitos EI, Hanke T, Karluss A, Hilker L, Stierle U, Sievers HH. New insights into bicuspid aortic valve disease: the elongated anterior mitral leaflet. *Eur J Cardio Thorac Surg.* 2013;43:367–370.
31. Ogawa S, Hayashi J, Sasaki H, et al. Evaluation of combined valvular prolapse syndrome by two-dimensional echocardiography. *Circulation.* 1982;65:174–180.
32. Lee AP, Jin CN, Fan Y, Wong RHL, Underwood MJ, Wan S. Functional implication of mitral annular disjunction in mitral valve prolapse: a quantitative dynamic 3D echocardiographic study. *JACC Cardiovasc Imaging.* 2017;10:1424–1433.
33. Dejgaard LA, Skjolsvik ET, Lie OH, et al. The mitral annulus disjunction arrhythmic syndrome. *J Am Coll Cardiol.* 2018;72:1600–1609.
34. Bennett S, Thamman R, Griffiths T, et al. Mitral annular disjunction: a systematic review of the literature. *Echocardiography.* 2019.
35. Hoen B, Duval X. Clinical practice. Infective endocarditis. *N Engl J Med.* 2013;368:1425–1433.
36. Harky A, Hof A, Garner M, Froghi S, Bashir M. Mitral valve repair or replacement in native valve endocarditis? Systematic review and meta-analysis. *J Card Surg.* 2018;33:364–371.
37. Lee HA, Cheng YT, Wu VC, et al. Nationwide cohort study of mitral valve repair versus replacement for infective endocarditis. *J Thorac Cardiovasc Surg.* 2018;156:1473–1483.e2.
38. Iung B, Vahanian A. Epidemiology of valvular heart disease in the adult. *Nat Rev Cardiol.* 2011;8:162–172.
39. Iung B, Baron G, Butchart EG, et al. A prospective survey of patients with valvular heart disease in Europe: the Euro Heart Survey on Valvular Heart Disease. *Eur Heart J.* 2003;24:1231–1243.
40. Dillon J, Yakub MA, Kong PK, Ramli MF, Jaffar N, Gaffar IF. Comparative long-term results of mitral valve repair in adults with chronic rheumatic disease and degenerative disease: is repair for "burnt-out" rheumatic disease still inferior to repair for degenerative disease in the current era? *J Thorac Cardiovasc Surg.* 2015;149:771–777; discussion 777–779.
41. Gujral DM, Lloyd G, Bhattacharyya S. Radiation-induced valvular heart disease. *Heart.* 2016;102:269–276.
42. Elmariah S, Budoff MJ, Delaney JA, et al. Risk factors associated with the incidence and progression of mitral annulus calcification: the multi-ethnic study of atherosclerosis. *Am Heart J.* 2013;166:904–912.
43. Saran N, Greason KL, Schaff HV, et al. Does mitral valve calcium in patients undergoing mitral valve replacement Portend Worse survival? *Ann Thorac Surg.* 2019;107:444–452.
44. Mihaila S, Muraru D, Miglioranza MH, et al. Normal mitral annulus dynamics and its relationships with left ventricular and left atrial function. *Int J Cardiovasc Imaging.* 2015;31:279–290.
45. Tang Z, Fan YT, Wang Y, Jin CN, Kwok KW, Lee AP. Mitral annular and left ventricular dynamics in atrial functional mitral regurgitation: a three-dimensional and Speckle-Tracking echocardiographic study. *J Am Soc Echocardiogr.* 2019;32:503–513.
46. Kim DH, Heo R, Handschumacher MD, et al. Mitral valve adaptation to isolated annular dilation: insights into the mechanism of atrial functional mitral regurgitation. *JACC Cardiovasc Imaging.* 2019;12:665–677.
47. Otsuji Y, Levine RA, Takeuchi M, Sakata R, Tei C. Mechanism of ischemic mitral regurgitation. *J Cardiol.* 2008;51:145–156.
48. Kalra K, Wang Q, McIver BV, et al. Temporal changes in interpapillary muscle dynamics as an active indicator of mitral valve and left ventricular interaction in ischemic mitral regurgitation. *J Am Coll Cardiol.* 2014;64:1867–1879.

49. Kumanohoso T, Otsuji Y, Yoshifuku S, et al. Mechanism of higher incidence of ischemic mitral regurgitation in patients with inferior myocardial infarction: quantitative analysis of left ventricular and mitral valve geometry in 103 patients with prior myocardial infarction. *J Thorac Cardiovasc Surg*. 2003;125:135–143.
50. Song JM, Qin JX, Kongsaerepong V, et al. Determinants of ischemic mitral regurgitation in patients with chronic anterior wall myocardial infarction: a real time three-dimensional echocardiography study. *Echocardiography*. 2006;23:650–657.
51. van Wijngaarden SE, Kamperidis V, Regeer MV, et al. Three-dimensional assessment of mitral valve annulus dynamics and impact on quantification of mitral regurgitation. *Eur Heart J Cardiovasc Imaging*. 2018;19:176–184.
52. Vergnat M, Jassar AS, Jackson BM, et al. Ischemic mitral regurgitation: a quantitative three-dimensional echocardiographic analysis. *Ann Thorac Surg*. 2011;91:157–164.
53. Yoshida S, Fukushima S, Miyagawa S, et al. The adaptive remodeling of the anterior mitral leaflet and chordae tendineae is associated with mitral valve function in advanced ischemic and nonischemic dilated cardiomyopathy. *Int Heart J*. 2018;59:959–967.
54. Zeng X, Nunes MC, Dent J, et al. Asymmetric versus symmetric tethering patterns in ischemic mitral regurgitation: geometric differences from three-dimensional transesophageal echocardiography. *J Am Soc Echocardiogr*. 2014;27:367–375.
55. Kron IL, Hung J, Overbey JR, et al. Predicting recurrent mitral regurgitation after mitral valve repair for severe ischemic mitral regurgitation. *J Thorac Cardiovasc Surg*. 2015;149:752–761. e1.
56. Daimon M, Saracino G, Gillinov AM, et al. Local dysfunction and asymmetrical deformation of mitral annular geometry in ischemic mitral regurgitation: a novel computerized 3D echocardiographic analysis. *Echocardiography*. 2008;25:414–423.
57. Nagasaki M, Nishimura S, Ohtaki E, et al. The echocardiographic determinants of functional mitral regurgitation differ in ischemic and non-ischemic cardiomyopathy. *Int J Cardiol*. 2006;108:171–176.
58. Acker MA, Gelijns AC, Kron IL. Surgery for severe ischemic mitral regurgitation. *N Engl J Med*. 2014;370:1463.
59. Acker MA, Dagenais F, Goldstein D, Kron IL, Perrault LP. Severe ischemic mitral regurgitation: repair or replace? *J Thorac Cardiovasc Surg*. 2015;150:1425–1427.
60. Wrobel K, Stevens SR, Jones RH, et al. Influence of baseline characteristics, operative conduct, and postoperative course on 30-day outcomes of coronary artery bypass grafting among patients with left ventricular dysfunction: results from the Surgical Treatment for Ischemic Heart Failure (STICH) trial. *Circulation*. 2015;132:720–730.
61. van Garsse L, Gelsomino S, Luca F, et al. Importance of anterior leaflet tethering in predicting recurrence of ischemic mitral regurgitation after restrictive annuloplasty. *J Thorac Cardiovasc Surg*. 2012;143:S54–S59.
62. Kongsaerepong V, Shiota M, Gillinov AM, et al. Echocardiographic predictors of successful versus unsuccessful mitral valve repair in ischemic mitral regurgitation. *Am J Cardiol*. 2006;98:504–508.
62a. Stone GW, Lindenfeld J, Abraham WT, et al. Transcatheter mitral-valve repair in patients with heart failure. *N Engl J Med*. 2018;379 (24):2307–2318.
63. Hensley N, Dietrich J, Nyhan D, Mitter N, Yee MS, Brady M. Hypertrophic cardiomyopathy: a review. *Anesth Analg*. 2015;120:554–569.
64. Gersh BJ, Maron BJ, Bonow RO, et al. ACCF/AHA guideline for the diagnosis and treatment of hypertrophic cardiomyopathy: a report of the American College of Cardiology Foundation/American Heart Association Task Force on Practice Guidelines. Developed in collaboration with the American Association for Thoracic Surgery, American Society of Echocardiography, American Society of Nuclear Cardiology, Heart Failure Society of America, Heart Rhythm Society, Society for Cardiovascular Angiography and Interventions, and Society of Thoracic Surgeons. *J Am Coll Cardiol 2011*. 2011;58:e212–e260.
65. Elliott PM, Anastasakis A, Borger MA, et al. 2014. ESC guidelines on diagnosis and management of hypertrophic cardiomyopathy: the Task Force for the Diagnosis and Management of Hypertrophic Cardiomyopathy of the European Society of Cardiology (ESC). *Eur Heart J*. 2014;35:2733–2779.
66. Patel P, Dhillon A, Popovic ZB, et al. Left ventricular outflow tract obstruction in hypertrophic cardiomyopathy patients without severe septal hypertrophy: implications of mitral valve and papillary muscle abnormalities assessed using cardiac magnetic resonance and echocardiography. *Circ Cardiovasc Imaging*. 2015;8. e003132.
67. Lang RM, Badano LP, Tsang W, et al. EAE/ASE recommendations for image acquisition and display using three-dimensional echocardiography. *J Am Soc Echocardiogr*. 2012;25:3–46.
68. Mahmood F, Hess PE, Matyal R, et al. Echocardiographic anatomy of the mitral valve: a critical appraisal of 2-dimensional imaging protocols with a 3-dimensional perspective. *J Cardiothorac Vasc Anesth*. 2012;269(5):777–784.
69. Hymel BJ, Townsley MM. Echocardiographic assessment of systolic anterior motion of the mitral valve. *Anesth Analg*. 2014;118:1197–1201.
70. Nishimura RA, Otto CM, Bonow RO, et al. 2014. AHA/ACC guideline for the management of patients with valvular heart disease: a report of the American College of Cardiology/American Heart Association Task Force on Practice Guidelines. *J Am Coll Cardiol*. 2014;63:e57–185.
71. Braunberger E, Deloche A, Berrebi A, et al. Very long-term results (more than 20 years) of valve repair with Carpentier's techniques in nonrheumatic mitral valve insufficiency. *Circulation*. 2001;104:I8–11.
72. David TE, David CM, Tsang W, Lafreniere-Roula M, Manlhiot C. Long-term results of mitral valve repair for regurgitation due to leaflet prolapse. *J Am Coll Cardiol*. 2019;74:1044–1053.
73. Perier P, Hohenberger W, Lakew F, et al. Toward a new paradigm for the reconstruction of posterior leaflet prolapse: midterm results of the "respect rather than resect" approach. *Ann Thorac Surg*. 2008;86:718–725; discussion 718-725.
74. Papadopoulos N, Steuer K, Doss M, Moritz A, Zierer A. Is removal of calcium bar during mitral valve surgery safe? Long-term clinical outcome of 109 consecutive patients. *J Cardiovasc Surg*. 2015;56:473–482.
75. Bouma W, Wijdh-den Hamer IJ, Koene BM, et al. Predictors of in-hospital mortality after mitral valve surgery for post-myocardial infarction papillary muscle rupture. *J Cardiothorac Surg*. 2014;9:171.
76. Fasol R, Lakew F, Pfannmuller B, Slepian MJ, Joubert-Hubner E. Papillary muscle repair surgery in ischemic mitral valve patients. *Ann Thorac Surg*. 2000;70:771–776; discussion 776–777.
77. Magne J, Senechal M, Dumesnil JG, Pibarot P. Ischemic mitral regurgitation: a complex multifaceted disease. *Cardiology*. 2009;112:244–259.
78. Nappi F, Lusini M, Avtaar Singh SS, Santana O, Chello M, Mihos CG. Risk of ischemic mitral regurgitation recurrence after combined valvular and subvalvular repair. *Ann Thorac Surg*. 2019;108:536–543.
79. Mihos CG, Pineda AM, Horvath SA, Santana O. Anterior mitral leaflet augmentation for ischemic mitral regurgitation performed via a right thoracotomy approach. *Innovat Tech Tech CardioThorac Vasc Surg*. 2016;11:298–300.
80. Obase K, Matsumaru I, Miura T, Eishi K. Echocardiographic visualization and quantification of mitral complex during mitral repair for severe functional mitral regurgitation. *J Thorac Cardiovasc Surg*. 2017;154:1252–1255.
81. Meyer MA, von Segesser LK, Hurni M, Stumpe F, Eisa K, Ruchat P. Long-term outcome after mitral valve repair: a risk factor analysis. *Eur J Cardio Thorac Surg*. 2007;32:301–307.
82. Suri RM, Schaff HV, Dearani JA, et al. Survival advantage and improved durability of mitral repair for leaflet prolapse subsets in the current era. *Ann Thorac Surg*. 2006;82:819–826.
83. Riegel AK, Busch R, Segal S, Fox JA, Eltzschig HK, Shernan SK. Evaluation of transmitral pressure gradients in the intraoperative echocardiographic diagnosis of mitral stenosis after mitral valve repair. *PLoS One*. 2011;6. e26559.
84. Kuperstein R, Spiegelstein D, Rotem G, et al. Late clinical outcome of transient intraoperative systolic anterior motion post mitral valve repair. *J Thorac Cardiovasc Surg*. 2015;149:471–476.
85. Varghese R, Anyanwu AC, Itagaki S, Milla F, Castillo J, Adams DH. Management of systolic anterior motion after mitral valve repair: an algorithm. *J Thorac Cardiovasc Surg*. 2012;143:S2–S7.
86. Ibrahim M, Rao C, Ashrafian H, Chaudhry U, Darzi A, Athanasiou T. Modern management of systolic anterior motion of the mitral valve. *Eur J Cardio Thorac Surg*. 2012;41:1260–1270.
87. Hsuan CF, Yu HY, Tseng WK, Lin LC, Hsu KL, Wu CC. Quantitation of the mitral tetrahedron in patients with ischemic heart disease using real-time three-dimensional echocardiography to evaluate the geometric determinants of ischemic mitral regurgitation. *Clin Cardiol*. 2013;36:286–292.

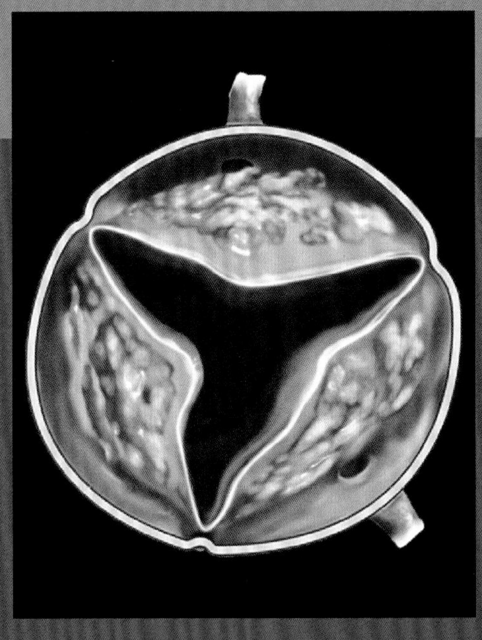

中文导读

第26章
经导管二尖瓣修复术

人口老龄化的发展导致二尖瓣反流的发病率呈逐年上升趋势。对于重度二尖瓣反流的临床治疗，在指征适宜的人群中，传统外科手术正在被非手术或杂交手术方式补充或替代。2020年AHA/ACC指南及2017年ESC指南推荐给予症状严重的二尖瓣反流患者临床干预，主要包括外科二尖瓣置换术、外科二尖瓣成形术和二尖瓣经皮介入缘对缘修复术。其中二尖瓣经皮介入缘对缘修复术（如MitraClip）与传统瓣膜手术相比，治疗临床症状严重的二尖瓣反流疗效类似。因此，指南推荐对于手术风险高或有禁忌证的患者，二尖瓣经皮介入缘对缘修复术可作为外科二尖瓣置换或成形的安全及有效的替代方法。研究共识表明超声心动图是评估二尖瓣反流机制、反流程度及其对于心脏结构、功能影响的基础。

本章主要介绍超声心动图在二尖瓣经皮介入缘对缘修复术患者的筛选（包括二尖瓣反流病因判断、反流程度评估、适应证超声参数评估等），介入超声引导规范流程（包括房间隔穿刺、输送装置进入及导航、瓣叶抓取、瓣膜释放、残余反流评估）以及效果评估的应用要点。

李　慧

26 Transcatheter Mitral Valve Repair

ERNESTO E. SALCEDO, MD | ROBERT A. QUAIFE, MD | JOHN D. CARROLL, MD

Despite the reduced incidence of rheumatic heart disease, the prevalence of mitral regurgitation (MR) is increasing and is anticipated to continue to increase as the population ages.[12] The management of advanced valvular heart disease, once the unique domain of cardiac surgery, is being supplemented or replaced in certain patient populations by nonsurgical or hybrid catheter-based interventions.[3–5] The 2020 AHA/ACC Guidelines for Management of Patients with Valvular Heart Disease[7] and the 2017 European Society of Cardiology Guidelines[6] for the management of valvular heart disease outline the appropriate interventions in patients with severe symptomatic MR, including recommendations for surgical mitral valve (MV) replacement, surgical MV repair, and mitral transcatheter edge-to-edge repair (TEER)[6,7] Comparisons of TEER (i.e., MitraClip, Abbott Vascular, Santa Clara, CA) with conventional valvular surgery for the treatment of severe symptomatic MR demonstrated no inferiority of the MitraClip as a treatment option.[8] In patients with high operative risk or contraindications for surgery, TEER has emerged as a feasible and safe alternative to surgical mitral valve replacement or repair.[9,10]

Consensus documents from the Mitral Valve Academic Research Consortium define the clinical trial design principles and end point definitions for TEER and replacement and emphasize the fact that echocardiography is fundamental in evaluating the causes, mechanisms, and severity of MR and its effects on cardiac structures and function.[11,12]

This chapter reviews the crucial role that echocardiography plays in patient selection, image guidance, and evaluation of outcomes in patients with MR undergoing TEER.

PERCUTANEOUS THERAPIES FOR MITRAL REGURGITATION

OVERVIEW

TEER is a feasible and safe alternative to surgical MV replacement or repair in patients with high operative risk or contraindications for surgery.[9,10] Multiple TEER technologies have been developed addressing each component of the mitral apparatus thought to be responsible for the MV dysfunction[13–16](Fig. 26.1). Each approach is tailored toward treating specific MV pathologies and regurgitation mechanisms. Transcatheter MV replacement has also become a reality.[17] Accurate and detailed evaluation of MV morphology and function is critical for the success of these interventions. Echocardiography plays a pivotal role in patient selection, procedural guidance, and evaluation of immediate and long-term results.[3,4,18]

Historically, reoperation was the only recourse for a failing bioprosthetic valve. Today, percutaneous options exist with the use of transcatheter valve implantation. Determining candidacy for this less invasive valve-in-valve option requires careful evaluation with echocardiography.[19] Transcatheter MV replacement and other novel approaches to TEER are being developed and are likely to expand the options to treat MV diseases percutaneously.[14,20–24] This chapter focuses on transcatheter repair using the edge-to-edge MitraClip technology (Fig. 26.2). Much of the knowledge and experience gained in selecting patients, guiding the intervention, and assessing the result of edge-to-edge repair can be applied to newer technologies as they enter clinical practice.

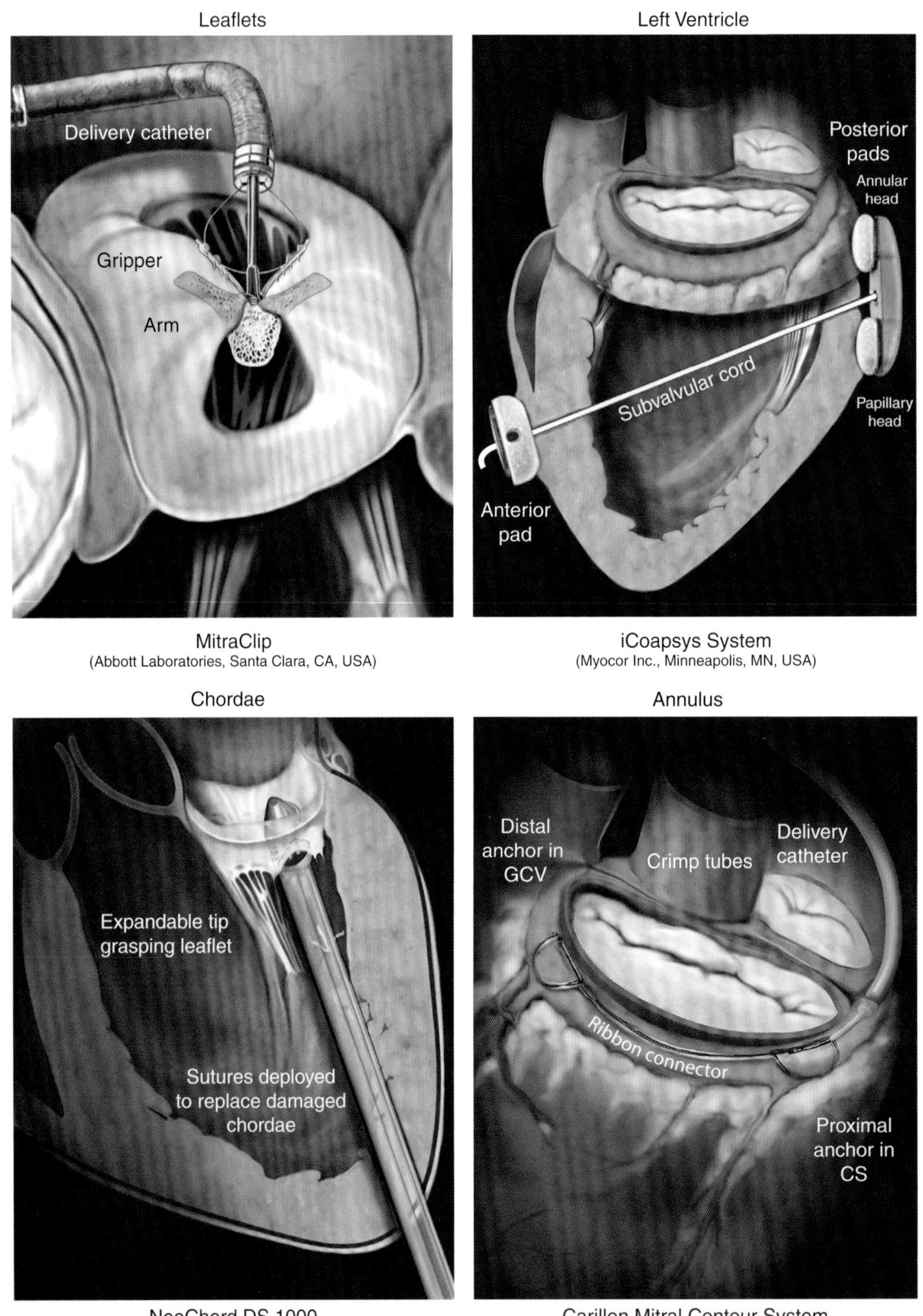

Fig. 26.1 Percutaneous mitral repair targets. All of the mitral apparatus components have been targeted in various ways for percutaneous mitral repair, including the leaflets, LV, chordae, and the mitral annulus. The most common procedure is edge-to-edge mitral repair with the MitraClip system. *CS*, Coronary sinus; *GCV*, great cardiac vein.

TEER is the general approach, with MitraClip edge-to-edge repair representing the major commercially available technology. MitraClip has achieved approval by the US Food and Drug Administration and the European Union CE Mark. The most recent generation of the MitraClip device, the MitraClip G4, puts new enhancements into the hands of physicians by delivering an expanded range of clip sizes, an alternative leaflet grasping feature, and procedure assessment in real time for treatment of MV disease.

EDGE-TO-EDGE MITRAL VALVE REPAIR

Of all available TEER procedures, the edge-to-edge MV repair has been used the most and has by far the largest number of treated patients. As of 2019, more than 80,000 patients had been treated with MitraClip therapy around the world. The first procedure was done in Venezuela in June 2003; this was quickly followed by the first procedure in the United States, which was performed on July 2, 2003, by Dr. Ted Feldman. The first procedure in Europe was performed on September 17, 2008, by

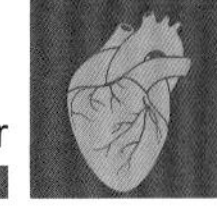

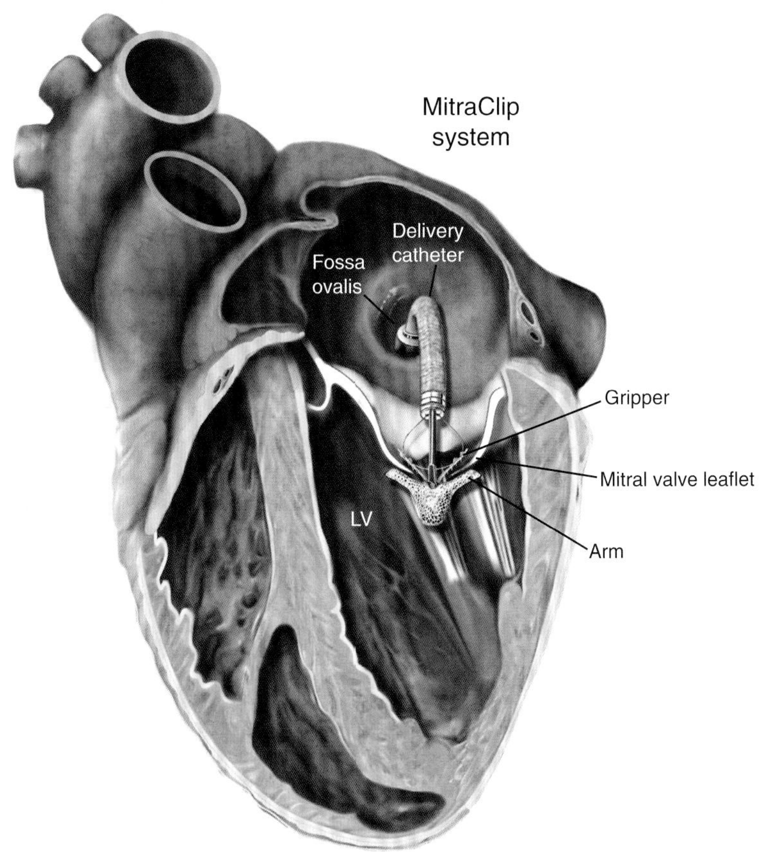

Fig. 26.2 The MitraClip system. Drawing of the MitraClip system shows the delivery catheter entering the LA through the fossa ovalis area and the clip with open arms in the LV near the tip of the mitral valve leaflets. (Image courtesy Abbott Vascular, Santa Clara, CA.)

Dr. Olaf Franzen. The use of TEER continues to expand, and a recent report highlights its potential application in nonagenarians.[25] In addition, there is growing interest in combining mitral and tricuspid edge-to-edge repairs in patients with severe MR and tricuspid regurgitation[26] and in using the MitraClip in the tricuspid valve for isolated severe tricuspid regurgitation.[27]

Multiple US and international prospective clinical trials and registries (Table 26.1) have demonstrated that in patients who are deemed to be at high risk for MV surgery, the percutaneous edge-to-edge mitral repair is feasible, safe, and effective in reducing mitral insufficiency, with resultant improvement of clinical symptoms, reduced frequency of hospitalizations for heart failure, improved quality of life, and significant left ventricular (LV) reverse remodeling.[10,28–43] Although the initial experience with the MitraClip was evaluated in primary MR, this has now been expanded to include patients with secondary mitral regurgitation.[44–47] Echocardiography has played a central role in these trials.[29,36,48–54] Three-dimensional (3D) transesophageal echocardiography (TEE) has expanded our understanding of the effects of the MitraClip procedure on the shape and size of the mitral annulus.[55,56] The applicability and use of 3D TEE among the various imaging modalities for the assessment and guidance of therapy for MV disorders was reviewed in 2018.[57]

USE OF ECHOCARDIOGRAPHY IN PATIENT SELECTION

Patients likely to benefit from TEER have moderate to severe (3+) or severe (4+) primary MR, suitable MV morphology, and high to prohibitive surgical risk. The 2020 AHA/ACC Valve Guidelines continue to recommend mitral valve surgery, with surgical valve repair when possible for primary MR unless surgical risk is prohibitive.[7] Two-dimensional (2D) transthoracic echocardiography (TTE) is recommended as the first-line imaging tool in MR and is often sufficient for diagnosis and characterization of the cause and severity of the MR. 2D TEE is used to better characterize mitral leaflet morphology and for guidance in preprocedural planning. 3D TEE provides realistic and intuitive anatomic images of the mitral leaflets and further aids in patient eligibility for TEER.

In addition to characterizing MV morphology and function, echocardiography is used for the quantitative assessment of LV diameters, volumes, and ejection fraction. The TTE 2D-based biplane method of disks is the recommended approach for the estimation of LV volumes and ejection fraction.[58] The MitraClip is contraindicated in patients with active endocarditis, rheumatic MV disease, small MV annulus, and evidence of intracardiac thrombus; echocardiography aids in excluding all of these problems. MV characteristics that potentially decrease the chance of a successful MitraClip repair include dense calcification of the mitral annulus, MV clefts, excessive leaflet flail gap or width, and inappropriate leaflet coaptation depth and length (Fig. 26.3). Finally, the location of the regurgitant jet or jets is best characterized by TEE and should be noted using the A1–A3/P1–P3 (Carpentier) nomenclature.

DETERMINING THE CAUSE OF MITRAL REGURGITATION

Most of the studies dealing with TEER have adopted the classification of MR as primary (i.e., intrinsic valvular disease, called primary, organic, or structural MR) or secondary (i.e., without evident structural abnormalities of the MV, called secondary or nonstructural MR). Secondary MR develops despite a structurally normal MV in the context of ischemic heart disease or dilated cardiomyopathy.

TABLE 26.1 MitraClip Trials and Registries: Role of Echocardiography.

Study	Design	Findings	Echo Parameters
EVEREST I[28] 2003–2006, USA *N* = 55 patients	Feasibility trial designed to evaluate the preliminary safety and effectiveness of the MitraClip device in the treatment of moderately severe (3+) or severe (4+) chronic MR	Percutaneous edge-to-edge MV repair can be performed safely, and MR can be reduced in a significant proportion of patients at 6 months.	MR severity 3+ or 4+ MVA > 4 cm^2 EF > 30% LVESD < 55 mm Appropriate mitral anatomy for device implantation
EVEREST II RCT[10,30,31,42] 2005–2008, USA *N* = 279 patients	RCT comparing the MitraClip for the reduction of MR with standard of care MV surgery Primary and secondary MR studied	Although percutaneous repair was less effective in reducing MR than conventional surgery, the procedure was associated with superior safety and similar improvements in clinical outcomes.	MR severity 3+ or 4+ MVA > 4 cm^2 EF > 30% LVESD < 55 mm Appropriate mitral anatomy for device implantation
EVEREST II HRR[73] 2007–2008, USA *N* = 78 patients	High-Risk Registry Primary and secondary MR studied	Percutaneous MV device significantly reduced MR, improved clinical symptoms, and decreased LV dimensions at 12 months in this high-surgical-risk cohort.	MR severity 3+ or 4+ MVA > 4 cm^2 EF > 30% LVESD < 55 mm Appropriate mitral anatomy for device implantation
REALISM HR[95] 2009–2013, USA *N* = 78 patients	Study evaluated treatment of MR in patients with severe primary MR at prohibitive surgical risk undergoing TEER	TEER in prohibitive-surgical-risk patients is associated with safety and good clinical outcomes, including decreases in rehospitalization, functional improvements, and favorable ventricular remodeling at 1 year.	TTE and TEE screening was used to establish protocol-based eligibility for the TEER procedure.
COAPT[45] 2012–2018, USA *N* = 614 patients	Randomization between MitraClip and medical therapy	TEER resulted in a lower rate of hospitalization for heart failure and lower all-cause mortality rate at 24 months of follow-up than medical therapy alone.	Secondary MR
MITRA_FR[43] 2015, France *N* = 288 patients	National RCT evaluated the benefits and safety of the MitraClip with medical therapy alone (control) in patients with severe symptomatic secondary MR	Among patients with severe secondary MR, the rate of death or unplanned hospitalization for heart failure at 1 year was not significantly different between patients who underwent percutaneous MV repair in addition to receiving medical therapy and those who received medical therapy alone.	Secondary MR
TRAMI Registry[34,96,97] 2010–2013, Germany *N* = 1064	Investigator-initiated multicenter national transcatheter MV interventions registry	Patients treated with MitraClip in Germany are mainly elderly with significant comorbidities and a high or unacceptable surgical risk. Most have secondary MR, and many have reduced LVEF.	Functional (two thirds of patients) vs. degenerative MR
GRASP-IT[33,98] 2013, Italy *N* = 117 patients	Report on the 30-day and 1-year outcomes of percutaneous MV repair with the MitraClip technique in patients with grade ≥ 3+ MR at high risk for conventional surgical therapy	Percutaneous MV repair with the MitraClip technique was safe and reasonably effective in 117 patients in a real-world setting.	The primary efficacy end point was freedom from death, surgery for MV dysfunction, or grade ≥ 3+ MR at 30 days and 1 year
CLASP[99] 2019, USA *N* = 62 patients	Trial evaluated the PASCAL system for treating 56% functional, 36% degenerative, and 8% mixed MR causes	The PASCAL repair system showed feasibility and acceptable safety in the treatment of patients with grade 3+ or 4+ MR severity regardless of cause.	At 30 days, the rate of major adverse events was 6.5%, with an all-cause mortality rate of 1.6%. Echocardiographic images were assessed by a core laboratory.

EF, Ejection fraction; *LVESD*, left ventricular end-systolic diameter; *MR*, mitral regurgitation; *MV*, mitral valve; *MVA*, mitral valve area; *RCT*, randomized, controlled trial; *TEER*, mitral transcatheter edge-to-edge repair.

The distinction between secondary and primary MR has practical implications related to TEER because there are specific echocardiographic exclusion criteria for each of these forms of MR (see Fig. 26.3), as well as mild differences in severity grading. An integrative clinical and echocardiographic approach to chronic MR, with a focus on the contrasts between primary and secondary MR, is essential for correct diagnosis, characterization, and management.[59]

PRIMARY MITRAL REGURGITATION

Primary MV disease is the most common cause of MR being treated with surgery[60] and has been the main MV pathology in many studies of TEER. Several forms of primary MR exist and have been well characterized by echocardiography.[61,62] These include the spectrum from mild single-scallop MV prolapse (usually fibroelastic deficiency) to multiscallop severe prolapse (Barlow disease) and ruptured chordae with flail leaflet (Fig. 26.4). Whereas the ideal TEER candidate will have central MR originating from prolapse affecting the A2-P2 scallops, the MitraClip can be implanted in patients with prolapse or flail of any of the scallops, with the caveat that potential Clip Delivery System entrapment in the chordae apparatus is increased.

SECONDARY MITRAL REGURGITATION

Unlike primary MR, for which repair therapy is clearly preferred, the optimal approach for secondary MR is still being defined. This has created growing interest in the potential application of TEER in patients with heart failure and secondary MR. Patients with both ischemic and non-ischemic secondary MR typically have structurally normal leaflets and mitral insufficiency due to poor leaflet coaptation (Fig. 26.5), leaflet tethering, tenting, and mitral annular dilation. In some patients, the posterior leaflet remains in a semi-open position throughout the cardiac cycle (restricted leaflet motion), and the anterior leaflet appears to be prolapsing during systole. The systolic restriction of posterior leaflet motion seen in secondary MR should not be confused with that seen in carcinoid or lupus valve disease or, more

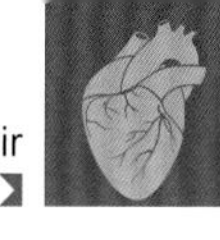

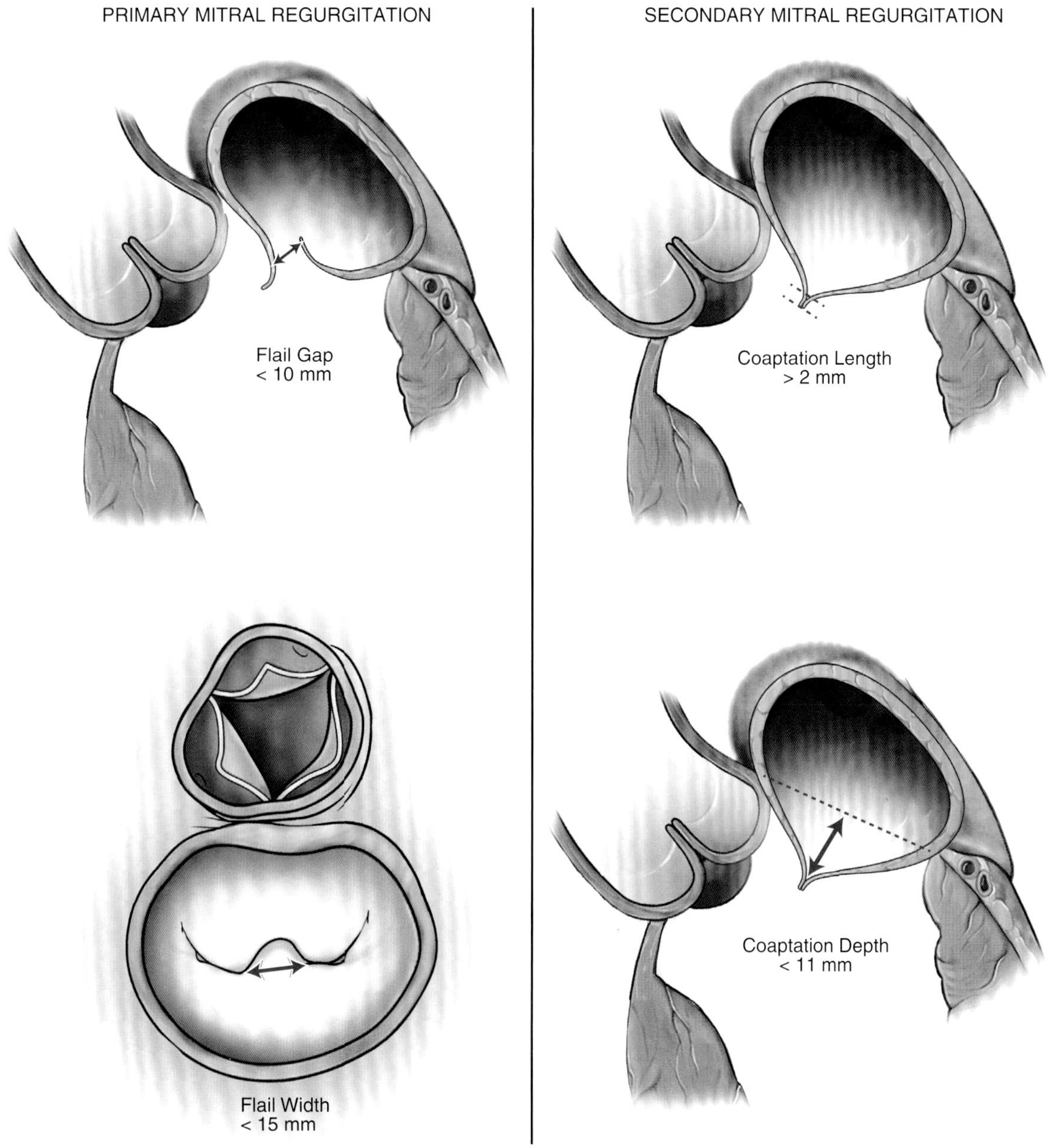

Fig. 26.3 Primary and secondary mitral regurgitation: morphologic qualifiers. In patients with primary mitral regurgitation (MR), qualifying morphologic mitral valve parameters for the MitraClip include a flail gap of less than 10 mm and a flail width of 15 mm. For patients with secondary MR, the coaptation length should be 2 mm or more, and the coaptation depth should be less than 11 mm. These measurements are based on the clip's arm length and the reaching length of the delivery catheter.

commonly, with rheumatic MR, where, in addition to systolic and diastolic leaflet motion restriction, there usually is leaflet thickening (especially at the tips), chordal thickening, and the key component of rheumatic involvement, commissural fusion. The 2020 AHA/ACC Valve Guidelines for secondary MR indicate that TEER is reasonable in patients with a low LVEF (<50%) with persistent symptoms on optimal guideline-directed medical therapy when mitral valve anatomy is favorable, LVEF is between 20% and 50%, LV end systolic diameter is less than 70 mm, and pulmonary systolic pressure is less than 70 mmHg.[7]

MIXED MITRAL REGURGITATION

Although the classification of secondary MR versus primary MR is well established and has helped in determining the appropriate therapeutic options, there exists a group of patients that can be better characterized as having mixed MR from a combination of primary and secondary causes. A good example would be a patient with MV prolapse who develops myocardial infarction (Fig. 26.6) or LV dilation and dysfunction, adding a secondary component to the MR. An attempt should be made to characterize the predominant type of MR as primary or secondary.

DETERMINING MITRAL REGURGITATION SEVERITY

Precise quantification of MR severity is essential for patient selection for TEER. Foster et al.[49] published the echocardiographic results from the first human trial of MitraClip and described a systematic and integrative approach to the analysis of MR severity at baseline and follow-up that included quantitative parameters.

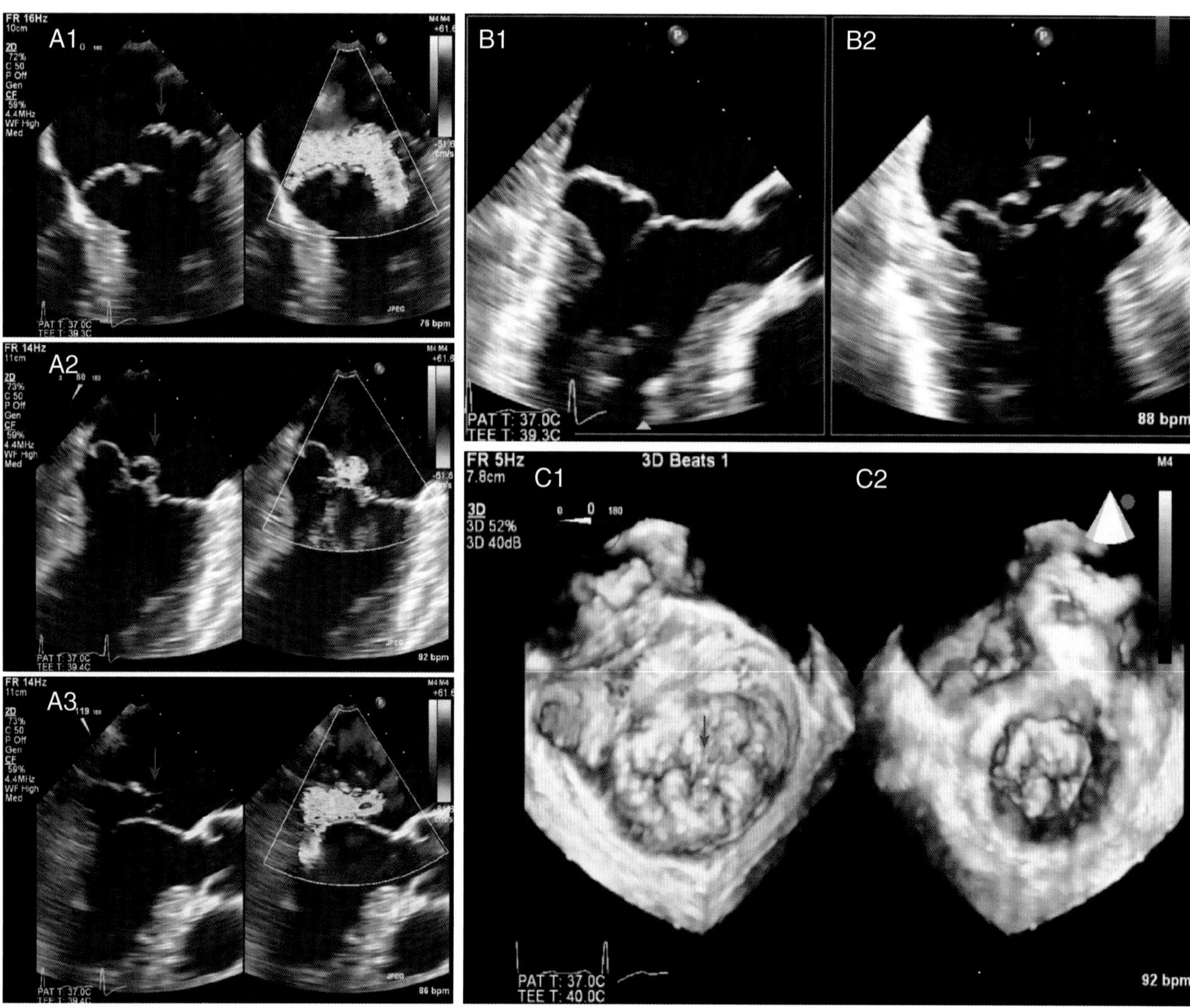

Fig. 26.4 Primary mitral regurgitation. Transesophageal 2D (A) and 3D (B and C) echocardiography in a patient with primary mitral regurgitation with ruptured chordae and a flail P2 scallop (see Videos 26.4A and 26.4C). Panels A1, A2, and A3 are mid-esophageal views at 0 degrees (4-chamber view), 60 degrees (bicommissural view), and 120 degrees (LV outflow tract view), respectively, depicting the flail P2 leaflet *(red arrows)* and the mitral regurgitant jet from different perspectives. Panels B1 and B2 represent biplane views of the mitral valve illustrating a flail segment of the P2 scallop *(red arrow)*. Panels C1 and C2 illustrate left atrial and left ventricular 3D perspectives of the mitral valve depicting the ruptured chordae and flail scallop *(red arrow)*.

This echocardiographic analysis showed the feasibility of a systematic standardized echocardiographic protocol to evaluate baseline entry criteria and efficacy of MR reduction in a multicenter clinical trial. This approach became the standard in subsequent trials and underscores the pivotal role played by echocardiography in the management of patients undergoing TEER. All of the TEER trials agree on the criterion of moderate to severe (3+) or severe (4+) MR for patients to be considered for therapy.

The American Society of Echocardiography and the European Association of Cardiovascular Imaging have published guidelines and recommendations for MR severity assessment.[63,64] These guidelines, as well as several review articles,[65,66] have emphasized an integrative and comprehensive approach that incorporates multiple variables for the quantification of MR, including qualitative findings (MV morphology, color flow jet size and shape, and spectral Doppler jet characteristics), semiquantitative measures (vena contracta width, pulmonary vein flow characteristics, and mitral inflow velocities), and quantitative parameters (effective regurgitant orifice area [EROA] and regurgitant volume). Evaluating the LV volumes and ejection fraction as well as pulmonary artery systolic pressure provides supportive information. There is increased interest in the use of 3D TEE measurement of the vena contracta area as a more robust parameter for quantification of MR.[67]

MR severity should be initially evaluated by TTE when the patient is clinically stable and awake because sedation and general anesthesia may alter the degree of regurgitation through manipulation of cardiac loading conditions. It is also important to register the blood pressure during the procedure and to consider the MR severity as it relates to this determinant (i.e., sedation and anesthesia) of loading conditions.

MODERATE TO SEVERE MITRAL REGURGITATION

Patients with moderately severe MR (i.e., the traditional 3+ score on a scale of 0 to 4+) have an MR jet of intermediate size on color-flow images. The leaflets may or may not show pathologic abnormalities, the flow convergence area is intermediate in size, the continuous-wave echocardiographic signal of the MR jet is dense and parabolic, the vena contracta is intermediate in size, the pulmonary vein flow shows systolic blunting, the EROA is 20 to 29 mm^2, and the regurgitant volume is 30 to 44 mL.

SEVERE MITRAL REGURGITATION

Patients with severe MR usually have a large color-flow MR jet (area > 40% of the left atrial [LA] area for central jets), a vena

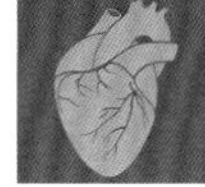

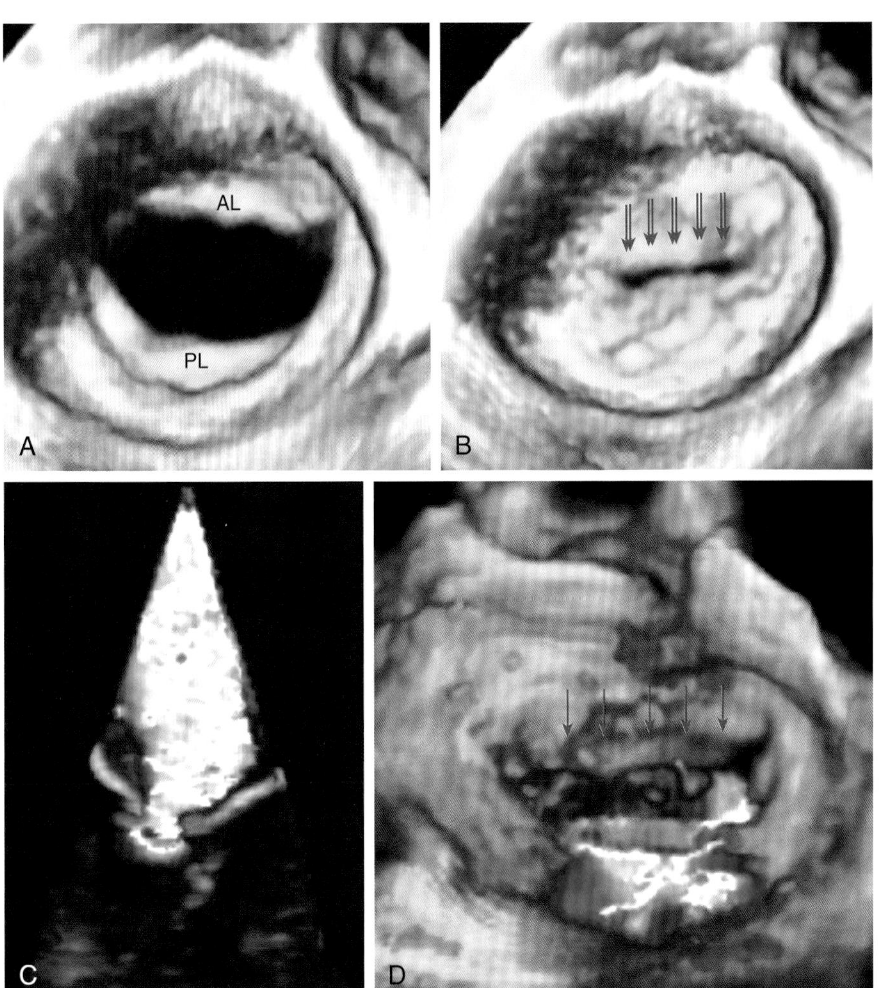

Fig. 26.5 Secondary mitral regurgitation. (A) The open mitral valve is seen from the LA during diastole. The anterior leaflet *(AL)* and posterior leaflet *(PL)* are fully opened (see Video 26.5A ▶). (B) During systole, the mitral leaflet is closed, but there is an area of non-coaptation along the coaptation line *(red arrows)*. (C) 3D color image of the regurgitant jet filling most of the LA. (D) 3D color en face view of the mitral regurgitation jet along the line of non-coaptation of the mitral valve *(red arrows)*.

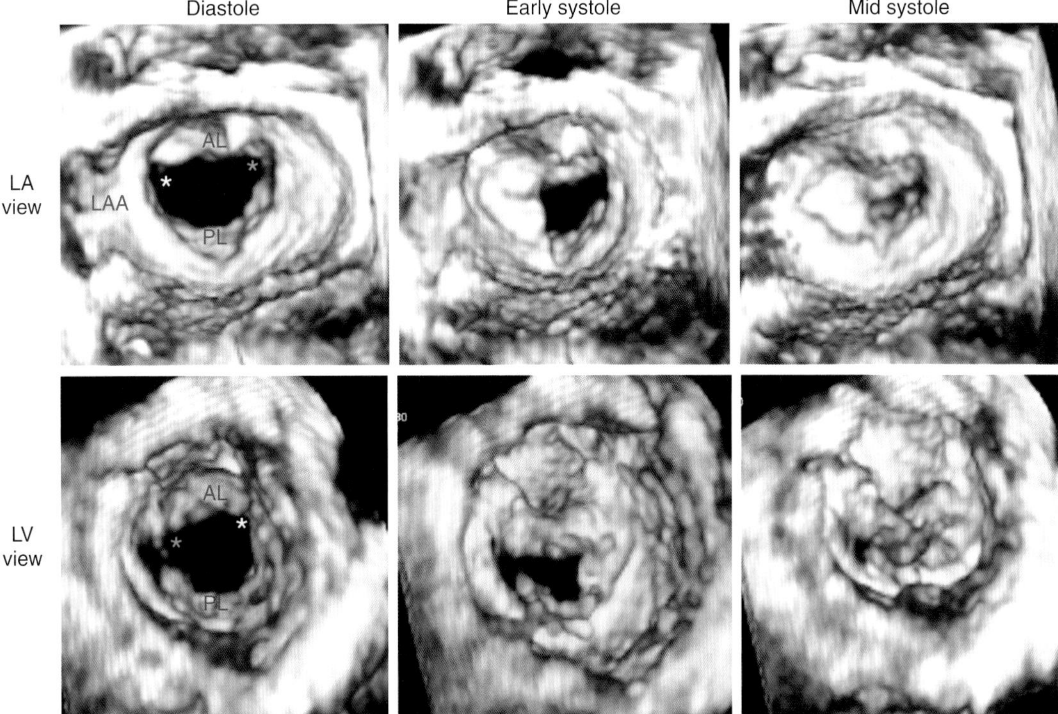

Fig. 26.6 Mixed mitral regurgitation. Patient with primary mitral valve disease with mitral valve prolapse of the A1-P1 scallops and restricted motion of the posterior leaflet *(PL)* caused by tethering of the P3 segment. The images in diastole depict the open anterior leaflet *(AL)* and the PL, as well as the uncompromised lateral commissure *(yellow asterisk)* next to the left atrial appendage *(LAA)* and the medial commissure *(green asterisk)*, from the LA and LV perspectives. In early systole, the lateral scallops close first, and it is not until mid-systole that the medial scallops coapt (see Videos 26.6A ▶ and 26.6B ▶).

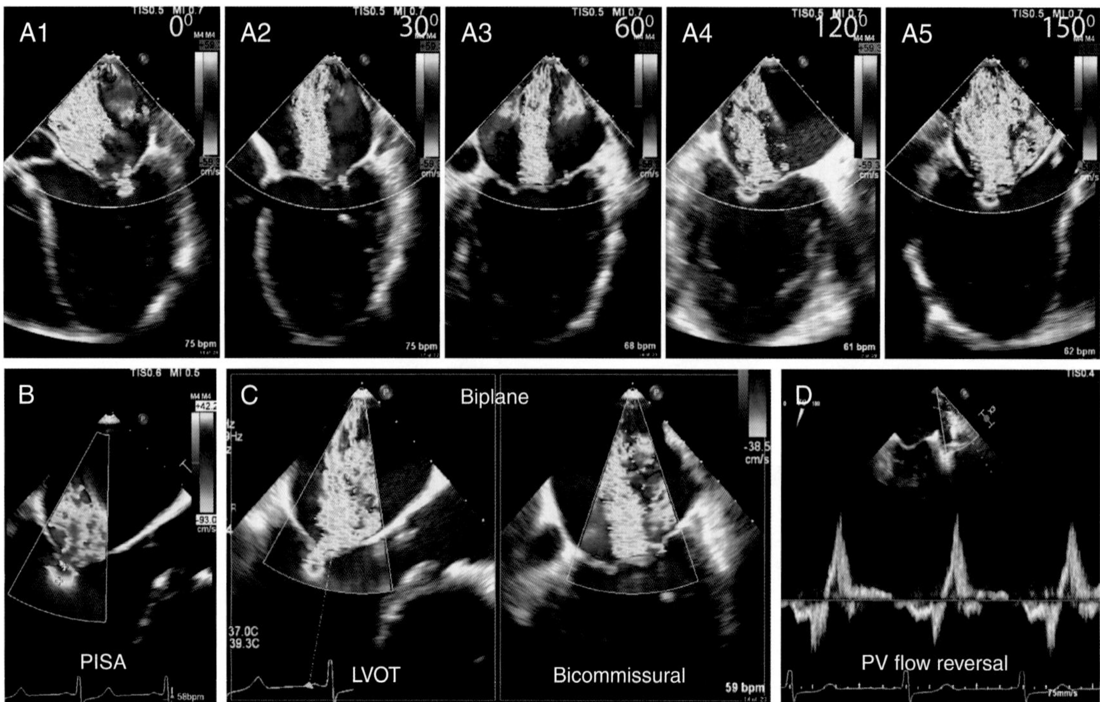

Fig. 26.7 Preprocedure mitral regurgitation characterization. Preprocedure TEE in a patient with severe secondary mitral regurgitation (MR). The upper panels (A1 through A5) depict multiple omniplane views from 0 to 150 degrees that characterize the severity and flow direction of the MR jet. (B) There is a large (9-mm) proximal isovelocity surface area *(PISA)*. (C) A simultaneous biplane (X-plane) image demonstrates the MR jet size and direction simultaneously from the LV outflow tract (LVOT) view and the bicommissural view. (D) Left upper pulmonary flow reversal indicates severe MR (see Videos 26.7A1, 26.7A2, 26.7A3, and 26.7C). *PV,* Pulmonary valve.

contracta of 7 mm or more, a large flow convergence zone (radius ≥ 9 mm), a dense and triangular CW signal of the MR jet, systolic flow reversal of the pulmonary veins, a dominant mitral inflow E wave of more than 1.5 m/s, an EROA greater than 40 mm^2, and a regurgitant volume equal to or greater than 60 mL. All of these parameters should be sought, and the more that are identified, the higher the chances that the MR is severe (Fig. 26.7).

ECHOCARDIOGRAPHIC PARAMETERS TO DETERMINE SUITABILITY FOR MITRAL TRANSCATHETER EDGE-TO-EDGE (TEER) REPAIR

The key echocardiographic points to consider in determining suitability for TEER include demonstration of moderately severe or severe MR and suitable MV morphology. Favorable valvular characteristics for TEER relate to the graspability of the leaflets in the area of regurgitation, and they relate to leaflet length and motility, the degree of thickening and calcification, the presence or absence of clefts, and an appropriate annulus size (>4 cm^2). Ideally, the posterior leaflet should be 10 mm or longer, and the MV annulus area should be 4 cm^2 or larger.

Suboptimal characteristics for TEER may not exclude a patient from consideration, but the chance of a successful procedure may be significantly reduced and technically more difficult to achieve. Unfavorable MV morphology that contraindicates a TEER includes mitral clefts or perforation, severe calcification in the grasping area, rheumatic MV disease, and mitral stenosis (Tables 26.2 and 26.3).

TABLE 26.2 Exclusion Criteria for TEER in Primary Mitral Regurgitation (EVEREST II Trial).

Severe LV dysfunction with ejection fraction < 25%
Severe LV dilation with LV end-systolic dimension > 55 mm
Mitral valve orifice area < 4 cm^2
Flail width > 15 mm; flail gap > 10 mm
Calcium in A2-P2 scallops grasping area
Significant cleft in A2-P2 scallops grasping area
Bileaflet flail or severe bileaflet prolapse
Lack of primary and secondary chordal support

TABLE 26.3 Exclusion Criteria for TEER in Secondary Mitral Regurgitation (COAPT Trial).

Transthoracic Echocardiography	*Transesophageal Echocardiography*
Mild or moderate mitral regurgitation	Presence of a second significant jet
LV ejection fraction < 20% or > 50%	Insufficient mobile leaflet available for grasping with the MitraClip device
LV end-systolic diameter > 70 mm	Calcification in the grasping area
Pulmonary artery systolic pressure > 70 mmHg	A significant cleft in the grasping area
Mitral valve orifice area < 4 cm^2	Lack of primary and secondary chordal support in the grasping area
Moderate or severe RV dysfunction	Leaflet mobility length < 1 cm
Tricuspid or aortic valve disease requiring surgery or intervention	Echocardiographic evidence of intracardiac mass, thrombus, or vegetation

PROCEDURAL GUIDANCE

The MitraClip G4 system has recently been introduced, providing enhancements to MitraClip's technology.[68] In addition to offering advanced steering during implantation, the new delivery system offers four clip sizes, including two wider clips, providing a greater variety of treatment options that can be tailored to a patient's unique mitral valve anatomy. The newest-generation device also offers independently controlled grippers, if needed, that allow physicians to grasp one or both mitral valve leaflets at a time during the MitraClip procedure.

A successful MitraClip TEER depends on a well-organized heart team with experienced interventionalists, imagers, and support personnel and on a clearly defined and well-orchestrated protocol. The echocardiographer providing the imaging support needs to be well informed about the details and steps of the entire procedure.[48,69] The echocardiographer needs to be cognizant of the physical, fluoroscopic, and echocardiographic appearance of the guide wires, catheters, and devices (Figs. 26.8–26.10) and to have a working knowledge of the nuances of the procedural steps so as to anticipate the imaging needs of the interventionalist.

While the interventionalist performs the baseline cardiac catheterization and obtains hemodynamic data, the echocardiographer obtains an updated baseline TEE characterizing the MV pathology, severity of the MR from multiple views, the presence or absence of pulmonary flow reversal, baseline MV gradients, LV size and function, and absence of contraindications to proceeding with the MitraClip repair (e.g., left atrial appendage thrombus, evidence of infective endocarditis). The echocardiographer defines the best possible views to be used for the intraprocedural echocardiographic guidance. Table 26.4 and Figs. 26.11 and 26.12 summarize the procedural steps for echocardiographic guidance of the TEER.

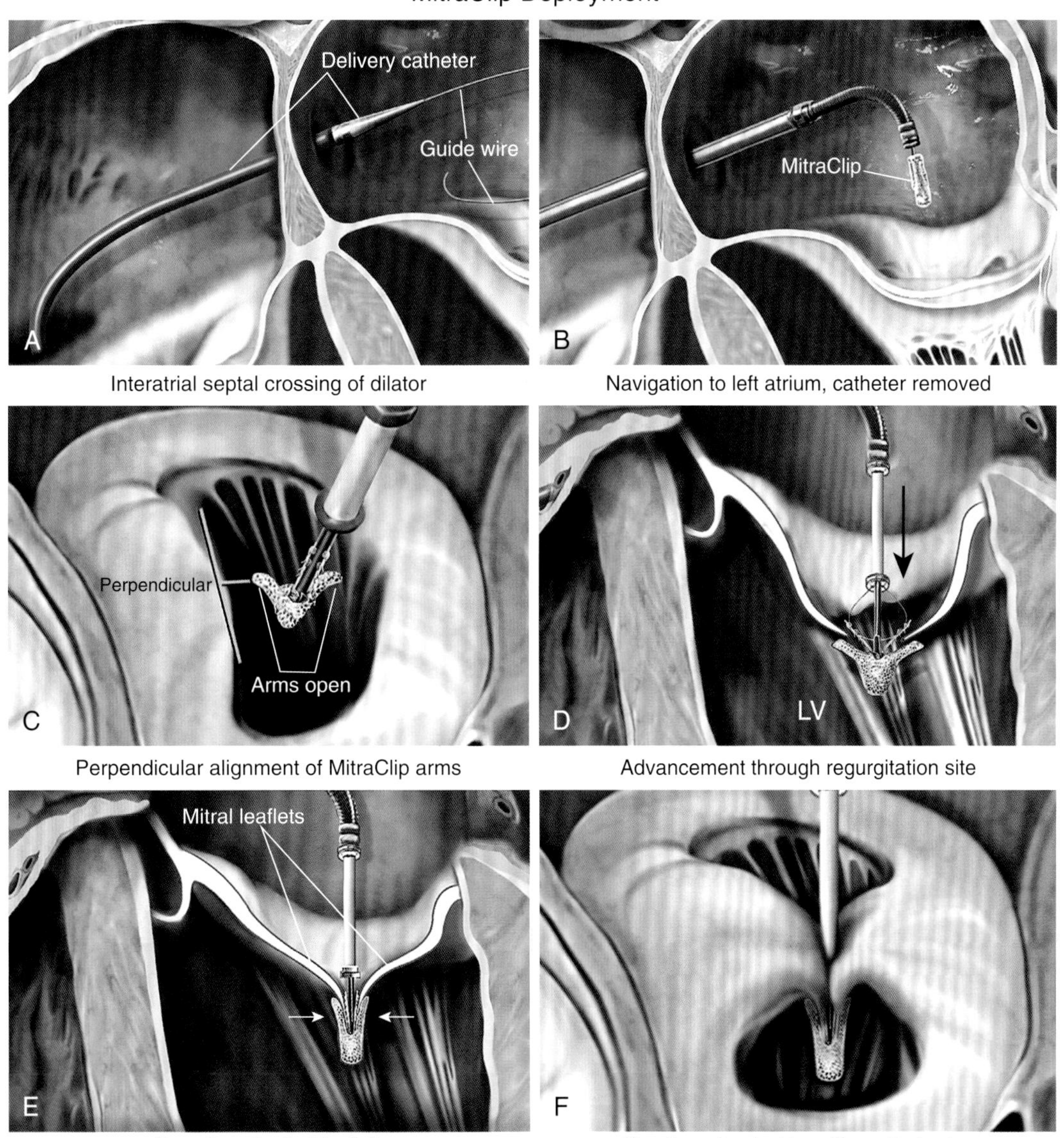

Fig. 26.8 MitraClip deployment. Diagrammatic illustration depicts the main steps in MitraClip deployment. (A) Interatrial septal crossing of the dilator, delivery catheter, and guide wire. (B) The MitraClip is out of the delivery catheter as it is navigated in the LA. (C) The MitraClip with arms opened is being aligned perpendicular to the coaptation line of the mitral valve. (D) The MitraClip has been advanced into the LV through the region of maximal mitral regurgitation. (E) The mitral leaflets are being grasped. (F) The leaflets have been grasped, and a double-orifice mitral valve is seen from the LA view. (Images courtesy Abbott Vascular, Santa Clara, CA.)

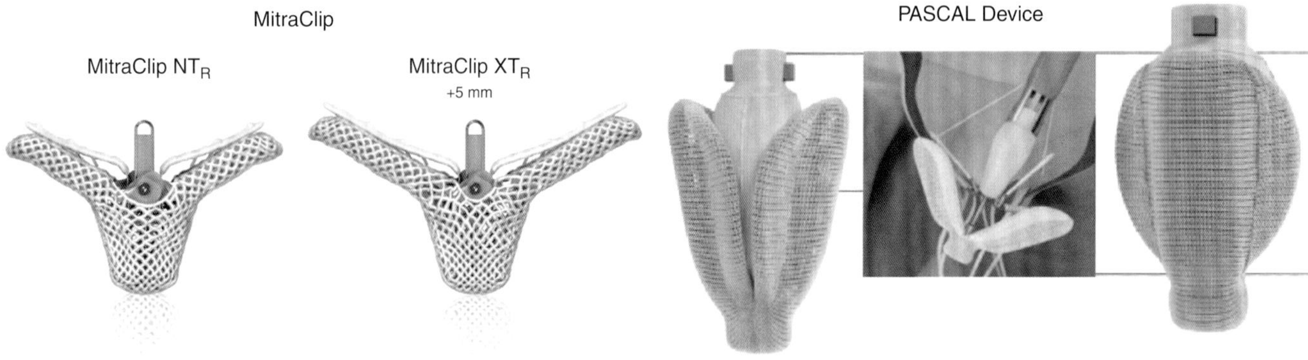

Fig. 26.9 Clip devices. The MitraClip device (Abbott) comes in two formats, the NTR and the newer XTR with extended arms and graspers. The PASCAL device (Edwards) has broad paddles to optimize leaflet coaptation and a central spacer that fills the regurgitant orifice area. Recently a new delivery system has been introduced, the Abbott G4 device, which offers four clip sizes, including two wider clips, providing a greater variety of treatment options that can be tailored to a patients' unique mitral valve anatomy. (Images courtesy Abbott Vascular, Santa Clara, CA, and Edwards Lifesciences, Nyon, Switzerland.)

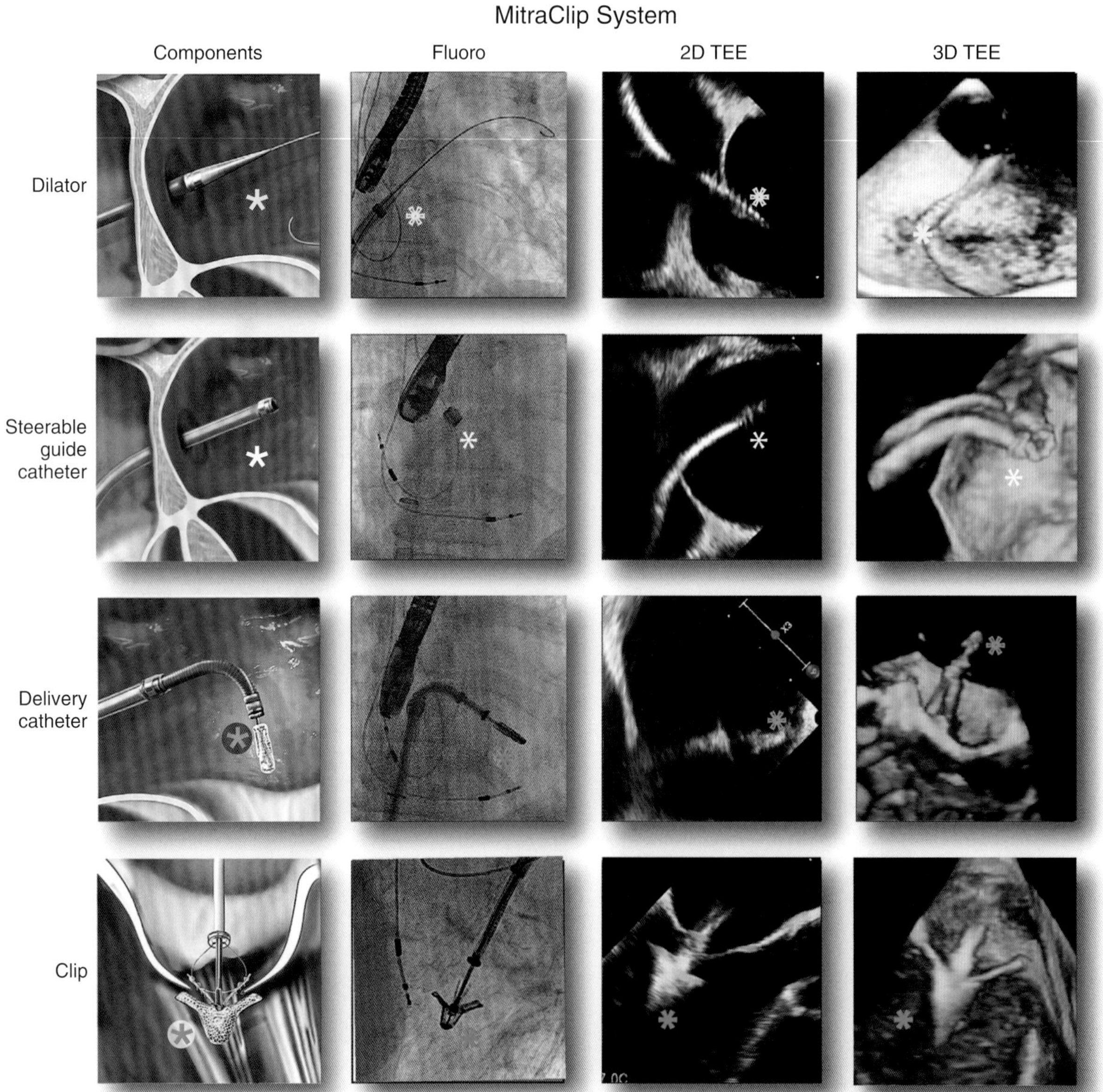

MitraClip System

Components | Fluoro | 2D TEE | 3D TEE

Dilator

Steerable guide catheter

Delivery catheter

Clip

Fig. 26.10 Visualizing the MitraClip system components. This composite figure illustrates the fluoroscopic, 2D TEE, and 3D TEE appearance of the components of the MitraClip system. The dilator *(yellow asterisks)* is recognized by its corkscrew appearance on echocardiography. The ring at the end of the steerable catheter *(white asterisks)* appears as two distinct parallel lines; the distance from these lines to the septum shows how much of the steerable catheter is in the LA. After the clip *(blue asterisks)* exits the delivery catheter, it appears as a very echo-bright target, frequently with multiple reverberations. After the clip is opened and aligned perpendicular to the line of mitral valve coaptation *(green asterisks)*, it appears in the LV outflow tract view as an arrowhead.

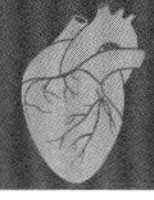

TABLE 26.4 MitraClip Procedural Guidance.

Task	*Steps*	*Echocardiographic Tools and Views*	*Comments*
Septal puncture	Choose puncture site. Perch catheter/needle. Tent septum. Puncture septum.	2D/3D TEE 0–degree mid-esophageal view 3D X-plane: bicaval and short-axis aortic valve	A superior and posterior puncture site in the fossa ovalis is preferred. Puncture site should be about 4 cm above MV coaptation.
Navigation in LA	Guide wire to LUPV. Advance dilator and steerable guide assembly across septum. Remove dilator and guide wire. Advance Clip Delivery System through steerable guide. Navigate clip around the Coumadin ridge.	2D/3D TEE	Confirm that steerable guide catheter is 1–2 cm into the LA. Ensure tip of clip is visualized at all times as it is advanced in the LA.
Guiding catheter and Clip Delivery System steering	Delivery catheter and Clip Delivery System can be steered to achieve a straight trajectory of the Clip Delivery System from above the MV to the leaflet location for clip placement and then into the LV.	2D/3D TEE	2D and 3D TEE to optimize the lateral-medial and anterior-posterior location of this trajectory path.
Device alignment to MV	Direct clip to area of maximal MR Adjust anterior-posterior and lateral-medial diving direction. Align open clip arms perpendicular to leaflets coaptation line.	3D X-plane color: LVOT and bicommissural views 3D TEE en face LA MV view	In the LVOT view, the open clip appears as an arrowhead.
Device advancement into LV	The clip is advanced through the MV into the LV inflow.	3D X-plane LVOT and bicommissural views	Be aware of changing clip orientation as it dives into the LV.
Leaflet grasping and verification of grasp	With the clip open at 180 degrees, the clip is retracted to grab both leaflets. After both leaflets are grabbed, the clip is closed and tightened. Bileaflet capture is confirmed from multiple views.	2D TEE LVOT view Confirm grasping with live 3D TEE	Maintain TEE plane so that the clip appears as an ar; this maintains the appropriate plane at all times. Live 3D is used to better visualize and confirm adequate leaflet grasping.
Evaluation of residual MR	Residual MR is evaluated before and after clip is tightened. In addition to pre-clip view of the most severe MR, multiple views are used.	Multiple 2D TEE color views 3D TEE X-plane 3D TEE with color	The origin of MR may shift after clip insertion, and multiple views are required for residual MR evaluation. SBP should be ≈ 140 mmHg.
MV gradients	Mean and peak MV gradients in each mitral orifice	CW Doppler from bicommissural view	Align CW Doppler velocities parallel to color Doppler inflow signal.
Consideration for additional clip	If residual MR is more than mild and the transmitral gradients are less than 7 mmHg, consider additional clip.	2D/3D TEE color	Consider moving clip medially or laterally before placing an additional clip.
Clip release	After clip position, stability, and MR reduction are established, the clip is released.	2D/3D TEE	Reevaluate MR after clip release; MR severity and jet direction may change.
Retrieval of delivery catheter	Under continuous fluoroscopic and echocardiographic guidance, the delivery catheter is pulled back to the RA.	2D/3D TEE	Monitor position of the delivery catheter tip as it is retracted, to prevent soft tissue injury.
Atrial septal defect check	Evaluate position, shape, size, and flow direction of ASD in area of septal puncture.	2D/3D TEE with and without color Pulsed-wave Doppler to determine flow direction	Consider using an ASD occluder if shunt is large and bidirectional.
Evaluation of possible complications	Search for these: Pericardial effusion/tamponade Chordal entanglement/rupture MV leaflet injury Clip embolization Single-leaflet device attachment	2D/3D TEE with and without color Pulsed-wave and CW Doppler	A fairly complete intraprocedural baseline study is useful to compare unexpected procedural findings.

ASD, Atrial septal defect; *LUPV*, left upper pulmonary vein; *LVOT*, left ventricular outflow tract; *MR*, mitral regurgitation; *MV*, mitral valve; *SBP*, systolic blood pressure.

TRANSSEPTAL PUNCTURE

After vascular access has been obtained from the right femoral vein, transseptal puncture (TSP) is the usual first (and arguably the most important) step in the MitraClip procedure. A relatively superior and posterior puncture site in the fossa ovalis is preferred. The puncture site should ideally be located approximately 4 cm above the line of MV coaptation (see Fig. 26.11).

The height of the TSP may vary, depending on the existing MV pathology. For example, in cases of a flail leaflet, TSP height is typically greater (4.2–4.5 cm) to allow for adequate retraction of the clip during grasping. Choosing the correct puncture site enormously facilitates device navigation down to the MV, and spending adequate time to choose the precise location for the puncture pays off at the end.

The use of biplane 3D TEE imaging significantly aids finding the correct spot by looking at the tenting point of the septum in the anterior-posterior and superior-inferior planes. We find that using the bicaval view and an orthogonal plane displaying the 4-chamber view facilitates measurement of the

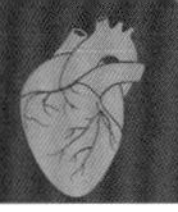

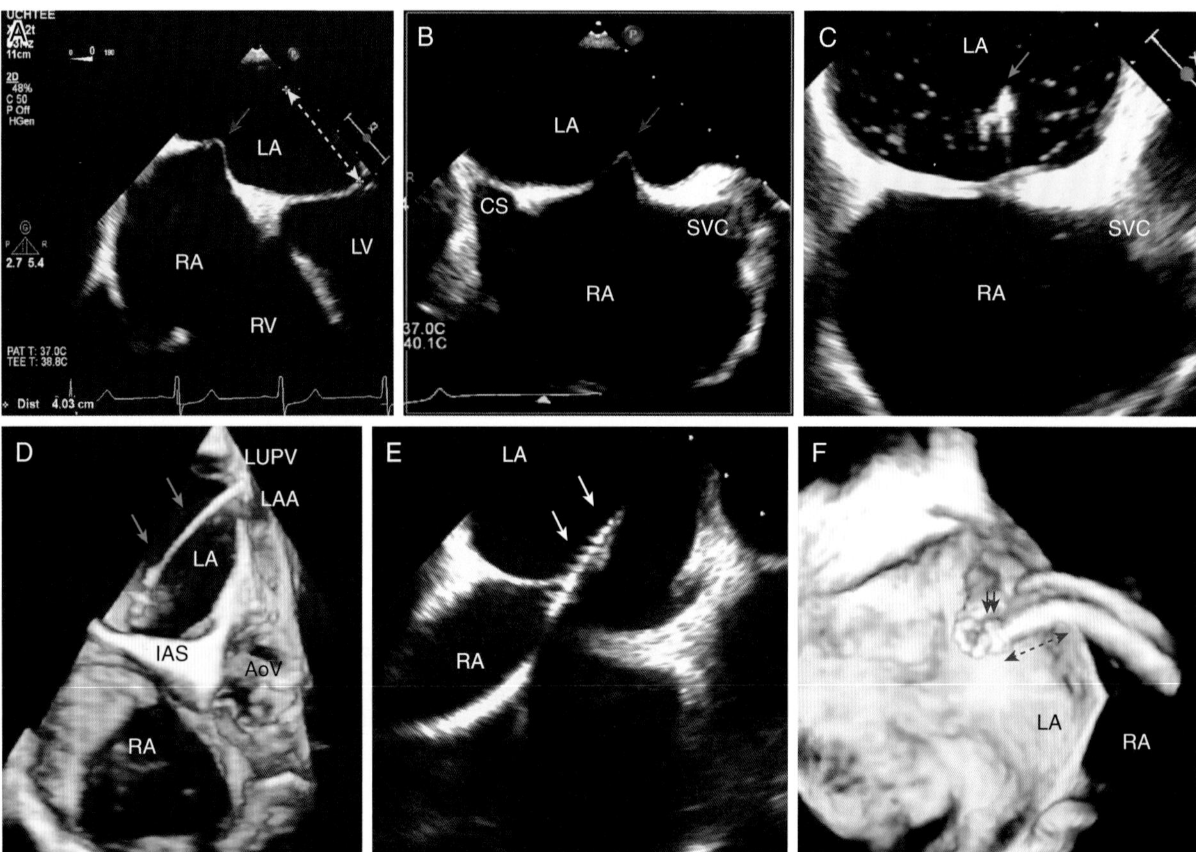

Fig. 26.11 Transseptal puncture. (A) The 4-chamber view depicts the preferred septal puncture point *(red arrow)* situated about 4 cm from the mitral coaptation line *(double-headed yellow arrow)*. (B) Bicaval view shows tenting *(red arrow)* in the middle of the interatrial septum in the superior-inferior plane (see Video 26.11B). (C) The catheter *(green arrow)* is in the LA immediately after transseptal puncture, when multiple bubbles can be seen (see Video 26.11C). (D) A guide wire *(green arrows)* has been advanced to the LUPV to serve as support for the catheters. (E) The dilator-sheath combination *(white arrows)* with the typical corkscrew appearance enters the LA. (F) The delivery catheter is about 2 cm into the LA *(double-headed red arrow)*, and the two metal rings appear as two parallel lines on the echocardiogram *(small red arrows)*. *AoV*, Aortic valve; *CS*, coronary sinus; *IAS*, interatrial septum; *LAA*, left atrial appendage; *LUPV*, left upper pulmonary vein; *SVC*, superior vena cava.

annulus-to-puncture distance. Because fluoroscopic guidance of TSP is often used, there has been early successful use of image guidance technologies that register x-ray and ultrasound images and use image overlay to perform the puncture.

DEVICE NAVIGATION IN THE LA

After the septum has been punctured, a dilator–sheath combination is advanced into the LA. Subsequently, a guide wire is positioned in the left upper pulmonary vein to provide stability and guidance to the upcoming insertion of the large delivery catheter used in the MitraClip procedure. TEE guidance is useful while the interventionalist is steering the guide wire into the pulmonary vein and avoiding the left atrial appendage.

The steerable guide catheter is advanced about 2 cm into the LA, a measure that is confirmed by echocardiography as the distance from the distinct ring at the tip of the catheter to the interatrial septum (see Fig. 26.11F). The delivery catheter with the MitraClip at its tip is then advanced into the LA, bypassing the Coumadin ridge, and navigated close to the MV in the lower aspect of the LA. Continued visualization of the tip of the MitraClip helps to avoid laceration or puncture of the atrial walls as the clip is navigated through the LA.

GUIDING CATHETER AND CLIP DELIVERY SYSTEM STEERING

The delivery catheter and the clip delivery system can be steered to achieve a straight trajectory from above the MV to the leaflet location for clip placement and then into the LV below the MV. This involves multiple small steering adjustments guided by 2D and 3D TEE to optimize the lateral-medial and anterior-posterior location of this trajectory path.

DEVICE ALIGNMENT TO MITRAL VALVE

After trajectory alignment, the clip arms are opened in the LA above the intended location of the clip. The open clip is advanced to the area where the mitral regurgitant jet is most prominent on color Doppler (see Fig. 26.12A and B). Through the use of an en face 3D TEE view of the MV, the clip is oriented perpendicular to the line of coaptation of the mitral leaflets (see Fig. 26.12E) by rotating the Clip Delivery System handle in a clockwise or counterclockwise direction.

DEVICE ADVANCEMENT INTO LV

After proper clip alignment is accomplished and with the clip arms open to 180 degrees, the clip is advanced through the MV into the LV. When properly oriented, the opened clip, slightly

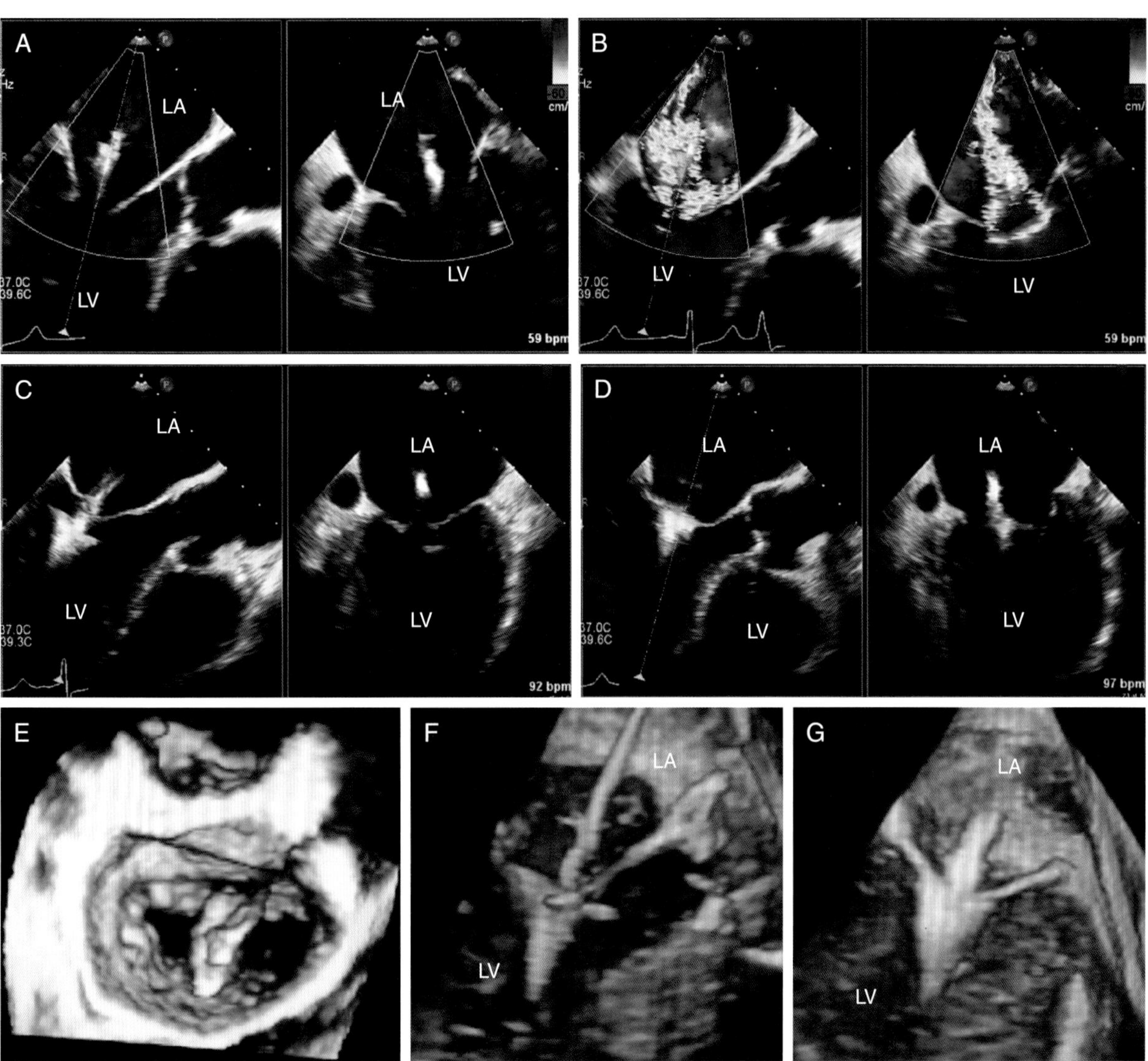

Fig. 26.12 Device advancement into the LV and leaflet grasping. Simultaneous biplane (X-plane) views of the clip being positioned just above the center of the mitral valve (A), in the area of maximal mitral regurgitation (B) (see Video 26.12B), being advanced with the arms open into the LV (C), and grasping the leaflets (D). The clip with open arms as seen from the LA perspective (E), in the LV near the mitral leaflets (F), and grasping the leaflets (G).

closed to an angle less than 180 degrees, has the echocardiographic appearance of an ar on the LV outflow tract view (see Fig. 26.12C). On the bicommissural view, the clip can be seen in profile, providing information regarding the position of the clip in the medial and lateral domain. The 3D biplane view provides simultaneous visualization of these two planes and is the preferred tool for this part of the procedure.

LEAFLETS GRASPING

With the clip in the LV and the arms opened to 120 degrees, the LV outflow tract view is used to guide grasping of the leaflets. As the clip is pulled back toward the LA, continuous visualization of the arms in relation to the anterior and posterior leaflets is monitored to ensure that the target portions of the leaflets are up against the open arms (i.e., each leaflet ceases to move at the point of capture; see Fig. 26.12D).

After proper positioning is confirmed, the grippers are lowered to secure the leaflets to the open arms, and the arms are then closed halfway. At this point, echocardiographic assessment is performed to determine adequate leaflet capture. There are two components: there must be an adequate length of each leaflet embedded into the semiclosed clip arms, and there should be minimal residual movement of the leaflets where they are grasped.

After capture is confirmed, attention is directed to the degree of reduction of MR. A residual jet is frequently seen at this stage. The clip arms are then closed completely, and frequently, the regurgitant jet immediately decreases further. If the residual MR is significant, the clip is not released. The clip arms are opened, and the grippers are raised; the Clip Delivery System is again advanced into the LV with return of leaflet opening. An assessment of where the clip might be better placed is made, and the controls of the Clip Delivery System and/or guiding catheter are adjusted appropriately.

DEVICE RELEASE AND DETERMINATION OF RESIDUAL MITRAL REGURGITATION

After clip stability is confirmed with adequate leaflet insertion, absence of mitral stenosis, and appropriate reduction in MR,

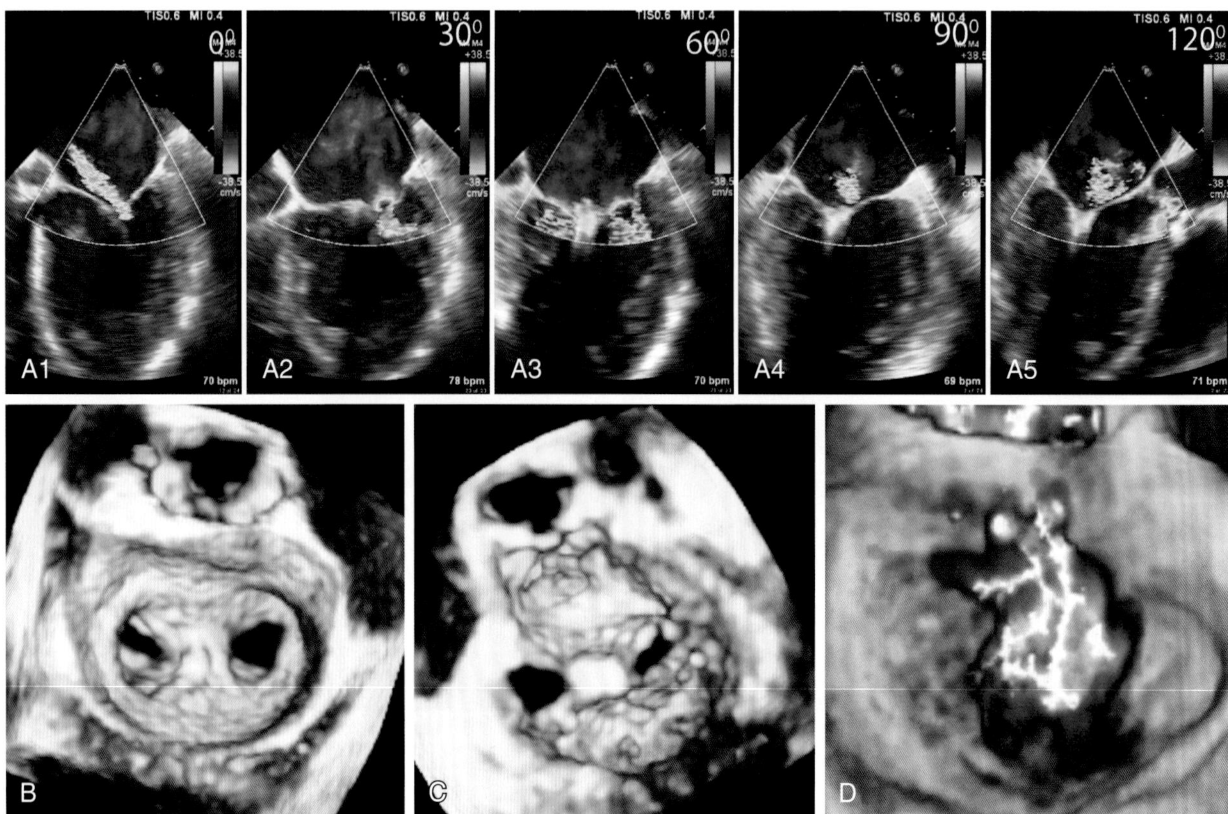

Fig. 26.13 Postprocedure mitral regurgitation characterization. Postprocedure TEE in same patient as in Fig. 26.12. (A1–A5) Multiple omniplane views from 0 to 120 degrees illustrate the significant reduction (from 4+ to 1+) in (MR) jet size after clip deployment (see Videos 26.13A1, 26.13A3, and 26.13A4). (B) The resulting double-orifice mitral valve is viewed from the LA. (C) The double-orifice mitral valve is viewed from the LV. (D) The residual MR jet *(narrow orange jet)* is seen from the LA with color 3D TEE.

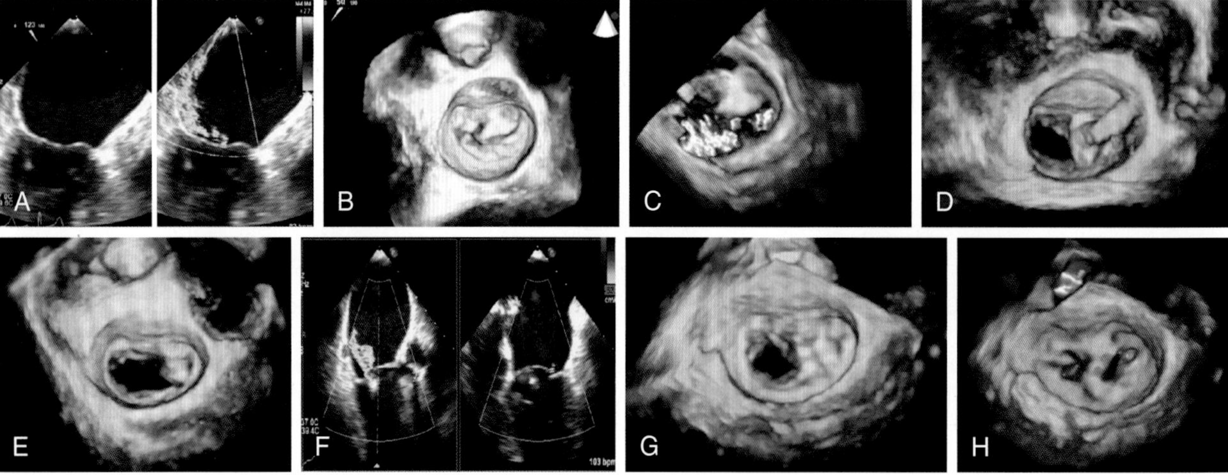

Fig. 26.14 Second MitraClip deployment in patient with A2-A3 mitral valve prolapse. This patient has a very eccentric mitral regurgitation (MR) jet (A) due to prolapse of the A2 (see Video 26.14A) and A3 segments (B) and two MR jets originating at the medial commissure and the A2-P2 area (C) (see Video 26.14C). (D) The clip is being positioned perpendicular to the coaptation line near the medial commissure (see Video 26.14D). (E) The clip has been deployed. (F) Residual MR is observed, requiring consideration of a second clip (see Video 26.14F). (G) A second clip is seen immediately lateral to the initial clip (see Video 14G). (H) Two very small residual MR jets after deployment of clips (see Video 26.14H).

the clip is released under fluoroscopic and TEE guidance. After the clip is released, the final assessment of residual MR is evaluated from multiple views (Fig. 26.13) and compared with the preprocedure MR. For this comparison to be valid, it must be confirmed that afterload is similar by having a similar systolic blood pressure.

CONSIDERATION FOR ADDITIONAL CLIPS

Deployment of an additional clip or clips is considered if the residual MR is more than 2+, the anatomy favors placement of an additional clip, and there is no significant device-induced mitral stenosis (usually defined as a mean MV gradient of 6–8 mm Hg) (Fig. 26.14).

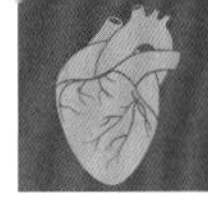

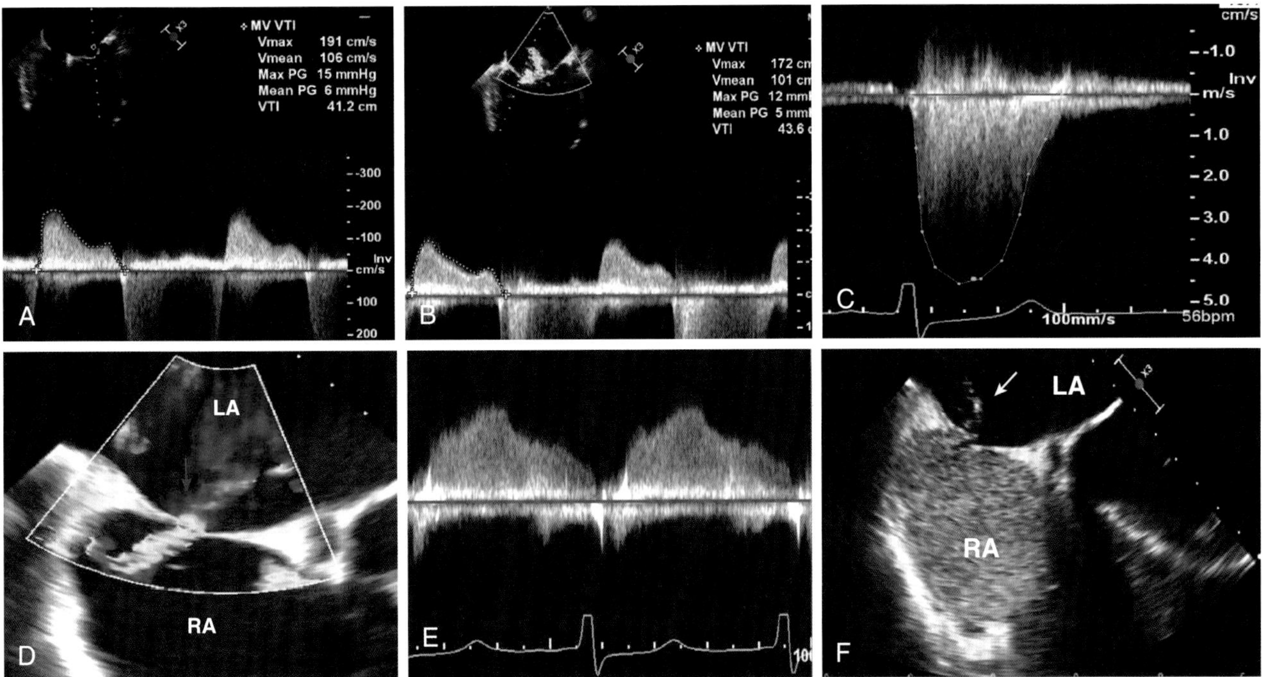

Fig. 26.15 Postprocedure hemodynamic assessment. After deployment of the clip or clips, the transmitral gradients are assessed with CW Doppler through the lateral (A) and medial (B) orifices, where the mean gradients were seen to be 6 and 5 mmHg, respectively. (C) Persistence of pulmonary hypertension is estimated from the tricuspid regurgitation jet velocity. (D–F) Postprocedure evaluation of the iatrogenic atrial septal defect in the area of septal puncture. The color Doppler jet (D, *red arrow*) demonstrates a small to moderate atrial septal defect with predominant left-to-right shunt (see Video 26.15D). (E) CW Doppler shows the left-to-right shunt with predominant systolic flow. (F) A few microbubbles of agitated saline injection are passing into the LA *(yellow arrow)*, demonstrating a small degree of right-to-left shunting.

RETRIEVAL OF DELIVERY CATHETERS

After the clip has been released, the delivery catheter (which at this point has a sharp end) is retrieved under continuous TEE and fluoroscopic guidance to minimize chances of injuring the soft tissues in the LA. This is followed by removal of the steerable guide catheter, which inevitably leaves an iatrogenic atrial septal defect (iASD) in the area from which the catheter is removed.

ATRIAL SEPTAL DEFECT CHECK

All patients have an iASD in the area of the septal puncture due to placement of the large (24 Fr or 8.7 mm) delivery catheter (Fig. 26.15). In most patients, the iASD is relatively small, presents no hemodynamic problems, and will close spontaneously within months. However, in a small number of patients, the residual iASD size is significant and may require percutaneous closure at the end of the procedure.

Echocardiography aids in determining which patients require iASD closure by measuring its size and determining direction of flow. If the iASD flow is predominantly left to right, the iASD usually requires no closure, but if the shunt is bidirectional or predominantly right to left, considerations for closure should be entertained to avoid systemic hypoxemia. The patients most at risk for this are those with elevated right atrial (RA) pressure and lowered LA pressure by successful reduction of MR.

iASD occurs in about 25% of patients who undergo the MitraClip procedure, and its presence 1 year after the procedure is associated with right-sided heart enlargement, worse tricuspid regurgitation, and a higher rate of rehospitalization for heart failure.[70] In the setting of poor baseline RV function, an iASD may result in significant shunting and may precipitate acute right ventricular (RV) failure. In these situations, the iASD needs to be treated with immediate closure using an Amplatzer device.[71]

EVALUATION OF POSSIBLE COMPLICATIONS

Throughout the procedure, the echocardiographer needs to be on the lookout for potential complications such as pericardial effusion or tamponade, thrombus formation on equipment, and leaflet damage. At the end of the procedure, it is a good time to systematically search for all potential complications that may not have been obvious. Before completing the case and before reversing anticoagulation with protamine, the echocardiographer needs to confirm the absence of a pericardial effusion, the size and flow direction of the iASD, the absence of significant mitral stenosis, and the absence of thrombus and stability of the clip. Unusual clip motion is suspicious for single-leaflet detachment (i.e., the closed clip no longer holds both leaflets but only one).

Prolonged use of TEE during TEER (i.e., procedure time > 60 min) increases the risk of esophageal damage. An increased leucocyte count after TEER may raise suspicion of new esophageal damage.[72] In prolonged cases, we routinely add lubricant gel to the esophagus to decrease esophageal dryness.

EVALUATION OF OUTCOMES

The role of echocardiography for evaluation of outcomes of patients with MR undergoing TEER with the MitraClip device is well established. This section summarizes the short- and long-term results of clinical trials of TEER with the MitraClip (see

Table 26.1). In all of these studies, echocardiography played a central role in determining LV size and function, measuring LA volumes, and characterizing MR cause and severity.

In the initial trials, TEER with the MitraClip produced a sustained decrease in MR severity (to moderate or less) for 6 to 12 months.[28,49,73] Echocardiographic and hemodynamic measurements after TEER with the MitraClip showed an expected decrease in MV area with no evidence of clinically significant mitral stenosis immediately after clip deployment or after 12 months of follow-up.[29,74]

TEER with the MitraClip system can be accomplished with low rates of morbidity and mortality, with acute MR reduction to less than 2+ in most patients, and with sustained freedom from surgery and recurrent MR in a substantial proportion of patients.[30] Although percutaneous repair has been less effective at reducing MR than conventional surgery, the procedure is associated with superior safety and similar improvements in clinical outcomes.[10] Patients undergoing TEER can later undergo surgical clip removal and mitral repair or replacement surgery with good results. Echocardiography has also defined the mitigation of MR by using one rather than two clips and the impact of a thicker anterior mitral leaflet on the degree of residual MR.[52]

The magnitude of reduction in LV and LA volumes is associated with the degree of MR reduction to 1+ or 2+.[75] Patients treated with TEER occasionally required surgery to treat residual MR in the early clinical trials; however, after the first year of follow-up, few operations were required. It is well documented that the reduction in MR is sustained in most patients at 4 years.[35]

A comprehensive 2D and 3D TTE analysis allows investigation of changes after TEER. In high-risk patients undergoing TEER, postprocedural heart remodeling involves all cardiac chambers, occurs in the short term, and further improves at midterm follow-up.[76]

ALTERNATIVE IMAGING TECHNIQUES

The standard imaging modalities for preprocedure assessment, image guidance, and post-intervention assessment of patients undergoing TEER include fluoroscopy and 2D or 3D TTE and TEE. Cardiac magnetic resonance (CMR) and multidetector computed tomography (MDCT) can provide complementary preprocedure and postprocedure information for patients undergoing TEER.[77–81] Both modalities provide excellent volumetric estimates of LV size and function and LA volume.

CMR can achieve precise quantification of MR, with quantification of EROA and regurgitant volume in patients with secondary MR equivalent, and it is potentially superior to 3D echocardiography.[82–85] However, this modality is rarely used for MR quantification. CMR is appealing for guiding complex cardiac procedures because it is free of ionizing radiation and offers flexible soft tissue contrast. Interventional CMR promises to improve existing procedures and to enable new procedures for complex arrhythmias and congenital and structural heart disease.[86]

MDCT has proved useful in delineating MV morphology.[87,88] However, it is rarely used in clinical practice. The use of intracardiac echocardiography for structural heart interventions, including TEER, has been reported.[89–91]

RECENT ADVANCES AND FUTURE DIRECTIONS

TEER requires echocardiographic image support during patient selection, procedural guidance, and evaluation of results. 2D and 3D TTE and TEE echocardiography and spectral and color Doppler are used, and they have become indispensable during different phases of the procedure. Because of the added anatomic characterization, 3D TEE guidance has become part of the routine echocardiographic guidance for TEER.

Several advances in echocardiographic imaging technology will further improve the management of patients with MR requiring TEER. Echocardiographic advances that are likely to positively impact TEER include imaging fusion of 3D TEE and fluoroscopy (EchoNavigator system, Philips Healthcare, Andover, MA), which allows real-time 3D TEE images to be overlaid on real-time fluoroscopic images, providing detailed soft tissue visualization of the area of interest superimposed on the fluoroscopic image[92,93] (Fig. 26.16). It also offers the possibility of demarcating a point of interest in the 3D echocardiographic domain with simultaneous markings appearing in the fluoroscopic image. Real-time fusion of echocardiography and fluoroscopy has proved to be as safe and successful as standard best practice for TSP. Moreover, efficacy was improved through significant reduction of time until TSP.[94]

Offline 3D image processing allows modeling of the mitral annulus and leaflets, providing further insights into the morphology of the MV apparatus (Fig. 26.17). It is likely that this tool will further assist in assessment of the different types of MR being considered for TEER and in understanding the deformations in the mitral apparatus that occur with MitraClip and other TEER techniques.

The use of 3D color Doppler will further enhance characterization of the size and origin of regurgitant jets. Miniaturization of the TEE probes with 3D and color capabilities will facilitate and simplify the use of echocardiography for transcatheter guidance of mitral repair.

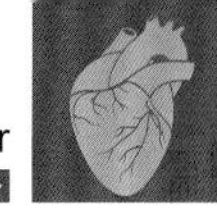

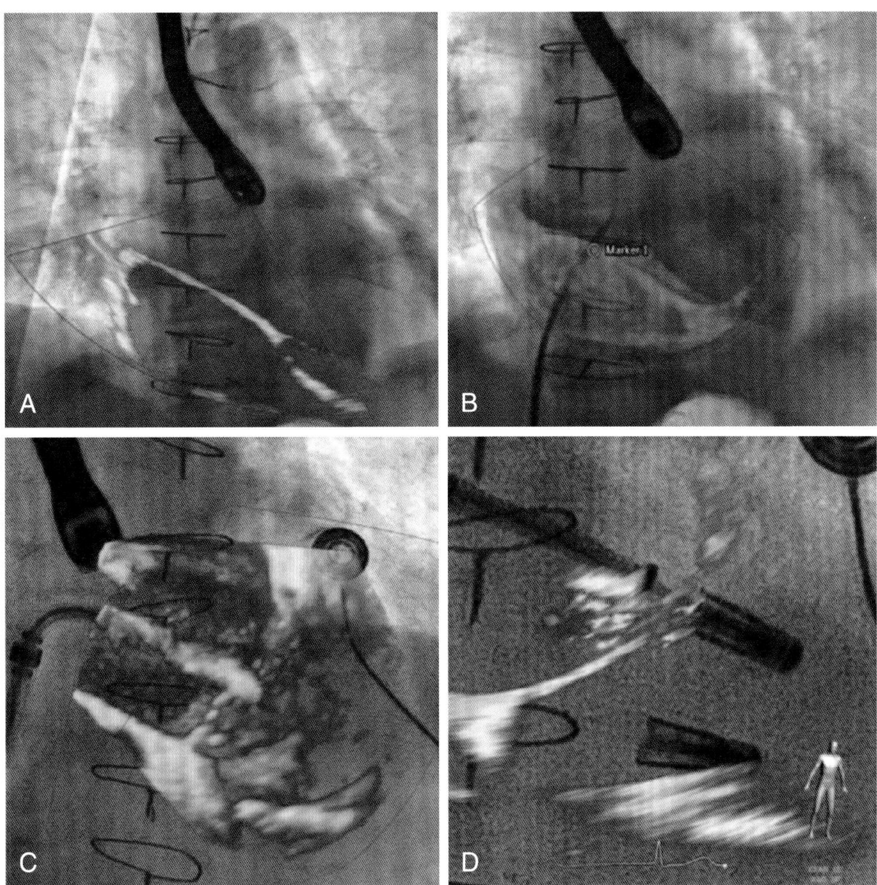

Fig. 26.16 3D TEE fluoroscopy fusion. (A) EchoNavigator (Philips Healthcare, Andover, MA) is used to show the position of the interatrial septum and the plane of the mitral valve orifice. Understanding these relationships is key in preparing for the transseptal puncture. (B) EchoNav has been used to facilitate the transseptal puncture with attention to placing the puncture at the exact spot for performance of the MitraClip. Shown are the overlay of the 3D ultrasound image of the RA and interatrial septum and a marker that corresponds to guiding catheter placement to achieve a distance of 4.0 cm to the plane of the mitral valve. (C) Overlay image of fluoroscopy and the ultrasound visualization of the mitral valve leaflets. Navigation and optimal alignment of the Clip Delivery System are facilitated with this advanced image guidance system. (D) A second clip is being placed with the assistance of a color-flow Doppler overlay to localize the residual mitral regurgitant jet.

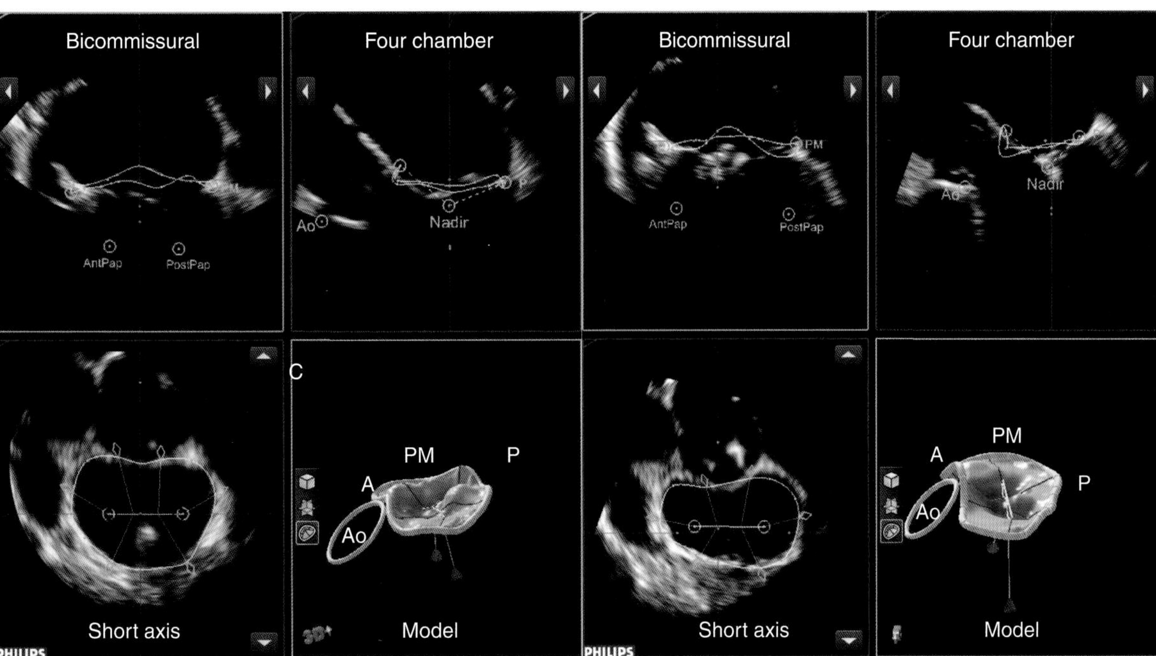

Fig. 26.17 Mitral valve modeling. An offline 3D model of the mitral valve apparatus can be created. By demarcating multiple points of the mitral annulus and mitral leaflets in three orthogonal planes (bicommissural, 4-chamber, and short-axis), a 3D model of the mitral leaflets, mitral annulus, and aortic annulus is created. Shown are the changes in mitral annulus morphology in a patient with primary mitral regurgitation who underwent TEER. Notice the significant shortening in the anteroposterior annular dimension that occurs with MitraClip repair. This change is evident on the short-axis and model views. The bulge of the P2 prolapsing scallop is apparent on the pre-MitraClip short-axis view and model but absent on the post-MitraClip views. *A*, Anterior; *Ao*, aorta; *P*, posterior; *PM*, posteromedial.

SUMMARY Transcatheter Mitral Valve Repair.

Topic	Details	Comments
Types of TEER[a]	Leaflets: MitraClip Chordae: NeoChord DS Annulus: Carillion LV: iCoapsys	MitraClip is by far the most common type of TEER and the only one approved by the FDA.
Patients likely to benefit from TEER (patient selection)	Secondary or primary moderate/severe (3+) or severe (4+) MR and high surgical risk	Echocardiography plays a central role in determining type and severity of MR and candidacy for TEER.
Procedural guidance	Transseptal puncture Device navigation in LA Device alignment to MV Advancement into LV Leaflets grasping Device release Residual MR assessment Additional clip? Retrieval of catheters	2D and 3D TEE with and without color is used throughout the procedure. Simultaneous 3D-derived biplane views are particularly helpful.
Evaluation of results	Confirmation of MR reduction Clip stability Absence of complications	2D and 3D TEE with color and spectral Doppler is preferentially used.
Search for complications	Pericardial effusion Size and flow direction in the ASD Absence of significant mitral stenosis Absence of thrombus Stability of the clip	The echocardiographer is on the lookout for these possible complications throughout the procedure.
Evaluation of outcomes	Multiple US and international prospective clinical trials and registries have been completed with the edge-to-edge PMVR in patients deemed to be at high risk for MV surgery.	The role of echocardiography for evaluation of outcomes in patients with MR undergoing TEER is well established.
Alternative imaging techniques	Cardiac magnetic resonance imaging Cardiac computed tomography	These techniques provide additional information but are rarely used.
Future directions	MV 3D modeling Imaging fusion of 3D TEE and fluoroscopy (EchoNav[b]) Improved 3D color Doppler TEE probe miniaturization	These techniques are in various stages of development and clinical use.

[a]MitraClip (Abbott Vascular, Santa Clara, CA); NeoChord DS (NeoChord, Inc., Minneapolis, MN); Carillon Mitral Contour System (Cardiac Dimensions, Kirkland, WA); iCoapsys system (Myocor, Inc., Maple Grove, MN [no longer being studied]).
[b]EchoNavigator system (Philips Healthcare, Andover, MA).
ASD, Atrial septal defect; *FDA*, US Food and Drug Administration; *MR*, mitral regurgitation; *MV*, mitral valve; *TEER*, mitral transcatheter edge-to-edge repair.

REFERENCES

1. Nkomo VT, Gardin JM, Skelton TN, Gottdiener JS, Scott CG, Enriquez-Sarano M. Burden of valvular heart diseases: a population-based study. *Lancet*. 2006;368:1005–1011.
2. Iung B, Baron G, Butchart EG, et al. A prospective survey of patients with valvular heart disease in Europe: the Euro Heart Survey on valvular heart disease. *Eur Heart J*. 2003;24:1231–1243.
3. Salcedo E, Carroll J. Echocardiography in patient assessment and procedural guidance in structural heart disease interventions. In: Carroll J, Webb J, eds. *Structural Heart Disease Interventions*. Philadelphia, PA: Lippincott Williams & Wilkins; 2012:79–96.
4. Schoenhagen P, Bax J. Transcatheter repair of valvular heart disease and periprocedural imaging. *Int J Cardiovasc Imaging*. 2011;27:1113.
5. Carroll JD, Edwards FH, Marinac-Dabic D, et al. The STS-ACC transcatheter valve therapy national registry: a new partnership and infrastructure for the introduction and surveillance of medical devices and therapies. *J Am Coll Cardiol*. 2013;62:1026–1034.
6. Baumgartner H, Falk V, Bax JJ, et al. 2017. ESC/EACTS guidelines for the management of valvular heart disease. *Eur Heart J*. 2017;38:2739–2791.
7. Otto CM, Nishimura RA, Bonow O, et al. 2020 ACC/AHA guideline for the management of patients with valvular heart disease: a report of the American College of Cardiology/American Heart Association Joint Committee on Clinical Practice Guidelines. *Circulation*. 2021;143:(5):e72-e227. https://doi.org/10.1161/CIR.0000000000000923.
8. Wan B, Rahnavardi M, Tian DH, et al. A meta-analysis of MitraClip system versus surgery for treatment of severe mitral regurgitation. *Ann Cardiothorac Surg*. 2013;2:683–692.
9. Al Amri I, van der Kley F, Schalij MJ, Ajmone Marsan N, Delgado V. Transcatheter mitral valve repair therapies for primary and secondary mitral regurgitation. *Future Cardiol*. 2015;11:153–169.
10. Feldman T, Foster E, Glower DD, et al. Percutaneous repair or surgery for mitral regurgitation. *N Engl J Med*. 2011;364:1395–1406.
11. Stone GW, Vahanian AS, Adams DH, et al. Clinical trial design principles and endpoint definitions for transcatheter mitral valve repair and replacement: Part 1: clinical trial design principles: a consensus document from the Mitral Valve Academic Research Consortium. *J Am Coll Cardiol*. 2015;66:278–307.
12. Stone GW, Adams DH, Abraham WT, et al. Clinical trial design principles and endpoint definitions for transcatheter mitral valve repair and replacement: Part 2: Endpoint definitions: a consensus document from the Mitral Valve Academic Research Consortium. *J Am Coll Cardiol*. 2015;66:308–321.
13. Goldberg SL, Feldman T. Percutaneous mitral valve interventions: overview of new approaches. *Curr Cardiol Rep*. 2010;12:404–412.
14. Feldman T, Young A. Percutaneous approaches to valve repair for mitral regurgitation. *J Am Coll Cardiol*. 2014;63:2057–2068.
15. Sarraf M, Feldman T. Percutaneous intervention for mitral regurgitation. *Heart Fail Clin*. 2015;11:243–259.
16. Figulla HR, Webb JG, Lauten A, Feldman T. The transcatheter valve technology pipeline for treatment of adult valvular heart disease. *Eur Heart J*. 2016;37:2226–2239.
17. Abdul-Jawad Altisent O, Dumont E, Dagenais F, et al. Initial experience of transcatheter mitral valve replacement with a novel transcatheter mitral valve: procedural and 6-month follow-up results. *J Am Coll Cardiol*. 2015;66:1011–1019.
18. Zamorano J, Goncalves A, Lancellotti P, et al. The use of imaging in new transcatheter interventions: an EACVI review paper. *Eur Heart J Cardiovasc Imaging*. 2016.
19. Mankad SV, Aldea GS, Ho NM, et al. Transcatheter mitral valve implantation in degenerated bioprosthetic valves. *J Am Soc Echocardiogr*. 2018. https://doi.org/10.1016/j.echo.2018.03.008.
20. Guerrero M, Dvir D, Himbert D, et al. Transcatheter mitral valve replacement in native mitral valve disease with severe mitral annular calcification: results from the first multicenter global registry. *JACC Cardiovasc Interv*. 2016;9:1361–1371.
21. Polomsky M, Koulogiannis KP, Kipperman RM, et al. Mitral valve replacement with SAPIEN 3 transcatheter valve in severe mitral annular calcification. *Ann Thorac Surg*. 2017;103:e57–e59.
22. Muller DW, Farivar RS, Jansz P, et al. Transcatheter mitral valve replacement for patients with symptomatic mitral regurgitation: a global feasibility trial. *J Am Coll Cardiol*. 2017;69:381–391.
23. Hachinohe D, Latib A, Montorfano M, Colombo A. Transcatheter mitral valve implantation in rigid mitral annuloplasty rings: potential differences between complete and incomplete rings. *Catheter Cardiovasc Interv*. 2018. https://doi.org/10.1002/ccd.27658.
24. Gualis J, Estevez-Loureiro R, Alonso D, Martinez-Comendador JM, Martin E, Castano M. Transapical transcatheter mitral valve-in-valve implantation using an Edwards SAPIEN 3 valve. *Heart Lung Circ*. 2018;27:e23–e24.
25. Elbadawi A, Elgendy IY, Megaly M, et al. Temporal trends and outcomes of transcatheter mitral valve repair among nonagenarians. *JACC Cardiovasc Interv*. 2020. https://doi.org/10.1016/j.jcin.2019.11.026.
26. Besler C, Blazek S, Rommel KP, et al. Combined mitral and tricuspid versus isolated mitral valve transcatheter edge-to-edge repair in patients with symptomatic valve regurgitation at high surgical risk. *JACC Cardiovasc Interv*. 2018;11:1142–1151.
27. Nickenig G, Kowalski M, Hausleiter J, et al. Transcatheter treatment of severe tricuspid regurgitation with the edge-to-edge MitraClip technique. *Circulation*. 2017;135:1802–1814.
28. Feldman T, Wasserman HS, Herrmann HC, et al. Percutaneous mitral valve repair using the edge-to-edge technique: six-month results of the EVEREST Phase I Clinical Trial. *J Am Coll Cardiol*. 2005;46:2134–2140.
29. Herrmann HC, Rohatgi S, Wasserman HS, et al. Mitral valve hemodynamic effects of percutaneous edge-to-edge repair with the MitraClip device for mitral regurgitation. *Catheter Cardiovasc Interv*. 2006;68:821–828.
30. Feldman T, Kar S, Rinaldi M, et al. Percutaneous mitral repair with the MitraClip system: safety and midterm durability in the initial EVEREST (Endovascular Valve Edge-to-Edge REpair Study) cohort. *J Am Coll Cardiol*. 2009;54:686–694.
31. Mauri L, Garg P, Massaro JM, et al. The EVEREST II Trial: design and rationale for a randomized study of the evalve mitraclip system compared with mitral valve surgery for mitral regurgitation. *Am Heart J*. 2010;160:23–29.
32. Baldus S, Schillinger W, Franzen O, et al. MitraClip therapy in daily clinical practice: initial results from the German transcatheter mitral valve interventions (TRAMI) registry. *Eur J Heart Fail*. 2012;14:1050–1055.
33. Grasso C, Capodanno D, Scandura S, et al. One- and twelve-month safety and efficacy outcomes of patients undergoing edge-to-edge percutaneous mitral valve repair (from the GRASP Registry). *Am J Cardiol*. 2013;111:1482–1487.
34. Schillinger W, Hunlich M, Baldus S, et al. Acute outcomes after MitraClip therapy in highly aged patients: results from the German TRAnscatheter Mitral valve Interventions (TRAMI) Registry. *EuroIntervention*. 2013;9:84–90.
35. Mauri L, Foster E, Glower DD, et al. 4-year results of a randomized controlled trial of percutaneous repair versus surgery for mitral regurgitation. *J Am Coll Cardiol*. 2013;62:317–328.
36. Foster E, Kwan D, Feldman T, et al. Percutaneous mitral valve repair in the initial EVEREST cohort: evidence of reverse left ventricular remodeling. *Circ Cardiovasc Imaging*. 2013;6:522–530.
37. Armoiry X, Brochet E, Lefevre T, et al. Initial French experience of percutaneous mitral valve repair with the MitraClip: a multicentre national registry. *Arch Cardiovasc Dis*. 2013;106:287–294.
38. Yeo KK, Yap J, Yamen E, et al. Percutaneous mitral valve repair with the MitraClip: early results from the MitraClip Asia-Pacific Registry (MARS). *EuroIntervention*. 2014;10:620–625.
39. Nickenig G, Estevez-Loureiro R, Franzen O, et al. Percutaneous mitral valve edge-to-edge repair: in-hospital results and 1-year follow-up of 628 patients of the 2011–2012 Pilot European Sentinel Registry. *J Am Coll Cardiol*. 2014;64:875–884.
40. Glower DD, Kar S, Trento A, et al. Percutaneous mitral valve repair for mitral regurgitation in high-risk patients: results of the EVEREST II study. *J Am Coll Cardiol*. 2014;64:172–181.
41. Cameron HL, Bernard LM, Garmo VS, Hernandez JB, Asgar AW. A Canadian cost-effectiveness analysis of transcatheter mitral valve repair with the MitraClip system in high surgical risk patients with significant mitral regurgitation. *J Med Econ*. 2014;17:599–615.
42. Glower D, Ailawadi G, Argenziano M, et al. EVEREST II randomized clinical trial: predictors of mitral valve replacement in de novo surgery or after the MitraClip procedure. *J Thorac Cardiovasc Surg*. 2012;143:S60–S63.
43. Obadia JF, Armoiry X, Iung B, et al. The MITRA-FR study: design and rationale of a randomised study of percutaneous mitral valve repair compared with optimal medical management alone for severe secondary mitral regurgitation. *EuroIntervention*. 2015;10:1354–1360.
44. Mendirichaga R, Singh V, Blumer V, et al. Transcatheter mitral valve repair with MitraClip for symptomatic functional mitral valve regurgitation. *Am J Cardiol*. 2017;120:708–715.
45. Stone GW, Lindenfeld J, Abraham WT, et al. Transcatheter mitral-valve repair in patients with heart failure. *N Engl J Med*. 2018;379:2307–2318.
46. Obadia JF, Messika-Zeitoun D, Leurent G, et al. Percutaneous repair or medical treatment for secondary mitral regurgitation. *N Engl J Med*. 2018;379:2297–2306.
47. Pibarot P, Delgado V, Bax JJ. MITRA-FR vs. COAPT: lessons from two trials with diametrically opposed results. *Eur Heart J Cardiovasc Imaging*. 2019;20:620–624.

48. Silvestry FE, Rodriguez LL, Herrmann HC, et al. Echocardiographic guidance and assessment of percutaneous repair for mitral regurgitation with the Evalve MitraClip: lessons learned from EVEREST I. *J Am Soc Echocardiogr.* 2007;20:1131–1140.
49. Foster E, Wasserman HS, Gray W, et al. Quantitative assessment of severity of mitral regurgitation by serial echocardiography in a multicenter clinical trial of percutaneous mitral valve repair. *Am J Cardiol.* 2007;100:1577–1583.
50. Pleger ST, Schulz-Schonhagen M, Geis N, et al. One year clinical efficacy and reverse cardiac remodelling in patients with severe mitral regurgitation and reduced ejection fraction after MitraClip implantation. *Eur J Heart Fail.* 2013;15:919–927.
51. Wunderlich NC, Siegel RJ. Peri-interventional echo assessment for the MitraClip procedure. *Eur Heart J Cardiovasc Imaging.* 2013;14:935–949.
52. Armstrong EJ, Rogers JH, Swan CH, et al. Echocardiographic predictors of single versus dual MitraClip device implantation and long-term reduction of mitral regurgitation after percutaneous repair. *Catheter Cardiovasc Interv.* 2013;82:673–679.
53. Attizzani GF, Ohno Y, Capodanno D, et al. Gender-related clinical and echocardiographic outcomes at 30-day and 12-month follow up after MitraClip implantation in the GRASP Registry. *Catheter Cardiovasc Interv.* 2015;85:889–897.
54. Grayburn PA, Sannino A, Packer M. Proportionate and disproportionate functional mitral regurgitation: a new conceptual framework that reconciles the results of the MITRA-FR and COAPT trials. *JACC Cardiovasc Imaging.* 2019;12:353–362.
55. Patzelt J, Zhang Y, Magunia H, et al. Improved mitral valve coaptation and reduced mitral valve annular size after percutaneous mitral valve repair (PMVR) using the MitraClip system. *Eur Heart J Cardiovasc Imaging.* 2018;19:785–791.
56. Donmez E, Salcedo EE, Quaife RA, Burke JM, Gill EA, Carroll JD. The acute effects of edge-to-edge percutaneous mitral valve repair on the shape and size of the mitral annulus and its relation to mitral regurgitation. *Echocardiography.* 2019;36:732–741.
57. Wunderlich NC, Beigel R, Ho SY, et al. Imaging for mitral interventions: Methods and efficacy. *JACC Cardiovasc Imaging.* 2018;11:872–901.
58. Kou S, Caballero L, Dulgheru R, et al. Echocardiographic reference ranges for normal cardiac chamber size: results from the NORRE study. *Eur Heart J Cardiovasc Imaging.* 2014;15:680–690.
59. El Sabbagh A, Reddy YNV, Nishimura RA. Mitral valve regurgitation in the contemporary era: insights into diagnosis, management, and future directions. *JACC Cardiovasc Imaging.* 2018;11:628–643.
60. Delling FN, Vasan RS. Epidemiology and pathophysiology of mitral valve prolapse: new insights into disease progression, genetics, and molecular basis. *Circulation.* 2014;129:2158–2170.
61. Anyanwu AC, Adams DH. Etiologic classification of degenerative mitral valve disease: Barlow's disease and fibroelastic deficiency. *Semin Thorac Cardiovasc Surg.* 2007;19:90–96.
62. Adams DH, Anyanwu AC, Sugeng L, Lang RM. Degenerative mitral valve regurgitation: surgical echocardiography. *Curr Cardiol Rep.* 2008;10:226–232.
63. Zoghbi WA, Enriquez-Sarano M, Foster E, et al. Recommendations for evaluation of the severity of native valvular regurgitation with two-dimensional and Doppler echocardiography. *J Am Soc Echocardiogr.* 2003;16:777–802.
64. Lancellotti P, Tribouilloy C, Hagendorff A, et al. Recommendations for the echocardiographic assessment of native valvular regurgitation: an executive summary from the European Association of Cardiovascular Imaging. *Eur Heart J Cardiovasc Imaging.* 2013;14:611–644.
65. Grayburn PA, Weissman NJ, Zamorano JL. Quantitation of mitral regurgitation. *Circulation.* 2012;126:2005–2017.
66. Zamorano JL, Fernandez-Golfin C, Gonzalez-Gomez A. Quantification of mitral regurgitation by echocardiography. *Heart.* 2015;101:146–154.
67. Goebel B, Heck R, Hamadanchi A, et al. Vena contracta area for severity grading in functional and degenerative mitral regurgitation: a transoesophageal 3D colour Doppler analysis in 500 patients. *Eur Heart J Cardiovasc Imaging.* 2018;19:639–646.
68. Rottbauer WD. Contemporary clinical outcomes with MitraClip (NTR/XTR) System: Core-lab Echo results from +1000 patients. The Global EXPAND Study. Data presented at PCR 2020. Available at https://www.pcronline.com/Cases-resources-images/Resources/Course-videos-slides/2020/Mitral-interventions-part-2-Global-EXPAND-registry.
69. Zamorano JL, Badano LP, Bruce C, et al. EAE/ASE recommendations for the use of echocardiography in new transcatheter interventions for valvular heart disease. *Eur Heart J.* 2011;32:2189–2214.
70. Toyama K, Rader F, Kar S, et al. Iatrogenic atrial septal defect after percutaneous mitral valve repair with the MitraClip system. *Am J Cardiol.* 2018;121:475–479.
71. Yeh L, Mashari A, Montealegre-Gallegos M, Mujica F, Jeganathan J, Mahmood F. Immediate closure of iatrogenic ASD after MitraClip procedure prompted by acute right ventricular dysfunction. *J Cardiothorac Vasc Anesth.* 2017;31:1304–1307.
72. Ruf TF, Heidrich FM, Sveric KM, et al. ELM-STREET (esophageal Lesions during MitraClip uSing TRansEsophageal echocardiography trial). *EuroIntervention.* 2017;13:e1444–e1451.
73. Whitlow PL, Feldman T, Pedersen WR, et al. Acute and 12-month results with catheter-based mitral valve leaflet repair: the EVEREST II (Endovascular valve edge-to-edge repair) high risk study. *J Am Coll Cardiol.* 2012;59:130–139.
74. Herrmann HC, Kar S, Siegel R, et al. Effect of percutaneous mitral repair with the MitraClip device on mitral valve area and gradient. *EuroIntervention.* 2009;4:437–442.
75. Grayburn PA, Foster E, Sangli C, et al. Relationship between the magnitude of reduction in mitral regurgitation severity and left ventricular and left atrial reverse remodeling after MitraClip therapy. *Circulation.* 2013;128:1667–1674.
76. Gripari P, Tamborini G, Bottari V, et al. Three-dimensional transthoracic echocardiography in the comprehensive evaluation of right and left heart chamber remodeling following percutaneous mitral valve repair. *J Am Soc Echocardiogr.* 2016. https://doi.org/10.1016/j.echo.2016.06.009.
77. Delgado V, Kapadia S, Marsan NA, Schalij MJ, Tuzcu EM, Bax JJ. Multimodality imaging before, during, and after percutaneous mitral valve repair. *Heart.* 2011;97:1704–1714.
78. Van de Heyning CM, Magne J, Vrints CJ, Pierard L, Lancellotti P. The role of multi-imaging modality in primary mitral regurgitation. *Eur Heart J Cardiovasc Imaging.* 2012;13:139–151.
79. Lopez-Mattei JC, Ibrahim H, Shaikh KA, et al. Comparative assessment of mitral regurgitation severity by transthoracic echocardiography and cardiac magnetic resonance using an integrative and quantitative approach. *Am J Cardiol.* 2016;117:264–270.
80. Khalique OK, Hahn RT. Multimodality imaging in transcatheter mitral interventions: Buzzword or modern age toolbox? *Circ Cardiovasc Imaging.* 2016;9.
81. Naoum C, Blanke P, Cavalcante JL, Leipsic J. Cardiac computed tomography and magnetic resonance imaging in the evaluation of mitral and tricuspid valve disease: implications for transcatheter interventions. *Circ Cardiovasc Imaging.* 2017;10.
82. Marsan NA, Westenberg JJ, Ypenburg C, et al. Quantification of functional mitral regurgitation by real-time 3D echocardiography: comparison with 3D velocity-encoded cardiac magnetic resonance. *JACC Cardiovasc Imaging.* 2009;2:1245–1252.
83. Gaasch WH, Meyer TE. Secondary mitral regurgitation (part 1): volumetric quantification and analysis. *Heart.* 2018;104:634–638.
84. Gaasch WH, Meyer TE. Secondary mitral regurgitation (part 2): deliberations on mitral surgery and transcatheter repair. *Heart.* 2018;104:639–643.
85. Delgado V, Hundley WG. Added value of cardiovascular magnetic resonance in primary mitral regurgitation. *Circulation.* 2018;137:1361–1363.
86. Campbell-Washburn AE, Tavallaei MA, Pop M, et al. Real-time MRI guidance of cardiac interventions. *J Magn Reson Imaging.* 2017;46:935–950.
87. Shanks M, Delgado V, Ng AC, et al. Mitral valve morphology assessment: three-dimensional transesophageal echocardiography versus computed tomography. *Ann Thorac Surg.* 2010;90:1922–1929.
88. Delgado V, Tops LF, Schuijf JD, et al. Assessment of mitral valve anatomy and geometry with multislice computed tomography. *JACC Cardiovasc Imaging.* 2009;2:556–565.
89. Saji M, Rossi AM, Ailawadi G, Dent J, Ragosta M, Lim DS. Adjunctive intracardiac echocardiography imaging from the left ventricle to guide percutaneous mitral valve repair with the MitraClip in patients with failed prior surgical rings. *Catheter Cardiovasc Interv.* 2016;87:E75–E82.
90. Patzelt J, Seizer P, Zhang YY, et al. Percutaneous mitral valve edge-to-edge repair with simultaneous biatrial intracardiac echocardiography: first-in-human experience. *Circulation.* 2016;133:1517–1519.
91. Basman C, Parmar YJ, Kronzon I. Intracardiac echocardiography for structural heart and electrophysiological interventions. *Curr Cardiol Rep.* 2017;19:102.
92. Jone PN, Haak A, Ross M, et al. Congenital and structural heart disease interventions using echocardiography-fluoroscopy fusion imaging. *J Am Soc Echocardiogr.* 2019;32:1495–1504.
93. Jone PN, Haak A, Petri N, et al. Echocardiography-fluoroscopy fusion imaging for guidance of congenital and structural heart disease interventions. *JACC Cardiovasc Imaging.* 2019;12:1279–1282.
94. Afzal S, Veulemans V, Balzer J, et al. Safety and efficacy of transseptal puncture guided by real-time fusion of echocardiography and fluoroscopy. *Neth Heart J.* 2017;25:131–136.

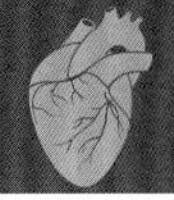

95. Lim DS, Reynolds MR, Feldman T, et al. Improved functional status and quality of life in prohibitive surgical risk patients with degenerative mitral regurgitation after transcatheter mitral valve repair. *J Am Coll Cardiol*. 2014;64:182–192.
96. Schillinger W, Senges J. [TRAMI (transcatheter mitral valve interventions) register. The German mitral register]. *Herz*. 2013;38:453–459.
97. Wiebe J, Franke J, Lubos E, et al. Percutaneous mitral valve repair with the MitraClip system according to the predicted risk by the logistic EuroSCORE: preliminary results from the German Transcatheter Mitral Valve Interventions (TRAMI) Registry. *Catheter Cardiovasc Interv*. 2014;84:591–598.
98. Adamo M, Capodanno D, Cannata S, et al. Comparison of three contemporary surgical scores for predicting all-cause mortality of patients undergoing percutaneous mitral valve repair with the MitraClip system (from the multicenter GRASP-IT registry). *Am J Cardiol*. 2015;115:107–112.
99. Lim DS, Kar S, Spargias K, et al. Transcatheter valve repair for patients with mitral regurgitation: 30-day results of the CLASP study. *JACC Cardiovasc Interv*. 2019;12:1369–1378.

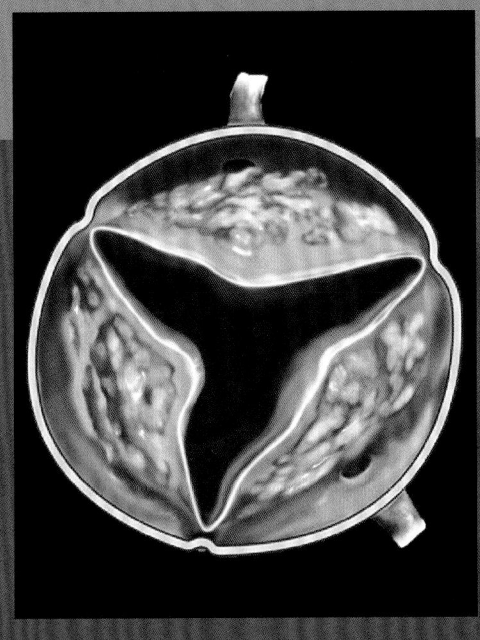

中文导读

第27章 二尖瓣狭窄

二尖瓣狭窄的主要病因是风湿性心脏病，风湿性心脏病在发展中国家的发病率很高，儿童发病率是2%～3%，而在风湿热流行的国家，单纯二尖瓣狭窄占中青年瓣膜病患者的5%～10%，联合心脏瓣膜病和反流占20%～30%，同时二尖瓣狭窄会影响瓣膜解剖结构，进而加重老年性瓣膜病退行性变的严重程度。退行性二尖瓣狭窄是二尖瓣环狭窄延伸至瓣叶的结果，二尖瓣环狭窄主要见于老年人，75岁后患病率超过25%。

本章主要概述了超声心动图诊断二尖瓣狭窄的各种方法、瓣膜解剖结构特点、血流动力学改变、瓣膜病变严重程度、二尖瓣狭窄相关情况（如肺动脉高压、左心房血栓），以及手术方式选择和手术疗效评价。本章最后介绍了超声新技术在诊断二尖瓣狭窄中的应用价值和局限性。

田莉莉

27 Mitral Stenosis

BERNARD IUNG, MD | CLAIRE BOULETI, MD, PhD | ALEC VAHANIAN, MD

Echocardiography plays a key role in the assessment of the severity and consequences of mitral stenosis (MS). Echocardiographic analysis of valve anatomy is used to differentiate rheumatic heart disease from other causes and to select the most appropriate intervention, particularly with regard to balloon mitral commissurotomy (BMC) in cases of rheumatic MS and transcatheter mitral valve replacement (TMVR) in cases of degenerative MS. The large experience acquired with BMC has improved guidelines for the type and timing of intervention for rheumatic MS, although the indications for intervention in degenerative MS remain challenging.

BACKGROUND

Unlike for other valve diseases, the main cause of MS is rheumatic heart disease.[1] The burden of rheumatic heart disease is high in developing countries, where its estimated prevalence is between 1 and 10 cases per 1000 school-age children when using clinical screening and between 20 and 30 cases per 1000 when using systematic echocardiographic screening.[2] In countries where rheumatic fever remains endemic, pure MS accounts for 5% to 10% of valvular diseases in patients between 20 and 50 years of age, and mixed stenosis and regurgitation accounts for 20% to 30%.[3]

In the 2001 EuroHeart Survey, rheumatic heart disease accounted for 22% and MS for 9% of all native valve disease in Europe. The corresponding figures were 11.8% and 4.5%, respectively, in the Valvular Heart Disease II (VHDII) Survey performed in 2017.[4,5] In Western countries, MS is more likely to affect older patients who have more severe impairment of valve anatomy than in countries where rheumatic fever remains endemic.

Degenerative MS is the consequence of mitral annular calcification (MAC) extending to the leaflets. MAC is mainly encountered in the elderly, with a prevalence of more than 25% after the age of 75, and it is favored by cardiovascular risk factors and impaired renal function.[6,7]

BASIC PRINCIPLES AND ECHOCARDIOGRAPHIC APPROACH

The aims of echocardiographic examination of MS patients include diagnosis, evaluation of the severity and consequences of valve lesions, assessment of valve anatomy, and assessment of associated diseases.

DIAGNOSIS

Transthoracic echocardiography (TTE) is mandatory if there is any clinical suspicion of MS. Given the decreased awareness of MS in Western countries and the difficulties of auscultatory diagnosis, MS may be diagnosed when TTE is performed to establish the cause of unexplained dyspnea or thromboembolic events.

The diagnosis of rheumatic MS relies mainly on two-dimensional (2D) echocardiography, which shows leaflet thickening with decreased mobility, commissural fusion, and involvement of the subvalvular apparatus with thickened, fused, and shortened chordae as assessed with parasternal and apical views. The parasternal short-axis view is particularly important for assessing commissural fusion and the location of leaflet thickening and calcification. Anatomic evaluation of the leaflets and subvalvular apparatus is detailed later. Anatomic analysis also plays an important role in the diagnosis of other causes of MS, which typically are not suitable for BMC.

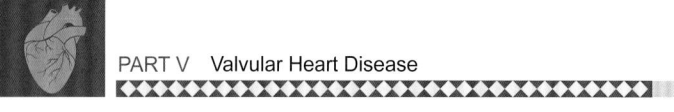

TABLE 27.1 **Approaches to Evaluation of Mitral Stenosis.**[a]

Measurement	*Units*	*Formula/Method*	*Concept*	*Advantages*	*Disadvantages*
Valve area					
• Planimetry by 2D echoardiography	cm^2	Tracing mitral orifice using 2D echocardiography	Direct measurement of anatomic MVA	Accuracy Independence from other factors	Experience required Not always feasible (poor acoustic window, severe valve calcification)
• Pressure half-time	cm^2	$220/t_{1/2}$	Rate of decrease of transmitral flow is inversely proportional to MVA	Easy to obtain	Dependence on other factors (e.g., AR, LA compliance, LV diastolic function)
• Continuity equation	cm^2	$MVA = CSA_{LVOT} \bullet VTI_{Aortic}/VTI_{Mitral}$	Volume flows through mitral and aortic orifices are equal	Independence from flow conditions	Multiple measurements (sources of errors) Not valid if significant AR or MR
• PISA	cm^2	$MVA = \pi r^2 \bullet (V_{Aliasing}/\text{peak } V_{Mitral})(\alpha/180°)$	MVA assessed by dividing mitral volume flow by the maximum velocity of diastolic mitral flow	Independence from flow conditions	Technically difficult
• Mean gradient	mmHg	$\Delta P_{Mitral} = 4v^2_{Mitral}$	Pressure gradient calculated from velocity using the Bernoulli equation	Easy to obtain	Depends on heart rate and flow conditions
Systolic pulmonary artery pressure	mmHg	$sPAP = 4v^2_{Tricuspid}$ + RA pressure	Addition of RA pressure and maximum gradient between RV and RA	Obtained in most patients with MS	Arbitrary estimation of RA pressure No estimation of pulmonary vascular resistance
Mean gradient and sPAP	mmHg	$\Delta P_{Mitral} = 4v^2_{Mitral}$ $sPAP = 4v^2_{Tricuspid}$ + RA pressure	Assessment of gradient and sPAP for increasing workload	Incremental value in assessment of tolerance	Experience required Lack of validation for decision making
Valve resistance	dyne sec^{-1} cm^{-5}	$MVres = \Delta P_{Mitral}/(CSA_{LVOT} \bullet VTI_{Aortic}/DFT)$	Resistance to flow caused by MS	Initially suggested to be less flow-dependent but not confirmed	No prognostic value No clear threshold for severity No additional value vs. valve area

[a]Level of recommendations: 1 *(yellow)* = appropriate in all patients; 2 *(green)* = reasonable when additional information is needed in selected patients; 3 *(blue)* = not recommended.
AR, Aortic regurgitation; *CSA*, cross-sectional area; *DFT*, diastolic filling time; *LVOT*, left ventricular outflow tract; *MR*, mitral regurgitation; *MS*, mitral stenosis; *MVA*, mitral valve area; *MVres*, mitral valve resistance; *ΔP*, pressure gradient; *PISA*, proximal isovelocity surface area; *sPAP*, systolic pulmonary artery pressure; *r*, radius of the convergence hemisphere; $t_{1/2}$, pressure half-time; *v*, velocity; *VTI*, velocity–time integral.
From Baumgartner H, Hung J, Bermejo J, et al. Echocardiographic assessment of valve stenosis: EAE./ASE recommendations for clinical practice. *J Am Soc Echocardiogr*. 2009;22:1–23.

Congenital MS is rare. It can be caused by a variety of lesions of the leaflets and the subvalvular apparatus, such as a parachute valve with a single papillary muscle.

Drug-induced valvular diseases most frequently cause valvular regurgitations. Patients may also present with thickening, reduced mobility and pliability of mitral leaflets, and chordal shortening. Taking into account these morphologic features improves the diagnosis of drug-induced valvular heart disease based on US Food and Drug Administration criteria.[8] Drug-induced valvular disease can manifest as MS, including commissural fusion.[9]

Inflammatory diseases also result in restrictive mitral valve disease. It often involves stenosis without commissural fusion and regurgitation.

In degenerative MS, MAC is the cause of significant MS in less than 10% of patients. It is caused by the extension of calcification to mitral leaflets, which reduces leaflet motion without commissural fusion.

It may be difficult to accurately identify a cause, particularly in elderly patients with superimposed calcification.

EVALUATION OF THE SEVERITY

Assessment of the severity of rheumatic MS is based on the estimation of valve area (Table 27.1).[10] Planimetry of the mitral orifice using the TTE parasternal short-axis view is the reference measurement because it is the only direct measurement of valve area and correlates closely with anatomic findings.[10,11] Planimetry does not incorporate hypotheses concerning loading conditions, compliance of cardiac chambers, or associated valve disease. Planimetry requires particular expertise to ensure that the cross-sectional area corresponds to the leaflet tips. The mitral orifice should be traced in mid-diastole, and the gain setting should not be too high to avoid underestimation of valve area.[10]

The *pressure half-time method* is frequently used because it is easy to perform, provided the Doppler signal of transmitral flow is of good quality with a well-defined linear slope of the Doppler E wave. When the deceleration slope is bimodal, the pressure half-time should be calculated in mid-diastole rather than using the early deceleration slope. The pressure half-time depends on valve area, chamber compliance, and associated aortic regurgitation, and it should not be used as the only method for assessing MS severity.[10]

The *continuity equation* is based on the ratio between stroke volume in the left ventricular outflow tract (LVOT) or right ventricular outflow tract and the velocity–time integral of the mitral flow. Its accuracy is limited by potential errors in taking the numerous measurements and in hypotheses regarding the circularity of the LVOT and mitral annulus.[10] It is valid only in the absence of significant mitral regurgitation (MR), and it tends to give smaller estimations of valve area compared with planimetry.

The *proximal isovelocity surface area (PISA) method* is based on the hemispherical shape of the convergence of mitral flow as shown by color Doppler imaging. This method can be used in the setting of significant MR. However, it is technically demanding and requires multiple measurements. The use of M-mode improves its accuracy, enabling simultaneous measurement of flow and velocity.[10] The assessment of MS severity is more difficult in degenerative MS.

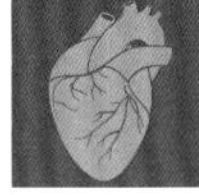

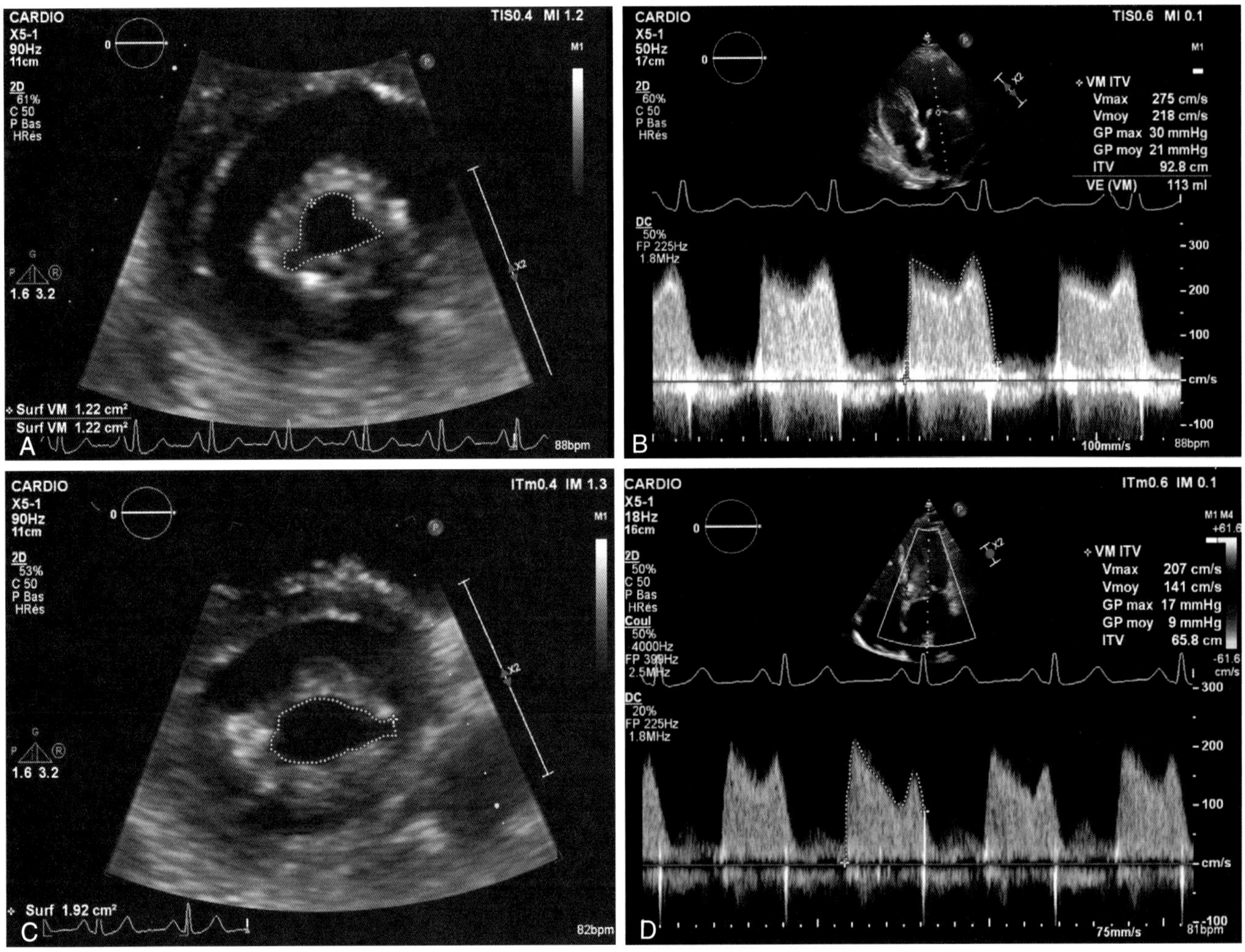

Fig. 27.1 Balloon mitral commissurotomy (BMC) for severe mitral stenosis in a pregnant woman. (A) Parasternal short-axis view before BMC shows a thickened, noncalcified valve with a valve area of 1.2 cm² (see Video 27.1A). (B) CW Doppler before BMC. Mean gradient is 21 mmHg. (C) Parasternal short-axis view after BMC shows complete opening of the anterolateral portion of the valve with a valve area of 1.9 cm² (see Video 27.1C). (D) CW Doppler. Mean gradient is 9 mmHg. High mitral gradient values are caused by the physiologic increase in cardiac output during pregnancy.

ASSESSMENT OF HEMODYNAMIC CONSEQUENCES

Mean mitral gradient as assessed by pulsed-wave or continuous-wave (CW) Doppler is not a reliable marker of MS severity because it depends on heart rate and flow conditions (Fig. 27.1). The mean gradient gives information on the consequences of MS, and it has strong prognostic value after BMC. The sample volume of pulsed-wave Doppler should be placed at the level of or just after the leaflet tips.

The Doppler gradient is assessed using the apical window in most cases. CW Doppler ensures that maximal velocities are recorded. The Doppler beam should be oriented to avoid underestimation of velocities. In the case of atrial fibrillation, the mean gradient should be averaged over five cycles as close as possible to normal heart rate. The heart rate at which gradients are measured should always be reported.

Systolic pulmonary artery pressure (sPAP) is estimated from the velocity of Doppler tricuspid flow. Diastolic and mean pulmonary artery pressures can be derived from pulmonary flow. Doppler-derived estimations of sPAP correlate well with measurements using right heart catheterization, which remains the reference method.[12]

ASSESSMENT OF CONSEQUENCES ON THE LA

Time–motion measurement may be inaccurate because enlargement does not follow a spherical pattern in most cases. The assessment of left atrial (LA) volume using the biplane area–length method is preferred because it is more accurate and is strongly related to other markers of thromboembolic risk.[13]

ASSESSMENT OF VALVE ANATOMY

A detailed analysis of the components of the mitral valve is necessary for diagnosis and contributes to the choice of intervention type (Fig. 27.2):

- Leaflet mobility is particularly well analyzed using the long-axis parasternal view.
- Leaflet thickening is considered significant if it is greater than or equal to 5 mm.
- Leaflet calcification is suspected in the setting of increased echo-brightness.
- The extent of commissural fusion is analyzed using the short-axis parasternal view.
- Impairment of the subvalvular apparatus is analyzed from long-axis parasternal and apical views, which show thickening, fusion, or shortening of chordae.

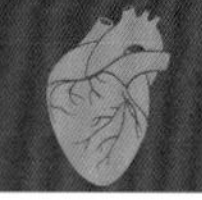

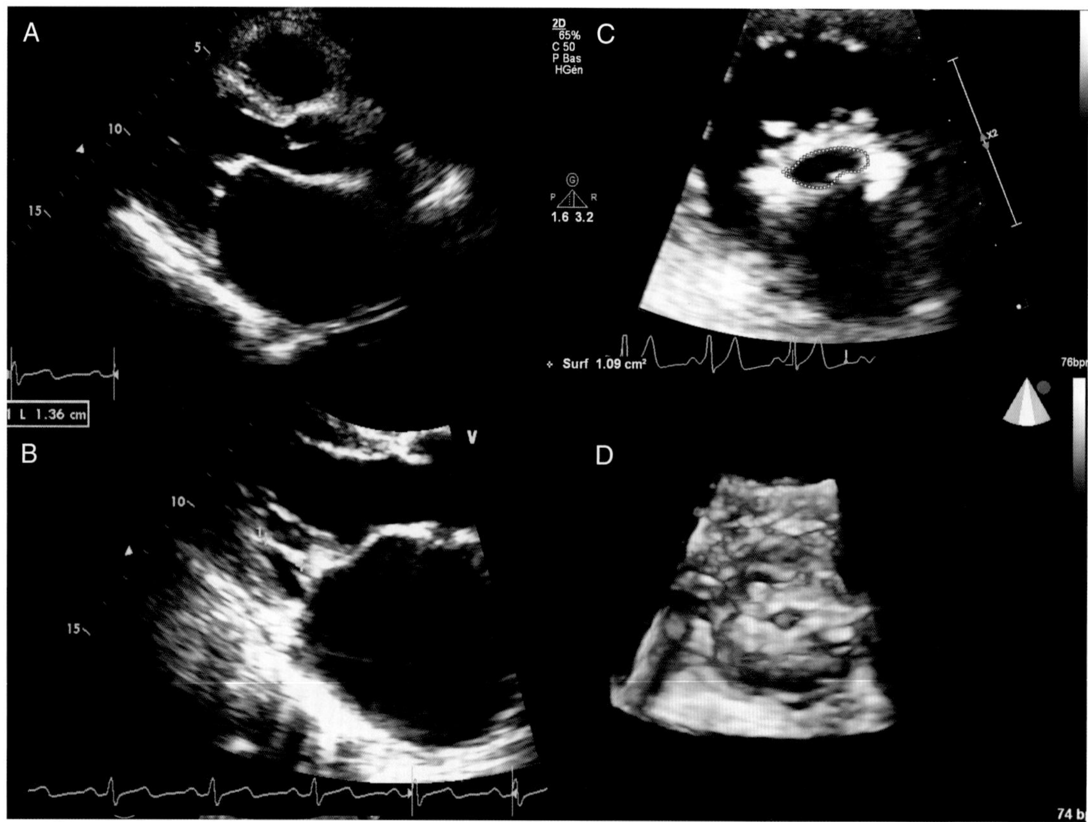

Fig. 27.2 Evaluation of valvular anatomy before balloon mitral commissurotomy. TTE. (A) Parasternal long-axis view shows thickened, noncalcified, and pliable valve (see Video 27.2A). (B) Parasternal long-axis view shows moderate impairment of subvalvular apparatus (length of chordae, 13.6 mm). (C) Parasternal short-axis view shows thickening of the leaflet tips and fusion of both commissures (see Video 27.2C). (D) 3D parasternal short-axis view shows valve thickening and fusion of both commissures (see Video 27.2D).

The echocardiographic report should accurately describe the extent and location of each abnormality, particularly with regard to commissural areas.

The assessment of commissural fusion is important to differentiate rheumatic MS from other causes, particularly degenerative MS. Complete fusion of both commissures usually indicates severe rheumatic MS.[10] Conversely, the lack of commissural fusion does not exclude significant MS due to other causes nor rheumatic MS caused by restenosis due to valve rigidity with persistent commissural opening.

The definition of calcification using ultrasonographic criteria may be debated. Only acoustic shadowing is specific to calcification alone; localized brightness can also be caused by fibrosis. For this reason, certain teams require the confirmation of calcification using fluoroscopic examination.[14] Computed tomography (CT) accurately assesses the location and severity of valve calcification, but its usefulness in the assessment of valve anatomy in rheumatic MS has not been studied (Fig. 27.3).

Different scoring systems combine the various features of mitral valve anatomy. Their value and limitations in predicting the results of BMC and use for patient selection are addressed later.

MITRAL REGURGITATION

Detection and quantitation of associated MR have important implications for the choice of intervention in MS. Quantitative measurements should be combined and are preferred over methods that use color-flow mapping of the regurgitant jet in the LA.[15] The existence of MR does not alter the validity of the quantitation of MS except in regard to the continuity equation.

ASSOCIATED LESIONS

Tricuspid regurgitation (TR) is frequently associated with MS and most often is caused by pulmonary hypertension, which leads to right ventricular dilation and lack of coaptation of the tricuspid leaflets despite normal valve anatomy. Quantitation of TR depends on loading conditions. Indications for tricuspid surgery are based more on the measurement of the tricuspid annulus than on the quantitation of TR.[16] Rheumatic tricuspid disease is far less common and is characterized by thickening and decreased mobility of the tricuspid leaflets. Quantitation of tricuspid stenosis relies mainly on the mean gradient.[10]

Associated rheumatic aortic valve disease is quantitated using standard techniques. Calculation of valve area is needed because low-gradient aortic stenosis may be encountered due to reduced stroke volume in MS.

Left ventricular (LV) enlargement and systolic dysfunction are unusual in MS. The first reaction should be to search for an associated valvular regurgitation or coronary artery disease.

THROMBOEMBOLIC COMPLICATIONS

The diagnosis of LA thrombosis relies on transesophageal echocardiography (TEE), particularly for location in the left atrial appendage. CT may also be used with specific techniques to avoid artifacts that may cause misdiagnosis.[17]

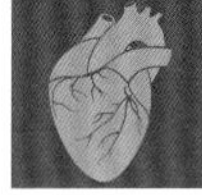

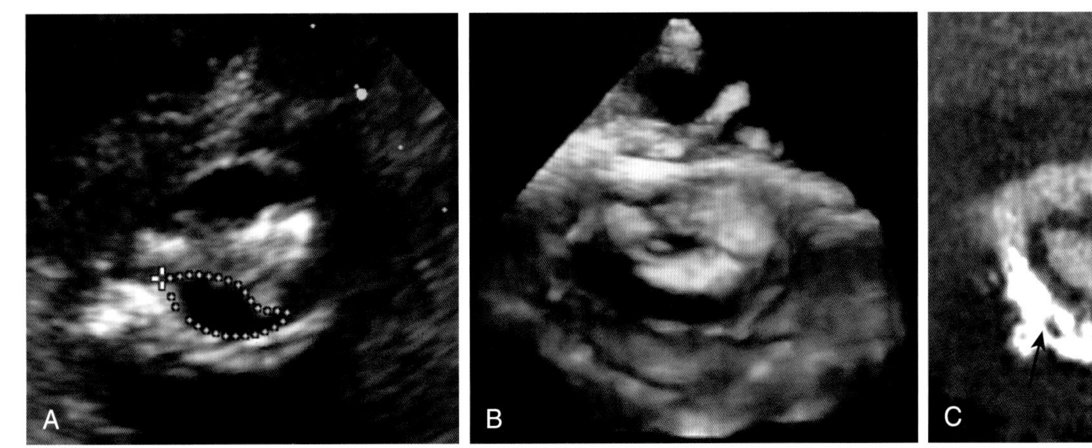

Fig. 27.3 Rheumatic mitral stenosis with valvular calcification. TTE 2D (A) and TTE 3D (B) parasternal short-axis views show thickened leaflets with dense and bright areas on the posterior leaflet and both commissural areas (see Videos 27.3A and 27.3B). (C) CT scan with iodine injection, short-axis view. These views show the added value of CT scanning over TTE for the characterization and location of valvular calcification. Calcification is located on the posterior leaflet *(arrow)* but does not involve the commissures.

Echocardiography is used in risk stratification of thromboembolism. LA enlargement is a risk factor for thromboembolism. An LA volume greater than 60 mL/m^2 of body surface area is associated with surrogate markers of thromboembolic risk.[13] The pattern of LA remodeling seems to be related to the thromboembolic risk, which is increased in cases of spherical rather than ellipsoidal LA shape.[18] LA spontaneous echocardiographic contrast is a strong predictor of thromboembolic risk for patients with MS.

USE OF THE DIFFERENT ECHOCARDIOGRAPHIC TECHNIQUES

A comprehensive evaluation of MS can be performed using TTE in most cases. TTE also plays an important role during the BMC procedure to monitor valve opening and quantitate MR.

In the rare cases in which TTE is of poor quality, TEE may be required. However, the main indication for TEE is detection of LA thrombosis before BMC. The main indication for stress echocardiography is exercise echocardiography to assess objective evaluation of functional tolerance for asymptomatic patients.

TECHNIQUE, QUANTITATION, AND DATA ANALYSIS

The respective features analyzed differ according to whether echocardiography is performed as an initial evaluation of rheumatic MS or to assess the results of BMC. The role of echocardiography is more limited in the assessment of degenerative MS.

BEFORE BALLOON MITRAL COMMISSUROTOMY

Valve Function

There is a consensus for considering intervention when the mitral valve area (MVA) is less than 1.5 cm^2 because this is the value above which hemodynamics are not affected at rest.[19,20] The patient's body size should be taken into account, although no cutoff value indexed to body surface area can be firmly established from the literature.

The main pitfall when using planimetry is overestimation of the valve area because of inappropriate positioning of the measurement plane above the leaflet tips. The best way to avoid this is to scan slowly from the apex to the base and to select the narrowest orifice. Real-time three-dimensional (3D) echocardiography is helpful to optimize positioning of the measurement, which improves the reproducibility and accuracy of planimetry, especially for less experienced echocardiographers.[21] Real-time 3D TEE provides accurate and reproducible measurements of MVA and can be used in patients with poor transthoracic windows.[22]

Technical difficulties inherent to planimetry justify systematic use of the pressure half-time method, keeping in mind its limitations due to confounding factors. In our experience, the most important discrepancies between the pressure half-time method and planimetry are observed for patients older than 60 years of age and those in atrial fibrillation, both before and after BMC.[23]

In current practice, 2D planimetry and the pressure half-time method are recommended for the standard evaluation of MS. Other methods are used only if the usual measurements are inconclusive or inconsistent with clinical data (see Table 27.1).[10,24]

Valve Anatomy

Different approaches have been developed to assess the anatomic features of MS, with the aim of predicting the results of BMC and improving patient selection.

The most widely used scoring system is the semiquantitative Wilkins score, in which four components are graded from 1 to 4: leaflet mobility, thickness, calcification, and impairment of the subvalvular apparatus (Table 27.2). The scores for the four components are added together, producing a final score between 4 and 16.[25]

The Cormier score is another approach based on a global assessment of mitral valve anatomy; three groups are identified according to the best surgical alternative. Patients in group 1 are optimal candidates for closed heart commissurotomy; patients in group 2 are more likely to be candidates for open heart commissurotomy; and patients in group 3 are usually treated with prosthetic valve replacement (Table 27.3). The corresponding ranges of the Wilkins score are 7 to 9 for group 1, 8 to 12 for group 2, and 10 to 15 for group 3.[26]

These two scores were formulated at the beginning of the development of BMC, and their association with immediate and long-term results of BMC has been widely studied. A common limitation of the two scoring systems is a lack of information

TABLE 27.2 Assessment of Mitral Valve Anatomy According to the Wilkins Score.[a]

Grade	*Mobility*	*Thickening*	*Calcification*	*Subvalvular Thickening*
1	Highly mobile valve with only leaflet tips restricted	Leaflets near normal in thickness (4–5 mm)	A single area of increased echo-brightness	Minimal thickening just below the mitral leaflets
2	Leaflet middle and base portions have normal mobility	Midleaflets normal, considerable thickening of margins (5–8 mm)	Scattered areas of brightness confined to leaflet margins	Thickening of chordal structures extending to one of the chordal lengths
3	Valve continues to move forward in diastole, mainly from the base	Thickening extending throughout the entire leaflet (5–8 mm)	Brightness extending into the middle portions of the leaflets	Thickening extended to distal third of the chords
4	No or minimal forward movement of the leaflets in diastole	Considerable thickening of all leaflet tissue (>8–10 mm)	Extensive brightness throughout much of the leaflet tissue	Extensive thickening and shortening of all chordal structures extending down to the papillary muscles

[a]Each component is given a score from 1 to 4. The total score is the sum of the four component scores and ranges between 4 and 16.
From Wilkins GT, Weyman AE, Abascal VM, Block PC, Palacios IF. Percutaneous balloon dilatation of the mitral valve: an analysis of echocardiographic variables related to outcome and the mechanism of dilatation. *Br Heart J.* 1988;60:299–308.

TABLE 27.3 Assessment of Mitral Valve Anatomy According to the Cormier Score.

Echocardiographic Group	*Mitral Valve Anatomy*
Group 1	Pliable noncalcified anterior mitral leaflet and mild subvalvular disease (i.e., thin chordae ≥ 10 mm long)
Group 2	Pliable noncalcified anterior mitral leaflet and severe subvalvular disease (i.e., thickened chordae <10 mm long)
Group 3	Calcification of mitral valve to any extent, as assessed by fluoroscopy, whatever the state of the subvalvular apparatus

From Iung B, Cormier B, Ducimetière P, et al. Immediate results of percutaneous mitral commissurotomy: a predictive model on a series of 1514 patients. *Circulation.* 1996;94:2124–2130.

about the location of leaflet thickening and calcification, particularly in relation to the commissures, which may influence the results of BMC.[27–29] Another drawback of the current scoring systems is that the respective importance of each abnormality may be debated. In particular, the significance of subvalvular apparatus impairment is probably underestimated.[30]

Commissural morphology was included in a score aimed at predicting the occurrence of severe MR after BMC. However, its predictive value in regard to immediate valve opening and late results has not been studied.[31] This score lacks validation in large series and is not widely used in practice. A score including the assessment of commissural anatomy was described in 2014 and had good predictive performance for immediate results of BMC.[32]

There are no large-scale comparative evaluations of predictive value on which to base recommendations of the use of a particular scoring system. For the echocardiographer, the best solution is to use a method of analysis with which he or she is familiar and to include valve anatomy along with other clinical and echocardiographic findings. The echocardiographic report should include a comprehensive description of mitral anatomy and not simply a summary using a score alone.[24]

Exercise Echocardiography

Semisupine exercise echocardiography enables the mitral gradient and sPAP to be recorded for increasing levels of exercise. Stroke volume and valve area are more difficult to obtain during exercise, and they are analyzed only for research purposes. Current guidelines recommend the use of exercise echocardiography to evaluate mean gradient and sPAP, in addition to functional tolerance when there is a discrepancy between resting echocardiography and clinical findings.[19,20] However, no thresholds of mean gradient and sPAP at exercise are recommended for consideration of intervention in asymptomatic patients. Our experience suggests that the type of limiting symptom (i.e., dyspnea or fatigue) is more related to the pattern of increase in mitral gradient than to the level of mean gradient or sPAP at peak exercise.[33]

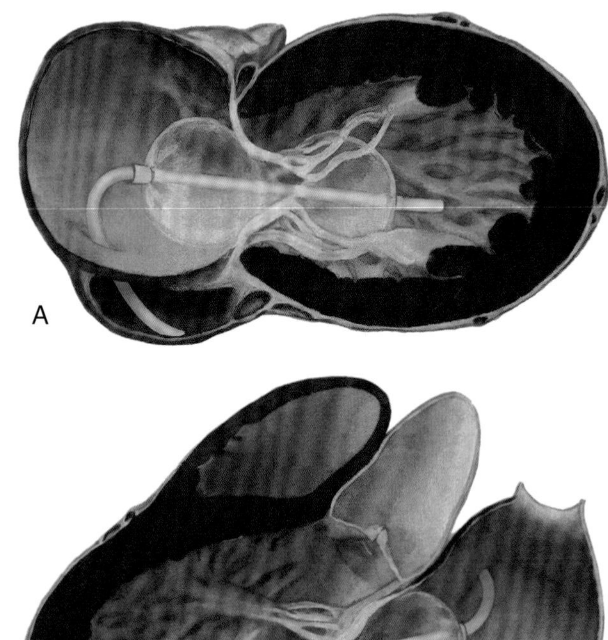

Fig. 27.4 Catheter balloon mitral commissurotomy using the Inoue balloon. The catheter is inserted through the atrial septum, and the balloon is inflated across the mitral valve. The waist of the balloon is positioned in the mitral orifice, and continuing inflation ensures commissural opening. (A) Right anterior oblique view. (B) Left anterior oblique view.

DURING BALLOON MITRAL COMMISSUROTOMY

Echocardiography plays an important role in the catheterization laboratory, particularly with the Inoue technique, which uses stepwise inflations with a progressive increase in balloon diameter (Fig. 27.4).[24] TTE enables assessment of valve area,

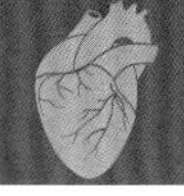

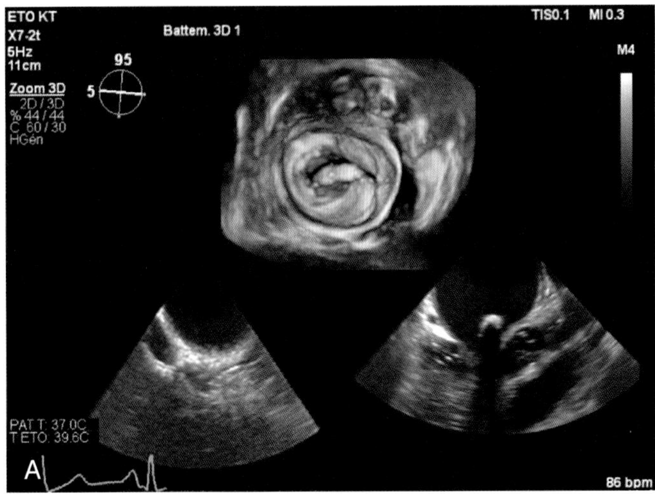

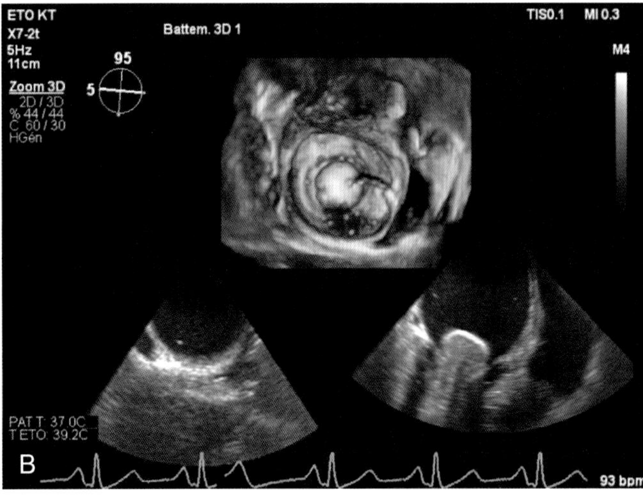

Fig. 27.5 TEE performed during balloon mitral commissurotomy. (A) Inoue balloon positioning across the mitral orifice (see Video 27.5A). (B) Balloon inflation in the mitral orifice. 3D TEE views from the LA *(top)* and 2D views *(bottom)* are shown (see Video 27.5B). (Courtesy Dr. Brochet, Bichat Hospital, Paris.)

degree of commissural opening, mean gradient, and MR after each balloon inflation, followed by continued balloon inflation or stopping the procedure. Planimetry should be used to monitor BMC because the pressure half-time method is not reliable in this context and mean gradient is influenced by changes in loading conditions or heart rate.

Echocardiography is also helpful in the catheterization laboratory to promptly detect pericardial effusion, which is a rare but severe complication of transseptal catheterization. In rare instances, TEE can be required during BMC, mainly to guide transseptal catheterization in difficult situations (Fig. 27.5). Given the discomfort for the patient, the procedure is usually conducted under general anesthesia when TEE is used.

EARLY AFTER BALLOON MITRAL COMMISSUROTOMY

Even more than in other situations, planimetry using 2D echo is the reference for measurement of MVA immediately after BMC. It enables the commissural opening to be visualized. Valvular area tracing should include opened commissures. The pressure half-time method is inaccurate in this setting, possibly because of acute changes in cardiac chamber compliance or the setting of right-to-left shunt at the site of the transseptal puncture.[10] However, the pressure half-time method has a good specificity (but low sensitivity) for identifying good valve opening, which may be helpful in technically difficult examinations.[23]

The echocardiographic assessment of the degree of opening of each commissure is strongly related to the quality of the immediate results of BMC and to late functional results.[34] It is also useful as a baseline evaluation for the interpretation of findings on echocardiographic follow-up. Assessment of the degree of commissural opening is improved by real-time 3D echocardiography.[21,22]

The mean gradient should be assessed after BMC because of its prognostic value in regard to late functional results. For patients who had initial pulmonary hypertension, there is frequently an early decrease in sPAP, although it is usually more pronounced after several months.[35]

In most cases, there is little or no increase in MR after BMC. Moderate MR is often related to incomplete closure of free edges or commissures because of thickening and rigidity.[36] In these cases, color Doppler shows central and/or commissural small jets, and 2D echocardiography does not suggest traumatic lesion. If MR is severe, its mechanism should be carefully assessed, using TEE if needed, looking for traumatic lesions. Traumatic MR is mainly caused by a tear of the noncommissural leaflet and is frequently associated with an absence of commissural opening, as shown by echocardiographic findings and confirmed by surgery (Fig. 27.6).[36] Lesions of the subvalvular apparatus are also common in traumatic MR. The most common is rupture of the chordae; partial or total papillary muscle rupture is rare. These lesions cause particularly severe MR in patients with pliable leaflets.

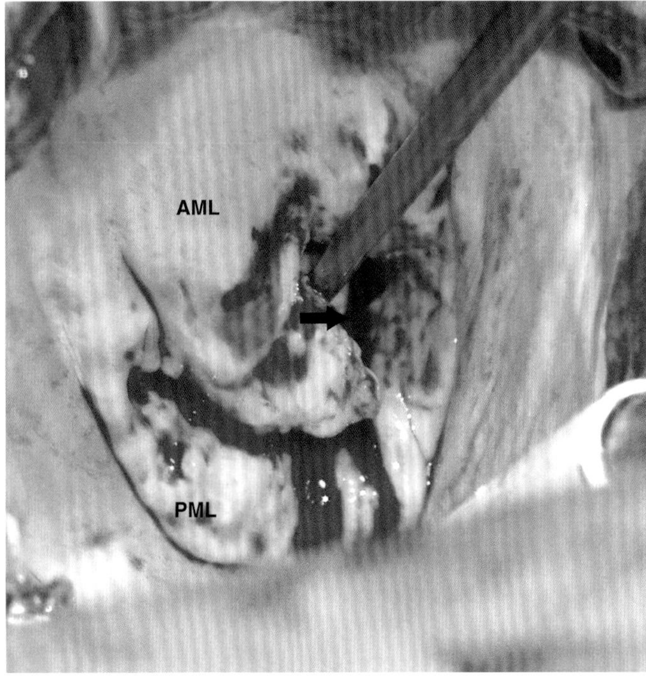

Fig. 27.6 Severe mitral regurgitation complicating balloon mitral commissurotomy. The mechanism of mitral regurgitation was a tear of the anterior leaflet *(arrow)*. Intraoperative surgical view of the mitral valve. *AML*, Anterior mitral leaflet; *PML*, posterior mitral leaflet. (Courtesy Dr. Raffoul, Bichat Hospital, Paris.)

Other findings from postprocedural echocardiography have less important consequences for patient management. Interatrial shunts are frequently visualized using TEE at the

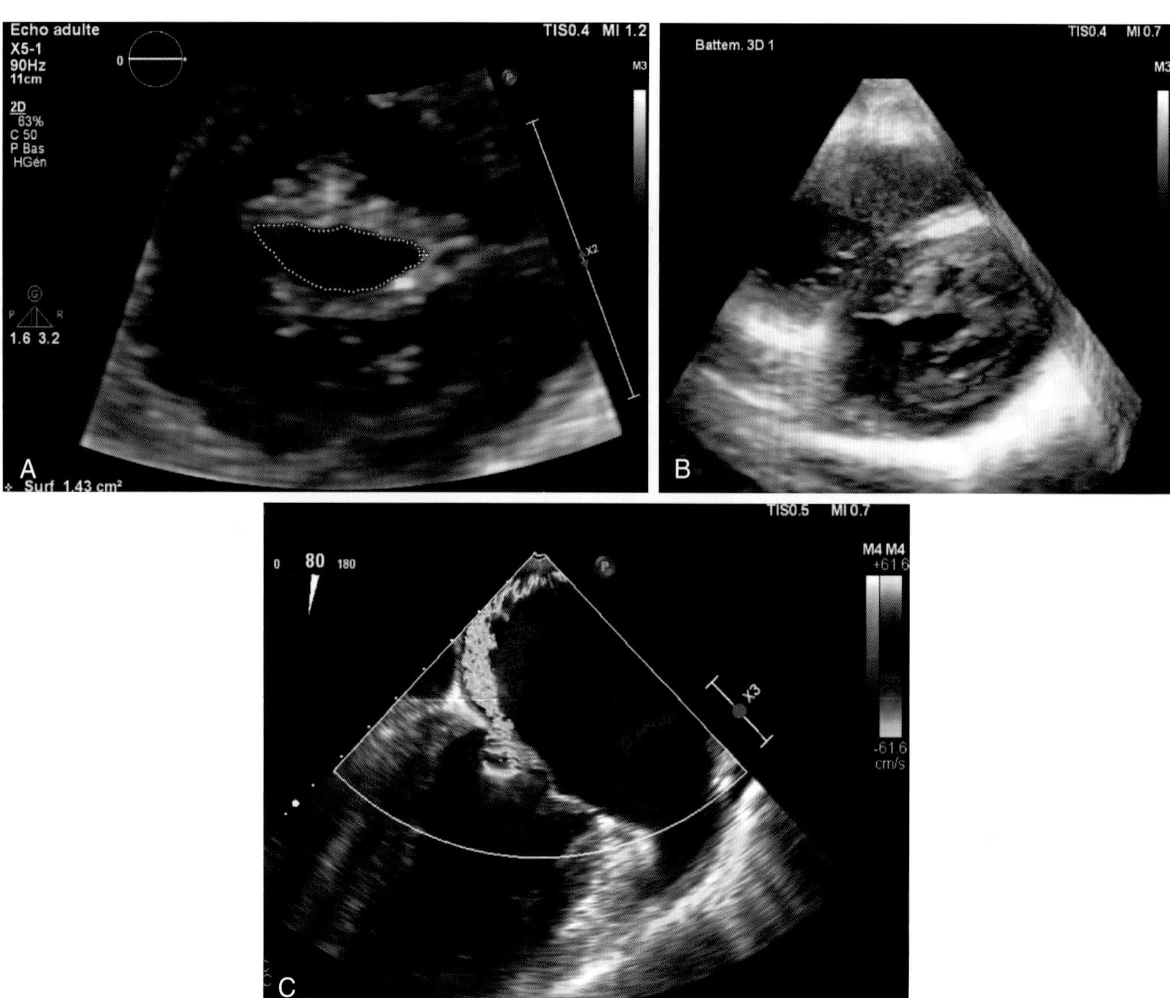

Fig. 27.7 **Mitral restenosis after previous balloon mitral commissurotomy.** TTE, 2D (A) and 3D (B) parasternal short-axis views show noncalcified, thickened leaflets with persistent opening of the posteromedial commissure, which is better visualized on the 3D view (see Videos 27.7A and 27.7B). (C)TEE, mitral regurgitation with eccentric jet. This patient was not a candidate for repeat BMC due to persistent opening of one commissure and more than mild mitral regurgitation (see Video 27.7C).

transseptal puncture site.[37] Usually, they are small shunts that progressively disappear in most cases. Six months after BMC, small residual shunts are observed in less than 10% of patients.[37] The intensity of LA spontaneous contrast frequently decreases after successful BMC, and there is a further decrease until the sixth month.[38]

DURING FOLLOW-UP AFTER BALLOON MITRAL COMMISSUROTOMY

Echocardiographic follow-up assesses the usual features of valve function and its consequences. The most common event is the occurrence of restenosis, which is often defined as a valve area smaller than 1.5 cm^2 and a greater than 50% loss of the initial gain in valve area, although there is no standardized definition.[39] For patients with restenosis, the assessment of valve anatomy should focus on the degree of commissural fusion because it contributes to the choice between repeat BMC and surgery (Fig. 27.7).

ASSESSMENT OF DEGENERATIVE MITRAL STENOSIS

Echocardiography diagnoses degenerative MS by showing an extensive MAC between the posterior leaflet and the posterior wall with acoustic shadowing in the parasternal short-axis view and without commissural fusion. MS is the consequence of thickening and restriction of both mitral leaflets.[7,40]

Direct planimetry is difficult in degenerative MS, and pressure half-time is influenced by confounding factors, particularly compliance of cardiac chambers in elderly patients. Measurement of the MVA by the continuity equation is the recommended method for degenerative MS (see Table 27.1).[10,40] Despite its flow dependence, the mean gradient is useful in degenerative MS because of the difficulties in the assessment of valve area.

The feasibility of TMVR depends in particular on mitral annulus size and the extension and thickness of calcifications to provide anchoring of the prosthesis. This requires a comprehensive assessment using echocardiography and electrocardiography-gated CT scans with intravenous contrast and 3D reconstruction (Fig. 27.8).[6,24] The risk of LVOT obstruction is a common contraindication to TMVR. This risk is best assessed using CT with software that simulates the position of the prosthesis and its interaction with the anterior mitral leaflet and the LVOT.

CLINICAL UTILITY

The clinical utility of BMC, including immediate and late results up to 20 years, has been analyzed in a number of series.

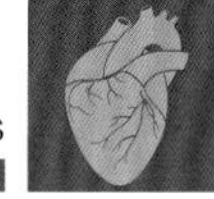

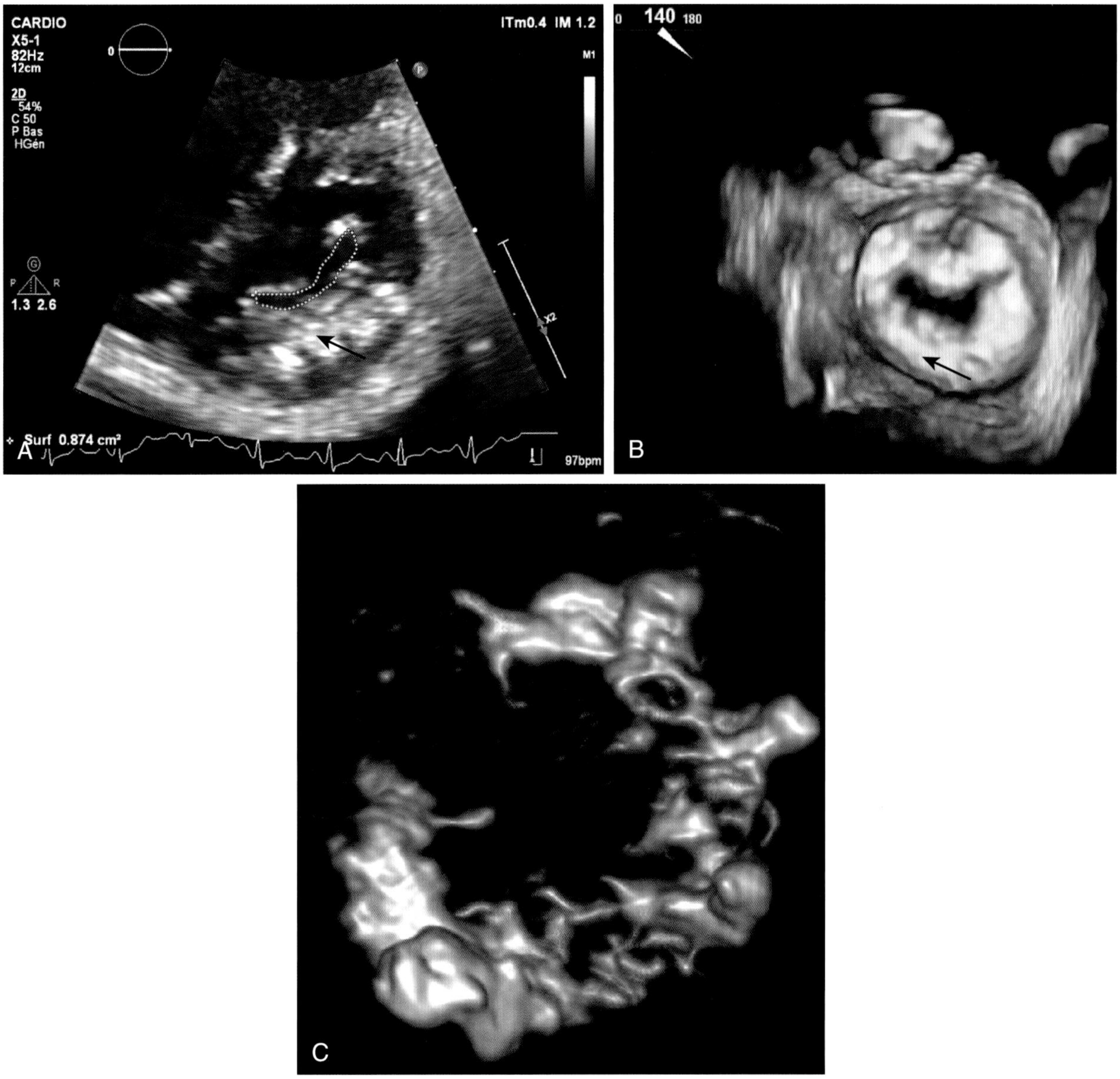

Fig. 27.8 Mitral stenosis due to degenerative calcific mitral valve disease. 2D TTE parasternal short-axis view (A), and 3D TEE view from the LA (B), demonstrate extensive calcification of the mitral annulus *(arrows)* extending to the leaflets without commissural fusion (see Videos 27.8A and 27.8B). (C) CT scan with 3D reconstruction shows extensive calcification of the mitral annulus.

BALLOON MITRAL COMMISSUROTOMY IN RHEUMATIC MITRAL STENOSIS

Results of Balloon Mitral Commissurotomy

Failure and Complications

The two main causes of failure of BMC are the impossibility of performing transseptal puncture and failure to position the balloon across the mitral orifice. The failure rate is approximately 1% in series from experienced teams.[39,41–44]

Severe complications are rare (Table 27.4).[39,41–51] In-hospital death occurs for less than 1% of patients, who are frequently in very poor clinical condition because of advanced age and severe hemodynamic impairment. Tamponade is a consequence of perforation by the transseptal needle or metallic guide wires. The risk of thromboembolic events is typically less than 2%. Embolic sequelae mainly result from fibrinothrombotic clots. Technical simplifications inherent in the Inoue technique contribute to low complication rates, particularly tamponade, and partly account for the wide use of this technique.

Severe traumatic MR is the most frequent severe complication of BMC. It occurs in 1% to 10% of cases and remains difficult to predict.[31] Severe MR is more common in patients with very tight MS and in those with severe impairment of leaflets and subvalvular apparatus, especially when there is a heterogeneous distribution of leaflet abnormalities.[30] Severe acute MR frequently requires surgery but is seldom an emergency.

Procedural complications are more common in low-volume centers, and they are highly dependent on the experience of the interventional cardiologist.[45,52] These findings highlight the need for BMC to be performed by experienced operators in high-volume centers.[19,20]

Immediate Results

After BMC, there is approximately a doubling of MVA (Table 27.5).[29,41–44,46–51,53–55] Series including heart catheterization demonstrated significant decreases in LA and pulmonary artery pressures and an increase in cardiac output. However, invasive

TABLE 27.4 **Severe Complications of Balloon Mitral Commissurotomy.**

Study	*N*	*Age (y)*	*In-Hospital Death (%)*	*Tamponade(%)*	*Embolic Events (%)*	*Severe Mitral Regurgitation (%)*
Arora et al.[43] (1987–2000)	4850	27	0.2	0.2	0.1	1.4
Chen et al.[41] (1985–1994)[a]	4832	37	0.1	0.8	0.5	1.4
Iung et al.[44] (1986–2001)	2773	47	0.4	0.2	0.4	4.1
Neumayer et al.[49] (1989–2000)	1123	57	0.4	0.9	0.9	6.0
Palacios et al.[48] (1986–2000)	879	55	0.6	1.0	1.8	9.4
NHLBI Registry[45] (1987–1989)[a]	738	54				
$n < 25$			2	6	4	4
$25 \leq n < 100$			1	4	2	3
$n \geq 100$			0.3	2	1	3
Ben-Farhat et al.[42] (1987–1998)	654	33	0.5	0.6	1.5	4.6
Hernandez et al.[39] (1989–1995)	620	53	0.5	0.6	—	4.0
Fawzy et al.[50] (1989–2006)	578	32	0	0.9	0.5	1.6
Meneveau et al.[46] (1986–1996)	532	54	0.2	1.1	—	3.9
Tomai et al.[51] (1991–2010)	527	55	0.4	0.4	0.2	4.9
Stefanadis et al.[47] (1988–1996)[a]	441	44	0.2	0	0	3.4

[a]Multicenter series.

TABLE 27.5 **Immediate Results of Balloon Mitral Commissurotomy: Increase in Mitral Valve Area.**

Study	*N*	*Age (y)*	*Mitral Valve Area (cm²)*		*Technique*
			Before BMC	*After BMC*	
Arora et al.[43]	4850	27	0.7	1.9	Inoue, double-balloon, metallic commissurotome
Chen et al.[41]	4832	37	1.1	2.1	Inoue balloon
Iung et al.[44]	2773	47	1.0	1.9	Inoue, single-, or double-balloon
Meneguz-Moreno et al.[53]	1582	36	0.9	2.0	Inoue, double-balloon, metallic commissurotome, multitrack
Neumayer et al.[49]	1123	57	1.1	1.8	Inoue balloon
Palacios et al.[48]	879	55	0.9	1.9	Inoue or double-balloon
Ben-Farhat et al.[42]	654	33	1.0	2.1	Inoue or double-balloon
Hernandez et al.[39]	561	53	1.0	1.8	Inoue balloon
Fawzy et al.[50]	547	32	0.9	2.0	Inoue balloon
Meneveau et al.[46]	532	54	1.0	1.7	Inoue or double-balloon
Tomai et al.[51]	527	55	1.0	1.9	Inoue balloon
Eltchaninoff et al.[54]	500	34	0.9	2.1	Metallic commissurotome
Stefanadis et al.[47]	441	44	1.0	2.1	Modified single-, double-, or Inoue ballon (retrograde)
Lee et al.[55] (randomized comparison)	152 150	42 40	0.9 0.9	1.8 1.9	Inoue balloon Double-balloon

BMC, Balloon mitral commissurotomy.

investigations are now unlikely to be performed in routine assessment. To simplify the interpretation and comparison of series, immediate results are also expressed with the use of a binary end point, which is most often a final valve area of 1.5 cm² or greater without MR greater than grade 2/4.

Mitral valve anatomy, as assessed by echocardiography regardless of the scoring system used, is a strong predictor of immediate results of BMC.[14,42,46–50] The discriminant cutoff point of the Wilkins score has been set at 8 according to analyses of immediate results of BMC. However, all scoring systems have limited predictive value, as is shown by the low correlation ($r = -0.15$) between the Wilkins score and final valve area.[56] Other factors strongly influence immediate results of BMC.[14,56,57] Older age and smaller valve area are significant predictors of poor immediate results and have similar or greater predictive strengths than valve calcification.[14,57]

There were less consistent associations between poor immediate results and previous commissurotomy or baseline MR. In our experience, the interaction between age and previous commissurotomy means that previous commissurotomy is a factor in poor immediate results only for patients older than 50 years of age.[14] Consistent with the predictors identified, series including a majority of young patients with favorable anatomic conditions report particularly good immediate results.[41–43,50]

Late Results

The assessment of late outcome after BMC is based on clinical end points in most series because standardized echocardiographic follow-up has obvious difficulties when a number of patients are followed over a long period. Late results should be interpreted according to the quality of the immediate results. Most patients with residual stenosis or severe MR after BMC require surgery. Conversely, cardiovascular events seldom occur after successful BMC, and most patients experience sustained functional improvement (Fig. 27.9). Mitral restenosis is the most frequent cause of late clinical deterioration after BMC, as it is after successful surgical commissurotomy.[39,58,59]

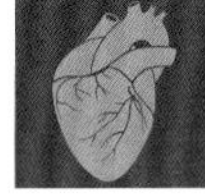

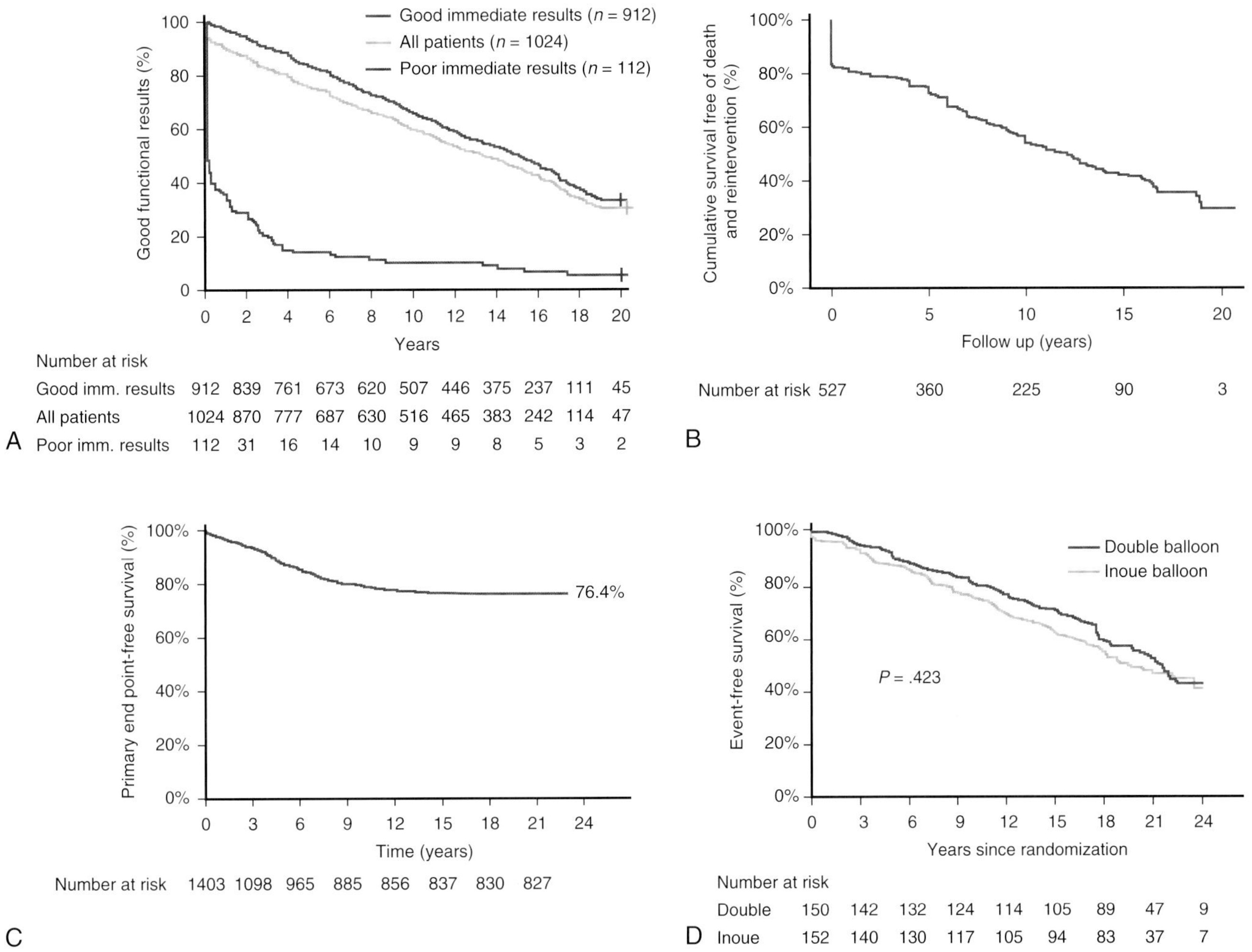

Good functional results (%)

— Good immediate results (n = 912)
— All patients (n = 1024)
— Poor immediate results (n = 112)

Years

Number at risk

Years	0	2	4	6	8	10	12	14	16	18	20
Good imm. results	912	839	761	673	620	507	446	375	237	111	45
All patients	1024	870	777	687	630	516	465	383	242	114	47
Poor imm. results	112	31	16	14	10	9	9	8	5	3	2

A

Cumulative survival free of death and reintervention (%)

Follow up (years)

Follow up (years)	0	5	10	15	20
Number at risk	527	360	225	90	3

B

Primary end point-free survival (%)

76.4%

Time (years)

Time (years)	0	3	6	9	12	15	18	21
Number at risk	1403	1098	965	885	856	837	830	827

C

Event-free survival (%)

— Double balloon
— Inoue balloon

P = .423

Years since randomization

Number at risk

Years since randomization	0	3	6	9	12	15	18	21	24
Double	150	142	132	124	114	105	89	47	9
Inoue	152	140	130	117	105	94	83	37	7

D

Fig. 27.9 Long-term results after good immediate results of balloon mitral commissurotomy. (A) Good functional results (cardiovascular survival without intervention and in New York Heart Association [NYHA] functional class I or II) for 912 patients. (B) Event-free survival (freedom from cardiovascular death, mitral surgery, and repeat BMC) rates for 482 patients. (C) Event-free survival (freedom from all-cause death, mitral surgery, and repeat BMC) rates for 1582 patients. (D) Event-free survival (freedom from all-cause death, mitral surgery, repeat BMC, and NYHA class ≥III) rates for 302 patients. (Data from [A] Bouleti C, Iung B, Laouénan C, et al. Late results of percutaneous mitral commissurotomy up to 20 years: development and validation of a risk score predicting late functional results from a series of 912 patients. *Circulation.* 2012;125:2119–2127; [B] Tomai F, Gaspardone A, Versaci F, et al. Twenty year follow-up after successful percutaneous balloon mitral valvuloplasty in a large contemporary series of patients with mitral stenosis. *Int J Cardiol.* 2014;177:881–885; [C] Meneguz-Moreno RA, Costa JR Jr, Gomes NL, et al. Very long term follow-up after percutaneous balloon mitral valvuloplasty. *JACC Cardiovasc Interv.* 2018;11:1945–1952; [D] Lee S, Kang DH, Kim DH, et al. Late outcome of percutaneous mitral commissurotomy: Randomized comparison of Inoue versus double-balloon technique. *Am Heart J.* 2017;194:1–8.)

The wide range in clinical outcome in different series (Table 27.6)[a] is related to differences in patient characteristics. Series from developing countries include younger patients with more favorable anatomic conditions than in Western countries and report higher rates of event-free survival.

European series that include patients with a mean age of approximately 50 years reported 20-year rates of survival without intervention between 30% and 40%.[51,60,63] Better outcomes were reported in series from Brazil and Korea that included patients with a mean age between 36 and 41 years.[53,55]

Valve anatomy is only one of the predictive factors of outcome (Fig. 27.10).[b] Besides impaired valve anatomy, baseline predictors of poor late outcome are higher age and the consequences of MS, such as a high functional class and atrial fibrillation (Table 27.7).

The degree of valve opening has an impact on late outcome.[39,51,60,61] Besides postprocedural valve area, the mean mitral gradient after BMC is also a strong predictor of late clinical results, suggesting that it provides additional information.[60] The degree of commissural opening is strongly linked with postprocedural valve area and mitral gradient but does not have an incremental prognostic value for late outcome.[34] The different predictive factors of late functional results can be combined using a scoring system developed by Bouleti et al. that enables good functional results to be estimated in an individual patient according to baseline characteristics and the immediate result of BMC (Fig. 27.11; see Table 27.7).[60]

Series that included serial echocardiographic examinations showed a progressive decrease in mean MVA over time after BMC that followed a linear pattern.[39,58] The yearly decrease in valve area varies among the series according to differences in patient characteristics, producing inhomogeneous estimations of restenosis rates. Conversely, there is typically no increase in mild-to-moderate MR.[39]

[a] References 39, 42, 46–48, 50, 51, 53, 55, 60–62.

[b] References 39, 42, 46–48, 50, 51, 53, 60–63.

Particular Subgroups

Restenosis After Previous Commissurotomy

In patients with restenosis after prior closed or open heart commissurotomy, BMC is feasible and has the attraction of avoiding iterative surgery, provided that restenosis is related to bicommissural fusion.[64,65] Surgery consists in prosthetic valve replacement in most patients with restenosis. Even if the results of BMC are less satisfying after previous commissurotomy than in native valves, the possibility of deferring surgery by at least 10 years in one half of patients enables prosthesis-related complications to be postponed. Young patients are likely to derive the greatest benefit from BMC for restenosis.[65]

Restenosis after previous BMC is becoming more common. Repeat BMC can be performed in selected patients and gives good mid-term clinical results, particularly in young patients with mild or no calcification,[64,66] whereas its efficacy is less convincing in older patients with calcified valves.[67] The possibility of repeat BMC enables surgery to be further postponed. Patients younger than 50 years of age at their first BMC derive particular benefit from repeat BMC (Fig. 27.12).[66]

Echocardiographic analysis of valve anatomy should carefully consider the extent of commissural re-fusion. Results of repeat BMC are less satisfying for patients who have incomplete commissural fusion. Whatever the type of initial commissurotomy, BMC should not be considered if there is complete opening of one or both commissures (see Fig. 27.7).

TABLE 27.6 Late Results (>5 y) After Balloon Mitral Commissurotomy.

Study	*N*	*Age (y)*	*Maximum Follow-Up (y)*	*Event-Free Survival (%)*
Meneguz-Moreno et al.[53]	1582	36	23	76[a]
Bouleti et al.[60]	1024	49	20	34[a] 30[b]
Palacios et al.[48]	879	55	12	33[b]
Ben-Farhat et al.[42]	654	34	10	72[b]
Hernandez et al.[39]	561	53	7	69[b]
Fawzy et al.[50,c]	547	32	19	28[b]
Meneveau et al.[46]	532	54	7.5	52[b]
Tomai et al.[51,c]	482	55	20	36[a] 21[b]
Stefanadis et al.[47]	441	44	9	75[b]
Song et al.[61]	402	44	9	90[a]
Lee et al.[55] (randomized comparison)	152 150	42 40	24 24	41[b] 43[b]
Orrange et al.[62]	132	44	7	65[a]

[a]Survival without intervention (mitral valve replacement or repeat balloon mitral commissurotomy).
[b]Survival without intervention and for New York Heart Association class I or II.
[c]Patients with good immediate results.

The Elderly

Theoretically, elderly patients are not good candidates for BMC because they combine predictive factors for poor immediate and poor late outcome; besides old age, valve calcification, atrial fibrillation, and severe symptoms are common. Despite unfavorable anatomic conditions, good immediate results are often obtained, but subsequent deterioration occurs more rapidly than in younger patients.[68–71] However, these results should be weighed against the risk of surgery. Echocardiographic examination should confirm the rheumatic origin of the MS and distinguish it from degenerative MS.

Young Patients

Severe rheumatic MS may be encountered in young patients in countries where rheumatic fever is endemic. Two series have reported consistent results of BMC for patients younger than 20 years of age who were followed for 12 years.[72,73] Results tended to be better than for adults, and late functional results did not differ from those for adults, with event-free survival rates ranging from 70% to 80% at 10 years. BMC is also a valid treatment of MS in children younger than 12 years of age.[74]

Pregnant Women

Hemodynamic changes during pregnancy worsen the clinical tolerance of MS, which may compromise the prognosis of the mother and fetus, particularly at delivery.[75] Intervention is required during pregnancy for women who remain symptomatic despite medical therapy (see Fig. 27.1).[76] BMC can be safely performed during pregnancy, and fetal tolerance is good.[76]

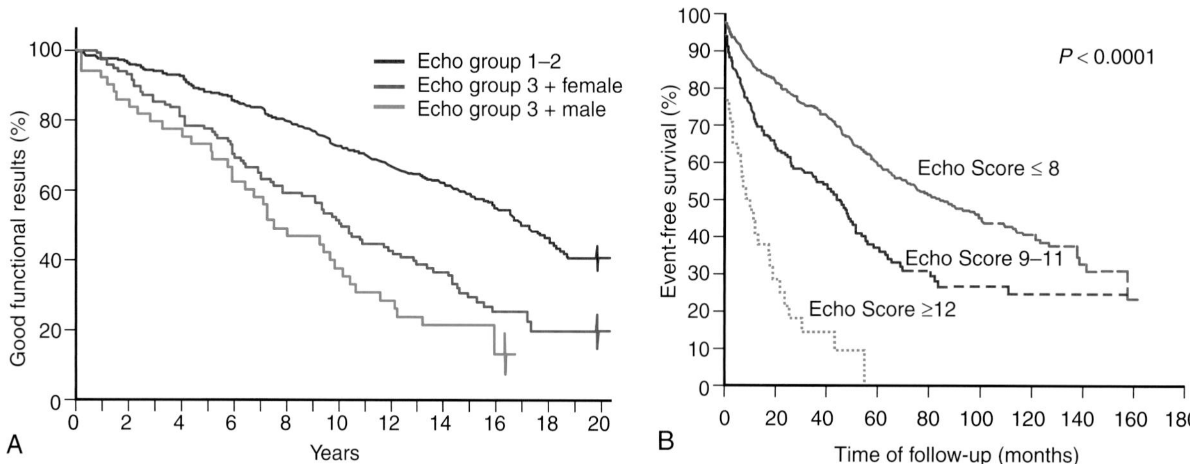

Fig. 27.10 Influence of valve anatomy on long-term results after balloon mitral commissurotomy. (A) Influence of Cormier echocardiographic group. (B) Influence of the Wilkins score. (Adapted from [A] Bouleti C, Iung B, Laouénan C, et al. Late results of percutaneous mitral commissurotomy up to 20 years: development and validation of a risk score predicting late functional results from a series of 912 patients. *Circulation.* 2012;125:2119–2127; [B] Palacios IF, Sanchez PL, Harrell LC, Weyman AE, Block PC. Which patients benefit from percutaneous mitral balloon valvuloplasty? Prevalvuloplasty and postvalvuloplasty variables that predict long-term outcome. *Circulation.* 2002;105:1465–1471.)

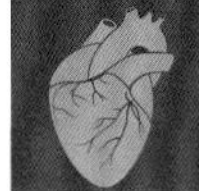

Implications for Patient Selection

Contraindications

Contraindications to BMC are summarized in Table 27.8. Although cases of BMC using the Inoue balloon have been reported for patients with thrombosis located in the left atrial appendage, the experience remains limited. The potential hazards related to thrombus migration should lead to consideration of persistent thrombus of the LA, even when localized to the left atrial appendage, as a contraindication to BMC in most cases.[19,20] However, if the patient is in stable condition, the decision should be postponed until after repeat TEE is performed following at least 2 months of optimal anticoagulant therapy.[77]

More than mild MR, or MR with a grade greater than 2/4 when using a semiquantitative approach, is a contraindication to BMC.[19,20] For patients with borderline MR, BMC is more likely to be considered if valve anatomy is favorable. Valve calcification contraindicates BMC in the rare cases in which it is massive or localized in both commissures.[19,20]

Other contraindications are related to associated heart diseases that require surgical correction. Underestimation of the degree of aortic stenosis should be avoided. Conversely, associated moderate aortic regurgitation without consequences for the LV does not contraindicate BMC because its progression is

TABLE 27.7 Predictive Factors of Poor Late Functional Results After Good Immediate Results of Balloon Mitral Commissurotomy (Valve Area ≥1.5 cm² With No Regurgitation >2/4).[a]

Parameter	*Adjusted Hazard Ratio [95% CI]*	*P*	*Points for Score (/13)*
Age (y) and final mitral valve area (cm²)			
<50 and MVA ≥ 2.00	1		0
<50 and MVA 1.50–2.00 *or* 50–70 and MVA > 1.75	2.1 [1.6–2.9]	<0.0001	2
50–70 and MVA 1.50–1.75 *or* ≥70 and MVA ≥ 1.50	5.1 [3.5–7.5]	<0.0001	5
Valve anatomy and sex			
No valve calcification	1		0
Valve calcification			
Female	1.2 [0.9–1.6]	0.18	0
Male	2.3 [1.6–3.2]	<0.0001	3
Rhythm and NYHA class			
Sinus rhythm *or* Atrial fibrillation and NYHA class I–II	1		0
Atrial fibrillation and NYHA class III–IV	1.8 [1.4–2.3]	<0.0001	2
Final mean mitral gradient (mmHg)			
≤3	1		0
3–6	[1.0–1.8]	0.05	1
≥6	2.5 [1.8–3.5]	<0.0001	3

[a]Multivariable analysis and definition of a predictive score of long-term results. The correspondence between the score and predicted long-term outcome is shown in Fig. 27.11.
CI, Confidence interval; *NYHA*, New York Heart Association.
From Bouleti C, Iung B, Laouénan C, et al. Late results of percutaneous mitral commissurotomy up to 20 years: development and validation of a risk score predicting late functional results from a series of 912 patients. *Circulation.* 2012;125:2119–2127.

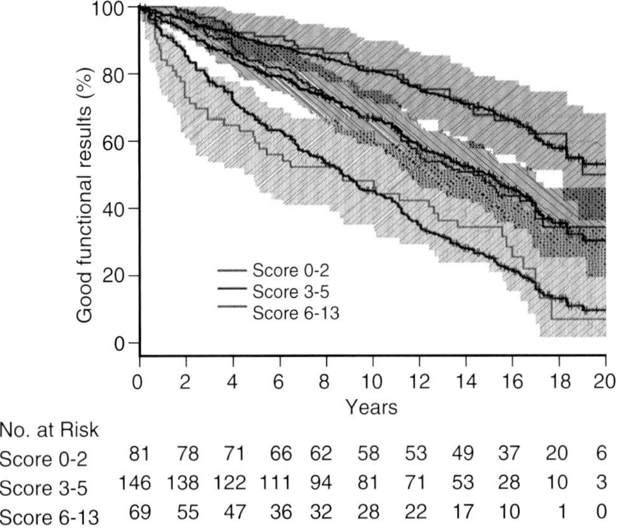

Fig. 27.11 Prediction of good late functional results after balloon mitral commissurotomy. A score is used for the prediction of cardiovascular survival without intervention and in New York Heart Association functional class I or II (see Table 27.7). Observed rates *(colored lines)* with their 95% confidence intervals and predicted rates *(black lines)*. (From Bouleti C, Iung B, Laouénan C, et al. Late results of percutaneous mitral commissurotomy up to 20 years: development and validation of a risk score predicting late functional results from a series of 912 patients. *Circulation.* 2012;125:2119–2127.)

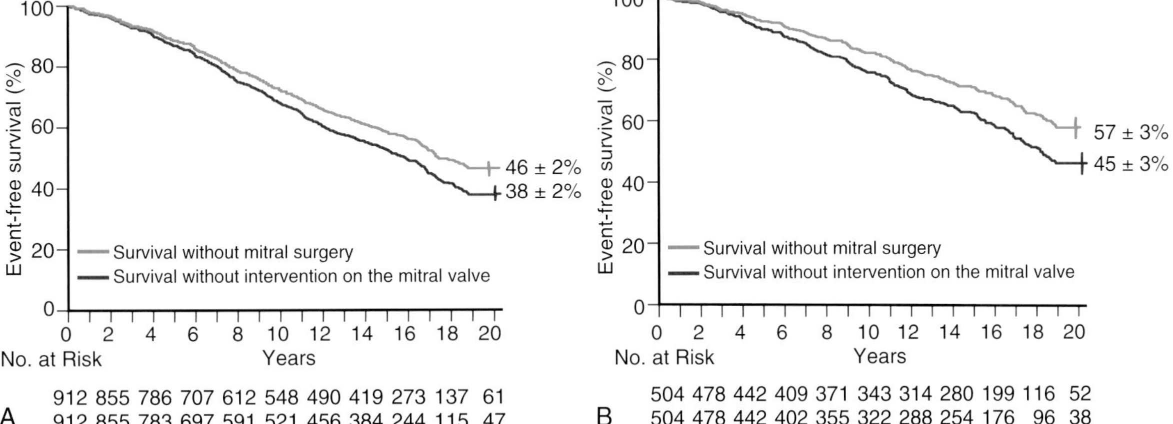

Fig. 27.12 Cardiovascular survival without reintervention after balloon mitral commissurotomy (BMC). Comparison of cardiovascular survival without mitral surgery or without any reintervention (surgery or repeat BMC) after good immediate results of BMC: in the whole population of 912 patients (A) and in the 504 patients aged less than 50 years at the time of initial BMC (B). (From Bouleti C, Iung B, Himbert D, et al. Reinterventions after percutaneous mitral commissurotomy during long-term follow-up, up to 20 years: the role of repeat percutaneous mitral commissurotomy. *Eur Heart J.* 2013;34:1923–1930.)

slow. Surgery is preferred if there is severe associated organic tricuspid disease or severe functional TR with major enlargement of the tricuspid annulus. In other cases, severe functional TR can decrease after BMC.

Choice of Procedure

There is now evidence supporting BMC as the procedure of choice in young patients. Randomized trials conducted with homogeneous populations showed that mid-term and long-term results of BMC were as good as those obtained with open heart commissurotomy and similar to or better than those after closed heart commissurotomy.[78–81] There are no differences in late outcome between the Inoue and the double-balloon techniques.[55]

To avoid iterative surgical interventions, the possibility of repeating BMC is particularly attractive in young patients. However, a number of good candidates in developing countries cannot afford BMC. This justifies attempts to lower the cost of the device, such as using a multitrack system or the metallic commissurotome.[54]

The decision is more difficult for older patients, who frequently have impairment of the anatomy of the leaflets and subvalvular apparatus, including calcification, and who represent the majority and a growing proportion of patients with MS in Western countries.[69,82] They form a heterogeneous group for whom no randomized studies are available.[83] Patients should not be denied BMC only on the basis of unfavorable valve anatomy, given the low predictive value of valve anatomy alone. Good immediate and mid-term results can be obtained in patients with unfavorable mitral anatomy, even with calcified valves.[70,82,84]

For patients with impaired valve anatomy, BMC can be considered if their other characteristics are favorable, particularly young age, MVA between 1.0 and 1.5 cm^2, moderate symptoms (New York Heart Association [NYHA] class II), and sinus rhythm. Predictive models show a high likelihood of good immediate and late results in these patients.[14,57,60]

Except in patients with large valve calcifications, BMC may provide sustained functional improvement in calcific MS. Results are particularly good for patients younger than 50 years of age, 57% of whom experience good functional results and NYHA class I–II after 10 years and 21% after 20 years.[84] Differences in long-term outcomes after BMC are less marked when comparing propensity-matched subgroups of patients with noncalcified and calcified valves to account for the impact of confounding factors (Fig. 27.13).[84]

BMC enables surgery, most often valve replacement, to be postponed for several years in selected patients with rheumatic MS and calcified valves. Conversely, there is a much lower likelihood of sustained long-term improvement in old patients who have unfavorable mitral anatomy, tight stenosis, severe symptoms, and atrial fibrillation. For these patients, mitral surgery, which is often combined with tricuspid repair, can be considered as the first-line treatment provided the operative risk is acceptable. The choice between BMC and surgery in these difficult situations should also take into account the local expertise of interventional cardiologists and surgeons and the wishes of the informed patient.

In Western countries, there is a trend for BMC to be performed in older patients who have more severe impairment of valve anatomy (Fig. 27.14).[82] In the VHDII Survey, surgical commissurotomy accounted for only 4% of the interventions performed for MS in 2017, whereas BMC was used in 45% of patients and prosthetic valve replacement in 51%.[5] In a nationwide administrative database accounting for 20% of US hospitals, there was a decrease in the number of BMC procedures between 1998 and 2010, and the mean patient age increased from 58 years in 1998 to 63 years in 2010.[52]

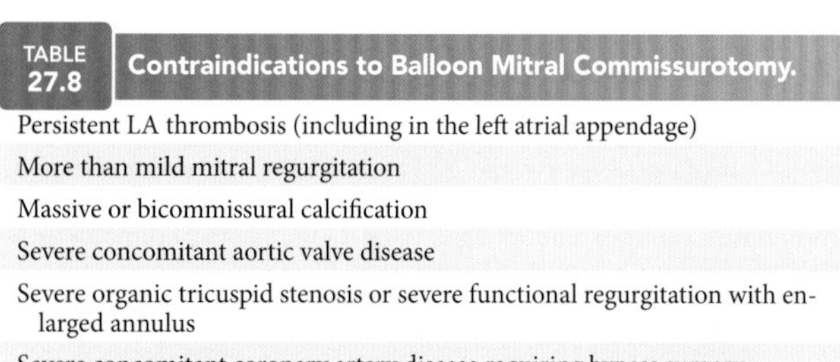

TABLE 27.8 Contraindications to Balloon Mitral Commissurotomy.
Persistent LA thrombosis (including in the left atrial appendage)
More than mild mitral regurgitation
Massive or bicommissural calcification
Severe concomitant aortic valve disease
Severe organic tricuspid stenosis or severe functional regurgitation with enlarged annulus
Severe concomitant coronary artery disease requiring bypass surgery

Timing of the Procedure

There is a consensus to advise intervention, whether it is percutaneous or surgical, for patients who have MS with a valve area smaller than 1.5 cm^2 and symptoms.[19,20] Better insights into the prognosis of MS, particularly regarding the risk of thromboembolic complications or hemodynamic decompensation, and the availability of low-risk intervention have led to consideration of the indications for BMC at an earlier stage in selected patients. A comparative prospective series reported higher rates

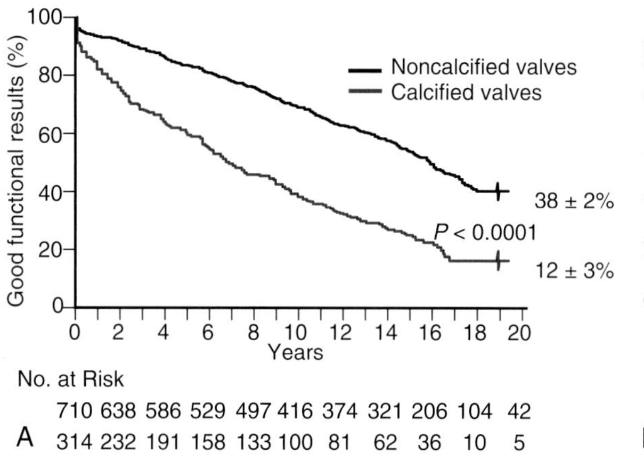

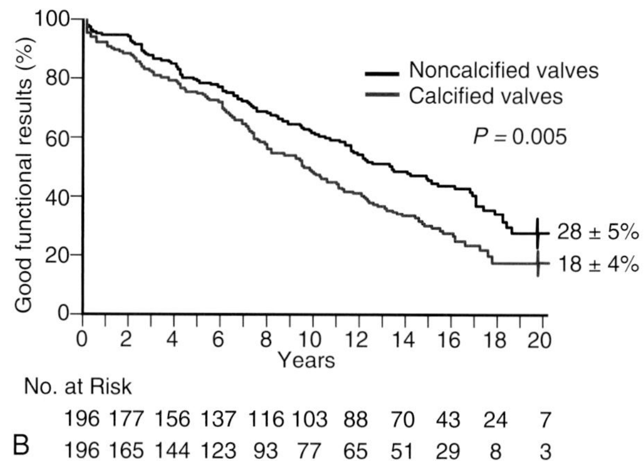

Fig. 27.13 Long-term results of balloon mitral commissurotomy in patients with or without fluoroscopic valve calcification. (A) In the whole population of 1024 patients. (B) In two propensity-matched subgroups of 196 patients each. (From BouletiC, Iung B, Himbert D, et al. Relationship between valve calcification and long-term results of percutaneous mitral commissurotomy for rheumatic mitral stenosis. *Circ Cardiovasc Interv.* 2014;7:381–389.)

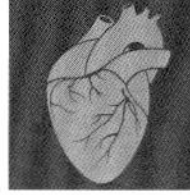

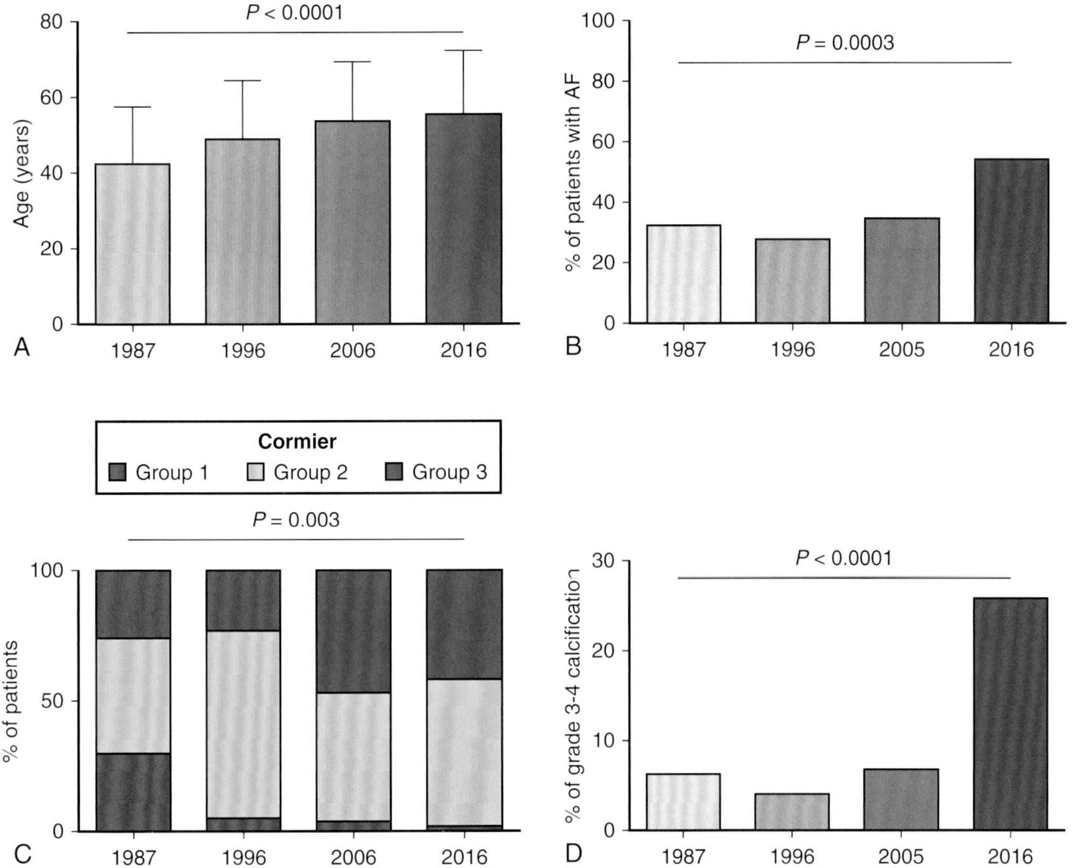

Fig. 27.14 Evolution of the characteristics of patients treated by BMC over 30 years. Evolution of patient population in regard to age (A), atrial fibrillation *(AF)* (B), valve anatomy as assessed by Cormier class (C), and severe calcification as assessed by fluoroscopy (D). (From Desnos C, Iung B, Himbert D, et al. Temporal trends on percutaneous mitral commissurotomy: 30 years of experience. *J Am Heart Assoc.* 2019;8:e012031.)

of event-free survival at 11 years for patients undergoing BMC with NYHA class I–II versus class III–IV indications, and the difference remained significant after propensity matching.[85] There was a particular benefit for patients at risk for thromboembolic events (i.e., with atrial fibrillation or previous embolic events).[85]

Intervention is generally not considered in MS with a valve area greater than 1.5 cm^2 because the variations in progression do not support prophylactic BMC.[19,20] BMC can be considered for patients with borderline valve area who have symptoms or pulmonary hypertension.

The efficacy of BMC has been demonstrated using various markers of thromboembolic risk in MS: LA spontaneous contrast, LA size and contractility, left atrial appendage flow velocity, and activation of coagulation in the LA. Although the efficacy of BMC in regard to thromboembolic risk has not been demonstrated by randomized studies, a retrospective and a prospective series showed that the performance of BMC was associated with decreased thromboembolic risk for patients with MS and atrial fibrillation.[86,87]

It is more difficult to evaluate the risk of acute hemodynamic complications in MS, apart from particular cases such as pregnancy. Exercise echocardiography can provide additional information compared with baseline evaluation, although no threshold of mitral gradient or sPAP can be proposed to recommend intervention.

It is difficult to provide recommendations for interventional antiarrhythmic therapy in MS. The particularities of anatomic and electric LA remodeling in MS should be taken into account.[88] However, there are few data in the literature that are specific for MS. Antiarrhythmic therapy should not be considered without treatment of the MS.[88] Recommendations on BMC according to current guidelines are summarized in Table 27.9.

TRANSCATHETER MITRAL VALVE REPLACEMENT FOR DEGENERATIVE CALCIFIC MITRAL STENOSIS

The search for alternatives to surgery is relevant in degenerative MS because of the high morbidity and mortality rates associated with surgical valve replacement. Because there is no commissural fusion, degenerative MS is not amenable to BMC.

TMVR for degenerative MS is an off-label use in which a transcatheter aortic valve is implanted in the calcified mitral annulus using a transapical or a transseptal approach (Fig. 27.15). Experience with TMVR in MAC remains limited. Preliminary experience shows that morbidity and mortality rates are higher when TMVR is performed in high-risk patients for MAC rather than for deterioration of a bioprosthesis or valve repair.[89] In the largest experience from a registry of 116 patients with a mean Society of Thoracic Surgeons (STS) score of 15.3%, the all-cause mortality rates were 25% at 30 days and 54% at 1 year.[90] The most frequent procedural complication leading to early death was LVOT obstruction, followed by prosthesis migration and perforation.[90] This highlights the need for careful patient selection based on multimodality imaging.

TABLE 27.9 Recommendations for Balloon Mitral Commissurotomy in Patients With Mitral Stenosis.

2020 ACC/AHA Guidelines	*2017 ESC/EACTS Guidelines*
Symptomatic Patients	
In symptomatic patients (NYHA class II, III or IV) with severe rheumatic mitral stenosis (mitral valve area ≤ 1.5 cm², stage D) and favorable valve morphology with less than moderate (2+) MR in the absence of left atrial thrombus PBMC is recommended if it can be performed at a Comprehensive Valve Center. **(1A)** In severely symptomatic patients (NYHA class III or IV) with severe rheumatic mitral stenosis (mitral valve area ≤ 1.5 cm², stage D) who (1) are not candidate to PBMC, (2) have failed a previous PBMC, (3) require other cardiac procedures, or (4) do not have access to PBMC, mitral valve surgery (repair, commissurotomy or valve replacement) is indicated. **(1B-NR)** In symptomatic patients (NYHA class II, III or IV) with severe rheumatic mitral stenosis (mitral valve area >1.5 cm², if there is evidence of hemodynamically significant MS on the basis of a pulmonary wedge pressure > 25 mmHg or mean mitral valve gradient >15 mmHg during exercise, PBMC may be considered if it can be performed at a Comprehensive Valve Center. **(2b C-LD)** In severely symptomatic patients (NYHA class III or IV) with severe rheumatic mitral stenosis (mitral valve area ≤ 1.5 cm², stage D) who have a suboptimal valve anatomy and who are not candidates for surgery or at high risk for surgery, PBMC may be considered if it can be performed at a Comprehensive Valve Center. **(2b B-NR)**	Patients with mitral stenosis and valve area ≤ 1.5 cm²: • Symptomatic patients without unfavorable characteristics[a] for percutaneous mitral commissurotomy. **(IB)** • Symptomatic patients with a contraindication or a high risk for surgery. **(IC)** • As initial treatment in symptomatic patients with suboptimal anatomy but no unfavorable clinical characteristics for percutaneous mitral commissurotomy.[a] **(IIaC)**
Asymptomatic Patients	
In asymptomatic patients with severe rheumatic mitral stenosis (mitral valve area ≤ 1.5 cm², stage C) and favorable valve morphology with less than 2+ MR in the absence of left atrial thrombus who have elevated pulmonary pressures (pulmonary artery systolic pressure >50 mmHg), PBMC is reasonable if it can be performed at a Comprehensive Valve Center. **(2a B-NR)** In asymptomatic patients with severe rheumatic mitral stenosis (mitral valve area ≤ 1.5 cm², stage C) and favorable valve morphology with less than 2+ MR in the absence of left atrial thrombus who have new onset of atrial fibrillation, PBMC may be considered if it can be performed at a Comprehensive Valve Center. **(2a B-NR)**	Asymptomatic patients with mitral stenosis and valve area ≤ 1.5 cm², without unfavorable clinical and anatomical characteristics for percutaneous mitral commissurotomy[a] *and:* • High thromboembolic risk (history of systemic embolism, dense spontaneous contrast in the left atrium, new-onset or paroxysmal atrial fibrillation). **(IIaC)** *and/or* • High risk of haemodynamic decompensation (systolic pulmonary pressure > 50 mmHg at rest, need for major non-cardiac surgery, desire for pregnancy). **(IIaC)**

[a]Unfavorable characteristics for percutaneous mitral commissurotomy can be defined by the presence of several of the following characteristics:
• Clinical characteristics: old age, history of commissurotomy, NYHA class IV, permanent atrial fibrillation, severe pulmonary hypertension.
• Anatomic characteristics: echo score >8, Cormier score 3 (calcification of mitral valve of any extent, as assessed by fluoroscopy), very small mitral valve area, severe tricuspid regurgitation.

ACC, American College of Cardiology; *AHA,* American Heart Association; *EACTS,* European Association for CardioThoracic Surgery; *ESC,* European Society of Cardiology; *NYHA,* New York Heart Association; *MR,* mitral regurgitation; *PBMC,* percutaneous balloon mitral commissurotomy.

From Otto CM, Nishimura RA, Bonow RO, et al. 2020 ACC/AHA guideline for the management of patients with valvular heart disease: a report of the American College of Cardiology/American Heart Association Joint Committee on Clinical Practice Guidelines. *Circulation.* 2021;143(5):e72-e227. https://doi.org/10.1161/CIR.0000000000000923; Baumgartner H, Falk V, Bax JJ, et al. 2017 ESC/ EACTS guidelines for the management of valvular heart disease. The Task Force for the Management of Valvular Heart Disease of the European Society of Cardiology (ESC) and the European Association for Cardio-Thoracic Surgery (EACTS). *Eur Heart J.* 2017;38:2739–2791.

RESEARCH APPLICATIONS

STRESS ECHOCARDIOGRAPHY

Exercise echocardiography is the most physiologic approach to assess changes in hemodynamic conditions. Mean gradient and sPAP increase at submaximal effort or peak effort but with an important heterogeneity that does not relate to baseline severity of MS. A possible explanation comes from differences in the evolution of MVA, as assessed by the continuity equation, and differences in stroke volume. The increase in MVA with exercise is associated with an increase in stroke volume. Conversely, stroke volume does not increase if there is no significant change in valve area during exercise.[91,92] These two different patterns are not related to MS severity but to the impairment of valve anatomy.[91] The pattern of increase in sPAP with exercise is related to the type of limiting symptoms (i.e., dyspnea or fatigue). Besides valvular function, lung function, chronotropic incompetence, stroke volume reserve, and peripheral factors contribute to impaired exercise tolerance.[93]

Dobutamine stress echocardiography is a less physiologic approach than exercise echocardiography for MS. It is also associated with significant increases in the mean gradient and sPAP compared with resting values, and the increases have prognostic value for clinical events.[94] Another study using dobutamine stress echocardiography showed a more important valve reserve (i.e., more important increase in valve area) in patients who had previously undergone commissurotomy compared with patients who had native valve MS.[95]

The implications of exercise echocardiography in decision making should be assessed by additional prospective studies. Studies are particularly needed to propose thresholds or progression patterns of mitral gradient and sPAP that may lead to considering intervention in asymptomatic patients with MS.

EVALUATION OF ATRIOVENTRICULAR COMPLIANCE

The decrease in upstream pressure observed in MS during diastole depends on valve area and the combined compliance of the LA and LV. Noninvasive assessment by Doppler echocardiography has been validated and combines the MVA as determined by planimetry and the E-wave downslope obtained from the Doppler signal of transmitral flow.[92,96] Net atrioventricular compliance (in mL/mmHg) is the product of 1270 × (MVA/E-wave downslope), where MVA is expressed in cm² and the E-wave downslope in cm/s².

Net atrioventricular compliance is a strong determinant of pulmonary artery pressure at rest and has an incremental predictive value over MVA and mean gradient.[92] Differences in atrioventricular compliance account for the wide range of pulmonary artery pressures that can be observed for a given level of MS severity in terms of MVA. Low atrioventricular compliance is mainly

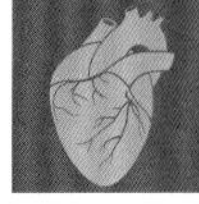

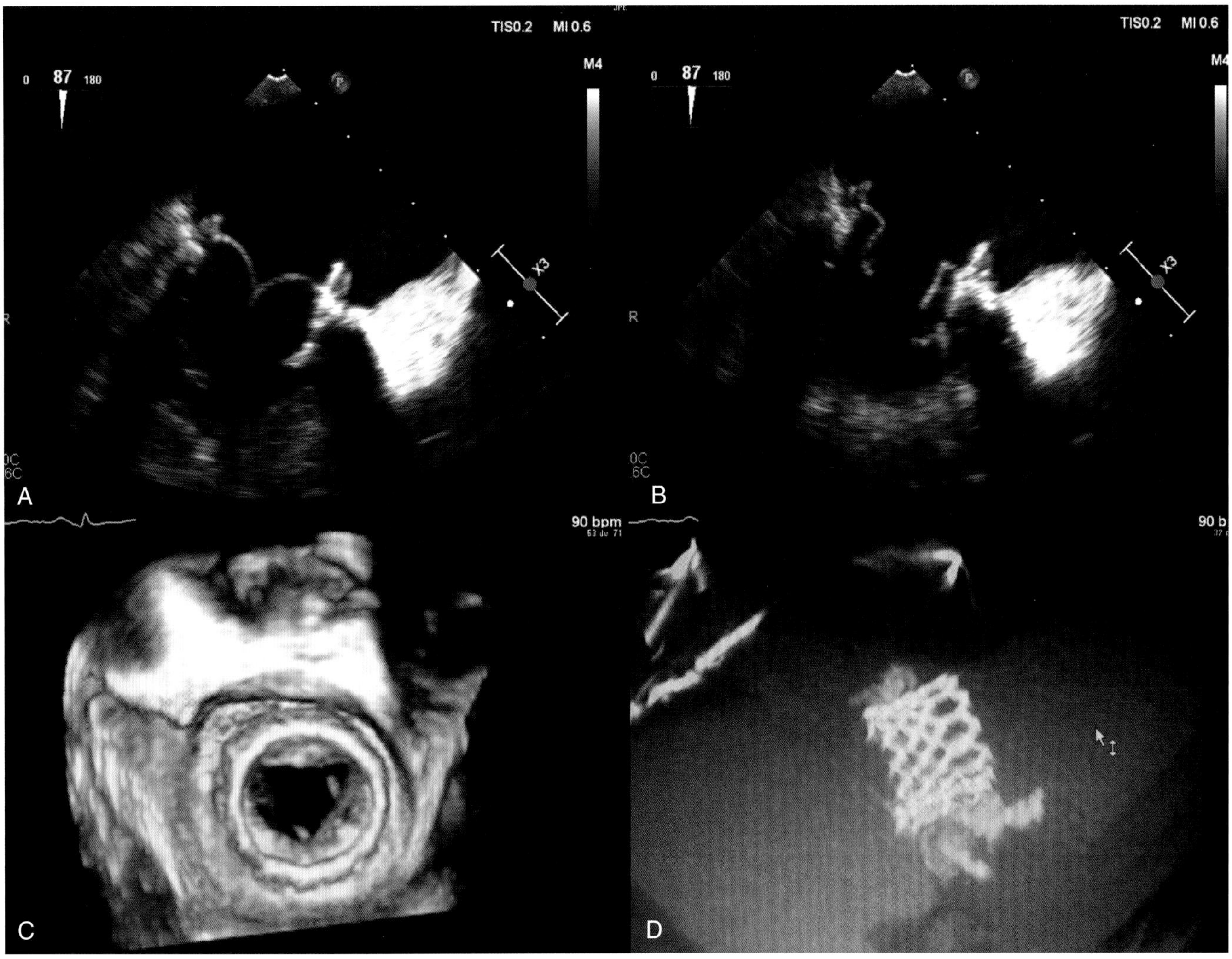

Fig. 27.15 Mitral annulus calcification treated by transcatheter mitral valve replacement of a Sapien prosthesis. (A) TEE shows the Sapien prosthesis in systole with closed leaflets (see Video 27.15A). (B) Sapien prosthesis in diastole with opened leaflets. (C) 3D TEE, Sapien prosthesis in diastole (see Video 27.15C). (D) CT scan with 3D reconstruction shows the prosthesis inserted in the mitral annular calcification. (Courtesy Dr. Himbert, Bichat Hospital, Paris.)

the consequence of low compliance of the LA, and it is associated, even more than the values at rest, with a higher pulmonary artery pressure during exercise and with more severe symptoms.[92]

Atrioventricular compliance has an effect on survival without intervention in conjunction with NYHA class and MVA before BMC.[96] Atrioventricular compliance of 4 mL/mmHg or lower identifies a subgroup of patients at high risk for subsequent intervention.[96]

Although atrioventricular compliance is not part of the routine assessment of MS, it may be useful for evaluating patients who present with discordance between symptoms and MS severity as assessed by valve area. Its usefulness for decision making about asymptomatic patients deserves further investigation.

EVALUATION OF VALVE ANATOMY

Given the limitations of commonly used scoring systems for predicting the results of BMC, alternative approaches have been developed, particularly taking into account the location of valve abnormalities in relation to the commissures. Serial studies have shown that the commissural location of valve thickening and calcification influences immediate results of BMC[27–29] and may contribute to increasing the risk of severe MR complicating BMC.

A recently developed score takes into account four echocardiographic measurements. Three of them are quantitative[32] (Table 27.10): MVA, maximum leaflet displacement, commissural area ratio quantifying the asymmetry of commissural thickening, and subvalvular involvement. This score was found to be reproducible and improved the prediction of immediate results of BMC compared with the Wilkins score, including in an independent population. However, validation remains limited.[97]

Various alternative approaches can refine the assessment of valve anatomy by combining more detailed scoring systems and evaluations of valvular mechanical properties. However, more complex analyses raise concerns regarding their applicability in current practice and their reproducibility. Moreover, it will be necessary to demonstrate their incremental predictive value for outcomes compared with current validated multifactorial approaches.

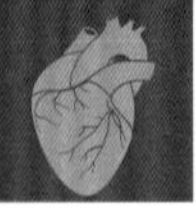

TABLE 27.10 Score Using Quantitative Echocardiographic Assessment for the Prediction of Immediate Outcome After Balloon Mitral Commissurotomy.[a]

Variable	*Prevalence (n, %)*	*Odds Ratio [95% CI]*	*P*	*Points for Score*
Mitral valve area ≤ 1 cm^2	73 (36)	2.73 [1.32–5.66]	0.007	2
Maximum leaflet displacement ≤ 12 mm	71 (35)	3.40 [1.65–6.99]	0.001	3
Commissural area ratio ≥ 1.25	75 (37)	3.10 [1.51–6.38]	0.002	3
Subvalvular involvement[b]	37 (18)	3.23 [1.35–7.71]	0.008	3

[a]Three risk groups are defined according to the total score: 0–3, low risk (17% suboptimal results); 5, intermediate risk (56% suboptimal results); 6–11, high risk (74% suboptimal results).

[b]Absent vs. mild or extensive thickening.

From Nunes MCP, Tan TC, Elmariah S, et al. The echo score revisited: impact of incorporating commissural morphology and leaflet displacement to the prediction of outcome for patients undergoing percutaneous mitral valvuloplasty. *Circulation*. 2014;129;886–895.

POTENTIAL LIMITATIONS AND FUTURE DIRECTIONS

Despite technical refinements, there remain limitations in the feasibility and relevance of certain echocardiographic analyses in MS. Although planimetry is the reference measurement, it may not be feasible in patients with poor echocardiographic windows or severe valve deformity, even with experienced operators. Other methods of measurement should be used, and their interpretation should consider their limitations.[10,24]

Doppler echocardiography cannot reliably assess capillary wedge pressure or, consequently, pulmonary vascular resistance. Pulmonary hypertension is passive in most patients because of an increase in LA pressure with normal pulmonary vascular resistance. However, in certain patients, who often have long-standing disease, pulmonary vascular resistance is increased because of pulmonary vascular disease. The risk of surgery is higher for these patients, and BMC should be favored when feasible because it provides functional improvement and progressive improvement of hemodynamics.[35] Estimation of pulmonary vascular resistance using right-sided heart catheterization is useful for patients who present with severe pulmonary hypertension that seems out of proportion with the degree of MS or pulmonary congestion as assessed by chest radiography.

The limitations of anatomic scoring systems for prediction of immediate and late results of BMC were previously reviewed. Given the multiple determinants of the results of BMC, there is a low likelihood that any echocardiographic scoring system can ensure optimal prediction of BMC results. A combined assessment using CT scanning to quantitate valve calcification may provide an interesting approach.

Future improvements in patient selection will probably come from the incorporation of improved anatomic evaluation using echocardiography and other imaging techniques and with other variables such as stress hemodynamics indices in multivariate models rather than from optimization of a single scoring system.

TMVR is an appealing treatment, but experience is limited, and a number of challenges remain, especially in patient selection, to decrease mid-term morbidity and mortality rates.

ALTERNATIVE APPROACHES

Right- and left-sided heart cardiac catheterization enables evaluation of the MVA using the Gorlin formula. The Gorlin formula is sometimes considered the reference method, but this is mainly for historical reasons. Experimental and clinical data raise concerns regarding the validity of the Gorlin formula in cases of low output and immediately after BMC.[98] This explains why guidelines advise limiting invasive evaluation of the severity of MS to the rare situations in which echocardiography is inconclusive or there are discrepancies between different measurements and clinical evaluation.[19,20] Right heart catheterization is indicated in cases of suspected vascular pulmonary hypertension. In current practice, the main indication for invasive investigations is the assessment of associated coronary disease using coronary angiography.

Magnetic resonance imaging (MRI) and CT scanning are valid alternative, noninvasive methods used to perform planimetry of the mitral valve.[99,100] These methods can be useful when planimetry using 2D echo is not feasible or reliable. Mitral gradient may also be assessed using velocity-encoded phase-contrast cine MRI, but the reliability of this estimation is not certain.

The experience with intracardiac echocardiography is limited. It is helpful to rule out LA thrombosis and to monitor transseptal puncture in difficult cases, thereby avoiding the use of TEE under general anesthesia. However, the high cost of the single-use device limits its use.

Experience acquired with BMC for more than 20 years has confirmed its efficacy in a wide range of patients. Most potential candidates for BMC live in developing countries, where the challenge is timely diagnosis and treatment of rheumatic heart disease in the face of restrictions due to cost. In Western countries, rheumatic MS often occurs with suboptimal anatomic conditions, and the issue is selection of the most appropriate intervention. Patient selection should not overstress the role of valve anatomy but should rely on a complete assessment that combines clinical and echocardiographic findings.

Continuing evaluation of the results of BMC in large series or in selected subgroups is needed to improve decision making about the choice of the most appropriate procedure and its timing at different stages of the disease. Degenerative MS is the subject of growing attention due to population aging and therapeutic innovations, but further evaluation of interventions is needed to identify patients who are likely to derive clinical benefits.

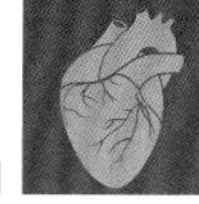

SUMMARY Approach to Echocardiographic Data Acquisition and Analysis in Mitral Stenosis.

Component	Modality	View	Measurement	Interpretation	Limitations/Comments
Severity	2D/3D TTE	Parasternal short-axis	Planimetry	Significant MS if VA < 1.5 cm^2	Reference measurement, but determination of the smallest orifice may be difficult
	CW Doppler[a]	Apical	Pressure half-time	VA = 220/pressure half-time Significant MS if VA < 1.5 cm^2	Easier than planimetry but influenced by confounding factors
	CW Doppler[a]	Apical	Mean gradient	Severe MS likely if > 10 mmHg	Highly depends on flow conditions; low reliability for severity assessment but prognostic value Average measurements if atrial fibrillation (all measures)
Anatomy	2D TTE	Parasternal long- and short-axis	Valve thickening, pliability	Consider maximum thickness and heterogeneity. Localize bright zones (fibrous nodules or calcification), in particular with regard to commissures.	Calcification may be difficult to differentiate from dense fibrosis Usual anatomic scores do not consider the location of abnormalities
		Apical 4-chamber Parasternal long-axis Apical 2-chamber	Subvalvular apparatus	Assess thickening, shortening, and fusion of chordae.	Frequent underestimation of subvalvular lesions
	3D TTE	Parasternal long- and short-axis	Commissural fusion	Visualization of the whole commissure.	Better accuracy than 2D echocardiography; particular importance for restenosis
	2D/3D TEE	0–180 degrees	Valve thickening, pliability, commissural fusion	Same assessment as with 2D echocardiography.	Mainly when transthoracic windows are of poor quality
Associated regurgitation	TTE color-flow imaging	Parasternal long-axis, apical 4- and 2-chamber	Vena contracta Effective regurgitant orifice Regurgitant volume	Contraindication for BMC if effective regurgitant orifice > 0.20 cm^2 and/or regurgitant volume >30 mL.	Quantitation may be influenced by loading conditions TEE is useful for analysis of the mechanism of regurgitation after BMC
	TEE color-flow imaging	0–180 degrees	Same measurements	Analyze the mechanism of regurgitation after BMC (search for leaflet tear).	
Left atrium	2D TTE	Parasternal short-axis	LA diameter	Enlarged if LA volume > 34 mL/m^2 BSA	Low reliability of diameter;
	2D TTE	Apical 4-chamber	LA area	LA volume > 60 mL/m^2	Preferably assessment of area or volume
	2D TTE	Apical 4- and 2-chamber	LA volume	BSA associated with other markers of embolic risk	TEE mandatory before BMC (low sensitivity of TTE)
	TEE	0–180 degrees	LA thrombus	Examination of the whole LA and left atrial appendage, where most thrombi are located	Thrombus may be difficult to differentiate from spontaneous contrast

SUMMARY Approach to Echocardiographic Data Acquisition and Analysis in Mitral Stenosis—cont'd

Component	Modality	View	Measurement	Interpretation	Limitations/Comments
Pulmonary artery pressure	CW Doppler	Apical	Maximum velocity of tricuspid regurgitant jet + estimated RA pressure	Elevated if > 35 mmHg Severe pulmonary hypertension if > 60 mmHg	Less reliable than cardiac catheterization; pulmonary vascular resistance cannot be assessed

[a]Intercept angle should be optimized when using CW Doppler.
BMC, Balloon mitral commissurotomy; *BSA*, body surface area; *MS*, mitral stenosis; *MVA*, mitral valve area.

REFERENCES

1. Iung B, Vahanian A. Epidemiology of acquired valvular heart disease. *Can J Cardiol.* 2014;30:962–970.
2. Rothenbühler M, O'Sullivan CJ, Stortecky S, et al. Active surveillance for rheumatic heart disease in endemic regions: a systematic review and meta-analysis of prevalence among children and adolescents. *Lancet Glob Health.* 2014;2. e717-726.
3. Zühlke L, Engel M, Karthikeyan G, et al. Characteristics, complications, and gaps in evidence-based interventions in rheumatic heart disease: the Global Rheumatic Heart Disease Registry (the REMEDY study). *Eur Heart J.* 2015;36:1115–1122.
4. Iung B, Baron G, Butchart EG, et al. A prospective survey of patients with valvular heart disease in Europe: the Euro Heart Survey on valvular heart disease. *Eur Heart J.* 2003;24:1231–1243.
5. Iung B, Delgado V, Rosenhek R, et al. Contemporary presentation and management of valvular heart disease: the EURObservational Research Programme Valvular Heart Disease II Survey. *Circulation.* 2019 ;140:1156–1169.
6. Abramowitz Y, Jilaihawi H, Chakravarty T, Mack MJ, Makkar RR. Mitral annulus calcification. *J Am Coll Cardiol.* 2015;66:1934–1941.
7. Faletra FF, Leo LA, Paiocchi VL, et al. Anatomy of mitral annulus insights from non-invasive imaging techniques. *Eur Heart J Cardiovasc Imaging.* 2019;20:843–857.
8. Marechaux S, Rusinaru D, Jobic Y, et al. Food and Drug Administration criteria for the diagnosis of drug-induced valvular heart disease in patients previously exposed to benfluorex: a prospective multicentre study. *Eur Heart J Cardiovasc Imaging.* 2015;16:158–165.
9. Jobic Y, Etienne Y, Bruneval P, Ennezat PV. Benfluorex-induced mitral stenosis: a misknown etiology. *Int J Cardiol.* 2014;177. e174-175.
10. Baumgartner H, Hung J, Bermejo J, et al. Echocardiographic assessment of valve stenosis: EAE/ASE recommendations for clinical practice. *J Am Soc Echocardiogr.* 2009;22:1–2.
11. Faletra F, Pezzano Jr A, Fusco R, et al. Measurement of mitral valve area in mitral stenosis: four echocardiographic methods compared with direct measurement of anatomic orifices. *J Am Coll Cardiol.* 1996;28:1190–1197.
12. Sohrabi B, Kazemi B, Mehryar A, et al. Correlation between pulmonary artery pressure measured by echocardiography and right heart catheterization in patients with rheumatic mitral valve stenosis (A prospective study). *Echocardiography.* 2016;33:7–13.
13. Keenan NG, Cueff C, Cimadevilla C, et al. Usefulness of left atrial volume versus diameter to assess thromboembolic risk in mitral stenosis. *Am J Cardiol.* 2010;106:1152–1156.
14. Iung B, Cormier B, Ducimtière P, et al. Immediate results of percutaneous mitral commissurotomy. A predictive model on a series of 1514 patients. *Circulation.* 1996;94:2124–2130.
15. Zoghbi WA, Adams D, Bonow RO, et al. Recommendations for noninvasive evaluation of native valvular regurgitation: a report from the American Society of Echocardiography developed in collaboration with the Society for Cardiovascular Magnetic Resonance. *J Am Soc Echocardiogr.* 2017;30:303–371.
16. Antunes MJ, Rodríguez-Palomares J, Prendergast B, et al. Management of tricuspid valve regurgitation: position statement of the European Society of Cardiology Working Groups of Cardiovascular Surgery and Valvular Heart Disease. *Eur J Cardio Thorac Surg.* 2017;52:1022–1030.
17. Choi BH, Ko SM, Hwang HK, et al. Detection of left atrial thrombus in patients with mitral stenosis and atrial fibrillation: retrospective comparison of two-phase computed tomography, transoesophageal echocardiography and surgical findings. *Eur Radiol.* 2013;23:2944–2953.
18. Nunes MC, Handschumacher MD, Levine RA, et al. Role of LA shape in predicting embolic cerebrovascular events in mitral stenosis: mechanistic insights from 3D echocardiography. *JACC Cardiovasc Imaging.* 2014;7:453–461.
19. Nishimura RA, Otto CM, Bonow RO, et al. 2014 AHA/ACC guideline for the management of patients with valvular heart disease: a report of the American College of Cardiology/American Heart Association Task Force on Practice Guidelines. *J Am Coll Cardiol.* 2014;63. e57-185.
20. Baumgartner H, Falk V, Bax JJ, et al. 2017 ESC/EACTS guidelines for the management of valvular heart disease. The Task Force for the Management of Valvular Heart Disease of The European Society of Cardiology (ESC) and the European Association for Cardio-Thoracic Surgery (EACTS). *Eur Heart J.* 2017;38:2739–2791.
21. Messika-Zeitoun D, Brochet E, Holmin C, et al. Three-dimensional evaluation of the mitral valve area and commissural opening before and after percutaneous mitral commissurotomy in patients with mitral stenosis. *Eur Heart J.* 2007;28:72–79.
22. Min SY, Song JM, Kim YJ, et al. Discrepancy between mitral valve areas measured by two-dimensional planimetry and three-dimensional transoesophageal echocardiography in patients with mitral stenosis. *Heart.* 2013;99:253–258.
23. Messika-Zeitoun D, Meizels A, Cachier A, et al. Echocardiographic evaluation of the mitral valve area before and after percutaneous mitral commissurotomy: the pressure half-time method revisited. *J Am Soc Echocardiogr.* 2005;18:1409–1414.
24. Wunderlich NC, Beigel R, Ho SY, et al. Imaging for mitral interventions methods and efficacy. *JACC Cardiovasc Imaging.* 2018;11:872–901.
25. Wilkins GT, Weyman AE, Abascal VM, Block PC, Palacios IF. Percutaneous balloon dilatation of the mitral valve: an analysis of echocardiographic variables related to outcome and the mechanism of dilatation. *Br Heart J.* 1988;60:299–308.
26. Iung B, Cormier B, Ducimètiere P, et al. Functional results 5 years after successful percutaneous mitral commissurotomy in a series of 528 patients and analysis of predictive factors. *J Am Coll Cardiol.* 1996;27:407–414.
27. Fatkin D, Roy P, Morgan JJ, Feneley MP. Percutaneous balloon mitral valvotomy with the Inoue single-balloon catheter: commissural morphology as a determinant of outcome. *J Am Coll Cardiol.* 1993;21:390–397.
28. Cannan CR, Nishimura RA, Reeder GS, et al. Echocardiographic assessment of commissural calcium: a simple predictor of outcome after percutaneous mitral balloon valvotomy. *J Am Coll Cardiol.* 1997;29:175–180.
29. Sutaria N, Shaw TR, Prendergast B, Northridge D. Transoesophageal echocardiographic assessment of mitral valve commissural morphology predicts outcome after balloon mitral valvotomy. *Heart.* 2006;92:52–57.
30. Bhalgat P, Karlekar S, Modani S, et al. Subvalvular apparatus and adverse outcome of balloon valvotomy in rheumatic mitral stenosis. *Indian Heart J.* 2015;67:428–433.
31. Padial LR, Freitas N, Sagie A, et al. Echocardiography can predict which patients will develop severe mitral regurgitation after per-

cutaneous mitral valvulotomy. *J Am Coll Cardiol.* 1996;27:1225–1231.

32. Nunes MC, Tan TC, Elmariah S, et al. The echo score revisited: impact of incorporating commissural morphology and leaflet displacement to the prediction of outcome for patients undergoing percutaneous mitral valvuloplasty. *Circulation.* 2014;129:886–895.
33. Brochet E, Detaint D, Fondard O, et al. Early hemodynamic changes versus peak values: what is more useful to predict occurrence of dyspnea during stress echocardiography in patients with asymptomatic mitral stenosis? *J Am Soc Echocardiogr.* 2011;24:392–398.
34. Messika-Zeitoun D, Blanc J, Iung B, et al. Impact of degree of commissural opening after percutaneous mitral commissurotomy on long-term outcome. *JACC Cardiovasc Imaging.* 2009;2:1–7.
35. Krishnamoorthy KM, Dash PK, Radhakrishnan S, Shrivastava S. Response of different grades of pulmonary artery hypertension to balloon mitral valvuloplasty. *Am J Cardiol.* 2002;90:1170–1173.
36. Essop MR, Wisenbaugh T, Skoularigis J, Middlemost S, Sareli P. Mitral regurgitation following mitral balloon valvotomy. Differing mechanisms for severe versus mild-to-moderate lesions. *Circulation.* 1991;84:1669–1679.
37. Manjunath CN, Panneerselvam A, Srinivasa KH, et al. Incidence and predictors of atrial septal defect after percutaneous transvenous mitral commissurotomy - a transesophageal echocardiographic study of 209 cases. *Echocardiography.* 2013;30:127–130.
38. Cormier B, Vahanian A, Iung B, et al. Influence of percutaneous mitral commissurotomy on left atrial spontaneous contrast of mitral stenosis. *Am J Cardiol.* 1993;71:842–847.
39. Hernandez R, Banuelos C, Alfonso F, et al. Long-term clinical and echocardiographic follow-up after percutaneous mitral valvuloplasty with the Inoue balloon. *Circulation.* 1999;99:1580–1586.
40. Eleid MF, Foley TA, Said SM, Pislaru SV, Rihal CS. Severe mitral annular calcification: multimodality imaging for therapeutic strategies and interventions. *JACC Cardiovasc Imaging.* 2016;9:1318–1337.
41. Chen CR, Cheng TO. Percutaneous balloon mitral valvuloplasty by the Inoue technique: a multicenter study of 4832 patients in China. *Am Heart J.* 1995;129:1197–1203.
42. Ben-Farhat M, Betbout F, Gamra H, et al. Predictors of long-term event-free survival and of freedom from restenosis after percutaneous balloon mitral commissurotomy. *Am Heart J.* 2001;142:1072–1079.
43. Arora R, Kalra GS, Singh S, et al. Percutaneous transvenous mitral commissurotomy: immediate and long-term follow-up results. *Catheter Cardiovasc Interv.* 2002;55:450–456.
44. Iung B, Nicoud-Houel A, Fondard O, et al. Temporal trends in percutaneous mitral commissurotomy over a 15-year period. *Eur Heart J.* 2004;25:701–707.
45. Complications and mortality of percutaneous balloon mitral commissurotomy. A report from the National Heart, Lung, and Blood Institute Balloon Valvuloplasty Registry. *Circulation.* 1992;85:2014–2024.
46. Meneveau N, Schiele F, Seronde MF, et al. Predictors of event-free survival after percutaneous mitral commissurotomy. *Heart.* 1998;80:359–364.
47. Stefanadis CI, Stratos CG, Lambrou SG, et al. Retrograde nontransseptal balloon mitral valvuloplasty: immediate results and intermediate long-term outcome in 441 cases—a multicenter experience. *J Am Coll Cardiol.* 1998;32:1009–1016.
48. Palacios IF, Sanchez PL, Harrell LC, Weyman AE, Block PC. Which patients benefit from percutaneous mitral balloon valvuloplasty? Prevalvuloplasty and postvalvuloplasty variables that predict long-term outcome. *Circulation.* 2002;105:1465–1471.
49. Neumayer U, Schmidt HK, Fassbender D, et al. Early (three-month) results of percutaneous mitral valvotomy with the Inoue balloon in 1,123 consecutive patients comparing various age groups. *Am J Cardiol.* 2002;90:190–193.
50. Fawzy ME. Long-term results up to 19 years of mitral balloon valvuloplasty. *Asian Cardiovasc Thorac Ann.* 2009;17:627–633.
51. Tomai F, Gaspardone A, Versaci F, et al. Twenty year follow-up after successful percutaneous balloon mitral valvuloplasty in a large contemporary series of patients with mitral stenosis. *Int J Cardiol.* 2014;177:881–885.
52. Badheka AO, Shah N, Ghatak A, et al. Balloon mitral valvuloplasty in the United States: a 13-year perspective. *Am J Med.* 2014;127:1126 e1–12.
53. Meneguz-Moreno RA, Costa Jr JR, Gomes NL, et al. Very long term follow-up after percutaneous balloon mitral valvuloplasty. *JACC Cardiovasc Interv.* 2018;11:1945–1952.
54. Eltchaninoff H, Koning R, Derumeaux G, Cribier A. Percutaneous mitral commissurotomy by metallic dilator. Multicenter experience with 500 patients. *Arch Mal Coeur.* 2000;93:685–692.
55. Lee S, Kang DH, Kim DH, et al. Late outcome of percutaneous mitral commissurotomy: randomized comparison of Inoue versus double-balloon technique. *Am Heart J.* 2017;194:1–8.
56. Multicenter experience with balloon mitral commissurotomy. NHLBI Balloon Valvuloplasty Registry Report on immediate and 30-day follow-up results. The National Heart, Lung, and Blood Institute Balloon Valvuloplasty Registry participants. *Circulation.* 1992;85:448–461.
57. Cruz-Gonzalez I, Sanchez-Ledesma M, Sanchez PL, et al. Predicting success and long-term outcomes of percutaneous mitral valvuloplasty: a multifactorial score. *Am J Med.* 2009;122:581 e11–9.
58. Wang A, Krasuski RA, Warner JJ, et al. Serial echocardiographic evaluation of restenosis after successful percutaneous mitral commissurotomy. *J Am Coll Cardiol.* 2002;39:328–334.
59. Hickey MS, Blackstone EH, Kirklin JW, Dean LS. Outcome probabilities and life history after surgical mitral commissurotomy: implications for balloon commissurotomy. *J Am Coll Cardiol.* 1991;17:29–42.
60. Bouleti C, Iung B, Laouénan C, et al. Late results of percutaneous mitral commissurotomy up to 20 years: development and validation of a risk score predicting late functional results from a series of 912 patients. *Circulation.* 2012;125:2119–2127.
61. Song JK, Song JM, Kang DH, et al. Restenosis and adverse clinical events after successful percutaneous mitral valvuloplasty: immediate post-procedural mitral valve area as an important prognosticator. *Eur Heart J.* 2009;30:1254–1262.
62. Orrange SE, Kawanishi DT, Lopez BM, Curry SM, Rahimtoola SH. Actuarial outcome after catheter balloon commissurotomy in patients with mitral stenosis. *Circulation.* 1997;95:382–389.
63. Jorge E, Pan M, Baptista R, et al. Predictors of very late events after percutaneous mitral valvuloplasty in patients with mitral stenosis. *Am J Cardiol.* 2016;117:1978–1984.
64. Fawzy ME, Hassan W, Shoukri M, et al. Immediate and long-term results of mitral balloon valvotomy for restenosis following previous surgical or balloon mitral commissurotomy. *Am J Cardiol.* 2005;96:971–975.
65. Bouleti C, Iung B, Himbert D, et al. Long-term efficacy of percutaneous mitral commissurotomy for restenosis after previous mitral commissurotomy. *Heart.* 2013;99:1336–1341.
66. Bouleti C, Iung B, Himbert D, et al. Reinterventions after percutaneous mitral commissurotomy during long-term follow-up, up to 20 years: the role of repeat percutaneous mitral commissurotomy. *Eur Heart J.* 2013;34:1923–1930.
67. Kim JB, Ha JW, Kim JS, et al. Comparison of long-term outcome after mitral valve replacement or repeated balloon mitral valvotomy in patients with restenosis after previous balloon valvotomy. *Am J Cardiol.* 2007;99:1571–1574.
68. Iung B, Cormier B, Farah B, et al. Percutaneous mitral commissurotomy in the elderly. *Eur Heart J.* 1995;16:1092–1099.
69. Sutaria N, Elder AT, Shaw TR. Long term outcome of percutaneous mitral balloon valvotomy in patients aged 70 and over. *Heart.* 2000;83:433–438.
70. Shaw TR, Sutaria N, Prendergast B. Clinical and haemodynamic profiles of young, middle aged, and elderly patients with mitral stenosis undergoing mitral balloon valvotomy. *Heart.* 2003;89:1430–1436.
71. Chmielak Z, Klopotowski M, Demkow M, et al. Percutaneous mitral balloon valvuloplasty beyond 65 years of age. *Cardiol J.* 2013;20:44–51.
72. Gamra H, Betbout F, Ben Hamda K, et al. Balloon mitral commissurotomy in juvenile rheumatic mitral stenosis: a ten-year clinical and echocardiographic actuarial results. *Eur Heart J.* 2003;24:1349–1356.
73. Fawzy ME, Stefadouros MA, Hegazy H, et al. Long term clinical and echocardiographic results of mitral balloon valvotomy in children and adolescents. *Heart.* 2005;91:743–748.
74. Kothari SS, Ramakrishnan S, Kumar CK, Juneja R, Yadav R. Intermediate-term results of percutaneous transvenous mitral commissurotomy in children less than 12 years of age. *Catheter Cardiovasc Interv.* 2005;64:487–490.
75. van Hagen IM, Thorne SA, Taha N, et al. Pregnancy outcomes in women with rheumatic mitral valve disease: results from the registry of pregnancy and cardiac disease. *Circulation.* 2018;137:806–816.
76. Regitz-Zagrosek V, Roos-Hesselink JW, Bauersachs J, et al. 2018 ESC Guidelines for the management of cardiovascular diseases during pregnancy. *Eur Heart J.* 2018;39:3165–3241.
77. Silaruks S, Thinkhamrop B, Kiatchoosakun S, Wongvipaporn C, Tatsanavivat P. Resolution of left atrial thrombus after 6 months of anticoagulation in candidates for percutaneous transvenous mitral commissurotomy. *Ann Intern Med.* 2004;140:101–105.

78. Reyes VP, Raju BS, Wynne J, et al. Percutaneous balloon valvuloplasty compared with open surgical commissurotomy for mitral stenosis. *N Engl J Med*. 1994;331:961–967.
79. Turi ZG, Reyes VP, Raju BS, et al. Percutaneous balloon versus surgical closed commissurotomy for mitral stenosis. A prospective, randomized trial. *Circulation*. 1991;83:1179–1185.
80. Ben Farhat M, Ayari M, Maatouk F, et al. Percutaneous balloon versus surgical closed and open mitral commissurotomy: seven-year follow-up results of a randomized trial. *Circulation*. 1998;97:245–250.
81. Rifaie O, Abdel-Dayem MK, Ramzy A, et al. Percutaneous mitral valvotomy versus closed surgical commissurotomy. Up to 15 years of follow-up of a prospective randomized study. *J Cardiol*. 2009;53:28–34.
82. Desnos C, Iung B, Himbert D, et al. Temporal trends on percutaneous mitral commissurotomy: 30 years of experience. *J Am Heart Assoc*. 2019;8. e012031.
83. Song JK, Kim MJ, Yun SC, et al. Long-term outcomes of percutaneous mitral balloon valvuloplasty versus open cardiac surgery. *J Thorac Cardiovasc Surg*. 2010;139:103–110.
84. Bouleti C, Iung B, Himbert D, et al. Relationship between valve calcification and long-term results of percutaneous mitral commissurotomy for rheumatic mitral stenosis. *Circ Cardiovasc Interv*. 2014;7:381–389.
85. Kang DH, Lee CH, Kim DH, et al. Early percutaneous mitral commissurotomy vs. conventional management in asymptomatic moderate mitral stenosis. *Eur Heart J*. 2012;33:1511–1517.
86. Chiang CW, Lo SK, Ko YS, et al. Predictors of systemic embolism in patients with mitral stenosis. A prospective study. *Ann Intern Med*. 1998;128:885–889.
87. Liu TJ, Lai HC, Lee WL, et al. Percutaneous balloon commissurotomy reduces incidence of ischemic cerebral stroke in patients with symptomatic rheumatic mitral stenosis. *Int J Cardiol*. 2008;123:189–190.
88. Iung B, Leenhardt A, Extramiana F. Management of atrial fibrillation in patients with rheumatic mitral stenosis. *Heart*. 2018;104:1062–1068.
89. Urena M, Brochet E, Lecomte M, et al. Clinical and haemodynamic outcomes of balloon-expandable transcatheter mitral valve implantation: a 7-year experience. *Eur Heart J*. 2018;39:2679–2689.
90. Guerrero M, Urena M, Himbert D, et al. 1-year outcomes of transcatheter mitral valve replacement in patients with severe mitral annular calcification. *J Am Coll Cardiol*. 2018;71:1841–1853.
91. Dahan M, Paillole C, Martin D, Gourgon R. Determinants of stroke volume response to exercise in patients with mitral stenosis: a Doppler echocardiographic study. *J Am Coll Cardiol*. 1993;21:384–389.
92. Schwammenthal E, Vered Z, Agranat O, et al. Impact of atrioventricular compliance on pulmonary artery pressure in mitral stenosis: an exercise echocardiographic study. *Circulation*. 2000;102:2378–2384.
93. Laufer-Perl M, Gura Y, Shimiaie J, et al. Mechanisms of effort intolerance in patients with rheumatic mitral stenosis: combined echocardiography and cardiopulmonary stress protocol. *JACC Cardiovasc Imaging*. 2017;10:622–633.
94. Reis G, Motta MS, Barbosa MM, et al. Dobutamine stress echocardiography for noninvasive assessment and risk stratification of patients with rheumatic mitral stenosis. *J Am Coll Cardiol*. 2004;43:393–401.
95. Okay T, Deligonul U, Sancaktar O, Kozan O. Contribution of mitral valve reserve capacity to sustained symptomatic improvement after balloon valvulotomy in mitral stenosis: implications for restenosis. *J Am Coll Cardiol*. 1993;22:1691–1696.
96. Nunes MC, Hung J, Barbosa MM, et al. Impact of net atrioventricular compliance on clinical outcome in mitral stenosis. *Circ Cardiovasc Imaging*. 2013;6:1001–1008.
97. Gajjala OR, Durgaprasad R, Velam V, Kayala SB, Kasala L. New integrated approach to percutaneous mitral valvuloplasty combining Wilkins score with commissural calcium score and commissural area ratio. *Echocardiography*. 2017;34:1284–1291.
98. Segal J, Lerner DJ, Miller DC, et al. When should Doppler-determined valve area be better than the Gorlin formula? Variation in hydraulic constants in low flow states. *J Am Coll Cardiol*. 1987;9:1294–1305.
99. Helvacioglu F, Yildirimturk O, Duran C, et al. The evaluation of mitral valve stenosis: comparison of transthoracic echocardiography and cardiac magnetic resonance. *Eur Heart J Cardiovasc Imaging*. 2014;15:164–169.
100. Messika-Zeitoun D, Serfaty JM, Laissy JP, et al. Assessment of the mitral valve area in patients with mitral stenosis by multislice computed tomography. *J Am Coll Cardiol*. 2006;48:411–413.

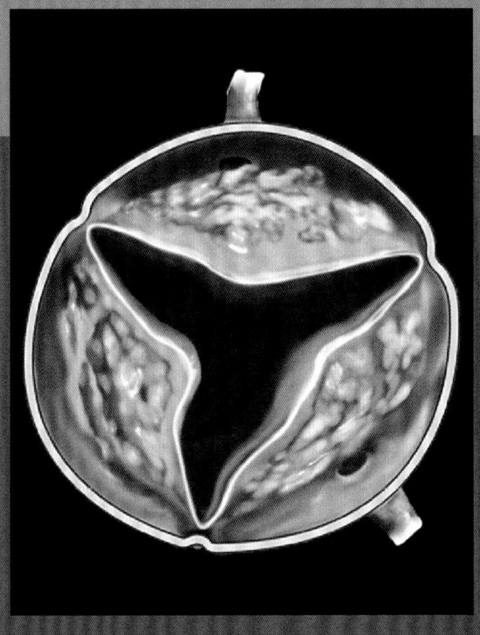

中文导读

第28章 成人右心瓣膜病

几十年以来，右心瓣膜疾病的重要性一直被低估，这主要是因为三尖瓣和肺动脉瓣疾病在出现明显症状之前有较长的潜伏期，三尖瓣反流通常继发于引起主要临床症状的其他疾病。研究者越来越认识到三尖瓣和肺动脉瓣疾病与发病率和死亡率增加是独立密切相关的，这引起了其对右心瓣膜功能障碍的机制以及这些病变对右心室功能影响的兴趣。

新兴的经皮结构性心脏介入治疗可因较少的并发症成为一种替代传统手术的新方案。超声心动图在诊断和量化三尖瓣和肺动脉瓣疾病中发挥着关键作用。本章详细讲解了三尖瓣、肺动脉瓣的解剖结构，以及超声对其结构的具体观察与测量评估；详细描述了右心瓣膜狭窄或反流的原因及分析相关联的疾病，并介绍了超声的成像原理及评估量化分级，超声心动图对于指导右心瓣膜疾病患者的临床诊疗及护理起到了至关重要的作用。

李晓妮

28 Right-Sided Valve Disease in Adults

ERIN A. FENDER, MD | WILLIAM R. MIRANDA, MD

The importance of right-sided valve disease was underappreciated for decades, largely because tricuspid and pulmonary valve diseases have a prolonged latency phase before the onset of overt symptoms. Tricuspid regurgitation (TR) is frequently caused by another predisposing disease process that may dominate the clinical presentation.

There is a growing recognition that tricuspid valve (TV) and pulmonary valve (PV) diseases are independently associated with increased morbidity and mortality. This has generated interest in understanding the mechanisms of valvular dysfunction and the physiologic impact of these lesions on right ventricular (RV) function.

Emerging percutaneous structural heart interventions may offer alternatives to traditional surgery with less morbidity. Echocardiography plays a critical role in diagnosing and quantifying TV and PV disease, and it is essential to guiding the clinical care of these patients (Table 28.1).

TRICUSPID VALVE DISEASE

TRICUSPID VALVE ANATOMY

The TV is composed of three leaflets: septal, anterior, and posterior (Fig. 28.1). They create a triangular orifice flanked by the ostium of the coronary sinus, the right coronary artery, and the atrioventricular node. The noncoronary sinus of Valsalva lies immediately behind the anterior and septal leaflet commissure.

The TV leaflets are asymmetric; the largest and most mobile is the anterior leaflet, whereas the septal leaflet is the smallest and least mobile.[1] Typically, the anterior and posterior leaflets are attached to the anterior papillary muscle, and the posterior and septal leaflets insert into the posterior papillary muscle. However, variations are common, and a third rudimentary papillary muscle may exist at the chordal insertion into the ventricular septum.[1,2]

The TV annulus is large, with an average orifice area of 7 to 9 cm^2 and an average diastolic diameter of 2.5 ± 0.5 cm. The elliptical annulus is shaped like a saddle. The posteroseptal portion is tipped toward the RV apex, and the anteroseptal portion angles up toward the right atrium (RA).[1,3,4] The coaptation length is between 5 and 10 mm, which allows moderate annular dilation to occur before the development of TR. Coaptation occurs at the level of the annulus or slightly ventricular to the annulus. The TV annulus has relatively little fibrous tissue, which allows for significant changes in the annular area and regurgitate orifice to occur with the cardiac and respiratory cycle and with variations in loading conditions.[2,5]

TRICUSPID REGURGITATION

Background

TR affects 80% of the population. Moderate-severe or worse TR affects approximately 1.6 million Americans.[6,7] As shown in Table 28.2, TR has many causes. Primary TR due to leaflet abnormalities occurs in approximately 10% of patients with TR and is most commonly caused by congenital heart disease, carcinoid syndrome, rheumatic valve disease, infective endocarditis, toxic drug exposure, or flail leaflet after blunt chest trauma.

A growing patient population has primary isolated TR due to endomyocardial biopsy or intracardiac device leads.[8,9] The true incidence of TR after endomyocardial biopsy is unknown, but moderate or worse TR has been reported for 14% to 33% of orthotopic heart transplant patients undergoing repeated biopsies over long-term follow-up.[10,11] Device leads are an underappreciated cause of primary isolated TR. In a series of 239 patients undergoing de novo ventricular lead implantation, 38% developed new TR of 2+ or greater.[9]

Ninety percent of severe TR cases are secondary (i.e., functional), meaning that the TR is mediated by RV and/or RA enlargement.[8] The most common cause of secondary TR is pulmonary hypertension (PH) resulting from intrinsic pulmonary vascular disease or elevation of the pulmonary artery wedge pressure due to left-sided heart disease. Over time, chronic pressure overload causes the RV to dilate, resulting in papillary muscle displacement and lateral annular dilation with resultant leaflet malcoaptation (Fig. 28.2).[12] As the annulus dilates, the TV loses its normal tipped-down elliptical shape and assumes a planar orientation with a circular orifice.[3,12] Recirculation of the regurgitant volume (RVol) creates chronic RV volume overload, causing the RV to further dilate and creating a cycle in which severe TR begets more severe TR.

An emerging population of adult patients has isolated TR in the absence of left-sided heart disease, PH, or congenital abnormalities. Most cases of isolated TR result from direct leaflet displacement or damage from RV pacemaker or defibrillator leads or from TV annular dilation due to RA enlargement caused by long-standing atrial fibrillation.[13,14] Isolated TR is associated with a poor long-term prognosis, even in the absence of other cardiopulmonary comorbidities.[15,16]

TABLE 28.1 Echocardiographic Assessment of the Tricuspid and Pulmonary Valves: Right-Sided Stenotic and Regurgitant Lesions.

Valve	*Modality*	*Valve Anatomy*	*Modality*	*Quantification*
Tricuspid valve	2D	Anatomic assessment: PSS, PSL, A4C, and SC TV annular diameter: A4C	CW	PSS, PSL, A4C and para-apical
	3D	PSS, PSL, A4C, SC	PW	Hepatic reversals: SC
	TEE	Mid/distal esophagus 4-chamber Transgastric 0–30 degrees	Color	TR jet area: A4C or para-apical Vena contracta: A4C PISA: A4C or para-apical
Pulmonary valve	2D	Anatomic assessment: PSS, PSS with anterior/superior angulation (RV outflow view), anterior angulation from 4-chamber SC or basal short-axis SC	CW	PSS and modified PSS (RV inflow view) Basal short-axis SC 4-chamber SC
	3D	PSS and modified PSS (RV inflow view) Basal short-axis SC 4-chamber SC	PW	PSS and modified PSS (RV inflow view) Basal short-axis SC 4-chamber SC
	TEE	Mid-esophageal 45–60 and 110–130 degrees High esophageal 0–30 degrees Transgastric 60 degrees	Color	PSS and modified PSS (RV inflow view) Basal short-axis SC 4-chamber SC

A4C, Apical 4-chamber view; *PISA*, proximal isovelocity surface area; *PSL*, parasternal long-axis view; *PSS*, parasternal short-axis view; *PW*, pulsed wave; *SC*, subcostal view; *TR*, tricuspid regurgitation; *TV*, tricuspid valve.

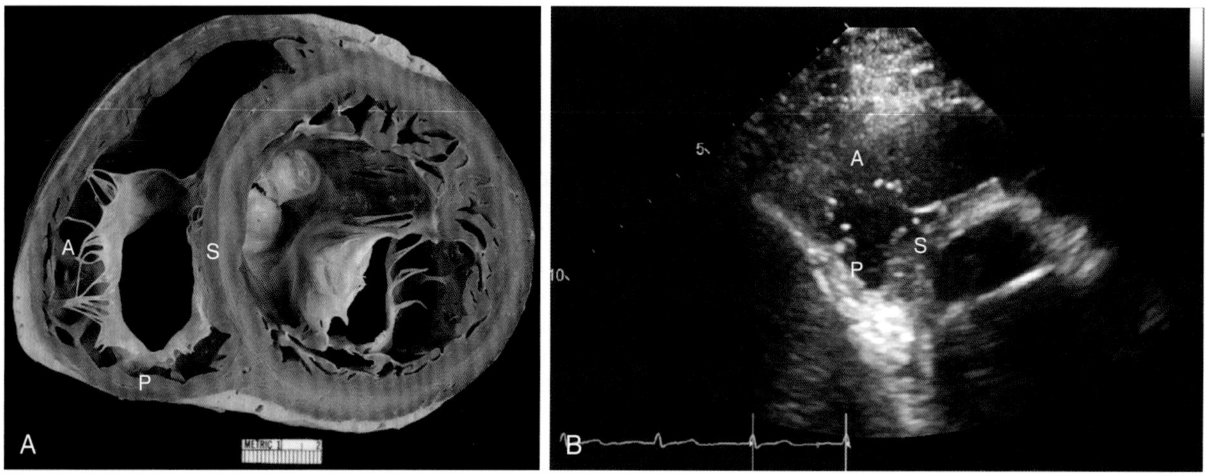

Fig. 28.1 Tricuspid valve anatomy. (A) Gross anatomy specimen illustrates the tricuspid valve anatomy. The short-axis format demonstrates all three leaflets: anterior *(A)*, posterior *(P)*, and septal *(S)*. (B) Transthoracic parasternal short-axis echocardiographic image shows an analogous view of the three tricuspid valve leaflets.

Basic Echocardiographic Imaging Principles

The symptoms and physical examination findings of TR can be nonspecific, and as a result, most cases of TR are diagnosed during echocardiography. When more than mild TR is appreciated on transthoracic echocardiography (TTE), a more thorough assessment of the mechanism and severity of TR is mandatory. Defining the mechanism and severity of TR is essential for determining the appropriate treatment. Patients with primary or isolated TR may benefit from surgical correction, whereas many patients with secondary TR are best served by treating the predisposing disease process[17–19] (Table 28.3).

Assessing the Mechanism and Severity of Tricuspid Regurgitation

A comprehensive TTE assessment of the TV should be performed in all patients with more than mild TR. TTE has several goals:

1. Define the mechanism of TR
2. Quantify the severity of regurgitation
3. Screen for PH and left-sided heart disease
4. Assess RV size and function

Echocardiographic assessment of the TV involves a systematic and stepwise interrogation of the TV from four main views; the parasternal short- and long-axis views, the apical 4-chamber view, and the subcostal windows. The RV inflow view from the parasternal long axis (Fig. 28.3A) allows visualization of the RA and the base of the RV. Rotating the probe 90 degrees brings in the parasternal short-axis view at the level of the aortic valve (see Fig. 28.3B), from which the RA, RV outflow tract (RVOT), TV, and PV can be viewed.

The apical 4-chamber view is best for visualization of the RV (see Fig. 28.3C) and is the view from which quantitative measurements of RV size and strain are performed. When functional TR due to significant aortic or mitral valve disease is suspected, the TV annular diameter should be measured from the apical 4-chamber view (see Fig. 28.3D). A diastolic diameter of more than 4 cm (or diameter indexed to body surface area of ≥ 21 mm/m^2) indicates an increased risk for persistent TR after mitral valve surgery if concomitant TV repair is not performed.[17,20,21]

From the parasternal short-axis and apical 4-chamber views, it is possible to visualize the septal and anterior leaflets.[1] The posterior leaflet is best viewed from the apical 4-chamber or subcostal windows by sweeping the probe posteriorly until the

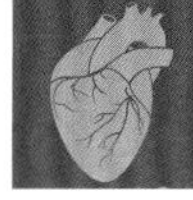

TABLE 28.2 Causes of Tricuspid Regurgitation.[a]

Lesion	*Causes*
Primary Tricuspid Regurgitation	
Congenital	Ebstein anomaly Leaflet prolapse Congenitally corrected transposition Atrioventricular septal defect Tricuspid dysplasia
Infectious or inflammatory	Rheumatic fever Radiation exposure Carcinoid Infective endocarditis Marantic endocarditis
Leaflet damage	Endomyocardial biopsy Device leads
Drug-induced	Fenfluramine Ergots Pergolide
Secondary Tricuspid Regurgitation	
Pulmonary hypertension	Pulmonary vascular disease Congestive heart failure Aortic valve disease Mitral valve disease
RV dysfunction	RV infarction Arrhythmogenic RV cardiomyopathy
RV volume overload	Left-to-right shunt High-output states
Idiopathic	Atrial fibrillation

[a]Classically, tricuspid regurgitation is categorized as primary, meaning that regurgitation results from a primary anatomic abnormality, or secondary, meaning that regurgitation is a secondary consequence of another disease process.

coronary sinus is brought into view. However, even with these techniques, correct identification of the individual leaflets is challenging because of anatomic variation. Although it is sometimes forgotten, a short-axis view of the TV on the parasternal short axis should always be attempted because, similar to 3D echocardiography, it provides simultaneous assessment of all three RV leaflets (see Fig. 28.1B). This can be obtained by tilting the probe inferiorly from the level of the mitral valve; with practice, it can be obtained in a large proportion of patients.

3D echocardiography provides superior visualization of the TV leaflets (Fig. 28.4) by overcoming the challenges of imaging the nonplanar TV annulus.[22] Optimal 3D imaging should include the surrounding anatomic landmarks in the acquisition volume to aid in recognition of the individual leaflets and to define the mechanism of TR. 3D echocardiography is the most accurate method of localizing focal anatomic disease such as infective endocarditis, intracardiac device lead impingement, or flail leaflet. Transthoracic 3D volumes can be obtained in the parasternal, apical, or subcostal window, but the apical window is typically best because of the anterior location of the RV near the chest wall and the perpendicular orientation of the TV relative to the ultrasound probe. Parasternal short- or long-axis views may also provide high-quality 3D images, and they allow improved spatial resolution because the TV lies in the parasternal near field.

Anatomic assessment of the leaflets is essential for identifying the cause of TR (Fig. 28.5) and referring patients for appropriate therapy.[17–19] Flail leaflet may result from myxomatous degeneration, infective endocarditis, blunt chest trauma, cardiac lead device extraction, or endomyocardial biopsy. Infective endocarditis may also result in leaflet perforation or leaflet destruction, or a large vegetation may interrupt coaptation. Rheumatic heart disease commonly causes combined regurgitation and stenosis due to commissural fusion with shortening and retraction of the leaflets and chordae. Carcinoid syndrome and serotonergic or dopaminergic drugs induce fibroproliferative leaflet thickening and reduce leaflet mobility (Fig. 28.6).

Ebstein anomaly is characterized by in utero failure of leaflet delamination, with subsequent apical displacement of the septal and posterior leaflets into the ventricle (Fig. 28.7). When a congenital cause such as Ebstein anomaly is identified, it is important to screen for associated cardiac defects such as patent foramen ovale, atrial septal defect, and LV noncompaction.

Intracardiac devices can induce TR through leaflet impingement, perforation, or adhesions; however, 2D TTE may be insensitive for lead-induced TR. In a series of 41 patients with surgically confirmed lead-induced TR, only 12% of patients were accurately identified by TTE preoperatively.[14] The use of 3D echocardiography and TEE imaging may substantially improve accurate detection of lead-mediated TR.

When TTE does not reveal a primary anatomic cause of TR, it is necessary to screen for predisposing disease processes such as left-to-right shunt, PH, and left-sided heart disease. Echocardiographic assessment of these disease processes is covered in depth in other chapters.

In approximately 10% of patients with secondary TR, a predisposing cause cannot be identified.[8,16,23] These patients tend to be elderly and female and have a high prevalence of atrial fibrillation.[13,16,24] Echocardiographic assessment of isolated TR in patients with atrial fibrillation and no other cardiopulmonary comorbidities has identified a unique pattern of RA enlargement and annular dilation out of proportion to RV enlargement, suggesting that atrial fibrillation may be a cause rather than a consequence of TR.[25]

Quantification of Regurgitant Severity

Determination of the severity of TR relies on integration of multiple qualitative and quantitative measures (Table 28.4). Some degree of TR is found in up to 80% of the population, and in many cases, visual assessment of the color Doppler jet area is sufficient to screen for trivial TR.[6] However, with more than mild TR, when the leaflets appear anatomically abnormal, the regurgitant jet is eccentric, or there is significant PH or left-sided heart disease, a more thorough assessment is warranted.

The TR jet area is assessed from a sector that allows visualization of the entire RA, which is typically the apical 4-chamber or para-apical window. Severe TR is suggested by a jet area that is greater than 10 cm^2 or a ratio of jet area to RA area of more than 30%.[26] The accuracy of this method is significantly limited by factors such as RA dilation, eccentric jet orientation, suboptimal instrument settings, and dependence on hemodynamic loading conditions. As a result, the correlation of jet area with TR severity is poor, and alternative methods are preferred when more than mild TR is suspected.

Color-flow Doppler is used to quantify TR by measurement of the vena contracta and calculation of the effective regurgitant orifice area and RVol using the proximal isovelocity surface area (PISA) method. To obtain the highest velocity and best continuous-wave (CW) signal requires alignment with the angle of insonation; because regurgitant jets may be eccentric, the CW signal should be assessed from all windows.

The 2D vena contracta is measured at the narrowest diameter of color flow seen immediately beyond the area of flow convergence. The vena contracta is usually best measured with the apical 4-chamber view during mid-systole. The image is optimized by narrowing the sector width to enhance the frame rate, zooming

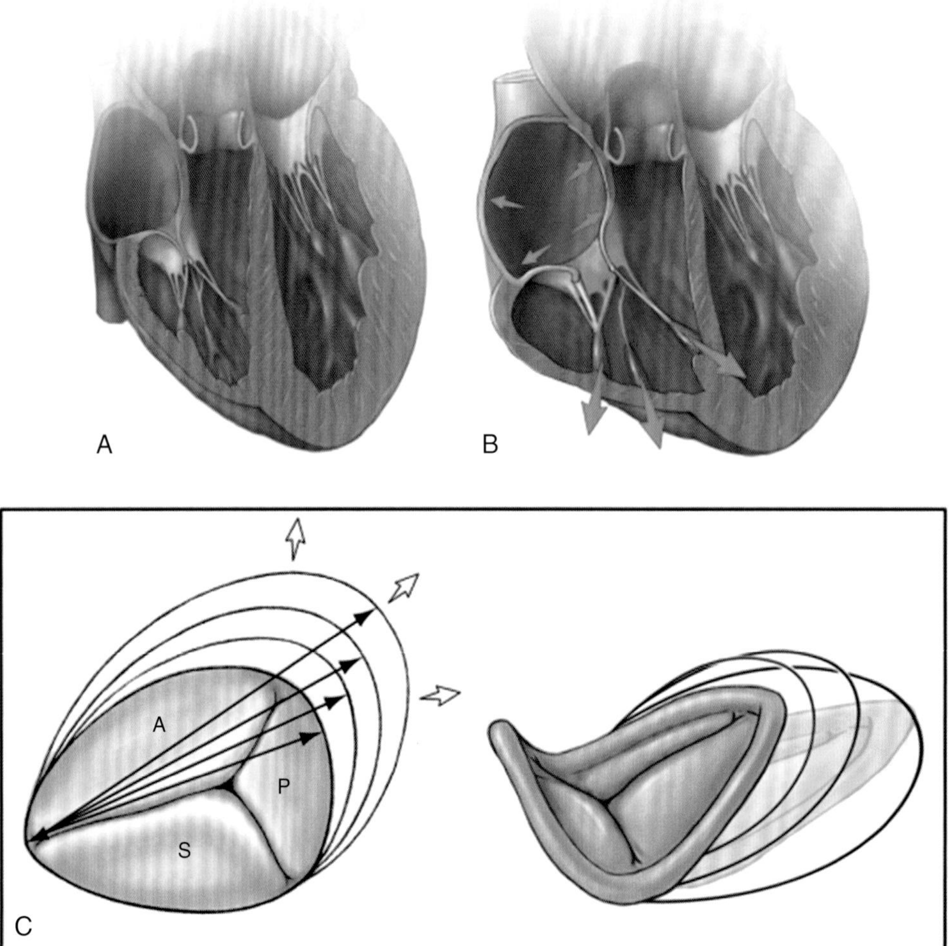

Fig. 28.2 Mechanism of secondary tricuspid regurgitation. A, Normal architecture of the right ventricle, papillary muscles, and tricuspid valve. B, Chronically elevated pulmonary pressure or RV volume overload causes the right atrium and ventricle to dilate. Ventricular enlargement results in annular dilation and displacement of the papillary muscles (*large arrows*), with resultant tenting of the tricuspid leaflets downward and right atrial dilation (*small arrows*). C, This remodeling distorts the normal three-dimensional orientation of the tricuspd valve. As remodeling occurs, the tricupsid valve annulus dilates outward toward the posterior leaflet (*left, black arrows*) and begins to flatten, losing its normal saddle-shaped configuration (*right*). *A*, Anterior leaflet; *P*, posterior leaflet; *S*, septal leaflet. (From Fender EA, Zack CJ, Nishimura RA. Isolated tricuspid regurgitation: outcomes and therapeutic interventions. *Heart*. 2018;104:798–806.)

in on the area of interest, and maximizing the color gain to the highest level that does not introduce color artifact. Because TR is highly load dependent and there are significant variations in right-sided venous return with the respiratory cycle, the vena contracta should be measured as an average of individual measurements obtained during four consecutive cardiac cycles. A vena contracta that is larger than 6.5 mm has an 89% sensitivity and 93% specificity for severe TR; however, current society guidelines use 7 mm as the threshold to optimize specificity.[27]

The PISA method is commonly used for assessing mitral valve regurgitation, but when it is used for quantification of the TR angle, correction is required to account for the funnel shape of the TV (Fig. 28.8). From the apical or para-apical windows, the transducer is adjusted to ensure coaxial alignment between the transducer and the area of flow convergence. The sector is zoomed to the area of interest, and the color gain is increased while the baseline is shifted downward to maximize visualization of the PISA shell. The radius *(r)* of the flow convergence is measured in mid-systole along with the corresponding aliasing velocity *(Vr)*. Next, TV angle correction *(alpha)* is performed by measuring the angle of the TV leaflets during systole. Classically, alpha is measured with the use of a protractor, but 220 degrees can be used as a rough approximation. Instantaneous regurgitant flow (Rflow) is then calculated:

$$\text{Rflow} = \left(2\pi \times r^2 \times Vr\right) \times \left(\frac{\text{alpha}}{180}\right)$$

The effective regurgitant orifice (ERO) area is

$$\text{ERO} = \text{Rflow}/V$$

where V is the peak TR velocity obtained from the CW Doppler signal. After the ERO is calculated, the regurgitant volume (RVol) is calculated:

$$\text{RVol} = \text{ERO} \times \text{TVI}$$

where TVI is the time–velocity integral of the tricuspid regurgitant CW Doppler signal. Severe TR is identified when the ERO is 0.4 cm^2 or greater and the RVol is 45 mL or greater.[28,29]

Quantification of TR using PISA methods has been validated, but it is less commonly performed in clinical practice because angle correction is time intensive and prone to error.[30] As with all echocardiographic methods that rely on mathematical derivation of flow, the impacts of minor variations in the

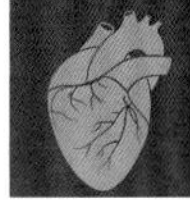

TABLE 28.3 **Guidelines for the Surgical Treatment of Tricuspid Regurgitation.**

European Society of Cardiology Recommendations	*American Heart Association/American College of Cardiology Recommendations*[17]
Class I	
Severe primary or secondary TR at the time of surgery for left-sided valve disease (LOE C)	Severe primary or secondary TR (stages C or D) undergoing left-sided valve surgery (LOE B)
Isolated symptomatic severe primary TR with preserved RV function (LOE C)	
Class IIa	
Surgery may be appropriate to treat moderate primary TR at the time of left-sided valve surgery (LOE C)	Surgery may be appropriate to treat severe primary TR when signs and symptoms of right-sided heart failure are present (LOE B)
Surgery may be appropriate for mild or worse secondary TR at the time of left-sided valve surgery if severe annular dilation exists (≥40 mm or or diameter indexed to body surface area ≥21 mm/m^2) (LOE C)	Surgery may be appropriate to alleviate symptoms in patients with progressive TR (stage B) undergoing left-sided valve surgery when there is severe annular dilation (end diastolic annular diameter >4 cm) or signs or symptoms of right-sided heart failure are present (LOE B)
Surgery may be appropriate for asymptomatic patients with severe isolated primary TR and evidence of progressive RV dilation or decreased RV function (LOE C)	Surgery may be appropriate to alleviate symptoms in patients with severe isolated secondary TR due to annular dilation (in the absence of significant left-sided heart disease or pulmonary hypertension) who have an inadequate response to medical therapy (stage D) (LOE B)
In patients with previous left-sided valve surgery; isolated TV surgery may be appropriate for those with severe secondary TR and with symptoms or evidence of RV dilation or dysfunction in the absence of left-sided valve dysfunction, severe RV or LV dysfunction, and severe pulmonary hypertension (LOE C)	
Class IIb	
	For patients with previous left-sided valve surgery, surgery may be appropriate for patients with symptomatic severe TR (stage D) in the absence of severe pulmonary hypertension or severe RV systolic dysfunction (LOE B)
	Surgery may be appropriate for patients with asymptomatic severe primary TR (stage C) and progressive RV dilation or systolic dysfunction (LOE C)

Stage B: Progressive TR (physical exam without signs of elevated venous pressure and no clinical symptoms; TTE findings of central TR jet <50% RA diameter, VC < 0.7 cm, ERO < 0.4cm^2, RV < 45 mL).
Stage C: Asymptomatic severe TR (physical exam with signs of elevated venous pressure but without clinical symptoms; TTE findings of central TR jet ≥50% RA area, VC ≥ 0.7 cm, ERO ≥ 0.4 cm^2, RV ≥ 45 mL, dense triangular CW signal, hepatic vein systolic reversal, dilated RA and RV, RA with "c-V" wave).
Stage D: Symptomatic severe TR (physical exam with signs of elevated venous pressure and patient with right-sided heart failure symptoms; TTE findings of central TR jet ≥50% RA, VC ≥ 0.7 cm, ERO ≥ 0.4 cm^2, RV ≥ 45 mL, dense triangular CW signal, hepatic vein systolic reversal, dilated RA and RV, RA with "c-V" wave, clinical signs of elevated venous pressure).
LOE, Level of evidence; *TR*, tricuspid regurgitation; *TV*, tricuspid valve.

measurement of radius, angle, or velocity are magnified. Careful attention to sector width, frame rate, and color gain are essential for accurate and reproducible quantification.

CW Doppler provides quantitative and qualitative information regarding the severity of TR, and it is used to estimate pulmonary pressure. The CW signal allows measurement of the maximal regurgitant velocity, which is required for calculation of the ERO. In severe TR, the CW signal is dense and has a dagger-shaped appearance due to rapid pressure equalization between the RA and RV (Fig. 28.9). Severe TR also results in increased TV inflow velocity (≥1 m/s) and hepatic vein systolic reversals, which can be visualized by pulsed-wave (PW) or color-flow Doppler (Fig. 28.10).[31]

The peak CW velocity can be used to calculate RV systolic pressure (RVSP):

$$RVSP = 4V^2 + RAP$$

where RAP is the estimated RA pressure. RAP is calculated by assessing the inferior vena cava (IVC) in the subcostal window at end-expiration.[32] The IVC is measured 0.5 to 3 cm proximal to the hepatic vein–IVC junction. A normal RAP value is estimated to be 3 mmHg when the IVC diameter is 2.1 cm or less and collapses by more than 50% during a brisk sniff (i.e., sniff test). When the IVC is dilated more than 2.1 cm and there is less than 50% IVC collapse during the sniff, the RAP is estimated to be elevated at 15 mmHg. When the IVC diameter and collapse do not fit into these patterns, an intermediate value of 8 mmHg is assigned.

Estimation of RVSP with these methods is fraught with challenges. As the severity of TR increases, the RA and RV act as a single chamber that reduces the pressure gradient and results in a lower peak CW velocity. Because of the lack of a restrictive orifice, the validity of the Bernoulli equation and the accuracy of noninvasive assessment of pulmonary pressures in these patients has been questioned.[33,34]

The correlation between invasively measured RAP and IVC diameter and inspiratory collapse is modest.[35] In patients with severe TR and severely elevated RA pressures, the noninvasive assessment of RVSP can lead to significant underestimation of the true RV pressures, even if an estimated RA pressure of 15 mmHg is used.

TEE

Transesophageal echocardiography (TEE) can provide detailed anatomic information about the TV, particularly in patients with suspected endocarditis or device infection or those undergoing assessment for novel percutaneous therapies. The American Society of Echocardiography (ASE) has provided guidelines for a comprehensive TEE assessment of the TV.[36] The location of the right heart within the anterior mediastinum places it far from the mid-esophageal window, with the left heart structures lying between the probe and the TV. As a result, the TV is best visualized from the middle to distal esophagus and using transgastric views.[1]

The 4-chamber mid-esophageal view allows visualization of the septal and anterior leaflets; biplane imaging can confirm which leaflets are in view because the aorta is next to the anterior leaflet. In the distal esophageal view, the RA lies immediately adjacent to the esophagus, creating a view that is unobstructed by the LA and permitting a comprehensive 2D and 3D assessment of all three leaflets. Assessment of the TV by 2D TEE using the transgastric view at 0 to 30 degrees is also of great value because it allows simultaneous visualization of all three TV leaflets. Hemodynamic interrogation of the TV (e.g., after tricuspid repair) is typically obtained from 45 to 60 degrees at the mid-esophageal level because it allows better alignment for CW Doppler imaging acquisition.

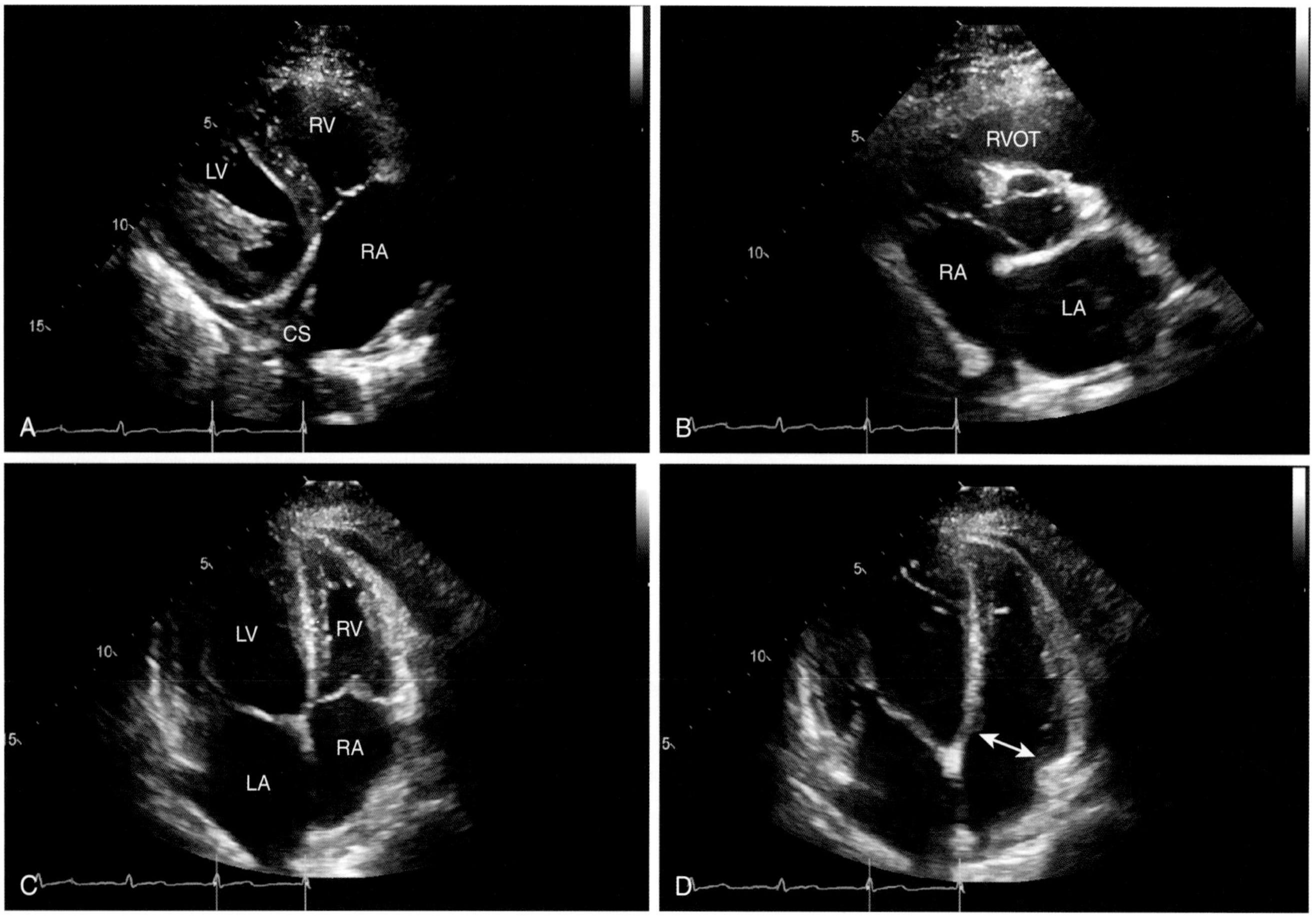

Fig. 28.3 **TTE assessment of the tricuspid valve.** (A) RV inflow view from the parasternal long axis allows visualization of the RA and the base of the RV. (B) Rotating the probe 90 degrees brings in the parasternal short-axis view at the level of the aortic valve, from which the RA, RV outflow tract *(RVOT)*, tricuspid valve, and pulmonary valve can be visualized. (C) The apical 4-chamber view provides the best visualization of RV and RA chamber size. (D) The diastolic annular dimension should also be assessed in this view *(double-headed arrow)*. *CS*, Coronary sinus.

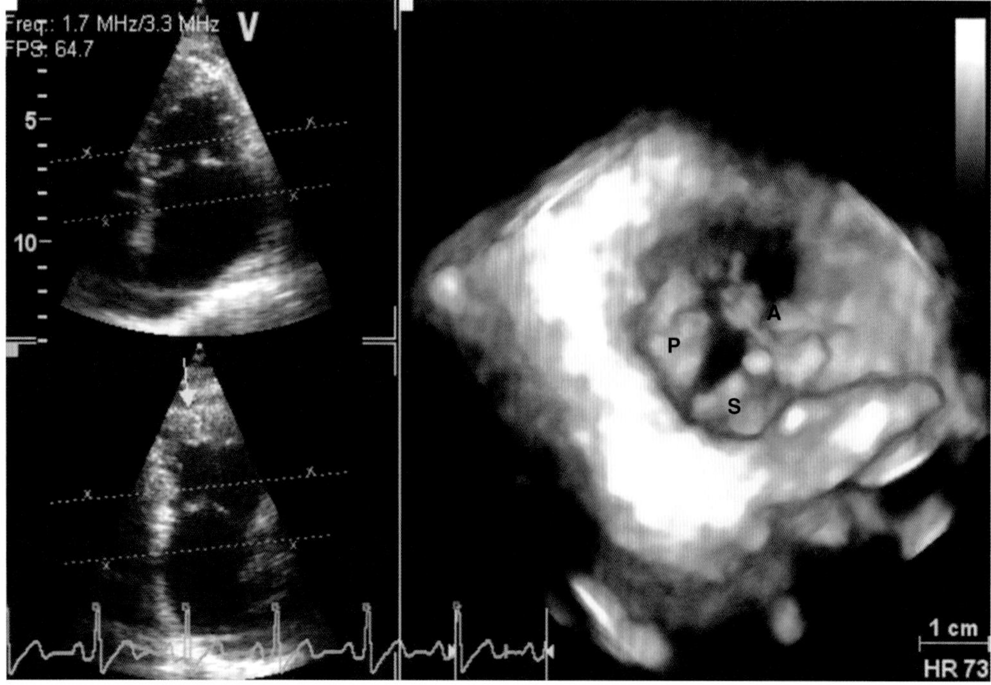

Fig. 28.4 **3D assessment of tricuspid valve anatomy.** Normal tricuspid anatomy demonstrates three leaflets: anterior *(A)*, posterior *(P)*, and septal *(S)* (see Video 28.4).

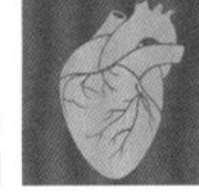

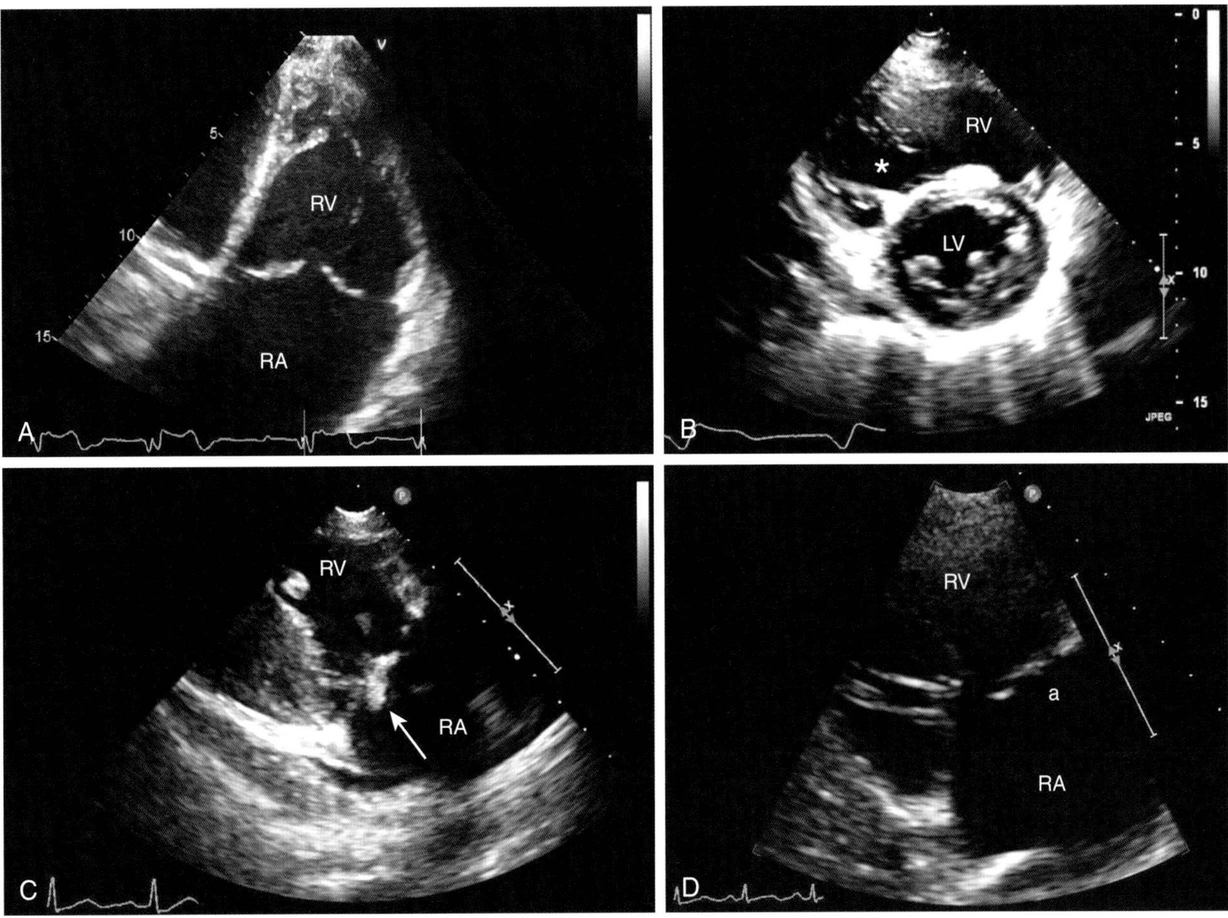

Fig. 28.5 Illustrative cases of tricuspid valve pathology. (A) Secondary tricuspid valve regurgitation. Notice the dilation of the RV and RA leading to tricuspid leaflet malcoaptation. (B) Parasternal short-axis view demonstrates impingement of the septal tricuspid leaflet by a pacemaker lead *(asterisk)* in a patient with device lead–induced TR. Tricuspid annular dilation is also seen. (C) RV inflow view shows a case of tricuspid valve endocarditis with a large vegetation attached to the anterior tricuspid valve leaflet *(arrow)* (see Video 28.5C). (D) Follow-up echocardiogram of the same patient as in C shows resolution of the vegetation with interval development of a flail tricuspid anterior leaflet *(a)*.

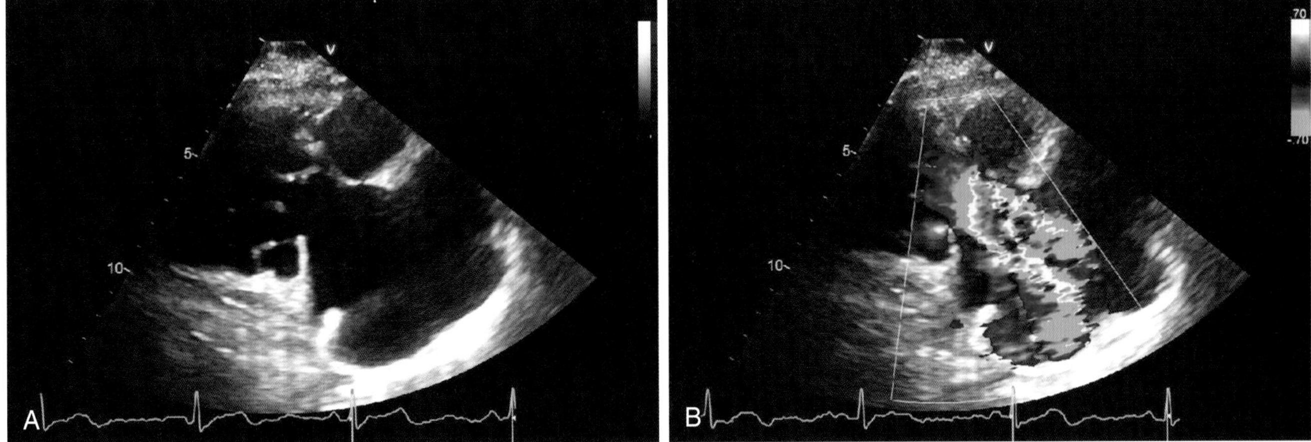

Fig. 28.6 Carcinoid tricuspid valve disease. (A) 2D echocardiography shows the typical appearance of carcinoid involvement of the tricuspid valve, with thickened, immobile leaflets (see Video 28.6). (B) Color Doppler shows torrential tricuspid valve regurgitation.

TEE 3D imaging typically provides lower-quality images compared with 3D TTE views because of the location of the TV in the far field, which results in beam widening and attenuation. Volumes can be acquired from a 0- to 30-degree midesophageal 4-chamber view or from a 40-degree transgastric view with anteflexion.[22,36] Imaging at the distal esophagus, where there are no left heart structures in the field of view and the right heart rests on the diaphragm, can improve image quality, but there are trade-offs with visualizing the TV throughout the cardiac cycle.

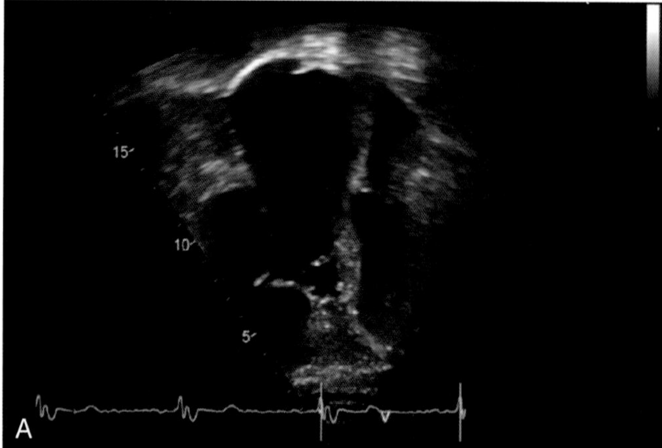

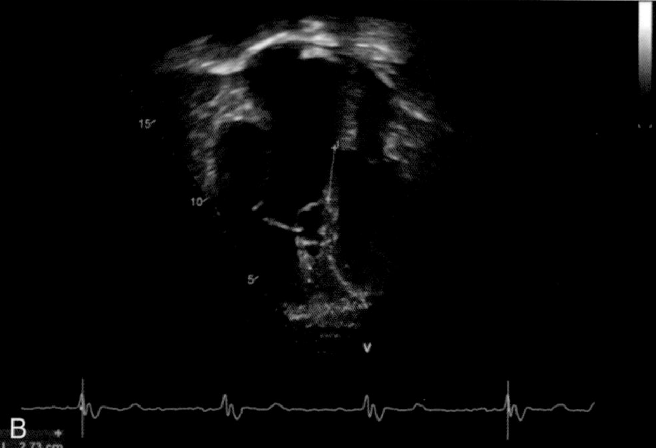

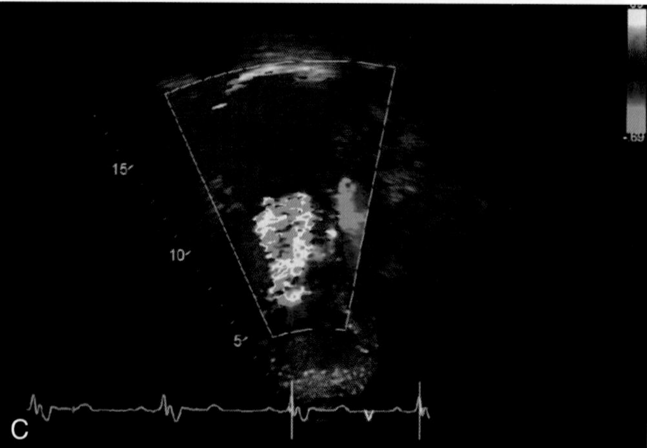

Fig. 28.7 Ebstein anomaly. (A and B) 2D TTE apical 4-chamber view shows the typical marked apical displacement of the tricuspid septal leaflet (displacement index of 17 mm/m^2) (see Video 28.7A). (C) Color Doppler demonstrates severe tricuspid regurgitation (TR). Notice the apical displacement of the origin of TR jet, which is another clue to the diagnosis of Ebstein anomaly (see Video 28.7C).

From the distal esophageal position, the TV leaflets are best viewed during systole, when they are perpendicular to the probe. During diastole, the leaflets open and become parallel to the angle of insonation, making visualization difficult. A similar principle applies to 3D volumes obtained from the transgastric position. The leaflets are best viewed during diastole, when they are perpendicular to the probe, and they are poorly seen during systole. Each TEE view has limitations, and as a result, an adequate TEE interrogation relies on obtaining multiple 3D data sets from several different positions.

TABLE 28.4 Echocardiographic Criteria for Establishing the Severity of Tricuspid Regurgitation.

Severity	*Criteria*
Mild tricuspid regurgitation	• Central jet area < 5.0 cm^2 • Vena contracta < 0.3 cm • Normal RA size • Normal IVC diameter • PISA ≤ 0.5 cm at Nyquist limit of 30–40 cm/s • Regurgitant volume < 30 mL • CW signal less dense with parabolic contour • Normal RV size and systolic function • Systolic-predominant hepatic vein flow • Tricuspid inflow A-wave dominant • ERO < 0.2 cm^2
Moderate tricuspid regurgitation	• Central jet area 5–10 cm^2 • Vena contracta 0.3–0.69 cm • Normal or mildly enlarged RA • Increased IVC diameter < 2.5 cm with normal respirophasic variation • PISA < 0.6–0.9 cm at Nyquist limit of 30–40 cm/s • Increased density of CW signal, varied contour • Mild or less RV enlargement with preserved function • Blunting of hepatic vein systolic flow • Variable tricuspid inflow • ERO 0.2–0.39 cm^2 • Regurgitant volume 30–44 mL
Severe tricuspid regurgitation	• Central jet area > 10 cm^2 or > 50% right atrial diameter • Vena contracta > 0.7 cm • RA enlargement • IVC diameter > 2.5 cm with reduced or absent respirophasic variation • PISA > 0.9 cm at Nyquist limit of 30–40 cm/s • Dense triangular CW signal with early peak • RV dilation with diminished systolic function • Systolic flow reversal in hepatic veins • Tricuspid inflow E wave > 1.0 m/s • ERO ≥ 0.4 cm^2 • Regurgitant volume ≥ 45 mL

CW, Continuous-wave Doppler signal; *ERO*, effective regurgitant orifice; *IVC*, inferior vena cava; *PISA*, proximal isovelocity surface area; *TR*, tricuspid regurgitation.

Role of Echocardiography in Clinical Care

Despite the negative impact TR has on survival, therapeutic interventions are largely limited to diuretics and optimizing treatment for the predisposing disease process. Surgery is rare and has traditionally been reserved for the minority of patients with severe TR due to congenital heart disease or primary TR or patients with secondary TR undergoing concomitant left-sided valvular surgery.[7,37] The role of stand-alone surgery in patients with TR due to atrial fibrillation, PH, or ventricular dysfunction is less clear.

In mitral regurgitation, there are well-established echocardiographic parameters to guide the timing of surgical referral. These criteria are based on intervening before LV dysfunction develops. Data on the optimal timing of TR surgery are sparse, but they suggest that RA pressure and RV size and function are inversely associated with outcomes.[23,24,38–40]

The mortality rate for stand-alone TV surgical treatment is significantly higher than for other forms of cardiac surgery, perhaps in part because referral is often delayed until the advanced stages of these disease, when patients become refractory to diuretic therapy.[19,41,42] Severe TR reduces RV afterload by unloading into the low-impedance RA, which can make RV systolic function appear artificially normal. It is possible that operative mortality rates could be improved if patients were treated before the onset of irreversible RV failure, but further research is needed to identify more sensitive echocardiographic markers of early RV dysfunction.[43]

For patients with TR and severe mitral or aortic valve disease, the role of surgery is well established. Current guidelines

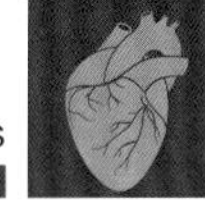

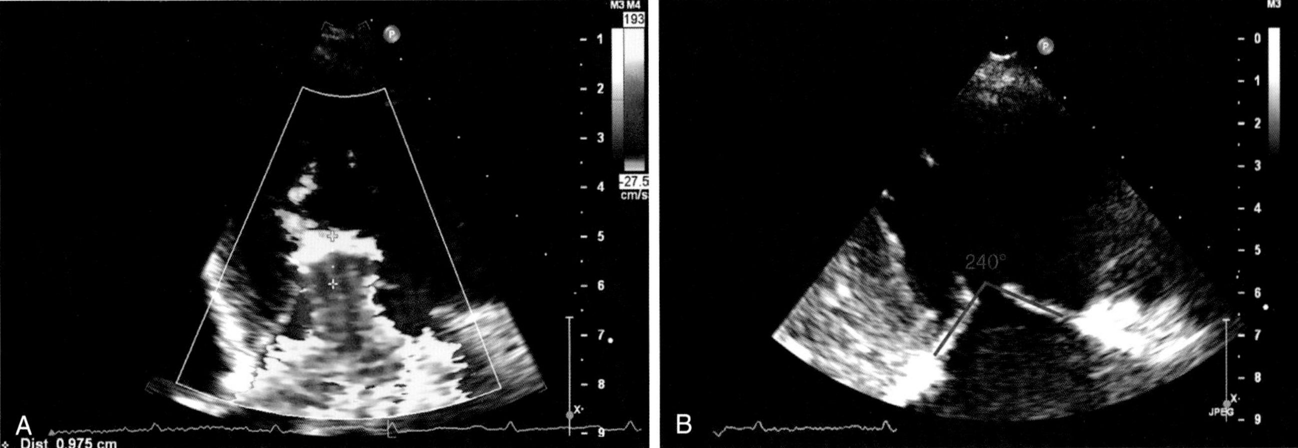

Fig. 28.8 Proximal isovelocity surface area method for the assessment of tricuspid regurgitation. (A) Measurement of proximal isovelocity area (PISA) radius; the baseline has been shifted down to optimize visualization of the isovelocity sphere. (B) When the PISA method is used for quantification of tricuspid regurgitation, angle correction is required to account for the funnel shape of the tricuspid leaflets.

recommend surgical TV intervention for patients undergoing left-sided valve surgery if there is severe TR (stage C or D) or progressive TR (stage B) when annular dilation is present (end-diastolic diameter > 4 mm) or when signs or symptoms of right-sided heart failure are present.

Intraoperative TEE assessment of TR severity is not a sensitive predictor of postoperative TR severity, particularly because patients undergoing general anesthesia and cardiopulmonary bypass may demonstrate less severe TR due to acute alterations in RV loading conditions. Preoperative TTE measurement of the diastolic annular diameter is preferred, and annular dilation rather than TR severity should guide the decision to combine a TV repair with mitral or aortic surgery.[45] Concomitant TV surgery improves clinical outcomes and survival of patients undergoing left-sided valve surgery, and reoperation for isolated TR has a high morbidity rate, making it preferable to address TR during the index operation.[20,21,44,46,47] Despite these recommendations, TV repair is rarely performed at the time of MV surgery, which represents a major area for practice improvement.[7,37]

Transcatheter interventions represent an emerging therapeutic option for all forms of valvular heart disease. No devices are currently approved for the TV, but many novel products are being developed and show promise in reducing the severity of regurgitation and improving clinical symptoms.[48,49] Off-label use of the MitraClip has improved TR severity and the outcomes of patients undergoing combined transcatheter tricuspid and mitral clipping procedures.[50,51] TTE and TEE play a critical role in identifying candidates for intervention and offer intraoperative procedural guidance during device placement.[49]

TRICUSPID STENOSIS

Native tricuspid valve stenosis (TS) is rarely seen in current clinical practice, and most cases of TS encountered today are iatrogenic (e.g., occurring after TV repair or replacement). Worldwide, rheumatic heart disease still accounts for most TS cases, even though it occurs in less than 5% of patients with rheumatic heart disease.[52,53] Rheumatic TS typically occurs with concomitant TR and left-sided valvular involvement.[54]

Other causes of native TS include carcinoid heart disease, congenital dysplasia, pacemaker lead–related valve fibrosis, and rarely, a large TV vegetation. TV inflow obstruction can result from RA tumors or thrombi, and it may be related to extrinsic compression of the TV annulus due to pericardial masses or intrapericardial hematoma.

Similar to more common valvular lesions, the echocardiographic assessment of TS includes 2D evaluation of the TV leaflets. As is typically seen in mitral valve rheumatic disease, rheumatic TS shows thickening of the leaflets with commissural fusion, diastolic doming, and various degrees of involvement of the subvalvular apparatus. Albeit rare, the detection of concomitant TS in patients with rheumatic heart disease and TR is important because it influences the candidacy for TV repair at the time of treatment for left-sided valve disease.

Hemodynamic assessment of TS includes measurement of the diastolic transtricuspid gradient and the TV area using the pressure half-time method. In severe TS, the TV Doppler pressure half-time is 190 ms or greater, and the calculated valve area is 1.0 cm^2 or less (for the TV, 190 ms instead of 220 ms should be used as the numerator when estimation of valve area by the half-time method is being performed[55]). Because of respiratory variation, the transtricuspid gradient should be measured over several consecutive beats to avoid miscalculation of the true degree of obstruction. A mean diastolic gradient of more than 5 mmHg has been suggested as diagnostic for severe TS.

Current practice guidelines[56] recommend TV surgery in patients with severe TS who are undergoing surgery for left-sided valve disease and for patients with isolated symptomatic severe TS. Percutaneous TV balloon valvuloplasty can be considered in selected cases of TS in the absence of significant TR, but data on outcomes (particularly in the long term) are lacking.

PULMONARY VALVE DISEASE

PULMONARY VALVE ANATOMY

PV abnormalities are the least commonly encountered of all cardiac valve pathologies. Unfortunately, the combination of low prevalence and less fluency among general sonographers and echocardiographers in assessing the PV by TTE leads to underappreciation and underdiagnosis of PV disease in clinical practice.

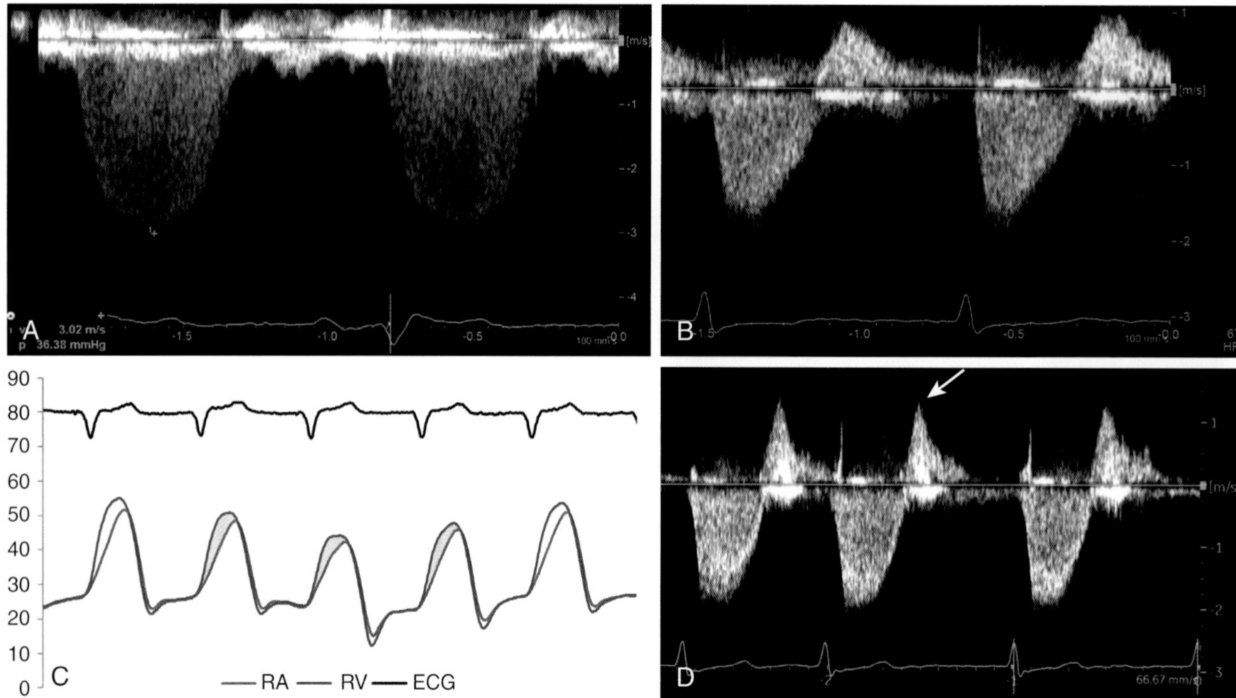

Fig. 28.9 Doppler assessment of tricuspid regurgitation. (A) CW Doppler imaging of mild tricuspid regurgitation (TR) shows minimal CW signal density and a parabolic shape. (B) In severe TR, the CW signal is dense and has a triangular shape with an early peak due to rapid pressure equalization between the RA and the RV. (C) *Shaded area* represents the RV-RA systolic gradient. *ECG*, Electrocardiographic tracing. (D) Increased tricuspid inflow velocity *(arrow)* is seen in a case of severe TR.

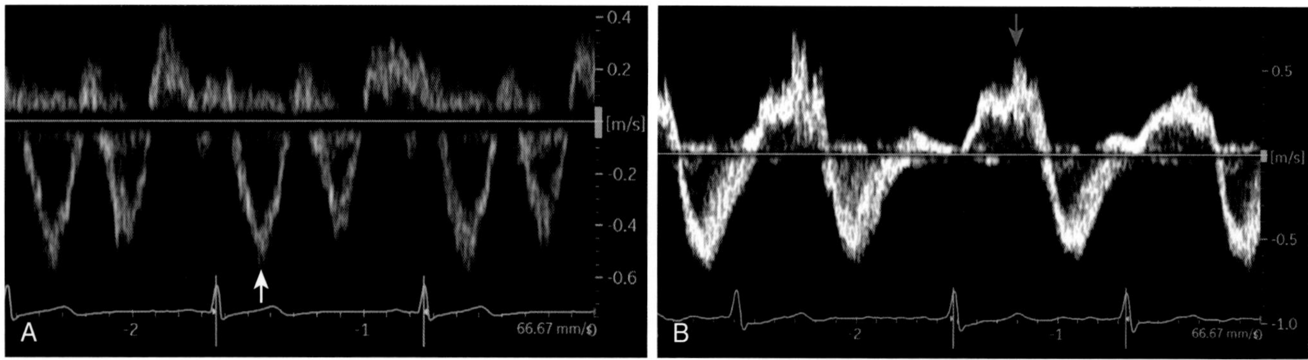

Fig. 28.10 Hepatic vein Doppler imaging in severe tricuspid regurgitation. (A) Normal hepatic venous pulsed-wave Doppler imaging shows a predominance of systolic forward flow *(white arrow)*. (B) High RA pressure coupled with a large reflux of blood during systole causes the typical systolic flow reversal *(red arrow)* seen in severe tricuspid regurgitation.

The PV is located anteriorly and leftward of the aortic valve and root, and it is the most anterior of the cardiac valves. Similar to the aortic valve, it has three cusps (i.e., anterior, right, and left) with three associated commissures. Although the valve itself shares similarities with the left semilunar valve, the pulmonary subvalvular apparatus is markedly different from the LV outflow tract (LVOT). Unlike the aortomitral curtain, there is no continuity between the PV and the TV, and the RVOT is muscular. The discontinuity between the PV and TV is one of the defining morphologic features of the RV.

The position of the PV in the chest facilitates its visualization by TTE, making TTE the imaging modality of choice in suspected PV disease. The PV is primarily imaged from the parasternal short-axis view, which provides great anatomic delineation of the valve cusps, the RVOT, and the main pulmonary artery and its proximal branches. Angulation of the probe superiorly and anteriorly from a typical parasternal long-axis view allows visualization of the PV, including the subvalvular and supravalvular components (i.e., RVOT view). In this view, the right pulmonary artery is on the right of the screen (i.e., opposite from its position in the short-axis view). Anterior angulation of the probe from a 4-chamber or basal short-axis subcostal view also leads to visualization of the RVOT and PV, analogous to the typical views obtained from a parasternal window.

The parasternal short-axis, RVOT, and subcostal views provide morphologic delineation of the PV and enable Doppler interrogation of the PV and RVOT. As is routinely done in cases of aortic valve pathology, color and CW Doppler evaluation of the PV should be performed from multiple angles. Visualization of the PV from the apical window is also possible, although it tends to be the most challenging window and is therefore less commonly used.

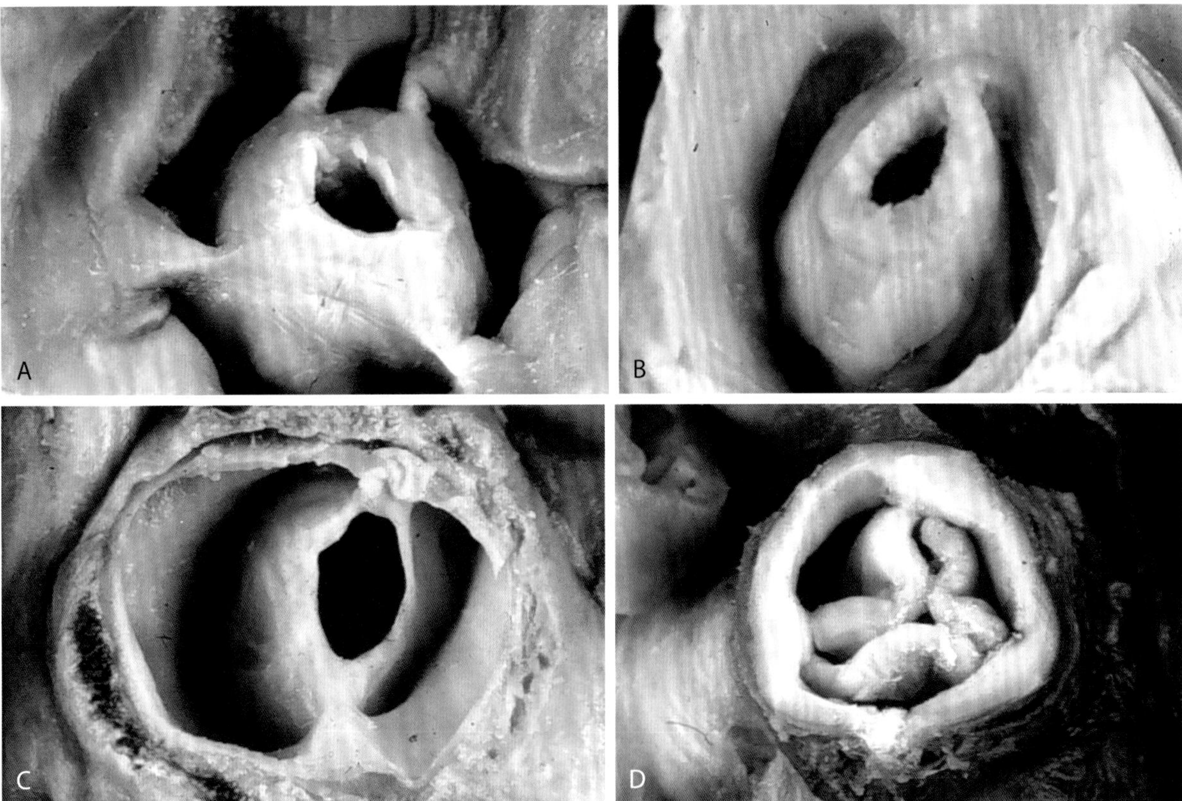

Fig. 28.11 Congenital pulmonic valve disease. The abnormal pulmonic valve can be classified as acommissural (A), with prominent systolic doming of the valve cusps and an eccentric orifice; unicommissural (B); bicuspid with fused commissures (C); or dysplastic (D), with severely thickened and deformed valve cusps. (Courtesy Dr. William D. Edwards, Department of Laboratory Medicine and Pathology, Mayo Clinic College of Medicine, with permission from Otto CM, Bonow RO. *Valvular Heart Disease*. 3rd ed. Philadelphia: WB Saunders; 2009.)

As opposed to TTE, visualization of the PV by TEE is less optimal because the valve is located in the far field. The valve may be obscured by acoustic shadowing arising from the left bronchus. Morphologic and color Doppler assessment of the PV is typically done from the mid-esophageal level (45- to 60-degree angulation). However, because of the almost perpendicular orientation in relation to the probe, this view provides poor angulation for CW Doppler assessment. Interrogation of the PV and RVOT can be performed from a high esophageal level at 0 to 30 degrees (particularly helpful intraoperatively) or from the transgastric view at approximately 60 degrees. The degree of angulation varies according to the position of the heart and the degree of right heart enlargement.

PULMONARY VALVE STENOSIS

Valvular pulmonary stenosis (PS) most commonly occurs in isolation. It can also occur as part of more complex congenital heart disease, such as tetralogy of Fallot and single ventricle, or in patients with genetic disorders. Less common causes of PS include carcinoid and rheumatic heart disease.

The abnormal PV in patients with PS can be categorized as acommissural, unicommissural, bicuspid, or dysplastic (Fig. 28.11). A dysplastic PV is typically seen in patients with Noonan syndrome, an autosomal dominant disorder associated with various degrees of abnormal facies, short stature, and intellectual or behavioral abnormalities.

In patients with PS, 2D assessment of the valve shows thickened cusps with reduced excursion and the typical systolic doming (Fig. 28.12). Patients with a dysplastic PV show more prominent degrees of cusp thickening with associated restricted motion. Identification of a dysplastic PV also has management implications because percutaneous balloon valvuloplasty tends to yield suboptimal relief of obstruction in this population.

2D assessment of the RV provides indirect hemodynamic assessment of PV stenosis because patients with moderate or severe PS show evidence of RV hypertrophy. RV enlargement and systolic dysfunction are not expected in adults with isolated severe PS, and their presence in the setting of PS should prompt the search for a concomitant hemodynamic lesion leading to RV volume overload, such as an atrial-level shunt or pulmonary regurgitation (PR).

Various degrees of pulmonary artery dilation are an almost universal finding in patients with PS. The degree of pulmonary artery dilation is unrelated to the hemodynamic significance of the PV obstruction.

Quantification of Pulmonary Stenosis Severity

The degree of PS is determined by CW Doppler interrogation of the PV. The exclusion of PV or RVOT obstruction should be mandatory for patients with increased estimated RV systolic pressures because patients with PS often are initially diagnosed as having PH. The severity of PS is normally determined based on the CW maximal instantaneous gradient calculated using the Bernoulli equation (Fig. 28.13).

The definition of severe PS has varied in the literature. According to the current Adult Congenital Heart Disease Practice Guidelines,[57,58] severe PS is defined by a maximal instantaneous gradient greater than 64 mmHg (peak velocity > 4 m/s), moderate PS by a maximal instantaneous gradient of 36 to 64

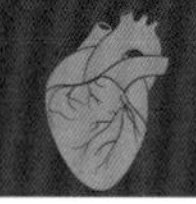

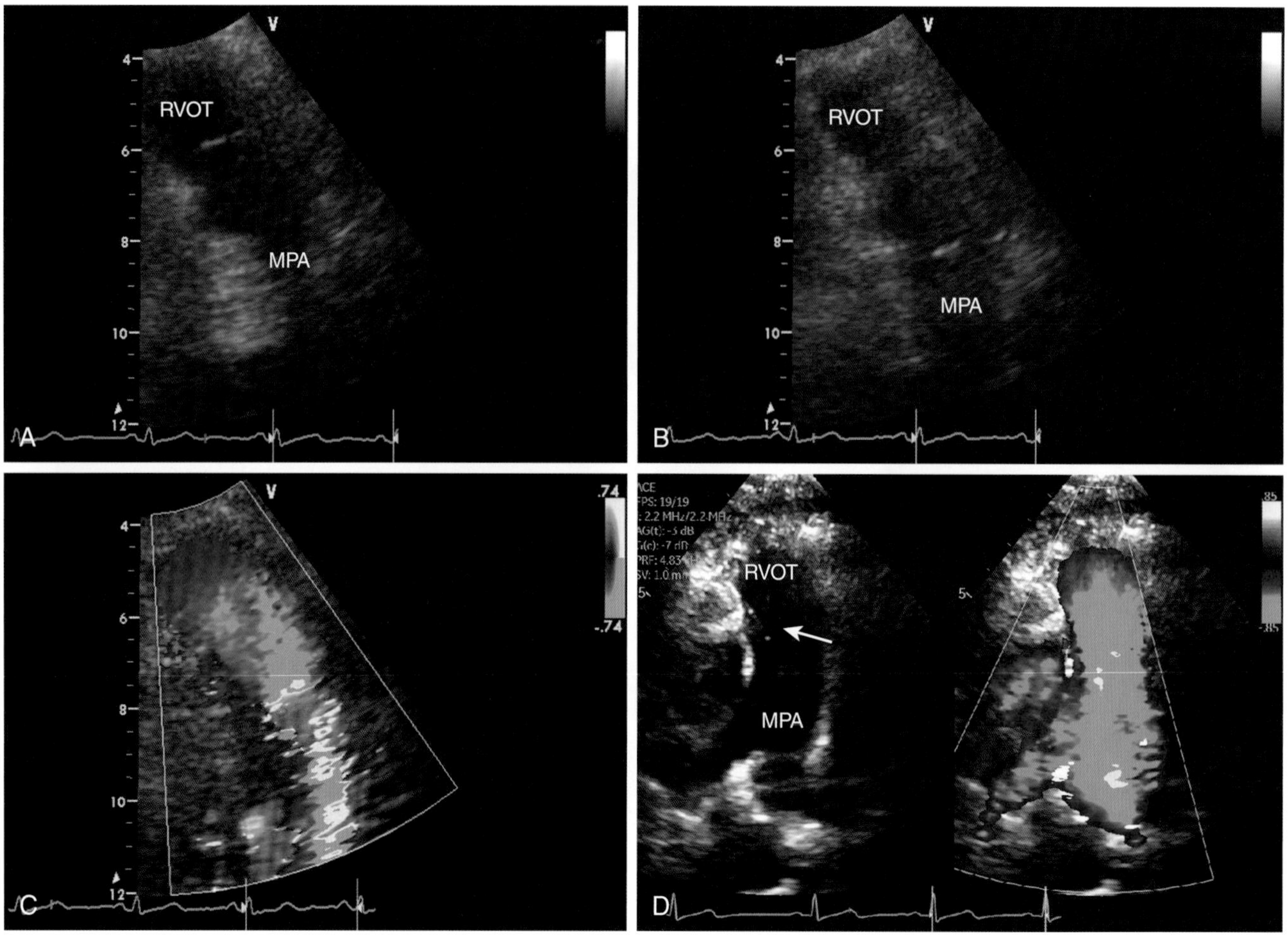

Fig. 28.12 2D and color Doppler echocardiography for imaging pulmonary stenosis. (A) 2D echocardiography shows mild thickening of the pulmonary valve cusps. (B) There is systolic doming of the pulmonary cusps during systole (see Video 28.12A), in contrast to the linear excursion of the normal pulmonary valve (D, *white arrow*). (C) Color Doppler imaging shows aliasing at the level of the tip of the pulmonary cusps rather than the laminar flow seen in a normal individual (see Video 28.12B). *MPA*, Main pulmonary artery; *RVOT*, RV outflow tract.

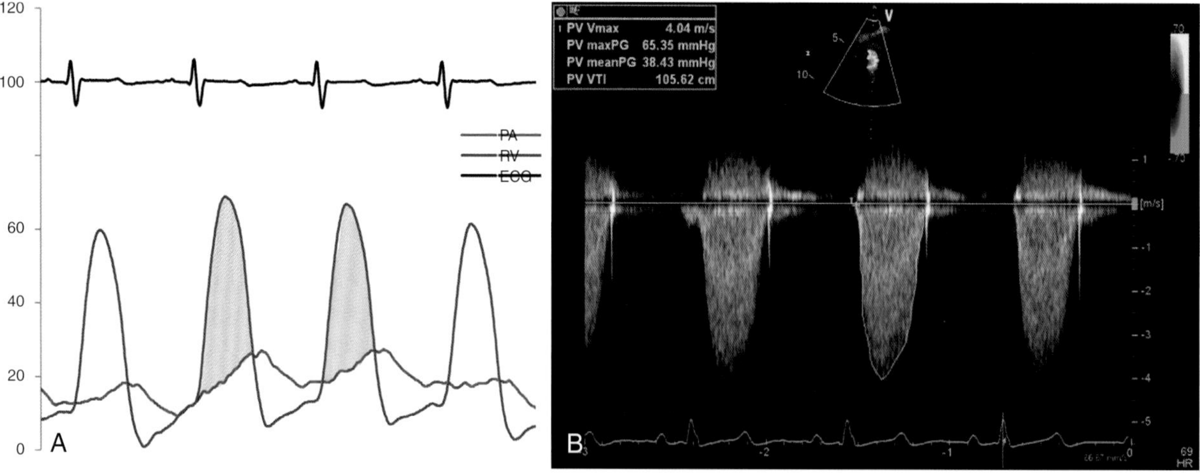

Fig. 28.13 Invasive and noninvasive hemodynamics in patients with severe pulmonary stenosis. (A) *Shaded areas* represent the systolic gradient on simultaneous RV and pulmonary artery (PA) tracings in patient with severe pulmonary stenosis. Notice the dampened appearance of the PA tracings, typical of significant RV outflow tract obstruction. (B) CW Doppler imaging of the same patient shows findings consistent with severe pulmonary stenosis (i.e., systolic mean gradient > 35 mmHg and maximal instantaneous gradient > 64 mmHg). *ECG*, Electrocardiographic tracing.

mmHg (peak velocity 3–4 m/s), and mild PS by a gradient of less than 36 mmHg (peak velocity > 4 m/s). A systolic mean gradient greater than 35 mmHg has also been suggested as diagnostic of severe PS.[58]

Despite the widely used maximal instantaneous gradient (i.e., peak gradient) for the diagnosis and management of patients with PS, the mean PV gradient appears to correlate with the peak-to-peak gradient obtained by cardiac catheterization.[59] Hemodynamic assessment of the PS should also include PW Doppler of the RVOT. If elevated (>1 m/s) RVOT velocities are identified, the modified Bernoulli equation $[P = 4(V_{distal}^2 - V_{proximial}^2)]$ should be applied.

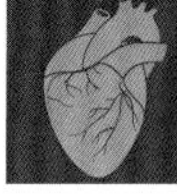

TABLE 28.5 Guidelines for the Treatment of Pulmonary Stenosis.

European Society of Cardiology Recommendations	*American Heart Association/ American College of Cardiology Recommendations*
Class I	
RV outflow tract obstruction at any level should be repaired regardless of symptoms when Doppler peak gradient is > 64 mmHg (peak velocity > 4 m/s), provided that RV function is normal and no valve substitute is required (LOE B).	For adults with more than moderate valvular PS and otherwise unexplained symptoms of HF, cyanosis from interatrial right-to-left communication, and/or exercise intolerance, balloon valvuloplasty is recommended (LOE B).
In valvular PS, balloon valvotomy should be the intervention of choice (LOE B).	For adults with more than moderate valvular PS and otherwise unexplained symptoms of HF, cyanosis, and/or exercise intolerance who are ineligible for or have failed balloon valvuloplasty, surgical repair is recommended (LOE B).
Class IIa	
Intervention in patients with gradient < 64 mmHg should be considered when at least one of the following is present: • Symptoms related to PS • Decreased RV function • Double-chambered RV (which is usually progressive) • Important arrhythmias • Right-to-left shunting through an ASD or VSD (LOE C)	For asymptomatic adults with severe valvular PS, intervention is reasonable (LOE C).

ASD, Atrial septal defect; *HF*, heart failure; *LOE*, level of evidence; *PS*, pulmonary stenosis; *TR*, tricuspid regurgitation; *VSD*, ventricular septal defect.

Role of Echocardiography in Clinical Care

The decision to intervene depends on clinical and hemodynamic information about the patient. Echocardiography is instrumental in the management of PS. Patients with mild to moderate PS are usually asymptomatic, whereas patients with severe PS can present with dyspnea, fatigue, decreased exercise tolerance, syncope, or exertional lightheadedness.

PS has a favorable natural history, with a reported 25-year survival rate of greater than 95%.[60] However, individual prognosis is determined by the severity of PS. Mild PS has a benign course, and it rarely progresses to moderate or severe PS or requires therapeutic intervention. In contrast, severe PS can lead to progressive RV diastolic dysfunction, arrhythmias, and right heart failure, and patients may require intervention in infancy or childhood. Moderate PS has a varied natural history and prognosis, and patients may not be diagnosed until adulthood.[58]

Current recommendations for management of PS are shown in Table 28.5.[57,58] Relief of PS is recommended for patients with moderate or severe PS who have unexplained symptoms, right-to-left shunt at the atrial level, and/or exercise intolerance. Intervention can be considered for those with asymptomatic severe PS. Pulmonary balloon valvuloplasty is the treatment of choice for patients with severe PS, and surgical intervention is reserved for selected cases such as failed percutaneous valvuloplasty (most commonly in patients with dysplastic PV), previous surgical valvotomy, concomitant mild or worse PR, and carcinoid or rheumatic PS.

Percutaneous pulmonary balloon valvuloplasty relieves PV obstruction by splitting the commissures. Procedural morbidity and mortality rates are low. The procedure typically leads to mild degrees of postprocedural PV obstruction with low rates of restenosis.[61] Percutaneous balloon valvuloplasty is effective and safe, even when performed in older adults.[62]

Follow-up of patients with PS is dictated by disease severity.[58] Patients with mild degrees of PS can have clinical and echocardiographic evaluation every 5 years, whereas most patients with moderate PS are seen every 2 to 5 years. The longitudinal care of patients after relief of PS should incorporate the degree of PR. PR after surgical or pulmonary balloon intervention is a well-established complication, and moderate or worse PR was reported for more than 50% of patients in early series.[63,64]

PULMONARY REGURGITATION

Although trivial or mild PR is common in the general population,[65] the prevalence of significant PR in general clinical practice is very low. Most cases of moderate or worse PR are observed in patients who underwent percutaneous or surgical PV intervention or those with repaired tetralogy of Fallot.

As in other regurgitant valvular disorders, PR can be divided into primary and secondary types. Noncongenital causes of primary PR include rheumatic disease and carcinoid disease, and concomitant TV involvement is the norm. PR due to infective endocarditis is rare; PV involvement occurs in up to 1% of endocarditis cases.[66]

Secondary PR occurs in patients with dilation of the PV annulus in the setting of ectatic or aneurysmal pulmonary arteries, typically caused by severe PH. More than mild PR in those with idiopathic or other pulmonary artery aneurysm suggests that an underlying abnormality of the PV is present.[67] In this population, PV morphology should be assessed carefully, avoiding the presumptive diagnosis of secondary PR.

Severe PR is most commonly iatrogenic and is seen in patients with congenital PS who have undergone surgical pulmonary valvotomy or balloon valvuloplasty. Severe PR is one of the most common long-term complications of repair of tetralogy of Fallot, particularly repairs in which an RVOT or pulmonary annulus transannular patch was placed. Expression of congenital PR in patients without prior intervention is rare, and it typically occurs in conjunction with some degree of pulmonary stenosis.

The hemodynamic consequence of PR is RV overload with progressive RV enlargement and, in more advanced cases, RV systolic dysfunction. The effect of PR on RV diastolic function is unknown, and controversy exists regarding the impact of PR with an underlying noncompliant RV (i.e., restrictive RV physiology in patients with severe PR). Progressive RV enlargement can be complicated by secondary TR; more than moderate TR is identified in 20% to 30% of those undergoing PV replacement.[68,69] If left untreated, chronic RV volume in those with PR can lead to atrial or ventricular arrhythmias, decreased exercise capacity, and increased morbidity and mortality rates due to right-sided heart failure.

Echocardiographic Evaluation of Pulmonary Regurgitation

TTE is the main echocardiographic modality for the assessment of patients with PR.[65] Echocardiographic assessment of PR should include a comprehensive 2D and Doppler evaluation. The 2D assessment includes determination of the underlying anatomy of the PV and the mechanism of regurgitation (e.g., flail, absent or surgically resected cusps, restricted mobility or thickening, annular dilation, associated vegetation).

Unlike the result for left-sided infective endocarditis, the diagnostic yield of TEE for infective endocarditis involving the PV is limited, and the echocardiographic evaluation includes TTE and TEE as complementary diagnostic tests.[70]

TABLE 28.6 **Echocardiographic Assessment of Pulmonary Regurgitation.**

Parameter	*Mild PR*	*Moderate PR*	*Severe PR*	*Advantages*	*Pitfalls*
RV size	Normal	Normal/mildly enlarged	Enlarged	Normal RV essentially excludes hemodynamically significant long-standing PR	Not specific because concomitant lesion can cause RV enlargement (TR, left-to-right shunt)
Jet width	Narrow	Intermediate but < 50% of PV annulus	Wide; > 50% of PV annulus	Simple	Challenging in case of eccentric jets
Doppler density	Faint	Dense but less than systolic forward flow	As dense as systolic forward flow	Simple	Subjective
PR signal pressure half-time by CW Doppler	Prolonged, holodiastolic	Prolonged, holodiastolic	Short (<100 ms)	Simple, reproducible	Not specific for PR (influenced by RV filling pressures or diastolic dysfunction)

PR, Pulmonary regurgitation; *TR*, tricuspid regurgitation.

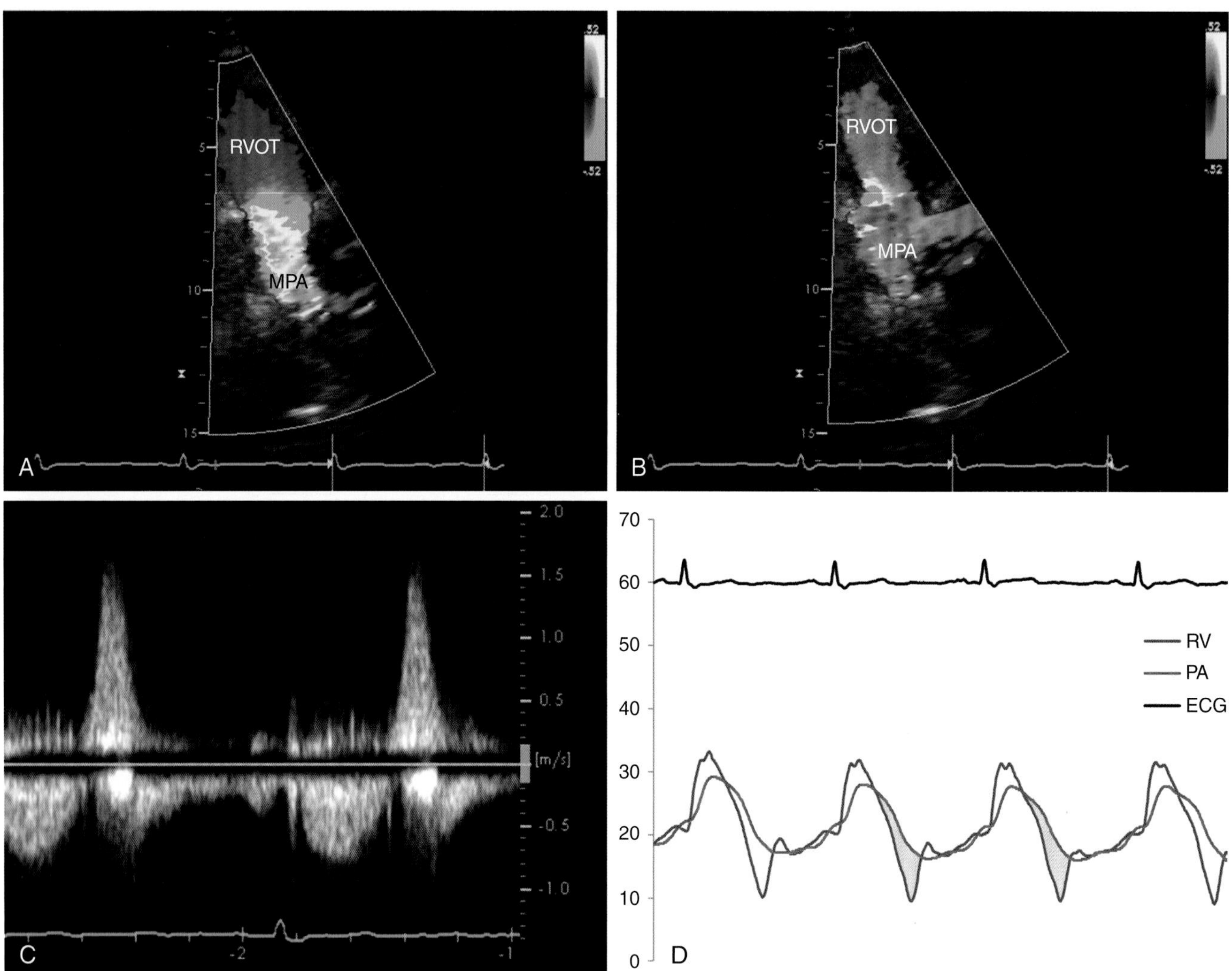

Fig. 28.14 Echocardiographic Doppler findings in severe pulmonary regurgitation. (A and B) Color Doppler parasternal short-axis views show a regurgitating jet that occupies essentially the entire pulmonary valve annulus in systole and diastole, respectively (see Video 28.14A), which is consistent with severe pulmonary regurgitation. (C and D) CW Doppler and simultaneous RV and pulmonary artery (PA) tracings, respectively, from the same patient. There was very short deceleration time of the pulmonary regurgitation signal, reflecting the early equalization of RV and PA pressures in early diastole (*shaded areas* represent the PA-RV pressure gradient). Notice the similar density between the systolic and diastolic components of the Doppler signal. *ECG*, Electrocardiographic tracing; *MPA*, main pulmonary artery; *RVOT*, RV outflow tract.

Similar to the 2D assessment of patients with PS, morphologic evaluation of the PV should include the parasternal short-axis view, the RVOT view, and the subcostal window. These views also provide appropriate alignment for Doppler interrogation of the PV.

Several criteria have been proposed for grading PR[71] (Table 28.6):

1. Jet width: In patients with severe PR, the regurgitant jet (vena contracta) occupies more than 50% of the pulmonary annulus[72,73] and sometimes the entire annular dimension in those with free PR (Fig. 28.14). In contrast,

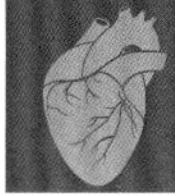

TABLE 28.7 **Guidelines for the Treatment of Pulmonary Regurgitation.**

	European Society of Cardiology Recommendations	*American Heart Association/American College of Cardiology Recommendations*
Class I	Pulmonary valve replacement should be performed in symptomatic patients with severe PR and/or stenosis (RV systolic pressure > 60 mmHg, TR velocity > 3.5 m/s) (LOE C).	For symptomatic patients with at least moderate PR resulting from treated isolated PS with RV dilation or RV dysfunction, pulmonary valve replacement is recommended (LOE C). Pulmonary valve replacement (surgical or percutaneous) for relief of symptoms is recommended for patients with repaired TOF and at least moderate PR with cardiovascular symptoms not otherwise explained (LOE C).
Class IIa	Pulmonary valve replacement should be considered in asymptomatic patients with severe PR and/or PS when at least one of the following is present: • Decrease in objective exercise capacity • Progressive RV dilation • Progressive RV systolic dysfunction • Progressive TR (at least moderate) • RV outflow tract obstruction with RV systolic pressure > 80 mmHg (TR velocity > 4.3 m/s) • Sustained atrial/ventricular arrhythmias	Pulmonary valve replacement (surgical or percutaneous) is reasonable for preservation of ventricular size and function in asymptomatic patients with repaired TOF and ventricular enlargement or dysfunction and at least moderate PR (LOE C).
Class IIb		For asymptomatic patients with at least moderate PR resulting from treatment of isolated PS with progressive RV dilation and/or RV dysfunction, pulmonary valve replacement may be reasonable (LOE C). Surgical pulmonary valve replacement may be reasonable for adults with repaired TOF and at least moderate PR with other lesions requiring surgical interventions (LOE C). Pulmonary valve replacement in addition to arrhythmia management may be considered for adults with repaired TOF and at least moderate PR and ventricular tachyarrhythmia (LOE C).

LOE, Level of evidence; *PR*, pulmonary regurgitation; *PS*, pulmonary stenosis; *TOF*, tetralogy of Fallot; *TR*, tricuspid regurgitation; *TV*, tricuspid valve.

those with mild PR tend to have a narrow and small jet (length < 10 mm[74]), and individuals with moderate PR have intermediate values.

2. Deceleration time: In patients with severe PR, there is equalization of diastolic RV and pulmonary artery pressures (see Fig. 28.14). Because CW Doppler imaging of the PR jet reflects the RV–pulmonary artery pressure gradient, patients with mild or moderate PR have holodiastolic Doppler signals, whereas patients with severe PR have short deceleration times. A pressure half-time of less than 100 ms is thought by some to correlate well with severe PR by cardiac magnetic resonance imaging (CMR).[75] Others have suggested that a cutoff of 167 ms is more sensitive for severe PR.[76] A short deceleration time is not a specific finding for PR. Patients with severe RV diastolic dysfunction, such as those with severe myocardial disease or pericardial disease, also have short deceleration times.
3. Doppler signal density: Albeit subjective, the density of the PR CW Doppler signal also provides qualitative information about severity. Patients with severe PR typically have dense diastolic CW Doppler signals (i.e., as dense as the systolic signal [forward flow]). This is particularly helpful for patients with short deceleration time due severe diastolic dysfunction from restrictive cardiomyopathy or constrictive pericarditis.

Other supportive findings of severe PR include markedly pulsatile pulmonary arteries and diastolic flow reversals in the branch pulmonary arteries; this is identified by color or PW Doppler and has been shown to have a high specificity for severe PR compared with magnetic resonance data.[73,76] Quantitation of the RV stroke volume and regurgitation fraction using PW Doppler imaging has been proposed as another tool for PR assessment, but this method is limited by the challenges in measuring the RVOT diameter accurately by 2D echocardiography and lack of validation.

Because RV volume overload is the hemodynamic hallmark of chronic significant PR, a normal RV size argues against more than moderate PR. However, some patients with severe PR may fail to show significant dilation of the RV despite a large regurgitant fraction (e.g., significant PR as a complication of treatment for isolated congenital PS).

Role of Echocardiography in Clinical Care

Thorough assessment of PR is mandatory in patients with previous PV intervention and those with prior repair of tetralogy of Fallot. It is important to rule out severe PR when patients present with atrial or ventricular arrhythmias because electrical instability may provide a clue to the underlying hemodynamic abnormality. Detailed evaluation of the PV hemodynamics should be undertaken for all patients with carcinoid heart disease because the PV is abnormal in most of those with TV disease. Undiagnosed PR can cause persistent symptoms and RV enlargement in carcinoid patients after TV surgery.

Recommendations for the management of PR are presented in Table 28.7.[57,58] Surgical or percutaneous PV replacement is a class I indication for patients with at least moderate PR and RV dilation or systolic dysfunction whose symptoms can be attributed to their PV disease. They typically experience fatigue, shortness of breath, reduced exercise tolerance, and/or atrial or ventricular arrhythmias.

PV replacement is considered reasonable for asymptomatic individuals with at least moderate PR after prior relief of PS who have evidence of progressive RV dilation and/or dysfunction. For patients with repaired tetralogy of Fallot and at least moderate PR, PV intervention may be considered (class IIa indication)

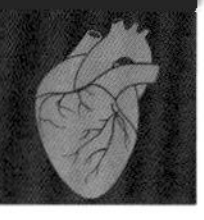

for those with two of following criteria[58]: mild or moderate RV or LV systolic dysfunction, severe RV dilation (RV end-diastolic volume index ≥ 160 mL/m^2, RV end-systolic volume index ≥ 80 mL/m^2, or RV end-diastolic pressure ≥ 2 × LV end-diastolic volume), RV systolic pressure that is two thirds or more of the systemic systolic pressure, or progressive reduction in objective exercise tolerance.

CMR is an integral component in the care of patients with significant residual PR after PV or RVOT surgical or percutaneous intervention. CMR provides an objective assessment of RV size and systolic function in patients with PR. The benefit of CMR in this patient population underscores the inherent pitfalls in assessment of RV size and function by TTE, including the additional imaging challenges in selected patients, such as those with repaired tetralogy of Fallot because of multiple prior cardiac operations or cardiac malposition.

CMR can assess the severity of PR in patients with incomplete TTE studies and provide supplemental information such as assessment of the pulmonary arteries (e.g., size, branch pulmonary artery stenosis), coronary artery anatomy (i.e., concomitant coronary artery anomalies), and sinus of Valsalva and ascending aortic measurements (e.g., aortic dilation). CMR has been used extensively for evaluating patients with PR, particularly those with conotruncal abnormalities. The RV volumes determined by CMR before PV replacement have been shown to predict favorable remodeling of the RV after relief of RV volume overload,[77,78] but data on the survival benefit solely based on CMR cutoffs are lacking.

The preprocedural echocardiographic evaluation of candidates for PV intervention should include assessment of the degree of TR. In our practice, concomitant TV repair in those with more than mild TR and a dilated TV annulus is typically performed at the time of PV replacement. The degree of TR improved in 65% of patients undergoing transcatheter PV replacement, and more than 50% of patients had mild or no TR at discharge.[69]

Serial echocardiographic evaluation of patients with PR after treatment of PS or repair of tetralogy of Fallot is also supported by the guidelines.[58] For those with asymptomatic severe PR, repeat TTE should be performed every 12 to 24 months. Those with less severe degrees of PR can have repeat imaging every 3 to 5 years.

REFERENCES

1. Hahn RT. State-of-the-art review of echocardiographic imaging in the evaluation and treatment of functional tricuspid regurgitation. *Circ Cardiovasc Imaging*. 2016;9(12). https://doi.org/10.1161/CIRCIMAGING.116.005332.
2. Dahou A, Levin D, Reisman M, Hahn RT. Anatomy and physiology of the tricuspid valve. *JACC Cardiovasc Imaging*. 2019;12(3):458–468.
3. Fukuda S, Saracino G, Matsumura Y, et al. Three-dimensional geometry of the tricuspid annulus in healthy subjects and in patients with functional tricuspid regurgitation: a real-time, 3-dimensional echocardiographic study. *Circulation*. 2006;114(1 Suppl):I492–I498.
4. Fukuda S, Gillinov AM, Song JM, et al. Echocardiographic insights into atrial and ventricular mechanisms of functional tricuspid regurgitation. *Am Heart J*. 2006;152(6):1208–1214.
5. Topilsky Y, Tribouilloy C, Michelena HI, Pislaru S, Mahoney DW, Enriquez-Sarano M. Pathophysiology of tricuspid regurgitation: quantitative Doppler echocardiographic assessment of respiratory dependence. *Circulation*. 2010;122(15):1505–1513.
6. Singh JP, Evans JC, Levy D, et al. Prevalence and clinical determinants of mitral, tricuspid, and aortic regurgitation (the Framingham Heart Study). *Am J Cardiol*. 1999;83(6):897–902.
7. Stuge O, Liddicoat J. Emerging opportunities for cardiac surgeons within structural heart disease. *J Thorac Cardiovasc Surg*. 2006;132(6):1258–1261.
8. Mutlak D, Lessick J, Reisner SA, Aronson D, Dabbah S, Agmon Y. Echocardiography-based spectrum of severe tricuspid regurgitation: the frequency of apparently idiopathic tricuspid regurgitation. *J Am Soc Echocardiogr*. 2007;20(4):405–408.
9. Hoke U, Auger D, Thijssen J, et al. Significant lead-induced tricuspid regurgitation is associated with poor prognosis at long-term follow-up. *Heart*. 2014;100(12):960–968.
10. Berger Y, Har Zahav Y, Kassif Y, et al. Tricuspid valve regurgitation after orthotopic heart transplantation: prevalence and etiology. *J Transplant*. 2012;2012:120702.
11. Chan MC, Giannetti N, Kato T, et al. Severe tricuspid regurgitation after heart transplantation. *J Heart Lung Transplant*. 2001;20(7):709–717.
12. Ton-Nu TT, Levine RA, Handschumacher MD, et al. Geometric determinants of functional tricuspid regurgitation: insights from 3-dimensional echocardiography. *Circulation*. 2006;114(2):143–149.
13. Yamasaki N, Kondo F, Kubo T, et al. Severe tricuspid regurgitation in the aged: atrial remodeling associated with long-standing atrial fibrillation. *J Cardiol*. 2006;48(6):315–323.
14. Lin G, Nishimura RA, Connolly HM, Dearani JA, Sundt TM 3rd, Hayes DL. Severe symptomatic tricuspid valve regurgitation due to permanent pacemaker or implantable cardioverter-defibrillator leads. *J Am Coll Cardiol*. 2005;45(10):1672–1675.
15. Nath J, Foster E, Heidenreich PA. Impact of tricuspid regurgitation on long-term survival. *J Am Coll Cardiol*. 2004;43(3):405–409.
16. Topilsky Y, Maltais S, Medina Inojosa J, et al. Burden of tricuspid regurgitation in patients diagnosed in the community setting. *JACC Cardiovasc Imaging*. 2019;12(3):433–442.
17. Otto CM, Nishimura RA, Bonow RO, et al. 2020 ACC/AHA guideline for the management of patients with valvular heart disease: a report of the American College of Cardiology/American Heart Association Joint Committee on Clinical Practice Guidelines. *Circulation*. 2021;143(5):e72-e227. https://doi.org/10.1161/CIR.0000000000000923.
18. Joint Task Force on the Management of Valvular Heart Disease of the European Society of Cardiology (ESC); European Association for Cardio-Thoracic Surgery (EACTS). Guidelines on the management of valvular heart disease (version 2012). *Eur Heart J*. 2012;33(19):2451–2496.
19. Fender EA, Zack CJ, Nishimura RA. Isolated tricuspid regurgitation: outcomes and therapeutic interventions. *Heart*. 2018;104(10):798–806.
20. Van de Veire NR, Braun J, Delgado V, et al. Tricuspid annuloplasty prevents right ventricular dilatation and progression of tricuspid regurgitation in patients with tricuspid annular dilatation undergoing mitral valve repair. *J Thorac Cardiovasc Surg*. 2011;141(6):1431–1439.
21. Benedetto U, Melina G, Angeloni E, et al. Prophylactic tricuspid annuloplasty in patients with dilated tricuspid annulus undergoing mitral valve surgery. *J Thorac Cardiovasc Surg*. 2012;143(3):632–638.
22. Muraru D, Hahn RT, Soliman OI, Faletra FF, Basso C, Badano LP. 3-Dimensional echocardiography in imaging the tricuspid valve. *JACC Cardiovasc Imaging*. 2019;12(3):500–515.
23. Topilsky Y, Nkomo VT, Vatury O, et al. Clinical outcome of isolated tricuspid regurgitation. *JACC Cardiovasc Imaging*. 2014;7(12):1185–1194.
24. Fender EA, Petrescu I, Ionescu F, et al. Prognostic importance and predictors of survival in isolated tricuspid regurgitation: a growing problem. *Mayo Clin Proc*. 2019;94(10):2032–2039.
25. Utsunomiya H, Itabashi Y, Mihara H, et al. Functional tricuspid regurgitation caused by chronic atrial fibrillation: a real-time 3-dimensional transesophageal echocardiography study. *Circ Cardiovasc Imaging*. 2017;10(1):e004897.
26. Gonzalez-Vilchez F, Zarauza J, Vazquez de Prada JA, et al. Assessment of tricuspid regurgitation by Doppler color flow imaging: angiographic correlation. *Int J Cardiol*. 1994;44(3):275–283.
27. Tribouilloy CM, Enriquez-Sarano M, Bailey KR, Tajik AJ, Seward JB. Quantification of tricuspid regurgitation by measuring the width of the vena contracta with Doppler color flow imaging: a clinical study. *J Am Coll Cardiol*. 2000;36(2):472–478.

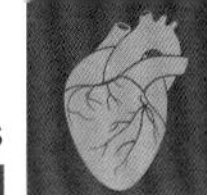

28. Tribouilloy CM, Enriquez-Sarano M, Capps MA, Bailey KR, Tajik AJ. Contrasting effect of similar effective regurgitant orifice area in mitral and tricuspid regurgitation: a quantitative Doppler echocardiographic study. *J Am Soc Echocardiogr*. 2002;15(9):958–965.
29. Simpson IA, Shiota T, Gharib M, Sahn DJ. Current status of flow convergence for clinical applications: is it a leaning tower of "PISA"? *J Am Coll Cardiol*. 1996;27(2):504–509.
30. Grossmann G, Stein M, Kochs M, et al. Comparison of the proximal flow convergence method and the jet area method for the assessment of the severity of tricuspid regurgitation. *Eur Heart J*. 1998;19(4):652–659.
31. Sakai K, Nakamura K, Satomi G, Kondo M, Hirosawa K. Evaluation of tricuspid regurgitation by blood flow pattern in the hepatic vein using pulsed Doppler technique. *Am Heart J*. 1984;108(3 Pt 1):516–523.
32. Rudski LG, Lai WW, Afilalo J, et al. Guidelines for the echocardiographic assessment of the right heart in adults: a report from the American Society of Echocardiography endorsed by the European Association of Echocardiography, a registered branch of the European Society of Cardiology, and the Canadian Society of Echocardiography. *J Am Soc Echocardiogr*. 2010;23(7):685–713; quiz 786–788.
33. Hioka T, Kaga S, Mikami T, et al. Overestimation by echocardiography of the peak systolic pressure gradient between the right ventricle and right atrium due to tricuspid regurgitation and the usefulness of the early diastolic transpulmonary valve pressure gradient for estimating pulmonary artery pressure. *Heart Ves*. 2017;32(7):833–842.
34. Ozpelit E, Akdeniz B, Ozpelit EM, et al. Impact of severe tricuspid regurgitation on accuracy of echocardiographic pulmonary artery systolic pressure estimation. *Echocardiography*. 2015;32(10):1483–1490.
35. Beigel R, Cercek B, Luo H, Siegel RJ. Noninvasive evaluation of right atrial pressure. *J Am Soc Echocardiogr*. 2013;26(9):1033–1042.
36. Hahn RT, Abraham T, Adams MS, et al. Guidelines for performing a comprehensive transesophageal echocardiographic examination: recommendations from the American Society of Echocardiography and the Society of Cardiovascular Anesthesiologists. *J Am Soc Echocardiogr*. 2013;26(9):921–964.
37. Vassileva CM, Shabosky J, Boley T, Markwell S, Hazelrigg S. Tricuspid valve surgery: the past 10 years from the Nationwide Inpatient Sample (NIS) database. *J Thorac Cardiovasc Surg*. 2012;143(5):1043–1049.
38. Kuwaki K, Morishita K, Tsukamoto M, Abe T. Tricuspid valve surgery for functional tricuspid valve regurgitation associated with left-sided valvular disease. *Eur J Cardio Thorac Surg*. 2001;20(3):577–582.
39. Kim JB, Jung SH, Choo SJ, Chung CH, Lee JW. Clinical and echocardiographic outcomes after surgery for severe isolated tricuspid regurgitation. *J Thorac Cardiovasc Surg*. 2013;146(2):278–284.
40. Kim YJ, Kwon DA, Kim HK, et al. Determinants of surgical outcome in patients with isolated tricuspid regurgitation. *Circulation*. 2009;120(17):1672–1678.
41. Marquis-Gravel G, Bouchard D, Perrault LP, et al. Retrospective cohort analysis of 926 tricuspid valve surgeries: clinical and hemodynamic outcomes with propensity score analysis. *Am Heart J*. 2012;163(5):851–858 e851.
42. Zack CJ, Fender EA, Chandrashekar P, et al. National trends and outcomes in isolated tricuspid valve surgery. *J Am Coll Cardiol*. 2017;70(24):2953–2960.
43. Ling LF, Obuchowski NA, Rodriguez L, Popovic Z, Kwon D, Marwick TH. Accuracy and interobserver concordance of echocardiographic assessment of right ventricular size and systolic function: a quality control exercise. *J Am Soc Echocardiogr*. 2012;25(7):709–713.
44. Dreyfus GD, Corbi PJ, Chan KM, Bahrami T. Secondary tricuspid regurgitation or dilatation: which should be the criteria for surgical repair? *Ann Thorac Surg*. 2005;79(1):127–132.
45. Kim JB, Yoo DG, Kim GS, et al. Mild-to-moderate functional tricuspid regurgitation in patients undergoing valve replacement for rheumatic mitral disease: the influence of tricuspid valve repair on clinical and echocardiographic outcomes. *Heart*. 2012;98(1):24–30.
46. Pagnesi M, Montalto C, Mangieri A, et al. Tricuspid annuloplasty versus a conservative approach in patients with functional tricuspid regurgitation undergoing left-sided heart valve surgery: a study-level meta-analysis. *Int J Cardiol*. 2017;240:138–144.
47. Chikwe J, Itagaki S, Anyanwu A, Adams DH. Impact of concomitant tricuspid annuloplasty on tricuspid regurgitation, right ventricular function, and pulmonary artery hypertension after repair of mitral valve Prolapse. *J Am Coll Cardiol*. 2015;65(18):1931–1938.
48. Rodes-Cabau J, Hahn RT, Latib A, et al. Transcatheter therapies for treating tricuspid regurgitation. *J Am Coll Cardiol*. 2016;67(15):1829–1845.
49. Hahn RT, Nabauer M, Zuber M, et al. Intraprocedural imaging of transcatheter tricuspid valve interventions. *JACC Cardiovasc Imaging*. 2019;12(3):532–553.
50. Besler C, Blazek S, Rommel KP, et al. Combined mitral and tricuspid versus isolated mitral valve transcatheter Edge-to-Edge repair in patients with symptomatic valve regurgitation at high surgical risk. *JACC Cardiovasc Interv*. 2018;11(12):1142–1151.
51. Braun D, Rommel KP, Orban M, et al. Acute and short-term results of transcatheter Edge-to-Edge repair for severe tricuspid regurgitation using the MitraClip XTR System. *JACC Cardiovasc Interv*. 2019;12(6):604–605.
52. Daniels SJ, Mintz GS, Kotler MN. Rheumatic tricuspid valve disease: two-dimensional echocardiographic, hemodynamic, and angiographic correlations. *Am J Cardiol*. 1983;51(3):492–496.
53. Hauck AJ, Freeman DP, Ackermann DM, Danielson GK, Edwards WD. Surgical pathology of the tricuspid valve: a study of 363 cases spanning 25 years. *Mayo Clin Proc*. 1988;63(9):851–863.
54. Yousof AM, Shafei MZ, Endrys G, Khan N, Simo M, Cherian G. Tricuspid stenosis and regurgitation in rheumatic heart disease: a prospective cardiac catheterization study in 525 patients. *Am Heart J*. 1985;110(1 Pt 1):60–64.
55. Perez JE, Ludbrook PA, Ahumada GG. Usefulness of Doppler echocardiography in detecting tricuspid valve stenosis. *Am J Cardiol*. 1985;55(5):601–603.
56. Baumgartner H, Falk V, Bax JJ, et al. 2017 ESC/EACTS guidelines for the management of valvular heart disease. *Eur Heart J*. 2017;38(36):2739–2791.
57. Baumgartner H, Bonhoeffer P, De Groot NM, et al. ESC guidelines for the management of grown-up congenital heart disease (new version 2010). *Eur Heart J*. 2010;31(23):2915–2957.
58. Stout KK, Daniels CJ, Aboulhosn JA, et al. 2018 AHA/ACC guideline for the management of adults with congenital heart disease: a report of the American College of Cardiology/American Heart Association Task Force on Clinical Practice Guidelines. *J Am Coll Cardiol*. 2019;73(12):e81–e192.
59. Silvilairat S, Cabalka AK, Cetta F, Hagler DJ, O'Leary PW. Echocardiographic assessment of isolated pulmonary valve stenosis: which outpatient Doppler gradient has the most clinical validity? *J Am Soc Echocardiogr*. 2005;18(11):1137–1142.
60. Hayes CJ, Gersony WM, Driscoll DJ, et al. Second natural history study of congenital heart defects. Results of treatment of patients with pulmonary valvar stenosis. *Circulation*. 1993;87(2 Suppl):I28–I37.
61. Rao PS. Percutaneous balloon pulmonary valvuloplasty: state of the art. *Catheter Cardiovasc Interv*. 2007;69(5):747–763.
62. Taggart NW, Cetta F, Cabalka AK, Hagler DJ. Outcomes for balloon pulmonary valvuloplasty in adults: comparison with a concurrent pediatric cohort. *Catheter Cardiovasc Interv*. 2013;82(5):811–815.
63. Garty Y, Veldtman G, Lee K, Benson L. Late outcomes after pulmonary valve balloon dilatation in neonates, infants and children. *J Invasive Cardiol*. 2005;17(6):318–322.
64. Voet A, Rega F, de Bruaene AV, et al. Long-term outcome after treatment of isolated pulmonary valve stenosis. *Int J Cardiol*. 2012;156(1):11–15.
65. Choong CY, Abascal VM, Weyman J, et al. Prevalence of valvular regurgitation by Doppler echocardiography in patients with structurally normal hearts by two-dimensional echocardiography. *Am Heart J*. 1989;117(3):636–642.
66. Prieto-Arevalo R, Munoz P, Cuerpo G, et al. Pulmonary infective endocarditis. *J Am Coll Cardiol*. 2019;73(21):2782–2784.
67. Reisenauer JS, Said SM, Schaff HV, Connolly HM, Maleszewski JJ, Dearani JA. Outcome of surgical repair of pulmonary artery aneurysms: a single-center experience with 38 patients. *Ann Thorac Surg*. 2017;104(5):1605–1610.
68. Egbe AC, Miranda WR, Said SM, et al. Risk stratification and clinical outcomes after surgical pulmonary valve replacement. *Am Heart J*. 2018;206:105–112.
69. Jones TK, Rome JJ, Armstrong AK, et al. Transcatheter pulmonary valve replacement reduces tricuspid regurgitation in patients with right ventricular volume/pressure overload. *J Am Coll Cardiol*. 2016;68(14):1525–1535.
70. Miranda WR, Connolly HM, DeSimone DC, et al. Infective endocarditis involving the pulmonary valve. *Am J Cardiol*. 2015;116(12):1928–1931.
71. Zoghbi WA, Adams D, Bonow RO, et al. Recommendations for noninvasive evaluation of native valvular regurgitation: a report from the American Society of Echocardiography developed in collaboration with the Society for Cardiovascular Magnetic Resonance. *J Am Soc Echocardiogr*. 2017;30(4):303–371.
72. Puchalski MD, Askovich B, Sower CT, Williams RV, Minich LL, Tani LY. Pulmonary regurgitation: determining severity by echocardiography and magnetic resonance imaging. *Congenit Heart Dis*. 2008;3(3):168–175.

73. Renella P, Aboulhosn J, Lohan DG, et al. Two-dimensional and Doppler echocardiography reliably predict severe pulmonary regurgitation as quantified by cardiac magnetic resonance. *J Am Soc Echocardiogr*. 2010;23(8):880–886.
74. Takao S, Miyatake K, Izumi S, et al. Clinical implications of pulmonary regurgitation in healthy individuals: detection by cross sectional pulsed Doppler echocardiography. *Br Heart J*. 1988;59(5):542–550.
75. Silversides CK, Veldtman GR, Crossin J, et al. Pressure half-time predicts hemodynamically significant pulmonary regurgitation in adult patients with repaired tetralogy of fallot. *J Am Soc Echocardiogr*. 2003;16(10):1057–1062.
76. Van Berendoncks A, Van Grootel R, McGhie J, et al. Echocardiographic parameters of severe pulmonary regurgitation after surgical repair of tetralogy of Fallot. *Congenit Heart Dis*. 2019;14(4):628–637.
77. Lee C, Kim YM, Lee CH, et al. Outcomes of pulmonary valve replacement in 170 patients with chronic pulmonary regurgitation after relief of right ventricular outflow tract obstruction: implications for optimal timing of pulmonary valve replacement. *J Am Coll Cardiol*. 2012;60(11):1005–1014.
78. Oosterhof T, van Straten A, Vliegen HW, et al. Preoperative thresholds for pulmonary valve replacement in patients with corrected tetralogy of Fallot using cardiovascular magnetic resonance. *Circulation*. 2007;116(5):545–551.

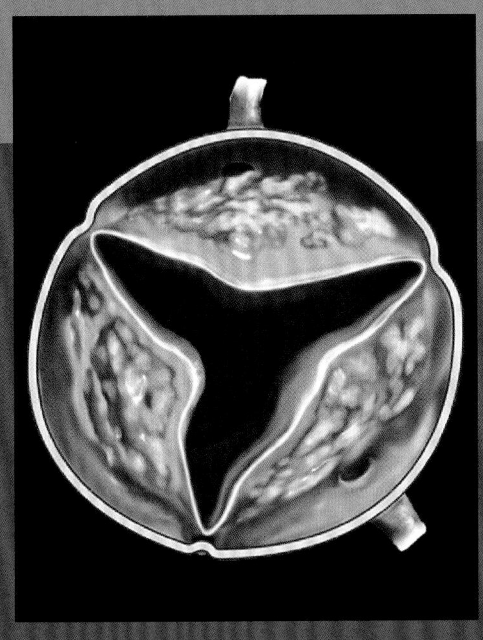

中文导读

第29章 感染性心内膜炎

感染性心内膜炎是心内膜和心脏瓣膜的非传染性感染疾病，发病率为2.6～11.6例／100万例。好发年龄为60岁左右，男女比例约为2：1。感染性心内膜炎的主要诱因是潜在的退行性瓣膜病，致病菌最常见的是金黄色葡萄球菌。随着二维超声心动图和经食管超声心动图的广泛应用，超声心动图已成为所有疑似感染性心内膜炎患者的首选诊断方式。

本章主要介绍了感染性心内膜炎的Duke诊断标准、感染性心内膜炎经胸超声心动图表现及临床意义、ACC/AHA提出关于经食管超声心动图对已知或可疑感染性心内膜炎的实践指南和诊断标准，以及外科手术适应证。经食管超声心动图分辨率高，图像显示更清晰，可以发现更细小的赘生物（<2 mm）。对于有心脏起搏器置入的患者，经食管超声心动图优于经胸超声心动图。如果临床怀疑感染性心内膜炎或其并发症发生率很高时（如人工心脏瓣膜或新发的房室传导阻滞），经胸超声心动图结果阴性不能排除感染性心内膜炎或其可能的并发症，应首选经食管超声心动图，其对赘生物和瓣周脓肿的检出具有更高的灵敏度。实时三维经食管超声心动图能精确地确定解剖结构，以及赘生物特征和位置。

本章同时介绍了不同心脏成像模式在诊断感染性心内膜炎中的价值，对于感染性心内膜炎的心内膜受累或并发症的显示，超声心动图的临床价值不可替代。

刘思岐

29 Endocarditis

ZAINAB SAMAD, MD | ANDREW WANG, MD

Infective endocarditis (IE), a noncontagious infection of the endocardium and heart valves, has an incidence of 2.6 to 11.6 cases per 1 million people.[1] The high in-hospital mortality rate remains approximately 20% despite medical and surgical advances.

The contemporary epidemiology of IE, particularly host and microbiologic characteristics, has changed compared with earlier eras, and these changes have an important influence on the evaluation and outcome of this condition. In the large, prospective, multinational International Collaboration on Endocarditis (ICE) registry, the age at diagnosis of definite IE is in the sixth decade, with an approximately 2:1 male predominance. It often occurs in the setting of comorbid conditions such as kidney disease and diabetes mellitus.[2]

The major predisposition for IE is underlying degenerative valvular disease (particularly mitral valve disease), which occurs in approximately 30% of cases, but there is a very low prevalence of underlying rheumatic heart disease.[2] The microbiology of the condition has shifted toward more virulent organisms, particularly to *Staphylococcus aureus* as the most common cause, which reflects the growing influence of health care–associated infection as a cause of bacteremia.

Diagnosis and management of IE has greatly improved with the advent of echocardiography. The first diagnostic use of echocardiography was described in 1973 by Dillon et al.,[3] who applied M-mode echocardiography to visualize vegetations. The high-frequency oscillations of vegetative lesions and destruction of aortic or mitral leaflet integrity could be documented using this technique (Fig. 29.1). M-mode, however, did not allow estimation of lesion size, morphology, and localization of specific leaflet involvement, information that was provided by the real-time, two-dimensional (2D) echocardiography first described by Gilbert et al.[4]

Over time, with the widespread use of 2D echocardiography and the improved spatial resolution offered by transesophageal echocardiography (TEE),[5] it has become the diagnostic modality of choice in all cases with suspected IE. Echocardiography provides noninvasive evidence of endocardial infection and offers important hemodynamic information regarding the presence and severity of valvular regurgitation and other structural complications, findings that are key to clinical management. For these reasons, echocardiography is considered essential in all suspected cases of IE.[6]

BASIC PRINCIPLES AND ECHOCARDIOGRAPHIC APPROACH

Clinical characteristics may identify the host at risk for IE and guide the use of echocardiography for diagnostic confirmation. IE is associated with fever in more than 90% of cases, and a similar percentage of patients have positive blood cultures for an associated microorganism.[2] Most patients present for evaluation after a symptom duration of less than 1 month.[2] Approximately 50% of patients show evidence of a new or changing heart murmur, reflecting valvular regurgitation or other endocardial damage, but a few have peripheral manifestations of classic, subacute IE (e.g., Osler nodes, Janeway lesions, splinter hemorrhages, Roth spots).[2]

The association between infective lesions on the endocardium and the clinical manifestations of IE has been recognized for more than a century. However, the clinical manifestations of the disease remained nonspecific and challenged accurate clinical diagnosis of the disease antemortem.[7] In 1977, Pelletier and Petersdorf proposed case definitions for IE that relied mainly on clinical characteristics and specifically on the demonstration of continuous bacteremia.[8] Although the case definitions provided a first step in standardization of the diagnosis of IE, the criteria were highly specific but lacked sensitivity. In 1981, von Reyn et al. expanded the clinical criteria and offered levels of diagnostic certainty (i.e., rejected, possible, probable, and definite) for suspected IE.[9] These modifications improved sensitivity and specificity, but they did not incorporate evidence of endocardial involvement by application of echocardiography, which was relatively novel at the time.

In 1994, the Duke criteria proposed by Durack et al.[10] incorporated visualization of endocardial involvement by echocardiography with microbiologic and clinical criteria for the first time. Evidence of endocardial involvement, which was visualized as new valvular regurgitation, intracardiac vegetation, periannular abscess, or new dehiscence of a prosthetic valve, became one of the two major diagnostic criteria for IE by the Duke case definition, along with microbiologic criteria. Several

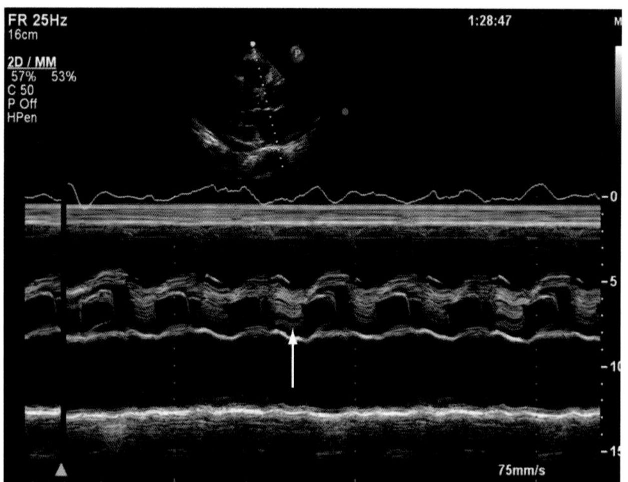

Fig. 29.1 M-mode echocardiography of aortic valve vegetation. The M-mode echocardiogram shows a mass of shaggy echoes suggesting a vegetation *(arrow)* in diastole in a patient with aortic valve endocarditis.

studies comparing the von Reyn and Duke criteria in various cohorts established the superior sensitivity of the Duke criteria compared with earlier case definitions.[11–18] The negative predictive value of these criteria was greater than 92%, with a high sensitivity (100%) and high specificity (88%).[19,20] Subsequent modifications of the Duke criteria (Table 29.1) have added greater specificity.[21]

TECHNICAL DETAILS, QUANTITATION, AND DATA ANALYSIS

Echocardiographic features of IE include vegetation, abscess, aneurysm, fistula, leaflet perforation, and valvular dehiscence (Table 29.2).[22] *Vegetations* occur at a region of endocardial denudation that often results from preexisting valvular disease (Figs. 29.2 and 29.3). Disruption of the endocardial surface results in platelet adhesion and fibrin deposition, to which microorganisms adhere during transient bacteremia to form an infected vegetation.

Vegetations are visualized in almost 90% of patients with definite IE.[2] Using echocardiography, vegetations appear as irregularly shaped, discrete, oscillating, echogenic masses that are adherent to valves, chordae, or other endocardial surfaces in the path of turbulent jets passing through regurgitant valves or septal defects. They are typically located on the low-pressure side of high-velocity jets, and in cases of regurgitation, they are located on the atrial aspect of the mitral and tricuspid valves or on the ventricular aspect of the aortic and pulmonic valves. They often display the same echogenicity as mid-myocardial structures and may be heterogeneous with echodense or echolucent areas. Vegetations may also be found on noncardiac structures such as intracardiac devices. In the setting of a vegetation, *perforation* of a valve leaflet may be visualized as a defect in the body of a valve leaflet along with evidence of flow through the defect (Fig. 29.4).

Machine settings such as frame rate, sector arc size, gray scale, and focal zones must be optimized, and a careful examination that includes nonstandard views should be conducted to exclude the possibility of vegetations. Increased gain settings and improper focal zones can make vegetations appear larger than their actual size. Color-flow Doppler imaging may change pulse repetition frequency and impair visualization of

TABLE 29.1 The Modified Duke Criteria and Case Definitions of Infective Endocarditis.

Modified Duke Criteria	*Case Definitions*
Major Criteria	**Definitive Infective Endocarditis**
Blood Culture Positive for IE	*Pathologic Criteria*
Typical microbes consistent with IE from 2 separate blood cultures: viridans group streptococci, *Streptococcus bovis*, HACEK group, *Staphylococcus aureus*; community-acquired enterococci in the absence of another focus *or* microrganisms consistent with IE from persistently positive blood cultures, defined as at least 2 blood cultures drawn > 12 hours apart or all of 3 or a majority of 4 or more separate blood cultures.	1. Microorganisms demonstrated by culture or histologic examination of a vegetation, a vegetation that has embolized, or an intracardiac abscess specimen *or* 2. Pathologic lesions; vegetation or intracardiac abscess confirmed by histologic examination that shows active endocarditis
Single positive blood culture for *Coxiella burnetti* or antiphase IgG antibody titer > 1:800	*Clinical Criteria* 1. 2 major criteria *or* 2. 1 major and 3 minor criteria *or* 3. 5 minor criteria
Evidence of Endocardial Involvement	
Echo-positive for IE, defined as follows: - Oscillating intracardiac mass on valve or supporting structure - Abscess - New partial dehiscence of prosthetic valve - New valvular regurgitation	
Minor Criteria	
Predisposition; predisposing heart condition or injection drug use	
Fever, temperature > 38°C	
Vascular phenomena, major arterial emboli, septic pulmonary infarctions, mycotic aneurysm, intracranial hemorrhage, conjunctival hemorrhage, and Janeway lesions	
Immunologic phenomena: glomerulonephritis, Osler nodes, Roth spots, rheumatoid factor	
Microbiologic evidence: blood cultures positive but do not meet a major criterion as noted above, or serologic evidence of active infection with an organism that causes IE	

IE, Infective endocarditis; *HACEK*, group of gram-negative bacteria that include *Haemophilus*, *Aggregatibacter* (previously *Actinobacillus*), *Cardiobacterium*, *Eikenella*, and *Kingella*; *IgG*, immunoglobulin G.
Data from Li JS, Sexton DJ, Mick N, et al. Proposed modifications to the Duke criteria for the diagnosis of infective endocarditis. *Clin Infect Dis*. 2000;30:633–638.

the vegetation. The size of the vegetations should be measured within the resolution characteristics of the transducer so that machine settings can be duplicated for future comparative studies if clinically indicated.

Vegetations need to be differentiated from other masses with a similar appearance on echocardiography such as Libman–Sacks endocarditis (i.e., noninfective or nonbacterial thrombotic endocarditis [NBTE]), degenerative change, Lambl excrescences, thrombus, or tumors. Because there are no echocardiographic features that can reliably differentiate infective from NBTE lesions, the key to a diagnosis lies in integrating imaging data and clinical information, particularly the microbiologic results. Visualization of a distinct vegetation may be impaired by severe underlying valvular degeneration, particularly a prominent calcification of valve leaflets.

Tissue destruction in IE may result in other structural complications that can be identified on echocardiography. *Paravalvular abscess* complicated 30% to 40% of IE cases in earlier reports,[5] and the lesion was found in 14% of patients with

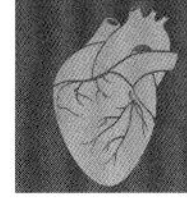

TABLE 29.2 Pathologic Features of Infective Endocarditis: Echocardiographic Appearance and Clinical Significance.

Finding	*Pathology*	*Appearance and Measurements*	*Pitfalls*	*Clinical Significance*
Vegetation	Collection of microorganisms embedded in platelets, fibrin, and other inflammatory cellular material adherent to an endothelial surface in the heart	Irregularly shaped, discrete echogenic mass Adherent to but distinct from cardiac surface Oscillation of mass is supportive but not mandatory Measure maximum size	*False negative:* Small size; sessile, not oscillating; degenerated valve; inappropriate gain setting *False positive:* Postoperative changes; valve calcification; Libman–Sacks disease; Lambl excrescence; thrombus; tumor	Size and location associated with embolic risk Large size can suggest lower likelihood of cure with antibiotics alone
Abscess	A cavity with purulent exudates formed by liquefactive necrosis	Thickened area or mass in the myocardium or annular region Appearance is nonhomogenous with echogenic and echolucent characteristics	*False negative:* Absence of flow; early in abscess formation; gain settings; posterior mitral valve annulus when calcification is present *False positive:* Postoperative change after valve replacement, including paravalvular regurgitation; gain settings	Possibly associated with new conduction abnormality Indication for surgery
Fistula	Abnormal connection between two distinct cardiac blood spaces through a nonanatomic channel	Left-to-right shunt visible on color Doppler imaging Recorded loops should contain sweeps of the region of interest CW Doppler to show high-velocity jet across defect	*False negative:* Small defect; masking by valvular regurgitation or flow turbulence *False positive:* Valvular regurgitation or other turbulent flow; no confirmation by high Doppler jet velocity across defect	Heart failure due to left-to-right shunting Indication for surgery
Leaflet perforation	Defect in body of a valve leaflet with evidence of flow through the defect	Color Doppler to document regurgitant flow through perforation Multiple views to differentiate perforation from leaflet regurgitation 3DE may help locate precise location preoperatively Quantify regurgitation	*False negative:* High gain setting; small defect; regurgitant jet masks flow through perforation *False positive:* Echo dropout; commissure or cleft	Increases severity of regurgitation and possibility of heart failure
Prosthetic valve dehiscence	Rocking motion of prosthetic valve with excursion > 15 degrees in at least one direction	Regurgitant jets visible by color Doppler imaging Quantify regurgitation	*False negative:* No paravalvular regurgitation visualized *False positive:* Normal annulus motion during cardiac cycle	Paravalvular regurgitation may result in heart failure, hemolysis Urgent indication for surgery
Cardiac implantable electronic device infection	Mobile mass seen on intracardiac device (lead) in setting of fever, bacteremia, and/or embolic events	Vegetation seen adherent to device lead Careful search for vegetations throughout intracardiac course of device Evaluate for concomitant valve infection	*False negative:* Vegetation on extracardiac region of device *False positive:* Thrombus	Usually treated with device extraction plus antibiotic therapy

3DE, Three-dimensional echocardiography.

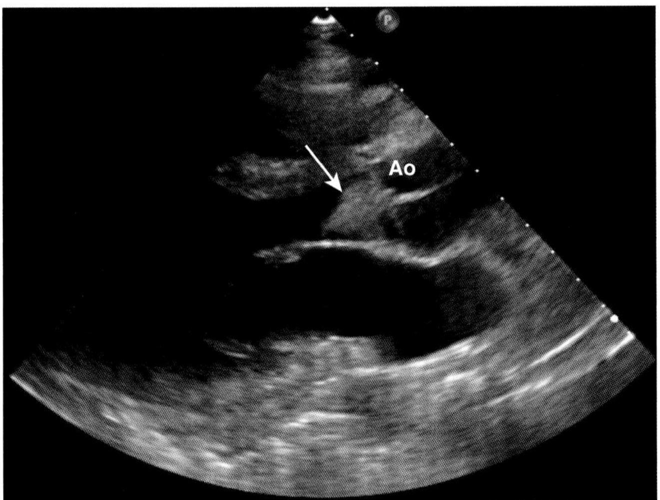

Fig. 29.2 2D TTE of an aortic valve vegetation. In the parasternal long-axis view, a heterogeneous, irregularly shaped mass *(arrow)* is attached to the aortic *(Ao)* valve noncoronary leaflet that is prolapsing into the LV outflow tract (see Video 29.2).

definite IE in a larger, more recent study.[2] An abscess results from an invasive infection that typically spreads along contiguous tissue planes, particularly in cases of aortic valve infection. Development of a new atrioventricular conduction abnormality, a worsening clinical picture, persistent bacteremia or fever in the setting of aortic valve endocarditis, injection drug use, infection with an invasive pathogen (staphylococcal), and prosthetic valves should prompt a search for an aortic root abscess.[23]

TEE is the diagnostic tool of choice when an abscess is suspected clinically. An abscess is diagnosed by TEE as the visualization of a thickened area or mass with a heterogeneous echogenic or echolucent appearance within the myocardium or annular region[5] (Fig. 29.5). On color Doppler imaging, flow within the area supports the diagnosis (Fig. 29.6). Abscesses complicating native valve IE most commonly involve the aortic valve annulus at the junction of the aortic root and anterior mitral valve leaflet. They may extend into the adjacent interventricular septum, right ventricular (RV) outflow tract, interatrial septum, or anterior mitral valve leaflet. Location of the abscess, particularly in the posterior annulus of the mitral valve when there is calcification, may limit visualization by echocardiography.[24]

In the ICE cohort, 22% of cases of definite aortic valve IE were complicated by a periannular abscess.[23] These patients were more likely to have prosthetic valves and coagulase-negative staphylococcal infections. Surgical experience suggests an even higher prevalence of abscess formation that is not visualized by TEE.[24] New paravalvular regurgitation around a prosthetic valve may also suggest an abscess or infected sewing ring of the prosthesis. Because mild paravalvular regurgitation is more common after transcatheter aortic valve replacement (TAVR) than after surgical aortic valve replacement, the extent

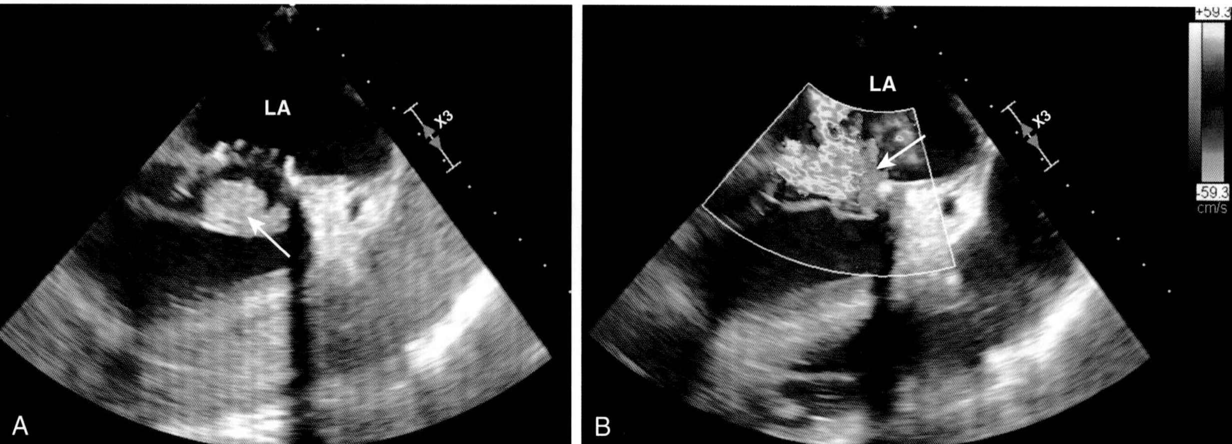

Fig. 29.3 2D TEE of a mitral valve vegetation. (A) On the long-axis TEE view, the mitral valve vegetation *(arrow)* is seen as a large heterogeneous mass on the anterior leaflet. There is a mitral valve annuloplasty ring from a previous mitral valve repair (see Video 29.3A ▶). (B) In the same long-axis TEE view during systole with color Doppler, the mitral valve vegetation *(arrow)* prolapses back into the LA, and a severe, wide jet of mitral valve regurgitation is seen (see Video 29.3B ▶).

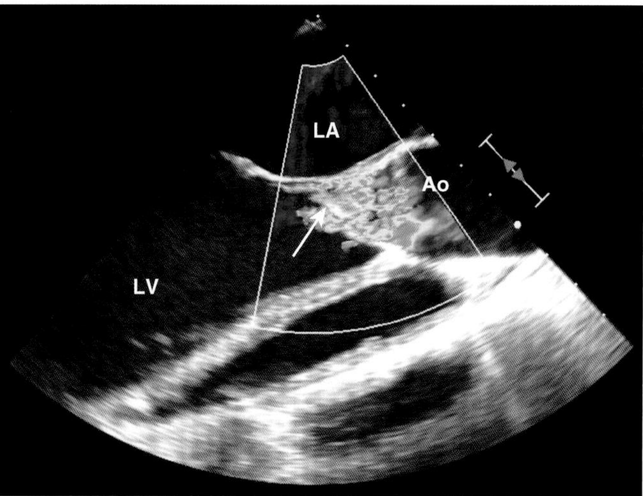

Fig. 29.4 2D TEE with color Doppler of an aortic valve perforation. On the long-axis TEE view, color Doppler shows multiple origins of aortic regurgitant jets, including through an aortic valve leaflet *(Ao)* with a large vegetation *(arrow)* prolapsing into the LV outflow tract (see Video 29.4 ▶).

and size of the regurgitant orifice should be compared with postimplantation imaging.

If an abscess is identified, a careful examination is required to rule out extension into adjacent areas because this additional information has considerable implications for the type of reparative surgery to be undertaken. Loss of structural integrity of the valve, valvular regurgitation and vegetations, and thickening of adjacent tissues help differentiate a native aortic valve abscess from fluid in the transverse pericardial sinus. These associated findings are also helpful in evaluating an abscess in patients with prosthetic valves in the aortic position. Postoperative changes, including an echolucent space between prosthetic valve sewing ring and the aortic root with or without paravalvular regurgitation, may pose a diagnostic dilemma for a patient with a prosthetic valve and fever. In this case, comparison with an intraoperative TEE, if available, may help in documenting the chronicity of the abnormality.

Interobserver variability in the identification of IE findings by TEE has been assessed. For most IE findings, including the identification and location of a vegetation, abscess, and leaflet perforation, interobserver variability was low (weighted kappa ≥ 0.8).[25] However, there was greater variability in evaluating characteristics of vegetations such as mobility (kappa = 0.72) and size (kappa = 0.74).[25]

In rare cases, exposure of abscesses to high intravascular pressures and progressive burrowing infection may lead to *pseudoaneurysm formation*; color-flow imaging demonstrates flow in an echolucent space that is contiguous with the bloodstream. Because of further tissue invasion, these paravalvular cavities or pseudoaneurysms can form aortoatrial or aortoventricular fistulous connections, leaflet perforations, and even myocardial perforations. *Fistula formation* complicated 1.6% cases of native valve IE and 3.5% cases of prosthetic valve endocarditis in a cohort of 4681 cases of definite IE[26] (Fig. 29.7). The fistulas occurred with similar frequency in each of the three sinuses of Valsalva. Fistulas from the right or noncoronary sinus usually track or exit into the RV, whereas fistulas from the left sinus exit to the LA.[27]

TEE is the modality of choice to investigate these structural complications. Color-flow Doppler imaging demonstrates flow turbulence, abnormal flow in echolucent spaces, and shunting of blood flow in cases of fistulous connections between cardiac chambers (see Fig. 29.7).

Progressive tissue destruction due to infection can also result in mitral chordal rupture in native valve IE and valve dehiscence in prosthetic valve endocarditis. *Valvular dehiscence* of a prosthetic valve is an uncommon but serious complication, and it portends a poor outcome for the patient. On echocardiography, valvular dehiscence is seen as a rocking motion of the prosthetic valve with excursion of 15 degrees or more in at least one direction (Fig. 29.8). This structural deterioration is often accompanied by severe paravalvular regurgitation.

In addition to these complications, it is important to recognize that new valvular regurgitation may represent endocardial infection and is a major diagnostic Duke criterion for IE. Determining the mechanism of regurgitation and quantifying its severity are important; severe regurgitation is poorly tolerated clinically due to an acute onset without time for ventricular compensation, and it is an indication for surgical intervention.

For patients with prosthetic valves, a complete examination requires a combination of TTE and TEE imaging modalities.

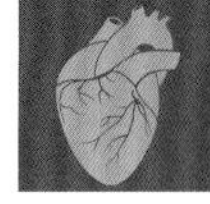

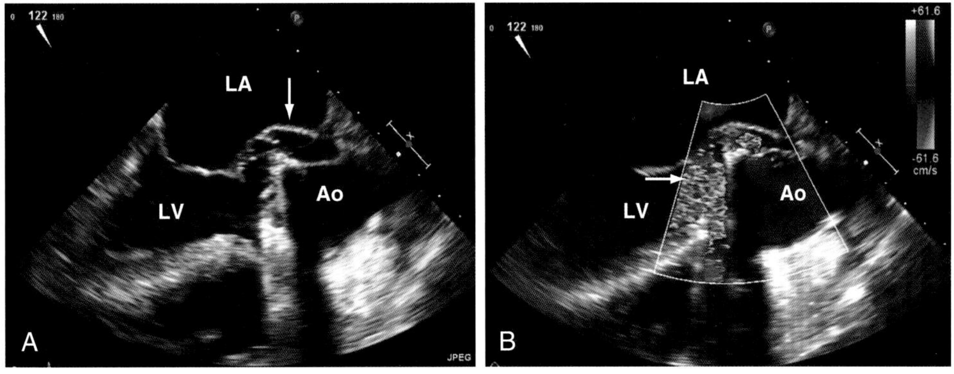

Fig. 29.5 Prosthetic valve paravalvular abscess. (A) 2D TEE long-axis view of a mechanical aortic *(Ao)* valve recorded in systole. Notice the large, echolucent space posterior to the valve *(arrow)*. (B) 2D color Doppler TEE image of the mechanical aortic valve demonstrates severe paravalvular regurgitation *(arrow)* due to valve dehiscence (see Video 29.5).

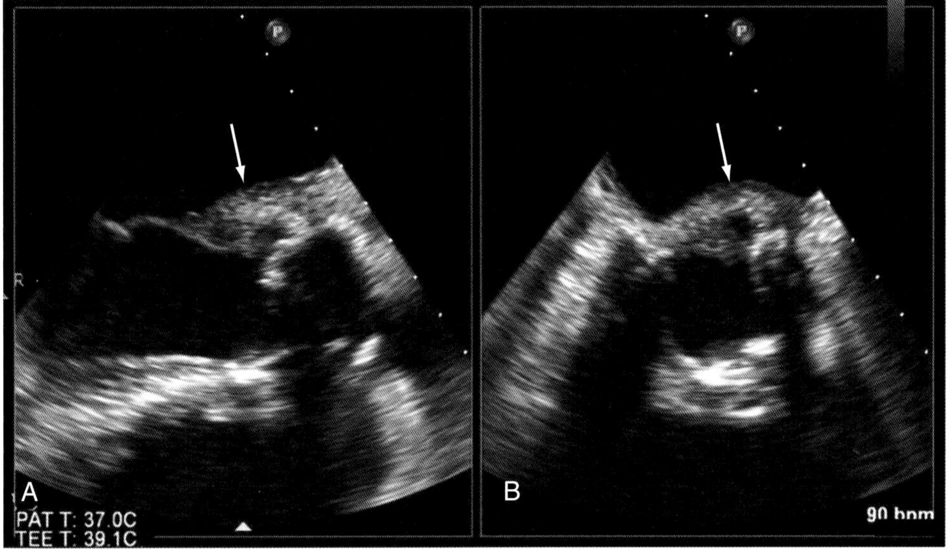

Fig. 29.6 Aortic root abscess. (A and B) 2D TEE orthogonal views of the aortic valve demonstrate thickening and heterogeneous echodensity *(arrows)* of the aortic annulus. This is most prominent at the junction of the anterior mitral valve leaflet and aortic valve.

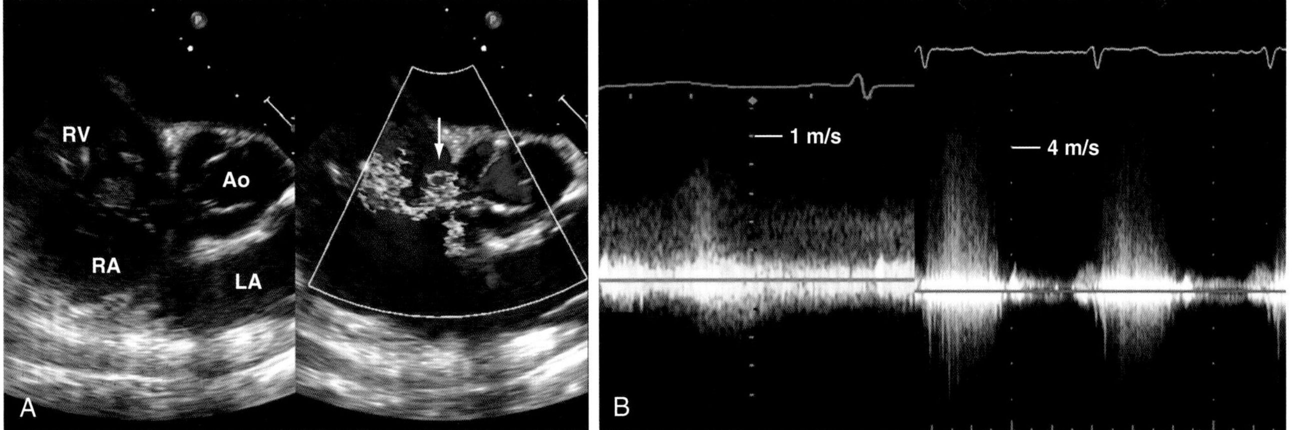

Fig. 29.7 Abscess with an aorta-to-RV fistula. (A) 2D *(left)* and color Doppler *(right)* TEE short-axis views of the aortic valve demonstrate a left-to-right shunt between the aorta *(Ao)* and the RV. Large vegetations are visible on the tricuspid valve *(arrow)*, and bright echoes of an intracardiac device are seen in the RA. (B) CW Doppler recordings demonstrate the difference in flow characteristics between an aorta-to-RV fistula *(left)*, which shows continuous systolic and diastolic flow, and a high-velocity systolic jet that is consistent with a perimembranous ventricular septal defect in a different patient *(right)*.

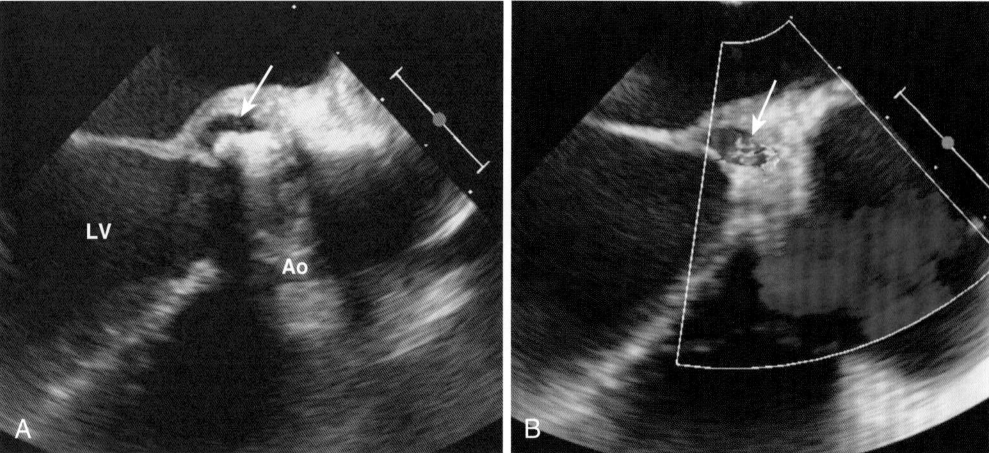

Fig. 29.8 Dehiscence of a prosthetic aortic valve replacement. (A) 2D long-axis TEE view shows the paravalvular echolucent space (*arrow*) posterior to the biologic prosthetic aortic valve replacement. The paravalvular abscess has led to partial dehiscence of the sewing ring from the aortic annulus (see Video 29.8A). (B) 2D long-axis TEE view with color Doppler demonstrates systolic flow into the area of annular dehiscence (*arrow*) of the prosthetic aortic valve (see Video 29.8B).

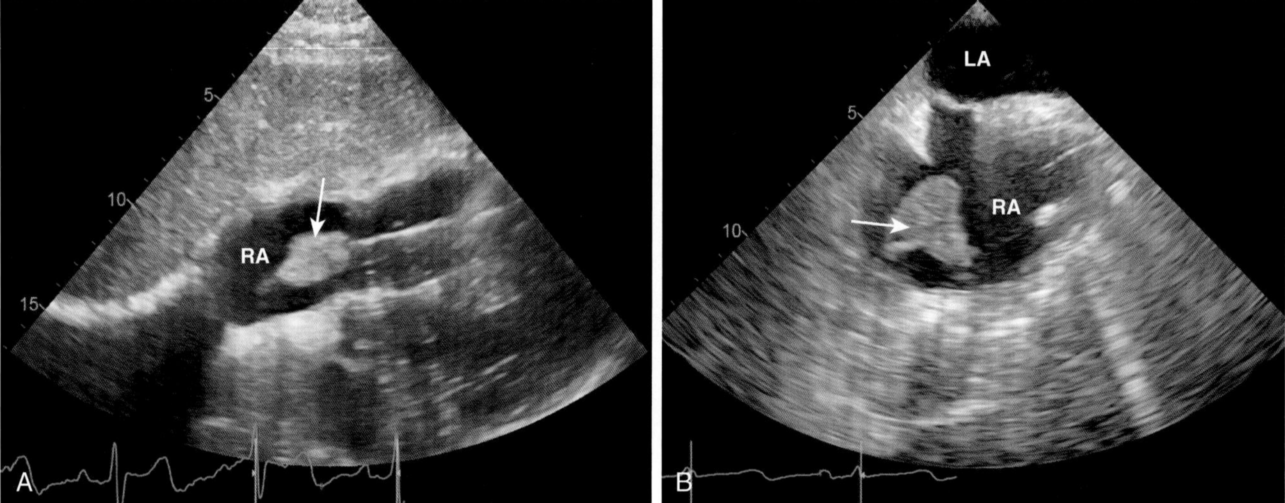

Fig. 29.9 Infected cardiac implantable electronic device lead. (A) 2D subcostal TTE view of an infected cardiac implantable electronic device (CIED) lead in the RA shows a large vegetation attached to the lead (*arrow*) (see Video 29.9A). (B) TEE short-axis view of an infected CIED shows a heterogeneous, irregular mass (*arrow*) attached to the intracardiac lead in the RA. The tricuspid valve is not involved (see Video 29.9B).

TTE allows visualization of the ventricular aspect of the valve but is limited for examining the atrial aspect because of beam attenuation and shadowing. For the same reason, assessment of valvular regurgitation in mitral and tricuspid valve prostheses is problematic with a TTE approach. Doppler echocardiography may be used to interrogate prosthetic valves for regurgitation using the velocity–time integral. TEE allows a much better assessment of valvular regurgitation and evaluation for vegetations on the atrial aspect of valve prostheses. For patients with TAVRs, the more extensive height of the stent frames and native leaflet and annular calcification may limit echocardiographic imaging.

In patients with cardiac implantable electronic devices (CIEDs), there is substantial artifact generation, and TEE is superior to TTE in cases of suspected CIED infection.[28-30] TEE visualization of the lead in the proximal superior vena cava may identify vegetations attached to CIED leads that are difficult to visualize by other modalities. During the examination, it is important to visualize the entire course of the prosthetic device throughout the vasculature and cardiac structures. Careful evaluation of the cardiac valves is also important because of the high rate of concomitant valve infection, particularly of the tricuspid valve (Fig. 29.9).

CLINICAL UTILITY AND OUTCOMES DATA

UTILITY IN DIAGNOSIS

General Considerations

The diagnostic yield of echocardiography depends on several variables, including the echocardiographic modality, vegetation size and location, native or prosthetic valve disease, valve calcification (which increases the sensitivity but reduces the specificity of identifying vegetations), and preexisting valvular degeneration. With TTE, in approximately 15% of cases, variations in sound transmission due to patient-related factors (e.g., obesity, lung disease, chest wall deformities) can limit diagnostic capability.

Although vegetations as small as 2 to 5 mm can be detected, the sensitivity of TTE is low (≈40%) for such small lesions.[31] The sensitivity of TTE is highest for tricuspid valve infection

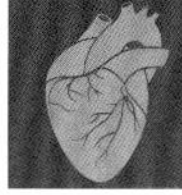

because of the proximity to the chest wall. In a study of injection drug users with suspected right-sided IE, TTE detected vegetations at the same rate as TEE; however, TEE was more effective in characterizing the vegetations.[32] The diagnostic utility of TTE for suspected IE is highest for patients with an intermediate to high likelihood of this disease[33] (e.g., patient with a new or changed heart murmur and bacteremia). The limited sensitivity of TTE for the visualization of an intracardiac vegetation or abscess precludes ruling out the diagnosis of IE based on a negative study result.

Despite its poor sensitivity, TTE is often performed as the initial diagnostic study to locate and evaluate valvular lesions and to determine ventricular function. The negative predictive value of TTE for the diagnosis of IE can be improved by adequate image quality and several criteria:

1. Absence of intracardiac catheters or other prosthetic material
2. No stenosis and no more than trivial regurgitation of cardiac valves
3. No morphologic abnormality of heart valves
4. No cardiac congenital abnormalities at the time of the initial examination and absence of pericardial effusion
5. No vegetations or mobile targets seen on TTE[34]

In a patient with a low pretest probability for IE and a normal TTE examination, a diagnosis other than IE should be pursued rather than proceeding to a TEE examination. TTE is also recommended for the reassessment of high-risk IE patients who develop clinical deterioration, persistent or recurrent fever, new murmur, persistent bacteremia, or recurrent embolic events.

Although TTE and TEE have concordant results for approximately one half of patients with suspected IE, TEE results in additional diagnostic information for a high percentage of these patients.[35] TEE has several major advantages over TTE for the assessment of IE, including better spatial resolution due to a higher-frequency transducer, lack of acoustic interference from adjacent structures such as the lungs and chest wall, and proximity to posterior structures such as the mitral valve and LA. TEE can detect vegetations as small as 1 to 2 mm and can detect vegetations of 2 to 5 mm with a sensitivity of almost 100%.[31] TEE should be performed for patients with a high clinical probability of IE and a negative TTE study.[36] An algorithm for the use of TTE and TEE in cases of suspected IE is shown in Fig. 29.10.

Specific subsets of patients for whom TEE should be performed, even as the primary imaging modality (without preceding TTE) for diagnosis of IE, include (1) those with prosthetic heart valves and suspected IE, (2) those with persistent staphylococcal or enterococcal bacteremia without a known source or with nosocomial staphylococcal bacteremia, and (3) those with suspected CIED infection. Evidence suggests that TEE is also better than TTE for diagnosing native pulmonic valve IE,[37] although it is the least commonly infected valve and is typically associated with congenital heart disease as a predisposing condition. For patients with suspected culture-negative IE (approximately 10% of all definite IE cases), TEE has higher sensitivity than TTE for visualizing diagnostic findings of endocardial involvement.[38]

Cost-effective analyses also support a diagnostic approach that uses echocardiography, particularly TEE. In cases of suspected IE, a diagnostic strategy that focuses on TEE as the initial imaging modality is more cost-effective than a staged procedure with TTE and is superior to empiric antibiotic therapy alone. In one study, TEE was optimal for patients who had a prior

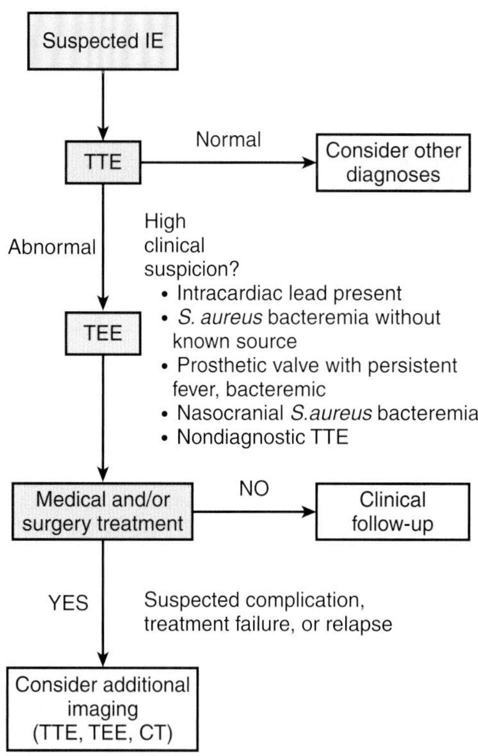

Fig. 29.10 Clinical applications of echocardiography. Echocardiography is used for the evaluation and management of infective endocarditis *(IE)*. *CT,* Computed tomography.

probability (4% to 60%) of IE, which is commonly observed in clinical practice, and the cost was modestly reduced compared with the use of TTE as the initial study.[39]

Appropriate use criteria for TTE and TEE in IE are shown in Tables 29.3 and 29.4. The utility of a diagnostic tool such as echocardiography is optimal in the appropriate clinical context or pretest probability of disease (i.e., >2% or 3%). Although there are few empiric data with which to quantify the pretest probability of disease, the general consensus is that certain characteristics increase the likelihood of disease (Table 29.5).

The literature suggests that imaging technologies such as echocardiography can be overused in certain clinical scenarios, such as the evaluation of suspected IE. Kurupuu et al. showed that 53% of echocardiograms could be avoided without loss of diagnostic accuracy by using an algorithm for patients with a low pretest probability of disease. Similarly, Greaves et al. showed that the absence of five clinical criteria was associated with a zero probability of a TTE demonstrating evidence of IE: (1) vasculitic or embolic phenomena, (2) central venous access, (3) recent history of injection drug use, (4) prosthetic heart valve, and (5) positive blood cultures.[40] Collectively, these studies have shown that for patients with a very low pretest probability of disease, echocardiography can be avoided without loss of diagnostic accuracy. The evaluation of possible IE in specific clinical scenarios is discussed next.

Evaluation of the Patient With Bacteremia

The clinical history of IE depends on the causative organism and the presence or absence of predisposing factors. Early suspicion is essential for an early diagnosis. A history of predisposing factors, including prosthetic valves, a previous episode of endocarditis, congenital heart disease, and heart failure or other

TABLE 29.3 ACC/AHA Practice Guidelines and Appropriateness Criteria for TTE in Known or Suspected Infective Endocarditis.

Indications	*Level of Evidence*
Class I: TTE should be performed in all cases of suspected IE.	B
Class IIa: TTE at the time of antimicrobial therapy completion to establish baseline features is reasonable.	C
Appropriateness Criteria	*Appropriateness Score (1–9)*
Initial evaluation of suspected IE with positive blood cultures or a new murmur	A (9)
Transient fever without evidence of bacteremia or a new murmur	I (2)
Transient bacteremia with a pathogen not typically associated with IE and/or a documented nonendovascular source of infection	I (3)
Re-evaluation of IE at high risk for progression or complication or with a change in clinical status or cardiac examination	A (9)
Routine surveillance of uncomplicated IE when no change in management is contemplated	I (2)

A, Appropriate use; *ACC*, American College of Cardiology; *AHA*, American Heart Association; *I*, inappropriate use; *IE*, infective endocarditis.
Data from Baddour LM, Wilson WR, Bayer AS, et al. Infective endocarditis in adults: diagnosis, antimicrobial therapy, and management of complications: a scientific statement for healthcare professionals from the American Heart Association. *Circulation.* 2015;132:1435–1486; Douglas PS, Garcia MJ, Haines DE, et al. 2011 Appropriate use criteria for echocardiography: a report of the American College of Cardiology Foundation Appropriate Use Criteria Task Force, American Society of Echocardiography, American Heart Association, American Society of Nuclear Cardiology, Heart Failure Society of America, Heart Rhythm Society, Society for Cardiovascular Angiography and Interventions, Society of Critical Care Medicine, Society of Cardiovascular Computed Tomography, and Society for Cardiovascular Magnetic Resonance. *J Am Coll Cardiol.* 2011:57:1126–1166.

stigmata of endocarditis with fever lasting longer than 72 hours, should prompt a search for the diagnosis with blood cultures and imaging.

Bacteremia with typical organisms, including viridans group streptococci, *Streptococcus bovis*, HACEK group organisms (i.e., gram-negative bacteria that include *Haemophilus*, *Aggregatibacter* [previously *Actinobacillus*], *Cardiobacterium*, *Eikenella*, and *Kingella*), *S. aureus,* and community-acquired enterococci, in the absence of a primary focus constitutes a major criterion for IE. Bacteremia with typical organisms should be investigated for endocardial involvement with TTE. If the TTE result is technically inadequate, nondiagnostic, or negative, a TEE study should be obtained.

S. aureus bacteremia of any origin or in any setting is a risk factor for IE, and the diagnosis should be ruled out by careful clinical evaluation and diagnostic testing. With a virulent organism such as *S. aureus,* which is capable of causing IE on apparently normal cardiac valves, the incidence of IE is high (≈30%).[41,42] Among 59 prospectively identified patients with *S. aureus* IE, the presumed source of the bacteremia was an intravascular catheter in 39%. Similarly, in a prospectively identified cohort of 922 patients with definite IE from 39 sites in 16 countries, *S. aureus* was the most common cause of IE, accounting for 35.7% of all cases, and it was associated with a presumed intravascular catheter source in 39%.[43,44] These studies underscore the association between catheter-associated bacteremia and IE.

Sohail et al. proposed a two-stage algorithm with which to evaluate *S. aureus* bacteremia with TEE using a clinical score at day 1 and day 5. On day 1, a score of 4 or greater (i.e., community-acquired *S. aureus* bacteremia with an intracardiac

TABLE 29.4 ACC/AHA Practice Guidelines and Appropriateness Criteria for TEE in Known or Suspected Infective Endocarditis.

Class I Indications	*Level of Evidence*
TEE should be done if initial TTE results are negative or inadequate for patients for whom there is an ongoing suspicion of IE or when there is concern about intracardiac complications in patients with an initial positive TTE study.	B
If there is a strong suspicion of IE despite an initial negative TEE study, a repeat TEE is recommended in 3 to 5 days, or sooner if clinical findings change.	B
Repeat TEE should be done after an initially positive TEE study if clinical features suggest new development of intracardiac complications.	B
Appropriateness Criteria	*Appropriateness Score (1–9)*
Evaluation of valvular structure and function to assess suitability for, and assist in planning of, an intervention	A (9)
To diagnose IE with a low pretest probability (e.g., transient fever, known alternative source of infection, or negative blood cultures or atypical pathogen for endocarditis)	I (3)
To diagnose IE with a moderate or high pretest probability (e.g., *Staphyloccus* bacteremia, fungemia, prosthetic heart valve, intracardiac device)	A (9)

A, Appropriate use; *ACC*, American College of Cardiology; *AHA*, American Heart Association; *I*, inappropriate use; *IE*, infective endocarditis.
Data from Baddour LM, Wilson WR, Bayer AS, et al. Infective endocarditis in adults: diagnosis, antimicrobial therapy, and management of complications: a scientific statement for healthcare professionals from the American Heart Association. *Circulation.* 2015;132:1435–1486; Douglas PS, Garcia MJ, Haines DE, et al. 2011 Appropriate use criteria for echocardiography: a report of the American College of Cardiology Foundation Appropriate Use Criteria Task Force, American Society of Echocardiography, American Heart Association, American Society of Nuclear Cardiology, Heart Failure Society of America, Heart Rhythm Society, Society for Cardiovascular Angiography and Interventions, Society of Critical Care Medicine, Society of Cardiovascular Computed Tomography, and Society for Cardiovascular Magnetic Resonance. *J Am Coll Cardiol.* 2011:57:1126–1166.

TABLE 29.5 Pretest Probability Estimates for Infective Endocarditis According to Patient Characteristics.

Clinical Feature	*Pretest Probability Estimate*
Viridans group streptococcal bacteremia	14% (95% CI: 6 %–22%)
Unexplained bacteremia	5%–40%
Bacteremia and recent injection drug use	31% (95% CI: 19%–44%)
Admission with fever and recent injection drug use	13% (95% CI: 7%–19%)
Persistently positive blood cultures and predisposing heart disease	>50%
Persistently positive blood cultures and a new regurgitant murmur	>90%
Enterococcus faecalis bacteremia	26.1% (95% CI: 21.5%–30.7%)
Collective absence of the following: vasculitic or embolic phenomena, central venous access, recent history of injection drug use, a prosthetic valve, and positive blood cultures	0%
Firm alternative diagnosis or resolution of endocarditis syndrome within 4 days	<2%
Gram-negative bacteremia with clear noncardiac source of infection	<2%

Data from Heidenreich PA, Masoudi FA, Maini B, et al. Echocardiography in patients with suspected endocarditis: a cost-effectiveness analysis. *Am J Med.* 1999;107:198–208; Greaves K, Mou D, Patel A, Celermajer DS. Clinical criteria and the appropriate use of transthoracic echocardiography for the exclusion of infective endocarditis. *Heart.* 2003;89:273–275; Dahl, A, Iverson, K, Tonder N, et al. Prevalence of infective endocarditis in *Enterococcus faecalis* bacteremia. *J Am Coll Cardiol.* 2019;74:193–201.

prosthesis *or* health care–associated *S. aureus* bacteremia plus a CIED) in the model had a low sensitivity (21%) but high specificity (96%), and TEE was recommended to optimize sensitivity. In contrast, on day 5, a score of less than 2 (i.e., health care–associated or nosocomial *S. aureus* bacteremia without an intracardiac prosthesis and bacteremia for < 72 hours) was associated with a higher sensitivity (98.8%) and a negative predictive value of 98.5%, suggesting that TEE could be deferred.[45] When there is low clinical suspicion and blood culture data suggest skin contaminants (e.g., coagulase-negative *Staphylococcus*), a technically adequate TTE should be sufficient to exclude IE, and other diagnoses should be considered.

Similarly, in a study of 344 consecutive patients with *Enterococcus faecalis* bacteremia examined with echocardiography (TEE in 74% of cases), definite IE was identified in 90 patients (26%). Risk factors for IE were a prosthetic heart valve, community acquisition, unknown portal of entry, three or more positive blood cultures, and immunosuppression.[46]

Evaluation of the Patient With Prosthetic Valves

Prosthetic valves are a predisposing factor for IE and inevitably place the patient in a high-risk group. Although prosthetic valve endocarditis was previously thought to account for only 1% to 5% of all IE cases, a prospective, multinational, observational cohort study showed that approximately 20% of 2670 patients with IE had definite PVE. Compared with native valve IE, the in-hospital mortality rate was high (23%) for this group of patients despite similar rates of complications and surgical intervention as other patient groups.[47]

After TAVR, a large, multicenter registry comprising 7944 patients reported a 0.67% incidence of IE (0.50% within the first year).[48] When TAVR was compared with surgical aortic valve replacement, the incidence of IE is similar for these two treatments at approximately 1% per year but onset occurred earlier after TAVR.[49] Important differences exist in the echocardiographic findings of TAVR IE compared with surgical prosthetic IE, including a much lower percentage of vegetations visualized (<50%), a higher percentage of negative TEE studies, and more subtle changes including TAVR leaflet thickening and higher transvalvular gradients.[50–52]

Although cases of IE after percutaneous edge-to-edge repair using the MitraClip device (Abbott Vascular, Santa Clara, CA) are uncommon, most are caused by *S. aureus* infection soon after the procedure.[53] Even with surgical intervention performed in most cases, the mortality rate is very high (42%).[53]

These data emphasize the aggressive nature of PVE and underscore the need for an early diagnosis and intervention. Fever not otherwise explained in a patient with a prosthetic valve along with risk factors such as bacteremia and indwelling catheters should heighten clinical suspicion and prompt an aggressive search for IE. *S. aureus* is the most common causative organism in cases of PVE. Among patients with a prosthetic valve and *S. aureus* bacteremia, 50% were found to have endocarditis regardless of the time since prosthetic valve implantation.[54] Similarly, after TAVR, the most common causes of IE are staphylococcal and enterococcal organisms, particularly nosocomial acquisition. Risk factors for PVE include male sex, liver and renal disease, and a CIED.[49]

TEE is preferred for the evaluation of suspected prosthetic valve IE, and it has greater sensitivity for detecting vegetations than TTE.[55,56] Because of the greatly improved accuracy with TEE, it is recommended as a first-line diagnostic study to diagnose PVE and assess for complications.[57]

In a prospective study of 72 patients with suspected PVE who underwent clinical, microbiologic, and echocardiographic evaluation and cardiac ^{18}fluorodeoxyglucose positron emission tomography/computed tomography (FDG-PET/CT), abnormal FDG uptake was seen around the prosthetic valve in 50% of cases. The addition of abnormal FDG uptake at the site of the prosthetic valve as a novel major diagnostic criterion significantly increased the sensitivity of the modified Duke criteria established at admission from 70% to 97% for definite PVE due to a significant reduction in the number of possible PVE cases. FDG-PET/CT may prove to be a useful adjunctive test in suspected PVE.[58]

Echocardiographic differentiation of tissue degeneration from small vegetations is sometimes not possible, even with TEE. Periprosthetic strands, which can be observed during the early postoperative months, can cause false-positive interpretations.[59,60] After TAVR, the diastolic blood flow and thickened, calcified native valve leaflets in the sinuses of Valsalva may be difficult to differentiate from abscess, and paravalvular regurgitation occurs more frequently than after surgical aortic valve replacement (Fig. 29.11).

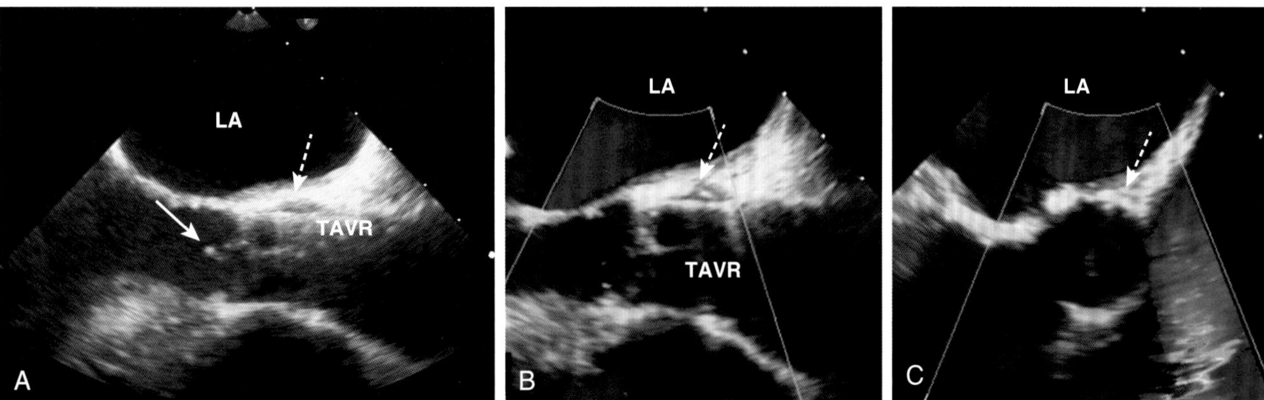

Fig. 29.11 Prosthetic valve infective endocarditis after transcatheter aortic valve replacement. (A) Long-axis TEE view of the transcatheter aortic valve replacement *(TAVR)* shows a small vegetation *(solid arrow)* on a leaflet prolapsing into the LV outflow tract. There is increased echocardiographic density and lucency *(dashed arrow)* posterior to the TAVR in the native sinus of Valsalva (see Video 29.11A). Long-axis (B) and short-axis (C) TEE views with color Doppler imaging of the TAVR show no diastolic flow in the paravalvular echolucent space posterior to the prosthetic valve *(dashed arrows)* (see Video 29.11B).

Evaluation of Patients With Cardiac Implantable Electronic Devices

An increase in the infection rate of cardiac devices (i.e., permanent pacemakers, implantable cardioverter-defibrillators, prosthetic heart valves or material, and ventricular assist devices) has been observed in recent years. Cabell et al. reported an increase from 0.94 to 2.11 cases per 1000 Medicare beneficiaries between 1990 and 1999.[61] The rate of native valve IE, however, remained stable over that period (0.26 to 0.36 cases per 1000 beneficiaries).

Imaging with echocardiography, particularly TEE, is essential for evaluating patients with suspected infection of a CIED.[28–30] TEE examination is particularly useful for patients with *S. aureus* bacteremia and a CIED because the rate of underlying IE is significant.[41,45]

Failure to visualize a mass adherent to a lead with TEE does not exclude lead infection.[29] Conversely, echocardiographic visualization of a mass adherent to a cardiac lead may indicate a thrombus or an infected vegetation. Because it is impossible to distinguish between these two entities by echocardiography alone, and recognizing that 5% of adherent masses were deemed thrombus in one retrospective survey,[62] careful clinical judgment must be employed for the diagnosis of CIED infection. Masses that are detected in patients without positive blood cultures (particularly staphylococcal) or other suggestive features for infection are likely to represent thrombus and, in isolation, may not require lead extraction or antibiotic treatment unless there is clinical suspicion of infection. Because of its poor sensitivity, TTE is less useful for ruling out the diagnosis of CIED infection, particularly in adults. Fig. 29.12 shows a suggested approach to the diagnosis and management of CIED infection using TEE.

UTILITY IN MANAGEMENT

Prompt diagnosis, initiation of appropriate antibiotics, consideration of surgical intervention, and a cohesive, multidisciplinary approach form the basis of management. From determining the duration of antibiotic therapy to identifying complications that may be indications for early surgery, echocardiography has an important role in the management of this complex disease, particularly with regard to prognostic factors that may require surgical intervention rather than medical therapy alone. Appropriate use criteria for TTE and TEE in IE are shown in Tables 29.3 and 29.4, respectively.

The Duke criteria were developed to provide a more sensitive case definition of IE, and their possible prognostic influence was evaluated in a single-center study. For 267 patients with definite or possible IE established by Duke criteria, early echocardiographic findings of IE, such as a vegetation and new valvular regurgitation used as categorical variables, were not associated with in-hospital mortality rates.[63]

Diagnostic imaging for evidence of IE typically occurs within the first few days after hospital admission for suspected IE. A delay in diagnostic imaging may delay appropriate treatment and has been associated with greater valve destruction, embolic events, and the need for surgical therapy.[64] Approximately 90% of patients with definite IE have vegetations visualized, and vegetation characteristics such as size, mobility, attachment site, and shape have been extensively studied as tools for risk stratification of patients with IE, particularly the risk of embolic events.

Vegetation size greater than 10 mm and increased mobility were shown in several series to predict embolic events.[65,66] Embolic events in IE are a strong, independent predictor of in-hospital death.[63] In one multicenter, prospective study of 384 consecutive patients with definite IE according to Duke University criteria, a vegetation length of more than 15 mm was independently associated with a 1-year mortality rate of 20.6%.[67] In another observational study of 132 patients with left-sided IE, approximately 40% of whom had a vegetation length of 15 mm or greater, early surgery within 7 days of diagnosis was associated with a significantly lower risk of embolic events compared with conventional treatment in which surgery was deferred until complications occurred.[68]

This reduction in embolic events with early surgery in left-sided IE was confirmed in a small, randomized trial of early surgery versus conventional treatment. Patients who underwent surgery within 48 hours of randomization had no embolic events at 6 weeks compared with 21% of those in the conventional treatment arm. There was no difference in in-hospital or 6-month mortality rates between treatment groups.[69] A retrospective, observational study found an association between early surgery and lower mortality rates for patients with left-sided IE and vegetation size larger than 10 mm[70] (Fig. 29.13).

Current American College of Cardiology/American Heart Association (ACC/AHA) guidelines recognize that surgery for native valve IE may be considered for patients who present with mobile vegetations larger than 10 mm[70] with or without emboli (class IIb recommendation, level of evidence B).[57] However, the risk of embolism decreases rapidly within the first week of antibiotic therapy[71] (Fig. 29.14), a beneficial effect of medical therapy that should be reflected in the decision to delay surgery for prevention of IE-related embolic events.

After an embolic event has occurred, the residual vegetation poses a risk of recurrent embolism.[72] However, routine surveillance for embolism in IE has demonstrated that approximately 50% of cases are associated with embolic events (typically to brain, spleen, kidney, or lungs), and that most of these events are clinically silent or asymptomatic. In this situation, the decision about whether to proceed with cardiac surgery is challenged by the subclinical nature of these events and the progressively lower risk of embolic events over time with antibiotic therapy (see Fig. 29.14). Conversely, asymptomatic brain infarcts have been associated with a poorer prognosis in IE and generally do not increase the risk of cardiac surgery in the absence of cerebral hemorrhage, abscess, or major neurologic impairment.[73]

Compared with TTE, TEE can better detect complications of IE such as paravalvular abscess[5] or regurgitation, valvular perforation,[74] intracardiac shunt, and secondary involvement of the mitral-aortic intervalvular fibrosa.[75] Many of these echocardiographic complications are indications for early surgery in the treatment of IE (Table 29.6) because they are unlikely to be cured with antibiotic therapy alone.

The diagnosis of an abscess has significant prognostic and management implications. Rarely, antibiotic therapy may be used to treat an intracardiac abscess, although this treatment alone typically is reserved for patients who are poor surgical candidates. Most patients with an intracardiac abscess require cardiac surgery for debridement (class I recommendation, level of evidence C), and failure to diagnose an abscess by echocardiography is associated with delayed time to surgery.[24]

In one study, the impact of early surgery on survival of patients with native valve IE was evaluated using a propensity score and instrumental variable methods to adjust for treatment

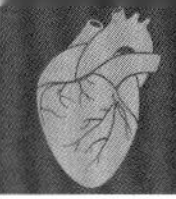

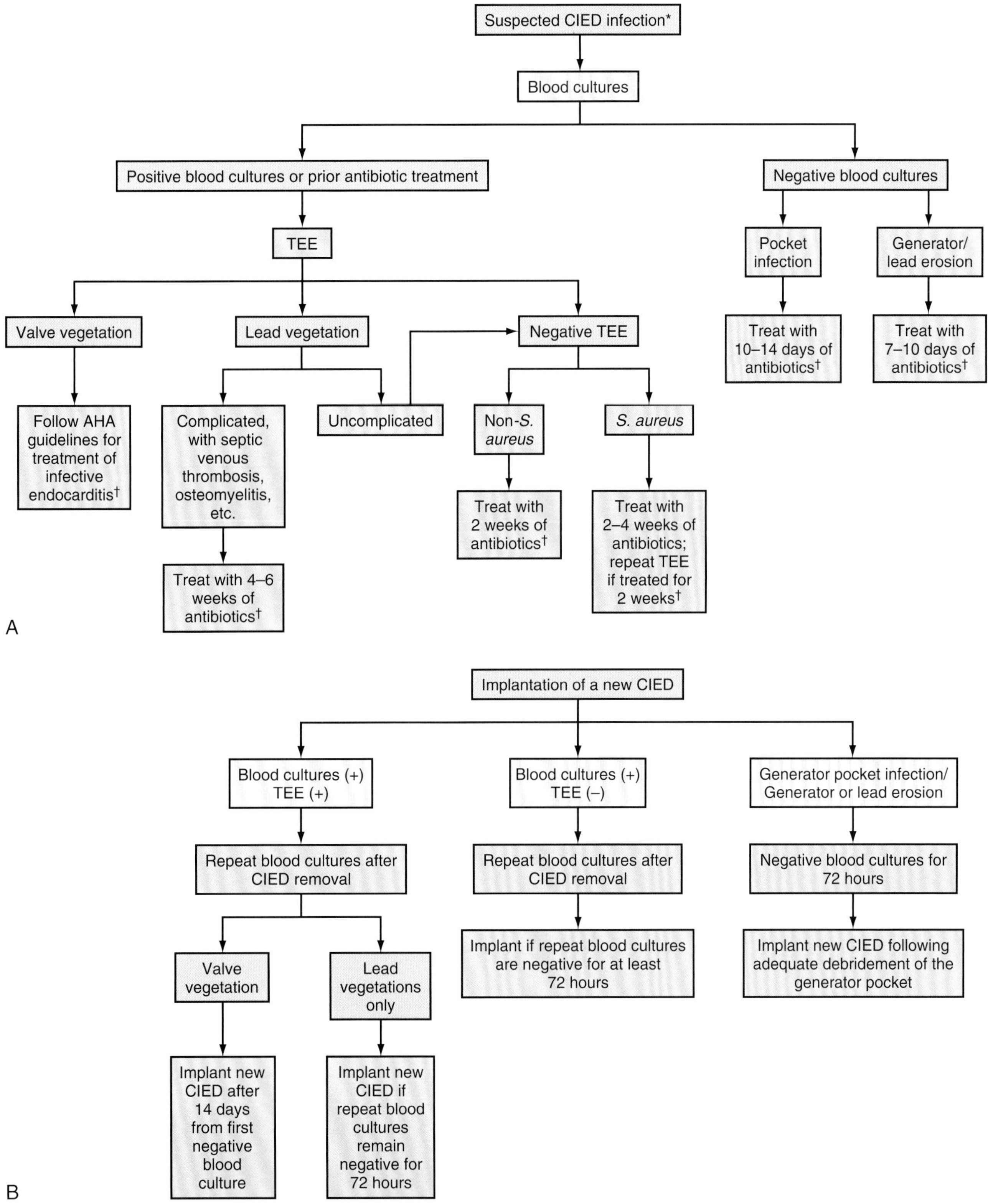

- Suspected CIED infection*
  - Blood cultures
    - Positive blood cultures or prior antibiotic treatment
      - TEE
        - Valve vegetation
          - Follow AHA guidelines for treatment of infective endocarditis†
        - Lead vegetation
          - Complicated, with septic venous thrombosis, osteomyelitis, etc.
            - Treat with 4–6 weeks of antibiotics†
          - Uncomplicated → Negative TEE
        - Negative TEE
          - Non-*S. aureus*
            - Treat with 2 weeks of antibiotics†
          - *S. aureus*
            - Treat with 2–4 weeks of antibiotics; repeat TEE if treated for 2 weeks†
    - Negative blood cultures
      - Pocket infection
        - Treat with 10–14 days of antibiotics†
      - Generator/ lead erosion
        - Treat with 7–10 days of antibiotics†

A

- Implantation of a new CIED
  - Blood cultures (+) TEE (+)
    - Repeat blood cultures after CIED removal
      - Valve vegetation
        - Implant new CIED after 14 days from first negative blood culture
      - Lead vegetations only
        - Implant new CIED if repeat blood cultures remain negative for 72 hours
  - Blood cultures (+) TEE (–)
    - Repeat blood cultures after CIED removal
      - Implant if repeat blood cultures are negative for at least 72 hours
  - Generator pocket infection/ Generator or lead erosion
    - Negative blood cultures for 72 hours
      - Implant new CIED following adequate debridement of the generator pocket

B

Fig. 29.12 Management of infected cardiac implantable electronic devices. (A) Approach to management of infected cardiac implantable electronic devices *(CIEDs)* in adults. (B) Approach to implantation of a new device in a patient after removal of an infected CIED. *AHA*, American Heart Association. *History, physical examination, chest radiography, and device interrogation are considered standard procedures before CIED removal. †Duration of antibiotics should be counted from the day of device extraction. (From Baddour LM, Epstein AE, Erickson CC, et al. Update on cardiovascular implantable electronic device infections and their management: a scientific statement from the American Heart Association. *Circulation*. 2010;121:458–477.)

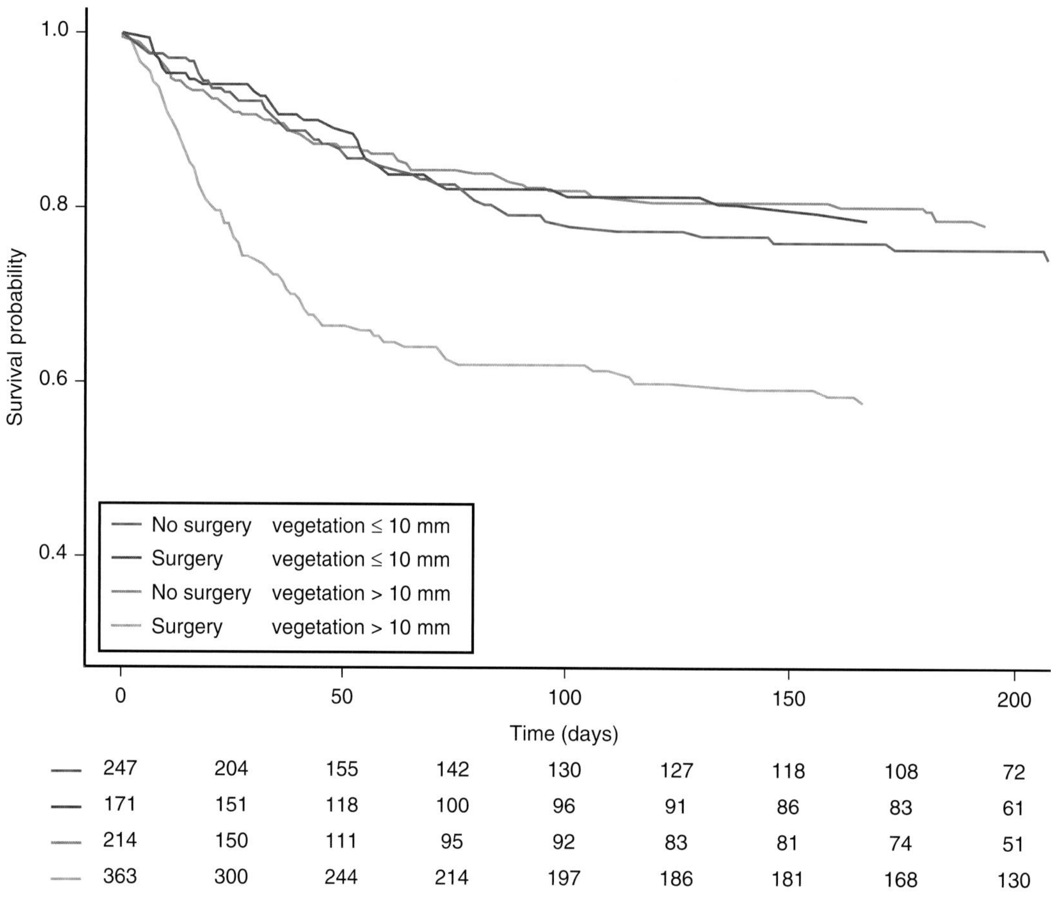

—	247	204	155	142	130	127	118	108	72
—	171	151	118	100	96	91	86	83	61
—	214	150	111	95	92	83	81	74	51
—	363	300	244	214	197	186	181	168	130

Fig. 29.13 Survival probabilities for infective endocarditis stratified by vegetation size and surgical treatment. Early surgery was associated with lower 6-month mortality in patients with left-sided infective endocarditis and vegetation size larger than 10 mm. (Data from Fosbol EL, Park LP, Chu VH, et al. The association between vegetation size and surgical treatment on 6-month mortality in left-sided infective endocarditis. *Eur Heart J.* 2019;40[27]:2243–2251.)

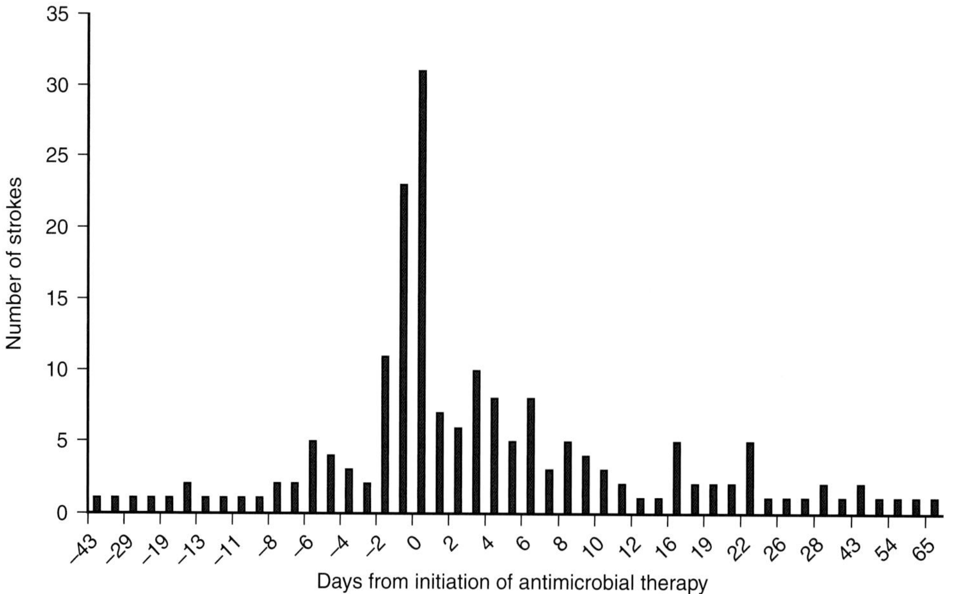

Fig. 29.14 Incidence of stroke versus days from initiation of antibiotic therapy for infective endocarditis. The risk of embolism decreases rapidly within the first week of antibiotic therapy. (From Dickerman SA, Abrutyn E, Barsic B, et al. The relationship between the initiation of antimicrobial therapy and the incidence of stroke in infective endocarditis: an analysis from the ICE Prospective Cohort Study (ICE-PCS). *Am Heart J* 2007;154:1086–1094.)

TABLE 29.6 Echocardiographic Findings That Represent Indications for Early Surgical Intervention in Infective Endocarditis.

Echocardiographic Finding	*ACC/AHA Class of Indication for Early Surgery*
Severe valve dysfunction causing heart failure	I
Abscess	I
Large (>10 mm), mobile vegetation on native valve	IIb
Recurrent emboli with persistent vegetation while on appropriate antibiotic therapy	IIa
Valve dehiscence, perforation or fistula	I
Infection of CIED lead	I

ACC, American College of Cardiology; *AHA*, American Heart Association; *CIED*, cardiac implantable electronic device.

selection bias.[75a] For the prospective, multinational cohort, the investigators found a significant in-hospital mortality rate benefit for those undergoing early surgery compared with medical therapy alone (12.1% vs. 20.7%) and for those with paravalvular complications such as intracardiac abscess or fistula formation determined by echocardiography (absolute risk reduction of −17.3%, $P < 0.001$). Surgery represents the gold standard for the confirmation of abscess visualized by echocardiography.

In IE complicated by fistula formation, the left-to-right shunting of blood flow usually augments the risk and severity of heart failure complicating IE. As a result, the in-hospital mortality rate is very high (41%) despite the use of surgical therapy in almost all cases.[23] Development of cavitary fistulas heralds a poor outcome and should prompt urgent surgical intervention.

Quantification of regurgitation severity and determination of its impact on heart failure as a complication of IE are important prognostic factors. Acute regurgitation in IE that develops without the compensatory eccentric hypertrophy seen in chronic regurgitation is poorly tolerated clinically, potentially resulting in life-threatening pulmonary edema and cardiogenic shock. Acute, aortic valve regurgitation is a complication associated with a high mortality rate, and it is an accepted criterion for surgical intervention. For patients with advanced heart failure symptoms (i.e., NYHA functional class III or IV) complicating left-sided native valve IE, surgical therapy has improved survival compared with medical therapy (Fig. 29.15), whereas surgery for patients with no or mild heart failure appears to have little benefit for overall survival.[76] Even for patients without overt evidence of heart failure, severe regurgitation of either left-sided heart valve is a poor prognostic finding and an indication for surgical intervention. If severe mitral or aortic valve regurgitation is evident by echocardiography, close observation of the patient's hemodynamic status should be performed, often in an intensive care unit setting, because clinical deterioration may occur abruptly.

Assessment of left ventricular (LV) function remains an important prognostic indicator in IE. For patients with left-sided native valve IE due to *S. aureus* infection, an LV ejection fraction of less than 40% was independently associated with higher in-hospital mortality rates.[77] Similarly, a higher global longitudinal strain (GLS) value (>15.4%) was associated with increased 1-year mortality rates in cases of left-sided IE.[78]

In IE cases complicated by mechanical complications such as abscess, fistula, severe valvular regurgitation, or valve dehiscence, intraoperative TEE is indicated to assess complete repair of these defects and is considered a standard of care in most centers. Shapira et al. analyzed the impact of TEE for 59 patients diagnosed with IE. The investigators found that intraoperative TEE before

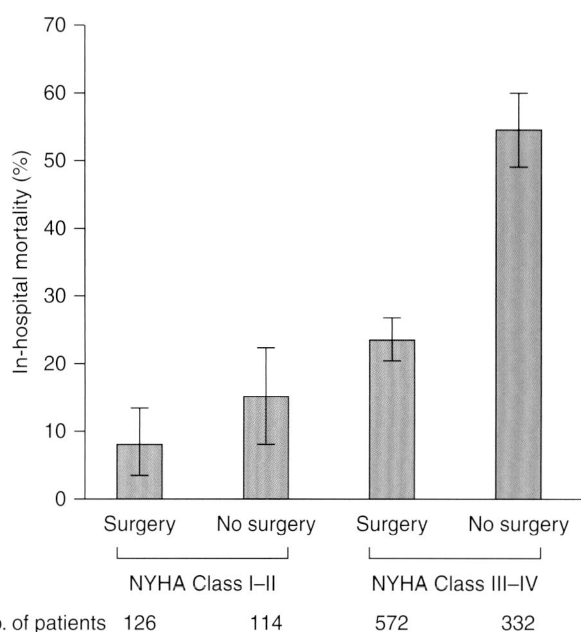

Fig. 29.15 Association between surgical therapy for native, left-sided infective endocarditis and survival in the setting of heart failure severity. For patients with advanced heart failure symptoms complicating left-sided, native valve endocarditis, the absolute survival benefit of surgery is significantly higher than for less severe degree of heart failure. *NYHA*, New York Heart Association (From Kiefer T, Park L, Tribouilloy C, et al: Association between valvular surgery and mortality among patients with infective endocarditis complicated by heart failure. *JAMA* 306:2239–2247, 2011.)

cardiopulmonary bypass led to modification of the surgical plan in 11.5% of cases.[79,80] Intraoperatively, echocardiographic goals include assessment of the obviously dysfunctional valve and the other valves and contiguous structures. Images after cardiopulmonary bypass should confirm the adequacy of the repair or replacement and document the successful closure of fistulous tracts. Paravalvular leaks related to technical factors should be recognized and documented to avoid future uncertainty about whether the leaks may be the result of recurrent infection.

During imaging after cardiopulmonary bypass, it is often necessary to augment afterload to reach representative ambulatory levels to avoid underestimation of regurgitant jet size and significance and to ensure that abnormal communications have been closed. Afterload augmentation, however, may not always mimic actual awake physiology and may still lead to an inaccurate evaluation of the conscious postoperative state.[6,81]

In suspected CIED endocarditis, differentiation between infection (i.e., vegetation) on the CIED intracardiac lead and vegetation on the tricuspid valve can be challenging. However, in native or prosthetic valve IE with an existing CIED, removal of the device is indicated even without other IE complications or definite CIED involvement because of the high probability of relapse. Patients with CIED IE who do not undergo device extraction have a high rate of mortality within 6 months of diagnosis (Fig. 29.16).[82]

Echocardiography has been used to analyze cost-effectiveness in establishing the duration of treatment in the setting of acute IE and for determining the need for surgical intervention. Rosen et al.[82a] evaluated the cost-effectiveness of TEE in establishing the duration of therapy for catheter-associated bacteremia. In this study, three management strategies were compared: (1) empiric treatment with 4 weeks of antibiotics (long course), (2) empiric treatment with 2 weeks of antibiotic therapy, and (3)

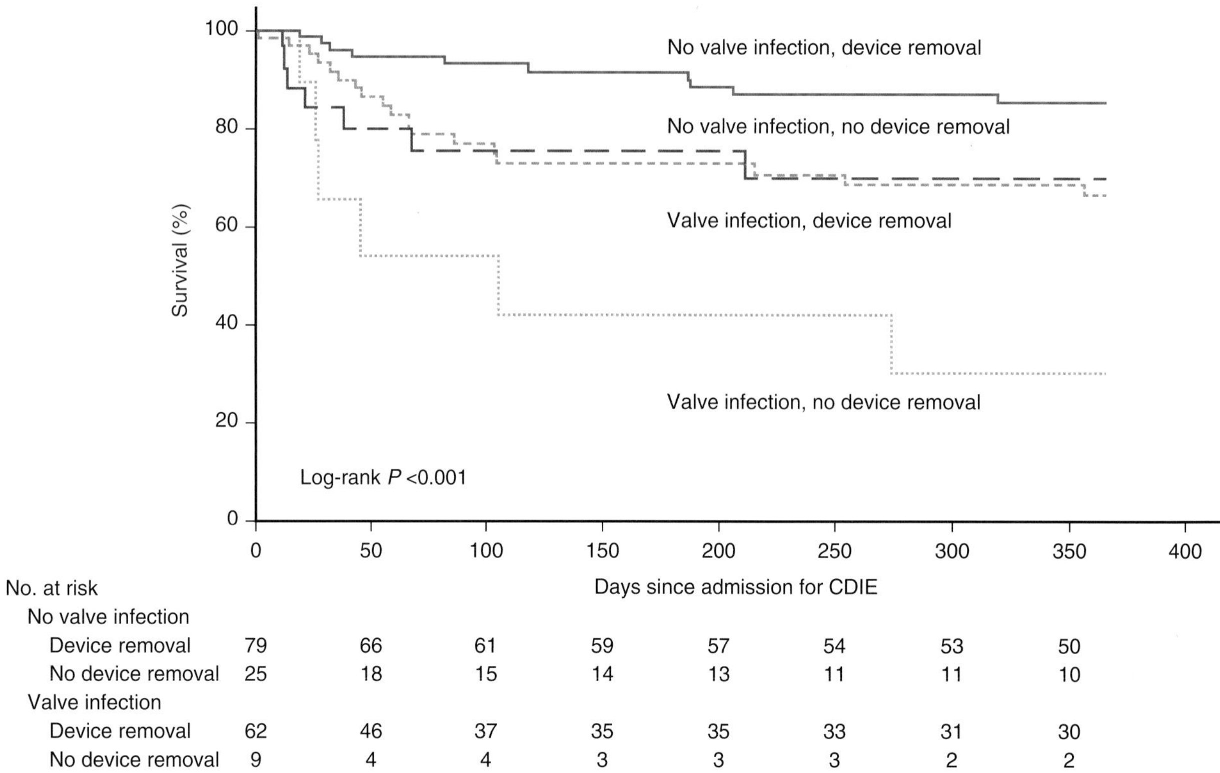

No. at risk	0	50	100	150	200	250	300	350
No valve infection								
Device removal	79	66	61	59	57	54	53	50
No device removal	25	18	15	14	13	11	11	10
Valve infection								
Device removal	62	46	37	35	35	33	31	30
No device removal	9	4	4	3	3	3	2	2

Fig. 29.16 Cardiac implantable electronic device removal in cases of infective endocarditis. Patients with cardiac implantable electronic device infective endocarditis *(CDIE)* who do not undergo device extraction have a high mortality rate within 6 months of diagnosis. Prognosis is worse with concomitant valve infection. (Data from Athan E, Chu VH, Tattevin P, et al. Clinical characteristics and outcome of infective endocarditis involving implantable cardiac devices. *JAMA*. 2012;307:1727–735.)

TEE-guided therapy. In the TEE-guided strategy, a positive TEE study dictated a long course of antibiotic therapy, and a negative TEE study dictated a short course of therapy. The empiric long-course strategy and the TEE-guided strategy were both superior to the empiric short-course therapy.

When costs were taken into account, the TEE-guided strategy was superior to the empiric long-course strategy, which costs more than $1,500,000 per quality-adjusted life-year (QALY) saved. In a similar study that used a decision tree and Markov analysis, Liao et al.[83] showed that echocardiography-guided risk stratification for assessing complications that might benefit from early surgical intervention was a cost-attractive treatment strategy and improved outcome for an incremental cost of less than $50,000/QALY.

Approximately 50% of patients with IE undergo cardiac valve surgery during their index hospitalization. After the decision to proceed to surgery is made, it is important to provide the surgeon with an accurate assessment of valve anatomy for the purpose of operative planning. Preoperative assessment may be especially valuable when repair, rather than replacement, of a diseased mitral valve is considered. For patients with an aortic abscess, consideration of a homograft replacement may be facilitated by accurate measurement of the annulus diameter. After valve surgery for IE, TTE is indicated for outpatients soon after surgery. Results of the TTE study serve as a useful baseline assessment of the replaced or repaired valve's function and ventricular function for future comparisons when clinically indicated.

UTILITY IN FOLLOW-UP

The data do not support serial echocardiographic examinations for surveillance in cases of uncomplicated IE. The diagnostic value of TEE in monitoring the clinical course was evaluated in[83] patients with echocardiographic evidence of IE by Rohmann et al.[84] Each patient received at least two consecutive TEE studies. The investigators found that patients with an increase or no change in vegetation size had a higher incidence of complications after diagnosis and initiation of therapy, including valve replacement, embolic events, paravalvular abscess formation, and death, compared with the cohort that demonstrated a decrease in vegetation size.[84] Although these data suggest that multiple echocardiographic evaluations may be useful in determining the prognosis of patients with IE, there is great potential for inappropriate overuse of the test.

Vieira et al. evaluated the diagnostic contribution of repeated TTE and TEE examinations for patients with suspected IE.[85] Over a 3-year period, they evaluated 262 patients with 266 episodes of suspected IE referred for echocardiography. They found that repeat echocardiography was common. TTE studies were repeated at least once in 192 (72.2%) of the patients, and TEE studies were repeated in 49 (18.4%). A mean of 2.4 TTE and 1.2 TEE examinations were performed for each episode of suspected IE. The second and third TTE studies added diagnostic information in 34 (26.7%) of 127 episodes of definite IE, and the second and third TEE studies added diagnostic information in 25 (19.7%). After the third TTE or TEE study, no additional diagnostic information was obtained.[85]

TTE or TEE used for routine surveillance of uncomplicated IE when no change in management is contemplated is deemed inappropriate according to published appropriateness criteria for echocardiography. For patients with an established diagnosis of IE who develop worrisome clinical features such as a new atrioventricular block, persistent fever or bacteremia, progression of heart failure symptoms, or a change in cardiac murmur during or after the course of therapy, repeat TTE or TEE to evaluate structural

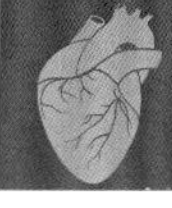

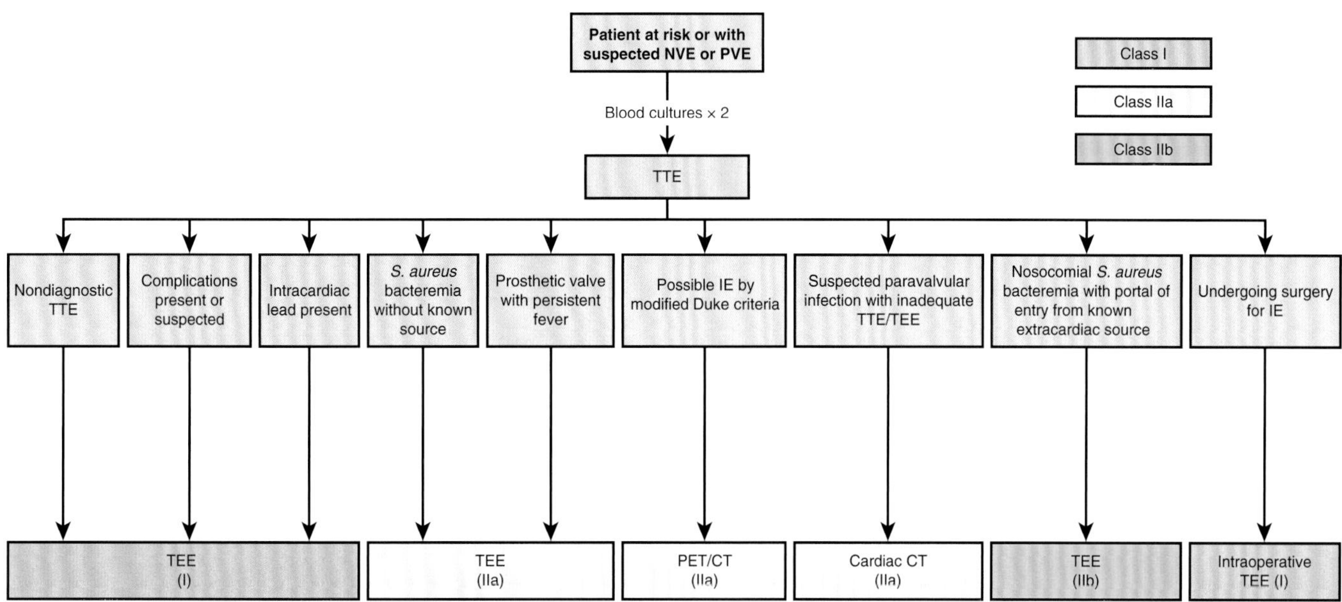

Fig. 29.17 Approach to diagnostic imaging in suspected endocarditis Recommendations for different cardiac imaging modalities in cases of native valve endocarditis *(NVE)*, prosthetic valve endocarditis *(PVE)*, and cardiac implantable electronic device *(CIED)* infective endocarditis *(IE)* (Adapted from Adapted from Otto CM, Nishimura RA, Bonow RO, et al. 2020 ACC/AHA guideline for the management of patients with valvular heart disease: a report of the American College of Cardiology/American Heart Association Joint Committee on Clinical Practice Guidelines. *Circulation*. 2021;143(5):e72-e227. doi: 10.1161/CIR.0000000000000923.)

complications is warranted (class I recommendation, level of evidence A). Because all patients with a history of IE remain at high risk for recurrent infection indefinitely, a TTE examination should be conducted to establish a new baseline for valve morphology and cardiac function after completion of antimicrobial therapy (class IIb recommendation, level of evidence C).

RESEARCH APPLICATIONS

With the advent of real-time 3D TEE, which allows acquisition of full-volume data, it is possible to precisely define anatomic structures and vegetation characteristics and location. Cropping images may reveal structures or flows not visualized with TEE or TTE. It appears to be a promising technique for examining patients with prosthetic valves and those with intracardiac devices. Initial experience using 3D TEE in patients with prosthetic valve endocarditis suggests that the modality may provide information not readily appreciated on standard 2D TEE imaging.[86]

Liu et al. performed 2D and real-time 3D TTE in 46 patients with definite IE.[86a] The sensitivity of both modalities was 91.6%, but specificity using real-time 3D TTE was higher (100% vs. 88.2%). Although these data are encouraging, further research is needed to define the role of 3D echocardiography for the diagnosis and management of IE. From a clinical perspective, additional studies are needed to better define the prognostic influence of echocardiographic findings and their severity over time after treatment.

POTENTIAL LIMITATIONS AND FUTURE DIRECTIONS

Use of echocardiography as a diagnostic tool is important in determining the correct clinical scenario and appropriate pretest probability of disease. Overuse is associated with avoidable costs. False-positive results can lead to unnecessary treatment, complications, and increased medical costs. With an invasive procedure such as TEE, there is a small but definable risk to the patient of complications related to sedation and probe insertion, including aspiration, esophageal perforation, induction of cardiac arrhythmia, respiratory compromise, and patient discomfort.

Approximately 10% of patients with IE do not have evidence of vegetation or other endocardial involvement at the time of diagnosis, perhaps due to the limitations of imaging previously described. Treatment of these patients should be guided by the clinical suspicion of IE, particularly in those patients with prosthetic heart valves and those who meet criteria for definite IE by other major and minor criteria.

ALTERNATIVE APPROACHES

Recommendations for the use of different cardiac imaging modalities in IE are shown in Fig. 29.17. A PET/CT scan may improve the sensitivity of the modified Duke criteria for IE in patients with bacteremia and prosthetic valves or CIEDs and may be helpful in the setting of possible IE by modified Duke criteria. Other imaging modalities, such as cardiac magnetic resonance imaging with contrast, appear promising for the detection of paravalvular abscesses, thrombus associated with vegetations, valvular complications, and aortocameral fistulas, although temporal resolution may limit its use for detection of vegetation (level of evidence C). Its role is limited in the evaluation of patients with CIEDs, and the procedure is often not feasible in critically ill patients.

Cardiac CT has been used to detect aortic root abscess, but the radiation risk and temporal resolution are factors limiting its widespread use. In a study comparing CT with TEE for diagnosing IE, TEE was superior for the diagnosis of small vegetations, valve perforation, and fistula, and CT was superior for the diagnosis of abscess.[87]

Clinical experience with these techniques in IE patients is limited, and their operating characteristics (i.e., sensitivity and specificity) compared with echocardiography are not well defined.[88-90] As a result, no other imaging modality for the visualization of endocardial involvement or complications of IE is an acceptable alternative to echocardiography in clinical practice, but adjunctive tests may be clinically useful.

SUMMARY Echocardiographic Data Acquisition, Measurement, and Interpretation.

- Machine settings such as frame rate, sector arc size, gray scale, and focal zones must be optimized, and a careful examination that includes nonstandard views should be conducted to exclude the presence of vegetations.
- The size of the vegetations should be measured within the resolution characteristics of the transducer so that machine settings can be duplicated for future comparative studies if clinically indicated.
- Visualization of a distinct vegetation may be impaired by severe, underlying valvular degeneration, and particularly by prominent calcifications of valve leaflets.
- TEE is the diagnostic test of choice when an abscess is suspected clinically. An abscess is diagnosed by visualization of a thickened area with a heterogeneous echogenic or echolucent appearance within the myocardium or annular region.
- If an abscess is identified, a careful examination is required to rule out extension into adjacent areas because this additional information has considerable implications for the type of reparative surgery to be undertaken. Loss of structural integrity of the valve, valvular regurgitation and vegetations, and thickening of adjacent tissues help differentiate a native aortic valve abscess from fluid in the transverse pericardial sinus.
- After prosthetic surgical or transcatheter valve implantation, anatomic changes, including an echolucent space between prosthetic valve sewing ring and the aortic root with or without paravalvular regurgitation, may pose a diagnostic dilemma for a patient with a prosthetic valve and fever. Comparison with an intraoperative TEE, if available, may help to document the chronicity of the abnormality.
- In patients with mechanical prosthetic valves, a complete examination requires using a combination of TTE and TEE approaches.
- In patients with cardiac implantable electronic devices (CIEDs), there is substantial artifact generation, and TEE is superior to TTE in cases of suspected CIED infection.[28–30] Visualization of the lead in the proximal superior vena cava on TEE views may identify vegetations attached to CIED leads that are difficult to visualize by other modalities. During the examination, it is important to visualize the entire course of the prosthetic device throughout the vasculature and cardiac structures. A careful evaluation of the cardiac valves is also important because of the high rate of concomitant valve infection, particularly infection of the tricuspid valve.

REFERENCES

1. Delahaye F, Goulet V, Lacassin F, et al. Characteristics of infective endocarditis in France in 1991. A 1-year survey. *Eur Heart J.* 1995;16:394–401.
2. Murdoch DR, Corey GR, Hoen B, et al. Clinical presentation, etiology, and outcome of infective endocarditis in the 21st century: the International Collaboration on Endocarditis-Prospective Cohort Study. *Arch Intern Med.* 2009;169:463–473.
3. Dillon JC, Feigenbaum H, Konecke LL, Davis RH, Chang S. Echocardiographic manifestations of valvular vegetations. *Am Heart J.* 1973;86:698–704.
4. Gilbert BW, Haney RS, Crawford F, et al. Two-dimensional echocardiographic assessment of vegetative endocarditis. *Circulation.* 1977;55:346–353.
5. Daniel WG, Mugge A, Martin RP, et al. Improvement in the diagnosis of abscesses associated with endocarditis by transesophageal echocardiography. *N Engl J Med.* 1991;324:795–800.
6. Baddour LM, Wilson WR, Bayer AS, et al. Infective endocarditis: diagnosis, antimicrobial therapy, and management of complications: a statement for healthcare professionals from the Committee on Rheumatic Fever, Endocarditis, and Kawasaki Disease, Council on Cardiovascular Disease in the Young, and the Councils on Clinical Cardiology, Stroke, and Cardiovascular Surgery and Anesthesia, American Heart Association: Endorsed by the Infectious Diseases Society of America. *Circulation.* 2005;111:e394–e434.
7. Osler W. Gulstonian lectures on malignant endocarditis: Lectures 1-3. *Lancet.* 1885;1:415–418.
8. Pelletier Jr LL, Petersdorf RG. Infective endocarditis: a review of 125 cases from the University of Washington Hospitals, 1963-72. *Medicine (Baltim).* 1977;56:287–313.
9. Von Reyn CF, Levy BS, Arbeit RD, Friedland G, Crumpacker CS. Infective endocarditis: an analysis based on strict case definitions. *Ann Intern Med.* 1981;94:505–518.
10. Durack DT, Lukes AS, Bright DK. New criteria for diagnosis of infective endocarditis: utilization of specific echocardiographic findings. *Duke Endocarditis Service. Am J Med.* 1994;96:200–209.
11. Andres E, Baudoux C, Noel E, Goichot B, Schlienger JL, Blickle JF. The value of the von Reyn and the Duke diagnostic criteria for infective endocarditis in internal medicine practice. A study of 38 cases. *Eur J Intern Med.* 2003;14:411–414.
12. Perez-Vazquez A, Farinas MC, Garcia-Palomo JD, Bernal JM, Revuelta JM, Gonzalez-Macias J. Evaluation of the Duke criteria in 93 episodes of prosthetic valve endocarditis: could sensitivity be improved? *Arch Intern Med.* 2000;160:1185–1191.
13. Stockheim JA, Chadwick EG, Kessler S, et al. Are the Duke criteria superior to the Beth Israel criteria for the diagnosis of infective endocarditis in children? *Clin Infect Dis.* 1998;27:1451–1456.
14. Heiro M, Nikoskelainen J, Hartiala JJ, Saraste MK, Kotilainen PM. Diagnosis of infective endocarditis. Sensitivity of the Duke vs von Reyn criteria. *Arch Intern Med.* 1998;158:18–24.
15. Sekeres MA, Abrutyn E, Berlin JA, et al. An assessment of the usefulness of the Duke criteria for diagnosing active infective endocarditis. *Clin Infect Dis.* 1997;24:1185–1190.
16. Martos-Perez F, Reguera JM, Colmenero JD. Comparable sensitivity of the Duke criteria and the modified Beth Israel criteria for diagnosing infective endocarditis. *Clin Infect Dis.* 1996;23:410–411.
17. Olaison L, Hogevik H. Comparison of the von Reyn and Duke criteria for the diagnosis of infective endocarditis: a critical analysis of 161 episodes. *Scand J Infect Dis.* 1996;28:399–406.
18. Hoen B, Selton-Suty C, Danchin N, et al. Evaluation of the Duke criteria versus the Beth Israel criteria for the diagnosis of infective endocarditis. *Clin Infect Dis.* 1995;21:905–909.
19. Cecchi E, Parrini I, Chinaglia A, et al. New diagnostic criteria for infective endocarditis. A study of sensitivity and specificity. *Eur Heart J.* 1997;18:1149–1156.
20. Dodds GA, Sexton DJ, Durack DT, Bashore TM, Corey GR, Kisslo J. Negative predictive value of the Duke criteria for infective endocarditis. *Am J Cardiol.* 1996;77:403–407.
21. Li JS, Sexton DJ, Mick N, et al. Proposed modifications to the Duke criteria for the diagnosis of infective endocarditis. *Clin Infect Dis.* 2000;30:633–638.
22. Sachdev M, Peterson GE, Jollis JG. Imaging techniques for diagnosis of infective endocarditis. *Cardiol Clin.* 2003;21:185–195.

23. Anguera I, Miro JM, Cabell CH, et al. Clinical characteristics and outcome of aortic endocarditis with periannular abscess in the International Collaboration on Endocarditis Merged Database. *Am J Cardiol*. 2005;96:976–981.
24. Hill EE, Herijgers P, Claus P, Vanderschueren S, Peetermans WE, Herregods MC. Abscess in infective endocarditis: the value of transesophageal echocardiography and outcome: a 5-year study. *Am Heart J*. 2007;154:923–928.
25. Lauridsen TK, Selton-Suty C, Tong S, et al. Echocardiographic agreement in the diagnostic evaluation for infective endocarditis. *Int J Cardiovasc Imaging*. 2016;32:1041–1051.
26. Anguera I, Del Rio A, Miro JM, et al. Staphylococcus lugdunensis infective endocarditis: description of 10 cases and analysis of native valve, prosthetic valve, and pacemaker lead endocarditis clinical profiles. *Heart*. 2005;91:e10.
27. Kang N, Wan S, Ng CS, Underwood MJ. Periannular extension of infective endocarditis. *Ann Thorac Cardiovasc Surg*. 2009;15:74–81.
28. Victor F, De Place C, Camus C, et al. Pacemaker lead infection: echocardiographic features, management, and outcome. *Heart*. 1999;81:82–87.
29. Baddour LM, Epstein AE, Erickson CC, et al. Update on cardiovascular implantable electronic device infections and their management: a scientific statement from the American Heart Association. *Circulation*. 2010;121:458–477.
30. Chu VH, Bayer AS. Use of echocardiography in the diagnosis and management of infective endocarditis. *Curr Infect Dis Rep*. 2007;9:283–290.
31. Khandheria BK. Suspected bacterial endocarditis: to TEE or not to TEE. *J Am Coll Cardiol*. 1993;21:222–224.
32. San Roman JA, Vilacosta I, Zamorano JL, Almeria C, Sanchez-Harguindey L. Transesophageal echocardiography in right-sided endocarditis. *J Am Coll Cardiol*. 1993;21:1226–1230.
33. Lindner JR, Case RA, Dent JM, Abbott RD, Scheld WM, Kaul S. Diagnostic value of echocardiography in suspected endocarditis. An evaluation based on the pretest probability of disease. *Circulation*. 1996;93:730–736.
34. Sivak JA, Vora AN, Navar-Boggan AM, Crowley AL, Kisslo J, Velazquez EJ, Samad Z. Negative predictive value of transthoracic echocardiography for infective endocarditis in the modern era. *Circulation*. 2014;130. 10-S.
35. Roe MT, Abramson MA, Li J, et al. Clinical information determines the impact of transesophageal echocardiography on the diagnosis of infective endocarditis by the Duke criteria. *Am Heart J*. 2000;139:945–951.
36. Erbel R, Rohmann S, Drexler M, et al. Improved diagnostic value of echocardiography in patients with infective endocarditis by transoesophageal approach. A prospective study. *Eur Heart J*. 1988;9:43–53.
37. Shapiro SM, Young E, Ginzton LE, Bayer AS. Pulmonic valve endocarditis as an underdiagnosed disease: role of transesophageal echocardiography. *J Am Soc Echocardiogr*. 1992;5:48–51.
38. Kupferwasser LI, Darius H, Muller AM, et al. Diagnosis of culture-negative endocarditis: the role of the Duke criteria and the impact of transesophageal echocardiography. *Am Heart J*. 2001;142:146–152.
39. Heidenreich PA, Masoudi FA, Maini B, et al. Echocardiography in patients with suspected endocarditis: a cost-effectiveness analysis. *Am J Med*. 1999;107:198–208.
40. Greaves K, Mou D, Patel A, Celermajer DS. Clinical criteria and the appropriate use of transthoracic echocardiography for the exclusion of infective endocarditis. *Heart*. 2003;89:273–275.
41. Fowler Jr VG, Li J, Corey GR, et al. Role of echocardiography in evaluation of patients with *Staphylococcus aureus* bacteremia: experience in 103 patients. *J Am Coll Cardiol*. 1997;30:1072–1078.
42. Abraham J, Mansour C, Veledar E, Khan B, Lerakis S. *Staphylococcus aureus* bacteremia and endocarditis: the Grady Memorial Hospital experience with methicillin-sensitive *S aureus* and methicillin-resistant S aureus bacteremia. *Am Heart J*. 2004;147:536–539.
43. Fowler Jr VG, Sanders LL, Kong LK, et al. Infective endocarditis due to *Staphylococcus aureus*: 59 prospectively identified cases with follow-up. *Clin Infect Dis*. 1999;28:106–114.
44. Fowler Jr VG, Miro JM, Hoen B, et al. *Staphylococcus aureus* endocarditis: a consequence of medical progress. *JAMA*. 2005;293:3012–3021.
45. Palraj BR, Baddour LM, Hess EP, et al. Predicting Risk of Endocarditis Using a Clinical Tool (PREDICT): scoring system to guide use of echocardiography in the management of *Staphylococcus aureus* bacteremia. *Clin Infect Dis*. 2015;61:18–28.
46. Dahl A, Iversen K, Tonder N, et al. Prevalence of infective endocarditis in Enterococcus faecalis bacteremia. *J Am Coll Cardiol*. 2019;74:193–201.
47. Wang A, Athan E, Pappas PA, et al. Contemporary clinical profile and outcome of prosthetic valve endocarditis. *JAMA*. 2007;297:1354–1361.
48. Amat-Santos IJ, Messika-Zeitoun D, Eltchaninoff H, et al. Infective endocarditis after transcatheter aortic valve implantation: results from a large multicenter registry. *Circulation*. 2015;131:1566–1574.
49. Butt JH, Ihlemann N, De Backer O, et al. Long-term risk of infective endocarditis after transcatheter aortic valve replacement. *J Am Coll Cardiol*. 2019;73:1646–1655.
50. Salaun E, Sportouch L, Barral PA, et al. Diagnosis of infective endocarditis after TAVR: value of a multimodality imaging approach. *JACC Cardiovasc Imaging*. 2018;11:143–146.
51. Mangner N, Woitek F, Haussig S, et al. Incidence, predictors, and outcome of patients developing infective endocarditis following transfemoral transcatheter aortic valve replacement. *J Am Coll Cardiol*. 2016;67:2907–2908.
52. Mangner N, Leontyev S, Woitek FJ, et al. Cardiac surgery compared with antibiotics only in patients developing infective endocarditis after transcatheter aortic valve replacement. *J Am Heart Assoc*. 2018;7. e010027.
53. Asmarats L, Rodriguez-Gabella T, Chamandi C, et al. Infective endocarditis following transcatheter edge-to-edge mitral valve repair: a systematic review. *Catheter Cardiovasc Interv*. 2018;92:583–591.
54. El-Ahdab F, Benjamin Jr DK, Wang A, et al. Risk of endocarditis among patients with prosthetic valves and *Staphylococcus aureus* bacteremia. *Am J Med*. 2005;118:225–229.
55. Birmingham GD, Rahko PS, Ballantyne 3rd F. Improved detection of infective endocarditis with transesophageal echocardiography. *Am Heart J*. 1992;123:774–781.
56. Mugge A, Daniel WG, Frank G, Lichtlen PR. Echocardiography in infective endocarditis: reassessment of prognostic implications of vegetation size determined by the transthoracic and the transesophageal approach. *J Am Coll Cardiol*. 1989;14:631–638.
57. Otto CM, Nishimura RA, Bonow RO, et al. 2020 ACC/AHA guideline for the management of patients with valvular heart disease: a report of the American College of Cardiology/American Heart Association Joint Committee on Clinical Practice Guidelines. *Circulation*. 2021;143(5):e72-e227. https://doi.org/10.1161/CIR.0000000000000923.
58. Saby L, Laas O, Habib G, et al. Positron emission tomography/computed tomography for diagnosis of prosthetic valve endocarditis: increased valvular 18F-fluorodeoxyglucose uptake as a novel major criterion. *J Am Coll Cardiol*. 2013;61:2374–2382.
59. Lengyel M. The impact of transesophageal echocardiography on the management of prosthetic valve endocarditis: experience of 31 cases and review of the literature. *J Heart Valve Dis*. 1997;6:204–211.
60. Rozich JD, Edwards WD, Hanna RD, Laffey DM, Johnson GH, Klarich KW. Mechanical prosthetic valve-associated strands: pathologic correlates to transesophageal echocardiography. *J Am Soc Echocardiogr*. 2003;16:97–100.
61. Cabell CH, Heidenreich PA, Chu VH, et al. Increasing rates of cardiac device infections among Medicare beneficiaries: 1990-1999. *Am Heart J*. 2004;147:582–586.
62. Lo R, D'Anca M, Cohen T, Kerwin T. Incidence and prognosis of pacemaker lead-associated masses: a study of 1,569 transesophageal echocardiograms. *J Invasive Cardiol*. 2006;18:599–601.
63. Chu VH, Cabell CH, Benjamin Jr DK, et al. Early predictors of in-hospital death in infective endocarditis. *Circulation*. 2004;109:1745–1749.
64. Young WJ, Jeffery DA, Hua A, et al. Echocardiography in patients with infective endocarditis and the impact of diagnostic delays on clinical outcomes. *Am J Cardiol*. 2018;122:650–655.
65. Di Salvo G, Habib G, Pergola V, et al. Echocardiography predicts embolic events in infective endocarditis. *J Am Coll Cardiol*. 2001;37:1069–1076.
66. Tischler MD, Vaitkus PT. The ability of vegetation size on echocardiography to predict clinical complications: a meta-analysis. *J Am Soc Echocardiogr*. 1997;10:562–568.
67. Thuny F, Di Salvo G, Belliard O, et al. Risk of embolism and death in infective endocarditis: prognostic value of echocardiography: a prospective multicenter study. *Circulation*. 2005;112:69–75.
68. Dae-Hee Kim D-HK, Lee M-Z, Yun S-C, et al. Impact of early surgery on embolic events in patients with infective endocarditis. *Circulation*. 2010;122:S17–S22.
69. Kang DH, Kim YJ, Kim SH, et al. Early surgery versus conventional treatment for infective endocarditis. *N Engl J Med*. 2012;366:2466–2473.
70. Fosbol EL, Park LP, Chu VH, et al. The association between vegetation size and surgical treatment on 6-month mortality in left-sided infective endocarditis. *Eur Heart J*. 2019. https://doi.org/10.1093/eurheartj/ehz204.
71. Dickerman SA, Abrutyn E, Barsic B, et al. The relationship between the initiation of antimicrobial therapy and the incidence of stroke in infective endocarditis: an analysis from the ICE Prospective Cohort Study (ICE-PCS). *Am Heart J*. 2007;154:1086–1094.
72. Ostergaard L, Dahl A, Fosbol E, et al. Residual vegetation after treatment for left-sided infective endocarditis and subsequent risk of stroke and recurrence of endocarditis. *Int J Cardiol*. 2019. https://doi.org/10.1016/j.ijcard.2019.06.059.
73. Cooper HA, Thompson EC, Laureno R, et al. Subclinical brain embolization in left-sided infective endocarditis: results from the Evaluation by MRI of the Brains of Patients with Left-sided Intracardiac Solid Masses (EMBOLISM) pilot study. *Circulation*. 2009;120:585–591.

74. De Castro S, Cartoni D, d'Amati G, et al. Diagnostic accuracy of transthoracic and multiplane transesophageal echocardiography for valvular perforation in acute infective endocarditis: correlation with anatomic findings. *Clin Infect Dis*. 2000;30:825–826.
75. Karalis DG, Bansal RC, Hauck AJ, et al. Transesophageal echocardiographic recognition of subaortic complications in aortic valve endocarditis. Clinical and surgical implications. *Circulation*. 1992;86:353–362.
75a. Lalani T, Cabell CH, Benjamin DK, et al. Analysis of the impact of early surgery on in-hospital mortality of native valve endocarditis: use of propensity score and instrumental variable methods to adjust for treatment-selection bias. *Circulation*. 2010;121(8):1005–1013.
76. Vikram HR, Buenconsejo J, Hasbun R, Quagliarello VJ. Impact of valve surgery on 6-month mortality in adults with complicated, left-sided native valve endocarditis: a propensity analysis. *J Am Med Assoc*. 2003;290: 3207–3214.
77. Lauridsen TK, Park L, Tong SY, et al. Echocardiographic findings predict in-hospital and 1-year mortality in left-sided native valve *Staphylococcus aureus* endocarditis: analysis from the International Collaboration on Endocarditis-Prospective Echo Cohort Study. *Circ Cardiovasc Imaging*. 2015;8. e003397.
78. Lauridsen TK, Alhede C, Crowley AL, et al. Two-dimensional global longitudinal strain is superior to left ventricular ejection fraction in prediction of outcome in patients with left-sided infective endocarditis. *Int J Cardiol*. 2018;260:118–123.
79. Shanewise JS, Cheung AT, Aronson S, et al. ASE/SCA guidelines for performing a comprehensive intraoperative multiplane transesophageal echocardiography examination: recommendations of the American Society of Echocardiography Council for Intraoperative Echocardiography and the Society of Cardiovascular Anesthesiologists Task Force for Certification in Perioperative Transesophageal Echocardiography. *J Am Soc Echocardiogr*. 1999;12:884–900.
80. Shapira Y, Vaturi M, Weisenberg DE, et al. Impact of intraoperative transesophageal echocardiography in patients undergoing valve replacement. *Ann Thorac Surg*. 2004;78:579–583. discussion 583-584.
81. Mestres CA, Fita G, Azqueta M, Miro JM. Role of echocardiogram in decision making for surgery in endocarditis. *Curr Infect Dis Rep*. 2010;12:321–328.
82. Athan E, Chu VH, Tattevin P, et al. AL, Wang A and Investigators I-P. Clinical characteristics and outcome of infective endocarditis involving implantable cardiac devices. *J Am Med Assoc*. 2012;307:1727–1735.
82a. Rosen AB, Fowler VG Jr, Corey GR, et al. Cost-effectiveness of transesophageal echocardiography to determine the duration of therapy for intravascular catheter-associated Staphylococcus aureus bacteremia. *Ann Intern Med*. 1999;130:810–820.
83. Liao L, Kong DF, Samad Z, et al. Echocardiographic risk stratification for early surgery with endocarditis: a cost-effectiveness analysis. *Heart*; 2007. https://doi.org/10.1136/hrt.2006.106716.
84. Rohmann S, Erbel R, Darius H, et al. Prediction of rapid versus prolonged healing of infective endocarditis by monitoring vegetation size. *J Am Soc Echocardiogr*. 1991;4:465–474.
85. Vieira ML, Grinberg M, Pomerantzeff PM, Andrade JL, Mansur AJ. Repeated echocardiographic examinations of patients with suspected infective endocarditis. *Heart*. 2004;90:1020–1024.
86. Kort S. Real-time 3-dimensional echocardiography for prosthetic valve endocarditis: initial experience. *J Am Soc Echocardiogr*. 2006;19:130–139.
86a. Liu YW, Tsai WC, Lin CC, et al. Usefulness of real-time three-dimensional echocardiography for diagnosis of infective endocarditis. *Scand Cardiovasc J*. 2009;43:318–323.
87. Kim IC, Chang S, Hong GR, et al. Comparison of cardiac computed tomography with transesophageal echocardiography for identifying vegetation and intracardiac complications in patients with infective endocarditis in the era of 3-dimensional images. *Circ Cardiovasc Imaging*. 2018;11. e006986.
88. Cowan JC, Patrick D, Reid DS. Aortic root abscess complicating bacterial endocarditis. Demonstration by computed tomography. *Br Heart J*. 1984;52:591–593.
89. Allum C, Knight C, Mohiaddin R, Poole-Wilson P. Images in cardiovascular medicine. Use of magnetic resonance imaging to demonstrate a fistula from the aorta to the right atrium. *Circulation*. 1998;97:1024.
90. Akins EW, Slone RM, Wiechmann BN, Browning M, Martin TD, Mayfield WR. Perivalvular pseudoaneurysm complicating bacterial endocarditis: MR detection in five cases. *AJR Am J Roentgenol*. 1991;156:1155–1158.

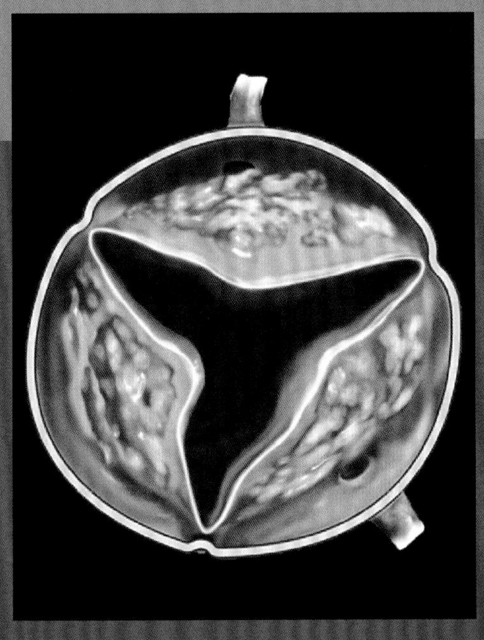

中文导读

第30章 人工心脏瓣膜的流体动力学

多普勒超声心动图使无创检查人工心脏瓣膜功能成为临床现实，但遗憾的是，其仍存在许多不完善的地方，这主要是由于人工心脏瓣膜的声影、反射和超声技术的局限性。但是超声检查可以通过计算或估计一些重要的参数来帮助评估人工心脏瓣膜的功能和性能。

人工心脏瓣膜植入后，其功能主要由其血流动力学特性决定。要了解人工心脏瓣膜的血流动力学性能，就必须对相应的物理学知识有深刻的了解。本章向读者介绍了流体动力学的基本原理、关于人工心脏瓣膜评估的相关公式和各种人工心脏瓣膜的流体力学特性。其主要内容如下：①流体动力学原理内容，包括质量守恒定律、伯努利原理、机械能损失机制、狭窄中的机械能转换和损失等；②人工心脏瓣膜中流体动力学的应用，包括压力下降、压差、有效瓣口面积、反流量、机械能的损失和人工心脏瓣膜的体内评价；③自体瓣膜的血流动力学；④不同人工心脏瓣膜的血流动力学改变，包括机械瓣、生物瓣和经导管植入瓣膜。

卫 青

30 Fluid Dynamics of Prosthetic Valves

AJIT P. YOGANATHAN, PhD | VRISHANK RAGHAV, PhD

Doppler echocardiography has made noninvasive examination of prosthetic heart valve function a clinical reality. Unfortunately, there are still many imperfections in echocardiographic examinations due to acoustic shadowing, reflections caused by implanted valves, and limitations in ultrasound technology. Nevertheless, a number of important parameters can be calculated or estimated to aid in the assessment of prosthetic heart valve function and performance.

After a valve has been implanted, its function is governed primarily by its hemodynamic characteristics. To understand the hemodynamic performance of prosthetic heart valves, it is necessary to have a solid background in the physical laws that govern their function. This chapter introduces cardiologists to the governing principles of fluid dynamics, relevant formulations used in prosthetic valve assessment, and fluid mechanical characteristics of specific prosthetic heart valves.

PRINCIPLES OF FLUID DYNAMICS

CONSERVATION OF MASS

The principle of conservation of mass is important in evaluating valve effective orifice area (EOA). Conservation of mass, or the continuity principle, is a mass balance over the boundaries of a volume of fluid. For example, a volume can be made to coincide with a section of an artery, with the left ventricle (LV), or with the surface of a blood cell, and it also can be made to move over time. This is the *control volume*, and its boundaries are usually chosen to give information regarding an unknown flow rate, average velocity, or surface area flow into or out of the volume based on more easily measurable quantities. Examples of control volumes useful for determining aortic and mitral valve areas with conservation of mass are shown in Fig. 30.1.

Conservation of mass within the control volume can be expressed as follows:

$$\text{Rate of mass accumulation} = \text{Rate of mass input} - \text{Rate of mass output} \quad \text{(Eq. 30.1)}$$

In cardiovascular applications, we can assume that the density of blood is constant because blood is composed mostly of water, which is almost incompressible, and thermal expansion or contraction is insignificant due to the narrow range of body temperature. Mass is the product of density and volume, and mass conservation can be expressed as volume conservation:

$$\text{Rate of volume accumulation} = \text{Rate of volume input} - \text{Rate of volume output} \quad \text{(Eq. 30.2)}$$

In mathematical form, this is

$$\frac{(V_f - V_i)}{t} = Q_{in} - Q_{out} \quad \text{(Eq. 30.3)}$$

where Q_{in} is the total flow rate into the control volume, Q_{out} is the total flow rate out of the control volume, V_i is the size of the control volume at the beginning of the observation, and V_f is the size of the control volume after an observation at time t. There can be multiple sources of flow inlets and outlets:

$$\frac{1}{t}(V_f - V_i) = (Q_{in(1)} + Q_{in(2)} + Q_{in(3)}) - (Q_{out(1)} + Q_{out(2)} + Q_{out(3)}) \quad \text{(Eq. 30.4)}$$

If we further assume that the volume of the control volume does not change with time, the left-hand side of Eq. 30.3 is zero, and conservation of mass can be expressed as follows:

$$Q_{in} = Q_{out} \quad \text{(Eq. 30.5)}$$

This is approximately true in most blood vessels if we neglect expansion vessels under elevated pressure. Often, flow rate in circular, nonbranching vessels can be decomposed into an average axial velocity *({vbar})* and a cross-sectional area *(A)*. Eq. 30.5 becomes

$$\dot{v}_{in}A_{in} = \dot{v}_{out}A_{out} \quad \text{(Eq. 30.6)}$$

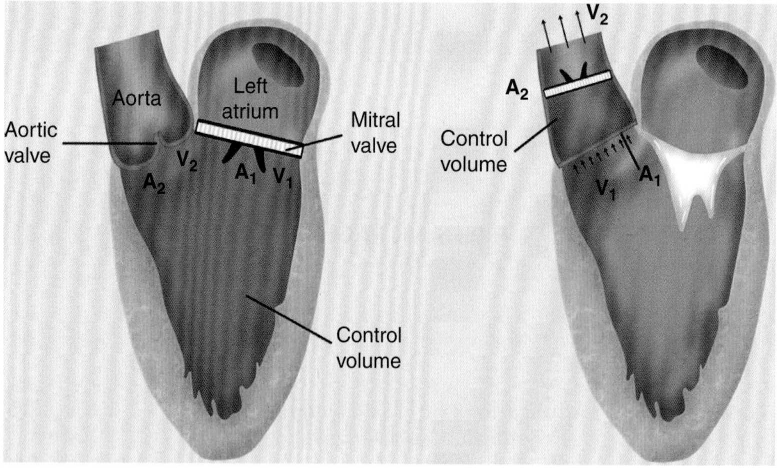

Fig. 30.1 Control volume analysis to determine valve area. Control volumes are used for determining mitral *(left)* and aortic *(right)* valve areas with conservation of mass. V_1 and V_2 represent average velocities of the blood flowing over areas *A1* and *A2*, respectively.

Flow through a prosthetic aortic valve is an example of this situation. The rate of fluid mass moving toward the valve from upstream has to equal the rate of fluid mass moving through the vena contracta or further downstream of the aorta. This principle is the basis of the equations for calculating EOA using Doppler echocardiography.

MECHANICAL ENERGY

Mechanical energy can be described as the ability to accelerate a mass of material over a certain distance. Energy per unit volume has the same dimensions as pressure. It is perhaps best to report energy in cardiovascular applications on a per-unit-volume basis because most members of the medical field are accustomed to working with units of pressure. However, it is important to consider pressure as only one of several forms of mechanical energy.

Pressure *(p)* can be shown to be a form of mechanical energy per unit volume by recognizing that it represents a force (F_p) per unit area *(A)*. If a force is applied to move a mass over a distance *(d)*, it performs work, expending pressure energy (E_p). The area that the force acts on multiplied by the distance over which it moves represents a volume *(V)*:

$$\frac{E_p}{V} = \frac{F_p d}{Ad} = \frac{F_p}{A} = p \qquad \text{(Eq. 30.7)}$$

Pressure is not the only form of mechanical energy in the circulation. Acceleration due to gravity *(g)* creates another form of mechanical energy per unit volume. Gravity can accelerate a mass *(m)* with a force (F_g). If this force moves the mass over a vertical distance *(h)*, it too performs work and expends gravitational energy (E_g). The energy per unit volume is obtained by substituting density (ρ) for mass per unit volume.

$$\frac{E_g}{V} = \frac{F_g h}{V} = \frac{mgh}{V} = \rho gh \qquad \text{(Eq. 30.8)}$$

Mechanical energy per unit volume exists in the circulation in the form of kinetic energy, or energy of movement. If a mass *(m)* is moving at a velocity *(v)*, it contains kinetic energy, equivalent to half the product of the mass and the square of the velocity:

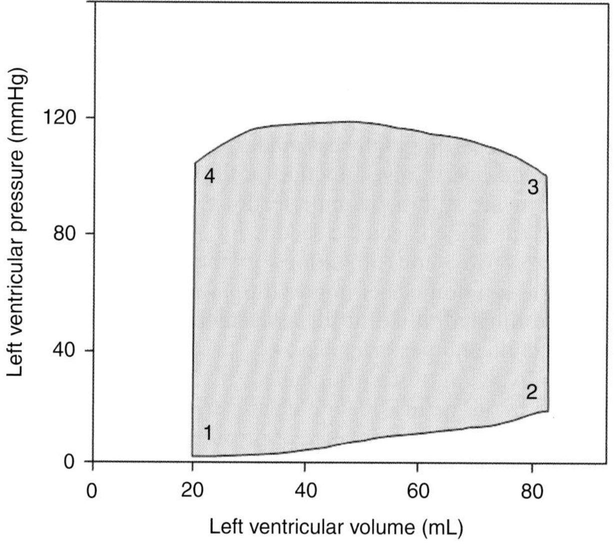

Fig. 30.2 The pressure-volume curve. Pressure-volume diagram for the LV. The *shaded area* represents the energy given to the flow by one stroke of the ventricle.

$$\frac{E_k}{V} = \frac{\frac{1}{2}mv^2}{V} = \frac{1}{2}\rho v^2 \qquad \text{(Eq. 30.9)}$$

The energy per unit volume is obtained by substituting density for mass per unit volume. There are three forms of mechanical energy in the circulation.

The primary source of mechanical energy in the circulation is the work performed by the LV. Contraction of the ventricle creates an increase in pressure inside the ventricle. As Eq. 30.7 implies, subsequent movement of a volume of fluid by this pressure results in the generation of mechanical energy. The energy generated by the ventricle during one cardiac cycle is illustrated in Fig. 30.2. This diagram represents the pressure and volume within the ventricle during the course of one cardiac cycle. The curve between points 1 and 2 represents the period of diastolic filling, when the mitral valve is open and the ventricle fills. The mitral valve shuts at point 2, and the period of isovolumic contraction begins. Between points 2 and 3, the volume of blood in the ventricle remains constant, but the pressure rises considerably. The aortic valve opens at point 3. This starts the period of systolic ejection, during which blood is moved by the ventricle into the aorta. At point 4, the aortic valve closes and the period of isovolumic relaxation begins. During this period, the ventricular volume remains constant, but the pressure falls, returning the ventricle to its state at point 1.

The energy generated by the ventricle during one cardiac cycle is equivalent to the integral of the pressure-volume diagram (the shaded area in Fig. 30.2). The energy per unit volume generated by the ventricle is equivalent to the integral of the pressure with respect to volume divided by the stroke volume. This is roughly equivalent to the average increase in LV pressure from diastole to systole. The ventricle creates energy in the form of pressure, but this energy is converted to gravitational and kinetic energy elsewhere in the circulation.

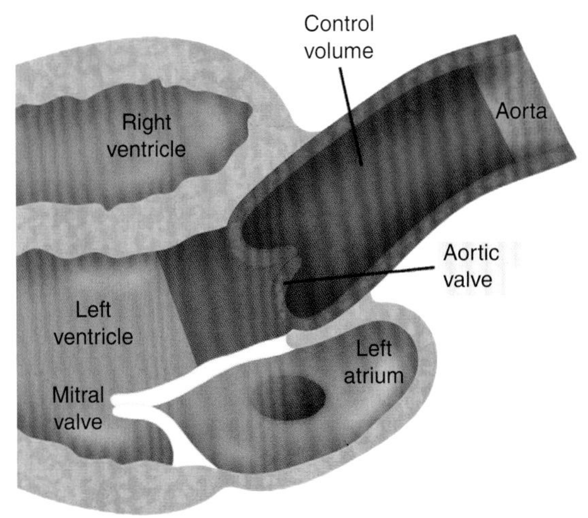

Fig. 30.3 Control volume analysis for the aortic valve. Example of control volume *(purple-shaded area)* for the analysis of energy loss in the aortic valve.

BERNOULLI'S EQUATION

Pressure, gravitational, and kinetic energies in the circulation can be freely converted from one to another without energy loss. Bernoulli's equation for steady flow illustrates this. The Bernoulli equation relates the relative amounts of pressure, gravitational energy, and kinetic energy per unit volume between two spatial locations along the path of a flow (locations 1 and 2, where location 2 is downstream of location 1), assuming that no energy is lost:

$$\frac{1}{2}\rho v_1^2 + \rho g h_1 + p_1 = \frac{1}{2}\rho v_2^2 + \rho g h_2 + p_2 \quad \text{(Eq. 30.10)}$$

The Bernoulli equation for steady flow states that the total mechanical energy per unit volume at locations 1 and 2 are the same but can exist in different forms. It shows that a decrease in pressure from location 1 to location 2 may be balanced by an increase in fluid velocity or height without loss of energy. A pressure drop is not mechanical energy loss if it is accompanied by an increase in gravitational or kinetic energy; these energies can be converted back to pressure energy later.

Additional variables may be added to the equation to account for the effects of unsteady flow and mechanical energy loss:

$$\frac{1}{2}\rho v_1^2 + \rho g h_1 + p_1 = \frac{1}{2}\rho v_2^2 + \rho g h_2 + p_2 + \int_1^2 \rho \frac{\partial v}{\partial t}\partial s + \Phi \quad \text{(Eq. 30.11)}$$

where s represents the distance of the path between locations 1 and 2, and Φ represents loss of mechanical energy per unit volume. The added terms represent the contribution of acceleration of the fluid to flow energy and the conversion of mechanical energy to heat, respectively, between locations 1 and 2. Rearranging Eq. 30.11 to express energy loss in terms of the other parameters yields the following:

$$\Phi = (p_1 - p_2) + \frac{1}{2}\rho\left(v_1^2 - v_2^2\right) + \rho g\left(h_1 - h_2\right) - \int_1^2 \rho \frac{\partial v}{\partial t}\partial s \quad \text{(Eq. 30.12)}$$

CONTROL VOLUME ENERGY ANALYSIS

A more detailed analysis of the energy of fluid flow through a valve can be conducted using the control volume approach. Bernoulli's equation describes energy conversion and loss along a streamline (line of fluid flow), and it is a useful, simplified approach to analyze fluid energy in valves, whereas the control volume approach provides three-dimensional (3D) analysis of fluid energy at any time in the cardiac cycle. If the control volume is the blood volume around the valve, as shown in Fig. 30.3, manipulation of the Navier-Stokes governing equations of fluid flow gives the following equation[1]:

$$\int S_{ij}T_{ij}dV = \int -P\left(u_i \cdot \dot{n}_i\right)dA - \int \rho u_i g_i dV - \frac{d}{dt}\int \frac{1}{2}\rho u_i^2 dV \quad \text{(Eq. 30.13)}$$

where S is the shear stresses, T is the shear deformation, P is pressure, u is velocity, A is the surface of the control volume, n is the normal direction at the surface of the control volume, g is the gravitational force, and V is the control volume. The subscripts i and j refer to any of the three Cartesian coordinate axes, in accordance to Einstein's notation. Eq. 30.13 can be described in words as follows:

Energy dissipation = Energy supplied by pressure gradient − Energy converted to gravitational potential energy − Energy converted into kinetic energy (Eq. 30.14)

The pressure gradient across the valve, which is supplied by the heart muscles, is partially converted into kinetic energy (used to accelerate fluid) and partially used to counter the effects of gravity. The remaining energy is lost as heat and sound.

MECHANISMS OF MECHANICAL ENERGY LOSS

Mechanical energy can be converted to heat and sound through friction between blood volumes moving at different velocities and between blood and the vessel walls. Heat and sound generated through friction is not readily converted back to mechanical energy, and this energy is said to be lost to the cause of blood circulation. The frictional losses take one of two forms: viscous losses and turbulent losses. Additional energy can be effectively

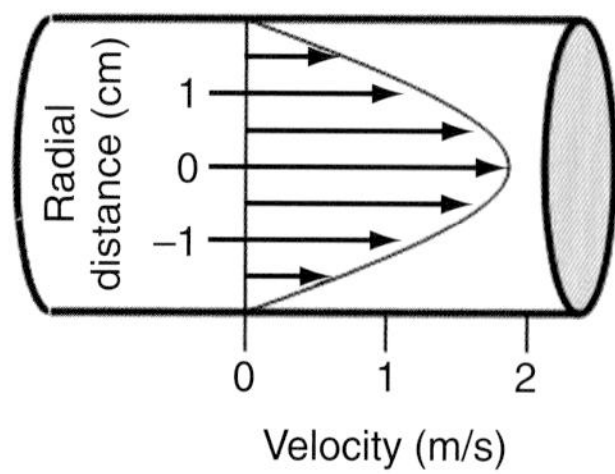

Fig. 30.4 Velocity profile in a blood vessel. The fluid velocity varies with respect to radial distance in a blood vessel. These variations are a result of viscous forces.

lost in the circulation due to valvular leakage. These forms of energy loss are described in the following sections.

Viscous Losses

As a result of frictional forces, fluid immediately adjacent to a solid boundary moves with the same velocity as the boundary. In the case of a stationary vessel, this means that fluid immediately adjacent to the vessel wall does not move, no matter how fast the surrounding flow is moving. As the distance increases from the solid boundary, the velocity may increase. This leads to differences in fluid velocity with respect to radial distance within the vessel (Fig. 30.4).

Fluid viscosity, the tendency of the fluid components or molecules to stick to each other, creates friction between fluid components that are close to one another if they move at different velocities. This is the mechanism of viscous energy loss. Viscous losses typically increase with flow rate, and they decrease dramatically with increasing vessel radius. This is why vasodilators are effective in relieving LV workload.

Turbulent Losses

Turbulent losses usually do not occur in the circulation but can be greater in magnitude than viscous losses when they do. Turbulence is characterized by chaotic spatial and temporal fluctuations in the direction and magnitude of fluid velocity. It is a result of the inertia of the flow being too great for frictional forces to stabilize fluid movement or to dampen unsteady secondary motions. Chaotic spatial and temporal velocity fluctuations result in excessive mixing of fluid; individual tiny pockets of fluid experience very high shear stresses with other pockets of fluid everywhere in the flow. Consequently, there are high overall frictional energy losses, which is the essence of turbulent losses.

In a straight vessel, fluid inertia disturbances may be initiated by small irregularities, or roughness, in the surface of the vessel. In laminar flow, these small inertia disturbances are quickly dampened by viscous forces, and unsteady secondary flow and fluid mixing are minimal. In turbulent flow, the inertia changes become amplified because viscous forces are not strong enough to dampen them. The analogy is being tripped while walking versus running. It is harder to maintain balance when tripped during running than during walking because the inertia of the body's motion is difficult to control.

The tendency toward turbulence in a fluid flow is determined by the ratio of inertial forces to frictional forces in the flow. The inertial force of a moving flow is the force required to bring the flow to rest; the frictional force of such a flow is created by viscous shear stress acting on solid surfaces. In vessel flow, this ratio is approximated by the Reynolds number:

$$N_{\mathrm{Re}} = \frac{D\bar{v}\rho}{\mu} \qquad \text{(Eq. 30.15)}$$

where D is the inner diameter of the vessel, $\bar{v}$ is the average velocity of the flow, ρ is the fluid density, and μ is the fluid viscosity.

A low Reynolds number results in laminar flow, whereas a high Reynolds number results in turbulent flow. The point of transition between the two states, the critical Reynolds number, varies for different flow systems. For flow through a straight pipe, the critical Reynolds number is approximately 2000, and flow becomes fully turbulent at a Reynolds number of approximately 6000.[2]

Flow through small, circular orifices creates a phenomenon known as a *free jet*. For steady free jet flows, the critical Reynolds number is approximately 1000, with fully turbulent flow occurring at Reynolds numbers greater than 3000.[3,4] This transition point is lowered by sharp corners and bends in the flow or rough solid surfaces. For turbulence to occur, sufficient time must be allowed for the unsteadiness to amplify and grow. In pulsatile flows, if the frequency of pulses is too high, there may be insufficient time for turbulence to fully develop, making it harder to achieve turbulence. The critical Reynolds number increases.[5]

Valvular Regurgitation

When valvular regurgitation occurs, the heart must compensate by expending more energy to pump additional blood through the valve during the forward flow phase, so that the net sum of forward flow and regurgitation flow remains sufficient for the body. Blood that leaks back through the valve does not contribute to circulation, and the energy used to pump that blood through the valve during forward flow can be viewed as being lost.

In prosthetic valves, valvular regurgitation consists of the closing volume, paravalvular regurgitation, and perivalvular regurgitation. The closing volume is the amount of blood that leaks backward through the valve at the end of forward flow before the valve can properly close. Paravalvular regurgitation is blood leakage through the valve orifice. In the bioprosthetic valve, calcification of the leaflets can lead to improper coaptation and paravalvular regurgitation. In mechanical valves, paravalvular regurgitation can occur through gaps in the closed valve. Perivalvular regurgitation occurs because of improper attachment of the prosthetic valve to the heart tissues. For example, when prosthesis dehiscence occurs, blood leaks through the gap opened up by the dehiscence.

MECHANICAL ENERGY CONVERSION AND LOSS IN A STENOSIS

To show how mechanical energy may be changed from one form to another or lost, it is good to refer to an illustration depicting the changes in mechanical energy across an aortic stenosis. Fig. 30.5 shows the overall energy conversion and losses, pressure energy, and kinetic energy as blood flow traverses the contraction, throat, and expansion sections of the stenosis.

The first section of the stenosis (1–2) is the flow contraction section. Because, according to the continuity equation, the velocity at location 2 must be higher than that at location 1, kinetic energy increases from 1 to 2. This increase in kinetic energy occurs at the expense of a large amount of pressure energy; a relatively small amount of total energy is lost in the flow contraction. Most of the lost energy in flow contraction consists of viscous losses. However, there may be a small amount of flow separation immediately after abrupt contractions.

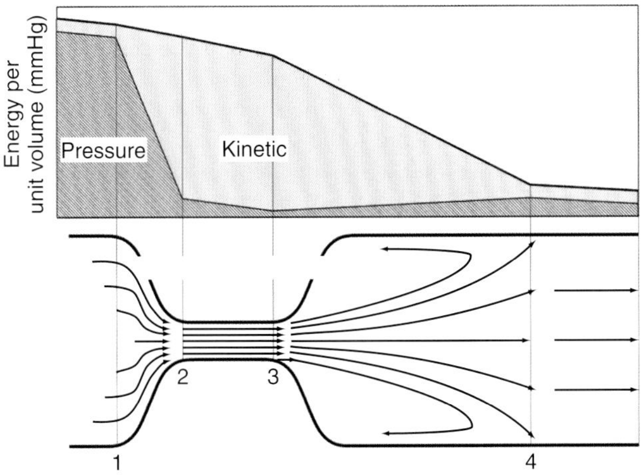

Fig. 30.5 **Conservation of energy through a stenosis.** Schematic shows the pressure and kinetic energy loss and conversion as flow traverses a stenosis. The flow undergoes contraction from location 1 to location 2. The throat of the stenosis lies between locations 2 and 3, and the flow suddenly expands from location 3 to location 4.

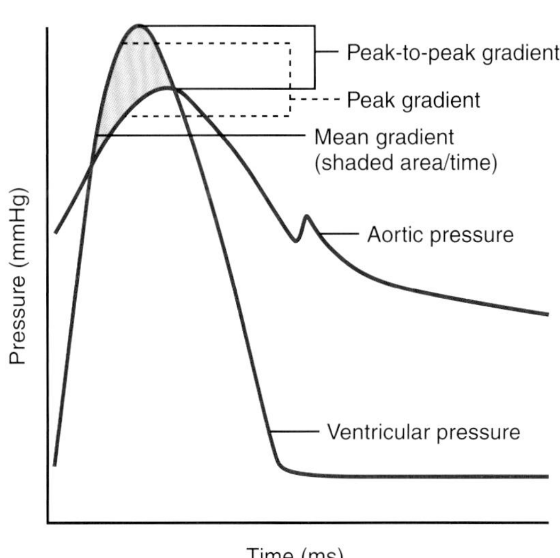

Fig. 30.6 **Transvalvular pressure gradients.** Mean, peak, and peak-to-peak pressure differences across an aortic valve.

Flow separation occurs because the momentum of the flow causes it to continue to converge for a short period after the anatomic contraction point (see Fig. 30.5). Such abrupt contractions have considerably more energy loss than gradual ones.

The second section of the stenosis (2–3) represents a throat of constant cross-sectional area. In this section, the continuity equation states that the velocity at locations 2 and 3 is the same. There is no loss in kinetic energy; the total energy lost in this section is completely pressure energy. However, only in non-branching vessels of constant cross-sectional area is the pressure gradient equivalent to the total energy loss per unit volume, and usually only a small amount of total energy is lost in the stenosis throat. This energy loss is viscous in nature if the flow is laminar and completely turbulent in nature if the flow has enough momentum to enable its transition to turbulence.

In the expansion section of the stenosis (3–4), a large amount of total energy is lost. All of this lost energy is kinetic in nature, which explains why the Doppler gradient correlates strongly with total mechanical energy loss. However, the Doppler gradient does not completely specify total energy loss because a portion of the kinetic energy is converted into pressure. This is the cause of the *pressure recovery* phenomenon. The expansion section of the stenosis illustrates why pressure gradients can be misleading when estimating the lost driving force for flow. Although the pressure does increase in the expansion section, the total energy loss is very large.

APPLICATIONS OF FLUID DYNAMICS TO PROSTHETIC HEART VALVES

PRESSURE DROP

The pressure drop across a heart valve is commonly used to estimate the amount of energy lost by the flow in traversing the valve. Pressure drops can be directly measured with invasive catheter techniques. Eq. 30.16 shows that the pressure drop across a heart valve is equivalent to energy loss per unit volume provided that the changes in kinetic energy, gravitational energy, and local acceleration of the flow can be ignored. Because of the law of conservation of mass (Eq. 30.6), changes in kinetic energy are negligible if the diameters of the vessels are the same at the points of upstream and downstream pressure measurements and if the downstream measurements are obtained at a location far enough from the valve to allow for pressure recovery.

Changes in gravitational energy are negligible if the patient is supine because there is little height difference between upstream and downstream measurement locations. If the patient is upright, every 5-cm difference in vertical height results in a pressure drop of approximately 3.9 mmHg.

Changes in local acceleration of the flow are negligible if measurements are obtained during peak flow rate across the valve (often called the *peak gradient*). At the peak flow rate, velocity is at its maximum turning point and is momentarily experiencing no acceleration. Effects of acceleration are also negligible if measurements are averaged over the forward flow portion of the valve cycle (i.e., the mean gradient). This occurs because fluid first accelerates and then decelerates back to the initial state over the forward flow phase; therefore, when the acceleration term is integrated over time, it becomes zero.

The peak gradient describes the energy loss during the peak flow phase, whereas the mean gradient describes the average energy lost over the entire forward flow period. For this reason, the peak gradient is always higher than the mean gradient. The pressure drop is often reported in terms of a *peak-to-peak gradient* for convenience, as an approximation of the peak gradient. Differences between peak and peak-to-peak gradients are shown in Fig. 30.6.

DOPPLER GRADIENT

Although energy lost by the flow in traversing the valve can be estimated more directly with catheterization, these losses are now typically estimated noninvasively with the help of echocardiography. A version of Eq. 30.12 is used to estimate the amount of pressure converted to kinetic energy as the flow contracts from well upstream of the valve to the point of maximum flow contraction; the equation is simplified by neglecting the small energy conversions to gravitational potential energy:

$$\Delta p = 4\left(v_{\max}^2 - v_{\text{ups}}^2\right) \quad \text{(Eq. 30.16)}$$

where Δp is the pressure drop $(p_1 - p_2)$ during flow contraction (in mmHg), v_{ups} is the velocity upstream of the contraction during forward flow (in cm/s), and v_{max} is the velocity at the point of maximum flow contraction during forward flow (in cm/s). The constant 4 is used to account for the density of blood and unit conversions. This simplification assumes that mechanical energy loss and changes in gravitational energy and local acceleration are negligible as the flow contracts. Assumptions regarding changes in kinetic energy, effects of accelerations, the use of mean gradient versus peak gradient, and gravitational potential energy are the same as those discussed earlier (see Pressure Drop).

The conversion from pressure to kinetic energy within the flow contraction section (see Fig. 30.5) is the quantity measured when estimating the pressure gradient with Doppler echocardiography. Most of this converted energy is lost after the expansion because the kinetic energy upstream and downstream of the expansion is about the same according to Eq. 30.6. Because the Doppler gradient is measured between the upstream point and the vena contracta point, it does not account for the pressure recovery, which occurs downstream of the vena contracta, and may overestimate energy lost by the flow.

Another problem with the use of the Doppler gradient is placement of the transducer. If the transducer is placed obliquely with respect to the jet axis, the measured velocity will underestimate the true velocity of the jet,[7] and the pressure gradient will be underestimated. Because the errors resulting from pressure recovery and oblique transducer placement tend to offset each other, Doppler ultrasound can sometimes match pressure measurements obtained from catheterization quite precisely. Nonetheless, there are instances when the Doppler gradient has significant errors.

Additional complications with the use of the Doppler gradient to evaluate the total energy loss across mechanical prostheses arise because these valves have more than one orifice and the resistance that each orifice offers to flow can be different. Velocity measurements made in the one orifice are not representative of the gradient in pressure or total energy as flow traverses the valve. The difference between Doppler and catheter gradients has been so notable for mechanical prostheses that empirically derived correction factors, depending on valve design, have been suggested to the US Food and Drug Administration (FDA).[6]

Some studies claim that there is negligible difference between pressure gradients measured with a catheter and with Doppler echocardiography, particularly with regard to mean gradients.[7] However, because of its potential problems, the use of Doppler to evaluate the performance of mechanical prostheses should be approached with caution. Often, Eq. 30.16 is simplified further by assuming that upstream velocity is very small relative to the maximum velocity within the contraction:

$$\Delta p = 4v_{max}^2 \qquad \text{(Eq. 30.17)}$$

For a very stenotic orifice, this equation works well because the velocity within the stenosis is much higher compared with the velocity upstream of the stenosis. This approximation should be used only for heavily calcified bioprosthetic valves.

EFFECTIVE ORIFICE AREA

Evaluation of valve performance by pressure drop and Doppler gradient depends on the flow rate across the valve. The EOA does not represent the anatomic orifice area. Instead, it represents the cross-sectional area of the jet issuing from the valve at the point of its greatest contraction (i.e., vena contracta). The size of the EOA depends on the nature of the contraction and the size of the orifice. A sudden contraction has a smaller EOA than a gradual contraction of the same orifice area. Although EOA has been considered to be a parameter for evaluation of valve performance that is independent of cardiac output and heart rate, in vivo[8,9] and in vitro[1] experiments have shown that it varies somewhat with the flow rate.

For bioprosthetic valves, higher flow causes the valve to open a bigger valve orifice area by stretching the valve leaflets outward, allowing the jet flow area and the EOA to increase. For mechanical valves, changes in volumetric flow rate can result in changes in the distribution of velocities across the diameter of the vena contracta,[10] leading to minor changes in the computed EOA. However, the variation of EOA with flow is small, and errors associated with the assumption of EOA invariance to flow rate are manageable.[11]

The EOA can be estimated by applying the continuity equation (Eq. 30.18) to echocardiography measurements of the upstream vessel area (A_{ups}), the temporal average of the velocity upstream of the contraction during forward flow (v_{ups}), and the temporal average of the velocity at the point of maximum flow contraction during forward flow (v_{max}):

$$EOA = \frac{A_{ups} v_{ups}}{v_{max}} \qquad \text{(Eq. 30.18)}$$

Pulsed-wave Doppler imaging is used to measure the upstream velocity, whereas continuous-wave Doppler is used to measure the maximum velocity or the velocity within the vena contracta. If EOA and A_{ups} are assumed to be constant over systole, the velocity–time integral (VTI) can be used instead of velocities; the VTI is the area under the curve of the velocity versus time plot. The upstream area is estimated with planimetry using B-mode echocardiography. The clinically implemented equation is

$$EOA = \frac{A_{ups} VTI_{ups}}{VTI_{max}} \qquad \text{(Eq. 30.19)}$$

The Gorlin formula can also be used to estimate EOA with catheter measurements. The Gorlin formula is a combination of Eq. 30.6 and either Eq. 30.16 or Eq. 30.17:

$$EOA = \frac{Q}{51.6\sqrt{\Delta p}} \qquad \text{(Eq. 30.20)}$$

where EOA is the effective orifice area (in cm^2), Q is the temporal average of the flow rate during forward flow (in cm^3/s), and Δp is the mean pressure drop across the valve during forward flow (in mmHg). The constant 51.6 is used to account for the density of blood and unit conversions.

The EOA differs from the aortic valve area initially described by Gorlin,[12] which is the geometric area of the valve orifice as traced by the free edge of the leaflets. EOA is the area of flow slightly downstream of the aortic valve area, where flow is contracted slightly. Whereas the factor of 44.3 is used in the computation of aortic valve area, a factor of 51.6 should be used for the EOA. The EOA can be obtained through this method with invasive cardiac catheterization or noninvasive echocardiographic examination. With the catheter approach, Δp is directly measured with fluid-filled or sensor-mounted catheters, and Q is estimated by measuring cardiac output (CO) by the Fick method (thermodilution and dye dilution),[13] the heart rate (HR), and the systolic duration (SD):

$$Q = \frac{CO}{HR \cdot SD} \quad \text{(Eq. 30.21)}$$

The catheter approach can be expected to overestimate the EOA due to the pressure recovery phenomenon. However, the catheter formulation, dubbed the *energy loss coefficient*, may be useful as a separate entity in evaluating the severity of aortic stenosis.

With the noninvasive echocardiography approach, Q is estimated by multiplying the upstream vessel area (A_{ups}) by the upstream velocity time integral (VTI_{ups}), and Δp is estimated by the Doppler gradient using Eq. 30.16 or 30.17:

$$EOA = \frac{A_{ups} \cdot VTI_{ups}}{51.6\sqrt{\Delta p}} \quad \text{(Eq. 30.22)}$$

The use of Eq. 30.16 or 30.17 makes the same simplifying assumptions as those previously described (see Doppler Gradient and Pressure Gradient) and should be adapted for use with caution.

When applying Eqs. 30.20 and 30.22, one subtlety should be kept in mind: all variables in the equations are averages obtained during the systolic or diastolic forward flow period through the heart valve. Instantaneous values of pressure and flow rate cannot be used in these equations unless they are taken at the peak flow rate. The Gorlin formula is derived from Bernoulli's equation for steady flow and is therefore invalid in situations in which there is a large net temporal acceleration or deceleration in the flow. For example, in the estimation of Δp using the echocardiography method, the cardiologist should use the average of a few pressure gradients spaced equally over the forward flow phase or the time-integration average of the pressure gradient data. For the estimation of Q in the echocardiography method, the VTI, which accounts for the velocities over the entire forward flow phase, is recommended.

Averages over the entire cycle may not be relevant, especially if aortic regurgitation occurs concurrently.[14] Estimations of forward flow rate that do not involve echocardiography (i.e., Fick's method, thermal dilution, and dye dilution) are averages over the entire cardiac cycle (Q_{net}). If there is no regurgitation, these methods can be used to estimate the average forward flow rate during systole. However, if aortic regurgitation exists, direct application of the Gorlin formula results in underestimation of EOA:

$$Q = \frac{Q_{net}}{(1 - RF)} \quad \text{(Eq. 30.23)}$$

where RF represents the regurgitant fraction of the aortic valve.

In the in vitro setting, prosthetic valve EOA is measured with the Gorlin equation because direct measurements of pressures and flow are very easily achieved. The volumetric flow rate can be measured at high temporal resolution with commercial flow probes, and pressures can be measured through catheter-like tubes directly upstream and downstream of the valve with the use of commercial pressure gauges. In vitro testing of prosthetic valves uses the following equation for calculating EOA[15]:

$$EOA = \frac{Q_{RMS}}{51.6\sqrt{\Delta p_{mean}}} \quad \text{(Eq. 30.24)}$$

where EOA is in units of cm^2, Q_{RMS} is the square root of the temporal mean of the square of volumetric flow rate (in mL/s) during the forward flow phase, and Δp_{mean} is the temporal mean of the pressure drop across the valve during the forward flow phase (in mmHg).

A measure of a valve's resistance to forward flow that is based on EOA is the *performance index*. This is the ratio of EOA to the valve sewing ring area (A_{sew}):

$$PI = \frac{EOA}{A_{sew}} \quad \text{(Eq. 30.25)}$$

The performance index provides a measure of how well a valve design uses its total mounting area, which is the area the flow would experience without the valve. Whereas EOA depends on valve size, the performance index effectively normalizes EOA for valve size.

REGURGITANT VOLUME

Pressure drop, Doppler gradient, and EOA give quantitative estimates of the energy lost by the flow in traversing a valve during forward flow. Flow energy can also be lost due to leakage across the valve when the pressure gradient across the valve reverses. A small amount of flow leaks across the valve during valve closure. Mechanical prosthetic valves are unable to form tight seals when closed, and regurgitant jets occur in these valves under normal conditions.

Normal regurgitant flow is characterized by a closing volume during valve closure and leakage after closure. The regurgitant volume is the total volume of fluid that moves through the valve per beat due to the retrograde flow. It is equal to the sum of the closing volume and the leakage volume. The closing volume is the volume of fluid flowing retrograde through the valve during valve closure. Any fluid volume accumulation after valve closure results from leakage and is referred to as the *leakage volume*.

Regurgitant volume of prosthetic valves is governed by valve type, size, and position. Bioprostheses have a small closing volume but do not leak if functioning properly. Bileaflet mechanical designs tend to have greater regurgitant volume than tilting disc designs.[16] Larger valves leak more than smaller ones. Regurgitant volume is most problematic in positions in which the pressure gradient during closure and leakage is high and the duration of leakage is long. Energy losses due to regurgitant flow can exceed forward flow energy losses in large mitral prostheses.[16] Although prosthetic valves normally exhibit a very small amount of regurgitant flow, they can cause substantial regurgitation when they malfunction.

To distinguish normal from abnormal valve function, it is important to differentiate normal regurgitant volume from additional regurgitation due to disease. For in vitro evaluation of prosthetic valves, regurgitation volumes can be easily evaluated with commercial flow probes or velocimetry techniques such as particle image velocimetry or laser Doppler velocimetry. The direct calculation of energy loss due to regurgitation can be estimated using Eq. 30.29 (discussed later).

Most means of quantifying regurgitant volume use some form of a control volume and conservation of mass. For noninvasive quantification of regurgitation flow with echocardiography, the most commonly used method is the proximal isovelocity surface area (PISA) method,[17-20] which is applicable for bioprosthetic valves. The principle of the PISA technique is based on the fact that a fluid entering a regurgitant orifice must accelerate to reach a peak velocity at the throat of the orifice. If the orifice is circular, this acceleration region should be axisymmetric about the center of the orifice. Upstream of the regurgitant orifice, a series of hemispherical isovelocity contours can be defined within the flow field. Eq. 30.5 states that for a control volume that does not change in size, the same amount of fluid that enters the volume must also exit it. If the control volume is constructed to coincide with a hemispherical contour and the regurgitant orifice,

$$RV = 2\pi r^2 v_{ups} t \quad \text{(Eq. 30.26)}$$

where v_{ups} represents the temporal average of the velocity at a radial distance r upstream of the regurgitant orifice during forward flow and t represents the time during which regurgitation takes place during a single beat. The expression $2\pi r^2$ in this equation represents the surface area of the hemispherical shell surrounding the control volume.

MECHANICAL ENERGY LOSSES

Pressure gradient and EOA parameters are indicative of the energy loss in valves. However, they are not direct measures of mechanical energy losses, which should be measured in joules per cycle or watts.

Direct measurement of mechanical energy loss is possible in vitro with Eq. 30.12 (i.e., Bernoulli equation analysis) and Eq. 30.15 (i.e., control volume analysis). When Eq. 30.12 is integrated over one cardiac cycle, the final term becomes zero due to the periodicity or repetitive nature of fluid flow through the valve. The gravitational potential energy term (i.e., second-last term) is usually small and can be neglected. The remaining terms can be simplified to the following:

$$\Phi_{cycle} = \int_{cycle} Q\left[\left(P_1 + \frac{1}{2}\rho v_1^2\right) - \left(P_2 + \frac{1}{2}\rho v_2^2\right)\right] dt \quad \text{(Eq. 30.27)}$$

where Φ_{cycle} is the energy loss per cycle, Q is the volumetric flow rate, and the subscripts 1 and 2 refer to locations upstream and downstream of the valve, respectively. Heinrich et al. measured the energy loss per cardiac cycle for the St. Jude Medical bileaflet mechanical valve and the Medtronic Hall tilting-disc mechanical valve and showed that there was no significant difference in energy loss between these two valves.[21] Energy loss escalated with increased stroke volume and heart rate.

Eq. 30.13 can be simplified to the following form by assuming that energy conversion to gravitational potential energy is small:

$$\Phi_{inst} = Q \cdot (P_1 - P_2) - \frac{dKE}{dt} \quad \text{(Eq. 30.28)}$$

where Φ_{inst} is the instantaneous energy loss, KE is the kinetic energy within the control volume, and the subscripts 1 and 2 refer to the control volume boundaries upstream and downstream of the valve, respectively. By making suitable assumptions of the flow profile, Yap et al. measured the instantaneous energy losses for a trileaflet valve and showed that most of the energy is lost during late systole, when there is an adverse pressure gradient to decelerate forward flow, and excessive mixing of fluid occurs from flow reversals.[1] Energy loss also increased with stroke volume and heart rate.

To calculate energy loss as a result of valvular regurgitation, we assume that all of the mechanical energy causing the regurgitation is lost:

$$\Phi_{regurg} = \int_{regurg} Q \cdot (P_1 - P_2)\, dt \quad \text{(Eq. 30.29)}$$

where Φ_{regurg} is the total regurgitation energy loss over one cardiac cycle, Q is the regurgitation volumetric flow rate, and the subscripts 1 and 2 refer, respectively, to locations upstream and downstream of the regurgitation orifice (i.e., the valve). Azadani et al. used this approach to estimate the regurgitation energy losses occurring in transcatheter valves and found that regurgitation energy loss can be as high one third of the total energy loss associated with the valve.[22]

Energy loss through valves during forward flow depends on the volumetric flow rate, the density of the fluid, the viscosity of the fluid, the size of the valve (which can be represented by the body surface area), and the shape of the valve (e.g., whether it is stenotic). Rigorous analysis with the Buckingham pi theorem indicates that energy loss can be nondimensionalized using density, the cube of flow rate, and the square of body surface area.[23] When normalized by these scaling parameters, the energy loss is directly dependent on the Reynolds number and the shape of the valve:

$$\varepsilon \propto \rho \frac{Q^3}{BSA^2} \quad \text{(Eq. 30.30)}$$

$$\frac{\varepsilon}{\rho \frac{Q^3}{BSA^2}} = f(N_{Re}, S) \quad \text{(Eq. 30.31)}$$

where ε is energy dissipation, ϱ is density, Q is flow rate, BSA is body surface area, N_{Re} is the Reynolds number, and S is the dimensionless shape factor.

Clinically, the direct measurement of energy loss is not widely used for assessment of heart valves in vivo. However, energy efficiency parameters have the advantage of being a direct measure of the contribution of valve fluid dynamics to heart failure (i.e., heart failure can be interpreted as failure of the heart to generate sufficient energy to overcome energy losses in the circulation). For example, as discussed by Dasi et al., patients with end-stage aortic stenosis failure who have low flow and low gradients can have deceivingly normal EOAs, but with energy loss analysis, it becomes apparent that these patients have failing hearts.[23] Atkins et al. provided a review of mechanical energy loss analysis in heart valves.[24]

NOVEL ENERGY LOSS PARAMETERS

As Fig. 30.5 implies, much more mechanical energy is lost in flow expansion than in flow contraction or in the throat regions of prosthetic valves. This is particularly true in tissue valves due to the gradual nature of the flow contraction and the small throat region. Localization of energy loss to the flow expansion region simplifies the problem considerably by allowing energy losses occurring in aortic valve stenoses to be modeled by an abrupt expansion. The total energy loss per unit volume across an abrupt expansion can be derived using Eq. 30.6, Eq. 30.12, and a form of conservation of momentum[25]:

$$\Phi = 4v_{max}^2\left(1 - \left(\frac{EOA}{A_{aorta}}\right)\right)^2 \quad \text{(Eq. 30.32)}$$

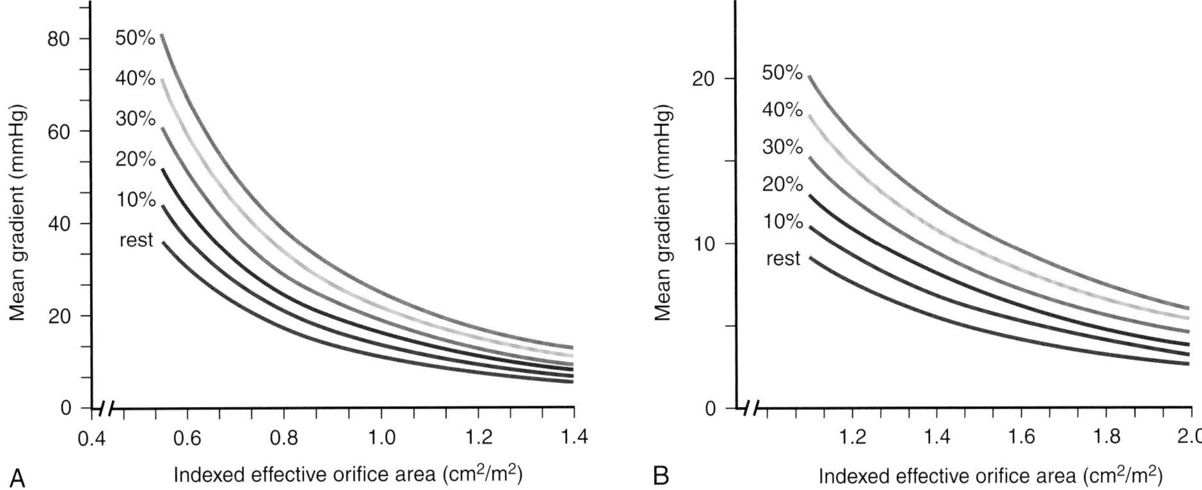

Fig. 30.7 Relationship between transvalvular pressure gradient and indexed effective orifice area. Mean transprosthetic pressure gradient and indexed effective orifice area are compared for aortic bioprostheses (A) and mitral bioprostheses (B) studied in vitro in a physiologic pulse duplicator system, assuming a normal cardiac index of 3.0 L/min/m² at rest and a 10% to 50% increase in stroke volume (as can occur during exercise). (Adapted from Dumesnil JG, Yoganathan AP. Valve prosthesis hemodynamics and the problem of high transprosthetic pressure gradients. *Eur J Cardiothorac Surg*. 1992;6[suppl 1]S34–S37; discussion S38.)

where Φ is measured in mmHg and v_{max} is the temporal average of the velocity at the point of maximum flow contraction (in cm/s). Eq. 30.32, like recovered pressure, is a strong function of the EOA and the cross-sectional area of the aorta. As this area ratio approaches zero, the energy loss per unit volume in the expansion region approaches the Doppler gradient. In cases of severe valvular stenosis, the Doppler gradient is therefore equivalent to mechanical energy loss per unit volume.

The advantage of using Eq. 30.32 rather than the pressure drop or Doppler gradient is that the equation allows estimation of the energy lost by the flow in traversing the valve by means of noninvasive echocardiography while compensating for pressure recovery. When this formulation is used in the aorta, the cross-sectional area of the expansion should be taken as the cross-sectional area of the aorta at the sinotubular junction because the separated flow disappears after the flow has traversed the sinuses of Valsalva.

The energy loss in Eq. 30.32, like the pressure drop and Doppler gradient, depends on flow rate. It is desirable to have a parameter that is closely related to energy loss but relatively independent of flow rate for the evaluation of prosthesis function. Such a parameter can be derived by substituting Eq. 30.32 for the Doppler gradient in Eq. 30.20. This parameter has been dubbed the *energy loss coefficient* (ELCo)[26]:

$$\text{ELCo} = \frac{A_{\text{aorta}}\,\text{EOA}}{(A_{\text{aorta}} - \text{EOA})} \qquad \text{(Eq. 30.33)}$$

where EOA is measured by echocardiography using Eq. 30.18 or Eq. 30.20. The energy loss coefficient is equivalent to Eq. 30.23 if Δp in Eq. 30.23 is measured with pressure transducers that are placed far enough downstream to account for energy recovery. The advantage of using the energy loss coefficient rather than EOA is that the energy loss coefficient is based on recovered pressure.

IN VIVO EVALUATION OF PROSTHETIC VALVES

The in vivo evaluation of prosthetic valves is done clinically when patients with prosthetic valve implants suffer from abnormal cardiac function. Prosthetic valve implants are all mildly stenotic, because the prosthetic valves are usually implanted within the aortic lumen space, all of which was previously available for flow. In some cases, unusually high gradients are observed despite normal prosthesis function.[27] These are most likely cases of patient-prosthesis mismatch, in which the implanted valve is too small to accommodate the cardiac output required by the large size of the patient. Patients with hypertrophic hearts or calcific aortic stenosis are especially prone to patient-prosthesis mismatch because it is difficult to insert large prostheses into constricted sites. Patient-prosthesis mismatch affects the patient's physical capacity and postoperative mortality risk.[28]

To detect patient-prosthesis mismatch, echocardiographic evaluation of the EOA of the prosthesis should be performed and the findings compared with literature values for the EOA of the same model and size of prosthesis. If the EOA is lower than that reported in the literature, it is likely that there is prosthesis dysfunction. If the EOA is similar to that reported in the literature but a high pressure gradient exists, it is likely that there is a patient-prosthesis mismatch. In vitro investigation has shown that the indexed EOA is inversely related to the mean pressure gradient, as shown in Fig. 30.7. In the case of a mismatch, when small indexed EOAs exist, exercising will lead to greater elevation in the mean gradient than when there is no mismatch.

HEMODYNAMICS OF NATIVE VALVES

To effectively analyze flow through prosthetic heart valves in the mitral or aortic positions, it is important to understand the conditions under which natural valves function. Fig. 30.8 shows the typical pressure and flow waveforms for healthy individuals at the aortic and mitral valves. During systole, the pressure difference required to drive the blood through the aortic valve is on the order of a few millimeters of mercury. Diastolic pressure differences across the aortic valve are much larger than systolic differences; the pressure usually is about 80 mmHg. The valve closes near the end of the deceleration phase of systole with very little reverse flow.

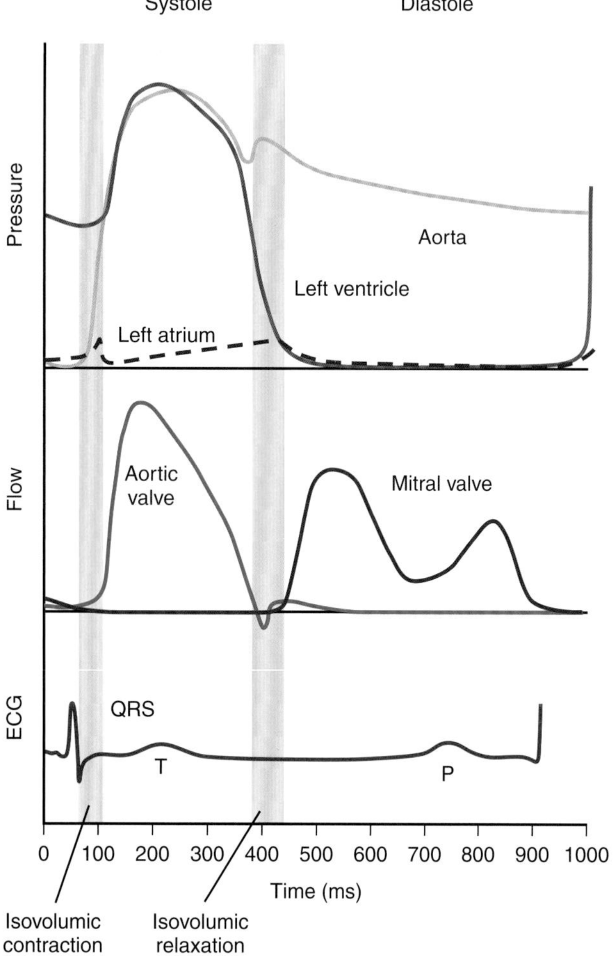

Fig. 30.8 Pressure and flow waveforms. Pressure and flow waveforms for the left heart. *ECG*, Electrocardiographic tracing.

Blood flow through the mitral valve is biphasic during diastole (see Fig. 30.8). The first peak, the E wave, is caused by ventricular relaxation, whereas the second peak, the A wave, is caused by contraction of the left atrium. This means that all valves in the mitral position open and close twice during each cardiac cycle. All cardiac valves are closed during isovolumic contraction and isovolumic relaxation.

Measurements of the velocity profile just distal to the aortic valve have been performed with Doppler echocardiography in normal subjects.[26] The peak systolic velocity was 1.35 ± 0.35 m/s, and the velocity profile at the level of the aortic valve annulus was relatively flat. However, there is usually a slight skew toward the septal wall (<10% of the centerline velocity) caused by the orientation of the aortic valve relative to the long axis of the LV. This skew in the velocity profile has been shown by many experimental techniques, including hot film anemometry,[29,30] Doppler ultrasound,[31] and magnetic resonance imaging.[32]

The flow patterns distal to the aortic valve also play an important role in proper valve function. During systole, vortices form behind each leaflet in the sinus region. In vitro studies have attempted to relate these vortices to effective valve closure.[33,34] As they have shown, the ventricular vortices are unnecessary for valve closure but do ensure that the valve closes quickly, reducing leakage.[35]

The velocity profile at the mitral valve has been determined in detail in pigs and should be comparable to the velocity profile in humans because of their similar cardiac anatomy.[36] There is a slight skew to the profile, but there does not seem to be a preferred orientation. The orientation depends on the particular geometry of the mitral valve, the diastolic flow patterns within the LV, and the location at which the pulsed-wave Doppler sample volume is placed. When the sample volume was placed at the mitral annulus, the peak early diastolic velocity was 63.6 ± 16.1 cm/s, and the late diastolic peak velocity was 53.7 ± 10.8 cm/s. When the sample volume was at the tip of the mitral valve leaflets, the peak early diastolic velocity was 82.9 ± 30.8 cm/s, and the peak late diastolic velocity was 39.6 ± 14.2 cm/s.

Vortices develop in the LV during diastole as blood enters through the mitral valve. Bellhouse[34] proposed that the vortices help to close the mitral valve at the end of diastole. Later work showed that the vortices play a role in early closing of the mitral valve, whereas late closure is dominated by LV pressure.[37]

Because of the restrictive area of prosthetic valves, the peak velocities are usually higher, and the spatial velocity profiles are dramatically different from those in natural valves. The shear stresses in prosthetic valves are also much larger because of the higher velocities and turbulence compared with native valves. The magnitude of the shear stress varies greatly according to the type of prosthetic valve. The differences and similarities between valve types in terms of shear stress magnitudes, peak velocities, and flow patterns are important to the performance of an effective assessment of prosthetic valve function.

HEMODYNAMICS OF SPECIFIC PROSTHETIC VALVE DESIGNS

Prosthetic heart valves have been successfully used in heart valve replacement for more than 50 years. Heart valve prostheses are categorized as mechanical valves, biologic valves, or transcatheter valves.

Mechanical valves are prosthetic valves manufactured from nonbiologic tissues. There are three basic designs or classifications: tilting-disc, bileaflet, and ball-and-cage valves. Biologic valves are prosthetic valves manufactured from animal tissues; they can be further classified as stented, unstented, or homograft valves. Transcatheter valves are the newest addition to the prosthetic valve market. Although they are essentially biologic valves delivered through a catheter, these valves deserve a separate classification because of the novelty of their implantation mechanism. Fig. 30.9 shows examples of each type of prosthesis, and Fig. 30.10 shows examples of major transcatheter valve designs that are currently in use or in clinical trials in the United States and Europe.

Although significant progress has been made in the development of better prostheses through new materials and more physiologic valve designs, several problems associated with prosthetic valves have not been eliminated. Existing problems related to valve hemodynamics or local fluid mechanics are (1) thrombosis and thromboembolism, (2) hemolysis, (3) tissue overgrowth, (4) damage to the endothelial lining, and (5) regurgitation.

High shear stresses can result in damage to formed blood elements, platelet activation, and initiation of biochemical processes affecting coagulation. Lethal damage to red cells can occur with fluid shear stresses as low as 800 dynes/cm^2.[38] However, shear stress levels can be significantly lower, in the range of 10 to 100 dynes/cm^2, in the setting of foreign surfaces such as valve prostheses.[39,40] Platelet activation and damage can occur with shear stresses ranging from 100 to 500 dynes/cm^2.[41]

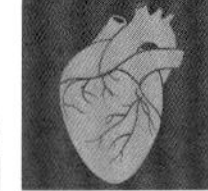

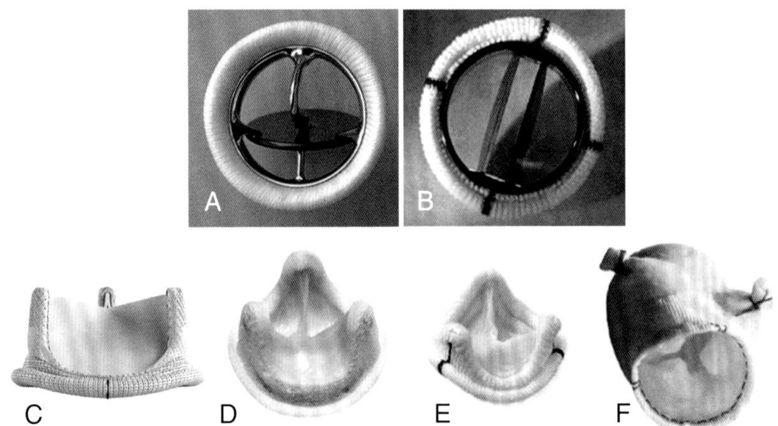

Fig. 30.9 Types of prosthetic heart valves. Major types of prosthetic heart valves: (A) tilting-disc valve, (B) bileaflet valve, (C–E), stented bioprostheses, (F) stentless bioprosthesis. The stented Carpentier-Edwards Perimount Magna (C), Medtronic Hancock 2 (D), and St. Jude Medical Biocor (E) valves are shown.

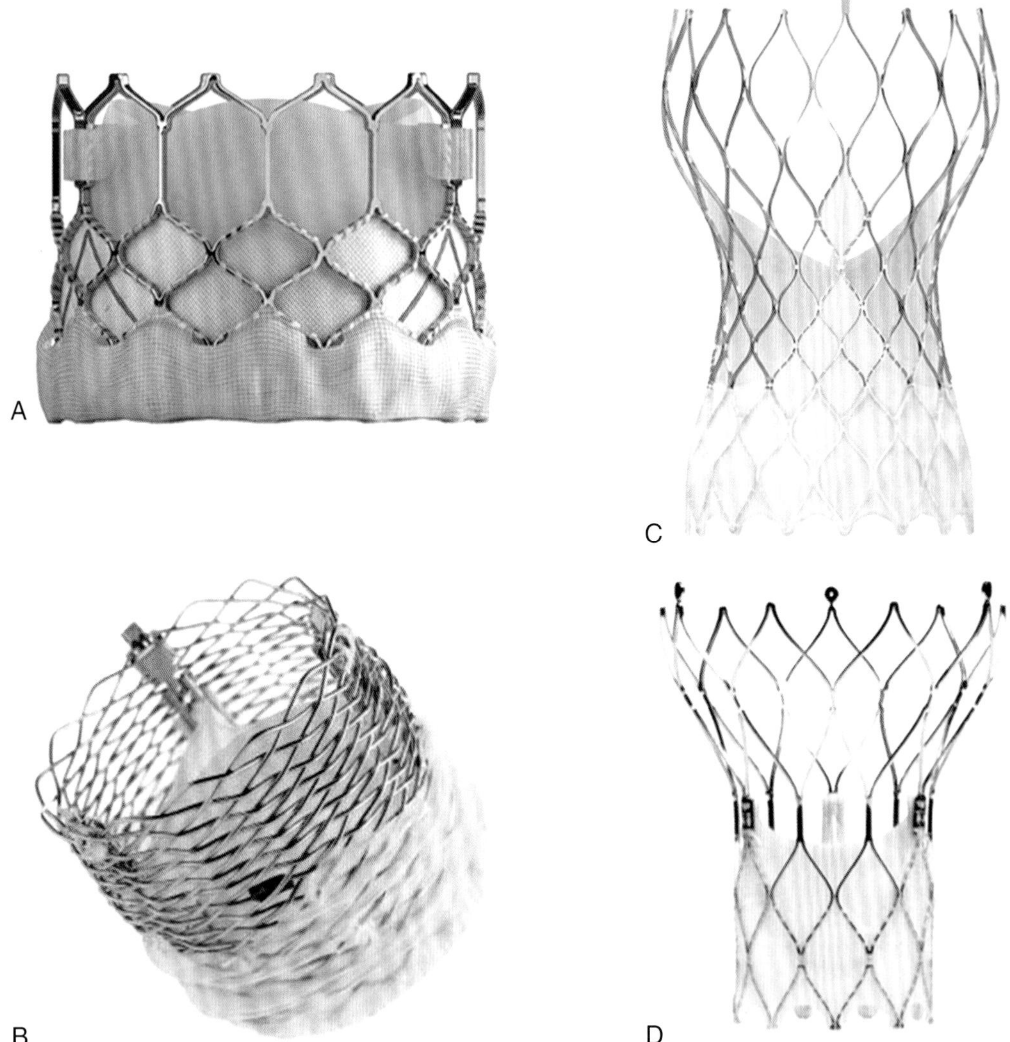

Fig. 30.10 Percutaneous valve designs. Major designs of transcatheter valves that have been approved by the US Food and Drug Administration (A–C) or are in clinical trials (D). The Edwards Sapien 3 (A), Medtronic CoreValve Evolut PRO (B), Boston Scientific Lotus Edge (C), and Abbott (formerly St. Jude Medical) Portico (D) valves are shown.

TABLE 30.1 Peak Systolic Velocity and Turbulent Shear Stress Levels for Common 27-mm Aortic Valve Prostheses.[a]

Valve Type	*Valve*	*Measurement Location*	*Peak Velocity (cm/s)*	*Peak Turbulent Shear Stress (dynes/cm²)*
Bileaflet	Abbott[b] Standard	13 mm downstream	210	1500
	DuraMedics	13 mm downstream	210	2300
	CarboMedics	12 mm downstream	228	1520
Stented bioprosthesis	Carpentier-Edwards Porcine 2625	15 mm downstream	370	4500
	Carpentier-Edwards Porcine 2650	15 mm downstream	200	2000
	Carpentier-Edwards Pericardial 2900	17 mm downstream	180	1000
	Hancock MO Porcine 250	10 mm downstream	330	2900
	Hancock II Porcine 410	18 mm downstream	260	2500
	Ionescu-Shiley Standard Pericardial	27 mm downstream	230	2500
	Hancock Pericardial	18 mm downstream	170	2100
Nonstented bioprosthesis	Medtronic Freestyle[c]	Leaflet tips	125	—
		10 mm from tips	100	—
	Toronto Stentless Porcine Valve (TSPV)[b]	Leaflet tips	150	—
		10 mm from tips	125	—

[a]Heart rate = 70 beats/min; cardiac output = 5 L/min; aortic pressure = 120/80 mmHg.
[b]Formerly St. Jude Medical.
[c]Data obtained from in vitro Doppler ultrasound measurements.

The residence time of the cell in the damaging fluid environment is a significant factor in determining lethal stress levels and further complicates the mechanism for damage. Regions of flow separation and stagnation form local environments that are suitable for accumulation and growth of thrombi and fibrous or pannus tissue.[42]

The fluid mechanical performance of prosthetic heart valves is often assessed through in vitro testing to determine transvalvular pressure drops, closure and leakage regurgitant volumes, distal and proximal velocity fields, and the locations and levels of turbulent stresses. The relationship between valve fluid mechanics and development of problematic function has been studied by numerous investigators over the past 2 decades. In vitro studies have concentrated on quantifying local fluid stress levels through flow measurement techniques such as laser Doppler anemometry, hot film anemometry, and ultrasound velocimetry.

Table 30.1 summarizes the peak velocity and turbulent shear stress levels for many of the 27-mm aortic valves; EOA and performance indices for these valves are provided in Tables 30.2 and 30.3. Data on ball-and-cage and tilting-disc valves can be found in previous versions of this textbook and in a review article.[43]

The fluid mechanics of the various prosthetic valve designs are discussed in the following sections. Many articles have been published dealing with the assessment of individual valves and can be consulted for comparison of valve designs within each classification. The antegrade and retrograde flow fields are described here. All flow characteristics are referenced from in vitro experiments conducted in our laboratory unless otherwise specified. In most citations, the data are representative of 25- or 27-mm aortic prostheses tested under physiologic pulsatile flow conditions that provided a cardiac output of 5.0 to 6.0 L/min and a heart rate of 70 beats/min. Exact test conditions (i.e., valve size, cardiac output, heart rate, and pressures) are described for each citation.

MECHANICAL VALVES

The three major mechanical valve designs or classes are the tilting-disc, bileaflet, and ball-and-cage valves. They differ primarily in the type and function of the occluder. Although the different designs influence the valvular fluid mechanics, all three share common flow structures such as well-defined jet flows, wakes with some degree of flow reversal, and turbulent shear layers.

The most widely used type of mechanical heart valves is the bileaflet valve. The antegrade flow and regurgitant flow characteristics for these mechanical valve designs are discussed in Table 30.4. More information on tilting-disc and ball-and-cage valve designs is available in previous editions of this textbook and a review article.[43]

BIOPROSTHETIC VALVES

The three major tissue valve designs or classes are the stented xenograft, unstented xenograft, and homograft. These valves differ primarily in tissue type and structure. Tissue valves are less thrombogenic compared with mechanical valves and do not require anticoagulant treatment. However, the valves suffer from calcification of the leaflets and material fatigue leading to valve failure due to leaflet rupture or tearing. Calcification of the tissue is often a precursor to leaflet rupture and tearing, which are often observed adjacent to calcified lesions.

All bioprosthetic valve designs share the characteristics of flexible leaflets, a single orifice, and little or no leakage after valve closure. The antegrade flow, regurgitant flow, and pressure drop characteristics for each valve type are summarized in Table 30.5.

TRANSCATHETER VALVES

The newest additions to the prosthetic valve family are the transcatheter valves. Transcatheter valves are essentially bioprosthetic aortic valves that are mounted onto a collapsible stent so that the valve can be collapsed onto a catheter and delivered through the catheter in a minimally invasive manner. These valves were introduced to target high-risk groups, such as elderly or diabetic patients, who are much less likely than others to survive an open heart valve replacement procedure. The catheter delivery approach avoids cross-clamping and cardiopulmonary bypass and reduces procedure duration, which reduces risks.

Transcatheter valves can be delivered by a transfemoral or transapical technique. In the former method, the catheter gains

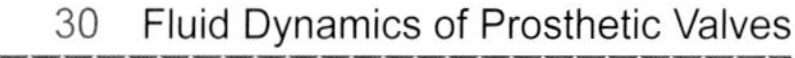

TABLE 30.2 **In Vitro Hemodynamic Data for Common Aortic Valve Prostheses.**[a]

Valve Type	*Valve*	*Size*	*Regurgitant Volume (mL/beat)*	*EOA*[b] *(cm²)*	*PI*
Bileaflet	St. Jude Standard	27	10.8	4.09	0.71
		25	9.9	3.23	0.66
		23	8.3	2.24	0.54
		21	6.8	1.81	0.52
		19	6.8	1.21	0.43
	St. Jude Regent	29	13.5	4.98	0.75
		27	12.3	4.40	0.77
		25	11.2	3.97	0.81
		23	10.3	3.47	0.83
		21	9.0	2.81	0.81
		19	7.6	2.06	0.73
		17	6.3	1.56	0.69
	CarboMedics	27	7.5	3.75	0.65
		25	6.1	3.14	0.64
		23	6.51	2.28	0.55
		21	3.4	1.66	0.48
		19	3.0	1.12	0.40
Stented bioprosthesis	Carpentier-Edwards Porcine 2625	27	<3	1.95	0.34
		25	<2	1.52	0.31
		21	<2	1.28	0.37
	Carpentier-Edwards Porcine 2650	27	<2	2.74	0.48
		25	<2	2.36	0.48
		21	<2	1.38	0.40
		19	<2	1.17	0.41
	Carpentier-Edwards Pericardial 2900	27	<3	3.70	0.64
		25	<2	3.25	0.66
		21	<2	1.88	0.54
		19	<2	1.56	0.55
	Hancock Porcine 242	27	<3	2.14	0.37
		25	<2	1.93	0.39
		23	<2	1.73	0.42
		21	<2	1.31	0.38
		19	<2	1.15	0.41
	Hancock MO Porcine 250	25	<2	2.16	0.44
		23	<2	1.94	0.47
		21	<2	1.43	0.41
		19	<2	1.22	0.43
	Hancock II Porcine 410	27	<2	2.36	0.41
		25	<2	2.10	0.43
		23	<2	1.81	0.44
		21	<2	1.48	0.43
	Ionescu-Shiley Standard Pericardial	27	<3	2.35	0.41
	Medtronic Mosaic Porcine	29	<3	3.15	0.48
		27	<2	2.81	0.49
		25	<2	2.11	0.43
		23	<2	1.74	0.42
		21	<1	1.54	0.44
	CarboMedics Mitroflow Pericardial	29	<4	3.71	0.56
		23	<3	2.12	0.51
		19	<2	1.34	0.47
Nonstented bioprosthesis	Medtronic Freestyle Porcine	27	<4	3.75	0.65
		25	<4	3.41	0.69
		23	<3	2.69	0.65
		21	<2	2.17	0.63
		19	<2	1.84	0.65

[a]Heart rate = 70 beats/min; cardiac output = 5 L/min typical; aortic pressure = 120/80 mmHg.
[b]EOA computed from Eq. 30.6.
EOA, Effective orifice area; *PI*, performance index.

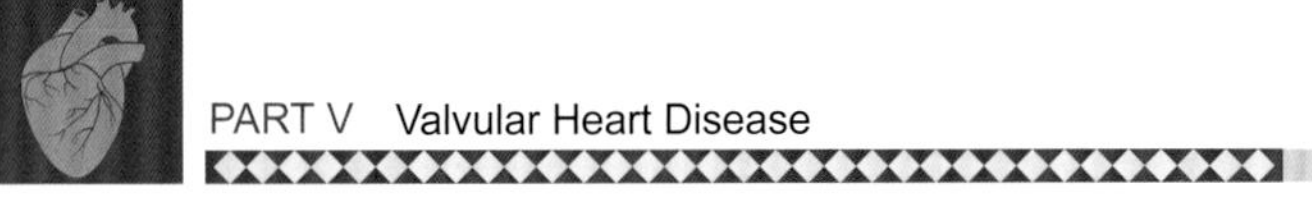

TABLE 30.3 In Vitro Hemodynamic Data for Common Mitral Valve Prostheses.[a]

Valve Type	*Valve*	*Size*	*Regurgitant Volume (mL/beat)*	*EOA[b] (cm²)*	*PI*
Bileaflet	Abbott[c] Standard	31	13.1	3.67	0.48
		29	10.9	3.40	0.51
		27	9.7	2.81	0.49
Stented bioprosthesis	Hancock Porcine 342	35	<4	2.72	0.28
		33	<4	2.54	0.30
		31	<4	2.36	0.31
		29	<4	2.11	0.32
		27	<2	1.77	0.31
		25	<2	1.63	0.33
	Hancock II Porcine	33	<4	2.66	0.31
		31	<3	2.29	0.30
		29	<3	2.05	0.31
		27	<2	1.78	0.31
		25	<2	1.59	0.32
	Carpentier-Edwards Porcine 6650	27	<2	2.03	0.35
	Carpentier-Edwards Porcine 6900	27	<2	2.68	0.47
	Carpentier-Edwards Porcine 6625	31	<4	2.58	0.39
	Edwards SAV	33	—	1.60	—
		31	—	1.58	—
		29	—	1.56	—
		27	—	1.32	—
		25	—	1.20	—
	Edwards Perimount	33	—	2.80	—
		31	—	2.76	—
		29	—	2.70	—
		27	—	1.92	—
		25	—	1.76	—
	Ionescu-Shiley Standard Pericardial	31	<5	3.00	0.40
		27	<2	1.77	0.31
		25	<2	1.61	0.33
	Mosaic Porcine	33	<4	2.38	0.28
		31	<3	2.26	0.30
		29	<3	2.02	0.31
		27	<2	1.71	0.30
		25	<2	1.55	0.32
	St. Jude Biocor Pericardial	31	—	2.53	—
		29	—	1.48	—
		33	—	2.04	—
		29	—	1.96	—
Nonstented bioprosthesis	Mitral Valve Allograft[d]	25	—	3.38	0.69
		23	—	1.80	0.43

[a]Heart rate = 70 beats/min; cardiac output = 5 L/min typical.
[b]EOA computed from Eq. 30.6.
[c]Formerly St. Jude Medical.
[d]In vitro measurements at 5 L/min.
EOA, Effective orifice area; *PI*, performance index.

access to the diseased valve by entering through the femoral artery and backtracking through the aorta to the heart. In the latter method, the catheter enters the LV directly from the apex of the heart. Balloon valvuloplasty is first applied to the calcified aortic valve to open it up. The ventricle is then induced into a state of rapid pacing, and the valve is deployed by expanding a second balloon from within the valve.

There are many transcatheter valve designs (see Fig. 30.10). The leading designs that are approved for clinical use by the FDA are the Edwards Sapien 3 and Sapien 3 Ultra, the Medtronic CoreValve Evolut R and CoreValve Evolut PRO, and the Boston Scientific Lotus Edge valves. Several other designs are undergoing clinical trials and awaiting FDA approval.

The Sapien transcatheter valves are trileaflet bovine pericardial valves mounted onto a stainless steel or cobalt-chromium frame. The CoreValve transcatheter valves are trileaflet porcine pericardial valves mounted onto a Nitinol frame. The profile of the CoreValve series stent is longer than that of the Sapien valves because it extends slightly proximally and is flared (like an hourglass) in the distal portions to anchor into the ascending aorta.

The Boston Scientific Lotus Edge valve is also a trileaflet bovine pericardial valve mounted on a braided Nitinol frame. It is the first percutaneous valve device that is fully repositionable and retrievable before release. The Abbott (formerly St. Jude Medical) Portico valve is a trileaflet bovine pericardial valve mounted on a Nitinol frame that is similar in geometry to the CoreValve. This valve is also repositionable until fully deployed.

TABLE 30.4 Mechanical Valve Types, Function, and Fluid Mechanics: Bileaflet Valves.

Characteristics
Consists of two semicircular leaflets typically made of pyrolytic carbon that are hinged to the valve housing (see Fig. 30.9B). The leaflets divide the flow into three regions: two lateral major orifices and a central minor orifice. Pressure drops and effective orifice areas are comparable to those of tilting-disc valves. The opening angle of leaflets varies from 75 to 90 degrees among different designs.
Antegrade Flow
Three jets emanate from the orifice (Figs. 30.11 and 30.12). Greater flow emerges from the lateral orifices than from the central orifice in most valves. Shear stress fields downstream of the St. Jude Medical bileaflet valve are shown in Fig. 30.13A.[59] Much of the shear stresses occur directly downstream of the leaflets due to uneven velocities between the central and lateral orifices. Reynolds shear stress analysis showed turbulence in the same region (see Fig. 30.13B).
Normal Regurgitant Flow
The bileaflet design shows slightly larger regurgitant volumes than the tilting-disc valve. Leakage flow occurs primarily through the hinges of the leaflets (see Fig. 30.12) and persists throughout diastole. Some leakage occurs through the gap between the two leaflets. Studies suggest that hinge leakage flow is mainly responsible for thrombosis.[54] Regurgitation flow is 2–3 m/s with very high turbulence stresses exceeding 3000 dynes/cm^2.[60,61] There are multiple hinge designs with varying flow features, summarized in Fig. 30.14.
Orientation
For the mitral position, there are two possible orientations: the anatomic position, with the gap between the leaflets perpendicular to the line between the aortic outflow and mitral inflow tracts, and the anti-anatomic position, in which the leaflet gap is parallel to the aortomitral line. In vivo studies showed that the anti-anatomic position results in diastolic flow that moves toward the ventricular outflow tract, whereas the anatomic position results in diastolic flow that moves back toward the valve.

Other than their fluid dynamic performance, there are significant concerns in the biomechanics community about the long-term durability of transcatheter devices compared with surgically implanted prosthetic valves. Recent investigations have reported leaflet thrombosis leading to reduced leaflet motility.[43a]

Antegrade Flow

Bench testing of transcatheter valves showed that they have EOAs of about 1.8 cm^2 and mean pressure gradients of 8.3 mmHg, which is comparable to the values for stented bioprostheses.[22] Clinically, the EOA of valves was shown to be between 1.5 and 1.8 cm^2, and pressure gradients were about 10 mmHg.[44,45] The antegrade velocity fields at peak systole of a transcatheter valve similar to the Medtronic CoreValve are presented in Fig. 30.16 for two cardiac output conditions and two positioning levels of the valve.

Normal Regurgitant Flow

In transcatheter valves, unlike bioprosthetic valves, regurgitation is very common. Mild to moderate regurgitation occurs in more than 50% of the cases, and severe regurgitation occurs in 5%.[44–47] Regurgitation in the transcatheter valve is mostly paravalvular, occurring between the valve and the native tissues rather than through the valve orifice. Because the implanted valve is merely pressed onto native tissues due to pressure exerted by the stents, a complete seal cannot be achieved in most cases, especially when the native aortic valve is heavily calcified and presents a very uneven surface for the transcatheter valve to fit onto.

This form of regurgitation (typically acute and not chronic) can lead to heart failure due to increased diastolic stiffness of the LV resulting from chronic aortic stenosis.[48] Assessment of LV diastolic stiffness is critical to estimate the ability of patients to

TABLE 30.5 Bioprosthesis Valve Types, Function, and Fluid Mechanics.

Characteristics	*Antegrade Flow*	*Normal Regurgitant Flow*	*Pressure Drops*
Stented Xenograft			
Most common valve Consists of three leaflets made from the porcine aortic valve or bovine pericardium and mounted on a metal or polymeric stented ring Various fixation methods are used.	All porcine stented valves are mildly stenotic in larger sizes and moderate to severely stenotic in small sizes. All valves have strong central jets (Fig. 30.15). Newer-generation valves have flatter velocity profiles then earlier designs.	Regurgitant volumes are on the order of 1 mL/beat for most tissue valves. Regurgitation jets are normally nonexistent, and their presence indicates abnormal valve incompetence.	Newer-generation pericardial valves have pressure drops similar to those of bileaflet mechanical valves.
Unstented Xenograft			
Fashioned from porcine, bovine, or equine tissue, they do not have rigid stents due to the complexity of the design, Optimal performance depends on patient geometry and sizing of the valve.	The flow accelerates uniformly through the valve, and downstream flow has a flat profile.[64] There is no appearance of a jet with steep velocity gradients, as is observed in stented bioprostheses.	Tests in our laboratory showed that unstented valves have closing volumes comparable to unfixed natural valves tested in the same flow loop. Good coaptation was observed with no leakage. The function of mitral heterografts strongly depends on the implantation technique.	The lack of stents and sewing cuffs allows larger valve sizes to be implanted for the same aorta size. Pressure drops are similar to those of mechanical prosthesis.[64–66]
Homograft			
Cryopreserved human valves have been used for more than 2 decades in the aortic position. Aortic valve homografts are usually implanted as a complete aortic root, whereas mitral homografts are implanted with the leaflets, annulus, papillary muscles, and chordae tendineae intact.	Similar to that of natural valves, although peak velocities are slightly higher due to reduced EOAs resulting from the smaller area of the outflow tract.	They exhibit small closing volumes and little or no regurgitation due to leakage. The hemodynamics of mitral homografts have the same dependency on implantation technique. For example, proper alignment of papillary muscles with the valve annulus can eliminate regurgitation.	Lower pressure drops and larger EOAs than mechanical and stented valves

EOA, Effective orifice area.

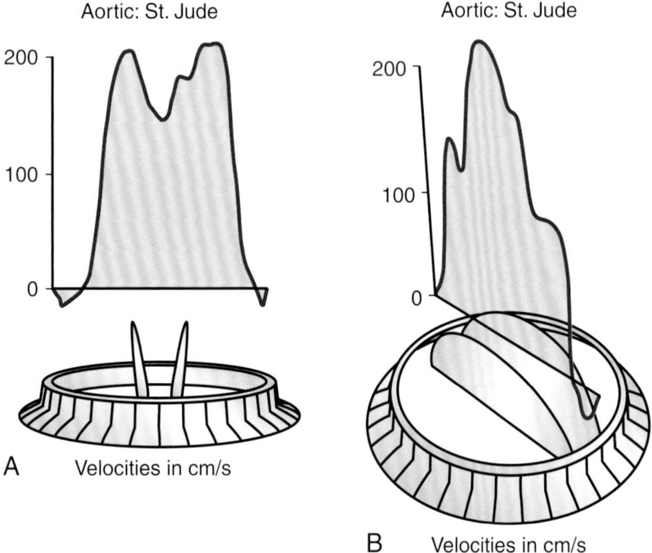

Fig. 30.11 Antegrade flow field. Velocity profiles downstream of a 27-mm St. Jude Medical bileaflet valve at peak systole, at the centerline 13 mm downstream (A), and traversing the lateral and central orifices 13 mm downstream (B).

tolerate postprocedural paravalvular leakage. Perivalvular leakage can exert high shear stress on regurgitating blood and cause clots, which may explain the high incidence of vascular complications (10%–15% of cases).[45,49]

Thrombosis

The unexpected discovery of thrombosis in transcatheter heart valves has led to increased concerns about long-term valve durability and stroke.[44,50] Thrombosis occurs at the base of the leaflets in a region called the *neosinus* (Fig. 30.17).[51] Based on Virchow's triad and current clinical data, the central hypothesis is that flow stagnation in the vicinity of the leaflets could be the primary cause.

Quantitative studies have shown that a supra-annular neosinus may reduce the risk of thrombosis due to reduced flow stasis.[51] This is evident in Fig. 30.18, which illustrates the influence of valve positioning on the volume of thrombus formed on the leaflets of transcatheter heart valves. Some studies have demonstrated the significance of 3D flow studies to thoroughly quantify the extent of flow stagnation in the neosinus.[52] The magnitude of coronary flow has an influence on the amount of flow stagnation in the neosinus and may influence the risk of thrombosis in transcatheter heart valves.[53]

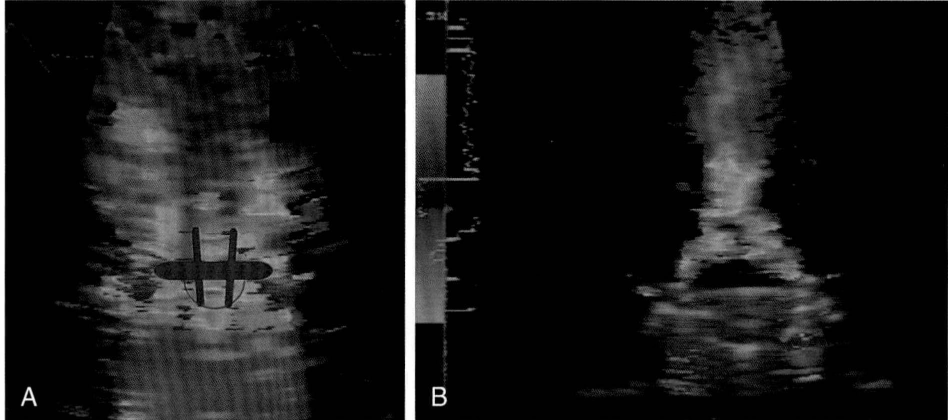

Fig. 30.12 Flow fields from 2D color Doppler echocardiography. (A) Antegrade flow mapping of the downstream triple-jet flow fields of a bileaflet valve design under physiologic pulsatile flow conditions. (B) Retrograde flow mapping of the leakage jet flow fields of a bileaflet valve design under physiologic pulsatile flow conditions.

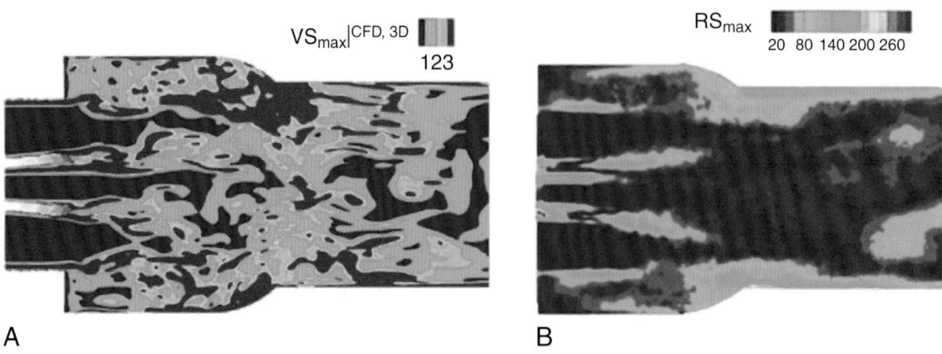

Fig. 30.13 Antegrade flow field. (A) Viscous shear stresses downstream of the bileaflet mechanical valve at the peak flow time point (in N/m^2) obtained through 3D computational fluid dynamics simulations. (B) Turbulence shear stresses downstream of the bileaflet mechanical valve at the peak flow time point (in N/m^2) obtained through experimental measurements using a physiologic pulse duplicator system. *RS*, Reynolds shear stresses; *VS*, viscous shear stresses. (From Ge L, Dasi LP, Sotiropoulos F, Yoganathan AP. Characterization of hemodynamic forces induced by mechanical heart valves: Reynolds vs. viscous stresses. *Ann Biomed Eng.* 2008;36[2]:276–297.)

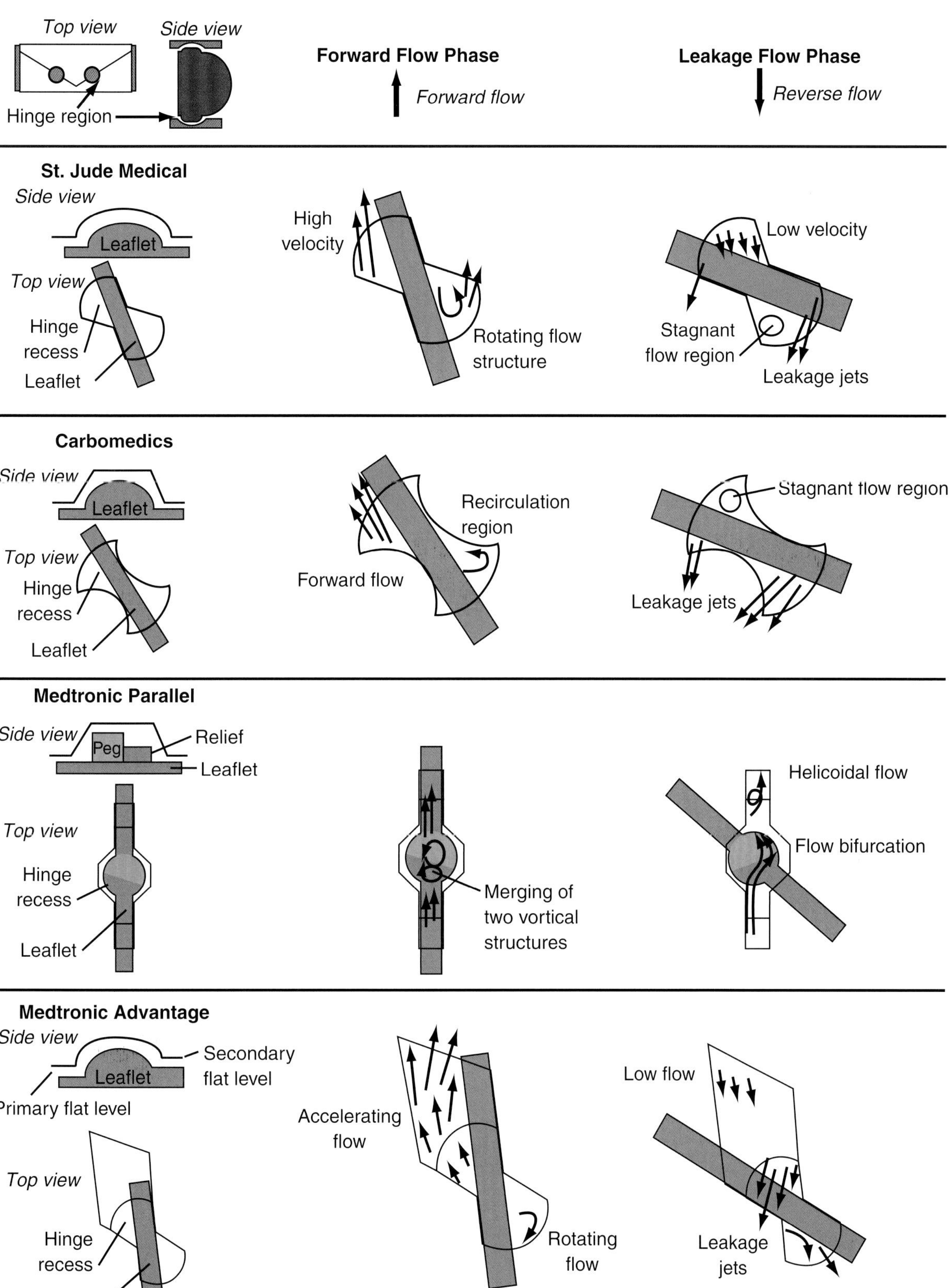

Fig. 30.14 Retrograde flow field. Flow characteristics within the hinges of various bileaflet mechanical heart valves.[54–58]

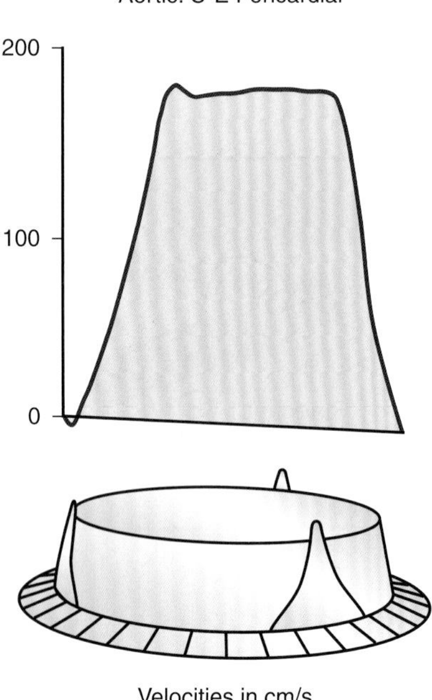

Fig. 30.15 Antegrade flow field. Centerline velocity profile 17 mm downstream of a 27-mm Carpentier-Edwards pericardial valve at peak systole.

Clinical studies have highlighted the potential relationship between thrombosis and transcatheter heart valve durability. There is a need for additional prospective studies to further quantify and minimize the thrombus burden; the current studies are important to identify patients at higher risk for thrombosis and could aid in the development of next-generation devices with low thrombogenic potential.

FUTURE DIRECTIONS

Future prosthetic valve research will likely include development of polymeric prostheses, tissue-engineered valves, invention of novel tissue fixation techniques, improved designs and materials for mechanical valves, and improved transcatheter valve technologies (i.e., delivery devices and valve design).

Polymeric prostheses may offer patients durable alternatives to mechanical valves and bioprostheses with little tendency for calcification or thromboembolic complications. However, the goal of tissue engineering research is to grow living aortic valves in the laboratory, preferably using the patient's own cells or tissues. Potential advantages include complete acceptance of the living tissue, with hemodynamic and cellular functions that are similar to those of the normal human aortic valve and result in a longer functional lifetime.

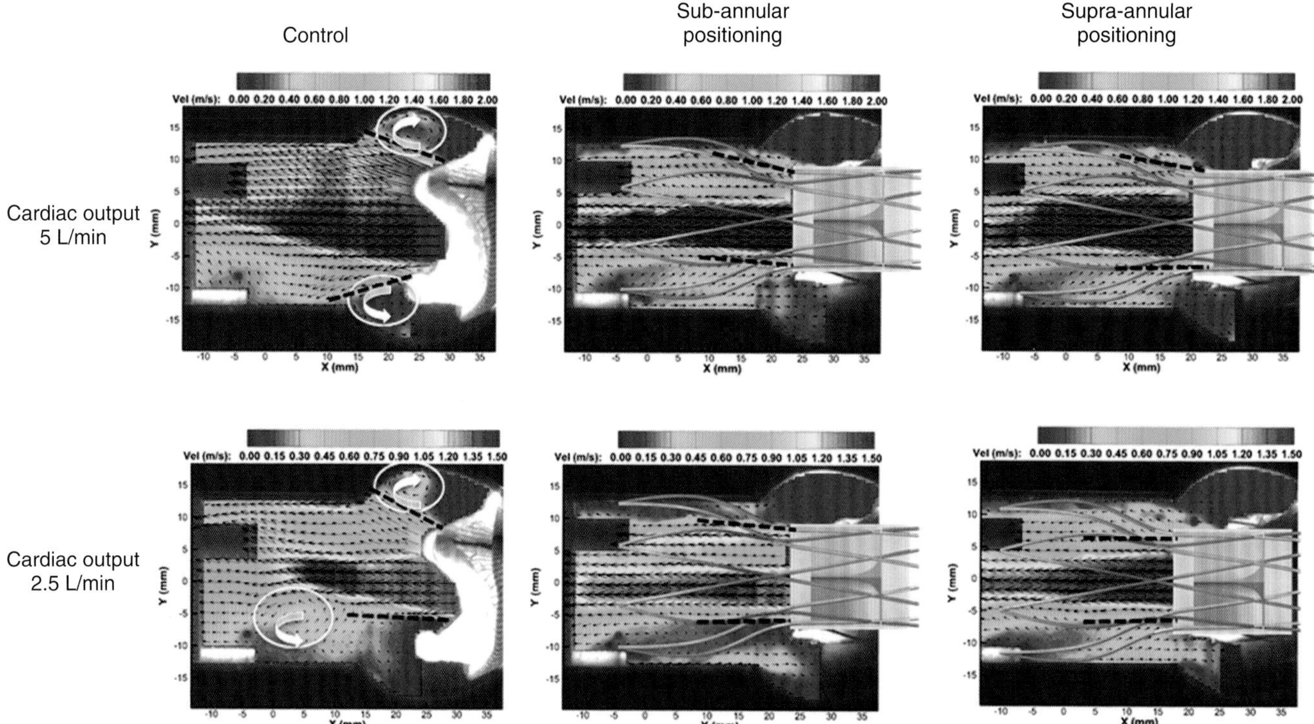

Fig. 30.16 Antegrade flow field for a percutaneous valve. Particle image velocimetry (PIV) flow fields at peak systole. *Dashed lines* indicate velocity equal to 0.5 m/s and show the extent of the systolic jet. *White circles* indicate the locations of vortices, and the *arrows* indicate direction of rotation. (From Kumasr G, Raghav V, Lerakis S, et al. High transcatheter valve replacement may reduce washout in the aortic sinuses: an in-vitro study. *J Heart Valve Dis.* 2015; 24:22–29.)

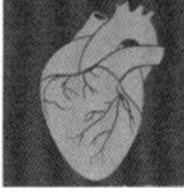

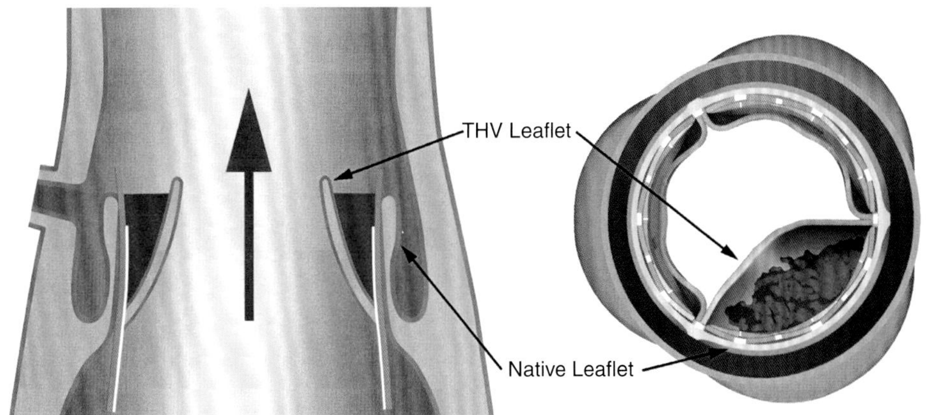

Fig. 30.17 Neosinus in transcatheter heart valve. Thrombus forms at the base of the neosinus, and the native aortic sinus decreases in size. *THV*, Transcatheter heart valve. (From Midha PA, Raghav V, Sharma R, et al. The fluid mechanics of transcatheter heart valve leaflet thrombosis in the neosinus. *Circulation*, 2017;136[17]:1598–1609.)

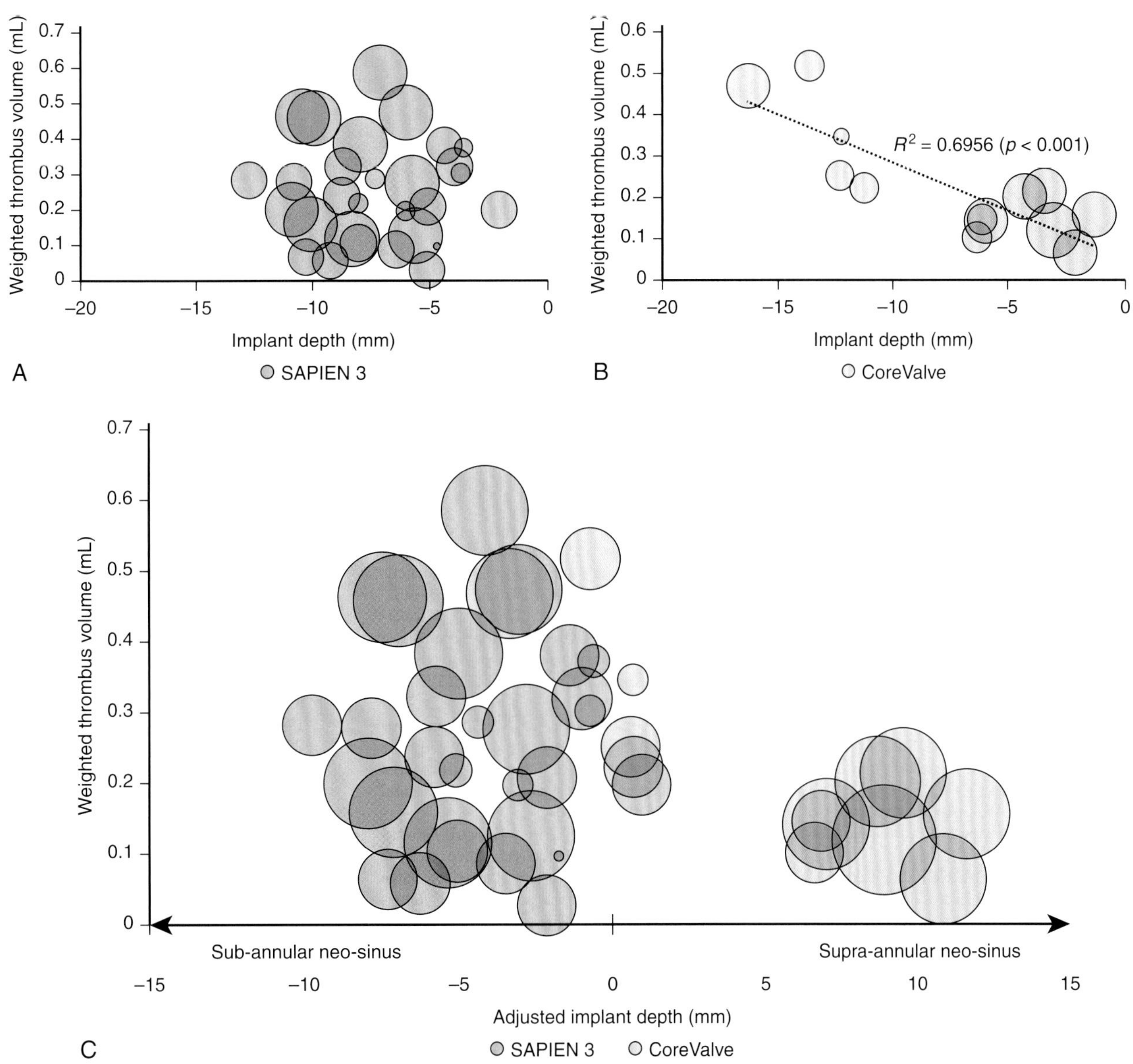

Weighted thrombus volume (mL)
Implant depth (mm)
A
SAPIEN 3

Weighted thrombus volume (mL)
$R^2 = 0.6956$ ($p < 0.001$)
Implant depth (mm)
B
CoreValve

Weighted thrombus volume (mL)
Sub-annular neo-sinus
Supra-annular neo-sinus
Adjusted implant depth (mm)
C
SAPIEN 3 CoreValve

Fig. 30.18 Effect of valve positioning on thrombus volume. Influence of supra-annular valve positioning on the volume of thrombus after transcatheter heart valve implantation. Data are presented for the Sapien 3 (A) and CoreValve (B) transcatheter heart valves according to depth of implantation and for both valves according to positioning of the neosinus (C). (From Midha PA, Raghav V, Sharma R, et al. The fluid mechanics of transcatheter heart valve leaflet thrombosis in the neosinus. *Circulation*. 2017;136[17]:1598–1516.)

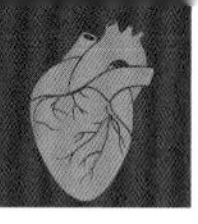

Tissue xenografts are currently fixed in glutaraldehyde, which stiffens the tissue and impedes hemodynamic performance. Other fixative techniques may improve hemodynamic performance and increase the durability and functional lifetime of xenografts. For mechanical valves, the focus will be on reducing their thrombogenic characteristics. This may be accomplished by development of biocompatible surface coatings and materials, new materials based on nanotechnologies, or changes in valve geometry that improve closure and leakage flow through these valves. A first step in this research should be improved understanding of blood element damage, platelet activation, and thrombus formation.

Although transcatheter valves enable minimally invasive valve replacement, there are still concerns about long-term durability, paravalvular leakage, and thromboembolic complications, including strokes. With FDA approval of the use of transcatheter heart valves in patients who are at low surgical risk, it is a critical and time-sensitive issue to evaluate and quantify the long-term durability of these valves. We believe that the use of these valves for low-risk patients should be cautiously considered after significant deliberation. Use of this valve as an alternative therapy for high-risk patients is the appropriate path forward, until the long-term durability concerns are addressed. Similar significant challenges exist in another area of transcatheter valve application, mitral valve position. Substantial effort is being dedicated to the development of transcatheter mitral and tricuspid valves.

ACKNOWLEDGMENTS

The work on prosthetic heart valves was performed in our Cardiovascular Fluid Mechanics Laboratory at Georgia Tech University and was supported by grants from the US Food and Drug Administration, the American Heart Association, the heart valve industry, and generous gifts from Tom and Shirley Gurley and the Lilla Boz Foundation.

SUMMARY Fluid Dynamics of Prosthetic Valves.

Application of conservation of mass to a control volume allows calculation of unknown flow rates, average velocities, or surface areas into or out of the volume based on measurable quantities.

Mechanical energy per unit volume is a measure of the work available to drive flow.

Pressure is one of several forms of mechanical energy, but there are others (kinetic and gravitational). These forms can be freely converted from one to another without loss. Pressure loss and mechanical energy loss per unit volume are not equivalent because pressure can be recovered from a fall in gravitational or kinetic energy.

Effective means of reducing mechanical energy loss in the circulation include ensuring that any expansions in flow occur gradually, ensuring that bends and corners in the flow path are not sudden or sharp, and increasing vessel radius.

The Doppler gradient measures the conversion of pressure to kinetic energy in the flow across a valvular prosthesis. It does not measure mechanical energy loss, although it can be closely related to it.

The effective orifice area (EOA) of a valvular prosthesis represents the cross-sectional area of a flow at its smallest contraction. It is equal to or smaller than the anatomic orifice area.

Mechanical energy losses occur because of regurgitant flow and forward flow. Losses due to regurgitant flow can be greater than losses due to forward flow in large mitral mechanical prostheses.

REFERENCES

1. Yap CH, Dasi LP, Yoganathan AP. Dynamic hemodynamic energy loss in normal and stenosed aortic valves. *J Biomech Eng*. 2010;132(2). 021005.
2. Batchelor G. *An Introduction to Fluid Mechanics*. Cambridge: Cambridge University Press; 1994.
3. Blevins R. *Applied Fluid Dynamics Handbook*. New York: Van Nostrand Reinhold Company; 1984.
4. McNaughton KJ, Sinclair CG. Submerged jets in short cylindrical flow vessels. *J Fluid Mech*. 1966;25(02):367–375.
5. Nerem RM, Seed WA. An in vivo study of aortic flow disturbances. *Cardiovasc Res*. 1972;6(1):1–14.
6. Stewart SF, Herman BA, Nell DM, Retta SM. Effects of valve characteristics on the accuracy of the Bernoulli equation: a survey of data submitted to the U.S. FDA. *J Heart Valve Dis*. 2004;13(3):461–466.
7. Knebel F, Gliech V, Walde T, et al. High concordance of invasive and echocardiographic mean pressure gradients in patients with a mechanical aortic valve prosthesis. *J Heart Valve Dis*. 2005;14(3):332–337.
8. Stewart WJ, Jiang L, Mich R, Pandian N, Guerrero JL, Weyman AE. Variable effects of changes in flow rate through the aortic, pulmonary and mitral valves on valve area and flow velocity: impact on quantitative Doppler flow calculations. *J Am Coll Cardiol*. 1985;6(3):653–662.
9. Burwash IG, Pearlman AS, Kraft CD, Miyake-Hull C, Healy NL, Otto CM. Flow dependence of measures of aortic stenosis severity during exercise. *J Am Coll Cardiol*. 1994;24(5):1342–1350.
10. DeGroff CG, Shandas R, Valdes-Cruz L. Analysis of the effect of flow rate on the Doppler continuity equation for stenotic orifice area calculations: a numerical study. *Circulation*. 1998;97(16):1597–1605.
11. Garcia D, Pibarot P, Landry C, et al. Estimation of aortic valve effective orifice area by Doppler echocardiography: effects of valve inflow shape and flow rate. *J Am Soc Echocardiogr*. 2004;17(7):756–765.
12. Gorlin R, Gorlin SG. Hydraulic formula for calculation of the area of the stenotic mitral valve, other cardiac valves, and central circulatory shunts. *I. Am Heart J*. 1951;41(1):1–29.
13. Fagard R, Conway J. Measurement of cardiac output: Fick principle using catheterization. *Eur Heart J*. 1990;11(Suppl I):1–5.
14. Scotten LN, Walker DK, Dutton JW. Modified gorlin equation for the diagnosis of mixed aortic valve pathology. *J Heart Valve Dis*. 2002;11(3):360–368; discussion 368.
15. Yoganathan AP, He Z, Casey Jones S. Fluid mechanics of heart valves. *Annu Rev Biomed Eng*. 2004;6:331–362.
16. Struber M, Campbell A, Richard G, Laas J. Hydrodynamic function of tilting disc prostheses and bileaflet valves in double valve replacement. *Eur J Cardio Thorac Surg*. 1996;10(6):422–427.
17. Recusani F, Bargiggia GS, Yoganathan AP, et al. A new method for quantification of regurgitant flow rate using color Doppler flow imaging of the flow convergence region proximal to a discrete orifice. An in vitro study. *Circulation*. 1991;83(2):594–604.
18. Utsunomiya T, Doshi R, Patel D, Nguyen D, Mehta K, Gardin JM. Regurgitant volume estimation in patients with mitral regurgitation: initial studies using color Doppler "proximal isovelocity surface area" method. *Echocardiography*. 1992;9(1):63–70.
19. Utsunomiya T, Ogawa T, Doshi R, et al. Doppler color flow "proximal isovelocity surface area" method for estimating volume flow rate: effects of orifice shape and machine factors. *J Am Coll Cardiol*. 1991;17(5):1103–1111.

20. Utsunomiya T, Ogawa T, Tang HA, et al. Doppler color flow mapping of the proximal isovelocity surface area: a new method for measuring volume flow rate across a narrowed orifice. *J Am Soc Echocardiogr*. 1991;4(4):338–348.
21. Heinrich RS, Fontaine AA, Grimes RY, et al. Experimental analysis of fluid mechanical energy losses in aortic valve stenosis: importance of pressure recovery. *Ann Biomed Eng*. 1996;24(6):685–694.
22. Azadani AN, Jaussaud N, Matthews PB, et al. Energy loss due to paravalvular leak with transcatheter aortic valve implantation. *Ann Thorac Surg*. 2009;88(6):1857–1863.
23. Dasi LP, Pekkan K, de Zelicourt D, et al. Hemodynamic energy dissipation in the cardiovascular system: generalized theoretical analysis on disease states. *Ann Biomed Eng*. 2009;37(4):661–673.
24. Akins CW, Travis B, Yoganathan AP. Energy loss for evaluating heart valve performance. *J Thorac Cardiovasc Surg*. 2008;136(4):820–833.
25. Garcia D, Pibarot P, Dumesnil JG, Sakr F, Durand LG. Assessment of aortic valve stenosis severity: a new index based on the energy loss concept. *Circulation*. 2000;101(7):765–771.
26. Garcia D, Jean GD, Louis-Gilles D, Lyes K, Philippe P. Discrepancies between catheter and Doppler estimates of valve effective orifice area can be predicted from the pressure recovery phenomenon: practical implications with regard to quantification of aortic stenosis severity. *J Am Coll Cardiol*. 2003;41(3):435–442.
27. Dumesnil JG, Yoganathan AP. Valve prosthesis hemodynamics and the problem of high transprosthetic pressure gradients. *Eur J Cardio Thorac Surg*. 1992;6(suppl 1). S34-S37; discussion S38.
28. Pibarot P, Dumesnil JG. Hemodynamic and clinical impact of prosthesis-patient mismatch in the aortic valve position and its prevention. *J Am Coll Cardiol*. 2000;36(4):1131–1141.
29. Paulsen PK, Hasenkam JM. Three-dimensional visualization of velocity profiles in the ascending aorta in dogs, measured with a hot-film anemometer. *J Biomech*. 1983;16(3):201–210.
30. Paulsen PK. Use of a hot-film anemometer system for cardiovascular studies, with special reference to the ascending aorta. *Dan Med Bull*. 1989;36(5):430–443.
31. Rossvoll O, Samstad S, Torp HG, et al. The velocity distribution in the aortic anulus in normal subjects: a quantitative analysis of two-dimensional Doppler flow maps. *J Am Soc Echocardiogr*. 1991;4(4):367–378.
32. Kilner PJ, Yang GZ, Mohiaddin RH, Firmin DN, Longmore DB. Helical and retrograde secondary flow patterns in the aortic arch studied by three-directional magnetic resonance velocity mapping. *Circulation*. 1993;88(5 Pt 1):2235–2247.
33. Bellhouse B, Bellhouse F. Fluid mechanics of model normal and stenosed aortic valves. *Circ Res*. 1969;25(6):693–704.
34. Bellhouse BJ. Velocity and pressure distributions in the aortic valve. *J Fluid Mech*. 1969;37(03):587–600.
35. Reul H, Talukder N. In: Hwang NHC, Gross DR, Patel DJ, eds. *Quantitative Cardiovascular Studies, Clinical and Research Applications of Engineering Principles*. Baltimore: University Park Press; 1979:527–564.
36. Kim WY, Bisgaard T, Nielsen SL, et al. Two-dimensional mitral flow velocity profiles in pig models using epicardial Doppler echocardiography. *J Am Coll Cardiol*. 1994;24(2):532–545.
37. Reul H, Talukder N, Muller EW. Fluid mechanics of the natural mitral valve. *J Biomech*. 1981;14(5):361–372.
38. Lu PC, Lai HC, Liu JS. A reevaluation and discussion on the threshold limit for hemolysis in a turbulent shear flow. *J Biomech*. 2001;34(10):1361–1364.
39. Mohandas N, Hochmuth RM, Spaeth EE. Adhesion of red cells to foreign surfaces in the presence of flow. *J Biomed Mater Res*. 1974;8(2):119–136.
40. Blackshear PL. Hemolysis at prosthetic surfaces. In: Hair MR, ed. *Chemistry of Biosurfaces*. New York: Marcel Dekker; 1972:523–561.
41. Klaus S, Korfer S, Mottaghy K, Reul H, Glasmacher B. In vitro blood damage by high shear flow: human versus porcine blood. *Int J Artif Organs*. 2002;25(4):306–312.
42. Yoganathan AP, Wick TM, Reul H. In: Butchart EG, Bodnar W, eds. *Thrombosis, Embolism and Bleeding*. London: ICR Publishers; 1992.
43. Yoganathan AP, He Z, Casey Jones S. Fluid mechanics of heart valves. *Annu Rev Biomed Eng*. 2004;6:331–362.
43a. Makkar RR, Fontana G, Jilaihawi H, et al. Possible subclinical leaflet thrombosis in bioprosthetic aortic valves. *N Engl J Med*. 2015;373(21):2015–2024.
44. Webb JG, Pasupati S, Humphries K, et al. Percutaneous transarterial aortic valve replacement in selected high-risk patients with aortic stenosis. *Circulation*. 2007;116(7):755–763.
45. Vahanian A, Alfieri OR, Al-Attar N, et al. Transcatheter valve implantation for patients with aortic stenosis: a position statement from the European Association of Cardio-Thoracic Surgery (EACTS) and the European Society of Cardiology (ESC), in collaboration with the European Association of Percutaneous Cardiovascular Interventions (EAPCI). *Eur Heart J*. 2008;29(11):1463–1470.
46. Clavel MA, Webb JG, Pibarot P, et al. Comparison of the hemodynamic performance of percutaneous and surgical bioprostheses for the treatment of severe aortic stenosis. *J Am Coll Cardiol*. 2009;53(20):1883–1891.
47. Grube E, Buellesfeld L, Mueller R, et al. Progress and current status of percutaneous aortic valve replacement: results of three device generations of the CoreValve Revalving system. *Circ Cardiovasc Interv*. 2008;1(3):167–175.
48. Okafor I, Raghav V, Midha P, Kumar G, Yoganathan A. The hemodynamic effects of acute aortic regurgitation into a stiffened left ventricle resulting from chronic aortic stenosis. *Am J Physiol Heart Circ Physiol*. 2016;310(11):H1801–H1807.
49. Vetter HO, Yoganathan AP, Fontaine AA, Erhorn A, Reichart B. Hydrodynamic characteristics of a new stentless mitral valve allograft: in vitro results. In: Leipschs D, ed. *3rd International Symposium on Biofluid Mechanics*. Munich, Germany: VDI-Verlag GmbH Publishers; 1994:287–294.
50. Kapadia SR, Goel SS, Svensson L, et al. Characterization and outcome of patients with severe symptomatic aortic stenosis referred for percutaneous aortic valve replacement. *J Thorac Cardiovasc Surg*. 2009;137(6):1430–1435.
51. Midha PA, Raghav V, Sharma R, et al. The fluid mechanics of transcatheter heart valve leaflet thrombosis in the neosinus. *Circulation*. 2017;136(17):1598–1609.
52. Raghav V, Clifford C, Midha P, Okafor I, Thurow B, Yoganathan A. Three-dimensional extent of flow stagnation in transcatheter heart valves. *J R Soc Interface*. 2019;16(154): 20190063.
53. Trusty PM, Sadri V, Madukauwa-David ID, et al. Neosinus flow stasis correlates with thrombus volume post-TAVR: a patient-specific in vitro study. *JACC Cardiovasc Interv*. 2019;12(13):1288–1290.
54. Ellis JT, Travis BR, Yoganathan AP. An in vitro study of the hinge and near-field forward flow dynamics of the St. Jude Medical Regent bileaflet mechanical heart valve. *Ann Biomed Eng*. 2000;28(5):524–532.
55. Saxena R, Lemmon J, Ellis J, Yoganathan A. An in vitro assessment by means of laser Doppler velocimetry of the medtronic advantage bileaflet mechanical heart valve hinge flow. *J Thorac Cardiovasc Surg*. 2003;126(1):90–98.
56. Leo HL, He Z, Ellis JT, Yoganathan AP. Microflow fields in the hinge region of the CarboMedics bileaflet mechanical heart valve design. *J Thorac Cardiovasc Surg*. 2002;124(3):561–574.
57. Gross JM, Shu MC, Dai FF, Ellis J, Yoganathan AP. A microstructural flow analysis within a bileaflet mechanical heart valve hinge. *J Heart Valve Dis*. 1996;5(6):581–590.
58. Ellis JT, Yoganathan AP. A comparison of the hinge and near-hinge flow fields of the St Jude medical hemodynamic plus and regent bileaflet mechanical heart valves. *J Thorac Cardiovasc Surg*. 2000;119(1):83–93.
59. Ge L, Dasi LP, Sotiropoulos F, Yoganathan AP. Characterization of hemodynamic forces induced by mechanical heart valves: Reynolds vs. viscous stresses. *Ann Biomed Eng*. 2008;36(2):276–297.
60. Simon HA, Dasi LP, Leo HL, Yoganathan AP. Spatio-temporal flow analysis in bileaflet heart valve hinge regions: potential analysis for blood element damage. *Ann Biomed Eng*. 2007;35(8):1333–1346.
61. Ellis JT, Healy TM, Fontaine AA, et al. An in vitro investigation of the retrograde flow fields of two bileaflet mechanical heart valves. *J Heart Valve Dis*. 1996;5(6):600–606.
62. Travis BR, Heinrich RS, Ensley AE, Gibson DE, Hashim S, Yoganathan AP. The hemodynamic effects of mechanical prosthetic valve type and orientation on fluid mechanical energy loss and pressure drop in in vitro models of ventricular hypertrophy. *J Heart Valve Dis*. 1998;7(3):345–354.
63. Kleine P, Perthel M, Nygaard H, et al. Medtronic Hall versus St. Jude Medical mechanical aortic valve: downstream turbulences with respect to rotation in pigs. *J Heart Valve Dis*. 1998;7(5):548–555.
64. Yoganathan AP, Eberhardt CE, Walker PG. Hydrodynamic performance of the medtronic Freestyle aortic root bioprosthesis. *J Heart Valve Dis*. 1994;3(5):571–580.
65. Nagy ZL, Fisher J, Walker PG, Watterson KG. The effect of sizing on the in vitro hydrodynamic characteristics and leaflet motion of the Toronto SPV stentless valve. *J Thorac Cardiovasc Surg*. 1999;117(1):92–98.
66. Eriksson MJ, Brodin LA, Dellgren GN, Radegran K. Rest and exercise hemodynamics of an extended stentless aortic bioprosthesis. *J Heart Valve Dis*. 1997;6(6):653–660.

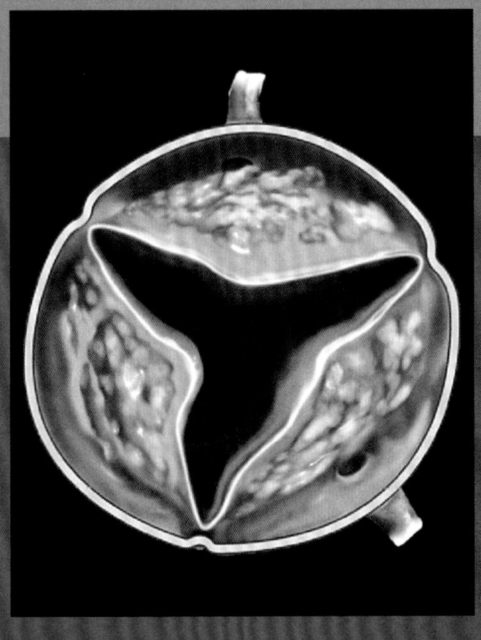

中文导读

第31章 人工心脏瓣膜功能障碍的超声心动图识别和定量分析

多普勒超声心动图是评估和随访主动脉、二尖瓣、三尖瓣或肺动脉瓣置换术后瓣膜功能及发现瓣膜并发症的首选检查方法。常见的人工心脏瓣膜功能障碍的原因包括人工心脏瓣膜不匹配、人工心脏瓣膜血栓形成和血管翳、瓣膜损毁和感染性心内膜炎。

人工心脏瓣膜的评估遵循与自体瓣膜评估相同的原则，但人工心脏瓣膜有一些重要的特殊之处和注意事项。人工心脏瓣膜置换术后的超声心动图检查应包括人工心脏瓣膜的二维成像，评估瓣膜瓣叶的形态和活动能力，测量跨人工心脏瓣膜压力梯度，测量有效瓣口面积，估计反流的位置和程度，评估左心室大小和收缩功能，计算收缩期肺动脉压力。本章详细介绍了超声心动图人工心脏瓣膜狭窄的识别与定量分析、人工心脏瓣膜反流的识别与定量分析、人工肺动脉瓣和三尖瓣的功能评价，以及超声心动图在处理人工心脏瓣膜相关并发症中的应用，包括人工心脏瓣膜血栓形成和人工心脏瓣膜置换术后心内膜炎的表现及诊断。

卫　青

31 Echocardiographic Recognition and Quantitation of Prosthetic Valve Dysfunction

PHILIPPE PIBAROT, DVM, PhD | MARIE-ANNICK CLAVEL, DVM, PhD

PROSTHETIC VALVE COMPLICATIONS AND DYSFUNCTION

Doppler echocardiography remains the cornerstone for evaluation and follow-up of prosthetic valve function and detection of valve complications after aortic, mitral, tricuspid, or pulmonary valve replacement (Fig. 31.1). Evaluation follows the same principles used for evaluation of native valves, although with some important particularities and caveats specific to the prosthetic valves, which are discussed in this chapter.

PATIENT-PROSTHESIS MISMATCH

Patient-prosthesis mismatch (PPM) is not an intrinsic dysfunction of the prosthesis. This problem occurs when the effective orifice area (EOA) of a normally functioning prosthesis is too small in relation to the patient's body size and cardiac output requirements, resulting in abnormally high postoperative gradients.

The most widely accepted and validated parameter for identifying a PPM is the *indexed EOA*, which is the EOA of the prosthesis divided by the patient's body surface area.[1–5] Table 31.1 shows the indexed EOA cutoff values used to identify a PPM and quantify its severity and its prevalence according to severity and prosthesis position.[5,6] Lower cutoff values of indexed EOAs should be used to define PPMs for obese patients (see Table 31.1). Transthoracic echocardiography (TTE) is essential to differentiate PPM from intrinsic prosthetic valve dysfunction.[5]

PROSTHETIC VALVE THROMBOSIS AND PANNUS

Obstruction of prosthetic valves may be caused by thrombus formation (see Fig. 31.1A), pannus ingrowth (see Fig. 31.1B), or a combination of both.[6] Pannus ingrowth alone may be encountered in bioprostheses and mechanical valves. It can manifest as a slowly progressive obstruction caused by a subvalvular annulus, in which case it may be difficult to visualize and distinguish from progressive structural valve deterioration (SVD). Pannus is usually encountered in patients with a normal anticoagulation profile and with subacute or chronic symptoms.[7,8]

Valve thrombosis should be suspected in a patient with any type of prosthetic valve who has had a recent increase in dyspnea or fatigue. Suspicion should be stronger if there has been a period of interrupted or subtherapeutic anticoagulation in the recent past. In such cases, echocardiography should be done promptly and should include transesophageal (TEE) studies, particularly if the prosthesis is in the mitral position. Valve thrombosis is most often encountered in patients with mechanical valves and inadequate antithrombotic therapy. Thrombosis may also be seen in surgical or transcatheter bioprosthetic valves, in which it most often occurs in the early postoperative period (3–6 months) (see Fig. 31.1E).[9,10]

Subclinical thrombosis (i.e., valve leaflet thickening not associated with valve dysfunction or clinical symptoms) can occur in 5% to 25% of patients within the first year after transcatheter aortic valve replacement (TAVR), and it appears to be more common than after surgical aortic valve replacement (SAVR).[9–12] In the PARTNER 3 randomized trial,[12a] the rate of subclinical thrombosis was 13% for the TAVR group versus 5% for the SAVR group ($P = 0.03$) at 30 days and 27% versus 20%, respectively, at 1 year ($P = 0.19$). Moreover, 50% of the positive cases at 30 days had spontaneously (i.e., without anticoagulation) regressed by 1 year, whereas a large proportion of the positive cases at 1 year were negative at 30 days.

The clinical significance of subclinical thrombosis is unclear. Some studies reported no association with clinical events,

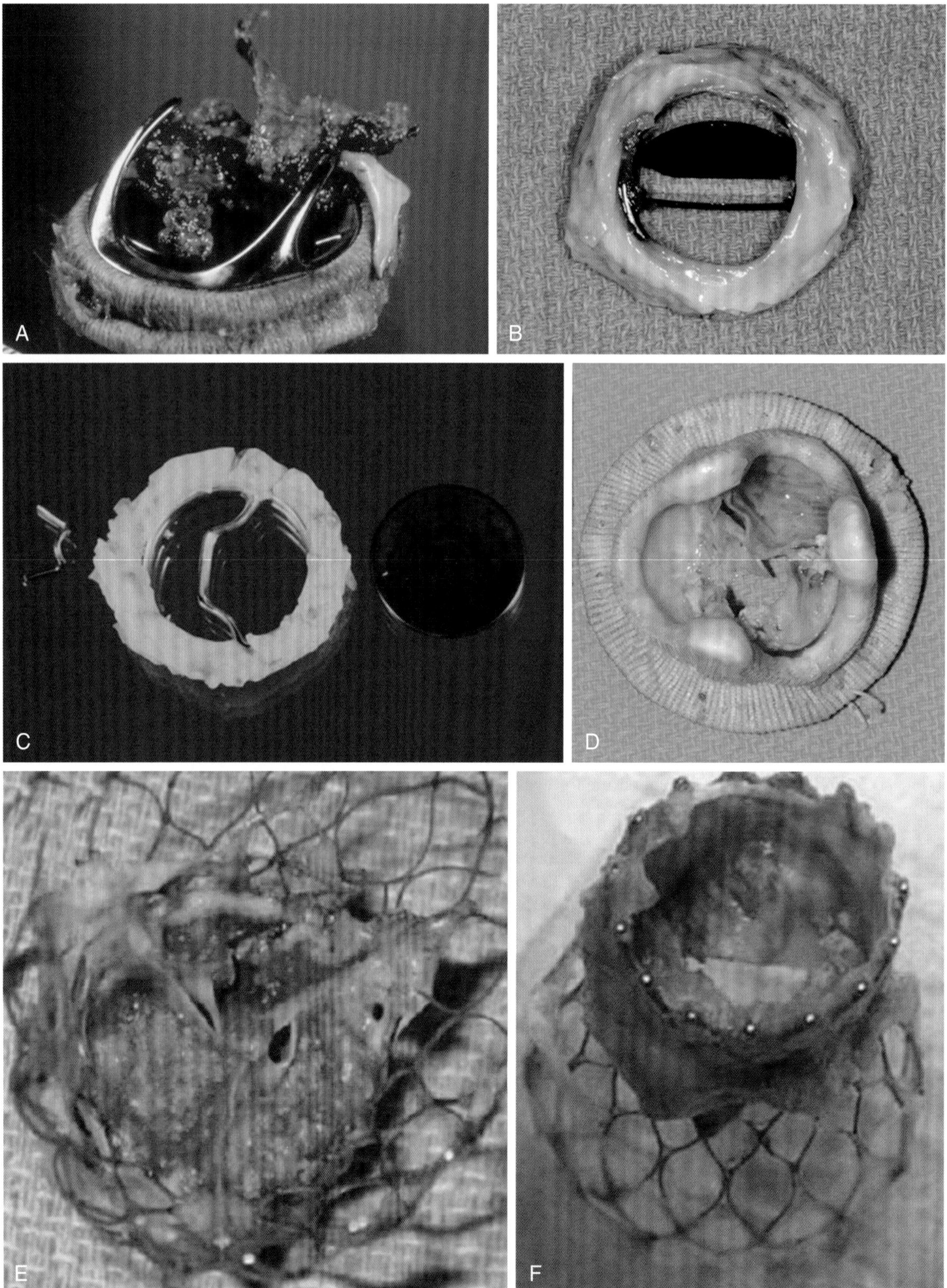

Fig. 31.1 Prosthetic valves explanted because of severe dysfunction. (A) Obstructive thrombosis of a Lillehei-Kaster prosthesis. (B) Pannus ingrowth hinders leaflet opening in a St. Jude Medical bileaflet valve. (C) Rupture of the outlet strut and leaflet escape in a Björk-Shiley prosthesis. (D) Leaflet calcific degeneration and tear in a porcine bioprosthesis. (E) Thrombosis in a self-expanding transcatheter aortic valve. (F) Leaflet calcific degeneration and stenosis in a self-expanding transcatheter aortic valve. (Courtesy Drs. Jacques Métras [A and C]; Christian Couture [B], Québec Heart & Lung Institute, Québec; and Gosta Petterson, Cleveland Clinic, Cleveland [D]). (E, From Latib A, Naganuma T, Abdel-Wahab M, et al. Treatment and clinical outcomes of transcatheter heart valve thrombosis. *Circ Cardiovasc Interv*. 2015;8:1–8. F, From Seeburger J, Weiss G, Borger MA, Mohr FW. Structural valve deterioration of a CoreValve prosthesis 9 months after implantation. *Eur Heart J*. 2013;34:1607)

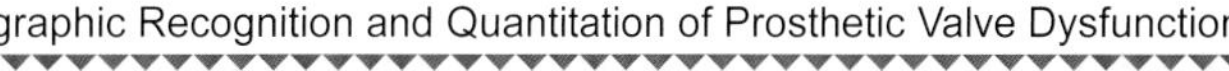
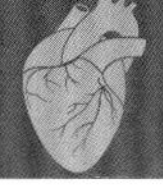

TABLE 31.1 **Doppler Echocardiographic Criteria for Identification and Quantitation of Patient-Prosthesis Mismatch.**

Parameter	*Mild or Not Clinically Significant PPM*	*Moderate PPM*	*Severe PPM*
Prosthetic Aortic Valves			
Indexed EOA (projected or measured)			
BMI < 30 kg/m^2	>0.85	0.85–0.66	≤0.65
BMI ≥ 30 kg/m^2	>0.70	0.70–0.56	≤0.55
Difference (measured EOA − reference EOA) (cm^2)[a,b]	<0.30	<0.30	<0.30
Valve structure and motion	Usually normal	Usually normal	Usually normal
Prosthetic Mitral Valves			
Indexed EOA (projected or measured)			
BMI < 30 kg/m^2	>1.2	1.2–0.91	≤0.90
BMI ≥ 30 kg/m^2	>1.0	1.0–0.76	≤0.75
Difference (measured EOA − reference EOA) (cm^2)[a,b]	<0.30	<0.30	<0.30
Valve structure and motion	Usually normal	Usually normal	Usually normal

[a]The criteria proposed for these parameters are valid for near-normal or normal stroke volume (50–90 mL).
[b]See Tables 31.4 and 31.5 for the normal reference values of the EOA for the different models and sizes of prostheses.
BMI, Body mass index; *EOA*, effective orifice area; *PPM*, patient-prosthesis mismatch.

whereas others reported an association with cerebrovascular events. A meta-analysis of observational studies reported that subclinical thrombosis detected by multidetector computed tomography (MDCT) was associated with a 3.38-fold increase in the risk of cerebrovascular events.[13]

STRUCTURAL VALVE DETERIORATION

Mechanical prostheses have excellent durability, and SVD is rare with contemporary valves, although mechanical failure (e.g., strut fracture, leaflet escape, occluder dysfunction due to lipid adsorption) has occurred with some models in the past (see Fig. 31.1C). Bioprosthetic SVD is expressed clinically by the development of a progressive stenosis due to leaflet calcification or by regurgitation due to leaflet tear (see Figs. 31.1D and F).[14–16] SVD is the major cause of bioprosthetic valve failure, and the rate of reoperation for SVD has been as high as 30% at 15 years.[15,17]

The traditional definition of SVD is based on the composite of valve reintervention or death related to structural valve failure. This definition, however, underestimates the true incidence of SVD because it captures only the most severe cases of SVD associated with heart failure symptoms. A substantial proportion of patients with severe SVD may not undergo valve reintervention because they are considered to be at high risk for poor outcomes with reoperation or a valve-in-valve procedure. Some deaths may not be classified as valve related even though SVD might have directly or indirectly contributed to the death.

More sensitive and granular definitions of SVD based on echocardiography have been proposed,[18,19] and they include four stages: stage 0, no SVD; stage 1, morphologic SVD (i.e., morphologic abnormalities consistent with SVD but with no deterioration in valve hemodynamic function); stage 2, moderate hemodynamic SVD (i.e., occurrence of moderate prosthetic valve stenosis or transvalvular regurgitation during follow-up); and stage 3, severe hemodynamic SVD. In one study, the rate of stage 2 or greater SVD was 41%, whereas the rate of reintervention was 3.5% at 10 years after SAVR.[14]

INFECTIVE ENDOCARDITIS

Prosthetic valve endocarditis is the most severe form of infective endocarditis. It occurs in 1% to 6% of patients with valve prostheses and accounts for 10% to 30% of all cases of infective endocarditis.[20] Prosthetic valve endocarditis (PVE) is an extremely serious condition with high mortality rates (30%–50%).

Echocardiography, particularly TEE, plays a key role in the diagnostic and prognostic assessment of PVE because the diagnosis relies predominantly on the combination of positive blood cultures and echocardiographic evidence of prosthetic infection, such as vegetations, paraprosthetic abscesses, or a new paravalvular regurgitation.[20–22] The diagnosis and management of PVE remains difficult, and a multidisciplinary approach is increasingly considered to be best practice. The team includes a consultant in cardiology and echocardiography with specialist competencies in valve disease. The incidence of PVE after TAVR is 1.1% per patient-year, which is similar to that after SAVR.[23]

DOPPLER ECHOCARDIOGRAPHIC EVALUATION OF PROSTHETIC VALVE FUNCTION

Doppler echocardiography is the method of choice for evaluating prosthetic valve function. The evaluation follows the same principles used for the evaluation of native valves, with some important caveats that are described later. A complete echocardiographic study includes two-dimensional (2D) imaging of the prosthetic valve, evaluation of valve leaflet/occluder morphology and mobility, measurement of the transprosthetic gradients and EOA, estimation of the location and degree of regurgitation, evaluation of left ventricular (LV) size and systolic function, and calculation of systolic pulmonary arterial pressure,[6,24–26]

TIMING OF ECHOCARDIOGRAPHIC FOLLOW-UP

An initial TTE examination performed 6 weeks to 3 months after prosthetic valve implantation is recommended to assess the results of surgery and serve as a baseline for comparison if complications or deterioration occurs later.[6,24] Repeat TTE along with TEE is recommended for patients with prosthetic valves if there is a change in clinical symptoms or signs suggesting valve dysfunction.[21,22]

The American College of Cardiology/American Heart Association (ACC/AHA) guidelines[21] suggest performing a TTE at 5 and 10 years and then annually thereafter, even in the absence of a change in clinical status. However, about 25% to 35% of patients with a bioprosthesis implanted for less than 10 years in the aortic position have some degree of valve degeneration or dysfunction at the Doppler echocardiographic examination.[14,17,28–31] The data support more frequent echocardiographic follow-up studies 5 years after implantation, as recommended in the 2009 American Society of Echocardiography (ASE) guidelines.[24] For patients with mechanical valves, routine annual echocardiography is not indicated in the absence of a change in clinical status.[21] Routine follow-up TTE

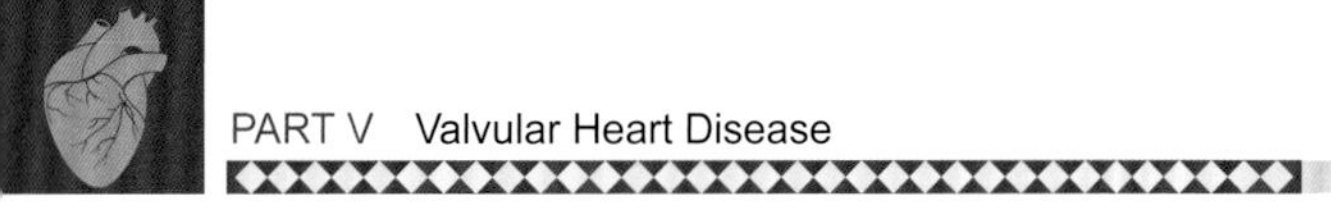

TABLE 31.2 Doppler Echocardiographic Criteria for Detection and Quantitation of Prosthetic Aortic Valve Stenosis.

Parameter	*Normal*	*Mild to Moderate Stenosis*	*Significant Stenosis*
Valve Structure and Motion			
Mechanical or bioprosthetic valve	Normal	Often abnormal[a]	Abnormal[a]
Doppler Quantitative Parameters			
Peak velocity (m/s)[b,c]	<3	3–4	≥4
Mean gradient (mmHg)[b,c]	<20	20–35	≥35
Doppler velocity index[b]	≥0.35	0.25–0.35	<0.25
Effective orifice area (cm^2)[b]	>1.1	0.8–1.1	<0.8
Difference (measured EOA – reference EOA) (cm^2)[b,d]	<0.30	0.30–0.6	≥0.60
Contour of the transprosthetic jet[e]	Triangular, early peaking	Triangular to intermediate	Rounded, symmetric
Acceleration time (ms)[e]	<80	80–100	>100
Acceleration time/LV ejection time ratio	<0.32	0.32–0.37	>0.37
Changes in Echocardiographic Parameters During Follow-Up			
Increase in mean gradient (mmHg)	<10	10–19	≥20
Decrease in EOA (mmHg)	<0.3	0.3–0.59	≥0.60
Decrease in Doppler velocity index	<0.10	0.10–0.19	≥0.20

[a]Valve leaflet that is immobile or with restricted mobility, thrombus, or pannus; abnormal biologic valves: leaflet thickening or calcification, thrombus, or pannus. The mobility and morphology of the leaflet is assessed by TTE, TEE, and cinefluoroscopy (for mechanical valves).
[b]The criteria proposed for these parameters are valid for a near-normal or normal stroke volume (50–90 mL).
[c]These parameters are more affected by low- or high-flow states, including low LV output and concomitant prosthetic valve regurgitation.
[d]Table 31.4 shows the normal reference EOA values for the various models and sizes of prostheses.
[e]These parameters are affected by LV function and chronotropy.
EOA, Effective orifice area.
Adapted from Lancellotti P, Pibarot P, Chambers J, et al. Recommendations for the imaging assessment of prosthetic heart valves: a report from the European Association of Cardiovascular Imaging endorsed by the Chinese Society of Echocardiography, the Inter-American Society of Echocardiography, and the Brazilian Department of Cardiovascular Imaging. *Eur Heart J Cardiovasc Imaging.* 2016;17:589–590.

after TAVR should include a baseline study (ideally within 30 days) at 1 year, and annually thereafter.[32]

CLINICAL DATA

The reason for the echocardiographic study and the patient's symptoms should be clearly documented. Because the interpretation of Doppler echocardiographic findings depends on the type and size of the prosthesis, this information and the date of implantation should be incorporated in the report. The exact type and model of prosthesis should be recorded because the design and hemodynamic performance may differ substantially from one model generation to another. The approach used for surgical (e.g., standard sternotomy, ministernotomy, right anterior thoracotomy) or transcatheter (e.g., transfemoral, transaxillary, transcarotid, transapical, transaortic, transcaval) valve replacement should also be collected.

Blood pressure and heart rate should be measured at the time of echocardiogram. The patient's height, weight, body surface area, and body mass index should be recorded to assess for the presence and severity of PPM and to index LV dimensions.

RECOGNITION AND QUANTITATION OF PROSTHETIC VALVE STENOSIS

The appearance of a new murmur with new congestive heart failure symptoms in a patient with prosthetic aortic valve should prompt an urgent TTE study and, if indicated, a TEE study. However, the initial suspicion of prosthetic valve stenosis may be the incidental finding of abnormally high flow velocities and gradients detected during a routine examination. Tables 31.2 and 31.3 show the Doppler echocardiographic criteria for the recognition and quantitation of prosthetic valve stenosis.[6,24,32]

Leaflet Morphology and Mobility

Echocardiographic imaging should identify the sewing ring, the valve occluder, and the surrounding area. Imaging of the ball or disc of mechanical valves is often difficult to obtain because of reverberations and shadowing caused by the valve components. Left parasternal short-axis views and especially off-axis views are useful for assessing mitral prosthetic valve leaflet mobility. The leaflets of bioprosthetic valves normally appear to be thin, with unrestricted motion and no evidence of prolapse. Stentless homograft or autograft valves may be indistinguishable from native valves.

Prosthetic valve stenosis generally is associated with abnormal valve morphology and/or mobility (Figs. 31.2–31.4; see Tables 31.2 and 31.3). In the case of mechanical valves, the mobility of the occluder is usually reduced or absent (see Fig. 31.2A). Thrombus, pannus, or vegetations are often visualized at the level of the prosthesis ring or hinge mechanism (Fig. 31.3D). In the case of bioprosthetic valves, prosthetic valve stenosis is most often associated with thickening, calcification, and reduced mobility of the leaflets (see Fig. 31.2B). Valve leaflet thickening is considered significant when the thickness of at least one leaflet is greater than 2 mm. Obstruction of bioprostheses may also be caused by thrombus, pannus, or vegetation (see Fig. 31.1).

Two- (2D) and three-dimensional (3D) TEE can improve assessment of leaflet mobility and detection of cusp calcification and thickening, valvular vegetations due to endocarditis, thrombus or pannus, and reduced leaflet, disc, or ball mobility (see Fig. 31.3).[33] In the case of mechanical prostheses, evaluation of occluder mobility can be attempted with some degree of success, but in our experience, valve cinefluoroscopy is definitely the best, most economical, and least invasive technique that can be used for this purpose (see Fig. 31.4A).[6] MDCT may also be used to evaluate leaflet mobility of mechanical and

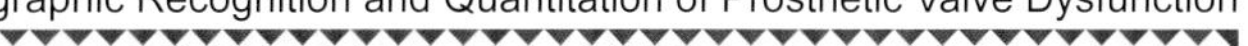

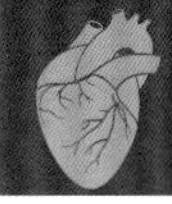

TABLE 31.3 Doppler Echocardiographic Criteria for Detection and Quantitation of Prosthetic Mitral Valve Stenosis.

Parameter	*Normal*	*Mild to Moderate Stenosis*	*Significant Stenosis*
Valve Structure and Motion			
Mechanical or bioprosthetic valve	Normal	Often abnormal[a]	Abnormal[a]
Doppler Quantitative Parameters			
Peak velocity (m/s)[b,c]	<1.9	1.9–2.5	≥2.5
Mean gradient (mmHg)[b,c]	≤5	6–10	≥10
Doppler velocity index [b]	<2.2	2.2–2.5	>2.5
Effective orifice area (cm^2)[b]	≥2	1–2	<1
Difference (measured EOA – reference EOA) (cm^2)[b,d]	<0.30	0.30–0.6	≥0.60
Pressure half-time (in ms)[e]	<130	130–200	>200
Changes in Echocardiographic Parameters During Follow-Up			
Increase in mean gradient (mmHg)	<3	3–5	>5
Decrease in EOA (mmHg)	<0.3	0.3–0.59	≥0.60
Decrease in Doppler velocity index	<0.10	0.10–0.19	≥0.20

[a]Valve leaflet that is immobile or with restricted mobility, thrombus, or pannus; abnormal biologic valves: leaflet thickening or calcification, thrombus, or pannus. The mobility and morphology of the leaflet is assessed by TTE, TEE, cinefluoroscopy (mechanical valves), or multidetector computed tomography.
[b]The criteria proposed for these parameters are valid for a near-normal or normal stroke volume (50–90 mL).
[c]These parameters are more affected by low- or high-flow states, including low LV output and concomitant prosthetic valve regurgitation.
[d]Table 31.5 shows the normal reference EOA values for the various models and sizes of prostheses.
[e]These parameters are affected by LV function and chronotropy.
EOA, Effective orifice area.
Adapted from Lancellotti P, Pibarot P, Chambers J, et al. Recommendations for the imaging assessment of prosthetic heart valves: a report from the European Association of Cardiovascular Imaging endorsed by the Chinese Society of Echocardiography, the Inter-American Society of Echocardiography, and the Brazilian Department of Cardiovascular Imaging. *Eur Heart J Cardiovasc Imaging*. 2016;17:589–590.

bioprosthetic valves and to assess for pannus or thrombus in all types of valves and for valve leaflet thickening and calcification in bioprosthetic valves (Fig. 31.4B–F).[6]

TTE lacks sensitivity to detect subclinical thrombosis of bioprosthetic valves. Contrast MDCT is superior to TTE for this purpose and is useful for identifying markers of leaflet thrombosis, such as hypoattenuated leaflet thickening (HALT) and reduced leaflet motion (RLM) (see Fig. 31.4C–E).[34] Given the dynamic nature of subclinical leaflet thrombosis and its absence of or weak association with clinical events, routine screening with contrast MDCT is not recommended. Noncontrast MDCT may be useful to identify bioprosthetic valve leaflet calcification, which is a marker of SVD (see Fig. 31.4F).[29,35]

Quantitative Parameters

Quantitative parameters of prosthetic valve function include flow velocity, pressure gradients, EOA, and Doppler velocity index.

Transprosthetic Velocity and Gradient

The principles of interrogation and recording of flow velocity through prosthetic valves are similar to those used in evaluating native valve stenosis. This includes pulsed-wave (PW) and continuous-wave (CW) Doppler and color Doppler, using several windows for optimal recording and minimizing angulation between the Doppler beam and flow direction. CW Doppler evaluation of aortic prostheses must be performed from multiple transducer positions, including apical, right parasternal, right supraclavicular, and suprasternal notch. Measurements of prosthetic valve velocity and gradients are made from the transducer position, yielding the highest velocities.[6,24]

The fluid dynamics of mechanical valves may differ substantially from those of the native valve (Fig. 31.5). The flow is eccentric in the monoleaflet valves and composed of three separate jets in the bileaflet valves. Because the direction of the jets across prosthetic valves may be eccentric, multiwindow CW interrogation is essential to obtain the highest transprosthetic velocity signal. Occasionally, an abnormally high jet gradient corresponding to a localized high velocity may be recorded by CW Doppler interrogation through the smaller central orifice of bileaflet mechanical prostheses in the aortic or mitral position (see Fig. 31.5).[36,37] This phenomenon may lead to overestimation of gradient, underestimation of the EOA, and therefore a false suspicion of prosthesis dysfunction.

Pressure gradient is calculated with the use of the simplified Bernoulli equation as follows: $\Delta P = 4 \times V_{Pr}^2$, where V_{Pr} is the velocity of the transprosthetic flow jet (in m/s). In patients with aortic prostheses and a high flow rate or narrow LV outflow tract (LVOT), the velocity proximal to the prosthesis may be increased and therefore not negligible. If proximal velocity (V_{LVOT}) is greater than 1.5 m/s, estimation of the pressure gradient is more accurately determined by including V_{LVOT} in the following equation:

$$\Delta P = 4 \times \left(V_{Pr}^2 - V_{LVOT}^2\right)$$

Because of the pressure recovery phenomenon, the gradients measured by Doppler echocardiography may be higher and EOAs smaller compared with the values obtained by cardiac catheterization (see Fig. 31.5). The extent of pressure recovery is more pronounced in patients with a small aorta.[37–40] It is important to distinguish between the pressure recovery phenomenon that may occur with any type of native or prosthetic aortic valve and the localized high gradient phenomenon that occurs in bileaflet mechanical valves (see Fig. 31.5).

Prosthetic valve stenosis is usually associated with increased transprosthetic peak flow velocity or mean gradient (≥3 m/s or ≥20 mmHg for aortic prostheses and ≥1.9 m/s or ≥6 mmHg for mitral prostheses) (see Tables 31.2 and 31.3).[6,24,32] However, a high velocity or gradient alone is not proof of intrinsic prosthetic valve obstruction and may be caused by PPM, high-flow conditions, prosthetic valve regurgitation, or localized high central jet velocity in bileaflet mechanical valves (data interpretation and

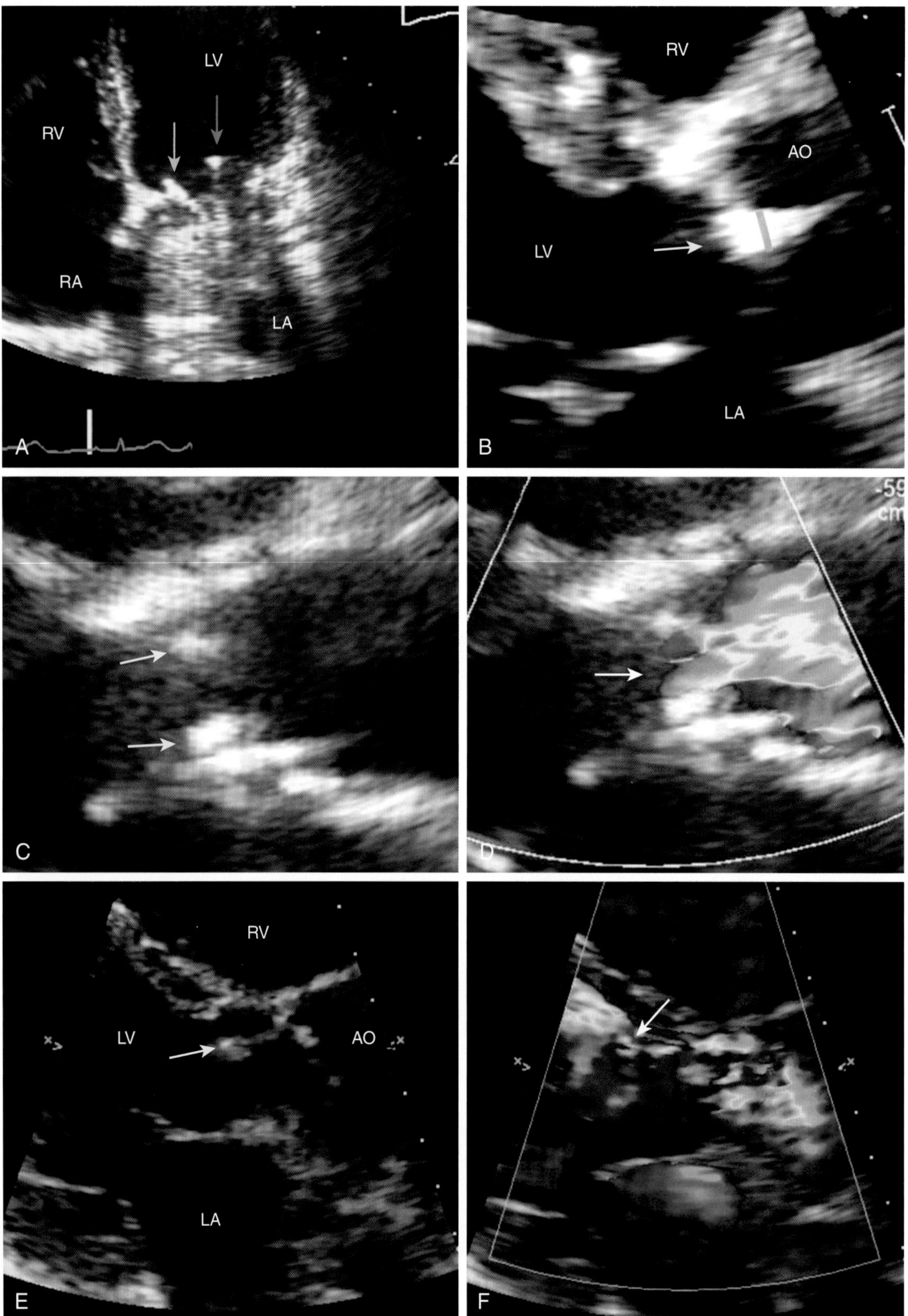

Fig. 31.2 Evaluation of prosthetic valve leaflet morphology and mobility. (A) Mitral bileaflet mechanical prosthesis in diastole has a fixed leaflet *(green arrow)*; the other leaflet remains mobile *(blue arrow)* (see Video 31.2A). (B) Thickening and reduced mobility of aortic bioprosthetic valve cusps *(yellow arrow)* in systole. The leaflet thickness is 4.6 mm *(orange line)*. (C and D) Thickening and reduced mobility of aortic bioprosthetic valve leaflets *(yellow arrows)* and narrowing of the transvalvular flow on color Doppler *(white arrow)* (see Video 31.2CD). (E and F) Avulsed cusp (*yellow arrow*) and resulting transvalvular regurgitant jet (*white arrow*) in an aortic bioprosthetic valve (see Videos 31.2E and 31. 2F).

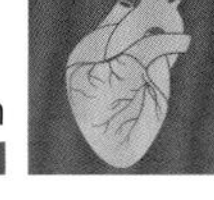

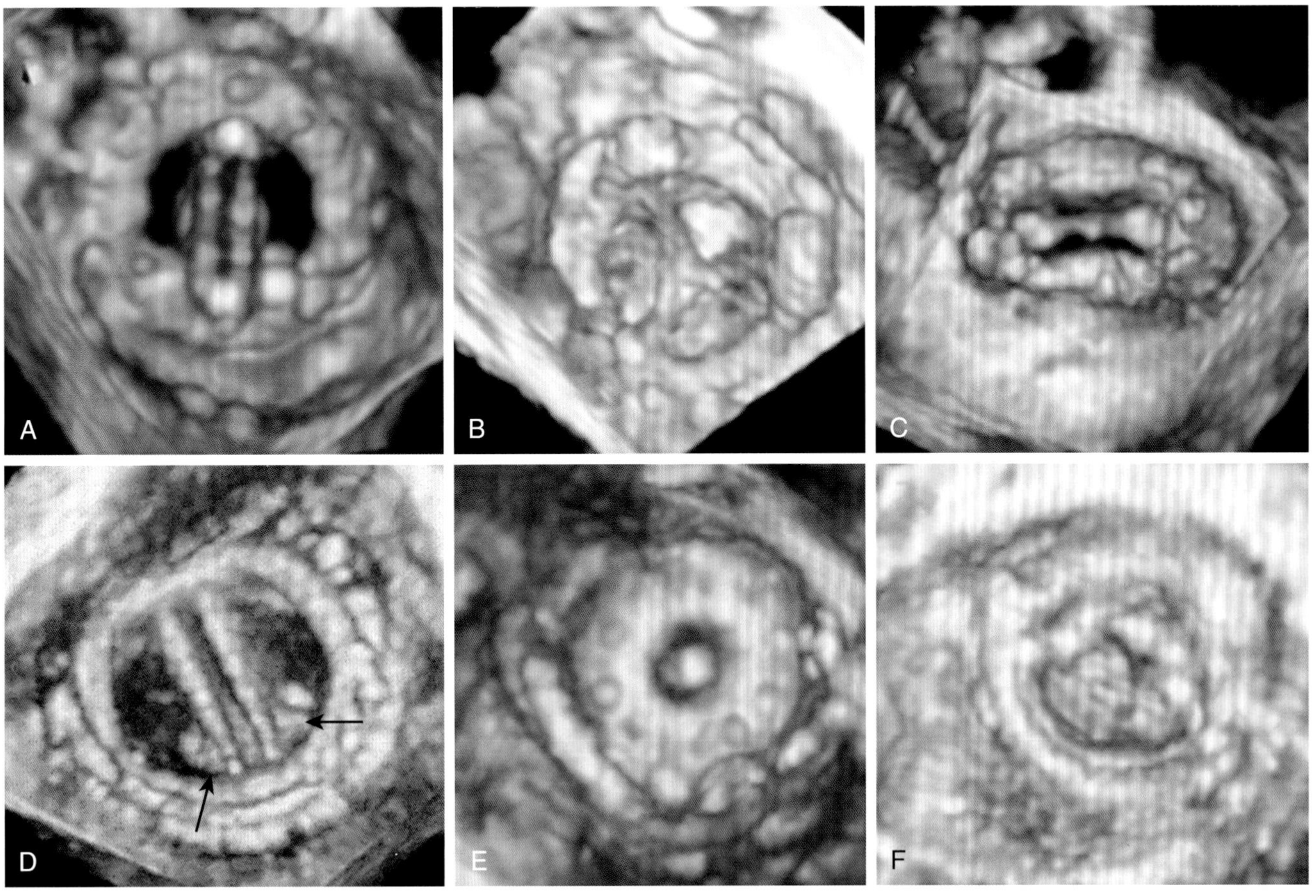

Fig. 31.3 3D transesophageal views of prosthetic valves and rings. Zoomed 3D TEE images of prosthetic valves. (A) Bileaflet mechanical mitral valve as viewed from the LA. (B) Bioprosthetic mitral valve as viewed from the LV. (C) Mitral annuloplasty ring from the LA. (D) Mitral bileaflet mechanical valve from the LA; small thrombi *(black arrows)* are attached to the hinge mechanism of the valve, and the motion of the leaflets is not impaired. (E) En face view from the LA of a ball-and-cage valve implanted in the mitral annulus. (F) Single tilting-disc valve in the mitral position as viewed from the LA. (Adapted from Lang RM, Tsang W, Weinert L, Mor-Avi V, Chandra S. Valvular heart disease: the value of 3-dimensional echocardiography. *J Am Coll Cardiol.* 2011;58:1933–1944.)

differential diagnosis are discussed later). Significant prosthetic valve regurgitation may cause the flow rate across the prosthesis to increase, resulting in increased velocities and gradients.

Transprosthetic Jet Contour and Flow Ejection Dynamics

The contour of the velocity through the prosthesis is a qualitative index that may be used to assess prosthetic aortic valve function in conjunction with the other quantitative indices. In a normal valve, the contour of the CW flow velocity usually has triangular shape, with early peaking of the velocity and a short acceleration time (AT), which is the time from the onset of flow to maximal velocity (AT < 80 ms) (Fig. 31.6). With prosthetic valve obstruction, a more rounded velocity contour is seen, with the velocity peaking almost in mid-ejection and prolonged AT (>100 ms) (see Fig. 31.6 and Tables 31.2 and 31.3).[6,24]

The main limitation of the AT is that it highly depends on chronotropy. To overcome this limitation, AT should be indexed to the LV ejection time (LVET); a ratio greater than 0.37 suggests prosthetic aortic valve stenosis.[41] The advantage of these indices is that they are independent of Doppler beam angulation in relation to flow direction. They are, however, influenced by LV systolic function. For example, a patient with normally functioning aortic prosthesis and concomitant depressed myocardial contractility may nonetheless exhibit a rounded velocity contour with late velocity peaking, as has been witnessed in patients with severe PPM.

Effective Orifice Area

The EOA of prosthetic aortic valves is calculated with the continuity equation, similar to calculating the native aortic valve area (Fig. 31.7).[42–44]

$$EOA = (CSA_{LVOT} \times VTI_{LVOT})/VTI_{PrAv}$$

where CSA_{LVOT} is the cross-sectional area of the LVOT, VTI_{LVOT} is the velocity–time integral (VTI) obtained by PW Doppler in the LVOT, and VTI_{PrAv} is the VTI obtained by CW Doppler though the aortic prosthesis. When measuring the EOA of prosthetic aortic valves, some caveats should be taken into consideration:

1. The cross-sectional area of the LVOT is derived from the diameter measurement just underneath the apical border of the prosthesis stent or ring from the parasternal long-axis zoomed view, assuming a circular geometry (see Fig. 31.7A–C). This measurement is often difficult because of the reverberations and artifacts caused by the prosthesis stent or sewing ring. The inner border of the prosthesis stent or ring should not be mistaken for the inner edge of the LVOT. Modified views (e.g., lower parasternal) can be used to keep the artifact from the prosthetic valve away from the LVOT. Substitution of the LVOT diameter by the labeled prosthesis size in the continuity equation is *not* a valid method to determine the EOA of aortic prostheses.[45]

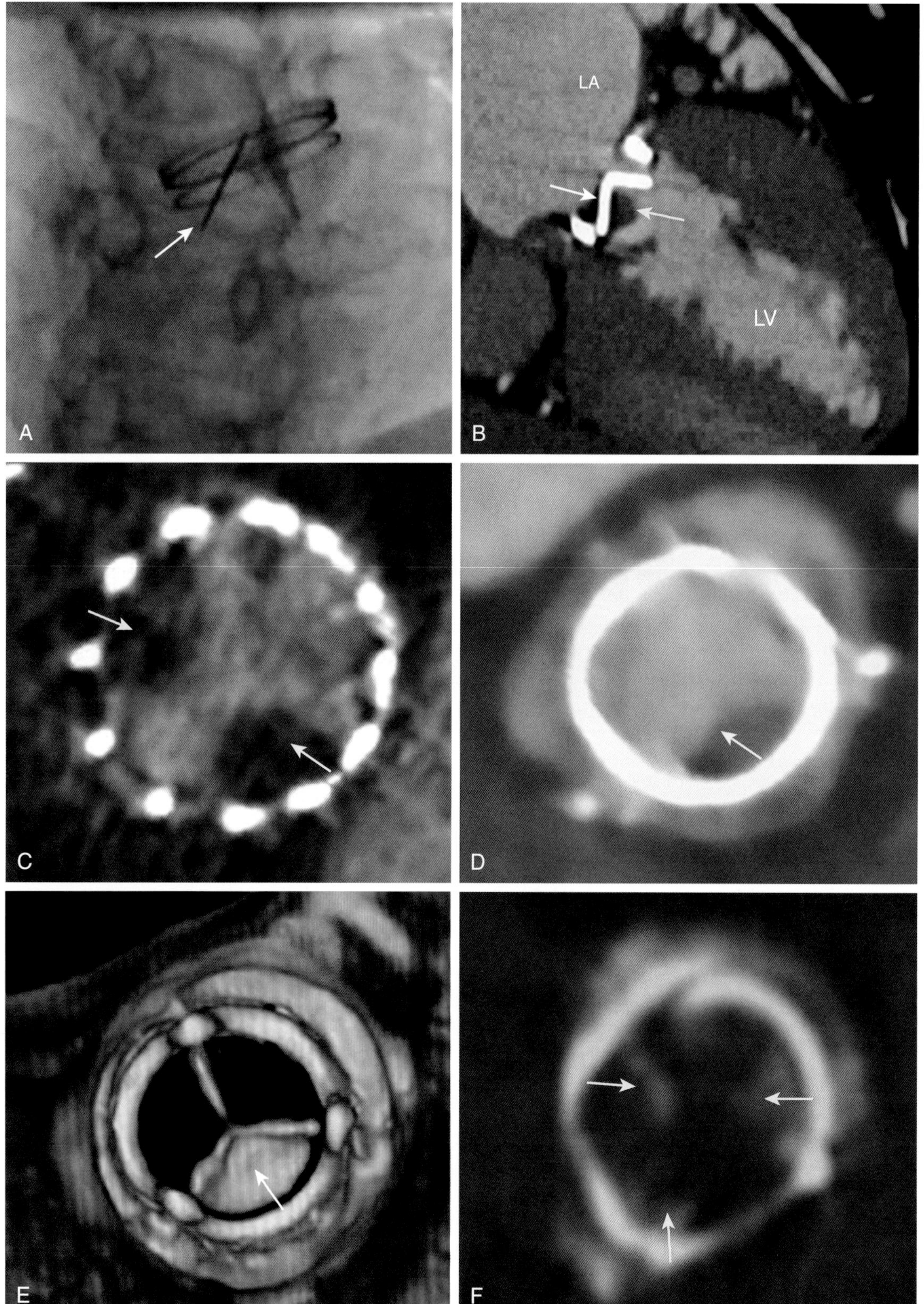

Fig. 31.4 Alternative imaging modalities to detect prosthetic valve dysfunction. (A) Cinefluoroscopy used for assessment of mechanical valve leaflet mobility shows an immobile leaflet in a mitral bileaflet mechanical valve *(arrow)* (see Video 31.4A). (B) Multislice computed tomography used for assessment of mechanical valve leaflet mobility shows an immobile leaflet *(white arrow)* and a thrombus *(yellow arrow)* (see Video 31.4B). (C and D) Contrast-enhanced multidetector computed tomography (MDCT) used to detect subclinical thrombosis *(arrows)* in transcatheter (C) and surgical (D) aortic bioprosthetic valves. (E) 4D MDCT identifies reduced leaflet mobility *(arrow)* (see Video 31.4E). (F) MDCT detects mineralization of bioprosthetic valve leaflets *(arrows)*, which is a marker of structural valve deterioration. (B, Courtesy Dr. Steven A. Goldstein, Washington Hospital Center.)

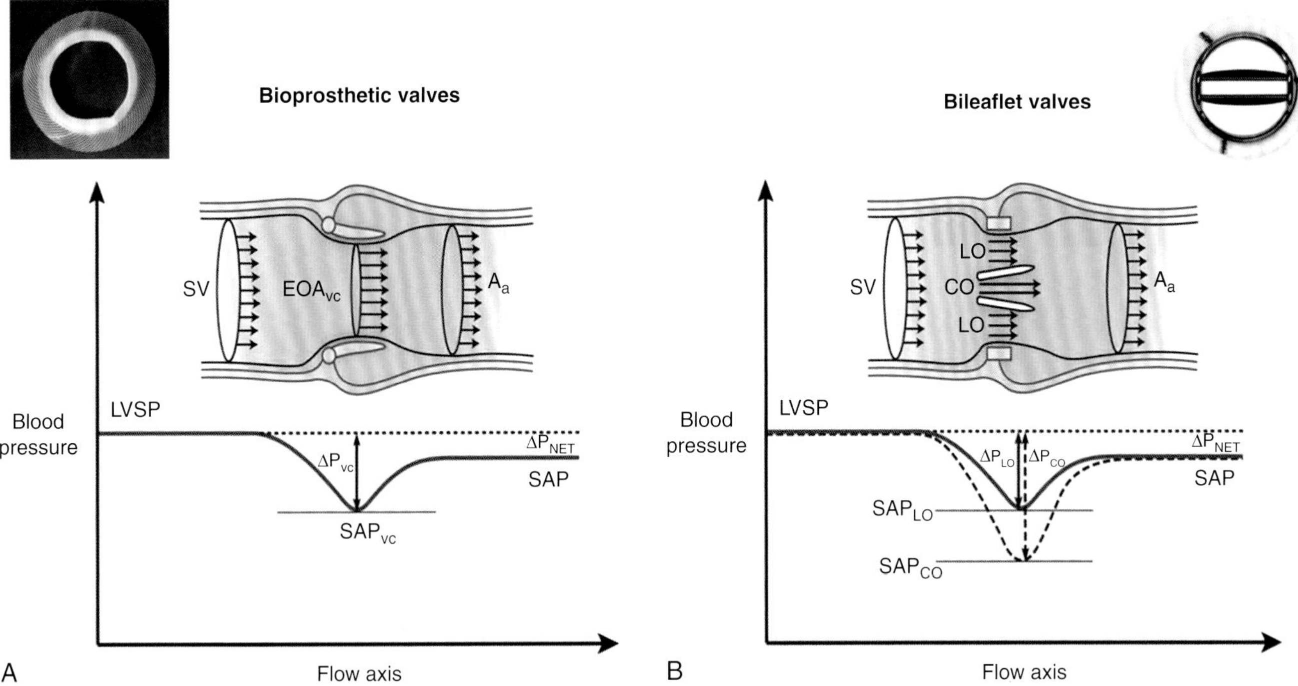

Fig. 31.5 Velocity and pressure changes. Schematic representation of velocity and pressure changes from the LV outflow tract to the ascending aorta (A_a) in the setting of a stented bioprosthesis (A) and a bileaflet mechanical valve (B) illustrate the phenomena of pressure recovery and localized high gradient. Because of pressure recovery, velocities are lower, and the systolic arterial pressure *(SAP)* is higher at the distal aorta than at the level of the vena contracta *(VC)*. This phenomenon can occur with any type of prosthetic aortic valve and is more pronounced in patients with a smaller (<30 mm) ascending aorta. In the case of a bileaflet valve, the velocity is locally higher in the central orifice *(CO)*, and the pressure gradient *(ΔP)* is higher at that level. This phenomenon of localized high velocity and gradient that is specific to bileaflet mechanical valves should be distinguished from the pressure recovery phenomenon that may occur downstream of the VC in native or prosthetic aortic valves. Doppler gradients are estimated from maximal velocity at the level of the VC and represent the maximal pressure drop, whereas invasive estimation of gradients usually reflect net pressure difference *(ΔP_{NET})* between the LV systolic pressure *(LVSP)* and ascending aorta. *EOA*: Effective orifice area; *LO*, lateral orifice; *SV*, stroke volume in the LV outflow tract. (Adapted from Zoghbi WA, Asch FM, Bruce C, et al. Guidelines for the evaluation of valvular regurgitation after percutaneous valve repair or replacement: a report from the American Society of Echocardiography developed in collaboration with the Society for Cardiovascular Angiography and Interventions, Japanese Society of Echocardiography, and Society for Cardiovascular Magnetic Resonance. *J Am Soc Echocardiogr.* 2019;32:431–475.)

2. When recording the LVOT velocity signal, care should be exercised to locate the PW Doppler sample volume adjacent to the prosthesis while avoiding the region of subvalvular acceleration (see Fig. 31.7D and F). The PW Doppler sample is positioned just below the apical border of the prosthesis stent or ring.[24,46] Color Doppler may be useful to guide the positioning of the PW Doppler sample. An effort should be made to measure the LVOT VTI and LVOT diameter at about the same location. In balloon-expandable transcatheter heart valves (THVs), the leaflets are attached close to the apical border of the stent, and placing the PW Doppler sample volume within the inflow portion of the stent results in overestimation of stroke volume and EOA because of subvalvular flow acceleration.[46] In self-expanding THVs, the leaflets are attached higher in the stent, and there is no or minimal flow acceleration at the level of the apical end of the stent.[47] For self-expanding valves when the stent landing zone is low in the LVOT, it may be preferable to measure the LVOT diameter and velocity within the apical (first 5 mm) portion of the stent.
3. The VTI across the prosthesis is obtained from the same signals that are used for measurement of prosthesis peak velocity and gradient.
4. The continuity equation method is also valid in the setting of concomitant prosthetic aortic valve regurgitation because the numerator and denominator of the equation are increased in a similar proportion.

The EOA of a mitral prostheses is calculated by the continuity equation using the stroke volume measured in the LVOT (see Fig. 31.7).[48]

$$EOA = (CSA_{LVOT} \times VTI_{LVOT}) / VTI_{PrMv}$$

where VTI_{PrMv} is the VTI obtained by CW Doppler though the mitral prosthesis (see Fig. 31.6). A few important caveats should be taken into consideration for the estimation of EOA of prosthetic mitral valves:

1. The continuity equation method cannot be applied when there is more than mild concomitant mitral or aortic regurgitation.
2. The pressure half-time (PHT) method (similar to that used for native mitral valve stenosis) is not valid to estimate the valve EOA of mitral prostheses.[48] The PHT is highly influenced by chronotropy, left atrial (LA) compliance, and LV compliance. Patients with tachycardia or reduced atrioventricular compliance may exhibit a normal PHT despite having significant prosthetic valve stenosis. Nonetheless, the PHT may be useful if it is significantly delayed (>200 ms) (see Table 31.3 and Fig. 31.6D) or shows significant lengthening from one follow-up visit to another despite similar heart rates.

Valve EOAs between 0.8 and 1.1 cm² and between 1.0 and 2.0 cm² suggest possible stenosis of aortic and mitral prostheses, respectively (see Tables 31.2 and 31.3), whereas values of less than 0.8 cm² (aortic) or less than 1.0 cm² (mitral) indicate significant

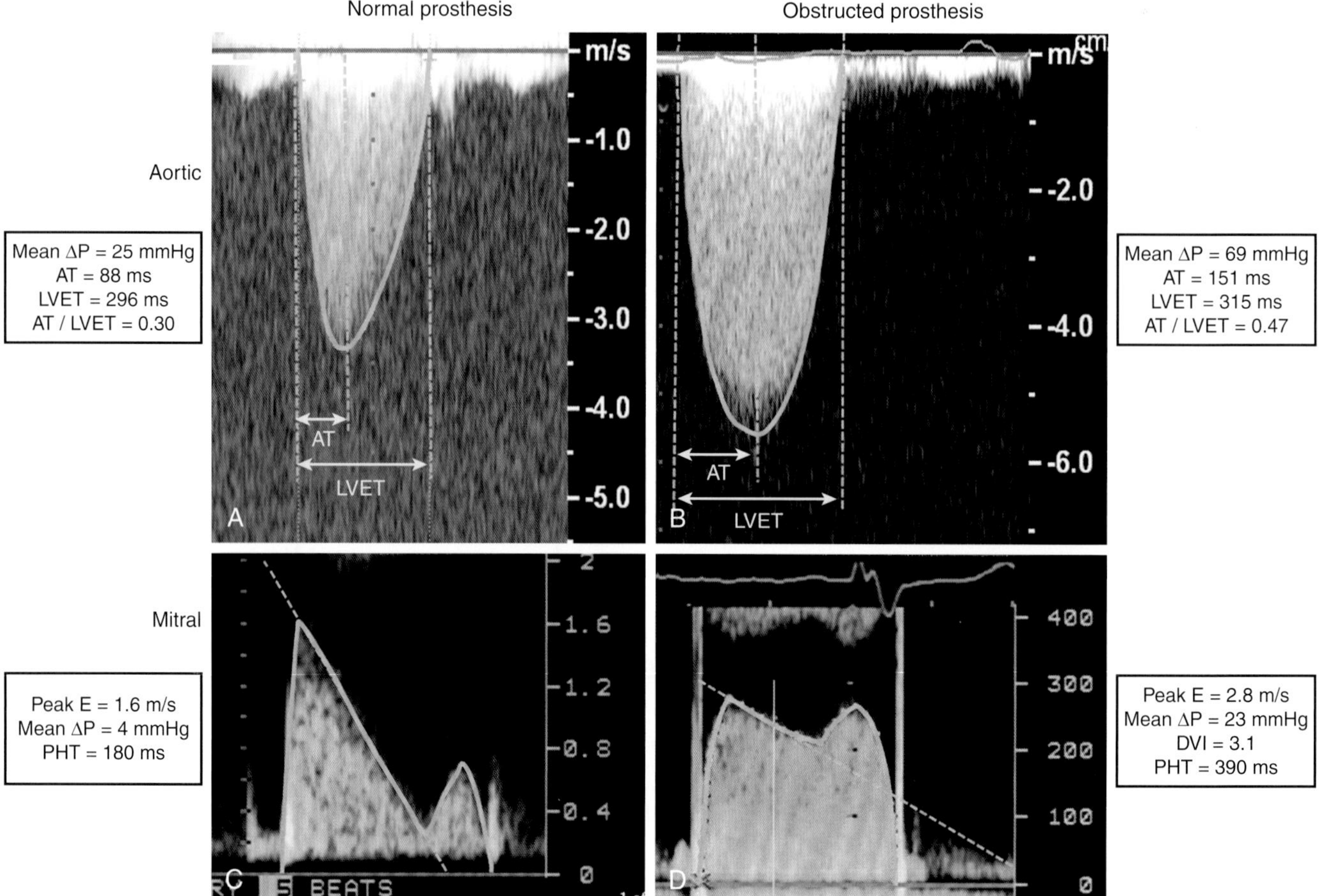

Fig. 31.6 CW Doppler velocity recordings in normal and obstructed prosthetic valves. (A and B) CW Doppler signal of the transaortic flow in a normal and an obstructed aortic valve prosthesis. Notice the rounded flow velocity curve for the obstructed prosthetic valve (B) and the early peaking of the velocity in the normal valve (A). A ratio of acceleration time *(AT)* to LV ejection time *(LVET)* of more than 0.37 suggests severe prosthetic valve stenosis. (C and D) CW Doppler signal of the transmitral flow in a normal and an obstructed mitral valve prosthesis. The peak E velocity, mean gradient, and pressure half-time are higher in the obstructed prosthesis. *ΔP*, Transprosthetic pressure gradient; *PHT*, pressure half-time.

stenosis.[6,24] These cutoff values proposed in the ASE and European Association of Cardiovascular Imaging (EACVI) recommendations[6,24] have an important limitation given that they overlap substantially with the normal reference values of EOA of several prostheses models. The recognition of prosthetic valve stenosis is better achieved by comparing the measured EOA with the normal reference value of the EOA for the model and size of prosthesis implanted in the patient rather than applying fixed cutoff values to all patients regardless of the characteristics of their prosthesis.[6,47,49]

Tables 31.4 and 31.5 show the normal reference values for EOA for the most commonly used prosthetic valves in the aortic and mitral position, respectively. If the difference between the normal reference EOA and the measured EOA is more than 0.30 cm^2, stenosis should be suspected, and if it is more than 0.60 cm^2, significant stenosis is likely (see Tables 31.2 and 31.3).[6,50,51]

Doppler Velocity Index

The Doppler velocity index is a dimensionless ratio of the proximal VTI in the LVOT to the VTI through the aortic prosthesis: Doppler velocity index = VTI_{LVOT}/VTI_{PrAv}. Peak velocities may be used in place of VTIs to calculate the index (V_{LVOT}/V_{PrAv}). In the case of prosthetic mitral valves, the Doppler velocity index is calculated by dividing the VTI of the transprosthetic flow by that of LVOT flow: Doppler velocity index = VTI_{PrMv}/VTI_{LVOT}. These parameters can be helpful to screen for valve obstruction, particularly when the cross-sectional area of the LVOT cannot be obtained.[6,52]

The Doppler velocity index is reduced (≤0.35) in the setting of prosthetic aortic valve stenosis (see Table 31.2),[6,24] whereas it is increased (≥2.2) in the setting of prosthetic mitral valve stenosis (see Table 31.3). In the setting of significant prosthetic valve stenosis, the Doppler velocity index usually is less than 0.25 for aortic prostheses and more than 2.5 for mitral prostheses. For aortic prosthetic valves, a cutoff of less than 0.35 improves sensitivity for the detection of mild to moderate dysfunction (see Table 31.2).[50,51]

RECOGNITION AND QUANTITATION OF PROSTHETIC VALVE REGURGITATION

The approach to detecting and grading prosthesis regurgitation is similar to that for native valves. It involves multiple color Doppler views and measurements of several Doppler echocardiographic indices.[6,25] However, care is needed to separate physiologic from pathologic prosthesis regurgitation. Mechanical prostheses have a normal regurgitant volume known as *leakage backflow*. This form of regurgitation theoretically prevents blood stasis and thrombus formation using a washing effect. Unlike pathologic regurgitant jets, the normal leakage backflow jets are characterized by being short in duration, narrow, and symmetric. Bioprosthetic valves also often have a minor degree of central transvalvular regurgitation. The stented pericardial bioprostheses and the stentless substitutes, which include the stentless bioprostheses, the aortic homografts, and the

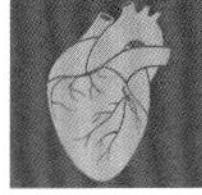

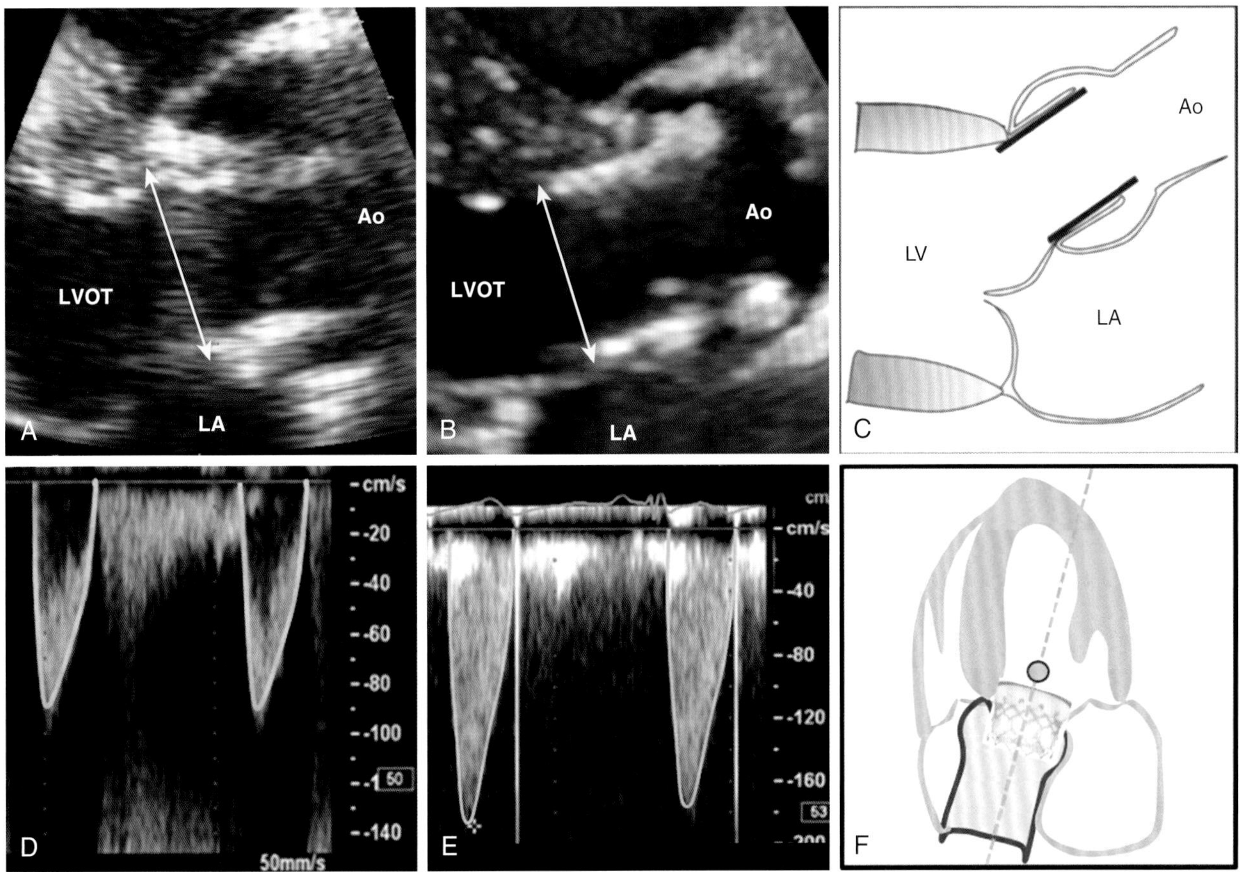

Fig. 31.7 **Doppler echocardiographic measurements for the calculation of the aortic prosthetic valve area by the continuity equation.** The stroke volume across the prosthetic aortic valve is calculated by multiplying the LV outflow tract *(LVOT)* area by the velocity–time integral of the LVOT flow measured by pulsed-wave Doppler. The LVOT diameter is measured from the external border to external border of the sewing ring for surgical prostheses (A) or the stent for transcatheter prostheses (B and C). The LVOT velocity is measured by placing the pulsed-wave Doppler sample just underneath the apical aspect of the prosthesis sewing ring or stent (D and F). The effective orifice area of the aortic prosthesis is calculated by dividing the stroke volume by the velocity–time integral of the transprosthetic flow obtained with CW Doppler (E).

pulmonary autografts (i.e., Ross operation), are more likely have minor transvalvular regurgitant jets.

In the case of pathologic regurgitation, it is important to localize the origin of the regurgitant jets to distinguish paravalvular from transvalvular regurgitation. In the late postoperative follow-up period, the most frequent cause of pathologic transvalvular regurgitation is calcific degeneration with tears of valve leaflets in bioprosthetic valves and thrombus or pannus in mechanical valves. Stentless substitutes are more likely than stented bioprostheses or mechanical valves to develop functional central aortic insufficiency due to continued dilation of the aortic root.

Paravalvular regurgitation is much more common after TAVR compared with SAVR or mitral valve replacement (MVR).[53–57] With surgical prostheses, residual paravalvular jets are rare, and if significant, they are usually corrected immediately during the initial operation. However, significant paravalvular regurgitation may develop during the late postoperative period, and it is often the result of endocarditis.

Prosthetic Aortic Valve Regurgitation

Imaging Considerations

For TEE and TTE evaluations of prosthetic valve regurgitation, particularly of paravalvular regurgitation, it is essential to obtain color Doppler images in multiple views and multiple planes (Fig. 31.8). The optimal views for the TTE assessment of prosthetic aortic regurgitation include the parasternal long-axis and short-axis views and the apical long-axis 5-chamber and 3-chamber views. Off-axis views may be helpful in determining the origin of the jets. The most important views for the assessment of prosthetic mitral valve regurgitation include the same views as for aortic prostheses and the apical 4-chamber and subcostal views.

Acoustic shadowing and occulting of regurgitant jets is less of an issue for aortic prostheses than for mitral prostheses.[24] However, posterior paravalvular jets of transcatheter aortic valves may be masked partially or totally in the parasternal views. Paravalvular regurgitant jets are often multiple, eccentric, and have irregular shapes (Figs. 31.9 and 31.10; see Fig. 31.8).[6,25,26] They are confined along the LVOT wall, and they may be masked partially or totally by acoustic shadowing from the calcifications of the native aortic annulus or from the THV stent. These features render the TTE imaging, detection, and quantification of paravalvular regurgitation particularly challenging.

TEE may be useful to identify the origin (i.e., paravalvular or transvalvular) of the regurgitant jets in technically difficult TTE studies and to identify the mechanism of regurgitation and associated complications such as flail bioprosthetic cusp, pannus, thrombus, vegetations or masses interacting with occluder closure, abscess formation, prosthesis dehiscence, or underdeployment or malapposition of the THV stent (see Figs. 31.3 and 31.9).[33,58]

Acoustic shadowing in the anterior region may limit the performance of TEE for evaluation of prosthetic aortic regurgitation in the mid-esophageal level. A concomitant mitral

TABLE 31.4 Normal Reference Values of the Effective Orifice Areas for Prosthetic Aortic Valves.[a]

	Prosthetic Valve Size					
Surgical Prosthetic Aortic Valves	*19 mm*	*21 mm*	*23 mm*	*25 mm*	*27 mm*	*29 mm*
Stented Bioprosthetic Valves						
Mosaic	1.1±0.2	1.2±0.3	1.4±0.3	1.7±0.4	1.8±0.4	2.0±0.4
Hancock II	—	1.2±0.2	1.3±0.2	1.5±0.2	1.6±0.2	1.6±0.2
Carpentier-Edwards Perimount	1.1±0.3	1.3±0.4	1.50±0.4	1.80±0.4	2.1±0.4	2.2±0.4
Carpentier-Edwards Magna	1.3±0.3	1.5±0.3	1.8±0.4	2.1±0.5	—	—
Biocor (Epic)	1.0±0.3	1.3±0.5	1.4±0.5	1.9±0.7	—	—
Trifecta	1.41±0.3	1.63±0.4	1.8±0.4	2.02±0.5	2.20±0.6	2.35±0.6
Mitroflow	1.1±0.2	1.2±0.3	1.4±0.3	1.6±0.3	1.8±0.3	—
Stentless Bioprosthetic Valves						
Medtronic Freestyle	1.2±0.2	1.4±0.2	1.5±0.3	2.0±0.4	2.3±0.5	—
St. Jude Medical Toronto SPV	—	1.3±0.3	1.5±0.5	1.7±0.8	2.1±0.7	2.7±1.0
Prima Edwards	—	1.3±0.3	1.6±0.3	1.9±0.4	—	—
Mechanical Valves						
Medtronic-Hall	1.2±0.2	1.3±0.2	—	—	—	—
St. Jude Medical Standard	1.0±0.2	1.4±0.2	1.5±0.5	2.1±0.4	2.7±0.6	3.2±0.3
St. Jude Medical Regent	1.6±0.4	2.0±0.7	2.2±0.9	2.5±0.9	3.6±1.3	4.4±0.6
MCRI On-X	1.5±0.2	1.7±0.4	2.0±0.6	2.4±0.8	3.2±0.6	3.2±0.6
Carbomedics Standard and Top Hat	1.0±0.4	1.5±0.3	1.7±0.3	2.0±0.4	2.5±0.4	2.6±0.4
ATS Medical[b]	1.1±0.3	1.6±0.4	1.8±0.5	1.9±0.3	2.3±0.8	—
Transcatheter Prosthetic Aortic Valves	*20 mm*	*23 mm*	*26 mm*	*29 mm*	*31 mm*	
Sapien	NA	1.6±0.4	1.8±0.5	—	—	—
Sapien XT	NA	1.4±0.3	1.7±0.4	2.1±0.5	—	—
Sapien 3	1.2±0.2	1.5±0.3	1.7±0.4	1.9±0.4	—	—
CoreValve	—	1.1±0.4	1.7±0.5	2.0±0.5	2.2±0.7	—
Evolut R	—	1.10±0.3	1.7±0.5	2.0±0.5	2.6±0.8	—

[a]Effective orifice area is expressed as the mean values available in the literature.
[b]For the ATS medical valve, the label valve sizes are 18, 20, 22, 24, and 26 mm.
NA, Not applicable.
Adapted from Lancellotti P, Pibarot P, Chambers J, et al. Recommendations for the imaging assessment of prosthetic heart valves: a report from the European Association of Cardiovascular Imaging endorsed by the Chinese Society of Echocardiography, the Inter-American Society of Echocardiography, and the Brazilian Department of Cardiovascular Imaging. *Eur Heart J Cardiovasc Imaging.* 2016;17:589–590.

TABLE 31.5 Normal Reference Values of the Effective Orifice Areas for Prosthetic Mitral Valves.[a]

	Prosthetic Valve Size				
Prosthetic Mitral Valves	*25 mm*	*27 mm*	*29 mm*	*31 mm*	*33 mm*
Stented Bioprosthetic Valves					
Medtronic Mosaic	1.5±0.4	1.7±0.5	1.9±0.5	1.9±0.5	—
Hancock II	1.5±0.4	1.8±0.5	1.9±0.5	2.6±0.5	2.6±0.7
Carpentier-Edwards Perimount	1.6±0.4	1.8±0.4	2.1±0.5	—	—
Mechanical Valves					
St. Jude Medical Standard	1.5±0.3	1.7±0.4	1.8±0.4	2.0±0.5	2.0±0.5
MCRI On-X[b]	2.2±0.9	2.2±0.9	2.2±0.9	2.2±0.9	2.2±0.9

[a]Effective orifice area is expressed as mean values available in the literature. Further studies are needed to validate these reference values.
[b]The ON-X valve has just one size for 27 to 29 mm and 31 to 33 mm prostheses. The strut and leaflets are identical for all sizes (25 to 33 mm); only the size of the sewing cuff is different.
Adapted from Lancellotti P, Pibarot P, Chambers J, et al. Recommendations for the imaging assessment of prosthetic heart valves: a report from the European Association of Cardiovascular Imaging endorsed by the Chinese Society of Echocardiography, the Inter-American Society of Echocardiography, and the Brazilian Department of Cardiovascular Imaging. *Eur Heart J Cardiovasc Imaging.* 2016;17:589–590.

prosthesis causes significant shadowing and obscures the LVOT. In these cases, it is crucial to evaluate the prosthesis from transgastric transducer positions.

Parameters of the Severity of Prosthetic Aortic Valve Regurgitation

The same principles and methods used for grading severity of native aortic valve regurgitation can be used for prosthetic aortic regurgitation.[6,25] However, there are limited data on the application and validation of semiquantitative and quantitative parameters such as the width of the regurgitant jet or of the vena contracta, the effective regurgitant orifice area, and the regurgitant volume and fraction in the context of prosthetic valves. Given that all parameters of aortic regurgitation have important limitations and may be subject to measurement errors, a comprehensive, multiparametric integrative approach is highly

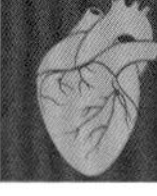

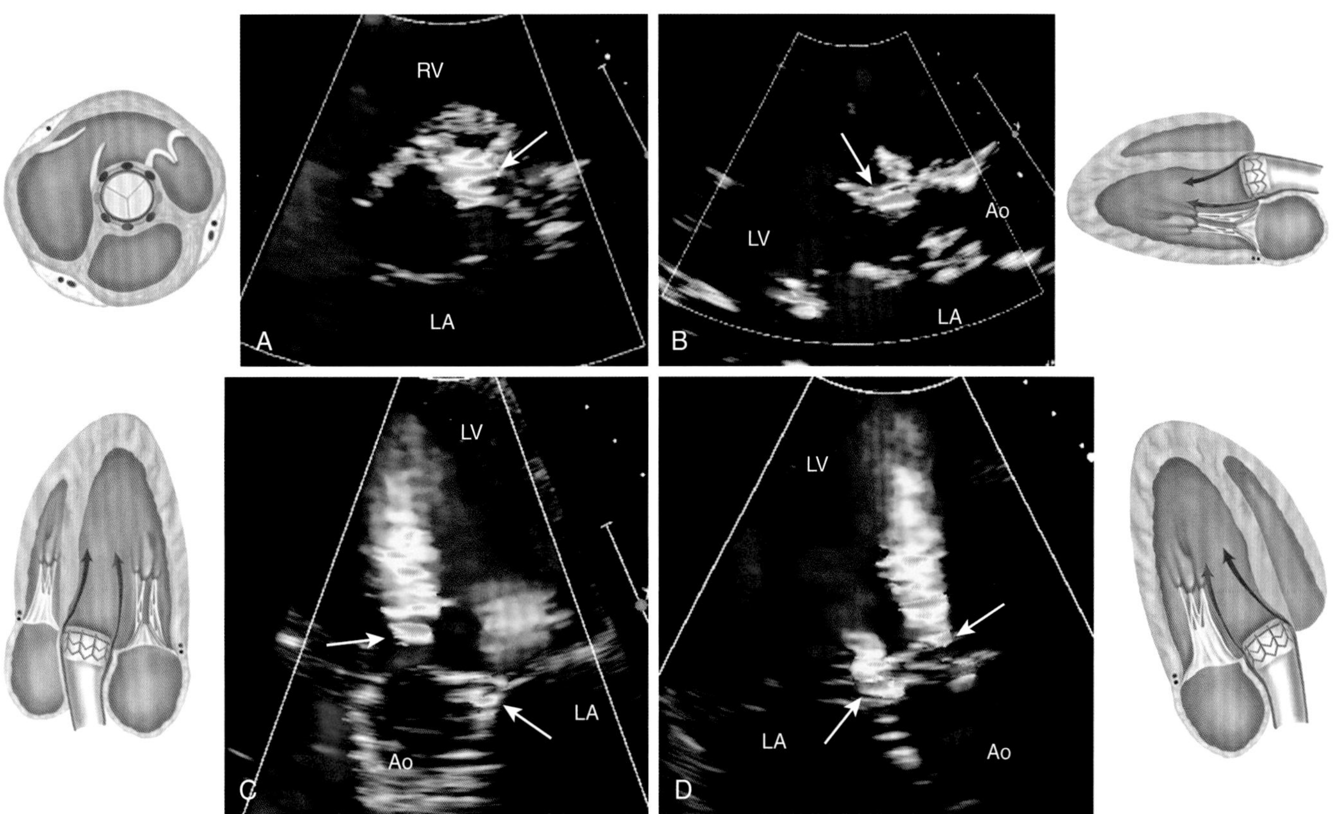

Fig. 31.8 Paravalvular regurgitation after transcatheter aortic valve replacement. (A–D) TTE parasternal short- and long-axis views and apical 5-chamber and 3-chamber views of a moderate paravalvular regurgitation in a transcatheter aortic valve (see Videos 31.8A, 31.8B, 31.8C, and 31.8D). There is a large anterior jet and a smaller posterior jet *(arrows)*. The posterior jet is not visible in the parasternal views (see Videos 31.8A and 31.8B). The circumferential extent of the anterior jet on the short-axis view (see Video 31.8A) is 15% to 20%, but the jet is wide.

recommended (Table 31.6). The guidelines suggest grading prosthetic valve regurgitation according to a three-class scheme: mild, moderate, and severe.[6,25] However, some investigators have suggested the use of a more granular grading scheme (i.e., five classes instead of three), in which the mild class is subdivided into two subclasses (i.e., mild and mild to moderate) and the moderate class is subdivided into two subclasses (i.e., moderate and moderate to severe).[26,59]

Color Doppler Parameters

The color Doppler Nyquist limit should be set between 40 and 70 cm/s. The width of the vena contracta of the regurgitant jet (if visualized) and/or the width of the regurgitant jet at its origin can be measured directly with a caliper from the parasternal and apical views. In contrast to native valves, the width of the vena contracta may be difficult to accurately measure in the parasternal long-axis view due to the shadowing caused by the prosthesis ring or stent (see Fig. 31.9). The ratios of the regurgitant jet diameter to the LVOT diameter from the parasternal long-axis view and of the jet area to the LVOT area from the parasternal short-axis view just below the prosthesis can be calculated or estimate visually to assess the severity of transvalvular regurgitation (see Table 31.6 and Figs. 31.8 and 31.9).

Unlike native aortic regurgitation or transvalvular prosthetic regurgitation, the vena contracta of paravalvular regurgitation is not circular and is often irregular (see Figs. 31.8–31.10). 3D echocardiography may eventually overcome the limitations of 2D and standard Doppler measurements for quantifying paravalvular regurgitation. Studies using 3D TTE have shown the feasibility of measuring the 3D vena contracta of paravalvular regurgitation (see Table 31.6).[60,61]

Circumferential extent of paravalvular regurgitation should be assessed. For semiquantitative evaluation of the severity of paravalvular regurgitation, careful imaging of the neck of the jet in a short-axis view, at the level of the prosthesis sewing ring (i.e., surgical prostheses), or the lower portion of stent (i.e., transcatheter bioprostheses) allows determination of the circumferential extent of paravalvular regurgitant jets. This parameter is assessed by estimating visually the approximate number of minutes occupied by the paravalvular regurgitant jets according to the face of a clock (with 9-o'clock set at the insertion of the tricuspid valve leaflet) and by dividing this number by 60 minutes (see Table 31.6 and Fig. 31.10).

The circumferential extent is expressed as a percentage. A value between 10% and 30% corresponds to moderate paravalvular regurgitation, and a value greater than 30% corresponds to severe paravalvular regurgitation.[6,25,26] However, the circumferential extent of paravalvular regurgitation can vary substantially depending on the plane of interrogation. It is important to scan the entire height of the prosthesis stent and use the short-axis plane where the vena contracta of the jet is the smallest. An image plane that is too high (above the stent or upper portion of the stent) may underestimate the regurgitation, whereas a plane that is too low in the LVOT may overestimate the regurgitation severity due to rapid broadening of the jet downstream of the vena contracta.

The circumferential extent of the jet becomes even more complex and less reliable when assessing multiple or eccentric jets.

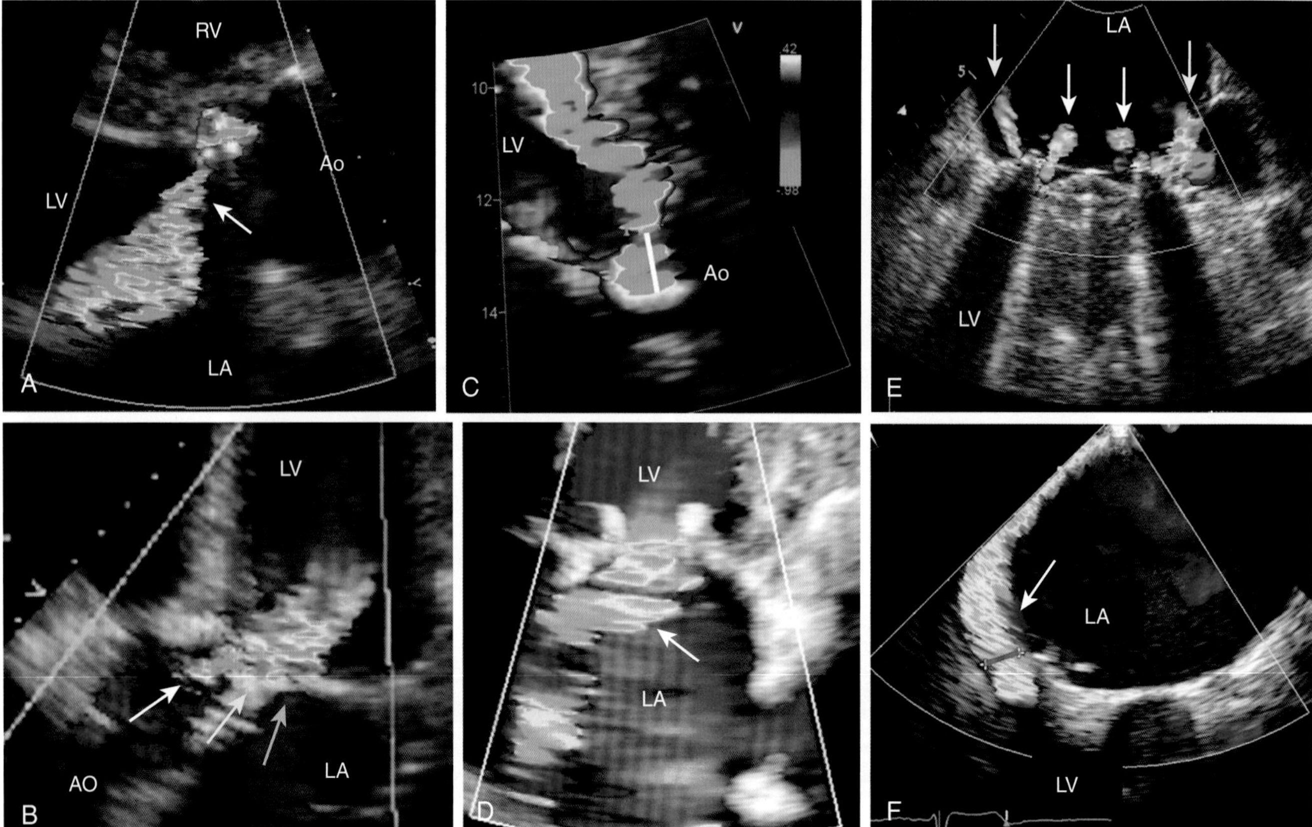

Fig. 31.9 Color Doppler images of prosthetic valve regurgitation. (A) Moderate paravalvular eccentric regurgitant jet in a surgical bioprosthetic aortic valve. (B) Color Doppler TTE image of a central regurgitation *(thin white arrow)* and a posterior paravalvular regurgitation *(thin yellow arrow)* in a transcatheter aortic valve. The posterior jet merges with the systolic mitral flow *(blue arrow)* make difficult visualization of the origin of this jet and grading of paravalvular regurgitation severity (see Video 31.9B). (C) Severe central regurgitation in a surgical bioprosthetic aortic valve (see Video 31.9C). The Nyquist limit has been decreased (42 cm/s) to allow optimal visualization of the proximal isovelocity area (PISA); the *white line* represents the radius of the PISA (7.7 mm). The effective regurgitant orifice area is 38 mm^2, and the regurgitant volume is 68 mL. (D) Severe transvalvular regurgitation with eccentric jet *(arrow)* in a bioprosthetic mitral valve (see Video 31.9D). (E) Mild paravalvular regurgitant jets *(yellow arrows)* and normal physiologic regurgitant jets *(thin arrows)* in a mitral bileaflet mechanical valve. (F) Severe posterolateral paravalvular regurgitation in a mitral bioprosthetic valve (see Video 31.9F); diastolic flow through the paravalvular leak from the LA to LV is visible. (Courtesy Dr. Arsène Basmadjan, Montreal Heart Institute, Montreal, Canada.)

In the case of multiple-jet paravalvular regurgitation, the vena contracta may be at different levels depending on the jets, and this may require several image planes to assess the overall circumferential extent of paravalvular regurgitation. The regurgitant jets, particularly the anterior jets, may be very eccentric (see Fig. 31.9A), in which case the jet may be directed across the short-axis plane, and this can lead to an overestimation of the circumferential extent and severity of paravalvular regurgitation. The severity of paravalvular regurgitation may be underestimated when a jet does not occupy a large circumferential extent but has a greater radial width (see Fig. 31.10). Some studies revealed that this parameter correlates poorly with the severity of paravalvular regurgitation measured by cardiac magnetic resonance.[62,63]

Grading of paravalvular regurgitation should not rely solely on examination of the short-axis view and estimation of circumferential extent. This measure should be integrated with other views and parameters.

Spectral Doppler Parameters

Doppler parameters, including the signal intensity and PHT of the CW envelope of the regurgitant jets and the timing and velocity of the diastolic flow reversal in the descending aorta, can be determined to corroborate prosthetic valve regurgitation severity (Fig. 31.11; see Table 31.6).[64] However, the accuracy of these parameters is limited in the early postprocedural period due to the acute nature of regurgitation and the frequent coexistence of moderate to severe diastolic dysfunction. The PHT strongly depends on heart rate.

Flow reversal in the descending aorta and the end-diastolic velocity measured by PW Doppler may be used to corroborate prosthetic valve regurgitation severity. Holodiastolic flow reversal in the descending thoracic aorta suggests at least moderate aortic regurgitation; severe regurgitation is suspected when the VTI of the reverse flow approximates that of the forward flow and when the end-diastolic velocity is greater than 20 cm/s (see Fig. 31.11 and Table 31.6).[65] Flow reversal in the descending aorta is strongly influenced by aortic compliance, and increased arterial stiffness may result in false-positive results. Several studies reported that holodiastolic and rapid flow reversal can occur in elderly patients with a stiff aorta, even in the absence of significant aortic regurgitation.[66] This considerably limits the usefulness of aortic flow reversal in the population undergoing AVR, particularly TAVR, because these patients typically are old and most have markedly reduced arterial compliance.

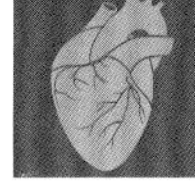

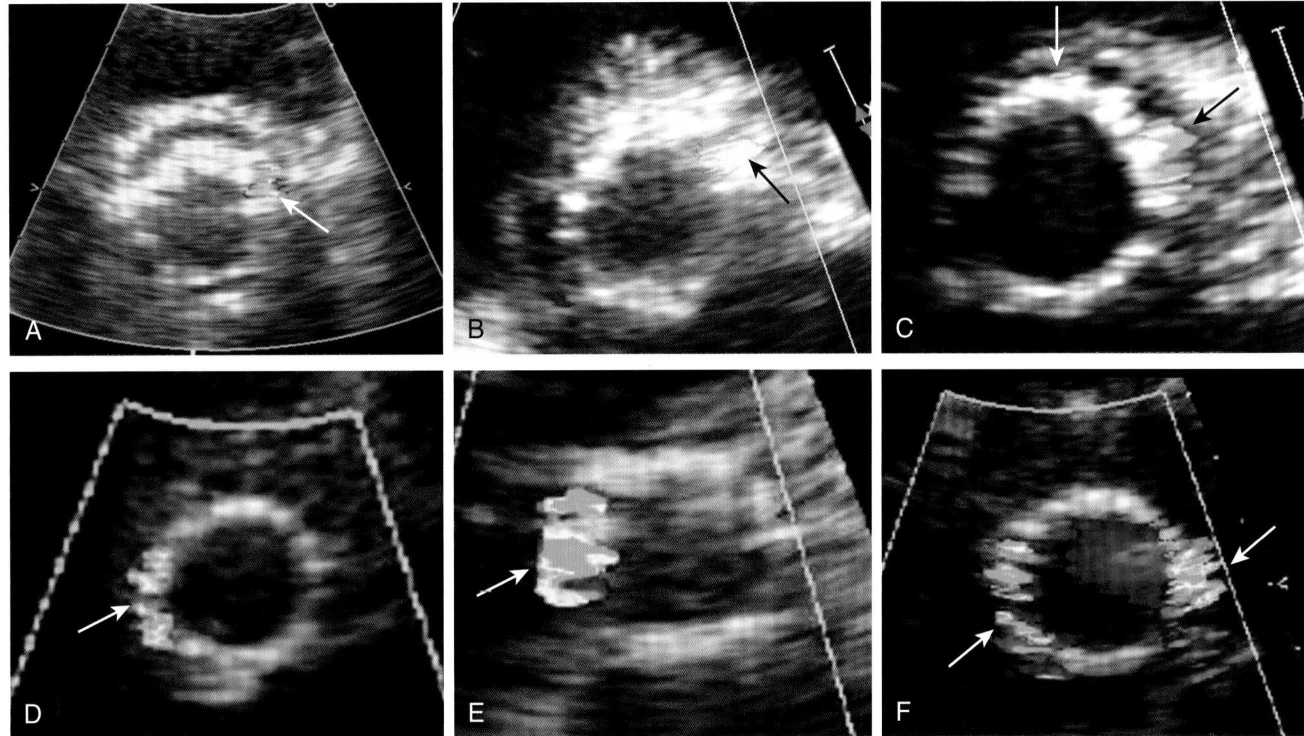

Fig. 31.10 Circumferential extent of paravalvular regurgitant jets for assessment of paravalvular regurgitation severity. TTE short-axis images show the circumferential extent of regurgitant jets *(white or black arrows)* and paravalvular regurgitation severity. (A) Less than 5%: trace paravalvular regurgitation. (B) Between 5% and 15%: mild regurgitation. (C and D) Between 15% and 25%: mild to moderate regurgitation. (E) Between 15% and 25% but with a larger jet width: moderate regurgitation. (F) More than 30%: moderate to severe regurgitation. (Adapted from Salaun E, Zenses AS, Clavel MA, et al. Valve-in-valve procedure in failed transcatheter aortic valves. *JACC Cardiovasc Imaging*. 2019;12:198–202.)

TABLE 31.6 Doppler Echocardiographic Criteria for Severity of Prosthetic Aortic Valve Central and Paravalvular Regurgitation.

Parameters	*Mild Regurgitation*	*Moderate Regurgitation*	*Severe Regurgitation*
Qualitative Parameters			
Valve structure and motion[a]	Usually normal	Usually abnormal	Usually abnormal
Jet features			
Extensive/wide jet origin	Absent	Often present	Present
Multiple jets	Possible	Possible	Often present
Jet path visible along the stent[b]	Usually absent	Usually present	Usually present
Proximal flow convergence visible	Absent	Possible	Often present
Semiquantitative Parameters			
Jet width at its origin (% LVOT diameter): color Doppler	Narrow (≤30)	Intermediate (31–60)	Large (>60)
Vena contracta width (mm): color Doppler	<4	4–6	>6
Vena contracta area (mm^2): 3D color Doppler	<20	20–40	>40
Jet density: CW Doppler	Incomplete or faint	Dense	Dense
Jet deceleration rate (PHT [ms]): CW Doppler[c]	Slow (>400)	Varies (200–400)	Steep (<200)
LV outflow vs. RV outflow ratio: PW Doppler (ratio of stroke volumes or velocity–time integrals)	Slightly increased (>1.2)	Intermediate (>1.5)	Greatly increased (>1.8)
Diastolic flow reversal in the descending aorta: PW Doppler[d]	Absent or brief early diastolic	Intermediate	Prominent holodiastolic (end-diastolic velocity > 20 cm/s)
Circumferential extent of paravalvular regurgitation (%)[b]	<10	10–30	>30
Quantitative Parameters			
Regurgitant fraction (%)	<30	30–50	>50
Indirect Signs			
LV size[e]	Normal	Normal/mildly dilated	Dilated

[a]Abnormal mechanical valves: immobile occlude (transvalvular regurgitation), dehiscence, or rocking (paravalvular regurgitation); abnormal bioprosthetic valves: leaflet thickening/calcification or prolapse (transvalvular regurgitation), dehiscence, or rocking (paravalvular regurgitation); abnormal transcatheter valves: abnormalities of stent position, deployment, and/or circularity (paravalvular or transvalvular regurgitation).
[b]Applies only to paravalvular regurgitation.
[c]Parameters are influenced by LV compliance. The low transvalvular end-diastolic aorta to LV pressure gradient due to concomitant moderate/severe LV diastolic dysfunction may lead to false-positive results.
[d]This parameter is influenced by aortic compliance and may yield to false-positive results in the elderly population with noncompliant aortas.
[e]Applies to chronic, late postoperative prosthetic aortic valve regurgitation in the absence of other causes.
LVOT, LV Outflow tract; *PHT*, pressure half-time; *PW*, pulsed wave.
Adapted from Lancellotti P, Pibarot P, Chambers J, et al. Recommendations for the imaging assessment of prosthetic heart valves: a report from the European Association of Cardiovascular Imaging endorsed by the Chinese Society of Echocardiography, the Inter-American Society of Echocardiography, and the Brazilian Department of Cardiovascular Imaging. *Eur Heart J Cardiovasc Imaging*. 2016;17:589–590.

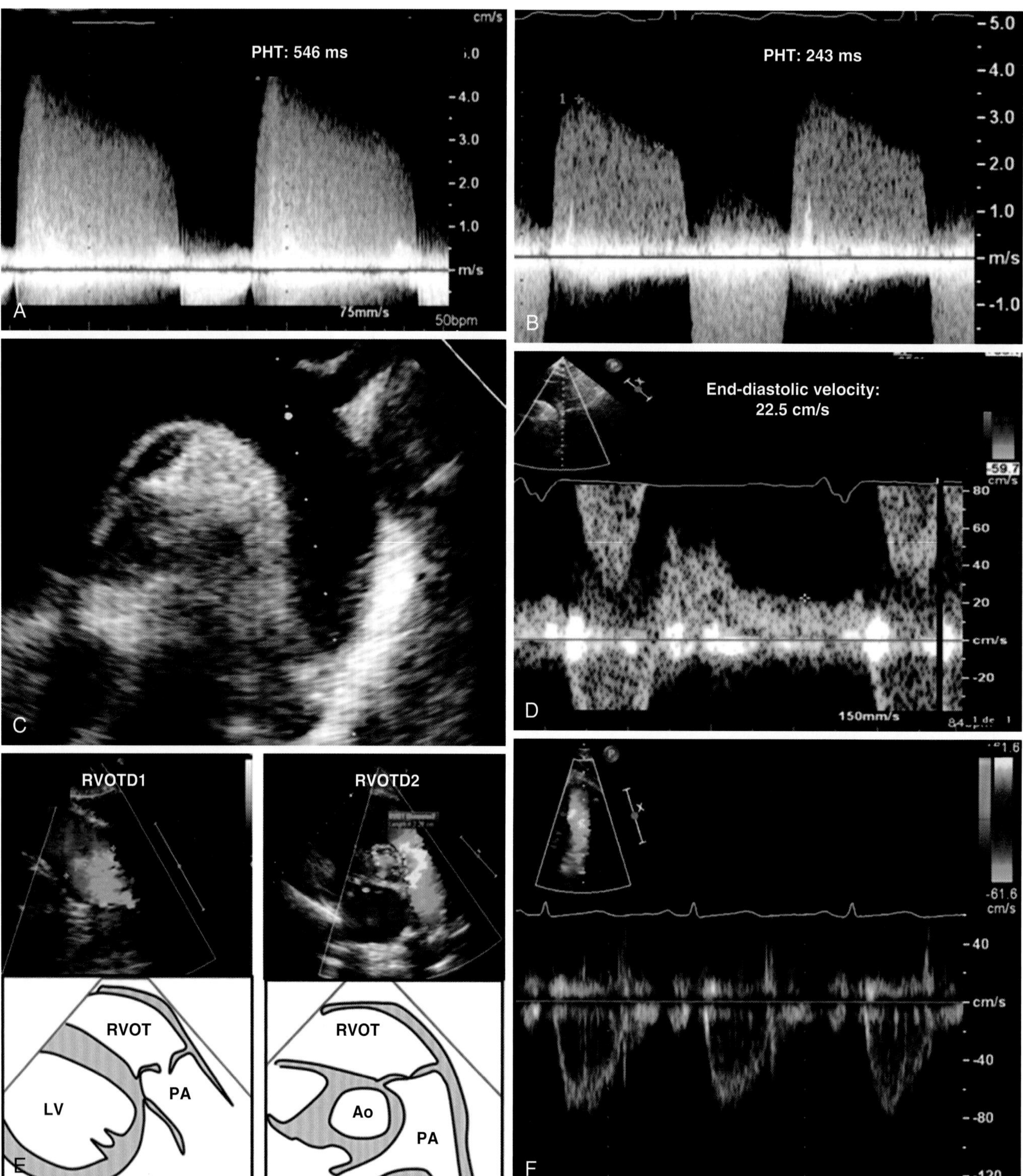

Fig. 31.11 Doppler parameters for the assessment of paravalvular regurgitation. (A and B) The pressure-half time *(PHT)* measured on the CW Doppler aortic regurgitant signal can be used to corroborate the prosthetic valve regurgitation severity. In the example shown in A, the PHT is long (546 ms), suggesting nonsignificant regurgitation, whereas in B, the PHT is short (243 ms), which is consistent with severe regurgitation. (C) Pulsed-wave Doppler sample in the descending aorta. (D) The flow reversal and end-diastolic velocity obtained by pulsed-wave Doppler in the descending aorta can be used to differentiate moderate from severe aortic regurgitation. In the example shown, there is holodiastolic flow reversal with a high end-diastolic velocity (22.5 cm/s), consistent with severe regurgitation. (E and F) A quantitative assessment of the aortic regurgitant volume can be obtained by calculating the difference of the stroke volume measured in the LV outflow tract (see Figs. 31.10 and 31.11) minus the stroke volume measured in the RV outflow tract *(RVOT)*. To measure the RVOT diameter, the RVOT view and the short-axis views are recommended (E). Color Doppler may be used to better delineate the borders of the RVOT. (Adapted from Pibarot P, Hahn RT, Weissman NJ, Monaghan MJ. Assessment of paravalvular regurgitation following TAVR: a proposal of unifying grading scheme. *JACC Cardiovasc Imaging*. 2015;8:340–360.)

Quantitative Parameters

Quantitative methods such as the proximal isovelocity surface area (PISA) method are rarely applicable to prosthetic aortic valve regurgitation (see Fig. 31.9).[6,25,26] However, the regurgitant volume may be estimated by calculating the difference between the LV and right ventricular (RV) stroke volumes, providing there is no significant pulmonary regurgitation (see Fig. 31.11 and Table 31.6). This parameter is subject to significant interobserver and intraobserver measurement variability, which is largely related to the difficulty of measuring the RVOT diameter by TTE.

Integrative, Multiparametric Approach to the Evaluation of Prosthetic Aortic Valve Regurgitation

Assessment of severity of prosthetic aortic valve regurgitation is usually much more complex than in native valves because of the high prevalence of paravalvular regurgitation and eccentric jets (see Figs. 31.8–31.10). The process of grading regurgitation severity should be comprehensive, integrative, and based on a multiparametric approach that includes the qualitative and semiquantitative parameters shown in Table 31.6.[6,24–26] If the regurgitation is classified as mild or less using these parameters, no further measurement is needed. If parameters suggest more than mild regurgitation and the quality of the data enables quantitation, quantitative parameters of regurgitation should be measured, including the vena contracta width and the regurgitant volume and fraction.

When the different parameters are concordant, it is easy to confirm the severity of the regurgitation. When there are discordances among the different parameters, the echocardiographer must look carefully for physiologic or technical reasons to explain the discrepancies and rely on the parameters that have the best quality in terms of image or signal and that are the more accurate and reliable in the context of prosthetic valves. The indirect signs of prosthetic valve dysfunction also should be examined. In the setting of severe chronic prosthetic valve regurgitation, a dilated LV is likely.

Cardiac magnetic resonance may be considered to corroborate severity of prosthetic valve regurgitation when TTE grading is uncertain or there is discordance between TTE grading of regurgitation and a patient's symptomatic status.[6,25,63] Same cut-point values of regurgitation fraction should be used for cardiac magnetic resonance imaging compared with TTE to grade prosthetic regurgitation (i.e., ≥30% is moderate, and ≥50% is severe).[6,26,63]

Prosthetic Mitral Valve Regurgitation

Imaging Considerations

Assessment of prosthetic mitral regurgitation by TTE is problematic because the LV is largely occulted by the acoustic shadowing due to the metallic components of the prosthesis.[24] This problem is more common in mechanical valves than in bioprosthetic valves. In contrast, TEE provides excellent visualization of the LV and mitral regurgitant jet, but acoustic shadowing limits visualization of the LV (see Fig. 31.9E and F). A comprehensive assessment of prosthetic mitral valve function often requires TTE and TEE when valve dysfunction is suspected.

At TTE examination, occult mitral prosthesis regurgitation should be suspected when the following signs are found: flow convergence on the LV side of the prosthesis during systole; increased mitral peak E-wave velocity (>2 m/s) and mean gradient (>6 mmHg); Doppler velocity index greater than 2.2; unexplained or new and worsening pulmonary arterial hypertension; and a dilated and hyperkinetic LV (Table 31.7).[6,25,67] TEE should be systematically performed when there is clinical or TTE suspicion of pathologic mitral regurgitation.[6,24] TEE is superior to TTE for detecting prosthetic mitral regurgitation and determining its localization and mechanism.[6]

On color Doppler, paravalvular leaks have a typical appearance of a jet that passes from the LV into the LA outside the prosthesis ring and often projects into the atrium in an eccentric direction (see Fig. 31.9E and F). Multiple-plane examination is essential to determine the origin and extent of the regurgitant jets. A 3D en face TEE view from the LA may be useful to assess the localization and cause of prosthetic mitral regurgitation (see Fig. 31.3).[58]

Parameters of the Severity of Prosthetic Mitral Valve Regurgitation

Assessment of the severity of prosthetic mitral regurgitation is complex because all quantitative parameters have important limitations and cannot be applied consistently in all patients. A comprehensive approach that integrates the different findings and parameters obtained by TTE and TEE is recommended (see Table 31.7).[6,25]

Estimation of regurgitant jet area in the LA is often difficult due to the shadowing and artifacts created by the prosthesis. A small, thin jet (jet area <4 cm^2, <20% of the LA) usually reflects mild mitral regurgitation but can be grossly underestimated and should not be used to exclude severe regurgitation, whereas a large, wide jet (≥8 cm^2, >40% of the LA) is most often consistent with moderate or severe regurgitation.[6,25] A width of the vena contracta of less than 3, 3 to 6, and more than 6 mm denotes mild, moderate, and severe regurgitation, respectively (see Table 31.7).[6,25,68]

Significant swirling of the jet within the atrium and retrograde systolic flow in one or more of the pulmonary veins are specific for significant mitral regurgitation. The density and contour of the regurgitant jet CW Doppler signal also may be helpful to corroborate regurgitation severity (see Table 31.7).

The radius of the proximal flow convergence (with the PISA method) can be used in combination with recordings of mitral regurgitation velocity by CW Doppler to estimate effective regurgitant orifice area.[6,25] However, because mitral prosthetic regurgitation is often characterized by eccentric or multiple jets, the PISA method is difficult to achieve and may grossly underestimate or overestimate regurgitation severity. Given these important limitations, the volumetric method is often preferred to the PISA method for quantitation of mitral prosthesis regurgitation.[6,25] In light of the important challenges and limitations posed by quantitation of prosthetic mitral regurgitation, a comprehensive, multiparametric, and integrative approach should always be used (see Table 31.7).

Indirect Signs and Consequences of Prosthetic Valve Regurgitation

The size and function of the LV and LA chambers and the level of systolic pulmonary arterial pressure can be used to corroborate the severity of prosthesis dysfunction, especially that of prosthetic valve regurgitation (see Tables 31.6 and 31.7). These measurements can be compared with previous measurements and are often the first alert when the regurgitation is difficult to visualize.

LV dilation is expected in the setting of hemodynamically significant prosthetic aortic or mitral valve regurgitation. If LV volumes fail to decrease after valve replacement for aortic or mitral regurgitation or tend to increase after valve replacement for aortic or mitral stenosis and particularly if the LV is hyperdynamic, a hemodynamically significant leak should be suspected

TABLE 31.7 Doppler Echocardiographic Criteria for Severity of Prosthetic Mitral Valve Central and Paravalvular Regurgitation.

Parameters	*Mild Regurgitation*	*Moderate Regurgitation*	*Severe Regurgitation*
Valve Structure and Motion			
Mechanical or bioprosthesis[a]	Usually normal	Usually abnormal	Usually abnormal
Doppler Qualitative or Semiquantitative Parameters			
Vena contracta width (mm)	<3	3–5.9	≥6
Color flow jet area[b]	Small, central jet (usually < 4 cm² or < 20% of LA area)	Varies	Large central jet (usually > 8 cm² or > 40% of LA area) or various sizes of wall-impinging jet swirling in LA
Flow convergence	None or minimal	Intermediate	Large
MR jet density: CW Doppler	Incomplete or faint	Dense	Dense
MR jet contour: CW Doppler[c]	Parabolic	Usually parabolic	Early peaking, triangular
Pulmonary venous flow: PW Doppler	Systolic dominance	Systolic blunting	Systolic flow reversal
Doppler velocity index: PW Doppler	<2.2	2.2–2.5	>2.5
Doppler Quantitative Parameters			
Regurgitant volume (mL/beat)	<30	30–59	>60
Regurgitant fraction (%)	<30	30–50	>50
Effective regurgitant orifice area (mm²)	<20	20–39	≥40
Indirect Signs			
LV size[d]	Normal	Normal or mildly dilated	Dilated
LA size	Normal	Normal or mildly dilated	Dilated
Pulmonary hypertension (SPAP ≥ 50 mmHg at rest and ≥ 60 mmHg at exercise)	Usually absent	Varies	Usually present

[a]Abnormal mechanical valves: immobile occluder, dehiscence, or rocking (paravalvular regurgitation); abnormal biologic valves: leaflet thickening/calcification or prolapse, dehiscence, or rocking (paravalvular regurgitation).
[b]Parameter applicable to central jets and is less accurate in eccentric jets.
[c]This parameter is influenced by LV compliance.
[d]Applies to chronic, late postoperative prosthetic aortic valve regurgitation in the absence of other causes.
Adapted from Lancellotti P, Pibarot P, Chambers J, et al. Recommendations for the imaging assessment of prosthetic heart valves: a report from the European Association of Cardiovascular Imaging endorsed by the Chinese Society of Echocardiography, the Inter-American Society of Echocardiography, and the Brazilian Department of Cardiovascular Imaging. *Eur Heart J Cardiovasc Imaging.* 2016;17:589–590.

among other factors. In the context of chronic aortic or mitral prosthesis regurgitation, the absence of dilation of LV and LA chambers during follow-up suggests a nonsignificant leak.

PROSTHETIC PULMONARY AND TRICUSPID VALVES

Prosthetic Tricuspid Valves

Prosthetic tricuspid valve stenosis should be assessed. The tricuspid prosthesis flow velocities vary with the duration of the cycle and with respiration. A minimum of 5 cardiac cycles should be averaged for estimation of the Doppler echocardiographic indices, whether the patient is in sinus rhythm or atrial fibrillation. Prosthetic tricuspid valve stenosis should be suspected when prosthetic valve leaflet morphology and mobility are abnormal, peak velocity is greater than 1.9 m/s, mean gradient is 6 mmHg or greater, and/or PHT time is 130 ms or longer (Table 31.8).[6,24,25]

The criteria for assessing severity of prosthetic tricuspid regurgitation are similar to those for native tricuspid valves (see Table 31.9).[6,24,25] TEE should be considered for all patients with clinical or TTE evidence of tricuspid prosthesis obstruction or regurgitation.

Color Doppler imaging is useful for screening prosthetic tricuspid valve regurgitation. The assumption is that larger color jets that extend deep into the right atrium represent more tricuspid regurgitation than smaller thin jets that are seen just beyond the tricuspid valve. The vena contracta width of the tricuspid regurgitation is typically imaged in the apical 4-chamber view using the same settings as for mitral regurgitation. A vena contracta of 7 mm or greater favors severe regurgitation, and a diameter of less than 6 mm indicates mild or moderate tricuspid regurgitation. Due to the shadowing caused by the prosthetic material, the vena contracta width may be difficult to assess. It is inaccurate in cases of multiple jets or an irregular orifice shape.

TABLE 31.8 Doppler Echocardiographic Criteria for Severity of Prosthetic Tricuspid Valve Stenosis.

Parameters	*Normal*	*Possible Stenosis[a]*
Qualitative Parameters		
Valve structure and motion	Normal	Often abnormal[b]
Semiquantitative Parameters		
Pressure half-time (ms)	<130	≥130
Doppler velocity index	<2	≥2
Doppler Quantitative Parameters		
Peak velocity (m/s)[c]	<1.9	≥1.9
Mean gradient (mmHg)[c]	<6	≥6

[a]Because of respiratory variation, average of 3 to 5 cycles in sinus rhythm.
[b]Cusp thickening or immobility.
[c]May be increased also with valvular regurgitation.
Adapted with permission of European Association of Cardiovascular Imaging from Lancellotti P, Pibarot P, Chambers J, et al. Recommendations for the imaging assessment of prosthetic heart valves: a report from the European Association of Cardiovascular Imaging endorsed by the Chinese Society of Echocardiography, the Interamerican Society of Echocardiography, and the Brazilian Department of Cardiovascular Imaging. *Eur Heart J Cardiovasc Imaging.* 2016;17:589–590.

Prosthetic Pulmonary Valves

Findings suspicious for prosthetic pulmonary valve stenosis include leaflet thickening or immobility, narrowing of a

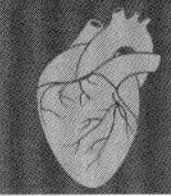

TABLE 31.9 Doppler-Echocardiographic Criteria for Severity of Prosthetic Tricuspid Valve Regurgitation.

	Mild	*Moderate*	*Severe*
Valve Structure and Motion			
Mechanical or bioprosthesis[a]	Usually normal	Usually abnormal	Usually abnormal
Doppler Parameters (Qualitative or Semi-Quantitative)			
Vena contracta width (mm)	ND	<7	≥7
Color flow TR jet	Small	Variable	Large central or eccentric wall impinging jet
Flow convergence	None or minimal	Intermediate	Large
TR jet density: CW Doppler	Incomplete or faint	Dense	Dense
Hepatic venous flow: PW Doppler	Systolic dominance	Systolic blunting	Systolic flow reversal
Indirect Signs			
RV size[b]	Normal	Normal/mildly dilated	Dilated
RA size	Normal	Normal/mildly dilated	Dilated

[a]Abnormal mechanical valves: immobile occluder, dehiscence or rocking (paravalvular regurgitation); abnormal biologic valves: leaflet thickening/calcification or prolapse.
[b]Applies to chronic, late postoperative prosthetic tricuspid valve regurgitation in the absence of other etiologies.
TR, Tricuspid regurgitation.
Adapted with permission of European Association of Cardiovascular Imaging from Lancellotti P, Pibarot P, Chambers J. et al. Recommendations for the imaging assessment of prosthetic heart valves: a report from the European Association of Cardiovascular Imaging endorsed by the Chinese Society of Echocardiography, the Interamerican Society of Echocardiography, and the Brazilian Department of Cardiovascular Imaging. *Eur Heart J Cardiovasc Imaging.* 2016;17:589–590.

forward color-flow map, transvalvular peak velocity greater than 3.2 m/s for a bioprosthesis or more than 2.5 m/s for a homograft, increase in peak velocity on serial studies, impaired RV function, or elevated RV systolic pressure (Table 31.10).[6,24,25] The severity of pulmonary prosthetic valve regurgitation is usually subjectively graded using an integrative approach similar to that for native pulmonary regurgitation (Table 31.11).[6,24,25]

INTERPRETATION OF DOPPLER ECHOCARDIOGRAPHIC DATA

Interpretation of High Transprosthetic Gradients

It is relatively common to measure a high gradient across a prosthetic valve, and the differential diagnosis is much more complex than for native valves. An elevated transprosthetic gradient has several causes. PPM is a common cause of a high gradient after valve replacement. Other potential causes are intrinsic valve dysfunction (due to thrombosis, SVD, or endocarditis), a central jet artifact in bileaflet prostheses, high flow states, and technical errors.[5,6,24] Figs. 31.12 and 31.13 show algorithms that help to assess high gradients (see Fig. 31.6) or symptoms that suggest prosthetic valve stenosis after AVR and MVR.[6]

Prosthetic Aortic Valves

A crucial step in the algorithm for assessment of prosthetic aortic valves is thorough evaluation of leaflet morphology and mobility (see Fig. 31.12). In the case of mechanical valves,

TABLE 31.10 Doppler Echocardiographic Criteria for Severity of Prosthetic Pulmonary Valve Stenosis.

Parameters	*Normal*	*Possible Stenosis*
Qualitative Parameters		
Valve structure and motion	Normal	Often abnormal[a]
Color flow	Normal	Narrowing of forward color map
Doppler semiquantitative parameters		
Pressure-half time (ms)	<230	≥230
Doppler Quantitative Parameters		
Flow dependent		
Peak velocity (m/s)[b,c]	<3.2 bioprosthesis <2.5 homograft	≥3.2 bioprosthesis ≥2.5 homograft
Mean gradient (mmHg)	<20 bioprosthesis <15 homograft	≥20 bioprosthesis ≥15 homograft

[a]Cusp thickening or immobility.
[b]The criterion is valid for near-normal or normal stroke volume (50–90 mL) and flow rate (200–300 mL/s).
[c]Increase in peak velocity on serial studies is the more reliable parameter.
Adapted with permission of European Association of Cardiovascular Imaging from Lancellotti P, Pibarot P, Chambers J, et al. Recommendations for the imaging assessment of prosthetic heart valves: a report from the European Association of Cardiovascular Imaging endorsed by the Chinese Society of Echocardiography, the Interamerican Society of Echocardiography, and the Brazilian Department of Cardiovascular Imaging. *Eur Heart J Cardiovasc Imaging.* 2016;17:589–590.

TABLE 31.11 Doppler-Echocardiographic Criteria for Severity of Prosthetic Pulmonary Valve Regurgitation.

	Mild	*Moderate*	*Severe*
Valve Structure and Motion			
Mechanical or bioprosthesis[a]	Usually normal	Usually abnormal	Usually abnormal
Doppler Parameters (Qualitative or Semi-Quantitative)			
Color flow PR jet width (mm)	Small	Intermediate	Large (>50-65% RVOT diameter)
PR jet density: CW Doppler	Incomplete or faint	Dense	Dense
PR jet deceleration rate: CW Doppler	Slow	Variable	Steep
Diastolic flow reversal in the pulmonary artery	None	Present	Present
Pulmonary vs. systemic flow by PW Doppler	Slightly increased	Intermediate	Greatly increased
Indirect Signs			
RV size[b]	Normal	Normal/mildly dilated	Dilated

[a]Abnormal mechanical valves: immobile occluder, dehiscence or rocking (paravalvular regurgitation); abnormal biologic valves: leaflet thickening/calcification or prolapse.
[b]Applies to chronic, late postoperative prosthetic tricuspid valve regurgitation in the absence of other etiologies.
PR, Pulmonary regurgitation; *RVOT,* right ventricular outflow tract.
Adapted with permission of European Association of Cardiovascular Imaging from Lancellotti P, Pibarot P, Chambers J, et al. Recommendations for the imaging assessment of prosthetic heart valves: a report from the European Association of Cardiovascular Imaging endorsed by the Chinese Society of Echocardiography, the Interamerican Society of Echocardiography, and the Brazilian Department of Cardiovascular Imaging. *Eur Heart J Cardiovasc Imaging* 2016;17:589–90.

TTE and even TEE often do not allow adequate visualization of leaflet motion, and cinefluoroscopy should be performed in addition to echocardiography (see Fig. 31.4).[6,69] In the case of bioprosthetic or mechanical valves, MDCT may be useful to complement TTE or TEE and assess valve thrombosis, calcification, vegetation, or pannus (see Fig. 31.4).[6]

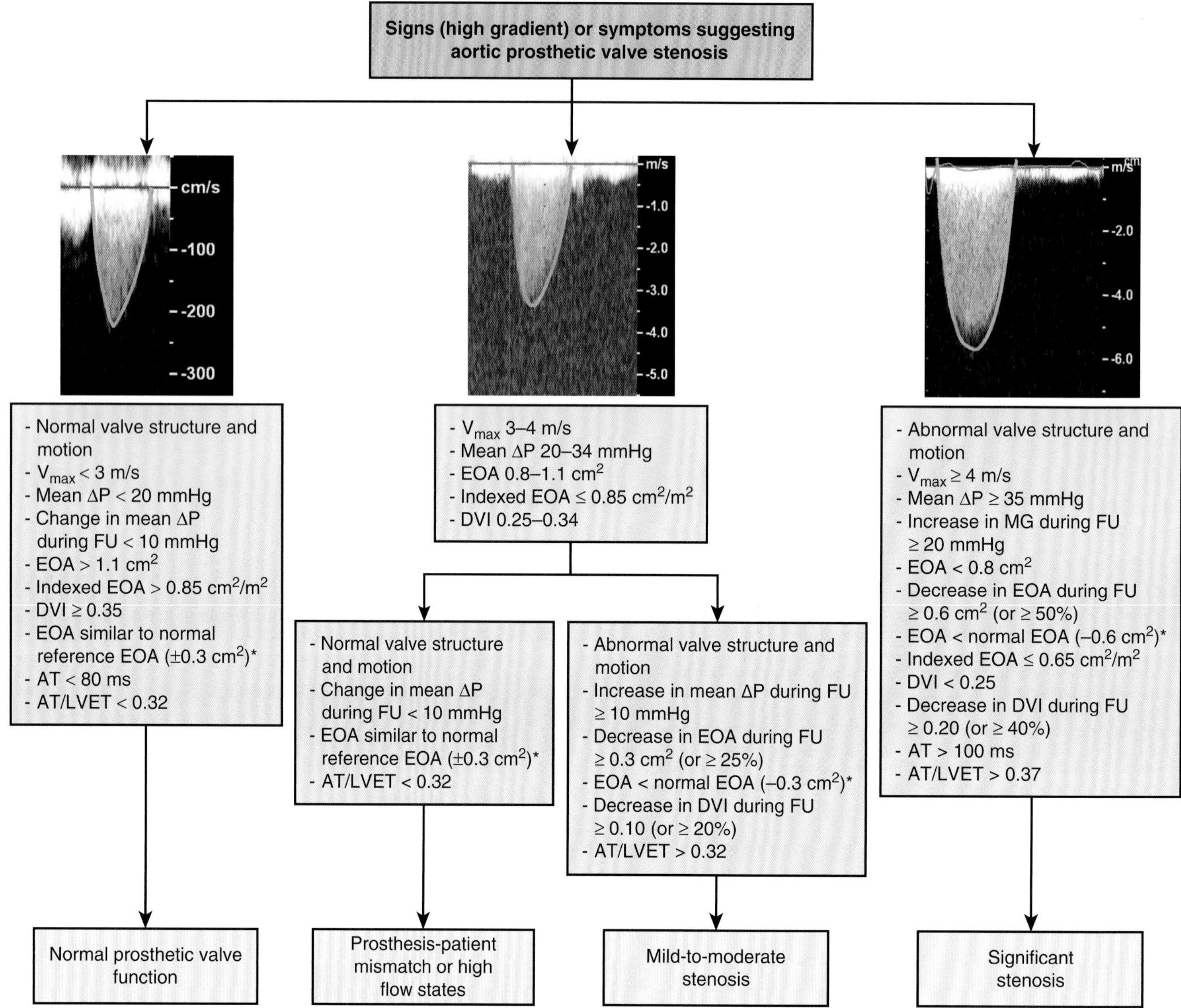

Fig. 31.12 High transprosthetic pressure gradients after aortic valve replacement. Algorithm for interpreting abnormally high transprosthetic pressure gradients after aortic valve replacement. Table 31.4 provides normal reference values *(asterisk)* for prosthetic aortic valves. *AT*, Acceleration time; *EOA*, effective orifice area; *DVI*, Doppler velocity index; *FU*, follow-up; *LVET*, left ventricular ejection time; *ΔP*, transprosthetic pressure gradient; *PPM*, patient-prosthesis mismatch; V_{max}, peak transprosthetic velocity.

If leaflet mobility is abnormal (Figs. 31.14 and 31.15; see Figs. 31.2–31.4), prosthetic valve stenosis should be suspected, and it can be corroborated by these findings: (1) the EOA measured by echocardiography is much lower than the normal reference value for the same type and size of prosthesis, and (2) the transprosthetic velocity and gradients have increased significantly during follow-up and the EOA and Doppler velocity index have decreased (see Table 31.2 and Figs. 31.12 and 31.15). If leaflet morphology and mobility are normal and the EOA and Doppler velocity index are within normal ranges (see Tables 31.2 and 31.4) but the indexed EOA is less than 0.85 cm^2/m^2 (see Table 31.1), the high transprosthetic gradient is most likely related to PPM (severe if <0.65 cm^2/m^2). If the indexed EOA is greater than 0.85 cm^2/m^2, the high gradient is probably related to high flow states, subvalvular obstruction, or technical errors (e.g., mistaking mitral regurgitation flow for prosthetic aortic valve flow).

Significant prosthetic aortic valve regurgitation may indirectly increase the flow across the prosthesis and lead to an increase in the gradient with a normal EOA and Doppler velocity index. If the prosthesis is a bileaflet valve, the high gradient may be caused by a central jet artifact, such as a localized high jet velocity through the central orifice (see Fig. 31.5B). The net gradient is less in patients with a small aortic diameter (<3.0 cm) due to pressure recovery, and it may be useful in these cases to calculate the energy loss index (see Fig. 31.5).[38,70]

Prosthetic Mitral Valves

A similar algorithm can be used when confronted with a high gradient (see Fig. 31.6) or symptoms suggesting mitral prosthetic valve stenosis (see Fig. 31.13).[6] However, the cutoff values of the indexed EOA and Doppler velocity index are different from those used for aortic prostheses (see Table 31.3). If the leaflet mobility is considered to be normal or is undetermined and the Doppler velocity index is less than 2.2, occult mitral transvalvular or paravalvular regurgitation should be suspected, and TEE should be performed (see Fig. 31.9). This situation

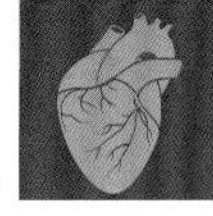

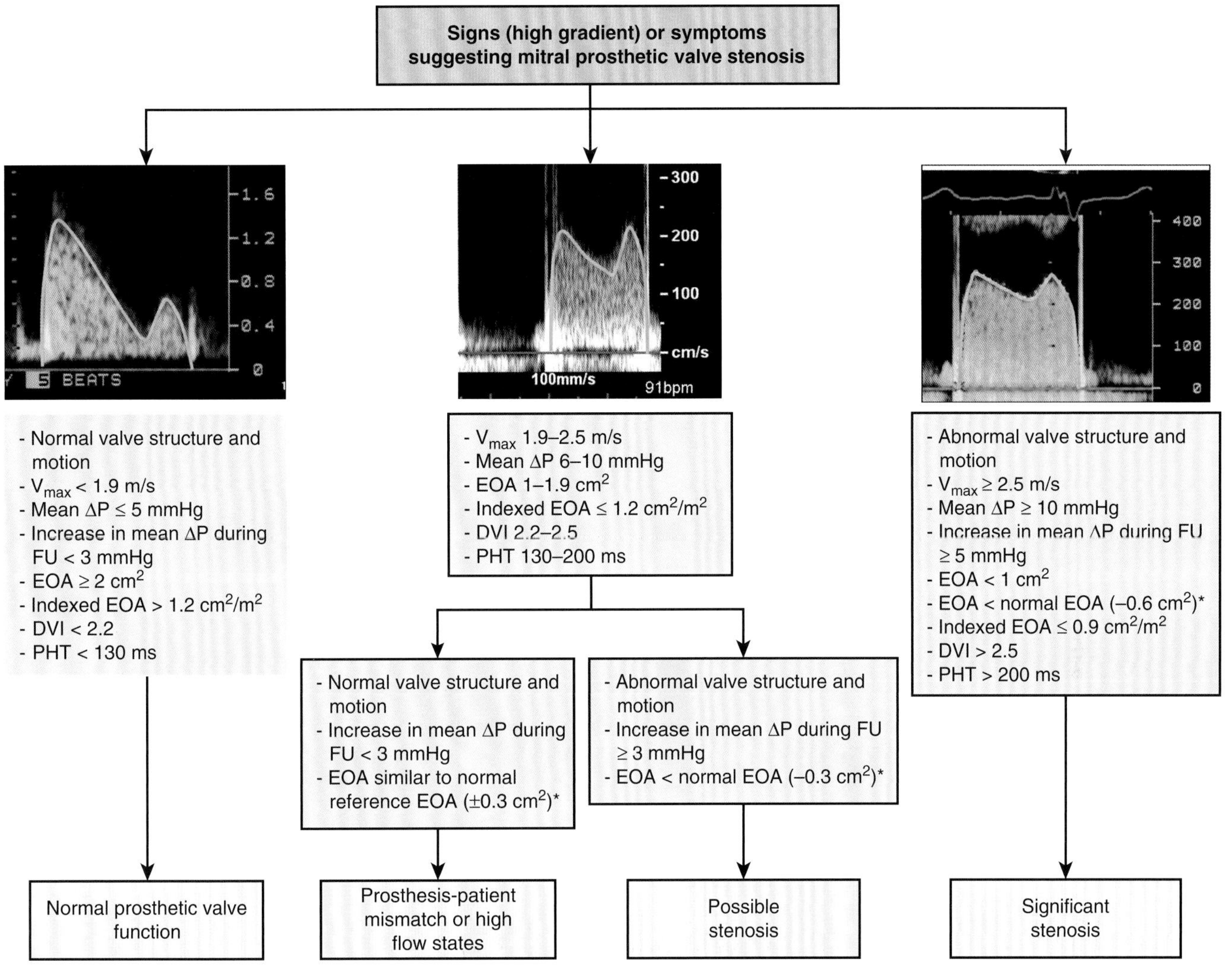

Signs (high gradient) or symptoms suggesting mitral prosthetic valve stenosis

- Normal valve structure and motion
- V_{max} < 1.9 m/s
- Mean ΔP ≤ 5 mmHg
- Increase in mean ΔP during FU < 3 mmHg
- EOA ≥ 2 cm^2
- Indexed EOA > 1.2 cm^2/m^2
- DVI < 2.2
- PHT < 130 ms

→ Normal prosthetic valve function

- V_{max} 1.9–2.5 m/s
- Mean ΔP 6–10 mmHg
- EOA 1–1.9 cm^2
- Indexed EOA ≤ 1.2 cm^2/m^2
- DVI 2.2–2.5
- PHT 130–200 ms

→

- Normal valve structure and motion
- Increase in mean ΔP during FU < 3 mmHg
- EOA similar to normal reference EOA (±0.3 cm^2)*

→ Prosthesis-patient mismatch or high flow states

- Abnormal valve structure and motion
- Increase in mean ΔP during FU ≥ 3 mmHg
- EOA < normal EOA (–0.3 cm^2)*

→ Possible stenosis

- Abnormal valve structure and motion
- V_{max} ≥ 2.5 m/s
- Mean ΔP ≥ 10 mmHg
- Increase in mean ΔP during FU ≥ 5 mmHg
- EOA < 1 cm^2
- EOA < normal EOA (–0.6 cm^2)*
- Indexed EOA ≤ 0.9 cm^2/m^2
- DVI > 2.5
- PHT > 200 ms

→ Significant stenosis

Fig. 31.13 High transprosthetic pressure gradients after mitral valve replacement. Algorithm for interpreting abnormally high transprosthetic pressure gradients after mitral valve replacement. Table 31.5 provides the normal reference values for prosthetic aortic valves *(asterisk). AT*, Acceleration time; *ET*, ejection time; *BSA*, body surface area; *EOA*, effective orifice area; *DVI*, Doppler velocity index; *FU*, follow-up; *ΔP*, trans prosthetic pressure gradient; *PHT*, pressure half-time; *PPM*, patient-prosthesis mismatch; V_{max}, peak transprosthetic velocity.

may also be related to the recording of a localized high gradient within the central orifice in the case of bileaflet mechanical valves (see Fig. 31.5).

Low-Flow States

In patients with LV dysfunction, transprosthetic gradients may be only slightly or moderately elevated despite the significant PPM or prosthesis dysfunction.[6] Gradients are highly flow dependent and may be pseudonormalized in the setting of low-flow states. Conversely, the valve EOA may be pseudosevere in the setting of a low-flow state. Measurement of a low gradient and a small EOA (see Tables 31.2 and 31.3) should prompt further evaluation.

For the management of low-flow, low-gradient native aortic or mitral stenosis, dobutamine stress echocardiography may be useful to differentiate true stenosis from pseudostenosis or mismatch in patients with prosthetic valves and low cardiac output.[6] In the case of pseudostenosis or pseudo-PPM, the resting transprosthetic flow rate and force applied on the leaflets is too low to completely open the valve. On dobutamine stress echocardiography, these patients nonetheless have a substantial increase in valve EOA and no or minimal elevation in gradients with increasing flow rate.

True stenosis or PPM is associated with no or minimal increase in EOA, a marked increase in gradient (absolute change > 20 mmHg in the aortic position), and most often the occurrence of indirect signs (e.g., LV dysfunction, marked elevation in pulmonary arterial pressure) and symptoms. However, dobutamine stress echocardiography cannot differentiate prosthesis stenosis from PPM. For this purpose, the algorithm presented in Figs. 31.12 and 31.13 should be applied to the EOA and Doppler velocity index values obtained after normalization of cardiac output on stress echocardiography.

DOPPLER ECHOCARDIOGRAPHY FOR MANAGING PROSTHETIC VALVE–RELATED COMPLICATIONS

PROSTHETIC VALVE THROMBOSIS

If prosthetic valve thrombosis is suspected, echocardiography should be performed promptly and should include TEE (Fig. 31.16; see Figs. 31.14 and 31.15).[7] A comprehensive TTE study is performed first, with particular attention directed at evaluation of leaflet mobility and valve hemodynamic function and

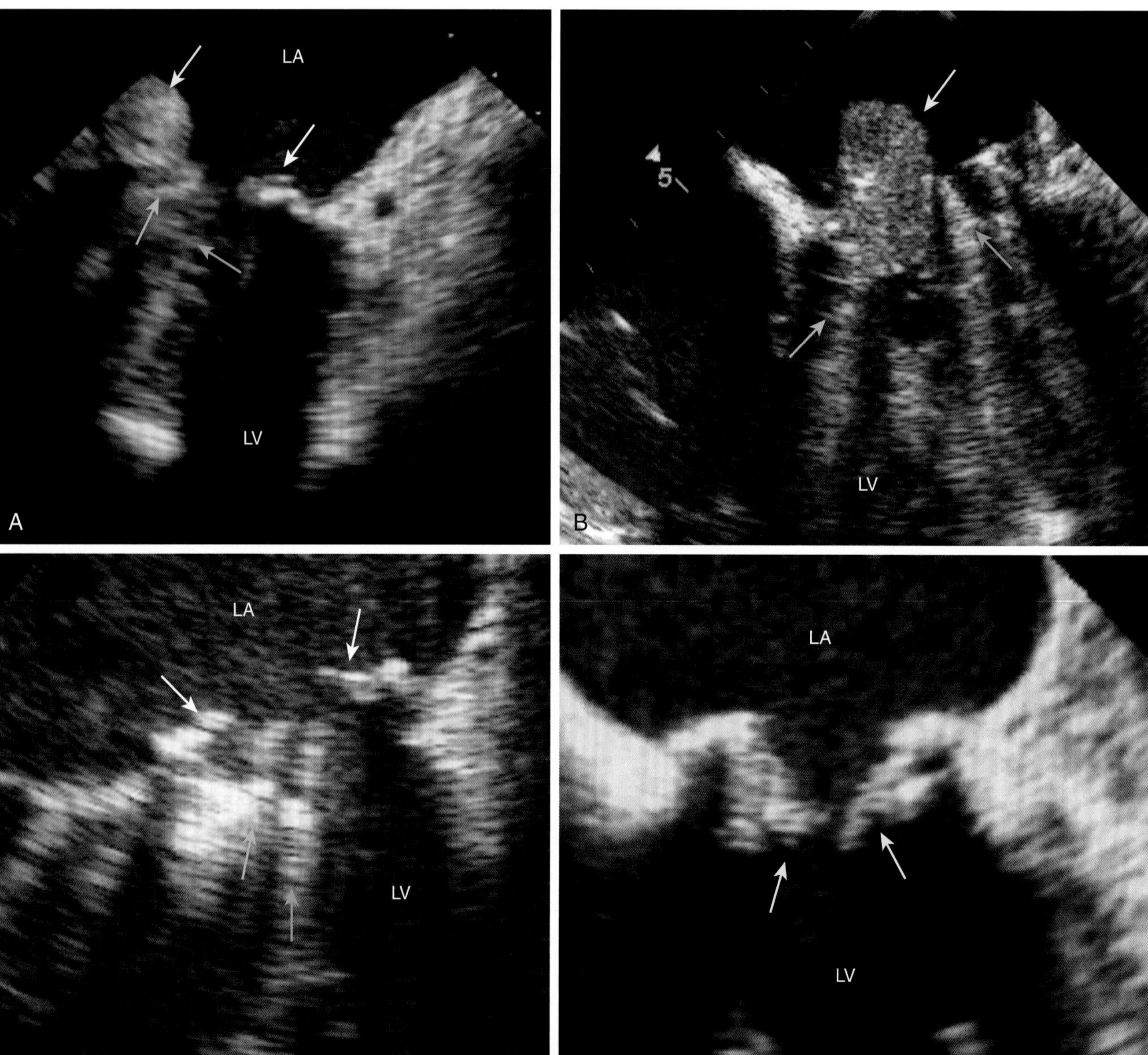

Fig. 31.14 Utility of TEE for diagnosis and treatment of prosthetic valve thrombosis. (A) Obstructed mitral bileaflet mechanical valve. TEE shows a large thrombus *(yellow arrow)*, pannus *(white arrow)*, mobile leaflet *(blue arrow)*, and immobile leaflet *(green arrow)*. (B) Mitral bileaflet mechanical valve obstructed by a very large thrombus *(yellow arrow)* (see Video 31.14B). TEE shows the reverberation of the immobile leaflet surrounded by the thrombus *(green arrow)* and the mobile leaflet with reverberation underneath *(blue arrow)*. (C) Pannus *(white arrows)* in a mitral bileaflet mechanical valve (see Video 31.14C). One leaflet *(green arrow)* has restricted motion. (D) Mitral bioprosthetic valve with severely thickened leaflets and very high peak and mean transprosthetic gradients (29/18 mmHg) due to thrombosis (see Video 31.14D). Valve obstruction resolved after aspirin therapy. (A, Courtesy Dr. Steven A Goldstein, Washington Hospital Center. B and C, Courtesy Dr. John Chambers, Guy's and St. Thomas Hospitals, London, UK. D, Courtesy Dr. Bibiana Cujec, Mazankowski Heart Institute, Edmonton, Canada.)

the identification of thrombus and pannus. In the rare case of massive prosthetic valve thrombosis with hemodynamic instability, TEE is not needed because this dramatic presentation constitutes a surgical emergency.[7] In most other cases, TEE can provide important incremental diagnostic information, which can guide therapeutic management (see Figs. 31.14, 31.15, and 31.16).

3D echocardiography can help to obtain more complete visualization of the different aspects of the prosthesis and therefore enhance the detection and description of pannus and thrombi (see Fig. 31.3D).[71] TEE has some limitations. Unlike TTE, aortic prostheses are more difficult to assess than mitral prostheses with TEE, and the ventricular side of a mitral prosthesis is more difficult to visualize than the atrial side.

Direct signs of prosthetic valve thrombosis include immobility or reduced leaflet mobility and thrombus on either side of the prosthesis, with or without obstruction (see Figs. 31.2A, 31.14, and 31.15). It is important to differentiate thrombi from a fibrous pannus, which is usually annular in location and typically appears as a very dense immobile echo (see Fig. 31.14). Pannus formation is more common on aortic than on mitral prostheses, and when observed on mitral prosthetic valves,

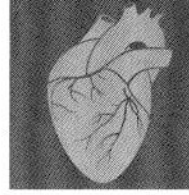

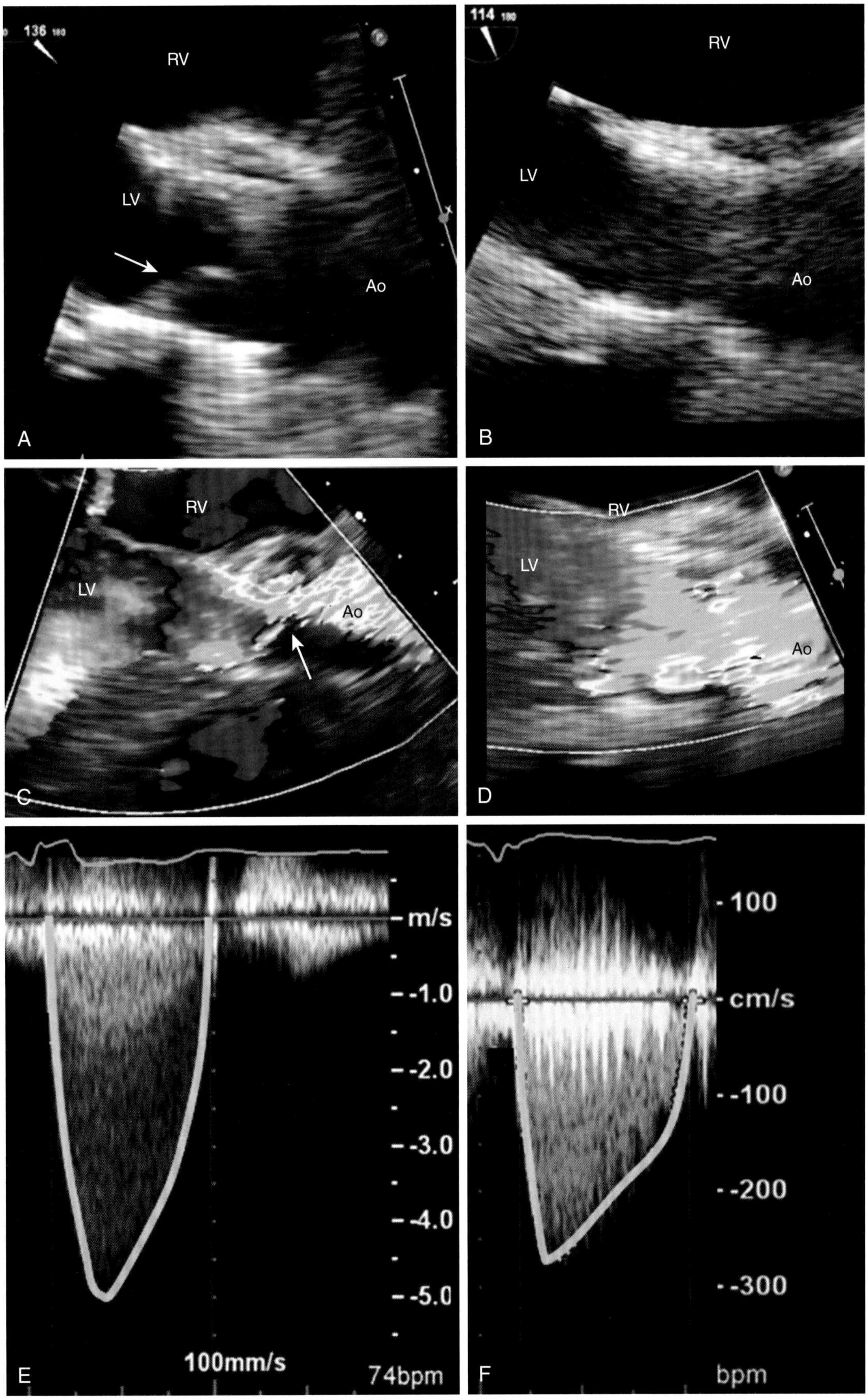

Fig. 31.15 Valve thrombosis after transcatheter aortic valve replacement. TEE shows thickening and reduced mobility of valve leaflets in a transcatheter aortic valve (A) with restricted transvalvular flow (C) and a very high peak/mean transprosthetic gradient of 100/61 mmHg and a small effective orifice area (EOA) of 0.91 cm^2 (E) (see Videos 31.15A and 31.15C). This patient was treated with warfarin and had a complete regression of the valve obstruction. The TTE and TEE examinations performed 2 months later show normal valve leaflet morphology and mobility (B), no evidence of thrombus, no flow restriction (D), and normal valve hemodynamics, including peak/mean gradients of 30/6 mmHg and an EOA of 1.72 cm^2 (F) (see Videos 31.15B and 31.15D).

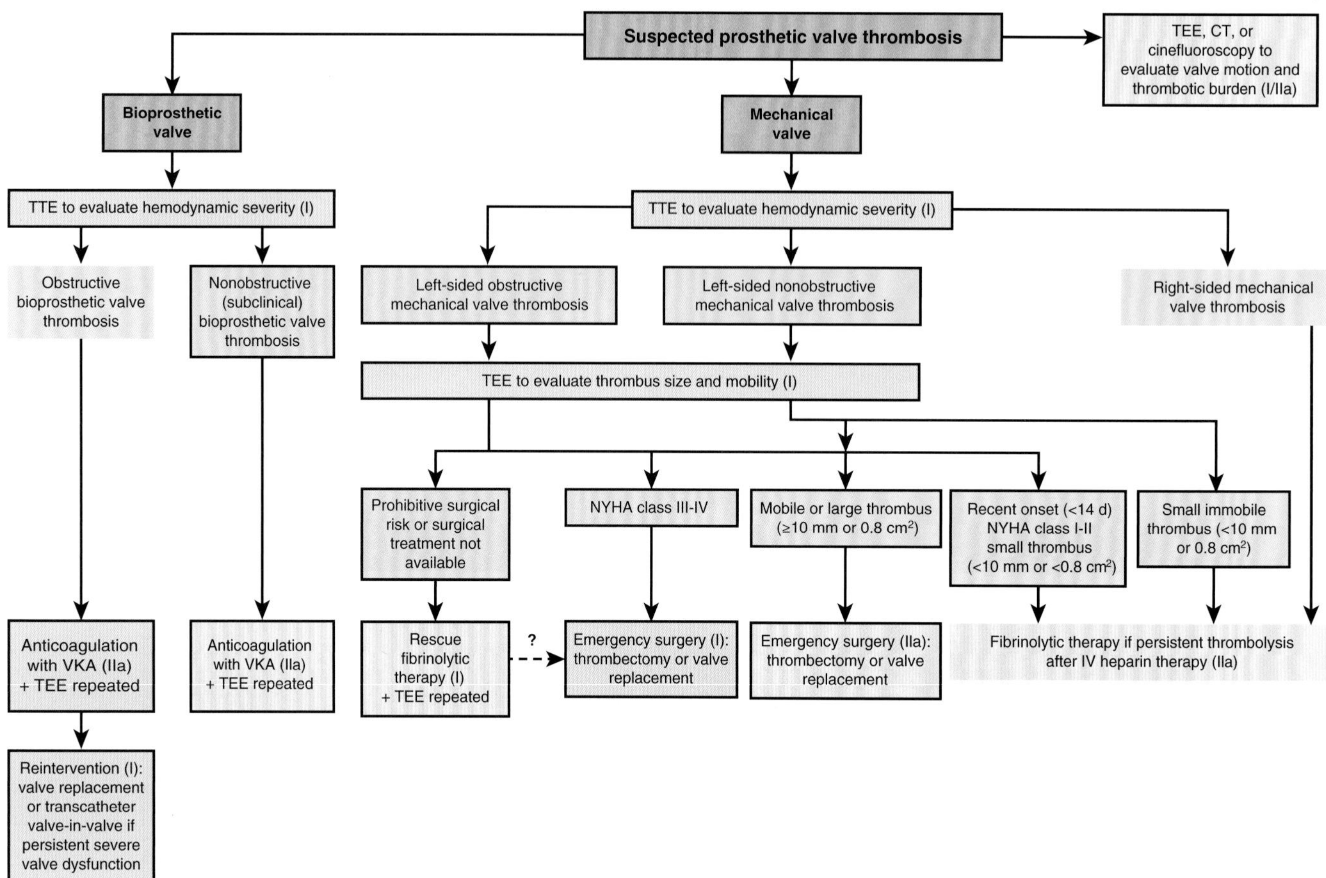

Fig. 31.16 Suspected prosthetic valve thrombosis. Algorithm for the evaluation and management of suspected prosthetic valve thrombosis. *PVT*, Prosthetic valve thrombosis; *NYHA*, New York Heart Association; *VKA*, vitamin K antagonist. (Adapted from Otto CM, Nishimura RA, Bonow RO, et al. 2020 AHA/ACC guideline for the management of patients with valvular heart disease: a report of the American College of Cardiology/American Heart Association Task Force on Clinical Practice Guidelines. *Circulation*. 2021;143. doi: 10.1161/CIR.0000000000000923.)

pannus most often occurs on the atrial side of the prosthesis (see Fig. 31.14).

Small thrombi should be differentiated from strands or sutures. Strands are thought to be fibrin filaments, which appear as fine (1 mm), filamentous, mobile echoes of various lengths (5–15 mm) and are most often observed on the atrial side of mitral prostheses.[7] Although the clinical relevance of these strands remains undetermined, there is no evidence that they are associated with an increased embolic risk.[7]

Cinefluoroscopy and multidetector computed tomography (MCDT) provide accurate information on the mobility of the leaflets of mechanical prostheses and can be helpful when TEE in inconclusive. MCDT is also useful for differentiating thrombus from pannus (see Fig. 31.4).[6,72]

The most important factors to consider for therapeutic decision making are (1) surgical prosthetic valve obstruction, (2) size and mobility of the thrombus, and (3) the clinical and hemodynamic condition of the patient (see Figs. 31.14 and 31.15).[8,22,74] Fig. 31.16 shows a recommended algorithm based on the 2020 AHA/ACC and 2017 ESC/EACTS guidelines for the evaluation and management of prosthetic valve thrombosis.[21,22]

For patients with a mechanical valve, the decision between emergency reoperation and fibrinolysis is based on the prosthesis position (i.e., left-or right-sided), symptom status, operative risk, existence and severity of prosthetic valve obstruction assessed by TTE, and size and mobility of the thrombus assessed by TEE. For patients with obstructive bioprosthetic valve thrombosis, anticoagulation with a vitamin K antagonist or unfractionated heparin is recommended before considering valve reintervention (i.e., surgical replacement of the prosthesis or a transcatheter valve-in-valve procedure[8,10,22,74] (see Fig. 31.16). For patients with subclinical bioprosthetic valve stenosis, close clinical and echocardiographic follow-up is recommended, and anticoagulation may be considered.

PROSTHETIC VALVE ENDOCARDITIS

Echocardiographic findings are major criteria in the diagnosis of infective endocarditis, and TEE is mandatory in PVE because of its better sensitivity (90%–100%) for the detection of vegetations, abscesses, and paravalvular lesions (Fig. 31.17).[20] Compared with native valve endocarditis, PVE is characterized by a lower incidence of vegetations and higher incidence of abscesses and paravalvular complications.

TEE is recommended (class I) for patients with a prosthetic valve and suspicion of endocarditis.[20] However, the sensitivity and specificity of TTE and TEE are lower for PVE than native valve endocarditis. Components of the prosthetic valve may hinder the detection of vegetations and abscesses. Moreover, it may be difficult to differentiate a thrombus from a vegetation or bioprosthetic valve degeneration from infective lesions. Consequently, a negative echocardiographic result is often observed in cases of PVE and does not rule out the diagnosis of infective endocarditis. If the initial TEE study is negative but suspicion for infective endocarditis remains, TEE should be repeated in 5 to 7 days and an

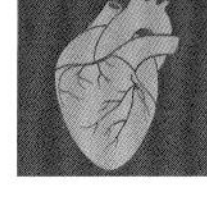

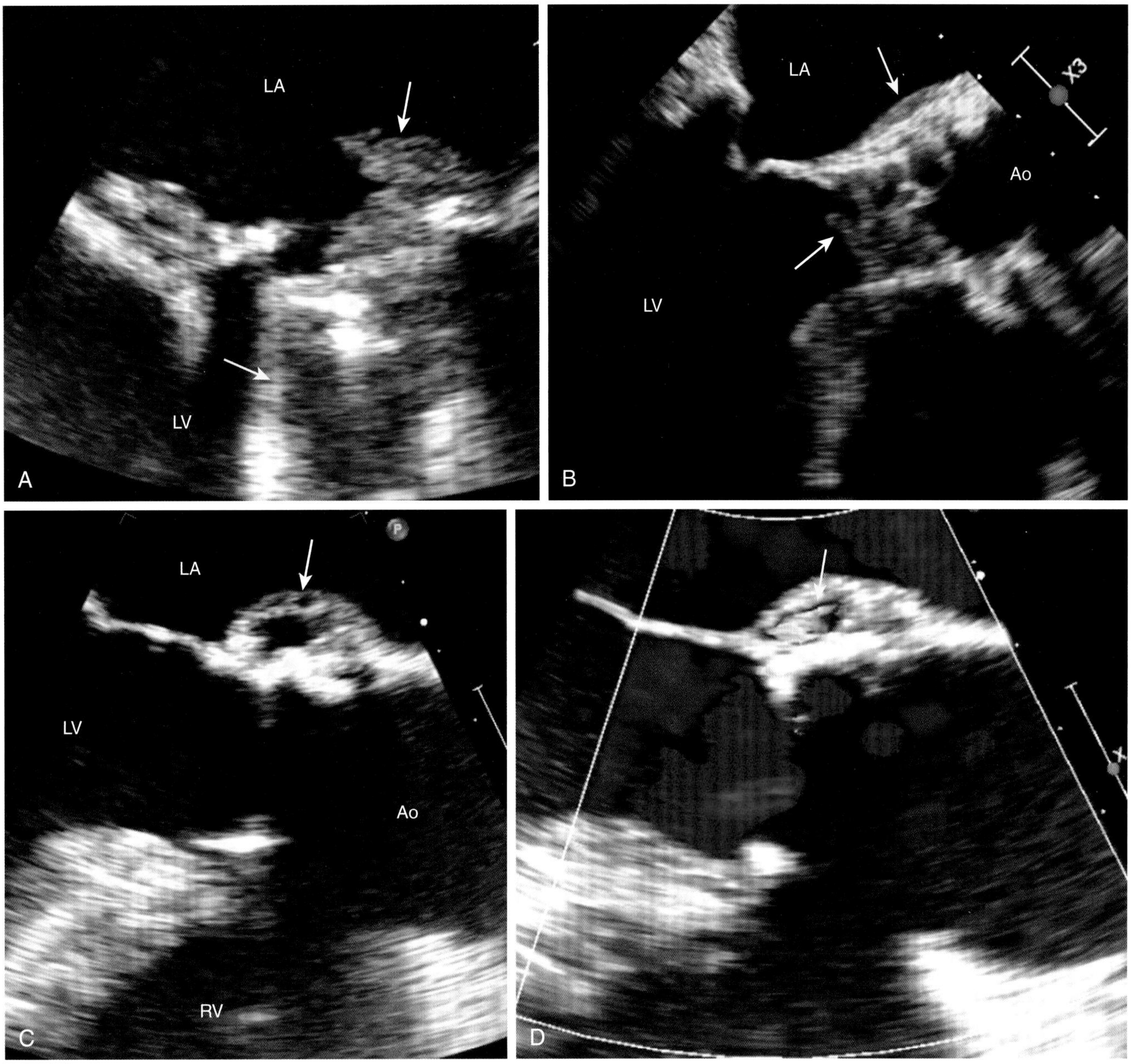

Fig. 31.17 Utility of TEE for diagnosis and treatment of prosthetic valve endocarditis. (A) Large vegetation *(yellow arrow)* is attached to a mitral bioprosthetic valve cusp and can be seen prolapsing into the LA *(white arrow)* during systole (see Video 31.17A). (B) The vegetation attached to one of the cups of a transcatheter aortic bioprosthetic valve *(white arrow)* and thickening of the noncoronary sinus *(yellow arrow)* suggest an abscess (see Video 31.17B). (C and D) The *white arrow* indicates a pseudoaneurysm (C) of the aortic root in a patient with bioprosthetic aortic valve, and color Doppler shows the flow *(yellow arrow)* entering in the pseudoaneurysm (D) (see Video 31.17D). (A, C, and D, Courtesy Dr. Gilbert Habib, Hôpital La Timone, Marseille, France.)

alternative imaging modality such as positron emission tomography/computed tomography (PET/CT) should be used.[20,75]

Infective endocarditis must be suspected in the setting of new paraprosthetic regurgitation, even in the absence of a vegetation or abscess. TEE has a better sensitivity than TTE for this diagnosis, especially in mitral PVE. Paravalvular complications are more common in aortic PVE.[20] The anatomic involvement of infective endocarditis depends on the type and timing of contamination and the type of prosthetic valve. In mechanical valves, the infection usually involves the junction between the sewing ring and the annulus, leading to paravalvular abscess, dehiscence, pseudoaneurysms, and fistula, whereas in bioprosthetic valves, infection is more often located on the leaflets, leading to cusp tear, perforation, and vegetations (see Fig. 31.17).

In PVE occurring in the early postoperative phase due to perioperative contamination, the infection predominantly involves the paraprosthetic tissues, whereas in late bioprosthetic valve endocarditis, it involves the valve leaflets. In transcatheter aortic valves, the Doppler echocardiographic features of PVE are often limited to valve leaflet thickening and obstruction with an absence of vegetation and regurgitation.[76] This mode of presentation is more insidious and makes the differential diagnosis with patient-prosthesis mismatch, prosthetic valve thrombosis, or SVD more difficult.

CONCLUSIONS

Doppler echocardiography is the primary imaging modality to identify and quantitate prosthetic valve dysfunction and to assess repercussions on cardiac function. A comprehensive approach that integrates several direct and indirect parameters of valve function measured by TTE and TEE is key to assessing prosthetic valve function. The particular context of prosthetic valves, however, poses several major challenges in terms of imaging and flow dynamics that push Doppler echocardiography to its limits. Other imaging modalities such as cineangiography, MDCT, cardiac magnetic resonance, and PET may be useful to complement or corroborate echocardiography for the detection and quantitation of prosthetic valve dysfunction and complications, but these modalities should not be used in isolation.

SUMMARY Imaging of Prosthetic Valve Dysfunction or Complications.

Valve Dysfunction or Complications	Imaging Approach	Echocardiographic Findings
Patient-prosthesis mismatch	2D/3D TTE/TEE: assess valve leaflet morphology/mobility CW Doppler through the prosthetic valve PW Doppler in the LVOT Calculate EOA: $D_{LVOT} \times VTI_{LVOT}/VTI_{Pr}$ Obtain normal EOA for model and size of implanted valve Calculate DVI: aortic VTI_{LVOT}/VTI_{Pr} Mitral: VTI_{Pr}/VTI_{LVOT} Other imaging modalities: cinefluoroscopy (mechanical valves), MDCT	Normal leaflet morphology/mobility High transprosthetic velocity/gradient EOA within normal range Small indexed EOA Intermediate DVI Aortic: intermediate AT/LVET
Prosthetic valve stenosis	Same as above	Abnormal leaflet morphology/mobility High transprosthetic velocity/gradient EOA < normal range Small indexed EOA Low DVI (aortic); high DVI (mitral) Increased AT/LVET ratio (aortic) Prolonged pressure half-time (mitral)
Prosthetic valve regurgitation	Color Doppler in multiple views and planes Measure regurgitant vena contracta width if feasible Visual assessment of regurgitant jet width at its origin Visual estimation of circumferential extent of paravalvular regurgitant jets in the PSAX view CW Doppler of regurgitant flow PISA method if feasible PW Doppler in LVOT and 2D TTE to measure LVOT diameter (aortic) PW Doppler in RVOT and 2D TTE to measure RVOT diameter (aortic) Calculate regurgitant volume: $SV_{LVOT} - SV_{RVOT}$ (aortic) Calculate regurgitant fraction: RV/SV_{LVOT} (aortic) PW in descending aorta (aortic)	Transvalvular or paravalvular regurgitation Criteria of prosthetic regurgitation severity: • Large regurgitant jet vena contracta and/or width at its origin • High percentage of circumferential extent for paravalvular regurgitation • Dense regurgitant jet CW Doppler signal • Large regurgitant volume and fraction • Short pressure half-time (aortic) • Holodiastolic flow reversal with high end-diastolic velocity
Prosthetic valve thrombosis	2D/3D TTE/TEE: assess leaflet mobility and morphology and localization and size of thrombus CW Doppler: assess valve stenosis Color Doppler: assess valve regurgitation Other imaging modalities: cinefluoroscopy (mechanical valves), MDCT	Abnormal leaflet morphology and mobility Thrombus Prosthetic valve stenosis and/or regurgitation
Prosthetic valve endocarditis	2D/3D TTE/TEE: assess leaflet integrity and paravalvular region CW Doppler: assess valve stenosis Color Doppler: assess valve regurgitation Other imaging modalities: PET-CT, MDCT	Vegetations, leaflet destruction, paravalvular abscess Prosthetic valve dehiscence, prosthetic valve stenosis and/or regurgitation

AT, Acceleration time; *CW*, continuous wave; *DVI*, Doppler velocity index; *EOA*, effective orifice area; *LVET*, LV ejection time; *LVOT*, LV outflow tract; *MDCT*, multidetector computed tomography; *PET*, positron emission tomography; *PISA*, proximal isovelocity area; *PSAX*, parasternal short-axis view; *PW*, pulsed wave; *RVOT*, RV outflow tract; *SV*, stroke volume; *VTI*, velocity-time integral; VTI_{LVOT}, LV outflow tract flow VTI; VTI_{PR}, prosthetic valve flow VTI.

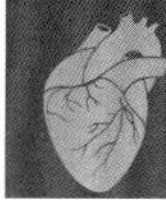

REFERENCES

1. Pibarot P, Dumesnil JG. Prosthesis-patient mismatch: definition, clinical impact, and prevention. *Heart.* 2006;92:1022–1029.
2. Pibarot P, Dumesnil JG. Valve prosthesis-patient mismatch, 1978 to 2011: from original concept to compelling evidence. *J Am Coll Cardiol.* 2012;60:1136–1139.
3. Durko AP, Head SJ, Pibarot P, et al. Characteristics of surgical prosthetic heart valves and problems around labeling: a document from the European Association for Cardio-thoracic Surgery (EACTS)-The Society of Thoracic Surgeons (STS)-American Association for Thoracic Surgery (AATS) Valve Labelling Task Force. *J Thorac Cardiovasc Surg.* 2019. https://doi.org/10.1093/ejcts/ezz034.
4. Head S, Mokhles M, Osnabrugge R, et al. The impact of prosthesis-patient mismatch on long-term survival after aortic valve replacement: a systematic review and meta-analysis of 34 observational studies comprising 27,186 patients with 133,141 patient-years. *Eur Heart J.* 2012;33:1518–1529.
5. Pibarot P, Magne J, Leipsic J, et al. Imaging for predicting and assessing prosthesis-patient mismatch after aortic valve replacement. *JACC Cardiovasc Imaging.* 2019;12:149–162.
6. Lancellotti P, Pibarot P, Chambers J, et al. Recommendations for the imaging assessment of prosthetic heart valves: a report from the European Association of Cardiovascular Imaging Endorsed by the Chinese Society of Echocardiography, the Inter-American Society of Echocardiography and the Brazilian Department of Cardiovascular Imaging. *Eur Heart J Cardiovasc Imaging.* 2016;17:589–590.
7. Roudaut R, Serri K, Lafitte S. Thrombosis of prosthetic heart valves: diagnosis and therapeutic considerations. *Heart.* 2007;93:137–142.
8. Dangas GD, Weitz JI, Giustino G, Makkar R, Mehran R. Prosthetic heart valve thrombosis. *J Am Coll Cardiol.* 2016;68:2670–2689.
9. Yanagisawa R, Hayashida K, Yamada Y, et al. Incidence, predictors, and mid-term outcomes of possible leaflet thrombosis after TAVR. *JACC Cardiovasc Imaging.* 2017;10:1–4.
10. Nakatani S. Subclinical leaflet thrombosis after transcatheter aortic valve implantation. *Heart.* 2017;103:1942–1946.
11. Makkar RR, Fontana G, Jilaihawi H, et al. Possible subclinical leaflet thrombosis in bioprosthetic aortic valves. *N Engl J Med.* 2015;373:2015–2024.
12. Chakravarty T, Søndergaard L, Friedman J, et al. Subclinical leaflet thrombosis in surgical and transcatheter bioprosthetic aortic valves: an observational study. *Lancet.* 2017. https://doi.org/10.1016/S0140-6736(17)30757-2.

12a. Makkar RR, Blanke P, Leipsic J, et al. Subclinical leaflet thrombosis in transcatheter and surgical bioprosthetic valves: PARTNER 3 Cardiac Computed Tomography Substudy. *J Am Coll Cardiol.* 2020;75(24):3003–3015.

13. Rashid HN, Gooley RP, Nerlekar N, et al. Bioprosthetic aortic valve leaflet thrombosis detected by multidetector computed tomography is associated with adverse cerebrovascular events: a meta-analysis of observational studies. *EuroIntervention.* 2018;13. e1748-e1755.
14. Salaun E, Clavel MA, Rodés-Cabau J, Pibarot P. Bioprosthetic aortic valve durability in the era of transcatheter aortic valve implantation. *Heart.* 2018;104:1323–1332.
15. Rodriguez-Gabella T, Voisine P, Dagenais F, et al. Long-term outcomes following surgical aortic bioprosthesis implantation. *J Am Coll Cardiol.* 2018;71:1401–1412.
16. Rodriguez-Gabella T, Voisine P, Puri R, Pibarot P, Rodés-Cabau J. Aortic bioprosthetic valve durability incidence, mechanisms, predictors, and management of surgical and transcatheter valve degeneration. *J Am Coll Cardio.* 2017;70:1013–1028.
17. Salaun E, Mahjoub H, Girerd N, et al. Rate, timing, correlates, and outcomes of hemodynamic valve deterioration after bioprosthetic surgical aortic valve replacement. *Circulation.* 2018;138:971–985.
18. Capodanno D, Petronio AS, Prendergast B, et al. Standardized definitions of structural deterioration and valve failure in assessing long-term durability of transcatheter and surgical aortic bioprosthetic valves: a consensus statement from the European Association of Percutaneous Cardiovascular Interventions(EAPCI) endorsed by the European Society of Cardiology (ESC) and the European Association for Cardio-Thoracic Surgery (EACTS). *Eur Heart J.* 2017;38:3382–3390.
19. Dvir D, Bourguignon T, Otto CM, et al. Standardized definition of structural valve degeneration for surgical and transcatheter bioprosthetic aortic valves. *Circulation.* 2018;137:388–399.
20. Habib G, Lancellotti P, Antunes MJ, et al. ESC Guidelines for the management of infective endocarditis: the Task force for the Management of Infective Endocarditis of the European Society of Cardiology (ESC) endorsed by: European Association for Cardio-Thoracic Surgery (EACTS), the European Association of Nuclear Medicine (EANM). *Eur Heart J.* 2015;36:3075–3128. 2015.
21. Otto CM, Nishimura RA, Bonow RO, et al. 2020 ACC/AHA guideline for the management of patients with valvular heart disease: a report of the American College of Cardiology/American Heart Association Joint Committee on Clinical Practice Guidelines. *Circulation.* 2021;143(5):e72–e227. doi: 10.1161/CIR.0000000000000923.
22. Baumgartner H, Falk V, Bax JJ, et al. 2017 ESC/EACTS guidelines for the management of valvular heart disease: the Task Force for the management of valvular heart disease of the European Society of Cardiology (ESC) and the European Association for Cardio-Thoracic Surgery (EACTS). *Eur Heart J.* 2017;38:2739–2791.
23. Regueiro A, Linke A, Latib A, et al. Association between transcatheter aortic valve replacement and subsequent infective endocarditis and in-hospital death. *Jama.* 2016;316:1083–1092.
24. Zoghbi WA, Chambers JB, Dumesnil JG, et al. Recommendations for evaluation of prosthetic valves with echocardiography and Doppler ultrasound: a report from the American Society of Echocardiography's Guidelines and Standards Committee and the Task Force on Prosthetic Valves, developed in conjunction with the American College of Cardiology Cardiovascular Imaging Committee, Cardiac Imaging Committee of the American Heart Association, the European Association of Echocardiography, a registered branch of the European Society of Cardiology, the Japanese Society of Echocardiography and the Canadian Society of Echocardiography, endorsed by the American College of Cardiology Foundation, American Heart Association, European Association of Echocardiography, a registered branch of the European Society of Cardiology, the Japanese Society of Echocardiography, and Canadian Society of Echocardiography. *J Am Soc Echocardiogr.* 2009;22:975–1014.
25. Zoghbi WA, Asch FM, Bruce C, et al. Guidelines for the evaluation of valvular regurgitation after percutaneous valve repair or replacement: a report from the American Society of Echocardiography developed in collaboration with the Society for Cardiovascular Angiography and Interventions, Japanese Society of Echocardiography, and Society for Cardiovascular Magnetic Resonance. *J Am Soc Echocardiogr.* 2019;32:431–475.
26. Pibarot P, Hahn RT, Weissman NJ, Monaghan MJ. Assessment of paravalvular regurgitation following TAVR: a proposal of unifying grading scheme. *JACC Cardiovasc Imaging.* 2015;8:340–360.
27. Reference deleted in review.
28. Lorusso R, Gelsomino S, Luca F, et al. Type 2 diabetes mellitus is associated with faster degeneration of bioprosthetic valve: results from a propensity score-matched Italian multicenter study. *Circulation.* 2012;125:604–614.
29. Mahjoub H, Mathieu P, Larose É, et al. Determinants of aortic bioprosthetic valve calcification assessed by multidetector CT. *Heart.* 2015;101:472–477.
30. Mahjoub H, Mathieu P, Sénéchal M, et al. ApoB/ApoA-I ratio is associated with increased risk of bioprosthetic valve degeneration. *J Am Coll Cardiol.* 2013;61:752–761.
31. Salaun E, Mahjoub H, Dahou A, et al. Hemodynamic deterioration of surgically implanted bioprosthetic aortic valves. *J Am Coll Cardiol.* 2018;72:241–251.
32. Kappetein AP, Head SJ, Généreux P, et al. Updated standardized endpoint definitions for transcatheter aortic valve implantation: the Valve Academic Research Consortium-2 consensus document. *Eur J Cardio Thorac Surg.* 2012;42. S45-S60.
33. Bach DS. Transesophageal echocardiographic (TEE) evaluation of prosthetic valves. *Cardiol Clin.* 2000;18:751–771.
34. Vollema EM, Kong WKF, Katsanos S, et al. Transcatheter aortic valve thrombosis: the relation between hypo-attenuated leaflet thickening, abnormal valve haemodynamics, and stroke. *Eur Heart J.* 2017;38:1207–1217.
35. Salaun E, Zenses AS, Clavel MA, et al. Valve-in-valve procedure in failed transcatheter aortic valves. *JACC Cardiovasc Imaging.* 2019;12:198–202.
36. Baumgartner H, Schima H, Kühn P. Discrepancies between Doppler and catheter gradients across bileaflet aortic valve prostheses. *Am J Cardiol.* 1993;71:1241–1243.
37. Aljassim O, Svensson G, Houltz E, Bech-Hanssen O. Doppler-catheter discrepancies in patients with bileaflet mechanical prostheses or bioprostheses in the aortic valve position. *Am J Cardiol.* 2008;102:1383–1389.
38. Garcia D, Pibarot P, Dumesnil JG, Sakr F, Durand LG. Assessment of aortic valve stenosis severity: a new index based on the energy loss concept. *Circulation.* 2000;101:765–771.
39. Abbas AE, Hanzel G, Shannon F, et al. Post-TAVR trans-aortic valve gradients: echocardiographic versus invasive measurements: the role of pressure recovery. *Structural Heart.* 2019;3:348–350.
40. Abbas AE, Mando R, Hanzel G, et al. Invasive versus echocardiographic evaluation of transvalvular gradients immediately post-transcatheter aortic valve replacement. *Circ Cardiovasc Interv.* 2019;12. e007973.
41. Ben Zekry S, Saad RM, Ozkan M, et al. Flow acceleration time and ratio of acceleration time to ejection time for prosthetic aortic valve function. *JACC Cardiovasc Imaging.* 2011;4:1161–1170.

42. Otto CM, Pearlman AS, Comess KA, Reamer RP, Janko CL, Huntsman LL. Determination of the stenotic aortic valve area in adults using Doppler echocardiography. *J Am Coll Cardiol.* 1986;7:509–517.
43. Chafizadeh ER, Zoghbi WA. Doppler echocardiographic assessment of the St. Jude medical prosthetic valve in the aortic position using the continuity equation. *Circulation.* 1991;83:213–223.
44. Dumesnil JG, Honos GN, Lemieux M, Beauchemin J. Validation and applications of indexed aortic prosthetic valve areas calculated by Doppler echocardiography. *J Am Coll Cardiol.* 1990;16:637–643.
45. Pibarot P, Honos GN, Durand LG, Dumesnil JG. Substitution of left ventricular outflow tract diameter with prosthesis size is inadequate for calculation of the aortic prosthetic valve area by the continuity equation. *J Am Soc Echocardiogr.* 1995;8:511–517.
46. Shames S, Koczo A, Hahn R, Jin Z, Picard MH, Gillam LD. Flow characteristics of the SAPIEN aortic valve: the importance of recognizing in-stent flow acceleration for the echocardiographic assessment of valve function. *J Am Soc Echocardiogr.* 2012;25:603–609.
47. Hahn RT, Leipsic J, Douglas PS, et al. Comprehensive echocardiographic assessment of normal transcatheter valve function. *JACC Cardiovasc Imaging.* 2019;12:25–34.
48. Dumesnil JG, Honos GN, Lemieux M, Beauchemin J. Validation and applications of mitral prosthetic valvular areas calculated by Doppler echocardiography. *Am J Cardiol.* 1990;65:1443–1448.
49. Pibarot P, Dumesnil JG. Prosthetic heart valves: Selection of the optimal prosthesis and long-term management. *Circulation.* 2009;119:1034–1048.
50. Muratori M, Montorsi P, Maffessanti F, et al. Dysfunction of bileaflet aortic prosthesis: accuracy of echocardiography versus fluoroscopy. *J Am Coll Cardiol Img.* 2013;6:196–205.
51. Smadi O, Garcia J, Pibarot P, Gaillard E, Hassan I, Kadem L. Accuracy of Doppler-echocardiographic parameters for the detection of aortic bileaflet mechanical prosthetic valve dysfunction. *Eur Heart J Cardiovasc Imaging.* 2014;15:142–151.
52. Fernandes V, Olmos L, Nagueh SF, Quinones MA, Zoghbi WA. Peak early diastolic velocity rather than pressure half-time is the best index of mechanical prosthetic mitral valve function. *Am J Cardiol.* 2002;89:704–710.
53. Kodali SK, Williams MR, Smith CR, et al. Two-year outcomes after transcatheter or surgical aortic-valve replacement. *N Engl J Med.* 2012;366:1686–1695.
54. Mack MJ, Leon MB, Thourani VH, et al. Transcatheter aortic-valve replacement with a balloon-expandable valve in low-risk patients. *N Engl J Med.* 2019;380:1695–1705.
55. Leon MB, Smith CR, Mack MJ, et al. Transcatheter or surgical aortic-valve replacement in intermediate-risk patients. *N Engl J Med.* 2016;374:1609–1620.
56. Reardon MJ, Adams DH, Kleiman NS, et al. 2-year outcomes in patients undergoing surgical or self-expanding transcatheter aortic valve replacement. *J Am Coll Cardiol.* 2015;66:113–121.
57. Popma JJ, Deeb GM, Yakubov SJ, et al. Transcatheter aortic-valve replacement with a self-expanding valve in low-risk patients. *N Engl J Med.* 2019;380:1706–1715.
58. Lang RM, Tsang W, Weinert L, Mor-Avi V, Chandra S. Valvular heart disease: the value of 3-dimensional echocardiography. *J Am Coll Cardiol.* 2011;58:1933–1944.
59. Pibarot P, Hahn RT, Weissman NJ, et al. Association of paravalvular regurgitation with 1-year outcomes after transcatheter aortic valve replacement with the SAPIEN 3 valve. *JAMA cardiol.* 2017;2:1208–1216.
60. Goncalves A, Almeria C, Marcos-Alberca P, et al. Three-dimensional echocardiography in paravalvular aortic regurgitation assessment after transcatheter aortic valve implantation. *J Am Soc Echocardiogr.* 2012;25:47–55.
61. Altiok E, Frick M, Meyer CG, et al. Comparison of two- and three-dimensional transthoracic echocardiography to cardiac magnetic resonance imaging for assessment of paravalvular regurgitation after transcatheter aortic valve implantation. *Am J Cardiol.* 2014;113:1859–1866.
62. Orwat S, Diller GP, Kaleschke G, et al. Aortic regurgitation severity after transcatheter aortic valve implantation is underestimated by echocardiography compared with MRI. *Heart.* 2014;100:1933–1938.
63. Ribeiro HB, Orwat S, Hayek SS, et al. Cardiovascular magnetic resonance to evaluate aortic regurgitation after transcatheter aortic valve replacement. *J Am Coll Cardiol.* 2016;68:577–585.
64. Palau-Caballero G, Walmsley J, Gorcsan 3rd J, Lumens J, Delhaas T. Abnormal ventricular and aortic wall properties can cause inconsistencies in grading aortic regurgitation severity: a computer simulation study. *J Am Soc Echocardiogr.* 2016;29:1122–1130. e4.
65. Tribouilloy C, Avinee P, Shen W, Rey J, Slama M, Lesbre J. End diastolic flow velocity just beneath aortic isthmus assessed by pulsed Doppler echocardiography: a new predictor of aortic reurgitant fraction. *Br Heart J.* 1991;65:37–40.
66. Hashimoto J, Ito S. Aortic stiffness determines diastolic blood flow reversal in the descending thoracic aorta: potential implication for retrograde embolic stroke in hypertension. *Hypertension.* 2013;62:542–549.
67. Ruiz CE, Hahn RT, Berrebi A, et al. Clinical trial principles and endpoint definitions for paravalvular leaks in surgical prosthesis: an expert statement. *Eur Heart J.* 2018;39:1224–1245.
68. Vitarelli A, Conde Y, Cimino E, et al. Assessment of severity of mechanical prosthetic mitral regurgitation by transoesophageal echocardiography. *Heart.* 2004;90:539–544.
69. Muratori M, Montorsi P, Teruzzi G, et al. Feasibility and diagnostic accuracy of quantitative assessment of mechanical prostheses leaflet motion by transthoracic and transesophageal echocardiography in suspected prosthetic valve dysfunction. *Am J Cardiol.* 2006;97:94–100.
70. Bach DS, Schmitz C, Dohmen G, Aaronson KD, Steinseifer U, Kleine P. In vitro assessment of prosthesis type and pressure recovery characteristics: Doppler echocardiography overestimation of bileaflet mechanical and bioprosthetic aortic valve gradients. *J Thorac Cardiovasc Surg.* 2012;144:453–458.
71. Singh P, Inamdar V, Hage FG, et al. Usefulness of live/real time three-dimensional transthoracic echocardiography in evaluation of prosthetic valve function. *Echocardiography.* 2009;26:1236–1249.
72. Tanis W, Habets J, van den Brink RB, Symersky P, Budde RP, Chamuleau SA. Differentiation of thrombus from pannus as the cause of acquired mechanical prosthetic heart valve obstruction by non-invasive imaging: a review of the literature. *Eur Heart J Cardiovasc Imaging.* 2014;15:119–129.
73. Reference deleted in review.
74. Huang G, Schaff HV, Sundt TM, Rahimtoola SH. Treatment of obstructive thrombosed prosthetic heart valve. *J Am Coll Cardiol.* 2013;62:1731–1736.
75. Saby L, Laas O, Habib G, et al. Positron emission tomography/computed tomography for diagnosis of prosthetic valve endocarditis: increased valvular 18F-fluorodeoxyglucose uptake as a novel major criterion. *J Am Coll Cardiol.* 2013;61:2374–2382.
76. Salaun E, Sportouch L, Barral PA, et al. Diagnosis of infective endocarditis after TAVR: value of a multimodality imaging approach. *JACC Cardiovasc Imaging.* 2018;11:143–146.
77. Latib A, Naganuma T, Abdel-Wahab M, et al. Treatment and clinical outcomes of transcatheter heart valve thrombosis. *Circ Cardiovasc Interv.* 2015;8:1–8.
78. Seeburger J, Weiss G, Borger MA, Mohr FW. Structural valve deterioration of a Corevalve prosthesis 9 months after implantation. *Eur Heart J.* 2013;34:1607.

PART VI
第六部分

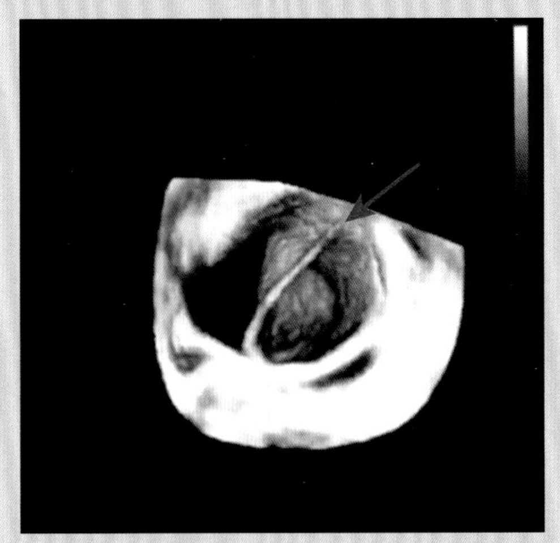

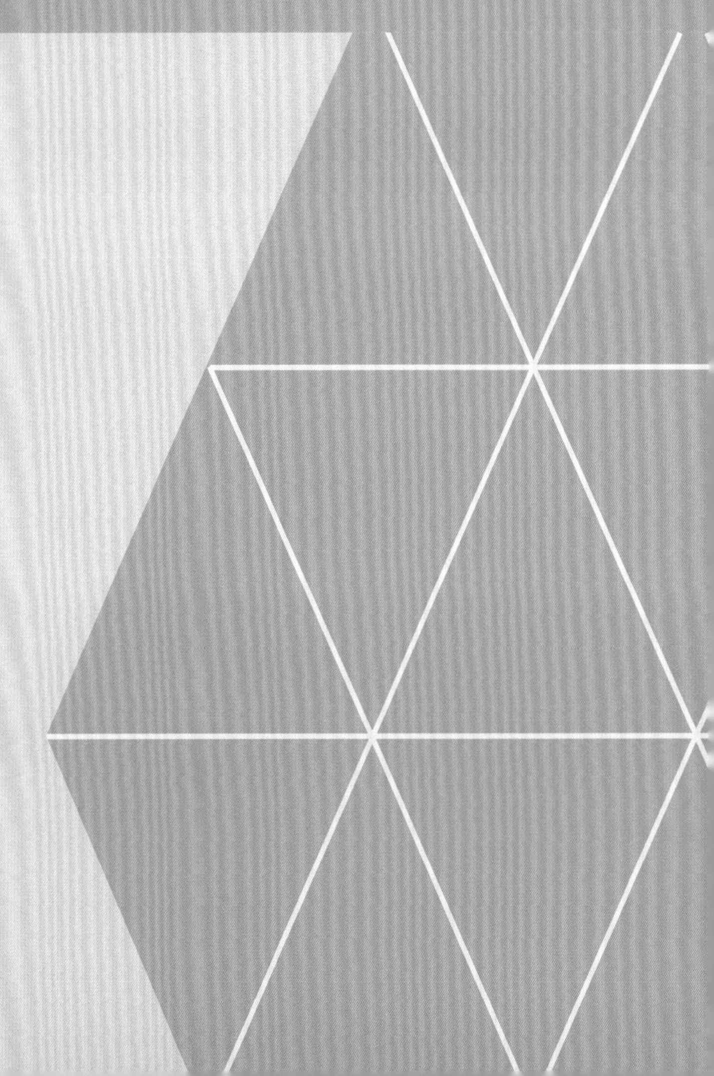

Vascular and Systemic Diseases
血管和全身疾病

中文导读

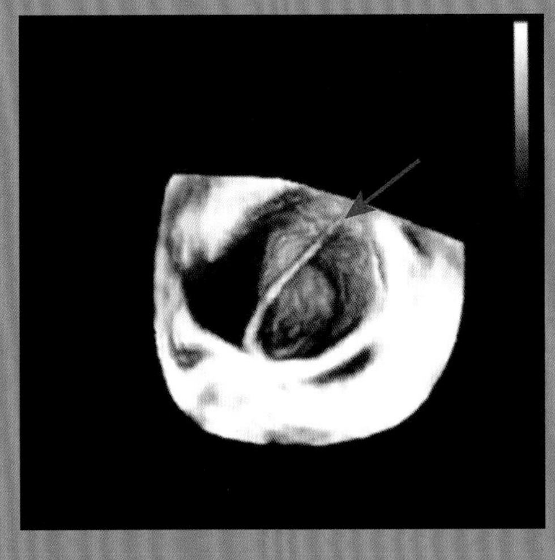

第32章 急性主动脉综合征

急性主动脉综合征是以急性胸痛为主要临床表现的一组疾病，包括主动脉夹层、主动脉壁内血肿、主动脉穿通性溃疡和创伤性主动脉损伤。其中主动脉夹层发生率最高（约占80%），其特征为主动脉内膜撕裂导致血流进入中层形成夹层。其次为主动脉壁内血肿（约占15%），两者通常分为A型（累及升主动脉）和B型（仅累及降主动脉）。AHA和ESC发布的急性主动脉综合征多模态成像指南均推荐超声心动图作为主要诊断方法。

本章主要介绍急性主动脉综合征常见病因、分型、病理生理表现、临床诊断规范流程；经胸超声心动图和经食管超声心动图应用多个切面评估急性主动脉综合征的直接征象：识别真假腔、定位破口、病变累及范围；评估并发症：左心室运动及收缩功能、主动脉瓣反流机制及程度、心包积液或心脏压塞征象、冠状动脉及主动脉分支受累情况；以及其在外科围手术期评估及术后随访中的诊断要点。

刘　偈

32

Acute Aortic Syndromes

CATHERINE M. OTTO, MD | DONALD C. OXORN, MD

BASIC PRINCIPLES

INCIDENCE AND PREDISPOSING FACTORS

Among patients with acute chest pain, a cardiac cause (most often acute myocardial infarction) is responsible for less than 20% of cases[1] (Fig. 32.1). Aortic disease accounts for less than 1% of patients with acute chest pain and is 20 times less common than acute myocardial infarction, with an estimated prevalence of only 3 to 4 cases per 100,000 persons per year.[2,3] However, aortic disease is important to recognize because prompt surgical intervention is lifesaving.[4]

Ascending aortic dissections have higher mortality rates than dissection limited to the descending thoracic aorta. Among patients with an acute aortic syndrome involving the ascending aorta, 20% to 40% suffer instant death, possibly accounting for up to 7% of out-of-hospital cardiac arrest cases[5–8] (Fig. 32.2). Among those who survive to hospital admission, outcomes remain poor, with an estimated mortality rate of 1% per hour for ascending aortic dissection, a surgical mortality rate between 5% and 20%, and continued excess deaths over longer-term follow-up.[1,9]

An acute aortic syndrome may be the initial presentation of a patient with no known cardiac or aortic disease, but it occurs more often in patients with underlying conditions associated with an increased risk of aortic aneurysm and dissection (see Chapter 33). In patients older than 40 years of age, the most common predisposing factors for an acute aortic syndrome are hypertension (72%), atherosclerosis (31%), and prior cardiac or aortic surgery. In younger patients, aortic dissection usually is related to an underlying connective tissue disorder (e.g., Marfan syndrome, Loeys-Dietz syndrome), bicuspid aortic valve disease, or drugs that acutely increase blood pressure (e.g., cocaine, methamphetamines) (Table 32.1).

PATHOPHYSIOLOGY

The most common type of acute aortic syndrome is aortic dissection (80% of cases). Less common presentations include aortic intramural hematoma (IMH; ≈15% of cases), penetrating ulcer in the aortic wall (≈5% of cases), and traumatic aortic injury.[10]

Anatomically, an aortic dissection is characterized by separation of the aortic intima from the adventitia, which results in two aortic lumens separated by a thin, mobile flap of tissue. It remains controversial whether dissection is initiated by a tear in the intima or by hemorrhage into the media with subsequent disruption of the intima, but blood flow through the intimal tear propagates downstream, with further separation of the flow into two lumens extending from the initiation site to the arch, descending thoracic, and abdominal aorta.[11,12]

An IMH occurs when there is hemorrhage into the aortic wall without an identifiable entry site, intimal flap, or false lumen, resulting in the appearance of a crescent-shaped thickening (≥5 mm) in the aortic wall on short-axis views. Among patients presenting with an IMH, progression to frank dissection with an intimal flap and/or aortic rupture is common.[10,13]

A penetrating ulcer is an atherosclerotic plaque that disrupts the aortic wall's elastic lamina, often with a localized IMH but without propagation distally.[14] Penetrating ulcers most often occur in the descending thoracic aorta and sometimes in the arch or abdominal aorta, but they rarely occur in the ascending aorta. Most patients with a penetrating ulcer are older (>70 years) and have extensive atherosclerotic vascular disease.

Blunt thoracic trauma, particularly a deceleration injury resulting from a motor vehicle accident, can cause aortic dissection or transection, typically at the aortic isthmus just distal to the left subclavian artery.

Iatrogenic causes of aortic dissection include direct injury to the aorta during cardiac surgery or injury related to catheter interventions for coronary disease, structural heart disease, and electrophysical procedures.

CLASSIFICATION

Acute aortic syndromes are classified as type A if the ascending aorta is involved and type B if the dissection or IMH is limited to the descending thoracic aorta. Other, more complex classifications of acute aortic syndromes are useful for surgical planning, but the key element in diagnosis and management is

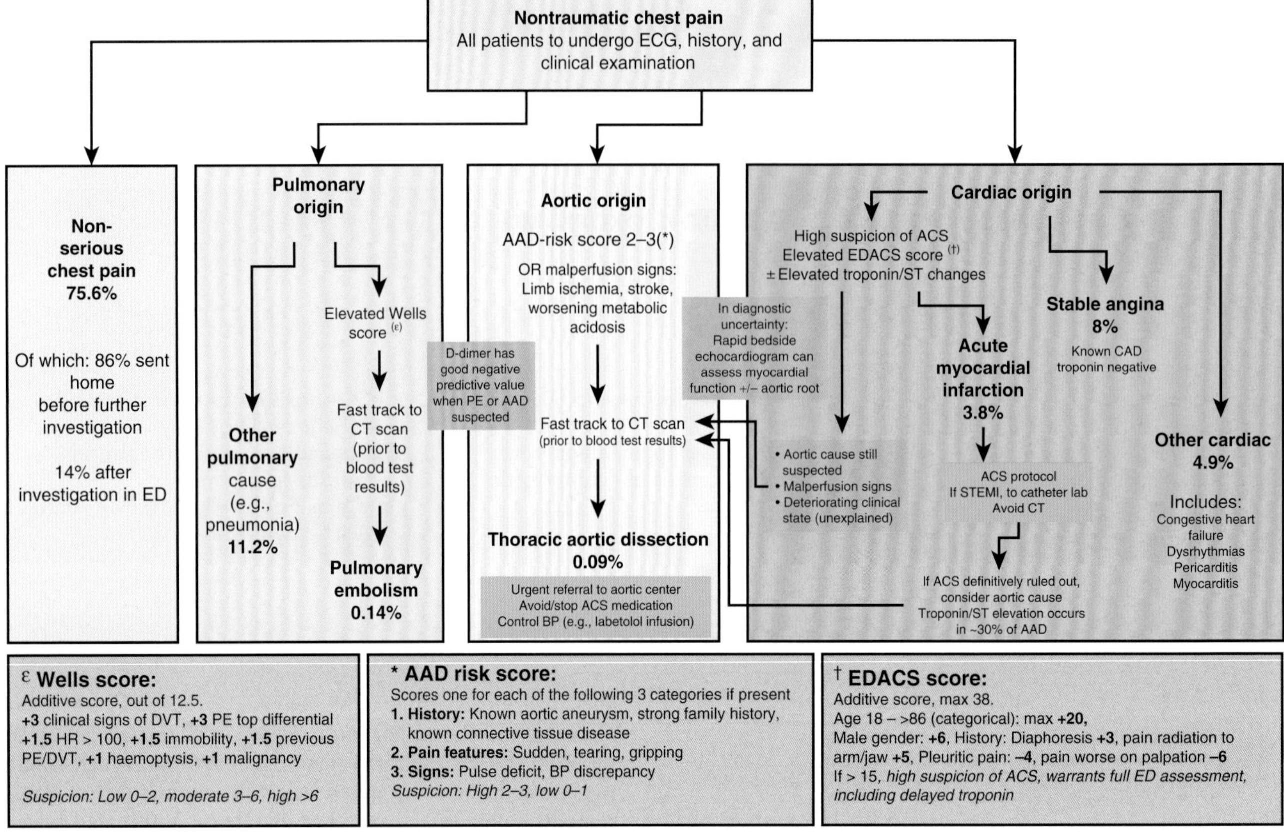

Fig. 32.1 Diagnostic processes for acute chest pain with targeted risk scoring and management. Quoted percentages are adapted from Kohn et al.[35] *AAD*, Acute aortic dissection; *ACS*, acute coronary syndrome; *BP*, blood pressure; *CAD*, coronary artery disease; *CT*, computed tomography; *DVT*, deep vein thrombosis; *ECG*, electrocardiography; *ED*, emergency department; *EDACS*, Emergency Department Assessment of Chest Pain Score; *HR*, heart rate; *PE*, pulmonary embolus; *STEMI*, ST-elevation myocardial infarction. (From Salmasi MY, Al-Saadi N, Hartley P, et al. The risk of misdiagnosis in acute thoracic aortic dissection: a review of current guidelines. *Heart.* 2020;106:885–891.)

whether the ascending aorta is involved in the disease process as the site of the initial tear or by retrograde dissection from a more distal intimal tear.

Management of type A dissection includes prompt surgical intervention with graft replacement of the ascending aorta. Type B dissections usually are treated medically with blood pressure control. Surgical or transcatheter intervention is considered only later in the disease course if needed for progressive changes in aortic size or branch vessel involvement.

COMPLICATIONS

Dissections can propagate retrogradely into the aortic sinuses, with rupture into the pericardium that produces tamponade physiology, distortion of normal aortic valve anatomy causing aortic regurgitation (AR), extension into a coronary artery resulting in acute infarction, or frank aortic rupture into the mediastinum[15] (Fig. 32.3). More often, the dissection extends distally into the descending thoracic aorta, the abdominal aorta, the iliofemoral arteries, and other branch vessels, resulting in vascular compromise and clinical symptoms (Fig. 32.4).

CLINICAL PRESENTATION AND DIAGNOSTIC APPROACH

Most patients present within 24 hours of the initiating event. Symptoms of severe chest or back pain occur in about 90% of patients. Pain is often described as "tearing," with radiation to the back or upper abdomen. Patients also can present with hypotension or shock due to partial rupture into the mediastinum or pleural cavities. The location of chest or back pain depends to some extent on the location of the dissection; the patient may notice the pain migrating to different locations as the dissection propagates downstream. For example, anterior chest pain may resolve and be replaced by upper back, then lower back, and then abdominal pain. A patient may present with only upper abdominal pain. For patients at risk for acute aortic dissection who present with atypical symptoms, it is important to consider this diagnosis and proceed with appropriate imaging.[1,6,16,17]

In patients with a suspected acute aortic syndrome, the first steps are based on the clinical history, physical examination findings, and serum D-dimer measurements. The number of high-risk clinical features determines the aortic dissection risk score, which ranges from 0 to 3 based on the predisposing conditions (i.e., Marfan, family history, and aortic valve disease), pain characteristics (i.e., abrupt onset, severity intensity, and tearing description), and physical examination findings (i.e., pulse deficit or differential, AR murmur, and hypotension). A score of 0 indicates a low risk, a score of 1 indicates an intermediate risk, and a score of 2 or greater is considered high risk.[18] Measurement of serum D-dimer levels is helpful for patients with a low risk score but for whom there is concern about an acute aortic syndrome.[19]

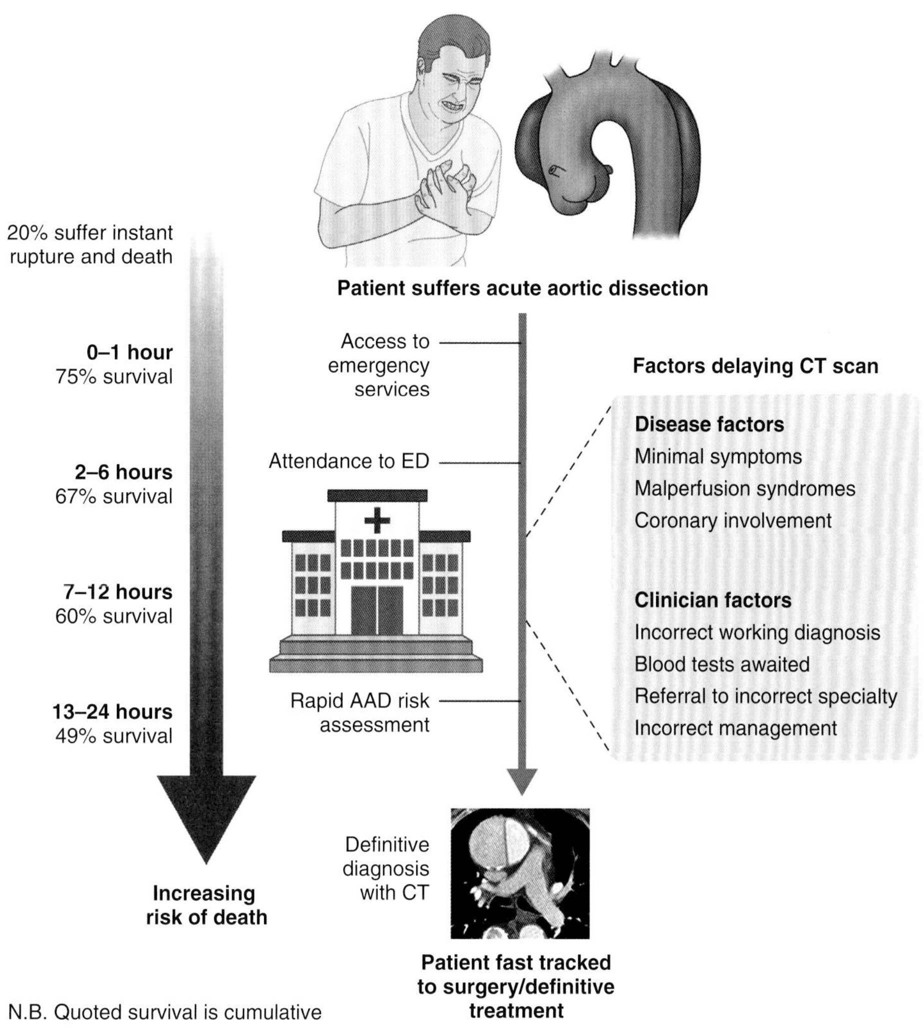

Fig. 32.2 Risk factors for misdiagnosis in aortic dissection. *AAD*, Acute aortic dissection; *CT*, computed tomography; *ED*, emergency department. (From Salmasi MY, Al-Saadi N, Hartley P, et al. The risk of misdiagnosis in acute thoracic aortic dissection: a review of current guidelines. *Heart.* 2020;106:885–891.)

Multimodality imaging is the key to diagnosis of acute aortic syndromes.[20] When clinical features suggest the possibility of an acute aortic syndrome, most centers use computed tomographic angiography (CTA) as the initial imaging approach.[6,16,21] CTA usually is the imaging modality of choice because of its accuracy for this diagnosis and the ability to obtain imaging quickly at any time in most emergency departments (Table 32.2).[22] CTA images should be gated to the electrocardiographic (ECG) tracing to avoid artifacts (Fig. 32.5) and can be reconstructed in 3D or with the centerline approach for surgical planning (Fig. 32.6).

Bedside transthoracic echocardiography (TTE) followed by transesophageal echocardiography (TEE) is recommended only if CTA is not available or is contraindicated due to patient instability or contrast allergy (Fig. 32.7).[21–25] However, some investigators suggest that more widespread use of point-of-care ultrasound would lead to the diagnosis of patients who might otherwise be missed.[26–28] Other imaging approaches, such as cardiac catheterization with aortic and coronary angiography, may be considered in some situations, depending on the other possible diagnoses for that patient. Currently, the major role for TEE evaluation of patients with acute aortic syndromes is for evaluation of the aortic valve and root in those undergoing emergency surgical intervention (discussed later). Imaging guidelines for patients with a suspected aortic dissection have been published by the American Heart Association (AHA) and the European Society of Cardiology (ESC)[6,16] (Table 32.3).

ECHOCARDIOGRAPHIC IMAGING FOR THE DIAGNOSIS OF ACUTE AORTIC SYNDROMES

Echocardiographic Views of the Aorta

TTE imaging often is the initial diagnostic approach in patients presenting with acute chest pain of unknown cause, and it may show direct findings that are specific for diagnosis of an acute aortic syndrome or indirect findings that raise concern for this diagnosis. Advantages of TTE include the ability to obtain images quickly at the bedside and to diagnosis other conditions that may account for the clinical presentation. However, only limited segments of the aorta are seen on TTE, and the diagnosis of an acute aortic syndrome cannot be excluded by this approach.

The sensitivity of TTE for diagnosis of an acute aortic syndrome ranges from 78% to 90% for a type A dissection but only 21% to 55% for a type B dissection. Specificity is higher, at 87% to 96% for type A and 60% to 80% for a type B dissection[21] (Table 32.4).

The standard TTE parasternal long-axis view (Fig. 32.8) allows visualization of the aortic root, defined as the aortic

TABLE 32.1 Patient Populations at Risk for Aortic Dissection.

Predisposing Factors	*Comments*
Degenerative Diseases	
Hypertension Atherosclerotic vascular disease • Aortic ulcer • Aortic aneurysm • Cysitc medial necrosis	Most common cause ascending aortic dissection in older adults
Genetic: Pathologic Single-Gene Variants	
Marfan syndrome Loeys-Dietz syndrome Familial aortic aneurysm Ehlers-Danlos syndrome, vascular form Osteogenesis imperfecta	Consider when there is effacement of the sinotubular junction and sinus dilation, a family history, or other phenotypic features (see Chapter 33)
Genetic: Chromosomal Defects	
Turner syndrome Noonan disease	Dissection can occur even without a BAV.
Congenital Conditions	
BAV Aortic coarctation	The population prevalence of BAV is 1%–2%, and it is associated with an increased risk of aortic dissection. Less than 10% of patients with BAV have an aortic coarctation, although 50%–75% of patients with a coarctation have a BAV (see Chapter 22).
Trauma	
Deceleration injury Penetrating injury	—
Cardiac Surgery	
Cannulation Cross-clamping Aortic valve replacement Catheter-based procedures Transcatheter aortic valve implantation	—
Systemic Inflammatory Disease	
Takayasu arteritis Giant cell arteritis Spondyloarthropathies Behçet disease	Dissection may be the first clinical manifestation of disease.
Infective Aneurysms	
Syphilis Bacterial, fungal, viral	Rare in Europe and the United States
Other Precipitating Factors	
Pregnancy Weightlifting Cocaine use Discontinuation of β-blockers Polycystic kidney disease	—

BAV, Bicuspid aortic valve.
Modified from Bolger AF. Aortic dissection and trauma: value and limitations of echocardiography. In: Otto CM, ed. *Practice of Clinical Echocardiography*. 5th ed. Philadelphia: Elsevier; 2017:677–691.

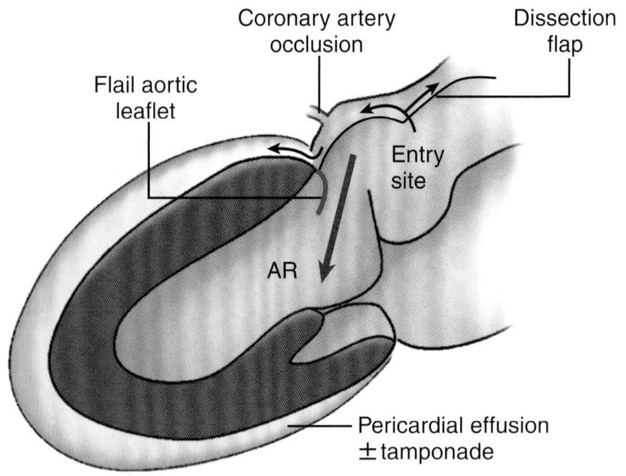

Fig. 32.3 Potential complications of dissection of the ascending aorta. If the dissection proceeds retrograde (and antegrade) from the entry site, the false lumen can cause (1) occlusion in the coronary artery ostium with resultant myocardial infarction, (2) loss of support of an aortic leaflet with consequent severe aortic regurgitation *(AR)*, or (3) rupture into the pericardium, which may result in tamponade physiology. (From Otto CM. *Textbook of Clinical Echocardiography.* 6th ed. Philadelphia: Elsevier; 2019.)

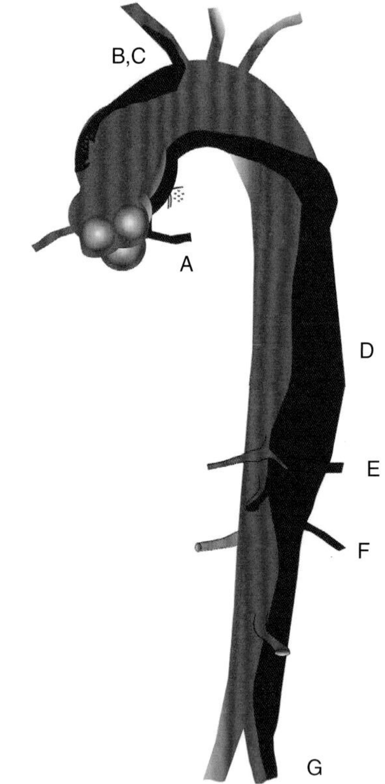

Fig. 32.4 Distal vessel involvement. Anatomic diagram of an evolving type A aortic dissection (DeBakey class I) and location of associated malperfusion syndromes affecting arteries arising from the aorta, including the coronary *(A)*, carotid *(B)*, subclavian *(C)*, spinal *(D)*, mesenteric *(E)*, renal *(F)*, and iliac and femoral arteries *(G)*. (From Salmasi MY, Al-Saadi N, Hartley P, et al. The risk of misdiagnosis in acute thoracic aortic dissection: a review of current guidelines. *Heart.* 2020;106:885–891.)

annulus, sinuses, and sinotubular junction. The ascending aorta is visualized by moving the transducer cephalad while maintaining a centered long-axis orientation of the aortic lumen. These views allow diameter measurements of the aortic annulus (e.g., LV outflow tract diameter) at the insertion of the valve leaflets in the closed position, the maximum diameter of the aortic sinuses, and the sinotubular junction.

Diameter measurements are made at end-diastole (i.e., onset of the QRS complex) and typically are made from the white-black interface anteriorly to the white-black interface along the posterior wall. Although some guidelines suggest a leading edge–to–leading edge measurement, this can be challenging when the aortic wall is thickened or not clearly defined. In clinical practice, luminal diameter measurements are more reproducible.

Care is needed to avoid including the right coronary artery ostium in the sinus measurement. Reverberation artifacts are common in the ascending aorta and must be distinguished from

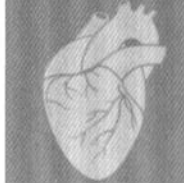

TABLE 32.2 American Society of Echocardiography Recommendations for Choice of Imaging Modality for Aortic Dissection.

Modality	*Recommendation*	*Advantages*	*Disadvantages*
CT	First-line	Initial study for > 70% of patients Widely available, quickest diagnostic times Very high diagnostic accuracy Relatively operator independent Allows evaluation of entire aorta, including arch vessels, mesenteric vessels, and renal arteries	Ionizing radiation exposure Requires iodinated contrast media Pulsation artifact in ascending aorta (can be improved with ECG gating)
TEE	First- and second-line	Very high diagnostic accuracy in thoracic aorta Widely available, portable, convenient, fast Excellent for pericardial effusion and for presence, degree, and mechanisms of AR and LV function Can detect involvement of coronary arteries Safely performed in critically ill patients, even those on ventilators Optimal procedure for guidance in OR	Depends on skill of operator Blind spot for upper ascending aorta, proximal arch Not reliable for cerebral vessels, celiac trunk, SMA, and others. Reverberation artifacts can potentially mimic dissection flap (can be differentiated from flaps in most cases) Semi-invasive
TTE	Second-line	Often initial imaging modality in ED Provides assessment of LV contractility, pericardial effusion, RV size and function, PA pressure Presence and severity of AR	Sensitivity not sufficient distal to aortic root Descending thoracic aorta imaged less easily and less accurately Misses IMH and PAU
MRI	Third-line	3D multiplanar and high resolution Very high diagnostic accuracy Does not require ionizing radiation or ICM Appropriate for serial imaging over many years	Less widely available Difficult monitoring in critically ill patients Not feasible in emergent or unstable clinical situations Longer examination time Caution with use of gadolinium in patients with renal failure
Angiography	Fourth-line	Rarely necessary	Often misses IMH (up to 10%–20% of ADs) Long diagnostic time Requires iodinated contrast media Increased morbidity Less sensitivity than CT, TEE, and MRI

AD, Aortic dissection; *AR*, aortic regurgitation; *CT*, computed tomography; *ECG*, electrocardiographic; *ED*, emergency department; *IMH*, intramural hematoma; *MRI*, magnetic resonance imaging; *OR*, operating room; *PA*, pulmonary artery; *PAU*, penetrating atherosclerotic ulcer; *SMA*, superior mesenteric artery.

From Goldstein SA, Evangelista A, Abbara S, et al. Multimodality imaging of diseases of the thoracic aorta in adults: from the American Society of Echocardiography and the European Association of Cardiovascular Imaging: endorsed by the Society of Cardiovascular Computed Tomography and Society for Cardiovascular Magnetic Resonance. *J Am Soc Echocardiogr.* 2015;28(2):119–182.

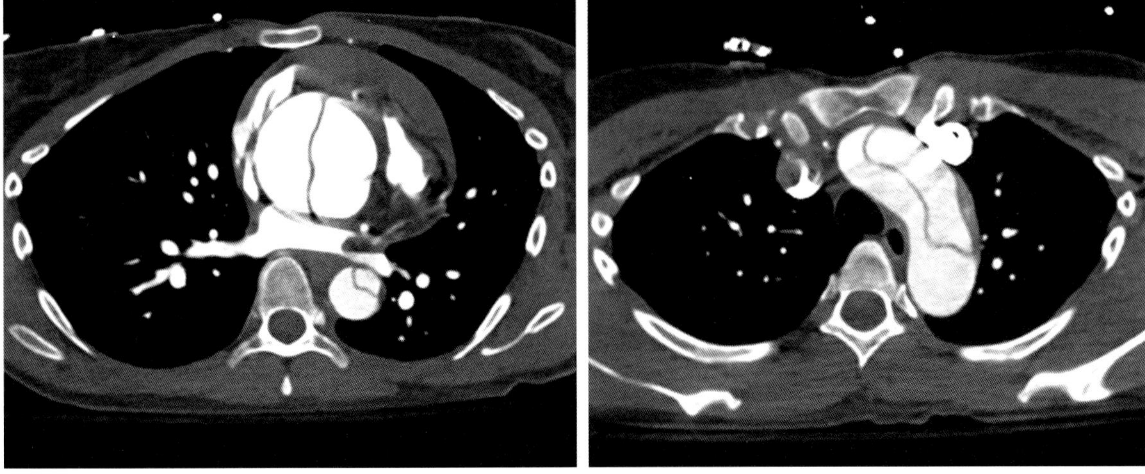

Fig. 32.5 Computed tomographic angiography. ECG-gated images at the level of the ascending aorta *(left)* and aortic arch *(right)* show a complex dissection flap that extends into the descending thoracic aorta.

an intimal flap based on appearance, motion pattern, and visualization in multiple views.

A segment of the descending thoracic aorta is seen posterior to the LV in the standard long-axis view, with more distal segments seen from an apical 2-chamber view angulated posteriorly. The aortic arch is visualized from the suprasternal notch in a view showing the ascending aorta, aortic arch, and proximal descending thoracic aorta. From the subcostal view, the proximal abdominal aorta is seen. Doppler flow velocities in the descending thoracic aorta can be recorded from the suprasternal notch and the subcostal views: there is a normal flow pattern for forward systolic ejection flow curve, with a peak velocity about 1 m/s, and then a brief early diastolic flow reversal, followed by low-velocity antegrade flow and brief reversal at end-diastole. Color Doppler imaging shows laminar systolic flow with a uniform color of flow away from the transducer (on suprasternal notch views) or toward the transducer (on subcostal views).

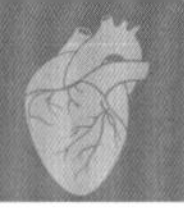

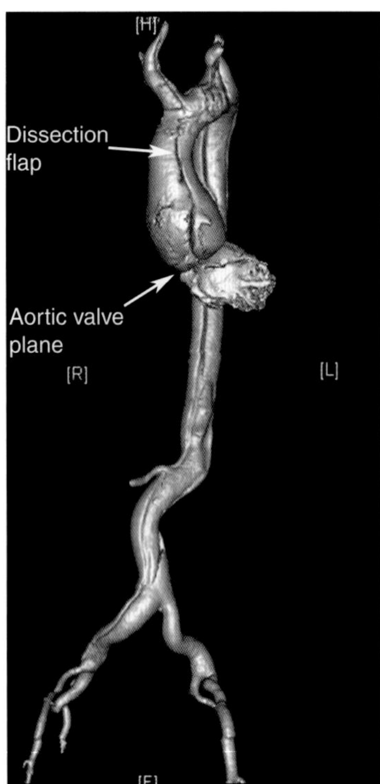

Fig. 32.6 3D reconstruction on computed tomographic imaging of the entire aorta in the same patient as Fig. 32.5. The 3D image can be rotated to view the aorta and dissection flap from different angles.

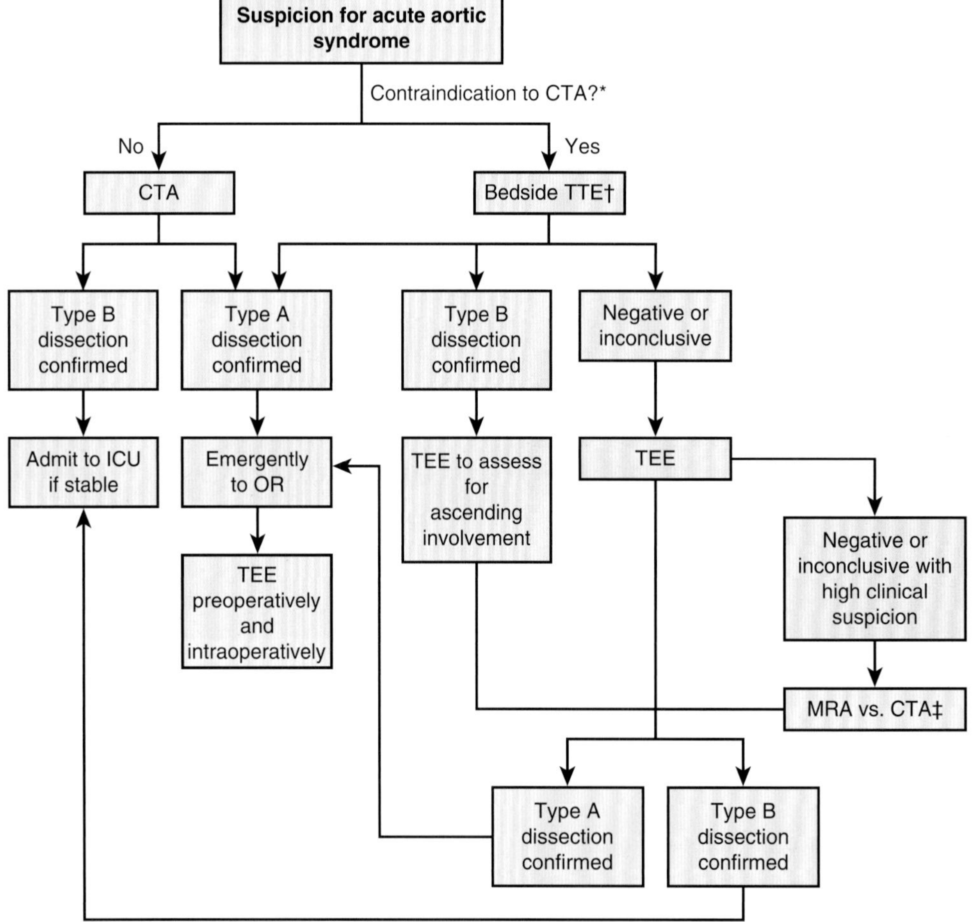

Fig. 32.7 Diagnostic imaging algorithm for suspected acute aortic syndrome. In patients with suspected acute aortic syndrome, computed tomographic angiography *(CTA)* is the imaging modality of choice. In patients who are at high risk for contrast-induced nephropathy or too unstable for a CTA *(asterisk)*, echocardiographic evaluation is appropriate. If TTE is rapidly available at the bedside *(dagger)*, it can be used to assess for a dissection while awaiting mobilization of TEE. Although a positive TTE result can prompt appropriate treatment, it is insufficient to exclude the diagnosis, and TEE should be performed if the TTE study is negative or inconclusive. For patients with very high suspicion and a negative TEE *(double dagger)*, magnetic resonance angiography *(MRA)* can be performed for those who are stable; if the patient is too unstable for MRA, CTA should be performed to confirm a negative TEE in consultation with the patient, even when a possible contraindication CTA exists. *ICU*, Intensive care unit; *OR*, operating room. (From Carroll BJ, Schermerhorn ML, Manning WJ. Imaging for acute aortic syndromes. *Heart.* 2020;106:182–189.)

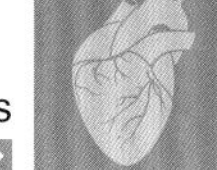

TABLE 32.3 Imaging Guidelines for Patients With a Clinical Presentation Suggesting Acute Aortic Syndrome.

Guideline	*AHA 2010*[6]	*ESC 2014*[16]
Acute Presentation		
Chest radiography	Chest radiography is indicated in patients with low to intermediate risk to evaluate alternative causes of symptoms or the need for prompt additional imaging (class I). A negative chest x-ray study should not delay definitive aortic imaging in high-risk patients (class III).	Chest radiography may be considered for low-risk patients (class IIb).
TTE	—	Recommended as the initial imaging investigation in patients with suspected acute aortic syndrome (class I)
Aortic imaging with TEE, CTA, or MRI	Urgent advanced imaging is recommended for all patients at high risk for aortic dissection (class I).	For unstable patients, TEE or CTA is recommended (class I).
	—	In stable patients, CTA, MRI (class 1), or TEE (class IIa) is recommended.
	A second imaging study should be obtained if initial imaging study is negative but clinical suspicion is high (class I).	A second imaging study should be obtained if initial imaging is negative but clinical suspicion is high (class I).
	—	CTA is recommended for diagnosis of traumatic aortic injury (class I) with TEE if CTA not available (class IIa).
	—	CTA is recommended for diagnosis of contained thoracic aortic rupture (class I).
Choicc of imaging modality	Imaging modality is based on patient variables, institutional capabilities, and immediate availability (class I).	Imaging modality is chosen based on local availability and expertise.
Intraoperative Study		
TEE	TEE monitoring is reasonable for all open surgical repairs and endovascular thoracic aortic procedures (class IIa).	—
Postprocedure Surveillance		
CT or MRI	Imaging of the thoracic aorta is reasonable after type A or B aortic dissection (class IIa).	—
Imaging interval	Imaging at 1, 3, 4, and 12 months after dissection is reasonable. Using the same modality at the same institution allows side-by-side comparison of images (class IIa).	—

AHA, American Heart Association; *ESC*, European Society of Cardiology.

TABLE 32.4 Studies Validating Imaging Diagnosis for Aortic Dissection

Study	*N*	*Approach*	*Sensitivity (%)*	*Specificity (%)*	*Prevalence of Dissection (%)*	*Standard of Reference* (n)
Victor et al., 1981[36]	42	TTE	80	96	36	Angiography
Erbel et al., 1987[37]	21	TTE	29	—	100	Surgery or angiography
		TEE	100			
Hashimoto et al., 1989[38]	22	TTE	71	—	100	Angiography (17) and/or surgery (12)
		TEE	100			
		CT	100			
Ballal et al., 1991[38]	61	TEE	97	100	56	Angiography, surgery, or autopsy
		CT	67	100		
Nienaber et al., 1992[40]	53	TTE	83	63	58	Surgery, autopsy, or angiography
		TEE	100	66		
		CMR	100	100		
Nienaber et al., 1993[41]	110	TTE	59	83	56	Surgery (62), autopsy (7), and/or angiography (64)
		TEE	98	98		
		CMR	98	87		
		CT	94	83		
Chirillo et al., 1994[42]	70	TEE	98	97	57	Surgery
Keren et al., 1996[43]	112	TEE	98	95	40	CT, CMR, aortography, surgery or autopsy
Evangelista et al., 1996[44]	13	TEE	99	100	49	Surgery, autopsy, and CMR
Silverman et al., 2000[45]	78	CMR	100	100	65	Surgery
Yoshida et al., 2003[46]	45	CT	100	100	78	Surgery
					Likelihood Ratio[a]	
Study	*N*	*Approach*	*Sensitivity (% and Range)*	*Specificity (% and Range)*	*Positive*	*Negative*
Shiga et al., 2006 (meta-analysis)[47]	1139	TEE	98 (95–99)	95 (92–97)	14.1 (6.0–33.2)	0.04 (0.02–0.08)
		CT	100 (96–100)	98 (87–99)	13.9 (4.2–46.0)	0.02 (0.01–0.11)
		CMR	98 (95–99)	98 (95–100)	25.3 (11.1–57.1)	0.05 (0.03–0.10)

[a]In most clinical settings, likelihood ratios > 10 (positive) or < 0.1 (negative) are considered, respectively, strong evidence for confirming or excluding a diagnosis.
CMR, Cardiac magnetic resonance imaging; *CT*, computed tomography.

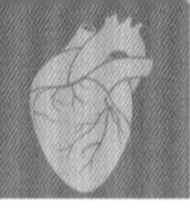

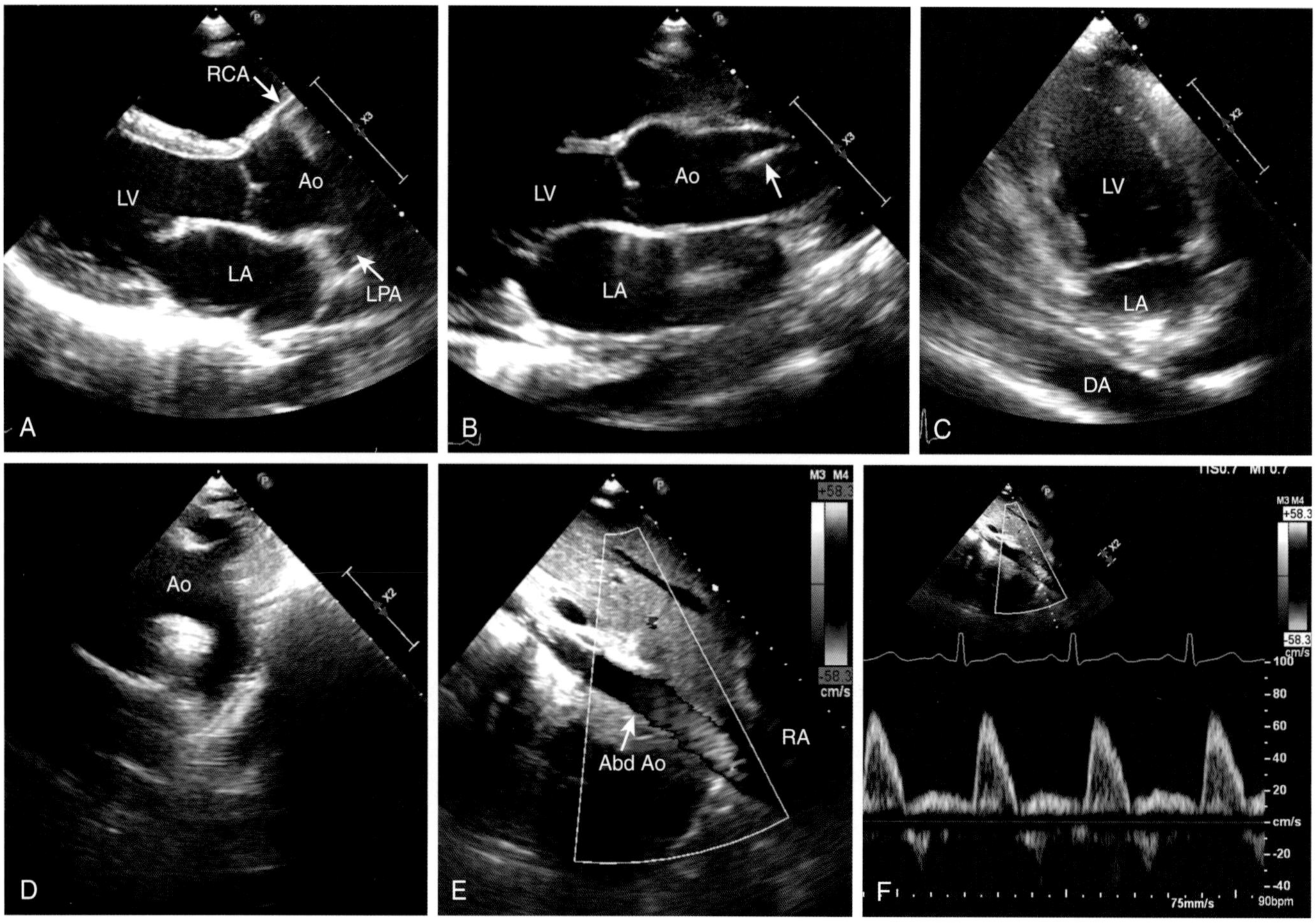

Fig. 32.8 TTE imaging of the aorta. The aortic sinuses are visualized in the standard parasternal long-axis view (A); the ascending aorta is seen by moving the transducer up an interspace (B). Linear artifacts *(arrow)* should not be mistaken for an intimal flap. The descending thoracic aorta *(DA)* is seen posterior to the LV in the apical 2-chamber view (C), the arch from the suprasternal notch window (D), and the proximal abdominal aorta from the subcostal window (E). Pulsed-wave Doppler imaging in the proximal abdominal aorta (F) shows an antegrade systolic ejection curve with brief reversal of flow at the beginning and end of diastole. *Abd*, Abdominal; *Ao*, aorta; *LPA*, left pulmonary artery; *RCA*, right coronary artery.

On TTE imaging, it is important to evaluate aortic valve anatomy and function using 2D and 3D imaging, color Doppler flow imaging, and continuous-wave Doppler velocity curves. For example, the presence of a bicuspid valve may provide an explanation for aortic dilation. In cases with a bicuspid or a trileaflet aortic valve, determining the degree and mechanism of aortic valve dysfunction is critical for surgical planning. For example, it may be possible to preserve an anatomically normal aortic valve if regurgitation is caused by aortic dilation resulting in stretched leaflets, whereas a flail aortic valve likely will require valve replacement. Additional standard elements of the TTE study include evaluation of LV size and systolic function, identification of any regional wall motion abnormalities, estimation of pulmonary systolic pressure, and detection of a pericardial effusion.

TEE imaging provides more complete visualization of the entire aorta with better image quality than TTE and has a higher sensitivity (98%) and specificity (95%) for the diagnosis of aortic dissection.[21] TEE can be performed at the bedside with sedation, but it may not be as quickly available as TTE or CT imaging at many medical centers. A small segment of the distal ascending aorta just before the arch may not be visualized, even by experienced operators. However, TEE is the modality of choice for evaluation of patients with acute aortic syndromes in the operating room at baseline and after surgical or thoracic endovascular aortic repair (TEVAR) procedures.

The aortic root and ascending aorta are visualized in a TEE long-axis view, initially with the aortic valve centered to evaluate leaflet anatomy and motion along with the anatomy and size of the sinuses and the sinotubular junction. Withdrawing the TEE probe slightly allows visualization of the middle and distal ascending aorta (Fig. 32.9). Short-axis views of the ascending aorta at each level are obtained by rotating the image plane to about 90 degrees. Color Doppler imaging in these views enhances identification of intimal flaps and helps distinguish artifact from pathology based on the associated flow pattern.

The aortic arch is seen in a high TEE long-axis view at about 0 degrees and in the short-axis view at about 90 degrees of rotation (Fig. 32.10). A simple way to obtain these views is to start with a view of the descending thoracic aorta in the short axis, withdraw the probe slowly until the proximal descending thoracic aorta is reached, and then turn the probe or image plane medially and inferiorly to visualize the arch and distal ascending aorta in the long axis. The short-axis view of the arch with the left subclavian artery take-off is seen in the orthogonal plane. These very high TEE views are best obtained in patients undergoing surgical procedures and may not be tolerated by patients receiving conscious sedation due to discomfort or a gag reflex.

The descending thoracic aorta is easily visualized in short-axis views by turning the probe posteriorly. The entire length

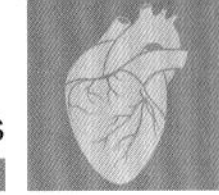

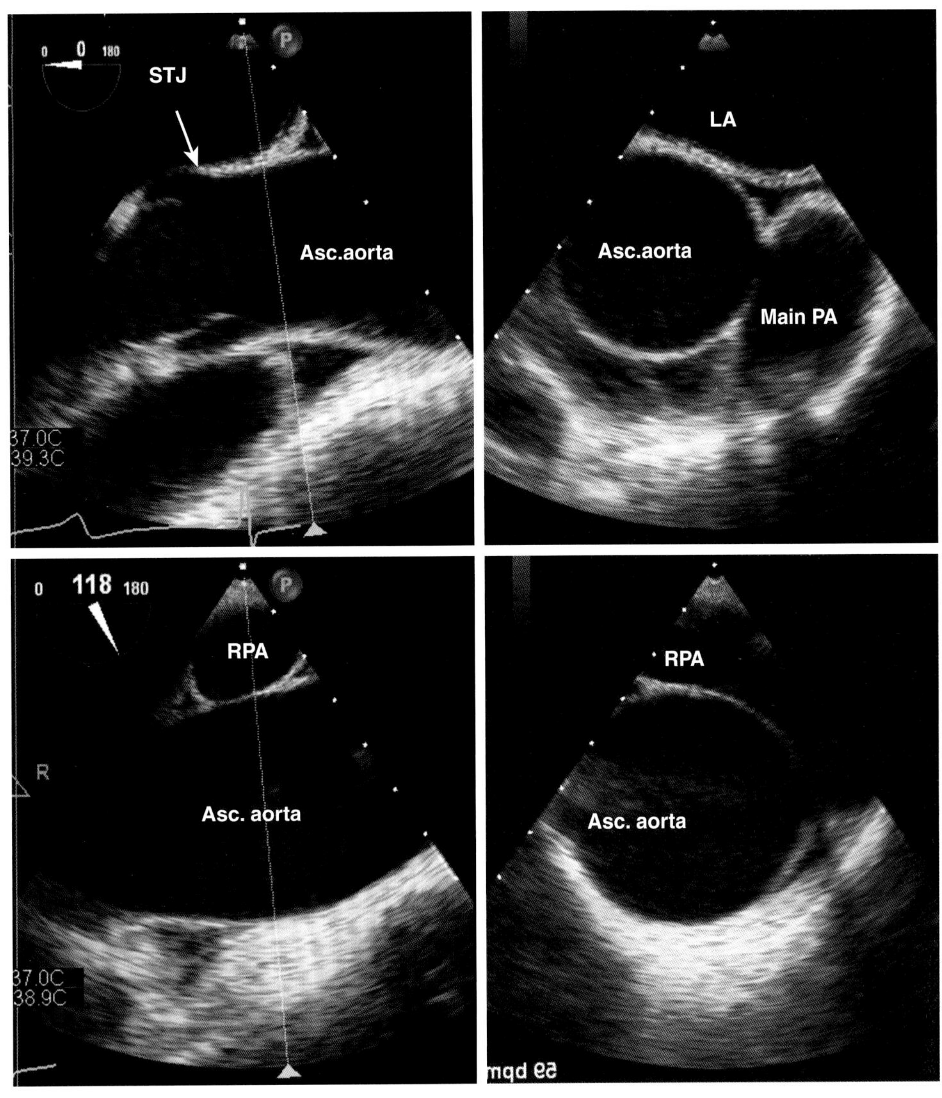

Fig. 32.9 TEE imaging of the ascending aorta. *Top row,* The ascending *(Asc.)* aorta can be seen in the mid-esophageal long-axis view. *Bottom row,* With slow withdrawal of the probe, the ascending aorta at the level of the right pulmonary artery *(PA)* often can be seen. *RPA,* Right pulmonary artery; *STJ,* sinotubular junction.

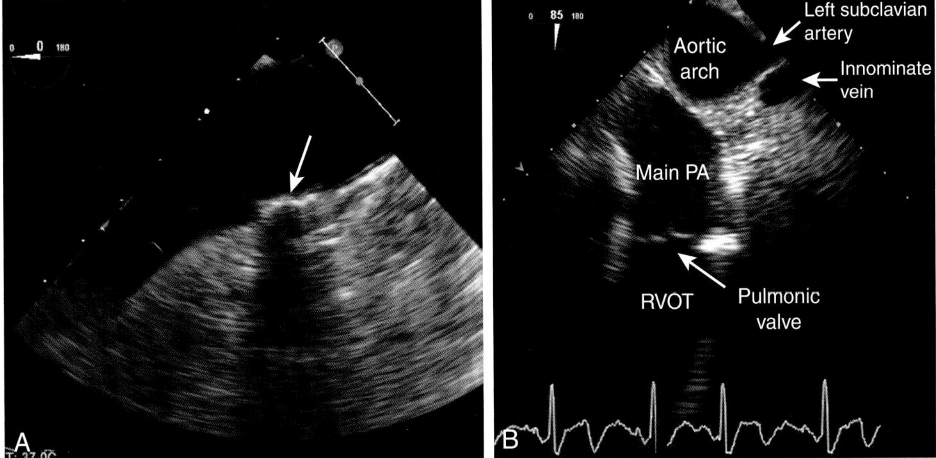

Fig. 32.10 TEE imaging of the aortic arch. (A) A long-axis view of the ascending aorta and arch is obtained from a high TEE position with the multiplane angle at 0 degrees. The *arrow* indicates an area of calcification in the aortic wall that leads to distal ultrasound dropout. *Right,* From the long-axis view of the descending aorta, the probe is withdrawn until the left subclavian artery is visualized. By turning the probe to the patient's right and increasing the depth setting, the pulmonary artery and pulmonic valve can be visualized. *RVOT,* Right ventricular outflow tract.

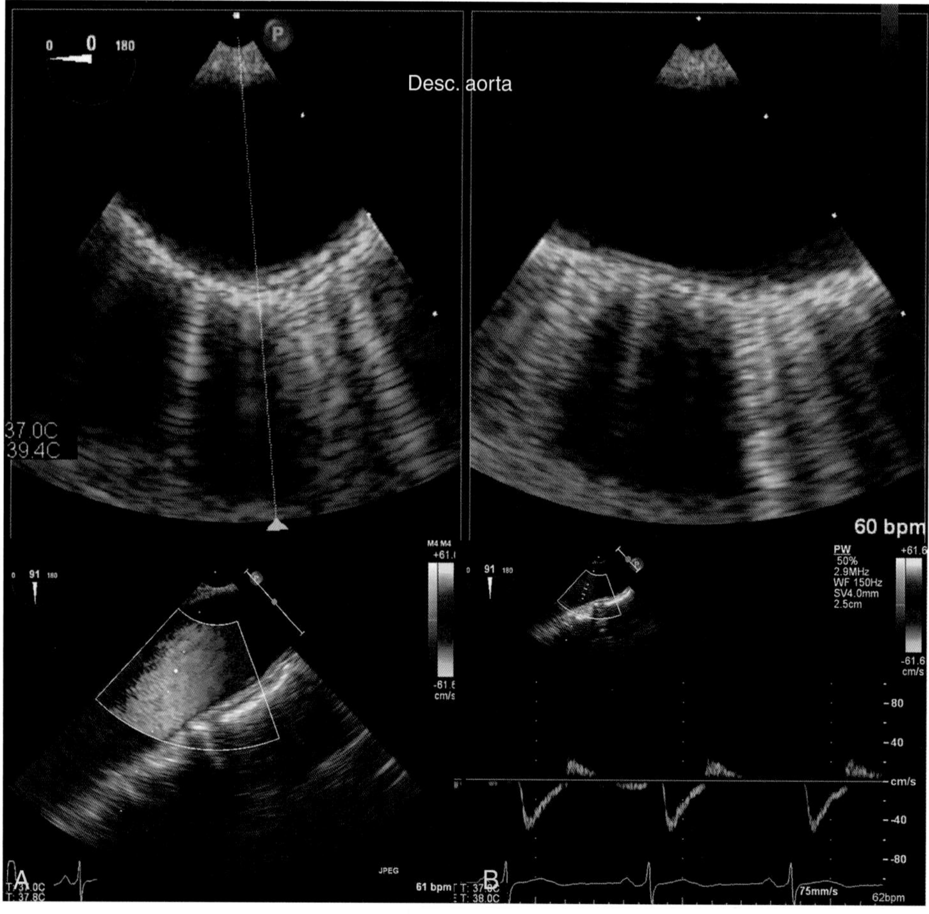

Fig. 32.11 **TEE view of descending thoracic aorta.** (A) With the TEE probe at the mid-esophageal level, by turning the probe posteriorly the descending *(Desc.)* aorta can be viewed in the long and short axis. (B) The probe is advanced distally to the point at which the angle of insonation is acceptable for Doppler interrogation. Aortic regurgitation can then be assessed.

of the descending aorta can be imaged in the short axis by advancing or withdrawing the probe, keeping the circular aorta centered in the image plane, or biplane imaging with a simultaneous long- and short-axis image can be recorded. In the long-axis view, color Doppler shows laminar flow, with pulsed-wave Doppler showing a normal arterial flow pattern (Fig. 32.11). Because the distal extent of imaging is limited to the length of the esophagus, more distal disease cannot be evaluated on TEE. Like TTE, imaging by TEE has limited utility for evaluation of branch vessels.

Acute Aortic Dissection

On TTE imaging, the most specific finding for a diagnosis of acute aortic syndrome is an enlarged aorta with an intimal flap and demonstration of flow in a true and a false lumen.[21,25] An intimal flap appears as a bright, thin, linear intraluminal structure with irregular, often undulating motion that does not parallel the motion of the aortic walls. Color Doppler shows flow on both sides of the intimal flap. Diagnosis is more challenging if the false lumen is thrombosed. Linear artifacts in the aortic lumen are common and are distinguished by moving with the aortic walls or not moving at all, by being seen only from one transducer position, and by color Doppler demonstration of an undisturbed flow pattern over the region of the artifact.

Nonspecific findings on TTE that should prompt advanced imaging include predisposing factors for dissection (e.g., bicuspid aortic valve, dilated aorta) and findings that may result from a complication of aortic dissection, such as new aortic valve regurgitation, a pericardial effusion, or regional wall motion abnormalities of the left ventricle (LV).

Point-of-care ultrasound has a low sensitivity (45%) for the diagnosis of an acute aortic syndrome when considering only the direct finding of an intimal flap, IMH, or penetrating ulcer.[27] However, if indirect findings on focused cardiac ultrasound (FoCUS) (i.e., aortic dilation, pericardial effusion, and AR) are included, sensitivity is much higher (89%), although specificity is low (75%).[26,27] Some investigators suggest that FoCUS has a role in the evaluation of patients at risk for an acute aortic syndrome, particularly if it is combined with a clinical risk score and measurement of serum D-dimer levels.[27,28]

Aortic dissection direct and indirect findings are better visualized on TEE, which shows the extent of the flap in more detail, particularly if there is involvement of the ascending aorta, and may show the entry site (Fig. 32.12). It is common to have multiple fenestrations between the true and false lumens with flow between the lumens seen on color Doppler imaging (Fig. 32.13).

Although imaging findings on TEE correlate well with those from other imaging modalities, most centers prefer CTA for evaluation of patients with a suspected acute aortic syndrome. CTA is widely available 24 hours a day, 7 days a week at most major medical centers, and imaging can be obtained rapidly because needed personnel are on duty in the medical center. The accuracy is very high, and CTA allows visualization of the entire aorta and branch vessels along with structures outside the

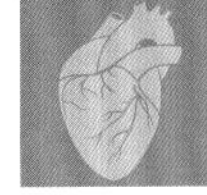

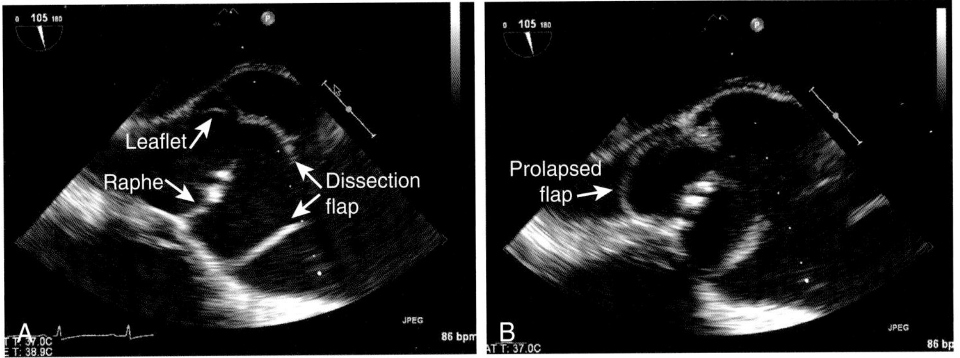

Fig. 32.12 Type A dissection in a patient with a bicuspid aortic valve. (A) A mobile linear intraluminal echodensity is seen in a TEE long-axis view. This is consistent with a dissection flap in systole, which prolapses into the LV outflow tract in diastole (B). Multiple imaging planes were used to differentiate the dissection flap from the bicuspid aortic valve leaflets, with a prominent raphe in the anterior leaflet.

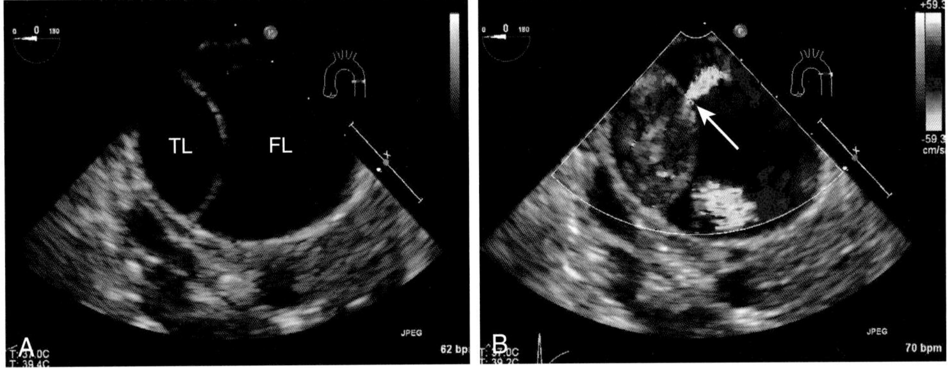

Fig. 32.13 TEE view of a descending aortic dissection. (A) A short-axis view of the descending thoracic aorta (A) shows the dissection flap bowing from the true lumen *(TL)* toward the false lumen *(FL)* in systole. (B) The flow through a small fenestration *(arrow)* from the TL to the FL is visible on color Doppler imaging (see Video 32.13).

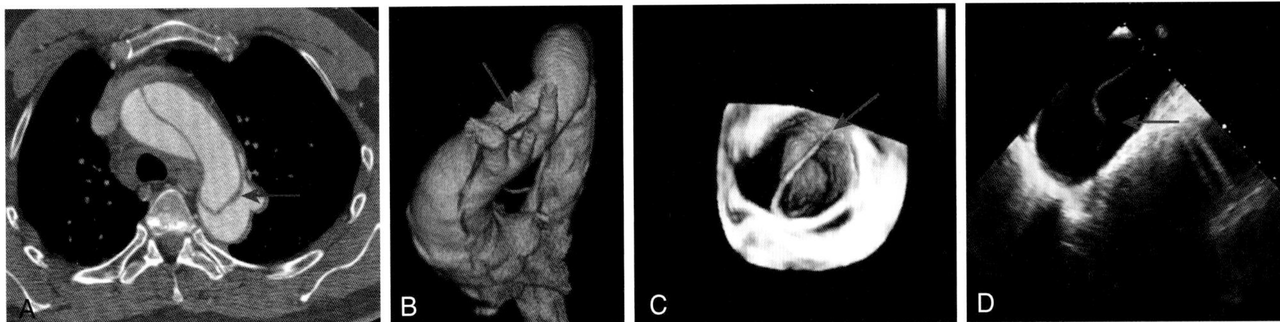

Fig. 32.14 Multimodality imaging of an aortic dissection. (A and B) Cardiac-gated contrast cross-sectional computed tomographic image demonstrates a prominent dissection flap *(arrow)* in the ascending aorta and arch that is well seen on the 3D reconstruction, allowing visualization of the full length of the aorta for surgical planning. (C and D) Intraoperative TEE shows the ascending aortic dissection flap *(arrow)* on 3D and 2D imaging (see Videos 32.14A and B).

aorta that may be involved by complications of aortic dissection (e.g., mediastinal hematoma, pleural effusion); it can also provide an alternative explanation for chest pain (e.g., pulmonary embolism) (Fig. 32.14).

Aortic Intramural Hematoma

Echocardiographic diagnosis of an aortic IMH is challenging. In short-axis views of the aorta, a crescent-shaped thickening of the aortic wall with a maximum diameter of 5 mm or more is diagnostic (Fig. 32.15). However, echocardiography primarily visualizes the aortic lumen; there is no intimal flap; intraluminal flow patterns are normal; and thickening of the aortic wall may not be appreciated.

A specific finding for IMH is displacement of intimal calcification due to the increased wall thickness, but this is better demonstrated by CT. The differential diagnosis for increased aortic wall thickening includes atherosclerotic changes or inflammatory aortic disease and IMH. Extraaortic tissues, such as adipose tissue or tumor, can be mistaken for the aortic wall on echocardiography, and they are better evaluated using a technique with a wide field of view, such as CT.

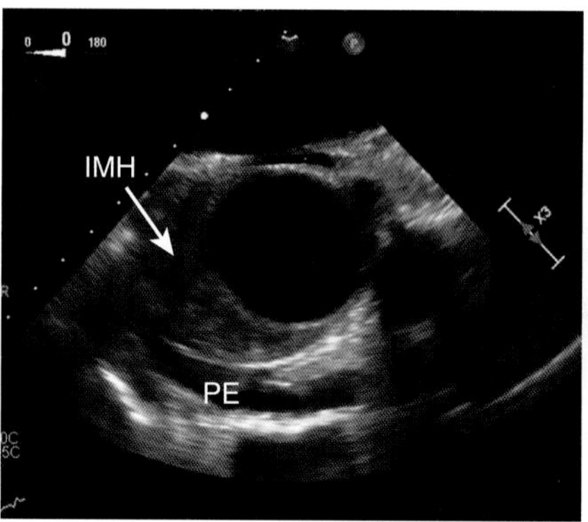

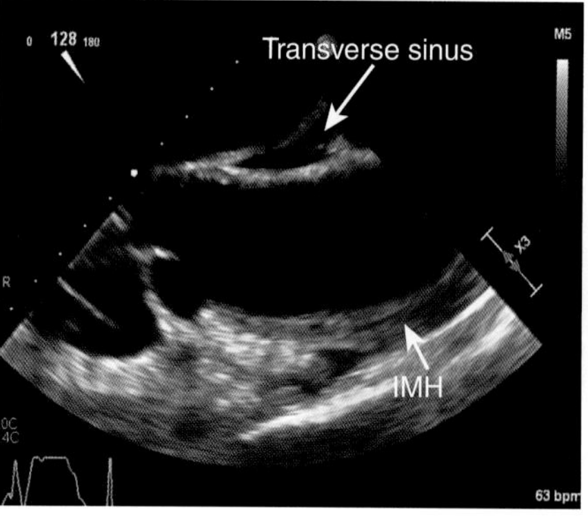

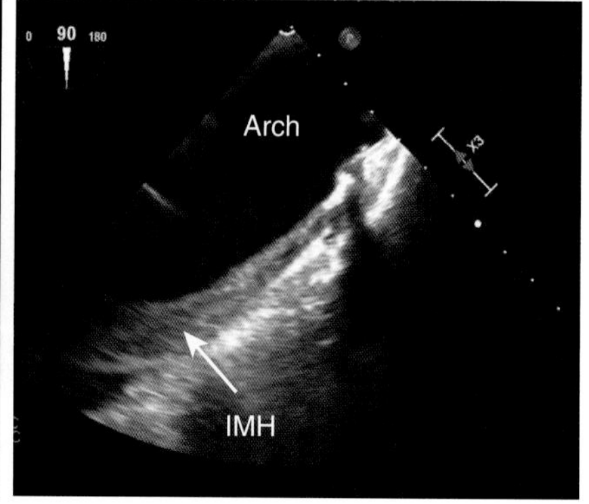

Fig. 32.15 Aortic intramural hematoma. An aortic intramural hematoma *(IMH)* appears as thickening of the aortic wall with a dimension greater than 5 mm, and not as two echo-lucent lumens. TEE short-axis views show the aortic root *(left)*, ascending aorta *(center)*, and arch *(right)*. A pericardial effusion *(PE)* extends into the transverse sinus of the pericardial space (see Video 32.15).

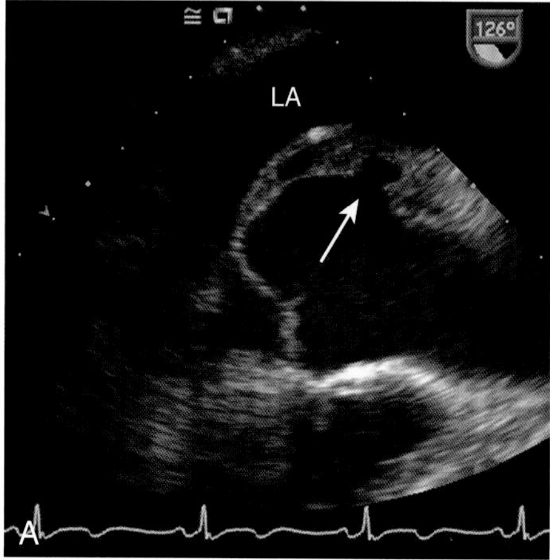

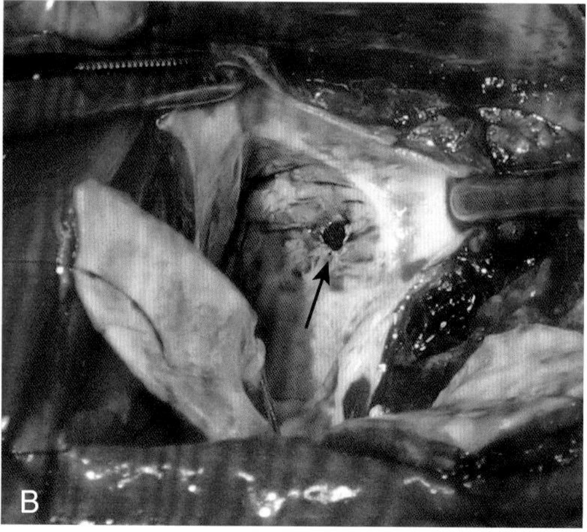

Fig. 32.16 Penetrating aortic ulcer. (A) The TEE long-axis view shows a discrete outpouching in the aortic lumen *(arrow)* surrounded by a localized intramural hematoma. Multiplane imaging was used to demonstrate that the normal coronary ostium was not being mistaken for a penetrating aortic ulcer (PAU). (B) The PAU was confirmed at surgery *(arrow)* (see Video 32.16).

Penetrating Aortic Ulcer

A penetrating aortic ulcer usually occurs in the setting of atherosclerotic changes and is typically seen in the arch or descending thoracic aorta. On echocardiographic imaging, the ulcer is a discrete outpouching in the aortic wall, often with a localized IMH but without an intimal flap or extension of the intramural thickening beyond the immediate region (Fig. 32.16). The edges of the ulcer may be irregular, and color Doppler shows flow into the outpouching. A normal branch vessel ostium should not be mistaken for a penetrating ulcer.

Traumatic Aortic Injury

Aortic injury due to blunt trauma is easily missed on TTE or TEE imaging because aortic disruption may not be evident on sequential tomographic views and 3D imaging has not been helpful in this situation (Fig. 32.17).[29] When an intimal flap is identified, the diagnosis is similar to that for other causes of aortic dissection. Iatrogenic aortic injury after surgery or a catheter-based procedure usually manifests as an aortic dissection with a typical intimal flap.[30–32]

DIAGNOSIS OF COMPLICATIONS BY ECHOCARDIOGRAPHY

In addition to direct diagnosis of an acute aortic syndrome, echocardiography has a key role in the diagnosis and evaluation of complications.

Aortic Regurgitation

Many patients with an acute aortic syndrome have had preexisting AR due to a bicuspid valve or chronic aortic dilation. However, new or worsening AR in a patient with chest pain raises concern about a possible acute aortic syndrome and should prompt further evaluation.

There are several potential mechanisms of AR in patients with an acute aortic syndrome. Aortic valve anatomy may be distorted by dilation of the aortic annulus, sinuses, or sinotubular junction with the aortic leaflets stretched across a larger orifice, resulting in non-coaptation at the center of the leaflets. As the leaflets are stretched, fenestrations or thin areas in the area of the leaflets that normally overlap may become weight bearing with localized leaflet rupture. Alternatively, aortic root dissection or IMH can extend directly into the aortic leaflet tissue with disruption of the commissural attachments and a flail valve leaflet (Figs. 32.18 and 32.19).

Coronary Artery Dissection

An aortic root dissection can extend into the coronary artery, resulting in myocardial ischemia that may be mistaken for an acute thrombotic coronary event (Fig. 32.20). The coronary dissection itself is unlikely to be imaged with TTE, and imaging is not always possible even with TEE, but it may be enhanced by 3D techniques in some cases.[33] However, the wall motion abnormality resulting from coronary ischemia can be easily and reliably detected by echocardiography.

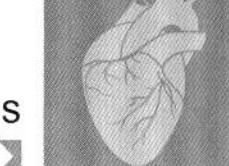

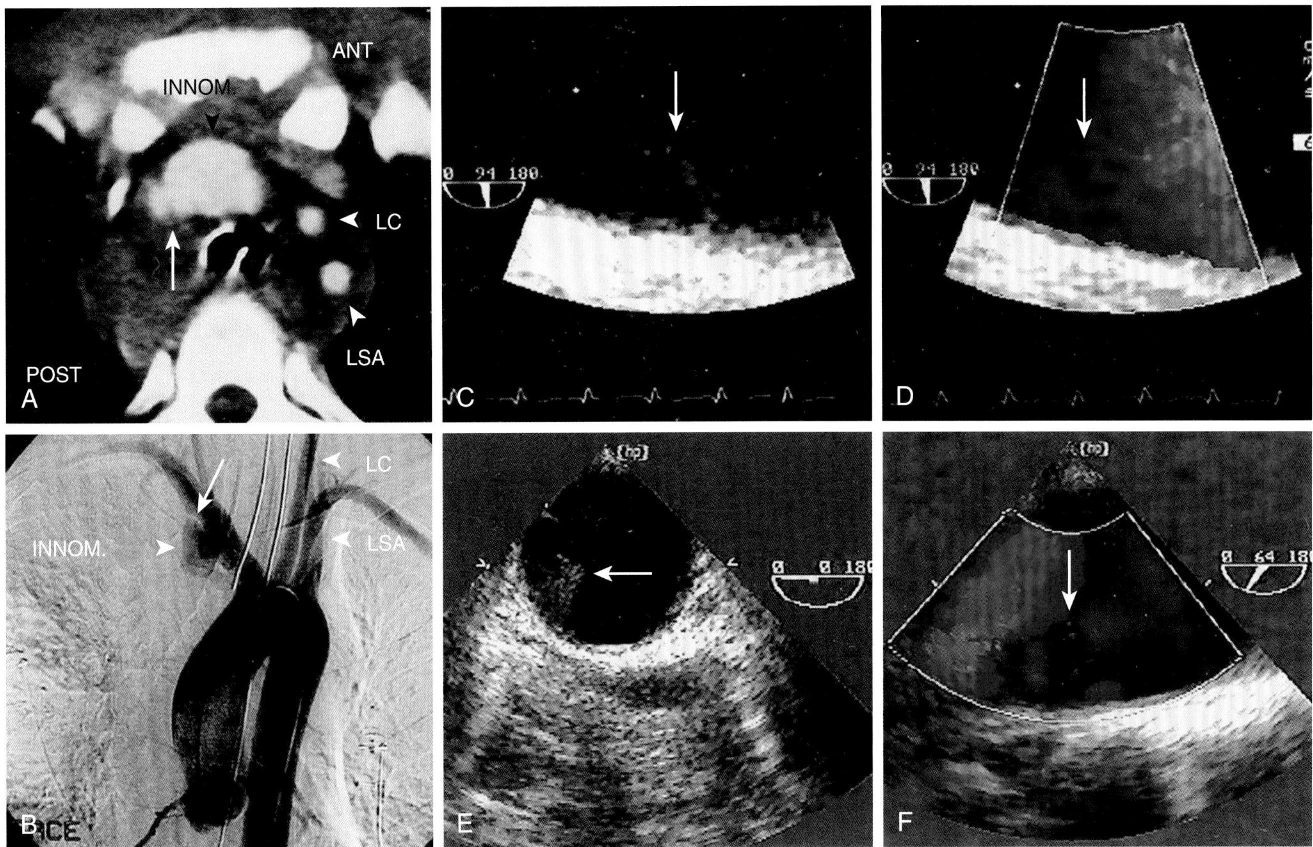

Fig. 32.17 **Traumatic aortic disruption.** Examples of traumatic disruption of the innominate artery (A and B) and superficial lesions of the aortic isthmus (C–F). (A) Helical computed tomography (CT) shows a laceration of the innominate artery *(arrow)* that was confirmed by angiography (B, *arrow*), whereas results of multiplane TEE were interpreted as normal. Conversely, TEE identified an aortic intimal tear (C and D, *arrows*) and mobile thrombi (E and F, *arrows*) that were not identified by chest CT. The superficial aortic lesions were too small to result in blood flow turbulence, as shown by color Doppler (D and F). *ANT*, Anterior; *INNOM*, innominate artery; *LC*, left common carotid artery; *LSA*, left subclavian artery; *POST*, posterior. (From Vignon P, Boncoeur MP, François B, et al. Comparison of multiplane transesophageal echocardiography and contrast-enhanced helical CT in the diagnosis of blunt traumatic cardiovascular injuries. *Anesthesiology.* 2001;94:615–622.)

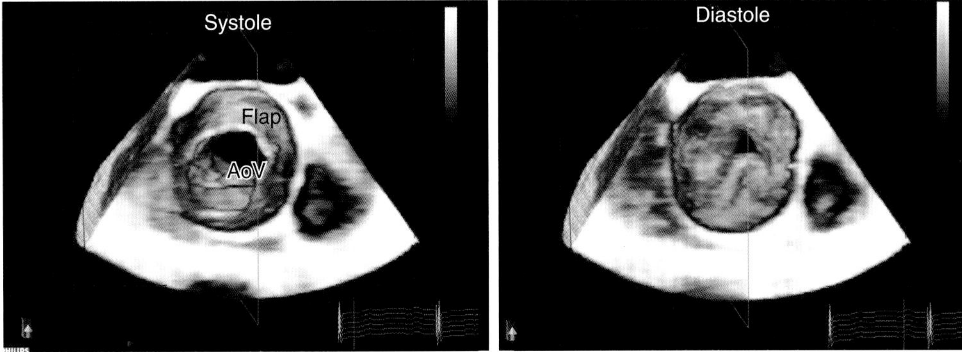

Fig. 32.18 **3D TEE of dissection flap in aortic sinuses.** For a dissection flap entry site very close to the aortic valve *(AoV)*, 3D imaging showed the relationship of the flap and valve leaflets. 3D imaging can also help to evaluate for extension of the flap into the coronary arteries. When the dissection is localized to the aortic root, the intimal flap may be mistaken for the valve leaflets by other imaging modalities. The rapid frame rates of TEE are useful for this distinction when CT images are not diagnostic (see Video 32.18).

Pericardial Effusion

Pericardial effusion is an ominous sign in patients with rupture of the dissection into the pericardial space (see Fig. 32.19). Tamponade physiology can occur with even a small effusion due to rapid accumulation of blood in the noncompliant pericardium. With a chronic effusion, the pericardium gradually expands as fluid accumulates, and tamponade physiology typically occurs with only a moderate to large effusion (see Chapter 17).

Distal Vessel Involvement

Distal vessel involvement with acute aortic syndrome cannot be reliably evaluated on echocardiographic imaging. Echocardiographers should be alert to simple physical examination findings, such as an absent peripheral pulse or different blood pressures in the right and left arms, and they should search more diligently for direct and indirect signs of an acute aortic syndrome in these patients. CT or direct angiography is preferred for evaluation of distal vessels in the acute setting.

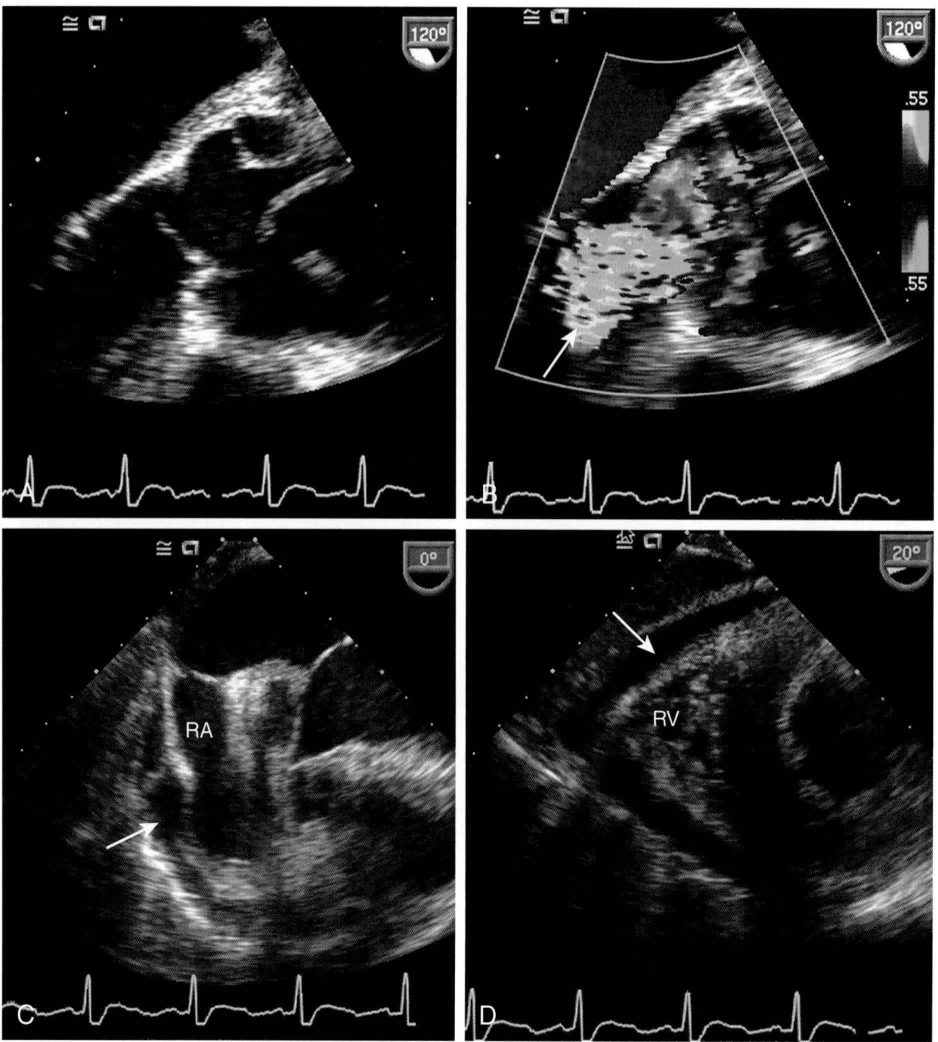

Fig. 32.19 Dissection with aortic regurgitation and pericardial tamponade. (A–B) In the same patient as in Fig. 32.18, severe aortic regurgitation *(arrow)* was caused by distortion of the valve and root anatomy (see Video 32.19A). (C–D) A pericardial effusion *(arrow)* is seen adjacent to the RA and RV, which indicated a possible early rupture into the pericardial space (see Videos 32.19C and 32.19D).

ECHOCARDIOGRAPHIC PROCEDURAL GUIDANCE

In patients undergoing intervention for an acute aortic syndrome, TEE done immediately before surgery assists in surgical planning (Table 32.5 and Fig. 32.21). The TEE study should first evaluate aortic anatomy, including vessel dimensions and the location and extent of the dissection flap. The degree of aortic root dilation determines whether replacement of the ascending aorta is appropriate or the aortic repair should also include the aortic sinuses.

Coronary artery involvement is most easily assessed by evaluation of LV regional and global systolic function in standard views of the LV. Imaging of the aortic valve is especially important for determining the number of valve leaflets, the mechanism of regurgitation, and the suitability of valve anatomy for a valve-sparing surgical approach.

IMAGING FOLLOW-UP AFTER AN ACUTE AORTIC SYNDROME

Several approaches are used for aortic repair in patients with a type A acute aortic syndrome. Accurate information about the exact procedure performed is needed for correct interpretation of the echocardiographic findings. In patients with a normal aortic root and normal valve function, the ascending aorta is replaced with a surgical fabric graft, sometimes with extension to the underside of the aortic arch (i.e., hemi-arch repair). The proximal end of the graft may be distal to the sinotubular junction, or it may be placed at the sinotubular junction with suturing of the aortic valve commissures to the graft to stabilize and align the aortic valve structures, preventing AR.[34] This type of valve-sparing procedure is often called *aortic valve resuspension* (Fig. 32.22). These patients have normal native sinuses and normal coronary artery ostia. In the future, some of these patients may be treated with a thoracic endovascular repair (TEVAR) approach rather than surgery.

In patients with a connective tissue disorder or dilated sinuses of unknown cause at the time of surgery, replacement of the entire aortic root along with stabilization of the aortic annulus and reimplantation of the coronary ostia is needed. In some patients with suitable valve anatomy and tissue, the aortic valve can be preserved and reimplanted inside the graft. This valve-sparing approach to root replacement, which was named after the surgeon who pioneered it, is called the *David procedure* or is generically referred to as *aortic valve reimplantation.*

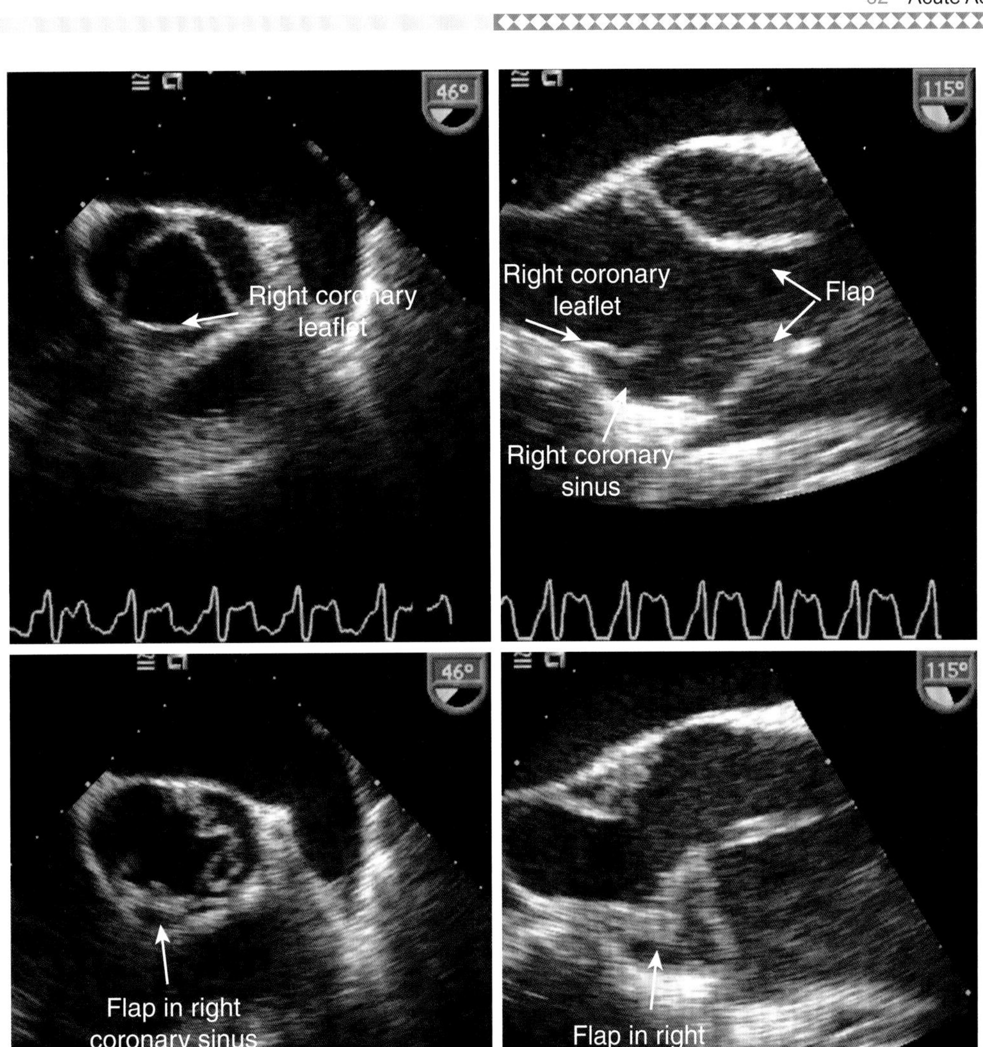

Fig. 32.20 Aortic dissection extending into the right coronary artery. *Top row,* In this patient with a trileaflet aortic valve, the intimal tear is close to the aortic valve leaflets. *Bottom row,* With the image plane moved cephalad and rightward, the flap is seen extending into the right coronary sinus (see Video 32.20).

Older aortic sinus grafts appeared to be tubular on echocardiographic imaging, but newer aortic root grafts are shaped more like native aortas, with sinuses visualized on follow-up imaging. When the aortic valve leaflet anatomy does not allow a valve-sparing procedure, a mechanical or bioprosthetic aortic valve is used inside the graft. This procedure is called a *Bentall procedure* or *conduit valve and root replacement*.

TEE imaging immediately after surgery for an acute aortic syndrome evaluates and documents aortic valve function, whether a reimplanted native valve or a prosthetic valve; images the aortic graft and any surrounding hematoma or postoperative changes; and assesses LV regional and global function. It also is prudent to image the distal aorta to serve as a future baseline (see Table 32.5).

Complications related to surgical repair for an acute aortic syndrome fall into three categories: (1) distal aortic or branch vessel disease, (2) native or prosthetic valve dysfunction, and (3) proximal coronary artery dilation due to the narrow ring of aortic tissue, often called the *aortic button*, needed for reimplantation of the coronary artery into the graft.

Periodic CTA or magnetic resonance angiography (MRA) of the entire aorta, from the valve to the bifurcation, is the standard approach for long-term follow-up. The frequency of imaging is based on surgical considerations and the underlying cause of aortic disease. These approaches also provide visualization of the coronary buttons. A persistent distal dissection flap is common, and chronic aortic disease is often managed by a team that includes specialists in cardiac surgery, cardiology, and vascular surgery.

The long-term roles of echocardiography include evaluation of aortic valve and LV function. The frequency of imaging depends on the type of valve, cause of disease, and concurrent cardiac conditions. On TTE, the distal dissection flap may be seen in the descending thoracic and proximal abdominal aorta, but it is better evaluated by CTA or MRA. TEE is not used routinely for acute aortic syndrome, but it may be useful to better visualize valve anatomy and function.

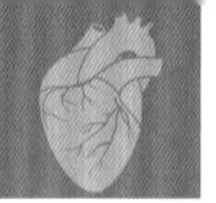

TABLE 32.5 Operative Uses of TEE in Cases of Aortic Dissection.

Assessment Before Cardiopulmonary Bypass

Aorta
- Intimal flap
  - Entry tear[a]
  - Intramural hematoma
  - Aortic rupture
  - Aortic pseudoaneurysm
  - Distal extent of extension
  - Additional tears
- False lumen flow patterns, including thrombus
- Branch vessel involvement[a]
  - Coronary situs and dissection
  - Involvement of origins of great vessels
- Underlying pathology
  - Atheromatous disease
  - Coarctation
  - Sites of previous repairs
- Cannulation and cross-clamp sites[a]

Aortic valve
- Regurgitation
- Suitability for repair versus replacement
- Sizing for allograft replacement

Mitral valve
- Regurgitation
- Suitability for repair versus replacement

LV and RV
- Wall motion abnormalities
- LV volumes and ejection fraction
- RV size and systolic function

Pericardium
- Effusion
- Signs of tamponade physiology

Assessment After Cardiopulmonary Bypass

Aorta
- Confirm competency of proximal anastomosis
- Establish baseline for false lumen flow and distal tears

Aortic valve
- Confirm competency of repaired or prosthetic valve

Mitral valve
- Confirm competency

LV and RV
- Wall motion abnormalities
- LV volumes and ejection fraction
- RV size and systolic function

[a]Epicardial and/or epiaortic scanning may be important in fully defining these features.

Modified from Bolger AF. Aortic dissection and trauma: value and limitations of echocardiography. In: Otto CM, ed. *Practice of Clinical Echocardiography*. 5th ed. Philadelphia: Elsevier; 2017:677–691.

TEE evaluation of aortic root for surgical planning

Sinotubular junction

- **Sinotubular junction dilation?**
  -ME AoV SAX, ME AoV LAX (biplane): Root measurement and focal sinus dilation
- **Proximal flap extension?**
  -ME AoV LAX (2D + 3D): Proximal extension of flap

Coronary arteries

- **Coronary artery involvement?**
  -LV chamber views (2D): Regional wall motion abnormalities
  -MV AoV SAX, ME AoV LAX (2D), MPR aortic root (3D): Coronary ostiaflap proximity/involvement

Aortic valve

- **Presence of aortic regurgitation?**
  -ME AoV LAX, ME AoV SAX (color Doppler): Regurgitation present, size, central vs. eccentric
- **Flap prolapse into LVOT?**
  -ME AoV LAX (2D): Location of flap in diastole
- **Leaflet prolapse?**
  -ME AoV SAX, ME AoV LAX (biplane): Leaflet tip location, coaptation integrity
  -En face of root and valve (3D): Circumferential extent of intimal dehiscence and AoV leaflet compromise

Fig. 32.21 TEE evaluation of the aortic root for surgical planning for type A dissections. A systematic approach should be followed to evaluate the aortic root, including location of the most proximal extent of the dissection and determination of coronary artery involvement and aortic valve integrity. Various views and use of biplane, 3D, and color Doppler are necessary for a full assessment. *AoV*, Aortic valve; *LAX*, long axis; *LVOT*, left ventricular outflow tract; *ME*, mid-esophageal; *MPR*, multiplane reconstruction; *SAX*, short axis. (From Carroll BJ, Schermerhorn ML, Manning WJ. Imaging for acute aortic syndromes. *Heart*. 2020;106:182–189.)

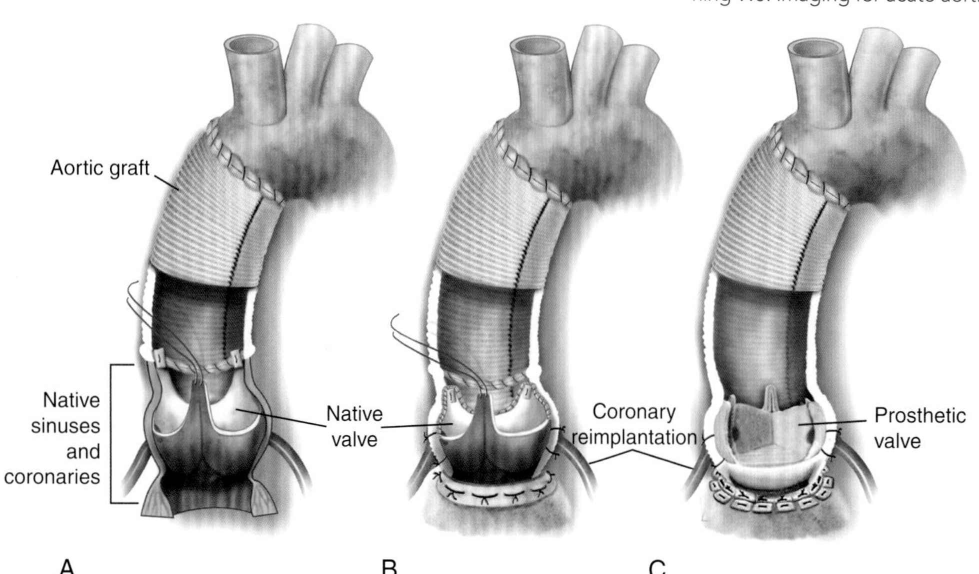

Fig. 32.22 Surgical procedures for an aortic dissection or aneurysm. (A) *Aortic valve resuspension* restores the aortic valve anatomy and function by attaching the three valve commissures to the ascending aortic graft. (B) *Aortic valve reimplantation (i.e., David procedure)* includes graft replacement of the aortic sinuses with reimplantation of the aortic valve and the coronary ostia in the sinus graft, which is then sutured to the ascending aortic graft. (C) *Aortic valve and root replacement (i.e., Bentall procedure)* uses a combined sinus graft for the sinuses, ascending aorta, and aortic prosthetic valve ((biologic or mechanical) with coronary reimplantation. (From Otto CM. *Textbook of Clinical Echocardiography*. 6th ed. Philadelphia: Elsevier; 2019.)

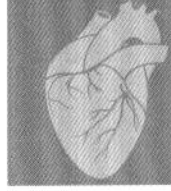

SUMMARY Echocardiographic Features of Acute Aortic Syndromes.[a]

TEE Feature	Dissection	Intramural Hematoma	Penetrating Aortic Ulcer	Traumatic Rupture
Intimal flap	Present	Absent	Absent	Medial rather than intimal flap may be seen.
Entry tear	Present	Absent	Absent	Present
Flow in a false lumen	Often present False lumen may fill with thrombus with elimination of visible flow.	Absent	Absent	Flow may be visible in the aortic wall outside the medial flap.
Coronary obstruction	May be present	Absent	Absent	Absent
Thrombus	In false lumen	In aortic wall	Surrounding ulcer	May protrude into the lumen or extend into the periadventitia
Pericardial effusion	May or may not represent acute extravasation TTE may be critical to assessment. Echocardiographic contrast may help assess acute extravasation. Tamponade physiology can occur with even a small effusion.	Absent	Absent	May or may not represent acute extravasation May be associated with other blunt thoracic trauma Tamponade physiology may exist with even a small effusion.
Aortic regurgitation severity and mechanism	Leaflet tear or flail Proximal aortic distortion Prolapse of an intimal flap	Absent	Absent	Valvular tear or dehiscence may be associated with other blunt thoracic trauma.
Branch vessel occlusion	May be present	Absent	Absent	May be present

[a]Clinically important associated findings: ventricular function, valvular competence, and other sources of chest pain or hemodynamic impairment.
Modified from Bolger AF. Aortic dissection and trauma: value and limitations of echocardiography. In: Otto CM, ed. *Practice of Clinical Echocardiography*. 5th ed. Philadelphia: Elsevier; 2017 :677–691.

REFERENCES

1. Salmasi MY, Al-Saadi N, Hartley P, et al. The risk of misdiagnosis in acute thoracic aortic dissection: a review of current guidelines. *Heart*. 2020;106:885–891.
2. LeMaire SA, Russell L. Epidemiology of thoracic aortic dissection. *Nat Rev Cardiol*. 2011;8:103–113.
3. Raghupathy A, Nienaber CA, Harris KM, et al. Geographic differences in clinical presentation, treatment, and outcomes in type A acute aortic dissection (from the International Registry of Acute Aortic Dissection). *Am J Cardiol*. 2008;102:1562–1566.
4. Chikwe J, Cavallaro P, Itagaki S, Seigerman M, Diluozzo G, Adams DH. National outcomes in acute aortic dissection: influence of surgeon and institutional volume on operative mortality. *Ann Thorac Surg*. 2013;95:1563–1569.
5. Tanaka Y, Sakata K, Sakurai Y, et al. Prevalence of type A acute aortic dissection in patients with out-of-hospital cardiopulmonary arrest. *Am J Cardiol*. 2016;117:1826–1830.
6. Hiratzka LF, Creager MA, Isselbacher EM, et al. Surgery for aortic dilatation in patients with bicuspid aortic valves: a Statement of Clarification from the American College of Cardiology/American Heart Association Task Force on Clinical Practice Guidelines. *J Am Coll Cardiol*. 2016;67:724–731.
7. Howard DP, Banerjee A, Fairhead JF, et al. Population-based study of incidence and outcome of acute aortic dissection and premorbid risk factor control: 10-year results from the Oxford Vascular Study. *Circulation*. 2013;127:2031–2037.
8. Olsson C, Thelin S, Stahle E, Ekbom A, Granath F. Thoracic aortic aneurysm and dissection: increasing prevalence and improved outcomes reported in a nationwide population-based study of more than 14,000 cases from 1987 to 2002. *Circulation*. 2006;114:2611–2618.
9. Meszaros I, Morocz J, Szlavi J, et al. Epidemiology and clinicopathology of aortic dissection. *Chest*. 2000;117:1271–1278.
10. Mussa FF, Horton JD, Moridzadeh R, Nicholson J, Trimarchi S, Eagle KA. Acute aortic dissection and intramural hematoma: a systematic review. *J Am Med Assoc*. 2016;316:754–763.
11. Pape LA, Awais M, Woznicki EM, et al. Presentation, diagnosis, and outcomes of acute aortic dissection: 17-year trends from the International Registry of Acute Aortic Dissection. *J Am Coll Cardiol*. 2015;66:350–358.
12. Hagan PG, Nienaber CA, Isselbacher EM, et al. The International Registry of Acute Aortic Dissection (IRAD): new insights into an old disease. *J Am Med Assoc*. 2000;283:897–903.
13. Dean JH, Woznicki EM, O'Gara P, et al. Cocaine-related aortic dissection: lessons from the International Registry of Acute Aortic Dissection. *Am J Med*. 2014;127:878–885.
14. Nathan DP, Boonn W, Lai E, et al. Presentation, complications, and natural history of penetrating atherosclerotic ulcer disease. *J Vasc Surg*. 2012;55:10–15.
15. Neri E, Toscano T, Papalia U, et al. Proximal aortic dissection with coronary malperfusion: presentation, management, and outcome. *J Thorac Cardiovasc Surg*. 2001;121:552–560.
16. Erbel R, Aboyans V, Boileau C, et al. 2014 ESC Guidelines on the diagnosis and treatment of aortic diseases: document covering acute and chronic aortic diseases of the thoracic and abdominal aorta of the adult. The Task Force for the Diagnosis and Treatment of Aortic Diseases of the European Society of Cardiology (ESC). *Eur Heart J*. 2014;35:2873–2926.

17. Chua M, Ibrahim I, Neo X, Sorokin V, Shen L, Ooi SB. Acute aortic dissection in the ED: risk factors and predictors for missed diagnosis. *Am J Emerg Med.* 2012;30:1622–1626.
18. Rogers AM, Hermann LK, Booher AM, et al. Sensitivity of the aortic dissection detection risk score, a novel guideline-based tool for identification of acute aortic dissection at initial presentation: results from the International Registry of Acute Aortic Dissection. *Circulation.* 2011;123:2213–2218.
19. Nazerian P, Mueller C, Soeiro AM, et al. Diagnostic accuracy of the aortic dissection detection risk score plus D-dimer for acute aortic syndromes: the ADvISED Prospective Multicenter study. *Circulation.* 2018;137:250–258.
20. Bhave NM, Nienaber CA, Clough RE, Eagle KA. Multimodality imaging of thoracic aortic diseases in adults. *JACC Cardiovasc Imaging.* 2018;11:902–919.
21. Carroll BJ, Schermerhorn ML, Manning WJ. Imaging for acute aortic syndromes. *Heart.* 2020;106:182–189.
22. Goldstein SA, Evangelista A, Abbara S, et al. Multimodality imaging of diseases of the thoracic aorta in adults: from the American Society of Echocardiography and the European Association of Cardiovascular Imaging: endorsed by the Society of Cardiovascular Computed Tomography and Society for Cardiovascular Magnetic Resonance. *J Am Soc Echocardiogr.* 2015;28:119–182.
23. Bossone E, LaBounty TM, Eagle KA. Acute aortic syndromes: diagnosis and management, an update. *Eur Heart J.* 2018;39:739–749d.
24. Evangelista A, Flachskampf FA, Erbel R, et al. Echocardiography in aortic diseases: EAE recommendations for clinical practice. *Eur J Echocardiogr.* 2010;11:645–658.
25. Evangelista A, Carro A, Moral S, et al. Imaging modalities for the early diagnosis of acute aortic syndrome. *Nat Rev Cardiol.* 2013;10:477–486.
26. Pare JR, Liu R, Moore CL, et al. Emergency physician focused cardiac ultrasound improves diagnosis of ascending aortic dissection. *Am J Emerg Med.* 2016;34:486–492.
27. Nazerian P, Mueller C, Vanni S, et al. Integration of transthoracic focused cardiac ultrasound in the diagnostic algorithm for suspected acute aortic syndromes. *Eur Heart J.* 2019;40:1952–1960.
28. Edvardsen T. Focused cardiac ultrasound examination is ready for use as a diagnostic tool of acute aortic syndromes in the emergency room. *Eur Heart J.* 2019;40:1961–1962.
29. Vignon P, Boncoeur MP, Francois B, Rambaud G, Maubon A, Gastinne H. Comparison of multiplane transesophageal echocardiography and contrast-enhanced helical CT in the diagnosis of blunt traumatic cardiovascular injuries. *Anesthesiology.* 2001;94:615–622. Discussion 5A.
30. Demetriades D. Blunt thoracic aortic injuries: crossing the rubicon. *J Am Coll Surg.* 2012;214:247–259.
31. Gosavi S, Tyroch AH, Mukherjee D. Cardiac trauma. *Angiology.* 2016;67:896–901.
32. Fogleman L, Caffery T, Gruner J, Tatum D. Thoracic aortic transection resulting in a type B dissection following blunt trauma. *BMJ Case Rep.* 2017;2017. https://doi.org/10.1136/bcr-2016-218766.
33. Sasaki S, Watanabe H, Shibayama K, et al. Three-dimensional transesophageal echocardiographic evaluation of coronary involvement in patients with acute type A aortic dissection. *J Am Soc Echocardiogr.* 2013;26:837–845.
34. David TE. Aortic valve sparing in different aortic valve and aortic root conditions. *J Am Coll Cardiol.* 2016;68:654–664.
35. Kohn MA, Kwan E, Gupta M, Tabas JA. Prevalence of acute myocardial infarction and other serious diagnoses in patients presenting to an urban emergency department with chest pain. *J Emerg Med.* 2005;29:383–390.
36. Victor MF, Mintz GS, Kotler MN, et al. Two dimensional echocardiographic diagnosis of aortic dissection. *Am J Cardiol.* 1981;48:1155–1159.
37. Erbel R, Börner N, Steller D, et al. Detection of aortic dissection by transoesophageal echocardiography. *Br Heart J.* 1987;58:45–51.
38. Hashimoto S, Kumada T, Osakada G, et al. Assessment of transesophageal Doppler echography in dissecting aortic aneurysm. *J Am Coll Cardiol.* 1989;14:1253–1262.
39. Ballal RS, Nanda NC, Gatewood R, et al. Usefulness of transesophageal echocardiography in assessment of aortic dissection. *Circulation.* 1991;84:1903–1914.
40. Nienaber CA, Spielmann RP, von Kodolitsch Y, et al. Diagnosis of thoracic aortic dissection. Magnetic resonance imaging versus transesophageal echocardiography. *Circulation.* 1992;85:434–447.
41. Nienaber CA, von Kodolitsch Y, Nicolas V, et al. The diagnosis of thoracic aortic dissection by noninvasive imaging procedures. *N Engl J Med.* 1993;328:1–9.
42. Chirillo F, Cavallini C, Longhini C, et al. Comparative diagnostic value of transesophageal echocardiography and retrograde aortography in the evaluation of thoracic aortic dissection. *Am J Cardiol.* 1994;74:590–595.
43. Keren A, Kim CB, Hu BS, et al. Accuracy of biplane and multiplane transesophageal echocardiography in diagnosis of typical acute aortic dissection and intramural hematoma. *J Am Coll Cardiol.* 1996;28:627–636.
44. Evangelista A, Garcia-del-Castillo H, Gonzalez-Alujas T, et al. Diagnosis of ascending aortic dissection by transesophageal echocardiography: utility of M-mode in recognizing artifacts. *J Am Coll Cardiol.* 1996;27:102–107.
45. Silverman JM, Raissi S, Tyszka JM, et al. Phase-contrast cine MR angiography detection of thoracic aortic dissection. *Int J Card Imaging.* 2000;16:461–470.
46. Yoshida S, Akiba H, Tamakawa M, et al. Thoracic involvement of type A aortic dissection and intramural hematoma: diagnostic accuracy—comparison of emergency helical CT and surgical findings. *Radiology.* 2003;228:430–435.
47. Shiga T, Wajima Z, Apfel CC, et al. Diagnostic accuracy of transesophageal echocardiography, helical computed tomography, and magnetic resonance imaging for suspected thoracic aortic dissection: systematic review and meta-analysis. *Arch Intern Med.* 2006;10(166):1350–1356.

中文导读

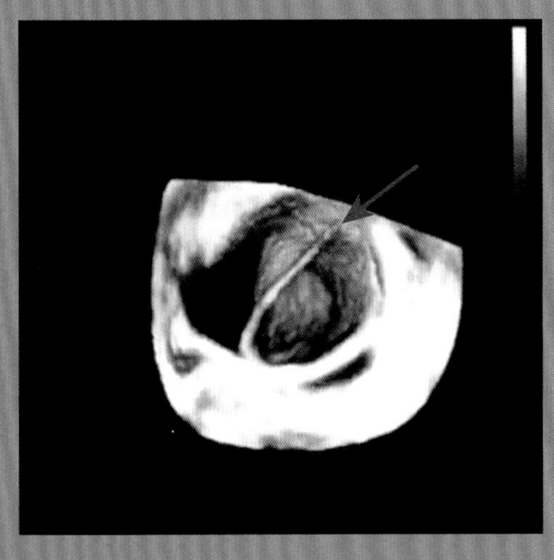

第33章 遗传性结缔组织疾病

结缔组织疾病主要包括马方综合征、Loeys-Dietz综合征、Ehlers-Danlos综合征、家族性胸主动脉瘤和夹层、主动脉二瓣化畸形和特纳综合征，其可累及全身多器官，其中心血管系统相关并发症最需关注，病理改变主要局限于二尖瓣、主动脉瓣和主动脉。主动脉的主要组织病理学改变为管壁弹性蛋白纤维断裂和丢失、平滑肌细胞丢失、胶原蛋白增加和蛋白多糖沉积。

超声心动图作为主要诊断方式，可显示主动脉扩张、主动脉夹层、主动脉弓降部并发症及二尖瓣脱垂，同时可对左心室收缩和舒张功能进行评估。由于该类患者存在出现主动脉并发症的风险，应根据主动脉大小、增长速度等进行连续监测。该类疾病治疗策略主要包括药物治疗，用以减少主动脉壁的结构变化，延迟主动脉扩张和后期的夹层或破裂；手术治疗，用以修复病变的主动脉。使用标准二维超声心动图可以评估遗传性结缔组织疾病瓣膜形态及主动脉大小，但仍存在一定局限性。目前已出现了替代诊断方法，如MRI、CT，可以对其进行更全面的评估。

本章主要介绍了遗传性结缔组织疾病的常见类型、组织病理、超声心动图表现、自然病程、治疗策略、评估方法及其局限性，以及替代诊断方法。

张　冰

33 Inherited Connective Tissue Disorders

ANDREW CHENG, MD | JONATHAN BUBER, MD

FORMS OF CONNECTIVE TISSUE DISORDERS

Connective tissue disorders can affect multiple organs, but the most feared sequelae are complications associated with the cardiovascular system. Although there is potential for left and right heart involvement, clinically important pathology is typically confined to the mitral valve, the aortic valve, and the aorta itself.

In contrast to other forms of cardiovascular disease, many patients first come to medical attention because of findings associated with the musculoskeletal system, lungs, or eyes. Cardiovascular pathology may be identified on screening cardiac assessment resulting from a defined or suspected connective tissue disorder in another family member.

Echocardiography is the mainstay of cardiac screening for the cardiac manifestations of connective tissue disorders. As in many other cardiac disorders, transesophageal echocardiography (TEE) complements transthoracic echocardiography (TTE) in diagnostic evaluation. Other noninvasive imaging modalities (i.e., computed tomography [CT] and magnetic resonance imaging [MRI]) contribute to diagnosis in selected circumstances. Marfan syndrome (MFS) is the most common connective tissue disorder leading to cardiovascular compromise, but other inherited and congenital conditions affect cardiac structures in similar ways (Table 33.1). Many of these conditions are described in this chapter. The spectrum of disease, therapeutic strategies, and methods of assessment are highlighted.

MARFAN SYNDROME

MFS is a well-described heritable connective tissue disorder with a broad phenotypic spectrum. Its prevalence is 1 case in 3000 to 5000 individuals, irrespective of gender or ethnicity. Mutations in the *FBN1* gene (locus 15q21.1), which encodes the extracellular matrix protein fibrillin-1, cause the disease. Major clinical manifestations are seen in the cardiovascular, ocular, and skeletal systems.

The diagnosis is based on the Ghent nosology, which was revised by an international expert panel in 2010[1] (Tables 33.2 and 33.3). The revised criteria place increased importance on the cardinal clinical features of aortic root dilation/dissection and ectopia lentis and on genetic test findings in the absence of a family history.

MFS is inherited in an autosomal dominant manner; 25% of patients have sporadic, new mutations without a family history. After an individual is diagnosed with MFS, first-degree relatives should be screened for the condition by physical examination, accompanied by ophthalmologic assessment and echocardiography if clinically appropriate. With advances in molecular genetic testing, a causative mutation in the *FBN1* gene can be found in more than 90% of individuals fulfilling the clinical diagnostic criteria for MFS.[2]

Over the past 25 years, more than 3000 *FBN1* mutations have been described. Despite a considerable effort to identify genotype-phenotype correlations for MFS, few definitive correlations have emerged,[2] and so far none have been specific enough to define clinical management. Of the identified associations, patients with the most severe phenotype (also called the *infantile Marfan syndrome*) harbor *FBN1* mutations in the central portion of the gene, between exons 24 and 32.[3–5] In contrast, mutations in *FBN1* that produce milder disease forms have included mutations in the C-terminus region, which result in only the skeletal manifestations of MFS.[6] Mutations in exons 59 to 65[7] and in exons 1 to 10[8] have been associated with phenotypes lacking significant aortic involvement or with only late-onset and relatively mild cardiovascular features. Researchers have also determined that the mutation type—one causing haploinsufficiency (resulting in less fibrillin protein) versus one with a dominant-negative effect (incorporating normal and mutated forms of fibrillin-1 in the extracellular matrix)—may affect clinical outcomes. Patients with haploinsufficiency have larger baseline aortic diameters, more rapid aortic growth, and higher risk of death and dissection.[9]

Approximately 60% to 80% of adult patients with MFS develop aortic root dilation, with a higher prevalence among

TABLE 33.1 Inherited and Congenital Disorders Associated With Aortic Dilation and/or Mitral Valve Prolapse.

- Marfan syndrome
- Loeys-Dietz syndrome
- Ehlers-Danlos syndrome
- Homocystinuria
- Familial thoracic aortic aneurysm and dissection (familial TAAD)
- MASS phenotype (i.e., mitral valve prolapse, aortic enlargement, skin and skeletal findings)
- Bicuspid aortic valve
- Coarctation of the aorta
- Mitral valve prolapse syndrome
- Turner syndrome
- Osteogenesis imperfecta

TABLE 33.2 Revised Ghent Criteria for the Diagnosis of Marfan Syndrome.

In the setting of a family history, any of the following make the diagnosis of MFS:

- Ectopia lentis
- Systemic score ≥7
- Aortic diameter at the sinus of Valsalva Z ≥ 2 for patients older than 20 years or Z ≥ 3 for those younger than 20 years

In the absence of family history and without discriminating features of another connective tissue disorder, any of the following make the diagnosis of MFS:

- Aortic diameter at the sinus of Valsalva (Z ≥ 2) and ectopia lentis
- Aortic diameter at the sinus of Valsalva (Z ≥ 2 for patients older than 20 years or Z ≥ 3 for those younger than 20 years) and *FBN1 (Fibrillin-1)* mutation
- Aortic diameter at the sinus of Valsalva (Z ≥ 2) and systemic score (≥7)
- Ectopia lentis and *FBN1* mutation with known aortic dilation

MFS, Marfan syndrome.
From Loeys BL, et al. The revised Ghent nosology for the Marfan syndrome. *J Med Genet.* 2010;47(7):476–485.

males. The mean rate of growth in the ascending aorta or root is 0.26 cm ± 0.05 cm/year, with annual rates up to 0.46 cm in individuals with an aneurysm larger than 6.0 cm.[10] One study followed individuals with initial normal aortic dimensions in the National Registry of Genetically Triggered Thoracic Aortic Aneurysms and Cardiovascular Conditions (GenTAC registry). Bicuspid aortic valve (BAV) (39%) and MFS (22%) were the leading diagnoses among participants. Over a 3-year period, the aortic dissection rate was 1.6%; 61% of the dissections occurred in individuals with MFS. The cumulative incidence of aortic dissection was sixfold higher among patients with MFS (4.5%) compared with other conditions. including BAV, for which the incidence was only 0.3%.[11]

Outcomes in patients with MFS have improved over the past decade, coinciding with surgical advancements. Since the emergence of composite graft aortic root surgery in the mid-1970s, life expectancy has almost doubled.[12] The mainstay of treatment is careful surveillance with echocardiography and other imaging modalities and elective aortic repair.

OTHER FIBRILLINOPATHIES

FBN1 mutations have been reported in distinct phenotypes that overlap with MFS but do not confer the high risk of aortic complications. They include mitral valve prolapse (MVP)

TABLE 33.3 Systemic Score in Marfan Syndrome.

Feature	*Score*
Wrist and thumb sign	3
Wrist or thumb sign	1
Pectus carinatum deformity	2
Pectus excavatum or chest asymmetry	1
Hindfoot deformity	2
Plain pes planus	1
Pneumothorax	2
Dural ectasia	2
Protrusio acetabuli	2
Reduced upper segment/lower segment ratio and increased arm/height ratio and no severe scoliosis	1
Reduced elbow extension	1
Scoliosis or thoracolumbar kyphosis	1
Facial feature (3/5: dolichocephaly, exophthalmos, downslanting palpebral fissures, malar hypoplasia, retrognathia)	1
Skin striae	1
Myopia >3 diopters	1
Mitral valve prolapse	1

syndrome, the MASS phenotype (*M*VP, borderline *a*ortic enlargement, nonspecific *s*kin and *s*keletal signs, and myopia), isolated ectopia lentis, and stiff skin syndrome.[13] Together, MFS and the Marfan-related phenotypes have been called *type 1 fibrillinopathies.*

Congenital contractural arachnodactyly (CCA, also known as Beals syndrome), another connective tissue disorder similar to MFS, is caused by fibrillin-2 gene (*FBN2*) mutations. It can be difficult to differentiate between these two syndromes because of the similar skeletal complications, including arachnodactyly, pectus deformities, and scoliosis. CCA usually manifests with multiple joint contractures and crumpled ear helices.[14]

LOEYS-DIETZ SYNDROME

Loeys-Dietz syndrome (LDS) is an autosomal dominant connective tissue disease associated with arterial aneurysms and dissections and with other systemic involvements.[15,16] LDS is characterized by the clinical triad of arterial tortuosity and aneurysms, hypertelorism, and bifid uvula or cleft palate. Aneurysms occur in the aortic root, but unlike in MFS, they are also commonly found in other arteries. The arterial tortuosity most commonly affects the head and neck vessels. Aortic dissection can occur at diameters smaller than those observed in MFS.

LDS is associated with deregulation in transforming growth factor-β (TGF-β) signaling; it is divided into six subtypes based on the pathologic gene variant (Table 33.4),[17] all of which encode proteins involved in the TGF-β signaling pathway. There is considerable overlap among the subtypes, and they are considered part of the same clinical continuum.

Specific diagnostic criteria for LDS have not been established. Typically, the diagnosis is rendered when a patient has findings for some of the commonly affected organ systems in addition to identification of a disease-causing mutation on genetic testing. The five main groups of clinical findings are vascular, skeletal, craniofacial, ocular, and cutaneous (Table 33.5). An important distinguishing feature between LDS and MFS is the lack of ectopia lentis in LDS.[17]

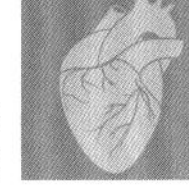

TABLE 33.4 Loeys-Dietz Syndrome Classification.

LDS Subtype	*Gene*	*Proportion (%)*
LDS type 1	*TGFBR1*	20–25
LDS type 2	*TGFBR2*	55–60
LDS type 3	*SMAD3*	5–10
LDS type 4	*TGFB2*	5–10
LDS type 5	*TGFB3*	1–5
LDS type 6	*SMAD2*	1–5

LDS, Loeys-Dietz syndrome.

We recommend genetic testing for LDS-associated gene mutations in patients with aortic root dilation and any suggestive clinical features, in patients who have had aortic dissection at diameters less than 5 cm without another identified causative condition, and in families in which multiple members have aortic or other arterial dilation. Some patients with aortic dilation and dissection have mutations in *TGF-β* pathway genes without physical features of LDS. These patients fall in the category of thoracic aortic aneurysms and dissections (discussed later).

The most important complication in LDS is aortic root dilation and dissection. The mean age at death in original case series was 26 years.[15] Almost all patients had aortic root aneurysms that led to dissection. Dissection can occur at aortic dimensions that are not considered high risk in MFS (<5.0 cm); dissections have been reported in infancy and early childhood. Approximately one half of patients with LDS have dilation or tortuosity in the arterial tree away from the aortic root, and these vascular features differentiate the vascular disease in LDS from that of MFS. These distal lesions are not detected by echocardiography. Additional cardiac malformations include patent ductus arteriosus, atrial septal defects, MVP, and BAV.

TABLE 33.5 Clinical Features of Loeys-Dietz Syndrome.

Vascular

- Aortic root dilation and dissection
- Arterial aneurysms and tortuosity affecting the head, neck, lung, lower extremities, and thoracic and abdominal aorta
- Dissection of the coronary artery, internal iliac, and superior mesenteric artery
- Cerebral hemorrhage
- Congenital abnormalities including bicuspid aortic valve, patent ductus arteriosus, and atrial septal defect

Skeletal Manifestations

- Pectus excavatum or carinatum
- Pes planus
- Scoliosis/kyphosis/symmetry of the costosternal junction and cervical spine malformation or instability
- Joint laxity/hypermobility
- Osteoporosis
- Arachnodactyly
- Talipes equinovarus

Craniofacial Features

- Ocular hypertelorism
- Bifid uvula (or uvula with a wide base or prominent ridge)
- Cleft palate
- Craniosynostosis

Cutaneous Features

- Translucent skin
- Easy bruising
- Dystrophic scars
- Striae atrophica

Ocular Features

- Blue sclerae
- Strabismus
- Retinal detachment
- Amblyopia, myopia

EHLERS-DANLOS SYNDROME

Ehlers-Danlos syndrome (EDS) is a heterogeneous group of hereditary connective tissue disorders characterized by joint hypermobility, skin hyperextensibility, and tissue fragility. It is marked by pathologic variants encoding collagen or collagen-modifying genes. Initially, EDS was categorized in six subtypes, but in 2017, classification of EDS was expanded to 13 subtypes based on clinical findings, inheritance patterns, and molecular defects. The estimated prevalence of EDS is 1 case in 5000 to 25,000 persons.[18] The classic and hypermobile forms account for more than 90% of EDS cases (involving hyperextensibility, fragile "cigarette paper" skin, scoliosis, and hernias). Between one fourth and one third of individuals with classic and hypermobile types of EDS have aortic dilation, but usually only to a mild degree. Aortic dissection is rare in the absence of significant preexisting dilation.[17]

Vascular EDS, which is considered the most malignant form of EDS given the increased susceptibility to spontaneous vascular dissection, represents less than 5% of cases.[17] Inheritance is autosomal dominant and involves the type III collagen gene *(COL3A1)*. The median age at death is 51 years. Large vessel dissections can involve the aorta, but the cerebral and abdominal large arteries are also at risk.[19]

The sites of arterial rupture are the thorax and abdomen (50%), head and neck (25%), and extremities (25%). Uncommonly, the vascular type of EDS is a cause of stroke in young adults. The mean age at intracranial aneurysmal rupture, spontaneous carotid-cavernous sinus fistula, or cervical artery aneurysm is 28 years.[20] Hyperelastic tissues and hyperextensible joints are less common manifestations, but easy bruising, poor wound healing, and rupture of the gastrointestinal tract are commonly seen.

There is no consensus regarding appropriate cardiovascular screening for patients with EDS. It is reasonable to obtain surveillance aortic imaging at least every 3 to 5 years for patients with vascular EDS and more frequently if there is evidence of aortic dilation. Mitral valve disease and aortic insufficiency may also exist. However, the fragile nature of the large vessels in the vascular form of EDS increases surgical morbidity and mortality rates. It is unclear whether early prophylactic repair of unruptured aneurysms in vascular EDS should be pursued.[21]

FAMILIAL THORACIC AORTIC ANEURYSM AND DISSECTION

Nonsyndromic familial thoracic aortic aneurysm and dissection (familial TAAD) is characterized by defects of the aorta without associated outward physical manifestations. The diagnosis of familial TAAD is based on progressive enlargement of the ascending aorta, positive family history of TAAD, and exclusion of syndromic causes of TAAD such as MFS, LDS, and EDS. Only 30% of patients with nonsyndromic TAAD have an

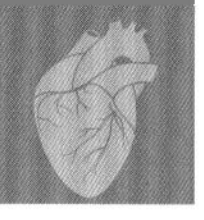

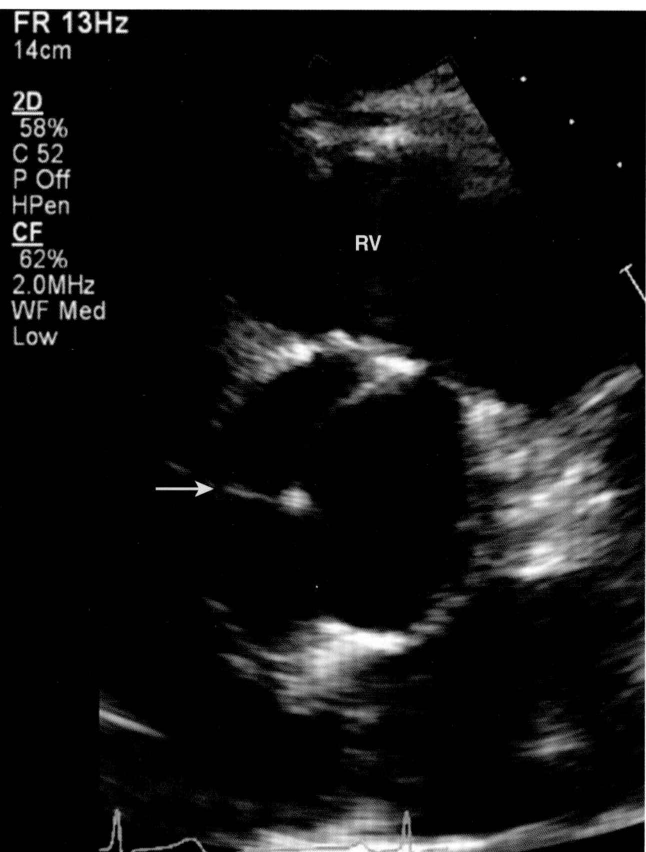

Fig. 33.1 Echocardiographic imaging of bicuspid aortic valve. Bicuspid aortic valve in parasternal short-axis view obtained from a 31-year-old patient. Notice the fish-mouth opening of the bicuspid valve with a raphe between the right and the left commissures *(arrow)* (see Video 33.1).

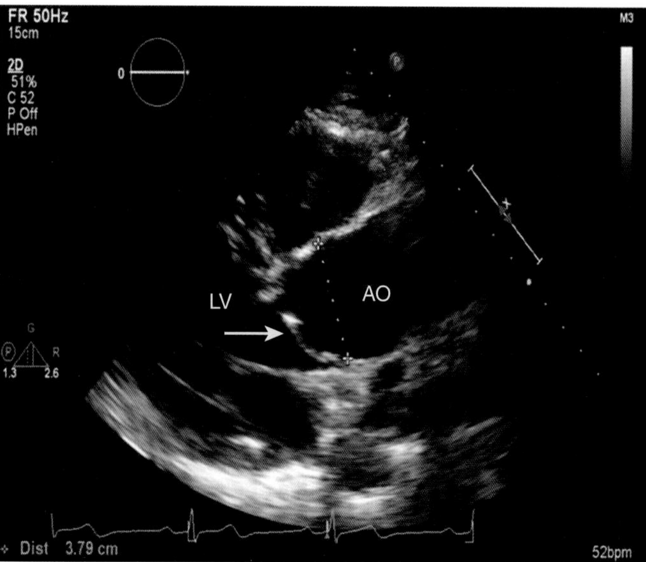

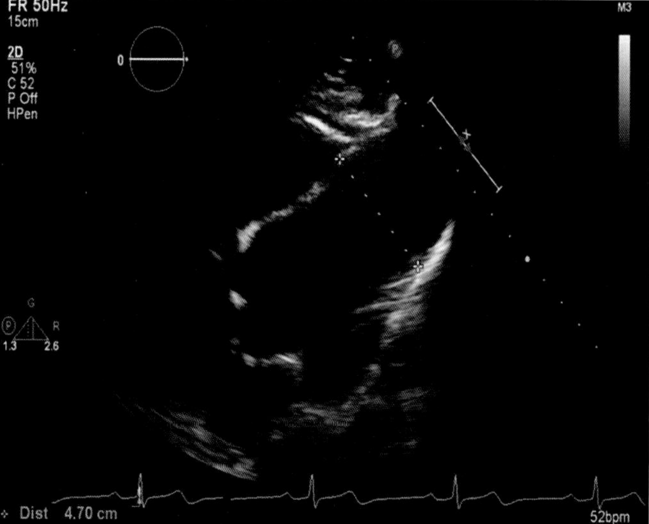

Fig. 33.2 Enlarged aorta with bicuspid aortic valve. Mildly dilated aortic root (3.8 cm, *top*) and more dilated ascending aorta (4.7 cm, *bottom*) in the same patient shown in Fig. 33.1. Notice the eccentric aortic valve leaflet closure *(arrow)* (see Videos 33.2A and 33.2B). *AO*, Aorta.

identified gene mutation, but new gene associations are discovered regularly. Most of the identified pathogenic mutations involve genes in the TGF-β pathway (i.e., *TGFBR1*, *TGFBR2*, *TGFB2* ligand, *TGFB3* ligand, *SMAD3*, and *SMAD6*) or genes involved in smooth muscle cell function: smooth muscle cell–specific myosin heavy chain 11 (*MYH11*), smooth muscle–specific alpha actin (*ACTA2*), myosin light chain kinase (*MYLK*), and cyclic guanosine monophosphate (cGMP)–dependent protein kinase 1 (*PRKG1*).[22]

Patients with familial TAAD typically come to medical attention earlier than patients with spontaneous dissections or dilation but later than those with MFS or LDS. As in LDS, dissections have been reported at smaller aortic dimensions than is typical for MFS.

BICUSPID AORTIC VALVE

BAV is the most common congenital heart disorder, affecting approximately 1% to 2% of the population with a 2:1 to 3:1 male to female ratio.[23] BAV is a heritable trait. Family studies report the prevalence of BAV in first-degree relatives of an individual with BAV to be 9% to 10%.[24,25] The inheritance of BAV is consistent with an autosomal dominant pattern with reduced penetrance.[24] Monozygotic twins do not necessarily both have BAV, highlighting the incomplete penetrance of this disorder.

The genetic causes of BAV remain elusive. Mutations in *NOTCH1* are associated with BAV and may result in aortic aneurysms and early aortic calcification.[23] Mutations in other single genes, such as *ACTA2*, *TGFB2*, *GATA5*, *NKX2-5*, and *SMAD6*, have been associated with BAV.[26] In most patients, no specific genetic variant is discovered. BAV is also prevalent among genetic conditions such as DiGeorge syndrome, LDS, Anderson syndrome (*KCNJ2* mutation), Turner syndrome, and complex congenital heart disease such as the Shone complex and hypoplastic left heart syndrome.[26,27]

Patients with a BAV are at increased risk for aortic aneurysm (Fig. 33.1). More than one half of those with BAV will have aortic enlargement greater than 2 standard deviations above the norm by 30 years of age. Compared with controls, patients who have a BAV have larger aortic annulus, sinus, and ascending aortic dimensions, even after adjusting for age, valvular lesions, and hypertension (Fig. 33.2).

Histologic examination shows pathologic changes in the aortic wall, including decreased fibrillin-1, loss of elastic fibers, increased apoptosis, and altered smooth muscle cell alignment.[28] There is uncertainty regarding the cause of BAV aortopathy, but genetic and hemodynamic contributions have been implicated.

Aortic dilation is greater in patients with aortic regurgitation than in those with stenotic or functionally normal BAVs.[23,29] However, dilation of the aorta (which can involve the root to the arch) frequently accompanies BAV even in the absence of aortic stenosis or aortic regurgitation. First-degree relatives of BAV patients who have a tricuspid aortic valve tend to have larger aortas than the control population, suggesting an inherited phenotype.[30] However, cardiac MRI flow patterns have revealed distinct aortic dilation patterns based on the variation in laminar blood flow and increased wall stress, underscoring the importance of flow hemodynamics.[31]

The rate of aortic growth among patients with BAV ranges from 0.2 to 2.3 mm/year and varies based on age, underlying valve disease (aortic regurgitation versus stenosis), location of the dilation, baseline aortic diameter, family history, and leaflet morphology.[32–34] The risk of aortic dissection in BAV populations is unclear. In historic necropsy studies, dissections were found in 6% to 15% of subjects with BAV.[35] Studies have shown that the absolute lifetime risk of aortic dissection for a BAV patient followed with routine surveillance imaging is quite low, with an incidence of 3.1 per 10,000 patient-years, and it depends most significantly on the size of the aorta and the patient's age.[36–39] Dissection rates are similar or only slightly higher than those for patients with a tricuspid valve but comparably sized aneurysms.[34,40] Some studies have reported that individuals with BAV experience dissection at larger dimensions than their counterparts with tricuspid aortic valve (62 vs. 53 mm).[41] The increased risk of aortic dissection in patients with a BAV seems limited to a small subset of the overall BAV population. We speculate that for this subsegment of the population, the concomitant finding of a BAV and aortic aneurysm and dissection indicates genetic underpinnings and is a manifestation of a systemic connective tissue disorder.

TURNER SYNDROME

Patients with Turner syndrome are at high risk for left heart pathology, particularly BAV and coarctation of the aorta.[42] Those with Turner syndrome have a higher incidence of systemic hypertension (even in the absence of anatomic cardiac pathology). Generalized vasculopathy in those with Turner syndrome is well described and is characterized by aortic wall stiffness, arterial dilation, vessel wall thickening, and abnormal pulse wave propagation.[43] Aortic dissection occurs in approximately 1.4% of patients with Turner syndrome,[44] and dissection often occurs at a young age (mean, 30 years).[45] Between 80% and 90% of those with aortic dissection have systemic hypertension or a BAV.

Criteria with which to assign risk have been difficult to ascertain, particularly because most criteria are based on somatic growth (i.e., height, weight, and body surface area). Patients with Turner syndrome have short stature, and the relationship between somatic growth and expected aortic dimension remains problematic. For this reason, the definition of normal aortic size, especially in light of the potentially confounding factors (i.e., hypertension, BAV, and coarctation of the aorta), is unclear. The American and European guidelines recommend indexing aortic dimensions to body surface area.[21] Whether the general adult guidelines for the prediction of heightened risk for aortic dissection can translate to adults with Turner syndrome remains undetermined. The relative aortic dimensions guiding when aggressive pharmacologic and/or surgical intervention should be instituted are unclear.

Study results on aortic size and growth rates in Turner syndrome have varied over the years. A cross-sectional study of girls younger than 18 years of age revealed that even in the absence of a BAV, Turner syndrome patients had a larger aorta at the levels of the aortic root, sinotubular junction, and ascending aorta, suggesting that Turner syndrome alone predicts aortic dilation. The effect of a BAV added incrementally to this independent effect.[46] However, a prospective cardiac MRI study showed no differences in absolute or indexed aortic growth rates between patients with Turner syndrome and age-matched heathy female controls at the aortic root and proximal aorta. There was larger variation in the Turner population, and the finding of BAV and coarctation was associated with accelerated growth rates.[47]

Nevertheless, aortic complications are more numerous in the Turner population. In a study that followed 198 Turner syndrome patients over a 23-year period, 9 suffered aortic dissection, a 12-fold increase compared with the general female population. Dissection risk was associated with aortic dilation, diagnosis of hypertension, BAV, and coarctation.[48]

Questions regarding aortic dilation and dissection risk in the setting of Turner syndrome remain. Better understanding of the relationship between dilation and dissection in this population will enable development of better treatment protocols.

HISTOPATHOLOGY

The fibrous structures of the heart are composed primarily of connective tissue proteins. These serve as a framework to support the contractile myocardial tissue. Connective tissue also supports the underlying structure of the large blood vessels and valves. Collagen and elastin fibrils underlie the endocardial cells of the heart and blood vessels. Type I collagen fiber bundles make up the support structure for the atrioventricular valves and constitute the primary elements of the valvular fibrous rings. The major structural support of the large blood vessels is elastin and collagen types I and III; lesser amounts of types IV, V, and VI collagen also contribute to vessel wall integrity.

The aorta comprises three layers: the intima, the media, and the adventitia. The medial layer consists of concentric layers of smooth muscle cells, collagen, and elastin with extracellular matrix proteoglycans. In connective tissue disorders such as MFS and in BAV, degenerative changes of the aorta result from disruption and loss of elastin fibers, loss of smooth muscle cells, increased collagen, and deposition of proteoglycans.

This process has historically been referred to as cystic medial necrosis. However, because there is no true necrosis or cyst formation, the preferred term is *medial degeneration*. Molecular studies have identified some mechanisms potentially underlying this process. Increased levels of matrix metalloproteinases (MMPs), particularly MMP-2 and MMP-9, that have elastolytic activity have been found in the medial layer of aortic aneurysms[34,49,50] (Fig. 33.3).

ECHOCARDIOGRAPHIC FINDINGS

NORMAL AORTIC MEASUREMENTS

The aorta is made up of five components, including the aortic root, the tubular portion of the ascending aorta, the aortic arch, the descending thoracic aorta, and the abdominal aorta. The aortic root consists of the aortic valve annulus, the sinus of Valsalva, the sinotubular junction, and the ascending aorta. By convention, echocardiographic measurements of these regions are performed from the parasternal long-axis view at early systole

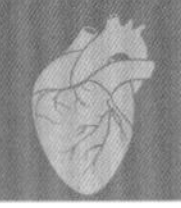

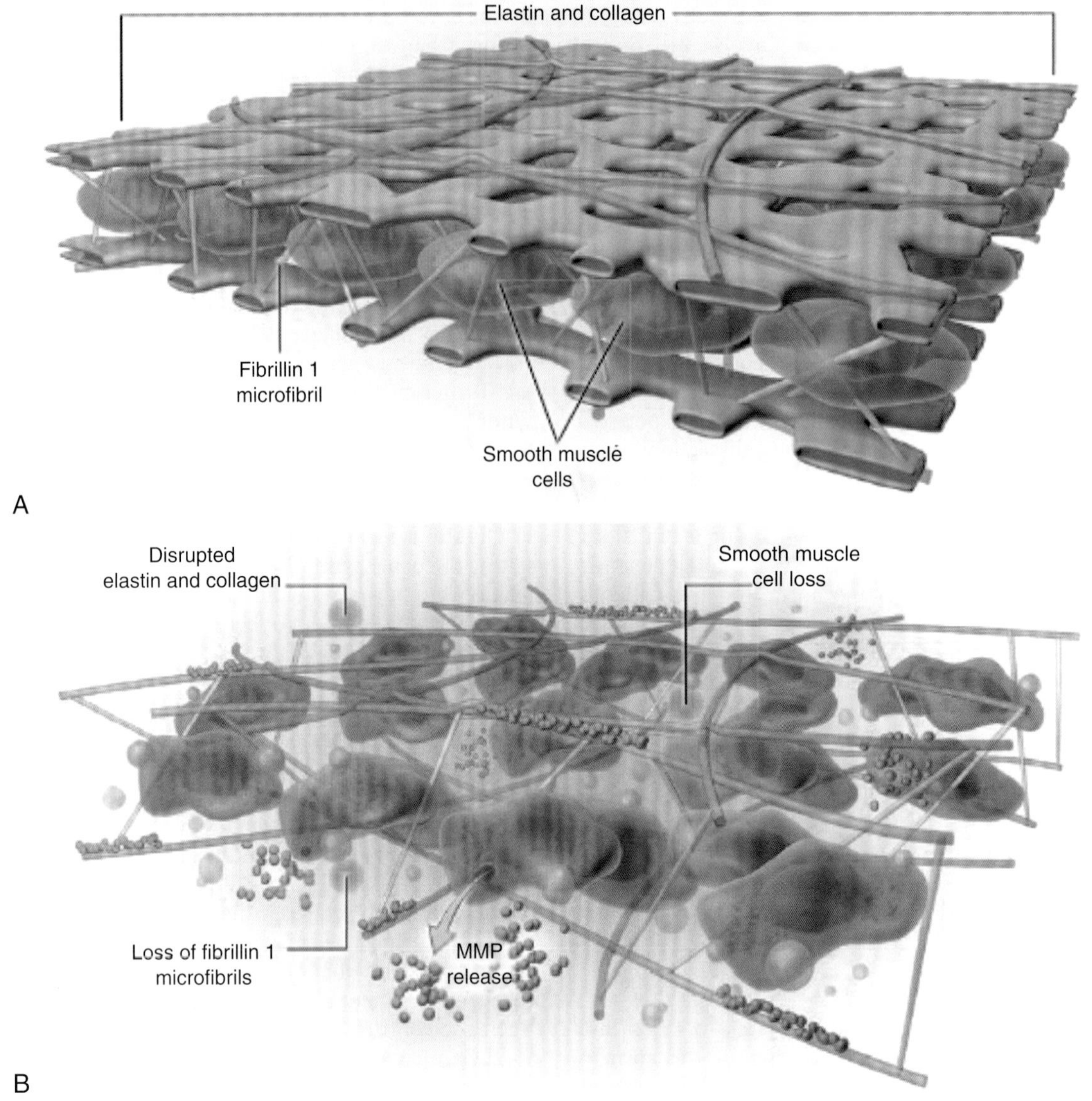

Fig. 33.3 Pathophysiologic features of normal aortas and in the setting of connective tissue disorders. The aorta's structural support and elasticity are conferred by alternating layers of elastic lamellae and smooth muscle cells. (A) At the histologic level, the smooth muscle cells are secured to the adjacent elastin and collagen matrix by fibrillin 1 microfibrils. (B) In connective tissue disorders, the aorta may be deficient in fibrillin 1. This deficiency culminates in a disrupted architecture in which smooth muscle cells detach, accompanied by a surge in matrix metalloproteinases *(MMPs)*, leading to loss of integrity in the extracellular matrix and accumulation of apoptotic cells. These events may lead to an aorta with weakened structural integrity and reduced elasticity. (From Verma S, Siu SC. Aortic dilatation in patients with bicuspid aortic valve. *N Engl J Med.* 2014;370(20):1920–1929.)

in pediatric patients and at end-diastole in adults (Fig. 33.4). The regions of the aortic arch are best viewed from the suprasternal notch (Fig. 33.5). The aortic valve and ascending aorta may be imaged in children from the subcostal imaging plane (Fig. 33.6).

In adults, aortic dimensions strongly correlate with gender, age, and body surface area. Normative values and reference ranges for aortic dimensions take into account these factors. Values for normative aortic root dimensions are based on the work of Roman et al.,[51] who reported normal aortic root diameters in three age groups and both genders. These benchmark values have been adopted by the various thoracic societies[21,53,54] (Fig. 33.7 and Table 33.6). For adults at the extremes of height and weight, normative values have not been well validated, and for this subpopulation, reference aortic root dimensions should be interpreted with caution.

The normal adult abdominal aorta measures 2.0 cm at the level of the celiac trunk and 1.8 cm just below the renal arteries. Most abdominal aortic aneurysms form between the renal and iliac arteries. Clinically significant abdominal aortic aneurysms measure greater than 4.0 cm in diameter. Excessive body habitus can hamper complete visualization with abdominal ultrasound or echocardiography. Abdominal aortic angiography, CT scanning, or aortic MRI can provide more complete visualization of this structure.

In the pediatric population, aortic dimensions are normalized to body surface area and reported as a Z score. The Z score represents the number of standard deviations of the measurement from the expected mean for body surface area based on large data sets for normal children.[55] By convention, values of 2 or more are considered outside the upper limits of normal.

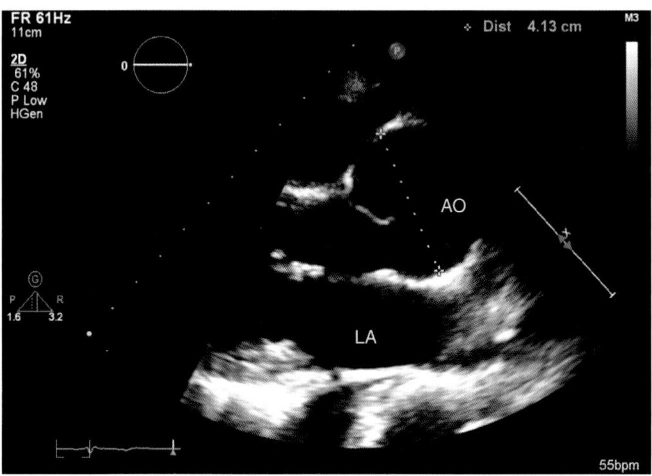

Fig. 33.4 **Sinus of Valsalva enlargement in Marfan syndrome.** Parasternal long-axis view of a 28-year-old woman with Marfan syndrome and known aortic root dilation at the sinus of Valsalva (see Video 33.4). *AO*, Aorta.

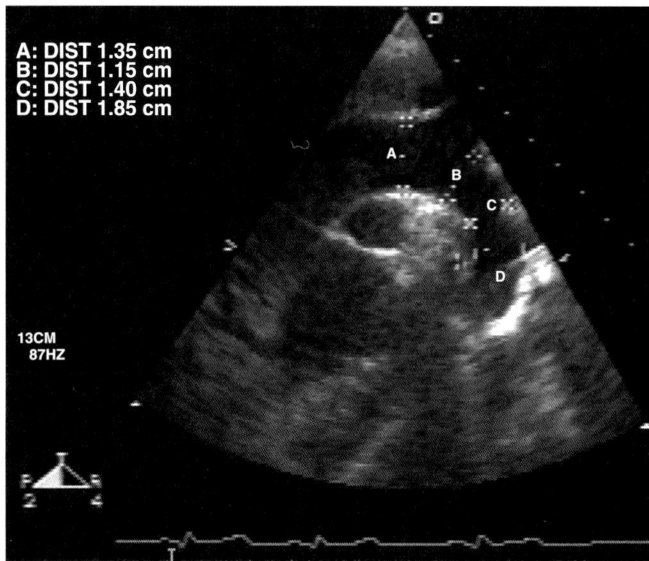

Fig. 33.5 **Echocardiographic imaging of the aortic arch.** Aortic arch viewed from the suprasternal long-axis imaging plane at end-systole demonstrates the appropriate locations at which to measure the distal ascending aorta just before the innominate artery (A), the transverse aorta between the innominate artery and the left carotid artery (B), the aortic isthmus just before the left subclavian artery (C), and the proximal descending aorta just beyond the left subclavian artery (D).

AORTIC DILATION

In the setting of connective tissue disorders, aortic dilation may occur at any position along the aortic root and throughout the descending thoracic and abdominal aorta. However, the most typical sites of dilation are the sinus of Valsalva, the sinotubular junction, and the proximal ascending aorta. Effacement of the sinotubular junction is a common finding in which the sinotubular junction and proximal ascending aorta develop a flattened appearance and have essentially the same diameter as the sinus of Valsalva (Fig. 33.8). As the severity of effacement progresses, there is a progressive transition to a morphologic pattern characterized by a constant caliber of vessel from the sinus of Valsalva through the proximal ascending aorta.

As the severity of aortic root dilation worsens, aortic insufficiency can develop. This is caused by asymmetric dilation of one or more cusps or by generalized dilation at the aortic valve annulus. Either mechanism has the potential to alter the geometry of the aorta in such a manner that insufficiency will develop (Figs. 33.9 and 33.10). In situations in which the thoracic aorta cannot be imaged completely with TTE, TEE or other modalities such as CT or aortic MR angiography (MRA) can be employed.

Aortic aneurysms are classified as true or false (i.e., pseudoaneurysm). A true aneurysm involves weakening and dilation of the entire vessel wall. A pseudoaneurysm occurs when a full-thickness defect in the aortic wall allows blood to circulate out of the confines of the artery. The circulating blood is contained by the surrounding soft tissues. The most common causes of a true aneurysm are atherosclerosis, medial degeneration, and aortic dissection. Pseudoaneurysms are often the result of trauma or infection (e.g., endocarditis). Sinus of Valsalva dilation or aneurysm is typically seen in MFS, whereas ascending aortic dilation is more common in BAV.

AORTIC DISSECTION

Patients with acute aortic root or proximal aortic dissection require emergent assessment and therapy. Prompt diagnosis is crucial to differentiate these patients from those presenting with more benign conditions. The mortality rate is estimated to be about 1% per hour in the first 48 hours for patients who survive to reach an acute care setting.[56] In addition to a diagnosis, the details of anatomy and physiology that are vital to care can be determined. These include classification of the dissection, definition of the site of rupture, detection of extravasation, assessment of pericardial effusion and tamponade, assessment of coronary artery involvement, assessment of aortic regurgitation, and assessment of side branch involvement.[57]

Whereas CT scanning is usually the first-line diagnostic test, TTE and/or TEE are alternative tools that can answer many of these questions. They may be preferred in situations such as pregnancy or poor renal function to avoid a CT scan with contrast (Fig. 33.11).

AORTIC ARCH AND DESCENDING THORACIC AORTIC COMPLICATIONS

Although aortic dilation in connective tissue disorders more commonly affects the aortic root or proximal aorta, complications involving the aortic arch and descending aorta may also occur. A study in which almost 1400 individuals with a connective tissue disorder were followed in the GenTAC registry found that 50% of resulting dissections were type B, originating at the arch or descending aorta.[11] In a study of patients with MFS, a multivariate analysis showed that previous elective aortic root surgery was associated with a fourfold increased risk of dilation of the descending aorta and subsequent higher risk for dissection.[58] Consequently, routine visualization of the entire aorta, including the arch and descending aorta, is important even after aortic graft placement.

MITRAL VALVE PROLAPSE

MVP is defined as the displacement of abnormally thickened and redundant mitral valve leaflets into the left atrium during systole. This geometric change in the integrity of the valve can lead to poor coaptation and resultant mitral regurgitation.

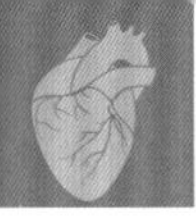

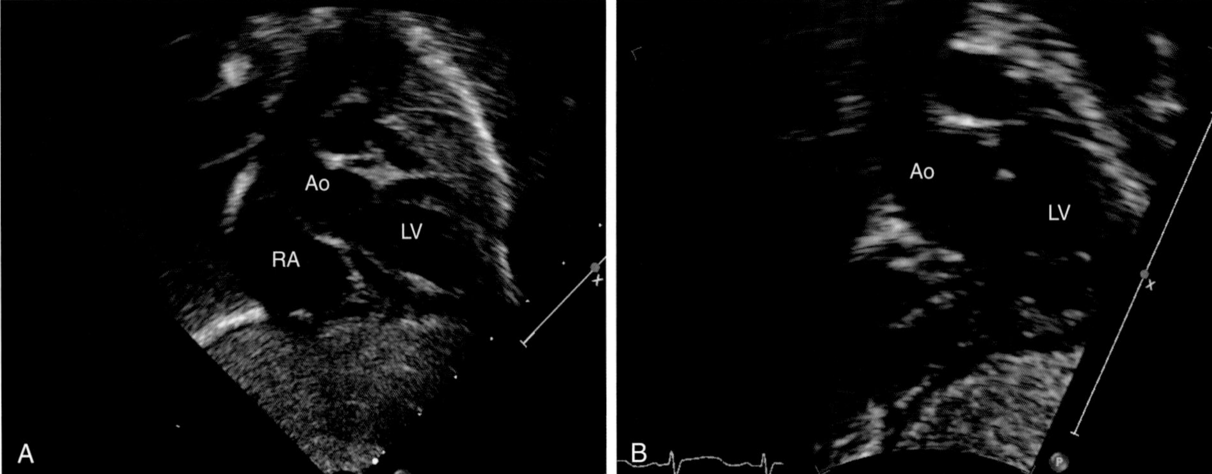

Fig. 33.6 Subcostal aortic imaging in a pediatric patient. (A) Subcostal coronal imaging plane allows visualization of the left ventricular outflow tract to the ascending aorta (see Video 33.6A). (B) Subcostal sagittal imaging plane (see Video 33.6B), *Ao*, Aorta.

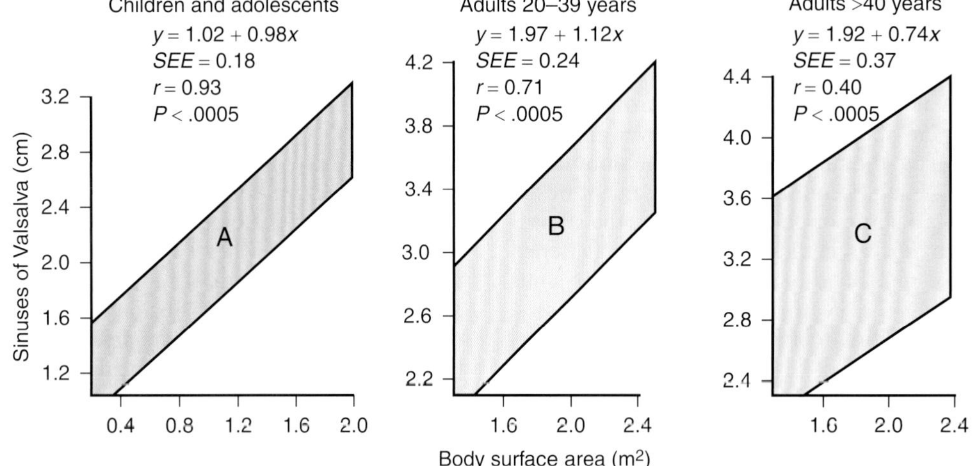

Fig. 33.7 Aortic root dimensions in normal children and adults. Aortic root diameter (y-axis) in relation to body surface area (x-axis). Normal range of aortic root dimensions is shown for individuals 20 years of age and younger (A), between 20 and 39 years of age (B), and for those 40 years of age and older (C). *P*, Probability; *r*, correlation coefficient; *SEE*, standard error of the estimate. (From Roman MJ, et al. Two-dimensional echocardiographic aortic root dimensions in normal children and adults. *Am J Cardiol.* 1989;64(8):507–512.)

TABLE 33.6 Normal Aortic Root Dimensions in Healthy Adults.[a]

	Absolute Values (cm)		Indexed Values (cm/m²)	
Aortic Root	*Men*	*Women*	*Men*	*Women*
Annulus	2.6 ± 0.3	2.3 ± 0.2	1.3 ± 0.1	1.3 ± 0.1
Sinuses of Valsalva	3.4 ± 0.3	3.0 ± 0.3	1.7 ± 0.2	1.8 ± 0.2
Sinotubular junction	2.9 ± 0.3	2.6 ± 0.3	1.5 ± 0.2	1.5 ± 0.2
Proximal ascending aorta	3.0 ± 0.4	2.7 ± 0.4	1.5 ± 0.2	1.6 ± 0.3

[a]Reference ranges for aortic dimensions by gender. Aortic root diameters are based on 2D echocardiography measurements taken at end-diastole using a leading-edge to leading-edge methodology.

Adapted from Roman MJ, Devereux RB, Kramer-Fox R, O'Loughlin J. Two-dimensional echocardiographic aortic root dimensions in normal children and adults. *Am J Cardiol.* 1989:64:507–512.

Echocardiography is the gold standard for the diagnosis and evaluation of MVP.

MVP is defined as displacement of one or both leaflets by greater than 2 mm above the mitral annulus in the parasternal long-axis or apical long-axis view; it also can be well visualized by TEE (Fig. 33.12). The connective tissue disorders are more commonly associated with redundancy of the mitral valve leaflets resulting in MVP, in distinction to MVP in the adult population, which is caused by calcific disease in which the leaflets are less redundant but more thickened.

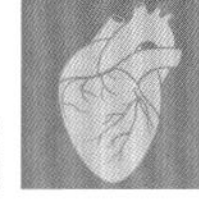

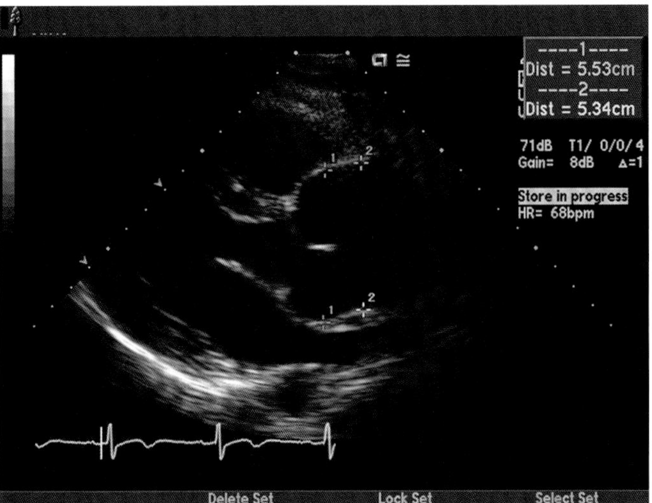

Fig. 33.8 Aortic effacement in a patient with Loeys-Dietz syndrome. Parasternal long-axis view of an 18-year-old man recently diagnosed with Loeys-Dietz syndrome. Image shows dilation of the aortic root resulting in effacement of the sinotubular junction. The aortic diameters at the sinus of Valsalva and at the sinotubular junction are almost equivalent (see Video 33.8).

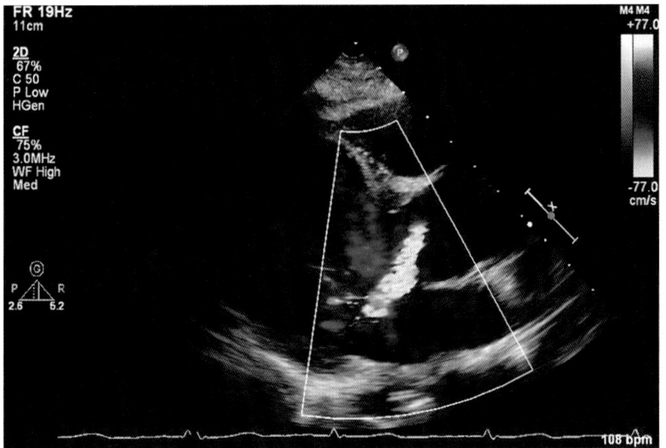

Fig. 33.9 Aortic regurgitation due to aortic root dilation. Parasternal long-axis color Doppler image of a 6-year-old child with a transforming growth factor-β (TGFB) mutation and a dilated aortic root (3.1 cm, Z score = 5) shows mild aortic regurgitation (see Video 33.9).

Although MVP is typically sporadic, it is also associated with connective tissue disorders. The common association of MFS and MVP has raised suspicion that isolated MVP might be due to a mutation of *FBN1*,[59] but this association has never been established.

MVP is the most prevalent valve abnormality in MFS, with a reported prevalence of greater than 35%.[60] Though it is less common than MFS, compared with the general population MVP is also seen more frequently with LDS and various forms of EDS, including the vascular type.[17] Surgical repair of mitral regurgitation can exacerbate aortic dilation postoperatively due to the increased hemodynamic stresses on the aorta.

LV FUNCTION

Whereas aortic abnormalities and mitral valve disease are most commonly seen in the setting of connective tissue disorders, abnormalities of LV systolic and diastolic function are beginning to be elucidated.

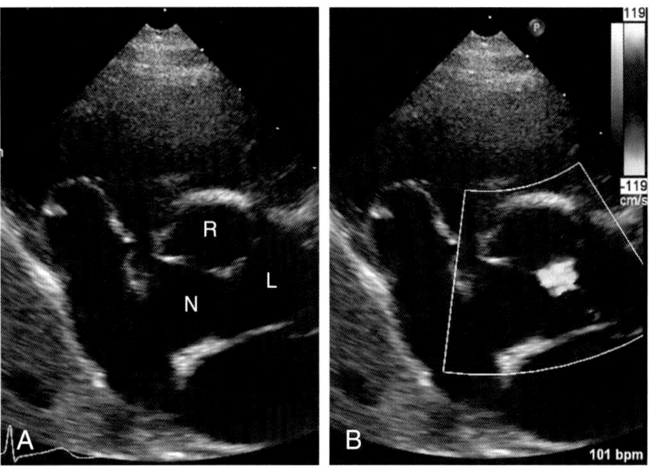

Fig. 33.10 Functional aortic valve regurgitation. (A) Parasternal short-axis image of the aortic valve in the same patient as in Fig. 33.9 shows the right *(R)*, left *(L)*, and noncoronary *(N)* leaflets in diastole. (B) Color Doppler image shows the central aortic regurgitation jet (see Video 33.10).

Diastolic Function

LV diastolic function has been evaluated in several small studies using cardiac MRI and echocardiography. Impaired LV diastolic function has been demonstrated with echocardiographic identification of an increase in deceleration time and an increase in isovolumic relaxation time; these findings were attributed to impaired elastic recoil.[61]

Further evidence of impaired diastolic function in MFS include findings demonstrating that the ratio of early diastolic mitral inflow velocity (E) to early relaxation in tissue Doppler (e') is higher in Marfan patients compared with control, and that the ratio of the E velocity to the A velocity (mitral inflow velocity during atrial contraction) is significantly lower.[62] Despite a preserved ejection fraction, levels of N-terminal pro B-type natriuretic peptide (NT-proBNP) are also higher in MFS, indicative of diastolic disturbances. Echocardiographic data obtained in children as young as 3 years of age with MFS demonstrate early LV diastolic (relaxation) impairment.

Systolic Function

Reduced systolic contractility in MFS was thought to be solely a secondary phenomenon caused by associated aortic and/or mitral valve regurgitation. However, even in the absence of valvular heart disease, subtle findings may suggest that LV systolic contractility is adversely affected. In a large-scale study of 234 adults with MFS, although none of the patients met criteria for dilated cardiomyopathy, a small subset of the patients did show increased LV end-systolic and end-diastolic dimensions, with an associated mild deterioration in ejection fraction.[63]

Using three-dimensional speckle tracking echocardiography (3D-STE), a study compared LV function in 45 asymptomatic patients with MFS and in aged-matched healthy controls. The Marfan patients had significant reductions in 3D-STE–derived LV ejection fraction, longitudinal strain, and circumferential strain.[64]

The pathogenesis of LV systolic and diastolic dysfunction in patients with MFS is incompletely understood but is likely due to the primary structural and functional disorder in the fibrillin-1 protein. Microfibrils, which act as scaffolding for the formation of elastic fibers and contribute to their function, play an important role in mediating elastic recoil. These microfibrils contain the protein fibrillin-1 as one of their primary components.

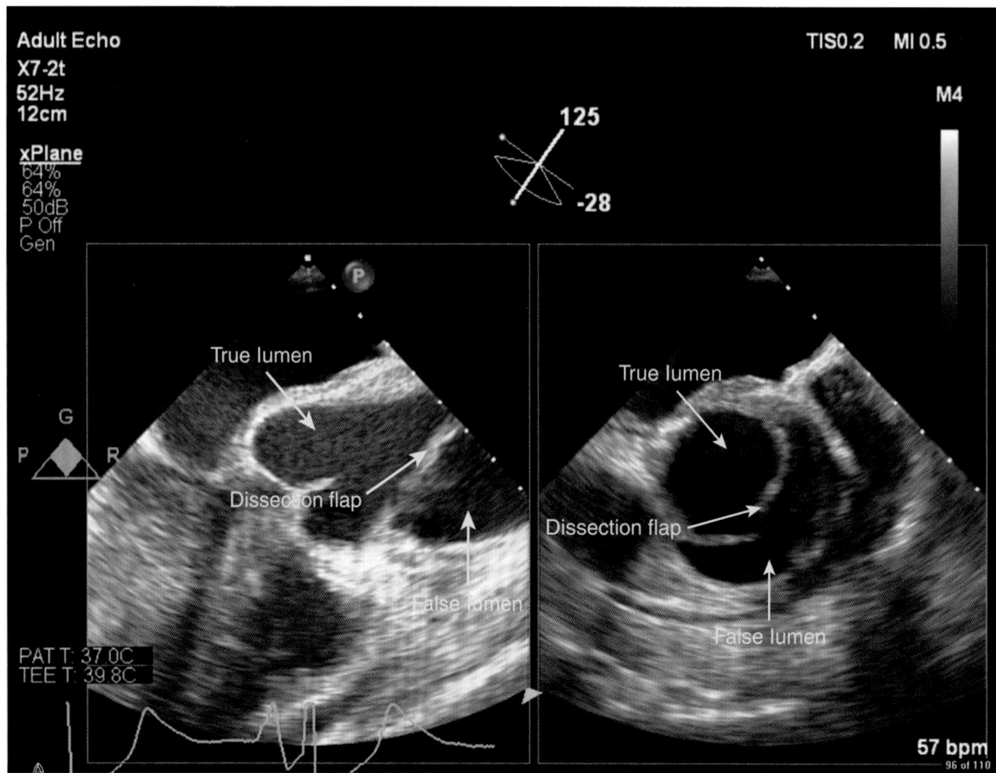

Fig. 33.11 TEE with aortic dissection. TEE imaging shows an acute type A aortic dissection in 29-year-old woman with thoracic aortic aneurysm and dissection (TAAD) syndrome and a myosin light-chain kinase (*MYLK*) mutation. *Left*, long-axis view of the aortic valve, aortic root, and ascending aorta; *right*, short-axis view of the ascending aorta.

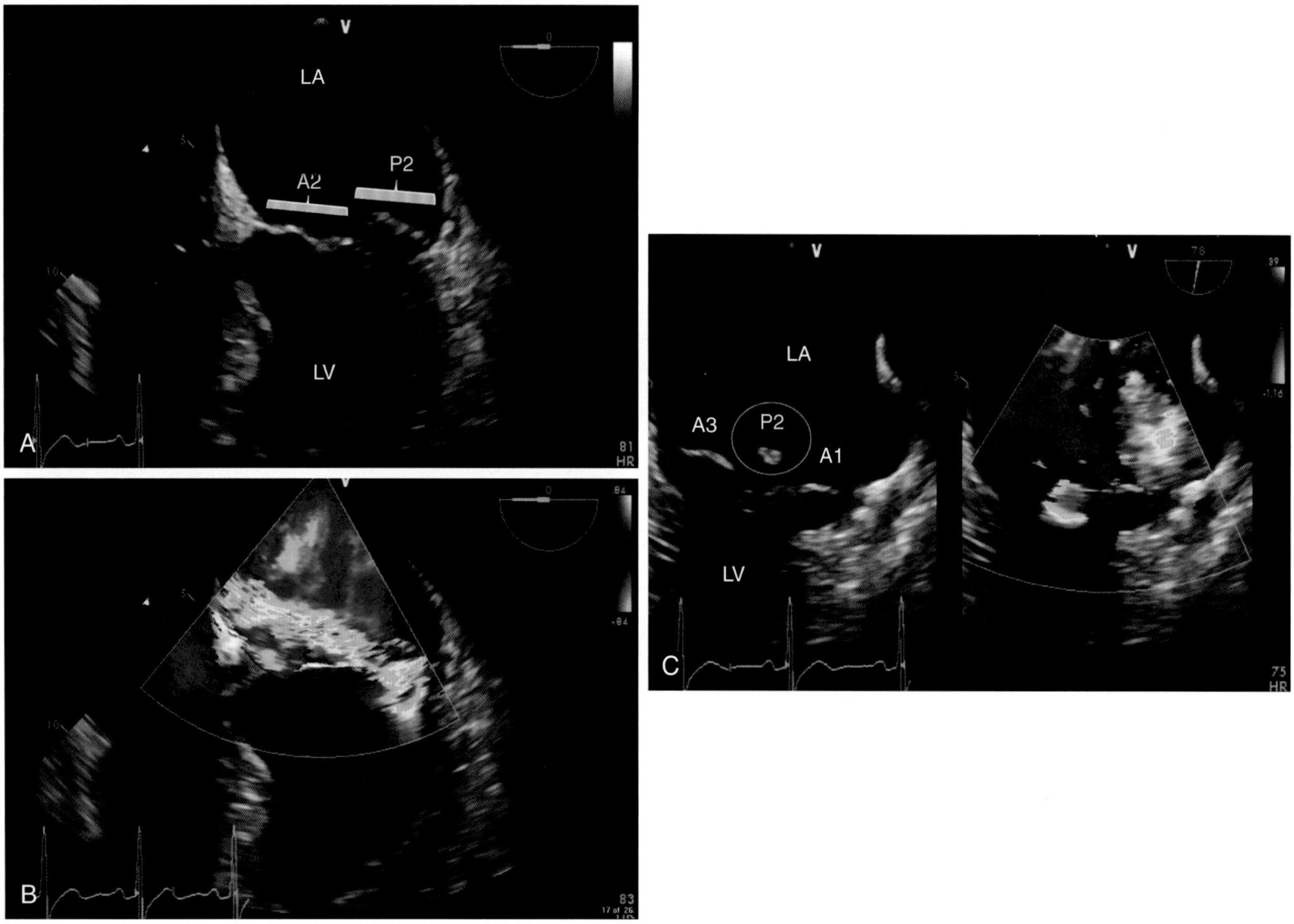

Fig 33.12 TEE with mitral valve prolapse and associated regurgitation. (A) TEE mid-esophageal 4-chamber view shows mitral valve prolapse of the posterior *(P2)* segment (see Video 33.12A). (B) Same view with color Doppler shows the eccentric mitral regurgitation (MR) jet (see Video 33.12B). (C) TTE mid-esophageal commissural view confirms P2 prolapse with significant MR (see Video 33.12C). A1 through A3, anterior segments of the mitral valve.

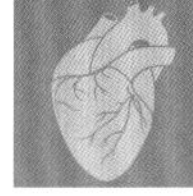

TABLE 33.7 Summary of Clinical and Echocardiographic Findings for the Most Common Forms of Connective Tissue Disorders.

Disorder	Affected Cardiac Structures	Characteristic Findings	Functional Sequelae	Prevalence
Marfan syndrome	MV TV Aortic root Ascending aorta	MVP TV prolapse Dilation of the sinus of Valsalva	Mitral regurgitation Aortic regurgitation Susceptibility to dissecting aortic aneurysm	1:3000–5000
Loeys-Dietz syndrome	MV PV Entire aorta Pulmonary artery	MVP (rare) Arterial tortuosity Aneurysm affecting aortic root to iliac arteries Pulmonary artery dilation	Mitral regurgitation Aortic regurgitation Pulmonic stenosis Aortic dissection (possibly at a smaller aortic diameter than in Marfan syndrome)	Unknown
Thoracic aortic aneurysm and dissection	Entire aorta	Dilation of the aortic root Aneurysm of the thoracic aorta	Aortic regurgitation Ascending aortic dissection Descending thoracic aortic dissection	Unknown: aortic aneurysm results in 15,000 US deaths/y
Bicuspid aortic valve	Aortic valve Ascending aorta Aortic arch	Aortic valve dysfunction Dilation of the ascending aorta/arch	Aortic regurgitation Aortic stenosis Ascending aortic dissection	≈1:100
Turner syndrome	Aortic valve Ascending aorta Thoracic aorta	Bicuspid aortic valve Coarctation of the aorta Dilation of the ascending aorta Hypertension	Aortic stenosis Aortic regurgitation Ascending aortic dissection	≈1:2000–5000 live-born females

MV, Mitral valve; *MVP*, mitral valve prolapse; *PV*, pulmonic valve; *TV*, tricuspid valve.

PULMONARY ARTERY

Compared with the well-defined left heart pathology, abnormalities of the right heart are less well recognized in connective tissue disorders. Dilation of the main pulmonary artery occurs more commonly, particularly in LDS. In severe forms of LDS, pulmonary stenosis can also occur. Serial echocardiographic measurements should be obtained. In the adult population, progressive dilation of the aortic root correlates well with that of the main pulmonary artery.[17] However, dangerous pathology due to pulmonary artery aneurysm or dissection has not been well defined, and the clinical significance of this finding requires further clarification.

Table 33.7 summarizes the clinical cardiac and echocardiographic features found in the most common connective tissue disorders.

NATURAL HISTORY

Of the connective tissue disorders described in this chapter, MFS is by far the best understood. Most patients with MFS present with ascending aortic dilation or dissection. There is a sharp increase in the risk of aortic complications at diameters of 5.5 to 6.0 cm.[10] Although less common than in LDS, complications can arise in MFS in the arch and descending aorta. For this reason, even in the absence of significant ascending aortic dilation, serial monitoring of the entire aorta (from the level of the aortic valve to the abdominal aorta) should occur.

The pregnant woman with MFS is at increased risk for aortic dissection, although the risk is low when the aorta is smaller than 4.0 cm in diameter. Dissection can occur at any time during gestation, and echocardiograms should be performed serially throughout the pregnancy.[65] Compared with MFS, the incidence of pregnancy complications in LDS is thought to be higher, and dissections may occur at aortic diameters smaller than 4.0 cm. Moreover, there is an increased risk of uterine rupture.[17]

As recommended by the 2010 ACC/AHA/AATS guidelines,[21] an echocardiogram should be performed at the time of diagnosis of MFS and 6 months later to evaluate aortic dimensions and the rate of enlargement. The frequency of surveillance imaging thereafter should be based on the patient's aortic size, age, interval change in aortic dimensions, and family history of aortic dissection. We typically perform aortic imaging assessment annually in patients with mild to moderate aortic dilation (<4.5 cm in adults) as long as these findings have been stable. Imaging consists of echocardiography alternating with aortic CT angiography (CTA) or aortic MRA to avoid frequent radiation exposure. More frequent imaging is performed as the aortic dimension exceeds 4.5 cm or if there is rapid aortic growth greater than 5 mm/year.

Fig. 33.13A provides a surveillance imaging strategy for the adult Marfan patient. We recommend a similar strategy for patients with LDS or familial TAAD, but because of reports of dissection at smaller aortic dimensions, our imaging frequency increases at lower thresholds (see Fig. 33.13B). For patients with LDS, we include an MRA from head to pelvis at least every 12 to 24 months, given the tendency of LDS to affect distal vascular beds.

THERAPEUTIC STRATEGIES

PHARMACOLOGIC APPROACHES

Pharmacologic strategies for the connective tissue diseases are based on studies of patients with MFS, but regardless of the cause and type of aortic disease, the main goals of medical therapy are to reduce the structural changes in the aortic wall and to delay aortic dilation and subsequent dissection or rupture. Lowering systolic blood pressure to less than 120 mmHg[21] and decreasing cardiac contractility are thought to be beneficial strategies for delaying progressive aortic dilation. Risk factors, particularly smoking and hypertension, should be aggressively addressed in all patients who have aortic disease. There are no specific cutoff values of aortic diameters above which initiation of medical therapy is recommended. Rather, data suggest that medical therapy should be initiated at a young age, potentially during the childhood years, to effectively modify vascular disease and delay aortic diameter growth.[66] No clinical trial has demonstrated that medical therapy alone decreases mortality rates for patients with MFS or other forms of inherited aortic diseases.

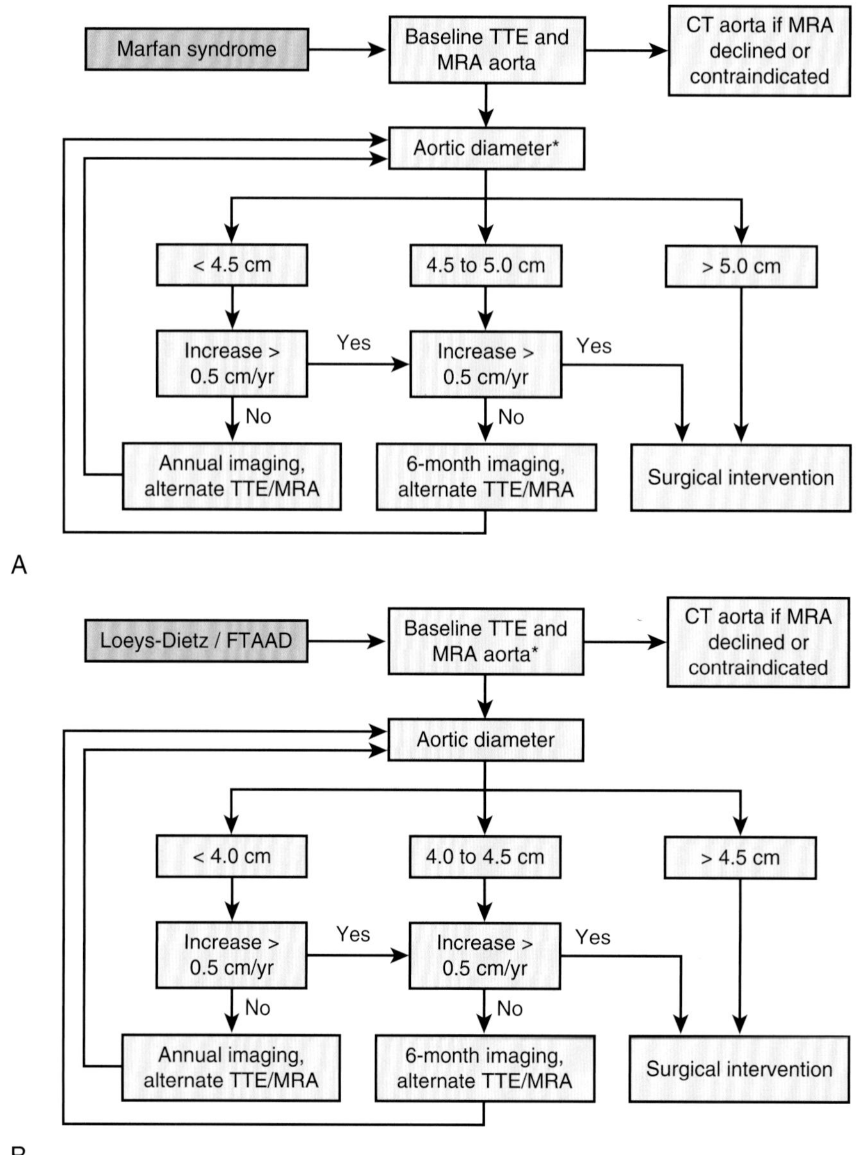

Fig. 33.13 Surveillance imaging strategies in Marfan syndrome and Loeys-Dietz syndrome. (A) Serial imaging and decision-making algorithm for adult patients with Marfan syndrome. If the patient is female and desires pregnancy *(asterisk)*, surgical intervention should be offered if the aortic diameter is greater than 4 cm. (B) Serial imaging and decision-making algorithms for adult patients with Loeys-Dietz syndrome or/and FTAAD. Obtain head and neck MFA every 1–2 years *(asterisk)*. *CT*, Computed tomography; *FTAAD*, familial thoracic aortic aneurysm and dissection; *MFA*, magnetic resonance angiography.

For the past 2 decades, the standard of care in the treatment of MFS with associated aortic dilation has been β-adrenergic blockade. This approach is based on longitudinal follow-up data assessing the progression of aortic dilation with and without β-blocker therapy, which demonstrated a beneficial response in a subset of these patients.[67] Treated patients showed predominantly slower aortic root growth and, in some studies, a reduced need for aortic surgery. This therapeutic strategy has been demonstrated in adults and children.[68] Although therapy does not necessarily result in avoidance of aortic surgery altogether, surgical intervention is usually forestalled.

Significant aortic dilation can render patients less responsive to β-blocker therapy compared with earlier treatment in patients with milder aortic dilation.[67] Some studies have demonstrated improved ascending aortic stiffness associated with β-blocker therapy in patients with MFS,[69,70] whereas others have shown no effect or worsening indices of aortic stiffness.[71] Only a handful of clinical trials involving β-blockers have been conducted in patients with non-MFS inherited aortic diseases. In one notable study of patients with vascular EDS, celiprolol, a β_1-adrenoceptor antagonist with a β_2-adrenoceptor agonist action, resulted in a significant reduction in cardiovascular morbidity and mortality rates for treated patients.[72]

β-Blockers are not administered to normotensive patients with aortic dilation associated with congenital heart diseases such as BAV or tetralogy of Fallot. Dosing of β-blockers can be challenging and should be adjusted based on the adequacy of their effect; a good surrogate is a heart rate of less than 100 beats/min after submaximal exercise. As with any other medical therapy, there are side effects that may be dose or type dependent. They include fatigue, erectile dysfunction, decrease in physical ability, depression, and an increase in body weight and should be discussed with the patient before initiation of treatment.

The second class of medications that has been extensively studied in patients with MFS in attempts to delay progressive aortic dilation is angiotensin receptor blockers (ARBs). Myxomatous mitral valve disease, aortic dilation, and impaired pulmonary alveolar septation—all features of the murine model of MFS—are thought to be mediated by excessive TGF-β signaling. It has been hypothesized that the ARB losartan may delay aortic dilation due to its inhibition of TGF-β signaling in the aortic wall. Treatment with losartan in a mouse model of MFS carrying a fibrillin-1 mutation demonstrated histologic improvement in aortic wall elastic matrix architecture. There was echocardiographic evidence of reduced aortic growth in the losartan-treated group.[73]

Randomized, controlled trials (RCTs) enrolling patients with MFS have provided discrepant results. In the Pediatric Heart Network Study, investigators compared losartan with atenolol in a large, double-blind RCT involving 608 children and young adults with MFS. Losartan was neither superior nor inferior to atenolol. Based on echocardiographic measurements, there were no differences in aortic growth or clinical outcomes over a 3-year period.[66] In the COMPARE trial (*Co*zaar in *M*arfan *Pa*tients *R*educes Aortic *E*nlargement), placebo or losartan (Cozaar) was added to baseline standard care (which included β-blockers for 74% of participants).[73a] After a median follow-up of 8 years, losartan significantly reduced the rate of aortic dilation compared with no losartan. However, in the Marfan Sartan trial, investigators studied the benefit of adding losartan to standard care for 292 MFS patients (86% were on β-blockers). There were no differences between losartan and no losartan treatment in aortic root dilation or clinical events.[74]

Similar to β-blocker therapy, the effects of ARBs have not been evaluated prospectively in patients with other forms of inherited aortic diseases, and the potential vascular protective effects must be inferred from data obtained from patients with MFS. Given the different mechanisms of action, combining ARBs and β-blockers may provide additional protective benefit against aortic growth and dissection, but data on the efficacy of such combinations are limited.

In a large, case-crossover study published in 2018, patients with an enlarged aorta who had taken fluoroquinolone antibiotics had an overall increased risk of aortic aneurysm progression or dissection within the subsequent 60 days.[75] The likely underlying mechanism for this unwarranted effect is increased MMP activity induced by fluoroquinolones. After this and other similar reports, the US Food and Drug Administration published a warning statement, stating that unless there are no other treatment options available, patients with any form of inherited aortic disease, aortic aneurysm, or connective tissue disorder should not be administered fluoroquinolones.

SURGICAL APPROACHES

Medical therapy alone is ineffective in halting aortic growth and preventing aortic dissection or rupture in patients with inherited aortic disease. The standard approach to preventing ascending aortic dissection in these patients remains the use of early surgical repair of aortic aneurysms. For adults with MFS, the threshold for consideration of aortic root replacement occurs when the diameter reaches 5.0 cm.[76,77] A clearly established risk exists when the aortic dimension exceeds 5.5 to 6.0 cm, with a fourfold increase in the cumulative risk of aortic dissection or rupture.[76]

Factors that are used to modify surgical parameters downward include rapid aortic growth (>0.5 cm/year), a family history of aortic dissection (particularly at <5 cm), patients considering pregnancy (prophylactic aortic root replacement if the diameter is >4.0 cm), and the associated finding of moderate or severe aortic regurgitation. However, some patients (even in the absence of factors that would place them at higher risk) develop aortic dissection at a diameter less than 5 cm.[77] For this reason, patient education regarding the symptoms of aortic dissection is crucial. Thresholds for surgical intervention are usually based on the external aortic diameter, as reported from MRI or CT studies, rather than the internal diameter typically reported with echocardiography. The external diameter is typically 0.2 to 0.4 cm larger than the internal diameter.

Surgical indications for non-Marfan connective tissue disorders are considerably less well understood and mostly based on small case series. Patients with LDS are at risk for aortic dissection at aortic diameters less than 5.0 cm. Current guidelines recommend aortic repair at ascending aortic measurements greater than 4.2 cm internal diameter in adults based on echocardiographic measurements or 4.4 to 4.6 cm based on CT/MRI.[21] For children with severe systemic manifestations of LDS, surgery should be considered when the aortic diameter exceeds the 99th percentile for age and the aortic valve annulus reaches 1.8 to 2.0 cm, which allows for placement of a graft that can accommodate future somatic growth.[21,78]

The optimal timing for prophylactic aortic surgical repair in patients with mutations in the smooth muscle apparatus (pathologic variants in *ACTA2, MYH11, MLCK, PRKG1)* is uncertain. There have been a few reported aortic dissections in patients with these mutations at diameters smaller than 5.0 cm. Surgical considerations for these patients may be reasonable at aortic diameters of 4.5 cm or greater. Given the high complication rate and tissue friability, it is unclear whether early prophylactic repair of aortic aneurysms in EDS type IV (vascular form) is indicated. Table 33.8 summarizes the recommendations published by the European Society of Cardiology[79] and the American Heart Association regarding aortic diameter thresholds for prophylactic surgery.

MFS patients undergoing prophylactic rather than nonelective aortic repair have dramatically improved outcomes. In a report by Gott et al. on 675 MFS patients who underwent aortic replacement, a 1.5% operative mortality rate was seen in elective cases, compared with 11.7% for emergency surgeries. The 5- and 10-year survival rates were 84% and 75%, respectively.[77]

Surgical intervention for aortic dilation typically takes the form of a composite graft and associated valve replacement (i.e., Bentall technique) or procedures performed when the aortic valve remains competent and the valve can be spared. A prospective study by Coselli et al. compared 1-year outcomes for patients with MFS who received aortic valve replacement (AVR) versus aortic valve–sparing aortic root replacement surgery; there was no difference in the rates of mortality or major valvular adverse events. However, 7% of patients with the valve-sparing procedure developed at least moderate aortic regurgitation, compared with none of the patients in the AVR group. Longer follow-up with periodic TTE is necessary to determine the durability of valve-sparing procedures.[80]

METHODS OF ASSESSMENT

Standard two-dimensional (2D) echocardiographic imaging for understanding of valve morphology and measurement of

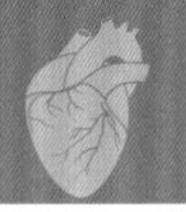

TABLE 33.8 Guideline Recommendations for Surgical Intervention.

Inherited Aortic Disease	*American Heart Association 2010, 2014*	*European Society of Cardiology 2014*
Marfan syndrome	>50 mm[a]	≥50
	>40 mm if contemplating pregnancy	≥45[b]
Loeys-Dietz syndrome thoracic aortic aneurysm/dissection	≥40–42 mm (echocardiogram) ≥44–46 mm (CT or MRI)	Treat patients with marfanoid manifestations as for Marfan syndrome thresholds
Turner syndrome	4.5–5 cm (aorta > 2.5 cm/m²)	>27.5 mm/m²[c]
Ehlers-Danlos syndrome (any type)	No specific data[d]	No specific data[d]
Nonsyndromic aortopathy	No specific data[d]	No specific data[d]
Bicuspid aortic valve	>55 mm	≥55 mm
	>50 mm[e]	≥50 mm[f]
	>45 mm[g]	
General population	≥55 mm	≥55 mm

[a]Repair if there is a family history of aortic dissection at <50 mm, severe aortic regurgitation, or rapid growth >5 mm/yr.
[b]If any of the following risk factors exist: family history of dissection, size increase >3 mm/yr, severe aortic regurgitation or mitral regurgitation, desire for pregnancy.
[c]Other data suggests a cutoff of >25 mm/m² should be used.
[d]Published data suggest that treatment should be based on family history.
[e]If any of the following risk factors exist: family history of dissection, growth ≥ 5 mm/yr.
[f]If any of the following risk factors exist: family history of dissection, hypertension, coarctation of the aorta, size increase >3 mm/yr.
[g]If having surgery for severe aortic stenosis or aortic regurgitation.
Data from American Heart Association 2010 (Hiratzka et al.[21]) and 2014 (Nashimura et al.[40]) and European Society of Cardiology 2014 (Erbel et al.[79]).

aortic dimensions is routinely obtained for all individuals coming through the echocardiography laboratory, and echocardiography remains the most frequently used screening tool for the assessment of these parameters. Measurements of the aortic dimensions are acquired from the parasternal long-axis view, the long axis of the suprasternal notch, and the subcostal plane. All measurements are typically made using 2D echocardiography, with data acquired at end-diastole for adults and early systole for children.

Some laboratories measure the sinus of Valsalva using M-mode; however, this may lead to overestimation of the region. The aortic valve annulus, sinus of Valsalva, and sinotubular junction (and proximal aspect of the ascending aorta) are imaged from the parasternal long-axis view, and the distal ascending aorta (just before the take-off of the innominate artery), transverse aortic arch, and aortic isthmus are measured from the suprasternal notch (Fig. 33.14). In some individuals, the proximal descending aorta can be imaged from the parasternal window. A short-axis view of the descending aorta can be obtained posterior to the LA in the parasternal long-axis view and in the 4-chamber view. By 90-degree rotation of the transducer, a long-axis view is obtained, and a median part of the descending thoracic aorta can be visualized.

The abdominal descending aorta can be easily visualized to the left of the inferior vena cava in sagittal (superior-inferior) subcostal views (Fig. 33.15). The precision of this assessment depends on the operator and on image quality (primarily due to issues of patient body habitus). Oblique measurements of the aorta can overestimate actual dimensions, as can an aortic diameter that is not drawn perpendicular to the aortic flow centerline.

Imaging of the valves can be enhanced by the acquisition of three-dimensional (3D) data. With the availability of real-time 3D echocardiography, we can obtain valve structure and function information such that immediate decisions can be made regarding the nature of the pathologic process. Although 3D imaging can also be used for acquisition of the thoracic aorta, the clinical application for this relatively novel technology is still unclear. It is possible that 3D technology with multiple imaging planes can help to minimize off-axis or oblique measurements of the aorta, which can occur with 2D imaging alone. Further experience is necessary to determine the relative utility of 3D

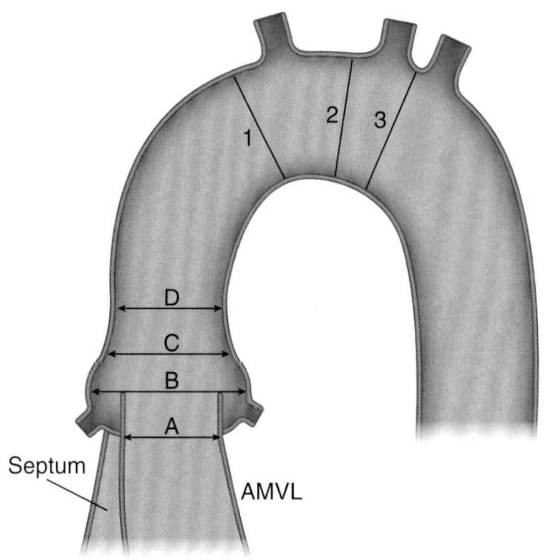

Fig. 33.14 Aortic root and arch measurements. Schematic shows the aortic valve annulus *(A)*, sinus of Valsalva *(B)*, sinotubular junction *(C)*, and proximal ascending aorta *(D)*. Measurements are obtained at early systole in children and at end-diastole in adults. In the suprasternal long-axis imaging plane, measurements are obtained of the distal ascending aorta *(1)* just before the innominate artery, the transverse arch *(2)* between the innominate artery and the left carotid artery, and the aortic isthmus *(3)* just before the left subclavian artery. *AMVL*, Anterior mitral valve leaflet.

echocardiography compared with standard 2D echocardiography, aortic CTA, and MRA.

Normalization of aortic measurements is an important aspect of accurate data interpretation. Dependence on the accuracy of normalized data is of particular importance in pediatric patients, in whom rapid changes occur during growth. Because of the prognostic significance of aortic measurements in patients with connective tissue disorders, aortic dimensions have been extensively studied with 2D echocardiography.

In a study of 52 normal infants and children (1 month to 15 years old) and 135 normal adults (20–74 years old), the aorta was measured at end-diastole in the parasternal long-axis view

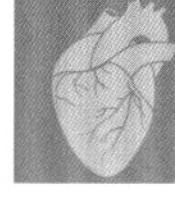

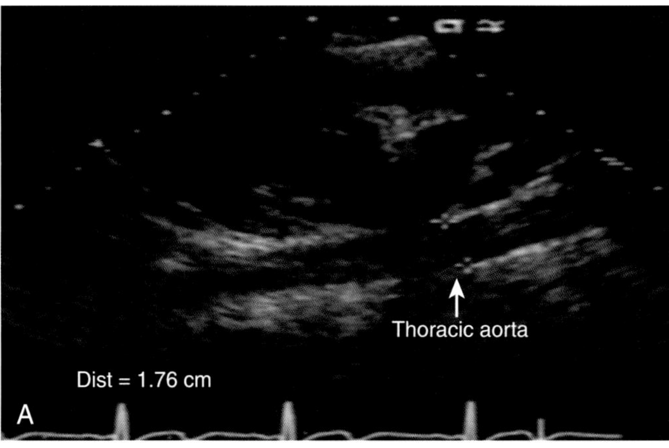

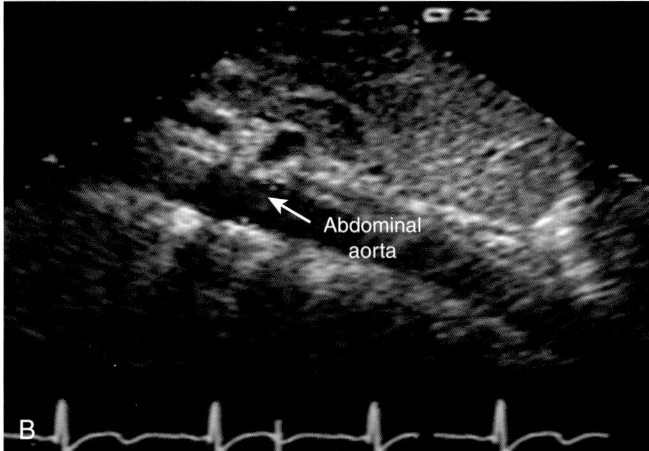

Fig. 33.15 Echocardiographic imaging of the thoracic and abdominal aorta. (A) Subcostal long-axis view shows the preferred location at which to measure the distal descending thoracic aorta. (B) Subcostal long-axis view. shows the preferred location at which to measure the descending aorta inferior to the diaphragm.

at four levels: aortic annulus, sinus of Valsalva, sinotubular junction, and proximal ascending aorta at its maximal dimension. In this study, 2D measurements at the sinus of Valsalva were larger than those obtained by M-mode echocardiography. When 2D values were normalized, M-mode nomograms falsely diagnosed aortic dilation in 40% of normal children and adults.[51]

There is still no formal consensus on methodology for measuring the ascending aortic diameter. The reference values derived from the work of Roman et al. are based on a leading edge-to-leading edge (LE) method and have been endorsed by the American Society of Echocardiography,[51,54] whereas the 2010 ACC/AHA thoracic aortic disease guidelines favor inner edge-to-inner edge (IE) measurement of the aortic diameter.[21] A 2D echocardiographic study in which both aortic measurement methods were applied in 218 healthy adults showed that ascending aortic measurements using the LE method were 2 mm larger on average than those obtained with the IE method.[53]

A consensus paper by the American Society of Echocardiography and the European Association of Cardiovascular Imaging compared the two approaches with CTA and MRA. The LE method used for 2D echocardiography was found to give, on average, a 2 mm larger measurement compared with the IE approach on CT.[54] In a study comparing TTE with CTA and MRA, the investigators found excellent agreement among modalities for diameter measurements of the sinuses of Valsalva, sinotubular junction, and tubular ascending aorta when parasternal long-axis images were measured perpendicular to the long axis of the aorta using the LE convention at end-diastole and when CTA and MRA data sets were reformatted in double-oblique fashion to create short-axis images and measured with IE (luminal edge–to–luminal edge) technique.[81]

Another study demonstrated that in patients with BAV, at the level of the sinuses of Valsalva, TTE short-axis LE diameters obtained at mid-diastole agreed best with CTA IE measurements obtained with double-oblique reformatting. At the tubular ascending aorta, TTE long-axis end-diastolic measurements obtained by the LE method agreed best with CTA IE measurements.[82] Regardless of the method used, the measurement technique should be specified in all reports.

Ideally, when following a patient with serial studies, images should be directly compared to determine whether there has been a meaningful change in aortic size. Rather than using published data sets, some groups have relied on internally derived normal controls or unpublished data obtained from large institutional studies.[83] When evaluating the aorta in patients with connective tissue diseases, the diameter alone, even when indexed to body size, reveals only part of the pathology involved in the disease because loss of elastic fibers in the arterial media is a key component in the pathogenesis of these conditions.[21]

Insights into the pathology and mechanical behavior of the thoracic aorta may be provided by STE analysis, which can demonstrate cyclic changes in length (i.e., longitudinal strain) and diameter (i.e., circumferential strain) and clockwise and counterclockwise twist of the ascending aorta.[84] Longitudinal strain of the ascending aorta is reduced in patients with MFS, BAV, or thoracic aortic aneurysms compared with patients who have three-cusp aortic valves.[85]

The aortic stiffness index is another reliable surrogate of aortic disease severity. It is a predictor of faster aortic growth rate and of several clinical outcomes, including aortic root surgery, dissection, and death, in patients with MFS.[86]

The TTE-derived aortic stiffness index, a surrogate for the severity of the aortic disease, was increased in a group of patients with MFS, BAV, and familial thoracic aneurysm compared with controls.[87] In an intraoperative TEE study of patients undergoing thoracic aortic aneurysm repair, the aortic stiffness index—calculated using STE measurements of circumferential strain—correlated with stiffness of the excised aortic wall on ex vivo mechanical testing.[88] The aortic stiffness can also be evaluated by 2D TTE and peripheral blood pressure measurement using the following formula[89]:

$$\text{Stiffness index} = [ln\ (\text{SBP/DBP})] / [(\text{Aorta}_{max} - \text{Aorta}_{min}) / \text{Aorta}_{min}]$$

where SBP is the systolic blood pressure, DBP is the diastolic blood pressure, Aorta_{max} is the highest aortic diameter, and Aorta_{min} is the lowest aortic diameter.

LIMITATIONS OF ASSESSMENT

Although transthoracic 2D and M-mode echocardiographic studies are the most common methods of assessing the mitral valve and aorta in patients with connective tissue disorders, these methods have limitations. Data acquisition is equipment and operator dependent. Measurements of aortic dimensions are affected by patient body habitus, and significant overestimates can occur if oblique measurements are obtained.

Although CTA and MRA are more commonly used, TEE is still a valuable tool for assessing the aorta in patients with

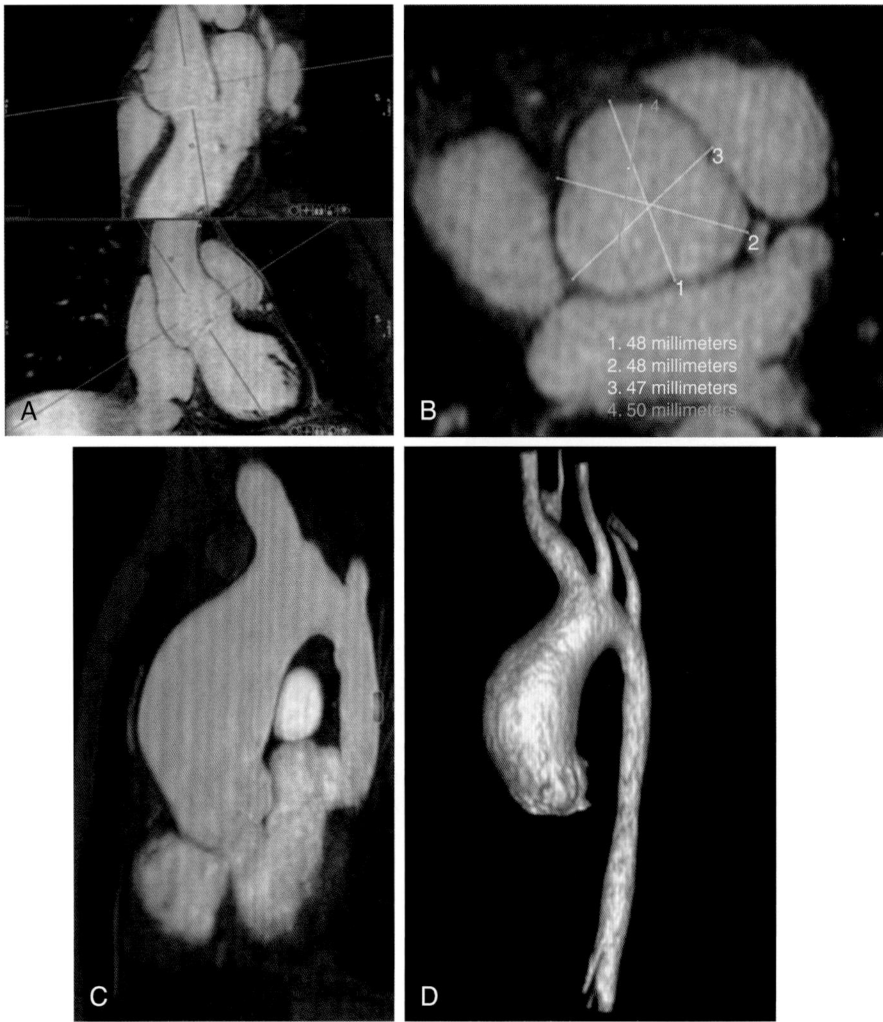

Fig. 33.16 Aortic magnetic resonance imaging in a patient with Marfan syndrome (A and B) and in a patient with a bicuspid aortic valve (C and D). (A) Oblique sagittal *(top)* and oblique coronal *(bottom)* images are used to obtain double-oblique planes. (B) Double-oblique measurements taken at the aortic sinuses are made from sinus to commissure *(yellow lines)* and sinus to sinus *(green line)*, which results in measurements that are often are larger by 1 to 3 mm. (C) Oblique sagittal "candy-cane" imaging showing marked dilation in mid-ascending aorta and proximal arch. (D) 3D volume-rendered MR angiogram showing dilation from the aortic sinuses through the proximal aortic arch.

difficult TTE acoustic images. In addition to routine use as a tool to obtain accurate measurements of the aortic root, TEE can be used to evaluate properties of aortic distensibility. Measurement of aortic distensibility, stiffness index, and pulsed-wave velocity can be obtained using M-mode data from the TEE short-axis view. Data derived from TEE imaging indicated that tissue Doppler imaging was complementary to M-mode; together, they served as a significant predictor of progressive aortic dilation and eventual dissection.[90] Although these measurement techniques are still largely limited to research purposes, the use of TEE and Doppler echocardiography to provide biophysical aortic properties can assist in identifying aortic pathology and prognosis.

ALTERNATIVE DIAGNOSTIC APPROACHES

MRI and cardiac CT can be used for patients who have limited acoustic images or require detailed assessment in situations with ambiguous data. This may include patients with unusual tortuosity of the aortic arch, those for whom there is a question of dilation extending into the carotid arteries or circle of Willis, and those for whom an aortic dissection cannot be entirely excluded. One of the strengths of MRI and cardiac CT is that these modalities allow visualization of the entire aorta, from the aortic root down to the iliac bifurcation and including the aortic arch branch vessels. However, as with echocardiographic assessment, the accuracy of CT and MRI evaluation relies on the availability of appropriate equipment and is operator dependent (Fig. 33.16).

Advances in MRI have allowed evaluation of aortic elasticity and stiffness, which are impaired in patients with MFS. Using velocity mapping of the aorta on MRI, aortic distensibility and elasticity during systole can be quantified and the pulsed wave propagation, which is increased in MFS patients, can be evaluated. Aortic circumferential and longitudinal aortic wall strain values are also surrogates of aortic wall stiffness and can be quantified on MRI. One study showed that longitudinal strain as measured on MRI is a reliable predictor of aortic root diameter growth rate and aortic events.[91,92]

In addition to the actual motion of the aortic wall, intraaortic blood flow patterns have been associated with formation and progression of aortic aneurysm. Four-dimensional MRA is a relatively new technique that is especially suitable for the assessment of aortic flow dynamics,[93,94] and data suggest that patients with aortopathies have aortic flow derangements.[95] These alternative techniques yield important information regarding the biophysical properties of the aorta in patients with connective tissue disorders and they may provide data to predict individual patient risk.

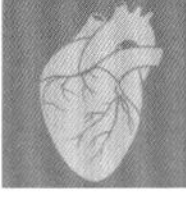

SUMMARY Transthoracic Echocardiographic Evaluation of a Patient With a Known or Suspected Connective Tissue Disorder[a]

Parameter	Views	Recording	Measurements
LV outflow tract/ aortic valve annulus diameter	Parasternal long axis	Decrease depth, narrow sector, zoom	At systole, measure outflow tract diameter between the anterior and posterior endocardium immediately below the attachments of the anterior and posterior aortic valve leaflets.
Sinus of Valsalva diameter	Parasternal long axis	Decrease depth, narrow sector, zoom	At end-diastole (adults) or end-systole (in children), measure maximum diameter between the anterior right coronary cusp and posterior (usually noncoronary) cusp, parallel to the aortic annulus and perpendicular to the ascending aorta. Measurement techniques vary among laboratories; LE or IE measurements can be made and should be consistent for all aortic measurements.
Sinotubular junction diameter	Parasternal long axis	Decrease depth, narrow sector, zoom	At end-diastole (adults) or end-systole (children), measure diameter at the junction between the anterior posterior coronary cusp and the ascending aorta.
Ascending aortic diameter	Parasternal long axis	Decrease depth, narrow sector, zoom	At end-diastole (adults) or end-systole (children), measure maximum visualized diameter parallel to the aortic annulus in the tubular portion of the ascending aorta.
Aortic arch diameter	Suprasternal notch	Careful positioning to obtain clearest image, zoom	Visualize the entire arch, including the take-off of the supraaortic vessels. Measure aortic arch diameter just proximal to the take-off of the innominate artery, between the innominate artery and the left carotid artery, and at the aortic isthmus just before the subclavian artery.
Abdominal aorta	Subcostal	Careful positioning to obtain clearest image	Visualize the abdominal aorta from the subcostal view. Measure aorta at largest diameter clearly visualized.

[a]For all patients, particularly during their initial evaluation, a complete echocardiographic evaluation should be performed with assessment of ventricular performance and special emphasis on valvular structure and function.

REFERENCES

1. Loeys BL, et al. The revised Ghent nosology for the Marfan syndrome. *J Med Genet.* 2010;47(7):476–485.
2. Loeys B. The search for genotype/phenotype correlation in Marfan syndrome: to be or not to be? *Eur Heart J.* 2016;37(43):3291–3293.
3. Dietz H, et al. The question of heterogeneity in Marfan syndrome. *Nat Genet.* 1995;9(3):228–231.
4. Schrijver I, et al. Cysteine substitutions in epidermal growth factor-like domains of fibrillin-1: distinct effects on biochemical and clinical phenotypes. *Am J Hum Genet.* 1999;65(4):1007–1020.
5. Wang M, et al. Recurrent mis-splicing of fibrillin exon 32 in two patients with neonatal Marfan syndrome. *Hum Mol Genet.* 1995;4(4):607–613.
6. Milewicz DM, et al. A mutation in FBN1 disrupts profibrillin processing and results in isolated skeletal features of the Marfan syndrome. *J Clin Invest.* 1995;95(5):2373–2378.
7. Palz M, et al. Clustering of mutations associated with mild Marfan-like phenotypes in the 3′ region of FBN1 suggests a potential genotype-phenotype correlation. *Am J Med Genet.* 2000;91(3):212–221.
8. Guo D, et al. Familial thoracic aortic aneurysms and dissections: genetic heterogeneity with a major locus mapping to 5q13-14. *Circulation.* 2001;103(20):2461–2468.
9. Franken R, et al. Relationship between fibrillin-1 genotype and severity of cardiovascular involvement in Marfan syndrome. *Heart.* 2017;103(22):1795–1799.
10. Saeyeldin A, et al. Natural history of aortic root aneurysms in Marfan syndrome. *Ann Cardiothorac Surg.* 2017;6(6):625–632.
11. Weinsaft JW, et al. Aortic dissection in patients with Genetically mediated aneurysms: incidence and predictors in the GenTAC registry. *J Am Coll Cardiol.* 2016;67(23):2744–2754.
12. Pyeritz RE. Marfan syndrome: improved clinical history results in expanded natural history. *Genet Med.* 2019;21(8):1683–1690.
13. Sakai LY, et al. FBN1: the disease-causing gene for Marfan syndrome and other genetic disorders. *Gene.* 2016;591(1):279–291.
14. Gupta PA, et al. FBN2 mutation associated with manifestations of Marfan syndrome and congenital contractural arachnodactyly. *J Med Genet.* 2004;41(5):e56.
15. Loeys BL, et al. Aneurysm syndromes caused by mutations in the TGF-beta receptor. *N Engl J Med.* 2006;355(8):788–798.
16. Loeys BL, et al. A syndrome of altered cardiovascular, craniofacial, neurocognitive and skeletal development caused by mutations in TGFBR1 or TGFBR2. *Nat Genet.* 2005;37(3):275–281.
17. Meester JAN, et al. Differences in manifestations of Marfan syndrome, Ehlers-Danlos syndrome, and Loeys-Dietz syndrome. *Ann Cardiothorac Surg.* 2017;6(6):582–594.
18. Takeda N, Komuro I. Genetic basis of hereditary thoracic aortic aneurysms and dissections. *J Cardiol.* 2019;74(2):136–143.
19. Pepin MG, et al. Survival is affected by mutation type and molecular mechanism in vascular Ehlers-Danlos syndrome (EDS type IV). *Genet Med.* 2014;16(12):881–888.
20. North KN, et al. Cerebrovascular complications in Ehlers-Danlos syndrome type IV. *Ann Neurol.* 1995;38(6):960–964.
21. Hiratzka LF, et al. ACCF/AHA/AATS/ACR/ASA/SCA/SCAI/SIR/STS/SVM guidelines for the diagnosis and management of patients with thoracic aortic disease: a report of the

American College of Cardiology Foundation/American Heart Association Task Force on Practice Guidelines, American Association for Thoracic Surgery, American College of Radiology, American Stroke Association, Society of Cardiovascular Anesthesiologists, Society for Cardiovascular Angiography and Interventions, Society of Interventional Radiology, Society of Thoracic Surgeons, and Society for Vascular Medicine. *Circulation.* 2010;121(13):e266–369. 2010.
22. Brownstein AJ, et al. Genes associated with thoracic aortic aneurysm and dissection: 2018 update and clinical implications. *Aorta (Stamford).* 2018;6(1):13–20.
23. Braverman AC, et al. The bicuspid aortic valve. *Curr Probl Cardiol.* 2005;30(9):470–522.
24. Cripe L, et al. Bicuspid aortic valve is heritable. *J Am Coll Cardiol.* 2004;44(1):138–143.
25. Hales AR, Mahle WT. Echocardiography screening of siblings of children with bicuspid aortic valve. *Pediatrics.* 2014;133(5):e1212–e1217.
26. Andreassi MG, Della Corte A. Genetics of bicuspid aortic valve aortopathy. *Curr Opin Cardiol.* 2016;31(6):585–592.
27. Prakash SK, et al. A roadmap to investigate the genetic basis of bicuspid aortic valve and its complications: insights from the International BAVCon (Bicuspid Aortic Valve Consortium). *J Am Coll Cardiol.* 2014;64(8):832–839.
28. Fedak PW, et al. Clinical and pathophysiological implications of a bicuspid aortic valve. *Circulation.* 2002;106(8):900–904.
29. Cecconi M, et al. Aortic dimensions in patients with bicuspid aortic valve without significant valve dysfunction. *Am J Cardiol.* 2005;95(2):292–294.
30. Biner S, et al. Aortopathy is prevalent in relatives of bicuspid aortic valve patients. *J Am Coll Cardiol.* 2009;53(24):2288–2295.
31. Guzzardi DG, et al. Valve-related hemodynamics mediate human bicuspid aortopathy: insights from wall shear stress mapping. *J Am Coll Cardiol.* 2015;66(8):892–900.
32. Adamo L, Braverman AC. Surgical threshold for bicuspid aortic valve aneurysm: a case for individual decision-making. *Heart.* 2015;101(17):1361–1367.
33. Avadhani SA, et al. Predictors of ascending aortic dilation in bicuspid aortic valve disease: a five-year prospective study. *Am J Med.* 2015;128(6):647–652.
34. Verma S, Siu SC. Aortic dilatation in patients with bicuspid aortic valve. *N Engl J Med.* 2014; 370(20):1920–1929.
35. Larson EW, Edwards WD. Risk factors for aortic dissection: a necropsy study of 161 cases. *Am J Cardiol.* 1984;53(6):849–855.
36. Tzemos N, et al. Outcomes in adults with bicuspid aortic valves. *J Am Med Assoc.* 2008;300(11): 1317–1325.
37. Michelena HI, et al. Natural history of asymptomatic patients with normally functioning or minimally dysfunctional bicuspid aortic valve in the community. *Circulation.* 2008;117(21): 2776–2784.
38. Michelena HI, et al. Incidence of aortic complications in patients with bicuspid aortic valves. *J Am Med Assoc.* 2011;306(10):1104–1112.
39. Kim JB, et al. Risk of aortic dissection in the moderately dilated ascending aorta. *J Am Coll Cardiol.* 2016;68(11):1209–1219.
40. Nishimura RA, et al. 2014. AHA/ACC guideline for the management of patients with valvular heart disease: executive summary: a report of the American College of Cardiology/American Heart Association Task Force on Practice Guidelines. *J Am Coll Cardiol.* 2014;63(22):2438–2488.
41. Etz CD, et al. Acute type A aortic dissection: characteristics and outcomes comparing patients with bicuspid versus tricuspid aortic valve. *Eur J Cardio Thorac Surg.* 2015;48(1):142–150.
42. Lin AE, et al. Aortic dilation, dissection, and rupture in patients with Turner syndrome. *J Pediatr.* 1986;109(5):820–826.
43. Ostberg JE, et al. Vasculopathy in Turner syndrome: arterial dilatation and intimal thickening without endothelial dysfunction. *J Clin Endocrinol Metab.* 2005;90(9):5161–5166.
44. Gravholt CH, et al. Clinical and epidemiological description of aortic dissection in Turner's syndrome. *Cardiol Young.* 2006;16(5):430–436.
45. Carlson M, Silberbach M. Dissection of the aorta in Turner syndrome: two cases and review of 85 cases in the literature. *J Med Genet.* 2007;44(12):745–749.
46. Lopez L, et al. Turner syndrome is an independent risk factor for aortic dilation in the young. *Pediatrics.* 2008;121(6):e1622–e1627.
47. Mortensen KH, et al. Aortic growth rates are not increased in Turner syndrome–a prospective CMR study. *Eur Heart J Cardiovasc Imaging.* 2019.
48. Thunström S, et al. Incidence of aortic dissection in Turner syndrome. *Circulation.* 2019;139(24):2802–2804.
49. LeMaire SA, et al. Severe aortic and arterial aneurysms associated with a TGFBR2 mutation. *Nat Clin Pract Cardiovasc Med.* 2007;4(3):167–171.
50. Segura AM, et al. Immunohistochemistry of matrix metalloproteinases and their inhibitors in thoracic aortic aneurysms and aortic valves of patients with Marfan's syndrome. *Circulation.* 1998;98(19 Suppl):II331–I337. Discussion II337–II338.
51. Roman MJ, et al. Two-dimensional echocardiographic aortic root dimensions in normal children and adults. *Am J Cardiol.* 1989;64(8):507–512.
52. Reference deleted in review.
53. Muraru D, et al. Ascending aorta diameters measured by echocardiography using both leading edge-to-leading edge and inner edge-to-inner edge conventions in healthy volunteers. *Eur Heart J Cardiovasc Imaging.* 2014;15(4):415–422.
54. Goldstein SA, et al. Multimodality imaging of diseases of the thoracic aorta in adults: from the American Society of Echocardiography and the European Association of Cardiovascular Imaging: endorsed by the Society of Cardiovascular Computed Tomography and Society for Cardiovascular Magnetic Resonance. *J Am Soc Echocardiogr.* 2015;28(2):119–182.
55. Pettersen MD, et al. Regression equations for calculation of Z scores of cardiac structures in a large cohort of healthy infants, children, and adolescents: an echocardiographic study. *J Am Soc Echocardiogr.* 2008;21(8):922–934.
56. Khan IA, Nair CK. Clinical, diagnostic, and management perspectives of aortic dissection. *Chest.* 2002;122(1):311–328.
57. Erbel R, et al. Diagnosis and management of aortic dissection. *Eur Heart J.* 2001;22(18): 1642–1681.
58. Engelfriet PM, et al. Beyond the root: dilatation of the distal aorta in Marfan's syndrome. *Heart.* 2006;92(9):1238–1243.
59. Dietz HC, et al. Marfan syndrome caused by a recurrent de novo missense mutation in the fibrillin gene. *Nature.* 1991;352(6333):337–339.
60. van Karnebeek CD, et al. Natural history of cardiovascular manifestations in Marfan syndrome. *Arch Dis Child.* 2001;84(2):129–137.
61. Savolainen A, et al. Left ventricular function in children with the Marfan syndrome. *Eur Heart J.* 1994;15(5):625–630.
62. Gehle P, et al. NT-proBNP and diastolic left ventricular function in patients with Marfan syndrome. *Int J Cardiol Heart Vasc.* 2016;12:15–20.
63. Meijboom LJ, et al. Evaluation of left ventricular dimensions and function in Marfan's syndrome without significant valvular regurgitation. *Am J Cardiol.* 2005;95(6):795–797.
64. Abd El Rahman M, et al. Left ventricular systolic dysfunction in asymptomatic Marfan syndrome patients is related to the severity of gene mutation: insights from the novel three dimensional speckle tracking echocardiography. *PLoS One.* 2015;10(4):e0124112.
65. Goland S, Elkayam U. Pregnancy and Marfan syndrome. *Ann Cardiothorac Surg.* 2017;6(6): 642–653.
66. Lacro RV, et al. Atenolol versus losartan in children and young adults with Marfan's syndrome. *N Engl J Med.* 2014;371(22):2061–2071.
67. Shores J, et al. Progression of aortic dilatation and the benefit of long-term beta-adrenergic blockade in Marfan's syndrome. *N Engl J Med.* 1994;330(19):1335–1341.
68. Rossi-Foulkes R, et al. Phenotypic features and impact of beta blocker or calcium antagonist therapy on aortic lumen size in the Marfan syndrome. *Am J Cardiol.* 1999;83(9):1364–1368.
69. Groenink M, et al. Changes in aortic distensibility and pulse wave velocity assessed with magnetic resonance imaging following beta-blocker therapy in the Marfan syndrome. *Am J Cardiol.* 1998;82(2):203–208.
70. Yin FC, et al. Arterial hemodynamic indexes in Marfan's syndrome. *Circulation.* 1989,79(4).854–862.
71. Haouzi A, et al. Heterogeneous aortic response to acute beta-adrenergic blockade in Marfan syndrome. *Am Heart J.* 1997;133(1):60–63.
72. Ong KT, et al. Effect of celiprolol on prevention of cardiovascular events in vascular Ehlers-Danlos syndrome: a prospective randomised, open, blinded-endpoints trial. *Lancet.* 2010;376(9751):1476–1484.
73. Habashi JP, et al. Losartan, an AT1 antagonist, prevents aortic aneurysm in a mouse model of Marfan syndrome. *Science.* 2006;312(5770):117–121.
73a. van Andel MM, Indrakusuma R, Jalalzadeh H, et al. Long-term clinical outcomes of losartan in patients with Marfan syndrome: follow-up of the multicenter randomized controlled COMPARE trial. *Eur Heart J.* 2020;41(43):4181–4187.
74. Milleron O, et al. Marfan Sartan: a randomized, double-blind, placebo-controlled trial. *Eur Heart J.* 2015.
75. Lee CC, et al. Oral fluoroquinolone and the risk of aortic dissection. *J Am Coll Cardiol.* 2018;72(12):1369–1378.
76. Davies RR, et al. Yearly rupture or dissection rates for thoracic aortic aneurysms: simple prediction based on size. *Ann Thorac Surg.* 2002;73(1):17–27. Discussion 27–28.
77. Gott VL, et al. Replacement of the aortic root in patients with Marfan's syndrome. *N Engl J Med.* 1999;340(17):1307–1313.
78. Williams JA, et al. Early surgical experience with Loeys-Dietz: a new syndrome of aggressive thoracic aortic aneurysm disease. *Ann Thorac Surg.* 2007;83(2):S757–S763. Discussion S785–S790.

79. Erbel R, et al. 2014. ESC guidelines on the diagnosis and treatment of aortic diseases: document covering acute and chronic aortic diseases of the thoracic and abdominal aorta of the adult. The Task Force for the Diagnosis and Treatment of Aortic Diseases of the European Society of Cardiology (ESC). *Eur Heart J.* 2014;35(41):2873–2926.
80. Coselli JS, et al. Early and 1-year outcomes of aortic root surgery in patients with Marfan syndrome: a prospective, multicenter, comparative study. *J Thorac Cardiovasc Surg.* 2014;147(6):1758–1766. 1767.e1–e4.
81. Rodríguez-Palomares JF, et al. Multimodality assessment of ascending aortic diameters: comparison of different measurement methods. *J Am Soc Echocardiogr.* 2016;29(9):819–826. e4.
82. Park JY, et al. Transthoracic echocardiography versus computed tomography for ascending aortic measurements in patients with bicuspid aortic valve. *J Am Soc Echocardiogr.* 2017;30(7):625–635.
83. Colan, S., Normal Echocardiographic Values in Infants and Children (Boston Children's Hospital; Unpublished Data).
84. Wittek A, et al. Cyclic three-dimensional wall motion of the human ascending and abdominal aorta characterized by time-resolved three-dimensional ultrasound speckle tracking. *Biomech Model Mechanobiol.* 2016;15(5):1375–1388.
85. Longobardo L, et al. Impairment of elastic properties of the aorta in bicuspid aortic valve: relationship between biomolecular and aortic strain patterns. *Eur Heart J Cardiovasc Imaging.* 2018;19(8):879–887.
86. Selamet Tierney ES, et al. Influence of aortic stiffness on aortic-root growth rate and outcome in patients with the Marfan syndrome. *Am J Cardiol.* 2018;121(9):1094–1101.
87. de Wit A, Vis K, Jeremy RW. Aortic stiffness in heritable aortopathies: relationship to aneurysm growth rate. *Heart Lung Circ.* 2013;22(1):3–11.
88. Alreshidan M, et al. Obtaining the biomechanical behavior of ascending aortic aneurysm via the use of novel speckle tracking echocardiography. *J Thorac Cardiovasc Surg.* 2017;153(4):781–788.
89. Hirai T, et al. Stiffness of systemic arteries in patients with myocardial infarction. A noninvasive method to predict severity of coronary atherosclerosis. *Circulation.* 1989;80(1):78–86.
90. Vitarelli A, et al. Aortic wall mechanics in the Marfan syndrome assessed by transesophageal tissue Doppler echocardiography. *Am J Cardiol.* 2006;97(4):571–577.
91. Bell V, et al. Longitudinal and circumferential strain of the proximal aorta. *J Am Heart Assoc.* 2014;3(6):e001536.
92. Guala A, et al. Proximal aorta longitudinal strain predicts aortic root dilation rate and aortic events in Marfan syndrome. *Eur Heart J.* 2019;40(25):2047–2055.
93. Markl M, et al. Advanced flow MRI: emerging techniques and applications. *Clin Radiol.* 2016;71(8):779–795.
94. Burris NS, Hope MD. 4D flow MRI applications for aortic disease. *Magn Reson Imaging Clin N Am.* 2015;23(1):15–23.
95. Bürk J, et al. Evaluation of 3D blood flow patterns and wall shear stress in the normal and dilated thoracic aorta using flow-sensitive 4D CMR. *J Cardiovasc Magn Reson.* 2012;14:84.

中文导读

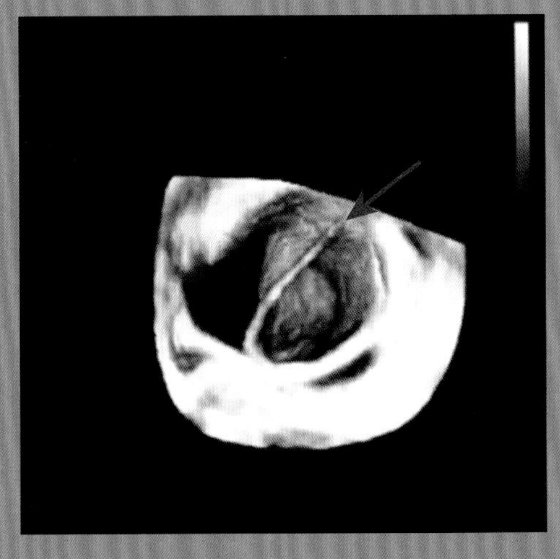

第34章 高血压性心脏病和营养代谢紊乱

高血压和营养代谢紊乱可以引起多种疾病，影响全身多个器官，其中最常出现的是心脏疾病，其致病率及病死率高，早期检测出心脏特异性改变，及时进行临床干预可以逆转心血管病的进程，减少治疗不及时导致代谢紊乱引起心肌纤维化进而发生不可逆心脏损伤。然而，此类疾病临床表现通常不特异，超声心动图等非侵入性检查在早期诊断中发挥重要作用。

本章主要将从临床流行病学、非特异性诊断方法介绍、超声心动图表现、检查方法及诊断指标、临床干预及预后等方面介绍高血压、肥胖、阻塞性睡眠呼吸暂停、Ⅱ型糖尿病和代谢综合征、内分泌疾病和肝脏疾病等。

李鸣瑶

34

Hypertensive Heart Disease and Nutritional and Metabolic Disorders

JASON P. LINEFSKY, MD, MS

Hypertensive, nutritional, and metabolic disorders have diverse presentations and adversely affect multiple organ systems. Heart disease is common, but it is often subclinical and detected only when noninvasive studies such as echocardiography are performed. Cardiovascular disease is a major source of morbidity and mortality in many metabolic disorders, and the ability to detect early cardiac changes is important. Early treatment of the underlying disorder can reverse the cardiac disease process (Table 34.1). However, when left untreated, these disorders lead to myocardial fibrosis that results in permanent cardiac dysfunction and increased mortality rates.

HYPERTENSION

BACKGROUND

Hypertension is the most prevalent modifiable risk factor for cardiovascular events. Almost one half of the US adult population has elevated blood pressure based on the 2017 US guidelines.[1] Elevated systemic arterial blood pressure leads to maladaptive changes in left ventricular (LV) size, geometry, and function. Prolonged exposure increases the risk of clinical heart failure and cardiovascular death.

Echocardiography is the most common imaging modality for evaluating changes in myocardial structure and performance. The benefit of routine echocardiography for all hypertensive patients without symptoms or signs of hypertensive heart disease is uncertain, and it may be costly due to the widespread burden of disease. The decision to pursue echocardiography should be guided by how the results will change management.[2] When patients have symptoms and signs that suggest hypertensive heart disease, an echocardiogram is appropriate.[3]

ECHOCARDIOGRAPHIC FINDINGS

The most notable change in cardiac structure from systemic arterial hypertension is an increase in LV mass. LV mass is calculated from M-mode measurements of the interventricular septal wall (IVS), the LV diastolic internal dimension (LVID), and the posterior wall (PW) using this well-validated formula[4]:

$$\text{LV mass} = \left[1.04 \times (\text{LVID} + \text{IVS} + \text{PW})^3 - \text{LVID}^3\right] \times 0.8 + 0.6$$

Modern image processing provides well-defined visualization of endocardial borders, allowing measurements to be made from the tissue-blood interface as opposed to the original leading edge–to–leading edge standard. When cardiac orientation does not allow M-mode measurements to be perpendicular to the LV long axis, two-dimensional (2D) echocardiography–guided linear measurements should be used. LV mass calculated from linear measurements is limited by several geometric assumptions about the three-dimensional (3D) heart. LV mass calculations subtract the ventricular cavity volume from the LV epicardial volume, and 2D and 3D techniques make fewer assumptions about the volume estimation (Fig. 34.1).[5] Although 3D techniques can overcome some limitations compared with the linear formula, 3D echocardiography relies more on image quality. The normal ranges for a 3D LV mass have not been as well validated as estimations made with the use of linear measurements. When making comparisons of changes between serial studies, measurements should be made with the same technique.

LV hypertrophy (LVH) can be categorized as different geometric patterns based on the relative wall thickness (RWT), body surface area, and gender (Table 34.2 and Fig. 34.2). RWT is calculated as 2 × PW/LVID or (PW + IVS)/LVID, but the latter is less accurate in the setting of a significant basal septal bulge. The most common remodeling pattern from hypertension is concentric hypertrophy. Geometric classifications can provide additional prognostic information beyond LV mass. Refinement in classification using LV volumes provides additional

TABLE 34.1 Cardiac-Relevant Clinical Guidelines and Scientific Statements for Management of Nutritional and Metabolic Disorders.

Year	*Name*	*Organizations*	*Content*
Hypertension			
2015	Recommendation on the Use of Echocardiography in Adult Hypertension[2]	European Association of Cardiovascular Imaging and American Society of Echocardiography	Echocardiography laboratory standards for adult hypertension
2017	Guideline for the Prevention, Detection, Evaluation, and Management of High Blood Pressure in Adults[1]	American College of Cardiology and American Heart Association	Practice recommendation for measurement and management of hypertension
Obesity Related			
2009	Clinical Guideline for the Evaluation, Management, and Long-Term Care of OSA in Adults[83]	American Academy of Sleep Medicine	Screening and diagnostic strategies for OSA Treatment options for OSA
2011	Bariatric Surgery and Cardiovascular Risk Factors[84]	American Heart Association	Types of bariatric surgery Complications of bariatric surgery Effect of bariatric surgery on CV risk factors and survival
2013	Management of Overweight and Obesity in Adults[14]	American College of Cardiology American Heart Association The Obesity Society	BMI cut points to determine risk Impact of weight loss on risk Dietary intervention strategies Bariatric surgery effectiveness
2015	Cardiac Chamber Quantification by Echocardiography in Adults[4]	American Society of Echocardiography European Association of Cardiovascular Imaging	Indexing for body size Chamber size and function measurements standards Normal ranges for echocardiographic parameters
Diabetes			
2015	Update on Prevention of Cardiovascular Disease in Adults with T2DM[85]	American Diabetes Association American Heart Association	New diagnostic criteria for T2DM Lifestyle management of T2DM Treatment targets in T2DM Screening for CV diseases in T2DM
2016	Contributory Risk and Management of Comorbidities of Hypertension, Obesity, Diabetes Mellitus, Hyperlipidemia, and Metabolic Syndrome in Chronic Heart Failure[86]	American Heart Association	Management of comorbidities in patients with heart failure
Liver Disease			
2012	Cardiac Disease Evaluation and Management Among Kidney and Liver Transplantation Candidates[69]	American College of Cardiology American Heart Association	CAD evaluation and management of transplant candidates Evaluation for pHTN for liver transplant candidates Medical management of CV risk in transplant candidates
2013	Evaluation for Liver Transplantation in Adults[72]	American Association for the Study of Liver Disease American Society of Transplantation	Indications for liver transplantation Cardiac evaluation for liver transplantation

BMI, Body mass index; *CAD*, coronary artery disease; *CV*, cardiovascular; *OSA*, obstructive sleep apnea; *pHTN*, pulmonary hypertension; *T2DM*, type 2 diabetes mellitus.

prognostic information. An increased LV mass-to-volume ratio has been associated with high rates of fibrosis, myocardial dysfunction, and adverse cardiovascular outcomes.[5]

LV function is adversely affected by hypertension and cardiac remodeling. Systolic function is most commonly assessed using EF, but in concentric hypertrophy, the EF is less accurate for systolic performance (see Chapter 4). A high systemic afterload impairs cardiac emptying, leading to a lower EF measurement without a change in myocardial contractility. Conversely, concentric hypertrophy with wall thickening increases the EF for any given level of contractility. When technically feasible, alternative measures can be made such as midwall fractional shortening or LV global longitudinal strain (Fig. 34.3).[6] Diastolic dysfunction more commonly occurs before changes in systolic function in hypertensive patients. Diastolic evaluation to include mitral inflow measurements, mitral annular tissue Doppler, and LA size should be performed in all studies (see Chapter 5).

CLINICAL INTERVENTIONS

The decision to begin antihypertensive therapy is based on clinical parameters, including cardiovascular risk and blood pressure measurements. Studies have shown that intensive blood pressure goals for people at elevated cardiovascular risk reduce cardiovascular events.[7] Although treatment recommendations for antihypertensive therapy may be affected in individuals with a reduced ejection fraction (EF), they otherwise do not depend on the more common hypertensive findings of LVH, diastolic dysfunction, or abnormal cardiac remodeling.[1]

Blood pressure lowering can lead to a reduction in LV mass. Initial recommended therapies with thiazide diuretics, calcium channel blockers, angiotensin-converting enzyme inhibitors, and angiotensin receptor blockers have demonstrated higher rates of LVH regression compared with β-blocker therapies.[8] However, observational registries have shown that LV regression is not as commonly observed in the general population as in clinical trials and may not have a large impact on clinical outcome.[9,10] This finding may in part result from LVH and diastolic dysfunction not being specific to hypertension, but there also may be an association with other common comorbidities such as obesity, obstructive sleep apnea, and diabetes. In a subanalysis from Anglo-Scandinavian Cardiac Outcomes, LV regression failed to correlate with improvement in diastolic parameters.[11] Echocardiography for evaluation of

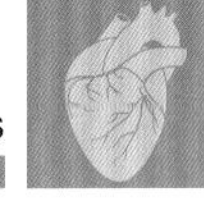

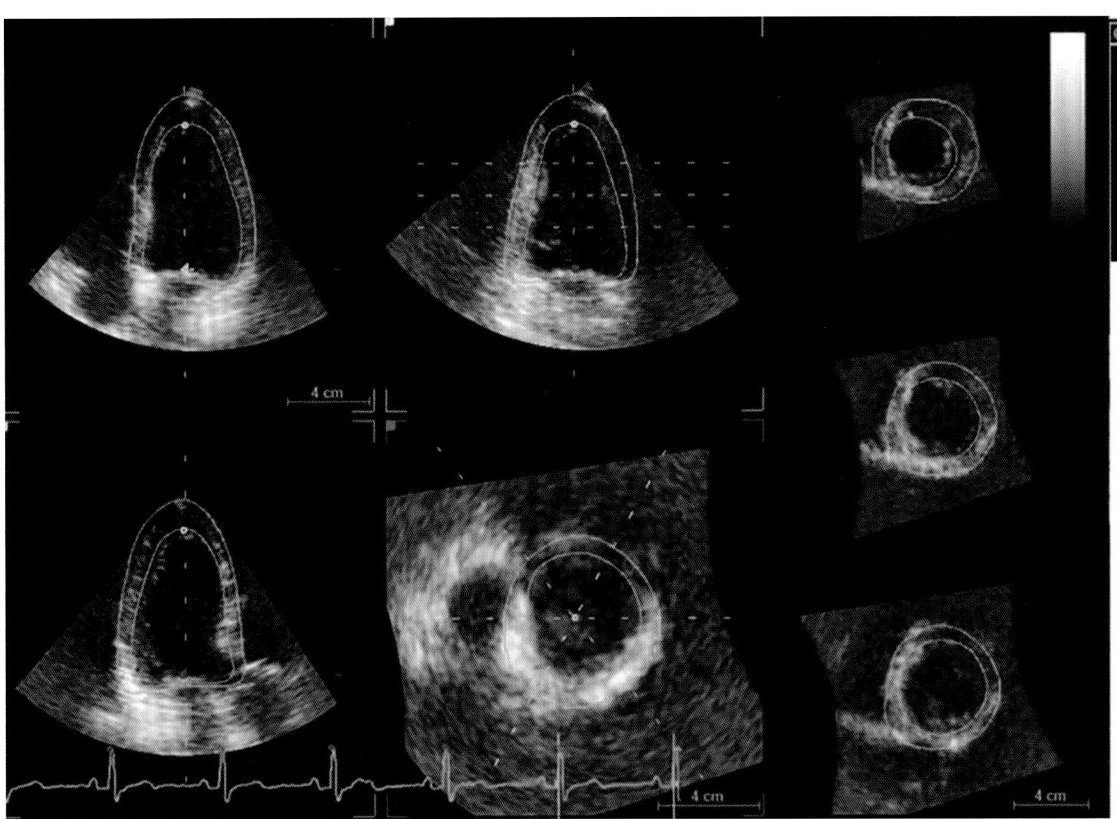

Fig. 34.1 **3D echocardiographic assessment of an LV mass.** *CO*, Cardiac output; *EDMass*, LV mass; *EDV*, LV end-diastolic volume; *EF*, LV ejection fraction; *ESV*, LV end-systolic volume; *HR*, heart rate; *LVM/EDV ratio*, LV mass/end-diastolic volume ratio; *Spl*, sphericity index; *SV*, stroke volume. (From Lembo M, Esposito R, Santoro C, et al. Three-dimensional echocardiographic ventricular mass/end-diastolic volume ratio in native hypertensive patients: relation between stroke volume and geometry. *J Hypertens.* 2018;36[8]:1697–1704.)

TABLE 34.2 **Left Ventricular Geometric Patterns.**

Geometry	*Mass*	*Regional Wall Thickness*
Normal	≤115 g/m² (men) ≤95 g/m² (women)	≤0.42
Concentric hypertrophy	>115 g/m² (men) >95 g/m² (women)	>0.42
Eccentric hypertrophy	>115 g/m² (men) >95 g/m² (women)	≤0.42
Concentric remodeling	≤115 g/m² (men) ≤95 g/m² (women)	>0.42

antihypertensive treatment effects on cardiac structure is not recommended.

OBESITY

BACKGROUND

Obesity is a chronic disease of excessive body fat. It is a worldwide epidemic with increasing global prevalence over the past 3 decades. In developed countries, most men are clinically categorized as overweight or obese.[12] Obesity has serious impact on overall health, with an increasing risk of cardiovascular comorbidities and a 40% increased risk of vascular mortality.[13] Medical providers commonly order echocardiographic evaluations for obese individuals with concerning symptoms (e.g., dyspnea on exertion) that may be related to underlying cardiac dysfunction or decreased cardiorespiratory fitness.

There are several measures of adiposity using anthropometric measurements or noninvasive imaging to directly measure visceral fat content; however, the most practical and recommended assessment of obesity remains the body mass index (BMI).[14] The BMI can be easily calculated by dividing body weight in kilograms by height in meters squared (kg/m²). BMI categories accurately stratify all-cause and cardiovascular mortality risks (Table 34.3).

BMI is a whole-body measure, and it may overestimate or underestimate adiposity in highly muscular individuals and Asian populations, respectively. Additional measures of abdominal obesity such as waist circumference and body fat percentage may provide complementary information in these situations. Computed tomography (CT) and magnetic resonance imaging (MRI) can determine visceral fat distribution and mass but remain too expensive for clinical use.

Direct pathophysiologic consequences of obesity on cardiac structure and function include hemodynamic, neurohormonal, and metabolic alterations.[15] Increased fat mass is associated with increased blood volume, cardiac output, and LV stroke work. A larger venous return increases LV filling pressures and wall stress, leading to cardiac remodeling with varied responses in LV geometry depending on the duration of obesity and comorbidities.

Animal and human studies have shown obesity-associated inflammatory responses from hypertrophied adipocytes. Epicardial fat deposits produce localized hypoxia leading to dysregulated adipocyte secretion of proinflammatory cytokines.[16] The increased triglyceride content and fatty acid use in cardiomyocytes with obesity can lead to myocardial dysfunction.

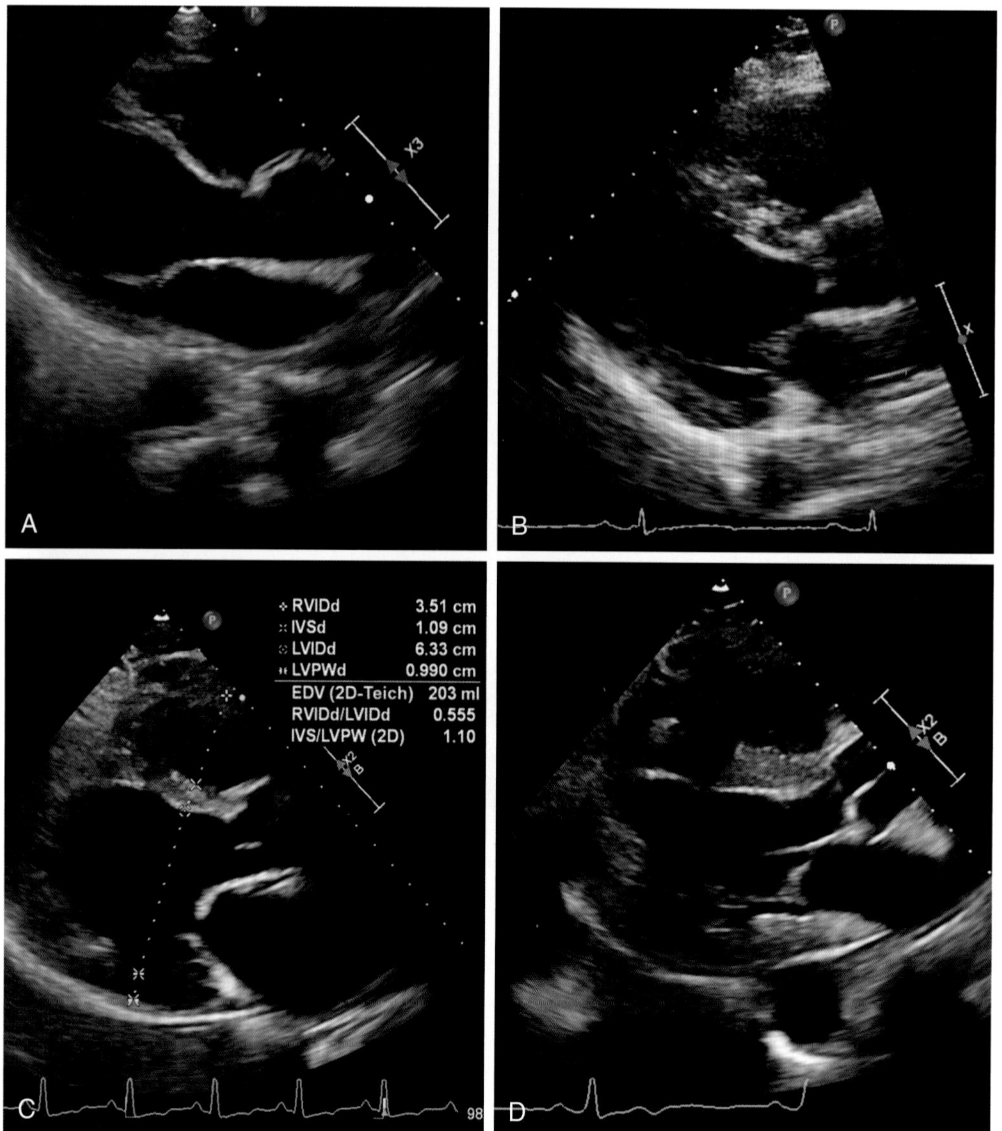

Fig. 34.2 Geometric patterns of LV hypertrophy. (A) Normal LV geometry in a 42-year-old woman with new-onset hypertension. (B) A 59-year-old hypertensive man with concentric remodeling (LV mass of 110 g/m^2 and RWT of 0.55). (C) A 63-year-old woman with eccentric hypertrophy (LV mass of 159 g/m^2 and RWT of 0.32). (D) A 57-year-old man with severe hypertension and concentric hypertrophy (LV mass of 137 g/m^2 and RWT of 0.65). *RWT*, Relative wall thickness.

These mechanisms are likely responsible for the development of an obesity cardiomyopathy and a doubling in the incidence of clinical heart failure.[17]

ECHOCARDIOGRAPHIC FINDINGS

TECHNICAL CONSIDERATIONS

Ultrasound image quality is adversely affected by obesity. Ultrasound energy is attenuated by excessive chest wall fat tissue and by the increased depth of insonation from large chest walls. Lower transducer frequencies, nontraditional views, proper patient positioning, and echocardiographic contrast can be used to improve image quality. Although echocardiographic image quality may be degraded more than in CT or MRI studies, these techniques may not be technically feasible for patients with severe obesity due to the weight and size limits of imaging tables. For patients undergoing bariatric surgery, technically difficult stress echocardiography is associated with worsening levels of obesity, but adequate studies can be almost universally achieved in experienced centers using contrast agents.[18]

Another important technical consideration is scaling of cardiac measurements for body size with obesity. The American Society of Echocardiography Chamber Quantification Guidelines recommend ratio-metric (linear) indexing of LV size and mass to body surface area (BSA).[4] Indexing measurements may allow normalization of parameters to refine the assessment of pathologic versus physiologic changes; however, in severe obesity, BSA may not adequately normalize measurements. Alternative indexing of LV mass with fat-free measurements such as height can better predict adverse events in obese populations. Allometric (exponential) scaling of LV measurements produces more accurate correction in obesity.[19] Similarly, indexing aortic valve area by BSA in obesity increases discordance between indexed and nonindexed valve area meeting criteria for severe aortic stenosis.[20]

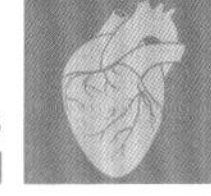

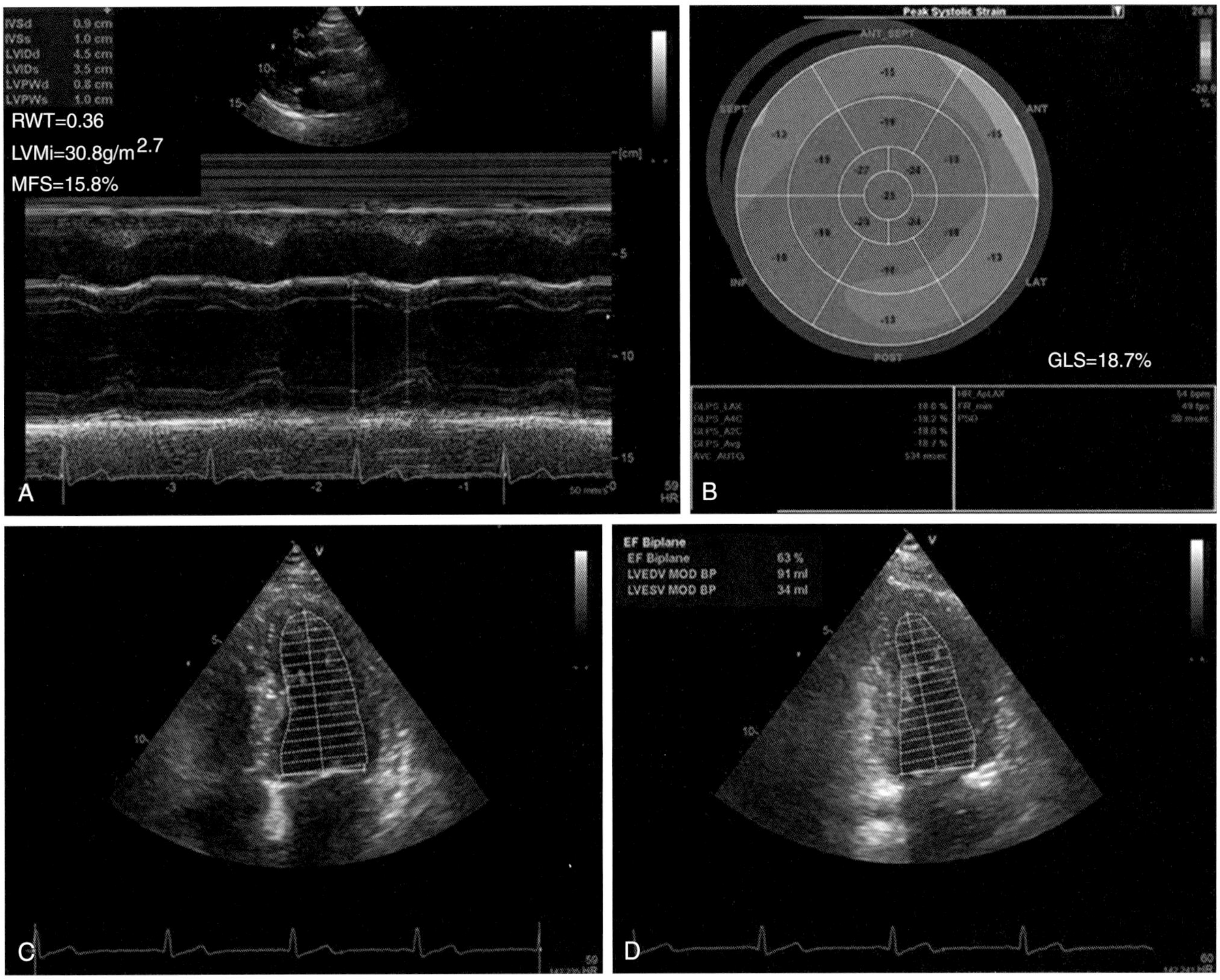

Fig. 34.3 **Measurements of systolic function in a hypertensive patient.** A 49-year-old hypertensive patient with normal ejection fraction *(EF)* but impairment in midwall fractional shortening *(MFS)* and global longitudinal strain *(GLS)*. (A) M-mode–derived LV quantitative analysis and computed MFS. (B) Bull's eye of LV GLS. (C and D) Assessment of biplane LVEF in the same patient. *HR*, Heart rate; *IVSd*, interventricular septum thickness at end-diastole; *IVSs*, interventricular septum thickness at end-systole; *LVEDV*, LV end-diastolic volume; *LVESV*, LV end-systolic volume; *LVIDd*, LV internal diameter at end-diastole; *LVIDs*, LV internal diameter at end-systole; *LVMi*, LV mass indexed for height to the power of 2.7; *LVPWTd*, LV posterior wall thickness at end-diastole; *LVPWTs*, LV posterior wall thickness at end-systole. (Adapted from Lembo M, Santoro C, Sorrentino R, et al. Interrelation between midwall mechanics and longitudinal strain in newly diagnosed and never-treated hypertensive patients without clinically defined hypertrophy. *J Hypertens*. 2020;38[2]:295–302.)

TABLE 34.3 All-Cause and Ischemic Heart Disease Adjusted Mortality Rates Stratified by Body Mass Index Classification.

WHO Category	*BMI (kg/m²)*	*All-Cause Mortality Rate (Men)*[a]	*All-Cause Mortality Rate (Women)*[a]	*IHD Mortality Rate*[a]
Underweight	<18.5	18.4	10.5	2.6
Normal weight	18.5–24.9	14.5	8.9	2.7
Overweight	25–29.9	16.9	10.4	3.5
Obesity class I	30–34.9	22.7	13.0	5.8
Obesity class II	35–39.9	28.2	17.0	7.8
Obesity class III (severe)	≥40	34.7	19.2	8.3

[a]Adjusted annual rates of cases per 1000 patients as calculated by Whitlock et al.[13]
BMI, Body mass index; *IHD*, ischemic heart disease; *WHO*, World Health Organization.

Structural Changes

Several changes in cardiac chamber sizes and geometry have been reported in obesity over the past 30 years. A significant association between obesity and LVH exists in almost all studies. The prevalence of LVH varies between 13% and 75% due to population characteristics of the study participants and the existence of common obesity-related comorbidities, such as hypertension or sleep apnea (Fig. 34.4).

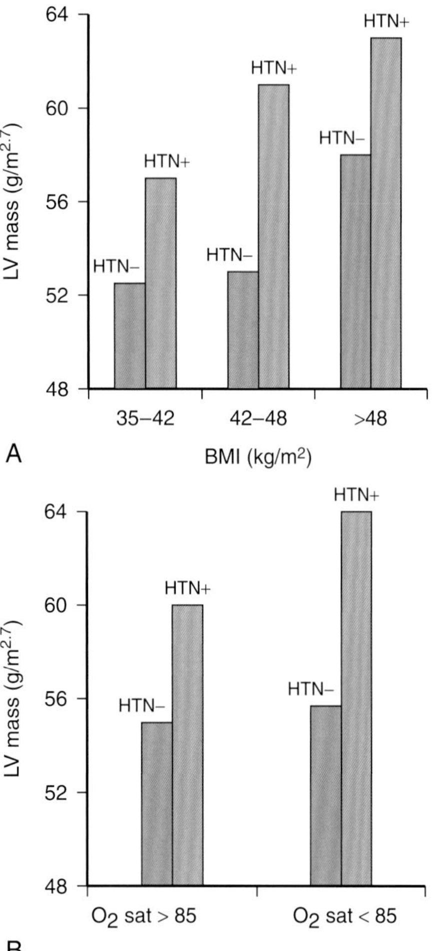

Fig. 34.4 Effect of the interaction of hypertension with obesity and nocturnal hypoxia on LV mass index. (A) LV mass index increases consistently as body mass index *(BMI)* increases. However, the increase in LV mass index is more pronounced in patients with hypertension *(HTN)* than in those without. Formal testing showed that the synergistic interaction of BMI and systolic blood pressure affected the LV mass index. (B) Relationship between the degree of nocturnal hypoxemia and LV mass index in subjects with or without HTN. The effects of nocturnal hypoxemia on LV mass index were amplified in those with HTN. (From Avelar E, Cloward TV, Walker JM, et al. Left ventricular hypertrophy in severe obesity: interactions among blood pressure, nocturnal hypoxemia, and body mass. *Hypertension*. 2007;49:34–39.)

Eccentric and concentric LVH patterns may be seen in obesity. Eccentric hypertrophy is associated with obesity measures because of the increased cardiac output and venous return.[21] However, increased wall thickness with concentric remodeling and hypertrophy are common and may be more likely in older patients with coexisting hypertension. Obese adolescents without comorbidities or significant obesity duration present with thicker LV walls and larger LV masses compared with age-matched, normal-weight teenagers, indicating there are direct consequences of obesity on LV remodeling.[22]

Diastolic Function

Diastolic function is commonly impaired in obese patients, and along with deconditioning, this leads to symptoms of dyspnea. Diastolic impairments have been demonstrated in relaxation and compliance of the LV; however, a grade I (i.e., impaired relaxation) mitral inflow filling pattern is most common. Tissue Doppler of the mitral annulus (e') as a load-independent measure of relaxation is reduced in obesity. Invasive hemodynamic studies reveal higher LV filling pressures in severe obesity. An echocardiographic correlate of elevated filling pressures (E/e') is also associated with higher BMI.

Although diastolic impairments are commonly related to LV structural changes in obesity, some studies have shown altered diastolic parameters with increasing BMI independent of LV mass and comorbidities.[23] Alterations in diastology are seen in all age groups, from obese children to obese elderly individuals, compared with their age-matched controls, but the changes are usually only mild, and the severity does not appear to change with duration of obesity.

Systolic Function

Systolic function is typically assessed by LVEF measurements. Despite obesity-related structural and hemodynamic changes, there is no solid evidence that severe obesity by itself causes a clinically significant reduced EF. Alternative pathologies should be sought in obese individuals with dilated cardiomyopathies.[24] Similar to hypertension-related LVH, obesity leads to increased endocardial shortening, preserving the EF, but midwall fractional shortening is modestly decreased.

Tissue Doppler and speckle tracking strain imaging provide load-independent measures of global and regional contractility. Reductions in systolic strain have been found with increasing BMI (Fig. 34.5).[25] Speckle tracking strain measurements, although promising, require high-quality 2D images, which can be difficult to obtain in obese patients and require further standardization between vendors before they will be acceptable for routine clinical practice.

Epicardial Fat

Patients with higher intraabdominal fat have increased epicardial fat stores. It is important to differentiate epicardial fat from pericardial fluid on echocardiography to prevent misdiagnosis of pericardial effusions. Epicardial fat is typically echogenic and brighter than myocardium and moves with the cardiac cycle, unlike echolucent pericardial fluid. The epicardial fat thickness can be measured by echocardiography (Fig. 34.6). Epicardial fat size serves as a marker for the development of cardiometabolic risk factors and coronary artery disease, possibly from paracrine effects on the vasculature from adipocytes near the coronary arteries.[26] Echocardiography techniques measuring epicardial fat are limited by its linear measurement at a single location, and fat thickness only moderately correlates with volume measurements from alternative imaging modalities such as CT or MRI.

A potential advantage of noninvasive measurements for visceral and epicardial fat deposition may be to identify increases in cardiovascular risk in cases of normal-weight obesity (i.e., increased body fat deposition with a normal BMI). MRI imaging enables improved tissue characterization when pronounced epicardial fat produces masslike features on echocardiography (Fig. 34.7).

CLINICAL INTERVENTIONS

The overwhelming cause of obesity is excess caloric intake and decreased caloric expenditure from limited physical activity. The primary intervention is lifestyle modification with a low-calorie diet and an increase in exertional activity. Weight loss, regardless of method, appears to cause favorable changes in cardiac structure and function.

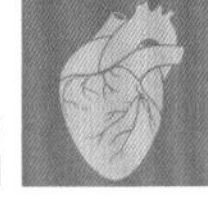

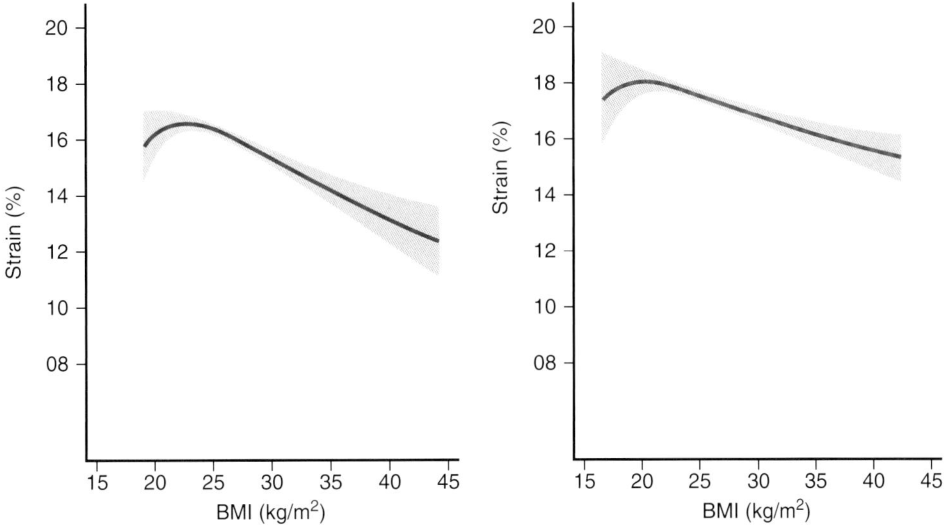

Fig. 34.5 Association of body mass index with longitudinal LV end-systolic strain. Age-adjusted fractional polynomial regression plot of global longitudinal LV end-systolic strain by body mass index *(BMI)*. Estimated mean *(line)* and 95% confidence interval *(shadow)* are displayed. *Blue lines* refer to men and *red lines* to women. (From Dalen H, Thorstensen A, Romundstad PR, et al. Cardiovascular risk factors and systolic and diastolic cardiac function: a tissue Doppler and speckle tracking echocardiographic study. *J Am Soc Echocardiogr.* 2011;24:322–332.e326.)

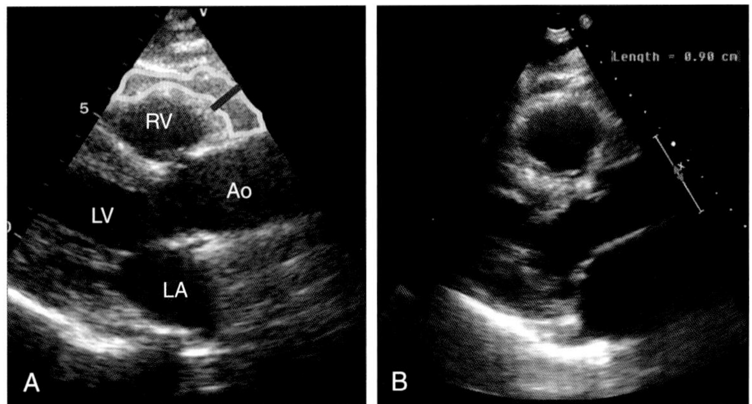

Fig. 34.6 Measurement of epicardial fat thickness with echocardiography. Maximal epicardial fat thickness *(red line)* from a parasternal long-axis view at end-systole as recommended by Iacobellis. (A) Thickness is measured within the epicardial fat *(yellow line border)* along the RV free wall perpendicular to the ultrasound beam and aortic *(Ao)* annulus (see Video 34.6A), (B) When the large epicardial thickness abruptly increases along the acute border of the RV as it approaches the ascending aorta in this 70-year-old, obese man, the largest epicardial fat thickness at or to the left of the aortic annulus should be measured. The epicardial fat thickness of 9 mm is higher than normal (<7 mm) and is associated with an excess risk of coronary artery disease. (From Iacobellis G. Local and systemic effects of the multifaceted epicardial adipose tissue depot. *Nat Rev Endocrinol.* 2015;11:363–371.)

Patients with long-standing severe obesity or class II obesity with comorbidities who have attempted previous lifestyle modifications may be candidates for bariatric surgery. Bariatric surgery has led to significant weight loss and reduction in cardiovascular risk factors compared with conservative lifestyle interventions. Consistently, investigators have demonstrated regression in LV mass, improvements in diastolic parameters, and reduction in LA volumes with bariatric surgery. The largest study followed 423 obese patients for 2 years after bariatric surgery who had on average lost 44 kg and compared them with 733 nonsurgical patients who experienced minimal weight loss.[27] Bariatric surgery reduced LV mass and wall thickness, increased midwall fractional shortening, and improved RV fractional area change values. Overall, regression of LV mass and normalization of LV diastolic filling patterns would be expected with bariatric surgery, but significant systolic recovery has been rarely described, likely due to surgical selection bias.

Pharmacotherapy has been less successful in treating obesity and related complications. Anorectic drugs such as fenfluramine and dexfenfluramine were discontinued by their manufacturer in 1997 after increased rates of mitral and aortic regurgitation were reported. A newer appetite suppressant, lorcaserin, has had a modest weight loss effect (approximately 4–6 kg) without any increased risk in echocardiographically confirmed valvulopathy.[28]

OBSTRUCTIVE SLEEP APNEA

BACKGROUND

Obstructive sleep apnea (OSA) is the most common sleep breathing disorder; the increasing prevalence correlates with the growing rate of obesity.[29] OSA is diagnosed using polysomnography to identify a minimum of five obstructive events per hour, known as the *apnea-hypopnea index,* with daytime

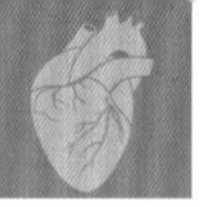

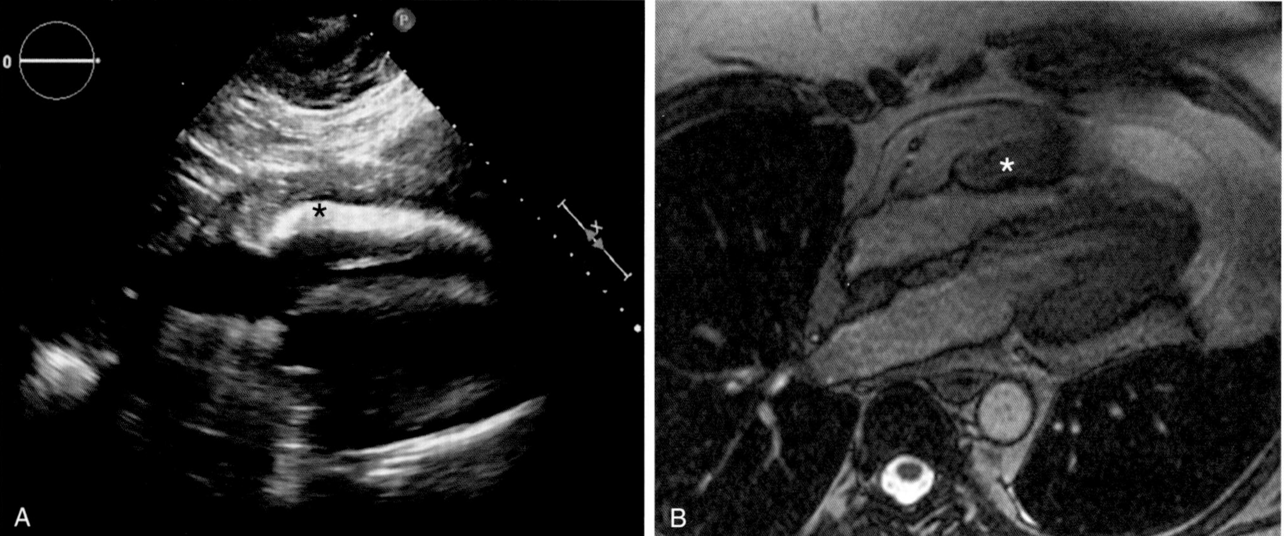

Fig 34.7 Severe epicardial fat. (A) Off-axis subcostal view with a prominent mass *(asterisk)* possibly infiltrating the RVs. (B) MRI study with a similar 4-chamber view demonstrates that the mass tissue *(asterisk)* is characteristic of epicardial fat and not a myocardial malignancy. The RV thickness is normal by MRI measurement.

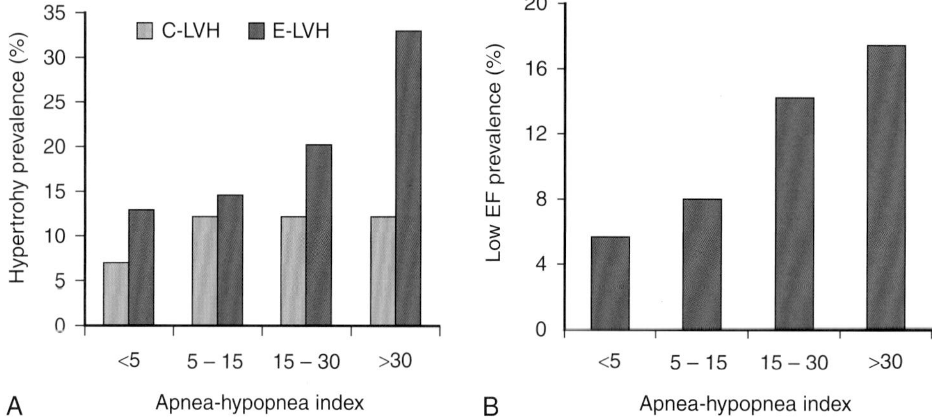

Fig. 34.8 Associations of obstructive sleep apnea severity with LV remodeling and systolic function in the Sleep Heart Health Study. (A) A higher apnea-hypopnea index is associated with a higher prevalence of eccentric LV hypertrophy. (B) The severity of obstructive sleep apnea correlates with a higher prevalence of ejection fraction values of less than 55%. *C-LVH,* Concentric LV hypertrophy; *E-LVH,* eccentric LV hypertrophy. (From Chami HA, Devereux RB, Gottdiener JS, et al. Left ventricular morphology and systolic function in sleep-disordered breathing: the Sleep Heart Health Study. *Circulation.* 2008;117:2599–2607.)

symptoms. An apnea-hypopnea index value of 15 or more events are considered diagnostic even without symptoms, and most studies consider an apnea hypopnea index of more than 30 to be severe.

Left untreated, severe OSA has been associated with increased cardiovascular events. Possible deleterious mechanisms of OSA on cardiac structure and function include raising LV afterload from high negative intrathoracic pressures, autonomic dysregulation with elevated sympathetic tone, apnea-related hypoxia activating inflammatory mediators, and thromboembolic susceptibility from a hypercoagulable state.[30] OSA patients have higher incidences of hypertension, coronary disease, heart failure, and atrial fibrillation than individuals without sleep-disordered breathing. OSA symptoms are often nonspecific (i.e., fatigue and daytime somnolence) and commonly lead to echocardiographic evaluations and high rates of associated cardiovascular risk factors.

ECHOCARDIOGRAPHIC FINDINGS

LVH is common in severe OSA and reported in approximately 40% of participants in community-based population studies. Similar to obesity, both concentric and eccentric geometric patterns of LVH have been demonstrated in OSA. However, the largest study with adjustment for confounders showed eccentric hypertrophy to be more strongly associated with increased severity of OSA (Fig. 34.8).[31] LV systolic and diastolic alterations also occur in OSA. There is a weak inverse correlation between OSA severity and EF measurements in community- and clinic-based samples without known symptomatic cardiovascular disease.

Diastolic parameters in OSA patients are similar to those for patients with hypertension and obesity when compared to healthy controls. OSA is associated with reduced mitral inflow velocity (E), higher E/*e*′, and lower ratios of peak transmittal early diastolic velocity to late diastolic velocity (E/A). LA

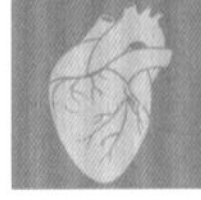

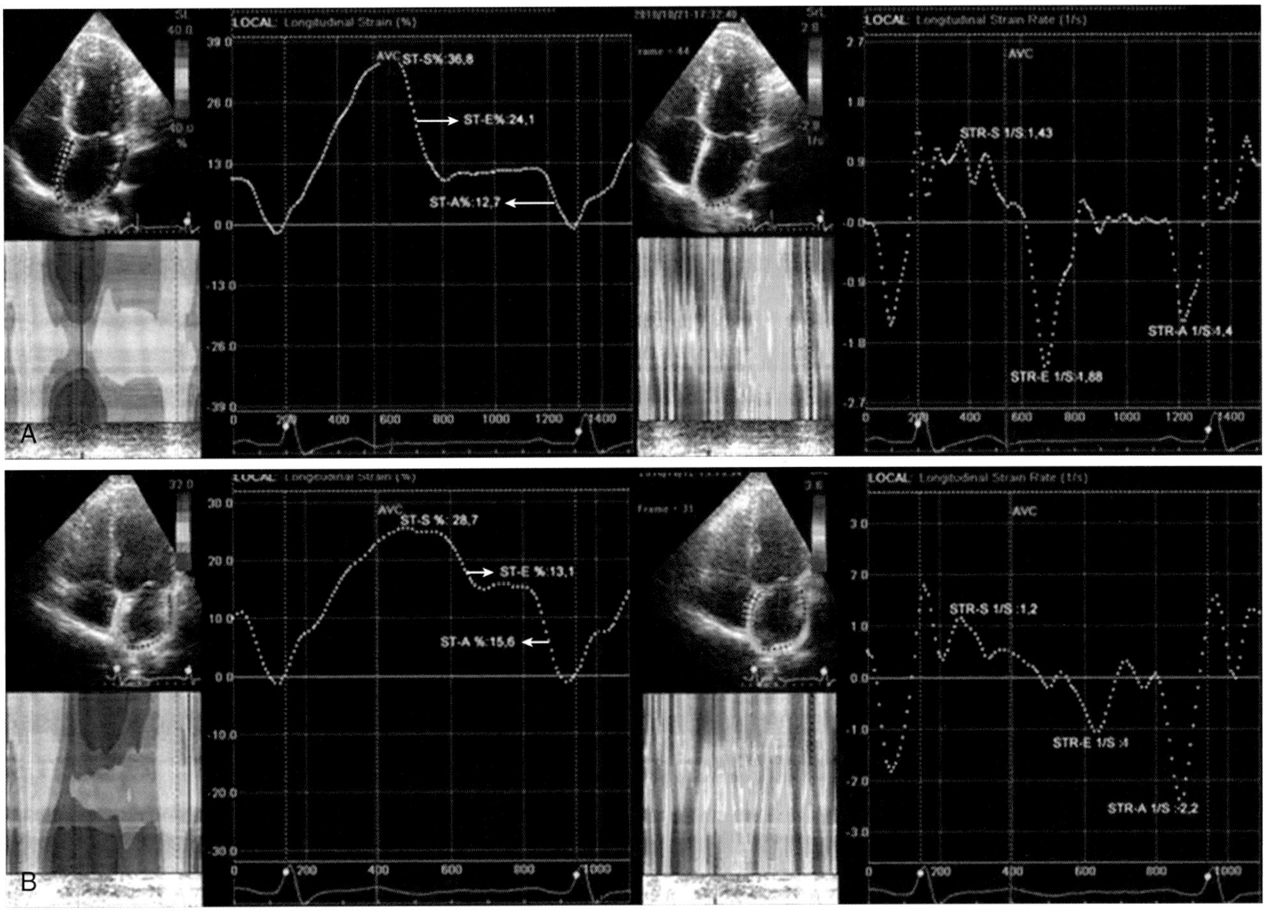

Fig. 34.9 LA strain in a patient with obstructive sleep apnea compared with a healthy control. Apical 4-chamber LA speckle tracking average longitudinal strain in a healthy individual (A) and a patient with severe obstructive sleep apnea (OSA) (B). Reduced peak LA strain rate *(ST-S)* and lower systole strain rate *(STR-S)* are consistent with reduced LA reservoir function in the patient with severe OSA. (From Altekin RE, Yanikoglu A, Karakas MS, et al. Assessment of left atrial dysfunction in obstructive sleep apnea patients with the two dimensional speckle-tracking echocardiography. *Clin Res Cardiol.* 2012;101:403–413.)

enlargement and decreased function also occur in OSA and may be independent of LV diastolic changes using traditional echocardiographic parameters.[32]

Fibrosis of the atrial wall has been suggested as a possible mechanism for reduced LA function in MRI studies. Deformation of the LA in OSA can be measured with strain and strain rate determined by speckle tracking echocardiography (Fig. 34.9). Decreased peak longitudinal strain of the atrium is associated with severe OSA and increased risk of cardiovascular events in the general population.[33]

Pulmonary pressures along with RV size and function are often specifically requested for patients with OSA. Pulmonary hypertension occurs in up to 20% of patients with OSA. Although intermittent hypoxia during sleep acutely alters pulmonary hemodynamics through vasoactive mediators, most OSA patients without underlying lung disease or obesity hypoventilation syndrome have normal daytime oxygen saturations. OSA-related hypoxia in combination with pulmonary venous hypertension from underlying LV dysfunction act synergistically to elevate pulmonary arterial pressure. However, the severity of pulmonary hypertension related to OSA is usually mild.

CLINICAL INTERVENTIONS

Weight loss by lifestyle modification or bariatric surgery can improve OSA as measured by the apnea-hypopnea index. Reduction of obesity also leads to improvements in cardiac function.

The mainstay treatment for OSA is positive airway pressure therapy, most often constant positive airway pressure (CPAP). CPAP definitively reduces the apnea-hypopnea index and improves daytime sleepiness and quality of life. Observational studies suggest CPAP-adherent OSA patients have reduced mortality rates compared with untreated or nonadherent patients, but randomized trials have yet to show a cardiovascular outcome benefit.[34] In the community, adherence to CPAP is poor, with use less than 4 hours per night by up to 40% of those prescribed therapy.

Cardiovascular risk factors may be improved with CPAP therapy for OSA. CPAP improves systolic blood pressure in OSA patients with hypertension, but only modest changes are usually seen, on average 2 to 3 mmHg.[35] Patients with systolic heart failure may improve their EF by an average of 5% with adherent use of CPAP.[36] Concordantly, improvements in LV diastolic parameters, LA volumes, and pulmonary pressure have been reported with nighttime positive airway pressure therapy.[37]

TYPE 2 DIABETES MELLITUS AND THE METABOLIC SYNDROME

BACKGROUND

Obesity-related insulin resistance is the foremost mechanism responsible for the type 2 diabetes mellitus (DM) epidemic.

TABLE 34.4 Metabolic Syndrome.[a]

Elevated waist circumference[b]	≥40 inches (102 cm) (males) ≥35 inches (88 cm) (females)
Elevated triglycerides	≥150 mg/dL (1.7 mmol/L) or drug treatment for triglycerides
Reduced high-density lipoprotein cholesterol	<40 mg/dL (1.03 mmol/L) (males) <50 mg/dL (1.3 mmol/L) (females)
Elevated blood pressure	≥130 mmHg systolic or ≥ 85 mmHg diastolic
Elevated fasting glucose	≥100 mg/dL or drug treatment of elevated glucose

[a]Requires three of the five characteristics.
[b]Smaller waist circumference may be appropriate for Asian populations (≥90 cm for males; ≥80 cm for females).

Resulting hyperinsulinemia and hyperglycemia lead to vascular dysfunction, high blood pressure, lipid dysregulation, and systemic inflammation. The milieu of diabetic and cardiovascular risk factors has been called the metabolic syndrome (MetS). The most widely used definition of MetS is based on minor modifications of the National Cholesterol Education Program Adult Treatment Panel III recommendations (Table 34.4).

It remains debatable whether the MetS is a distinct entity or the summation of coexisting risk factors for DM and cardiovascular disease. It is clear that DM and MetS share a spectrum of pathophysiologic mechanisms and are associated with an almost doubling of risk for cardiovascular events and death. Most of the risk is from vascular disease, including coronary and cerebral artery disease causing myocardial infarctions and strokes, respectively.[38] However, changes in cardiac structure and function are independent of coronary artery disease and BMI in these insulin-resistant disease states.

Hyperglycemia, lipotoxicity, and hyperinsulinemia cause cardiomyocytes to undergo cellular hypertrophy, stiffness, hypoxia, and death. Reactive interstitial and replacement fibrosis ensues, instigating diabetic cardiomyopathy with diastolic and sometimes systolic dysfunction.[39] These mechanisms may explain the poor clinical outcomes that are seen in heart failure patients with diabetes.

ECHOCARDIOGRAPHIC FINDINGS

Similar to obesity, patients with DM have LVH that may be from eccentric remodeling in a dilated cardiomyopathy phenotype or concentric remodeling with preservation of the EF. Although coexisting comorbidities in DM and MetS may influence cardiac structure and function, changes still exist when controlling for these risk factors. In a population study of 4419 participants without prevalent cardiovascular disease, DM was independently associated with significantly higher indexed LV mass and regional wall thickness, although the average increase in mass was only 3 g after adjustment.[40] Most studies have been limited by cross-sectional analysis; however, in the longitudinal MONICA/KORA cohort study, diabetic participants without a myocardial infarction followed over 10 years exhibited increases in LV mass and eccentric remodeling, with a 7% average enlargement of LV cavity size.[41]

DM and MetS are associated with diastolic abnormalities using conventional and tissue Doppler imaging. DM has been consistently associated with lower E/A ratios and reduced basal septal velocities. The magnitude of these diastolic changes correlates with the severity of insulin resistance.[42] Systolic function, as assessed by tissue Doppler longitudinal strain and strain rate, was similarly reduced despite preservation of the EF. Diabetic alterations in global longitudinal strain may serve as a risk marker for adverse cardiac remodeling over time; however, its prognostic ability for clinical outcomes has not been determined.[43]

CLINICAL INTERVENTIONS

Treatment for MetS and DM includes lifestyle modifications and pharmacotherapy to optimize cardiovascular risk factors. DM therapies focus on lowering hyperglycemia as measured by glycated hemoglobin (HbA1c) levels. Glycemic levels are known to be associated with microvascular and macrovascular complications, along with the incidence of symptomatic heart failure. HbA1c levels correlate with cardiac alterations in structure and with diastolic and systolic function by echocardiography (Fig. 34.10).

The HbA1c goal for most patients is below 7% to reduce vascular complications. However, for elderly individuals and long-term diabetics at high risk for cardiovascular disease, intensive therapy to lower HbA1c goals to normal levels increased mortality rates in the ACCORD trial.[44] Higher mortality rates may have resulted from medication side effects, such as hypoglycemia, and care should be taken in this population to consider liberalizing HbA1c goals to less than 8% to help prevent low blood glucose levels.

Various therapies can produce subtle improvements in cardiac function in diabetic cardiomyopathies. Diet and exercise directly reduce myocardial lipid content and can have favorable effects on cardiac function in experimental models, although adherence to lifestyle changes remains poor. A clinical trial on exercise intervention restricted to diabetic patients who maintained follow-up over 3 years showed attenuation of worsening diastolic dysfunction over the follow-up period. However, there was no improvement in diastolic function from baseline.[45] Current recommendations for 150 minutes of moderate aerobic activity per week are based on improvement in glycemic control and reduction of vascular events.[46]

Aside from lowering blood glucose levels, DM medication class–specific effects on cardiac function have been studied, and there have been clinical and structural improvements with sodium-glucose cotransporter 2 (SGT2) inhibitors. Empagliflozin has reduced LV mass in diabetics.[47] A large clinical trial demonstrated that dapagliflozin reduced the risk of worsening heart failure and cardiovascular death of patients with reduced EF.[48] The SGT2 inhibitors are preferred over thiazolidinediones and dipeptidyl peptidase-4 inhibitors, because the latter agents are associated with increased risk of heart failure and hospitalization.[49]

ENDOCRINOPATHIES

Endocrinopathies result in hormonal imbalances from dysregulated gland metabolism. The inability to maintain metabolic homeostasis results in systemic changes that depend on the hormone involved. Cardiac disease rarely exists exclusively; more often, various symptoms occur because of hormonal involvement of multiple organs. Cardiac changes usually result from a combination of alterations in systemic hemodynamics and direct hormonal effects on myocardial tissue.

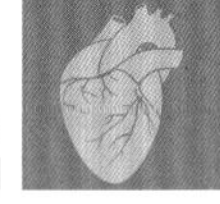

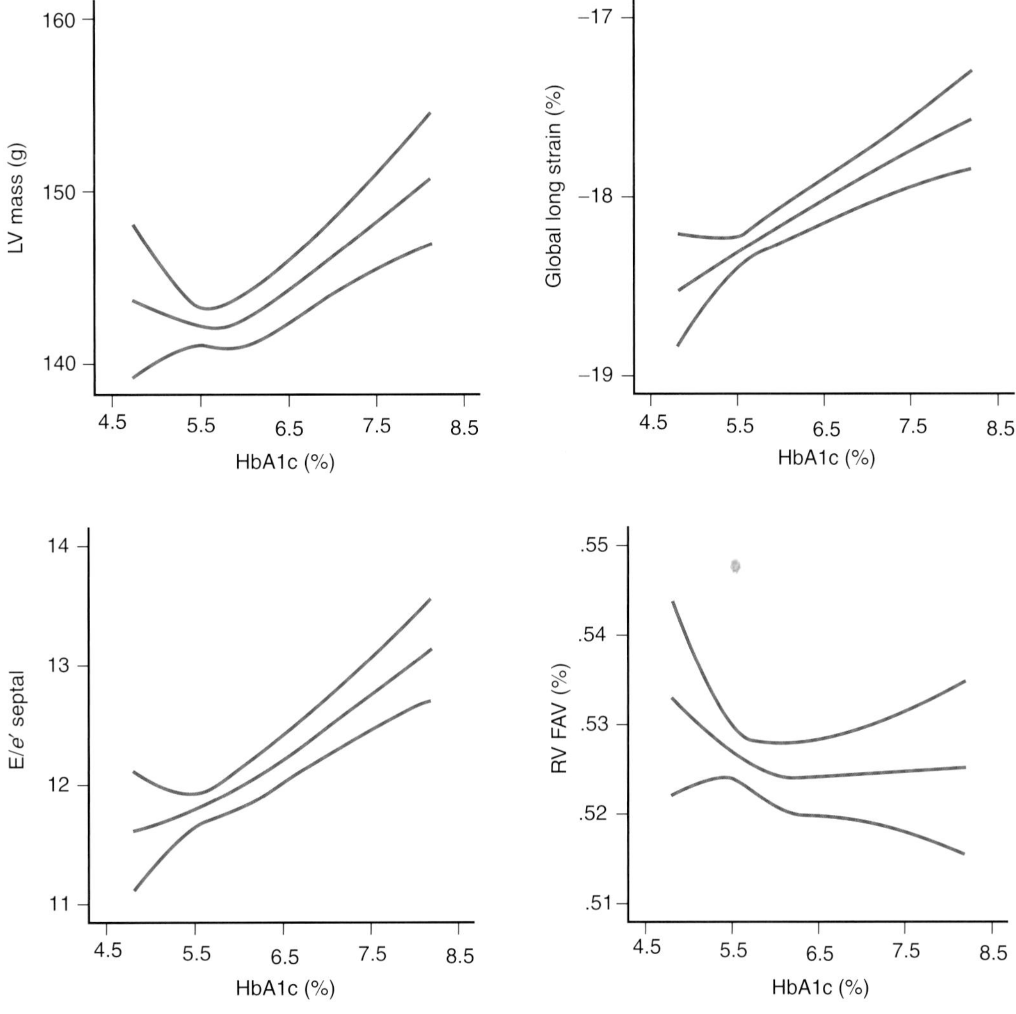

Fig. 34.10 Association between glycated hemoglobin and LV mass, LV systolic and diastolic function, and RV systolic function. The association between glycated hemoglobin (HbA1c) levels and echocardiographic measures of cardiac structure and function is displayed with multivariable-adjusted restricted cubic splines. The model is adjusted for age, sex, race, center, body surface area, body mass index, systolic blood pressure, heart rate, hypertension, current smoking, and chronic kidney disease. The *middle line* represents the cubic spline; the *upper* and *lower lines* represent the 95% confidence limits. *FAC,* Fractional area change; *Long,* longitudinal. (Adapted from Skali H, Shah A, Gupta DK, et al. Cardiac structure and function across the glycemic spectrum in elderly men and women free of prevalent heart disease: the atherosclerosis risk in the community study. *Circ Heart Fail.* 2015;8:448–454.)

It is important to recognize underlying endocrine disorders as a potential cause of cardiac disease because treatment can restore cardiac function. A complete review of all endocrinopathies is beyond the scope of this textbook, but the most relevant clinical disorders with defined cardiovascular manifestations are summarized (Table 34.5).

HYPERTHYROIDISM

Increased production of the thyroid hormones thyroxine (T_4) and triiodothyronine (T_3) leads to dramatic metabolic effects on almost every system in the human body. Cardiomyocytes have thyroid hormone nuclear receptors that when bound, alter gene transcription regulating intracellular calcium metabolism and myofilaments.[50] Nongenomic effects on cardiomyocytes include altering ion channel permeability, leading to tachycardia. Hyperthyroidism changes hemodynamic loading conditions, with increasing blood volume and decreasing systemic vascular resistance. The combination of cardiac and vascular changes leads to increasing cardiac output and cardiac remodeling over time.

Various studies with different levels of increased thyroid exposure have shown changes in LV morphology. LVH has been long associated with overt (symptomatic) hyperthyroidism. Even when thyroid levels are in the normal range, there was a correlation with concentric remodeling; higher free T_3 levels were associated with a decrease in LV end-diastolic diameters and increase in relative wall thickness in a large population-based study.[51]

Increases in contractility and preload produce higher EFs in hyperthyroid states. However, excessive prolonged tachycardia and atrial arrhythmias can lead to tachycardia-induced dilated cardiomyopathy if not treated. Initial hyperthyroid states enhance lusitropy, but volume loading and LVH can produce diastolic dysfunction over time. Pulmonary hypertension may result from hyperthyroidism. It may be caused by shared autoimmune mechanisms or the pulmonary vasculature not dilating in response to excess thyroid hormone and increasing

TABLE 34.5 Clinical Echocardiographic Correlates of Primary Endocrine Disorders.

Disorder	*Initial Diagnostic or Screening Test*	*Clinical Manifestations*	*Echocardiographic Findings*
Hyperthyroidism	↓TSH (<0.4 mU/L)	Heat intolerance Anxiety Palpitations Weight loss	↑EF ↑LVM ↓IVRT ↑PA pressure ↑HR Mitral valve prolapse
Hypothyroidism	↑TSH (>5 mU/L)	Cold intolerance Fatigue Constipation Myxedema Anemia	↓EF/GLS ↑IVRT ↓e′ ↓HR Pericardial effusion
Acromegaly	↑IGF-1 Followed by GH >1 ng/mL (2 hours after OGTT)	Increased skin thickness Macrognathia Macroglossia Arthropathy Hypertension	Biventricular hypertrophy Grade 1 diastolic dysfunction Mitral regurgitation Aortic regurgitation
GH deficiency	↓IGF-1 Followed by GH <4.1 ng/mL after provocative testing (GHRH-arginine)	Short stature (childhood) Osteopenia or fractures Low energy or fatigue Dyslipidemia ↓Lean body mass	↓EF ↓LVM
Cushing syndrome	↑24-hour urinary free cortisol and/or low dose (1 mg) dexamethasone suppression	Central obesity Purple striae Hypertension Menstrual irregularity Glucose intolerance Proximal muscle atrophy	Biventricular hypertrophy ↓EF/GLS Grade 1 diastolic dysfunction
Hyperparathyroidism	↑PTH (>65 pg/mL)	Nephrolithiasis Neuropsychiatric changes Bone pain/osteopenia Muscle weakness Nausea, vomiting	↑LVM Aortic valve calcification Mitral annular calcification Myocardial calcification Grade 1 diastolic dysfunction
Pheochromocytoma	↑24-hour urine fractionated catecholamines and metanephrines	Headaches Sweating Tachycardia Hypertension Orthostasis	LV hypertrophy Dilated cardiomyopathy Apical hypokinesis with hyperkinetic base (Takotsubo-type pattern)

e′, Peak early diastolic tissue-Doppler velocity; *EF*, ejection fraction; *GH*, growth hormone; *GHRH*, growth hormone–releasing hormone; *GLS*, global longitudinal strain; *HR*, heart rate; *IGF*, insulinlike growth factor; *IVRT*, isovolumic relaxation time; *LVM*, LV mass; *OGTT*, oral glucose tolerance test; *PA*, pulmonary artery; *TSH*, thyroid-stimulating hormone, ↓, reduced.

cardiac output. Mitral valve prolapse has a higher prevalence among patients with autoimmune hyperthyroidism (i.e., Graves disease).

HYPOTHYROIDISM

Unlike the hyperdynamic state of hyperthyroidism, converse cardiac effects occur with low T_4 and T_3 conditions. Slow heart rates, narrowed pulse pressure, and decreased contractility are found in hypothyroidism. Both systolic and diastolic dysfunction in overt hypothyroidism have been detected using tissue Doppler imaging and strain analysis.[52] Prolonged isovolumic relaxation and deceleration times occur with hypothyroidism. Global longitudinal strain and 3D EF in subclinical hypothyroidism are lower compared with healthy controls and improve with thyroid hormone supplementation. Fluid retention may occur from decreased water clearance and with associated accumulation of glycosaminoglycans, leading to skin myxedema, and to pericardial and pleural effusions.[53]

ACROMEGALY

Excessive production of growth hormone (GH), most commonly by pituitary adenomas, leads to stimulation of growth of various soft tissues and visceral organs. Cardiac structural and functional changes are mediated by a combination of direct GH effects, increased hepatic production of insulinlike growth factor-1 (IGF-1), and hypertensive hemodynamic changes.[54]

The clinical manifestation of acromegaly is usually insidious, occurring over many years and producing headaches, skin thickening, facial changes, swollen hands and feet, arthropathy, and hypertension. Mortality rates reflect the increased number of cardiovascular and cancer deaths, but the risk can be reduced with adequate hormonal control of the disease.

Acromegalic cardiomyopathy can occur, even with short-term exposure to excess GH. Biventricular LVH and diastolic dysfunction are common and correlate with duration of disease and resulting hypertension. A 29-year retrospective study from two centers involving 330 acromegaly patients showed that 3% eventually developed advance systolic heart failure despite GH-suppressive treatment.[55] LVH changes can be reversed in most patients with treatment by somatostatin analogs or tumor removal. GH effects on connective tissue leads to permanent valvular myxomatous thickening and increased prevalence of aortic and mitral regurgitation that does not resolve despite long-term treatment.

GROWTH HORMONE DEFICIENCY

GH deficiency may result from injury to the pituitary gland. Deficiency in childhood results in short stature, which is the most common reason for GH supplementation. Adults with new-onset GH deficiency experience osteopenia, reduced lean body mass with increased fat mass, less energy, and increased cardiovascular risk due to dyslipidemia and endothelial dysfunction. GH-deficient adults have a lower LV mass and EF, which can improve with supplementation.

GH deficiency is common in patients with heart failure and is associated with poor clinical outcomes. GH supplementation has been studied in randomized trials of heart failure patients. Mild improvement in peak oxygen consumption (12.9–14.5 mL/kg/min) and EF (34%–36%) was seen in one trial, but improvement in clinical end points has not been proved.[56] GH supplementation for patients with heart failure remains investigational and is not recommended at this time.

CUSHING SYNDROME

Excess chronic exposure to cortisol results in Cushing syndrome, which manifests as centripetal obesity, fragile and atrophied skin (e.g., purple striae), menstrual irregularity, proximal muscular weakness, hypertension, osteoporosis, and glucose intolerance. Increased cortisol secretion may result from adrenal tumors, adrenocorticotropin hormone–producing pituitary adenomas (i.e., Cushing disease), or malignant paraneoplastic syndromes. Individuals with Cushing syndrome are at an increased risk for death from cardiovascular diseases, primarily from myocardial infarction and stroke. Predictors of death include cortisol excess–related diabetes, hypertension, and obesity that may lead to a higher prevalence of atherosclerotic coronary disease.[57]

Cardiac remodeling with higher LV mass and regional wall thickness occurs in Cushing syndrome. As with other metabolic disorders, investigators have demonstrated a reduced E/A, decreased e' velocities, and lower global longitudinal strain values in Cushing patients compared with healthy controls. Although many patients with excess cortisol have hypertension, changes in cardiac function can occur in normotensive individuals. Glucocorticoids directly induce myocardial remodeling and affect calcium handling in rat models, and hypercortisolism may have direct clinical cardiac effects independent of vascular and hemodynamic load changes.

HYPERPARATHYROIDISM

Parathyroid hormone (PTH) is the principal regulator of calcium homeostasis. PTH may be elevated from primary overproduction in the parathyroid gland (leading to hypercalcemia) or secondary causes that stimulate PTH release, such as hypocalcemia. The primary action of PTH occurs in the skeletal and renal system to mobilize calcium stores into the serum and increase reabsorption of filtered calcium. Clinical signs and symptoms of hyperparathyroidism are related to the hypercalcemic state and parathyroid bone effects, including nephrolithiasis, polyuria, gastrointestinal distress, bone pain, osteopenia, and altered mental status.

In addition to bone mineral metabolism effects, PTH has direct cardiac and vascular effects. A 50% increase in cardiovascular events has been reported for patients with excess PTH.[58] The exact mechanism of PTH leading to cardiovascular events is unclear but may include trophic effects exerted on cardiomyocytes, impaired calcium handling and cellular overload, a hypertensive vascular effect, or may reflect early kidney damage that can lead to adverse cardiovascular outcomes. Direct consequences of elevated PTH are suggested by its association with increases in incident heart failure and LV mass independent of other cardiovascular risk factors and mineral metabolism biomarkers.[59]

The significance of cardiac dysfunction is related to the severity of the hyperparathyroidism. Older studies that included symptomatic patients with more significant perturbations in calcium and PTH levels demonstrated impaired diastolic function and an increased prevalence of valvular and myocardial calcification. Milder forms of asymptomatic hyperparathyroidism diagnosed only by biochemical analysis do not appear to cause significant cardiac dysfunction but do increase subclinical aortic valve calcification.[60]

Surgical treatment of primary hyperparathyroidism to prevent bone and kidney disease is based on symptoms or significantly high calcium levels. Regression of LV mass and halting of calcification have been demonstrated as outcomes after surgery for overt hyperparathyroidism, but mitigation of cardiovascular risk has not been proven in the treatment of less severe disease.

PHEOCHROMOCYTOMA

Catecholamine-secreting neuroendocrine tumors may arise from the adrenal medulla (i.e., pheochromocytoma) or from extraadrenal autonomic tissue (i.e., paragangliomas), including the heart and posterior mediastinum (Fig. 34.11). The tumors are most commonly benign but may be malignant in up to 10% of patients. The classic triad of symptoms includes paroxysmal headaches, sweating, and tachycardia. Up to 90% of patients with pheochromocytoma have hypertension, and treatment of hypertension should include combined α- and β-adrenergic blockade, with avoidance of sole use of β-blocker therapy.

Cardiac manifestations of pheochromocytomas vary. Normal cardiac findings are most common, but concentric LVH and diastolic dysfunction can occur from the associated hypertension, which may persist even after treatment.[61] Catecholamine excess is directly toxic to cardiomyocytes and may result in ischemia due to increasing myocardial oxygen demand with a decrease in oxygen supply caused by coronary vasoconstriction. LV systolic dysfunction in forms of dilated cardiomyopathy with global hypokinesis or a transient apical-ballooning (takotsubo) cardiomyopathy may be the initial presentation.[62]

LIVER DISEASES

Liver disorders commonly involve the heart due to vascular alterations, toxic injury from metabolic derangements, or common pathologies that may affect both organs, such as alcoholism. Echocardiography is the first-line noninvasive assessment for cardiopulmonary complications of cirrhosis (Table 34.6). Selection of candidates for liver transplantation or a transjugular intrahepatic portosystemic shunt (TIPS) depends on echocardiographic evaluation.

CIRRHOTIC CARDIOMYOPATHY

Progressive late-stage liver disorders result in hepatic fibrosis (i.e., cirrhosis) and distortion of the liver microcirculation, which leads to portal hypertension and ascites (Fig. 34.12). The high cardiovascular morbidity and mortality rates after liver transplantation or the TIPS procedure, suggest possible cardiac dysfunction related to cirrhosis (i.e., cirrhotic cardiomyopathy). The working definition is quite broad and has been modified to include deformation imaging changes: cardiac dysfunction

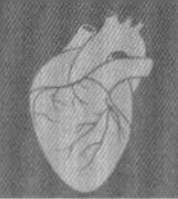

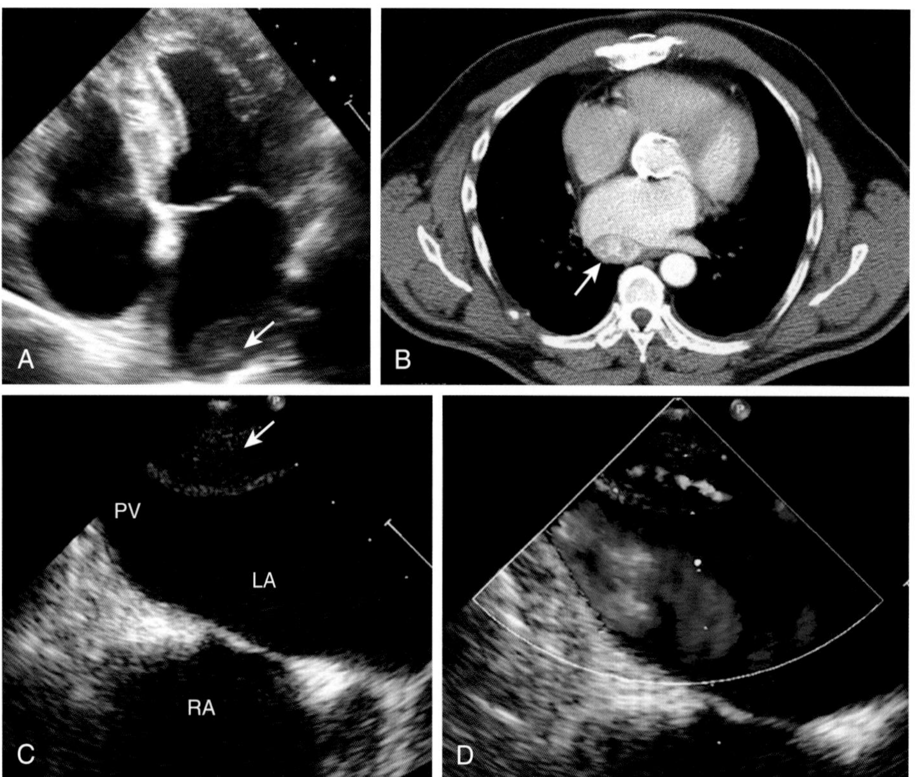

Fig. 34.11 Multimodality imaging of a functional cardiac paraganglioma. (A) Apical 4-chamber view from a TTE study of a 56-year-old man undergoing surveillance of an aortic valve replacement. The patient had difficult-to-treat hypertension, and imaging revealed an extracardiac mass at the base of the heart behind the LA *(arrow)* (see Video 34.11A). Further evaluation with chest computed tomography (B) and TEE (C and D) showed a well-encapsulated mass *(arrows)* with vascularity demonstrated by contrast enhancement (B) and color Doppler (D) (see Videos 34.11C and 34.11D). Results of biopsy of the mass confirmed an extraadrenal paraganglioma, and biochemical analysis revealed the tumor to be functional, with elevated serum and 24-hour urine metanephrine levels. *PV,* Pulmonary vein.

TABLE 34.6 Echocardiography Acquisition for Risk Assessment in Liver Disease.

Pathology	*Echocardiographic Finding*	*Clinical Prognosis*	*Studies*
Cirrhotic cardiomyopathy Diastolic dysfunction Systolic dysfunction	E/A ≤1 e′ septal <8 cm/s or lateral <10 cm/s Reduced cardiac index <1.5 L/min/m^2,[a] EF <55%	Death after TIPS (HR = 4.7, 95% CI: 1.1–20, P = 0.035) Independently associated with an 8.6% increased rate of death for liver cirrhosis (P = 0.017) Associated with developing hepatorenal syndrome (43% vs. 5%, P = 0.04) Uncommonly reported in the literature but commonly excludes OLT because abnormal hemodynamics are significantly associated with adverse outcomes	Rabie et al., 2009[87] Karagiannakis et al., 2014[88] Krag et al., 2010[89] Ripoll et al., 2008[90] Foaud et al., 2009[91]
Coronary artery disease	DSE negative for ischemia Chronotropic impairment during DSE <82% of target heart rate Peak rate–pressure product <16,333	NPV 89% for death and MI after OLT Increased CV events after OLT 22% vs. 6%, P = 0.01 17% vs. 5%, P = 0.02	Safadi et al., 2009[92] Umphrey et al., 2008[74]
Hepatic hydrothorax	Echolucent space posterior to the descending aorta (left-sided effusion) or the right of the RA and cephalad to the liver on the subcostal view (right-sided effusion)	63% mortality rate for 64 medically managed patients (median survival of 167 days) vs. 0% mortality rate for 5 patients undergoing OLT	Badillo and Rockey, 2014[71]
Hepatopulmonary syndrome	Transpulmonary shunting: agitated saline microbubbles appeared in LA 3 beats after RA opacification	Severe shunting with near LA opacification predicted death while awaiting OLT (P = 0.01)	Donovan et al., 1996[93]
LV hypertrophy	IVS thickness >1.1 cm	Increased risk of 30-day postoperative OLT death (OR = 2.84, 95% CI: 1.12–7.17, P = 0.027)	Safadi et al., 2009[92]
LVOT obstruction	Peak LVOT gradient >36 mmHg during DSE from CW Doppler in apical views	Elevated gradient in 43% of study participants; associated with intraoperative hypotension during OLT (P = 0.03)	Maraj et al., 2004[94]
Portopulmonary hypertension	PASP > 60 mmHg	High OLT mortality rate (42% at 9 mo, 71% at 36 mo); PASP > 45 mmHg by echocardiography should undergo right heart catheterization	Ramsay et al., 1997[95]

[a]Study used myocardial perfusion imaging, but cardiac output calculations may be estimated from TTE.

CI, Confidence interval; *CV,* cardiovascular; *DSE,* dobutamine stress echocardiography; *E/A,* peak transmitral early diastolic velocity/late diastolic velocity; *e′,* peak early diastolic tissue Doppler velocity of mitral annulus; *HR,* hazard ratio; *IVS,* interventricular septal thickness; *LVOT,* LV outflow tract; *MI,* myocardial infarction; *NPV,* negative predictive value; *OLT,* orthotopic liver transplant; *OR,* odds ratio; *PASP,* pulmonary artery systolic pressure; *TIPS,* transjugular intrahepatic portosystemic shunt.

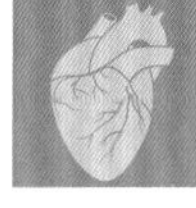

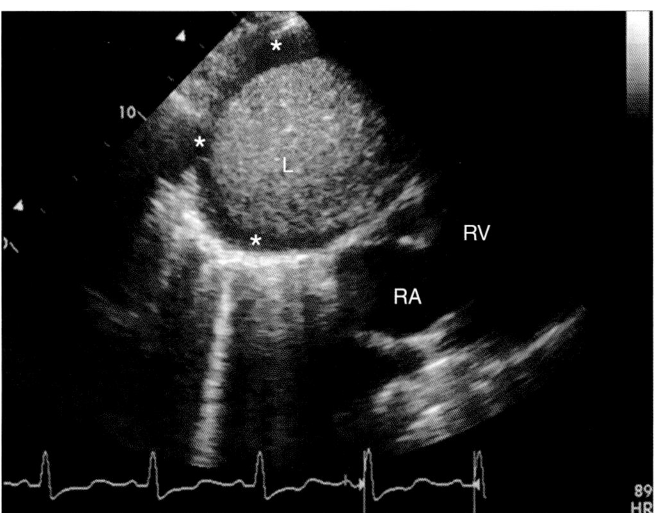

Fig. 34.12 Echocardiographic appearance of ascites. Subcostal view in a 49-year-old man with cirrhosis demonstrates ascites *(asterisks)* in the echolucent circumferential space around the speckled echodense liver *(L)* (see Video 34.12).

in cirrhosis not attributable to another process with systolic impairment (rest EF <55% or global longitudinal strain <18%) or advanced diastolic dysfunction with at least three of the following abnormalities: septal e' less than 7 cm/s, $E/e' \geq 15$, enlarged LA volume, or tricuspid regurgitation velocity greater than 2.8 m/s.[63]

Many pathogenic mechanisms have been suggested. The most important factor is pronounced systemic vasodilation leading to reduced systemic vascular resistance and a hyperdynamic circulation. Splanchnic blood pooling reduces central blood volume (i.e., preload), which then activates compensating neurohormonal reflexes, including the sympathetic nervous system and renin-angiotensin-aldosterone system. Prolonged activation of these systems, along with increases in circulating toxic mediators, leads to cardiac fibrosis, β-receptor downregulation, and impaired cell membrane signaling.

Echocardiographic studies of cirrhotic patients most commonly report a normal systolic function at rest with a normal or elevated EF. However, because of the underlying hyperdynamic circulation and a reduction in β-receptor density, systolic function is blunted with stress or exercise.[64] When the cardiac reserve is exhausted from extreme circulatory dysfunction, refractory ascites and hepatorenal syndrome may ensue.[65] Despite a normal EF, one study reported systolic dysfunction at rest compared with healthy controls using speckle tracking echocardiography. Averaged apical 4- and 2-chamber peak longitudinal strain values were lower for patients with cirrhosis than for matched healthy controls (−20% vs. −22%, respectively, $P = 0.003$).[66]

Diastolic dysfunction in cirrhosis is common; it was reported in 40% to 60% of patients when using the original 2005 working definition of cirrhotic cardiomyopathy. However, this description used transmitral flow parameters that are influenced by preload and heart rate, both of which are commonly abnormal in cirrhosis. Approximately 80% of the diastolic dysfunction in cirrhotic cardiomyopathy is classified as mild (grade 1) by transmitral flow patterns. Later studies have used tissue Doppler imaging of the mitral annulus to define diastolic dysfunction as recommended by American Society of Echocardiography (ASE) guidelines. Using the more specific ASE definition of diastolic dysfunction leads to lower rates (20%–40%) of a diastolic dysfunction diagnosis; however, it may be a better prognosticator for cirrhosis-related mortality.[67]

LIVER TRANSPLANTATION

Orthotopic liver transplantation (OLT) improves systolic and diastolic function in those with cirrhotic cardiomyopathy. However, cardiovascular complications after OLT are common and account for up to one fourth of perioperative deaths.[68] Echocardiography for risk assessment of OLT is recommended for all potential candidates.[69] Besides LV systolic and diastolic function, an echocardiographic examination should thoroughly evaluate for other common comorbid diseases such as pulmonary hypertension, transpulmonary shunts, effusions, and dynamic LV outflow obstruction.

Pulmonary hypertension (i.e., pulmonary systolic pressure >30 mmHg) may be seen in up to 20% of all patients with cirrhosis. Significant pulmonary hypertension with a mean pulmonary artery pressure above 35 mmHg is associated with a 50% OLT mortality rate and is a contraindication to OLT in most settings. Mild pulmonary hypertension may arise from the increased cardiac output with cirrhosis, but very significant pressure elevations that increase the risk of death are related to increased pulmonary vascular resistance from portopulmonary hypertension. When pulmonary systolic pressures exceed 45 mmHg by echocardiography, referral for right heart catheterization to evaluate pulmonary vascular resistance, mean pulmonary pressure, and LV filling pressures is recommended. Pulmonary vasodilators may be considered in selected candidates with severe disease and advanced heart failure symptoms.

A mild elevation in pulmonary pressures due to the high cardiac output with associated hypoxemia and dyspnea may result from hepatopulmonary syndrome. Hepatopulmonary syndrome is characterized by the triad of liver disease, intrapulmonary vascular dilation, and arterial hypoxemia.[70] Patients with hepatopulmonary syndrome commonly have progressive dyspnea that worsens with upright posture (i.e., platypnea) due to an increased ventilation-perfusion mismatch. Contrast echocardiography is a sensitive test for hepatopulmonary syndrome, and it should be performed for cirrhotic patients because OLT is curative (Fig. 34.13).

Pleural and pericardial effusions may be found by echocardiography in patients with cirrhosis. Hepatic hydrothorax normally occurs on the right side and most often causes dyspnea. Case series have shown pleural effusions in approximately 5% to 16% of patients with cirrhosis, but they may occur with atypical presentations, and a high degree of suspicion is needed. Fluid accumulation in the peritoneum from portal hypertension can translocate through diaphragmatic defects into the pleural space or rarely into the pericardial space to cause these conditions. Percutaneous drainage is recommended for symptomatic effusions, but hepatic hydrothorax is associated with dismal outcomes in those who do not undergo definitive treatment with OLT.[71]

Patients with coronary artery disease who undergo OLT may have up to a 50% mortality rate. OLT candidates with multiple risk factors, including diabetes, hypertension, age older than 60 years, LVH, smoking, and dyslipidemia, should undergo initial noninvasive testing for ischemia, most commonly using dobutamine stress echocardiography (DSE).[72] DSE has a high negative predictive value (almost 90%) for postoperative OLT outcomes in patients with low to moderate cardiovascular risk. However,

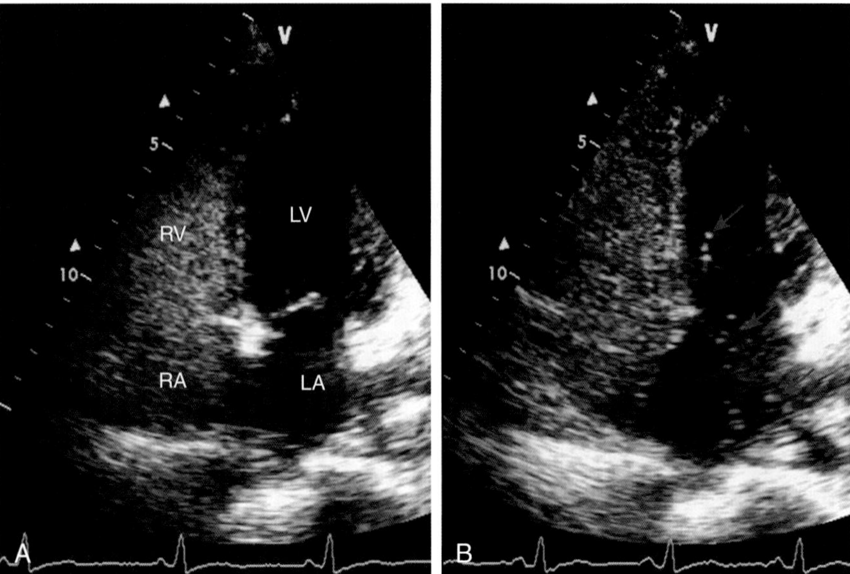

Fig. 34.13 Agitated saline contrast study of a patient with hepatopulmonary syndrome. Apical 4-chamber view from an agitated saline contrast echocardiogram in a 46-year-old man with advanced cirrhosis, dyspnea, and hypoxia. (A) Initial opacification of the right heart with saline microbubbles. (B) Late bubbles appeared *(red arrows)* in the LA and LV after 10 beats originating from the left pulmonary veins, consistent with intrapulmonary shunts in hepatopulmonary syndrome (see Video 34.13).

DSE has a low sensitivity for obstructive coronary artery disease in this setting, and angiography may be needed.[73] Additional adverse prognostic factors such as chronotropic incompetence, a low rate-pressure product, and inducible LV outflow tract gradient should be assessed during DSE in OLT candidates.[74]

ALCOHOL

Chronic alcohol abuse can directly lead to liver and heart disease. It is estimated that consumption of more than 90 g/day over 5 years can lead to an alcoholic cardiomyopathy, but a lower average daily intake of only 25 g/day over 10 to 12 years can produce liver cirrhosis.[75] Cardiac dysfunction may arise without cirrhosis, and liver dysfunction can develop without cardiac impairment. Variations in alcohol metabolism due to sex and genetic differences account for why some patients may be protected from organ dysfunction with high levels of chronic alcohol use.

Contrary to the cardiac dangers of heavy alcohol abuse, moderate alcohol use of 2 standard drinks per day or fewer has been associated with reduced cardiovascular events and death. Potential mechanisms include alcohol increasing high-density lipoprotein cholesterol and decreasing platelet aggregation and coagulation. However, unmeasured confounders between alcohol abstainers and low to moderate alcohol users may account for these findings.

Alcoholic cardiomyopathy is a diagnosis of exclusion for patients with at least 5 years of heavy alcohol use and no other identified cause of dilated cardiomyopathy. Reduced EF, increased LV mass, and higher LV volumes can occur before the development of overt heart failure symptoms.[76] Increased wall thickness, ventricular dilation, and impaired relaxation may appear before systolic dysfunction is evident. Diastolic changes such as lower E/A ratios and higher deceleration times are linearly correlated with the duration of alcohol abuse.

Women may be more susceptible to cardiac toxicity than men with equal amounts of alcohol consumption. At-risk heavy drinking is defined as more than 7 drinks per week for women or more than 14 drinks per week for men by the United States National Institute of Alcohol Abuse and Alcoholism.

Treatment for alcoholic cardiomyopathy should follow typical heart failure management for dilated cardiomyopathy. Studies have not found differences in medical management for alcoholic or nonalcoholic cardiomyopathy. However, alcohol cessation or reduction can improve cardiac function in patients with alcoholic cardiomyopathy. Older case series before routine use of angiotensin-converting enzyme inhibitors and β-blocker therapy demonstrated that abstinence could lead to normalization of the EF in some patients. In one study, 37% of patients with alcoholic cardiomyopathy (with an average baseline EF of 25%) followed over a median time of 59 months had recovery of LV function with an EF of at least 40%.[77] Improvements in EF were seen in patients who abstained from or reduced alcohol consumption to less than 80 g/day, but no improvement was seen with continued heavy alcohol use.

Alcoholic cardiomyopathy has a better prognosis than idiopathic dilated cardiomyopathies with moderation of drinking (Fig. 34.14). Patients with alcoholic cardiomyopathy are at risk for nutritional deficiencies of essential micronutrients (e.g., thiamine, selenium) that can lead to heart failure. Nutritional assessment should be performed, and vitamin and mineral supplementation should be provided if deficiencies exist.

NONALCOHOLIC FATTY LIVER DISEASE

Nonalcoholic fatty liver disease (NAFLD) is defined by fat deposition in the liver, with or without inflammation, after a known secondary cause is excluded. It is commonly associated with components of the MetS, and concordantly, NAFLD prevalence is rising in industrialized countries. NAFLD may progress to cirrhosis in patients with evidence of inflammation (i.e., nonalcoholic steatohepatitis), and obesity and DM are risk factors for nonalcoholic steatohepatitis progression. Cardiovascular events constitute the leading cause of death for NAFLD patients, but

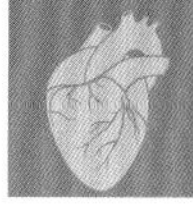

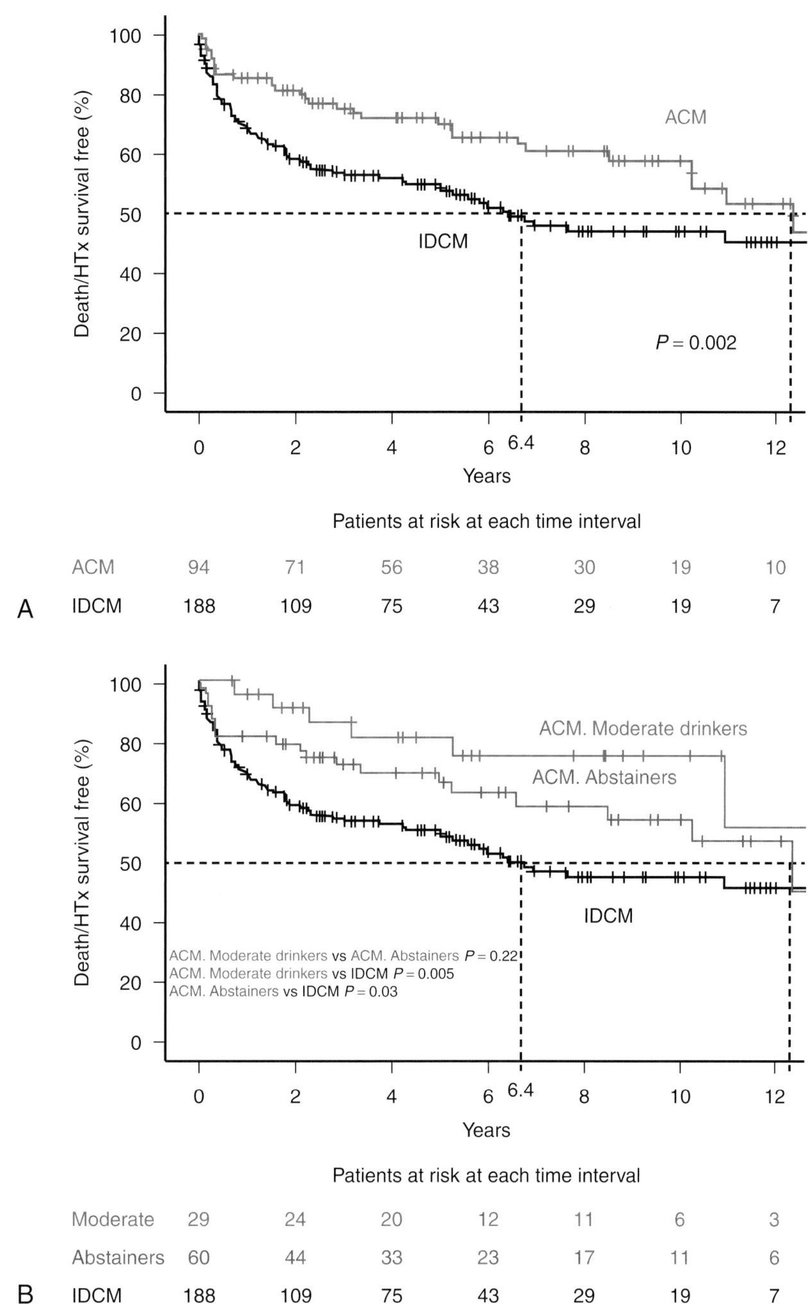

Fig. 34.14 Transplantation-free survival of idiopathic dilated cardiomyopathy and alcoholic cardiomyopathy cohorts according to alcohol consumption. (A) Survival curves for major cardiac events (e.g., cardiac death, heart transplantation *[HTx]*) in patients with alcoholic cardiomyopathy *(ACM) (blue curve)* and idiopathic dilated cardiomyopathy *(IDCM) (black curve)*. (B) Survival curves for cardiac events in patients with IDCM *(black curve)*, those with ACM with persistent moderate alcohol intake (<80 g/day) *(blue curve)*, and abstainers *(red curve)*. The number below the x-axis indicates patients at risk in each time interval. (From Guzzo-Merello G, Segovia J, Dominguez F, et al. Natural history and prognostic factors in alcoholic cardiomyopathy. *JACC Heart Fail.* 2015;3:78–86.)

whether NAFLD is an independent factor for cardiovascular events or a marker of the underlying adiposity disease processes remains unclear.[78]

Similar to obesity and MetS, case-controlled echocardiographic studies of patients with NAFLD and healthy controls have shown that NAFLD is associated with LVH, reduced longitudinal strain, diastolic dysfunction with lower E/A ratios and higher E/e′ values, and LA enlargement.[79,80] However, the impact of shared risk factors, obesity, hypertension, and MetS on these findings was not fully evaluated in these studies. Severity of fibrosis in nonalcoholic steatohepatitis has been independently associated with epicardial fat thickness, worsening cardiac geometry, and diastolic impairment.[81]

In a population analysis from the CARDIA study, NAFLD was independently associated with longitudinal strain values after adjustment for demographic, heart failure, and metabolic risk factors.[82] However, significant attenuation of associations with subclinical echocardiographic parameters were seen when adjusted for adiposity, suggesting obesity plays a role in the causal pathway of NAFLD-related cardiac dysfunction. Accordingly, patients with NAFLD should have aggressive modification of their metabolic risk factors.

SUMMARY Commonly Reported Findings in Cardiomyopathies From Nutritional and Metabolic Disorders.

Echocardiographic Parameter	Obesity Cardiomyopathy	Diabetic Cardiomyopathy	Cirrhotic Cardiomyopathy	Alcoholic Cardiomyopathy	Limitations
LV size	Increased volumes Increased wall thickness Older age, hypertension, sleep apnea lead to more concentric remodeling	Typically normal but may increase depending on duration of diabetes Very mild increase in LV thickness and mass (average, 3 g)	Normal but can be mildly dilated with long exposure to hyperdynamic circulation	Severely dilated Eccentric hypertrophy	Assumed geometric shapes for M-mode and 2D imaging 3D imaging requires high-quality images MRI is considered the gold standard
EF	Typically high-normal to elevated Reported 59%–74% Low normal (50%–55%) with comorbidities (hypertension, OSA)	Normal	Hyperdynamic EF commonly >60%	Significantly reduced EF <40%	Load dependent Associated comorbidities affect load conditions Requires endocardial border visualization
Global longitudinal strain	Reported averages approximately 1%–2% lower than non-obese subjects	Reduced 3% compared with nondiabetics	<18% or >22%	Not rigorously studied, probably reduced with reduced EF	Vendor dependent Prognostic significance unclear Normal values not fully established
Transmitral inflow pattern	E/A <1 Absolute velocities may be slightly higher than age-matched controls	Lower E/A Deceleration time prolonged	E/A <1 in up to 60% of patients Lower in decompensated cirrhosis	Varies greatly	Changes with age
Mitral annulus tissue Doppler (e')	Reduced	Reduced	Usually normal; may be mildly reduced	Likely reduced in dilated cardiomyopathy	Correct annulus placement Angle dependent
Pulmonary artery systolic pressure	Upper end of normal to mildly elevated Range of 25–40 mmHg Higher with sleep apnea	Normal	Commonly elevated May be severe	Elevated with cirrhosis	Underestimated in severe TR Inadequate spectral envelope Angle dependent
RV size	Dilated in setting of sleep apnea	Usually normal	Mildly dilated	Dilated	Irregular shape leads to varied quantification
Additional comments	Consider indexing by height in cases of severe obesity Use lower transducer frequency for better penetration Difficult visualization can be improved with echocardiographic contrast	Rule out ischemia. Risk factor modification Less commonly results in dilated cardiomyopathy phenotype	Consider exercise or stress testing to detect lack of systolic reserve and chronotropic incompetence	Obtain drinking history	Comorbidities must be considered Study population differences may account for variation in reported descriptions in the literature

E/A, Ratio of peak transmittal early diastolic velocity to late diastolic velocity; *EF*, ejection fraction; *OSA*, obstructive sleep apnea; *TR*, tricuspid regurgitation.

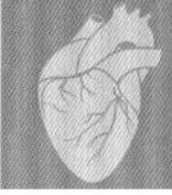

REFERENCES

1. Whelton PK, Carey RM, Aronow WS, et al. ACC/AHA/AAPA/ABC/ACPM/AGS/APhA/ASH/ASPC/NMA/PCNA guideline for the prevention, detection, evaluation, and management of high blood pressure in adults: a report of the American College of Cardiology/American Heart Association Task Force on clinical practice guidelines. *Circulation*. 2017;138(17):e484–e594.
2. Marwick TH, Gillebert TC, Aurigemma G, et al. Recommendations on the use of echocardiography in adult hypertension: a report from the European Association of Cardiovascular Imaging (EACVI) and the American Society of Echocardiography (ASE). *J Am Soc Echocardiogr*. 2015;28(7):727–754.
3. Doherty JU, Kort S, Mehran R, et al. ACC/AATS/AHA/ASE/ASNC/HRS/SCAI/SCCT/SCMR/STS 2019 appropriate use criteria for multimodality imaging in the assessment of cardiac structure and function in nonvalvular heart disease: a report of the American College of Cardiology Appropriate Use Criteria Task Force, American Association for Thoracic Surgery, American Heart Association, American Society of Echocardiography, American Society of Nuclear Cardiology, Heart Rhythm Society, Society for Cardiovascular Angiography and Interventions, Society of Cardiovascular Computed Tomography, Society for Cardiovascular Magnetic Resonance, and the Society of Thoracic Surgeons. *J Am Soc Echocardiogr*. 2019;32(5):553–579.
4. Lang RM, Badano LP, Mor-Avi V, et al. Recommendations for cardiac chamber quantification by echocardiography in adults: an update from the American Society of Echocardiography and the European Association of Cardiovascular Imaging. *J Am Soc Echocardiogr*. 2015;28(1):1–39. e14.
5. Lembo M, Esposito R, Santoro C, et al. Three-dimensional echocardiographic ventricular mass/end-diastolic volume ratio in native hypertensive patients: relation between stroke volume and geometry. *J Hypertens*. 2018;36(8):1697–1704.
6. Lembo M, Santoro C, Sorrentino R, et al. Interrelation between midwall mechanics and longitudinal strain in newly diagnosed and never-treated hypertensive patients without clinically defined hypertrophy. *J Hypertens*. 2020;38(2):295–302.
7. Wright JT, Williamson JD, Whelton PK, et al. A randomized trial of intensive versus standard blood-pressure control. *N Engl J Med*. 2015;373(22):2103–2116.
8. Fagard RH, Celis H, Thijs L, Wouters S. Regression of left ventricular mass by antihypertensive treatment: a meta-analysis of randomized comparative studies. *Hypertension*. 2009;54(5):1084–1091.
9. Lønnebakken MT, Izzo R, Mancusi C, et al. Left ventricular hypertrophy regression during antihypertensive treatment in an outpatient clinic (the Campania Salute Network). *J Am Heart Assoc*. 2017;6(3).
10. Johnson K, Oparil S, Davis BR, Tereshchenko LG. Prevention of heart failure in hypertension–disentangling the role of evolving left ventricular hypertrophy and blood pressure lowering: the ALLHAT study. *J Am Heart Assoc*. 2019;8(8). e011961.
11. Barron AJ, Hughes AD, Sharp A, et al. Long-term antihypertensive treatment fails to improve E/e' despite regression of left ventricular mass: an Anglo-Scandinavian cardiac outcomes trial substudy. *Hypertension*. 2014;63(2):252–258.
12. Ng M, Fleming T, Robinson M, et al. Global, regional, and national prevalence of overweight and obesity in children and adults during 1980-2013: a systematic analysis for the Global Burden of Disease Study 2013. *Lancet*. 2014;384(9945):766–781.
13. Whitlock G, Lewington S, Sherliker P, et al. Body-mass index and cause-specific mortality in 900 000 adults: collaborative analyses of 57 prospective studies. *Lancet*. 2009;373(9669):1083–1096.
14. Jensen MD, Ryan DH, Apovian CM, et al. AHA/ACC/TOS guideline for the management of overweight and obesity in adults: a report of the American College of Cardiology/American Heart Association Task Force on practice guidelines and the Obesity Society. *Circulation*. 2013;129(25 suppl 2):S102–S138. 2014.
15. Alpert MA, Omran J, Mehra A, Ardhanari S. Impact of obesity and weight loss on cardiac performance and morphology in adults. *Prog Cardiovasc Dis*. 2014;56(4):391–400.
16. Fitzgibbons TP, Czech MP. Epicardial and perivascular adipose tissues and their influence on cardiovascular disease: basic mechanisms and clinical associations. *J Am Heart Assoc*. 2014;3(2):e000582.
17. Aune D, Sen A, Norat T, et al. Body mass index, abdominal fatness, and heart failure incidence and mortality: a systematic review and dose-response meta-analysis of prospective studies. *Circulation*. 2016;133(7):639–649.
18. Supariwala A, Makani H, Kahan J, et al. Feasibility and prognostic value of stress echocardiography in obese, morbidly obese, and super obese patients referred for bariatric surgery. *Echocardiography*. 2014;31(7):879–885.
19. Carnevalini M, Deschle H, Amenabar A, et al. Evaluation of the size of cardiac structures in patients with high body mass index. *Echocardiography*. 2020;37(2):270–275.
20. Rogge BP, Gerdts E, Cramariuc D, et al. Impact of obesity and nonobesity on grading the severity of aortic valve stenosis. *Am J Cardiol*. 2014;113(9):1532–1535.
21. Hu T, Yao L, Gustat J, Chen W, Webber L, Bazzano L. Which measures of adiposity predict subsequent left ventricular geometry? Evidence from the Bogalusa Heart Study. *Nutr Metab Cardiovasc Dis*. 2015;25(3):319–326.
22. Mangner N, Scheuermann K, Winzer E, et al. Childhood obesity: impact on cardiac geometry and function. *JACC Cardiovasc Imaging*. 2014;7(12):1198–1205.
23. Russo C, Jin Z, Homma S, et al. Effect of obesity and overweight on left ventricular diastolic function: a community-based study in an elderly cohort. *J Am Coll Cardiol*. 2011;57(12):1368–1374.
24. Khan MF, Movahed MR. Obesity cardiomyopathy and systolic function: obesity is not independently associated with dilated cardiomyopathy. *Heart Fail Rev*. 2013;18(2):207–217.
25. Dalen H, Thorstensen A, Romundstad PR, et al. Cardiovascular risk factors and systolic and diastolic cardiac function: a tissue Doppler and speckle tracking echocardiographic study. *J Am Soc Echocardiogr*. 2011;24(3):322–332. e326.
26. Iacobellis G. Local and systemic effects of the multifaceted epicardial adipose tissue depot. *Nat Rev Endocrinol*. 2015;11(6):363–371.
27. Owan T, Avelar E, Morley K, et al. Favorable changes in cardiac geometry and function following gastric bypass surgery: 2-year follow-up in the Utah obesity study. *J Am Coll Cardiol*. 2011;57(6):732–739.
28. Bohula EA, Wiviott SD, McGuire DK, et al. Cardiovascular safety of lorcaserin in overweight or obese patients. *N Engl J Med*. 2018;379(12):1107–1117.
29. Peppard PE, Young T, Barnet JH, et al. Increased prevalence of sleep-disordered breathing in adults. *Am J Epidemiol*. 2013;177(9): 1006–1014.
30. Kasai T, Floras JS, Bradley TD. Sleep apnea and cardiovascular disease: a bidirectional relationship. *Circulation*. 2012;126(12):1495–1510.
31. Chami HA, Devereux RB, Gottdiener JS, et al. Left ventricular morphology and systolic function in sleep-disordered breathing: the Sleep Heart Health Study. *Circulation*. 2008;117(20):2599–2607.
32. Imai Y, Tanaka N, Usui Y, et al. Severe obstructive sleep apnea increases left atrial volume independently of left ventricular diastolic impairment. *Sleep Breath*. 2015;19(4):1249–1255.
33. Altekin RE, Yanikoglu A, Karakas MS, et al. Assessment of left atrial dysfunction in obstructive sleep apnea patients with the two dimensional speckle-tracking echocardiography. *Clin Res Cardiol*. 2012;101(6):403–413.
34. McEvoy RD, Antic NA, Heeley E, et al. CPAP for prevention of cardiovascular events in obstructive sleep apnea. *N Engl J Med*. 2016;375(10):919–931.
35. Gottlieb DJ, Punjabi NM, Mehra R, et al. CPAP versus oxygen in obstructive sleep apnea. *N Engl J Med*. 2014;370(24):2276–2285.
36. Sun H, Shi J, Li M, Chen X. Impact of continuous positive airway pressure treatment on left ventricular ejection fraction in patients with obstructive sleep apnea: a meta-analysis of randomized controlled trials. *PloS One*. 2013;8(5):e62298.
37. Kholdani C, Fares WH, Mohsenin V. Pulmonary hypertension in obstructive sleep apnea: is it clinically significant? A critical analysis of the association and pathophysiology. *Pulm Circ*. 2015;5(2):220–227.
38. Sarwar N, Gao P, Seshasai SR, et al. Diabetes mellitus, fasting blood glucose concentration, and risk of vascular disease: a collaborative meta-analysis of 102 prospective studies. *Lancet*. 2010;375(9733):2215–2222.
39. Seferović PM, Paulus WJ. Clinical diabetic cardiomyopathy: a two-faced disease with restrictive and dilated phenotypes. *Eur Heart J*. 2015;36(27):1718–1727.
40. Skali H, Shah A, Gupta DK, et al. Cardiac structure and function across the glycemic spectrum in elderly men and women free of prevalent heart disease: the Atherosclerosis Risk in the Community study. *Circ Heart Fail*. 2015;8(3):448–454.
41. Markus MR, Stritzke J, Wellmann J, et al. Implications of prevalent and incident diabetes mellitus on left ventricular geometry and function in the ageing heart: the MONICA/KORA Augsburg cohort study. *Nutr Metab Cardiovasc Dis*. 2011;21(3):189–196.
42. Hwang YC, Jee JH, Kang M, et al. Metabolic syndrome and insulin resistance are associated with abnormal left ventricular diastolic function and structure independent of blood pressure and fasting plasma glucose level. *Int J Cardiol*. 2012;159(2):107–111.

43. Ernande L, Bergerot C, Girerd N, et al. Longitudinal myocardial strain alteration is associated with left ventricular remodeling in asymptomatic patients with type 2 diabetes mellitus. *J Am Soc Echocardiogr*. 2014;27(5):479–488.
44. Gerstein HC, Miller ME, Byington RP, et al. Effects of intensive glucose lowering in type 2 diabetes. *N Engl J Med*. 2008;358(24):2545–2559.
45. Hare JL, Hordern MD, Leano R, et al. Application of an exercise intervention on the evolution of diastolic dysfunction in patients with diabetes mellitus: efficacy and effectiveness. *Circ Heart Fail*. 2011;4(4):441–449.
46. Hansen D, Niebauer J, Cornelissen V, et al. Exercise prescription in patients with different combinations of cardiovascular disease risk factors: a consensus statement from the EXPERT working group. *Sports Med*. 2018;48(8):1781–1797.
47. Verma S, Mazer CD, Yan AT, et al. Effect of empagliflozin on left ventricular mass in patients with type 2 diabetes mellitus and coronary artery disease: the EMPA-HEART CardioLink-6 randomized clinical trial. *Circulation*. 2019;140(21):1693–1702.
48. McMurray JJV, Solomon SD, Inzucchi SE, et al. Dapagliflozin in patients with heart failure and reduced ejection fraction. *N Engl J Med*. 2019;381(21):1995–2008.
49. Weir DL, McAlister FA, Senthilselvan A, Minhas-Sandhu JK, Eurich DT. Sitagliptin use in patients with diabetes and heart failure: a population-based retrospective cohort study. *JACC Heart Fail*. 2014;2(6):573–582.
50. Dillmann W. Cardiac hypertrophy and thyroid hormone signaling. *Heart Fail Rev*. 2010;15(2):125–132.
51. Roef GL, Taes YE, Kaufman JM, et al. Thyroid hormone levels within reference range are associated with heart rate, cardiac structure, and function in middle aged men and women. *Thyroid*. 2013;23(8):947–954.
52. Kong LY, Gao X, Ding XY, Wang G, Liu F. Left ventricular end-diastolic strain rate recovered in hypothyroidism following levothyroxine replacement therapy: a strain rate imaging study. *Echocardiography*. 2019;36(4):707–713.
53. Klein I, Danzi S. Thyroid disease and the heart. *Curr Probl Cardiol*. 2016;41(2):65–92.
54. Colao A, Grasso LFS, Di Somma C, Pivonello R. Acromegaly and heart failure. *Heart Fail Clin*. 2019;15(3):399–408.
55. Bihan H, Espinosa C, Valdes-Socin H, et al. Long-term outcome of patients with acromegaly and congestive heart failure. *J Clin Endocrinol Metab*. 2004;89(11):5308–5313.
56. Isgaard J, Arcopinto M, Karason K, Cittadini A. GH and the cardiovascular system: an update on a topic at heart. *Endocrine*. 2015;48(1):25–35.
57. Neary NM, Booker OJ, Abel BS, et al. Hypercortisolism is associated with increased coronary arterial atherosclerosis: analysis of noninvasive coronary angiography using multidetector computerized tomography. *J Clin Endocrinol Metab*. 2013;98(5):2045–2052.
58. van Ballegooijen AJ, Reinders I, Visser M, Brouwer IA. Parathyroid hormone and cardiovascular disease events: a systematic review and meta-analysis of prospective studies. *Am Heart J*. 2013;165(5):655–664.664.e651–655.
59. Bansal N, Zelnick L, Robinson-Cohen C, et al. Serum parathyroid hormone and 25-hydroxyvitamin D concentrations and risk of incident heart failure: the multi-ethnic study of atherosclerosis. *J Am Heart Assoc*. 2014;3(6). e001278.
60. Iwata S, Walker MD, Di Tullio MR, et al. Aortic valve calcification in mild primary hyperparathyroidism. *J Clin Endocrinol Metab*. 2012;97(1):132–137.
61. Weismann D, Liu D, Bergen T, et al. Hypertension and hypertensive cardiomyopathy in patients with a relapse-free history of phaeochromocytoma. *Clin Endocrinol*. 2015;82(2):188–196.
62. Park JH, Kim KS, Sul JY, et al. Prevalence and patterns of left ventricular dysfunction in patients with pheochromocytoma. *J Cardiovasc Ultrasound*. 2011;19(2):76–82.
63. Izzy M, VanWagner LB, Lin G, et al. Redefining cirrhotic cardiomyopathy for the modern era. *Hepatology*. 2020;71(1):334–345.
64. Pellicori P, Torromeo C, Calicchia A, et al. Does cirrhotic cardiomyopathy exist? 50 years of uncertainty. *Clin Res Cardiol*. 2013;102(12):859–864.
65. Nazar A, Guevara M, Sitges M, et al. LEFT ventricular function assessed by echocardiography in cirrhosis: relationship to systemic hemodynamics and renal dysfunction. *J Hepatol*. 2013;58(1):51–57.
66. Sampaio F, Pimenta J, Bettencourt N, et al. Systolic and diastolic dysfunction in cirrhosis: a tissue-Doppler and speckle tracking echocardiography study. *Liver Int*. 2013;33(8):1158–1165.
67. Cesari M, Frigo AC, Tonon M, Angeli P. Cardiovascular predictors of death in patients with cirrhosis. *Hepatology*. 2018;68(1):215–223.
68. Liu H, Jayakumar S, Traboulsi M, Lee SS. Cirrhotic cardiomyopathy: implications for liver transplantation. *Liver Transpl*. 2017;23(6):826–835.
69. Lentine KL, Costa SP, Weir MR, et al. Cardiac disease evaluation and management among kidney and liver transplantation candidates: a scientific statement from the American Heart Association and the American College of Cardiology Foundation. *J Am Coll Cardiol*. 2012;60(5):434–480.
70. Tumgor G. Cirrhosis and hepatopulmonary syndrome. *World J Gastroenterol*. 2014;20(10):2586–2594.
71. Badillo R, Rockey DC. Hepatic hydrothorax: clinical features, management, and outcomes in 77 patients and review of the literature. *Medicine (Baltim)*. 2014;93(3):135–142.
72. Martin P, DiMartini A, Feng S, Brown R, Fallon M. Evaluation for liver transplantation in adults: 2013 practice guideline by the American Association for the Study of Liver Diseases and the American Society of Transplantation. *Hepatology*. 2014;59(3):1144–1165.
73. Soldera J, Camazzola F, Rodríguez S, Brandão A. Cardiac stress testing and coronary artery disease in liver transplantation candidates: meta-analysis. *World J Hepatol*. 2018;10(11): 877–886.
74. Umphrey LG, Hurst RT, Eleid MF, et al. Preoperative dobutamine stress echocardiographic findings and subsequent short-term adverse cardiac events after orthotopic liver transplantation. *Liver Transpl*. 2008;14(6): 886–892.
75. Møller S, Bernardi M. Interactions of the heart and the liver. *Eur Heart J*. 2013;34(36):2804–2811.
76. Iacovoni A, De Maria R, Gavazzi A. Alcoholic cardiomyopathy. *J Cardiovasc Med*. 2010;11(12):884–892.
77. Guzzo-Merello G, Segovia J, Dominguez F, et al. Natural history and prognostic factors in alcoholic cardiomyopathy. *JACC Heart Fail*. 2015;3(1):78–86.
78. Stahl EP, Dhindsa DS, Lee SK, et al. Nonalcoholic fatty liver disease and the heart: JACC state-of-the-art review. *J Am Coll Cardiol*. 2019;73(8):948–963.
79. Sert A, Aypar E, Pirgon O, et al. Left ventricular function by echocardiography, tissue Doppler imaging, and carotid intima-media thickness in obese adolescents with nonalcoholic fatty liver disease. *Am J Cardiol*. 2013;112(3):436–443.
80. Karabay CY, Kocabay G, Kalayci A, et al. Impaired left ventricular mechanics in nonalcoholic fatty liver disease: a speckle-tracking echocardiography study. *Eur J Gastroenterol Hepatol*. 2014;26(3):325–331.
81. Petta S, Argano C, Colomba D, et al. Epicardial fat, cardiac geometry and cardiac function in patients with non-alcoholic fatty liver disease: association with the severity of liver disease. *J Hepatol*. 2015;62(4):928–933.
82. VanWagner LB, Wilcox JE, Colangelo LA, et al. Association of nonalcoholic fatty liver disease with subclinical myocardial remodeling and dysfunction: a population-based study. *Hepatology*. 2015;62(3):773–783.
83. Epstein LJ, Kristo D, Strollo PJ, et al. Clinical guideline for the evaluation, management and long-term care of obstructive sleep apnea in adults. *J Clin Sleep Med*. 2009;5(3): 263–276.
84. Poirier P, Cornier MA, Mazzone T, et al. Bariatric surgery and cardiovascular risk factors: a scientific statement from the American Heart Association. *Circulation*. 2011;123(15):1683–1701.
85. Fox CS, Golden SH, Anderson C, et al. Update on prevention of cardiovascular disease in adults with type 2 diabetes mellitus in light of recent evidence: a scientific statement from the American Heart Association and the American Diabetes Association. *Circulation*. 2015;132(8):691–718.
86. Bozkurt B, Aguilar D, Deswal A, et al. Contributory risk and management of comorbidities of hypertension, obesity, diabetes mellitus, hyperlipidemia, and metabolic syndrome in chronic heart failure: a scientific statement from the American Heart Association. *Circulation*. 2016;134(23):e535–e578.
87. Rabie RN, Cazzaniga M, Salerno F, Wong F. The use of E/A ratio as a predictor of outcome in cirrhotic patients treated with transjugular intrahepatic portosystemic shunt. *Am J Gastroenterol*. 2009;104(10):2458–2466.
88. Karagiannakis DS, Papatheodoridis G, Vlachogiannakos J. Recent advances in cirrhotic cardiomyopathy. *Dig Dis Sci*. 2015;60(5):1141–1151.
89. Krag A, Bendtsen F, Henriksen JH, Møller S. Low cardiac output predicts development of hepatorenal syndrome and survival in patients with cirrhosis and ascites. *Gut*. 2010;59:105–110.
90. Ripoll C, Catalina MV, Yotti R, et al. Cardiac dysfunction during liver transplantation: incidence and preoperative predictors. *Transplantation*. 2008;85:1766–1772.
91. Fouad TR, Abdel-Razek WM, Burak KW, et al. Prediction of cardiac complications after liver transplantation. *Transplantation*. 2009;87:763–770.

92. Safadi A, Homsi M, Maskoun W, et al. Perioperative risk predictors of cardiac outcomes in patients undergoing liver transplantation surgery. *Circulation*. 2009;120:1189–1194.
93. Donovan CL, Marcovitz PA, Punch JD, et al. Two-dimensional and dobutamine stress echocardiography in the preoperative assessment of patients with end-stage liver disease prior to orthotopic liver transplantation. *Transplantation*. 1996;61:1180–1188.
94. Maraj S, Jacobs LE, Maraj R, et al. Inducible left ventricular outflow tract gradient during dobutamine stress echocardiography: an association with intraoperative hypotension but not a contraindication to liver transplantation. *Echocardiography*. 2004;21:681–685.
95. Ramsay MA, Simpson BR, Nguyen AT, et al. Severe pulmonary hypertension in liver transplant candidates. *Liver Transpl Surg*. 1997;3:494–500.

中文导读

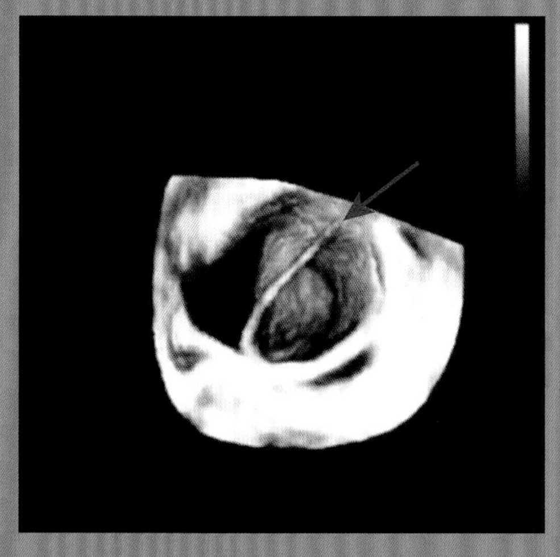

第35章
运动员心脏的超声心动图表现

运动员心脏是指运动员的心脏结构和功能通常会随着规律性的体能训练而发生改变，这种改变的程度和体育锻炼的种类与强度不一进而有所不同，因此反映心脏的各项结构功能如左、右心室的结构及功能、主动脉内径的参考值也会与普通人群产生差异，出现了与疾病所致的心脏结构改变等相似表现。应用超声心动图可以探查到运动员心脏各项参数的变化，有助于界定各项心脏参数的生理变化范围，同时区分这些参数变化是否为病理性。

本章介绍了运动员心脏的多种结构和功能特点，特别是在超声心动图方面的典型表现。列举了超声心动图在耐力性训练与瓣膜病或心肌病理性扩张的联系、力量和耐力训练和心肌肥厚的关系等评估中的应用。以及从超声心动图所获信息中心对运动员的心脏功能进行有效的管理，适时地评估运动员的职业寿命。

李羽加

35 The Athletic Heart on Echocardiography

DAVID PRIOR, MBBS, PhD | MARIA BROSNAN, MBBS, PhD

Regular athletic training causes changes in cardiac structure and function, commonly referred to as *athlete's heart.* The character and magnitude of these changes vary with the type and volume of training but may result in parameters of cardiac structure and function that fall outside the normal range for the general population. The echocardiographer should understand the characteristics of athlete's heart and the normal limits of these changes and, more importantly, understand how to differentiate these changes from those seen in cardiac disease.

This chapter outlines the structural and functional characteristics of the athlete's heart, particularly as it relates to echocardiographic examination; some of the key clinical dilemmas that may be evaluated using cardiac ultrasound; and how the echocardiographic information can be used to manage patients.

THE IMPACT OF EXERCISE ON CARDIAC STRUCTURE AND FUNCTION

Undertaking regular exercise can change cardiac structure and function to produce a phenotype known as athlete's heart. The intermittent volume and pressure loading of the heart during training activates gene pathways that result in physiologic cardiac hypertrophy and cardiac chamber enlargement in addition to changes in autonomic tone and cardiac conduction. Athlete's heart is not one distinct phenotype but a spectrum of changes that vary with the sporting discipline and the intensity with which it is undertaken.

In assessing whether echocardiographic findings are physiologic or pathologic, it is first necessary to decide whether the individual is performing sufficient exercise to produce the heart of an athlete. The changes of athlete's heart, such as bradycardia, increased aerobic capacity, and increased left ventricular (LV) mass, are usually seen only in individuals undertaking at least 3 hours of moderate-intensity exercise per week.[1] Greater volume and intensity of exercise results in greater degrees of change in cardiac structure and function, such that a fundamental question in the evaluation of an athlete is whether he or she is doing enough exercise of the appropriate volume and intensity to explain the changes seen during echocardiography.

The cardiac diseases that are of concern in athletes and must be distinguished from athlete's heart are influenced by age. Younger athletes are more likely to be affected by inherited cardiac abnormalities such as hypertrophic cardiomyopathy (HCM), arrhythmogenic cardiomyopathy, and coronary artery anomalies, whereas older athletes (e.g., >35 years of age) are more likely to suffer from acquired cardiac disease, such as coronary artery disease, in addition to the inherited diseases seen in younger athletes.

It is likely that the changes of athlete's heart are modulated by the effects of aging, but this is incompletely understood. The age at which intense exercise was commenced appears to influence the pattern and extent of the changes of athlete's heart.[2] Conversely, exercise may modulate the effect of normal aging on cardiac properties. Reduction in the normal age-related decline in LV compliance has been described and is a beneficial manifestation of lifelong exercise.[3]

EFFECT OF DIFFERENT EXERCISE TYPES

Sporting disciplines vary markedly in the degree of static (strength) and dynamic (endurance) loads imposed on the heart and the relative intensity of these loads. The concept that different forms of exercise have different effects on the cardiac phenotype produced is known as the Morganroth hypothesis.[4] This has led to classification of sporting disciplines based on the characteristics of the loads imposed. A simplified outline of this classification is presented in Table 35.1; a more complete classification is provided in the work of the task force led by Mitchell.[5]

Dynamic exercise places a volume load on the cardiovascular system, with marked increases in cardiac output required

TABLE 35.1 Sports Grouped by the Amount of Dynamic (Endurance) and Static (Strength) Components.

Static Component	Dynamic Component: Low	Medium	High
Low	Golf Cricket Bowling	Baseball Fencing Volleyball	Hockey Long-distance running Soccer
Medium	Archery Diving Equestrian events	American football Jumping events Sprinting Rugby	Middle-distance running Swimming Basketball Ice hockey Cross-country skiing
High	Throwing events Weight lifting Gymnastics Martial arts	Downhill skiing Body building Snowboarding Wrestling	Cycling Triathlon Rowing Canoeing/Kayaking

during exercise. This is achieved by increasing the heart rate and stroke volume and is accompanied by increased systolic blood pressure, reduced diastolic blood pressure, and only a small increase in mean arterial pressure. Static exercise places a more modest volume load on the cardiovascular system, with small increases in heart rate, but it is characterized by a significant pressure load resulting from elevation of systolic, diastolic, and mean blood pressures.

Traditional teaching aligned with the Morganroth hypothesis has been that endurance-trained athletes develop increased LV cavity volumes and dimensions with a normal wall thickness or with increased thickness in proportion to the LV cavity size (i.e., eccentric left ventricular hypertrophy [LVH]), whereas strength-trained athletes develop increased LV wall thickness (concentric LVH) with relatively normal LV cavity volumes and dimensions. The latter concept has been questioned because studies have failed to demonstrate concentric LVH in strength-trained athletes; LV wall thickness was within normal limits in purely strength-trained adolescents and adults, and LV cavity measures were similar to or only slightly larger than those of sedentary controls in cross-sectional and prospective studies.[6–10]

It is possible that understanding of the effects of strength training has been clouded by the use of anabolic agents in this athlete group (see Left Ventricle: Structure). The most profound changes in terms of chamber enlargement and increased cardiac mass have been consistently demonstrated in subjects who were engaged in activities involving a combination of significant static and dynamic components, such as rowing, canoeing, and cycling.[9,11,12] These types of athletes also have a higher prevalence of electrocardiographic (ECG) changes.[13]

Echocardiography has played a critical role in understanding the impact of exercise on the heart and in defining the normal changes in cardiac structure and function associated with athlete's heart. Precise cutoffs to differentiate between an athlete and a nonathlete are difficult to define because of the different amounts of remodeling seen in athletes with different training backgrounds and the overlap between athletes and nonathletes. Table 35.2 lists suggested normal ranges for quantification of cardiac structure in athletes by gender, age, and racial background.

LEFT VENTRICLE

STRUCTURE

Regular training increases LV mass, with the pattern determined in part by the type of training undertaken by the athlete, as described earlier. For the echocardiographer trying to differentiate physiologic remodeling from cardiac pathology, the key issue is whether the echocardiographic findings fall inside or outside the expected range for the type and intensity of exercise undertaken by the athlete being examined. Most studies that have determined normal ranges for LV structure have used M-mode to measure LV internal diameter at end-diastole and end-systole, septal wall thickness, and posterior wall thickness at end-diastole, with these values used to determine relative wall thickness and often mass.[14] Others have reported LV volume measurements obtained by echocardiography or cardiac magnetic resonance imaging (MRI).[15]

In pure dynamic exercise, LV mass, volume, dimensions, and wall thickness are all increased[14]; however, the extent of chamber enlargement and the increase in wall thickness tends to be in balance, such that relative wall thickness is similar to that in nonathletes in many studies. In pure static exercise training, LV dimensions are normal or mildly increased with normal or increased wall thickness. The commonly held view that a concentric pattern of hypertrophy is seen as a result of strength training is incorrect, and a smaller than normal LV cavity should raise the possibility of HCM.

The most profound changes are seen in athletes undertaking endurance and strength training, such as cyclists and rowers. Most studies have found these athletes to have the greatest LV mass and largest dimensions. Many studies are carried out in recreational athletes, and the changes seen in elite and professional athletes can be quite profound when compared with the ranges presented in many cross-sectional studies (Fig. 35.1).

The parameters of cardiac structure most commonly used to differentiate healthy athletes from those with inherited cardiac disease such as HCM have been measures of LV wall thickness and relative wall thickness. Wall thickness less than 13 mm in males or less than 11 mm in females is considered to be normal for an athlete (Fig. 35.2). Wall thicknesses greater than 15 mm in a black male athlete, 14 mm in a white male athlete, and 13 mm in a female athlete are considered to be abnormal. This leaves a "gray zone" between these values where differentiation of physiology from pathology may be necessary.

It is clear that gender, age, and race have effects on the athlete's heart phenotype. Although the direction of change with training is similar, dimensions, wall thickness, and LV mass are lower in females than in males, even when indexing for body surface area (BSA) is performed. However, published data on cardiac dimensions in female athletes, particularly elite female endurance athletes, are sparse. Whether female athletes undertaking high intensities and volumes of exercise similar to those

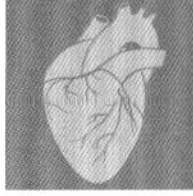

TABLE 35.2 Published Normal Ranges and Range of Values for Cardiac Structural and Functional Parameters in Athletes by Gender, Age, and Racial Background.[a]

Parameter	*Normal ASE/EACVI Values*	*Adolescent Caucasian Athlete*	*Adult Caucasian Athlete*	*Adolescent Afro-Caribbean Athlete*	*Adult Afro-Caribbean Athlete*
Males					
LVWT (mm)	6–10	6–13 (>12)	7–14 (>12)	6–14 (>12)	8–16 (>14)
LVIDd (mm)	42–58	45–60 (>60)	42–66 (>60)	35–62 (>60)	44–64 (>60)
RWT	0.34–0.37	0.27–0.43	0.37–0.48	0.30–0.58	—
LV mass (g), linear	88–224	42–465	113–489	109–329	113–618
LV mass (g), 2D	96–200	42–465	—	—	—
LVEDV (mL)	62–150	—	180–340 (>330)	65–153	—
LVEDVI (mL/m^2)	34–74	—	—	—	—
LVEF (%)	52–72	—	41–77 (<45)	50–76 (<50)	—
GLS (%)	—	—	14–21	—	—
LA diameter	—	25–41 (>40)	29–45 (>45)	25–44 (>40)	—
LAVi (mL/m^2)	16–34	—	25–57	—	—
RVEDV (mL)	—	—	200–390 (>375)	—	—
RVEF (%)	—	—	40–58 (<45)	—	—
Females					
LVWT (mm)	6–9	6–11 (>10)	7–11 (>10)	7–11 (>10)	6–13 (>11)
LVIDd (mm)	38–52	41–55 (>55)	40–66 (>55)	—	39–60 (>55)
LV mass (g), linear	67–162	54–268	67–261	—	95–322
LV mass (g), 2D	66–150	—	—	—	—
LVEDV (mL)	46–106	—	140–260 (>260)	—	—
LVEDVI (mL/m^2)	29–61	—	—	—	—
LVEF (%)	54–74	—	44–76 (<45)	—	41–78 (<45)
LA diameter		—	24–40 (>40)	—	21–41 (>40)
LAVi (mL/m^2)	16–34	—	17–39	—	—
RVEDV (mL)	—	—	150–290 (>280)	—	—
RVEF (%)	—	—	40–67 (<45)	—	—

[a]Athletes have not been separated by type of training undertaken. Values likely to be abnormal when further evaluation is indicated are shown in parentheses.

ASE, American Society of Echocardiography; *EACVI*, European Association of Cardiovascular Imaging; *GLS*, global longitudinal strain; *LAVi*, left atrial volume index; *LVEDV*, left ventricular end-diastolic volume; *LVEDVI*, left ventricular end-diastolic volume index; *LVEF*, left ventricular ejection fraction; *LVIDd*, left ventricular internal dimension at end-diastole; *LVWT*, left ventricular wall thickness; *RVEDV*, right ventricular end-diastolic volume; *RVEF*, right ventricular ejection fraction; *RWT*, relative wall thickness.

Data from References 14, 16, 17, 37, 39, 40, 84–94.

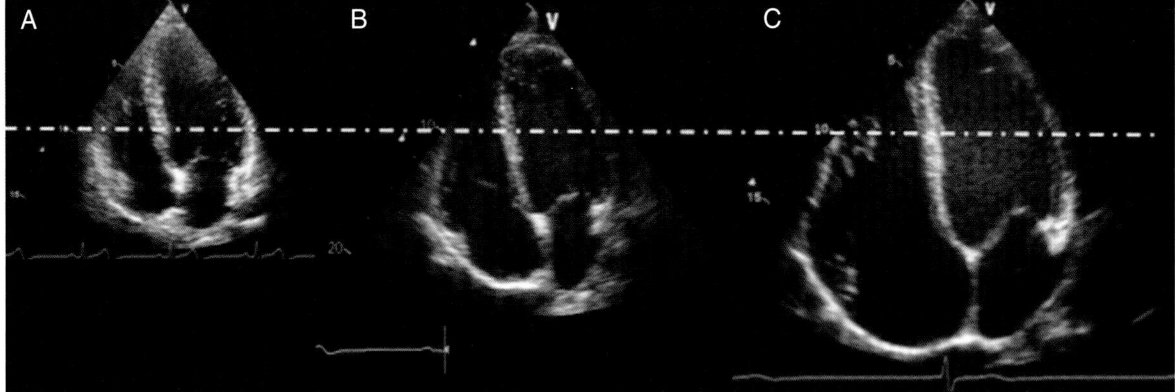

Fig. 35.1 Apical 4-chamber views of a normal young heart and the hearts of healthy athletes. The sectors have been aligned, and a line has been placed at the 10-cm sector depth mark to illustrate the heart of a normal young adult (A) and the extent of cardiac remodeling in the hearts of an endurance-trained professional football player (B) and a professional cyclist (C) with mixed strength and endurance training.

of male athletes may develop similarly profound adaptations is a question that requires further research. Different normal ranges are employed for female athletes (see Table 35.2).

Adolescent athletes tend to have less developed changes of athlete's heart that become more pronounced during maturation, leading to different published normal ranges for younger athletes (see Table 35.2). Whether these differences are truly attributable to cardiac maturation or simply to the lower volume of training exposure compared with adults is unknown. Adolescent cohorts in these publications have been largely subelite nonendurance athletes; data are lacking on the cardiac adaptations in populations of elite adolescent athletes, who may have already undergone 3 to 4 years of intensive endurance training.

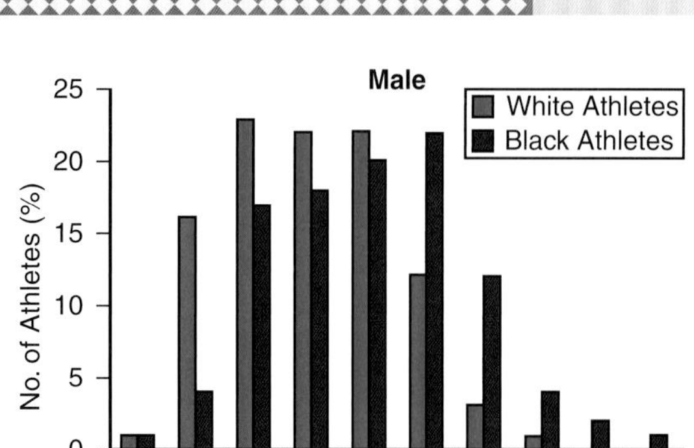

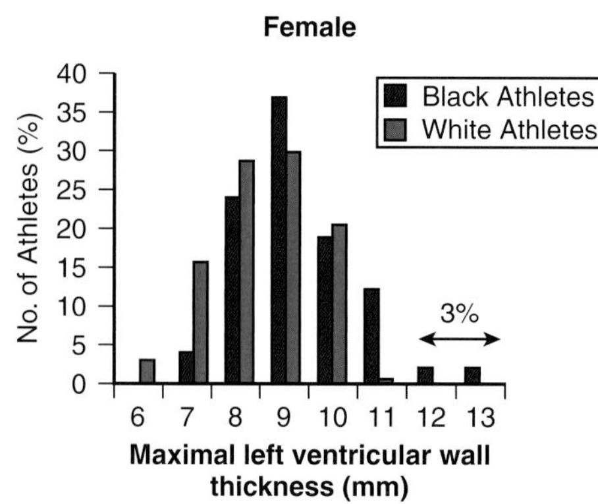

Fig. 35.2 Distribution of LV wall thickness in athletes according to gender and race. Male *(left panel)* and female *(right panel)* black athletes have greater wall thickness than their white counterparts. LV wall thickness is greater than 11 mm in 3% of black females and greater than 12 mm in 18% of black males. (From Basavarajaiah et al.[16] and Rawlins et al.[17])

Nonathlete

Cardiac output = 5.0 L/min
Heart rate = 75 beats/min
LVEDV = 100 mL
Stroke volume = 67 mL
LVEF = 67%

Endurance athlete

Cardiac output = 5.0 L/min
Heart rate = 50 beats/min
LVEDV = 220 mL
Stroke volume = 100 mL
LVEF = 45%

Fig. 35.3 Impact of LV dilation and heart rate on the LVEF required to maintain a normal cardiac output at rest. Despite identical cardiac output values, the LVEF for the endurance athlete's dilated ventricle is only 45%, which falls below the normal range for a nonathlete. *LVEDV*, left ventricular end-diastolic volume; *LVEF*, left ventricular ejection fraction (see Videos 35.3A and 35.3B).

Athletes of Afro-Caribbean background have increased wall thickness compared with white athletes, and different ranges are used to define normality. For example, the upper limit of normal wall thickness in a white male athlete is 12 mm, but it may be up to 15 mm in healthy Afro-Caribbean male athletes[16] (see Fig. 35.2). Wall thickness in black female athletes is also greater than in their white counterparts. Wall thickness greater than 11 mm is unusual in white female athletes, but wall thickness up to 13 mm is seen in black female athletes.[17]

Determining the impact of performance-enhancing drugs on cardiac structure and function is difficult because most athletes are reluctant to admit to their use. Studies using cardiac MRI and echocardiography have shown that strength-trained athletes who do not use anabolic steroids have LV wall thicknesses, ventricular volumes, and left ventricular ejection fractions (LVEFs) similar to those of nonathletes. In contrast, users of anabolic steroids have larger LV volumes, thicker walls, and lower LVEFs compared with nonathletes and with strength-trained athletes not using steroids.[18] Echocardiographic studies have also suggested that anabolic steroid use produces abnormalities in Doppler measures of LV systolic function[19] and diastolic function.[18] It is therefore likely that pure strength training is not truly associated with significant changes in measures of LV structure and that published normal cardiac findings for purely strength-trained athletes have been affected by undeclared use of anabolic steroids.

SYSTOLIC FUNCTION

Two large meta-analyses reported similar LVEF values for athletes and the general population.[6,14] However, lower than normal resting LVEF with preserved stroke volumes can be observed in healthy elite endurance athletes, in whom profound increases in volumes affect all four cardiac chambers.[20] In other words, a healthy enlarged LV needs less vigorous contraction and a lower LVEF to maintain normal cardiac output at rest (Fig. 35.3). The same finding has been observed in elite athletes with nondilated ventricles.[21] In cases of uncertainty, imaging of the heart during exercise may be helpful to differentiate a dilated athlete's heart from a dilated cardiomyopathy (DCM) (see Technical Considerations and Physiologic Differences).

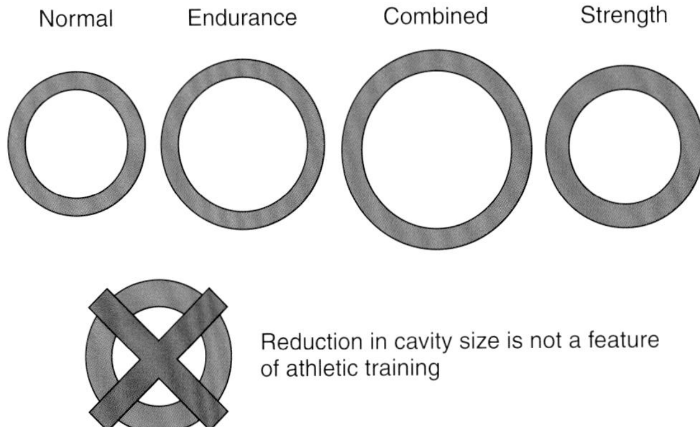

Fig. 35.4 Remodeling of the heart based on type of training. Schematic representation of the changes in LV cavity size and wall thickness in an athlete's heart by type of training undertaken.

Less is known about the effect of athletic activity on direct measures of myocardial function, such as tissue velocity, strain, and strain rate. Most studies have reported normal or supranormal LV myocardial systolic velocities at rest in athletes.[22,23] A cutoff value of 9 cm/s of systolic peak velocity (*s′*, averaged over four mitral annular sites) has been proposed as an accurate discriminator between pathologic LVH and athlete's heart.[24] However, athletes with HCM may have preserved myocardial velocities. Therefore, when there is a clinical suspicion of HCM, normal systolic myocardial velocities should not be used as a discriminator between HCM and athlete's heart.[25]

Resting global longitudinal strain measures have been reported to be lower in athletic cohorts compared with nonathletic controls.[26–28] In much the same way as LVEF may appear reduced at rest in healthy endurance athletes, these observations likely reflect the inadequacy of resting measures to assess functional reserve; lower strain velocities may be required at rest to maintain normal stroke volumes in physiologically enlarged hearts. This has been eloquently demonstrated in the right ventricle (RV), with lower RV strain rates at rest in endurance athletes than in controls but normal augmentation of these indices with exercise.[29] In the absence of normative values in large populations of athletes from a spectrum of sporting disciplines, these measures are not currently considered routine in the assessment of the athlete's heart but may prove to be useful in the future, particularly in the assessment of cardiac reserve with stress echocardiography (Fig. 35.4).

DIASTOLIC FUNCTION

Resting measures of LV diastolic function are typically normal or supranormal in athletes, who demonstrate higher LV chamber compliance than sedentary controls.[12,30] Increases in measures of early diastolic function (i.e., peak transmitral E-wave and E′ tissue velocities) and late diastolic indices (i.e., peak transmitral A-wave and A′ velocity) appear to be most marked in endurance athletes.[12] Although cutoffs for diastolic parameters (e.g., $E/e' > 7.3$) have been proposed for discrimination between athlete's heart and pathologic LVH,[31] normal diastolic parameters may be observed in athletes with HCM.[25] Although abnormal diastolic filling detected by echocardiography in an athlete is likely to reflect myocardial disease, diastolic filling in the normal range for nonathletes does not exclude disease.

RIGHT VENTRICLE

STRUCTURE

During exercise, the RV is subjected to the same volume load as the LV, but wall stress increases more in the RV[32] due to increases in pulmonary artery pressure that parallel the increased cardiac output. Compared with nonathletes, athletes have increased RV volume, increased RV linear dimensions, and increased wall thickness.[33] The magnitude of the increase in RV volume with training is similar to the increase in LV volume, and some reports suggest that it is slightly greater.[32] This has been seen with both strength- and endurance-trained athletes. The degree of RV remodeling increases with duration of training, with more profound changes seen in older athletes with longer participation.[34]

At a practical level, the use of a focused RV view is important for examining the RV, identifying the free wall and the trabeculae, and quantifying dimensions and area (Fig. 35.5).

FUNCTION

Most studies suggest that measures of RV function in athletes are similar to those in nonathletes, although some of the caveats that exist with the LV also apply to the RV. Athletes with the most dilated hearts may have mildly reduced LVEF as a normal finding. Right ventricular fractional area change (RVFAC) appears to be a reasonable surrogate for RVEF in many cases, as long as specific RV-focused views are used.

Measures of systolic function such as tricuspid annular plane systolic excursion (TAPSE) and peak systolic velocity of the tricuspid annulus (RV*s′*) are typically within the normal range. Mildly reduced basal RV free wall strain has been demonstrated in endurance athletes,[35] but this appears to normalize during exercise,[29] suggesting that it is a normal finding.

ATRIA

Athletes have larger atria than nonathletes (Fig. 35.6). Meta-analysis has shown that increased left atrial (LA) size is reflected in greater LA dimensions, when quantified using anteroposterior diameter by echocardiography from a parasternal view, and increased LA volume indexed for BSA (LAVi)[36] as measured by echocardiography from the apical views. LA dimension is an average of 4.1 mm greater, and LAVi is 7.0 mL/m^2 greater in elite athletes compared with sedentary controls, although many athletes still fall within the normal range. Pelliccia et al. found that 20% of competitive athletes had LA dimensions greater than 40 mm.[84] As with many measures of cardiac structure, the degree of enlargement is influenced by the type of sport and the duration of athletic training. A meta-analysis reported that LAVi was 37% higher in elite athletes than in sedentary controls.[37] There are currently more normative data for athletes available using LA dimension than LAVi, making it a more robust measure. LAVi is now considered the preferred method for quantification of LA size in the non-athletic population, and it is likely that more data for this measure in athletes will be become available.[38]

When 2 standard deviations from the mean is taken as the upper limit of normal findings in athletes, the upper limit for LA dimension is 45 mm in males and 40 mm in females, and the upper limit of LAVi is 57 mL/m^2 in males and 39 mL/m^2 in

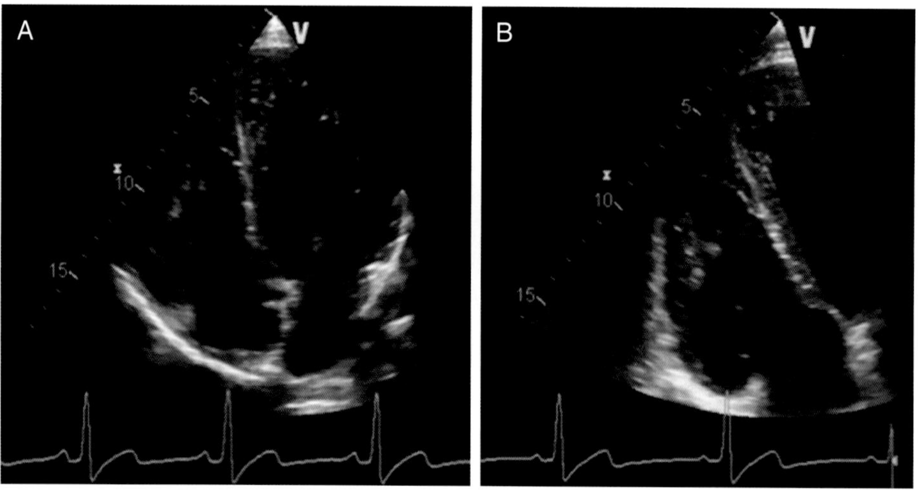

Fig. 35.5 Importance of an RV-focused apical view. A standard 4-chamber view (A; see Video 35.5A) and an RV-focused view (B; see Video 35.5B) obtained by shifting the transducer lateral to the true apex in a professional cyclist. Notice the difficulty in seeing the RV wall in the standard view. The RV wall and trabeculae are seen much better in the RV-focused view.

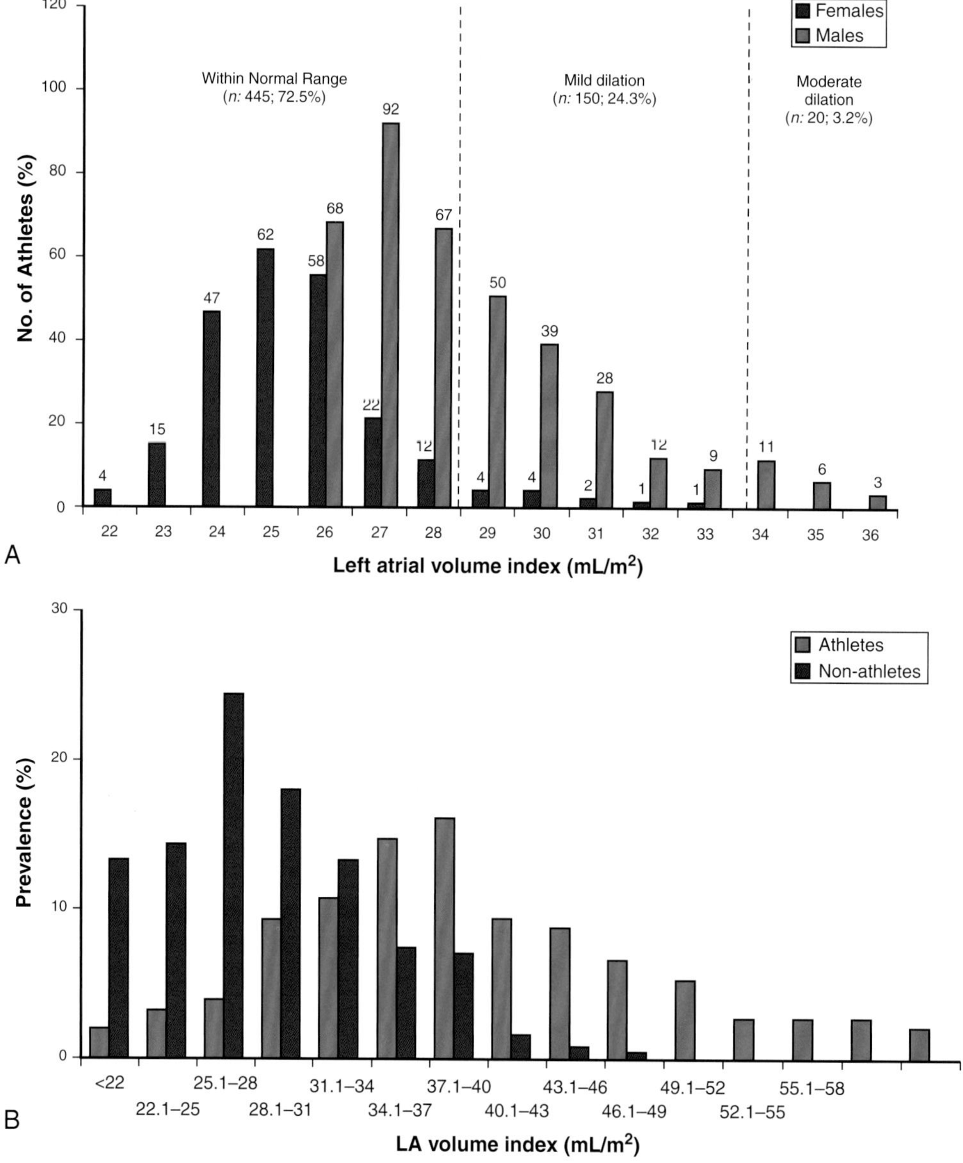

Fig. 35.6 LA size in athletes. Left atrial volume index (LAVi) in a cohort of male versus female athletes (A) and predominantly endurance-trained athletes versus nonathletes (B). LAVi is greater in males than in females and greater in athletes than in nonathletes. Athletes showed a much greater range of values and a higher 95% cutoff value. The mean LAVi in the athletes was 38.9 mL/m^2, compared with 28.4 mL/m^2 in the nonathletes. (A, From D'Andrea A, Riegler L, Cocchia R, et al. Left atrial volume index in highly trained athletes. *Am Heart J.* 2010;159:1155–11610. B, From Nistri S, Galderisi M, Ballo P, et al. Determinants of echocardiographic left atrial volume: implications for normalcy. *Eur J Echocardiogr.* 2011;12:826–833.)

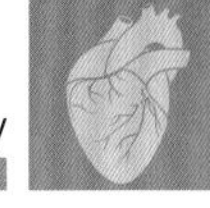

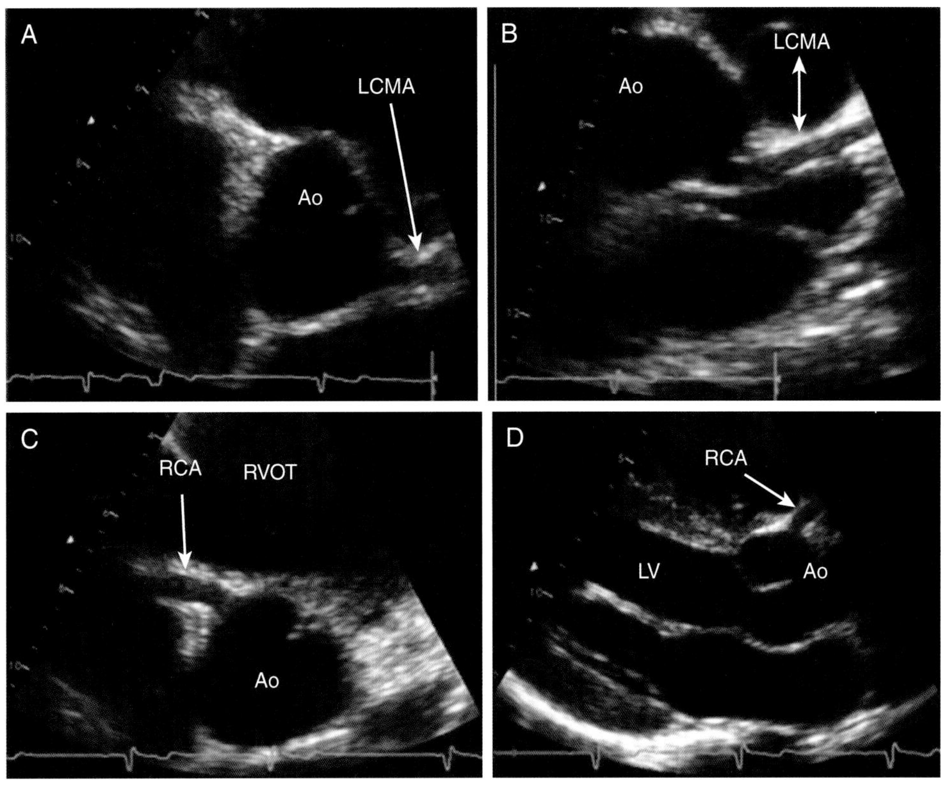

Fig. 35.7 Echocardiographic imaging of coronary arteries. Imaging of the coronary ostia by TTE from parasternal views. (A and B) Imaging of the left main coronary artery *(LMCA)* from a parasternal short-axis view. (C) Imaging of the proximal right coronary artery *(RCA)* from a parasternal short-axis view. (D) Imaging of the proximal RCA from a parasternal long-axis view. *Ao*, Aortic root; *RVOT*, right ventricular outflow tract.

females.[39] As with ventricular size, the largest LA sizes are seen in endurance athletes, but increased atrial size is also a feature of strength-trained athletes and those with combined strength and endurance training.[36] Mild to moderate enlargement of the LA should be considered a normal finding in athletes.[40] More significant enlargement should prompt consideration of underlying cardiac pathology.

Studies evaluating measures of atrial function by echocardiography in athletes have yielded conflicting results for atrial strain by speckle tracking, analogous to those seen with ventricular function. Meta-analysis suggests that LA reservoir strain may be marginally lower in athletes.[41] LA contractile function is lower in athletes, probably reflecting excellent early diastolic filling in this group, which leads to reduced reliance on atrial contraction to fill the ventricle. It may be that physiologic remodeling of the LA is accompanied by normal reservoir function, whereas reduced reservoir function suggests the possibility of underlying pathology, but the status of this proposal is unclear.[42]

Although right atrial size is increased in athletes,[43] there currently are insufficient normative data to make recommendations about quantification and normal ranges in athletes. Atrial enlargement may be important clinically because it is hypothesized that increased atrial size is a factor in the higher rate of atrial fibrillation seen in long-term endurance athletes.[44,45]

AORTA

Enlargement of the aorta and aortic dissection have been described as a cause of sudden cardiac death during exercise.[46] Features of Marfan syndrome, including tall stature and long arms, may offer a competitive advantage in sports such as basketball, and accurate identification of pathologic aortic enlargement that may lead to aortic dissection is an important clinical issue for these athletes. Although athletes have larger aortic root size at the level of the sinuses of Valsalva and the aortic annulus[47] compared with control subjects, the numeric difference is very small, with the sinuses measuring 3.2 mm larger and the aortic annulus 1.6 mm larger in athletes. The difference is not thought to be clinically significant. It is possible that the observed difference reflects differences in body habitus rather than a training effect because values have not been adjusted for body composition in most studies.

Other studies recommend scaling to height rather than BSA.[48] Enlargement of the aortic sinuses usually should be regarded as pathologic. Cutoff values for abnormality of 40 mm in males and 34 mm in females have been proposed.[49] One study suggested that 0.3% of young athletes had mildly increased aortic diameter, but medium-term follow-up did not show progressive enlargement.[50]

The coronary ostia can often be imaged by transthoracic and transesophageal echocardiography because they arise from the aortic root (Fig. 35.7). The efficacy of echocardiography in identification of the coronary ostia varies and is influenced by image quality and operator and interpreter experience. Therefore, a standardized imaging protocol should be used.[51,52] Often a short-axis view at the level of the coronary sinuses can be used to visualize the proximal portions of the left and right coronary arteries.

Anomalous coronary artery is an important cause of sudden cardiac death in athletes, particularly a left coronary artery arising from the right sinus or a right coronary artery arising from

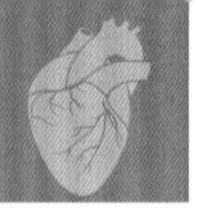

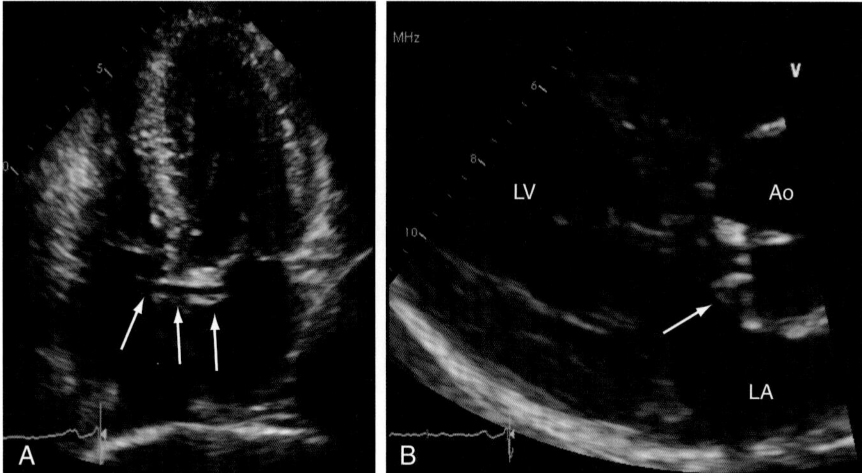

Fig. 35.8 Aberrant left circumflex coronary artery arising from the right coronary sinus with a retroaortic course. A double shadow seen at the mitral annular level on a 4-chamber view and highlighted with *arrows* (A) raises suspicion for this abnormality. The artery can be seen in cross-section *(arrow)* on a zoomed parasternal long-axis view (B) (see Video 35.8). *Ao*, Aortic root.

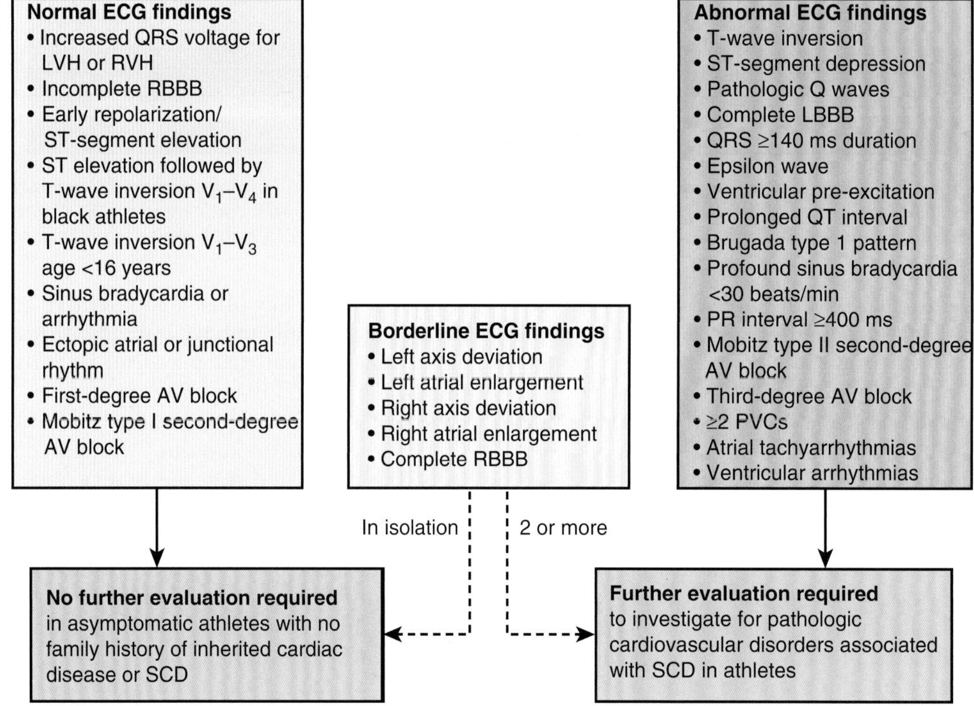

Fig. 35.9 International consensus standards for electrographic interpretation in an athlete. Findings are grouped into those considered normal in an asymptomatic athlete, which do not require further evaluation; those considered abnormal, which do require further evaluation; and those that are borderline and require evaluation only if more than one abnormality is present. *AV*, Atrioventricular; *ECG*, electrocardiographic; *LBBB*, left bundle branch block; *LVH*, left ventricular hypertrophy; *PVCs*, premature ventricular contractions; *RBBB*, right bundle branch block; *RVH*, right ventricular hypertrophy; *SCD*, sudden cardiac death. (From Sharma S, Drezner JA, Baggish A, et al. International recommendations for electrocardiographic interpretation in athletes. *J Am Coll Cardiol*. 2017;69[8]:1057–1075, Fig. 1.)

the left sinus. An anomalous left circumflex coronary artery arising from the right sinus with a retroaortic route may produce a typical double line at the level of the mitral annulus in an apical 4-chamber view (Fig. 35.8). In the appropriate clinical setting, the inability to image two ostia arising from the left and right sinuses of Valsalva may raise the possibility of an anomalous origin and lead to further investigations such as computed tomography coronary angiography (CTCA), which can provide a more definitive diagnosis and describe the course of the arteries in relation to the aortic wall and other great vessels.

ELECTRICAL REMODELING

Regular training changes the ECG findings, with some changes considered to be benign manifestations of athlete's heart and others associated with higher rates of cardiac abnormalities and worthy of further investigation. International recommendations exist for ECG interpretation in athletes.[53] They are summarized in Fig. 35.9. Sinus bradycardia, first-degree atrioventricular block, incomplete right bundle branch block, early repolarization, and isolated voltage criteria for LVH are accepted as normal findings in athletes[53] (Fig. 35.10).

Distinctly abnormal ECG findings in athletes include lateral T-wave inversion, ST-segment depression, Q waves, left bundle branch block, marked QT prolongation, changes of Brugada syndrome, and frequent ventricular premature beats (PVCs) (see Fig. 35.10B). These are not usually related to the typical pattern of benign cardiac remodeling seen in the athlete's heart and therefore are considered to be abnormal findings warranting further investigation, often with echocardiography as the next test. Right precordial T-wave inversion or T-wave inversion in the early V leads is among the diagnostic criteria for arrhythmogenic right ventricular cardiomyopathy (ARVC)[54] and is considered to be abnormal in white athletes (see Fig. 35.10C).

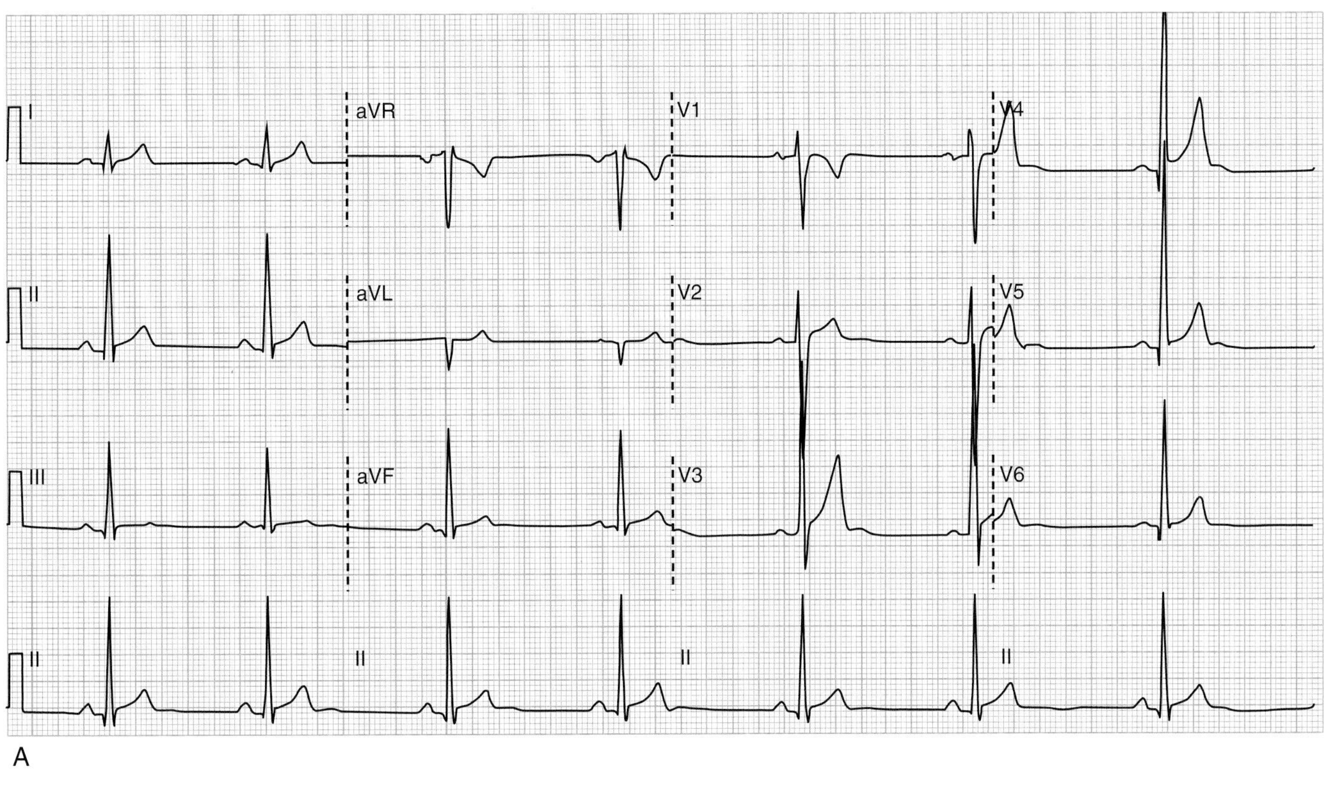

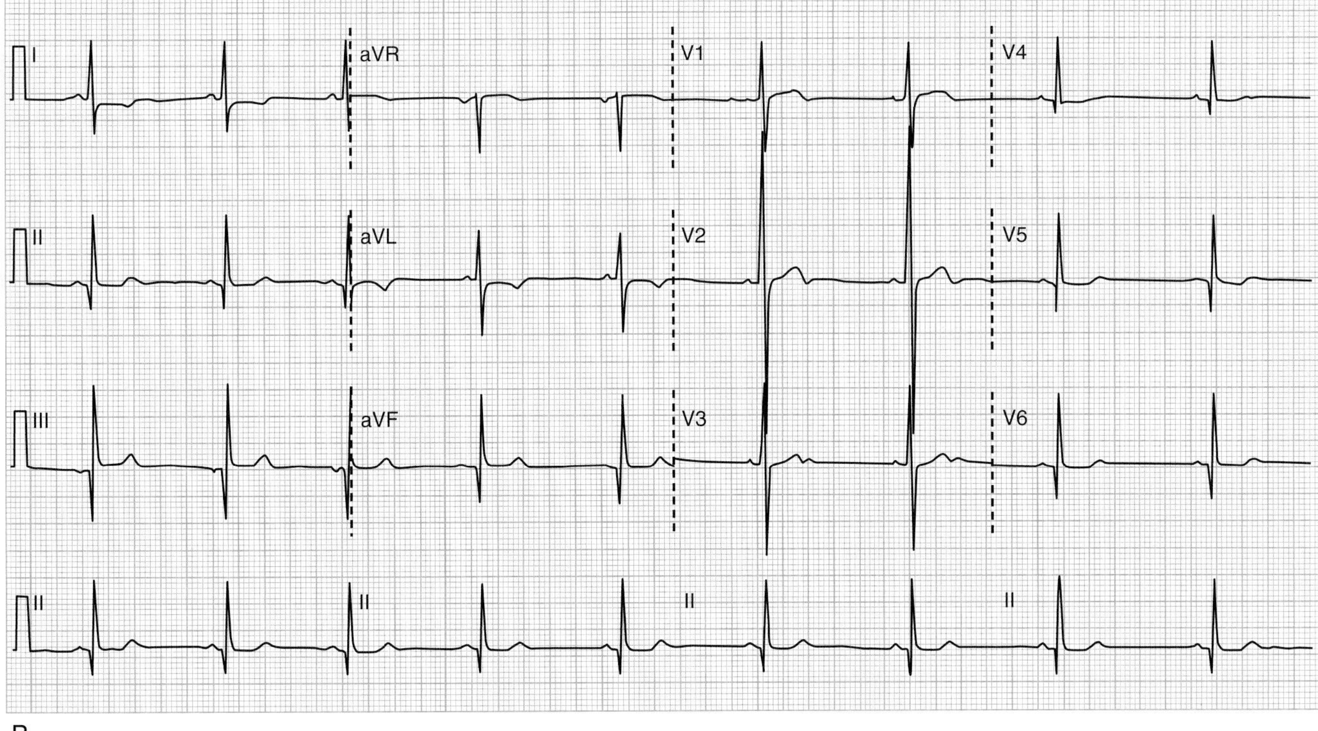

Fig. 35.10 Electrocardiographic findings in athletes. (A) Sinus bradycardia, left ventricular hypertrophy by voltage criteria without associated T-wave changes, and early repolarization are considered normal in athletes. (B) A tracing from an athlete with hypertrophic cardiomyopathy shows pathologic Q waves inferolaterally and lateral T-wave inversion and should prompt further investigation.

Continued

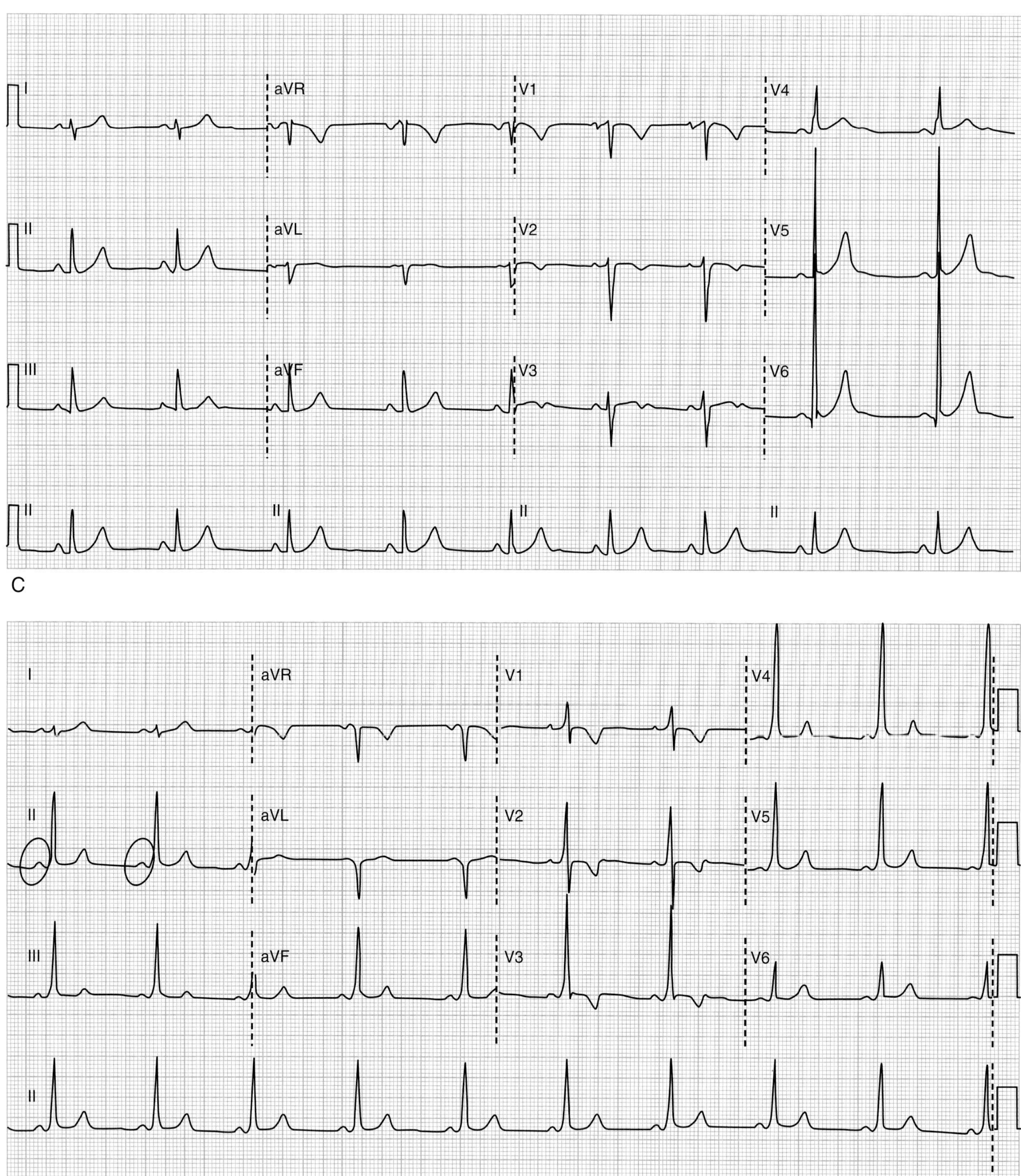

Fig. 35.10, cont'd (C) T-wave inversion in the early V leads and an epsilon wave are suggestive of arrhythmogenic right ventricular cardiomyopathy. (D) Wolff-Parkinson-White syndrome is generally associated with a normal echocardiogram and is usually detected from personal history or a screening electrocardiogram.

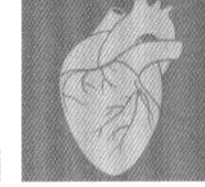

TABLE 35.3 Recommendations for Screening of Asymptomatic Athletes.

Parameter	*USA*[95]	*Italy*[96]	*Israel*[97]	*IOC*[98]
Personal history	Recommended	Mandated	Mandated	Recommended
Family history	Recommended	Mandated	Mandated	Recommended
Physical examination	Recommended	Mandated	Mandated	Recommended
Electrocardiogram	2nd line	Mandated	Mandated	recommended
Echocardiogram	2nd line	2nd line	2nd line	2nd line
Holter monitor/loop recorder	2nd line	2nd line	2nd line	2nd line
Cardiac MRI	2nd line	2nd line	2nd line	2nd line
Stress ECG/stress echocardiography	2nd line	2nd line	2nd line	2nd line
EP study	2nd line	2nd line	2nd line	2nd line
CTCA	2nd line	2nd line	2nd line	2nd line

CTCA, Computed tomography coronary angiography; *ECG*, electrocardiographic; *EP*, electrophysiology; *IOC*, International Olympic Committee; *MRI*, magnetic resonance imaging.

However, for uncertain reasons, healthy black athletes and sedentary controls of Afro-Caribbean descent frequently demonstrate T-wave inversion in V_1 through V_4, usually preceded by convex ST-segment elevation.[55] This has led to the inclusion of this ECG finding as normal in black athletes.

Right precordial T-wave inversion is not infrequently seen in elite endurance athletes. T-wave inversion extended beyond V_2 in 4% of subjects in one study, thereby meeting a major diagnostic criterion for ARVC.[13,56] This finding does not seem to be related purely to increased RV volumes in this population[57,58] but rather to the position of the RV apex with respect to the surface ECG leads, with lateral displacement of an enlarged heart resulting in more of the RV underlying the surface ECG leads V_2 through V_3.[57]

Echocardiography alone is often not sufficient to confirm or exclude a diagnosis of cardiomyopathy that has been suggested by an abnormal ECG. In some conditions of relevance to screening and sports participation such as ion channelopathies (i.e., long QT syndrome, Brugada syndrome, CPVT, or Wolff-Parkinson-White syndrome) (see Fig. 35.10D), the echocardiographic examination is expected to be normal. A normal echocardiographic study should not be viewed as adequate reassurance of the absence of pathology. The ECG and echocardiographic findings should always be interpreted along with the entire clinical picture, which should include thorough physical examination, personal and family history, and often further testing such as Holter monitoring, exercise ECG and stress echocardiography, signal-averaged electrocardiography (SAECG), cardiac MRI, and familial screening.

DETRAINING EFFECTS

Although no large, prospective studies have addressed reverse cardiac remodeling with detraining, the existing evidence suggests that the changes of athlete's heart begin to regress toward normal within about 6 weeks after complete cessation of athletic training.[10] LV wall thickness and mass have been reported to return to within normal limits, whereas reductions in LV cavity size appear to be more modest months to years after cessation of training.[10,59] The effects on the RV and atria have been even less well described.[60]

From a practical perspective, one of the major diagnostic dilemmas in echocardiographic assessment of athletes is the distinction between physiologic LVH and pathologic LVH, as seen in HCM. Case reports and small series have described regression of LVH with detraining in athletes with borderline wall thickness (13–15 mm), and this parameter has been suggested as a useful aid in the differentiation of athlete's heart from HCM.[60–62] However, this notion hinges on the assumption that in athletes with HCM, pathologic LVH will not be accentuated by exercise nor attenuated by detraining.

No prospective study has addressed the effect of athletic training or detraining on cardiac morphology in athletes with genotypically confirmed HCM. A single case report of an adolescent male soccer player with phenotypic expression of HCM (i.e., asymmetric septal and apical LVH) who underwent 6 months of enforced sports restriction described a reduction in LV wall thickness similar to that observed in healthy athletes with detraining.[63] Until the effects of detraining in athletic subjects with proven pathologic cardiac conditions such as HCM and ARVC are defined, reduction in LV wall thickness and cardiac dimensions with detraining cannot be considered a reliable sole differentiator of physiologic from pathologic cardiac adaptation in athletes with equivocal echocardiographic findings such as borderline LV wall thickness or ventricular dilation.

SCREENING ECHOCARDIOGRAPHY IN ATHLETES

The indications for echocardiography in athletes are essentially the same as for nonathletes[64]; the major differences are in how the findings are interpreted. There are, however, some indications that are more common in athletes than in the nonathletic population, such as frequent PVCs, atrial fibrillation, lightheadedness, presyncope, syncope, and a murmur. They are classified as appropriate indications for echocardiography in an athlete. In some cases, stress echocardiography is needed to evaluate the athlete with symptoms. Indications for stress echocardiography are outlined in the section entitled Stress Echocardiography in the Athlete.

In countries with preparticipation screening of athletes for underlying cardiac diseases that may predispose to sudden cardiac death during exercise, one common indication is for evaluation of cardiac structure and function after results of previous testing (e.g., clinical evaluation, ECG) raised concern about underlying structural heart disease. In some countries and for some elite sports, screening is mandatory for competitive athletes; in other countries, screening is simply recommended. The recommendations vary among countries depending on the level of the athlete, from recreational to elite to professional. Common screening recommendations are presented in Tables 35.3 and 35.4.

TABLE 35.4 Recommendations for Essential Components of an Echocardiographic Examination of the Athlete as Part of a Routine Echocardiogram.

Left Ventricle	*Right Ventricle*	*Other Structures*
LV end-diastolic dimension	RV free wall thickness	LA diameter LAVi
LV septal and posterior wall thickness	RV basal dimension Proximal RVOT dimension	RA area
LV mass index	RV fractional area change	Confirmation of normal coronary ostial locations
LV ejection fraction	TAPSE	
Mitral valve inflow Doppler	IVC size and collapsibility	
Mitral annular septal and lateral annular *s′* velocities		
Mitral annular septal and lateral annular *e′* velocities		
E/*e′* ratio		

IVC, Inferior vena cava; *LAVi*, left atrium volume index; *RVOT*, right ventricular outflow tract; *TAPSE*, tricuspid annular plane systolic excursion.

STRESS ECHOCARDIOGRAPHY IN THE ATHLETE

TECHNICAL CONSIDERATIONS AND PHYSIOLOGIC DIFFERENCES

Because symptoms such as palpitations, chest pain, or reduced performance, with or without abnormal shortness of breath, are not uncommon in athletes, stress echocardiograms are often performed to evaluate these symptoms. In younger athletes, abnormalities such as anomalous origin of coronary arteries can cause myocardial ischemia and are considered risk factors for sudden cardiac death during exercise; in older athletes. atherosclerotic coronary artery disease may develop, causing angina, myocardial infarction, and sudden cardiac death. In performing and interpreting these tests, the clinician should understand where similarities and differences exist between the athletic and nonathletic populations. Sometimes a stress echocardiogram for an athlete may evaluate more than just LV wall motion and myocardial ischemia. RV response to exercise can be very important, as can change in pulmonary artery systolic pressure (PASP), although some caution is needed in interpreting pulmonary artery pressure changes with exercise.

If possible, the type and intensity of exercise should be tailored to the athlete's normal activity or the activity that causes symptoms. Some athletes have fitness in particular muscle groups and can exercise to a greater intensity using a particular form of exercise stress. For example, a cyclist may reach a higher workload if a supine bike is used rather than a treadmill. An athlete is likely to take longer to reach maximal exercise than a nonathlete, and a modified protocol with more frequent increments in workload sometimes can be useful. It is vital to aim for maximal exercise and to achieve the level of exercise that produces an athlete's symptoms, a level that may be significantly higher than in the normal population.

ACUTE EFFECTS OF EXERCISE

As with nonathletes, there are expected normal findings during stress echocardiography in the athletic population. Blood pressure should increase during exercise stress. LV cavity size should decrease with a uniform increase in wall thickening of all wall segments in response to exercise. As a result, LVEF should increase; one study of professional American football players showed an average increase in LVEF from 58% to 76% with exercise.[65]

Augmentation of LVEF with exercise has been proposed as useful for differentiating athlete's heart from a DCM with a mildly reduced LVEF,[66] although evidence to support this guideline or defined cutoff values is sparse. One study used exercise cardiac MRI to demonstrate blunted improvement of LVEF in athletes with myocardial fibrosis and borderline LVEF and in subjects with DCM, compared with healthy athletes[67] (see Endurance Athlete or Dilated Cardiomyopathy).

RV function should be augmented with exercise, and reduced RV reserve in endurance athletes has been associated with RV arrhythmias,[68] suggesting possible utility in identifying abnormalities when resting function appears normal. Strict guidelines and cutoffs have not been well defined due to a lack of outcome data. Useful measures for quantifying RV function with exercise have included the right ventricular ejection fraction (RVEF), RVFAC, TAPSE, and systolic annular velocity of the tricuspid valve (RV*s′*).

There are some important differences in findings on stress echocardiography in athletes that mandate caution in interpretation. In a highly trained athlete, it is not unusual for PASP to increase to levels such as 70 mmHg during intense exercise; in other populations, this would be considered to indicate significant pulmonary hypertension, such as in the setting of mitral stenosis. This increase in PASP appears to be closely related to the workload and the cardiac output achieved.[69] It is a flow-induced phenomenon in a pulmonary vascular bed with limited vasodilatory capacity in the face of elevated flow, rather than a sign of pulmonary vascular dysfunction.

Invasive pulmonary artery pressure (PAP) measurements with exercise suggest that mean PAP should rise by 1.0 to 1.5 mmHg for every L/min of cardiac output increase.[70,71] This measurement needs to be interpreted in the context of the workload achieved. An increase in cardiac output from 5 to 30 L/min in an athlete with a resting mean PAP of 15 mmHg could result in a mean PAP of 40 to 52 mmHg at peak exercise as a normal phenomenon. Resting PASP measured by echocardiography is also slightly higher in athletes than in nonathletes; it may reach 40 mmHg and is thought to be caused by higher stroke volume, suggesting that this should be considered the upper limit of normal in athletes.[72]

ALTERNATIVE IMAGING MODALITIES

When echocardiography fails to provide sufficient information to reach an accurate diagnosis or additional prognostic information is required, additional imaging modalities, most commonly cardiac MRI, may be useful and may provide complimentary information to the echocardiography examination. When ventricular volumes and EF cannot be accurately quantified, cardiac MRI provides accurate measures of these parameters, although volumes measured by cardiac MRI tend to be larger than those measured by echocardiography.

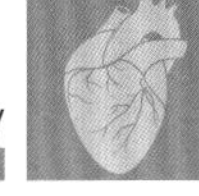

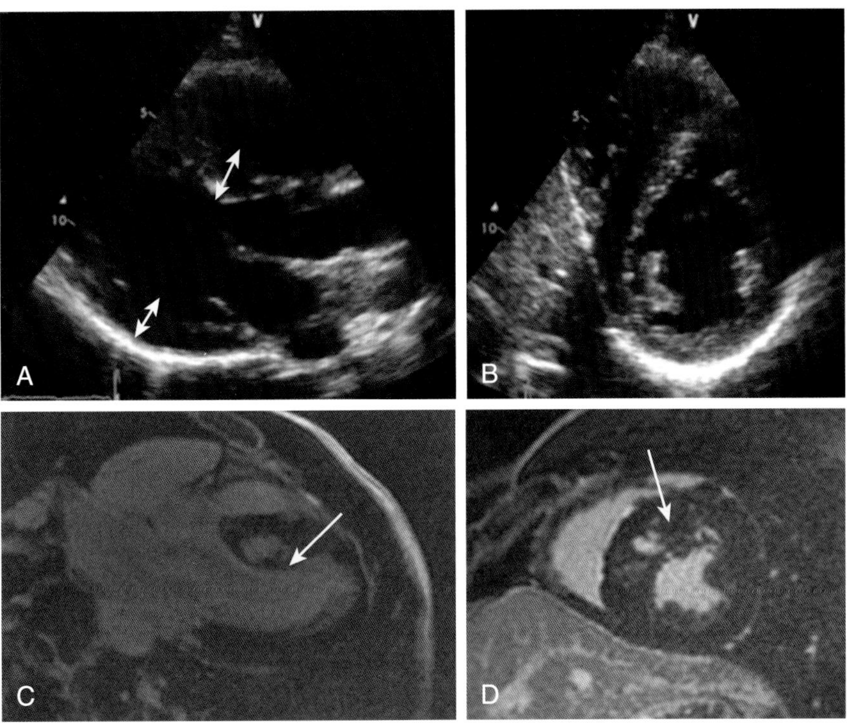

Fig. 35.11 **Typical hypertrophic cardiomyopathy in an asymptomatic football player.** Imaging findings in an asymptomatic professional male football player with an abnormal electrocardiogram who was found to have hypertrophic cardiomyopathy. (A) Parasternal long-axis view shows increased thickness of the basal anteroseptum *(double-headed arrows)*. (B) Short-axis view of the LV shows asymmetric septal hypertrophy. (C and D) Cardiac magnetic resonance images of the heart in views similar to those in A and B, respectively, after administration of gadolinium contrast. There is extensive late enhancement of the septum and anteroseptum *(arrows)*, consistent with extensive fibrosis.

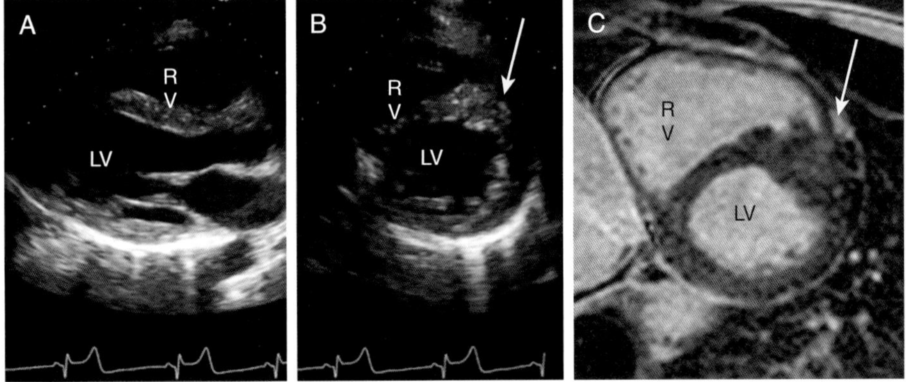

Fig. 35.12 **Hypertrophic cardiomyopathy with focal anteroseptal hypertrophy.** Imaging findings in an asymptomatic young female athlete with an abnormal electrocardiogram who was found to have hypertrophic cardiomyopathy. The parasternal long-axis view was normal (A), as were many standard views. Focal hypertrophy of the anteroseptum *(arrow)* was seen only with off-axis views during systematic examination of the entire LV (B). Cardiac magnetic resonance imaging (C) confirmed focal anteroseptal hypertrophy *(arrow)* with associated late enhancement after gadolinium administration.

Cardiac MRI can characterize myocardial structure more effectively than echocardiography, and LV mass measures are more reproducible by cardiac MRI. Myocardial edema and hyperemia can be imaged in suspected myocarditis using specific sequences, and T1 and T2 mapping sequences are also useful in this setting. Late gadolinium enhancement (LGE) identifies increased extracellular volume, which is most commonly caused by fibrosis but is also seen with edema and infiltration. This may provide additional diagnostic information and may have additional prognostic significance in cases of suspected HCM (Figs. 35.11 and 35.12).

In cases of suspected anomalous coronary artery or atherosclerotic coronary artery disease, CTCA can be diagnostic, providing information about the location of coronary ostia, the course of coronary arteries and their relationships to other thoracic structures, and the presence and location of atherosclerotic plaque. In some cases, this may lead to invasive coronary angiography.

COMMON CLINICAL DILEMMAS

In differentiating the normal athlete's heart from the pathologic heart, echocardiography provides only part of the puzzle required to reach an accurate assessment, and findings should not be taken in isolation. A complete and accurate history, including a detailed family history, a history of previous athletic training, a thorough physical examination, and a 12-lead ECG, forms the basis of the diagnostic assessment. In some cases, a resting echocardiogram may provide sufficient additional

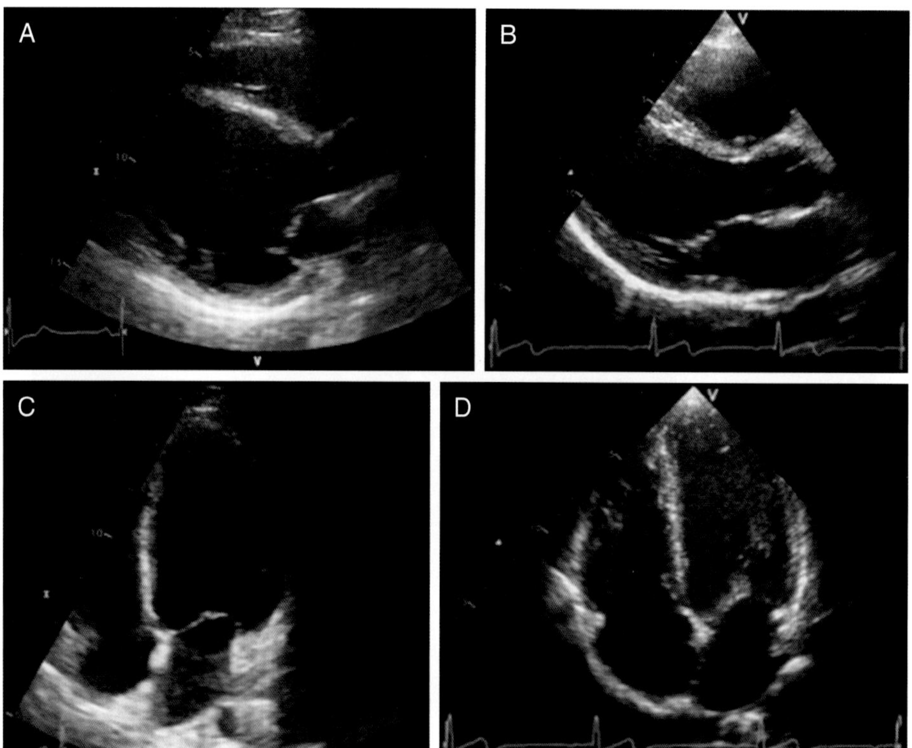

Fig. 35.13 Distinguishing athlete's heart from dilated cardiomyopathy with resting TTE measures. (A and C) Imaging findings in a young male subject with dilated cardiomyopathy secondary to Becker muscular dystrophy. The parasternal long-axis view (A) shows normal LV wall thickness, with the following measurements: interventricular septal thickness at end-diastole (IVSd), 0.7 cm; LV posterior wall thickness (LVPW), 0.8 cm; and LV internal dimension in diastole (LVIDd), 6.0 cm. The 4-chamber view (C) shows the following: LV end-diastolic volume (LVEDV), 160 mL; LV end-systolic volume (LVESV), 82 mL; stroke volume (SV), 78 mL; LV ejection fraction (LVEF), 49%; ratio of E-wave to A-wave velocity (E/A), 2.7; deceleration time of early mitral inflow velocity (MVDecT), 136 ms; peak early diastolic velocity lateral (E′ lateral), 20 cm/s; peak early diastolic velocity septal (E′ septal), 11 cm/s; septal E/E′ ratio, 6.8; and global longitudinal systolic peak strain (GLPS), −13%. (B and D) Comparison imaging findings in a young asymptomatic professional cyclist. The parasternal long-axis view (B) shows normal wall thickness (IVSd, 0.8 cm; LVPW, 0.8 cm) and an LVIDd of 5.1 cm. The 4-chamber view (D) shows LVEDV, 146 mL; LVESV, 76 mL; LVEF, 47%; E/A, 1.93; MVDecT, 155 ms; E′ lateral, 17 cm/s; E′ septal, 16 cm/s; septal E/E′, 3.05; and GLPS, −16.3%.

information for a diagnostic decision, but stress echocardiography, cardiac MRI, cardiac computed tomography, or cardiac catheterization may be required as additional imaging tests.

It is also worth considering that most evidence guiding practice in this area has been derived from comparisons of athletes without the disease of interest with nonathletes with the disease. In clinical practice, the task is to determine whether the patient is an athlete with a disease or a normal athlete, a more difficult task. Imaging parameters are likely to perform less well in this task, a concept that has been supported in HCM.[25]

VALVE DISEASE IN ATHLETES

Athletes may suffer from congenital and acquired valvular disease, and this may result in ventricular hypertrophy and/or dilation superficially similar to that seen from training. Little is known about teasing out the relative contributions of athletic training and valvular disease on cardiac structure and function. There are no prospective studies addressing whether exercise can accelerate progression of ventricular dilation or hypertrophy in athletes with stenotic or regurgitant valve lesions.

One small study compared LV dimensions in handball and football players who had mild aortic or mitral regurgitation ($n = 14$) with those in 14 players matched for body size and exercise exposure who were without valvular regurgitation.[73] They reported that LV end-diastolic diameter indexed to BSA was slightly higher in athletes with mild aortic or mitral regurgitation than in subjects without valvular regurgitation, but measures of exercise capacity were not different. Another study examined athletes and sedentary control subjects with bicuspid aortic valves and mild valvular dysfunction; there was progressive enlargement of the LV over 5 years of training in athletes, but all values remained within the normal range, suggesting a normal training effect rather than a pathologic effect.[74]

In the absence of systematic data, guidelines for sports participation in athletes with valvular heart disease are largely based on expert opinion.[75–77] Echocardiographic assessment of valvular disease plays a critical role in assessing the severity of valve disease and its impact on cardiac function.

ENDURANCE ATHLETE OR DILATED CARDIOMYOPATHY

Cardiac dilation can be profound in some endurance athletes (see Fig. 35.1), and it can be associated with measures of LV and RV systolic function that fall below the normal range for nonathletes. A dilated heart with a low LVEF in an athlete with an abnormal ECG or symptoms presents a significant diagnostic challenge (Fig. 35.13). Abnormal diastolic filling suggests that the cardiac enlargement is pathologic, as does functional atrioventricular valvular regurgitation, but otherwise differentiation of pathology from physiology on resting assessment can be difficult.

An example of the challenge in differentiating DCM from athlete's heart is shown in Fig. 35.13, which shows imaging findings for a young male subject with DCM due to Becker muscular dystrophy and for a professional cyclist. Measures of LV size and function, myocardial velocities, and diastolic dimensions are similar in subjects at rest. In the endurance athlete, there is dilation of all four cardiac chambers, with the RV and both atria more dilated than in the subject with DCM. In cases such as this, if there is clinical doubt, exercise measures are potentially useful in discriminating between physiologic adaptation and pathologic dilation.

Studies of exercise in patients with DCM have suggested that the low LVEF does not increase with exercise, although there is obviously a range of responses.[66] Claessen et al. compared a group of 19 healthy endurance athletes with 9 patients with mild DCM and 5 endurance athletes with arrhythmias and subepicardial fibrosis on cardiac MRI, all of whom demonstrated a borderline resting LVEF.[67] Exercise capacity (VO_2 max) and cardiac augmentation in response to maximal exercise were assessed using exercise cardiac MRI. Not surprisingly, healthy athletes and athletes with fibrosis had better exercise capacity than sedentary subjects with mild DCM. The most salient finding of the study was that improvement in LVEF with exercise was blunted in both comparison groups (5% ± 6% in the mild DCM group and 4% ± 3% in athletes with fibrosis) compared with 14% ± 3% improvement in the healthy athletes ($P < 0.005$). Exercise capacity alone did not differentiate healthy endurance athletes from athletes with myocardial fibrosis and arrhythmias, but reduced cardiac contractile reserve (i.e., increase in LVEF < 11.2%) with exercise did. Functional cardiac evaluation during exercise may emerge as the best discriminator in the differential diagnosis of DCM and athlete's heart, whereas supranormal exercise capacity should not be considered incompatible with underlying pathology in an athlete with suspected DCM.

STRENGTH-TRAINED ATHLETE OR HYPERTROPHIC CARDIOMYOPATHY

Increased LV wall thickness in athletes presents a common diagnostic dilemma, and echocardiography is often used as part of the diagnostic workup to differentiate physiologic from pathologic causes. If the echocardiographic findings are typical for a disease such as HCM, with wall thickness clearly outside the normal range and the gray zone and an unusual distribution of increased wall thickness, the study result can confidently be reported as abnormal. For cases in which parameters such as wall thickness fall into the gray zone and the pattern is global, additional information is required.

One key fact is useful in separating normal from abnormal: athletes do not normally develop a concentric pattern of hypertrophy with reduced cavity size. One study of athletes with increased wall thickness in the gray zone of 13 to 15 mm reported that a diastolic LV internal dimension (LVIDd) of less than 54 mm was the most reliable criterion with which to identify those with HCM, achieving 100% sensitivity and 100% specificity.[31] The study was small, but LV dimension has consistently emerged as a useful parameter to differentiate athlete's heart from HCM, although other investigators have suggested that a cutoff value of 5.0 cm is more reliable.[78] In this context, a simple dimension measurement performs better than measures of abnormal diastolic filling such as the E′ velocity or E/E′ ratio.

TABLE 35.5 Differentiation of Athlete's Heart From Hypertrophic Cardiomyopathy.

Features Suggesting Athlete's Heart	*Features Suggesting HCM*
LV cavity diastolic dimension >5.5 cm	LV cavity diastolic dimension <5.0 cm
	Unusual pattern of LVH
	Maximal wall thickness >16 mm
	Abnormal diastolic filling
	Mitral valve SAM
	Unusual ECG patterns such as deep T-wave inversion or widespread ST-T changes
	Family history of HCM
	Typical LGE on cardiac MRI

ECG, Electrocardiogram; *HCM*, hypertrophic cardiomyopathy; *LGE*, late gadolinium enhancement; *LVH*, left ventricular hypertrophy; *MRI*, magnetic resonance imaging; *SAM*, systolic anterior motion.

Adapted from Maron BJ. Distinguishing hypertrophic cardiomyopathy from athlete's heart: a clinical problem of increasing magnitude and significance. *Heart*. 2005;91:1380–1382.

In many cases, athletes with HCM may be more difficult to distinguish from normal athletes than sedentary patients with HCM, and much of our understanding is based on the latter comparison. Athletes with HCM appear to have larger LV cavities, less LVH, and more normal parameters of diastolic filling than sedentary patients with the disease[25] (Table 35.5). As discussed earlier (see Left Ventricle: Diastolic Function), the previously held notion that normal diastolic function can exclude a diagnosis of HCM does not hold true in athletic populations.

Figs. 35.11 and 35.12 show examples of asymptomatic athletes diagnosed with HCM after screening who had a markedly abnormal 12-lead ECG. In an asymptomatic football player (Fig. 35.11), fairly typical features of nonobstructive HCM with asymmetric hypertrophy of the basal and mid-anteroseptum were seen on standard echocardiographic views. Cardiac MRI provided confirmatory findings and showed fibrosis identified with LGE.

The case of a female athlete with an abnormal ECG (see Fig. 35.12) was more challenging because most standard echocardiographic views were unremarkable, and off-axis views were required to identify the presence of focal anteroseptal hypertrophy. Cardiac MRI confirmed this finding and identified patchy fibrosis in the same region. Further assessment uncovered a history of HCM in a first-degree relative. This case highlights the importance of a complete examination, which may involve off-axis views, particularly if the study is performed to further investigate an abnormal ECG.

The challenge of differentiating cases of generalized hypertrophy from athlete's heart based on structural features alone is illustrated in Fig. 35.14. Both the patient with hypertensive heart disease presenting to the emergency department in heart failure and the cyclist had mildly increased LV cavity size and wall thickness. Diastolic function assessment has been suggested as a method for reliably differentiating HCM from athlete's heart. It has been shown that measures of diastolic function in athletes with HCM are often within normal limits, with no diastolic parameter able to reliably distinguish those individuals from athletes with physiologic LVH.[25] Although abnormal diastolic parameters should raise concern about the possibility of cardiac pathology, normal diastolic parameters in athletes for whom a clinical suspicion of HCM has been raised should not be taken as reassurance.

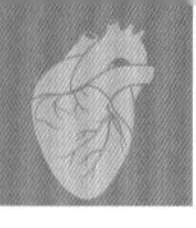

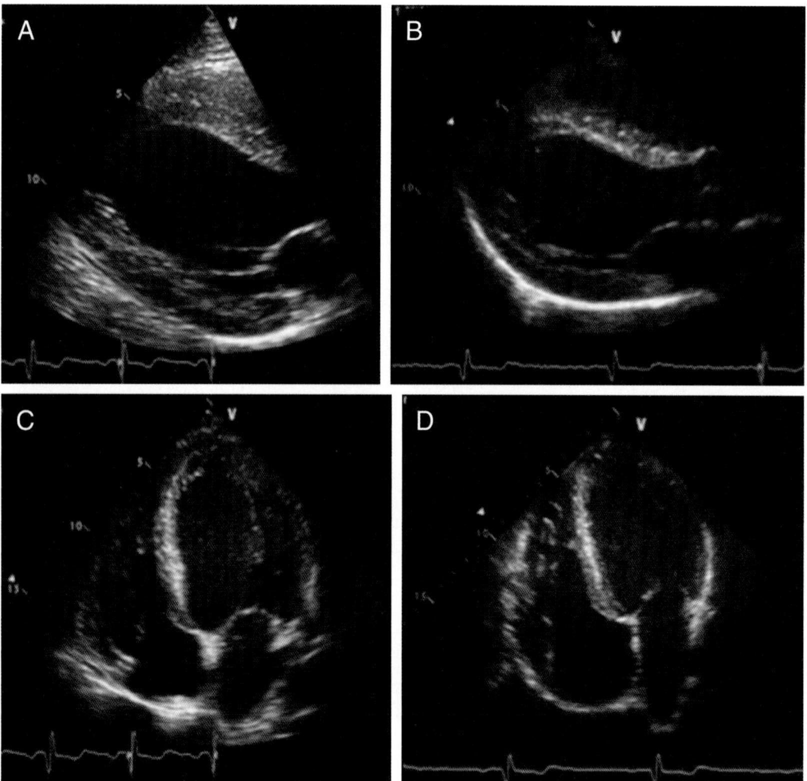

Fig. 35.14 Differentiating athlete's heart from hypertensive heart disease on echocardiographic parameters. Parasternal long-axis views (A and B) and apical 4-chamber views (C and D) are shown in a patient with hypertensive heart failure *(left panels)* and in a professional cyclist *(right panels)* using similar sector depths. Many findings were similar on 2D imaging. Both patients had mildly increased LV wall thickness and an LV cavity size at the upper limit of normal. LV ejection fraction was similar at approximately 55%. LA size was increased in the hypertensive patient, and RA size was increased in the cyclist (see Videos 35.14A, 35.14B, 35.14C, and 35.14D).

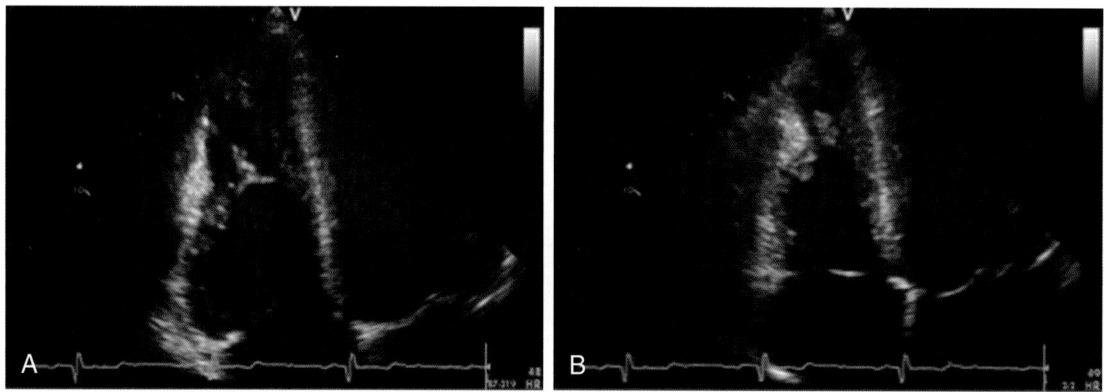

Fig. 35.15 Distinguishing ARVC from athlete's heart. Focused RV views of a professional cyclist demonstrate a prominent moderator band and a heavily trabeculated RV apex at end-diastole (A) and end-systole (B). Although hypertrabeculation is not a typical feature of ARVC, it can create the appearance of a regional wall motion abnormality (RWMA) with a hinge point at the moderator band (see Videos 35.15A and 35.15B). Given that RWMA and increased RV volumes are among the major diagnostic criteria for ARVC, this is a condition that can be overdiagnosed in elite endurance athletes. *ARVC*, Arrhythmogenic right ventricular cardiomyopathy.

ENDURANCE ATHLETE OR RV CARDIOMYOPATHY

Athletic training results in enlargement of the right heart, which can in some cases be more marked than the remodeling of the left heart (Fig. 35.15; see Right Ventricle: Structure). In an athlete with palpitations, a family history of sudden cardiac death, or ECG abnormalities suggesting ARVC (e.g., T-wave inversion in the early V leads), echocardiography can play an important role in differentiation of athlete's heart from ARVC.

Those modified task force criteria that can be evaluated by echocardiography are largely based on increased RV size, particularly in the RV outflow tract (regional RV akinesia, dyskinesia, or aneurysm), and reduced RVEF (≤33%).[54] They should be assessed if ARVC is suspected in an athlete, but echocardiographic assessment alone cannot make the diagnosis of ARVC and must be considered in the context of the clinical history, family history, 12-lead ECG findings, SAECG, and cardiac MRI.[79] As can be seen in Fig. 35.15 and Videos 35.15A and B, care needs to be taken when imaging the RV of endurance athletes because trabeculation along with constraint from a hypertrophied moderator band and the chest wall may produce the impression of a regional wall motion abnormality in a normal athlete.

TABLE 35.6 Differentiation of Athlete's Heart From Arrhythmogenic Right Ventricular Cardiomyopathy.

Features Suggesting Athlete's Heart	*Features Suggesting ARVC*
Symmetric cardiac enlargement	RV ejection fraction <45% or RVFAC <30%
Enlargement of the inflow portion of the RV only	Enlargement of inflow and outflow portions of the RV
Early repolarization on ECG	RV wall motion abnormalities
Voltage criteria for LV or RV hypertrophy on ECG	Q waves or precordial QRS amplitude <1.8 mV
	Delayed gadolinium enhancement on cardiac MRI
	>100 VPCs per 24 h
	PVCs or attenuated BP response during exercise testing

ARVC, Arrhythmogenic right ventricular cardiomyopathy; *BP*, blood pressure; *ECG*, electrocardiogram; *MRI*, magnetic resonance imaging; *PVCs*, premature ventricular contractions; *RVFAC*, right ventricular fractional area change; *VPCs*, ventricular premature complexes.
Adapted from Zaidi A, Sheikh N, Jongman JK, et al. Clinical differentiation between physiological remodeling and arrhythmogenic right ventricular cardiomyopathy in athletes with marked electrocardiographic repolarization anomalies. *J Am Coll Cardiol*. 2015;65:2702–2711.

One study examined the performance of clinical, ECG, echocardiographic, and cardiac MRI parameters to differentiate individuals with ARVC from athletes with and without right precordial or lateral T-wave inversion.[58] The subjects with ARVC were not athletes, and the results do not specifically address this clinical dilemma. However, features of asymmetric RV enlargement and reduced RV function measured by RVEF or RVFAC in the athletes suggested ARVC (Table 35.6). Other work has highlighted the frequency with which normal athletes fulfill some criteria for ARVC[79,80] (Fig. 35.16), which appears to be related to the extent of right heart enlargement.

Blunted augmentation of RV function with exercise has been demonstrated in athletes with ventricular arrhythmias arising from the RV. La Gerche et al.[68] assessed RV function with exercise echocardiography and exercise cardiac MRI in 10 healthy endurance athletes and 17 endurance athletes with ventricular arrhythmias. Resting measures of RV function did not differ between the two groups, but in the athletes with ventricular arrhythmias, the RV at peak exercise dilated and failed to contract adequately. Healthy endurance athletes demonstrated an RVFAC of 45% ± 6% at rest and 57% ± 5% at peak stress; endurance athletes with arrhythmias had an RVFAC of 41% ± 7% at rest and 44% ± 11% at peak stress. Stress echocardiography added additional information to resting echocardiography findings for subjects with suspected RV pathology but normal resting echocardiographic measures of function.[68]

An exercise-induced RV cardiomyopathy that may be associated with ventricular arrhythmias and sudden cardiac death has been described.[81] Although it is known that phenotypic expression of ARVC in those with recognized desmosomal mutations is accelerated by engaging in endurance exercise, athletes with the exercise-induced RV cardiomyopathy do not have a higher than expected rate of genetic polymorphisms[82] known to cause ARVC. This suggests that the cardiomyopathy is not caused by the common, currently known desmosomal mutations but by excessive exercise in susceptible individuals and that it possibly reflects cumulative episodes of minor RV injury due to endurance training and competition.[11]

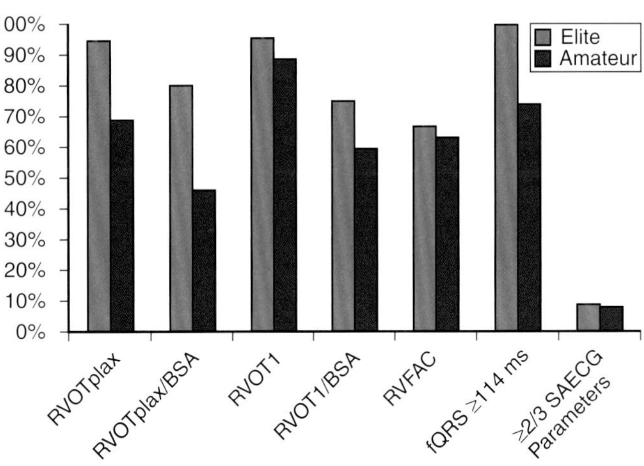

Fig. 35.16 Prevalence of positive ARVC criteria in normal athletes. A large proportion of elite athletes have RV dimensions in the abnormal category. Differentiation between ARVC and athlete's heart can be challenging, and the distinction cannot be made based on echocardiography alone. Correlation with electrocardiographic findings is essential, and often further investigations such as cardiac magnetic resonance imaging, Holter monitoring, SAECG, family history/screening, and follow-up imaging are required to exclude the diagnosis. This should occur in a center with experience with athlete's heart and ARVC. *ARVC*, Arrhythmogenic right ventricular cardiomyopathy; *SAECG*, signal-averaged electrocardiography. (From Jongman JK, Zaidi A, Muggenthaler M, Sharma S. Relationship between echocardiographic right-ventricular dimensions and signal-averaged electrocardiogram abnormalities in endurance athletes. *Europace*. 2015;17[9]:1441–1448; Fig. 2.)

TABLE 35.7 Key Questions to Be Addressed During Echocardiographic Examination of an Athlete.

1. Does this person exercise enough to produce cardiac changes typical of athlete's heart?
2. Does the pattern of cardiac change fit with the type and intensity of exercise being undertaken by the athlete?
3. Do the echocardiographic findings suggest significant cardiac disease when considered in the context of age, gender, and racial background?
4. Has the clinical question been adequately addressed, or are further investigations such as electrocardiography, cardiac magnetic resonance imaging, or computed tomography coronary angiography required?

CAN THIS ATHLETE CONTINUE TO COMPETE SAFELY?

In general, the athlete who has a diagnosis of structural cardiac disease known to be associated with an increased risk of sudden cardiac death, such as HCM, arrhythmogenic RV cardiomyopathy, DCM, Marfan syndrome with a dilated aorta, or anomalous coronary arteries, should be advised not to play competitive sports. Echocardiography plays a key role in ensuring an accurate diagnosis (Table 35.7) so that those with normal changes consistent with athlete's heart are not inappropriately excluded from competing and those who have diseases associated with significant risk of adverse events are given appropriate advice.

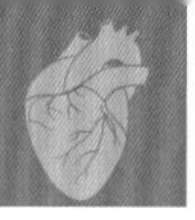

SUMMARY Evaluation of the Athlete's Heart[a]

Parameter	Modality	Views	Endurance	Strength	Mixed
LV size: LVIDd	M-mode or 2D	Parasternal long-axis	Increased ++	Normal or increased +	Increased +++
LV size: LV volume	2D or 3D	Apical	Increased ++	Normal or increased +	Increased +++
LV wall thickness	M-mode or 2D	Parasternal long-axis	Normal	Normal or increased[b]	Increased
LV ejection fraction	2D or 3D	Apical	Normal	Normal	Normal or mildly reduced (in those with markedly dilated hearts)
LA size: LA dimension or LAVi	2D	Parasternal long-axis and apical	Increased +	Normal or increased	Increased ++
RV size: basal dimension and RVOT dimension	2D	Apical and parasternal short-axis	Increased basal diameter (in proportion to LV)	Normal	Increased basal diameter (in proportion to LV)
Aortic sinuses	M-mode or 2D	Parasternal long-axis	Normal	Normal	Normal
LV diastolic filling	Doppler	Apical	Normal	Normal	Normal

[a]The extent of change is in proportion to the quantity of exercise performed.
[b]Values considered normal may be influenced by the use of performance-enhancing drugs.
LVIDd, Left ventricular internal dimension at end-diastole; *LAVi*, left atrial volume indexed to body surface area; *RVOT*, right ventricular outflow tract.

REFERENCES

1. Fagard R. Athlete's heart. *Heart*. 2003;89:1455–1461.
2. Ryffel CP, Eser P, Trachsel LD, et al. Age at start of endurance training is associated with patterns of left ventricular hypertrophy in middle-aged runners. *Int J Cardiol*. 2018;267:133–138.
3. Bhella PS, Hastings JL, Fujimoto N, et al. Impact of lifelong exercise "dose" on left ventricular compliance and distensibility. *J Am Coll Cardiol*. 2014;64:1257–1266.
4. Morganroth J, Maron BJ, Henry WL, et al. Comparative left ventricular dimensions in trained athletes. *Ann Intern Med*. 1975;82:521–524.
5. Mitchell JH, Haskell W, Snell P, et al. Task Force 8: classification of sports. *J Am Coll Cardiol*. 2005;45:1364–1367.
6. Utomi V, Oxborough D, Whyte GP, et al. Systematic review and meta-analysis of training mode, imaging modality and body size influences on the morphology and function of the male athlete's heart. *Heart*. 2013;99:1727–1733.
7. Utomi V, Oxborough D, Ashley E, et al. Predominance of normal left ventricular geometry in the male 'athlete's heart'. *Heart*. 2014;100:1264–1271.
8. Haykowsky M, Humen D, Teo K, et al. Effects of 16 weeks of resistance training on left ventricular morphology and systolic function in healthy men >60 years of age. *Am J Cardiol*. 2000;85:1002–1006.
9. Luijkx T, Cramer MJ, Prakken NH, et al. Sport category is an important determinant of cardiac adaptation: an MRI study. *Br J Sports Med*. 2012;46:1119–1124.
10. Spence AL, Naylor LH, Carter HH, et al. A prospective randomised longitudinal MRI study of left ventricular adaptation to endurance and resistance exercise training in humans. *J Physiol*. 2011;589:5443–5452.
11. La Gerche A, Burns AT, Mooney DJ, et al. Exercise-induced right ventricular dysfunction and structural remodelling in endurance athletes. *Eur Heart J*. 2012;33:998–1006.
12. Baggish AL, Yared K, Weiner RB, et al. Differences in cardiac parameters among elite rowers and subelite rowers. *Med Sci Sports Exerc*. 2010;42:1215–1220.
13. Brosnan M, La Gerche A, Kalman J, et al. Comparison of frequency of significant electrocardiographic abnormalities in endurance versus nonendurance athletes. *Am J Cardiol*. 2014;113:1567–1573.
14. Pluim BM, Zwinderman AH, van der Laarse A, et al. The athlete's heart. A meta-analysis of cardiac structure and function. *Circulation*. 2000;101:336–344.
15. Wernstedt P, Sjostedt C, Ekman I, et al. Adaptation of cardiac morphology and function to endurance and strength training. A comparative study using MR imaging and echocardiography in males and females. *Scand J Med Sci Sports*. 2002;12:17–25.
16. Basavarajaiah S, Boraita A, Whyte G, et al. Ethnic differences in left ventricular remodeling in highly-trained athletes relevance to differentiating physiologic left ventricular hypertrophy from hypertrophic cardiomyopathy. *J Am Coll Cardiol*. 2008;51:2256–2262.
17. Rawlins J, Carre F, Kervio G, et al. Ethnic differences in physiological cardiac adaptation to intense physical exercise in highly trained female athletes. *Circulation*. 2010;121:1078–1085.
18. Angell PJ, Chester N, Green DJ, et al. Anabolic steroid use and longitudinal, radial, and circumferential cardiac motion. *Med Sci Sports Exerc*. 2012;44:583–590.
19. D'Andrea A, Caso P, Salerno G, et al. Left ventricular early myocardial dysfunction after chronic misuse of anabolic androgenic steroids: a Doppler myocardial and strain imaging analysis. *Br J Sports Med*. 2007;41:149–155.
20. Abergel E, Chatellier G, Hagege AA, et al. Serial left ventricular adaptations in world-class professional cyclists: implications for disease screening and follow-up. *J Am Coll Cardiol*. 2004;44:144–149.
21. Boraita A, Sanchez-Testal MV, Diaz-Gonzalez L, et al. Apparent ventricular dysfunction in elite young athletes: another form of cardiac adaptation of the athlete's heart. *J Am Soc Echocardiogr*. 2019;32:987–996.
22. Zoncu S, Pelliccia A, Mercuro G. Assessment of regional systolic and diastolic wall motion velocities in highly trained athletes by pulsed wave Doppler tissue imaging. *J Am Soc Echocardiogr*. 2002;15:900–905.
23. Florescu M, Stoicescu C, Magda S, et al. "Supranormal" cardiac function in athletes related to better arterial and endothelial function. *Echocardiography*. 2010;27:659–667.
24. Vinereanu D, Florescu N, Sculthorpe N, et al. Differentiation between pathologic and physiologic

left ventricular hypertrophy by tissue Doppler assessment of long-axis function in patients with hypertrophic cardiomyopathy or systemic hypertension and in athletes. *Am J Cardiol*. 2001;88: 53–58.
25. Sheikh N, Papadakis M, Schnell F, et al. Clinical profile of athletes with hypertrophic cardiomyopathy. *Circ Cardiovasc Imaging*. 2015;8. e003454.
26. Matsumura Y, Elliott PM, Virdee MS, et al. Left ventricular diastolic function assessed using Doppler tissue imaging in patients with hypertrophic cardiomyopathy: relation to symptoms and exercise capacity. *Heart*. 2002;87:247–251.
27. Richand V, Lafitte S, Reant P, et al. An ultrasound speckle tracking (two-dimensional strain) analysis of myocardial deformation in professional soccer players compared with healthy subjects and hypertrophic cardiomyopathy. *Am J Cardiol*. 2007;100:128–132.
28. Vitarelli A, Capotosto L, Placanica G, et al. Comprehensive assessment of biventricular function and aortic stiffness in athletes with different forms of training by three-dimensional echocardiography and strain imaging. *Eur Heart J Cardiovasc Imaging*. 2013;14:1010–1020.
29. La Gerche A, Burns AT, D'Hooge J, et al. Exercise strain rate imaging demonstrates normal right ventricular contractile reserve and clarifies ambiguous resting measures in endurance athletes. *J Am Soc Echocardiogr*. 2012;25:253–262 e1.
30. Fagard R, Van den Broeke C, Amery A. Left ventricular dynamics during exercise in elite marathon runners. *J Am Coll Cardiol*. 1989;14:112–118.
31. Caselli S, Maron MS, Urbano-Moral JA, et al. Differentiating left ventricular hypertrophy in athletes from that in patients with hypertrophic cardiomyopathy. *Am J Cardiol*. 2014;114:1383–1389.
32. La Gerche A, Heidbuchel H, Burns AT, et al. Disproportionate exercise load and remodeling of the athlete's right ventricle. *Med Sci Sports Exerc*. 2011;43:974–981.
33. D'Andrea A, La Gerche A, Golia E, et al. Right heart structural and functional remodeling in athletes. *Echocardiography*. 2015;32(suppl 1):S11–S22.
34. Popple E, George K, Somauroo J, et al. Right ventricular structure and function in senior and academy elite footballers. *Scand J Med Sci Sports*. 2018;28:2617–2624.
35. Teske AJ, Prakken NH, De Boeck BW, et al. Echocardiographic tissue deformation imaging of right ventricular systolic function in endurance athletes. *Eur Heart J*. 2009;30:969–977.
36. Iskandar A, Mujtaba MT, Thompson PD. Left atrium size in elite athletes. *JACC Cardiovasc Imaging*. 2015;8:753–762.
37. Cuspidi C, Sala C, Tadic M, et al. Left atrial volume in elite athletes: a meta-analysis of echocardiographic studies. *Scand J Med Sci Sports*. 2019;29:922–932.
38. D'Andrea A, Riegler L, Cocchia R, et al. Left atrial volume index in highly trained athletes. *Am Heart J*. 2010;159:1155–1161.
39. Nistri S, Galderisi M, Ballo P, et al. Determinants of echocardiographic left atrial volume: implications for normalcy. *Eur J Echocardiogr*. 2011;12:826–833.
40. Baggish AL. Athletic left atrial dilation: size matters? *JACC Cardiovasc Imaging*. 2015;8:763–765.
41. Cuspidi C, Tadic M, Sala C, et al. Left atrial function in elite athletes: a meta-analysis of two-dimensional speckle tracking echocardiographic studies. *Clin Cardiol*. 2019;42:579–587.
42. D'Ascenzi F, Anselmi F, Focardi M, et al. Atrial enlargement in the athlete's heart: assessment of atrial function may help distinguish adaptive from pathologic remodeling. *J Am Soc Echocardiogr*. 2018;31:148–157.
43. Grunig E, Henn P, D'Andrea A, et al. Reference values for and determinants of right atrial area in healthy adults by 2-dimensional echocardiography. *Circ Cardiovasc Imaging*. 2013;6:117–124.
44. Aizer A, Gaziano JM, Cook NR, et al. Relation of vigorous exercise to risk of atrial fibrillation. *Am J Cardiol*. 2009;103:1572–1577.
45. Mont L, Elosua R, Brugada J. Endurance sport practice as a risk factor for atrial fibrillation and atrial flutter. *Europace*. 2009;11:11–17.
46. Harmon KG, Asif IM, Klossner D, et al. Incidence of sudden cardiac death in National Collegiate Athletic Association. *Circulation*. 2011;123:1594–1600.
47. Iskandar A, Thompson PD. A meta-analysis of aortic root size in elite athletes. *Circulation*. 2013;127:791–798.
48. Oates SA, Forsythe L, Somauroo JD, et al. Scaling to produce size-independent indices of echocardiographic derived aortic root dimensions in elite Rugby Football League players. *Ultrasound*. 2019;27:94–100.
49. Pelliccia A, Di Paolo FM, Quattrini FM. Aortic root dilatation in athletic population. *Prog Cardiovasc Dis*. 2012;54:432–437.
50. Gati S, Malhotra A, Sedgwick C, et al. Prevalence and progression of aortic root dilatation in highly trained young athletes. *Heart*. 2019;105:920–925.
51. Zeppilli P, dello Russo A, Santini C, et al. In vivo detection of coronary artery anomalies in asymptomatic athletes by echocardiographic screening. *Chest*. 1998;114:89–93.
52. Lorber R, Srivastava S, Wilder TJ, et al. Anomalous aortic origin of coronary arteries in the young: echocardiographic evaluation with surgical correlation. *JACC Cardiovasc Imaging*. 2015;8:1239–1249.
53. Sharma S, Drezner JA, Baggish A, et al. International recommendations for electrocardiographic interpretation in athletes. *J Am Coll Cardiol*. 2017;69:1057–1075.
54. Marcus FI, McKenna WJ, Sherrill D, et al. Diagnosis of arrhythmogenic right ventricular cardiomyopathy/dysplasia: proposed modification of the Task Force criteria. *Eur Heart J*. 2010;31:806–814.
55. Papadakis M, Carre F, Kervio G, et al. The prevalence, distribution, and clinical outcomes of electrocardiographic repolarization patterns in male athletes of African/Afro-Caribbean origin. *Eur Heart J*. 2011;32:2304–2313.
56. Wasfy MM, DeLuca J, Wang F, et al. ECG findings in competitive rowers: normative data and the prevalence of abnormalities using contemporary screening recommendations. *Br J Sports Med*. 2015;49:200–206.
57. Brosnan MJ, Claessen G, Heidbuchel H, et al. Right precordial T-wave inversion in healthy endurance athletes can be explained by lateral displacement of the cardiac apex. *JACC Clin Electrophysiol*. 2015;1:84–91.
58. Zaidi A, Sheikh N, Jongman JK, et al. Clinical differentiation between physiological remodeling and arrhythmogenic right ventricular cardiomyopathy in athletes with marked electrocardiographic repolarization anomalies. *J Am Coll Cardiol*. 2015;65:2702–2711.
59. Pelliccia A, Maron BJ, De Luca R, et al. Remodeling of left ventricular hypertrophy in elite athletes after long-term deconditioning. *Circulation*. 2002;105:944–949.
60. Weiner RB, Wang F, Berkstresser B, et al. Regression of "gray zone" exercise-induced concentric left ventricular hypertrophy during prescribed detraining. *J Am Coll Cardiol*. 2012;59:1992–1994.
61. Maron BJ, Pelliccia A, Spataro A, et al. Reduction in left ventricular wall thickness after deconditioning in highly trained Olympic athletes. *Br Heart J*. 1993;69:125–128.
62. Basavarajaiah S, Wilson M, Junagde S, et al. Physiological left ventricular hypertrophy or hypertrophic cardiomyopathy in an elite adolescent athlete: role of detraining in resolving the clinical dilemma. *Br J Sports Med*. 2006;40:727–729. discussion 729.
63. de Gregorio C, Speranza G, Magliarditi A, et al. Detraining-related changes in left ventricular wall thickness and longitudinal strain in a young athlete likely to have hypertrophic cardiomyopathy. *J Sports Sci Med*. 2012;11:557–561.
64. American College of Cardiology Foundation Appropriate Use Criteria Task F, American Society of E, American Heart A, et al. ACCF/ASE/AHA/ASNC/HFSA/HRS/SCAI/SCCM/SCCT/SCMR 2011 Appropriate Use Criteria for Echocardiography. A report of the American College of Cardiology Foundation Appropriate Use Criteria Task Force, American Society of Echocardiography, American Heart Association, American Society of Nuclear Cardiology, Heart Failure Society of America, Heart Rhythm Society, Society for Cardiovascular Angiography and Interventions, Society of Critical Care Medicine, Society of Cardiovascular Computed Tomography, Society for Cardiovascular Magnetic Resonance American College of Chest Physicians. *J Am Soc Echocardiogr*. 2011;24:229–267.
65. Abernethy WB, Choo JK, Hutter Jr AM. Echocardiographic characteristics of professional football players. *J Am Coll Cardiol*. 2003;41:280–284.
66. Holloway CJ, Dass S, Suttie JJ, et al. Exercise training in dilated cardiomyopathy improves rest and stress cardiac function without changes in cardiac high energy phosphate metabolism. *Heart*. 2012;98:1083–1090.
67. Claessen G, Schnell F, Bogaert J, et al. Exercise cardiac magnetic resonance to differentiate athlete's heart from structural heart disease. *Eur Heart J Cardiovasc Imaging*. 2018;19:1062–1070.
68. La Gerche A, Claessen G, Dymarkowski S, et al. Exercise-induced right ventricular dysfunction is associated with ventricular arrhythmias in endurance athletes. *Eur Heart J*. 2015.
69. La Gerche A, MacIsaac AI, Burns AT, et al. Pulmonary transit of agitated contrast is associated with enhanced pulmonary vascular reserve and right ventricular function during exercise. *J Appl Physiol*. 2010;109:1307–1317.
70. Lewis GD, Murphy RM, Shah RV, et al. Pulmonary vascular response patterns during exercise in left ventricular systolic dysfunction predict exercise capacity and outcomes. *Circ Heart Fail*. 2011;4:276–285.
71. Lau EM, Vanderpool RR, Choudhary P, et al. Dobutamine stress echocardiography for the assessment of pressure-flow relationships of the pulmonary circulation. *Chest*. 2014;146:959–966.
72. D'Andrea A, Naeije R, D'Alto M, et al. Range in pulmonary artery systolic pressure among highly trained athletes. *Chest*. 2011;139:788–794.

73. Langer C, Butz T, Mellwig KP, et al. Elite athletes with mitral or aortic regurgitation and their cardiopulmonary capability. *Acta Cardiol.* 2013; 68:475–480.
74. Stefani L, Galanti G, Innocenti G, et al. Exercise training in athletes with bicuspid aortic valve does not result in increased dimensions and impaired performance of the left ventricle. *Cardiol Res Pract.* 2014;2014:238694.
75. Pelliccia A, Fagard R, Bjornstad HH, et al. Recommendations for competitive sports participation in athletes with cardiovascular disease: a consensus document from the study group of Sports Cardiology of the working group of Cardiac Rehabilitation and Exercise Physiology and the working group of Myocardial and Pericardial Diseases of the European Society of Cardiology. *Eur Heart J.* 2005;26:1422–1445.
76. Mellwig KP, van Buuren F, Gohlke-Baerwolf C, et al. Recommendations for the management of individuals with acquired valvular heart diseases who are involved in leisure-time physical activities or competitive sports. *Eur J Cardiovasc Prev Rehabil.* 2008;15:95–103.
77. Bonow RO, Nishimura RA, Thompson PD, et al. Eligibility and disqualification recommendations for competitive athletes with cardiovascular abnormalities: Task Force 5: valvular heart disease: a scientific statement from the American Heart Association and American College of Cardiology. *Circulation.* 2015;132:e292–e297.
78. Pelliccia A, Maron MS, Maron BJ. Assessment of left ventricular hypertrophy in a trained athlete: differential diagnosis of physiologic athlete's heart from pathologic hypertrophy. *Prog Cardiovasc Dis.* 2012;54:387–396.
79. Prior D. Differentiating athlete's heart from cardiomyopathies - the right side. *Heart Lung Circ.* 2018;27:1063–1071.
80. Jongman JK, Zaidi A, Muggenthaler M, et al. Relationship between echocardiographic right-ventricular dimensions and signal-averaged electrocardiogram abnormalities in endurance athletes. *Europace.* 2015;17:1441–1448.
81. Heidbuchel H, Prior DL, La Gerche A. Ventricular arrhythmias associated with long-term endurance sports: what is the evidence? *Br J Sports Med.* 2012;46(suppl 1):i44–50.
82. La Gerche A, Robberecht C, Kuiperi C, et al. Lower than expected desmosomal gene mutation prevalence in endurance athletes with complex ventricular arrhythmias of right ventricular origin. *Heart.* 2010;96:1268–1274.
83. Pelliccia A, Maron BJ, Culasso F, et al. Athlete's heart in women. Echocardiographic characterization of highly trained elite female athletes. *J Am Med Assoc.* 1996;276:211–215.
84. Pelliccia A, Maron BJ, Di Paolo FM, et al. Prevalence and clinical significance of left atrial remodeling in competitive athletes. *J Am Coll Cardiol.* 2005;46:690–696.
85. Sheikh N, Papadakis M, Carre F, et al. Cardiac adaptation to exercise in adolescent athletes of African ethnicity: an emergent elite athletic population. *Br J Sports Med.* 2013;47:585–592.
86. Schmied C, Zerguini Y, Junge A, et al. Cardiac findings in the precompetition medical assessment of football players participating in the 2009 African Under-17 Championships in Algeria. *Br J Sports Med.* 2009;43:716–721.
87. Whyte GP, George K, Nevill A, et al. Left ventricular morphology and function in female athletes: a meta-analysis. *Int J Sports Med.* 2004;25:380–383.
88. Whyte GP, George K, Sharma S, et al. The upper limit of physiological cardiac hypertrophy in elite male and female athletes: the British experience. *Eur J Appl Physiol.* 2004;92:592–597.
89. D'Andrea A, Cocchia R, Riegler L, et al. Left ventricular myocardial velocities and deformation indexes in top-level athletes. *J Am Soc Echocardiogr.* 2010;23:1281–1288.
90. Lang RM, Badano LP, Mor-Avi V, et al. Recommendations for cardiac chamber quantification by echocardiography in adults: an update from the American Society of Echocardiography and the European Association of Cardiovascular Imaging. *J Am Soc Echocardiogr.* 2015;28:1–39 e14.
91. Prior DL, La Gerche A. The athlete's heart. *Heart.* 2012;98:947–955.
92. Iskandar A, Mujtaba MT, Thompson PD. Left atrium size in elite athletes. *JACC Cardiovasc Imaging.* 2015.
93. Pela G, Li Calzi M, Crocamo A, et al. Ethnicity-related variations of left ventricular remodeling in adolescent amateur football players. *Scand J Med Sci Sports.* 2015;25:382–389.
94. Prakken NH, Velthuis BK, Bosker AC, et al. Relationship of ventricular and atrial dilatation to valvular function in endurance athletes. *Br J Sports Med.* 2011;45:178–184.
95. Maron BJ, Douglas PS, Graham TP, et al. Task Force 1: preparticipation screening and diagnosis of cardiovascular disease in athletes. *J Am Coll Cardiol.* 2005;45:1322–1326.
96. Corrado D, Pelliccia A, Bjornstad HH, et al. Cardiovascular pre-participation screening of young competitive athletes for prevention of sudden death: proposal for a common European protocol. Consensus statement of the study group of Sport Cardiology of the working group of Cardiac Rehabilitation and Exercise Physiology and the working group of myocardial and pericardial diseases of the European Society of Cardiology. *Eur Heart J.* 2005;26:516–524.
97. Steinvil A, Chundadze T, Zeltser D, et al. Mandatory electrocardiographic screening of athletes to reduce their risk for sudden death proven fact or wishful thinking? *J Am Coll Cardiol.* 2011;57:1291–1296.
98. Ljungqvist A, Jenoure P, Engebretsen L, et al. The International Olympic Committee (IOC) consensus statement on periodic health evaluation of elite athletes March 2009. *Br J Sports Med.* 2009;43:631–643.
99. Maron BJ. Distinguishing hypertrophic cardiomyopathy from athlete's heart: a clinical problem of increasing magnitude and significance. *Heart.* 2005;91:1380–1382.

中文导读

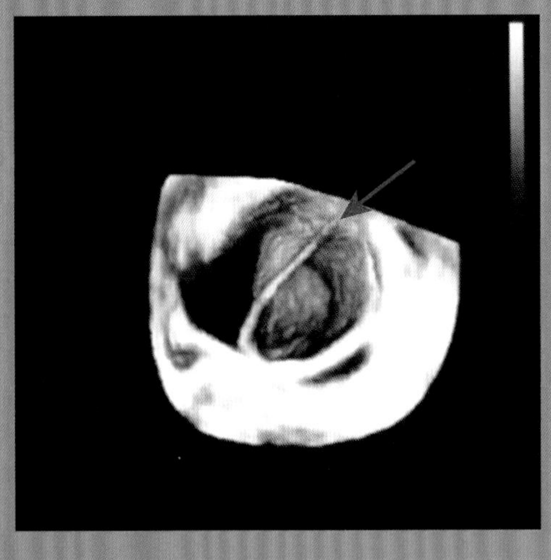

第36章 肺动脉高压

肺动脉高压常见病因分为5大类：①动脉性肺动脉高压；②左心疾病所致肺动脉高压；③肺部疾病和（或）低氧所致肺动脉高压；④慢性血栓栓塞性肺动脉高压；⑤未明确多因素机制所致肺动脉高压。呼吸困难通常是肺动脉高压的首发症状，当患者出现呼吸困难时应进行全面的超声心动图检查，为肺动脉高压的病因诊断及严重程度评估提供临床依据。超声心动图可根据三尖瓣反流及肺动脉瓣反流频谱对肺动脉压力进行估测，包括肺动脉收缩压、舒张压和平均压。不同类型肺动脉高压的超声心动图表现不同，应根据心脏大小和结构、肺动脉压力及其他相关检查等仔细辨认肺动脉高压机制。

同时应对右心室形态、内径、收缩、舒张功能及室间隔运动等进行准确评估，及时发现肺动脉高压患者右心室功能变化进而指导临床干预。必要时，运动负荷超声心动图能够帮助肺动脉高压患者进行更加全面的评估。肺动脉高压患者治疗后应定期应用超声心动图监测肺动脉压力和右心功能。

本章重点介绍了肺动脉高压的定义、临床分类、超声心动图在肺动脉高压诊断中的作用、运动负荷超声心动图对于疑似肺动脉高压患者的诊断流程及对肺动脉高压患者肺动脉压力和右心室反应的监测。

张　冰

36 Pulmonary Hypertension

DAVID PLAYFORD, MBBS, PhD | DAVID S. CELERMAJER, MD

GENERAL PRINCIPLES

Breathlessness is usually the first presenting symptom of pulmonary hypertension (PHT). Because breathlessness has a wide variety of causes, PHT is often not suspected initially by the patient or the physician. However, identification of PHT has important implications for the diagnosis and for morbidity, and mortality.[1,2] The diagnostic workup for breathlessness should include comprehensive echocardiography, which may provide the first objective evidence of PHT.

Comprehensive echocardiography includes rigorous assessment of pulmonary pressures, right and left heart function, and pulmonary vascular resistance (PVR), which requires right heart catheterization (RHC). PHT is diagnosed when elevated pulmonary artery pressures are identified, whereas *pulmonary arterial hypertension* (PAH) refers to PHT in the setting of normal left heart filling pressure and elevated PVR (Fig. 36.1). New diagnostic criteria have defined PHT as a mean pulmonary artery pressure (mPAP) greater than 20 mmHg at RHC[3]; it is identified echocardiographically as a right ventricular systolic pressure (RVSP) greater than approximately 30 mmHg.

PHT is not a diagnosis in itself; it is the observation of higher-than-normal pulmonary artery pressures. Whether the elevation is pathologic for that individual and the reason for PHT should be rigorously investigated. For example, a high cardiac output may result in pulmonary artery pressures above the reference range but not indicate cardiopulmonary pathology.

DEFINING PULMONARY HYPERTENSION

Since 1975, PHT has been defined by consensus view[4] on the basis of invasively measured elevation of an mPAP greater than 25 mmHg.[5] Based on hemodynamic data obtained from normal individuals at rest and in the supine position, the mPAP is 14.0 ± 3.3 mmHg,[6] with a slight increase for individuals older than 50 years of age. The upper limit of normal based on 2 standard deviations above the mean in a normally distributed sample is 20.6 mmHg. Based on this and other data from normal individuals, the updated clinical definition of PHT is an mPAP greater than 20 mmHg,[3] independent of age and gender. The mortality hazard ratio increases progressively above this upper limit of normal.[7]

The normal peak pulmonary artery systolic pressure (PASP) measured during RHC is 20.8 ± 4.4 mmHg, with an upper limit of normal of 29.8 mmHg.[6] Data from a very large, real-world echocardiographic database linked with mortality values showed a clear threshold for PASP of 30 mmHg,[8] above which mortality rates progressively and relentlessly increase. This threshold corresponds well with the new definition of abnormal hemodynamic findings at rest and in the supine position, and it assumes a normal right atrial (RA) pressure of 5 mmHg. From this large data set, there was no significant increase in estimated PASP with age, gender, or body mass index, and values were consistent with the hemodynamic definition previously described.

Table 36.1 summarizes clinical echocardiographic studies that examined the normal range of PASP. Different RA pressures have been reported in various studies (Table 36.2). To allow for meaningful comparisons, a fixed RA pressure of 5 mmHg has been provided in parentheses for each study. Evidence for treatment of PHT at a threshold of more than 20 mmHg is lacking because clinical trials on treatment of PAH typically have recruited based on an mPAP (measured at RHC) of greater than 25 mmHg.

DIFFERENTIATING PULMONARY HYPERTENSION FROM PULMONARY ARTERIAL HYPERTENSION

PHT is simply the identification of elevated pulmonary artery pressures; the term PAH is reserved for PHT in the setting of normal left heart filling pressure, defined as mean pulmonary

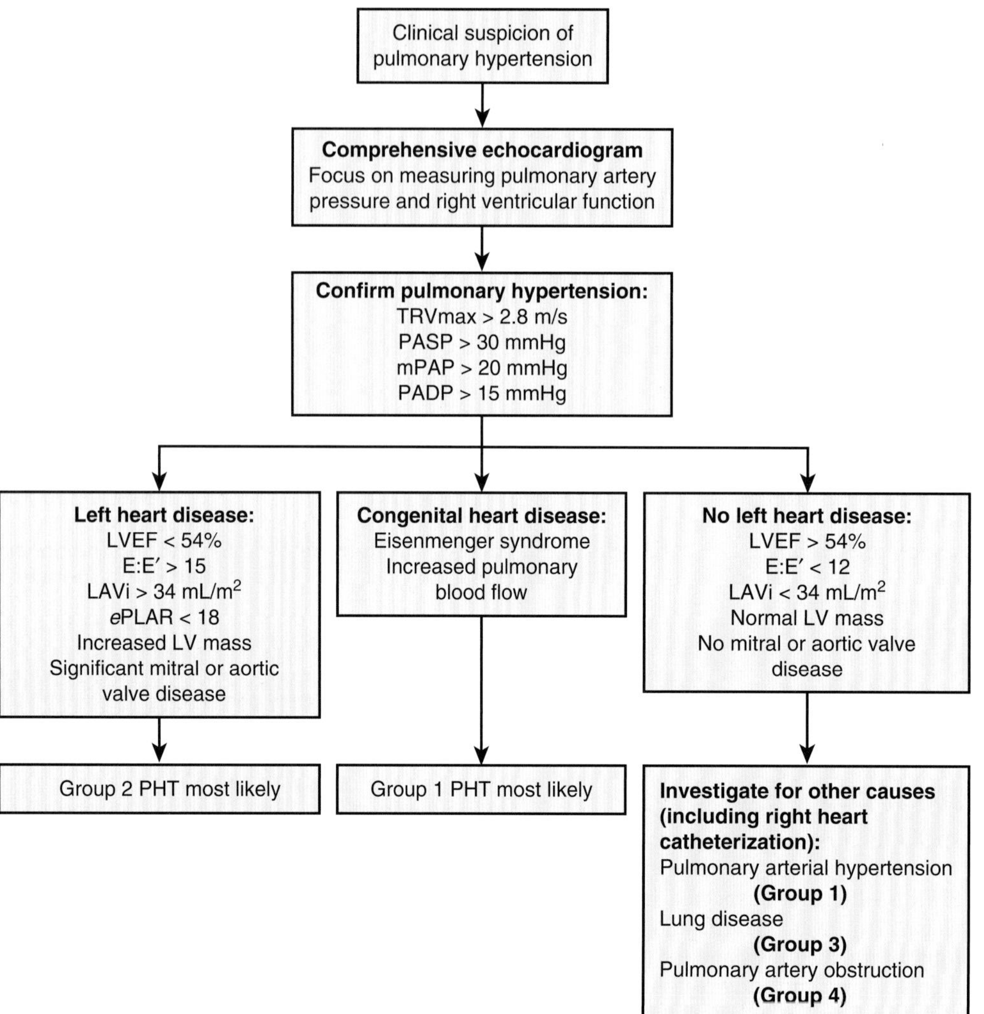

Fig. 36.1 A diagnostic approach to a patient with clinically suspected pulmonary hypertension. Pulmonary hypertension *(PHT)* is diagnosed when elevated pulmonary artery pressures are identified. The World Health Organization (WHO) has classified PHT into groups based on the underlying cause. *E:E′*, ratio of peak mitral inflow E velocity to the medial mitral annular tissue velocity; *ePLAR*, echocardiographic pulmonary-to-LA ratio; *LAVi*, left atrial volume index (maximal LA volume/body surface area); *LVEF*, left ventricular ejection fraction; *mPAP*, mean pulmonary artery pressure; *PADP*, pulmonary artery diastolic pressure; *PASP*, pulmonary artery systolic pressure; *TRVmax*, peak tricuspid regurgitation velocity.

TABLE 36.1 Large Studies Describing Normal Echocardiographic Values for Pulmonary Artery Systolic Pressure.[a]

Parameter	*McQuillan et al.[25] (N = 3790)*	*Lam et al.[85] (N = 778)*	*Grossman et al.[86] (N = 6598)*	*Strange et al.[8] (N = 90,950)*
Estimated RA pressure[b]	10 (5) mmHg	5 mmHg	5 mmHg	5 mmHg
Analyzable TR jet	69%	69%	29%	50.3%
PASP ± SD	28 ± 5 mmHg (23 ± 5 mmHg)[b]	27 ± 4 mmHg	31 ± 4 mmHg	25 ± 4 mmHg
Age[c]				
20–40 y	≤37 (32) mmHg	—	<34 mmHg	24 ± 4 mmHg
40–60 y	≤40 (35) mmHg	26 ± 4 mmHg	—	25 ± 4 mmHg
>60 y	≤43 (38) mmHg	28 ± 5 mmHg	—	26 ± 4 mmHg
BMI[d]				
<20 kg/m²	≤36 (31) mmHg	No change	No change	25 ± 4 mmHg
20–30 kg/m²	≤37 (32) mmHg	No change	No change	26 ± 3 mmHg
>30 kg/m²	≤40 (35) mmHg	No change	Excluded	26 ± 3 mmHg

[a]The data of Strange et al. (2019)[8] are from a nationwide study in Australia; additional analysis of the data set included age and BMI ranges. The population studied by McQuillan et al.[25] was from a tertiary referral center in Boston. The data of Lam et al.[85] were from a population sample in Olmstead County, MN. Data of Grossman et al.[86] were from young male Army recruits in Israel.
[b]The estimated RA pressure has been modified to 5 mmHg where marked in parentheses to allow for comparisons.
[c]Age range for normal PASP has been modified from the original publication to allow comparisons between studies. Smaller studies (<100 subjects) have not been included in this table.
[d]No change was reported among BMI ranges, although subjects with BMI greater than 30 kg/m² weere excluded from the Grossman study.
BMI, Body mass index; *PASP*, pulmonary artery systolic pressure; *SD*, standard deviation; *TR*, tricuspid regurgitation.

artery wedge pressure (mPAWP) of less than 15 mmHg and a PVR greater than 3 Wood units (WU), as calculated by the following formula:

$$PVR = \frac{mPAP - mPAWP}{CO}$$

where CO is the cardiac output (L/min).

Because the definition is based on hemodynamic assessment using RHC, all patients with clinically and echocardiographically suspected PHT should be considered for RHC confirmation. However, RHC is an invasive test, has some inherent risks, and is not universally available. Those patients most likely to have a pulmonary vascular cause for PHT are ideally suited to confirmation by RHC.

Echocardiography helps differentiate precapillary PHT, in which there is no left heart disease but PVR is increased, from postcapillary PHT, in which left heart disease is the dominant cause for the increased pulmonary artery pressures. Fig. 36.2 shows four broad possibilities when considering PHT from an echocardiographic perspective.

Several simple echocardiographic markers have been used to help differentiate precapillary from postcapillary PHT. Differentiation is important because identification of PAH early in the disease process can influence treatment choices. Echocardiography can help those in need of more invasive investigation and assist in the more appropriate use of health resources.

TABLE 36.2 ASE Recommendations for RA Pressure Estimation.

RAP Grading	*Estimated RAP*	*Echocardiographic Findings*
Normal	3 mmHg	IVC < 2.1 cm and IVC collapse >50% on sniff
Indeterminate	8 mmHg	If IVC findings indeterminate: Tricuspid E:E′ > 6 Hepatic vein D > S velocity
Increased	15 mmHg	IVC ≥ 2.1 cm and IVC collapse <50% on sniff

ASE, American Society of Echocardiography; *D*, diastolic; *E:E′*, ratio of peak mitral inflow E velocity to the medial mitral annular tissue velocity; *IVC*, inferior vena cava; *RAP*, RA pressure; *sniff*, inspiration; *S*, systolic.

From Rudski LG, Lai WW, Afilalo J, et al. Guidelines for the echocardiographic assessment of the right heart in adults: a report from the American Society of Echocardiography endorsed by the European Association of Echocardiography. *J Am Soc Echocardiogr*. 2010;23:685–713.

CLINICAL CLASSIFICATION OF PULMONARY HYPERTENSION

The World Health Organization (WHO) classified PHT into five groups according to the underlying cause. The most recent modification was made in 2019 by the Sixth World Symposium on Pulmonary Hypertension.[3] Group 1 represents PAH, in which the primary abnormality is increased PVR. Group 2 is PHT caused by left heart disease. Group 3 is PHT caused by lung disease and/or hypoxia. Group 4 is PHT caused by pulmonary artery obstruction (predominantly chronic thromboembolic pulmonary hypertension [CTEPH]). Group 5 is PHT caused by unclear or multifactorial mechanisms (Table 36.3).

Group 2 (left heart disease) is the largest, representing approximately 70% of all causes of PHT.[2] Table 36.4 presents clinical-echocardiographic correlates for each cause of PHT.

ECHOCARDIOGRAPHY IN THE DIAGNOSTIC WORKUP OF PULMONARY HYPERTENSION

ESTIMATING PULMONARY ARTERY PRESSURES

Determining the PASP depends on knowing (or estimating) the RA pressure, the RV-RA peak pressure gradient, and any RV outflow tract (RVOT) obstruction (in which case the RVSP will be higher than the PASP). Techniques and limitations for

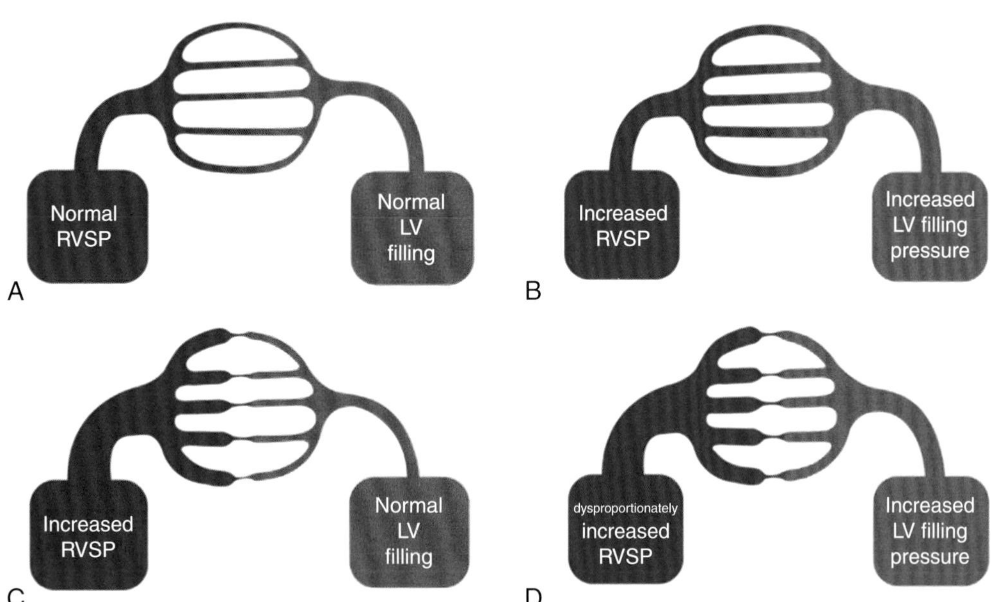

Fig. 36.2 Pulmonary hypertension due to left heart disease. (A) In the absence of congenital heart disease, normal LV filling pressures and normal pulmonary vascular resistance (PVR) are associated with normal pulmonary artery pressures. (B) Increased LV filling pressure or mitral stenosis causes proportional increases in LA and pulmonary venous pressures along with parallel increases in pulmonary capillary and pulmonary artery pressures. There is no significant rise in PVR. This is typical of group 2 pulmonary hypertension. (C) In the setting of pulmonary arterial hypertension (typically group 1 pulmonary hypertension), there is increased PVR and normal LV filling pressures. (D) Some individuals with group 2 pulmonary hypertension and elevated LV filling pressure also develop increased PVR. This results in a disproportionate rise in the pulmonary artery pressure, beyond that explained by the increased pulmonary venous pressure alone. *RVSP*, Right ventricular systolic pressure.

assessing the RA pressure and the RV-RA peak pressure gradient are discussed next.

Estimating the RV-RA Pressure Difference From the Tricuspid Regurgitation Profile

The most important echocardiographic finding in PHT is an elevation in the RVSP, based on the peak velocity of the tricuspid regurgitation (TR) profile (Fig. 36.3), according to the following equation[9,10]:

$$RVSP = \left(4 \times TRVmax^2\right) + RAP$$

where the RVSP is taken to be the PASP in the absence of RVOT obstruction or pulmonary valve stenosis, TRVmax is the peak TR velocity (m/s), and RAP is the estimated (or known) RA pressure.

Doppler interrogation of the TR jet should be undertaken from multiple views[11] to obtain the most direct alignment, and the position of the continuous-wave (CW) cursor should be placed to obtain the highest velocity. This usually requires the TR waveform to be acquired from parasternal RV inflow, basal short-axis, apical long-axis, and subcostal views. Because of the eccentric nature of the TR profile in some patients, off-axis two-dimensional (2D) views may be required to optimize alignment.

Care should be taken to measure only the well-defined spectral trace, avoiding measurement of an incomplete TR profile (Fig. 36.4). Avoidance of noise ("beard") around the spectral signal ("chin"), sometimes referred to as the *chin and beard approach*, is important to correctly measure the TRV,[12] particularly if contrast is used to enhance the TR signal.

The mPAP can be estimated from the TRV using the formula derived by Chemla et al.[13]:

$$mPAP = (0.61 \times RVSP) + 2$$

Alternatively, the mPAP can be estimated from the velocity–time integral of the TR trace[14–16] (see Fig. 36.3E). These estimations can be cross-checked with the mPAP estimated using the initial pulmonary regurgitation (PR) velocity.

Up to one third of patients attending the echocardiography laboratory have insufficient TR to accurately estimate the RVSP. Various techniques have been used to improve an incomplete TR profile. Agitated saline contrast and intravenous microbubble contrast agents can be used to intensify the TR signal.[17]

In the setting of RV dysfunction from PHT, incomplete tricuspid leaflet closure may occur, initially due to dysfunction and then to displacement of the subvalvular apparatus. The effect of this is an increase in TR severity (Fig. 36.5). Most patients with significant RV dysfunction have some measurable TRV.

In the setting of severe TR, there may be pressure equalization between the RV and RA during systole. This may result in blunting of the TRV profile and potential underestimation of the RVSP. Fig. 36.5D demonstrates this phenomenon.

TABLE 36.3 Classification of Pulmonary Hypertension.[a]

Pulmonary Hypertension Group	*Examples*	*Precapillary vs. Postcapillary[b]*
Group 1: PAH	Idiopathic PAH Heritable PAH Drug or toxin induced PAH associated with other diseases: Scleroderma HIV infection Portal hypertension Congenital heart disease	Precapillary
Group 2: PHT due to left heart disease	Myocardial disorders: Systolic dysfunction Diastolic dysfunction Congenital cardiomyopathy Inflow/outflow disorders: Valvular heart disease Congenital LV inflow or outflow obstruction	Postcapillary
Group 3: PHT due to lung disease	Obstructive lung disease Restrictive lung disease Chronic hypoxia	Precapillary
Group 4: pulmonary artery obstruction	Multiple chronic pulmonary emboli Pulmonary artery obstruction: Malignant tumors Parasites	Precapillary
Group 5: PHT with multifactorial causes	Hematologic disorders: Systemic and metabolic disorders Complex congenital heart disease	Precapillary and/or postcapillary

[a]This table was condensed to include the diseases most relevant to echocardiographers.
[b]Precapillary indicates PHT predominantly from increased vascular resistance; postcapillary indicates PHT predominantly from increased left heart filling pressures.
HIV, Human immunodeficiency virus; *PAH*, pulmonary arterial hypertension; *PHT*, pulmonary hypertension.
Adapted from Simonneau G, Montani D, Celermajer DS, et al. Haemodynamic definitions and updated clinical classification of pulmonary hypertension. *Eur Respir J.* 2019;53(1):180–191.

TABLE 36.4 Clinical-Echocardiographic Correlates for Causes of Pulmonary Hypertension.

Pulmonary Hypertension Group[a]	*Clinical Findings*	*Echocardiographic Findings*
Group 1: PAH	Unexplained breathlessness Absence of signs of systemic disease	Normal (or undervolumed) left heart; dilated RV with signs of pressure overload
Group 2: PHT due to left heart disease	Prior cardiac history (e.g., known coronary, valvular, or myocardial disease or arrhythmia) Clinical signs of left heart failure (e.g., cardiac dilation, atrial fibrillation, lung crepitations on auscultation, pleural effusions)	Abnormal LV systolic and/or diastolic function; mitral or aortic valve disease; LA dilation
Group 3: PHT due to lung disease	Clinical features of obstructive or restrictive lung disease History of asthma, smoking, or occupational exposure; chronic obstructive pulmonary disease	Echocardiographic features similar to group 1
Group 4: pulmonary artery obstruction	History of pulmonary embolus, risk factors for pulmonary embolus, or malignancy	Echocardiographic features similar to group 1
Group 5: PHT with multifactorial causes	History and signs of systemic disease	PHT without features most consistent with groups 1–4

[a]There may be multiple causes of hypertension for an individual patient, and some findings are not specific for the pulmonary hypertension group indicated.
PAH, Pulmonary arterial hypertension; *PHT*, pulmonary hypertension.

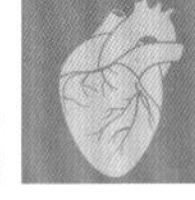

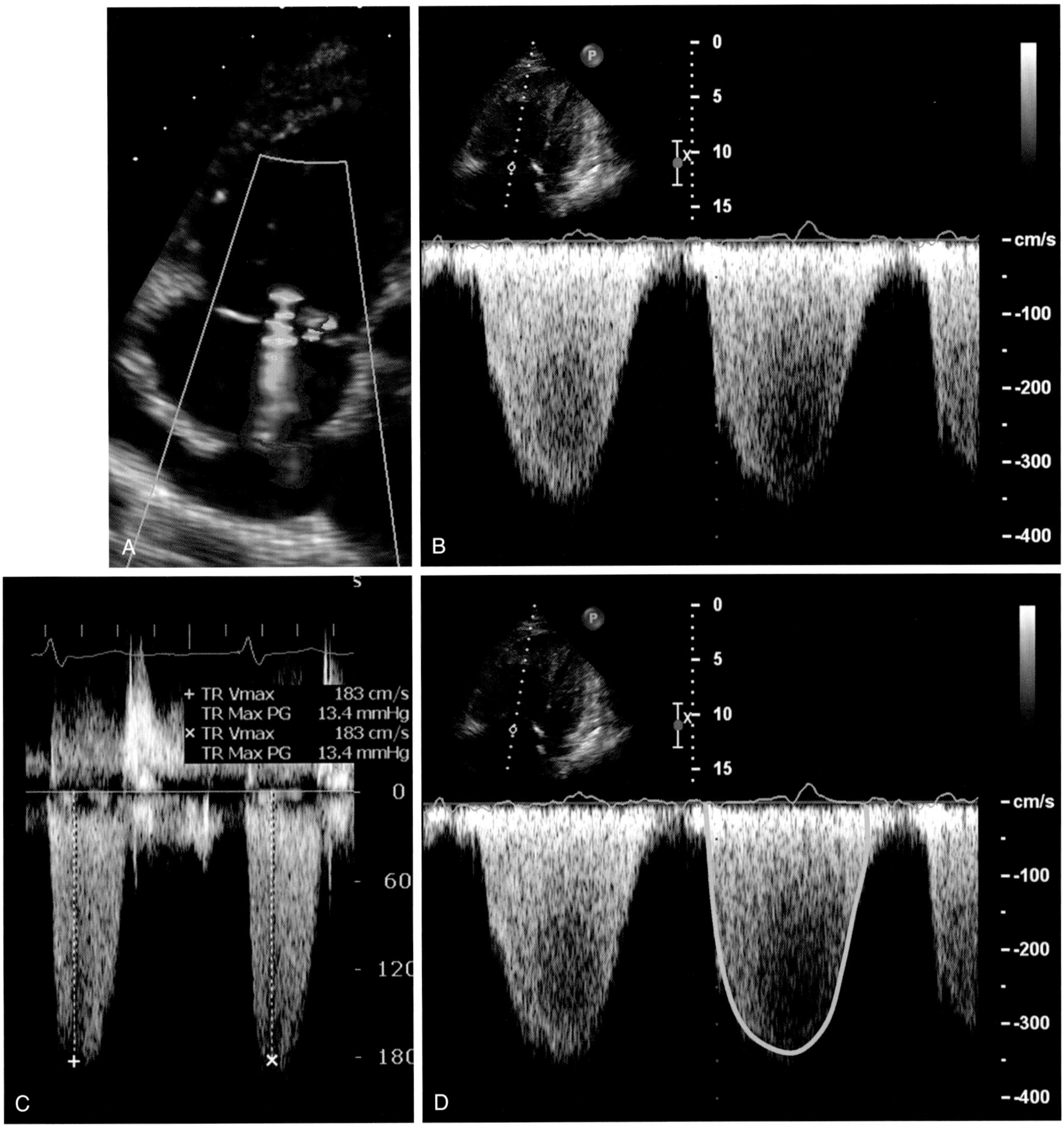

Fig. 36.3 Measurement of increased RV systolic pressure. (A) From an RV-focused apical 4-chamber view, the tricuspid regurgitation *(TR)* jet is identified using color Doppler. Care is taken to ensure that the TR jet direction is parallel to the ultrasound beam. (B) CW Doppler is applied over the vena contracta of the TR jet, and gain, range, and sweep speed are optimized. (C) The maximum velocity is then measured, which may be cross-checked using the nonimaging transducer. (D) The mean TR velocity can be estimated by tracing the Doppler envelope and applying the velocity–time integral.

PHT identified by the TRV requires confirmation by other measures, particularly if the TR profile is incomplete. Other measures, such as PR profile and pulmonary acceleration time, should be used along with surrogate markers of increased RV pressures. The final arbiter of increased pulmonary artery pressures is RHC.[18]

Estimating RA Pressure

An assumed RA pressure is routinely added to the RV-RA pressure difference to estimate the RVSP. Several techniques have been proposed for noninvasive estimation of RA pressure. Some laboratories have chosen a constant RA pressure (e.g., 10 mmHg) to avoid variation in the RA pressure estimation, but the problem with this approach is overestimation of RVSP in patients with normal RA pressure. For ease of comparison, Table 36.1 has modified the RA pressure to 5 mmHg in all studies. The American Society of Echocardiography (ASE) recommendation[19] for RA pressure estimation is based on inferior vena cava (IVC) diameter and degree of inspiratory collapse (Fig. 36.6; see Table 36.2). Clinical estimation of the jugular venous pressure

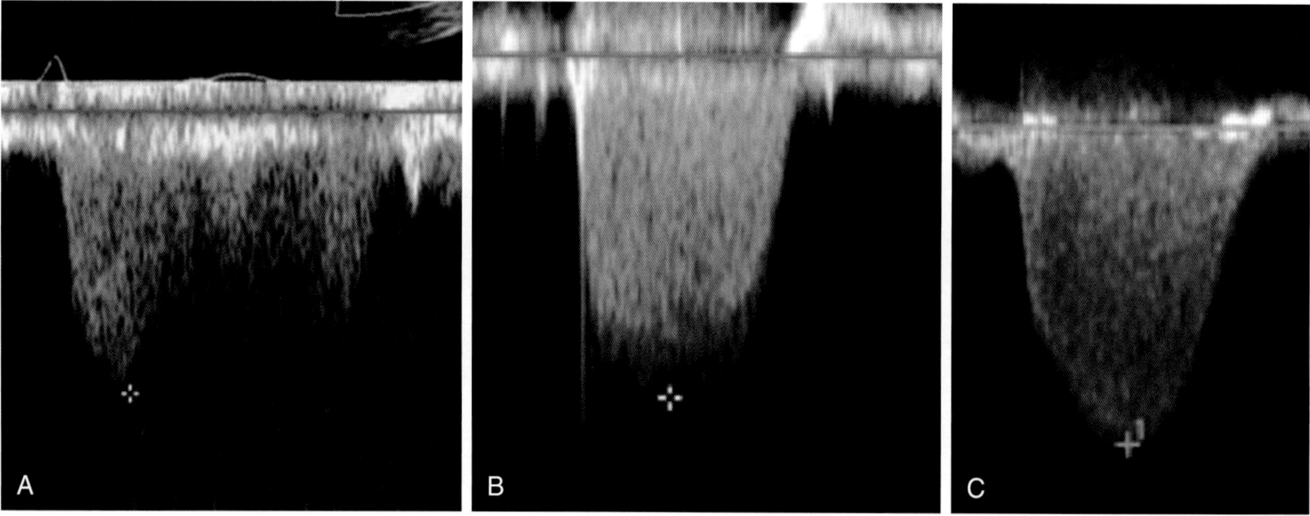

Fig. 36.4 Chin and beard estimation of peak tricuspid regurgitation velocity. The chin measurement (i.e., distinct TRVmax signal) rather than the beard measurement (i.e., higher, indistinct TRVmax signal) is used to correctly assess peak velocity from the tricuspid regurgitation (TR) spectral display. (A) Incomplete TR profile. TRV should not be estimated from this tracing because of inadequate visualization of the peak velocity. (B) Measurement of TRV at the beard does not accurately reflect the true pulmonary artery systolic pressure. (C) Measurement at the chin of the TR profile most accurately reflects the pulmonary artery pressure. *TRVmax*, Maximum tricuspid regurgitation velocity.

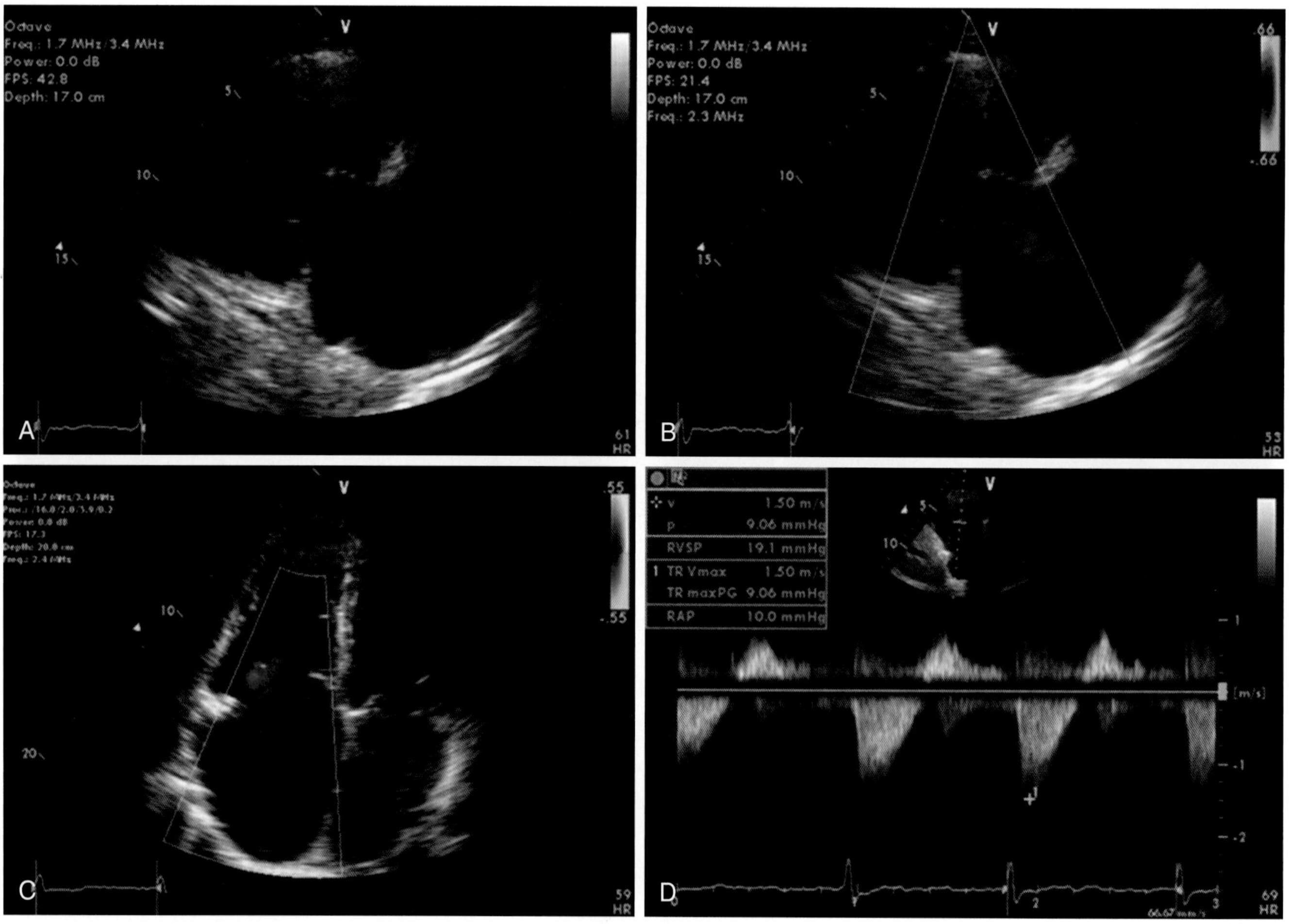

Fig. 36.5 Severe tricuspid regurgitation and incomplete tricuspid leaflet closure. The 2D RV inflow view (A), color Doppler RV inflow view (B), and color Doppler RV-focused 4-chamber view (C) demonstrate incomplete tricuspid leaflet closure. Displacement of the subvalvular apparatus resulted from RV dilation and tricuspid annular dilation, and there is significant tricuspid regurgitation (TR) (see Videos 36.5A, 36.5B, and 36.5C). (D) In severe TR, there may be equalization of RV and RA pressure in systole, which creates an early-peaking, knife-shaped velocity profile. This abrupt end to the systolic upstroke of the velocity profile limits applicability of the Bernoulli principle.

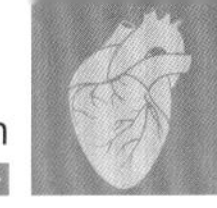

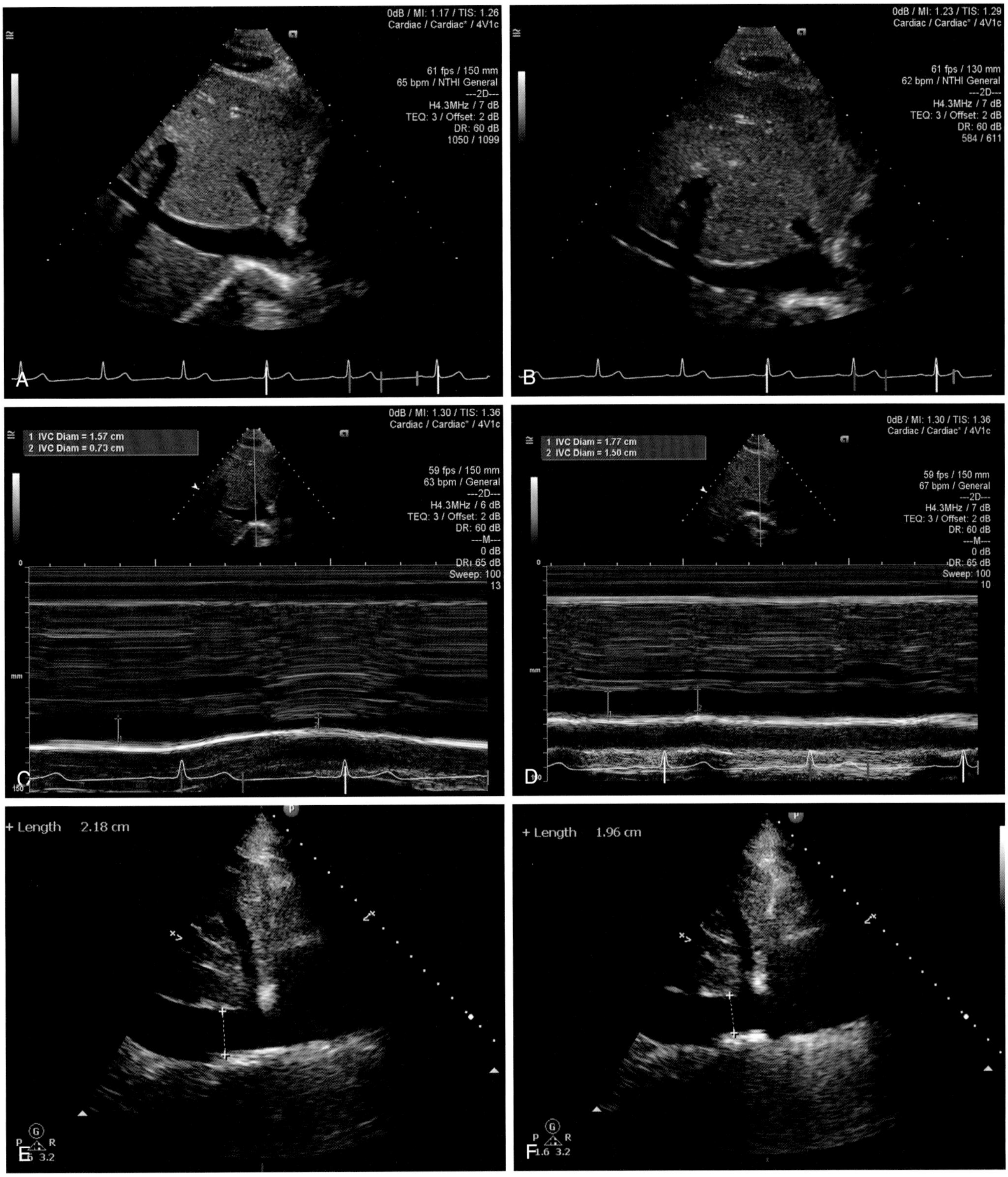

Fig. 36.6 RA pressure estimation. (A–C) When RA pressures are normal, there is a decrease in RA pressure with inspiration (i.e., sniff), causing more than 50% collapse of the inferior vena cava *(IVC)*. (D–F) With increased RA pressures, the IVC no longer collapses with inspiration and eventually dilates. (G) Lack of inspiratory collapse of the IVC during respiration. The IVC should be measured perpendicular to its long axis, inner edge to inner edge, and 1 to 2 cm proximal to the entrance of the IVC into the RA (see Video 36.6).

can help corroborate the echocardiographically estimated RA pressure.

RA dilation usually indicates exposure to chronic elevations in RA pressure due to tricuspid valve disease or increased RV filling pressure. RA dilation occurs when the RA area exceeds 18 cm^2 or the RA volume exceeds 28 mL/m^2. Chronic elevation of RA pressure (>8 mmHg) and corresponding RA dilation indicate increased risk of clinical events.[20]

Pulmonary Regurgitation Profile

Significant PR occurs in approximately 30% of patients with PHT.[21] The pulmonary artery diastolic pressure (PADP) can

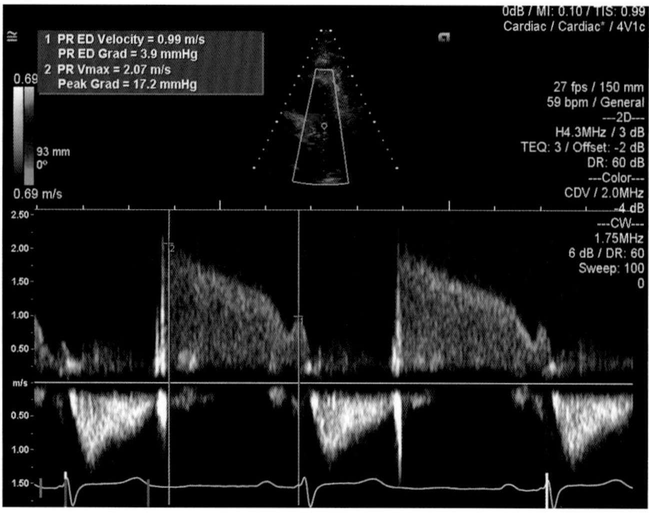

Fig. 36.7 Pulmonary artery pressure measurement made from the pulmonary regurgitation profile. The velocity at end-diastole is used to calculate the pulmonary artery (PA) diastolic pressure, and the early diastolic velocity is used to calculate the mean PA pressure (see Video 36.7).

be estimated from the PR profile using the modified Bernoulli equation and RAP estimation used in TRV measurements (Fig. 36.7).

$$\text{PADP} = 4 \times (\text{PR}_{\text{end}})^2 + \text{RAP}$$

and

$$\text{mPAP} = 4 \times (\text{PR}_{\text{in}})^2 + \text{RAP}$$

where PR_{end} is the end PR velocity and PR_{in} is the initial PR velocity.

Pulmonary Acceleration Time

In PHT, early pulmonary ejection may be enhanced, resulting in a short pulmonary acceleration time. A pulmonary acceleration time of less than 90 ms predicts a PVR greater than 3 WU[22] and PHT (Fig. 36.8).

Mid-Systolic Notching of the RV Outflow Doppler Signal

During pulsed-wave (PW) or CW Doppler assessment of the RVOT, a mid-systolic notch may be identified (see Fig. 36.8). The notch is presumed to be caused by a pressure wave reflection against the increased PVR that temporarily decreases the forward velocity.[23] A notch reliably indicates increased PVR. The presence of an RVOT notch has been used to improve the sensitivity of abnormal noninvasive PVR calculations[24] (see Estimating Pulmonary Vascular Resistance at Rest).

Factors Affecting Pulmonary Artery Pressure in Normal Individuals

There may be a small rise in pulmonary artery pressures with age,[25] although this has not been consistently demonstrated.[8] Similarly, the effect of body mass index on pulmonary artery pressures appears to be small. The PASP is approximately 1 mmHg higher in males than in females after adjusting for other variables. Systemic blood pressure and pulse pressure, along with echocardiography-derived left ventricular (LV) filling pressures, are also associated with higher PAP in otherwise normal individuals, and this association is also linked with increasing age.[1]

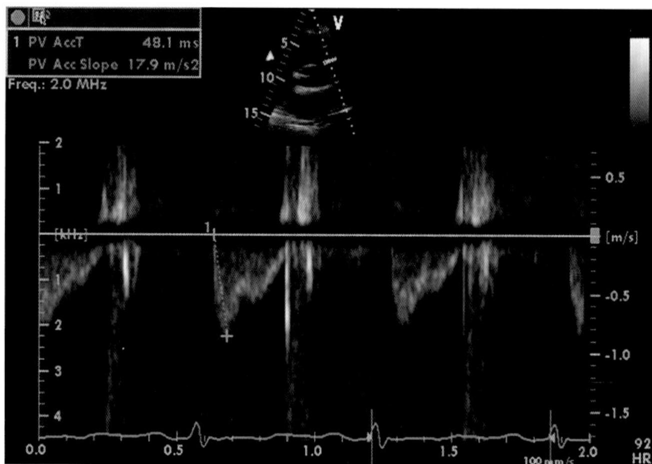

Fig. 36.8 Pulmonary acceleration time in pulmonary hypertension. Initial forward flow of blood may be increased, resulting in rapid acceleration of blood through the pulmonary valve, as measured by the pulmonary acceleration time (PAT). A PAT of less than 90 ms suggests increased pulmonary vascular resistance and pulmonary hypertension.

IDENTIFYING THE CAUSE OF PULMONARY HYPERTENSION USING ECHOCARDIOGRAPHY

Pulmonary Arterial Hypertension

PHT can be caused by specific abnormalities in the pulmonary vasculature; these are grouped under the term PAH and are represented as group 1 of the WHO classification. Idiopathic pulmonary arterial hypertension (iPAH), PAH due to connective tissue diseases, and PAH due to congenital heart disease are examples of group 1 PAH. Because PAH has been identified in approximately 10% of patients with scleroderma and in some patients with mixed connective tissue disease, regular echocardiographic screening has been recommended for these patients.[26] For other connective tissue diseases in which PHT is less prevalent, symptomatic patients (i.e., those with breathlessness) should undergo echocardiography.[27]

Patients with PAH have increased PVR with normal pulmonary venous pressures (i.e., normal LV filling pressures) (see Fig. 36.2C). This results in pulmonary arterial dilation and chronic right heart pressure loading in the setting of a normal left heart. Chronic RV pressure overload results in ventricular septal deviation toward the left (i.e., D-shaped LV in a short-axis view) and mild LV diastolic dysfunction. Some data have raised the possibility of LV myocyte dysfunction in patients with PAH.[28]

Treatment of group 1 PHT with pulmonary vasodilator drugs such as prostacyclin, endothelin receptor antagonists (ERAs), and phosphodiesterase type 5 (PDE-5) inhibitors decreases the rate of progression, decreases clinically relevant complications, and improve symptoms associated with PAH. The greatest benefits occurring when treatment is given early in the disease course.[29–33] Prescription of disease-specific therapy relies on early identification of the underlying cause of PHT.

Pulmonary Hypertension Due to Congenital Heart Disease

During the past 30 to 40 years, considerable advances in pediatric cardiology and cardiac surgery have resulted in an increasing number of adult survivors with congenital heart disease, many of whom survive with pressure and/or volume loads on their ventricles. A significant proportion of adult patients with congenital heart disease have coexisting PAH, which is associated

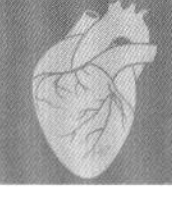

with worse functional status and a poorer prognosis for each type of congenital heart disease.[34] In some countries where this has been documented, adults with congenital heart disease can comprise up to one third of patients attending specialty PHT clinics.[35]

The overall prevalence of PAH complicating congenital heart disease in adults is approximately 5%.[35,36] However, it has been higher in certain series in which patients were drawn mainly from tertiary referral centers, where the prevalence of PAH in an adult congenital heart disease population is approximately 25%.[34]

PAH complicating congenital heart disease has been broadly classified in four categories[5]:

1. Eisenmenger syndrome, in which large congenital heart defects are complicated by a substantial rise in PVR and eventual reversal of the shunt flow through the defect so that blood is flowing right to left, with consequent arterial hypoxemia and secondary erythrocytosis
2. PAH due to left-to-right shunts with high PVR but without Eisenmenger syndrome
3. PAH associated with small defects with a natural history that more closely resembles that of idiopathic PAH
4. PAH that persists after corrective surgery (e.g., late correction of ventricular septal defect, overshunting from aortopulmonary shunts created surgically)

Some rare left heart obstructive lesions (e.g., severe supramitral stenosis) may be congenital and can be associated with severe PHT. They are analogous to type 2 PHT.

The risk of PAH in congenital heart disease is clearly related to the underlying lesion, although certain genetic factors are thought to play a role. For example, if truncus arteriosus is left uncorrected, severe pulmonary vascular disease usually occurs during the first year of life. With a large ventricular septal defect, severe pulmonary vascular disease usually occurs before age 2 years, and it is more likely if there is coexisting transposition of the great arteries. In contrast, the lifetime risk of severe PAH in patients with atrial septal defects is approximately 10% (higher for sinus venosus defects than for secundum-type defects), suggesting a pathogenetic role for factors other than the hemodynamic consequence of the congenital heart lesion in the development of PAH.

In terms of diagnostic categories, certain patients with complex, palliated congenital heart disease can have segmental PAH. For example, PAH might be present in only one lung, with the other lung oligemic and at low pressure. Preliminary reports have suggested that these patients may respond to specific pulmonary vasodilator therapy with initially gratifying results.[37]

Echocardiography plays a vital role in the assessment of PAH associated with congenital heart disease. The contribution of echocardiography is as follows.

1. The anatomy of defects can be carefully outlined, including the size, precise location, and relation of intracardiac and vascular structures to the congenital heart defect. Transesophageal echocardiography is often informative, particularly for atrial septal defects.
2. The physiologic consequences of the defect can be inferred from the direction and flow velocity of blood across a defect with the use of the Bernoulli equation to estimate right heart pressures (e.g., in the case of a ventricular septal defect with left-to-right shunting).
3. Traditional measurements of right heart pressure can be made in patients with congenital heart diseases, albeit with some special features (e.g., ventricular septal defects and TR jets can be closely positioned in certain circumstances). Measurement of TR and/or PR velocities can provide information about systolic and diastolic pressures in the RV.
4. The consequences for the right heart of pressure and volume loads from congenital heart disease and pulmonary vascular disease can be inferred by studying RV size and contractility, TR, and RA size and pressure.

TABLE 36.5 Left Heart Abnormalities Found in Group 2 Pulmonary Hypertension.

Parameter	*PHT From Left Heart Disease*	*PHT From Other Causes[a]*
Estimated PASP[b]	>30 mmHg	>30 mmHg
RVOT notching	Rare	Common
LV ejection fraction	<50%	>50%
LV GLS[c]	<−18%	>−18%
E:E′ ratio	>15	<12
LV mass index	>90 g/m² (females) >104 g/m² (males)	<89 g/m² (females) <103 g/m² (males)
LA volume index	>34 mL/m²	≤34 mL/m²
RA vs. LA size	LA > RA	RA > LA
Atrial septum	Bows toward the right	Bows toward the left
Left-sided valvular disease:		
Mitral regurgitation	Moderate or greater	Mild or less
Mitral stenosis	Any severity	Mild or less
Aortic regurgitation	Moderate or greater	Mild or less
Aortic stenosis	Moderate or greater	Mild or less

[a]Multiple causes may exist for an individual patient, and significant crossover may exist.
[b]Assuming an RA pressure of 5 mmHg.
[c]The greater than (>) symbol refers to a more positive number, closer to zero.
E:E′, Ratio of peak mitral inflow E velocity to the medial mitral annular tissue velocity; *GLS*, global longitudinal strain; *PASP*, pulmonary artery systolic pressure; *RVOT*, right ventricular outlet tract.

Pulmonary Hypertension Due to Left Heart Disease

Left heart disease (i.e., group 2 PHT) accounts for approximately 70% of all cases of PHT[2] (Table 36.5), and approximately 70% of patients with heart failure with a preserved ejection fraction (HFpEF) eventually develop PHT. The hallmark of PHT due to left heart disease is increased LV filling pressures (see Fig. 36.2B), and this is the focus of echocardiography in identifying group 2 PHT.

Abnormal LV myocardial relaxation is the most common of left heart causes, and it may be accompanied by systolic dysfunction. During diastolic LV filling, there is pressure equalization between the left atrium (LA) and the LV (assuming there is no mitral stenosis) along with equalization of LA and pulmonary venous pressures. If LV filling pressures increase, pulmonary venous pressures rise in parallel. Pulmonary veins contain no valves or other protective mechanisms against increased pulmonary venous pressures. Any increase in LV filling pressure translates directly into increased pulmonary capillary pressure and causes PHT. In this scenario, the PVR is normal (<3 WU) and the PAWP is increased (>15 mmHg).

In some individuals, the severity of the PHT is greater than would be expected from the left heart disease alone (i.e., combined precapillary and postcapillary PHT).[38] In this situation, there is increased PVR in addition to the passive component described previously, and it may be partially reversible (see Fig. 36.2D).

Some characteristics of PHT caused by left heart disease help in the initial echocardiographic assessment. They are summarized in Table 36.5. Although they are not always present, signs of increased LV filling pressure, an enlarged LA, impaired global longitudinal strain, and increased LV mass may be useful markers. Left-sided valvular disease can also increase LA pressures and amplify existing LV abnormalities, thereby increasing

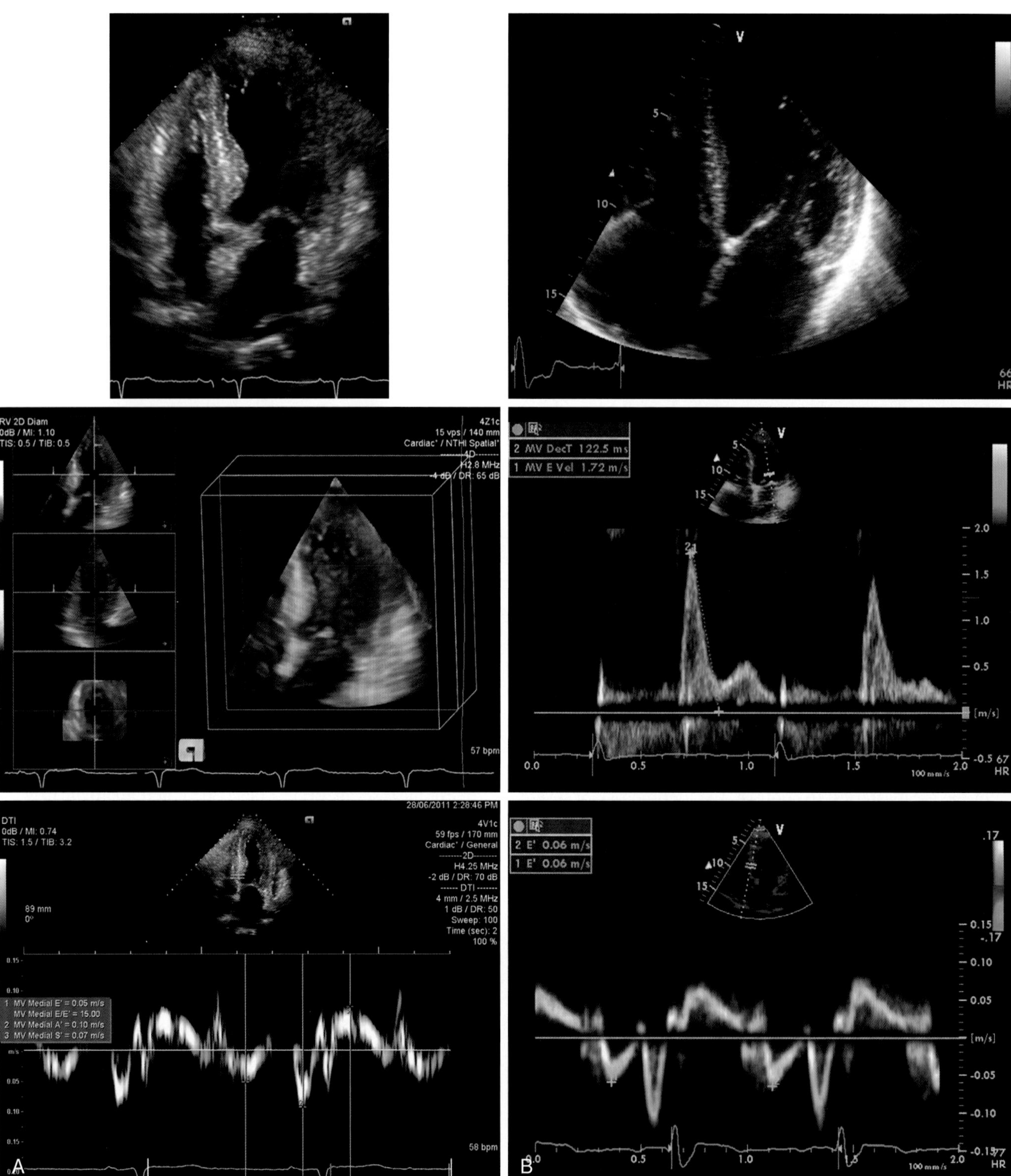

Fig. 36.9 Examples of pulmonary hypertension due to left heart disease. (A) Infiltration with amyloid protein results in severely increased LV mass, impaired myocardial relaxation, and increased LA volume (see Videos 36.9A1 and 36.9A2). (B) Severely impaired LV systolic function results in impaired myocardial relaxation and increased LA volume (see Video 36.9B).

pulmonary pressures. Because of its prognostic importance, RV dysfunction is an important marker of increased risk in left heart disease and should prompt further investigation, including RHC.[38] Examples of PHT due to left heart disease are provided in Fig. 36.9.

Treatment of group 2 PHT usually requires diuretics to decrease preload and effectively decrease the pressures across the pulmonary circuit. Treatment of the underlying left heart pathology may also improve pulmonary artery pressures. Trials of pulmonary vasodilator therapies such as endothelin receptor antagonists have been disappointing,[39–41] although phosphodiesterase inhibition with sildenafil may be beneficial in some of these patients,[42] particularly if there is a component caused by increased PVR (see Fig. 36.2D). However, a 2018 meta-analysis

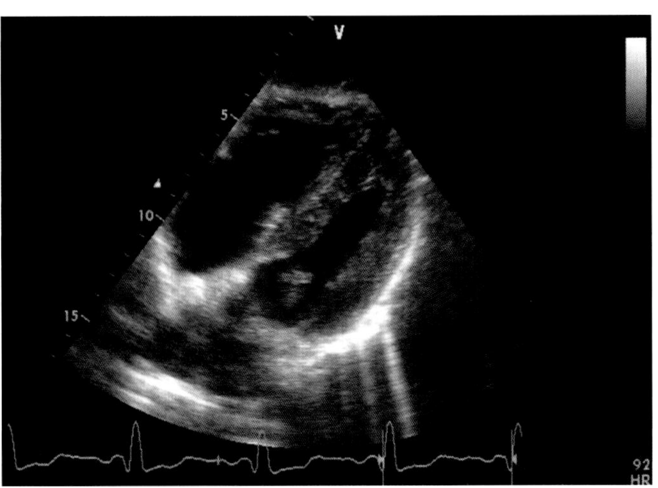

Fig. 36.10 Respirophasic variation in right heart filling caused by severe lung disease. During inspiration, there is increased blood flow to the right heart caused by negative intrathoracic pressure. This leads to dilation of the right heart and a transient shift of the ventricular septum to the left (see Video 36.10).

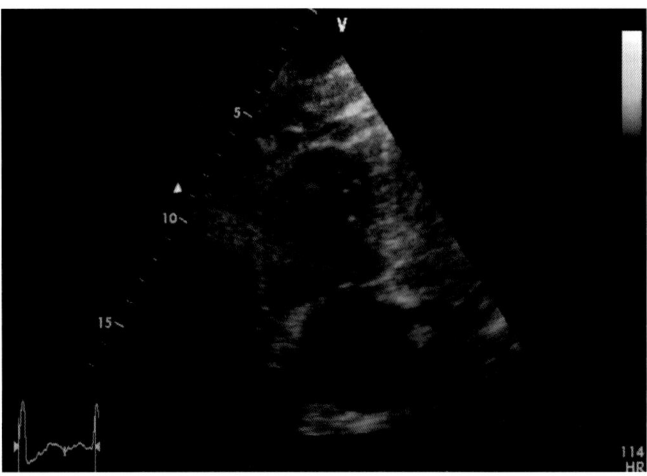

Fig. 36.11 Acute RV pressure overload in the setting of acute pulmonary embolus. There is relative sparing of size and function of the RV apex, whereas the remainder of the RV acutely dilates, causing impaired systolic function. The RA does not significantly dilate in acute pulmonary embolus (see Video 36.11).

suggested that, in general, pulmonary vasodilator therapies should not be used in group 2 PHT.[43]

Pulmonary Hypertension Due to Lung Disease

Abnormalities in lung structure, including loss of lung substance (e.g., in chronic obstructive pulmonary disease [COPD]) or lung fibrosis (e.g., interstitial pneumonitis), can result in increased PVR but with normal pulmonary capillary pressures (i.e., group 3 PHT). On echocardiography, the pulmonary artery and right heart changes are similar to those of PAH (see Fig. 36.2C); the diagnosis is based on significant, long-standing respiratory disease demonstrated on respiratory function testing and lung imaging.

Several technical difficulties can be encountered while obtaining good imaging windows in the setting of severe lung disease, including lung hyperinflation, displacement of the heart, and breathlessness limiting the imaging window during the cardiac cycle. Contrast echocardiography can be used to improve 2D and Doppler imaging in these circumstances. Because of marked variations in intrathoracic pressures with inspiration and expiration, there may be respirophasic variation in right heart filling in patients with severe lung disease (Fig. 36.10).

Hypoxia causes pulmonary arterial vasoconstriction, and chronic hypoxia can result in increased PVR that is only partly reversed by oxygen therapy. Pulmonary vasodilator therapy (e.g., sildenafil) may be helpful in selected patients.[44]

Pulmonary Hypertension Due to Pulmonary Artery Obstruction

Multiple acute pulmonary emboli occurring in different regions of the pulmonary circulation may eventually result in remodeling of the pulmonary arteries and a chronic increase in PVR. These pathologic changes occur in up to 2% of patients after acute pulmonary embolism.[45] Some echocardiographic features of group 4 PHT are shared with PAH and PHT due to lung disease (see Fig. 36.2C). The diagnosis is based on ventilation-perfusion mismatching in conjunction with respiratory function testing and lung imaging.

As in other forms of PHT, identification of chronic pulmonary thromboembolic disease has important implications for treatment and prognosis. Chronic thromboembolic PHT may respond to pulmonary vasodilator therapy,[46] but the most effective treatment is surgical pulmonary thromboendarterectomy. Although this major surgical procedure is gaining wider acceptance and in specialist centers is associated with excellent outcomes, many patients with chronic pulmonary thromboembolic disease remain undertreated, emphasizing the importance of an accurate diagnosis of the cause of PHT.

Balloon pulmonary angioplasty is another mechanical procedure that often has dramatic effects in suitable cases,[47,48] although the procedures involved can be long and require multiple, separate interventions. Ventilation-perfusion lung scans are particularly useful in the investigation of suspected chronic pulmonary thromboembolic disease.

Acute Pulmonary Hypertension

In patients experiencing acute pulmonary embolus, there is a sudden rise in PVR that often overwhelms the compensatory ability of the right heart, which is accustomed to a low-pressure system. There is an acute increase in RV size at the basal and middle regions, which is associated with impaired systolic function. There is relative sparing of the RV apical region, bounded by the insertion of the moderator band laterally, where systolic function is normal or increased. This sign, sometimes called the *McConnell's sign*, is less common in chronic RV pressure overload when compensation has occurred (Fig. 36.11).

In acute RV pressure overload, there is systolic bowing of the ventricular septum toward the left, an effect that is exaggerated by underfilling of the left heart due to low pulmonary flow. Acutely, the pulmonary artery diameter and RA volume remain normal.

Because each cause of PHT has a different pathophysiology, disease progression, and treatment, identification of the underlying cause is of great importance. The clinical-echocardiographic correlates for identifying the cause of each group of PHT are summarized in Table 36.4.

EFFECTS OF PULMONARY HYPERTENSION ON THE RIGHT HEART

In early PHT, RV systolic function remains normal, and there are minor if any shape changes, allowing for adaptation (or coupling with the pulmonary artery pressure) (Fig. 36.12). As pulmonary artery pressures rise further, RV shape changes become more pronounced, with limited capacity for the RV to respond to increased cardiac output requirements during exercise. These changes may be seen as a barometer of elevated downstream pressures.[49,50] RV-to–pulmonary artery coupling can be measured using the force-length relationship according to the following formula:

$$CR_{RV} = \frac{TAPSE}{RVSP}$$

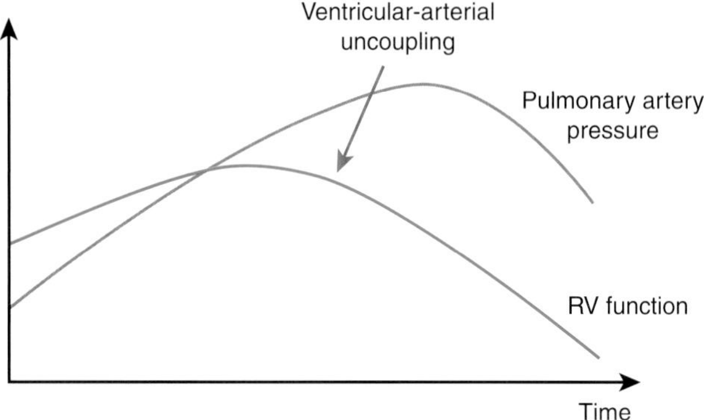

Fig. 36.12 Effects of elevated pulmonary artery pressure. RV-to–pulmonary artery coupling and eventual uncoupling occur as pulmonary artery pressure rises beyond the RV adaptive capacity. (Courtesy Professor Andrew La Gerche, St. Vincent's Hospital, Melbourne, Australia.)

where CR_{RV} is the coupling ratio of the RV, TAPSE is the tricuspid annular plane systolic excursion, and RVSP is the RV systolic pressure. CR_{RV} has been validated as a marker of uncoupling of the RV to the pulmonary artery in left heart disease[51]; a lower ratio (<0.35) is associated with an increased risk of hospitalization and death.

Eventually, as pulmonary artery pressures continue to rise, RV systolic function deteriorates, resulting in uncoupling of RV function from the pulmonary artery pressures. This causes a downward spiral of RV function and lower pulmonary artery pressures, which is demonstrated as a crossing of the curves in Fig. 36.12. Prognosis in patients with PHT is determined predominantly by its effects on RV function.[52] Estimation of pulmonary artery pressure alone has limited meaning unless it is accompanied by simultaneous assessment of RV function.

RV Shape Changes in the Setting of Pressure Loading

The RV has a complex shape and is structurally very different from the LV (see Chapter 4). Seen on 2D echocardiography, the normal shape of the RV is roughly triangular in the apical 4-chamber view and crescentic in a parasternal short-axis view (Fig. 36.13).

The unique shape of the RV is fully appreciated with three-dimensional (3D) echocardiography. Fig. 36.14A shows a multiplanar reconstruction of the right heart, and Fig. 36.14B shows a surface rendering of the internal contour of the RV using 3D

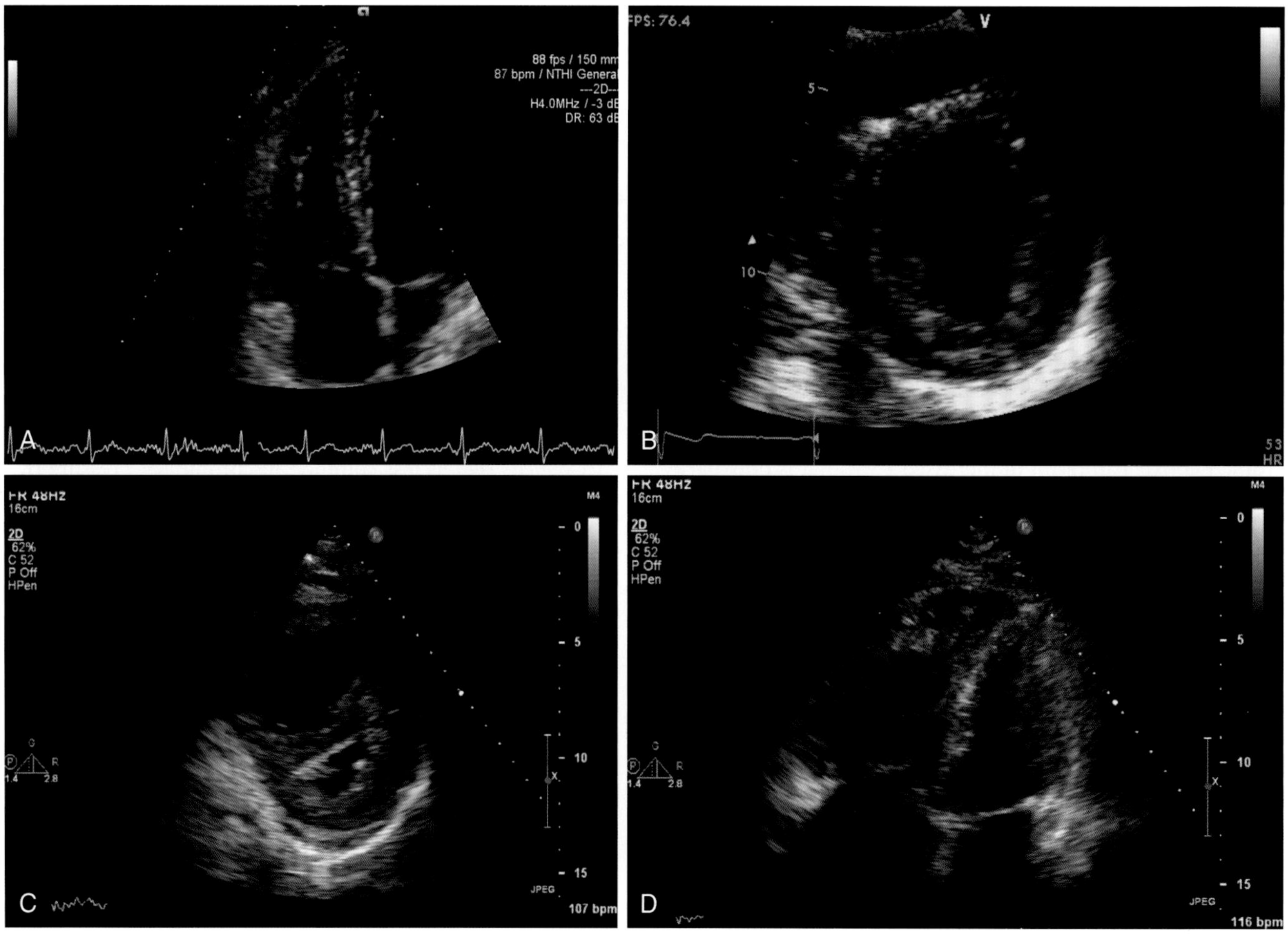

Fig. 36.13 Normal shape of the right heart. (A) Typical triangular shape of the RV when viewed from an RV-focused apical 4-chamber view (see Video 36.13A). (B) Normal crescent shape of the RV when viewed from the mid-ventricular short-axis view (see Video 36.13B). (C and D) In the setting of RV pressure overload, there is flattening of the ventricular septum toward the LV in systole (see Videos 36.13C and 36.13D).

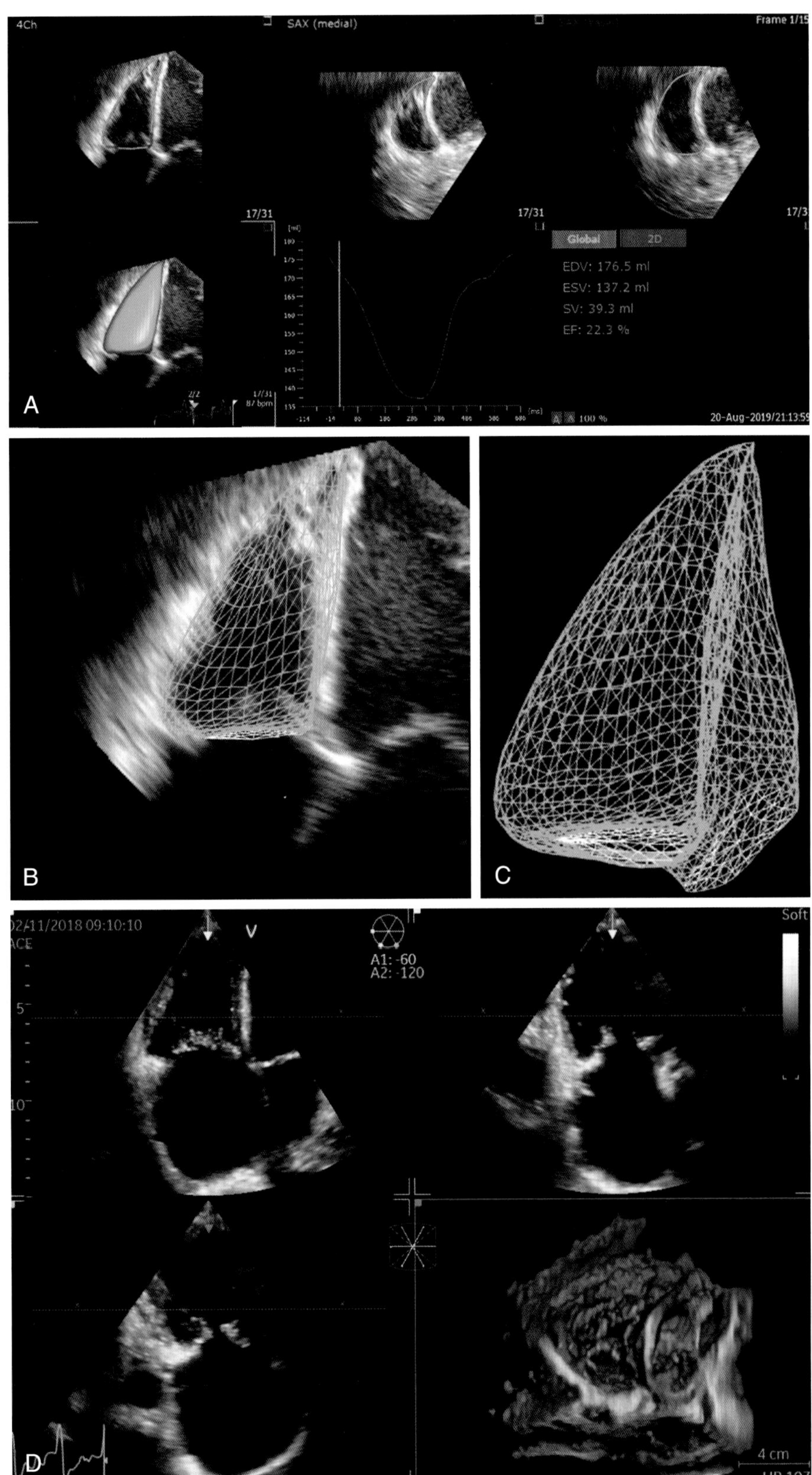

Fig. 36.14 3D echocardiography can help reveal changes to RV shape in the setting of pressure overload. (A) Multiplanar reconstruction of the right heart (see Video 36.14A). (B, C) Surface rendering of the internal contour of the RV using 3D echocardiography (see Videos 36.14B and 36.14C). (D) In pulmonary hypertension, the RV appears more rectangular when imaged from a 4-chamber view (see Video 36.14D).

echocardiography. In PHT, several structural and functional changes occur in the RV (Table 36.6; see Figs. 36.13C and D and Fig. 36.14C). The RV becomes more rectangular when imaged from a 4-chamber view, with the moderator band becoming prominent and directed more horizontally across the RV cavity. On short-axis views, the RV appears more circular as a result of RV dilation and compression of the ventricular septum. The increase in RV size and compression of the ventricular septum may impair filling of the LV in the pericardial space and create ventricular interdependence.

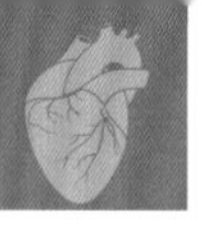

TABLE 36.6 Right Heart Abnormalities in Pulmonary Hypertension.

Measurement	*Abnormal Values*
TRV	>2.5 m/s
PASP[a]	>30 mmHg
PR initial velocity	2.0 m/s
PR end velocity	1.75 m/s
RV basal diameter	>42 mm
RV mid diameter	>35 mm
RVOT PSAX distal diameter	>27 mm
RA end-systolic area	>18 cm^2
TAPSE	<17 mm
RV S′	<10 cm/s
Pulsed-wave Doppler RIMP	≥0.44
Tissue Doppler RIMP	≥0.55
FAC (%)	<35%
3D RV assessment	
End-diastolic volume	≥87 mL/m^2 (male); ≥74 mL/m^2 (female)
End-systolic volume	≥45 mL/m^2 (male); ≥36 mL/m^2 (female)
Ejection fraction	<45%
RV subcostal wall thickness	>5 mm
RV shape	
PSAX	Circular
Apical 4-chamber	Rectangular
Ventricular septum	Concave to the right

[a]Assuming an RA pressure of 5 mmHg.
FAC, Fractional area change; *PASP*, pulmonary artery systolic pressure; *PR*, pulmonary regurgitation; *PSAX*, parasternal short axis; *RIMP*, RV index of myocardial performance; *RVOT*, RV outflow tract; *S′*, systolic tissue Doppler velocity measured at the lateral tricuspid annulus; *TAPSE*, tricuspid annular plane systolic excursion; *TRV*, tricuspid regurgitation velocity.

Ventricular Septal Motion

The shared association of the ventricular septum with the LV becomes more important when RVSP starts to rise. The systolic pressure difference between the RV and LV is diminished, causing flattening of the ventricular septum (see Fig. 36.15A–C). This results in a D-shaped LV and an O-shaped RV during systole. This sign is exaggerated in the setting of low systemic blood pressure, and it may be subtle or absent when systemic blood pressure is increased, even with significant PHT. In the setting of pressure overload, flattening of the ventricular septum occurs predominantly in systole.

When RV failure develops, abnormal RV diastolic function causes increased RV diastolic pressures. If RV filling pressures rise above LV filling pressures, the ventricular septum flattens during diastole (see Fig. 36.15D and E). Diastolic septal flattening may also occur in the setting of significant TR or PR and may become exaggerated in the setting of volume overload. Diastolic flattening is diminished when coexisting LV diastolic dysfunction or LV hypertrophy exists.

Ventricular septal flattening can be quantified using the eccentricity index, which is measured in the parasternal short-axis view at papillary muscle level (see Fig. 36.15F and G) and defined as the ratio of the anteroposterior to the septolateral LV dimension. It can be measured in systole and diastole. A ratio greater than 1.0 during diastole suggests elevated RV diastolic pressure, whereas a ratio greater than 1.0 during systole suggests RV pressure overload. Abnormal systolic and diastolic septal motion may also occur in the setting of a bundle branch block, with cardiac pacing, and after cardiac surgery. These signs of pressure loading in systole and diastole are important in the overall evaluation of the right heart in PHT and when there is insufficient TR to estimate the RVSP.

RV Dimensions

Standard RV dimensions can be evaluated from an RV-focused 4-chamber view or automatically using 3D echocardiography (Fig. 36.16).[53] A diameter of greater than 41 mm at the base and greater than 35 mm in the mid-RV indicates dilation (see Table 36.6). Because of tapering of the RV dimension when rotated views are obtained, 3D echocardiography can be used to ensure that the maximum width of the RV is being measured. Very large or small patients may have RV dimensions outside the normal range which normalize when indexed for body surface area.

RV Wall Thickness

Increased RV wall thickness may occur in PHT, but it is not specific to this diagnosis. It also occurs in patients with pulmonary valve stenosis or infiltrative cardiomyopathies. When measured along the RV free wall from a subcostal 4-chamber view, an RV wall thickness of more than 5 mm indicates RV hypertrophy. The trabecular muscle pattern of the RV endocardium, however, can occasionally make this assessment difficult.

RV Systolic Function

RV fractional area change (FAC) is measured using the same focused 4-chamber view as the RV dimensions, with an FAC of less than 35% suggesting impaired RV systolic function (Fig. 36.17).[53] RV FAC should be considered with other measures of RV function such as TAPSE and myocardial performance index (MPI).

TAPSE is a reliable measurement of RV longitudinal systolic function. It is measured by M-mode imaging of the lateral tricuspid annulus with the same focused 4-chamber view as is used for RV dimensions. Visualization of this motion can be enhanced by the addition of tissue color Doppler to the M-mode. Measurement of TAPSE does not require geometric assumptions and is simple to perform compared with other techniques.

Impaired RV systolic function is likely when TAPSE is less than 1.7 cm, and it strongly predicts an increased mortality risk when less than 1.5 cm.[54,55] In the setting of normal LV function, LV apical movement may pull the RV free wall toward the apex, resulting in an apparently greater TAPSE than would be expected from the observed RV function. Measures of regional RV free wall function (e.g., longitudinal strain) may be helpful.

The RV S′ measures the peak systolic tissue Doppler velocity of the lateral tricuspid annulus. Because of the angle dependency of tissue Doppler, care should be taken to ensure that the lateral tricuspid annulus is lined up with the center of the ultrasound beam before measurements are undertaken. Because of the intensity of the tissue Doppler signal, this marker is less reliant on image quality than other measures. As with other tissue Doppler measures, the modal velocity should be measured. Although RV S′ decreases with age,[56] an S′ of less than 10 cm/s indicates RV dysfunction, particularly when combined with an abnormal TAPSE value.

The RV index of myocardial performance (RIMP) is a marker of global RV performance. Using PW Doppler or myocardial velocities, the RV isovolumetric contraction time (IVCT), RV isovolumetric relaxation time (IVRT), and RVOT ejection time (ET) are measured (Fig. 36.18). RIMP may then be calculated using the following formula:

$$\text{RIMP} = \frac{\text{IVRT} + \text{IVCT}}{\text{ET}}$$

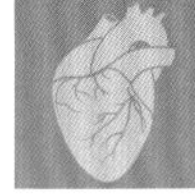

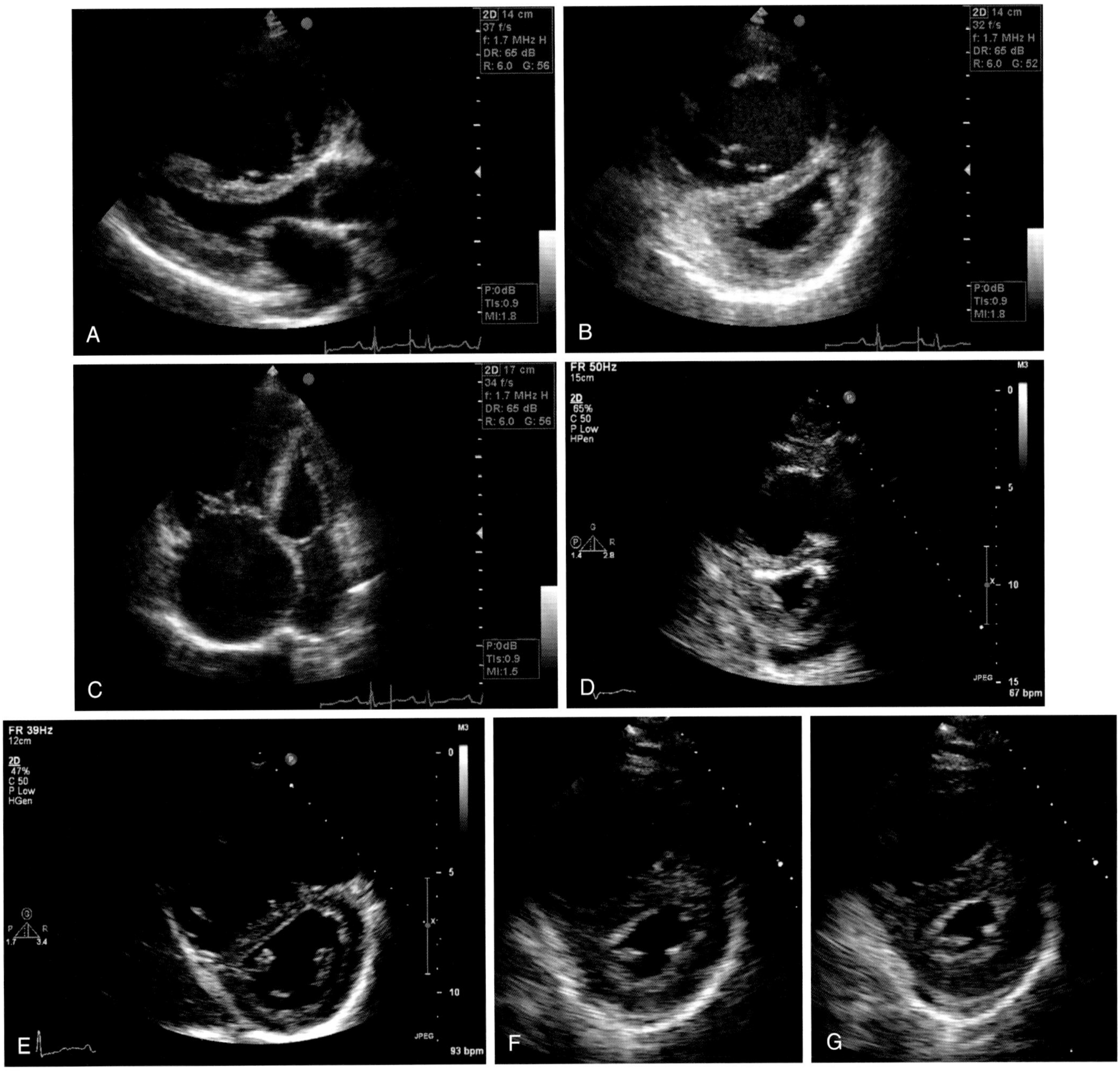

Fig. 36.15 **Motion of the ventricular septum in systole is a useful guide to RV pressure overload.** Ventricular septal compression during systole is consistent with RV systolic pressure overload. (A) Ventricular septal compression in systole in the parasternal long-axis view (see Video 36.15A). (B) The corresponding parasternal short-axis view (see Video 36.15B). (C) Apical 4-chamber view of the same patient shows severe RV dilation with the ventricular septum compressed toward the left predominantly in systole, limiting LV size. Motion of the ventricular septum in diastole can help identify increased RV diastolic filling pressures (see Video 36.15C). (D and E) Flattening of the ventricular septum in diastole caused by abnormally increased RV filling pressures. D also demonstrates some systolic septal flattening due to RV pressure overload (see Videos 36.15D and 36.15E). (F and G) Using the sphericity index, the anteroposterior dimension of the LV is compared with the septolateral dimension in systole and diastole.

in which IVRT + IVCT equals the total RV systolic time (from tricuspid closure to tricuspid opening) minus the ET (from RVOT PW Doppler). A normal RIMP value is less than 0.44 (see Table 36.6). The RV MPI may be limited by the absence of isovolumetric periods in a normal right ventricle.

RV Strain

Speckle tracking echocardiography has shown prognostic utility in evaluation and follow-up of patients with PHT (Fig. 36.19). Decreased RV free wall strain is associated with a threefold increased risk of death[57]; this measurement has possible performance advantages over TAPSE.[57–59]

In patients with PHT, abnormal RV free wall strain on cardiac magnetic resonance imaging (MRI) is associated with RV-arterial uncoupling,[60] and correlates with the degree of RV fibrosis.[61] Although there is only modest agreement between echocardiographic and cardiac MRI–measured RV strain,[62] echocardiographic RV free wall strain correlates well with cardiac MRI–measured ejection fraction, with ≥ −14% identifying a group at highest risk of progression to hospitalization or death.[62–65] Alterations in 3D strain and deformation patterns have been shown to predict death.[66]

Specific RV longitudinal strain measurement packages are required because LV strain software cannot be reliably applied

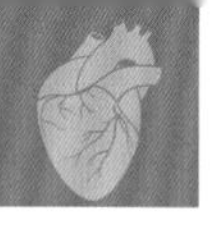

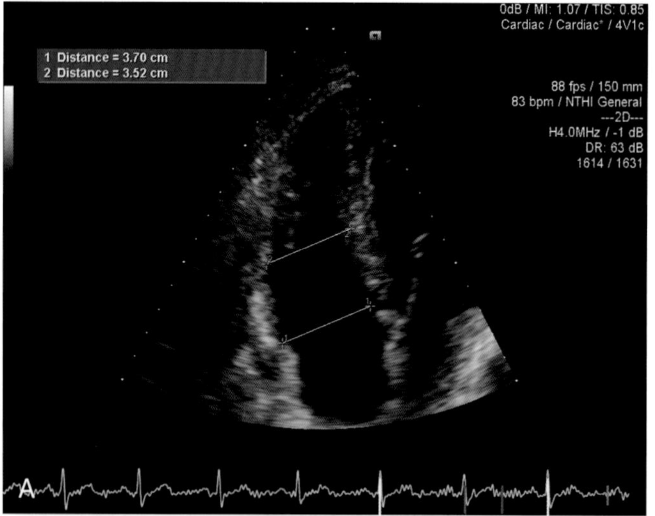

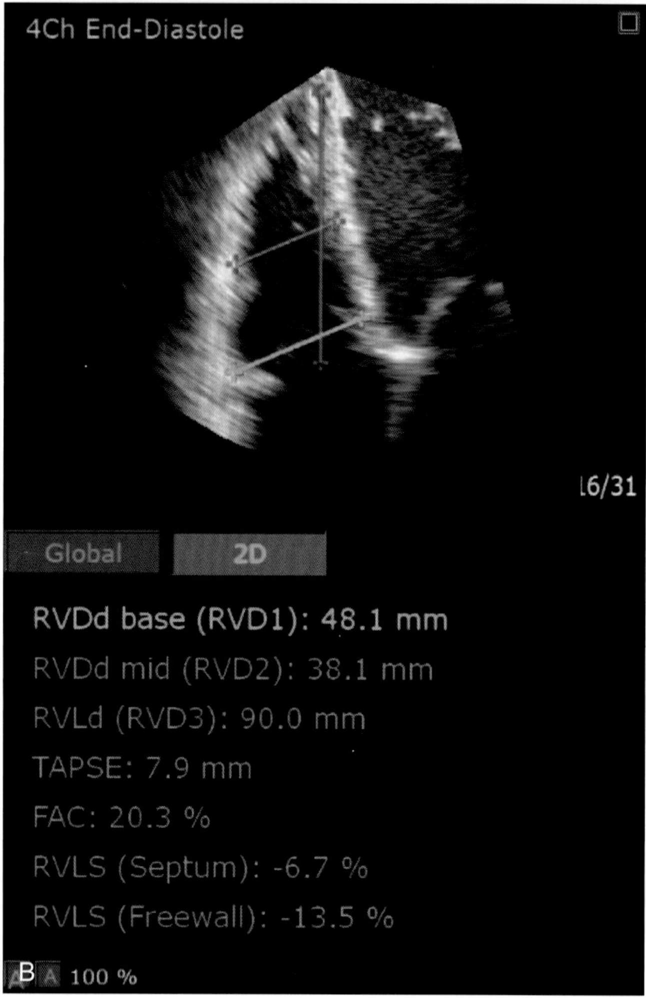

Fig. 36.16 Measurement of RV dimensions from an RV-focused apical 4-chamber view. Basal measurements are made on the RV side of the tricuspid annulus during diastole (A) and in the mid-RV just basal to the moderator band (B) (see Video 36.16B ▶).

to the RV to measure free wall strain. A narrow strain width is required because the RV is a thin-walled structure.

3D Analysis of RV Systolic Function

Because of the complex shape of the RV, 2D assessment cannot fully appreciate the changes in RV shape due to PHT. 3D echocardiography has several theoretical advantages over 2D echocardiography, particularly the ability to simultaneously view the RVOT and RV to create RV volumes (see Fig. 36.14).

In practice, there are challenges to RV volume acquisition. It is technically very difficult to visualize the RVOT and pulmonary valve from apical views alone, and parasternal acquisition may be needed, requiring off-line combining of volume data with inherent assumptions and risks. The anterior wall of the RV is often not well seen from apical views; algorithmic assumptions must be relied upon to complete volume assessments.

Most volume algorithms are based on normal RV templates, and analysis may be less accurate in the setting of an abnormal RV in PHT. Although 3D analysis of RV function is attractive, until these practical challenges can be overcome, we recommend a comprehensive assessment of RV function based predominantly on 2D assessments for most patients.

Table 36.6 summarizes the 3D echocardiographic findings for PHT. During 3D analysis of RV function, maximum and minimum RV volumes should be selected manually, and the trabeculations and moderator band should be included in the RV cavity.

RV Diastolic Function

Diastolic function of the RV is assessed using PW Doppler of the tricuspid inflow, tissue Doppler of the lateral tricuspid annulus, and 2D assessment of IVC size and collapsibility. These parameters are described in Chapter 6. Care should be taken to ensure that tissue Doppler assessment of the tricuspid annulus is performed from an RV-focused view, with the lateral tricuspid annulus descending directly toward the transducer in systole. Table 36.6 summarizes the right heart structural changes found in PHT.

Estimating Pulmonary Vascular Resistance at Rest

Normal pulmonary circulation is a low-pressure system with low vascular resistance and with PVR usually decreasing or remaining unchanged with exercise.[67] PVR may be considered to represent the degree of obstruction to flow, and it is a function of pulmonary pressure and cardiac output. The gold standard for estimation of PVR is RHC. As described earlier, PVR is calculated from the following formula:

$$\text{PVR (WU)} = \frac{\text{mPAP} - \text{PAWP}}{\text{CO}}$$

where mPAP is the mean pulmonary artery pressure, PAWP is the pulmonary artery wedge pressure, and CO is the cardiac output (i.e., pulmonary blood flow [Qp]).

Several methods have been proposed to estimate PVR using echocardiography. Each is based on the principle of pressure as a function of cardiac output (i.e., ratio of PAP to cardiac output). The following formula, proposed by Abbas et al.,[68] has been widely used:

$$\text{PVR} = 10 \times \frac{\text{TRV}}{\text{RVOT VTI}} + 0.16$$

where TRV is given in meters per second and the RVOT VTI in centimeters. A PVR greater than 2 WU suggests abnormally increased PVR.

In patients with a PVR greater than 6 WU, the original formula performs less well. A second equation has been proposed for those with a high PVR[69]:

$$\text{PVR} = 5.19 \times \frac{\text{TRV}^2}{\text{RVOT VTI}} - 0.4$$

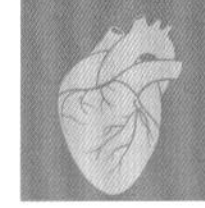

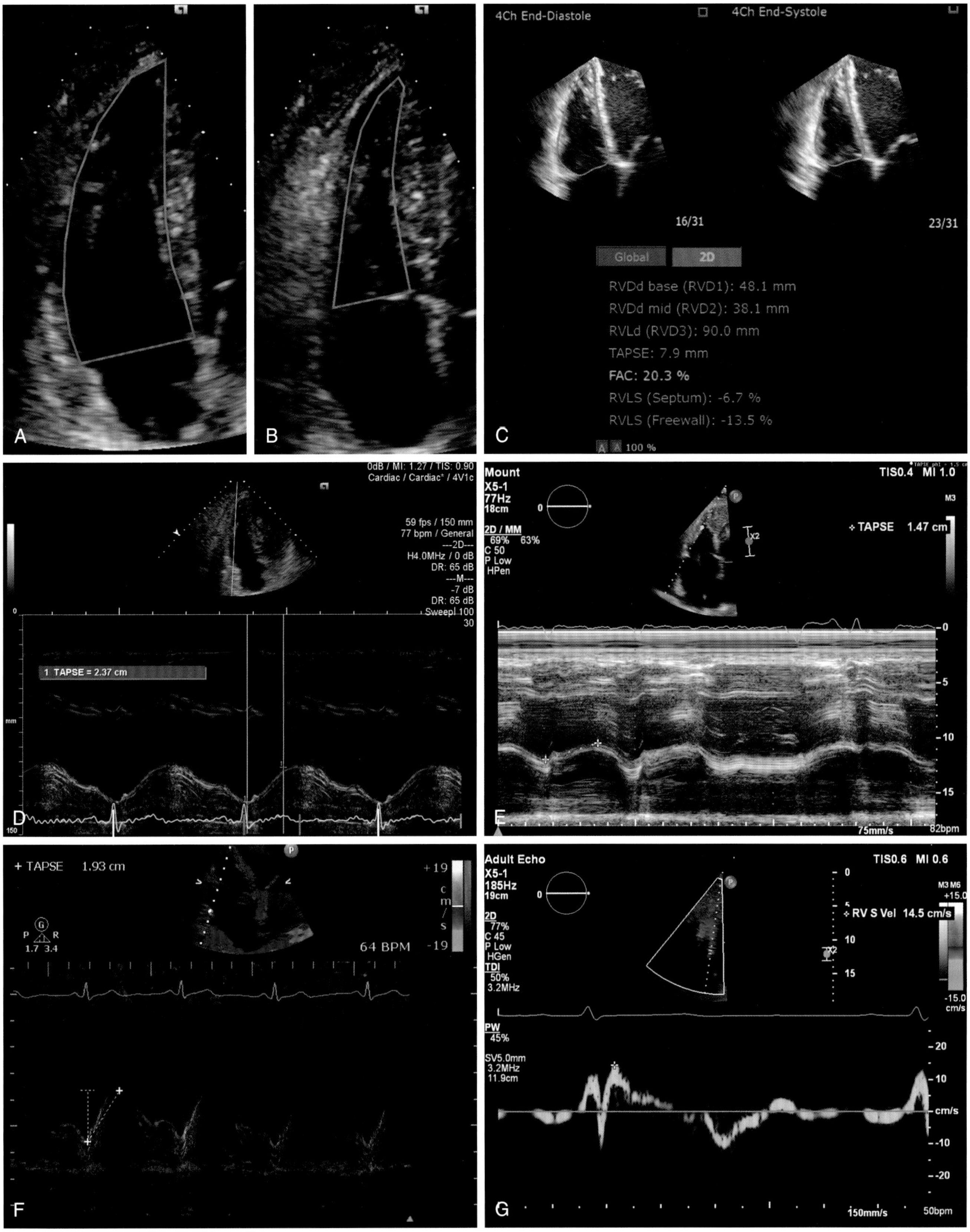

Fig. 36.17 Measurement of RV function from an RV-focused apical 4-chamber view. Fractional area change is measured by tracing the endocardial border in diastole (A) and in systole (B), calculating the ratio of these two measures and using 3D echocardiography (C) (see Video 36.17C). The tricuspid annular plane systolic excursion *(TAPSE)* is the distance the lateral tricuspid annulus travels in systole, measured using M-mode (D and E) or M-mode performed during color-coded tissue Doppler imaging (F). (G) Systolic function can also be measured using tissue Doppler systolic descent velocities of the tricuspid annulus (S′).

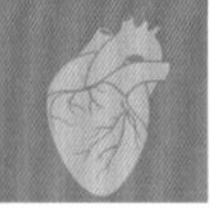

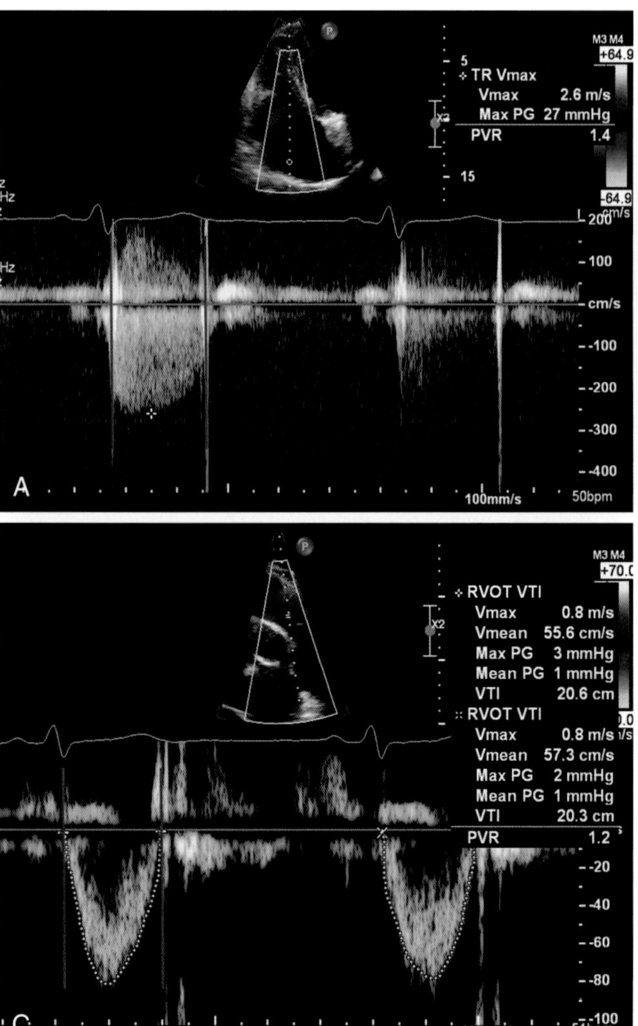

Fig. 36.18 Calculation of the RV index of myocardial performance and pulmonary vascular resistance. The time from tricuspid closure to tricuspid opening (i.e., TR duration) is measured (A), along with the RV outlet tract *(RVOT)* ejection time *(ET)* (B). The difference between these values is divided by the ET to create the RV index of myocardial performance (RIMP). Pulmonary vascular resistance *(PVR)* is measured using the tricuspid regurgitation velocity *(TRV)* (A) and the RVOT velocity–time integral *(VTI)* (C). The formulas used in calculating PVR are provided in the text.

However, this method does not take into account the left heart filling pressures. This is a potentially important limitation because increased LA pressure decreases PVR.[70] For example, a 5-mmHg increase in LA pressure causes a 1-WU decrease in PVR.[71] Increased LA pressure increases the pulsatile RV load relative to the resistive RV load and may contribute to RV dysfunction.[70]

Simple noninvasive measures of LV filling pressure (e.g., E:E′ ratio) may help separate PHT due to left heart disease from that due to increased PVR. A simple ratio of the TRV to a marker of LV filling pressure has been proposed to help distinguish these two broad groups of PHT:

$$ePLAR = \frac{TRVmax}{E:E'}$$

where *e*PLAR is the echocardiographic pulmonary-to-LA ratio (m/s), TRVmax is the peak TR velocity (m/s), and E:E′ is the ratio of peak mitral inflow E velocity to the medial mitral annular tissue velocity (unitless).

*e*PLAR is based on the assumption that the pulmonary pressure rises in parallel with increased LA pressure in the setting of left heart disease but is out of proportion to the LA pressure in the setting of pulmonary vascular disease (along with a rise in the transpulmonary gradient). Early results are consistent with this notion; the mean *e*PLAR for patients with precapillary PHT was 0.44 ± 0.22 m/s, compared with a group of left heart disease patients with postcapillary PHT, for whom the mean was 0.20 ± 0.11 m/s.[72] The main limitation of *e*PLAR is the lack of correction for cardiac output, an important determinant of PVR.

Fig. 36.18 summarizes echocardiographic methods for separating precapillary from postcapillary PHT. However, no specific echocardiographic methods are completely reliable for assessing PHT that is out of proportion to the degree of left heart disease.

When PVR appears to be increased on noninvasive assessment, other abnormal findings such as a systolic notch on RVOT Doppler imaging,[24] a short pulmonary acceleration time, and signs of RV pressure overload help provide confirmatory evidence.

EXERCISE STRESS ECHOCARDIOGRAPHY AND PULMONARY HYPERTENSION

Exercise-induced PHT is not considered a pathologic entity in its own right because there are no age-specific normative values for exercise-related pulmonary artery pressures, and a rise

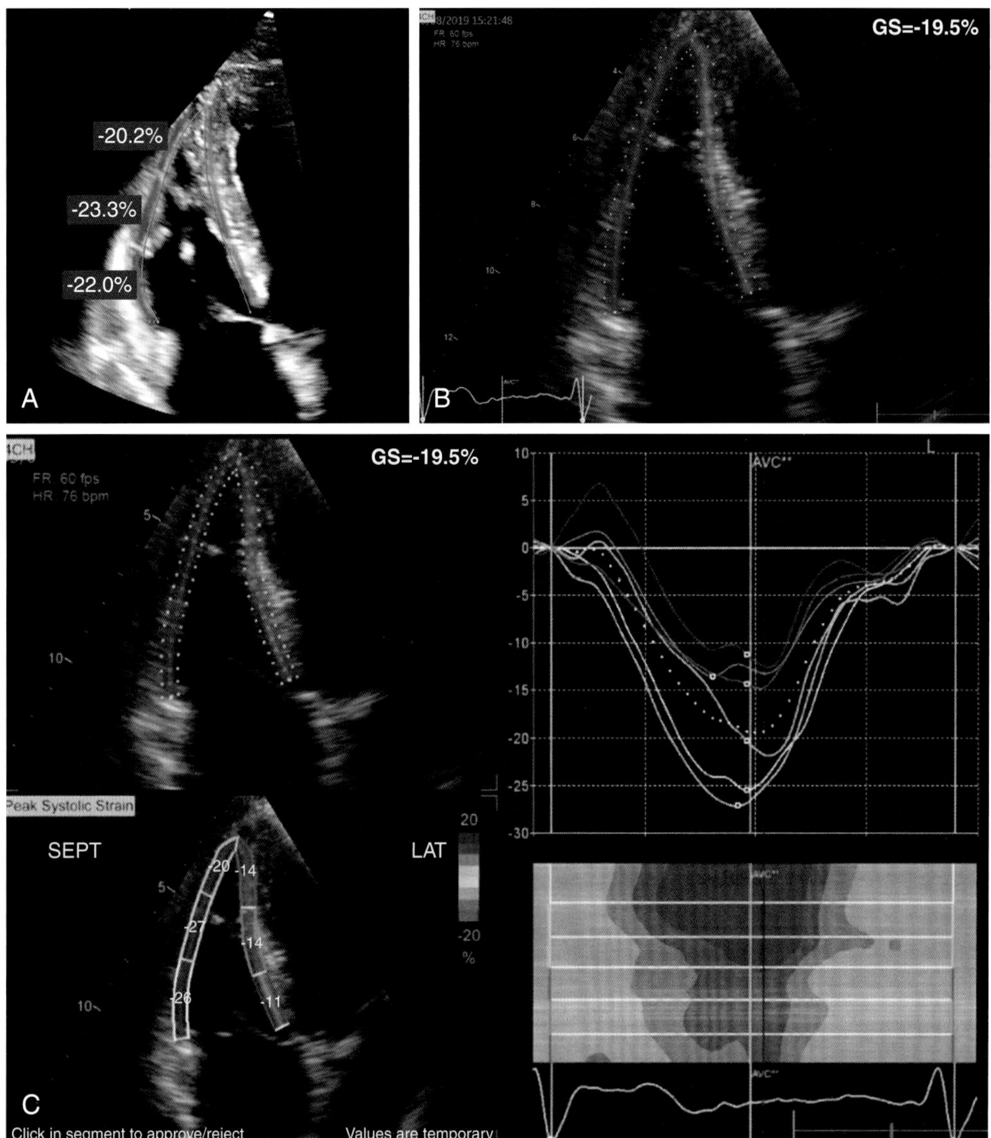

Fig. 36.19 Measurement of RV longitudinal strain. (A) Percentage deformation of the RV free wall using the Philips TomTec imaging system (see Video 36.19A). (B) Measurement using GE Healthcare IT technology (see Video 36.19B). (C) Individual walls can also be examined (see Video 36.19C).

in pressure without information on flow is meaningless. Athletes who have substantial increases in their cardiac output with exercise may have high pulmonary artery pressures but normal PVR, no symptoms, and excellent exercise tolerance.[73,74]

Some patients have unusually exaggerated increases in pulmonary artery pressure with low levels of exercise that are not associated with a substantial increase in the cardiac output or left heart filling pressure. This may represent a precursor to PHT with a corresponding poor prognosis.[50] Because a disproportionate rise in pulmonary artery pressure may result from mildly increased PVR,[75] diastolic dysfunction, or valvular heart disease, an exercise-related increase in pulmonary artery pressure does not necessarily indicate pulmonary vascular disease. Many of these patients also have an abnormal response of the right heart to exercise, uncovering impaired contractile reserve at rest. In symptomatic patients, there remains a role for noninvasive pulmonary artery pressure estimation during cardiovascular stress, such as exercise or dobutamine infusion, to better diagnose pulmonary vascular disease earlier in its natural history.

Because pulmonary artery pressures fall rapidly after cessation of exercise, it is important to estimate these pressures *during* exercise. Semisupine stationary ergometry, with side tilt to allow for optimal echocardiographic imaging, is ideal for this purpose. Despite this purpose-built equipment, it can be technically difficult to obtain all relevant measurements at peak exercise, particularly in a breathless patient, and only key measurements should be sought. We recommend performing measurements at baseline and at peak exercise to allow meaningful comparisons. The LV outflow diameter acquired at baseline can also be used to assess cardiac output with exercise.

In selected patients for whom exercise is difficult or echocardiographic windows are challenging, dobutamine echocardiography may be preferred as the method of increasing cardiac output, although the degree of augmentation of cardiac output is usually much less than that seen with moderate or greater exercise levels. Dobutamine is usually given at doses of 20 μg/kg /min or lower to minimize vasomotor effects on the pulmonary circulation.

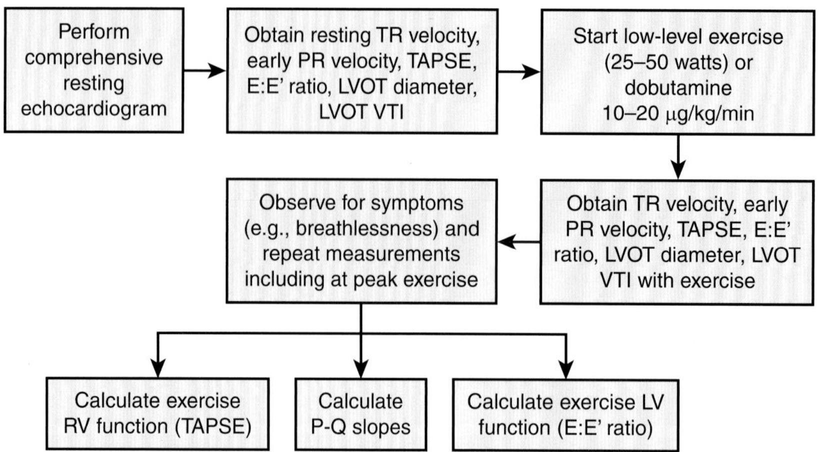

Fig. 36.20 Pulmonary hypertension stress test with a suggested flow chart. A patient with suspected pulmonary hypertension underwent comprehensive echocardiography followed by low levels of exercise or dobutamine stress testing. Changes to the LV, RV, and pulmonary artery pressure measurements were examined during and immediately after exercise. *E:E′*, Ratio of peak mitral inflow E velocity to the medial mitral annular tissue velocity; *LVOT*, left ventricular outlet tract; *P*, mean pulmonary artery pressure; *PR*, pulmonary regurgitation; *Q*, cardiac output; *TAPSE*, tricuspid annular plane systolic excursion; *TR*, tricuspid regurgitation; *VTI*, velocity–time integral.

A suggested PHT diagnostic workflow chart for stress echocardiography is shown in Fig. 36.20. The PASP should be estimated from the TRV, using the same RA pressure assumption as at baseline, followed by TAPSE measurement, evaluation of the left heart (including E:E′ ratio as a marker of acute LV diastolic filling pressure), and the LV outflow tract (LVOT) velocity–time integral (LVOT VTI). The cardiac output can then be calculated using the LVOT diameter obtained at rest and the peak heart rate at the time of LVOT VTI acquisition.

There is no consensus about whether the absolute RVSP with exercise or the degree of increase in RVSP is more important. E:E′ ratios in the intermediate range (8–12) at rest may not be reliable as a marker of increased LV filling pressure with exercise[76] or dobutamine stress.[77] As a rule, an increase in RVSP by more than 15 mmHg at low levels of exercise (5–6 METs on a treadmill[78] or 50 W on a cycle ergometer[79,80]) suggests increased PVR. Conversely, failure of the RVSP to augment with exercise (i.e., RVSP does not increase above 30 mmHg at 50–75 W) suggests impaired RV contractile reserve,[50] which may be associated with a worse prognosis. In patients with pulmonary thromboembolic PHT, uncoupling of RV function during exercise is associated with impaired contractile reserve, higher PVR, and more severe disease.[81]

To quantify the association between mean pulmonary artery pressure and cardiac output, it is possible to measure them during stress echocardiography using standard formulas:

$$P = \left(4 \times PR_{in}^2\right) + RAP$$

or

$$P = (0.61 \times RVSP) + 2$$

where P is the mean pulmonary artery pressure, PR_{in}^2 is the initial diastolic PR velocity squared, RAP is the estimated RA pressure, and RVSP is the estimated right ventricular systolic pressure using the peak TR velocity; and

$$Q = \frac{\pi D^2}{4} \times LVOT_{VTI} \times HR$$

where Q is the cardiac output (L/min), D is the LVOT diameter (cm), $LVOT_{VTI}$ is the LVOT velocity–time integral (cm), and HR is the heart rate (beats/min).

Assuming no shunts are present, the PVR is normalized for flow rate to determine the total pulmonary vascular resistance (PVRt):

$$PVRt = \frac{P\ (mmHg)}{Q\ (L/min)}$$

Pulmonary capillary wedge pressure is not taken into account in this formula and is not equivalent to the invasively measured PVR, which is determined as follows:

$$PVR = \frac{mPAP - PAWP}{CO}$$

where mPAP is the mean pulmonary artery pressure, mPAWP is the mean pulmonary artery wedge pressure, and CO is the cardiac output. Performing all of these measures during exercise is technically difficult, and dobutamine is often preferred over exercise to produce a more controlled environment and to allow each measurement to be performed accurately.

In young, normal individuals, mPAP rises by approximately 1 mmHg for each liter per minute of cardiac output increase (P/Q slope = 1), whereas with PAH, the rise in mPAP is approximately 5 mmHg for the same increase in cardiac output (P/Q slope = 5).[82,83] The suggested cutoff for abnormal of 3 mmHg/L/min or higher.[84] In older individuals (>60 years of age), the increase in mPAP with exercise is more marked, up to 3 mmHg for each 1 L/min of increase in cardiac output. A higher P/Q slope is associated with worse New York Heart Association functional status.

DIAGNOSTIC APPROACH FOR A PATIENT WITH SUSPECTED PULMONARY HYPERTENSION

Fig. 36.1 shows a suggested diagnostic approach for a patient with suspected PHT (e.g., impaired exercise tolerance, breathlessness). Evaluation of pulmonary artery pressures using the TRV and other approaches is required, followed by careful assessment for left heart disease. Detailed analysis of RV function and PVR is required if no left heart disease is identified.

The formulas used for PHT assessment are shown in Table 36.7. PHT may have more than one cause, especially with the aging population and improved treatment and prognosis of chronic respiratory, hematologic, and cardiac diseases.

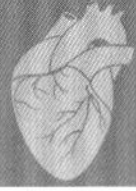

TABLE 36.7 Key Equations for Evaluation of Pulmonary Hypertension.

Pulmonary vascular resistance	$PVR = 10\times\frac{TRV}{RVOT\ VTI} + 0.16$
	$PVR = 5.19\times\frac{TRV^2}{RVOT\ VTI} - 0.4$
	$PVR = \left(\frac{mPAP - mPAWP}{CO}\right)$
Echocardiographic pulmonary-to-LA ratio (m/s)	$ePLAR = \frac{TRVmax}{E:E'}$
RV systolic pressure	$RVSP = \left(4\times TRVmax^2\right) + RAP$
Pulmonary artery diastolic pressure	$PADP = 4\times(PR_{end})^2 + RAP$
Mean pulmonary artery pressure	$mPAP = 4\times(PR_{in})^2 + RAP$
	$mPAP = (0.61\times RVSP) + 2$
RV performance index[a]	$RIMP = \frac{IVRT + IVCT}{ET}$
PVR normalized for flow rate	$PVRt = \frac{P\ (mmHg)}{Q\ (L/min)}$
Volume flow rate (Q) (mL^3/min)	$Q = \frac{\pi D^2}{4}\times LVOT_{VTI}\times HR$

CO, Cardiac output (L/min); *D*, LVOT diameter; *E:E′*, ratio of peak mitral inflow E velocity to the medial mitral annular tissue velocity (unitless); *ePLAR*, echocardiographic pulmonary-to-LA ratio (m/s); *ET*, ejection time; *HR*, heart rate; *IVCT*, RV isovolumetric contraction time; *IVRT*, RV isovolumetric relaxation time; *LVOT*, left ventricular outflow tract; *mPAP*, mean pulmonary artery pressure (mmHg); *mPAWP*, mean pulmonary artery wedge pressure (mmHg); *PADP*, pulmonary artery diastolic pressure; PR_{end}, end pulmonary regurgitation velocity; PR_{in}, initial pulmonary regurgitation velocity; *PVR*, pulmonary vascular resistance; *PVRt*, total pulmonary vascular resistance; *Q*, flow rate; *RAP*, estimated (or known) RA pressure; *RIMP*, RV index of myocardial performance; *RVOT*, RV outlet tract; *RVSP*, RV systolic pressure (taken to be the pulmonary artery systolic pressure in the absence of RVOT obstruction or pulmonary valve stenosis); *TRV*, tricuspid regurgitation velocity (m/s); *VTI*, velocity–time integral (cm).

[a]IVRT + IVCT = Total systole (from tricuspid closure to tricuspid opening) – Ejection time (from RVOT pulsed-wave Doppler).

It remains a significant challenge for an echocardiographer to identify PHT with multiple causes.

MONITORING PULMONARY HYPERTENSION AND RV RESPONSES

After prescription of disease-specific therapy for PAH, regular monitoring of pulmonary artery pressures and right heart function are required. For diseases that increase the risk of PAH (e.g., scleroderma), regular screening is also recommended. With repeated measurements and inherent inconsistencies, any echocardiographic parameter is likely to vary over time. Minimizing variations can help identify increases in pulmonary artery pressures and deterioration of RV function as they occur.

Regular education of those performing echocardiograms is important, including consensus examples of measurement points and regular feedback. Side-by-side comparison of previous studies can help to ensure that similar views are obtained from identical windows, and assumptions should be standardized for each patient.

Increased blood volume can adversely affect RV function in the setting of PHT, as can other clinical factors such as systemic hypertension and tachycardia. For this reason, we recommend the repeated evaluation of patients with PHT at approximately the same time of day, with standardized hydration and use of the same echocardiographer and equipment when possible.

SUMMARY Suspected Pulmonary Hypertension.[a]

Assessment	Measurements Performed	Method	Abnormal Values	Interpretation
Is there pulmonary hypertension?	RA pressure	IVC collapse from subcostal IVC long-axis view	>2.1 cm diameter <50% collapse with sniff	RA pressure >15 mmHg
	JVP height	Clinical assessment	>6 cm at 45 degrees	RA pressure >15 mmHg
	RA area	RV focused apical 4-chamber view	18 cm^2	Chronic RA pressure elevation
	RV-RA pressure difference	Maximum TRV from multiple views	2.5 m/s	Beware of incomplete traces and angle dependency
	PASP	$RVSP = 4\ (TRVmax)^2 + RAP$	>30 mmHg (assuming RAP = 5 mmHg)	Assumes no pulmonary stenosis
	PA-RV pressure difference	Initial PR velocity	>20 mmHg	Mean PAP estimation
	PA-RV pressure difference	End PR velocity	>10 mmHg	Diastolic PAP estimation
	Pulmonary acceleration time	Duration of upstroke in pulmonary valve CW Doppler wave	<90 ms	Predicts PVR >3 WU

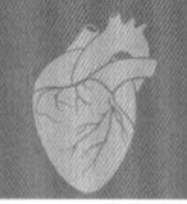

SUMMARY Suspected Pulmonary Hypertension.—cont'd

Assessment	Measurements Performed	Method	Abnormal Values	Interpretation
Why is there pulmonary hypertension?	Groups 1, 3, 4, and 5 PHT	PHT without signs of left heart disease	—	Investigation for underlying cause is required
	Group 1 due to congenital heart disease	Describe exact location of defect in relation to arteries and other cardiac structures. Determine the physiologic effects of the lesion using the Bernoulli equation. Use traditional measures of PHT. Assess volume and pressure effects on the right heart.	—	PAH with Eisenmenger syndrome PAH with left-to-right shunting and increased PVR but no Eisenmenger syndrome PAH with small defects PAH after corrective surgery
	Group 2 pulmonary hypertension: left heart disease	Measure LV ejection fraction from parasternal and apical views.	<50%	LV systolic dysfunction
		Measure diastolic function.	E:E′ ratio >15	Increased LV filling pressures
		Measure biplane LA volume from apical views.	LA volume >34 mL/m^2	
		Measure LV mass using the area-length method.	Males > 104 g/m^2 Females > 90 g/m^2	
		Assess for valvular disease.	—[b]	—[b]
What are the consequences for the right heart?	RV shape	Visual assessment using parasternal short-axis and apical 4-chamber views	PSAX: Ventricular septal systolic flattening Circular RV shape Apical 4-chamber view: Rectangular RV shape Horizontal RV moderator band	Suggests RV pressure overload
	Eccentricity index	Ratio of AP to septolateral LV dimension in mid-PSAX view	>1.0	Suggests RV pressure overload
	RV dimensions	RV-focused 4-chamber view	>41 mm RV base >35 mm RV middle	—
	RV wall thickness	RV free wall in subcostal 4-chamber view	>5 mm	RV hypertrophy seen in chronic pressure overload
	RV fractional area change	RV-focused 4-chamber view	<35%	Impaired RV systolic function
	TAPSE	M-mode of lateral tricuspid annulus in RV focused 4-chamber view	<17 mm	Impaired RV systolic function

Continued

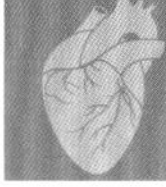

SUMMARY Suspected Pulmonary Hypertension—cont'd

Assessment	Measurements Performed	Method	Abnormal Values	Interpretation
	Tricuspid annular plane systolic velocity	Tissue Doppler imaging of lateral tricuspid annulus in RV focused 4-chamber view	<10 cm/s	Impaired RV systolic function
	RIMP	$\frac{IVRT + IVCT}{ET}$ using PW Doppler[b]	>0.44	Indicates systolic and diastolic RV dysfunction
	PVR	$10 \times \frac{TRV}{RVOT\ VTI} + 0.16$ *or* $5.19 \times \frac{TRV^2}{RVOT\ VTI} - 0.4$[b]	PVR > 3 WU Increased LA pressure decreases PVR	Suggests a precapillary PHT
	Stress echocardiography	RV-RA pressure gradient	>15-mmHg rise on low levels of exercise Failure to increase with exercise	Rapid rise of PASP with exercise suggests increased PVR. In patients with PHT, failure to increase with exercise suggests impaired RV contractile reserve.
		Measure P-Q slope[b]	Rise in RVSP > 3 mmHg/L/min	

[a]See Table 36.7 for formulas.
[b]Details are given in the text.
AP, Anteroposterior; *E:E′*, ratio of peak mitral inflow E velocity to the medial mitral annular tissue velocity; *ET*, ejection time; *IVC*, inferior vena cava; *IVCT*, isovolumetric contraction time; *IVRT*, isovolumetric relaxation time; *JVP*, jugular venous pulsation; *PAH*, pulmonary artery hypertension; *PAP*, pulmonary artery pressure; *PASP*, pulmonary artery systolic pressure; *PHT*, pulmonary hypertension; *PSAX*, parasternal short-axis view; *PVR*, pulmonary vascular resistance; *PW*, pulsed wave; *RAP*, estimated (or known) RA pressure; *RIMP*, RV index of myocardial performance; *RVOT VTI*, RV outlet tract velocity-time integral; *RVSP*, RV systolic pressure; *TAPSE*, tricuspid annular plane systolic excursion; *TRV*, tricuspid regurgitation velocity.

REFERENCES

1. Lam CS, Borlaug BA, Kane GC, Enders FT, Rodeheffer RJ, Redfield MM. Age-associated increases in pulmonary artery systolic pressure in the general population. *Circulation.* 2009;119:2663–2670.
2. Strange G, Playford D, Stewart S, et al. Pulmonary hypertension: prevalence and mortality in the Armadale echocardiography cohort. *Heart (British Cardiac Society).* 2012;98:1805–1811.
3. Simonneau G, Montani D, Celermajer DS, et al. Haemodynamic definitions and updated clinical classification of pulmonary hypertension. *Eur Respir J.* 2019;53(1):180–191.
4. Hatano SS, Strasser T, World Health Organization. *Primary Pulmonary Hypertension: Report on a WHO Meeting, Geneva, 15–17 October 1973.* World Health Organization; 1975.
5. Simonneau G, Gatzoulis MA, Adatia I, et al. Updated clinical classification of pulmonary hypertension. *J Am Coll Cardiol.* 2013;62:D34–D41.
6. Kovacs G, Berghold A, Scheidl S, Olschewski H. Pulmonary arterial pressure during rest and exercise in healthy subjects: a systematic review. *Eur Respir J.* 2009;34:888–894.
7. Maron BA, Hess E, Maddox TM, et al. Association of borderline pulmonary hypertension with mortality and hospitalization in a large patient cohort: insights from the Veterans Affairs clinical assessment, reporting, and tracking program. *Circulation.* 2016;133:1240–1248.
8. Strange G, Stewart S, Celermajer D, et al. Threshold of pulmonary hypertension associated with increased mortality. *J Am Coll Cardiol.* 2019;73(21):2660–2672.
9. Yock PG, Popp RL. Noninvasive estimation of right ventricular systolic pressure by Doppler ultrasound in patients with tricuspid regurgitation. *Circulation.* 1984;70:657–662.
10. Currie PJ, Seward JB, Chan K-L, et al. Continuous wave Doppler determination of right ventricular pressure: a simultaneous Doppler-catheterization study in 127 patients. *J Am Coll Cardiol.* 1985;6:750–756.
11. Abramson SV, Burke JB, Pauletto FJ, Kelly Jr JJ. Use of multiple views in the echocardiographic assessment of pulmonary artery systolic pressure. *J Am Soc Echocardiogr.* 1995;8:55–60.
12. Kyranis SJ, Latona J, Platts D, et al. Improving the echocardiographic assessment of pulmonary pressure using the tricuspid regurgitant signal—the "chin" vs the "beard. *Echocardiography.* 2018;35:1085–1096.
13. Chemla D, Castelain V, Humbert M, et al. New formula for predicting mean pulmonary artery pressure using systolic pulmonary artery pressure. *Chest.* 2004;126:1313–1317.
14. Parasuraman S, Walker S, Loudon BL, et al. Assessment of pulmonary artery pressure by echocardiography—a comprehensive review. *IJC Heart & Vasculature.* 2016;12:45–51.
15. Er F, Ederer S, Nia AM, et al. Accuracy of Doppler-echocardiographic mean pulmonary artery pressure for diagnosis of pulmonary hypertension. *PLoS One.* 2010;5. e15670.
16. Aduen JF, Castello R, Lozano MM, et al. An alternative echocardiographic method to estimate mean pulmonary artery pressure: diagnostic and clinical implications. *J Am Soc Echocardiogr.* 2009;22:814–819.
17. Jeon D-S, Luo H, Iwami T, et al. The usefulness of a 10% air-10% blood-80% saline mixture for contrast echocardiography: Doppler measurement of pulmonary artery systolic pressure. *J Am Coll Cardiol.* 2002;39:124–129.
18. Taleb M, Khuder S, Tinkel J, Khouri SJ. The diagnostic accuracy of Doppler echocardiography in assessment of pulmonary artery systolic pressure: a meta-analysis. *Echocardiography (Mount Kisco, NY).* 2013;30:258–265.
19. Rudski LG, Lai WW, Afilalo J, et al. Guidelines for the echocardiographic assessment of the right heart in adults: a report from the American Society of Echocardiography endorsed by the European Association of Echocardiography. *J Am Soc Echocardiogr.* 2010;23:685–713.
20. Boucly A, Weatherald J, Savale L, et al. Risk assessment, prognosis and guideline implementation in pulmonary arterial hypertension. *Eur Respir J.* 2017;50:1700889.

21. Berger M, Hecht SR, Van Tosh A, Lingam U. Pulsed and continuous wave Doppler echocardiographic assessment of valvular regurgitation in normal subjects. *J Am Coll Cardiol.* 1989;13:1540–1545.
22. Tossavainen E, Söderberg S, Grönlund C, et al. Pulmonary artery acceleration time in identifying pulmonary hypertension patients with raised pulmonary vascular resistance. *Eur Heart J Cardiovasc Imaging.* 2013;14:890–897.
23. Kitabatake A, Inoue M, Asao M, et al. Noninvasive evaluation of pulmonary hypertension by a pulsed Doppler technique. *Circulation.* 1983;68:302–309.
24. Opotowsky AR, Clair M, Afilalo J, et al. A simple echocardiographic method to estimate pulmonary vascular resistance. *Am J Cardiol.* 2013;112:873–882.
25. McQuillan BM, Picard MH, Leavitt M, Weyman AE. Clinical correlates and reference intervals for pulmonary artery systolic pressure among echocardiographically normal subjects. *Circulation.* 2001;104:2797–2802.
26. Phung S, Strange G, Chung LP, et al. Prevalence of pulmonary arterial hypertension in an Australian scleroderma population: screening allows for earlier diagnosis. *Intern Med J.* 2009;39:682–691.
27. Consensus statement on the management of pulmonary hypertension in clinical practice in the UK and Ireland. *Heart (British Cardiac Society).* 2008;94(suppl 1):i1–i41.
28. Manders E, Bogaard H-J, Handoko ML, et al. Contractile dysfunction of left ventricular cardiomyocytes in patients with pulmonary arterial hypertension. *J Am Coll Cardiol.* 2014;64:28–37.
29. Liu C, Chen J, Gao Y, Deng B, Liu K. Endothelin receptor antagonists for pulmonary arterial hypertension. *Cochrane Database Syst Rev.* 2013. Cd004434.
30. Channick RN, Sitbon O, Barst RJ, Manes A, Rubin LJ. Endothelin receptor antagonists in pulmonary arterial hypertension. *J Am Coll Cardiol.* 2004;43:62s–67s.
31. Raja SG. Endothelin receptor antagonists for pulmonary arterial hypertension: an overview. *Cardiovasc Ther.* 2010;28:e65–e71.
32. Pulido T, Adzerikho I, Channick RN, et al. Macitentan and morbidity and mortality in pulmonary arterial hypertension. *N Engl J Med.* 2013;369:809–818.
33. Galie N, Badesch D, Oudiz R, et al. Ambrisentan therapy for pulmonary arterial hypertension. *J Am Coll Cardiol.* 2005;46:529–535.
34. Engelfriet PM, Duffels MGJ, Möller T, et al. Pulmonary arterial hypertension in adults born with a heart septal defect: the Euro Heart Survey on adult congenital heart disease. *Heart (British Cardiac Society).* 2007;93:682–687.
35. van Riel ACMJ, Schuuring MJ, van Hessen ID, et al. Contemporary prevalence of pulmonary arterial hypertension in adult congenital heart disease following the updated clinical classification. *Int J Cardiol.* 2014;174:299–305.
36. Silversides CK, Salehian O, Oechslin E, et al. Canadian Cardiovascular Society 2009 Consensus Conference on the management of adults with congenital heart disease: complex congenital cardiac lesions. *Can J Cardiol.* 2010;26:e98–e117.
37. Schuuring MJ, Bouma BJ, Cordina R, et al. Treatment of segmental pulmonary artery hypertension in adults with congenital heart disease. *Int J Cardiol.* 2013;164:106–110.
38. Vachiéry J-L, Tedford RJ, Rosenkranz S, et al. Pulmonary hypertension due to left heart disease. *Eur Respir J.* 2019;53:1801897.
39. Kalra PR, Moon JC, Coats AJ. Do results of the ENABLE (Endothelin Antagonist Bosentan for Lowering Cardiac Events in Heart Failure) study spell the end for non-selective endothelin antagonism in heart failure? *Int J Cardiol.* 2002;85:195–197.
40. Bermejo J, Yotti R, Garcia-Orta R, et al. Sildenafil for improving outcomes in patients with corrected valvular heart disease and persistent pulmonary hypertension: a multicenter, double-blind, randomized clinical trial. *Eur Heart J.* 2018;39:1255–1264.
41. Hoendermis ES, Liu LC, Hummel YM, et al. Effects of sildenafil on invasive haemodynamics and exercise capacity in heart failure patients with preserved ejection fraction and pulmonary hypertension: a randomized controlled trial. *Eur Heart J.* 2015;36:2565–2573.
42. Lindman BR, Zajarias A, Madrazo JA, et al. Effects of phosphodiesterase type 5 inhibition on systemic and pulmonary hemodynamics and ventricular function in patients with severe symptomatic aortic stenosis. *Circulation.* 2012;125:2353–2362.
43. Cao JY, Wales KM, Cordina R, Lau EMT, Celermajer DS. Pulmonary vasodilator therapies are of no benefit in pulmonary hypertension due to left heart disease: a meta-analysis. *Int J Cardiol.* 2018;273:213–220.
44. Zhao L, Mason NA, Morrell NW, et al. Sildenafil inhibits hypoxia-induced pulmonary hypertension. *Circulation.* 2001;104:424–428.
45. Galiè N, Palazzini M, Leci E, Manes A. Current therapeutic approaches to pulmonary arterial hypertension. *Revista Española De Cardiología.* 2010;63:708–724.
46. Pepke-Zaba J, Ghofrani H-A, Hoeper MM. Medical management of chronic thromboembolic pulmonary hypertension. *Eur Respir Rev.* 2017;26:160107.
47. Lang I, Meyer BC, Ogo T, et al. Balloon pulmonary angioplasty in chronic thromboembolic pulmonary hypertension. *Eur Respir Rev.* 2017;26:160119.
48. Menon K, Sutphin PD, Bartolome S, Kalva SP, Ogo T. Chronic thromboembolic pulmonary hypertension: emerging endovascular therapy. *Cardiovasc Diagn Ther.* 2018;8:272–278.
49. La Gerche A, Claessen G. Right ventricular function: the barometer of all that *lies ahead. JACC Cardiovasc Imaging.* 2019;12(12):2386–2388.
50. Grünig E, Tiede H, Enyimayew EO, et al. Assessment and prognostic relevance of right ventricular contractile reserve in patients with severe pulmonary hypertension. *Circulation.* 2013;128:2005–2015.
51. Guazzi M, Dixon D, Labate V, et al. RV contractile function and its coupling to pulmonary circulation in heart failure with preserved ejection fraction: stratification of clinical phenotypes and outcomes. *JACC Cardiovasc Imaging.* 2017;10:1211–1221.
52. Tonelli AR, Arelli V, Minai OA, et al. Causes and circumstances of death in pulmonary arterial hypertension. *Am J Respir Crit Care Med.* 2013;188:365–369.
53. Lang RM, Badano LP, Mor-Avi V, et al. Recommendations for cardiac chamber quantification by echocardiography in adults: an update from the American Society of Echocardiography and the European Association of Cardiovascular Imaging. *Echocardiogr.* 2015;28:1–39. e14.
54. Forfia PR, Fisher MR, Mathai SC, et al. Tricuspid annular displacement predicts survival in pulmonary hypertension. *Am J Respir Crit Care Med.* 2006;174:1034–1041.
55. Ghio S, Klersy C, Magrini G, et al. Prognostic relevance of the echocardiographic assessment of right ventricular function in patients with idiopathic pulmonary arterial hypertension. *Int J Cardiol.* 2010;140:272–278.
56. Innelli P, Esposito R, Olibet M, Nistri S, Galderisi M. The impact of ageing on right ventricular longitudinal function in healthy subjects: a pulsed tissue Doppler study. *Eur J Echocardiogr.* 2009;10(4):491–498.
57. Shukla M, Park J-H, Thomas JD, et al. Prognostic value of right ventricular strain using speckle-tracking echocardiography in pulmonary hypertension: a systematic review and meta-analysis. *Can J Cardiol.* 2018;34:1069–1078.
58. van Kessel M, Seaton D, Chan J, et al. Prognostic value of right ventricular free wall strain in pulmonary hypertension patients with pseudo-normalized tricuspid annular plane systolic excursion values. *Int J Cardiovasc Imag.* 2016;32:905–912.
59. Sachdev A, Villarraga HR, Frantz RP, et al. Right ventricular strain for prediction of survival in patients with pulmonary arterial hypertension. *Chest.* 2011;139:1299–1309.
60. Tello K, Dalmer A, Vanderpool R, et al. Cardiac magnetic resonance imaging-based right ventricular strain analysis for assessment of coupling and diastolic function in pulmonary hypertension. *JACC Cardiovasc Imaging.* 2019;12(11 Pt 1):2155–2164.
61. Lisi M, Cameli M, Righini FM, et al. RV longitudinal deformation correlates with myocardial fibrosis in patients with end-stage heart failure. *Cardiovasc Imaging.* 2015;8:514–522.
62. Freed BH, Tsang W, Bhave NM, et al. Right ventricular strain in pulmonary arterial hypertension: a 2D echocardiography and cardiac magnetic resonance study. *Echocardiography (Mount Kisco, NY).* 2015;32:257–263.
63. da Costa Junior AA, Ota-Arakaki JS, Ramos RP, et al. Diagnostic and prognostic value of right ventricular strain in patients with pulmonary arterial hypertension and relatively preserved functional capacity studied with echocardiography and magnetic resonance. *Int J Cardiovasc Imag.* 2017;33:39–46.
64. Li Y, Wang Y, Meng X, Zhu W, Lu X. Assessment of right ventricular longitudinal strain by 2D speckle tracking imaging compared with RV function and hemodynamics in pulmonary hypertension. *Int J Cardiovasc Imag.* 2017;33:1737–1748.
65. Kemal HS, Kayikcioglu M, Kultursay H, et al. Right ventricular free-wall longitudinal speckle tracking strain in patients with pulmonary arterial hypertension under specific treatment. *Echocardiography (Mount Kisco, NY).* 2017;34:530–536.
66. Moceri P, Duchateau N, Baudouy D, et al. Three-dimensional right-ventricular regional deformation and survival in pulmonary hypertension. *Eur Heart J Cardiovasc Imaging.* 2018;19:450–458.
67. Kovacs G, Olschewski A, Berghold A, Olschewski H. Pulmonary vascular resistances during exercise in normal subjects: a systematic review. *Eur Respir J.* 2012;39:319–328.
68. Abbas AE, Fortuin FD, Patel B, Moreno CA, Schiller NB, Lester SJ. Noninvasive measurement of systemic vascular resistance using Doppler echocardiography. *Echocardiogr.* 2004;17:834–838.

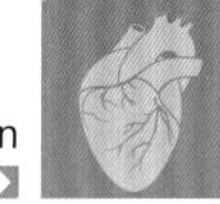

69. Abbas AE, Franey LM, Marwick T, et al. Noninvasive assessment of pulmonary vascular resistance by Doppler echocardiography. *J Am Soc Echocardiogr*. 2013;26:1170–1177.
70. Tedford RJ, Hassoun PM, Mathai SC, et al. Pulmonary capillary wedge pressure augments right ventricular pulsatile loading. *Circulation*. 2012;125:289–297.
71. Sorajja P, Nishimura RA. Measurement of pulmonary pressures and pulmonary resistance: is Doppler ready for prime time? *J Am Soc Echocardiogr*. 2013;26:1178–1179.
72. Scalia GM, Scalia IG, Kierle R, et al. ePLAR - the echocardiographic Pulmonary to Left Atrial Ratio - a novel non-invasive parameter to differentiate pre-capillary and post-capillary pulmonary hypertension. *Int J Cardiol*. 2016;212:379–386.
73. D'Andrea A, Naeije R, D'Alto M, et al. Range in pulmonary artery systolic pressure among highly trained athletes. *Chest*. 2011;139:788–794.
74. Argiento P. Exercise stress echocardiography of the pulmonary circulation: limits of normal and sex differences. *Chest*. 2012;142:1158–1165.
75. Collins N. Abnormal pulmonary vascular responses in patients registered with a systemic autoimmunity database: pulmonary hypertension assessment and screening evaluation using stress echocardiography (PHASE-I). *Eur J Echocardiogr*. 2006;7:439–446.
76. Talreja DR, Nishimura RA, Oh JK. Estimation of left ventricular filling pressure with exercise by Doppler echocardiography in patients with normal systolic function: a simultaneous echocardiographic-cardiac catheterization study. *J Am Soc Echocardiogr*. 2007;20:477–479.
77. Egstrup M, Gustafsson I, Andersen MJ, et al. Haemodynamic response during low-dose dobutamine infusion in patients with chronic systolic heart failure: comparison of echocardiographic and invasive measurements. *Eur Heart J Cardiovasc Imaging*. 2013;14:659–667.
78. Collins N, Bastian B, Quiqueree L, Jones C, Morgan R, Reeves G. Abnormal pulmonary vascular responses in patients registered with a systemic autoimmunity database: pulmonary hypertension assessment and screening evaluation using stress echocardiography (PHASE-I). *Eur J Echocardiogr*. 2006;7:439–446.
79. Ha JW, Choi D, Park S, et al. Determinants of exercise-induced pulmonary hypertension in patients with normal left ventricular ejection fraction. *Heart (British Cardiac Society)*. 2009;95:490–494.
80. Mahjoub H, Levy F, Cassol M, et al. Effects of age on pulmonary artery systolic pressure at rest and during exercise in normal adults. *Eur J Echocardiogr*. 2009;10:635–640.
81. Claeys M, Claessen G, La Gerche A, et al. Impaired cardiac reserve and abnormal vascular load limit exercise capacity in chronic thromboembolic disease. *JACC Cardiovasc Imaging*. 2019;12(8 Pt 1):1444–1456.
82. Lau EMT, Vanderpool RR, Choudhary P, et al. Dobutamine stress echocardiography for the assessment of pressure-flow relationships of the pulmonary circulation. *Chest*. 2014;146: 959–966.
83. Naeije R, Vanderpool R, Dhakal BP, et al. Exercise-induced pulmonary hypertension: physiological basis and methodological concerns. *Am J Respir Crit Care Med*. 2013;187:576–583.
84. Lewis GD, Bossone E, Naeije R, et al. Pulmonary vascular hemodynamic response to exercise in cardiopulmonary diseases. *Circulation*. 2013;128:1470–1479.
85. Lam CS. Age-associated increases in pulmonary artery systolic pressure in the general population. *Circulation*. 2009;119:2663–2670.
86. Grossman A, Prokupetz A, Benderly M, Wand O, Assa A, Kalter-Leibovici O. Pulmonary artery pressure in young healthy subjects. *J Am Soc Echocardiogr*. 2012;25:357–360.

中文导读

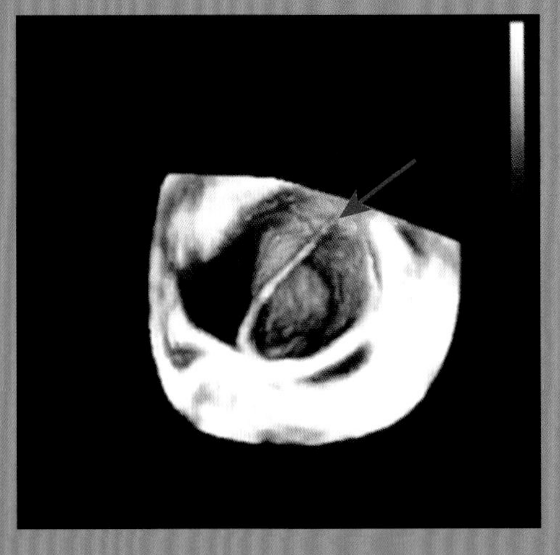

第37章 以免疫介导损伤为特征的系统性疾病

风湿免疫性疾病通过免疫介导机制引起继发性心血管损伤，尤其是自身免疫性结缔组织病、系统性血管炎累及心血管系统的发病率较高。常见风湿免疫性疾病主要有累及心内结构的系统性红斑狼疮、抗磷脂综合征、类风湿性关节炎、强直性脊柱炎、硬皮病和皮肌炎等自身免疫性结缔组织病；累及主动脉及主要分支的系统性血管炎，如多发性大动脉炎、巨细胞性动脉炎和贝赫切特综合征。此类疾病可引起心血管系统损伤，如无菌性心内膜炎（非炎症性疣状赘生物）、大动脉和冠状动脉粥样硬化、舒张性心力衰竭、无菌性心包炎、肺动脉高压和反复难治性大动脉炎等病变。该类疾病在超声心动图、CT、MRI和心血管造影等影像学上均具有独特的特点。本章详细描述了此类疾病特征的影像学特点及其形成的病理机制，与传统心血管疾病的影像学鉴别要点，并比较了以上几种影像技术在诊断中的优劣，简单介绍了疾病最新治疗方案、疾病转归和预后情况。

戴　莹

37 Systemic Diseases Characterized by Immune-Mediated Injury

CARLOS A. ROLDAN, MD

Rheumatologic diseases are chronic inflammatory states caused by autoimmunity. They are more common in women than in men (with the exception of ankylosing spondylitis and Behçet disease), and they usually manifest between the second and fifth decade.

Cardiovascular involvement is common in rheumatologic diseases and causes significant morbidity and mortality. Estimates of the prevalence of cardiovascular involvement vary widely because of differences in study design, study populations, and methods of cardiac evaluation (Table 37.1). Echocardiography plays a major role in understanding the prevalence, incidence, characteristics, severity, evolution, prognosis, and response to therapy of the cardiovascular diseases associated with rheumatologic diseases.

SYSTEMIC LUPUS ERYTHEMATOSUS

BACKGROUND

The most important and characteristic form of cardiac involvement in systemic lupus erythematosus (SLE) is Libman-Sacks endocarditis. Cardiovascular disease is the third most common cause of death in SLE, after infectious and renal disease. Independent predictors of cardiovascular disease include duration, age at onset, activity and severity of SLE, antiphospholipid antibodies, and corticosteroid therapy.

CARDIOVASCULAR INVOLVEMENT

Valve Disease and Thromboembolism

The typical valve disease in SLE is Libman-Sacks endocarditis, which is characterized by Libman-Sacks vegetations.[1] The pathogenesis of Libman-Sacks endocarditis includes an immune complex–mediated inflammation exacerbated by associated increased thrombogenesis.[1,2] Active Libman-Sacks vegetations have central myxoid degeneration, fibrinoid necrosis, and hemorrhages surrounded by polymorphonuclear cell inflammation; platelet and fibrin thrombi occur peripherally.

Healed vegetations are those with fibroblastic proliferation, central fibrosis, neovascularization, and minimal to no inflammation. Peripherally, there are organized and partially or fully endothelialized thrombi or no thrombi. Mixed vegetations have intermixed areas of activity and healing and superimposed thrombi with various degrees of organization and endothelialization (Fig. 37.1).

Echocardiographic studies using two-dimensional (2D) and three-dimensional (3D) transesophageal echocardiography (TEE) have characterized Libman-Sacks vegetations as predominantly affecting the mitral and aortic valves. They are usually smaller than 1 cm in diameter; are sessile, oval or tubular, protuberant, or coalescent; are more often heterogeneously echoreflectant; are located on the leaflets' coaptation point (atrial side of mitral leaflets and ventricular side of aortic cusps) but frequently extend through the leaflets into the opposite side; and usually are associated with some degree of leaflet thickening and valve regurgitation or rarely with valve stenosis[1] (Fig. 37.2; see Fig. 37.1). Rarely, vegetations are seen on the right-sided heart valves, atrial or ventricular endocardium, mitral or tricuspid subvalvular apparatus, or aortic root (Fig. 37.3).

The estimated prevalence of Libman-Sacks vegetations is less than 15% with transthoracic echocardiography (TTE) and 35% to 45% with TEE.[1,3] With TEE as the standard, TTE has a very low sensitivity and a low negative predictive value for detection of vegetations (11% and 57%, respectively).[3] Compared with 2D TEE, 3D TEE detects more vegetations and determines larger sizes of vegetations; better defines the location, extent, shape, and appearance of vegetations; more often detects associated valve commissural fusion; and detects a higher frequency of vegetations in patients with cerebrovascular disease (Table 37.2).[4]

TEE is the most accurate diagnostic method for detecting Libman-Sacks endocarditis, but it is semi-invasive and has potential risks. Preliminary data suggest that acute stroke or transient ischemic attack (TIA), SLE with a duration of 12 years

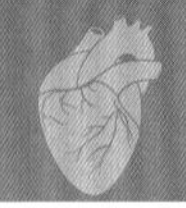

TABLE 37.1 Cardiovascular Involvement in Rheumatologic Diseases.

Disease	Type of Involvement	Frequency (%)[a]	Key Characteristics
Systemic lupus erythematosus (SLE)	Libman-Sacks vegetations	10–45	Characteristic of, but not exclusive to, SLE Inflammatory, thrombotic, or mixed vegetations commonly resolve or significantly improve with antithrombotic and antiinflammatory therapy. Vegetations are a high cardioembolic substrate, most commonly (50%–80%) to the brain.
	Leaflet fibrosis	30–50	Commonly diffuse Associated calcification is uncommon.
	Valve regurgitation (usually mild to moderate)	30–50	Can be severe with acute valvulitis or with overimposed infection Valve stenosis is rare (<3%).
	Coronary artery disease (CAD)		
	Functional	25–50	Involves small and medium-sized vessels Abnormal coronary vasodilation or microvascular disease Microvascular thrombosis is uncommon.
	Atherosclerotic	10–30	Nonobstructive or obstructive epicardial atherosclerosis, exacerbated by increased vasospasm or thrombosis
	Arteritis, coronary thromboembolism, or in situ thrombosis without atherosclerosis	Rare	Respectively, arteritis with severely active disease, Libman-Sacks vegetations, or increased levels of antiphospholipid antibodies
	Myocardial infarction	<10	From obstructive or nonobstructive epicardial atherosclerosis exacerbated by vasospasm and/or thrombogenesis, and rarely by embolism or arteritis
	Diastolic dysfunction[b]	15–35	Predominantly subclinical decreased global myocardial strain and strain rate and impaired LV relaxation
	Myocarditis or cardiomyopathy	1–20	Primary myocarditis is associated with cellular antigen Ro (SS-A) and La (SS-B) antibodies May mimic an acute coronary syndrome Chloroquine-induced type is rare.
	Pericarditis	10–50	Antinuclear antibodies in pericardial fluid are diagnostic but not always present. Tamponade or constriction is rare.
	Asymptomatic effusion	2–20	Caused by mild pericarditis, hypoalbuminemia, or cor pulmonale
	Pulmonary hypertension	5–15	Caused by interstitial lung disease, vasculitis, and thromboembolism
Primary antiphospholipid syndrome (PAPS)	Valve vegetations	10–30	All valve abnormalities, especially valve vegetations, have similar characteristics and evolution as those of SLE. They are predominantly thrombotic but can be inflammatory or mixed. Vegetations also change in appearance, resolve, or reappear over time.
	Valve thickening	40–60	Similar characteristics as those of SLE
	Valve regurgitation	30–40	Similar characteristics as those of SLE
	Pulmonary hypertension	20–25	More commonly the result of pulmonary emboli, but pulmonary vasoconstriction or obstructive vasculopathy can occur.
	CAD	20–30	Predominantly functional microvascular disease
	Myocardial disease	15–30	Rarely primary inflammatory Most commonly diastolic dysfunction from microvascular CAD
Rheumatoid arthritis	CAD	40–60	—
	Functional	25–50	Abnormal coronary vasodilation or microvascular CAD two to four times more common than in the general population. Predominantly subclinical
	Atherosclerotic	>40	Commonly subclinical as detected with electron-beam CT, but moderate to severe obstructive disease is common.
	Arteritis	Uncommon	Difficult to diagnose clinically
	Myocardial infarction	10–15	Most commonly the result of epicardial atherosclerosis; rarely, coronary vasospasm, in situ thrombosis, embolism, or arteritis
	Pericarditis	≤10	Occurs in patients with active disease, high rheumatoid factor level, and nodular disease Pericardial fluid can have rheumatoid factor.
	Asymptomatic effusion	≈25	—
	Leaflet fibrosis	>30	Indistinguishable from that of SLE.
	Valve nodules	≈10	Characteristic of rheumatoid arthritis
	Valve regurgitation, mild or worse	≥25%	—
	Myocarditis or cardiomyopathy	<10	Amyloid deposition and chloroquine-induced types are rare.
	Diastolic dysfunction[b]	30–75	Predominantly subclinical decreased global myocardial strain and strain rate and impaired LV relaxation
	Pulmonary hypertension	≈20	—
Ankylosing spondylitis	Proximal aortitis or valvulitis	20–60	Root sclerosis extending to base of anterior mitral leaflet and root dilation are characteristic.
	Aortic regurgitation, mild or worse	10–40	Decreased anterior mitral leaflet mobility, also causes mitral regurgitation
	Subaortic bump	10–40	Characteristic of the disease
	Conduction system disease	>20	Results from extension of aortic root/annulus sclerosis into the proximal septum and atrioventricular node
	Diastolic dysfunction[b]	10–45	Predominantly subclinical decreased global myocardial strain and strain rate and impaired LV relaxation

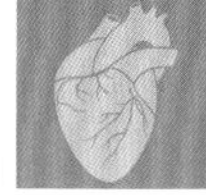

TABLE 37.1 **Cardiovascular Involvement in Rheumatologic Diseases.—cont'd**

Disease	*Type of Involvement*	*Frequency (%)*[a]	*Key Characteristics*
	Pericarditis	<5	Primary immune-mediated type is uncommon.
	Asymptomatic effusion	<5	—
	Myocarditis or cardiomyopathy	<5	Primary immune-mediated myocarditis is rare.
Scleroderma	CAD		
	Functional	≈60	Predominantly vasospastic or coronary Raynaud phenomenon
	Atherosclerotic	<30	—
	Myocarditis or cardiomyopathy	10–50	Most commonly related to recurrent intramyocardial ischemia/necrosis/fibrosis Inflammatory type is uncommon.
	Diastolic dysfunction[b]	30–50	Affects the LV and RV; predominates as subclinical decreased global myocardial strain and strain rate–impaired LV relaxation
	Pulmonary hypertension	35–50	Caused by pulmonary fibrosis, vasculitis, vasospasm, or left heart disease
	Pericarditis	5–20	—
	Asymptomatic effusion	30–40	—
	Valve disease	<10	Nonspecific
Polymyositis/ dermatomy-ositis	Myocarditis or cardiomyopathy	>25	Primary myocarditis is more common in patients with myositis. Diastolic dysfunction occurs in 10%–40% of patients.
	Pericarditis	≈10	More common in children and in overlap syndrome
	Asymptomatic effusion	5–25	—
	CAD	≈20	Microvascular disease is most common. Commonly nonobstructive, atherosclerotic Arteritis is rare.
	Valve disease	Unknown	Nonspecific. Libman-Sacks–like vegetations are rare.

[a]Rates may vary because of differences in patient population characteristics, study design, or diagnostic methods.
[b]Defined by Doppler and speckle-tracking echocardiographic criteria.

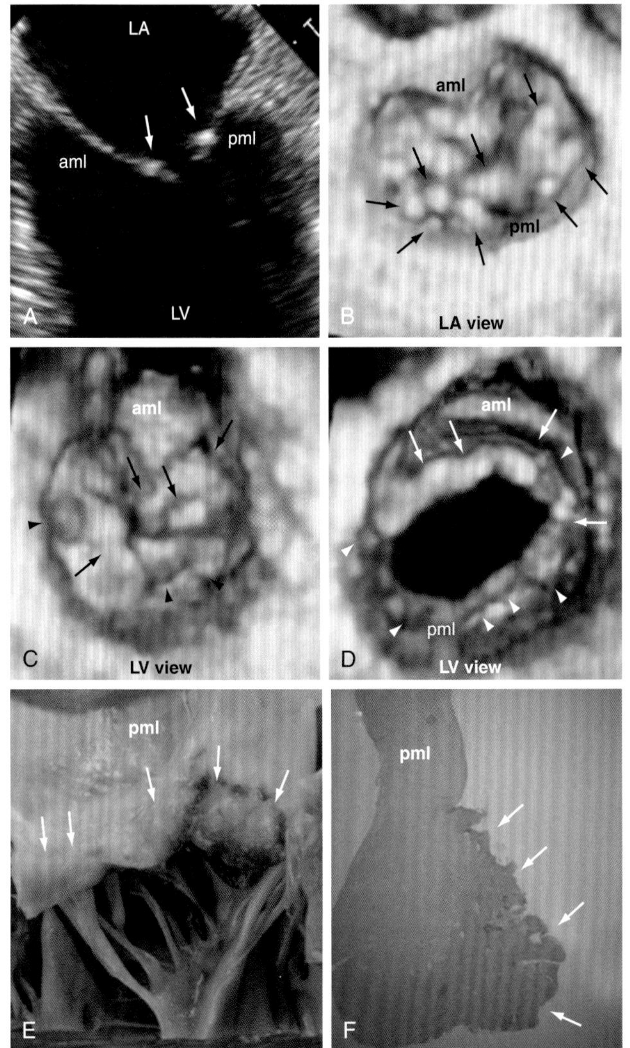

Fig. 37.1 Libman-Sacks endocarditis of the mitral valve. (A) 2D TEE close-up view of the mitral valve in a 26-year-old woman with systemic lupus erythematosus with past stroke and acute transient ischemic attack demonstrates small, sessile, and homogeneously hyperreflectant oval nodularities *(arrows)*, consistent with healed Libman-Sacks vegetations. They are located on the LA side and on the distal portions of the anterior *(aml)* and posterior *(pml)* mitral leaflets and are associated with mild leaflet thickening and severely decreased mobility, predominantly of the posterior mitral leaflet (see Video 37.1A). (B) 3D TEE LA view of the mitral valve during systole demonstrates small- to medium-sized, protruding, sessile, oval, and homogeneously echoreflectant nodularities *(arrows)*, located predominantly at the tips of both leaflets and involving all scallops (see Video 37.1B). (C) 3D TEE LV view of the mitral valve during systole demonstrates multiple, small- to medium-sized, homogeneously echoreflectant nodularities *(arrows)* protruding from the LA side into the LV side and located mainly at the tips of both mitral leaflets. It also shows three small to medium-sized, oval and tubular, sessile, and brown discolored vegetations located on the tip and commissural portions of the P3, tip of the P2, and tip of the P1 scallops *(arrowheads)*, suggestive of recently formed vegetations (see Video 37.1C). (D) 3D TEE LV view of the mitral valve during diastole demonstrates (1) multiple nodularities with homogeneous *(arrows)* and heterogeneous *(arrowheads)* echoreflectance along the tips of both mitral leaflets; (2) decreased mobility of both leaflets, with fixed P1 and P2 scallops; and (3) a mild degree of anterolateral commissural fusion *(horizontal arrow)* (see Video 37.1C). (E) The middle scallop of the posterior mitral leaflet demonstrates sessile, granular, protruding, grayish to brown discolored, clustered, and coalescent Libman-Sacks vegetations *(arrows)* located on the coaptation point, predominantly on the LA side and extending through the leaflet into the LV side. (F) Hematoxylin and eosin staining of a histopathologic section of the posterior mitral leaflet demonstrates diffuse thickening, predominantly of the leaflet tip, with a well-adhered vegetation mainly on the LA side *(arrows)* but also extending to the LV side, where it appears organized and endothelialized

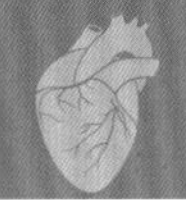

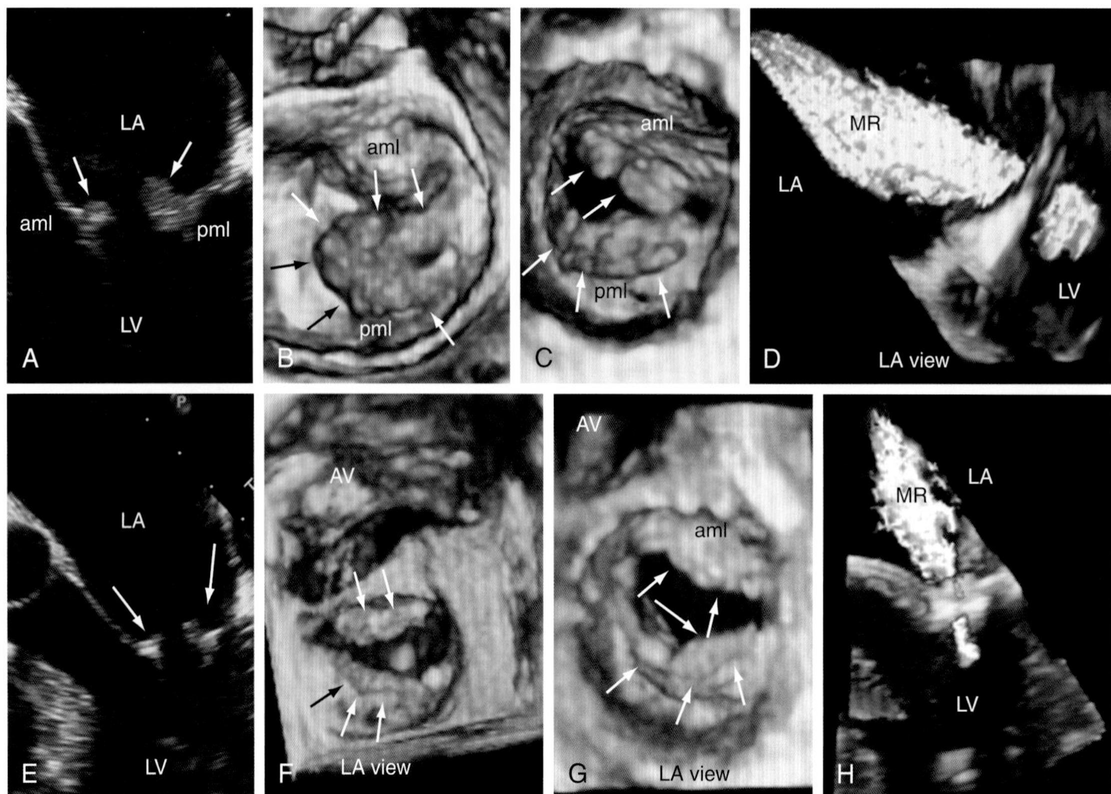

Fig. 37.2 Echocardiographic views of Libman-Sacks endocarditis of the mitral valve. (A) 2D TEE close-up view of the mitral valve demonstrates medium- to large-sized, oval-shaped, sessile, and homogeneously soft tissue echoreflectant Libman-Sacks vegetations on the LA side and on distal portions of the anterior *(aml)* and posterior *(pml)* mitral leaflets *(arrows)*, associated with mild leaflet tip thickening and decreased mobility. 3D TEE LA view during systole (B) and LV view during diastole (C) of the mitral valve demonstrate large, severely protruding vegetations with an irregular and nodular surface, a tubular and multilobed shape, and a roll-like motion (moving from the LA to the LV side during diastole), located on the LA side and tips of the entire anterior and posterior mitral leaflets *(arrows)*, with associated decreased mobility and incomplete coaptation of the leaflets. (D) Associated severe mitral regurgitation is demonstrated by color Doppler. Corresponding follow-up 2D (E), 3D LA (F), 3D LV (G), and color Doppler (H) images show remarkable improvement *(arrows)* in the size of the mitral valve vegetations and reduction in the degree of mitral regurgitation to mild to moderate after 6 months of immunosuppressive antiinflammatory and dual antiplatelet therapy (see Videos 37.2A–H).

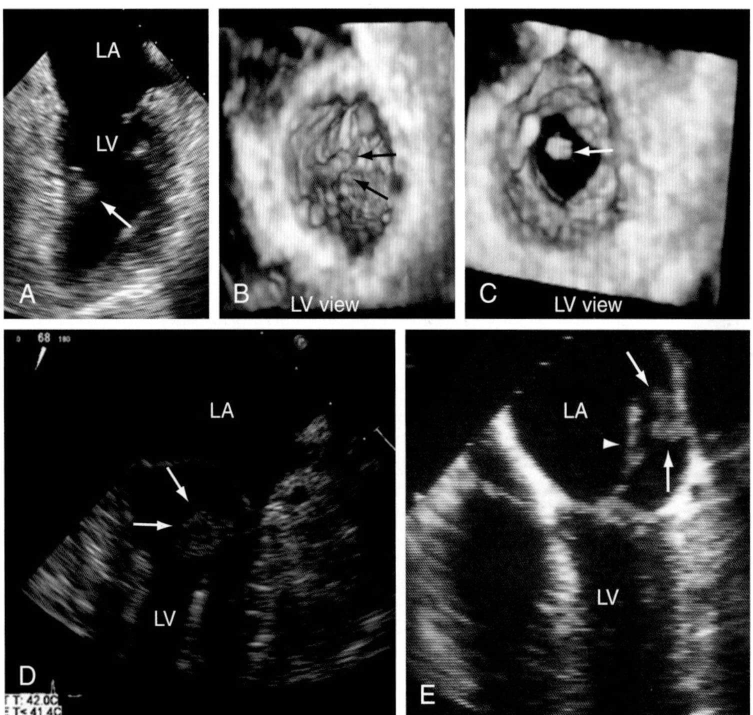

Fig. 37.3 Nonvalvular Libman-Sacks vegetations in systemic lupus erythematosus. (A) 2D TEE 2-chamber view in a 26-year-old woman with systemic lupus erythematosus (SLE), previous stroke, and acute transient ischemic attack demonstrates a large-sized, oval-shaped, and homogeneously soft tissue echoreflectant mass suggesting a recently formed vegetation *(arrow)* located on the posteromedial LV wall and apparently extending into the chordae tendineae. (B) 3D TEE LV view demonstrates a large-sized, tubular-shaped vegetation *(arrows)* attached to the posteromedial LV wall and extending toward the chordal apparatus. (C) 3D TEE LV view of the subvalvular mitral valve apparatus demonstrates a medium-sized chordal vegetation *(arrow)* in addition to multiple nodularities (probably healed and active vegetations) on the tip portions of both mitral leaflets. (D) 2D TEE commissural view in a 32-year-old woman with SLE and acute stroke demonstrates a large-sized, oval-shaped, homogeneously soft tissue echoreflectant vegetation *(arrows)* attached to the basal anterolateral wall of the LV. (E) 2D TEE 4-chamber view in a 23-year-old woman with SLE and acute stroke demonstrates a large vegetation with soft tissue echoreflectance and irregular borders attached to the LA lateral wall *(arrows)*. Notice also the very large, elongated, hypermobile, soft tissue echoreflectant vegetations *(arrowhead)* located at the coaptation point and on the atrial side of the anterior mitral leaflets (the video shows vegetations on the anterior and posterior mitral leaflets). Severe thickening and decreased mobility, predominantly of the leaflet tips, are also present (see Videos 37.3A–E).

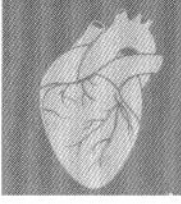

TABLE 37.2 Detection and Characterization of Libman-Sacks Vegetations by 3D and 2D TEE.

Valve	*3D TEE* N = *40*	*2D TEE* N = *40*	P *Value*
Studies With Vegetations			
Mitral valve	18 (45%)	14 (35%)	0.046[a]
Aortic valve	19 (48%)	12 (30%)	0.008[a]
Either valve	26 (65%)	20 (50%)	0.01[a]
Number of Vegetations			
Mitral valve	59 (1.48)	42 (1.05)	0.09[b]
Aortic valve	31 (0.78)	15 (0.38)	<0.001[b]
Either valve	90 (2.25)	57 (1.43)	0.001[b]
Size of Vegetations			
Mitral valve	9.16 ± 5.76	5.3 ± 4.15	0.03[c]
Aortic valve	5.59 ± 1.61	3.9 ± 1.26	0.005[c]
Location of Vegetations			
Anterior mitral leaflet	35 (0.88)	19 (0.48)	0.02[d]
Anterolateral (A1, P1) or posteromedial (A3, P3) scallops	26 (0.65)	12 (0.30)	0.046[d]
LV side or both atrial and ventricular sides of mitral leaflets (protruding through)	11 (0.28)	6 (0.15)	0.04[d]
Involving two or three contiguous scallops	15 (0.38)	7 (0.18)	0.03[d]
Left coronary cusp	9 (0.23)	3 (0.08)	0.05[d]
Noncoronary cusp	14 (0.35)	5 (0.13)	0.002[d]
Coronary cusps tip	18 (0.45)	8 (0.20)	0.009[d]
Coronary cusps margin	10 (0.25)	2 (0.05)	0.004[d]
Ventricular to aortic side (protruding through)	11 (28%)	1 (3%)	0.02[d]
Aortic side or both aortic and ventricular sides	16 (40%)	3 (8%)	0.01[d]
Commissural Fusion			
Anterolateral commissure	5 (13%)	2 (5%)	0.08
Posteromedial commissure	6 (15%)	1 (3%)	0.03
Either mitral valve commissure	8 (20%)	2 (5%)	0.01
Any aortic valve commissure	4 (10%)	0	0.08
Any mitral or aortic valve commissure	12 (30%)	2 (5%)	0.002

[a]Paired comparisons by the McNemar test; number and percentage of studies with vegetations.
[b]Paired comparisons by Poisson regression; number of vegetations and mean number per study.
[c]Paired comparisons by paired *t*-test; mean diameter (mm) ± standard deviation.
[d]Number of vegetations in each location and mean number of vegetations per study; all *P* values by Poisson regression.
Adapted from Roldan CA, Tolstrup K, Macias L, et al. Libman-Sacks endocarditis: detection, characterization, and clinical correlates by three-dimensional transesophageal echocardiography. *J Am Soc Echocardiogr*. 2015;28:770–779.

or longer without a stroke or TIA, or SLE with a duration of 5 years or longer and age of 32 years or older without stroke or TIA provides high sensitivity (85%), specificity (81%), and positive and negative predictive values (both 83%) for detection of Libman-Sacks endocarditis on TEE.[5]

Embolic cerebrovascular disease is the most common complication of Libman-Sacks endocarditis. A multimodality imaging study using 2D TEE demonstrated that patients with vegetations, compared with patients without vegetations, have more cerebromicroembolisms per hour, lower cerebral perfusion, greater brain injury, more strokes and TIAs, and greater neurocognitive dysfunction. Valve vegetations are a strong independent risk factor for stroke and TIA, neurocognitive dysfunction, focal brain lesions, and all three outcomes combined. Patients with vegetations also have reduced event-free survival time to stroke or TIA, cognitive disability, or death (Table 37.3 and Figs. 37.4 and 37.5; see Fig. 37.2).[6]

Left-sided vegetations embolize to peripheral arteries and rarely to the coronary and visceral arteries. Right-sided lesions can embolize to the lungs or cause paradoxical embolism. Libman-Sacks endocarditis can also be complicated by severe valve regurgitation that results from recurrent or acute valvulitis; noninfective valvulitic perforations, including bioprosthetic leaflets; noninfective mitral valve chordal rupture; or overimposed infective endocarditis.[7,8] Patients with moderate to severe valve dysfunction have a threefold to fourfold higher rate of valve surgery and death compared with patients without valve disease or only mild valve disease.

There is no expert consensus or guidelines about the medical treatment of Libman-Sacks endocarditis.[9] Recent data suggest that antiinflammatory and anti-thrombotic therapies resolve or significantly improve Libman-Sacks endocarditis and its associated embolic cerebrovascular disease[6,10] (Table 37.4; see Figs. 37.2, 37.4, and 37.5). Although valve surgery may be beneficial in selected cases, it is associated with three to five times higher morbidity and mortality rates than for non-SLE patients and should be deferred until failure of medical therapy.[11–13] However, medical therapy alone and medical versus surgical therapy needs to be studied in randomized, controlled trials.

Although Libman-Sacks endocarditis has a distinctive echocardiographic appearance, some of its characteristics may overlap with those of thrombotic and infective vegetations, acute or chronic rheumatic valve disease, degenerative valve disease, and Lambl excrescences (Table 37.5).[1,6,14]

TABLE 37.3 **Association of Libman-Sacks Vegetations With Cerebrovascular Disease.**

Abnormality	*Patients With Vegetations (N = 39)*	*Patients Without Vegetations (N = 37)*	*P Value*
Microembolism			
Right or left MCA microemboli	12 (31%) 21 events/56.6 h	5 (14%) 7 events/55 h	Adjusted hazard ratio[a] = 3.0. $P = 0.01$
NPSLE,[b] *n* (%)			
Acute stroke/TIA	22 (56%)	1 (3%)	<0.001
Acute overall NPSLE	26 (67%)	4 (11%)	<0.001
Neurocognitive Z Scores, Mean ± SD			
Attention	−2.36 ± 3.00	−0.82 ± 0.91	0.02[c]
Memory	−1.75 ± 1.27	−0.79 ± 1.00	0.001[c]
Processing speed	−1.90 ± 1.92	−0.90 ± 1.15	0.04[c]
Executive function	−3.31 ± 3.60	−1.68 ± 2.53	0.03[c]
Motor function	−4.38 ± 7.40	−1.40 ± 1.54	0.005[c]
Global	−2.42 ± 2.32	−1.17 ± 0.98	0.01[d]
Focal Brain Lesions, *n* (%)			
Focal brain lesions	28 (72%)	12/36 (34%)[e]	<0.001
Cerebral infarcts	14 (36%)	0/36	<0.001
White matter lesions	25/37 (68%)	12/36 (34%)	0.005

[a]Poisson regression with repeated measures adjusting for patent foramen ovale, interatrial septal aneurysm, carotid or aortic atherosclerosis, and antiphospholipid antibodies.
[b]NPSLE includes stroke, TIA, acute confusional state, cognitive dysfunction, or seizures.
[c]Wilcoxon Rank Sum test.
[d]$P = 0.02$ after simultaneously adjusting for age, depression index, premorbid intelligence, and education.
[e]One of the patients without vegetations had no MRI due to claustrophobia.
MCA, Middle cerebral artery; *NPSLE,* neuropsychiatric systemic lupus erythematosus; *TIA,* transient ischemic attack; *SD,* standard deviation.
Adapted from Roldan CA, Sibbitt WL Jr, Qualls CR, et al. Libman-Sacks endocarditis and embolic cerebrovascular disease. *JACC Cardiovasc Imaging.* 2013;6:973–983.

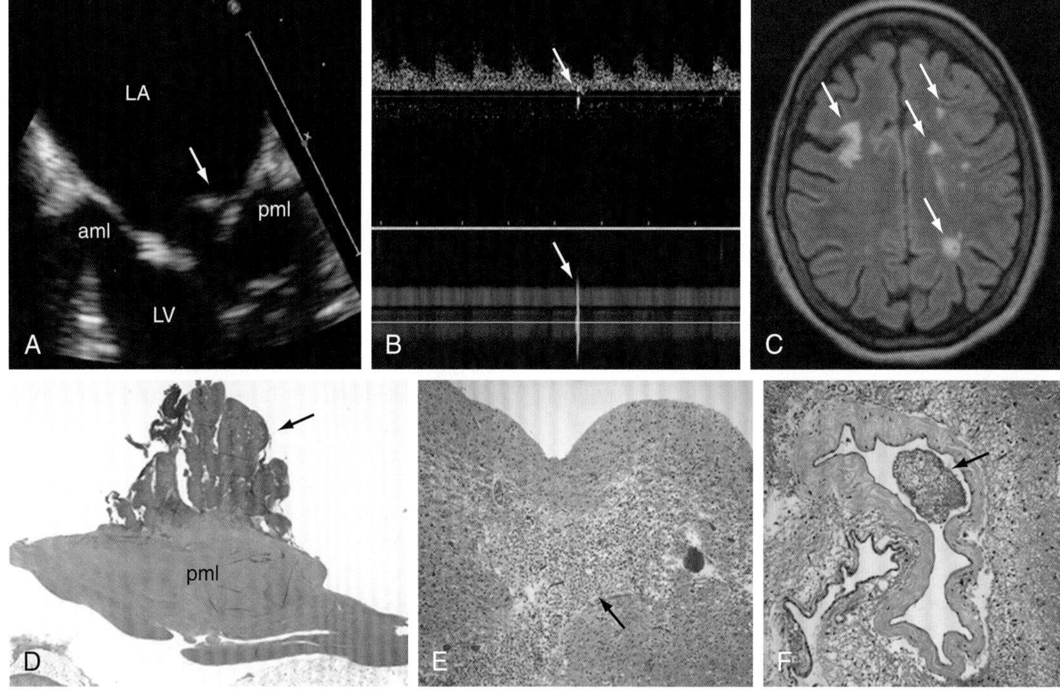

Fig. 37.4 Libman-Sacks endocarditis and embolic cerebrovascular disease. (A) 2D TEE view in a 55-year-old woman with systemic lupus erythematosus and transient ischemic attack demonstrates a moderate-sized, elongated, sessile, and heterogeneously echoreflectant Libman-Sacks vegetation *(arrow)* on the LA side of the posterior mitral leaflet *(pml)*. There is moderate thickening and sclerosis with decreased mobility of the middle and distal portions of the anterior *(aml)* and posterior mitral leaflets (see Video 37.4A). (B) Transcranial Doppler image demonstrates a microembolic signal on spectral Doppler *(upper arrow)* and within the vessel lumen *(lower arrow)* traveling through the left middle cerebral artery (red power M-mode) and anterior communicating artery (blue power M-mode). (C) Brain magnetic resonance imaging demonstrates multiple, bilateral, periventricular and deep white matter cerebral infarcts of various sizes *(arrows)*. The global neurocognitive Z score was indicative of severe neurocognitive dysfunction. (D) Hematoxylin and eosin staining (H&E 40×) demonstrates thickening and fibrosis of the posterior mitral leaflet with a well-adhered, verrucous, fibrinous vegetation *(arrow)*. (E) H&E staining (20×) reveals a subacute cerebral infarct at the junction of the white and gray matter with necrotic debris and moderate cellular infiltration *(arrow)*. (F) H&E staining (100×) demonstrates a large cerebral vessel with fibrin thrombi *(arrow)*. Multiple subacute and old microinfarcts were demonstrated in both cerebral hemispheres, along with a fibrin-thrombosed microvasculature with neoangiogenesis characteristic of chronic cardiothromboembolic disease.

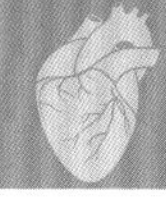

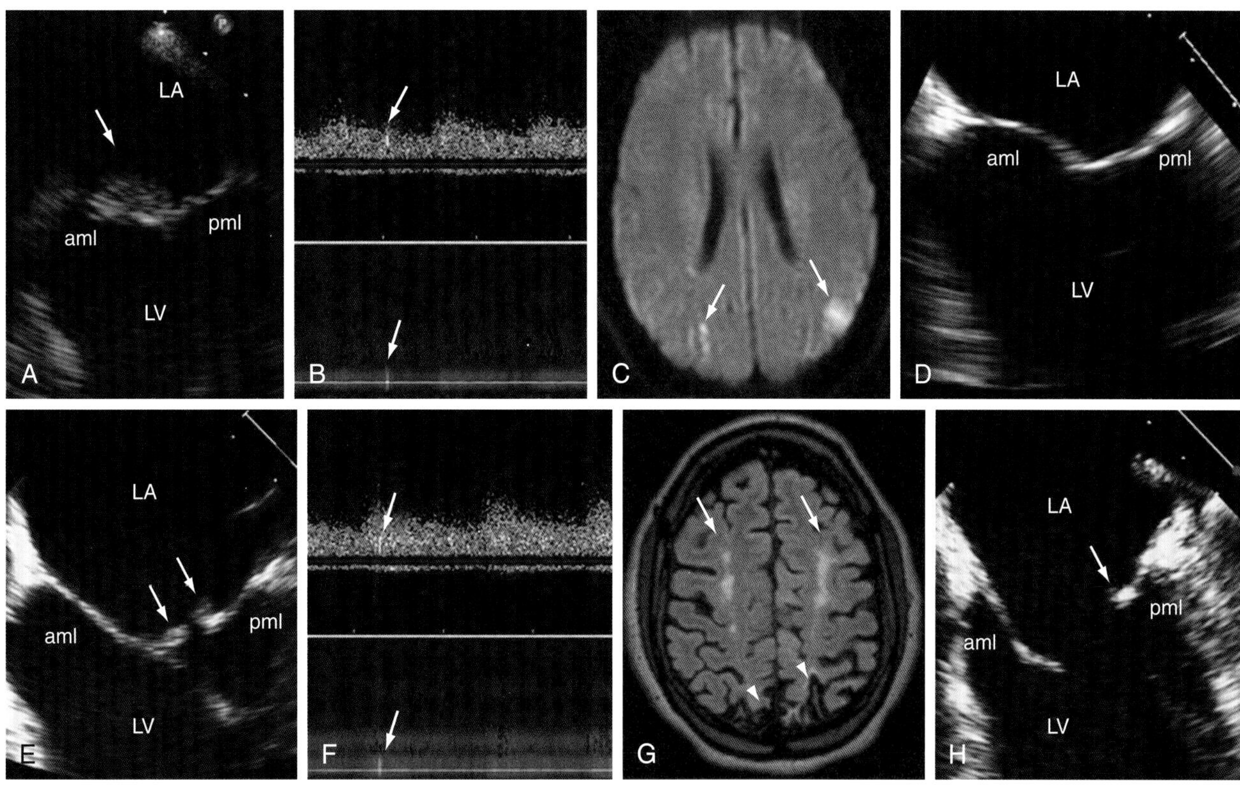

Fig. 37.5 Libman-Sacks endocarditis and embolic cerebrovascular disease: the effect of therapy. (A) TEE 4-chamber view in an 18-year-old woman with systemic lupus erythematosus (SLE) and acute homonymous hemianopsia, confusional state, and cognitive dysfunction demonstrates a large-sized, oval-shaped, sessile, and homogeneously soft tissue echoreflectant Libman-Sacks vegetation *(arrow)* on the LA and middle to distal portions of the anterior mitral leaflet *(aml)* (see Video 37.5A). (B) Transcranial Doppler image of the right middle cerebral artery demonstrates a microembolus on spectral Doppler *(upper arrow)* and within the vessel *(lower arrow)*. (C) Diffuse weighted imaging of the brain demonstrates bilateral acute parietal infarcts *(arrows)*. The global neurocognitive score was consistent with moderate neurocognitive dysfunction. (D) After 9 weeks of immunosuppressive therapy and anticoagulants, repeat imaging studies showed resolution of the mitral valve vegetation and the cerebromicroembolism, decreased brain lesions, and significant improvement in the global neurocognitive score to mild neurocognitive dysfunction (see Video 37.5D). (E) 2D TEE close-up view in a 21-year-old woman with SLE with a history of stroke and an acute transient ischemic attack demonstrates small- to moderate-sized, oval-shaped, sessile, and heterogeneously echoreflectant Libman-Sacks vegetations *(arrows)* on the LA side and on distal portions of the anterior and posterior *(pml)* mitral leaflets associated with leaflet thickening and decreased mobility (see Video 37.5E). (F) Transcranial Doppler image of the patient's left middle cerebral artery demonstrates a microembolus *(arrows)*. (G) Old cerebral infarcts *(arrowheads)* and multiple small white matter lesions *(arrows)* were demonstrated on MRI. The global neurocognitive score was consistent with severe neurocognitive dysfunction. (H) After 3 months of immunosuppressive antiinflammatory therapy and anticoagulation, repeat imaging demonstrated resolution of the anterior mitral valve vegetation, significant reduction in size *(arrow)* of the posterior mitral leaflet vegetation, reduction of cerebromicroembolism, decrease in white matter lesions, and significant improvement in global neurocognitive score (see Video 37.5H).

TABLE 37.4 Effect of Antiinflammatory and Antithrombotic Therapy on Libman-Sacks Vegetations and Correlates of Cerebrovascular Disease.

Finding	*Initial Study*	*Follow-Up Study*	*Δ% P Value*[a]
TEE, Mean ± SD			
Vegetations (*n*)	2.0 ± 1.41	1.33 ± 1.28	0.03
Vegetations (area, cm^2)	0.38 ± 0.46	0.18 ± 0.19	0.09
Transcranial Doppler, *n* (%)			
Right or left MCA microemboli	5 patients (28%) with 14 microemboli	0	0.007[b]
Neurocognitive Z score, Mean ± SD			
Attention	−3.55 ± 4.24	−2.26 ± 3.20	0.002
Memory	−1.62 ± 1.64	−0.88 ± 1.61	0.001
Motor function	−6.43 ± 10.46	−2.32 ± 2.70	0.002
Global cognitive dysfunction	−3.12 ± 3.08	−1.86 ± 2.32	<0.001
Brain Perfusion, Mean ± SD			
Overall gray matter	28.10 ± 18.04	33.87 ± 15.02	34%/0.02
Overall white matter	14.36 ± 9.73	17.47 ± 6.88	38%/0.02
Brain Lesion Load, Median (IQR)			
Whole-brain lesion load (cm^3)	0.68 (0.17, 3.93)	0.55 (0.07, 1.74)	0.03

[a]Wilcoxon Signed Rank test.
[b]Poisson regression with repeated measures.
IQR, Interquartile range; *MCA*, middle cerebral artery; *SD*, standard deviation.
Adapted from Roldan CA, Sibbitt WL Jr, Qualls CR, et al. Libman-Sacks endocarditis and embolic cerebrovascular disease. *JACC Cardiovasc Imaging*. 2013;6:973–983.

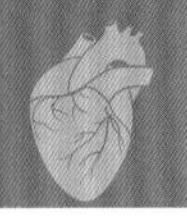

TABLE 37.5 Key Echocardiographic Features of Valve Lesions in Selected Conditions.

Disease	*Affected Structures*	*Key Characteristics*	*Functional Sequelae*
Systemic lupus erythematosus	Mitral and aortic valve predominantly affected; rarely chordae, tricuspid valve, and pulmonary valve; spares annuli	Libman-Sacks vegetations: masses usually < 1 cm in diameter, with heterogeneous echocardiographic reflectance (but not calcified) and with irregular borders; of varied shape (oval, tubular, protuberant, or coalescent) Attached to leaflet with a broad base Usually no independent motion Lesions are located at any portion of leaflets, on LA side of mitral valve, and LV side of aortic valve, but commonly extend through the leaflet into the opposite side. Diffuse leaflet thickening or sclerosis and a mild degree of commissural fusion are common; calcification is uncommon and mild.	Mild to moderate MR or AR is common, but stenosis is rare. High-risk embolic source
Primary antiphospholipid syndrome	Mitral valve and aortic valve leaflets predominantly affected; rarely chordae, tricuspid valve, and pulmonary valve; spares annuli	Libman-Sacks–like vegetations with characteristics similar to those described for SLE.	Mild to moderate MR or AR is common. High-risk embolic source
Rheumatoid arthritis	Mitral valve and aortic valve leaflets; rarely annuli and chordae; spares tricuspid valve and pulmonary valve	Rheumatoid nodules: masses usually < 1 cm in diameter, with homogeneous soft tissue echocardiographic reflectance and irregular border; usually round shape Any location within the leaflet; leaflet thickening/sclerosis generally mild or absent Libman-Sacks–like vegetations are uncommon.	More than mild MR or AR is rare. Rupture of a nodule may lead to severe valve regurgitation. Rarely associated with cardioembolism Associated with acute or recurrent valvulitis Characteristics similar to those associated with SLE High embolic potential Postvalvulitis stenosis is rare.
Ankylosing spondylitis	Proximal aorta, annulus and aortic valve, base of anterior mitral leaflet; posterior mitral leaflet, mitral annulus, and chordae are spared.	Sclerosis, stiffness, and dilation of aortic root extend to the annulus. Aortic valve leaflet sclerosis is generally mild. Subaortic bump: localized thickening of the base of the anterior mitral leaflet resulting from downward extension of aortic root and annular sclerosis	Mild to moderate AR or MR are common. Stenosis not reported
Rheumatic heart disease	90% involvement of mitral valve or aortic valve; 10% tricuspid valve or pulmonary valve Annuli of valves and aortic root spared	Mitral valve leaflet edges and chordae are most affected, and commissural fusion is common. With severe disease, sclerosis extends toward base of leaflet and may involve papillary muscles. Extensive calcification may occur. When localized, sclerosis may appear masslike, but very high echocardiographic reflectance is unlike other lesions, except degenerative. Aortic valve cusp edges are affected in a similar pattern.	Leaflet edge fusion and chordal shortening produce a tethered mitral leaflet motion. Analogous doming motion of the aortic cusps may be seen. If fusion predominates, stenosis results; if leaflet retraction predominates, regurgitation results.
Degenerative disorders	Mitral valve and aortic valve annuli and leaflets; commonly involves chordae and tips of papillary muscles.	Sclerosis is concentrated at base of leaflets and annulus, with progressive extension toward the leaflet midportion Tip is uncommonly involved. When localized, sclerosis may appear masslike or as nodules. Aortic valve nodules are more commonly located at the base and commissural portions.	Annular calcification predominates for the mitral valve, with leaflet sclerosis less common and usually limited to the posterior leaflet. MR is rarely more than mild. Stenosis is rare and subclinical or mild. Aortic valve leaflet sclerosis and fusion lead to stenosis, and leaflet distortion leads to AR, usually mild.
Infective endocarditis	Isolated native aortic valve endocarditis in 55%–60% of cases Isolated mitral valve endocarditis in 25% of cases Involvement of aortic and mitral valves in about 15% of cases Right-sided heart valve involvement in 5%–10% of cases	*Acute*: mass with homogeneous soft tissue reflectance and irregular borders; size and shape vary, usually with narrow base, often pedunculated Lesions usually exhibit motion independent of underlying structure and almost always oscillatory. Mitral valve and tricuspid valve lesions prolapse into atria in systole; aortic valve and pulmonary valve lesions prolapse into outflow tracts in diastole. Lesions are usually attached to distal third of leaflet. With aortic valve disease, additional vegetations may occur on anterior mitral leaflet and chordae. *Chronic*: localized thickening or increased reflectance of leaflet or chordae Lesion is not necessarily distal on leaflet. Fibrous tissue reflectance and calcification are common.	Valve regurgitation is common and typically severe; stenosis involving native valves is rare. Leaflet perforation or abscess formation occurs. Cardioembolism is common.
Valve or Lambl excrescences	Predominantly detected on the mitral and aortic valves with similar frequency. Rarely detected on the right heart valves	Detected with TEE, rarely with TTE Similarly high frequency (35%–40%) in healthy subjects, patients with connective tissue diseases, and patients with suspected cardioembolism The predominant filiform types are thin (0.6–2 mm), elongated (4–16 mm), hypermobile structures seen at or near the leaflet coaptation point, on the LA side during systole for the mitral and tricuspid valves and on the LV side during diastole for the aortic valve. The uncommon lamellar types are shorter in length and thicker in diameter and therefore may mimic vegetations. Multivalvular involvement is seen in 20%–25% of subjects.	Valve excrescences are not associated with and do not cause valvular dysfunction; persist unchanged over time; are not associated with aging or with clinical or laboratory parameters of atherogenesis, thrombogenesis, or inflammation; and are not associated with an increased risk of cardioembolism.

AR, Aortic regurgitation; *MR*, mitral regurgitation; *SLE*, systemic lupus erythematosus.

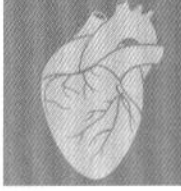

Atherosclerosis

Premature atherosclerosis is prevalent among patients with SLE, and it is a major cause of morbidity and mortality. After controlling for traditional atherogenic risk factors, the prevalence of subclinical and clinical atherosclerosis among SLE patients is two to four times higher than among matched controls.[15,16]

Early functional atherosclerosis, the most common form, manifests as decreased coronary flow reserve by dipyridamole or adenosine Doppler TTE, decreased peripheral arterial vasodilation, or increased carotid arteries or aortic stiffness (Fig. 37.6A–C).[17–19] Premature subclinical atherosclerosis also manifests as an increased prevalence (30%–45%) of aortic and coronary artery calcifications (with two to three times higher rates in the aorta than in the coronary arteries) on computed tomography (CT), increased carotid and aortic intima media thickening and plaques on carotid ultrasonography and TEE (see Fig. 37.6D–E), and a more diffuse coronary vessel wall inflammation by contrast magnetic resonance imaging (MRI).[20,21]

Imaging and pathologic studies of the aorta and coronary arteries demonstrate that adventitial thickening is greater in people with atherosclerosis and abnormal arterial stiffness compared with those who do not have these abnormalities, suggesting that adventitial thickening is associated with and may be a pathogenic factor for atherosclerosis and arterial stiffness in SLE (see Fig. 37.6D–E).[22,23] In SLE patients and in relation to age, atherosclerosis and stiffness progress within the aorta and within the carotid arteries in a parallel manner. However, aortic atherosclerosis and stiffness progress at two times the rate of carotid atherosclerosis and stiffness.[24] For SLE patients, premature subclinical atherosclerosis portends a 35% increased risk of myocardial infarction, percutaneous coronary interventions, coronary artery bypass grafting, stroke, and death.

In patients with active SLE, an acute coronary syndrome more often results from nonobstructive epicardial atherosclerosis exacerbated by increased vasomotor tone or thrombogenesis and rarely from coronary arteritis, embolism from a valve vegetation, or in situ thrombosis without atherosclerosis. Resting and exercise echocardiography may have decreased sensitivity and specificity for detecting epicardial coronary artery disease (CAD), and consequently, coronary angiography may be warranted in patients with acute coronary syndrome.

Although no randomized, controlled data exist, hydroxychloroquine therapy may have a protective effect against the development and progression of atherosclerosis.[25] Standard

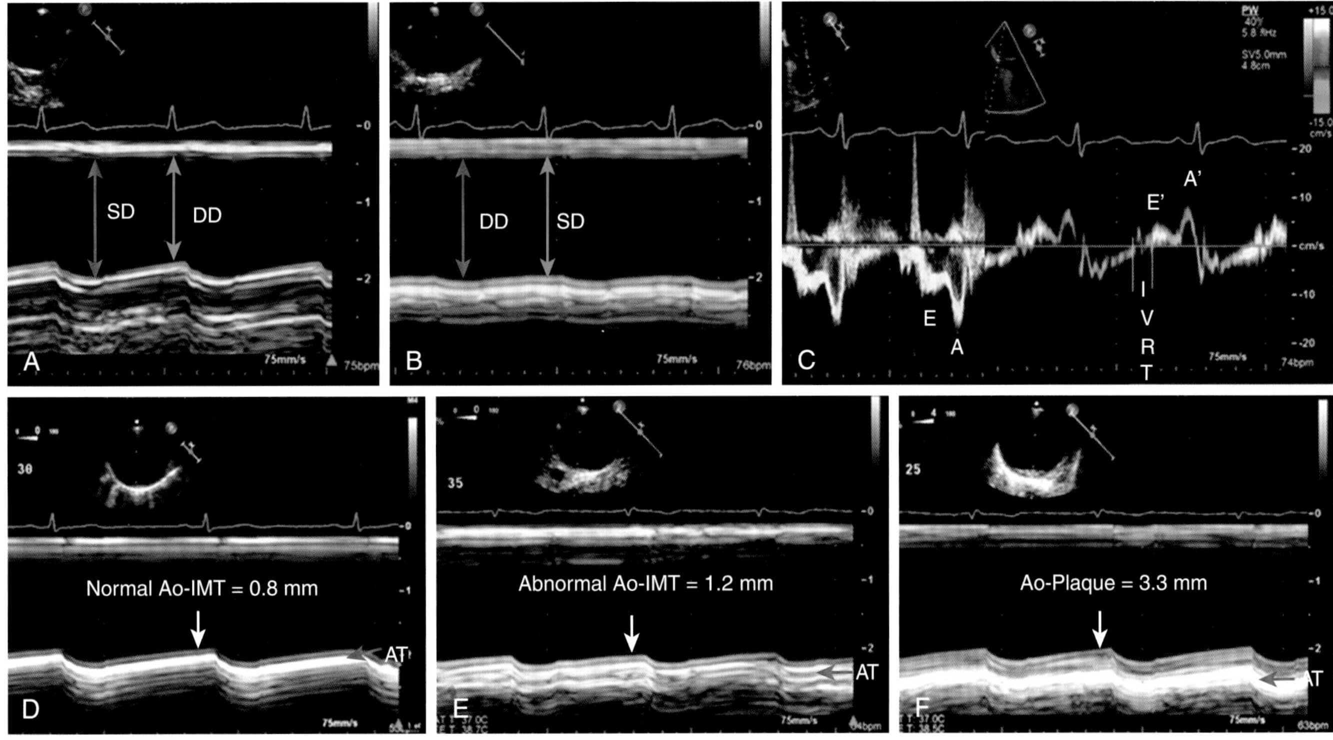

Fig. 37.6 Assessment of aortic stiffness and atherosclerosis by TEE in systemic lupus erythematosus. (A) Short-axis 2D TEE-guided M-mode image of the mid-descending thoracic aorta in a 27-year-old woman with systemic lupus erythematosus (SLE) shows end-systolic *(SD)* and end-diastolic *(DD)* aortic diameters of 17.3 and 16 mm, respectively. The calculated pressure-strain elastic modulus (PSEM), a well-validated parameter of static arterial stiffness, was 7.9 Pascal units (in the normal range). [PSEM = [k(sBP − dBP)/(sD − dD/dD)]/10,000, where k = 133.3 is the conversion factor from mmHg to Nm^{-2} (Pascal units); *sBP* is the brachial systolic blood pressure; and *dBP* is the brachial diastolic blood pressure.] (B) Short-axis 2D TEE-guided M-mode of the mid-descending thoracic aorta in a 38-year-old woman with SLE with abnormal aortic stiffness and LV diastolic dysfunction shows an aortic SD of 19 mm and a DD of 18 mm. The calculated PSEM was high at 11.04 Pascal units. (C) The patient's mitral inflow exhibited an abnormal E/A ratio of 0.57, a septal mitral annulus tissue Doppler low E′ peak velocity of 4.0 cm/s, E′/A′ ratio of 0.5, isovolumic relaxation time (IVRT) of 87 ms, and a mitral E/septal E′ ratio of 10.5. (D) Short-axis 2D TEE-guided M-mode image of the posterior wall at the midlevel (30–35 cm) of the descending thoracic aorta demonstrates a normal (≤1 mm) intima media thickness *(IMT, vertical white arrow)* of 0.8 mm and normal adventitial thickness (*AT, horizontal red arrow*) of 0.9 mm in a patient with SLE. (E and F) 2D TEE-guided M-mode images of a 48-year-old woman with SLE demonstrate an abnormal IMT of 1.2 mm *(vertical white arrow)* and an AT of 2.6 mm (*horizontal red arrow*) at the distal descending thoracic aorta (E) and a well-defined aortic plaque of 3.3 mm in thickness *(vertical white arrow)* with increased AT of 3.4 mm (*horizontal red arrow*) at the proximal (F) descending thoracic aorta. *Ao*, Aorta.

medical therapy in combination with immunosuppressive antiinflammatory therapy may be considered concomitantly with percutaneous coronary intervention in patients with active SLE and acute coronary syndrome.

Myocardial Disease

Myocardial disease, manifested predominantly in the form of subclinical ventricular diastolic dysfunction, is common in SLE patients. The predominant cause is microvascular CAD.[17,18] Arterial hypertension may be the second most common cause, with a prevalence of 25% to 35%. Premature peripheral arterial stiffness can cause left ventricular (LV) diastolic dysfunction. A controlled study in young patients with SLE who were undergoing TEE for simultaneous assessment of LV diastolic function and aortic stiffness demonstrated that patients have higher degrees of aortic stiffness independent of traditional atherogenic risk factors and aortic atherosclerosis; they also have higher LV mass and greater degrees of LV diastolic dysfunction. Aortic stiffness correlated with increased left atrial (LA) volume, LV mass, and LV diastolic dysfunction in this study, and aortic stiffness was independently associated with LV diastolic dysfunction (see Fig. 37.6A–C).[26] Acute myocarditis is uncommon; it rarely can be the initial manifestation of SLE, and it may manifest with heart failure and global or segmental LV dysfunction on echocardiography and MRI.[27,28] Small-vessel vasculitis and coronary arteritis are rare. Hydroxychloroquine sulfate–induced dilated or restrictive cardiomyopathy has been reported.

Controlled Doppler and speckle-tracking echocardiography (STE) in asymptomatic patients without systemic or pulmonary hypertension (PH) who have normal LV systolic function have shown a 15% to 35% prevalence of LV and right ventricular (RV) diastolic dysfunction. Longitudinal, circumferential, and radial myocardial strain and strain rate followed by tissue Doppler parameters provide a more sensitive measure than mitral inflow Doppler parameters for detecting subclinical ventricular diastolic and systolic dysfunction.[29] Similarly, STE has demonstrated impairment of LA conduit and storage functions with associated increased LA volumes but preserved pump function.[30]

Indicative of microvascular CAD, LV diastolic dysfunction is associated with reversible, fixed, and mixed myocardial perfusion defects in young patients with active SLE and normal coronary arteries. In contrast to ventricular diastolic dysfunction, the prevalence of systolic dysfunction is less than 20% among unselected patients. The clinical and prognostic implications of subclinical LV and RV diastolic and systolic dysfunction in SLE are undefined.

Pericardial Disease

As many as 50% of SLE patients have at least one episode of symptomatic pericarditis. Pericardial disease is associated with myocarditis and with valve and renal disease.[27,31,32] Cardiac tamponade and constrictive pericarditis are rare. Acute pericarditis and cardiac tamponade rarely may be the initial manifestation of SLE. Up to 20% of female patients younger than 50 years of age with acute pericarditis have SLE.[33] Asymptomatic pericardial effusions may result from mild pericarditis, hypoalbuminemia, or cor pulmonale.

Echocardiography is the standard method for evaluating suspected SLE pericarditis. A large pericardial effusion with or without indicators of tamponade in a patient with active SLE prompts an earlier echocardiography-guided pericardiocentesis, either diagnostic (i.e., aimed to exclude infection) or therapeutic (due to rapid progression or hemorrhagic transformation), followed by immunosuppressive antiinflammatory therapy. A pericardial window should be avoided because of the commonly associated peritonitis and pleuritis with increased risk of infection. Echocardiography is an effective screening method when constriction is under consideration. Cardiac MRI and CT are preferred methods for assessment of pericardial thickness when echocardiography suggests constriction.

Pulmonary Hypertension

PH, defined as pulmonary artery systolic pressure of 40 mmHg or more by Doppler echocardiography, occurs in 5% to 15% of patients with SLE and is associated with increased mortality rates independent of its cause.[34,35] The most common causes are thromboembolism, interstitial lung disease, left heart disease, and vasculitis. The association of PH with Raynaud phenomenon suggests a vasospastic cause.

Predictors of PH include ribonucleoprotein, soluble substance A, anticentromere and endothelin receptor type A antibodies, and SLE-scleroderma overlap syndrome.[35,36] STE detects early effects of PH on the right heart. Compared with patients without PH and with controls, patients with PH have decreased RV and right atrial (RA) free wall longitudinal peak systolic strain, systolic strain rate, and early and late diastolic strain rates, while they have increased maximum, preatrial contraction, and minimum RA volumes.[37,38] Doppler echocardiography at rest and, in selected cases, with exercise is commonly used for diagnosis and assessment of the cause, severity, response to therapy, and follow-up outcomes of SLE-associated PH.

PRIMARY ANTIPHOSPHOLIPID SYNDROME

BACKGROUND

Primary antiphospholipid syndrome (PAPS) is defined by (1) antiphospholipid antibodies; (2) venous or arterial thrombosis or complicated pregnancy (i.e., fetal loss, preeclampsia, or eclampsia); and (3) lack of diagnostic criteria for other rheumatologic disease. The diagnosis is established by one or more clinical criteria and one type of antiphospholipid antibodies on two or more occasions at least 6 weeks apart. Cardiovascular disease occurs in 50% to 75% of patients with PAPS.

CARDIOVASCULAR INVOLVEMENT

Valve Disease and Thromboembolism

Valve disease is the most common cardiac manifestation of PAPS. The prevalence, distribution, characteristics, and clinical implications of valve disease in PAPS mimic those of Libman-Sacks endocarditis in SLE (Fig. 37.7). Valve disease manifests as valve vegetations (consisting mainly of platelet or fibrin thrombi), valve thickening, and, uncommonly, valve regurgitation. Vegetations are uncommonly identified on the right heart valves and on the atrial or ventricular endocardium. Endocardial injury caused by intracardiac catheters, wires, or prostheses is associated with a higher rate of device-associated thrombosis and thromboembolism.

The prevalence of left-sided valve disease ranges from 30% to 40% by TTE and up to 60% by TEE, compared with less than 5% in controls. 3D TEE may provide superior detection and characterization of valve vegetations, but data are limited (see

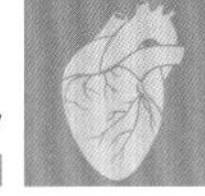

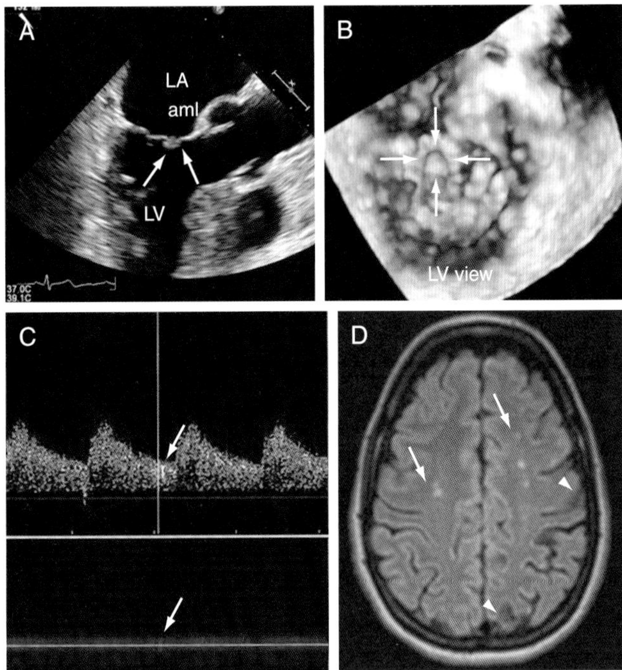

Fig. 37.7 Libman-Sacks–like vegetation and cerebroembolism in antiphospholipid syndrome. (A) 2D TEE long-axis view in a 43-year-old woman with antiphospholipid syndrome with a history of stroke and acute transient ischemic attack demonstrates a moderate-sized, oval-shaped, sessile, and homogeneously soft tissue echoreflectant Libman-Sacks–like vegetation *(arrows)* on the LV side and the middle to distal portions of the anterior mitral leaflet *(aml)* without associated leaflet thickening or decreased mobility (see Video 37.7A). (B) 3D TEE LV view of the mitral valve demonstrates a moderate-sized, oval-shaped, sessile, and homogeneously echoreflectant vegetation with well-defined borders on the middle to distal portion of the anterior mitral leaflet *(top three arrows)* with an additional brown discolored, smaller vegetation *(bottom arrow)* (probably recently formed). The rest of the anterior mitral leaflet has an irregular and nodular appearance (see Video 37.7B). (C) Transcranial Doppler image of the patient's right middle cerebral artery demonstrates a microembolus *(arrows)*. (D) MRI of the brain demonstrates old cerebral infarcts *(arrowheads)* and multiple, small, periventricular and deep white matter abnormalities *(arrows)*.

Fig. 37.7). As in patients with SLE, left-sided valve vegetations are associated with thromboembolism, most commonly to the brain, uncommonly to the peripheral and coronary arteries, and rarely to intraabdominal viscera. Right-sided valve, endocardial, or device-associated vegetations can cause pulmonary or paradoxical embolism. The effect of anticoagulation therapy on vegetations is beneficial, but the effect of immunosuppressive antiinflammatory therapy is undefined.

Pulmonary Hypertension

The prevalence of PH in a prospective echocardiographic series of patients with PAPS is at least 20% to 25%; it results predominantly from chronic and recurrent pulmonary embolism and uncommonly from vasospastic or in situ thrombotic vasculopathy. Doppler echocardiography has diagnostic and clinical implications for PAPS-associated PH similar to those for SLE.

Atherosclerosis

A high prevalence (20% to 35%) of myocardial infarction has been reported for patients with PAPS. It results from microvascular disease or rarely from in situ coronary thrombosis (Fig. 37.8A–D) or coronary thromboembolism. However, these patients have increased intima media thickness of the carotid arteries.[39] Resting or stress echocardiography for detection of epicardial CAD in patients with PAPS may have low sensitivity given the low prevalence of epicardial atherosclerosis.

Myocardial Disease

In controlled studies using Doppler and STE in asymptomatic patients, a high prevalence of mild LV and RV diastolic dysfunction has been reported, independent of arterial hypertension or PH, respectively.[40] The mechanisms of diastolic dysfunction include microvascular CAD, thrombotic microangiopathy, and, rarely, primary myocardial disease.

RHEUMATOID ARTHRITIS

BACKGROUND

Clinically apparent cardiovascular disease occurs in 25% to 40% of patients with rheumatoid arthritis and accounts for 40% to 50% of their deaths. Rheumatoid arthritis–related predictors of cardiovascular disease include active, long-standing (>10 years) disease and older age at onset of rheumatoid arthritis; elevated inflammatory markers; positive SS-A/SS-B antibodies and anticyclic citrullinated peptide antibodies; longer duration of corticosteroid therapy; active extraarticular, erosive polyarticular, and nodular disease; and vasculitis.[41] Epicardial adipose tissue thickness correlates positively with cardiovascular disease.[42]

CARDIOVASCULAR INVOLVEMENT

Atherosclerosis

After controlling for traditional atherogenic risk factors, the prevalence of atherosclerosis in patients with rheumatoid arthritis is two to three times higher than in matched controls. Among unselected patients, functional microvascular CAD is the predominant type (≈50%), followed by nonobstructive (≈25%) and obstructive (≈25%) epicardial CAD.[43] By age 65 to 70 years, 75% to 80% of patients with rheumatoid arthritis have angiographic evidence of CAD (30% with three-vessel CAD), and there is a high incidence of myocardial infarction (4.8 to 5.9 events per 1000 person-years). Coronary arteritis (Fig. 37.9), in situ coronary thrombosis without atherosclerosis or arteritis, and coronary embolism are rare.

Patients who have rheumatoid arthritis with an acute coronary syndrome have 30% to 40% higher rates of event recurrence and death at 1 year than matched controls.[44] Their morbidity and mortality rates after percutaneous or surgical coronary revascularization are two to four times higher than those of matched controls.

Resting and stress echocardiography are useful for detection of wall motion abnormalities in those with obstructive CAD but have decreased sensitivity for microvascular CAD or coronary arteritis. Dipyridamole or adenosine TTE is used to assess coronary flow reserve in those with microvascular disease. Symptomatic patients with rheumatoid arthritis who have evidence of ischemia on resting and exercise echocardiography have a two to three times higher risk of death than matched controls with negative resting or exercise study results.

For patients who have active rheumatoid arthritis with acute coronary syndromes, standard general medical therapy in combination with immunosuppressive antiinflammatory therapy may be considered concomitantly with high-risk percutaneous coronary revascularization (see Fig. 37.9).

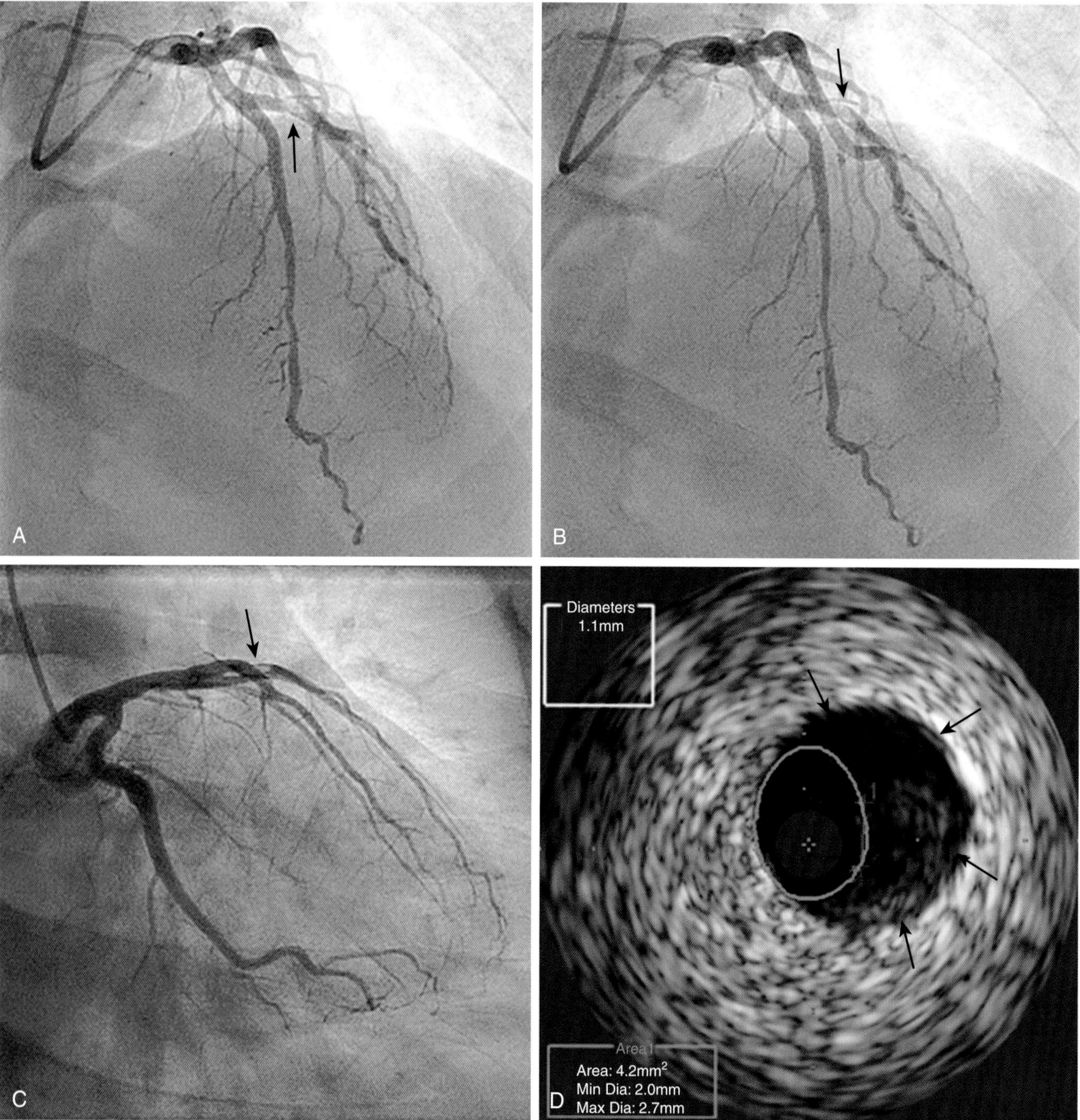

Fig. 37.8 Non–ST-segment elevation myocardial infarction in primary antiphospholipid syndrome. Left anterior (A), cranial (B), and right lateral (C) views of the left coronary system in a 45-year-old man with no risk factors for coronary artery disease who was admitted with a clinical syndrome of acute non–ST-segment elevation myocardial infarction demonstrate a filling defect *(arrows)*, suggesting a partially occlusive thrombus in the proximal portion of the principal diagonal branch. Intravascular ultrasound imaging (D) confirmed a partially occlusive thrombus *(arrows)* without underlying atherosclerotic disease. The *green oval* illustrates the vessel lumen (see Video 37.8D). The patient was continued on anticoagulation therapy in addition to standard therapy for acute coronary syndrome. An echocardiogram was unremarkable with no evidence of intracardiac thrombus, valve vegetations, or intracardiac shunting. A hypercoagulation workup demonstrated elevated levels of immunoglobulin G (IgG) and IgM anticardiolipin antibodies and positive β2-glycoprotein antibody and lupus anticoagulant. The diagnosis of primary antiphospholipid antibody syndrome complicated by in situ coronary artery thrombosis was made. The patient was discharged home on dual antiplatelet therapy and has had no recurrent cardiovascular or cerebrovascular events.

Pericardial Disease

In patients with acute pericarditis, the pericardial effusion is exudative and bloody with a low glucose level, and it may contain rheumatoid factor. Large pericardial effusion with typical tamponade, large focal masses of fibrinous deposition causing focal tamponade, and constriction are rarely reported.[45] Asymptomatic pericardial effusions, seen in about 25% of patients, are associated with renal disease, hypoalbuminemia, and cor pulmonale. The role of echocardiography in rheumatoid pericardial disease parallels its role in SLE.

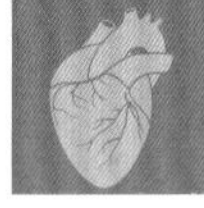

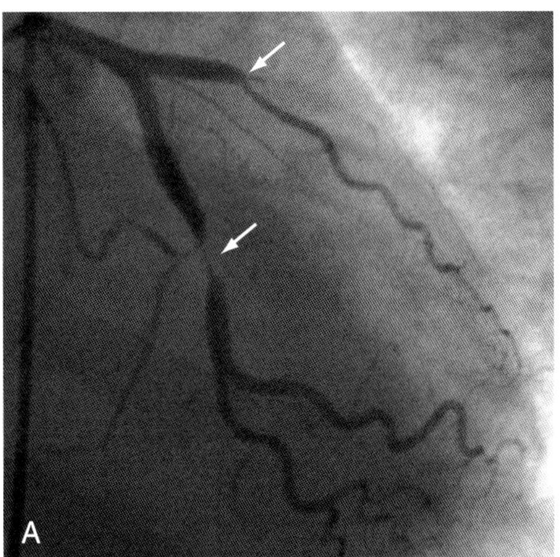

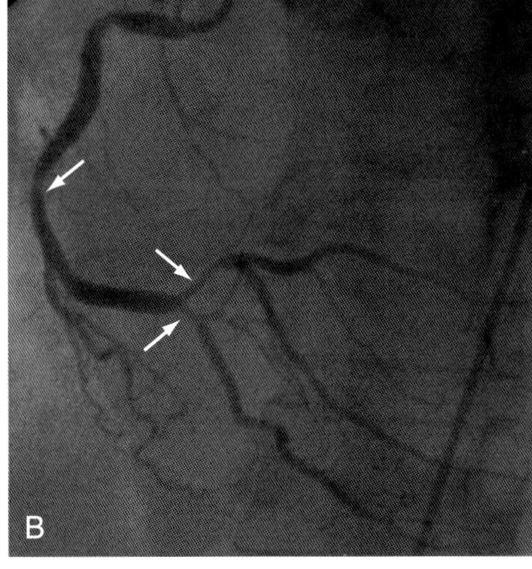

Fig. 37.9 Coronary arteritis in rheumatoid arthritis. (A) Left coronary angiogram of a 47-year-old woman with severely active rheumatoid arthritis who presented to the emergency room with 2 weeks of atypical chest pain associated with dyspnea of exertion, inferolateral nonspecific ST-T abnormalities on electrocardiography, and elevated creatine phosphokinase muscle band and troponin I demonstrates an occluded left anterior descending coronary artery *(upper arrow)* and a 90% stenosis of the circumflex artery *(lower arrow)*. (B) The right coronary angiogram demonstrates a 40% middle stenosis *(upper arrow)* and a 60% to 70% ostial stenosis of the posterior descending and posterolateral branches *(lower arrows)*. After initiation of standard therapy in combination with aggressive immunosuppressive antiinflammatory therapy (i.e., pulse corticosteroids and cyclophosphamide), successful percutaneous coronary interventions with stent placement in the anterior descending and circumflex arteries was performed. One week after discharge, the patient returned with a recurrent non–ST-segment elevation myocardial infarction with evidence on repeat angiography of severe stenosis (i.e., rapid progression from 40% to 90% stenosis) of the mid–right coronary artery, for which she underwent a successful stent placement. The clinical and serologic activity of her rheumatoid arthritis with multivessel and rapidly progressive coronary artery disease suggests coronary arteritis with or without underlying atherosclerotic disease. The patient also had associated severe mitral and aortic valvulitis with significant regurgitation (see Fig. 35.11). The patient had an uneventful clinical course and was discharged home in stable condition.

Valve Disease

The reported prevalence of valve abnormalities among unselected patients younger than 60 years of age is as low as 30% with TTE and almost 60% with TEE.[46] Valve disease occurs in four forms:

1. Valve nodules
2. Healed valvulitis with residual leaflet fibrosis and regurgitation, rarely stenosis
3. Acute valvulitis with Libman-Sacks–like vegetations and/or significant regurgitation
4. Superimposed infective endocarditis

Although acute and chronic valvulitis with leaflet thickening or fibrosis may have clinical and echocardiographic manifestations similar to those of SLE, rheumatoid arthritis–related valvulitis has a much lower prevalence and incidence of noninfective vegetations. In contrast, valve nodules appear to be unique to rheumatoid arthritis. These nodules can also be seen on valve rings, papillary muscles, and atrial or ventricular endocardium. Histologically, valve nodules resemble subcutaneous nodules and may result from focal vasculitis.

On TEE, rheumatoid valve nodules are detected in one third of patients; they are small (<0.5 cm^2), spheroid masses with homogeneous reflectance, typically appearing singly on any portion of the leaflet.[46] The adjacent leaflet appears normal or shows mild sclerosis. This picture is unlike that of Libman-Sacks vegetations (compare Fig. 37.10 with Figs. 37.1–37.5). Valve thickening is detected in one half of patients and is equally diffuse or localized; it is usually mild, involves the left heart valves equally, and rarely involves the annulus and subvalvular apparatus. Mild or worse valve regurgitation is seen in 20% to 25% of patients, but stenosis is rare.

Rheumatoid valve disease is typically mild and asymptomatic. However, several uncommon severe manifestations of the disease have been described[46–48]:

1. A mixed picture of nodular disease, active or healed valvulitis, and regurgitation (Fig. 37.10)
2. Acute or recurrent valvulitis resulting in severe valve regurgitation (Fig. 37.11)
3. Valve thrombus on top of a valve nodule, Libman-Sacks–like vegetations, or superimposed valve strands complicated by systemic embolism
4. Acute severe valve regurgitation due to rupture of a single or coalescent nodule or a large nodule that affects leaflet coaptation
5. Aortitis with aortic root dilation and aortic regurgitation
6. Superimposed infective endocarditis

The short- and long-term mortality rates of patients with rheumatoid valve disease are significantly higher than those of matched controls. The 30-day and 1-year morbidity and mortality rates for patients undergoing valve replacement or, rarely, valve repair are two to three times higher than those of patients without rheumatoid arthritis. Early diagnosis and immunosuppressive antiinflammatory therapy may improve or decrease the progression of valve disease and improve patient survival without high-risk valve surgery.

Myocardial Disease

Patients with rheumatoid arthritis have a high prevalence of subclinical and clinical LV (30%–76%) and RV (25%–45%) diastolic dysfunction compared with matched controls (>20%) by Doppler and STE.[49–52] In these patients, LV diastolic dysfunction progresses over time more rapidly than in matched controls. The prevalence of subclinical LV systolic

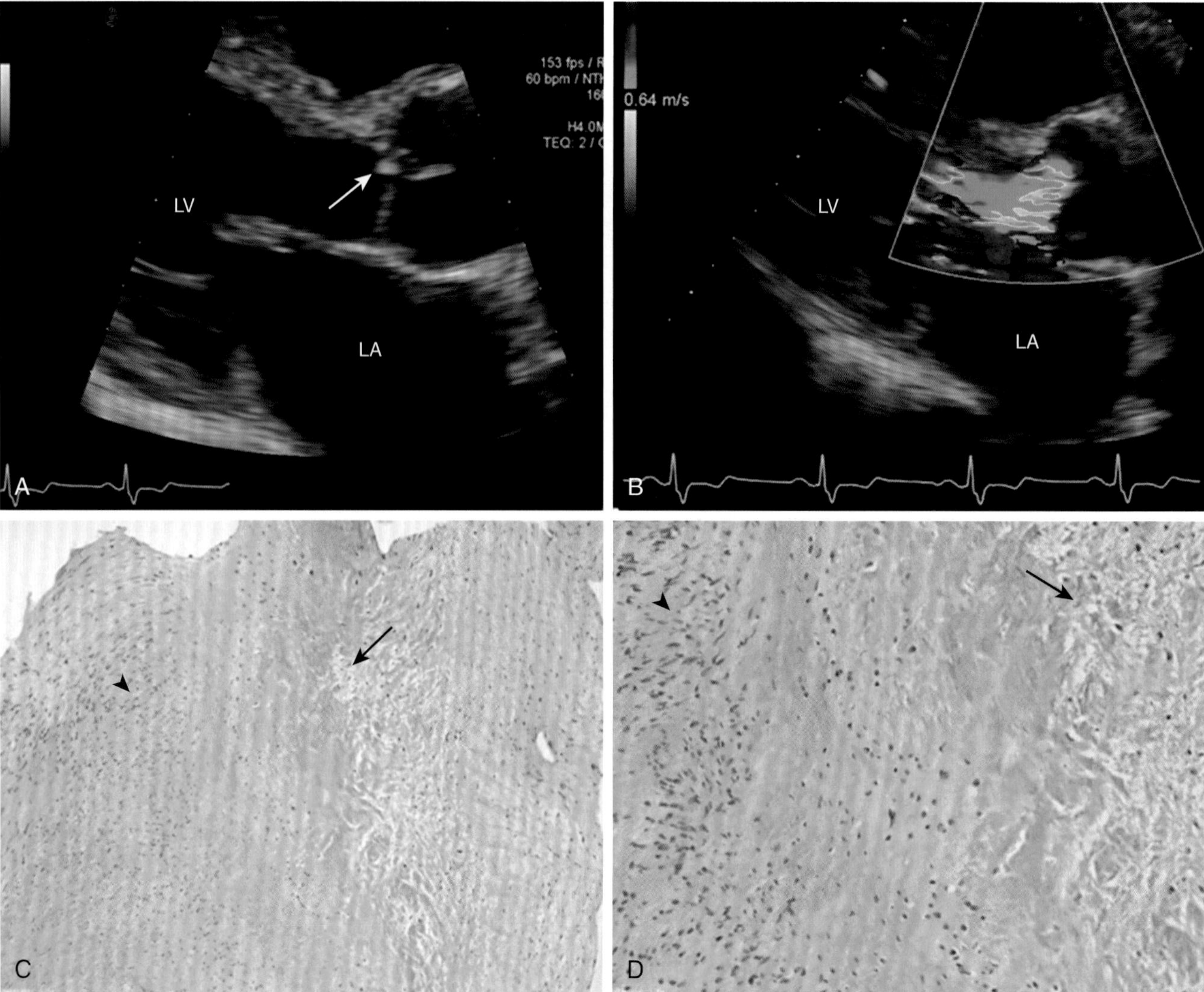

Fig. 37.10 Aortic valve nodular disease, valvulitis, and symptomatic moderate to severe aortic regurgitation in rheumatoid arthritis. (A) 2D parasternal long-axis view of the aortic valve in a 55-year-old man with rheumatoid arthritis and progressive dyspnea of exertion demonstrates small nodularities (*arrow*) on the tip of the noncoronary cusp (see Video 37.10A). The right coronary cusp showed mild thickening and retraction leading to eccentric valve closure. (B) 2D parasternal long-axis view with color Doppler of the aortic valve demonstrates a large and posteriorly directed regurgitant jet, consistent with moderate to severe aortic regurgitation (see Video 37.10B). Histopathology studies of the explanted aortic valve with hematoxylin and eosin staining at low (C) and high (D) magnification demonstrate a palisading or necrobiotic granuloma characterized by altered connective tissue with blurring and loss of detail in the collagen and increased eosinophilia (*arrows*) surrounded by spindle-shaped histiocytes (*arrowheads*). These histologic findings are consistent with a rheumatoid nodule.

dysfunction is low but higher than matched controls (10%–15% vs. ≤6%).

The most common pathogenic origins of ventricular diastolic dysfunction are functional microvascular CAD, peripheral arterial stiffness, hypertensive heart disease, and epicardial CAD. Clinically evident myocarditis is uncommon and can mimic acute coronary syndromes. Rare causes include myocardial nodules, vasculitis, and amyloidosis. A restrictive or dilated cardiomyopathy resulting from hydroxychloroquine therapy has been reported.[53] PH is the most common cause of RV diastolic dysfunction, but microvascular CAD may also play a role. Decreased longitudinal, circumferential, and radial diastolic and systolic myocardial strain and strain rates, low E′ and A′ velocities, increased E/E′ ratio, low color flow propagation velocity, and increased myocardial performance index are more sensitive than mitral or tricuspid inflow Doppler parameters. Associated reduced LA contractility, as determined by a decreased global LA strain with increased LA volume index, may occur.

Large series have shown a high incidence (35%–40%) of clinical diastolic heart failure independent of traditional pathogenic factors. Compared with matched controls, the mortality risk is doubled for patients with diastolic heart failure but no rheumatoid arthritis.

Pulmonary Hypertension

PH resulting from interstitial fibrosis, pulmonary vasculitis, obliterative bronchiolitis, or thromboembolism is more common than that caused by left heart disease.[54] In a controlled series of asymptomatic patients, the prevalence of PH determined by echocardiography was five times higher for patients with rheumatoid arthritis than for controls (21% vs. 4%); it was even higher for those with symptoms or evident pulmonary disease. The 1- and 3-year mortality rates for patients with PH are high (10%–15% and 40%–45%, respectively).[55]

Resting or exercise echocardiography is useful for detection and assessment of the severity and type of PH and its associated

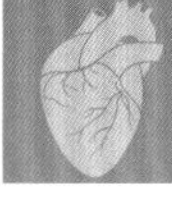

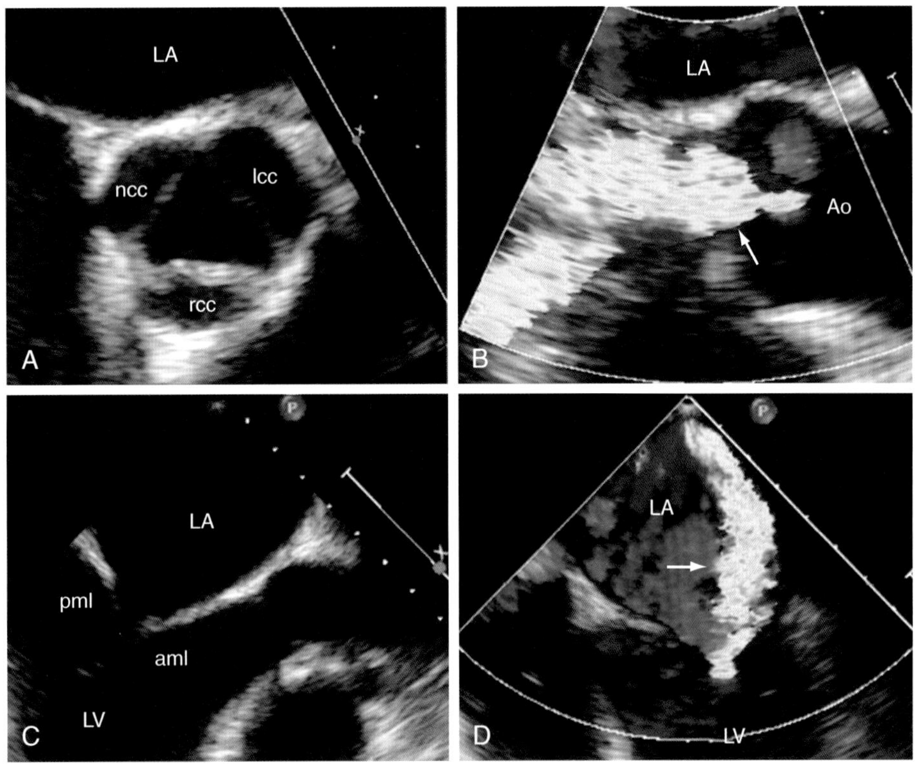

Fig. 37.11 Acute aortic and mitral valvulitis in rheumatoid arthritis. (A) 2D TEE basal short-axis view of the aortic valve in a 47-year-old woman with severely active rheumatoid arthritis who presented to the emergency room with rapidly progressive dyspnea of exertion and clinically evident heart failure (see Fig. 37.9) demonstrates severe diffuse thickening with soft tissue echoreflectance and decreased mobility of all cusps, predominantly the right coronary cusp *(rcc)*. (B) Color Doppler TEE view longitudinal to the aortic valve shows severe aortic regurgitation based on a greater than 65% ratio of regurgitant jet height to LV outflow tract height *(arrow)*. (C) TEE longitudinal view of the aorta shows diffuse thickening of soft tissue echoreflectance and marked decreased mobility of the anterior *(aml)* and posterior *(pml)* mitral leaflets. (D) Color Doppler 4-chamber TEE view demonstrates a large and posterolaterally directed mitral regurgitant jet *(arrow)* with a vena contracta width of at least 7 mm, consistent with severe mitral regurgitation. In the context of the patient's clinical data, these echocardiographic findings are consistent with severe acute rheumatoid mitral and aortic valvulitis complicated by severe mitral and aortic regurgitation and heart failure. In addition to standard therapy, the patient received aggressive immunosuppressive therapy (i.e., pulse corticosteroids and cyclophosphamide). Her valve regurgitation and clinical syndrome improved and stabilized, and she was discharged home in stable condition. *Ao*, Aorta; *lcc*, left coronary cusp; *ncc*, noncoronary cusp.

RV diastolic or systolic dysfunction. It is also valuable for assessment of the response to therapy.

ANKYLOSING SPONDYLITIS

BACKGROUND

Ankylosing spondylitis is characterized by inflammation of the vertebral and sacroiliac joints and uveitis. Associated proximal aortitis and aortic valvulitis and conduction disturbances are common. Cardiovascular disease in these patients is associated with age, disease activity and duration, aortic root and valve disease, and epicardial adipose tissue thickness.

CARDIOVASCULAR INVOLVEMENT

Aortitis and Valve Disease

Aortic root and valve disease in patients with ankylosing spondylitis is categorized as follows:

1. Proximal aortitis leading to aortic root thickening, stiffness, dilation, and rarely aneurysm formation, all of which contribute to aortic regurgitation (Fig. 37.12)
2. Aortic valvulitis resulting in cusp thickening and retraction leading to aortic regurgitation (see Fig. 37.12)
3. Thickening of the aortomitral junction (i.e., subaortic bump) causing anterior mitral leaflet retraction with decreased mobility and asymmetric or incomplete mitral leaflet coaptation leading to mitral regurgitation (see Fig. 37.12)
4. Extension of the subaortic fibrotic process into the basal septum, atrioventricular node, proximal bundle of His, and bundle branches or fascicles causing conduction disturbances[56]

The reason for selective injury of the proximal aorta is unknown. The prevalence of clinically manifested ascending aorta and aortic and mitral valve disease varies widely but is probably about 20%. Aortic or mitral regurgitation is usually mild to moderate. However, acute or healed aortitis or acute or healed aortic valvulitis can lead to severe aortic regurgitation.

On echocardiography, including TEE, the prevalences of aortic root thickening or sclerosis, increased stiffness, and dilation range from 20% to 60%.[56,57] On STE, decreased transverse strain of the anterior and posterior walls of the proximal aorta may be an early manifestation of aortic disease.[58] Aortic valve thickening, seen in up to 40% of patients, manifests mainly as nodularities of the aortic cusps. Associated aortic regurgitation is common, and the prevalence ranges from 20% to 40%; it is moderate in up to 25% and severe in less than 5% of patients.[56,59,60] Mitral valve thickening, seen in one third of patients, manifests as basal thickening of the anterior mitral leaflet, forming the characteristic subaortic bump. Mitral regurgitation, seen in almost one half of patients, is moderate in one third of them.

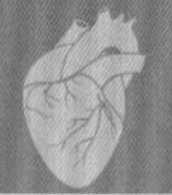

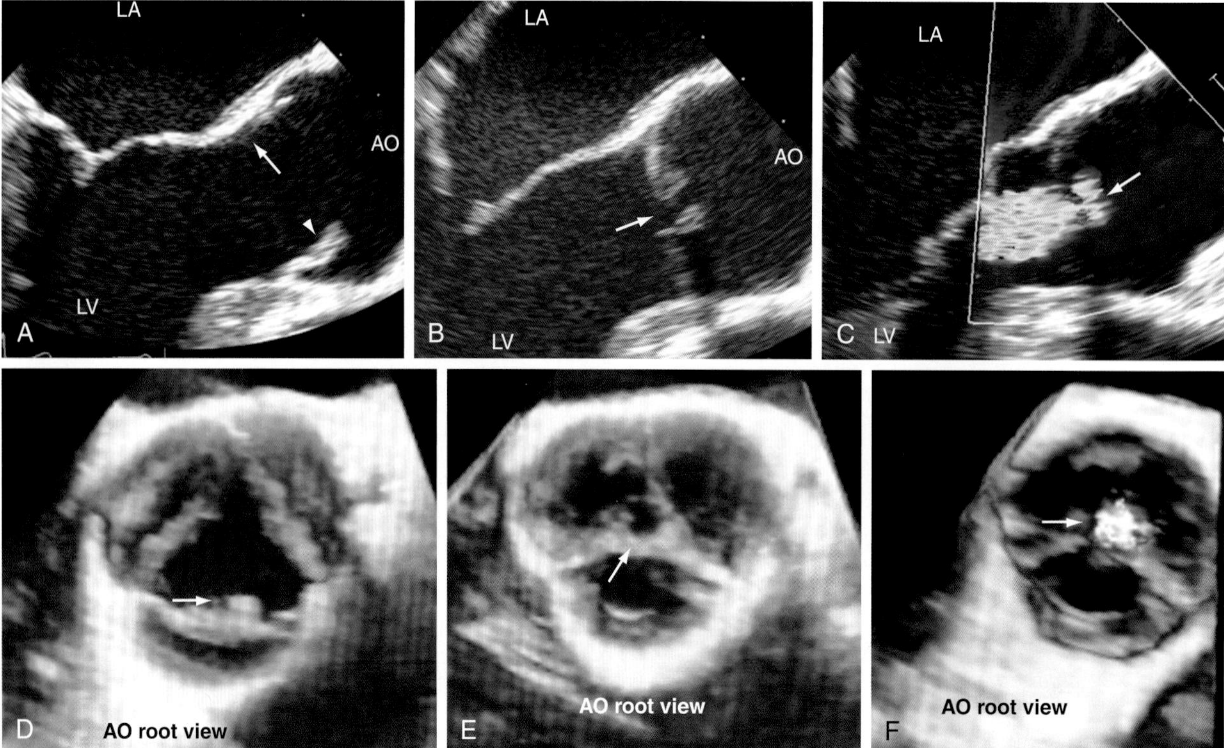

Fig. 37.12 Aortitis and aortic valvulitis in a 37-year-old man with ankylosing spondylitis. (A) 2D TEE long-axis view during systole shows cusp thickening, retraction, and decreased doming mobility, predominantly of the right coronary cusp (*arrowhead*). The aortic root sclerosis and mild thickening extend to the base of the anterior mitral leaflet (subaortic bump) (*arrow*). (B) 2D TEE long-axis view during diastole shows thickening, predominantly of the tip portions, and retraction of the aortic cusps leading to an incomplete coaptation (*arrow*). (C) 2D TEE long-axis view with color Doppler imaging shows moderate aortic regurgitation based on a flow convergence zone of 3 mm (*arrow*), a vena contracta of 4 mm, and a 40% ratio of jet height to LV outflow tract height. (D) 3D TEE image of the aortic valve viewed from the aortic (*AO*) root during systole better defines the moderate and diffuse thickening of the cusp tips and decreased mobility of all three cusps. There is a well-defined oval nodularity at the tip and ventricular side of the right coronary cusp (*arrow*). (E) During diastole, the cusp retraction leads to an incomplete central coaptation (*arrow*). (F) With 3D color Doppler TEE of the aortic valve viewed from the aorta, the effective regurgitant orifice area and vena contracta area were 0.18 and 0.19 cm^2 (*arrow*), respectively, confirming the severity of aortic regurgitation as moderate (see Videos 37.12A–F).

The effect of corticosteroids or disease-modifying antirheumatic drugs on aortic root and valve disease is uncertain. Due to absent multiorgan disease and uncommon use of immunosuppressive therapy in these patients, their mortality rate during valve replacement is probably similar to that of the general population. However, aortic valve replacement during active aortitis is associated with a higher risk of prosthetic valve dehiscence.

Conduction Abnormalities

Atrioventricular and intraventricular conduction blocks occur in 20% or more of patients with ankylosing spondylitis and are associated with aortic root thickening and subaortic bump, suggesting an extension of aortic root fibrosis into the proximal septum and atrioventricular node.

Myocardial and Pericardial Disease

The rate of myocardial disease for patients with ankylosing spondylitis is higher than for the general population; it is usually subclinical and is associated with aortic root and valve disease.[57] Associated aortic stiffness may also lead to increased LV afterload and LV mass and diastolic dysfunction. Subclinical diastolic dysfunction is associated with microvascular CAD in these patients. Controlled Doppler imaging and especially STE studies of asymptomatic young patients have reported a 9% to 45% prevalence of LV diastolic dysfunction, but systolic dysfunction is uncommon.[61]

The prevalence of pericardial disease in patients with ankylosing spondylitis is probably similar to that of the general population (<2%).

Atherosclerosis

Compared with matched controls, patients with ankylosing spondylitis have a higher prevalence of carotid intima-media thickening or plaques, increased carotid and aortic stiffness, coronary calcifications, and acute coronary syndromes or stroke.[62]

SCLERODERMA

BACKGROUND

In the diffuse type of scleroderma, symmetric fibrosis of the skin of the face, trunk, and extremities is seen, with frequent involvement of internal organs, including the heart. In the limited cutaneous type, the skin changes are restricted to the extremities and face; internal organs are commonly spared.

Cardiovascular disease occurs in as many as 60% of patients with scleroderma. The predominant findings are functional and structural microvascular CAD, myocarditis, pulmonary and systemic hypertension–related heart disease, and pericarditis. Cardiovascular disease is associated with the duration and severity of scleroderma, severity and duration of peripheral Raynaud phenomenon, anti–Scl-70 and anticentromere antibody positivity, higher levels of inflammatory markers, overlap syndrome with vasculitis, and peripheral myositis. Pulmonary arterial hypertension and pulmonary fibrosis with or without cor pulmonale, congestive heart failure, and arrhythmias are the leading causes of death of these patients.

CARDIOVASCULAR INVOLVEMENT

Atherosclerosis

In scleroderma, the intramyocardial coronary arteries and arterioles are predominantly affected by two mechanisms. The first is abnormally increased vasoconstriction resulting from an immune-mediated inflammatory endothelial dysfunction. In these patients, intramyocardial coronary arterial spasm is highly associated with peripheral Raynaud phenomenon. The second mechanism is obstructive microvascular disease resulting from endothelial proliferation, intimal hypertrophy, intimal smooth muscle cell migration, fibrinoid necrosis, fibrosis, and ultimately vessel narrowing. Increased avascularity and capillary ramifications on nailfold videocapillaroscopy correlate with decreased coronary flow reserve and suggest a diffuse microvascular remodeling process.[63] Consequently, focal or diffuse contraction band necrosis (resulting from ischemia and reperfusion) and myocardial fibrosis occur.

The prevalence of epicardial CAD is of less clinical relevance. Coronary angiography in asymptomatic patients with diffuse scleroderma commonly shows normal coronary arteries, with slow flow indicative of increased intramyocardial coronary resistance. Among those with angina, epicardial CAD is seen in less than 50% of patients, and among patients with myocardial infarction, normal epicardial arteries are seen in more than 30%. Typical acute coronary syndrome is uncommon in these patients. Ischemic heart disease most commonly manifests as subacute or chronic diastolic and uncommonly as systolic congestive heart failure.

Because of predominant microvascular disease, echocardiographic findings typical of transmural ischemia or myocardial infarction are uncommon. In asymptomatic young patients studied with dipyridamole or adenosine Doppler TTE, dobutamine stress echocardiography, and multidetector CT, reduction in coronary flow reserve (<2.5) and wall motion abnormalities (but no epicardial CAD) were detected in 60% to 75%, compared with less than 5% in matched controls.[63,64] As a result of microvascular CAD, LV and RV diastolic and, uncommonly, systolic dysfunction can occur. Occasionally, transmural myocardial infarction from epicardial coronary vasospasm can occur.

The cold pressor test with echocardiography and myocardial perfusion imaging shows transient wall motion abnormalities with corresponding reversible, fixed, or mixed perfusion abnormalities in patients with angiographically unremarkable epicardial coronary arteries.[65] Patients with microvascular CAD commonly have associated increased carotid artery and aortic stiffness, indicative of a diffuse microcirculatory disease. Symptoms and wall motion or myocardial perfusion abnormalities improve with coronary vasodilator and antiinflammatory therapy.

Myocardial Disease

Myocardial disease is more common in patients with diffuse cutaneous involvement, systemic and PH, or active peripheral myositis. In these patients, wall motion abnormalities plus T2-weighted hyperintensity (indicative of active inflammation) and delayed gadolinium enhancement (indicative of increased interstitial collagen deposition and fibrosis) by cardiac MRI are common.[66,67] Patchy myocyte contraction band necrosis (typical of ischemia and reperfusion) with myocardial fibrosis is characteristic of the disease and has been reported in up to 80% of patients in postmortem series. These data support functional or structural microvascular CAD as the most common cause of myocardial disease. A septal infarction pattern, ventricular arrhythmias, or conduction abnormalities on electrocardiography are associated with fixed septal or anteroseptal perfusion abnormalities and correspond to areas of myocardial fibrosis on gadolinium-enhanced MRI.[66,67]

Autoimmune-mediated myocarditis is uncommon, but when present, it is associated with microvascular CAD and peripheral myositis (Fig. 37.13). Elevation of troponin I and N-terminal pro-B-type natriuretic peptide (NT-proBNP) in unselected asymptomatic patients further supports intermittent myocardial ischemia, myocarditis, or fibrosis.[68] Hydroxychloroquine-induced restrictive cardiomyopathy has been reported in these patients. Independent of the pathogenesis, systolic heart failure is associated with a high mortality rate (up to 80% at 1 year).

Using Doppler and speckle-tracking TTE, a high prevalence (30%–50%) of subclinical LV and RV diastolic dysfunction and, less often, systolic dysfunction is seen among unselected middle-aged patients with diffuse or limited cutaneous disease, compared with less than 10% in controls.[69–71] Reductions of longitudinal, circumferential, and radial strain and strain rate are more sensitive than mitral and tricuspid inflow and tissue Doppler patterns (60% vs. 30%, respectively).

Type I LV diastolic dysfunction is twice as common as type II, and type III is rare. By 3D and STE, RV and RA increased volumes and areas and diastolic dysfunction are common in those with or without PH and indicate secondary pressure overload and primary myocardial disease, respectively.[69,70,72,73] Although subclinical LV and RV diastolic dysfunction may be associated with a higher incidence of heart failure,[69] the prognostic implications of subclinical myocardial dysfunction remain undefined. LV and RV diastolic dysfunction may improve with antiinflammatory and vasodilator therapy.

Pulmonary Hypertension

Interstitial lung disease and pulmonary arterial hypertension are major causes of death in scleroderma patients.[74] On Doppler echocardiography or right heart catheterization, PH at rest (i.e., pulmonary artery pressure ≥40 mmHg) is detected in 10% to 20% of patients, and exercise-induced PH (i.e., ≥50 mmHg) is detected in 35% to 50% of patients. PH may be similarly related to left heart disease (≈40%) or pulmonary arterial hypertension (≈30%–40%) and less often to lung disease or hypoxia (≈20%–30%). Pulmonary arterial hypertension from inflammatory vasculopathy or pulmonary vasospasm is associated with the limited cutaneous type, digital ulcers, pulmonary diffusion capacity of less than 60%, parameters of endothelial dysfunction, elevated NT-proBNP and endothelin-1 levels, and abnormal lung uptake of gallium and technetium 99m (^{99m}Tc) sestamibi.[75,76] From the time of diagnosis of scleroderma, the incidence of PH over a median follow-up of 3 years is about 25%. Independent of its cause, patients with PH have decreased survival: 81%, 63%, and 56% at 1, 2, and 3 years, respectively.

Resting or exercise Doppler echocardiography and cardiopulmonary exercise testing allow estimation of the systolic and mean pulmonary artery pressures, pulmonary vascular

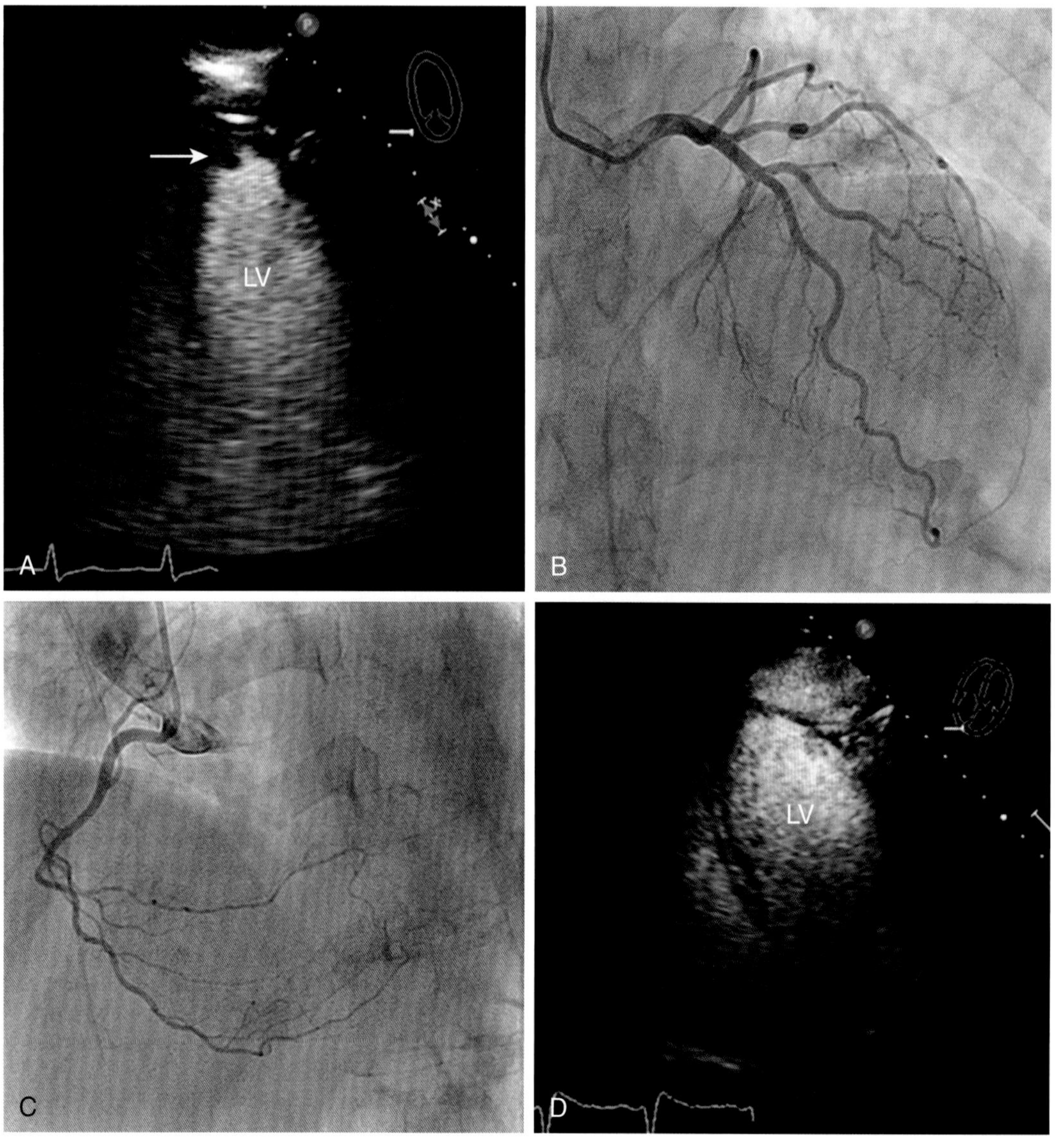

Fig. 37.13 **Myocarditis complicated by severe cardiomyopathy and LV thrombus in scleroderma.** (A) 2D chamber view with Definity contrast in a 43-year-old female patient with diffuse scleroderma and active myositis (i.e., elevated creatinine phosphokinase and aldolase serum levels and electromyogram consistent with diffuse myopathy), chest pain syndrome (with elevated levels of troponin I), and decompensated heart failure demonstrates a severely reduced ejection fraction of 29% and a small apical thrombus (*arrow*) (see Video 37.13A). Left (B) and right (C) coronary angiograms demonstrate narrow-caliber vessels with slow antegrade flow (Thrombolysis in Myocardial Infarction [TIMI] grade II flow) without intimal irregularities, consistent with microvascular coronary artery disease. After 3 months of intravenous immunoglobulin and pulsed intravenous and oral corticosteroid therapy (patient did not tolerate methotrexate or mofetil mycophenolate), standard therapy for heart failure, and warfarin, the patient's cardiomyopathy and heart failure resolved. (D) Follow-up 2D 4-chamber view with Definity contrast demonstrates a low-normal LV ejection fraction of 51% and resolution of the LV apical thrombus (see Video 37.13D).

resistance, and LV diastolic and systolic function. These modalities also help to differentiate precapillary from postcapillary PH and to select patients for right heart catheterization.[77,78] A significant increase (≥20 mmHg) from resting to peak exercise echocardiography is seen in up to 40% of patients with dyspnea of exertion or abnormal pulmonary function.

RA area and volume and peak longitudinal systolic strain at the RV apical lateral segment are independent predictors of pulmonary arterial hypertension.[79] Pulmonary artery systolic pressure and pulmonary vascular resistance are negatively associated with RV systolic performance as measured by the tricuspid annular plane systolic excursion, tissue Doppler tricuspid S′ velocity, and RV fractional area change. The severity of PH on echocardiography is a powerful independent predictor of death over 2 years of follow-up. Using a pulmonary artery systolic pressure of less than 30 mmHg as a reference, the hazard ratio for death is 1.67 for a pressure of 30 to 36 mmHg, 2.37 for 36 to 40 mmHg, 3.72 for 40 to 50 mmHg, and 9.75 for a pressure greater than 50 mmHg. The sensitivity of Doppler echocardiography for detecting PH compared with right heart catheterization is moderate (about 60%) but highly specific (98%).

For patients with suspected PH, the ultimate diagnosis and therapeutic decisions may be best determined with right heart catheterization. Expert consensus standards for performing right heart catheterization include one or more of the following: progressive dyspnea over 3 months, unexplained dyspnea, any finding on physical examination of elevated right heart pressures or right heart failure, pulmonary artery systolic pressure greater than 45 mmHg or RV dilation on echocardiography, and diffusion lung capacity for carbon monoxide of less than 50%.

Pericardial Disease

Symptomatic pericardial disease occurs in 4% to 17% of patients with scleroderma. It manifests as acute pericarditis and, rarely, as cardiac tamponade or pericardial constriction. Asymptomatic pericardial effusions on echocardiography are common in patients with cor pulmonale or hypoalbuminemia. Symptomatic pericardial disease is two to four times more common among patients with the diffuse form than among those with the limited cutaneous form of the disease.

Valve Disease

Scleroderma rarely causes primary valve disease. Reports describe Libman-Sacks–like vegetations, aortitis, and aortic regurgitation. Because of the high prevalence of PH and cor pulmonale, mild to moderate functional tricuspid regurgitation is common.

POLYMYOSITIS AND DERMATOMYOSITIS

BACKGROUND

Polymyositis and dermatomyositis are diseases characterized by autoimmune-mediated skeletal muscle inflammation that leads to symmetric proximal muscle weakness. Myocarditis, pericarditis, and functional or structural microvascular CAD are associated common cardiac manifestations. Although clinically manifested heart disease may occur in less than 25% of patients, it accounts for at least 10% of deaths.

CARDIOVASCULAR INVOLVEMENT

Myocardial Disease

Myocardial disease results from autoimmune-mediated myocarditis and, less often, from functional microvascular CAD. In postmortem series, as many as 50% of patients show histologic evidence of active or healed myocarditis. Multimodality imaging series show myocardial inflammation on cardiac MRI, increased myocardial uptake of ^{99m}Tc pyrophosphate on myocardial scintigraphy, and wall motion abnormalities or LV diastolic dysfunction on echocardiography.[80]

Although the clinical prevalence of myocarditis is unknown, approximately 10% to 20% of those who have myocarditis develop cardiomyopathy. Up to 50% of patients with myocarditis have active skeletal myositis, and vice versa. Rarely, a fulminant myocarditis with severe LV systolic dysfunction is the initial manifestation of the disease. Acute myocarditis can mimic an acute coronary syndrome. With 2D and 3D Doppler and STE, subclinical LV and RV diastolic dysfunction, predominantly impaired relaxation and reduction in LV and RV longitudinal systolic strain, is identified in 12% to 76% of patients, but a decreased ejection fraction is uncommon.[81]

Pericardial Disease, Atherosclerosis, Valve Disease, and Pulmonary Hypertension

With lower prevalences, the pathogenesis and clinical and echocardiographic characteristics of pericardial disease, atherosclerosis, valve disease, and PH associated with polymyositis and dermatomyositis are similar to those of other rheumatologic diseases (see Table 37.1).

SELECTED ARTERITIDES AFFECTING THE AORTA AND BRANCHES

TAKAYASU ARTERITIS

Background

Takayasu arteritis is a chronic vasculitis that affects large vessels and causes (1) focal or diffuse thickening of the vessel walls with consequent stenosis, occlusion, or thrombosis; (2) destruction of the elastic lamina and muscular media leading to aneurysmal or pseudoaneurysmal formation; and (3) vessel stiffness and accelerated atherosclerosis. Takayasu arteritis can be distinguished from other arteritides by identifying at least three of six cardinal clinical features (Table 37.6).

CARDIOVASCULAR INVOLVEMENT

Vascular Disease

Takayasu arteritis predominantly affects the aorta and its main branches. Although the thoracic aorta and abdominal aorta usually are affected, the disease more often clinically manifests with involvement of the left subclavian artery, followed by the carotid, brachiocephalic, and vertebral arteries. The pulmonary arteries are also commonly affected. Nonspecific manifestations of the disease such as fever, malaise, weight loss, and myalgias are commonly associated with or followed by an early nonobstructive vasculitis, and ultimately by an obstructive, pulseless vasculitis. The pulseless phase includes these manifestations:

1. Claudication symptoms with asymmetric, decreased pulses and bruits on the affected arteries
2. Occlusive subclavian artery disease leading to subclavian steal syndrome, in which collateral flow from the vertebral arteries to the poststenotic artery causes reduction of posterior cerebral blood flow and neurologic manifestations, including stroke or syncope[82]
3. Arterial dissections of the carotid, subclavian, vertebral, brachial, celiac, or femoral arteries or of the thoracic aorta and abdominal aorta with a characteristic diffuse and homogeneous wall thickening called the *macaroni sign* seen on ultrasonography[83]
4. Acute coronary syndromes resulting from ascending aortitis that cause coronary artery ostial narrowing, coronary arteritis, or coronary artery aneurysms[84]
5. Symptomatic chronic, subacute, or acute aortic regurgitation mainly resulting from aortic root and annular dilation, less often from primary valvulitis, and rarely from sinus of Valsalva aneurysms, which may rupture into the RA, RV, or LV
6. Hypertension due to aortic stiffness, obstruction, or renal artery disease[85]
7. Accelerated atherosclerosis
8. Chest pain, dyspnea, hemoptysis, and PH in those with aneurysms or stenosis of the pulmonary arteries[86]
9. Focal stenosis of the proximal ascending aorta, descending thoracic aorta, and main pulmonary artery mimicking supravalvular aortic stenosis, aortic pseudocoarctation, and supravalvular pulmonic stenosis, respectively (Table 37.7)[87,88]

Heart Disease

Primary heart disease is common (30%–40% of cases) in these patients. It more often affects the heart valves with regurgitation, uncommonly affects the myocardium or

TABLE 37.6 Distinguishing Characteristics of Selected Arteritides.

Characteristic	*Takayasu Arteritis*	*Giant Cell Arteritis*	*Behçet Disease*
Cardinal Clinical Characteristics			
Age at onset	≤40 years	>50 years	20–40 years
Main symptoms and physical findings	Claudication of upper and lower extremities Decreased pulses on one or both brachial arteries Bruit on one or both subclavian or carotid arteries or abdominal aorta Difference of ≥10 mmHg in systolic blood pressure between arms	New-onset and localized headache Tenderness or decreased pulse of the temporal artery (commonly associated with jaw claudication and visual disturbances, including blindness)	Genital aphthosis (2 points) Anterior or posterior uveitis, or retinal vasculitis (2 points) Oral aphthosis (1 point) Pseudofolliculitis or erythema nodosum (1 point) Superficial phlebitis, deep vein thrombosis, large vein thrombosis, arterial thrombosis, or aneurysms (1 point)
Diagnostic data	Narrowing or occlusion of the aorta and/or its primary branches on imaging	ESR > 50 mm/h Temporal artery biopsy reveals a necrotizing arteritis with mononuclear cell inflammation or granulomatous process with multinucleated giant cells	Pathergy: erythematous papular or pustular response (≥2 mm in diameter) to local skin injury (1 point)
Distinguishing diagnosis	≥3 of above 6 criteria with a sensitivity of 91% and specificity of 98%	≥3 of above 5 criteria with a sensitivity of 94% and specificity of 91%	≥3 of above 8 points with a sensitivity of 87%–97% and specificity of 89%–97%
Other General Characteristics			
Female-to-male ratio	7:1	3:2	1:1 (more common in women in United States)
Ethnicity	Asian	European	Eastern Asian and Mediterranean
Prevalence	1–3 cases/year per million population in United States and Europe	1 in 500 individuals >50 years old	1 in 15,000–500,000 in United States and Northern Europe
HLA association	HLA-Bw52, HLA-B39.2	HLA-DR4	HLA-B51
Affected vascular bed	Large vessels	Medium and large vessels	Small, medium, and large vessels
Histopathologic findings	Mononuclear and granulomatous inflammation	Mononuclear and granulomatous inflammation	Mononuclear and granulomatous inflammation
Inflammatory markers	ESR and CRP usually elevated	ESR and CRP usually elevated	ESR and CRP usually elevated
Mainstay pharmacotherapy	Corticosteroids	Corticosteroids	Corticosteroids
Percutaneous or surgical revascularization	Commonly needed	Uncommonly needed	Rarely needed

CRP, C-reactive protein; *ESR,* erythrocyte sedimentation rate; *HLA,* human leucocyte antigens.

coronary arteries, and rarely affects the pericardium (see Table 37.7).[89] Aortic regurgitation occurs in two thirds of patients with valve regurgitation, and in almost one half of them, aortic regurgitation is moderate to severe. Mitral valve regurgitation occurs in about one third of patients, and in most cases, it is mild.

Diagnostic Imaging

Multimodality imaging, which is usually required in the diagnosis and management of Takayasu arteritis, provides a diagnostic sensitivity and specificity of 95% or higher.[90] Echocardiography detects and characterizes aortic root and annular dilation, vessel wall thickening, and the presence, severity, and mechanism of aortic regurgitation (Fig. 37.14). TTE parasternal short-axis, subxiphoid, and suprasternal long-axis views can help to detect involvement of the left or right pulmonary arteries.[91] Computed tomography angiography (CTA) and MRI or magnetic resonance angiography (MRA) provide information on vessel lumen pathology (i.e., tapered, focally or diffusely narrowed vessels commonly associated with focal or diffuse aneurysmal dilation) and vessel wall thickening.

^{18}Fluorodeoxyglucose positron emission tomography (PET) in combination with CTA differentiates vessel wall thickening due to active inflammation or scarring and provides guidance for antiinflammatory therapy (see Fig. 37.14I). MRA with T2-weighted imaging detects vessel wall thickening due to edema, and gadolinium contrast MRA detects vessel wall scarring. Confirmatory invasive angiography is needed before revascularization procedures.

Therapy

Corticosteroids, frequently in combination with percutaneous transluminal angioplasty or stenting and vascular surgery, are the mainstays of therapy for Takayasu arteritis.[88,90,92]

GIANT CELL ARTERITIS

BACKGROUND

Giant cell arteritis is a chronic vasculitis that affects medium and large vessels and classically manifests clinically as temporal arteritis. Involvement of the aorta and its branches is common. Giant cell arteritis can be distinguished from other arteritides by at least three of five cardinal clinical characteristics (see Table 37.6). The mortality rate for giant cell arteritis is similar to that for Takayasu arteritis and predominantly results from aortic dissection and aneurysms and from ischemic and hypertensive heart disease.[93,94]

CARDIOVASCULAR INVOLVEMENT

Vascular Disease

Giant cell arteritis typically manifests as temporal arteritis, but involvement of the aorta and its proximal branches is common (Fig. 37.15). Involvement of the aorta and its branches with sparing of the temporal arteries can also occur.

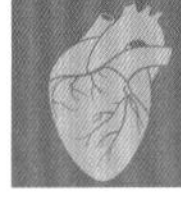

TABLE 37.7 Associated Cardiovascular Disease in Takayasu Arteritis, Giant Cell Arteritis, and Behçet Disease.

Vascular Disease

Aorta and Proximal Branches (25%–50% of Cases)

1. Aortitis
2. Ascending aortitis causing coronary ostial stenosis
3. Aneurysmal dilation of the ascending and/or thoracic and abdominal aorta
4. Aortic pseudoaneurysms
5. Aortic dissection
6. Aortic thrombosis
7. Aortic stiffness and atherosclerosis
8. Arteritis with stenosis, thrombosis, aneurysms or pseudoaneurysms, dilation of aortic branches

Pulmonary Arteries and Branches (15%–25% of Cases)

1. Pulmonary arteritis
2. Pulmonary artery stenosis
3. Pulmonary artery thrombosis
4. Pulmonary artery aneurysmal or pseudoaneurysmal formation

Primary Heart Disease (30%–40% of Cases)

Myocardial Disease

1. Subclinical diastolic and systolic dysfunction
2. Clinical diastolic dysfunction
3. Myocarditis with segmental or global systolic dysfunction
4. Dilated cardiomyopathy

Subendocardial Disease

1. Endomyocardial fibrosis
2. Endocardial calcification
3. Atrial or ventricular thrombosis (more common in the right heart)
4. Ventricular pseudoaneurysms

Heart Valve Disease

1. Aortic or pulmonic valve regurgitation due to aortic or pulmonary artery dilation
2. Aortic regurgitation due to aortic annular stiffness with decreased elastic diastolic recoiling
3. Aortic pseudoinfective endocarditis or Libman-Sacks–like endocarditis
4. Aortic regurgitation due to prosthetic valve dehiscence or pseudoaneurysm formation in those with active aortitis (≤50% of cases)

Coronary Artery Disease

1. Coronary artery ostial stenosis, occlusion, or thrombosis due to ascending aortitis
2. Coronary arteritis
3. Coronary artery aneurysmal and pseudoaneurysmal disease
4. Microvascular coronary artery disease

Pericardial Disease

1. Uncomplicated acute pericarditis
2. Acute pericarditis with cardiac tamponade
3. Myopericarditis

Heart Disease

Primary heart disease is common and clinically manifests as Takayasu arteritis (see Table 37.7). Ischemic heart disease is the predominant manifestation (10%–25%).[93,94] Myocarditis is rare (≤3%).

Diagnostic Imaging and Therapy

The applications and diagnostic value of multimodality imaging in giant cell arteritis are similar to those in Takayasu arteritis (see Fig. 37.15). Ultrasonography can demonstrate a hypoechogenic halo sign in the temporal artery vessel wall in addition to stenosis or occlusion. The diagnostic sensitivities and specificities, respectively, are 69% and 82% for the halo sign, 68% and 78% for stenosis or occlusion, and 78% and 88% for the presence of halo sign, stenosis, or occlusion.

Characteristic histopathology of a temporal artery biopsy is considered the standard for diagnosis, but its sensitivity ranges from 60% to 85%, and complementary MRI or MRA and/or PET are often needed. However, initiation of corticosteroids should not await confirmation by biopsy or imaging in patients with other diagnostic clinical and laboratory data. Corticosteroids in combination with other immunosuppressive therapy, percutaneous transluminal angioplasty, less frequently stenting, and rarely vascular surgery are the main therapies for giant cell arteritis.[94,95]

BEHÇET DISEASE

BACKGROUND

Behçet disease is a chronic vasculitis that affects small, medium, and large arteries and veins. The disease manifests clinically with recurrent and painful oral and genital aphthae; various cutaneous manifestations; asymmetric, nonerosive, and nondeforming arthritis of the knees, ankles, and wrists; recurrent and bilateral panuveitis; and parenchymal and nonparenchymal brain disease. The ocular, vascular, and neurologic manifestations carry the highest morbidity and mortality rates. Behçet disease can be distinguished from other arteritides by a score of at least three of eight points derived from five cardinal clinical characteristics (see Table 37.6).

CARDIOVASCULAR INVOLVEMENT

Vascular Disease

Behçet disease causes vessel wall thickening, stenosis, occlusion, and aneurysm formation. Vascular disease can be the initial manifestation of the disease in about 25% of cases; it is more prevalent among men (male-to-female ratio of 4:1) in their third decade of life and manifests more commonly with superficial or deep vein thrombosis. Arterial disease is also common, but it varies and usually involves small vessels. Involvement of medium and large vessels occurs in one third of cases (Fig. 37.16).[96] Arterial and venous diseases occur in 25% of cases.

Women may have more arterial disease and cardiac involvement than men. The aortic, iliac, femoral, popliteal, and carotid arteries are most commonly affected. Involvement of the cerebral, renal, and coronary arteries is uncommon. Involvement of the pulmonary arteries with formation of aneurysms carries a 25% mortality rate.

Heart Disease

Primary heart disease is common (≈30% of cases) and clinically manifests similar to Takayasu and giant cell arteritides. It can rarely precede vascular disease (see Table 37.7).

Moderate to severe aortic regurgitation is the most common manifestation[97,98] and in 30% of cases is associated with aortic root dilation, aneurysm, or pseudoaneurysm or with coronary sinus aneurysm.[99] In patients with moderate to severe aortic regurgitation, prolapse of aortic cusps, vegetation-like mobile lesions, an echo-free space mimicking aortic root abscess, and aortic aneurysm are common findings.[98,99]

Atrioventricular, bundle branch, and fascicular blocks are common (20%–25%) in patients with aortic root and valve disease. Decreased LV global longitudinal strain can be seen in up to 50% of patients with active disease. Intracardiac thrombosis (≥90% of cases on the right heart), coronary arterial pseudoaneurysm, pulmonary artery dilation and aneurysm, pericardial effusion, and dissections of the proximal interventricular septum are rare.

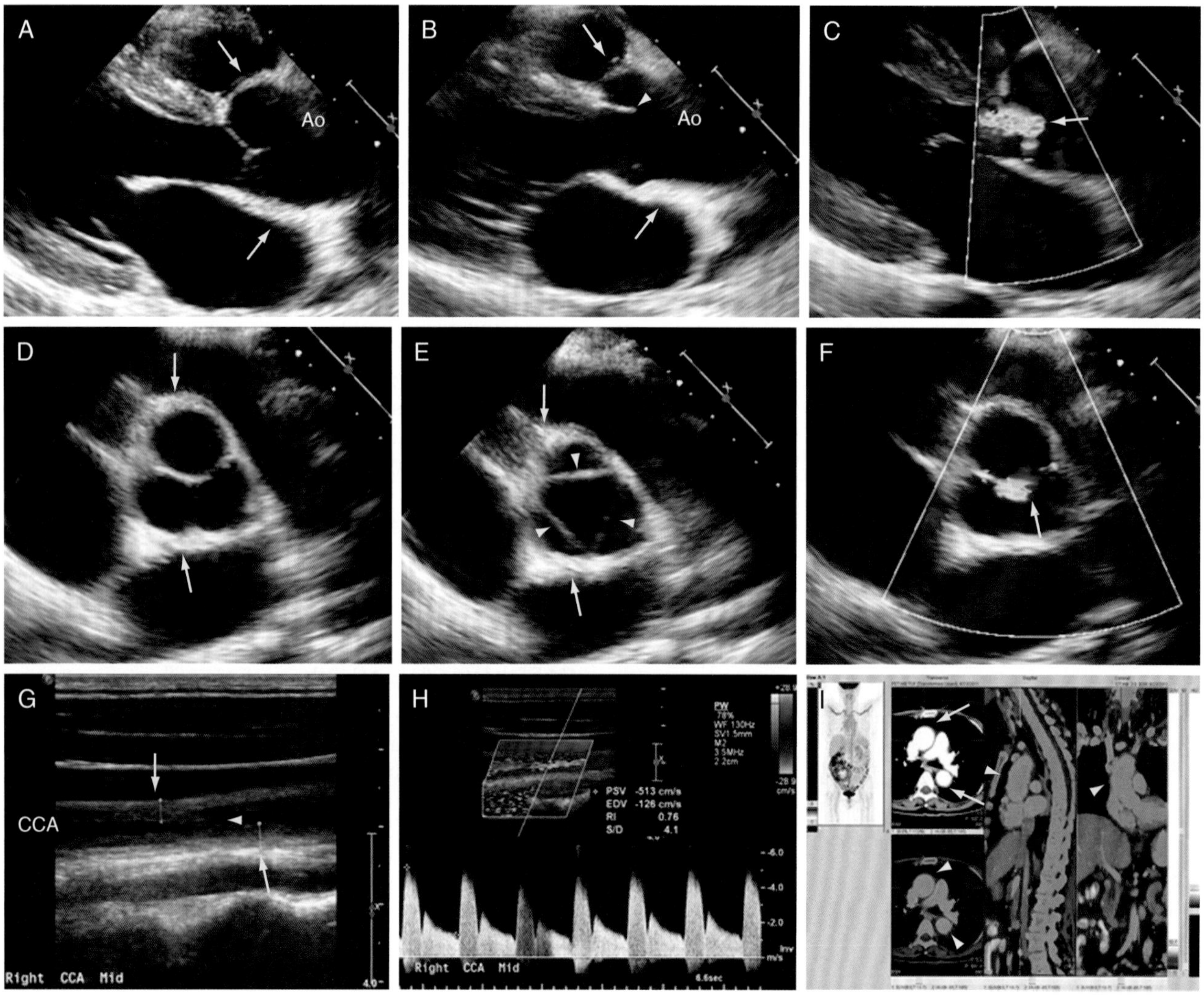

Fig. 37.14 Takayasu arteritis. Takayasu arteritis in a 22-year-old man manifested clinically with a diastolic heart murmur and a right carotid bruit. (A–F) 2D and color Doppler parasternal long-axis and short-axis views of the aortic root *(Ao)* and aortic valve demonstrate mild aortic root dilation, marked and circumferential thickening of the aortic root walls *(arrows)*, decreased mobility of all three aortic cusps (*arrowheads* in B and E), and incomplete coaptation of the cusps due to aortic root dilation and decreased elastic recoiling of the aortic annulus, resulting in moderate central aortic regurgitation (*arrows* in C and F). (G and H) Carotid ultrasonography demonstrates severe thickening (3–5 mm) of the middle, near, and far walls *(arrows)* of the right common carotid artery *(CCA)*, resulting in severe carotid stenosis *(arrowhead)* and very high systolic and diastolic flow velocities (H). (I) Transverse, sagittal, and coronal fused computed tomographic angiography–positron emission tomography (CTA-PET) images demonstrate circumferential thickening of the ascending and descending thoracic aorta *(arrows)* with significant increase in metabolic activity on the entire aorta *(arrowheads)*, indicating active aortitis (see Videos 37.14A and 37.14C–14F).

Diagnostic Imaging and Therapy

The diagnostic value of multimodality imaging in Behçet disease and its therapy are similar to those for Takayasu and giant cell arteritis (see Fig. 37.16).

Cardiovascular disease is common in rheumatologic diseases and noninfectious arteritides and is associated with high morbidity and mortality rates. Echocardiography helps in the selection of, timing of, and response to therapy for cardiovascular disease associated with rheumatologic diseases (see Tables 37.1–37.7). However, echocardiography has some limitations, and other complementary imaging modalities may be needed in specific conditions (Table 37.8).

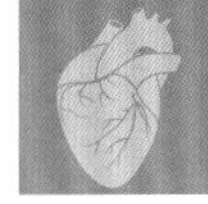

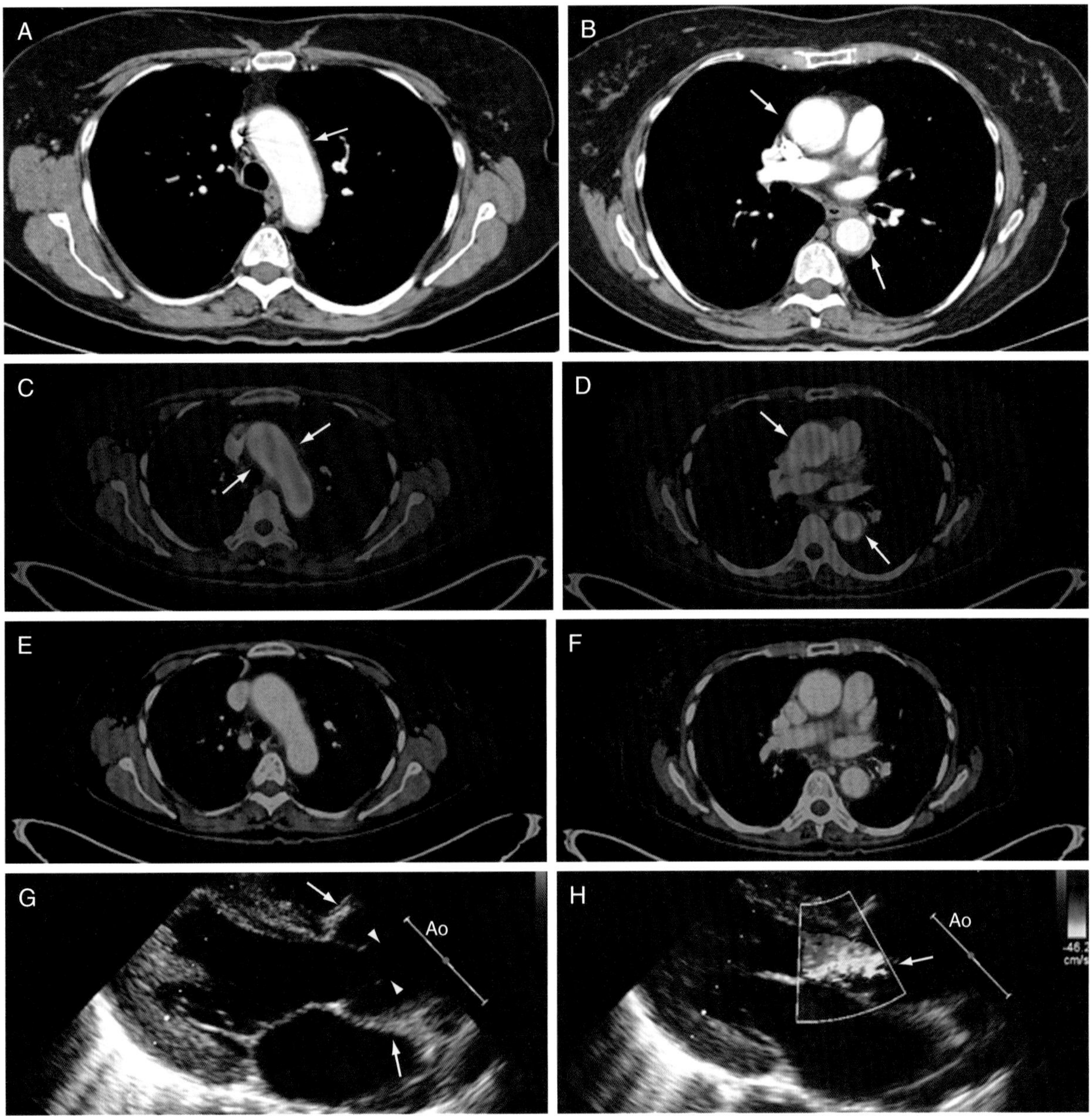

Fig. 37.15 Giant cell arteritis. Giant cell arteritis associated with aortic regurgitation in a 62-year-old man. (A and B) Transverse computed tomographic angiography (CTA) images of the chest demonstrate moderate circumferential and diffuse thickening of the thoracic aorta *(arrows)*. (C and D) Fused positron emission tomography–CTA (PET-CTA) images demonstrate diffuse increased metabolic activity within the walls of the entire aorta *(arrows)*, indicating active aortitis. (E and F) Fused PET-CTA images performed after corticosteroid therapy demonstrate resolution of the increased metabolic activity within the walls of the aorta, suggesting resolution of vascular inflammation. (G and H) Long-parasternal 2D (G) and color Doppler (H) images of the aortic *(Ao)* root and aortic valve before corticosteroid therapy demonstrate mild aortic root dilation, moderate thickening of the anterior and posterior root walls *(arrows)*, decreased mobility *(arrowheads)* of structurally normal-appearing aortic cusps (G), and moderate degree of central aortic regurgitation (*arrow* in H). Associated mild LV hypertrophy with moderate global LV hypokinesis and moderate LV systolic dysfunction due to associated myocarditis was also demonstrated (see Videos 37.15G and 37.15H ▶).

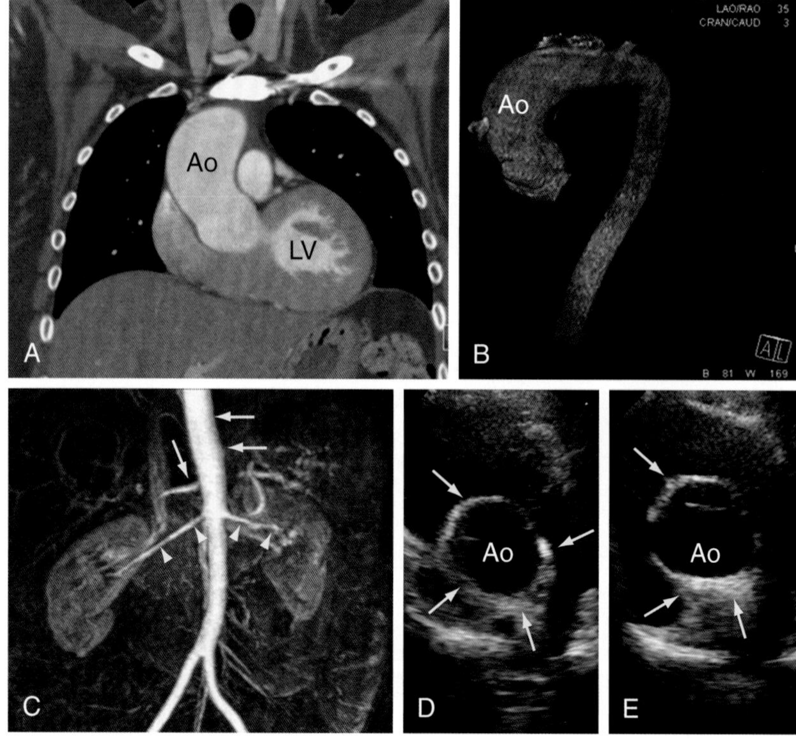

Fig. 37.16 Behçet disease. Behçet disease in a 30-year-old man with severe refractory hypertension. (A) Coronal computed tomographic angiogram (CTA) demonstrates aneurysmal dilation of the ascending aorta *(Ao)* and moderate concentric LV hypertrophy. (B) 3D-rendered CTA of the aorta confirms the aneurysmal dilation of the ascending aorta. (C) Contrast magnetic resonance angiography of the abdominal aorta demonstrates mild thickening of the aortic walls and its branch vessels *(arrows)*, suggestive of vasculitis. The renal arteries demonstrate diffuse and heterogeneous narrowing *(arrowheads)*. Lobulation of both kidneys suggests ischemic scarring. (D and E) 2D parasternal short-axis TTE views of the aortic root (at the level of the coronary sinus) during end-diastole (D) and end-systole (E) demonstrate mild dilation and moderate to severe heterogeneous thickening of the aortic walls *(arrows)*, predominantly of the posterior wall (see Video 37.16D). Mild aortic regurgitation was detected. Fused positron emission tomography (PET)-CTA imaging (not shown) confirmed wall thickening of the thoracic and abdominal aorta without increased metabolic activity, suggesting inactive or healed vasculitis.

TABLE 37.8 Limitations of Echocardiography in the Assessment of Cardiovascular Disease Associated With Rheumatologic Diseases and Arteritides.

Valve Disease, Intracardiac Thrombosis, and Thromboembolism

- Low rate of detection of noninfective vegetations by TTE (less than one third of those detected by 2D or 3D TEE)
- With TEE as the standard, TTE has very low sensitivity (<15%) and low negative predictive value (<60%) for detection of noninfective vegetations; has low sensitivity, specificity, and negative predictive values (<60%) for detecting valve thickening; and underestimates the severity of mitral and aortic regurgitation.
- The low rate of detection of noninfective vegetations by TTE precludes assessment of its specificity and positive predictive value for detection of this abnormality.
- TTE is limited in the characterization of noninfective endocarditis or valvulitis.
- TTE is limited in the assessment of patients with suspected embolic cerebrovascular disease or peripheral arterial embolism.
- TEE is semi-invasive and requires high expertise. There is a need for an algorithm of clinical and laboratory predictors that will allow performing a TEE with a high diagnostic yield for detecting noninfective endocarditis, especially in those with suspected cardioembolism.
- The echocardiographic features of noninfective and infective vegetations and sometimes of normal variants (e.g., Lambl excrescences, nodes of Arantius) may overlap on 2D and 3D TEE, and complementary clinical and laboratory data (including microbiology) may be required.

Myocardial Disease

- Although speckle tracking and tissue Doppler echocardiography are highly sensitive for detecting subclinical LV and RV diastolic and systolic dysfunction, specific cutoff values for defining abnormality and categorizing the degree of myocardial dysfunction have not been determined in these young and predominantly female patients.
- The clinical and prognostic implications of echocardiographically detected subclinical LV and RV diastolic and systolic dysfunction have not been determined.
- Echocardiography is also limited in defining the cause of subclinical or clinical myocardial disease as vasculitis, myocarditis, or ischemic epicardial coronary artery disease (CAD).

Coronary Artery Disease

- Resting and exercise echocardiography yield a low rate of abnormal results for patients with predominant functional or structural microvascular CAD.
- The resting and exercise echocardiographic features of primary myopericarditis or myocarditis overlap with those of an acute coronary syndrome due to epicardial atherosclerotic CAD or coronary arteritis.
- Coronary angiography may be warranted for patients with suspected acute coronary syndrome.

Pericardial Disease

- Asymptomatic small pericardial effusions are a common incidental finding (≈20%) in hospitalized patients with active rheumatologic diseases and may be caused by mild pericarditis, hypoalbuminemia, or pulmonary hypertension with or without cor pulmonale.
- Absence of a pericardial effusion is common in a patient with symptomatic acute pericarditis.
- Complementary clinical, electrocardiographic, and serology data are needed for the proper assessment of pericarditis in these patients.
- Echocardiography is insensitive for detection of mild or moderate pericardial thickening. Cardiac magnetic resonance imaging and computed tomography are important complementary imaging studies for assessment of pericardial thickening when pericardial constriction is suspected by echocardiography.

Pulmonary Hypertension

- With right heart catheterization as the standard, the sensitivity of Doppler echocardiography for detection of pulmonary hypertension is moderate (≈60%), although it is highly specific (98%).
- Echocardiography may be limited in the differentiation of a type or combination of types of pulmonary hypertension.
- For patients with suspected symptomatic pulmonary hypertension, the ultimate diagnosis and therapeutic decisions for pulmonary hypertension may require right heart catheterization.

Arteritides Affecting the Aorta and Its Branches

- TTE is limited to the assessment of the aortic root.
- TTE and TEE cannot differentiate aortic wall thickening due to active inflammation from that due to scarring.
- TEE is limited in the assessment of pathology of the aortic arch and its main branches.
- Contrast computed tomography angiography and contrast magnetic resonance angiography with ^{18}fluorodeoxyglucose positron emission tomography are the preferred diagnostic modalities for assessment of luminal and wall pathology of the aorta and its main branches in these conditions.

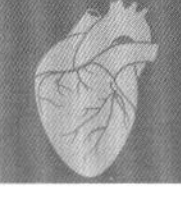

SUMMARY Rheumatologic Diseases and Arteritides: Clinical Presentations, Echocardiographic Correlates, and Therapeutic Caveats of Associated Cardiovascular Diseases

Clinical Presentations	Echocardiographic Findings	Therapeutic Caveats
Valve Disease and Thromboembolism		

• Cerebroembolism
  • Cerebromicroembolism
  • Stroke/TIA
  • Acute confusional state or seizures
• Decreased cerebral perfusion
• Focal ischemic brain injury
  • Cerebral infarcts
  • Small focal periventricular and deep white matter abnormalities
• Cognitive dysfunction and disability
• Peripheral arterial embolism including to the coronary arteries
• Rarely, pulmonary or paradoxical embolism from right heart valve vegetations or vegetations/thrombosis associated with right heart catheters or wires
• Acute valvulitis with or without perforations and severe valve regurgitation
• Superimposed infective endocarditis
	• Libman-Sacks vegetations in SLE
	• Libman-Sacks–like or thrombotic vegetations in PAPS
	• Rarely, atrial or ventricular endocardial vegetations in SLE and PAPS
	• Vegetations or thrombi associated with right heart catheters or wires
	• Valve nodules and Libman-Sacks–like vegetations in rheumatoid arthritis
	• Superimposed infective vegetations
	• Associated, various degrees of regurgitation; rarely stenosis
	• TEE should be considered in patients with (1) acute, recent (within 2–4 weeks), or recurrent stroke or TIA; (2) acute, recent, or recurrent confusional state, cognitive dysfunction, or seizures if focal brain lesions are seen on MRI or cerebromicroembolism on transcranial Doppler; (3) peripheral arterial embolism; (4) moderate or worse regurgitation by TTE; or (5) suspected superimposed infective endocarditis
		• Based on a specific clinical scenario and in consultation with rheumatology, medical therapy with immunosuppressive antiinflammatory (corticosteroids or cytotoxics) and antithrombotic therapy for noninfective endocarditis complicated by valve vegetations and cerebroembolism or valvulitis complicated by significant valve regurgitation may be considered before considering short-term and long-term high-risk valve surgery (if needed, repair may be preferable)

Coronary Artery Disease		

• Commonly asymptomatic or overshadowed by musculoskeletal inflammatory manifestations or misinterpreted as pleuritis or pericarditis
• Atypical chest pain is common in these predominantly young women
• Typical presentation as acute coronary syndrome, including unstable angina, non-STEMI, and STEMI occur
	• Decreased coronary flow reserve with dipyridamole or adenosine echocardiography in those with functional microvascular CAD
	• Resting or exercise or dobutamine stress-induced wall motion abnormalities or myocardial perfusion defects in patients with epicardial obstructive CAD or coronary arteritis
	• Correlates of CAD
	  • Decreased peripheral arterial vasodilation
	  • Increased carotid arteries and/or aortic stiffness
	  • Coronary artery calcifications on CT
	  • Increased carotid and aortic intima media thickening or plaques on carotid ultrasonography and TEE, respectively
		• Based on a specific clinical scenario and in consultation with rheumatology, standard medical therapy in combination with immunosuppressive antiinflammatory therapy and DMARDS may be considered concomitantly with high-risk PCI for acute coronary syndromes
		• Conventional and biologic DMARDS (e.g., TNF-α blocker, anti–B cell therapy) and vasodilators (e.g., endothelin antagonists) may be beneficial in patients with rheumatoid arthritis or scleroderma

Continued

SUMMARY Rheumatologic Diseases and Arteritides: Clinical Presentations, Echocardiographic Correlates, and Therapeutic Caveats of Associated Cardiovascular Diseases—cont'd

Clinical Presentations	Echocardiographic Findings	Therapeutic Caveats
Myocardial Disease		
• Subclinical LV and RV diastolic and systolic dysfunction • Atypical or typical chest pain in those with symptomatic microvascular CAD • Clinical diastolic and, uncommonly, systolic heart failure • Acute coronary syndrome–like syndrome, such as in those with myopericarditis or myocarditis • Rarely, severe global cardiomyopathy due to primary myocarditis • Rarely, transient and reversible stress-like cardiomyopathy and chloroquine-induced restrictive or dilated cardiomyopathy • Secondary atrial or ventricular arrhythmias	• Traditional parameters of diastolic dysfunction assessed by mitral inflow velocities, tissue Doppler, and STE • Infrequent resting or exercise-induced segmental wall motion abnormalities or myocardial perfusion defects in those with microvascular CAD • Common resting segmental or global wall motion abnormalities in those with myopericarditis or myocarditis or global cardiomyopathy	• Based on a specific clinical scenario and in consultation with rheumatology, immunosuppressive antiinflammatory therapy, conventional and biologic DMARDS, and vasodilators (e.g., endothelin antagonists) may be considered in addition to standard medical therapy
Pericardial Disease		
• Acute pericarditis • Moderate or large pericardial effusion without findings of cardiac tamponade • Cardiac tamponade • Transient effusive constrictive pericarditis • Constrictive pericarditis • Asymptomatic noninflammatory small pericardial effusions • Rare but important to exclude, superimposed or primary infective pericarditis	• Small pericardial effusion or no effusion • Thrombotic or inflammatory strands in the pericardial fluid • Pericardial thickening • Traditional parameters of cardiac tamponade and constrictive pericarditis	• In a patient with an active rheumatologic disease and a large pericardial effusion with or without indicators of tamponade, an earlier diagnostic (to exclude infection) or therapeutic (for rapid progression or hemorrhagic transformation) echocardiography-guided pericardiocentesis followed by intensive immunosuppressive antiinflammatory therapy and DMARDS may be considered • Avoid a pericardial window in these patients because of commonly associated serositis (peritonitis and pleuritis) and increased risk of infection
Pulmonary Hypertension		
• Asymptomatic RV structural abnormalities and subclinical diastolic and systolic dysfunction • Acute or chronic cor pulmonale with clinical right heart failure • Secondary atrial tachyarrhythmias	• Resting (≥40 mmHg) or exercise-induced (≥50 mmHg) pulmonary artery systolic pressure • Elevated pulmonary artery systolic pressure and pulmonary vascular resistance if associated normal LA pressure (type I or type III) or elevated LA pressure (type II) • Cor pulmonale (various degrees of right heart enlargement and RV diastolic and/or systolic dysfunction) • Associated tricuspid regurgitation of various degrees • Associated abnormal septal motion of RV pressure and/or volume overload	• Confirmatory right heart catheterization is usually required • Based on a specific clinical scenario and in consultation with rheumatology, immunosuppressive antiinflammatory therapy, DMARDS, and vasodilators should be considered in addition to standard medical therapy for type I and type III PH

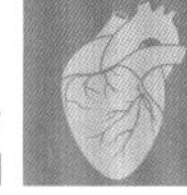

SUMMARY Rheumatologic Diseases and Arteritides: Clinical Presentations, Echocardiographic Correlates, and Therapeutic Caveats of Associated Cardiovascular Diseases—cont'd

Clinical Presentations	Echocardiographic Findings	Therapeutic Caveats
Arteritides Affecting the Aorta and Its Branches		
• Claudication symptoms with asymmetric and decreased pulses and bruits on affected arteries • Occlusive subclavian or carotid artery disease • Subclavian steal syndrome • Chest pain, dyspnea, hemoptysis, and PH in those with aneurysms or stenosis of the pulmonary arteries • Acute coronary syndromes from ascending aortitis causing coronary artery ostial narrowing or from coronary arteritis • Chronic, subacute, or acute aortic regurgitation • Hypertension due to aortic stiffness and/or renal artery disease • Accelerated atherosclerosis	• Aortic root and annular dilation, wall thickening, and stiffness by TTE and TEE • Ascending aorta, arch, and descending aorta aneurysmal or pseudoaneurysmal dilation, wall thickening, stiffness, and atherosclerosis by TEE • Detection, characterization, and determination of the mechanism of associated aortic regurgitation • Detection and characterization of associated myocardial, endocardial, and pericardial disease • Detection and characterization of PH, right heart thrombosis, and main pulmonary artery dilation by TTE • Detection and characterization of aortic branch disease requires CTA or MRA	• Based on a specific clinical scenario and in consultation with rheumatology, consider cardiothoracic or vascular surgery or interventional cardiology evaluations • Stabilization with oral or intravenous corticosteroid therapy for severe aortitis complicated by significant valve regurgitation, ostial CAD, coronary arteritis, and/or aortic branch vessel occlusive disease may be considered before proceeding with short-term and long-term high-risk valve, coronary artery, or branch vessel surgical or percutaneous revascularization due to the high rate of prosthetic valve dehiscence and bypass graft and stent closure or thrombosis

CAD, Coronary artery disease; *CT,* computed tomography; *CTA,* computed tomography angiography; *DMARDs,* disease-modifying antirheumatic drugs; *MRA,* magnetic resonance angiography; *MRI,* magnetic resonance imaging; *PAPS,* primary antiphospholipid antibody syndrome; *PCI,* percutaneous coronary intervention; *PH,* pulmonary hypertension; *SLE,* systemic lupus erythematosus; *STE,* speckled track echocardiography; *STEMI,* ST-segment elevation myocardial infarction; *TIA,* transient ischemic attack; *TNF-α,* tumor necrosis factor-α.

REFERENCES

1. Roldan CA, Shively BK, Crawford MH. An echocardiographic study of valvular heart disease associated with systemic lupus erythematosus. *N Engl J Med.* 1996;335:1424–1430.
2. Ruiz D, Oates JC, Kamen DL. Antiphospholipid antibodies and heart valve disease in systemic lupus erythematosus. *Am J Med Sci.* 2018;355:293–298.
3. Roldan CA, Qualls CR, Sopko KS, Sibbitt Jr WL. Transthoracic versus transesophageal echocardiography for detection of Libman-Sacks endocarditis: a randomized controlled study. *J Rheumatol.* 2008;35:224–229.
4. Roldan CA, Tolstrup K, Macias L, et al. Libman-sacks endocarditis: detection, characterization, and clinical correlates by three-dimensional transesophageal echocardiography. *J Am Soc Echocardiogr.* 2015;28:770–779.
5. Levin D, Snider R, Ratliff M, Qualls C, Roldan CA. Libman-sacks endocarditis: who should undergo TEE? *Circulation.* 2019;140:A12345.
6. Roldan CA, Sibbitt Jr WL, Qualls CR, et al. Libman-Sacks endocarditis and embolic cerebrovascular disease. *JACC Cardiovasc Imaging.* 2013;6:973–983.
7. Aby ES, Rosol Z, Simegn MA. Mitral valve perforation in Libman-Sacks endocarditis: a heart-wrenching case of lupus. *J Gen Intern Med.* 2016;31:964–969.
8. Roberts WC, Lee AY, Lander SR, Roberts CS, Hamman BL. Libman-Sacks endocarditis involving a bioprosthesis in the aortic valve position in systemic lupus erythematosus. *Am J Cardiol.* 2019;124:316–318.
9. Fanouriakis A, Kostopoulou M, Alunno A, et al. 2019. Update of the EULAR recommendations for the management of systemic lupus erythematosus. *Ann Rheum Dis.* 2019;78:736–745.
10. Roldan CA, Sibbitt WL, Greene ER, Qualls CR, Jung RE. Libman-Sacks endocarditis and associated cerebrovascular disease: the role of medical therapy. *PLoS One.* 2021;16(2):e0247052. https://doi: 10.1371/journal.pone.0247052. PMID: 33592060.
11. Bouma W, Klinkenberg TJ, van der Horst IC, et al. Mitral valve surgery for mitral regurgitation caused by Libman-Sacks endocarditis: a report of four cases and a systematic review of the literature. *J Cardiothorac Surg.* 2010;5(13).
12. Foroughi M, Hekmat M, Ghorbani M, et al. Mitral valve surgery in patients with systemic lupus erythematosus. *Scientific World Journal.* 2014;216291:2014.
13. Tejeda-Maldonado J, Quintanilla-González L, Galindo-Uribe J, Hinojosa-Azaola A. Cardiac surgery in systemic lupus erythematosus patients: clinical characteristics and outcomes. *Reumatol Clin.* 2018;14:269–277.
14. Roldan CA, Schevchuck O, Tolstrup K, et al. Lambl's excrescences: association with cerebrovascular disease and pathogenesis. *Cerebrovasc Dis.* 2015;40:18–27.
15. Giannelou M, Mavragani CP. Cardiovascular disease in systemic lupus erythematosus: a comprehensive update. *J Autoimmun.* 2017;82:1–12.
16. Kravvariti E, Konstantonis G, Tentolouris N, Sfikakis PP, Tektonidou MG. Carotid and femoral atherosclerosis in antiphospholipid syndrome: Equivalent risk with diabetes mellitus in a case-control study. *Semin Arthritis Rheum.* 2018;47:883–889.
17. Taraborelli M, Sciatti E, Bonadei I, et al. Endothelial dysfunction in early systemic lupus erythematosus patients and controls without previous cardiovascular events. *Arthritis Care Res.* 2018;70:1277–1283.
18. Kakuta K, Dohi K, Sato Y, et al. Chronic inflammatory disease is an independent risk factor for coronary flow velocity reserve impairment unrelated to the processes of coronary artery calcium deposition. *J Am Soc Echocardiogr.* 2016;29:173–180.
19. Roldan CA, Joson J, Qualls CR, et al. Premature aortic stiffness in systemic lupus erythematosus by transesophageal echocardiography. *Lupus.* 2010;19:1599–1605.
20. Roldan CA, Joson J, Sharrar J, et al. Premature aortic atherosclerosis in systemic lupus erythematosus: a controlled transesophageal echocardiographic study. *J Rheumatol.* 2010;37:71–78.
21. Hu L, Chen Z, Jin Y, et al. Incidence and predictors of aorta calcification in patients with systemic lupus erythematosus. *Lupus.* 2019;28:275–282.
22. Roldan LP, Roldan PC, Sibbitt WLJr, Qualls CR, Ratliff MD, Roldan CA. Aortic adventitial thickness as a marker of aortic atherosclerosis, vascular stiffness, and vessel remodeling in systemic lupus erythematosus. *Clin Rheumatol.* 2020 Oct 6. https://doi:10.1007/s10067-020-05431-7. Online ahead of print. PMID: 33025269.
23. Hollan I, Prayson R, Saatvedt K, et al. Inflammatory cell infiltrates in vessels with different susceptibility to atherosclerosis in rheumatic and non-rheumatic patients. *Circ J.* 2008;72:1986–1992.

24. Roldan PC, Greene ER, Qualls CR, Sibbitt Jr WL, Roldan CA. Progression of atherosclerosis versus arterial stiffness with age within and between arteries in systemic lupus erythematosus. *Rheumatol Int*. 2019;39:1027–1036.
25. Floris A, Piga M, Mangoni AA, et al. Protective effects of hydroxychloroquine against accelerated atherosclerosis in systemic lupus erythematosus. *Mediators Inflamm*. 2018: 2018:3424136.
26. Roldan CA, Alomari IB, Awad K, et al. Aortic stiffness is associated with left ventricular diastolic dysfunction in systemic lupus erythematosus: a controlled transesophageal echocardiographic study. *Clin Cardiol*. 2014;37:83–90.
27. Thomas G, Cohen Aubart F, Chiche L, et al. Lupus myocarditis: initial presentation and longterm outcomes in a multicentric series of 29 patients. *J Rheumatol*. 2017;44:24–32.
28. Mavrogeni S, Koutsogeorgopoulou L, Markousis-Mavrogenis G, et al. Cardiovascular magnetic resonance detects silent heart disease missed by echocardiography in systemic lupus erythematosus. *Lupus*. 2018;27:564–571.
29. Dedeoglu R, Şahin S, Koka A, et al. Evaluation of cardiac functions in juvenile systemic lupus erythematosus with two-dimensional speckle tracking echocardiography. *Clin Rheumatol*. 2016;35:1967–1975.
30. Dai M, Li KL, Qian DJ, et al. Evaluation of left atrial function by speckle tracking echocardiography in patients with systemic lupus erythematosus. *Lupus*. 2016;25:496–504.
31. Mohamed AAA, Hammam N, El Zohri MH, Gheita TA. Cardiac manifestations in systemic lupus erythematosus: clinical correlates of subclinical echocardiographic features. *BioMed Res Int*. 2019 Jan 10;2019:2437105.
32. Chang JC, Knight AM, Xiao R, Mercer-Rosa LM, Weiss PF. Use of echocardiography at diagnosis and detection of acute cardiac disease in youth with systemic lupus erythematosus. *Lupus*. 2018;27:1348–1357.
33. Assayag M, Abbas R, Chanson N, et al. Diagnosis of systemic inflammatory diseases among patients admitted for acute pericarditis with pericardial effusion. *J Cardiovasc Med*. 2017;18:875–880.
34. Kang KY, Jeon CH, Choi SJ, et al. Survival and prognostic factors in patients with connective tissue disease-associated pulmonary hypertension diagnosed by echocardiography: results from a Korean nationwide registry. *Int J Rheum Dis*. 2017;20:1227–1236.
35. Kim JS, Kim D, Joo YB, et al. Factors associated with development and mortality of pulmonary hypertension in systemic lupus erythematosus patients. *Lupus*. 2018;27:1769–1777.
36. Pérez-Peñate GM, Rúa-Figueroa I, Juliá-Serdá G, et al. Pulmonary arterial hypertension in systemic lupus erythematosus: prevalence and predictors. *J Rheumatol*. 2016;43:323–329.
37. Luo R, Cui H, Huang D, et al. Early assessment of right ventricular function in systemic lupus erythematosus patients using strain and strain rate imaging. *Arq Bras Cardiol*. 2018;111:75–81.
38. Sun L, Wang Y, Dong Y, et al. Assessment of right atrium function in patients with systemic lupus erythematosus with different pulmonary artery systolic pressures by 2-dimensional speckle-tracking echocardiography. *J Ultrasound Med*. 2018;37:2345–2351.
39. Ames PRJ, Margarita A, Sokoll KB, et al. Premature atherosclerosis in primary antiphospholipid syndrome: preliminary data. *Ann Rheum Dis*. 2005;64:315–317.
40. Tufano A, Lembo M, Di Minno MN, et al. Left ventricular diastolic abnormalities other than valvular heart disease in antiphospholipid syndrome: an echocardiographic study. *Int J Cardiol*. 2018;271:366–370.
41. Tanrıkulu O, Sarıyıldız MA, Batmaz İ, et al. Serum GDF-15 level in rheumatoid arthritis: relationship with disease activity and subclinical atherosclerosis. *Acta Reumatol Port*. 2017;42:66–72.
42. Temiz A1, Gökmen F, Gazi E, et al. Epicardial adipose tissue thickness, flow-mediated dilatation of the brachial artery, and carotid intima-media thickness: associations in rheumatoid arthritis patients. *Herz*. 2015;40:217–224.
43. Kakuta K, Dohi K, Sato Y, et al. Chronic inflammatory disease is an independent risk factor for coronary flow velocity reserve impairment unrelated to the Processes of coronary artery calcium deposition. *J Am Soc Echocardiogr*. 2016;29:173–180.
44. Mantel Ä, Holmqvist M, Jernberg T, Wållberg-Jonsson S, Askling J. Long-term outcomes and secondary prevention after acute coronary events in patients with rheumatoid arthritis. *Ann Rheum Dis*. 2017;76:2017–2024.
45. Cañas F, Lopez Ponce de León JD, Gomez JE, Cañas CA. A giant fibrinoid pericardial mass in a patient with rheumatoid arthritis: a case report. *Eur Heart J Case Rep*. 2019;3: pii: ytz061.
46. Roldan CA, DeLong C, Qualls CR, Crawford MH. Characterization of valvular heart disease in rheumatoid arthritis by transesophageal echocardiography and clinical correlates. *Am J Cardiol*. 2007;100:496–502.
47. Marques L, Moreno N, Seabra D, et al. Aortic regurgitation in rheumatoid arthritis: an uncommon presentation. *Int J Cardiovasc Imaging*. 2019;35:117–118.
48. Tennyson C, Kler A, Chaturvedi A, Paschalis A, Venkateswaran R. Rheumatoid nodule on the anterior mitral valve leaflet. *J Card Surg*. 2018;33:643–645.
49. Baktir AO, Sarli B, Cebıcı MA, et al. Preclinical impairment of myocardial function in rheumatoid arthritis patients. Detection of myocardial strain by speckle tracking echocardiography. *Herz*. 2015;40:669–674.
50. Lo Gullo A, Rodríguez-Carrio J, Aragona CO, et al. Subclinical impairment of myocardial and endothelial functionality in very early psoriatic and rheumatoid arthritis patients: association with vitamin D and inflammation. *Atherosclerosis*. 2018;271:214–222.
51. Geraldino-Pardilla L, Russo C, Sokolove J, et al. Association of anti-citrullinated protein or peptide antibodies with left ventricular structure and function in rheumatoid arthritis. *Rheumatology*. 2017;56:534–540.
52. Fatma E, Bunyamin K, Savas S, et al. Epicardial fat thickness in patients with rheumatoid arthritis. *Afr Health Sci*. 2015;15:489–495.
53. Yogasundaram H, Putko BN, Tien J, et al. Hydroxychloroquine-induced cardiomyopathy: case report, pathophysiology, diagnosis, and treatment. *Can J Cardiol*. 2014;30:1706–1715.
54. Panagiotidou E, Sourla E, Kotoulas SX, et al. Rheumatoid arthritis associated pulmonary hypertension: clinical challenges reflecting the diversity of pathophysiology. *Respir Med Case Rep*. 2017;20:164–167.
55. Kang KY, Jeon CH, Choi SJ, et al. Survival and prognostic factors in patients with connective tissue disease-associated pulmonary hypertension diagnosed by echocardiography: results from a Korean nationwide registry. *Int J Rheum Dis*. 2017;20:1227–1236.
56. Roldan CA, Chavez J, Weist P, et al. Aortic root disease and valve disease associated with ankylosing spondylitis. *J Am Coll Cardiol*. 1998;32:1397–1404.
57. Ozen S, Ozen A, Unal EU, et al. Subclinical cardiac disease in ankylosing spondylitis. *Echocardiography*. 2018;35:1579–1586.
58. Ozkaramanli Gur D, Ozaltun DN, Guzel S, et al. Novel imaging modalities in detection of cardiovascular involvement in ankylosing spondylitis. *Scand Cardiovasc J*. 2018;52:320–327.
59. Klingberg E, Sveälv BG, Täng MS, et al. Aortic regurgitation is common in ankylosing spondylitis: time for routine echocardiography evaluation? *Am J Med*. 2015;128:1244–1250.
60. Hwang HJ, Kim JI, Lee SH, Park CB, Sohn IS. Full-blown cardiac manifestations in ankylosing spondylitis. *Echocardiography*. 2016;33:1785–1787.
61. Midtbø H, Semb AG, Matre K, et al. Left ventricular systolic myocardial function in ankylosing spondylitis. *Arthritis Care Res*. 2019;71:1276–1283.
62. Surucu GD, Yildirim A, Yetisgin A, Akturk E. Epicardial adipose tissue thickness as a new risk factor for atherosclerosis in patients with ankylosing spondylitis. *J Back Musculoskelet Rehabil*. 2019;32:237–243.
63. Zanatta E, Famoso G, Boscain F, et al. Nailfold avascular score and coronary microvascular dysfunction in systemic sclerosis: a newsworthy association. *Autoimmun Rev*. 2019;18:177–183.
64. Kakuta K, Dohi K, Sato Y, et al. Chronic inflammatory disease is an independent risk factor for coronary flow velocity reserve impairment unrelated to the processes of coronary artery calcium deposition. *J Am Soc Echocardiogr*. 2016;29:173–180.
65. Papagoras C, Achenbach K, Tsifetaki N, et al. Heart involvement in systemic sclerosis: a combined echocardiographic and scintigraphic study. *Clin Rheumatol*. 2014;33:1105–1111.
66. Muresan L, Oancea I, Mada RO, et al. Relationship between ventricular arrhythmias, conduction disorders, and myocardial fibrosis in patients with systemic sclerosis. *J Clin Rheumatol*. 2018;24:25–33.
67. Hromádka M, Seidlerová J, Suchý D, et al. Myocardial fibrosis detected by magnetic resonance in systemic sclerosis patients - relationship with biochemical and echocardiography parameters. *Int J Cardiol*. 2017;249:448–453.
68. Nordin A, Svenungsson E, Björnådal L, et al. Troponin I and echocardiography in patients with systemic sclerosis and matched population controls. *Scand J Rheumatol*. 2017;46:226–235.
69. Saito M, Wright L, Negishi K, Dwyer N, Marwick TH. Mechanics and prognostic value of left and right ventricular dysfunction in patients with systemic sclerosis. *Eur Heart J Cardiovasc Imaging*. 2018;19:660–667.
70. Durmus E, Sunbul M, Tigen K, et al. Right ventricular and atrial functions in systemic sclerosis patients without pulmonary hypertension. *Speckle-tracking echocardiographic study, Herz*. 2015;40:709–715.
71. Vemulapalli S, Cohen L, Hsu V. Prevalence and risk factors for left ventricular diastolic dysfunction in a scleroderma cohort. *Scand J Rheumatol*. 2017;46:281–287.
72. Pigatto E, Peluso D, Zanatta E, et al. Evaluation of right ventricular function performed by 3D-echocardiography in scleroderma patients. *Reumatismo*. 2015;66:259–263.

73. Mukherjee M, Chung SE, Ton VK, et al. Unique abnormalities in right ventricular longitudinal strain in systemic sclerosis patients. *Circ Cardiovasc Imaging*. 2016;9. e003792.
74. Athanasiou KA, Sahni S, Rana A, Talwar A. Diagnosing and managing scleroderma-related pulmonary arterial hypertension. *JAAPA*. 2017;30:11–18.
75. Guillén-Del Castillo A, Callejas-Moraga EL, García G, et al. High sensitivity and negative predictive value of the DETECT algorithm for an early diagnosis of pulmonary arterial hypertension in systemic sclerosis: application in a single center. *Arthritis Res Ther*. 2017;19:135.
76. Coghlan JG, Wolf M, Distler O, et al. Incidence of pulmonary hypertension and determining factors in patients with systemic sclerosis. *Eur Respir J*. 2018;51 pii: 1701197.
77. Dumitrescu D, Nagel C, Kovacs G, et al. Cardiopulmonary exercise testing for detecting pulmonary arterial hypertension in systemic sclerosis. *Heart*. 2017;103:774–782.
78. Chin K, Mathai SC. Exercise echocardiography in connective tissue disease. *J Am Coll Cardiol*. 2015;66:385–387.
79. Hekimsoy V, Kaya EB, Akdogan A, et al. Echocardiographic assessment of regional right ventricular systolic function using two-dimensional strain echocardiography and evaluation of the predictive ability of longitudinal 2D-strain imaging for pulmonary arterial hypertension in systemic sclerosis patients. *Int J Cardiovasc Imaging*. 2018;34:883–892.
80. Diederichsen LP, Simonsen JA, Diederichsen AC, et al. Cardiac abnormalities in adult patients with polymyositis or dermatomyositis as assessed by noninvasive modalities. *Arthritis Care Res*. 2016;68:1012–1020.
81. Zhong Y, Bai W, Xie Q, et al. Cardiac function in patients with polymyositis or dermatomyositis: a three-dimensional speckle-tracking echocardiography study. *Int J Cardiovasc Imaging*. 2018;34:683–693.
82. Kim H, Barra L. Ischemic complications in Takayasu's arteritis: a meta-analysis. *Semin Arthritis Rheum*. 2018;47:900–906.
83. Wang J, Lee YZ, Cheng Y, et al. Sonographic characterization of arterial dissections in Takayasu arteritis. *J Ultrasound Med*. 2016;35:1177–1191.
84. Rigatelli G, Zuin M, Picariello C, Cardaioli P, Roncon L. Aortitis-related isolated bilateral coronary artery ostial stenosis in a young woman with acute coronary syndrome. *Int J Cardiol*. 2016;223:111–112.
85. Yang Y, Wang Z, Yuan LJ, et al. Aortic stiffness evaluated by echocardiography in female patients with Takayasu's arteritis. *Clin Exp Rheumatol*. 2017;35(suppl 103):134–138.
86. Sari A, Sener YZ, Firat E, et al. Pulmonary hypertension in Takayasu arteritis. *Int J Rheum Dis*. 2018;21:1634–1639.
87. Kim DY, Kim HW. Atypical initial presentation of Takayasu arteritis as isolated supra-valvular aortic stenosis. *J Cardiothorac Surg*. 2016;11(15) https://doi:10.1186/s13019-016-0408-0.
88. Dong H, Jiang X, Peng M, et al. Percutaneous transluminal angioplasty for symptomatic pulmonary stenosis in Takayasu arteritis. *J Rheumatol*. 2014;41:1856–1862.
89. Nishigami K. Role of cardiovascular echo in patients with Takayasu arteritis. *J Echocardiogr*. 2014;12:138–141.
90. Kim ESH, Beckman J. Takayasu arteritis: challenges in diagnosis and management. *Heart*. 2018;104:558–565.
91. Jiang W, Yang Y, Lv X, et al. Echocardiographic characteristics of pulmonary artery involvement in Takayasu arteritis. *Echocardiography*. 2017;34:340–347.
92. Mason JC. Surgical intervention and its role in Takayasu arteritis. *Best Pract Res Clin Rheumatol*. 2018;32:112–124.
93. Dagan A, Mahroum N, Segal G, et al. The association between giant cell arteritis and ischemic heart disease: a population based cross-sectional study. *Isr Med Assoc J*. 2017;19:411–414.
94. Li L, Neogi T, Jick S. Giant cell arteritis and vascular disease-risk factors and outcomes: a cohort study using UK Clinical Practice Research Datalink. *Rheumatology*. 2017;56:753–762.
95. Gagné-Loranger M, Dumont É, Voisine P, et al. Giant cell aortitis: clinical presentation and outcomes in 40 patients consecutively operated on. *Eur J Cardio Thorac Surg*. 2016;50:555–559.
96. Goliasch G, Hoke M. Large vessel vasculitis in Behçet's disease. *Eur Heart J Cardiovasc Imaging*. 2017;18:724.
97. Li R, Pu L, Sun Z, Wang Y, et al. Echocardiographic findings of cardiovascular involvement in Behçet's disease and post-operative complications after cardiac surgery. *Clin Exp Rheumatol*. 2018;36(6 suppl 115):103–109.
98. Abidov A, Alpert JS. Importance of echocardiographic findings in the acute presentation of Behçet's diseasediagnostic and prognostic considerations. *Echocardiography*. 2014;31:913–915.
99. Pu L, Li R, Xie J, et al. Characteristic echocardiographic manifestations of Behçet's disease. *Ultrasound Med Biol*. 2018;44:825–830.

中文导读

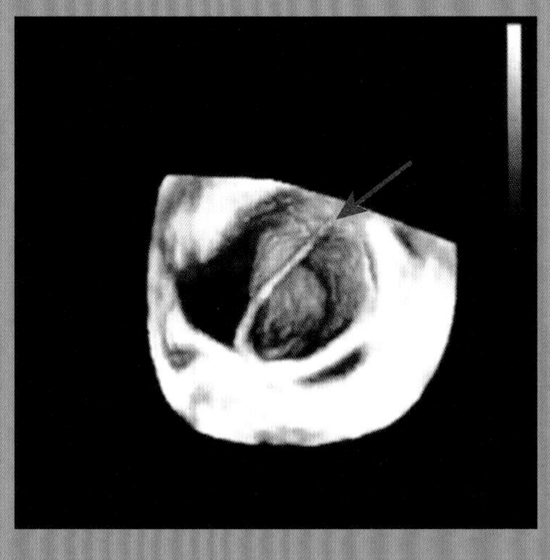

第38章
系统性栓塞事件的超声心动图评估

心脏和主动脉是体循环栓塞事件的主要来源，而栓子脱落的常见靶器官是脑部，微小的栓子脱落即可导致严重的功能障碍和后遗症，因此对栓塞事件发生后的患者筛查潜在的栓子来源具有重要临床意义。栓子最常见的分类有心肌梗死、心力衰竭后的左心室血栓形成；瓣膜的赘生物形成；心脏肿瘤；房颤后左心房和左心耳的血栓形成；主动脉近段的粥样斑块形成等。此外，卵圆孔未闭和房间隔膨凸瘤也被证实与脑卒中事件相关。常规的经胸超声心动图已经广泛应用于栓塞患者，对于相当一部分的栓子来源已经有很好的检出率，而且当医师怀疑卵圆孔未闭、左心耳血栓或对瓣膜病变和主动脉显示不足时，可以借助经食管超声心动图的高分辨率来增加诊断的敏感性。对于左心室心尖部的血栓，有时无法清楚显示时，可以使用超声对比剂左心室造影来帮助明确心腔和栓子边界，以更好地显示栓子的位置、大小和形态等。多种超声检查方法的结合对于栓子来源的综合诊断能力已非常强大，其他检查方法如CT和MRI作为补充，可以提供病变部位的组织学特性，以及提供心脏周围器官的受累情况。本章详细比较了每种超声检查手段的优缺点，并阐述了如何利用这些超声检查的特点，针对性的探查心血管系统中可能发生的各种栓子来源。

卢宏泉

38

Echocardiographic Evaluation of Patients With a Systemic Embolic Event

MARCO R. DI TULLIO, MD

BACKGROUND

CARDIAC EMBOLISM

The heart and the aorta are a potential source of embolism to the systemic circulation. Because the brain is the most frequent target, investigation of cardiac embolic sources is especially aggressive after a cerebral embolic event. Most data on outcome and prevention of recurrences come from the stroke literature. The same embolic sources and principles for investigating them also apply to peripheral embolic events, with the addition of the descending aorta.

CARDIOEMBOLIC AND CRYPTOGENIC STROKE

Stroke is the third leading cause of death in the United States, after cardiac diseases and cancer (pre-COVID-19 era). Approximately 7.0 million Americans 20 years of age or older have had a stroke.[1] Each year, approximately 795,000 people experience a stroke; it occurs as a first event in 75% of cases.[1] The estimated prevalence of silent cerebral infarction is 6% to 28%. That of transient ischemic attacks (TIAs), which are temporary episodes of neurologic dysfunction that have risk factors similar to those of stroke and often precede it, is 2.3%, which probably is an underestimation.[1] Most strokes (87%) have an ischemic origin, involving blockage of the blood supply to the affected territory. The remainder are accounted for by intracerebral (10%) or subarachnoid (3%) hemorrhage.[1]

Ischemic stroke has a cardioembolic source in approximately 20% of cases.[2] Cases that have no apparent cause (i.e., cryptogenic strokes) often have a clinical presentation and neurologic imaging findings that suggest an embolic event and are also known as *embolic strokes of undetermined source*, or ESUS. Identification of new cardioembolic sources has led to the involvement of cardiologists, especially echocardiographers, in stroke diagnosis and prevention. Their efforts have reduced the proportion of strokes labeled as cryptogenic[3] and changed treatment and secondary prevention strategies.

BASIC PRINCIPLES AND ECHOCARDIOGRAPHIC APPROACH

Transthoracic echocardiography (TTE) and especially transesophageal echocardiography (TEE) are widely used to investigate cardioembolic sources in patients with stroke or TIA. TTE is indicated for screening because it can detect some embolic sources (i.e., left ventricular [LV] apical thrombus in particular but also large valvular vegetations and intracardiac masses) and aid the decision whether to proceed to the more invasive TEE. TEE is preferred when TTE cannot clearly visualize the cardiac or aortic structures and in all instances in which high-resolution imaging of structures is needed.

TEE is superior to TTE for visualization of the atrial septum and cardiac valves. It allows a more accurate diagnosis of patent foramen ovale (PFO) or infective endocarditis (IE). TEE also provides accurate visualization of structures such as the left atrial appendage and the proximal thoracic aorta, which are important potential embolic sources. Table 38.1 shows a clinically useful classification of embolic sources and the most appropriate echocardiographic technique for each of them.

TECHNICAL ASPECTS: TEE VERSUS TTE IN CRYPTOGENIC CEREBRAL ISCHEMIA

TEE has greater sensitivity than TTE for detection of cardioembolic sources. Among 231 patients with cryptogenic stroke or TIA, a potential source of embolism was observed in 55% by TEE but in only 16% by TTE.[4] A major embolic source, with an absolute indication for anticoagulation, was found in 20% of patients by TEE and in only 4% by TTE.[4] The superior diagnostic yield of TEE was confirmed in 702 consecutive patients with ischemic stroke or TIA.[5] TEE produced relevant findings in 52.6% of the patients; PFO (21.7%) and previously undiagnosed valvular disease (15.8%) were the most common findings.[5]

TABLE 38.1 Echocardiographic Evaluation of Cardioaortic Embolic Sources.

Embolic Source	*Possibly Associated Conditions*	*Age Group*	*Best Diagnostic Study*
LV thrombus	Prior myocardial infarction, dilated cardiomyopathy	Any	TTE
LA thrombus or spontaneous echocardiographic contrast	Atrial fibrillation, mitral valve disease	Any	TEE
Valvular vegetations	Infective endocarditis (fever, murmur, systemic symptoms), lupus erythematosus	Any	TEE/TTE (less sensitive)
Valvular disease	Varies	Any	TTE for initial evaluation TEE for further assessment, especially for prosthetic valves
Cardiac tumors (myxoma, fibroelastoma, secondary malignancies)	None or nonspecific systemic symptoms	Any	TTE for screening TEE if suspicion is high despite nondiagnostic TTE
Patent foramen ovale	None	Any; more frequent in patients < 55 y	TTE with contrast for screening TEE if more detail is needed
Atrial septal aneurysm	None	Any; more frequent in patients < 55 y	TTE for screening TEE for better imaging
Valve strands	None	Any	TEE
Aortic plaques	Diffuse atherosclerosis	>60 y	TEE

TABLE 38.2 Therapeutic Changes Resulting From the Use of TEE to Investigate Cardiac Embolic Sources in Patients With Acute Ischemic Stroke or Transient Ischemic Attack.

	Patient Characteristics				Therapeutic Changes		
Study	N	M/F	Age	*Most Common Findings*	N	%	*Type of Change*
de Bruijn et al. (2006)[4]	231	N/A	39 pts ≤ 45 y; 192 pts > 45 y	Aortic plaques 30%; LAA thrombus 16%	46	20	Initiation of OAC
Harloff et al. (2006)[6]	212	125/87	58.2 ± 13.9 y	PFO 20.3%; aortic plaque 17.6%	65	22.6	Initiation of OAC
Khariton et al. (2014)[7]	1458	792/726	60.5 y (range, 17–93 y)	PFO 11.9%; IE 1.4%; aortic plaque 1%; tumor or mass 0.5%	243	16.7	Initiation of OAC, PFO closure, antibiotics for IE, cardiac surgery

IE, Infective endocarditis; *LAA*, left atrial appendage; *N/A*, information not available; *OAC*, oral anticoagulation; *PFO*, patent foramen ovale; *pts*, patients.

Several studies have shown that TEE findings directly affect the therapeutic choices for approximately 20% of cryptogenic stroke patients (Table 38.2).[4,6,7] Criteria for appropriate use of echocardiography in patients with a recent embolic event were issued in 2011 by the American College of Cardiology Foundation (from the consensus of the major imaging and medical societies in the United States).[8] More recently, guidelines on appropriate use were issued by the American Society of Echocardiography.[9] These guidelines, which have more emphasis on the inappropriateness of imaging in cases of low pretest probability or when the results are unlikely to affect management, are summarized in Table 38.3.

CLINICAL UTILITY AND OUTCOME DATA

MYOCARDIAL INFARCTION, LV DYSFUNCTION, AND THROMBUS

Myocardial infarction (MI) and dilated cardiomyopathy are frequently associated with LV thrombus formation. In the first month after an acute MI, the incidence of stroke is between 2% and 3%; 50% of the events occur in the first 5 days.[10] Among 2160 patients with incident MI, the incidence of stroke during the first month was increased 44-fold compared with controls.[11] The risk of stroke or TIA is elevated during the first 3 to 6 months and declines thereafter, but it is still twofold to threefold higher than for controls during the first 3 years after an MI.[11]

The risk of stroke or TIA is mainly related to the formation of thrombus in the infarcted area. In a meta-analysis, an echocardiographically demonstrated mural thrombus carried a more than fivefold increased risk of stroke.[12] The frequency of thrombus formation is higher after an anterior than an inferior MI. Among 642 patients with an anterior MI, LV thrombus formed in 6.2%.[13] Thrombus characteristics associated with embolic risk are a central lack of lucency, hyperkinesis of adjacent myocardial segments, and (possibly) thrombus size.[9]

TTE is commonly used for the detection of LV thrombus because of its excellent sensitivity (95%) and specificity (85%–90%).[9] With adequate images, TTE is preferred to TEE because most ventricular thrombi tend to form in the apex (Fig. 38.1), which may or may not be visualized by TEE. The use of a contrast agent for LV opacification (Fig. 38.2) decreases the number of uncertain findings. Among 123 patients with inconclusive TTE results, contrast revealed a thrombus in 14, allowing exclusion of its presence in all others.[14] Among 33 patients with suspected thrombus, contrast allowed its exclusion in 13 (39%). Overall, the use of contrast led to a therapeutic change for a large number of patients by guiding the initiation of anticoagulation or by avoiding it when unnecessary.[14]

Because most LV thrombi form in the apex, multiple TTE views of the apex should be obtained from different imaging windows (see Fig. 38.1). Thrombus size, protrusion, and mobility can be assessed, and these features may affect its thromboembolic potential. The use of higher-frequency transducers (3.5 or 5 MHz) can enhance the thrombus detection rate.

For patients with documented LV thrombus, prophylaxis with warfarin aiming for an international normalized ratio (INR) of 2.0 to 3.0 is recommended in addition to aspirin (75–162 mg) for secondary prevention of MI. At least 3 months of anticoagulation is recommended,[15] with continuation of treatment based on follow-up echocardiographic findings (e.g., persistence of LV thrombus, severity of LV dysfunction).

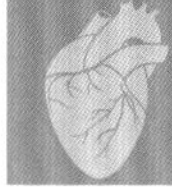

TABLE 38.3 Appropriate Use Criteria for Echocardiography in Evaluation of Cardiac Sources of Emboli.

Appropriate Use: TTE
Symptoms or conditions potentially related to suspected cardiac etiology, including but not limited to chest pain, shortness of breath, palpitations, TIA, stroke, or peripheral embolic event
Suspected cardiac mass
Suspected cardiovascular source of embolus
Initial evaluation of suspected IE with positive blood culture results or new murmur
Reevaluation of IE at high risk for progression or complication or with a change in clinical status or cardiac examination results
Known acute PE to guide therapy (e.g., thrombectomy and thrombolytic therapy)
Reevaluation of known PE after thrombolysis or thrombectomy for assessment of change in RV function and/or pulmonary artery pressure
Appropriate Use: TEE
As initial or supplemental test for evaluation for cardiovascular source of embolus with no identified noncardiac source
As initial or supplemental test to diagnose IE with a moderate or high pretest probability (e.g., staph bacteremia, fungemia, prosthetic heart valve, or intracardiac device)
As initial test for evaluation to facilitate clinical decision making with regard to anticoagulation, cardioversion, and/or radiofrequency ablation
Uncertain Indication for Use: TEE
Evaluation for cardiovascular source of embolus with a previously identified noncardiac source
Inappropriate Use: TTE
Transient fever without evidence of bacteremia or new murmur
Transient bacteremia with a pathogen not typically associated with IE and/or a documented nonendovascular source of infection
Routine surveillance of uncomplicated IE when no change in management is contemplated
Suspected PE to establish diagnosis
Routine surveillance of prior PE with normal RV function and pulmonary artery systolic pressure
Inappropriate Use: TEE
Evaluation for cardiovascular source of embolus with a known cardiac source in which TEE would not change management
Routine use of TEE when diagnostic TTE is reasonably anticipated to resolve all diagnostic and management concerns
Surveillance of prior transesophageal echocardiographic finding for interval change (e.g., resolution of thrombus after anticoagulation, resolution of vegetation after antibiotic therapy) when no change in therapy is anticipated
To diagnose IE with low pretest probability (e.g., transient fever, known alternative source of infection, negative blood culture results, or atypical pathogen for endocarditis)
Evaluation when a decision has been made to anticoagulate and not to perform cardioversion

IE, Infective endocarditis; *PE*, pulmonary embolism; *TIA*, transient ischemic attack.
From Saric M, Armour AC, Arnaout S, et al. Guidelines for the use of echocardiography in the evaluation of a cardiac source of embolism. *J Am Soc Echocardiogr.* 2016;29:1–42.

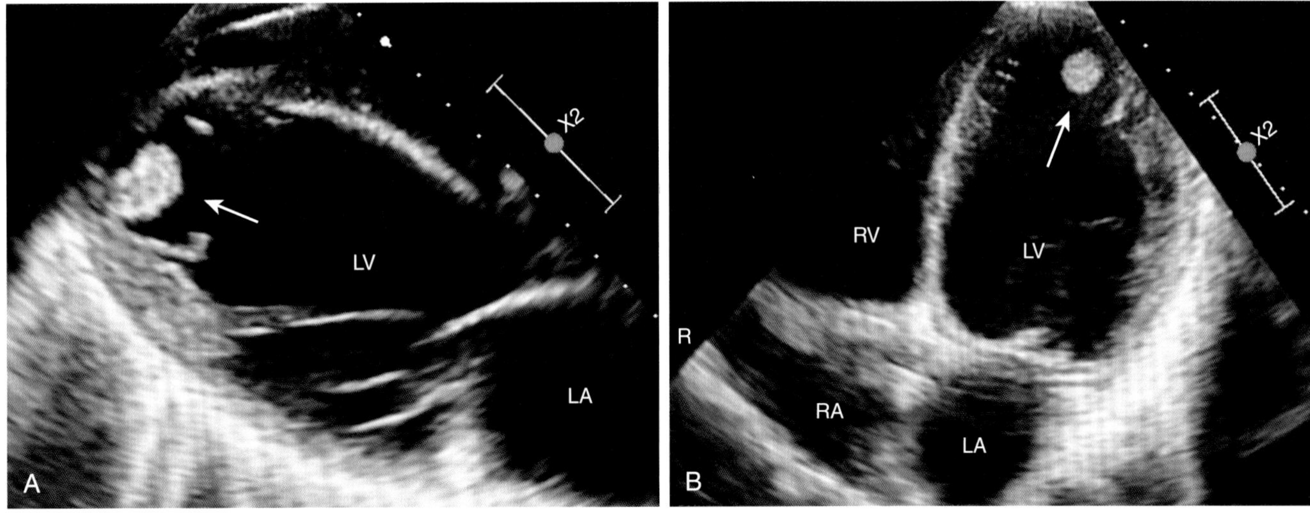

Fig. 38.1 Large apical thrombus imaged by TTE. The thrombus *(arrows)* was highly mobile in real-time imaging. (A) Parasternal long-axis view (see Video 38.1A). (B) Apical 4-chamber view (see Video 38.1B).

In a meta-analysis of 25,307 patients, warfarin treatment with an INR of 2 to 3 in addition to aspirin resulted in a sharp decrease in incident stroke compared with aspirin alone (odds ratio [OR] = 0.43, 95% confidence interval [CI]: 0.27–0.70, *P* = 0.0007), although with an increase in major bleeding (OR = 2.32, 95% CI: 1.63–3.29, *P* < 0.00001).[16] However, the usefulness of systemic anticoagulation in all patients with anterior MI appears questionable. For 2482 anterior MI survivors, the use of anticoagulation for up to 90 days after MI was not associated with a significant reduction in stroke risk over 4 years (hazard ratio [HR] = 0.68, 95% CI: 0.37–1.26), whereas treatment with angiotensin-converting enzyme inhibitors (HR = 0.65, 95% CI: 0.44–0.95) and β-blockers (HR = 0.60, 95% CI: 0.41–0.87) was.[17]

Sparse information is available on the frequency of thrombus and cerebral embolization among patients with dilated cardiomyopathy. The frequency of embolic events is thought to parallel the deterioration in LV function because of the increased frequency of blood stagnation and thrombus formation. Stroke incidence

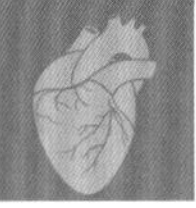

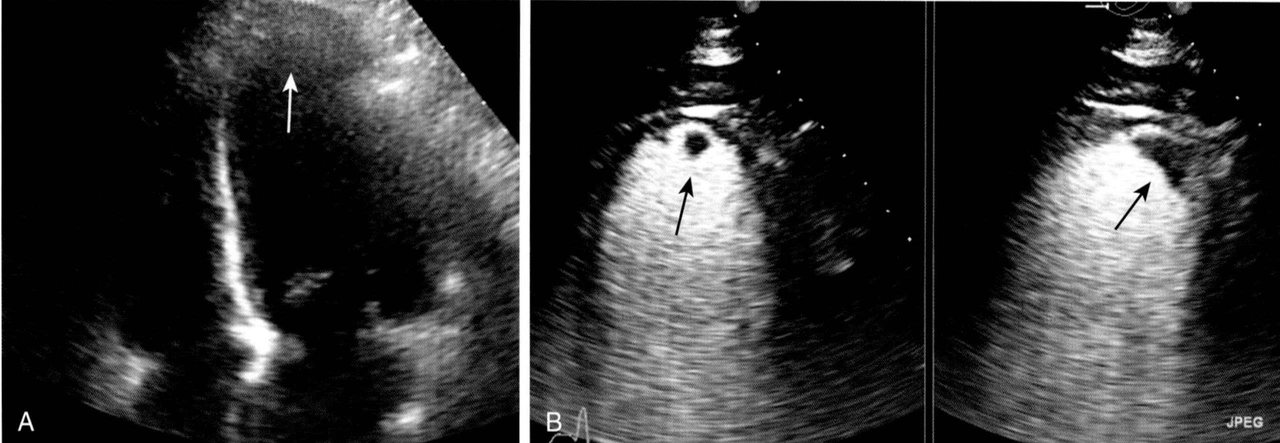

Fig. 38.2 Use of LV contrast for detecting an intraventricular thrombus. (A) A faint echogenicity *(arrow)* of uncertain significance is visualized by TTE in the LV apex (see Video 38.2A). (B) LV contrast injection demonstrates a thrombus *(arrows)* filling the apex. Orthogonal views allow a more accurate evaluation of the thrombus size (see Video 38.2B).

TABLE 38.4 Antithrombotic Treatment and Embolic Risk in Heart Failure: Results From the WATCH and WARCEF Trials.

WATCH[19] (N = 1587) Median F/U = 19 mo	Warfarin (n = 540)		Aspirin (n = 523)		Clopidogrel (n = 524)		*P* Value		
Parameter[a]	*N*	*Rate (%)*	*N*	*Rate (%)*	*N*	*Rate (%)*	*W vs. A*	*W vs. C*	*A vs. C*
Death	92	17.0	94	18.0	96	18.3	0.69	0.58	0.88
Ischemic stroke	3	0.6	12	2.3	12	2.3	0.02	0.02	1.0
Peripheral embolism	2	0.4	4	0.8	4	0.8	0.39	0.39	1.0
Pulmonary embolism	1	0.2	2	0.4	1	0.2	0.55	0.56	0.98
Major hemorrhage	28	5.2	19	3.6	11	2.1	0.22	0.007	0.14
Intracerebral hemorrhage	6	1.1	3	0.6	1	0.2	0.34	0.06	0.32

WARCEF[20] (N = 2305) Median F/U = 42 mo	Warfarin (n = 1142)		Aspirin (n = 1163)			
Parameter[a]	*N*	*Rate/y (%)*	*N*	*Rate/y (%)*	*Hazard Ratio*[b] *(95% CI)*	*P Value*
Death	268	6.63	263	6.52	1.01 (0.85–1.21)	0.91
Ischemic stroke	29	0.72	55	1.36	0.52 (0.33–0.82)	0.005
Peripheral embolism	5	0.015	3	0.007	N/A	0.46
Pulmonary embolism	5	0.015	6	0.014	N/A	0.79
Major hemorrhage	72	1.78	35	0.87	2.05 (1.36–3.12)	<0.001
Intracerebral hemorrhage	5	0.12	2	0.05	2.22 (0.43–11.66)	0.35

[a]Cumulative event rates are reported for WATCH; event rates per year are reported for WARCEF.
[b]Adjusted for demographics and cardiovascular risk factors.
F/U, Follow-up; *N/A*, information not available; *WATCH*, Warfarin and Antiplatelet Therapy in Chronic Heart Failure; *WARCEF*, Warfarin Versus Aspirin in Reduced Cardiac Ejection Fraction.

of up to 4% per year[18] has been reported for chronic heart failure, although this may partly reflect its frequent coexistence with atrial fibrillation. Because heart failure is often accompanied by hypercoagulability, antithrombotic treatment has been attempted to prevent embolic events. Although anticoagulation is definitely indicated in patients with concomitant atrial fibrillation, its role in patients in sinus rhythm is controversial.

Table 38.4 summarizes the results of the two major trials on this topic.[19,20] In both trials, warfarin treatment failed to reduce combined vascular events but appeared to decrease the risk of stroke compared with antiplatelet agents, while increasing major but not intracerebral hemorrhages.

VALVULAR VEGETATIONS AND STRANDS

Vegetations on the mitral and/or aortic valve often embolize to the brain and systemic circulation. Neurologic complications occur in 20% to 40% of patients with IE[21] (see Chapter 29). Silent brain infarcts visualized on magnetic resonance imaging (MRI) are found in approximately 50% of patients with IE.[22] Systemic embolism most commonly involves the spleen, the liver, the kidney, and the iliac or mesenteric arteries.[21]

Among 2781 patients, stroke (16.9%), peripheral embolism (22.6%), and heart failure (32.3%) were the most frequent complications of IE. The frequency decreased rapidly after the initiation of effective antimicrobial treatment.[21] For 1437 patients with left-sided IE, the stroke incidence fell from 4.82 cases per 1000 patient-days during the first week of treatment to 1.71 cases per 1000 patient-days during the second week, and it continued to decrease thereafter, regardless of the valve or organism involved.[23] Overall, only 3.1% of patients experienced a stroke after the first week of therapy.[23]

Early surgery may confer a survival benefit for patents who are at high risk for complications. For 1552 patients with native

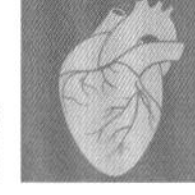

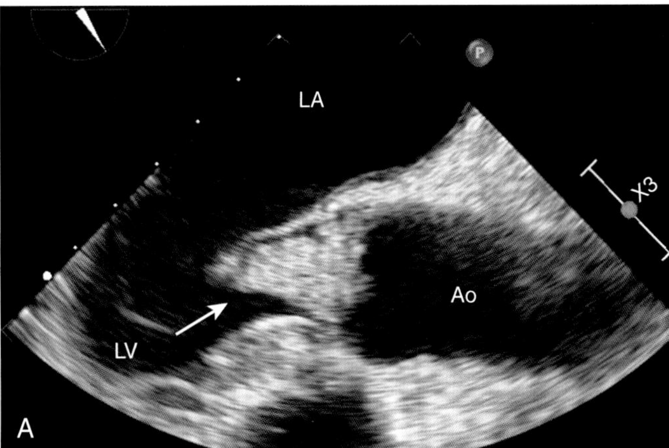

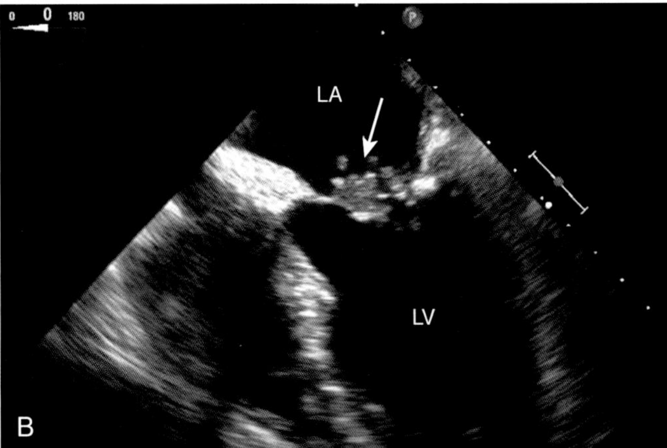

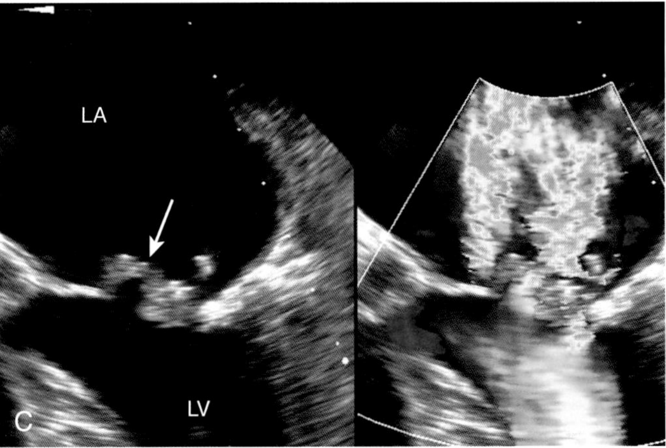

Fig. 38.3 **TEE visualization of a vegetation on left-sided valves.** (A) A large vegetation *(arrow)* is visualized on the ventricular aspect of the aortic valve (see Video 38.3A). (B) A vegetation is seen on the atrial aspect of the anterior leaflet of the mitral valve (see Video 38.3B). (C) Severe prolapse and possible perforation of the middle segment of the leaflet is visualized *(left, arrow)*; color-flow Doppler *(right)* shows two separate regurgitant jets, confirming the existence of a perforation (see Video 38.3C). *Ao*, Ascending aorta.

valve IE, surgery was associated with a significant reduction in the mortality rate (12.2% vs. 20.1%, $P < 0.001$).[24] Patients with stroke ($P = 0.02$) or peripheral embolization ($P = 0.002$) were among those who benefited most from surgical treatment.[24] Early identification of IE is especially important for patients with embolic events because of the potential influence on treatment.

TEE is the study of choice for the identification of valvular vegetations (Fig. 38.3). In one meta-analysis, the sensitivity of harmonic TTE for IE was only 61%, although its specificity was high (94%); a negative TTE result strongly predicted the absence of IE in patients with adequate images and no prosthetic valves, although not in other cases.[25]

The sensitivity of TEE is very high, as is its specificity (both > 90%).[9] Echocardiographic characteristics of the vegetation that affect its embolic potential are size (>10 mm increases the risk), extension (>1 leaflet or valve involved), and mobility.[26] A negative TEE result has a high negative predictive value for IE (86%–97%).[27] However, TEE performed early in the course of the disease may be negative because the vegetation is still forming; this finding has prompted the recommendation to consider repeating the test if clinical suspicion of IE remains high.[9,27]

Vegetations on prosthetic valves are even more difficult to detect by TTE because the prosthesis (especially mitral prostheses) may be interposed between the ultrasound beam and the vegetation (see Chapter 31). The sensitivity of TTE for prosthetic IE is therefore very low (20%–40%),[9] whereas TEE has a sensitivity and specificity between 80% and 90%.[9] TEE is recommended as the initial diagnostic study for all patients with suspected prosthetic valve endocarditis[28] (Fig. 38.4).

Valve vegetations or similar lesions may be found in patients without IE. Potential causes are listed in Table 38.5. Libman-Sacks endocarditis may be observed in up to 40% of patients with systemic lupus erythematosus.[9] Marantic endocarditis is frequently associated with malignancies.[9] Nonbacterial endocarditis may embolize in up to 50% of cases.[9] The clinical scenario and results of other diagnostic tests are crucial for a correct diagnosis and determining the need for cardiac imaging in these conditions.

Filamentous strands, also known as Lambl excrescences, are often observed by TEE on mitral and aortic valves (Fig. 38.5), especially in the elderly. They are more common on aortic than mitral valves and in women than men.[29] Often representing fibrinous material or hamartomatous growths on the valve's edge, the valve strands have been linked to an increased risk of stroke or TIA in case-control studies.[30] Patients with valve strands incidentally found on TEE had a stroke incidence of 1% to 2% over a follow-up period of 4 years.[31] However, embolic events were observed in 27% of patients in another study.[29]

The need for preventive treatment and what type should be used is unclear. For 619 patients with acute ischemic stroke undergoing TEE and randomized to warfarin or aspirin treatment, no increased risk of recurrent stroke was observed over a 2-year follow-up period (HR = 1.05, 95 CI: 0.70–1.57, $P = 0.82$).[32] Valve strands are often found on prostheses, especially in mitral position. Among 300 patients with left-sided prosthetic heart valves, strands were observed in 49%.[33] A lower level of anticoagulation (INR < 2.5) was significantly associated with their presence, suggesting that more aggressive anticoagulation may be necessary for these patients.[33]

INTRACARDIAC TUMORS

Primary intracardiac tumors are identified in less than 0.2% of unselected autopsy series,[34] and they are associated with a high frequency of embolic events (see Chapter 18). This is especially true for the two most common types: myxomas and papillary fibroelastomas. Approximately 75% of all cardiac tumors are benign, and 50% of them are myxomas.[35] Three of four myxomas originate from the left atrium (LA), especially the fossa ovalis of the interatrial septum (Fig. 38.6A and B), although they can originate from any endocardial surface (see Fig. 38.6C). An estimated 30% to 40% of all myxomas eventually embolize,[36] to the cerebral circulation in more than 50% of cases. Tumor

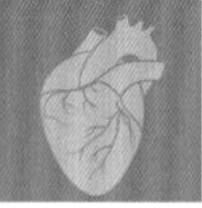

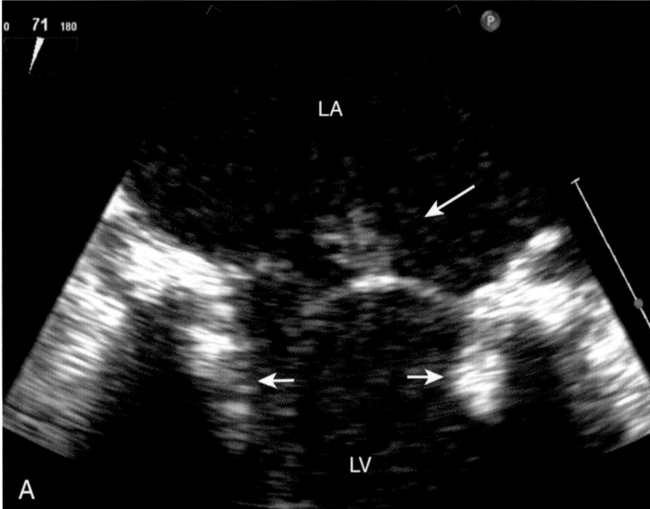

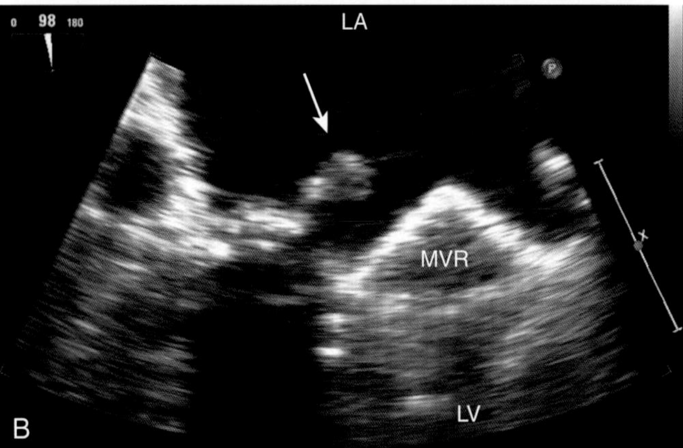

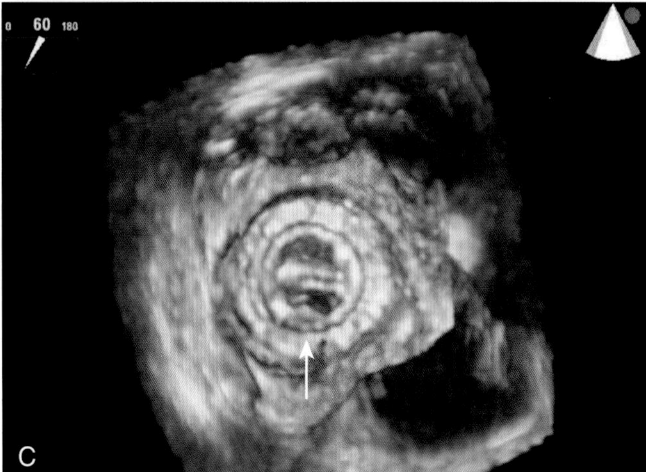

Fig. 38.4 TEE visualization of vegetations on mitral prostheses. (A) A vegetation *(upper arrow)* is visualized on the atrial aspect of a biologic prosthesis. Notice the native valve–like appearance of the leaflets and the valvular supporting struts *(lower arrows)* (see Video 38.4A). (B) Large vegetation *(arrow)* on the medial aspect of the annular ring of a mechanical prosthesis *(MVR)*. The two leaflets of the prosthesis are visualized in mid-opening (see Video 38.4B). (C) In the same patient as in B, 3D imaging shows the vegetation on the prosthetic ring *(arrow)* from an atrial (superior) view (see Video 38.4C).

fragmentation and embolization of superimposed thrombus are the purported embolic mechanisms.

The morphologic features of the myxoma are important determinants of embolic risk. Large, mobile myxomas and those with villous excrescences are more likely to embolize than more solid, polypoid tumors.[36] TEE can identify even small tumors and can help clarify morphologic aspects such as point of insertion into the cardiac wall and relation to adjacent structures. 3D imaging (see Fig. 38.6D) more closely resembles the surgical view and is useful for planning the surgical approach. Surgical resection is recommended in all cases, especially when there are high-risk morphologic features.

TABLE 38.5 Differential Diagnosis of Valve Masses: Causes of Noninfective Vegetations and Similar Lesions.

- Degenerative or myxomatous valve disease
- Systemic lupus erythematosus (Libman-Sacks endocarditis)
- Systemic inflammatory disease, antiphospholipid syndrome, malignancy (marantic endocarditis)
- Chordal rupture
- Small intracardiac tumors
- Lambl excrescences

Papillary fibroelastomas frequently are associated with cerebral embolism and are often the first clinical manifestation due to their preferential location on highly mobile valve leaflets. Most fibroelastomas are diagnosed in the fourth or fifth decade of life, often after an episode of cerebral or cardiac ischemia. In a review of 725 cases, the aortic valve was the most common location, followed by the mitral valve, and the LV was the most common extravalvular location.[37] Among the morphologic features, only mobility was an independent predictor of death or nonfatal embolization.[37]

Fibroelastomas are often located on the aortic side of the aortic valve (Fig. 38.7A and B), unlike valvular vegetations, which tend to grow on the ventricular side. A clinically significant papillary fibroelastoma may be only a few millimeters wide, which makes TEE a vastly better imaging option than TTE. An example of fibroelastoma on the mitral valve is provided in Fig. 38.7C and D.

Although no controlled studies of treatment are available, surgical resection appears to be indicated for all symptomatic patients. For asymptomatic patients, oral anticoagulation is often used for nonmobile tumors, and surgical resection should be strongly considered for mobile ones.[37]

Malignant primary cardiac tumors are rare (0.001%–0.03% of autopsies).[35] Sarcomas are the most common malignancies,[38] and they manifest with flow obstruction, systemic or cerebral embolization, or systemic and constitutional symptoms. Metastatic cardiac tumors occur 20 to 40 times more frequently than primary tumors[34]; the lungs are the most common primary location.[39] The same considerations made for benign tumors about the usefulness of TEE and TTE for assessment of embolic risk apply here. TEE is also invaluable in the assessment of tumor extension to adjacent structures and blood vessels, information that may be critical for the decision about surgical treatment.

LA THROMBUS AND SPONTANEOUS ECHOCARDIOGRAPHIC CONTRAST

Thrombus in the LA is associated with a significant risk of systemic embolization. LA thrombus, especially in the atrial appendage, frequently occurs with atrial fibrillation (see Chapter 39), although it is occasionally seen in patients in sinus rhythm with a recent cerebral ischemic event, especially when LV dysfunction coexists.[40]

Because of the proximity to the LA and the possibility of using high-frequency transducers, TEE is the study of choice for imaging the LA and especially its appendage, which is

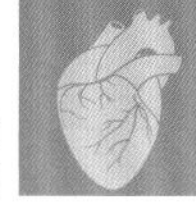

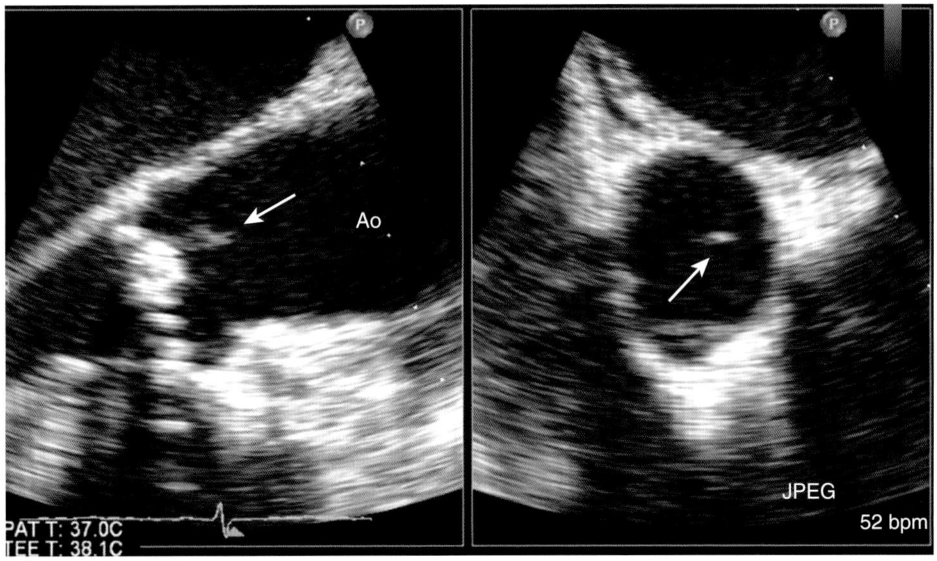

Fig. 38.5 Visualization of filamentous strand (Lambl excrescence) by TEE. Lambl excrescence *(arrow)* on the aortic side of the aortic valve *(left)* is confirmed by TEE in the orthogonal view *(right)*. The aortic valve is heavily calcified and restricted (see Video 38.5).

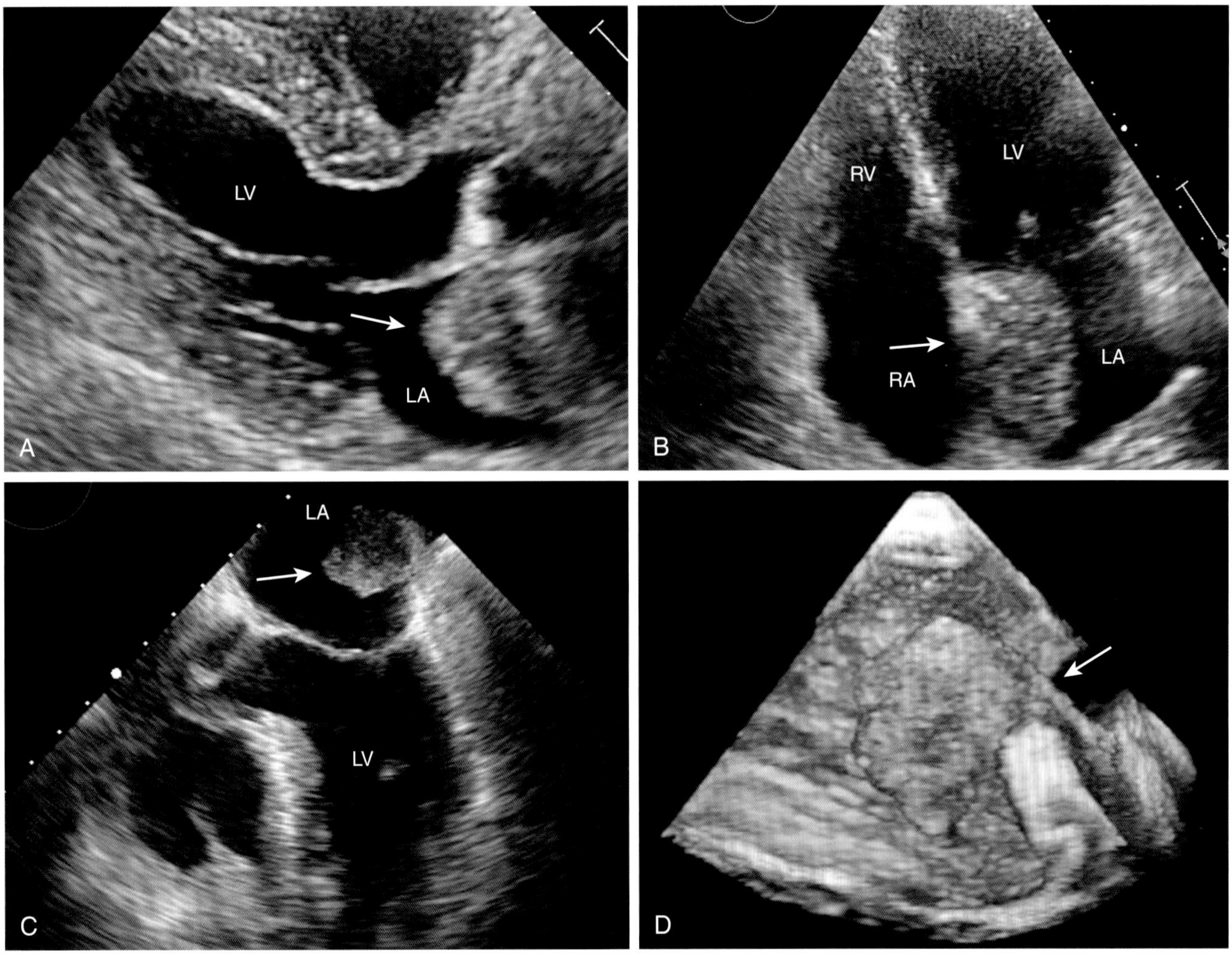

Fig. 38.6 LA myxoma. (A) TTE visualization of a myxoma *(arrow)* in the LA (see Video 38.6A). (B) In the same patient, imaging from the apical view identifies the connection of the myxoma to the atrial septum *(arrow)* (see Video 38.6B). (C) TEE visualization of a large myxoma *(arrow)* on the lateral wall of the LA (see Video 38.6C). (D) 3D imaging of the same tumor as in C shows the insertion point of the tumor into the partition of the wall near the entrance of the left upper pulmonary vein *(arrow)*. This information is helpful for planning the surgical resection (see Video 38.6D).

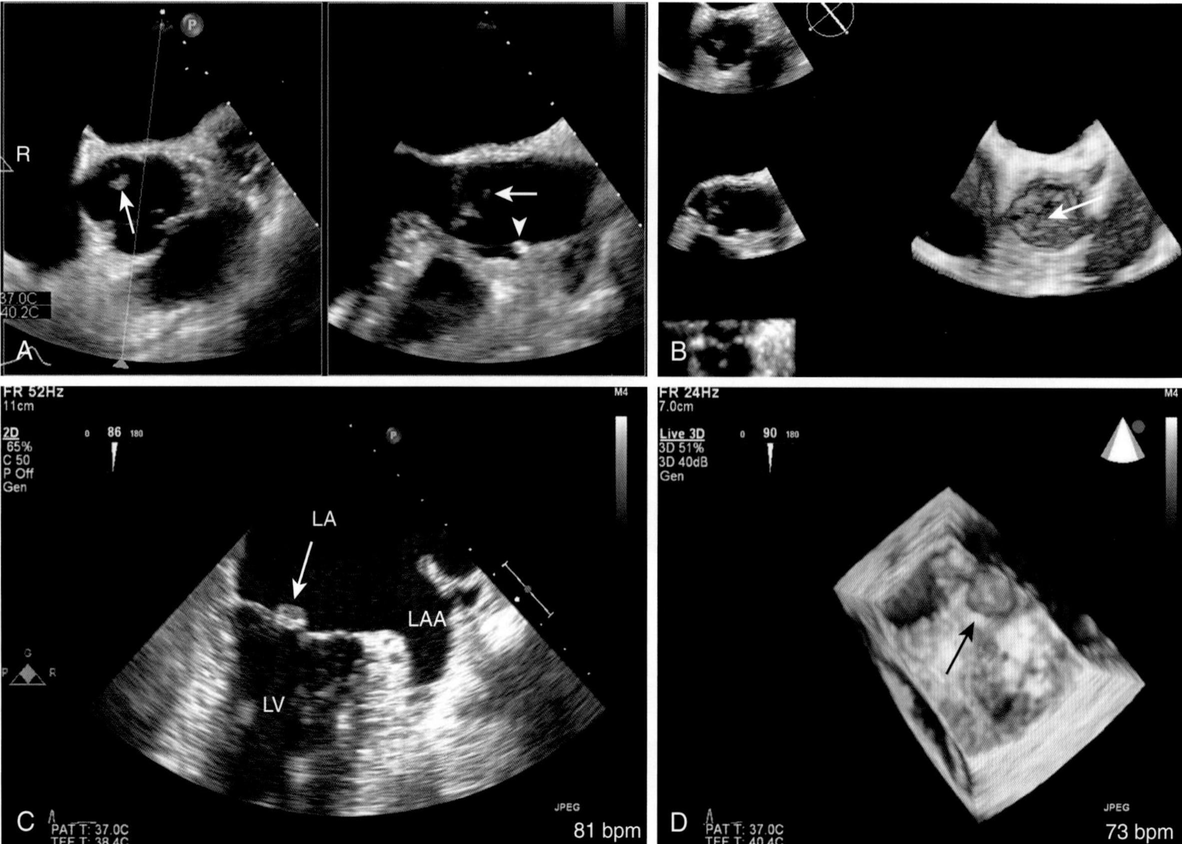

Fig. 38.7 TEE visualization of papillary fibroelastomas on left-sided valves. (A) Orthogonal views show a small, echolucent mass *(arrow)* consistent with a fibroelastoma on the aortic aspect of the noncoronary cusp of the aortic valve. A calcification *(arrowhead)* is seen on the aortic anterior wall, near the take-off of the right coronary artery (see Video 38.7A). (B) 3D imaging shows the small tumor *(arrow)* during diastolic closure of the valve. Simultaneously obtained orthogonal views of the valve and tumor are displayed on the *left* (see Video 38.7B). (C) In a longitudinal view of the left-sided chambers, a small fibroelastoma *(arrow)* is seen on the atrial aspect of the mitral valve during systolic closure of the valve. The left atrial appendage *(LAA)* is visible on the *right* (see Video 38.7C). (D) 3D imaging showed the same tumor *(arrow)* from a superior (atrial) view, looking down at the valve from a viewing point located in the body of the atrium. The dimensions and spatial location of the tumor can be better appreciated in this view, which is similar to the view the surgeon has after opening the atrial wall, and this is helpful for planning the surgical approach (see Video 38.7D).

infrequently visualized by TTE. With the use of modern omniplane transducers, the appendage can be imaged from a variety of angles, allowing a thorough investigation. The sensitivity of TEE is 90% to 95%, and the specificity is 95% to 100%.[41] An example of a left atrial appendage thrombus is shown in Fig. 38.8.

3D imaging may contribute to better thrombus visualization by providing different views (see Fig. 38.8). The frequency of LA thrombus in atrial fibrillation is estimated at more than 20%[42] and at 22% to 43% for patients with recent embolic events.[42,43] Although it is more common in chronic atrial fibrillation (27%), LA thrombus is often observed in atrial fibrillation of less than 3 days' duration (14%),[42] especially when accompanied by an embolic event (21%–43%).[42,43]

Decreased LV systolic function increases LA thrombus formation, even in patients in sinus rhythm. An LV ejection fraction of less than 35% was one of two independent predictors of thrombus in stroke patients; the other being a left atrial appendage flow velocity of 55 cm/s or less.[44] Flow velocity in the appendage is a useful clinical indicator of risk of thrombus. It is measured by pulsed-wave Doppler interrogation of the inlet of the appendage, which is possible in essentially all patients by TEE (see Fig. 38.8C) and occasionally by TTE.

With normal appendage function, velocities are 55 to 80 cm/s or higher. The risk of thrombus formation starts with a velocity of 55 cm/s or less[45] and increases as the velocity decreases. In the TEE substudy of the Stroke Prevention in Atrial Fibrillation III (SPAF-III) study, a velocity of 20 cm/s or less was associated with an increased frequency of thrombus (17% vs. 5% in patients with higher velocity, $P < 0.001$).[46]

Decreased LA flow velocity is also a determinant of spontaneous echocardiographic contrast (SEC). SEC is defined as dynamic, slowly swirling echoes resembling a smoky haze within the body of the atrium or its appendage (see Fig. 38.8A). SEC represents increased echogenicity due to blood cell aggregation at low shear rates, and it therefore indicates stagnant blood or low-flow states. SEC is associated with severely decreased (<25 cm/s) and with mildly or moderately decreased (<55 cm/s) appendage flow velocities.[45]

SEC can be occasionally seen by TTE in low-flow states, but it is better visualized by TEE because of the higher transducer frequency and proximity to the LA. Accurate gain and compression settings are necessary to optimize the view and increase detection. Relatively high gain settings may be necessary to maximize the detection rate, and white noise artifacts created by these settings are usually identified because of their fixed, nonswirling appearance.

The atrium and appendage should be imaged from different angles, and enough time should be spent to ensure visualization of an often transient phenomenon such as SEC. LA SEC occurs in more than 50% of patients with atrial fibrillation undergoing

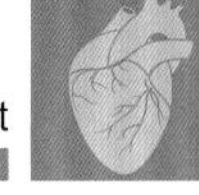

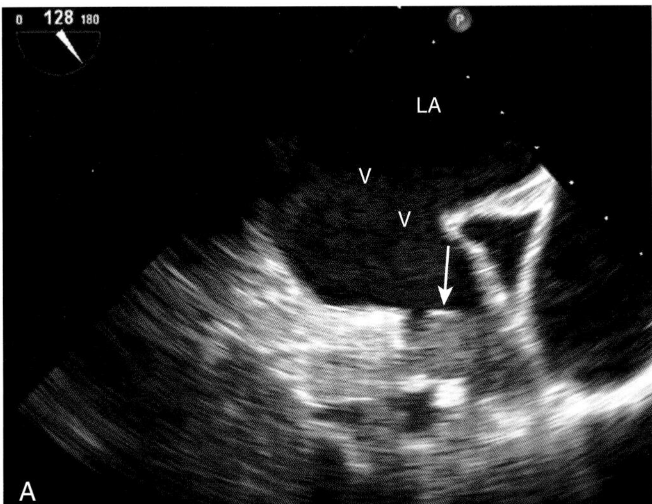

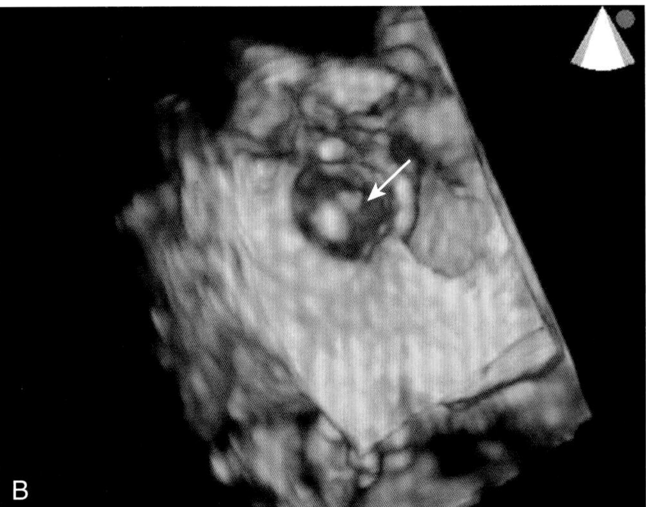

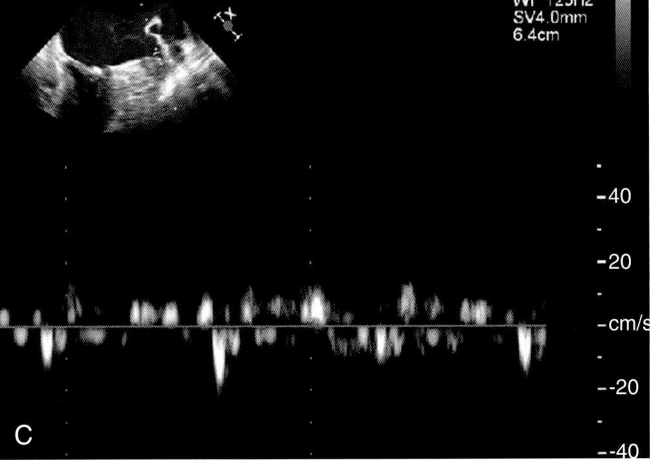

Fig. 38.8 Visualization of the left atrial appendage by TEE. (A) A thrombus *(arrow)* is seen on the appendage near its apex. Spontaneous echocardiographic contrast *(arrowheads)* is another important predictor of thrombus formation and embolic risk (see Video 38.8A). (B) 3D imaging from an atrial (superior) viewpoint for the same patient as in Fig. 38.9B; the view, which corresponds to looking down at the appendage from the body of the atrium, shows the protrusion of the thrombus *(arrow)* toward the atrial chamber (see Video 38.8B). (C) Pulsed-wave Doppler interrogation of the appendage. Because emptying of the appendage is directed toward the imaging transducer, velocities above the baseline represent emptying flow. Low emptying velocity (approximately 10–15 cm/s; see scale on the right of the screen) is demonstrated, which is associated with an increased risk of thrombus formation and increased embolic risk.

TEE. In a series of 272 patients, SEC was found in 161 (59%); during 17.5 months, the rate of stroke or other embolic events was increased by fourfold for patients with SEC (12%/y vs. 3%/y, $P = 0.002$).[47] SEC was also associated with an increased mortality rate (25 vs. 11 deaths, $P = 0.025$).[47] In SPAF-III, identification of SEC almost tripled the risk of stroke. For 295 patients with nonvalvular atrial fibrillation, atrial SEC or thrombus increased the likelihood of death by threefold over a 5-year follow-up period,[48] although it was not an independent predictor of stroke or death for anticoagulated patients (OR = 1.55, 95% CI: 0.50–4.83).

The TEE-derived variables previously described (i.e., left atrial appendage thrombus, reduced flow velocity, and SEC) can aid in deciding on the treatment to prevent thromboembolic events in patients with atrial fibrillation. Although prognostic scores such as $CHADS_2$ (Cardiac Failure, Hypertension, Age >75, Diabetes, Stroke or TIA [doubled]) and CHA_2DS_2–VASc (which adds vascular disease, age 65–74, female sex, and doubles the score for age > 75 y) have been devised to assess the probability of incident embolic events,[49] some gray areas still exist. In general, oral anticoagulation is recommended when the expected stroke risk is 2%/y or greater; aspirin or no treatment may be chosen when the expected stroke risk is less than 1%/y.

The intermediate risk group is more controversial. In the 2014 American College of Cardiology, American Heart Association, and Heart Rhythm Society (ACC/AHA/HRS) atrial fibrillation guideline, oral anticoagulation was recommended starting with a CHA_2DS_2–VASc score of 2 and no antithrombotic therapy for a score of 0.[50] The use of aspirin, oral anticoagulants, or no antithrombotic treatment was mentioned, although with a low level of evidence, for patients with a CHA_2DS_2–VASc score of 1. In the 2016 European Society of Cardiology (ESC) guidelines, a similar case-by-case approach was mentioned for men with a CHA_2DS_2–VASc score of 1 and women with a CHA_2DS_2–VASc score of 2.[51]

Use of TEE and detection of one of the high-risk echocardiographic indicators described earlier may direct the therapeutic choice toward anticoagulation. Among newer therapeutic options, oral thrombin inhibitors have proved at least as effective as warfarin in preventing stroke in patients with atrial fibrillation[52–55] (Table 38.6) without the need for frequent laboratory tests and with a lower risk of severe hemorrhagic complications.

The utility of TEE in atrial fibrillation goes beyond assessment of thrombus or SEC. In the SPAF-III TEE substudy, among multiple possible predictors, only SEC and complex aortic arch plaques were independently associated with recurrent vascular events. Adjusted-dose warfarin treatment decreased the event rates by 75% for patients with atrial fibrillation and complex arch plaques (4.0% vs. 15.8%, $P = 0.02$), whereas among patients without plaques, the event rate was low (1.1%–1.2%/y), regardless of treatment type.[46]

TEE may be used to exclude LA thrombus before cardioversion of atrial fibrillation, eliminating the need for several weeks of preprocedural anticoagulation. The safety and efficacy of a TEE-based strategy to shorten anticoagulation before electrical cardioversion was demonstrated in the Assessment of Cardioversion Using Transesophageal Echocardiography (ACUTE) study (Table 38.7).[56]

ATRIAL SEPTUM ABNORMALITIES: PATENT FORAMEN OVALE AND ATRIAL SEPTAL ANEURYSM

A PFO is associated with an increased risk of ischemic stroke, especially cryptogenic stroke. The foramen ovale, which is a component of the fetal circulation, usually closes after birth, but

TABLE 38.6 Clinical Trials Comparing Oral Systemic Anticoagulants With Warfarin for the Prevention of Stroke and Systemic Embolism in Nonvalvular Atrial Fibrillation.

Trials	Patients (n)	Event Rate (%/y)	Hazard Ratio	P Value	
				Noninferiority	Superiority
RE-LY[52]					
Dabigatran, 150 mg bid	6076	1.11	0.66	<0.001	<0.001
Dabigatran, 110 mg bid	6015	1.53	0.91	<0.001	0.34
Warfarin	6022	1.69	Reference	Reference	Reference
ROCKET AF[53]					
Rivaroxaban, 20 mg qd	7131	1.7	0.79	<0.001	0.12
Warfarin	713	2.2	Reference	Reference	Reference
ARISTOTLE[54]					
Apixaban, 5 mg bid	9120	1.27	0.79	<0.001	0.01
Warfarin	9081	1.60	Reference	Reference	Reference
ENGAGE-AF TIMI 48[55]					
Edoxaban, 60 mg qd	7035	1.18	0.79	<0.001	0.08
Edoxaban, 30 mg qd	7034	1.61	1.07	0.005	0.10
Warfarin	7036	1.50	Reference	Reference	Reference

ARISTOTLE, Apixaban for Reduction in Stroke and Other Thromboembolic Events in Atrial Fibrillation; *ENGAGE-AF TIMI 48*, Effective Anticoagulation with Factor Xa Next Generation in Atrial Fibrillation–Thrombolysis in Myocardial Infarction 48; *RE-LY*, Randomized Evaluation of Long-Term Anticoagulation Therapy; *ROCKET AF*, Rivaroxaban Once Daily Oral Direct Factor Xa Inhibition Compared with Vitamin K Antagonism for Prevention of Stroke and Embolism Trial in Atrial Fibrillation.

TABLE 38.7 Use of TEE Before Cardioversion in Atrial Fibrillation: the ACUTE Study.

Parameter	Conventional Treatment[a] (n = 603)	TEE-Guided Strategy (n = 609)	P Value
Time to cardioversion (days)	30.6	3.0	<0.001
Successful cardioversion (%)	65.2	71.1	0.03
Hemorrhagic events (%)	5.5	2.9	0.03
Embolic events within 8 weeks (%)	0.5	0.8	0.5

[a]Defined as 3 weeks of oral anticoagulation before cardioversion. Both treatment groups received 4 weeks of oral anticoagulation after cardioversion.

From Klein AL, Grimm RA, Murray RD, et al. Use of transesophageal echocardiography to guide cardioversion in patients with atrial fibrillation. *N Engl J Med*. 2001;344:1411–1420.

it remains partially open in 15% to 35% of normal people.[57] An atrial septal aneurysm (ASA), which is a localized protrusion of the septum into either atrial chamber, also has been associated with an increased embolic risk. ASA is infrequently observed in the general population (approximately 1% to 4% of subjects),[58,59] and it is associated with a PFO in more than 60% of cases.

Detection of Patent Foramen Ovale

A PFO is a functional opening that becomes patent when the pressure in the right atrium (RA) exceeds that in the LA. Diagnosis is based on the demonstration of a right-to-left shunt at rest or during maneuvers (e.g., coughing, Valsalva maneuver) that increase the RA pressure. TTE or TEE with contrast injection (i.e., aerated, agitated saline, or polygelatine agents) is used. Five injections under different conditions (e.g., rest, Valsalva maneuver, coughing) have been recommended.

TEE has up to 100% sensitivity and specificity for PFO detection when both color Doppler and contrast evaluation are performed. The prevalence of PFO in a TEE study that sampled the general population was 24.3%,[58] which is similar to that observed in autopsy studies. Using a longitudinal bicaval view, TEE often allows direct visualization and measurement of the PFO opening and visualization (Fig. 38.9A and B) and semiquantitative assessment of the shunt (by count of microbubbles) (see Fig. 38.9C). This technique can differentiate PFO from an intrapulmonary shunt by direct visualization of the pulmonary veins. 3D imaging may better evaluate the size of the PFO opening (Fig. 38.9D).

TEE is highly accurate in detecting an ASA (Fig. 38.10A), which is usually diagnosed by protrusion of the septum at least 10 mm from the midline into either atrium. An ASA can also be visualized by TTE (see Fig. 38.10B), although with lower sensitivity.

Because TEE is a semi-invasive study that requires conscious sedation, its use is appropriate in diagnostically equivocal cases or when morphologic characterization is necessary (e.g., when PFO closure is entertained). For screening purposes, TTE with contrast is used. Contrast TTE (Fig. 38.11A) has lower sensitivity than TEE (50%–60%, which has improved to > 80% in later studies).[60] In a sample of the general population, the PFO prevalence by contrast TTE was 14.9%.[59] Direct PFO visualization is not obtained by TTE, and differentiation from an intrapulmonary shunt is therefore based on the timing of the appearance of microbubbles in the left-sided chambers (i.e., within three cardiac cycles from RA opacification for PFO and delayed appearance for an intrapulmonary shunt).

Patent Foramen Ovale, Atrial Septal Aneurysm, and Stroke Risk

Paradoxical embolization (i.e., embolization to the systemic circulation of a thrombus originating in the venous circulation) is the embolic mechanism; it is confirmed by the occasional detection of thrombus lodged in the PFO (see Fig. 38.11B). The relationship between PFO and cryptogenic stroke was first described in patients younger than 55[61] or 40[62] years of age, and then extended to older patients.[63,64] Available evidence indicates an approximately fourfold increase in stroke risk from PFO for younger patients and a twofold increase for older patients (Table 38.8).

Possible Associated Factors

Anatomic atrial septal and RA characteristics have been suggested as potential cofactors in the PFO-related risk of stroke.

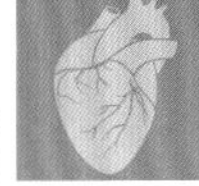

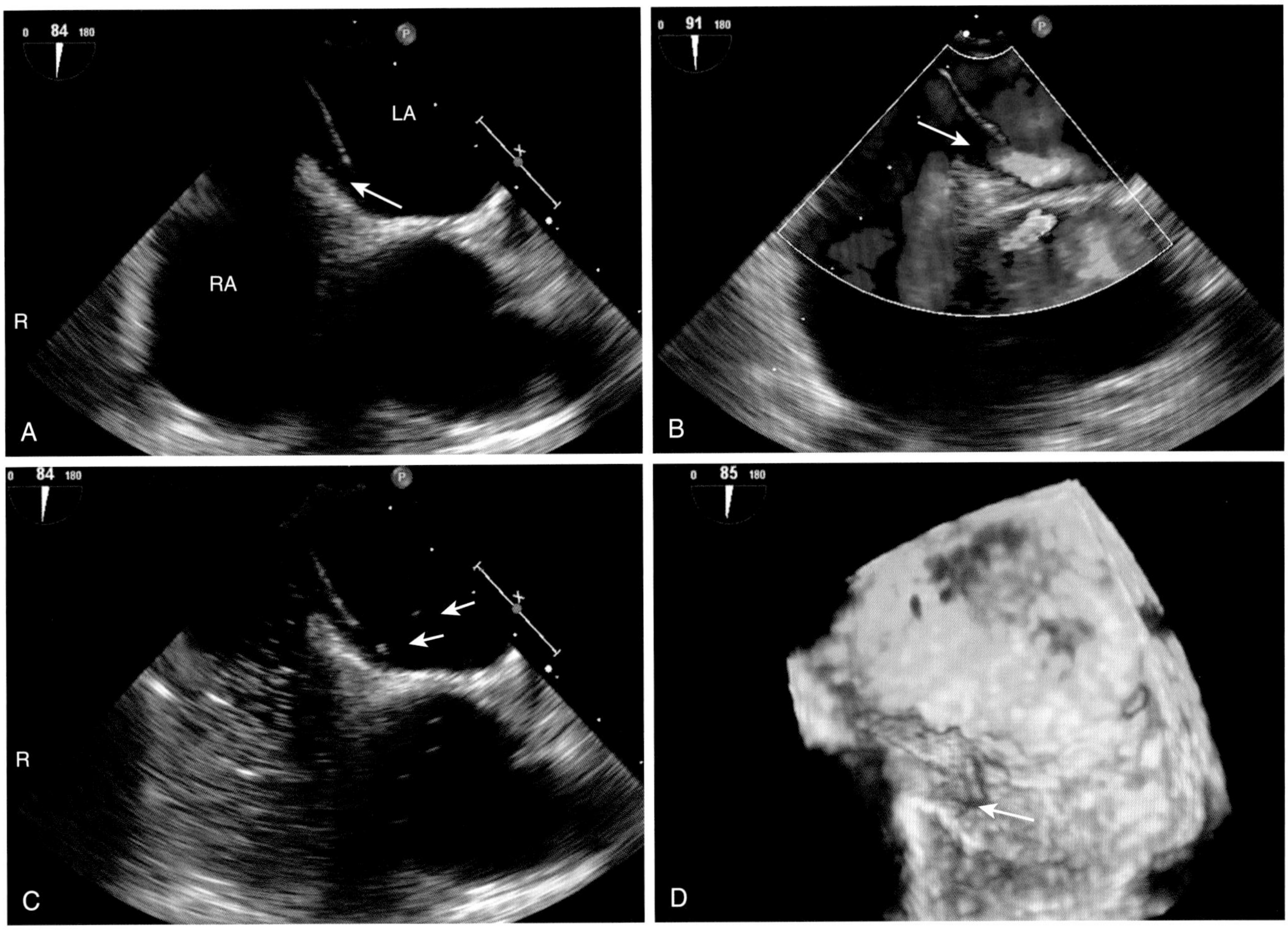

Fig. 38.9 **TEE visualization of a patent foramen ovale.** (A) A bicaval view shows the patent foramen ovale (PFO) opening *(arrow)*, with visualization of the smallest opening (see Video 38.9A). (B) Color-flow Doppler shows an interatrial shunt *(arrow)* (see Video 38.9B). (C) PFO visualization by contrast TEE. Contrast material fills the RA, and few microbubbles *(arrows)* are seen as they enter the LA. The study should be repeated after a Valsalva maneuver and cough to increase the pressure in the RA and maximize the likelihood of a right-to-left shunt (see Video 38.9C). (D) In the same patient, 3D imaging allows better visualization of the PFO opening *(arrow)* and funnel shape. This view is especially useful when PFO closure is contemplated because it aids in choosing the size of the closure device to be used (see Video 38.9D).

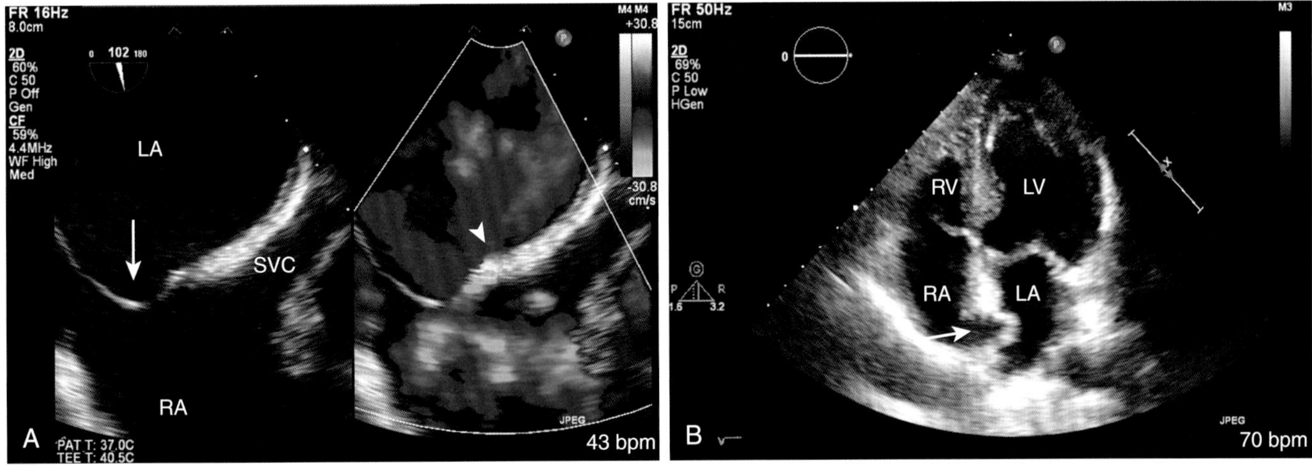

Fig. 38.10 **Echocardiographic visualization of an atrial septal aneurysm.** (A) TEE using a longitudinal (bicaval) view shows a large atrial septal aneurysm (ASA) *(arrow)* protruding into the RA *(left)*. A coexisting patent foramen ovale *(arrowhead)* is visualized by color-flow Doppler *(right)* (see Video 38.10A). (B) TTE shows a large ASA *(arrow)* protruding into the LA (see Video 38.10B). *SVC*, Superior vena cava.

The width of septal separation assessed by TEE (see Fig. 38.9) has been associated with an increased stroke risk. A PFO of 2 mm or larger was more frequently seen in patients with embolic stroke confirmed by MRI,[65] and a PFO larger than 4 mm may be an independent risk factor for recurrent cerebrovascular events.[66] The degree of shunt, determined by the number of shunting microbubbles counted in the LA by TEE in a still frame (i.e., large shunt > 25–30 microbubbles) appears to be a rather rough estimate of the embolic risk, although it has been used in some treatment trials.[67–70]

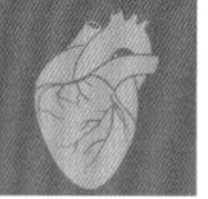

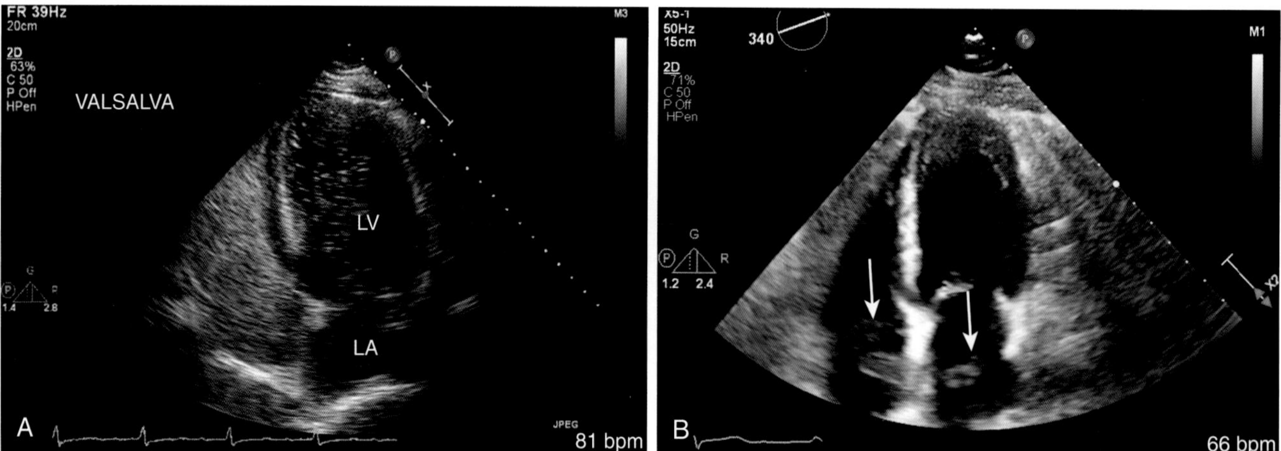

Fig. 38.11 Visualization of a patent foramen ovale by TTE. (A) Patent foramen ovale (PFO) visualization by saline contrast TTE. Contrast material fills the RA and RV, and a large right-to-left shunt is demonstrated (see Video 38.11A). (B) TTE shows a large thrombus *(arrows)* lodged in a PFO and protruding into both atria. Although infrequently observed, this condition should prompt emergent intervention (i.e., surgical removal or thrombolysis or anticoagulation) because of the extremely high risk of pulmonary, cerebral, or systemic embolic events (see Video 38.11B).

TABLE 38.8 Relationship Between Patent Foramen Ovale and Cryptogenic Stroke for Different Age Groups.

			Prevalence of PFO		
Study	*Patients (N)*	*Age*	*Cryptogenic*	*Control*	*P Value*
Younger Patients					
Lechat et al.[61]	26	<55	54% (14/26)	10% (10/100)	<0.001
Webster et al.[62]	34	<40	56% (19/34)	15% (6/40)	<0.001
Cabanes et al.[101]	64	<55	56% (36/64)	18% (9/50)	<0.001
De Belder et al.[102,a]	39	<55	13% (5/39)	3% (1/39)	—
Di Tullio et al.[63]	21	<55	47% (10/21)	4% (1/24)[b]	<0.001
Hausmann et al.[103]	18	<40	50% (9/18)	11% (2/18)	<0.05
Handke et al.[64]	82	<55	44% (36/82)	14% (7/49)[b]	<0.001
Total	285	—	45% (129/284)	11% (36/320)	<0.001
Older Patients					
De Belder et al.[102,a]	64	>55	20% (13/64)	5% (3/56)	<0.001
Di Tullio et al.[63]	24	>55	38% (9/24)	8% (6/77)[b]	<0.001
Hausmann et al.[103]	20	>40	15% (3/20)	23% (23/98)	NS
Jones et al.[104]	57	>50	18% (10/57)	16% (29/183)	NS
Handke et al.[64]	145	>55	44% (36/82)	14% (7/49)[b]	<0.001
Total	310	—	25% (76/310)	14% (89/646)	<0.001

[a]Includes different stroke subtypes.
[b]Controls were patients with stroke of known cause.
NS, Not significant; *PFO*, patent foramen ovale.

ASA (see Fig. 38.10) has been associated with an increased risk of stroke. Because ASA is often associated with a PFO and the PFO size tends to be larger in patients with ASA,[71] the risk is considered to result from the coexistent PFO. However, in a meta-analysis, the stroke risk was higher in patients with a PFO plus ASA than in those with either condition alone.[72] In stroke patients younger than 55 years of age treated with aspirin, the 4-year recurrent stroke rate was markedly higher (15.2%) for those with a combined PFO and ASA than for those with an isolated PFO (2.3%).[73] Patients with a PFO and ASA more often had multiple acute brain lesions on brain MRIs than did patients with a PFO alone (53% vs. 17%, $P = 0.01$), even after adjustment for PFO size, degree of shunt, and vascular risk factors.[74]

There may be more to the stroke risk of ASA than coexistence of a PFO. Other potential stroke mechanisms include in situ thrombosis, which appears to be uncommon, and a predisposition to atrial arrhythmias.

A prominent ASA valve (i.e., remnant of the right valve of the fetal sinus venosus that directs the blood from the inferior vena cava to the foramen ovale) and a Chiari network (threads and fibers variably connecting the eustachian valve to other atrial structures) have been proposed as cofactors in the risk of paradoxical embolism risk, but this has not been conclusively established. Pulmonary embolism, right ventricular infarction, severe tricuspid regurgitation, and the presence of an LV assist device have been associated with an increased degree of PFO shunting.

Deep venous thrombosis has been reported in patients with cryptogenic stroke and a PFO. Pelvic vein thrombi were found more frequently in young patients with cryptogenic stroke than in those with defined causes of stroke.[75]

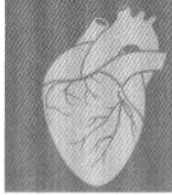

TABLE 38.9 Trials Comparing Patent Foramen Ovale Closure With Antithrombotic Treatment for Prevention of Recurrent Cerebrovascular Events.

Study	Follow-Up Duration	PFO Closure % (n)	Medical Treatment % (n)	P Value
CLOSURE 1[67]	**2 y**	**N = 447**	**N = 462**	
Stroke		3.1 (12)	3.4 (13)	0.77[a]
TIA		3.3 (13)	4.6 (17)	0.39[a]
Composite		5.9 (25)	7.7 (30)	0.30[a]
RESPECT[69]	**2.1 y (median)**	**N = 499**	**N = 481**	
Entire Cohort				
Stroke/early death (45 days from randomization or 30 days from implantation)		1.8 (9)	3.3 (16)	0.08[b]
Subgroups				
Large shunt		0.8 (2/247)	4.3 (10/231)	0.07[c]
PFO + ASA		1.1 (2/280)	5.3 (9/169)	0.10[c]
RESPECT–Long-term[70]	**5.9 y (median)**	**N = 499**	**N = 481**	
Entire Cohort				
Recurrent stroke		3.6 (18)	5.8 (28)	0.046
Recurrent cryptogenic stroke		2.0 (10)	4.8 (23)	0.007
Subgroups				
Large shunt		2.0 (5/247)	6.9 (16/231)	0.04[c]
PFO + ASA		1.7 (3/179)	7.6 (13/170)	0.04[c]
PC[68]	**4 y (mean)**			**0.34[d]**
Entire Cohort				
Stroke, death, TIA or peripheral embolism		3.4 (7)	5.2 (11)	0.34[d]
Subgroups				
Age < 45 y		1.1 (1/91)	6.2 (6/97)	0.10[c]
PFO + ASA		8.5 (4/47)	3.9 (2/51)	0.09[c]

[a]Cox proportional hazard model adjusting for age, ASA, prior TIA/CVA, smoking, hypertension, hypercholesterolemia.
[b]Log-rank test.
[c]*P* value for the interaction.
[d]Cox proportional hazard model.
ASA, Atrial septal aneurysm; *CLOSURE 1*, Evaluation of the STARFlex Septal Closure System in Patients With a Stroke and/or Transient Ischemic Attack due to Presumed Paradoxical Embolism Through a Patent Foramen Ovale; *CVA*, cerebrovascular accident; *PC*, Clinical Trial Comparing Percutaneous Closure of Patent Foramen Ovale Using the Amplatzer PFO Occluder with Medical Treatment in Patients with Cryptogenic Embolism; *PFO*, patent foramen ovale; *RESPECT*, Randomized Evaluation of Recurrent Stroke Comparing PFO Closure to Established Current Standard of Care Treatment; *TIA*, transient ischemic attack.

Prothrombotic states may increase the likelihood of thrombus formation and embolization. Frequent G20210A and factor V Leiden mutations have been reported in patients with cryptogenic stroke and PFO. The association of either genotype with a PFO increased the stroke risk by 4.7-fold.[76] Recent surgery, trauma, or oral contraceptive use may increase the likelihood of thrombus formation and paradoxical embolization.

Prevention of Recurrent Embolism

Because paradoxical embolization is the purported stroke mechanism, antithrombotic treatment (i.e., systemic anticoagulation with warfarin and antiplatelet agents such as aspirin) has been tested for preventive purposes. Transcatheter closure of the PFO has also been used. In the sole randomized, double-blind trial of medical treatments, 630 patients with noncardioembolic stroke were randomized to aspirin (325 mg) or warfarin (target INR of 1.4–2.8).[77] After 2 years, no significant differences were observed in the rates of recurrent stroke or death among patients with or without a PFO for the entire study group (14.8% vs. 15.4%, HR = 0.96, 95% CI: 0.62–1.48, $P = 0.84$) and for the subgroup of patients with cryptogenic stroke (14.3% vs. 12.7%; HR = 1.17, 95% CI: 0.60–2.37, $P = 0.65$). No significant differences in recurrent stroke or death were observed for patients treated with warfarin (9.5%) or aspirin (17.9%, HR = 0.52, 95% CI: 0.16–1.67, $P = 0.28$). PFO size and coexistence of an ASA did not significantly affect the stroke risk,[77] as was also confirmed in another study.[78]

Given the preventive efficacy of antithrombotic treatment, transcatheter closure of the PFO would appear to be indicated only if its efficacy were to be found to be superior in randomized clinical trials or in patients who failed or had contraindications to medical treatment. Three randomized trials comparing PFO closure with antithrombotic treatment were initially published (Table 38.9). Two studies (CLOSURE[67] and PC[68]) failed to demonstrate the superiority of PFO closure in preventing recurrent events. The third study (RESPECT) showed no significant difference at 2.1 years,[69] but superiority of PFO closure was found at 5.9 years for recurrent stroke and especially for cryptogenic stroke in an intention-to-treat analysis, although with a higher rate of venous thromboembolism. Patients with large shunts and/or ASAs showed the largest benefit.[70] More recently, the superiority of PFO closure plus antiplatelet therapy over antiplatelet therapy alone in preventing stroke recurrence was demonstrated in two studies, the Patent Foramen Ovale Closure or Anticoagulants versus Antiplatelet Therapy to Prevent Stroke Recurrence (CLOSE) study[78a] and the Gore REDUCE trial,[78b] although at the expense of device-related complications and more frequent atrial fibrillation.

After PFO closure, TTE can evaluate the correct position of the device (Fig. 38.12A) and possible complications (e.g., septal erosion, pericardial effusion). A contrast study is used to evaluate any residual shunt, which is relatively common during the first months after the procedure. TEE may be necessary for

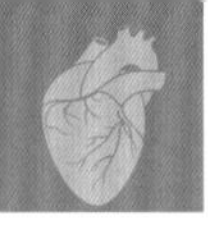

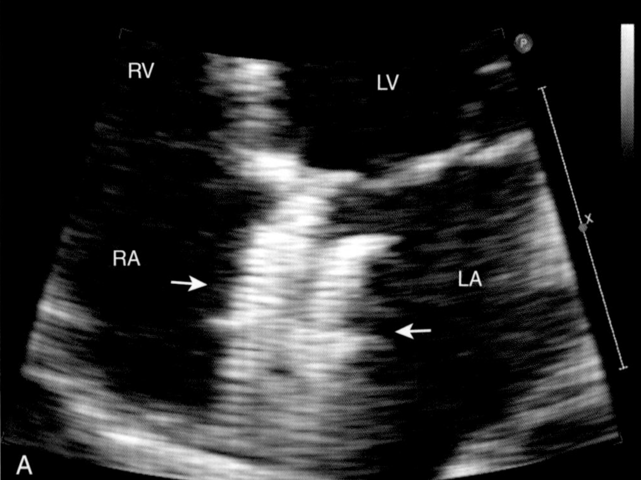

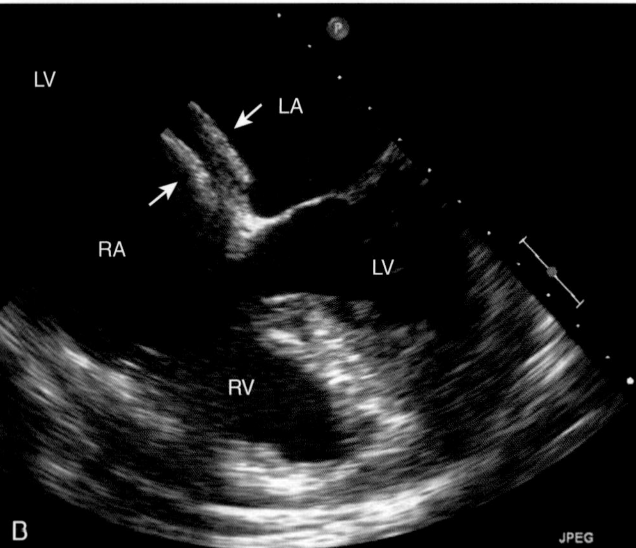

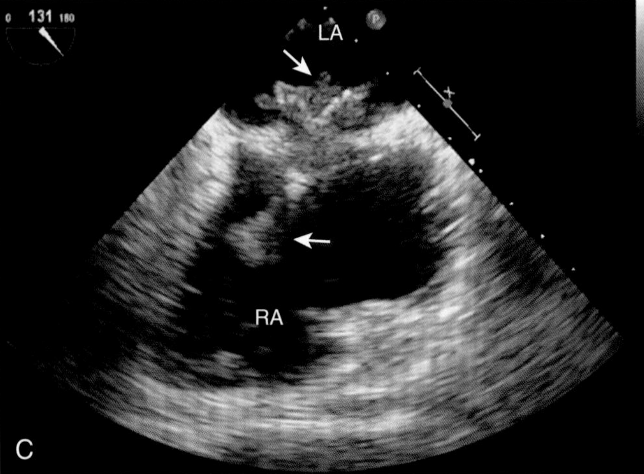

Fig. 38.12 Echocardiographic visualization of a patent foramen ovale closure device. (A) Visualization by TTE (apical 4-chamber view, cropped to visualize the atrial chambers). The arms of the device *(arrows)* are seen on each atrial side (see Video 38.12A). (B) Visualization by TEE in a 4-chamber (transverse) view. The device arms encase the septum *(arrows)* (see Video 38.12B). (C) TEE visualization of a patent foramen ovale closure complication. In a bicaval view, large echogenic masses *(arrow)* are seen on both sides of the device (see Video 38.12C). They were found at surgery to be infected thrombi.

better visualization of the device (see Fig. 38.12B) and complications such as thrombus or vegetation (see Fig. 38.12C).

ATHEROSCLEROTIC PLAQUES IN THE PROXIMAL AORTA

The association between proximal aortic plaques and ischemic stroke was first reported in a pathology study in which elderly patients who had died from a stroke showed much greater rates of ulcerated aortic plaques than patients who had died from other neurologic diseases (26% vs. 5%, age-adjusted OR = 4.0, 95% CI: 2.1–7.8).[79] The difference was especially significant for cryptogenic stroke (61% vs. 28%, adjusted OR = 5.7, 95% CI: 2.4–13.6), and it persisted after adjustment for atrial fibrillation and carotid artery disease.[79] Only 3% of patients with ulcerated plaques were younger than 60 years of age.

TEE provided a tool for visualization of atherosclerotic plaques in vivo. The proximity of the esophagus to the aorta and the absence of interposed structures allow the use of high-frequency ultrasound transducers, resulting in high-resolution images. The segment of aorta proximal to the take-off of the left subclavian artery is the focus of the examination, although retrograde diastolic flow has been demonstrated in the aorta, and the possibility of embolization to the brain from the initial segment of the descending aorta has been suggested[80] but not supported by a meta-analysis.[81] The aorta can be accurately visualized from the aortic valve level to the initial curvature of the arch. The middle and distal segments of the aortic arch are also visible in all patients, whereas a small portion of the proximal arch cannot be visualized due to the interposition of the trachea.

An accurate assessment of plaques and their thickness (Fig. 38.13A) and of ulcerations (see Fig. 38.13AB) or superimposed thrombus (see Fig. 38.13C) is possible. TEE has high sensitivity and specificity (>90%)[82] for aortic plaques and thrombus, although the sensitivity may be lower (≈75%) for small ulcerations. Reproducibility of TEE measurements of aortic plaque thickness is very good, with agreement of 84% to 88% for the diagnosis of large (≥4 mm) plaques,[83] which are thought to carry higher risk of stroke.[84]

Numerous TEE case-control[84–86] and prospective studies[87–89] have confirmed the role of proximal arch plaques as risk factors for stroke and other embolic events (Tables 38.10 and 38.11). The general consensus is that a plaque thickness of 4 mm or greater (i.e., measured perpendicular to the major vessel diameter; see Fig. 38.13A) is associated with a higher embolic risk. It is unclear, however, whether plaque thickness is directly related to the stroke mechanism or is a marker of diffuse atherosclerosis that portends a higher risk of stroke. Plaque thickness was associated with subsequent vascular events (i.e., stroke, TIA, MI, or death) in patients with stroke or TIA over a follow-up period of 1.7 years (51% vs. 11%, $P < 0.0001$).[90]

A plaque's complex morphology may be more directly related to the stroke mechanism than its thickness. Plaque ulceration and mobility have been linked to increased risk of stroke,[85] especially cryptogenic stroke. Conversely, plaque calcification seems to decrease the risk of events, possibly indicating a more stable lesion. The use of 3D imaging has added to the accuracy of TEE for plaque morphology assessment, allowing a more complete examination of the aortic walls (see Fig. 38.13B). Mobile components superimposed on an aortic plaque are infrequently identified, with a rate of 1.6% to 8.7% reported in different studies.[84,86,91] When present, they represent a very strong risk factor for brain embolization.[85]

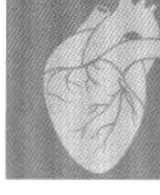

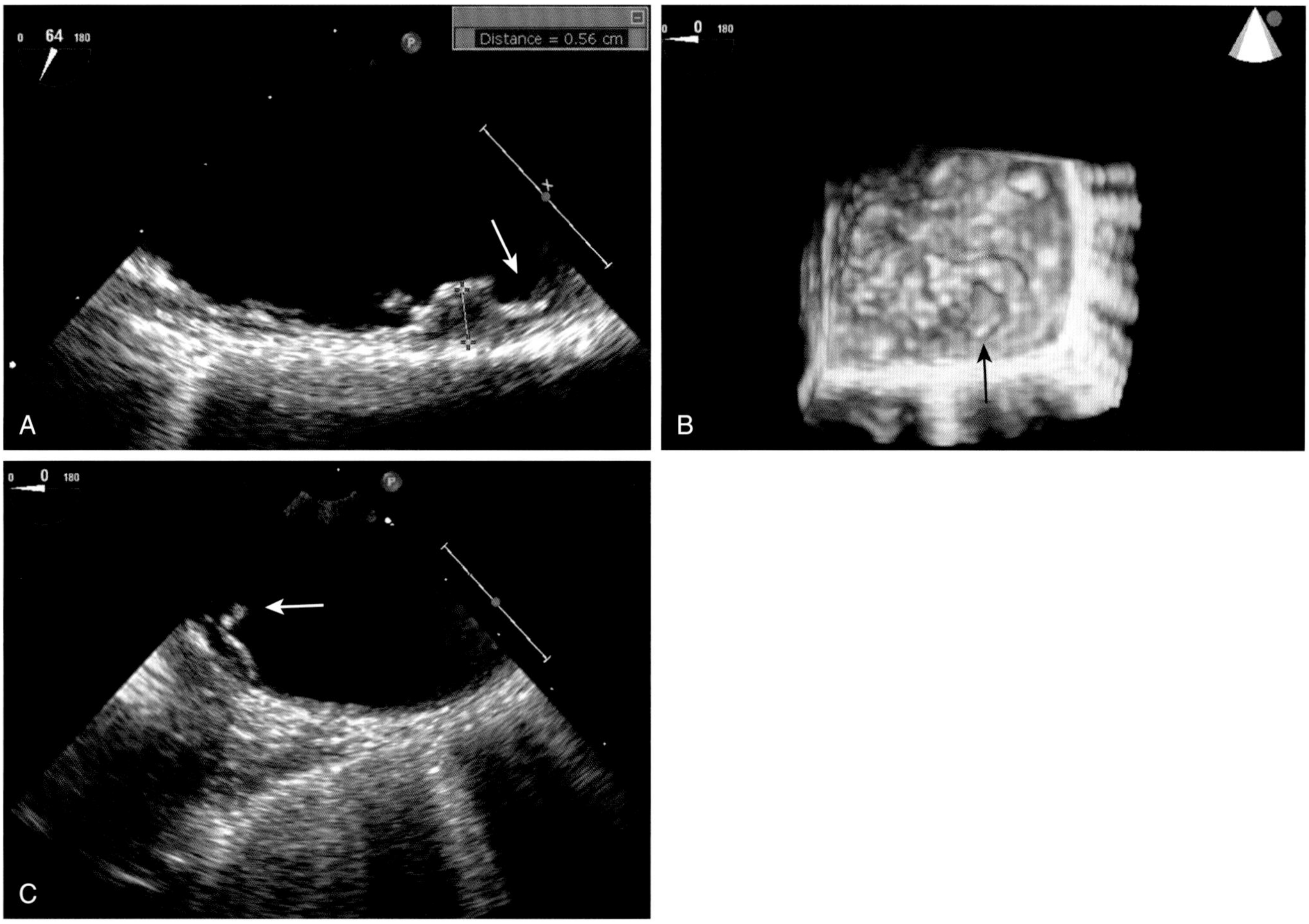

Fig. 38.13 TEE assessment of aortic arch plaques. (A) In a horizontal imaging plane, the middle to distal segment of the aortic arch is visualized. A large plaque is present in the distal arch; it is more than 5 mm thick *(upper right corner,* measurement perpendicular to the major axis of the vessel). A large ulceration *(arrow)* is seen at its intimal surface. The thickness (>4 mm) and ulceration are indicators of increased embolic potential of the plaque (see Video 38.13A). (B) 3D imaging allows a more accurate assessment of the plaque and its ulceration *(arrow)* (see Video 38.13B). (C) Large plaque in the middle segment of the aortic arch. A mobile component was seen in real-time imaging *(arrow)*. Although uncommon, mobile components of a plaque, which represent superimposed thrombus, confer an especially high embolic risk (see Video 38.13C).

Occasionally, mobile thrombi without severe atherosclerotic changes can be seen in younger patients with embolic events (23 cases of 27,855 TEE examinations in a multicenter cardiology study).[92] The thrombi usually originate on small atherosclerotic plaques (Fig. 38.14), possibly representing a rare variant of atherosclerosis in younger patients.[92]

Plaque-related stroke is a major risk for patients undergoing cardiac surgery or transcatheter procedures involving the proximal aorta. Aortic atherosclerosis predicted early and delayed strokes in 2972 patients undergoing cardiac surgery; 82% of early strokes and 71% of delayed strokes occurred in patients older than 65 years of age.[93] Modification of aortic cannulation or off-pump procedures can drastically decrease perioperative stroke.[94] Aortic plaques were an independent stroke predictor after transcatheter aortic valve replacement (TAVR).[95] Use of devices that allow cerebral embolic protection can decrease the stroke incidence by 70% (from 4.6% to 1.4%).[96] These data reinforce the need for preprocedural imaging in elderly patients and those with multiple atherosclerotic risk factors. TTE from a suprasternal window can be used for screening (Figs. 38.15 and 38.16). TEE or epiaortic ultrasound imaging of the aorta at the time of surgery may also be performed for this purpose.

In case of systemic embolism, the investigation should be extended to the descending aorta, where plaques are more common. Besides thromboembolism, aortic atherosclerosis can generate an atheroembolism, with cholesterol crystals usually lodging in small arterioles, spontaneously or after vascular surgery, arteriography, or anticoagulation.[97] Atheroembolism has a wide spectrum of manifestations, from silent episodes that are recognized only during diagnostic procedures to complex clinical pictures with multiple organ involvement. Simultaneous or consecutive involvement of different body segments may facilitate a correct diagnosis.

Therapy for and Prevention of Recurrent Events

Because most embolic events associated with aortic plaques are thromboembolic, systemic anticoagulation has been suggested to prevent recurrent events, and it appears to be indicated for patients with superimposed thrombus, although they are a small fraction of those affected. For patients with large but nonmobile plaque, the best preventive option is debated. For 516 stroke patients treated with aspirin or warfarin, large plaques (≥4 mm) remained associated with an increased risk of events (adjusted HR = 2.12, 95% CI: 1.04–4.32), especially for those with complex morphology (HR = 2.55, CI: 1.10–5.89). The risk was highest among cryptogenic stroke patients for large plaques (HR = 6.42, CI: 1.62–25.46) and for large complex plaques (HR = 9.50, CI: 1.92–47.10).[98]

TABLE 38.10 Aortic Arch Plaques and Risk of Ischemic Stroke: Case-Control Studies.

Study	*No. of Cases/Controls*	*Age (y)*	*Type of Plaque*	*Stroke Patients (%)*	*Controls (%)*	*Adjusted Odds Ratio[a] (95% CI)*
Amarenco et al.[84]	250/250	≥60	1–3.9 mm ≥4 mm	46 14	22 2	4.4 (2.8–6.8) 9.1 (3.3–25.2)
Jones et al.[105]	215/202	≥60	<5 mm, smooth ≥5 mm, complex	33 22	22 4	2.3 (1.2–4.2) 7.1 (2.7–18.4)
Di Tullio et al.[106]	106/114 30/36 76/78	≥40 <60 ≥60	≥5 mm ≥5 mm ≥5 mm	26 3 36	13 3 18	2.6 (1.1–5.9) 1.2 (0.7–20.2) 2.4 (1.1–5.7)
Di Tullio et al.[86]	255/209	≥55	≥4 mm	49	24	2.4 (1.3–4.6)

[a]Adjusted for conventional stroke risk factors.

TABLE 38.11 Aortic Arch Plaques and Risk of Ischemic Stroke: Prospective Studies.

Study	*No. of AP+/AP− Cases*	*Follow-Up (mo)*	*Type of Plaque*	*AP+ Events (%)*	*AP− Events (%)*	*Adjusted RR[a] (95% CI)*
Tunick et al.[107]	42/42	14	≥4 mm	33	7	4.3 (1.2–15.0)
Mitusch et al.[87]	47/136	16	≥5 mm/mobile vs. < 5 mm	13.7/y	4.1/y	4.3 (1.5–12.0)
Levy D et al.[88]	45/143	24–48	≥4 mm	11.9/y 26.0/y[b]	2.8/y 5.9/y[b]	3.8 (1.8–7.8) 3.5 (2.1–5.9)
Fujimoto et al.[89]	67/216	40	≥4 mm vs. < 4 mm	9.1	2.3	2.0 (0.9–4.2)
	51/232	40	≥4 mm, extending to arch branches	9.8	2.9	2.4 (1.1–5.2)

[a]Adjusted for traditional stroke risk factors.
[b]Recurrent stroke and other embolic events combined.
AP, Arch plaque; *RR*, relative risk.

Aspirin and clopidogrel were tested against adjusted-dose warfarin in stroke patients with large (≥4 mm) plaques in the Aortic Arch Related Cerebral Hazard (ARCH) trial. Unfortunately, insufficient enrollment and lower than expected event rates resulted in limited statistical power. Over a median follow-up period of 3.4 years, the primary end point (i.e., stroke, MI, peripheral embolism, vascular death, or intracranial hemorrhage) occurred for 7.6% of patients on combination therapy compared with 11.3% of those on warfarin therapy (adjusted HR = 0.76, 95% CI: 0.36–1.61, $P = 0.5$).[99]

Statins are commonly prescribed after a stroke, and they may help reduce the plaque-related risk of recurrent events. Surgical endarterectomy for high-risk plaques carries a significant risk of intraoperative stroke[100] and should be reserved for carefully selected cases.

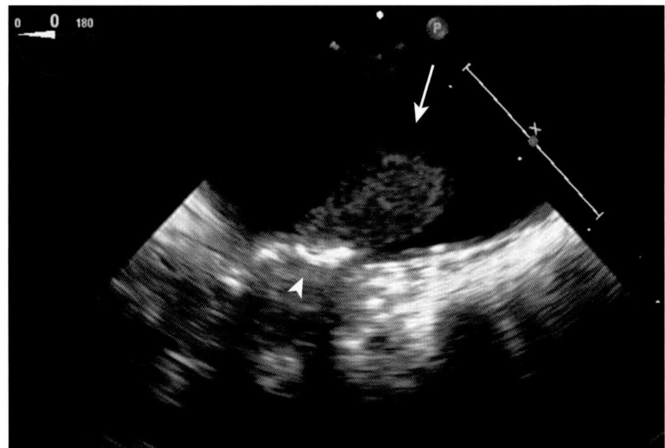

Fig. 38.14 TEE visualization of thrombus superimposed to small plaque. Large mobile thrombus *(arrow)* is visualized in the middle segment of the aortic arch by TEE. Its insertion on a calcified atherosclerotic plaque is visible *(arrowhead)* (see Video 38.14).

POTENTIAL LIMITATIONS AND ALTERNATIVE APPROACHES

TTE is limited by suboptimal visualization of cardiac structures distant from the chest wall. TEE limitations include its semi-invasive nature, use of conscious sedation, and suboptimal ability to provide tissue characterization (i.e., thrombus, vegetation, or tumor and lipid content vs. thrombotic components in a plaque). These aspects may be improved with future technical advancements.

When TEE cannot be performed because of esophageal pathology or other contraindications, the choice of imaging techniques depends on the pretest probability of a cardioembolic source. No real alternatives to echocardiography exist to identify valvular vegetations in IE, leaving the diagnosis to be made on clinical grounds. For intracardiac masses, computed tomography (CT) or MRI can be used and has the added capabilities of tissue characterization and imaging of chest structures surrounding the heart.[13] Transcranial Doppler with contrast injection and intracardiac echocardiography have been used to assess patients with suspected PFOs. MRI correlates well with TEE for aortic plaque determination and definition of fibrotic and lipid plaque components. Dual-helical CT showed good sensitivity, specificity, and overall accuracy for the detection of aortic plaques when compared with TEE.

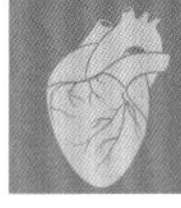

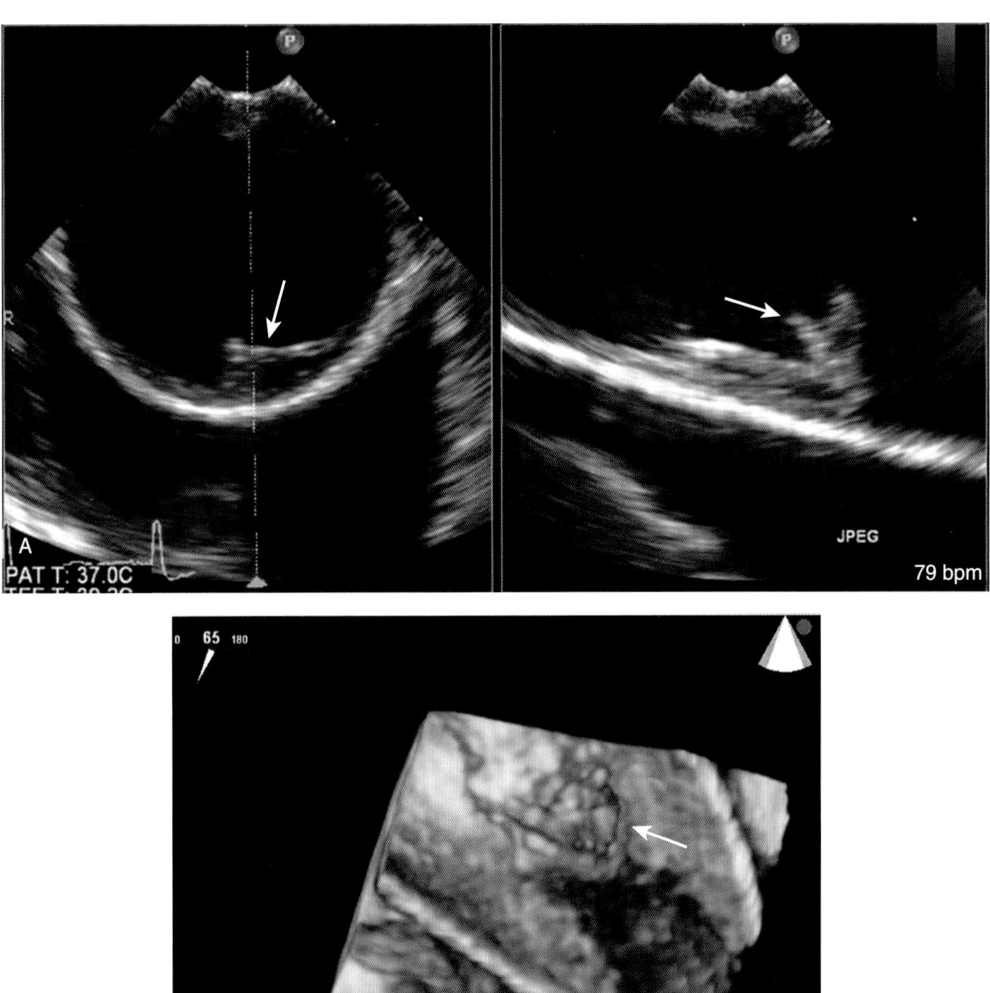

Fig. 38.15 Visualization of atherosclerotic plaque in the descending aorta. (A) A large plaque *(arrow)* is visualized *(left)*, and orthogonal imaging reveals a large, mobile component *(arrow)* on a slightly different plane *(right)* (see Video 38.15A). (B) 3D imaging allows a more accurate assessment of the mobile component *(arrow)* (see Video 38.15B).

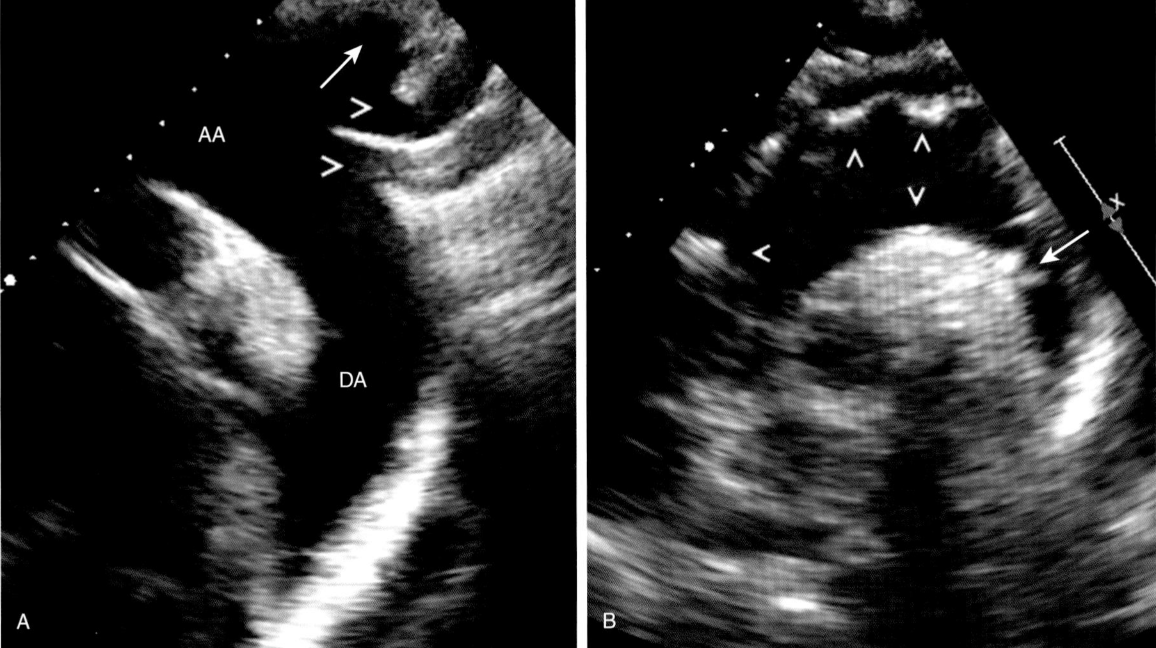

Fig. 38.16 Visualization of the aortic arch by suprasternal TTE. (A) Normal aortic arch. The take-off of the innominate artery *(arrow)* is shown, along with the take-off of the left carotid and left subclavian arteries *(arrowheads)* (see Video 38.16A). (B) A large, ulcerated atherosclerotic plaque *(arrow)* is visualized in the distal portion of the aortic arch. Multiple plaques *(arrowheads)* are visualized in the proximal and middle segments of the arch (see Video and 38.16B). *AA*, Aortic arch; *DA*, descending aorta.

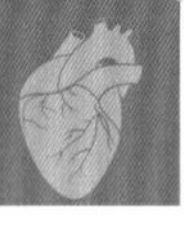

SUMMARY Echocardiographic Evaluation of Cardiac and Proximal Aortic Embolic Sources.

Embolic Source	Studies	Views	Measurements
LV apical thrombus	TTE, possibly with LV contrast; TEE in case of inadequate visualization by TTE	Apical 4-chamber and 2-chamber views; parasternal short-axis view	Measure dimensions Assess protrusion into the chamber and mobility (increased embolic risk)
Valvular vegetations, strands	TEE; TTE has low sensitivity (can identify large vegetations or be used in case of low clinical suspicion)	Transverse and longitudinal views of each valve	Measure vegetation size (embolic risk increases if >1 cm), number of leaflets affected, mobility
Cardiac tumors	TTE; TEE for small lesions	All standard TTE and TEE views	Assess size and mobility Assess for possible superimposed thrombus
LA thrombus, SEC	TEE	Left atrial appendage visualization from multiple views; adjustment of gain settings to minimize background noise	For thrombus, assess size and mobility Use PW Doppler to measure left atrial appendage emptying velocity (embolic risk increases at < 55 cm/s; highest risk is at < 25 cm/s)
PFO and ASA	TTE with aerated saline injection for screening; TEE for better definition and morphologic assessment	TTE: apical 4-chamber view; subcostal view when parasternal view is suboptimal TEE: bicaval view is most useful; 4-chamber view can also be used	TTE with saline: assess time of appearance of bubbles in LA (<3 cardiac cycles) TEE: measure minimum separation of septum primum and secundum, if visible; confirm with color-flow Doppler and aerated saline injection ASA: measure base width (at least 10 mm) and excursion (10 mm, adding excursions into either atrium)
Proximal aortic plaques	TEE; TTE for screening when TEE is contraindicated	Longitudinal view of the ascending aorta; transverse and longitudinal views of the arch and visible segment of the descending aorta; suprasternal view for TTE	Record number of plaques Measure maximum plaque thickness (perpendicular to the major axis of the vessel; ≥4 mm increases risk) Evaluate plaque morphology (hypoechoic plaque increases risk; calcification may decrease it) Search carefully for mobile components (thrombus; great increase in embolic risk)

ASA, Atrial septal aneurysm; *PFO*, patent foramen ovale; *PW*, pulsed wave; *SEC*, spontaneous echocardiographic contrast.

REFERENCES

1. Benjamin EJ, Muntner P, Alonso A, et al. American Heart Association Council on Epidemiology, Prevention Statistics Committee and Stroke Statistics Subcommittee. Heart Disease and Stroke Statistics-2019 Update: a report from the American Heart Association. *Circulation*. 2019;139:e56–e528.
2. Furie KL, Kasner SE, Adams RJ, et al. Guidelines for the prevention of stroke in patients with stroke or transient ischemic attack: a guideline for Healthcare Professionals from the American Heart Association/American Stroke Association. *Stroke*. 2011;42:227–276.
3. Ay H, Furie KL, Singhal A, Smith WS, Sorensen AG, Koroshetz WJ. An evidence-based causative classification system for acute ischemic stroke. *Ann Neurol*. 2005;58:688–697.
4. de Bruijn SF, Agema WR, Lammers GJ, et al. Transesophageal echocardiography is superior to transthoracic echocardiography in management of patients of any age with transient ischemic attack or stroke. *Stroke*. 2006;37:2531–2534.
5. Knebel F, Masuhr F, von Hausen W, et al. Transesophageal echocardiography in patients with cryptogenic cerebral ischemia. *Cardiovasc Ultrasound*. 2009;7:15.
6. Harloff A, Handke M, Reinhard M, Geibel A, Hetzel A. Therapeutic strategies after examination by transesophageal echocardiography in 503 patients with ischemic stroke. *Stroke*. 2006;37:859–864.
7. Khariton Y, House JA, Comer L, et al. Impact of transesophageal echocardiography on management in patients with suspected cardioembolic stroke. *Am J Cardiol*. 2014;114:1912–1916.
8. American College of Cardiology Foundation Appropriate Use Criteria Task Force, American Society of Epidemiology, American Heart Association, American Society of Nuclear Cardiology, Heart Failure Society of America, Heart Rhythm Society, Society for Cardiovascular Association, Interventions, Society of Critical Care Medicine, Society of Cardiovascular Computed Tomography, Society for Cardiovascular Magnetic Resonance, Douglas PS, Garcia MJ, et al. ACCF/ASE/AHA/ASNC/HFSA/HRS/SCAI/SCCM/SCCT/SCMR 2011 Appropriate Use Criteria for Echocardiography. A Report of the American College of Cardiology Foundation Appropriate Use Criteria Task Force, American Society of Echocardiography, American Heart Association, American Society of Nuclear Cardiology, Heart Failure Society of America, Heart Rhythm Society, Society for Cardiovascular Angiography and Interventions, Society of Critical Care Medicine, Society of Cardiovascular Computed Tomography, and Society for Cardiovascular Magnetic Resonance Endorsed by the American College of chest Physicians. *J Am Coll Cardiol*. 2011;57:1126–1166.
9. Saric M, Armour AC, Arnaout MS, et al. Guidelines for the use of echocardiography in the evaluation of a cardiac source of embolism. *J Am Soc Echocardiogr*. 2016;29:1–42.
10. Mooe T, Eriksson P, Stegmayr B. Ischemic stroke after acute myocardial infarction. A population-based study. *Stroke*. 1997;28:762–767.

11. Witt BJ, Brown Jr RD, Jacobsen SJ, Weston SA, Yawn BP, Roger VL. A community-based study of stroke incidence after myocardial infarction. *Ann Intern Med*. 2005;143:785–792.
12. Vaitkus PT, Barnathan ES. Embolic potential, prevention and management of mural thrombus complicating anterior myocardial infarction: a meta-analysis. *J Am Coll Cardiol*. 1993;22:1004–1009.
13. Osherov AB, Borovik-Raz M, Aronson D, et al. Incidence of early left ventricular thrombus after acute anterior wall myocardial infarction in the primary coronary intervention era. *Am Heart J*. 2009;157:1074–1080.
14. Siebelink HM, Scholte AJ, Van de Veire NR, et al. Value of contrast echocardiography for left ventricular thrombus detection postinfarction and impact on antithrombotic therapy. *Coron Artery Dis*. 2009;20:462–466.
15. O'Gara PT, Kushner FG, Ascheim DD, et al. 2013. ACCF/AHA guideline for the management of ST-elevation myocardial infarction: executive summary: a report of the American College of Cardiology Foundation/American Heart Association Task Force on Practice Guidelines. *J Am Coll Cardiol*. 2013;61:485–510.
16. Andreotti F, Testa L, Biondi-Zoccai GG, Crea F. Aspirin plus warfarin compared to aspirin alone after acute coronary syndromes: an updated and comprehensive meta-analysis of 25,307 patients. *Eur Heart J*. 2006;27:519–526.
17. Udell JA, Wang JT, Gladstone DJ, Tu JV. Anticoagulation after anterior myocardial infarction and the risk of stroke. *PloS One*. 2010;5. e12150.
18. Witt BJ, Brown Jr RD, Jacobsen SJ, et al. Ischemic stroke after heart failure: a community-based study. *Am Heart J*. 2006;152:102–109.
19. Massie BM, Collins JF, Ammon SE, et al. Randomized trial of warfarin, aspirin, and clopidogrel in patients with chronic heart failure: the Warfarin and Antiplatelet Therapy in Chronic Heart Failure (WATCH) trial. *Circulation*. 2009;119:1616–1624.
20. Homma S, Thompson JL, Pullicino PM, et al. Warfarin and aspirin in patients with heart failure and sinus rhythm. *N Engl J Med*. 2012;366:1859–1869.
21. Mylonakis E, Calderwood SB. Infective endocarditis in adults. *N Engl J Med*. 2001;345:1318–1330.
22. Cooper HA, Thompson EC, Laureno R, et al. Subclinical brain embolization in left-sided infective endocarditis: results from the evaluation by MRI of the brains of patients with left-sided intracardiac solid masses (EMBOLISM) pilot study. *Circulation*. 2009;120:585–591.
23. Dickerman SA, Abrutyn E, Barsic B, et al. The relationship between the initiation of antimicrobial therapy and the incidence of stroke in infective endocarditis: an analysis from the ICE Prospective Cohort Study (ICE-PCS). *Am Heart J*. 2007;154:1086–1094.
24. Lalani T, Cabell CH, Benjamin DK, et al. Analysis of the impact of early surgery on in-hospital mortality of native valve endocarditis: use of propensity score and instrumental variable methods to adjust for treatment-selection bias. *Circulation*. 2010;121:1005–1013.
25. Bai AD, Steinberg M, Showler A, et al. Diagnostic accuracy of transthoracic echocardiography for infective endocarditis findings using transesophageal echocardiography as the reference standard: a meta-analysis. *J Am Soc Echocardiogr*. 2017;30:639–646 e8.
26. Thuny F, Di Salvo G, Belliard O, et al. Risk of embolism and death in infective endocarditis: prognostic value of echocardiography: a prospective multicenter study. *Circulation*. 2005;112:69–75.
27. Evangelista A, Gonzalez-Alujas MT. Echocardiography in infective endocarditis. *Heart*. 2004;90:614–617.
28. Bonow RO, Carabello BA, Chatterjee K, et al. 2008. Focused update incorporated into the ACC/AHA 2006 guidelines for the management of patients with valvular heart disease: a report of the American College of Cardiology/American Heart Association Task Force on Practice Guidelines (Writing Committee to revise the 1998 guidelines for the management of patients with valvular heart disease). Endorsed by the Society of Cardiovascular Anesthesiologists, Society for Cardiovascular Angiography and Interventions, and Society of Thoracic Surgeons. *J Am Coll Cardiol*. 2008;52:e1–142.
29. Leitman M, Tyomkin V, Peleg E, Shmueli R, Krakover R, Vered Z. Clinical significance and prevalence of valvular strands during routine echo examinations. *Eur Heart J Cardiovasc Imaging*. 2014;15:1226–1230.
30. Roberts JK, Omarali I, Di Tullio MR, Sciacca RR, Sacco RL, Homma S. Valvular strands and cerebral ischemia. Effect of demographics and strand characteristics. *Stroke*. 1997;28:2185–2188.
31. Roldan CA, Shively BK, Crawford MH. Valve excrescences: prevalence, evolution and risk for cardioembolism. *J Am Coll Cardiol*. 1997;30:1308–1314.
32. Homma S, Di Tullio MR, Sciacca RR, Sacco RL, Mohr JP. Effect of aspirin and warfarin therapy in stroke patients with valvular strands. *Stroke*. 2004;35:1436–1442.
33. Kiavar M, Sadeghpour A, Bakhshandeh H, et al. Are prosthetic heart valve fibrin strands negligible? The associations and significance. *J Am Soc Echocardiogr*. 2009;22:890–894.
34. Reynen K. Frequency of primary tumors of the heart. *Am J Cardiol*. 1996;77:107.
35. Butany J, Nair V, Naseemuddin A, Nair GM, Catton C, Yau T. Cardiac tumours: diagnosis and management. *Lancet Oncol*. 2005;6:219–228.
36. Reynen K. Cardiac myxomas. *N Engl J Med*. 1995;333:1610–1617.
37. Gowda RM, Khan IA, Nair CK, Mehta NJ, Vasavada BC, Sacchi TJ. Cardiac papillary fibroelastoma: a comprehensive analysis of 725 cases. *Am Heart J*. 2003;146:404–410.
38. Neragi-Miandoab S, Kim J, Vlahakes GJ. Malignant tumours of the heart: a review of tumour type, diagnosis and therapy. *Clin Oncol*. 2007;19:748–756.
39. Ekmektzoglou KA, Samelis GF, Xanthos T. Heart and tumors: location, metastasis, clinical manifestations, diagnostic approaches and therapeutic considerations. *J Cardiovasc Med*. 2008;9:769–777.
40. Yahia AM, Shaukat A, Kirmani JF, Latorre JG, Qureshi AI. Prevalence and prediction of left atrial thrombus in patients with a recent cerebral ischemic event, who are in sinus rhythm: a single-center experience. *J Neuroimaging*. 2009;19:323–325.
41. Agmon Y, Khandheria BK, Gentile F, Seward JB. Echocardiographic assessment of the left atrial appendage. *J Am Coll Cardiol*. 1999;34:1867–1877.
42. Stoddard MF, Dawkins PR, Prince CR, Ammash NM. Left atrial appendage thrombus is not uncommon in patients with acute atrial fibrillation and a recent embolic event: a transesophageal echocardiographic study. *J Am Coll Cardiol*. 1995;25:452–459.
43. Manning WJ, Silverman DI, Waksmonski CA, Oettgen P, Douglas PS. Prevalence of residual left atrial thrombi among patients with acute thromboembolism and newly recognized atrial fibrillation. *Arch Intern Med*. 1995;155:2193–2198.
44. Handke M, Harloff A, Hetzel A, Olschewski M, Bode C, Geibel A. Predictors of left atrial spontaneous echocardiographic contrast or thrombus formation in stroke patients with sinus rhythm and reduced left ventricular function. *Am J Cardiol*. 2005;96:1342–1344.
45. Handke M, Harloff A, Hetzel A, Olschewski M, Bode C, Geibel A. Left atrial appendage flow velocity as a quantitative surrogate parameter for thromboembolic risk: determinants and relationship to spontaneous echocontrast and thrombus formationa transesophageal echocardiographic study in 500 patients with cerebral ischemia. *J Am Soc Echocardiogr*. 2005;18:1366–1372.
46. Echocardiography TSPiAFICo. Transesophageal echocardiographic correlates of thromboembolism in high-risk patients with nonvalvular atrial fibrillation. The Stroke Prevention in Atrial Fibrillation Investigators Committee on Echocardiography. *Ann Intern Med*. 1998;128:639–647.
47. Leung DY, Black IW, Cranney GB, Hopkins AP, Walsh WF. Prognostic implications of left atrial spontaneous echo contrast in nonvalvular atrial fibrillation. *J Am Coll Cardiol*. 1994;24:755–762.
48. Kleemann T, Becker T, Strauss M, Schneider S, Seidl K. Prevalence and clinical impact of left atrial thrombus and dense spontaneous echo contrast in patients with atrial fibrillation and low CHADS2 score. *Eur J Echocardiogr*. 2009;10:383–388.
49. Gage BF, Waterman AD, Shannon W, Boechler M, Rich MW, Radford MJ. Validation of clinical classification schemes for predicting stroke: results from the National Registry of Atrial Fibrillation. *J Am Med Assoc*. 2001;285:2864–2870.
50. January CT, Wann LS, Alpert JS, et al. 2014 AHA/ACC/HRS Guideline for the Management of Patients with Atrial Fibrillation: a Report of the American College of Cardiology/American Heart Association Task Force on Practice Guidelines and the Heart Rhythm Society. *J Am Coll Cardiol*. 2014;64:e1–76.
51. Kirchhof P, Benussi S, Kotecha D, et al. 2016 ESC guidelines for the management of atrial fibrillation developed in collaboration with EACTS. *Eur Heart J*. 2016;37:2893–2962.
52. Connolly SJ, Ezekowitz MD, Yusuf S, et al. Dabigatran versus warfarin in patients with atrial fibrillation. *N Engl J Med*. 2009;361:1139–1151.
53. Patel MR, Mahaffey KW, Garg J, et al. Rivaroxaban versus warfarin in nonvalvular atrial fibrillation. *N Engl J Med*. 2011;365:883–891.
54. Granger CB, Alexander JH, McMurray JJ, et al. Apixaban versus warfarin in patients with atrial fibrillation. *N Engl J Med*. 2011;365:981–992.
55. Giugliano RP, Ruff CT, Braunwald E, et al. Edoxaban versus warfarin in patients with atrial fibrillation. *N Engl J Med*. 2013;369:2093–2104.
56. Klein AL, Grimm RA, Murray RD, et al. Use of transesophageal echocardiography to guide cardioversion in patients with atrial fibrillation. *N Engl J Med*. 2001;344:1411–1420.
57. Hagen PT, Scholz DG, Edwards WD. Incidence and size of patent foramen ovale during the first 10 decades of life: an autopsy study of 965 normal hearts. *Mayo Clin Proc*. 1984;59:17–20.

58. Meissner I, Khandheria BK, Heit JA, et al. Patent foramen ovale: innocent or guilty? Evidence from a prospective population-based study. *J Am Coll Cardiol.* 2006;47:440–445.
59. Di Tullio MR, Sacco RL, Sciacca RR, Jin Z, Homma S. Patent foramen ovale and the risk of ischemic stroke in a multiethnic population. *J Am Coll Cardiol.* 2007;49:797–802.
60. Clarke NR, Timperley J, Kelion AD, Banning AP. Transthoracic echocardiography using second harmonic imaging with Valsalva manoeuvre for the detection of right to left shunts. *Eur J Echocardiogr.* 2004;5:176–181.
61. Lechat P, Mas JL, Lascault G, et al. Prevalence of patent foramen ovale in patients with stroke. *N Engl J Med.* 1988;318:1148–1152.
62. Webster MW, Chancellor AM, Smith HJ, et al. Patent foramen ovale in young stroke patients. *Lancet.* 1988;2:11–12.
63. Di Tullio M, Sacco RL, Gopal A, Mohr JP, Homma S. Patent foramen ovale as a risk factor for cryptogenic stroke. *Ann Intern Med.* 1992;117:461–465.
64. Handke M, Harloff A, Olschewski M, Hetzel A, Geibel A. Patent foramen ovale and cryptogenic stroke in older patients. *N Engl J Med.* 2007;357:2262–2268.
65. Steiner MM, Di Tullio MR, Rundek T, et al. Patent foramen ovale size and embolic brain imaging findings among patients with ischemic stroke. *Stroke.* 1998;29:944–948.
66. Schuchlenz HW, Weihs W, Horner S, Quehenberger F. The association between the diameter of a patent foramen ovale and the risk of embolic cerebrovascular events. *Am J Med.* 2000;109:456–462.
67. Furlan AJ, Reisman M, Massaro J, et al. Closure or medical therapy for cryptogenic stroke with patent foramen ovale. *N Engl J Med.* 2012;366:991–999.
68. Meier B, Kalesan B, Mattle HP, et al. Percutaneous closure of patent foramen ovale in cryptogenic embolism. *N Engl J Med.* 2013;368:1083–1091.
69. Carroll JD, Saver JL, Thaler DE, et al. Closure of patent foramen ovale versus medical therapy after cryptogenic stroke. *N Engl J Med.* 2013;368:1092–1100.
70. Saver JL, Carroll JD, Thaler DE, et al. Long-term outcomes of patent foramen ovale closure or medical therapy after stroke. *N Engl J Med.* 2017;377:1022–1032.
71. Homma S, Sacco RL, Di Tullio MR, Sciacca RR, Mohr JP. Atrial anatomy in non-cardioembolic stroke patients: effect of medical therapy. *J Am Coll Cardiol.* 2003;42:1066–1072.
72. Overell JR, Bone I, Lees KR. Interatrial septal abnormalities and stroke: a meta-analysis of case-control studies. *Neurology.* 2000;55:1172–1179.
73. Mas JL, Arquizan C, Lamy C, et al. Recurrent cerebrovascular events associated with patent foramen ovale, atrial septal aneurysm, or both. *N Engl J Med.* 2001;345:1740–1746.
74. Bonati LH, Kessel-Schaefer A, Linka AZ, et al. Diffusion-weighted imaging in stroke attributable to patent foramen ovale: significance of concomitant atrial septum aneurysm. *Stroke.* 2006;37:2030–2034.
75. Cramer SC, Rordorf G, Maki JH, et al. Increased pelvic vein thrombi in cryptogenic stroke: results of the Paradoxical Emboli from Large Veins in Ischemic Stroke (PELVIS) study. *Stroke.* 2004;35:46–50.
76. Botto N, Spadoni I, Giusti S, Ait-Ali L, Sicari R, Andreassi MG. Prothrombotic mutations as risk factors for cryptogenic ischemic cerebrovascular events in young subjects with patent foramen ovale. *Stroke.* 2007;38:2070–2073.
77. Homma S, Sacco RL, Di Tullio MR, Sciacca RR, Mohr JP. Effect of medical treatment in stroke patients with patent foramen ovale: patent foramen ovale in Cryptogenic Stroke Study. *Circulation.* 2002;105:2625–2631.
78. Serena J, Marti-Fabregas J, Santamarina E, et al. Recurrent stroke and massive right-to-left shunt: results from the prospective Spanish multicenter (CODICIA) study. *Stroke.* 2008;39:3131–3136.
78a. Mas JL, Durumeaux J, Guillon B, et al. Patent foramen ovale closure or anticoagulation vs. antiplatelets after stroke. *N Engl J Med.* 2017;377(11):1011–1021.
78b. Søndergaard L, Kasner SE, Rhodes JF, et al. Patent foramen ovale closure or antiplatelet therapy for cryptogenic stroke. *N Engl J Med.* 2017;377(11):1033–1042.
79. Amarenco P, Duyckaerts C, Tzourio C, Henin D, Bousser MG, Hauw JJ. The prevalence of ulcerated plaques in the aortic arch in patients with stroke. *N Engl J Med.* 1992;326:221–225.
80. Harloff A, Strecker C, Frydrychowicz AP, et al. Plaques in the descending aorta: a new risk factor for stroke? Visualization of potential embolization pathways by 4D MRI. *J Magn Reson Imaging.* 2007;26:1651–1655.
81. Katsanos AH, Giannopoulos S, Kosmidou M, et al. Complex atheromatous plaques in the descending aorta and the risk of stroke: a systematic review and meta-analysis. *Stroke.* 2014;45:1764–1770.
82. Vaduganathan P, Ewton A, Nagueh SF, Weilbaecher DG, Safi HJ, Zoghbi WA. Pathologic correlates of aortic plaques, thrombi and mobile "aortic debris" imaged in vivo with transesophageal echocardiography. *J Am Coll Cardiol.* 1997;30:357–363.
83. Weber A, Jones EF, Zavala JA, Ponnuthurai FA, Donnan GA. Intraobserver and interobserver variability of transesophageal echocardiography in aortic arch atheroma measurement. *J Am Soc Echocardiogr.* 2008;21:129–133.
84. Amarenco P, Cohen A, Tzourio C, et al. Atherosclerotic disease of the aortic arch and the risk of ischemic stroke. *N Engl J Med.* 1994;331:1474–1479.
85. Di Tullio MR, Sacco RL, Savoia MT, Sciacca RR, Homma S. Aortic atheroma morphology and the risk of ischemic stroke in a multiethnic population. *Am Heart J.* 2000;139:329–336.
86. Di Tullio MR, Homma S, Jin Z, Sacco RL. Aortic atherosclerosis, hypercoagulability and stroke: the aortic plaques and risk of ischemic stroke (APRIS) study. *J Am Coll Cardiol.* 2008;52:855–861.
87. Mitusch R, Doherty C, Wucherpfennig H, et al. Vascular events during follow-up in patients with aortic arch atherosclerosis. *Stroke.* 1997;28:36–39.
88. Levy D, Larson MG, Vasan RS, Kannel WB, Ho KK. The progression from hypertension to congestive heart failure. *J Am Med Assoc.* 1996;275:1557–1562.
89. Fujimoto S, Yasaka M, Otsubo R, Oe H, Nagatsuka K, Minematsu K. Aortic arch atherosclerotic lesions and the recurrence of ischemic stroke. *Stroke.* 2004;35:1426–1429.
90. Sen S, Hinderliter A, Sen PK, et al. Aortic arch atheroma progression and recurrent vascular events in patients with stroke or transient ischemic attack. *Circulation.* 2007;116:928–935.
91. Ueno Y, Kimura K, Iguchi Y, et al. Mobile aortic plaques are a cause of multiple brain infarcts seen on diffusion-weighted imaging. *Stroke.* 2007;38:2470–2476.
92. Laperche T, Laurian C, Roudaut R, Steg PG. Mobile thromboses of the aortic arch without aortic debris. A transesophageal echocardiographic finding associated with unexplained arterial embolism. The Filiale Echocardiographie de la Societe Francaise de Cardiologie. *Circulation.* 1997;96:288–294.
93. Hogue Jr CW, Murphy SF, Schechtman KB, Davila-Roman VG. Risk factors for early or delayed stroke after cardiac surgery. *Circulation.* 1999;100:642–647.
94. Trehan N, Mishra M, Kasliwal RR, Mishra A. Reduced neurological injury during CABG in patients with mobile aortic atheromas: a five-year follow-up study. *Ann Thorac Surg.* 2000;70:1558–1564.
95. Kataoka Y, Puri R, Pisaniello AD, et al. Aortic atheroma burden predicts acute cerebrovascular events after transcatheter aortic valve implantation: insights from volumetric multislice computed tomography analysis. *EuroIntervention.* 2016;12:783–789.
96. Seeger J, Gonska B, Otto M, Rottbauer W, Wohrle J. Cerebral embolic protection during transcatheter aortic valve replacement significantly reduces death and stroke compared with unprotected procedures. *JACC Cardiovasc Interv.* 2017;10:2297–2303.
97. Ben-Horin S, Bardan E, Barshack I, Zaks N, Livneh A. Cholesterol crystal embolization to the digestive system: characterization of a common, yet overlooked presentation of atheroembolism. *Am J Gastroenterol.* 2003;98:1471–1479.
98. Di Tullio MR, Russo C, Jin Z, Sacco RL, Mohr JP, Homma S. Aortic arch plaques and risk of recurrent stroke and death. *Circulation.* 2009;119:2376–2382.
99. Amarenco P, Davis S, Jones EF, et al. Clopidogrel plus aspirin versus warfarin in patients with stroke and aortic arch plaques. *Stroke.* 2014;45:1248–1257.
100. Stern A, Tunick PA, Culliford AT, et al. Protruding aortic arch atheromas: risk of stroke during heart surgery with and without aortic arch endarterectomy. *Am Heart J.* 1999;138:746–752.
101. Cabanes L, Mas JL, Cohen A, et al. Atrial septal aneurysm and patent foramen ovale as risk factors for cryptogenic stroke in patients less than 55 years of age. A study using transesophageal echocardiography. *Stroke.* 1993;24:1865–1873.
102. de Belder MA, Tourikis L, Leech G, Camm AJ. Risk of patent foramen ovale for thromboembolic events in all age groups. *Am J Cardiol.* 1992;69(16):1316–1320.
103. Hausmann D, Mugge A, Becht I, Daniel WG. Diagnosis of patent foramen ovale by transesophageal echocardiography and association with cerebral and peripheral embolic events. *Am J Cardiol.* 1992;70(6):668–672.
104. Jones EF, Calafiore P, Donnan GA, Tonkin AM. Evidence that patent foramen ovale is not a risk factor for cerebral ischemia in the elderly. *Am J Cardiol.* 1994;74(6):596–599.
105. Jones EF, Kalman JM, Calafiore P, et al. Proximal aortic atheroma. An independent risk factor for cerebral ischemia. *Stroke.* 1995;26(2):218–224.
106. Di Tullio MR, Sacco RL, Gersony D, et al. Aortic atheromas and acute ischemic stroke: a transesophageal echocardiographic study in an ethnically mixed population. *Neurology.* 1996;46(6):1560–1566.
107. Tunick PA, Perez JL, Kronzon I. Protruding atheromas in the thoracic aorta and systemic embolization. *Ann Intern Med.* 1991;115(6):423–427.

中文导读

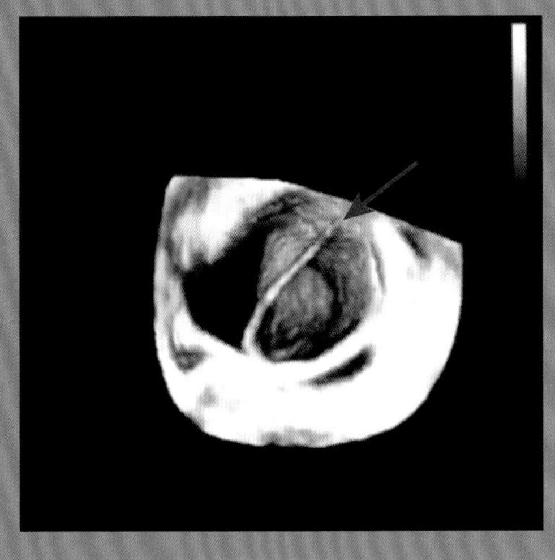

第39章 心房颤动和心房扑动患者的超声心动图

心房颤动是最常见的心律失常，发病率逐年升高，多个大型临床试验已经证实心房颤动是患者死亡的独立危险因素。由于心房颤动患者的心房细小血栓脱落可导致缺血性脑卒中，具有较高致残率，因此需要给予患者积极的临床干预。

超声对心房颤动患者心脏结构和功能的评估，根据仪器技术主要分为两大部分：一线的常规经胸超声心动图、相对有创的经食管超声心动图及心腔内超声。经胸超声心动图除了可以测量心房和心室的内径大小，还可以对心脏的结构和血流动力学进行整体评估，如是否合并瓣膜的狭窄或反流、是否存在心室或心房功能减低等。心房颤动患者接受治疗过程中（如射频消融术、左心耳封堵术），需要使用经食管超声心动图和心腔内超声，协助观察肺静脉、心耳形态和尺寸，以及是否合并血栓形成，并引导房间隔穿刺和左心耳封堵术。左心耳封堵术中的评估步骤包括观察有无血栓，测量心耳开口最大径；当引导房间隔穿刺后，封堵器置入时评估封堵器的深度、锚定牢固度和封堵的紧密程度；封堵器释放后再次评估上述内容，并观察有无心包积液等并发症。

卢宏泉

39 Echocardiography in Patients With Atrial Fibrillation and Flutter

NAZEM AKOUM, MD, MS | JORDAN M. PRUTKIN, MD, MHS

PREVALENCE AND IMPACT OF ATRIAL FIBRILLATION

Atrial fibrillation (AF) is the most common cardiac arrhythmia, with an estimated prevalence of more than 3 million Americans in 2012.[1] Although the true prevalence of atrial flutter (AFL) is not known, it is suspected that a large proportion of patients with cavotricuspid isthmus–dependent AFL, also known as typical flutter, have AF. Other forms of AFL, referred to as atypical, are encountered after cardiac surgery, in congenital heart disease, during treatment with class I antiarrhythmic agents, or after catheter ablation of AF. From an echocardiography perspective, management of AFL is largely similar to that of AF.

The prevalence of AF is expected to increase over the coming decades,[2] in part because of increasing longevity of the population, a greater prevalence of comorbidities, and improved mortality rates for ischemic heart disease and congestive heart failure. Advanced age is independently associated with the development of AF. In the United States, it is estimated that approximately 15% of the population older than 65 years is affected with AF. This percentage increases to about 25% among those older than 80 years. Other cardiovascular conditions are also associated with an increased prevalence of AF, including ischemic heart disease, valvular heart disease, hypertension, hypertrophic cardiomyopathy, and congestive heart failure. Heart failure with preserved systolic function is associated with a higher prevalence of AF compared with heart failure with reduced systolic function.[3] AF is also associated with obesity and obstructive sleep apnea, two conditions that are increasingly prevalent.

The Framingham Heart Study showed AF to be independently associated with increased mortality rates.[4] It is also associated with significant morbidity, most notably from ischemic stroke, and with increased office and emergency room visits and inpatient hospitalizations. All of these factors make AF a major contributor to health care expenditure in the United States.

ATRIAL REMODELING ASSOCIATED WITH ATRIAL FIBRILLATION

AF is associated with electrical and structural remodeling of the atria. Electrically, AF is associated with shortening of the atrial myocyte action potential duration and a reduced rate adaptation of calcium release.[5] Structurally, AF is associated with atrial myocyte loss, increased interstitial fibrosis, and collagen deposition.[6]

Autopsy studies have demonstrated that patients with a history of AF have higher rates of atrial fibrosis compared with patients without a history of AF, independent of age.[7] Other studies, which included patients undergoing cardiac surgery, have demonstrated that biopsies from the atria of patients with AF have a higher collagen content compared with those from patients without a history of the arrhythmia. Animal studies have shown that AF leads to progressive adverse atrial remodeling and worsening of the atrial substrate, a process often referred to as *AF begets AF*.[8] These ultrastructural changes of the atrial tissue are often accompanied by gross morphologic changes that can be seen on imaging, including increased atrial size measured by atrial diameter, surface area, and volume and reduced atrial contractile function.

ECHOCARDIOGRAPHY IN THE WORKUP OF PATIENTS WITH ATRIAL FIBRILLATION AND FLUTTER

The clinical presentation of patients with AF and AFL varies greatly. Some patients are minimally symptomatic, and the arrhythmia is discovered incidentally on physical examination or electrocardiographic evaluation. Clinical symptoms range from subtle effects, such as decreased stamina and exercise capacity; to palpitations, chest pain, and shortness of breath; to more serious symptoms such as syncope, stroke, or transient ischemic attack.

TABLE 39.1 Use of Echocardiography in Patients With Atrial Fibrillation as Recommended by Guidelines.

Study	When	Reason
TTE[95]	As part of the initial evaluation of all patients with AF	To assess for structural heart disease, ventricular function, valvular disease, and LA size
TEE[47,95]	If a cardioversion or ablation is planned when the duration of AF has been > 48 hours or is unknown and there has not been therapeutic anticoagulation for > 3 weeks. Some electrophysiologists perform a TEE on all patients before AF ablation regardless of anticoagulation status or presenting rhythm.	To rule out intracardiac thrombus with a focus on the LAA
ICE[47,96,97]	During AF ablation or possibly LAA closure	To aid in transseptal puncture, assess for complications, image the catheters, and visualize cardiac structures, including the pulmonary veins and LAA

AF, Atrial fibrillation; *ICE*, intracardiac echocardiography, *LAA*, left atrial appendage.

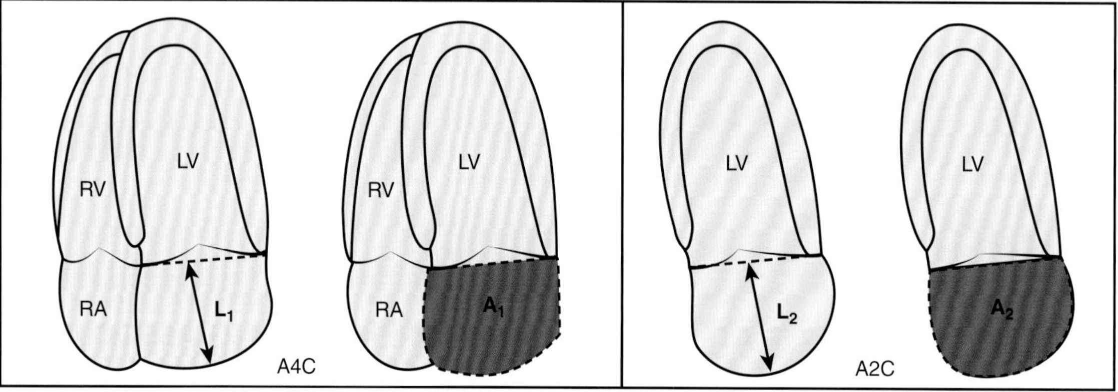

Fig. 39.1 Calculation of LA volume. LA volume (cm^3 or mL) is calculated from the measured LA length (*L*, cm) and LA area (*A*, cm^2) by the following formula: LA volume = $1.7\ (A_1 \times A_2)/0.5(L_1 + L_2)$, where A_1 and L_1 are measured from the apical 4-chamber *(A4C)* view and A_2 and L_2 from the apical 2-chamber *(A2C)* view. (Modified from Lang RM, Bierig M, Devereux RB, et al. Recommendations for chamber quantification: a report from the American Society of Echocardiography's Guidelines and Standards Committee and the Chamber Quantification Writing Group, developed in conjunction with the European Association of Echocardiography, a branch of the European Society of Cardiology. *J Am Soc Echocardiogr.* 2005;18:1440–1463.)

After the electrical abnormality is identified, echocardiographic evaluation plays a key role in the workup (Table 39.1). Initial questions are usually addressed with a transthoracic echocardiographic (TTE) study. Although AF and AFL are atrial arrhythmias, a comprehensive echocardiographic evaluation of the whole heart and hemodynamics is always warranted. This includes qualitative and quantitative assessment of atrial and ventricular sizes, valvular stenosis or regurgitation, and ventricular systolic function, diastolic filling pattern, and intravascular volume status. Some patients go on to more invasive echocardiographic examinations such as transesophageal echocardiography (TEE) and intracardiac echocardiography (ICE) during the course of their AF treatment.

ATRIAL SIZE

M-mode and two-dimensional (2D) TTE are commonly used to measure the left atrial (LA) diameter in the parasternal long-axis view.[9] This correlates with the atrial surface area measured in the apical long-axis view and with atrial volume measured using computed tomography (CT) or magnetic resonance angiography.[10,11] However, the LA diameter can underestimate atrial dilation, especially when dilation occurs in an asymmetric fashion. The American Society of Echocardiography (ASE) advocates the use of a 2D-derived LA volume (cm^3) measured by the Simpson or the biplane method from the apical 4-chamber (4C) and 2-chamber (2C) views using the following formula:

$$\text{LA volume} = 1.7\,(\text{A4C} \times \text{A2C})\ /\ 0.5\,(\text{L4C} + \text{L2C})$$

where *L* is length (cm) and *A* is surface area (cm^2) (Fig. 39.1). A normal LA volume derived from echocardiographic measurement ranges from 22 to 52 mL in women and from 18 to 58 mL in men, or 22 ± 6 mL/m^2 when normalized to body surface area (Table 39.2).[9]

ATRIAL FUNCTION

Atrial function includes two components: (1) a reservoir or conduit for blood returning from the vena cava and the pulmonary veins and (2) a contractile chamber that augments ventricular filling, similar to a supercharger on an internal combustion engine.

Assessment of atrial mechanical function includes complementary information derived from M-mode and transmitral Doppler echocardiography. M-mode enables measurement of the excursion of mitral valve leaflets, even in the setting of arrhythmia.[12] In the absence of mitral valve stenosis, normal mitral valve excursion is about 13 mm from a closed to a fully open position (Fig 39.2). Anterior leaflet excursion is sometimes used to assess LA function and is reduced in low cardiac output states, with elevated left ventricular (LV) filling pressure, and with atrial mechanical dysfunction.[12]

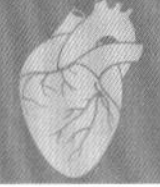

TABLE 39.2 **Reference Ranges for LA Size.**

Parameter	*Women*	*Men*
RA minor axis dimension (cm/m^2)	1.9 ± 0.3	1.9 ± 0.3
RA major axis dimension (cm/m^2)	2.5 ± 0.3	2.4 ± 0.3
2D echocardiographic RA volume (mL/m^2)[a]	21 ± 6	25 ± 7
AP dimension (cm)	2.7–3.8	3.0–4.0
AP dimension index (cm/m^2)	1.5–2.3	1.5–2.3
A4C area index (cm^2/m^2)	9.3 ± 1.7	8.9 ± 1.5
A2C area index (cm^2/m^2)	9.6 ± 1.4	9.3 ± 1.6
A4C volume index MOD (mL/m^2)	25.1 ± 7.2	24.5 ± 6.4
A4C volume index AL (mL/m^2)	27.3 ± 7.9	27.0 ± 7.0
A2C volume index MOD (mL/m^2)	26.1 ± 6.7	27.1 ± 7.9
A2C volume index AL (mL/m^2)	28.0 ± 7.3	28.9 ± 8.5
LA volume index (mL/m^2)[a]	Normal: 16–34 Mildly enlarged: 35–41 Moderately enlarged: 42–48 Severely enlarged: >48	Normal: 16–34 Mildly enlarged: 35–41 Moderately enlarged: 42–48 Severely enlarged: >48

[a]Recommended measurement to determine chamber size.

A2C, Apical 2 chamber; *A4C*, apical 4-chamber; *AL*, area length; *AP*, anteroposterior; *MOD*, method of disks.

From Lang RM, Badano LP, Mor-Avi V, et al. Recommendations for cardiac chamber quantification by echocardiography in adults: an update from the American Society of Echocardiography and the European Association of Cardiovascular Imaging. *J Am Soc Echocardiogr*. 2015;28:1–39.

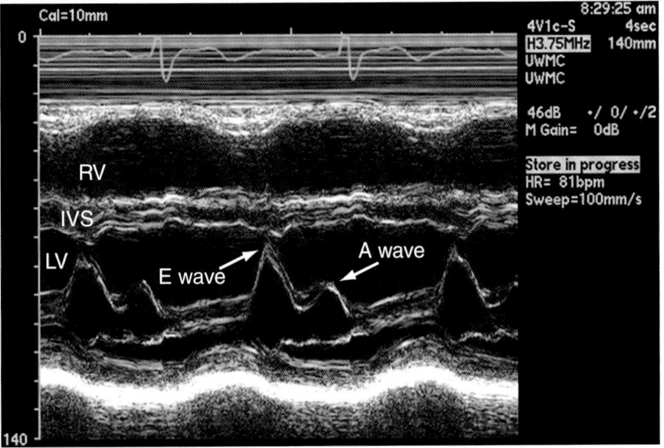

Fig. 39.2 Normal anterior mitral valve leaflet excursion. M-mode imaging in a parasternal long-axis view shows E and A waves of the anterior mitral valve leaflet during mitral valve opening. A normal A wave measures about 13 mm, and lesser values have been associated with reduced atrial mechanical function. The RV, interventricular septum *(IVS)*, and LV are also seen.

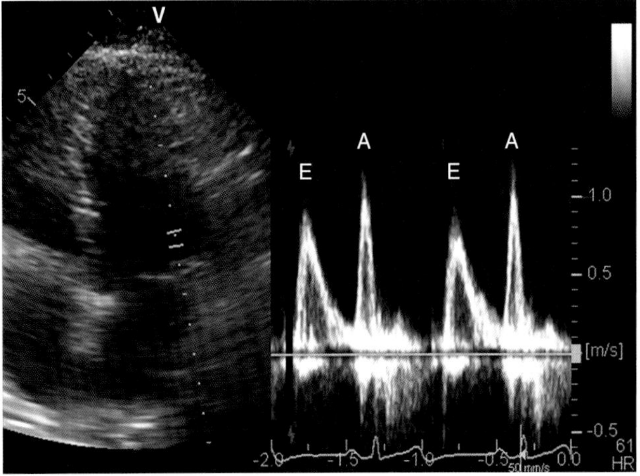

Fig. 39.3 TTE 2D–guided spectral display of transmitral pulsed-wave Doppler echocardiographic flow velocity. The size, envelope, and relationship of the E and A waves are influenced by heart rate, loading conditions, and the sample volume position on pulsed-wave Doppler interrogation. *A*, Atrial filling wave; *E*, early filling wave.

Transmitral Doppler is an accurate method to assess flow across the mitral valve during ventricular filling. Early diastolic passive ventricular filling is captured by the E wave, whereas active late filling, which includes the contribution from atrial contraction, is captured by the A wave. The size, envelope, and relationships of the E and A waves are influenced by heart rate, loading conditions, and the sample volume position on pulsed-wave (PW) Doppler interrogation. The most common pulse volume position is between the tips of the mitral valve leaflets (Fig. 39.3).

Common measures used to assess LA function include the height of the A wave, which can be used to calculate atrial contraction force,[13] and the atrial emptying fraction, which is derived from the calculated minimum (end of ventricular diastole) and maximum (end of ventricular systole) atrial volumes. The magnitude of the A wave depends on the loading conditions and is commonly absent when the echocardiogram is done during AF, resulting in significant limitations to this method of assessing atrial function.

Another echocardiographic method to estimate atrial function uses speckle tracking echocardiography to assess wall deformation. Longitudinal deformation of the atrial wall is assessed in the mid-septal and mid-lateral walls in the apical 4-chamber view. Wall strain and strain rate versus time curves are generated from these areas of interest (Fig. 39.4). Global peak atrial longitudinal strain of 42.2% ± 6.1% and global time to peak longitudinal strain of 368 ± 30 ms have been reported as reference indices of normal atrial myocardial deformation.[14]

Patients with AF imaged during sinus rhythm have a reduced LA emptying fraction and reduced lateral atrial wall strain

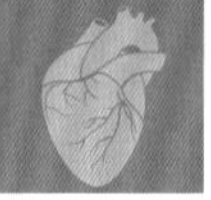

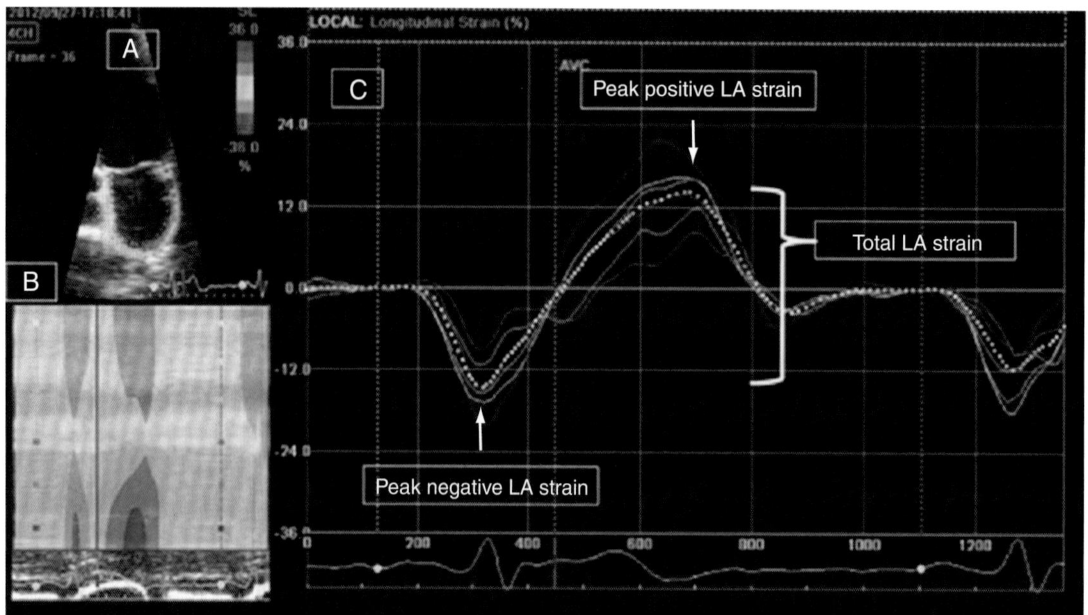

Fig. 39.4 2D LA speckle tracking echocardiography. (A) 4-Chamber view depicts the region of interest created by the speckle tracking software. (B) Color M-mode imaging shows LA deformation of all regions throughout the cardiac cycle. (C) The LA strain curve of the global deformation *(dashed line)* is obtained by averaging the six curves. (Adapted from Teixeira R, Vieira MJ, Goncalves L. Left atrial reservoir phase: deformation analysis. *Eur Heart J Cardiovasc Imaging.* 2013;14:500–501.)

TABLE 39.3 Association of Measured Echocardiographic Parameters and Risk of Incident Atrial Fibrillation or Recurrence After Catheter Ablation.

Echocardiographic Measure	*Associated Risk*
Increased E/A ratio on tissue Doppler imaging	Increased risk of AF[18]
Increased A-wave velocity	U-shaped association with risk of AF
Increased atrial diameter	Increased risk of AF[19]
Increased LV wall thickness	Increased risk of AF[19]
Decreased LV fractional shortening	Increased risk of AF[19]
Impaired ventricular relaxation, pseudonormal ventricular filling, and restrictive ventricular filling pattern	Increased risk of AF[21]
Increased LA volume	Increased risk of recurrence after catheter ablation[33]
Reduced LA wall strain	Increased risk of recurrence after catheter ablation[16]

AF, Atrial fibrillation.

compared with control subjects without AF.[15] Patients with AF and high levels of atrial fibrosis measured by magnetic resonance imaging (MRI) with late gadolinium enhancement also have a reduced atrial strain, indicating that atrial fibrosis is associated with reduced mechanical atrial function.[16,17]

Echocardiographic parameters, including atrial size and function and ventricular size and relaxation pattern, can predict incident AF. Data from the Framingham Heart Study showed that an increase in the E/A ratio was independently associated with incident AF.[18,19] Impaired LV relaxation has also been associated with incident AF in patients older than 65 years.[20] TTE evidence of LA enlargement by surface area and volume measurements also predicts incident AF,[21] independent of parameters such as age, diabetes, hypertension, congestive heart failure, coronary artery disease, and stroke (Table 39.3).

Right atrial (RA) size is increased in AF and AFL, but RA size and function have been less well studied than left-sided parameters. Conditions such as chronic lung disease, pulmonary emboli, and pulmonary hypertension preferentially affect the right heart and have been associated with AF and AFL. An apical 4-chamber view is preferred for the assessment of RA size on TTE (Fig. 39.5). From this view, the RA diameter, surface area, and volume can be measured.

RA reservoir and contractile function are less well studied and understood. Under normal hemodynamic conditions, the right heart pressures are significantly lower than the left, and early passive right ventricular (RV) filling is the norm. Pulmonary vascular resistance is also low, and a mild amount of tricuspid valve regurgitation is not uncommon. For the right heart, reduced tricuspid annular plane systolic excursion (TAPSE) has been associated with AF in patients with systolic heart failure.[7]

Atrial size and function can be assessed using TEE. TEE is not routinely used solely for this evaluation because it is more invasive and less comfortable for the patient than TTE. It does offer a distinct advantage in evaluating the left and right atrial appendages for function and existence of thrombus. TEE is most commonly performed in AF to answer the important question of whether a thrombus is present; the answer dictates the management of AF patients from the perspective of reducing stroke. The following sections address the relationship of AF and thromboembolization in more detail.

STROKE AND ATRIAL FIBRILLATION

The association between AF and ischemic stroke was established through multiple cohort studies. AF is associated with a fivefold increase in the risk of stroke,[22] and AF-related thromboembolization is implicated in about 20% of ischemic strokes.[23] This may be an underestimation because some strokes of uncertain origin (i.e., cryptogenic) are suspected to be related

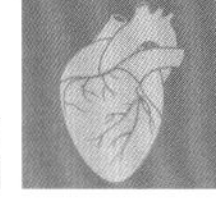

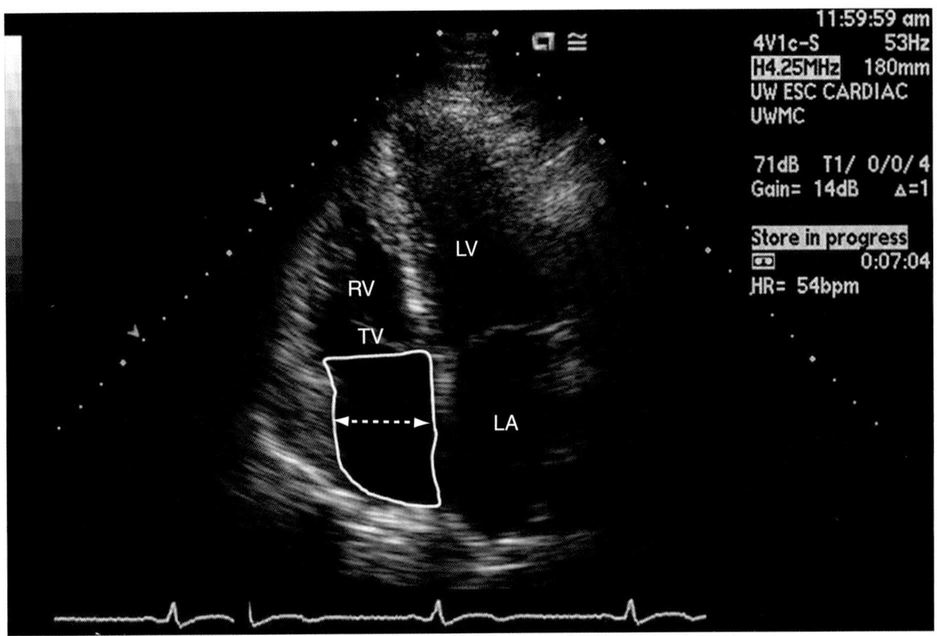

Fig. 39.5 **TTE imaging of the RA from an apical 4-chamber view.** Linear measurement of the minor axis of the RA between the mid-lateral RA wall and the mid-interatrial septum is shown *(dotted line with ar)*. The blood-tissue interface of the RA is traced at end-systole, with the area below the tricuspid valve *(TV)* excluded to define the RA area measurement.

to AF. AF-associated strokes are more devastating and lead to more disability and death than other ischemic strokes.[4] Stroke is therefore a major cause of mortality, morbidity, and health care expenditure in AF, and one of the initial steps in managing patients with AF is to estimate the thromboembolic risk and determine the best strategy to reduce it.

ROLE OF THE LEFT ATRIAL APPENDAGE

Stroke in AF is thought to result from thrombus formation within the LA chamber and subsequent embolization into the cerebral circulation. When thrombi are detected in the atria of patients with AF, they are found in the left atrial appendage (LAA) about 90% of the time.[24]

Thrombus formation in the LAA in AF patients is thought to be mediated through a combination of several factors forming the components of a Virchow triad: (1) structural and contractile changes leading to *blood stasis,* (2) atrial *tissue injury,* and (3) blood *hypercoagulability* from platelet and hemostatic activation.

Appendage Morphology

The LAA is an elongated, tubular, anatomic blind pouch that connects to the anterolateral aspect of the LA. Studies show that the appendage is the embryologic LA, serving as a reservoir for blood entering the developing LV. The LAA shape varies among individuals. Necropsy studies show that most LAAs have more than one lobe (range, one to four), and most patients have two lobes.[25] The inner surface of the LAA demonstrates extensive trabeculations due to the presence of pectinate muscle strands, which may play a role in contraction and emptying of the appendage. This contrasts with the smooth inner surface of the LA, which develops later from the coalescence of the developing pulmonary veins.[24]

Anatomic variations can present challenges to echocardiographic assessment of the LAA.[26] Retrospective studies have suggested that certain shape variations of the LAA (e.g., cauliflower) are associated with an increased risk of stroke compared with others (e.g., chicken wing) (Fig. 39.6).[27,28] Some change to the morphology of the LAA has been described in AF patients compared with patients without AF. Necropsy studies demonstrate that the volume of the LAA in patients with AF is three times larger than in patients without a history of AF. LAAs of patients with AF also had a larger surface area and a wider appendage orifice connecting to the LA.[24,29] Whether these variations contribute to the development of AF or are a consequence of the remodeling process associated with the arrhythmia is not well understood.

Appendage Function

LAA function is usually evaluated with TEE Doppler studies to assess blood flow velocities through the appendage orifice over the entire cardiac cycle. In a study of 50 patients with structurally normal hearts and clinically indicated TEE studies, the LAA contraction velocity was 60 ± 14 cm/s, and the filling velocity was 52 ± 13 cm/s.[30] Another echocardiography-based method uses tissue Doppler imaging to assess appendage tissue velocities. Reduced LAA contraction leads to blood stasis, which is suspected to contribute to thrombus formation.

Appendage Tissue Changes

AF is associated with fibroelastic change of the atrial endocardium. Electron microscopic studies of patients with AF and mitral valve disease (i.e., stenosis and regurgitation) have demonstrated that AF is likely to be associated with advanced endothelial tissue change. This change has been more commonly seen in the LAA than in the right atrial appendage (RAA), and it has been paralleled by an increase in levels of von Willebrand factor, a marker of endothelial injury.[31] Similar changes probably occur in patients with nonvalvular AF, but this has not yet been demonstrated. These observations were made on tissue samples obtained during valve surgery. A noninvasive method to assess atrial tissue changes would be more practical in AF patients.

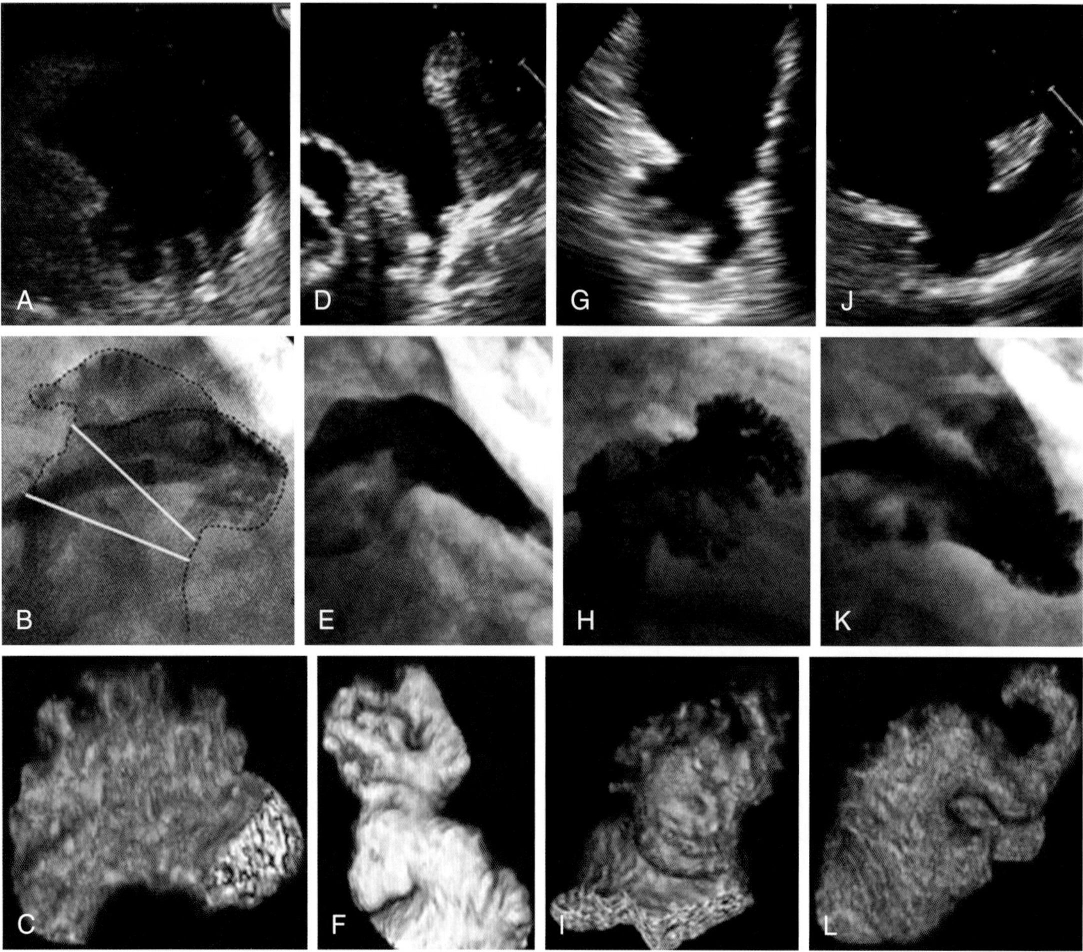

Fig. 39.6 Left atrial appendage morphologies. The left atrial appendage can be seen on TEE (A, D, G, and J) with correlates on angiography (B, E, H, and K) and computed tomography (C, F, I, and L). Each column represents a different patient with imaging from each modality. In column A–C, the patient's left atrial appendage has a so-called cauliflower shape; in column D–F, a windsock; in column G–I, a cactus, and in column J–L, a chicken wing. (From Beigel R, Wunderlich NC, Ho SY, Arsanjani R, Siegel RJ. The left atrial appendage: anatomy, function, and noninvasive evaluation. *JACC Cardiovasc Imaging.* 2014;7:1251–1265.)

HEMOSTATIC CHANGES

The formation of an LAA thrombus, which shares some pathophysiology with other thrombi that form throughout the vasculature, requires activation of the coagulation cascade and the contribution of platelet factors. For a thrombus to form, the balance between prothrombotic and antithrombotic factors must favor clotting. Over an extended period, some fluctuation in the balance of prothrombotic and antithrombotic factors is expected in a patient with AF. The thrombus identified on TEE is only a snapshot of this process. The cascade leading to thrombus formation and subsequent resolution and the time it takes for these processes to occur are not well understood.

Treatment with an oral anticoagulant dampens the variations in the direction of favoring the antithrombotic side. Lim et al. demonstrated that induced AF and rapid regular atrial pacing at 150 beats/min were associated with significant platelet and hemostatic activation after a period of 15 minutes in patients with a history of AF.[32] Factors studied included P-selectin as a marker of platelet activation, CD40 as a marker of platelet-derived inflammation, thrombin-antithrombin complexes as a marker of activation of the coagulation cascade, and asymmetric dimethylarginine as a marker of endothelial dysfunction.

TEE IN THE MANAGEMENT OF ATRIAL FIBRILLATION

When restoration of normal rhythm is deemed to be the best strategy for a patient, treatment options include direct current cardioversion, antiarrhythmic drugs, and catheter ablation. Before any of these interventions, it is imperative to ensure that the patient has not developed a thrombus, especially when the duration of the arrhythmia episode cannot be reliably ascertained.

Restoration of normal rhythm is followed by the return of normal LAA contraction, which is thought to expel the thrombus into the systemic circulation. Direct contact with an LAA thrombus in the setting of catheter ablation can also lead to its embolization. Patients with AF often undergo TEE to identify LAA thrombi before interventions to restore normal rhythm are performed when adequate oral anticoagulation cannot be verified (Fig. 39.7).[33]

TEE is the standard of care for evaluation of the LAA for thrombus[34] because thrombus is poorly visualized on TTE. TEE is an invasive procedure that requires hypopharyngeal anesthesia and conscious sedation followed by esophageal intubation for cardiac visualization. This can cause patient discomfort and

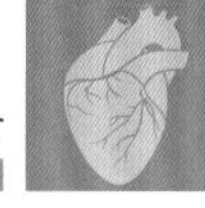

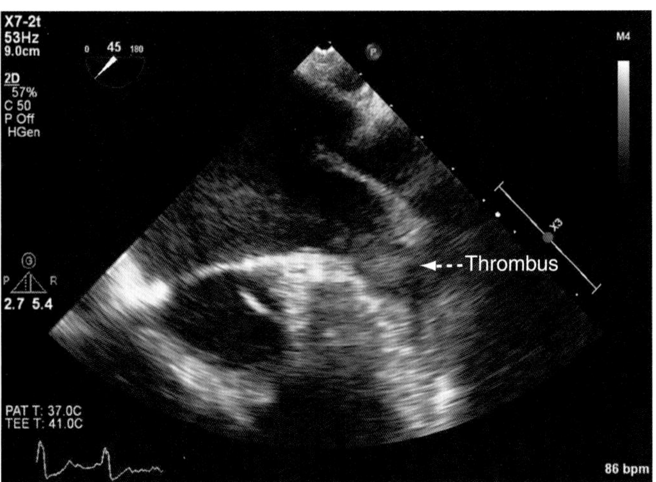

Fig. 39.7 Left atrial appendage thrombus seen on TEE imaging. To exclude artifact or trabeculae, the thrombus should be seen in multiple views, should have independent motion, and should be present throughout the cardiac cycle. Trabeculae are usually more linear and attached to the atrial wall. Using a higher-frequency transducer (7 MHz) with zoom mode is helpful (see Video 39.7).

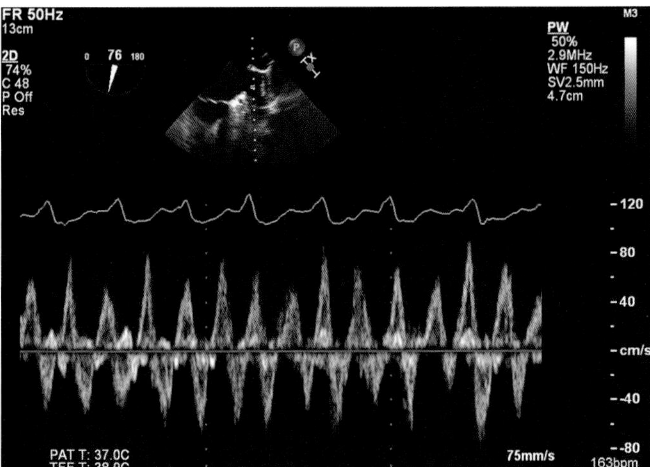

Fig. 39.8 Pulsed-wave Doppler imaging of the left atrial appendage in a patient with atrial fibrillation and a rapid ventricular response. In this example, with the sample volume measured approximately 1 cm from the ostium of the appendage, the velocity is 0.4 to 0.8 m/s with an average of 0.63 m/s over 10 beats. A normal value is more than 0.4 m/s. Velocities less than 0.4 m/s have been associated with an increased risk of stroke.

is rarely associated with complications such as esophageal perforation, aspiration pneumonia, or dysphagia.

Multiplane and three-dimensional (3D) TEE evaluation of the LAA helps elucidate anatomic variations, including the pectinate muscles and multiple lobes (see Fig. 39.6). PW Doppler is used to measure inflow and outflow velocities, which are typically reduced in long-standing, persistent AF (Fig. 39.8). A normal velocity is more than 0.4 m/s.

After restoration of normal rhythm, it is recommended to continue oral anticoagulation for at least 4 weeks because the post-cardioversion period is considered high risk for thrombus formation. This is thought to be a result of the delay in return of normal atrial contractile function after cardioversion, even in the absence of AF. The acute and short-term effects of cardioversion on the clotting milieu and tissue injury have not been studied.

TEE has several limitations, the most common of which is related to anatomic variation in the size and shape of the LAA, including trabeculations and multiple lobes. This leads to some uncertainty in conclusive assessment of the presence or absence of thrombus. AF patients may require repeated TEEs as part of their usual clinical care because AF is commonly a recurrent arrhythmia despite the interventions discussed previously.

An alternative strategy to TEE-guided cardioversion is 4 consecutive weeks of therapeutic oral anticoagulation. This strategy is viable when a patient's symptoms with the arrhythmia can be tolerated for this duration.[35]

VALVULAR VERSUS NONVALVULAR ATRIAL FIBRILLATION

AF often coexists with valvular heart disease of different levels of severity, and the term *valvular AF* is sometimes used. The definition of valvular AF, however, is a matter of debate among experts in the field. The most important implications in distinguishing valvular from nonvalvular AF are in thromboembolic risk assessment and the choice of oral anticoagulation. Guideline definitions of valvular AF intersect at worse-than-moderate mitral stenosis and artificial heart valves (along with valve repairs in the North American guidelines).[36–38] Patients with the aforementioned valvular conditions have a particularly elevated risk of thromboembolism, and vitamin K antagonists are recommended.

With the advent of non–vitamin K antagonist oral anticoagulants, some patients with valvular heart disease were excluded from clinical trials, producing a significant degree of heterogeneity in patient exclusion. In the Randomized Evaluation of Long-Term Anticoagulation Therapy (RE-LY) trial, which studied two doses of dabigatran versus warfarin, patients with prosthetic heart valves and "hemodynamically significant" valvular heart disease, which included aortic valve stenosis and regurgitation and mitral stenosis and regurgitation, were excluded.[39] The ROCKET AF, ARISTOTLE, and ENGAGE-AF trials studied rivaroxaban, apixaban, and edoxaban, respectively, versus warfarin, and they excluded only patients with prosthetic heart valves and hemodynamically significant mitral valve stenosis while permitting participation of patients with other valvular lesions.[40–42] Subgroup analyses from these studies showed no difference from overall study cohort findings, suggesting similar efficacy and safety of these agents in patients with and without these valvular lesions. Only dabigatran has been tested in patients with mechanical heart valves; it was found to be associated with an increased risk of thromboembolic and bleeding complications.[43]

Echocardiographic evaluations with TTE and TEE remain the standard for patients with various forms of valvular heart disease. This topic is thoroughly discussed in dedicated chapters in this textbook.

INTRAPROCEDURAL ECHOCARDIOGRAPHY

ATRIAL FIBRILLATION CATHETER ABLATION

The discovery that the trigger for AF in many patients is premature atrial contractions originating from within the pulmonary veins led to the concept that radiofrequency ablation of premature atrial contractions could prevent future AF episodes.[44] Current methodology targets the pulmonary vein antrum by radiofrequency or cryoballoon ablation to create

TABLE 39.4 Intraprocedural Use of Intracardiac Echocardiography to Assess Atrial Fibrillation Ablation Complications.

Complication	Technical Considerations	Limitations	Alternative Modalities
Pericardial effusion	If ICE is used, the catheter can be advanced into the RV and rotated clockwise to image the pericardial space around the RV. Further clockwise rotation shows the LV.	There are no validated measures of tamponade using ICE, but an effusion of ≥ 1 cm is usually considered significant. Catheter is sometimes difficult to enter into the RV.	TEE and TTE can be used and often are more helpful than ICE to guide pericardiocentesis.
Steam pop	Microbubble explosion at the tip of the catheter, which may occur even without an auditory pop.	Catheter should be in the field of view.	TEE could be used but would infrequently visualize the catheter tip.
Air or thromboembolus	Imaging of the LV with the ICE catheter in the RV can show a wall motion abnormality.	Imaging the LV other than the septum or lateral wall may be challenging.	TEE or TTE can image the LV, although TTE may be difficult, depending on where sterile drapes are located.
Phrenic nerve palsy	The ICE catheter is pulled back to the IVC-RA junction, and imaging of the diaphragm and liver is performed during phrenic nerve pacing. Absence of diaphragm movement indicates phrenic nerve palsy.	This method may not show a gradual reduction in phrenic nerve excursion. If the ICE image is run through a 3D mapping system, there may be a half-second delay between image acquisition and display.	Manual touching of the abdomen, fluoroscopy, or diaphragm electromyogram recording may be used.
LA thrombus	ICE may demonstrate thrombus in the LA or attached to sheaths.	Imaging of the entire sheath must be completed frequently because a thrombus may develop out of plane. Small thrombi may not be seen.	TEE may also be used.
Esophageal injury	The ICE catheter is placed within the RA and rotated clockwise to the posterior wall to visualize the esophagus.	Image quality of the esophagus may sometimes be poor.	For esophageal temperature monitoring, a 3D map made with a catheter in the esophagus or merging of the esophagus from a preprocedural CT/MRI, and a 3D mapping system can be used.
Mitral valve injury	Rarely, mitral valve damage from catheter entrapment may occur. With the ICE catheter in the RA, the mitral valve may sometimes be seen when rotating clockwise past the aortic valve. The catheter can also be advanced into the RV and rotated clockwise to image the LV and mitral valve.	Imaging of the mitral valve by ICE is often inadequate to achieve the correct angle to assess the extent of damage and/or regurgitation. Catheter entrapment may occur, but the location within the chordae may not be fully appreciated.	TEE can better assess the mitral valve and/or the presence of catheter entrapment.
Pulmonary vein stenosis	TEE can demonstrate PV size and flows. Pulsed-wave and color Doppler can identify an increased velocity and turbulent flow. TEE can also be used if balloon angioplasty or stent placement is performed.	TEE is invasive, and the right-sided pulmonary veins may be more difficult to image accurately.	CT or MRI is usually the first step to demonstrate PV size. Quantitative lung perfusion scanning can also be used to demonstrate flow reduction to a lung segment.

CT, Computed tomography; *ICE,* intracardiac echocardiography; *IVC,* inferior vena cava; *MRI,* magnetic resonance imaging; *PV,* pulmonary vein.

electrical isolation of the pulmonary veins. Some operators add additional ablation lines or isolation of other targets, such as the LAA or superior vena cava.[45]

Intracardiac Echocardiography

ICE is used routinely in the electrophysiology laboratory for real-time imaging of cardiac anatomy, transseptal puncture, catheter location and contact, venous occlusion for balloon-based technologies, ablation lesion formation, clot visualization, esophageal location, and surveillance for procedural complications (Table 39.4). ICE has taken on greater importance as more cases are addressed without fluoroscopy.[46,47]

The most commonly used ICE device is a sector-based phased array transducer on an 8- or 10-French catheter. This catheter can be steered anteriorly, posteriorly, leftward, and rightward. It allows 2D imaging, M-mode, and color, PW, continuous-wave, and tissue Doppler imaging. A newer model with 3D imaging is also available. A second type of ICE catheter, a 9-French radial transducer, is available, but it is nonsteerable and has a smaller depth of view.

The ICE catheter can be advanced through the venous system up to the RA without using fluoroscopy. A long-axis view of the vein should be continuously seen on the screen; if it is not present, the catheter can be advanced or pulled back, rotated, or angled to give this view. If another catheter or wire is in the same vein, it can help demonstrate the vein lumen.

Evaluation of cardiac anatomy can be done with the catheter placed in the RA. Starting from the tricuspid valve and RV and rotating the catheter clockwise from this position can demonstrate the aortic valve and LV outflow tract, followed by the mitral valve and LAA, left-sided pulmonary veins (Fig. 39.9), posterior LA wall with the esophagus, right inferior pulmonary vein, and right superior pulmonary vein.

ICE imaging is a very useful adjunct and can be a primary tool for transseptal puncture. ICE can clearly demonstrate the interatrial septum, including abnormalities such as lipomatous hypertrophy, aortic root dilation, or an aneurysmal septum that may make transseptal puncture more difficult (Fig. 39.10 and Video 39.10). The anatomic relationship of the septum to the aortic valve anteriorly and the LA wall posteriorly can be visualized. The sheath and needle tip can be seen to ensure proper positioning in the fossa ovalis. The needle tip is visualized directly or as the spot of maximum tenting of the septum. This allows accurate positioning of the sheath and needle in the desired location, which may differ according to the procedure used. For instance, a more posterior location with the needle tip directed toward the left pulmonary veins is usually preferred for radiofrequency ablation, but an anterior approach toward the LAA may be preferred for cryoballoon ablation. As the septum is crossed, the needle tip can often be seen jumping into the LA, and the septum relaxes a small amount.

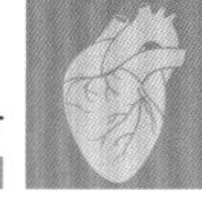

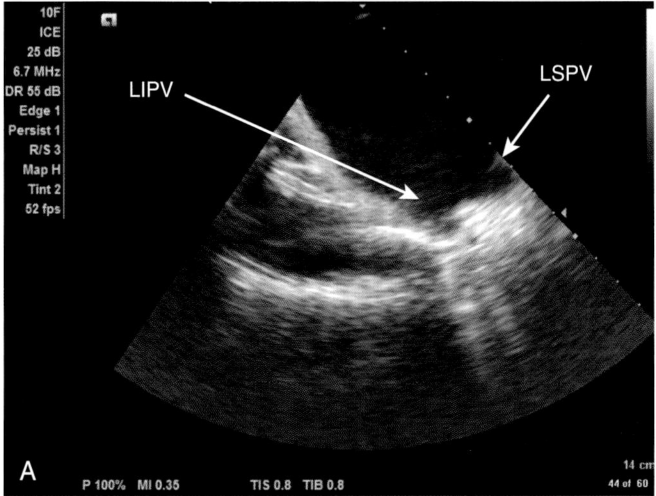

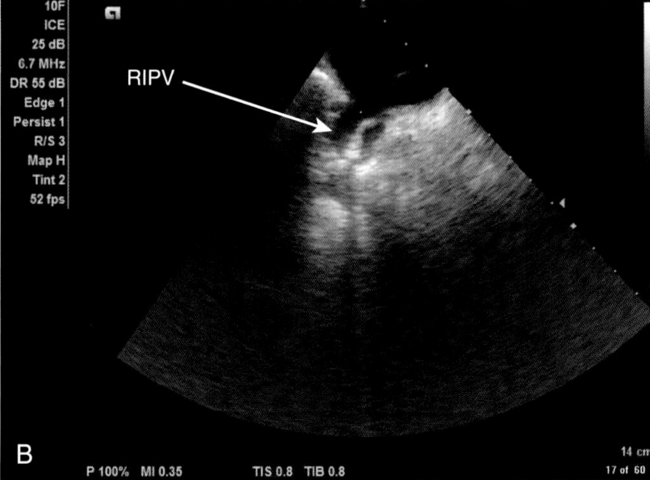

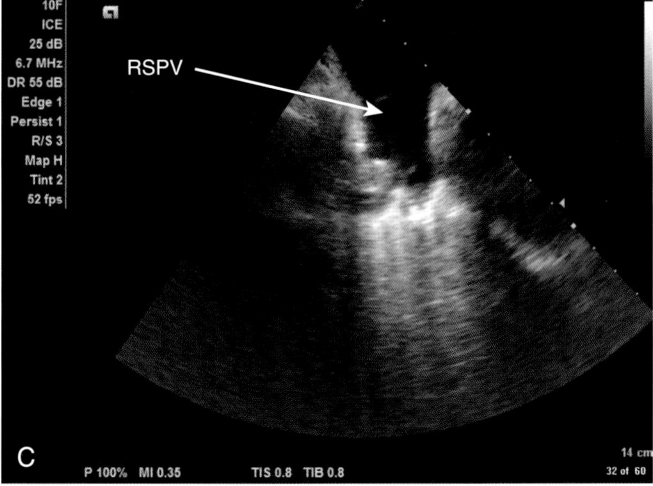

Fig. 39.9 **Pulmonary veins seen on ICE imaging.** (A) The intracardiac echocardiography (ICE) catheter is in the RA and initially faces the left inferior pulmonary vein *(LIPV)* and left superior pulmonary vein *(LSPV)*. (B) It is rotated clockwise to show the right inferior pulmonary vein *(RIPV)*. (C) It is then further rotated clockwise and advanced inward a small amount to show the right superior pulmonary vein *(RSPV)*.

In those with prior atrial septal defect patches or closure devices, ICE can indicate where to cross the septum. The best place is usually away from the patch or closure device, if possible, but the puncture can be made through these if needed.[48,49]

ICE can be used to assess thrombus in the LAA. Typically, a phased array catheter is used because it can be manipulated within the heart to provide the optimal views. The LAA can be viewed in several different manners, and it is typically necessary to image from each location to ensure that no LAA thrombus exists. The best view is from the RV outflow tract or pulmonary artery.[50,51] The catheter is maneuvered to that location and rotated clockwise, which can open a long-axis view of the LAA, including the orifice and side lobes. The catheter can then be advanced across the pulmonic valve and into the pulmonary artery, and with further manipulation inferomedially, a short-axis view or further side lobes can be seen. Clockwise rotation can further open the LAA orifice and show the relationship to the mitral valve.

Pulling the catheter back into the RA and rotating anteriorly can demonstrate the LAA orifice, although frequently with worse quality. The use of higher ultrasonic frequencies (7.5–8.5 MHz) may provide better imaging of the LAA to differentiate thrombus from spontaneous echocardiographic contrast.[51] Imaging of the LAA can also be completed by placing the ICE catheter in the coronary sinus.[52,53] It is possible to place the ICE catheter into the LA after a transseptal puncture, although care must be taken not to dislodge a thrombus, if one is present.[52]

One multicenter study suggested that ICE was equivalent to TEE for detecting spontaneous echocardiographic contrast in the LA or LAA, whereas ICE was superior for imaging thrombus in the body of the LA, and TEE was superior for imaging thrombus in the LAA.[54] Others have found that ICE had a higher diagnostic imaging quality than TEE for visualization of the LAA, especially with imaging of the distal LAA and if the ICE catheter could be advanced to the pulmonary artery (Fig. 39.11 and Video 39.11).[55] ICE can help to assess and prevent several complications during the procedure (see Table 39.4), including pericardial effusion, thrombus on a catheter,[56] steam pop occurrence, phrenic nerve palsy,[57] mitral valve injury, and esophageal injury.[58]

For cryoballoon ablation, some operators use color Doppler imaging to assess pulmonary vein occlusion.[59,60] If color flow is seen between the balloon and the atrial wall, there is incomplete occlusion, and balloon repositioning is needed (Fig. 39.12).

ICE imaging can be combined with a 3D electroanatomic mapping system (CartoSound, Biosense Webster, Diamond Bar, CA) to image anatomy on the mapping system without entering the LA.[61] This may improve merging of a preprocedure CT or MRI image, enhance the ability to see the catheter tip, document the esophageal location, and reduce LA dwell time.

Transesophageal Echocardiography

TEE may be used in lieu of ICE during AF ablation because there is already familiarity with its use in the intraoperative setting, although general anesthesia must be used instead of conscious sedation. It is common to use TEE to exclude LAA thrombus before AF ablation, especially if the patient is in AF at the time of the procedure and has not had adequate anticoagulation, or for a transseptal puncture.[62,63]

3D TEE may offer the advantage of improved visualization of the interatrial septum to make transseptal puncture easier. It may be helpful in assessing occlusion of the pulmonary veins while using the cryoballoon. Pulmonary vein occlusion can be seen with 3D TEE, but the inferior pulmonary veins may be more difficult to visualize.[64,65]

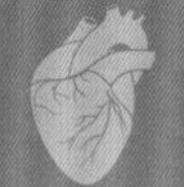

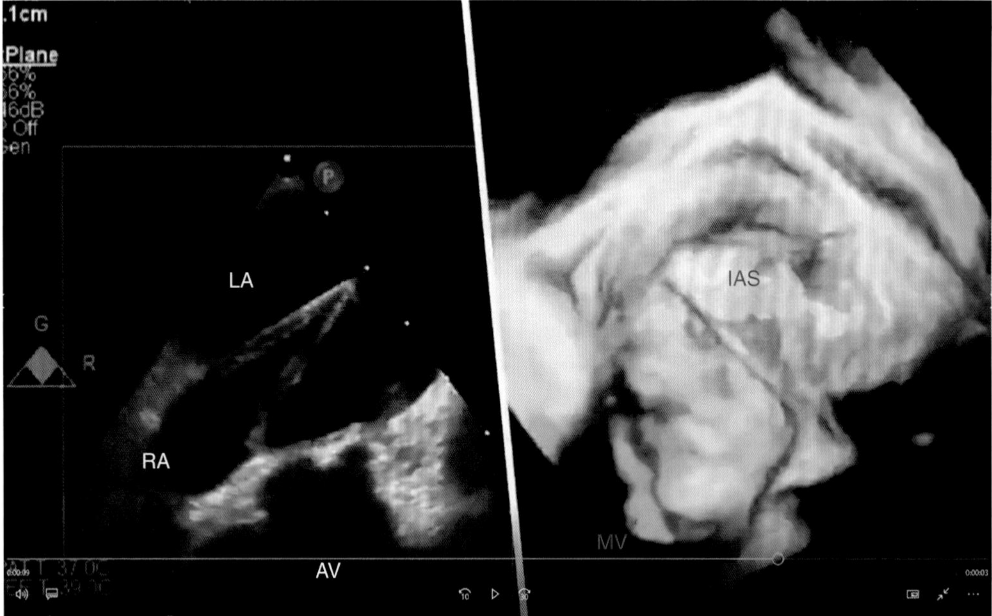

Fig. 39.10 Transseptal puncture. On 2D TEE *(left)* and 3D TEE *(right)*, the transseptal needle and sheath are seen in the RA with the needle tip seen tenting an aneurysmal interatrial septum *(IAS)* before entering the LA. *AV*, Aortic valve; *MV*, mitral valve (see Video 39.10). (Courtesy Richard Sheu, MD, University of Washington.)

There is some concern that use of TEE with the patient under general anesthesia may increase the risk of esophageal ulceration during AF ablation.[66] This can occur because of heating of the echocardiography probe from piezoelectric crystal vibration, absorption of ultrasound energy, mechanical trauma, or ischemia due to probe compression of the esophagus.[66,67]

Atrial esophageal fistula is one of the most feared complications of AF ablation. It manifests about 2 to 4 weeks after ablation with symptoms of stroke or other sequela of an air embolus, septic shock, or hematemesis, and it is a surgical emergency. If an atrial esophageal or atrial pericardial fistula is suspected, TEE should not be completed so that air is not pushed from the esophagus into the LA. A CT scan with intravenous contrast should be completed instead.[68]

Severe pulmonary vein stenosis occurs in about 1.3% of patients who undergo AF ablation,[69] but usually two veins must be stenotic for symptoms to occur.[70] When CT, MRI, or quantitative lung perfusion scanning is equivocal or unavailable, TEE imaging can be used to assess the severity of pulmonary vein stenosis with color and PW Doppler.[71] TEE can also guide balloon dilation or stent implantation, if needed, and assess in-stent restenosis.

ATRIAL FLUTTER ABLATION

ICE can sometimes be useful for ablation of AFL. The cavotricuspid isthmus is the critical region where ablation treats typical AFL. The anatomy in this area can vary, with pectinate muscles, trabeculae, and a eustachian valve that can cause difficulty for catheter manipulation and stability. ICE can be used to visualize any anatomic obstacles and to demonstrate catheter contact with the myocardium.[72–74] The best view has the catheter placed in the mid-RA and rotated to show the cavotricuspid isthmus, although sometimes a posterior tilt is needed.

LEFT ATRIAL APPENDAGE CLOSURE

LAA closure has been performed to reduce the risk of LAA thrombus and subsequent stroke. The traditional method has been surgical excision or exclusion of the LAA.[36] However, there is commonly incomplete exclusion, and TEE imaging has shown that surgical exclusion of the LAA may be successful only 23% of the time, compared with 73% for excision.[75] Those with unsuccessful surgical LAA exclusion are at significant risk for LAA thrombus.[75]

The Watchman device (Boston Scientific, Minneapolis, MN) is approved by the US Food and Drug Administration to reduce the risk of thromboembolism in patients with nonvalvular AF who do not wish to take anticoagulation. It is implanted endocardially in the LAA to exclude it from the LA. The Watchman contains a nitinol frame with 10 active fixation anchors around the outside that attach to the LAA wall to prevent migration. It is surrounded on one end by a polyethylene terephthalate cap, which endothelializes to cause LAA exclusion.

In a meta-analysis of two randomized trials and two registries, the Watchman device was compared with warfarin and was shown to reduce the rate of hemorrhagic stroke, cardiovascular/unexplained death, and nonprocedure-related bleeding.[76] There was a higher rate of ischemic stroke with Watchman, although this result was no longer significant when procedure-related strokes were excluded.

The Amplatzer Amulet (Abbott, St. Paul, MN) is undergoing evaluation in the United States (NCT02879448) but has a Conformité Européene (CE) mark of approval in Europe. This is a second-generation device derived from the Amplatzer Cardiac

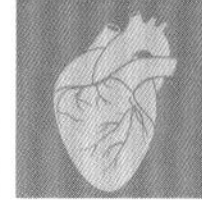

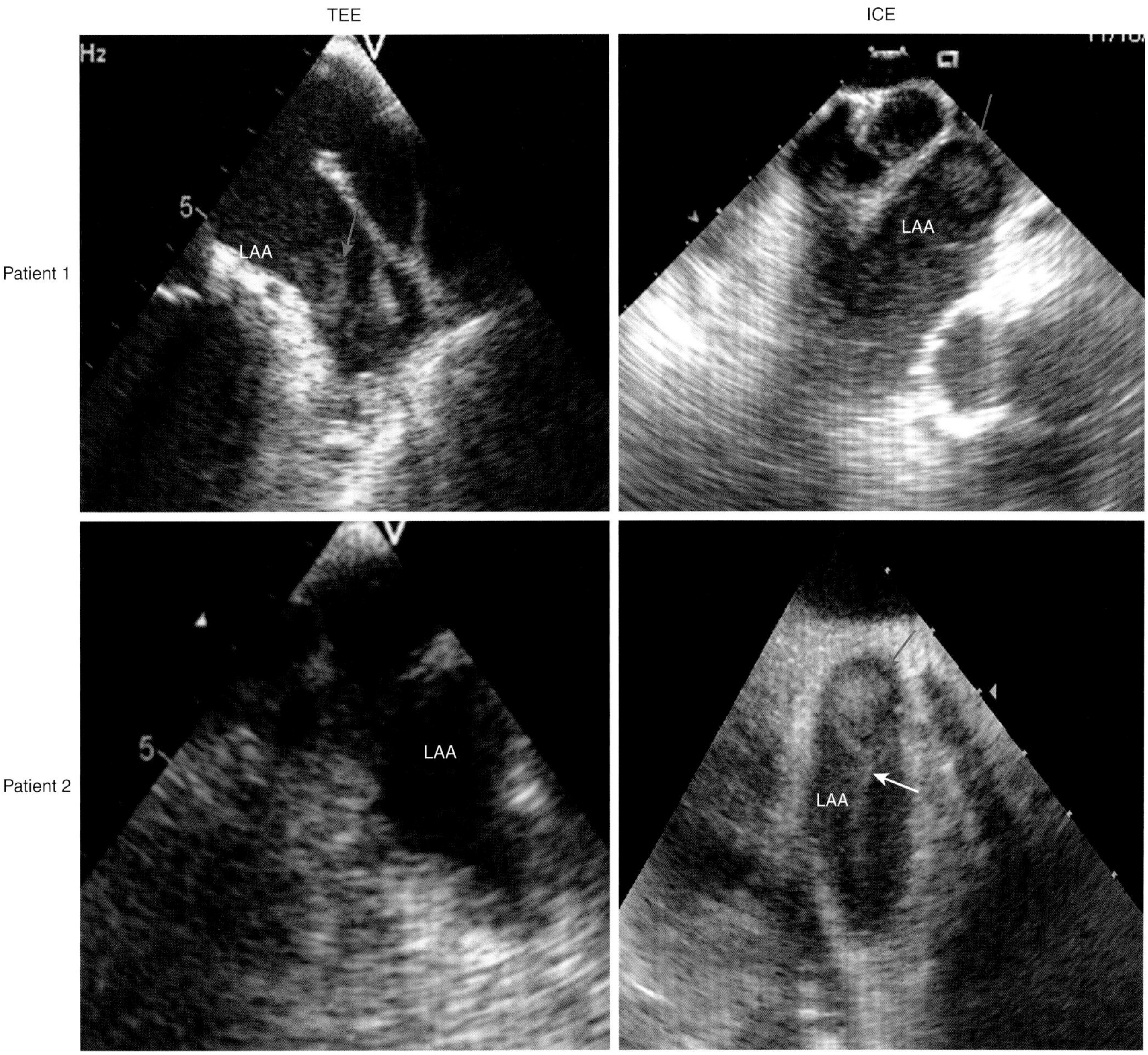

Fig. 39.11 Imaging of the left atrial appendage (LAA) on TEE and intracardiac echocardiography (ICE). In patient 1, thrombus was visible on TEE and ICE *(red arrows)*. In patient 2, a 0.8 cm^2 thrombus was not visualized on TEE because the distal LAA was not well seen, but it was present on ICE *(red arrow)* with spontaneous echocardiographic contrast *(white arrow)* (see Video 39.11). (From Anter E, Silversteen J, Tschabrunn CM, et al. Comparison of intracardiac echocardiography and TEE for imaging of the right and left atrial appendages. *Heart Rhythm*. 2014;11:1890–1897.)

Plug to isolate the LAA. It is made of nitinol with Dacron patches and a disc to seal off the LAA orifice, a lobe with stabilizing wires to allow attachment to the LAA inner wall, and a central waist between the two components.

TEE is completed before implantation to assess LAA size, which determines the best occluder device size. It is used to rule out LAA thrombus, which is a contraindication to the procedure.[77] Imaging of the LAA should be completed to determine LAA ostial size and depth (Fig. 39.13).[78] Depth is measured toward the back wall of the LAA for the Amulet or at the LAA apex for the Watchman.[79]

TEE guidance is used during the implantation procedure (Table 39.5).[80–82] ICE may be considered instead of TEE for some patients. Data are limited, but a meta-analysis of five studies demonstrated no difference in success rates, fluoroscopy time, procedure time, or complications between TEE and ICE.[83] Echocardiography is helpful for the transseptal puncture when the goal is to be in the inferior and posterior portion of the interatrial septum. TEE is also helpful for ensuring appropriate device seating in the LAA.

3D TEE is better than 2D TEE for estimating LAA orifice diameter because 2D tends to underestimate orifice size and 3D TEE gives more reproducible results.[84,85] TEE may be good enough to eliminate the need for contrast to assess LAA size.[86] Color Doppler or contrast can be used to assess for residual flow and appropriate device seal of the LAA, with a goal of

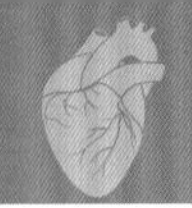

3 ± 2 mm or less.[79,87] TEE is used to assess complications such as pericardial effusion or development of thrombus on the sheath.

Contrast angiography is often used to determine LAA morphology, but the views may not be familiar to echocardiographers. A right anterior oblique (RAO) caudal view approximates 135 degrees, and an RAO cranial view approximates 45 degrees when the images are rotated 90 degrees counterclockwise (Fig. 39.14).[79]

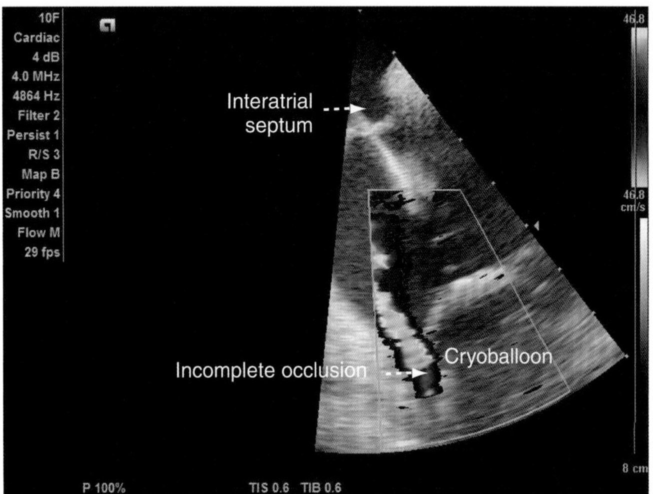

Fig. 39.12 Intracardiac echocardiographic image of a cryoballoon in the left inferior pulmonary vein. The cryoballoon is across the interatrial septum into the LA at the ostium of the left inferior pulmonary vein (LIPV), which is not well seen due to shadowing. Poor occlusion, or leak, is present because color Doppler demonstrates flow out of the inferior portion of the LIPV into the LA (see Video 39.12).

It is common practice to obtain a TTE before discharge to assess for device embolization and for pericardial effusion. A TEE is completed at 45 days to evaluate the LAA seal. The goal is a leak of 3 to 5 mm or less, but if it is greater, a repeat TEE can be completed at 6 to 12 months to reassess the seal.[88] There should also be assessment of thrombus on the device itself, especially if there has been a thrombotic event; if thrombus is identified, anticoagulation should be continued until it is gone.

The Lariat device (SentreHEART, Palo Alto, CA), although not specifically approved for LAA closure, is being used for that purpose to prevent thromboembolic events.[89,90] The Lariat implant procedure involves endocardial and epicardial LAA access to place a lasso-like epicardial suture around the LAA ostium. It has been deployed in more than 4500 patients in the United States, and data are emerging regarding efficacy and safety.[89] The largest study, which enrolled 712 patients from 18 centers, demonstrated a greater than 95% successful placement of the device and a complication rate of 2.2%, driven by a decrease in the rate of pericardial effusion using a micropuncture needle to access the pericardial space.[90] However, the Left Atrial Appendage Ligation and Ablation for Persistent Atrial Fibrillation (LAALA-AF) Registry demonstrated that 12% of patients had incomplete LAA ligation.[91]

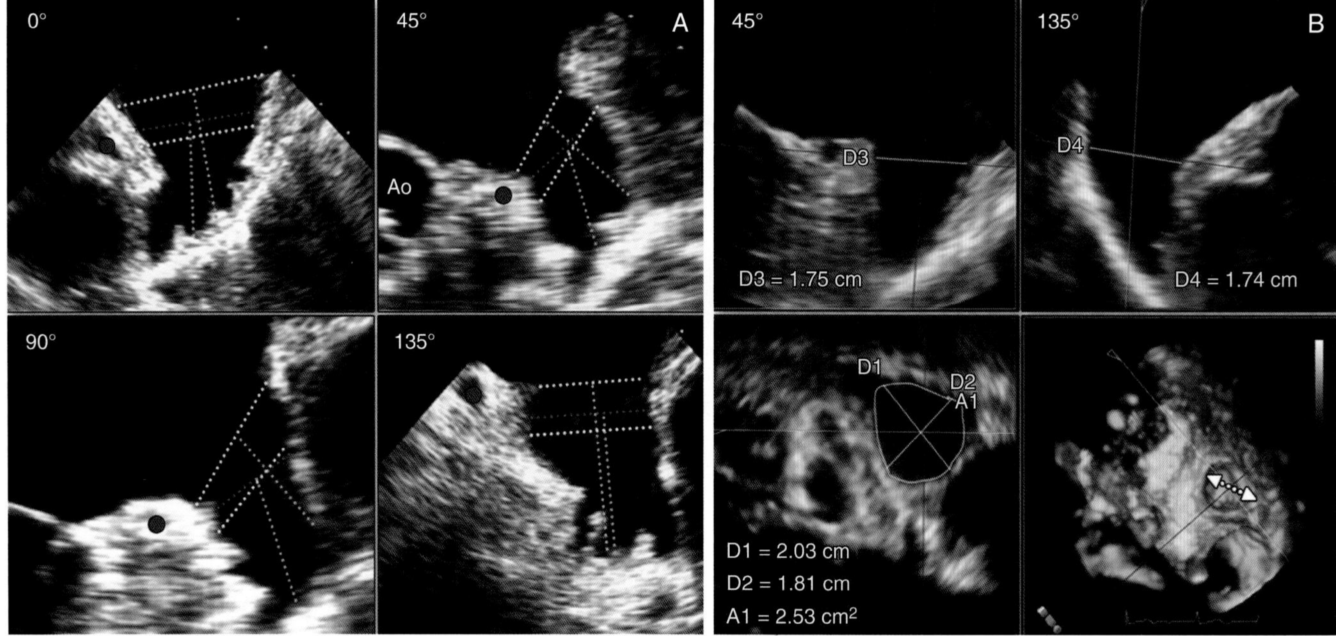

Fig. 39.13 TEE imaging to determine left atrial appendage size. (A) 2D TEE measurements of the landing zone diameters and the maximum length of the left atrial appendage (LAA) in the axis of the device are demonstrated in four 2D imaging planes (i.e., 0, 45, 90, and 135 degrees). For the Watchman occluder device, the landing zone *(dotted red line)* is measured from the inferior part of the LAA ostium at the level of the circumflex coronary artery *(red dot)* to a point 1 to 2 cm distal to the tip of the rim to the left superior pulmonary vein. The LAA depth *(dotted green line)* is measured perpendicular to that line. For the Amulet occluder device, the measurement of the landing zone diameter in the anchoring lobe is obtained about 10 mm distal from the ostial plane *(dotted yellow line)* into the lobe *(dotted white line)*. The depth of the main lobe *(dotted orange line)* is measured in the expected axis of the device. (B) The landing zone is measured by 3D TEE. In this postprocessing analysis, 45- and 135-degree views are shown at the upper left and upper right, respectively. The *yellow line* demarcates the landing zone measurement. An en face plane at the level of the landing zone is shown at the lower left. Diameters (D1 and D2) and the area (A1) are measured. An additional 3D en face view (lower right) shows the LAA orifice in relation to neighboring structures. The *white double arrowhead* marks the largest diameter that would be missed by measuring only along the red or green cropping line. (From Wunderlich NC, Beigel R, Swaans MJ, Ho SY, Siegel RJ. Percutaneous interventions for left atrial appendage exclusion: options, assessment, and imaging using 2D and 3D echocardiography. *JACC Cardiovasc Imaging* 2015;8[4]:472–488)

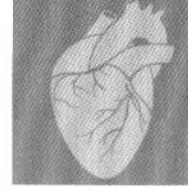

TABLE 39.5 Intraprocedural Transesophageal Echocardiographic Imaging for Implantation of the Left Atrial Appendage Occluder Devices.

Step	*Measurement*[a]	*Watchman Interpretation and/or Management*	*Amulet Interpretation and/or Management*
Evaluate for LA thrombus.	Image the LAA and entire LA for thrombus.	Do not implant if LAA thrombus is seen.	Do not implant if LAA thrombus is seen.
Determine maximal ostial size.	Image the LAA ostium and depth at 0, 45, 90, and 135 degrees. The long-axis measurement of the diameter is typically larger than in the short axis. Maximal size is usually seen at 135 degrees.	At 0 degrees, the LAA ostium diameter is measured from the left coronary artery to a point 2 cm from the tip of the LSPV limbus. Then imaged at 45, 90, and 135 degrees and measured from the mitral valve annulus to the LSPV limbus. A device should be chosen that is 10%–20% larger than the measured maximal ostial size. Available device sizes are 21, 24, 27, 30, and 33 mm and can be placed in LAA ostia of 17–31 mm.	At 0 degrees, the LAA ostium diameter is measured from the left circumflex artery to the pulmonary vein ridge, and then the landing zone diameter is measured 10–12 mm distal to the ostium and perpendicular to the neck axis. A device should be chosen that is about 10% larger than the measured maximal ostial size. Available device sizes are 16, 18, 20, 22, 25, 28, 31, and 34 mm and can be placed in LAA ostia of 14–32 mm.
Perform transseptal puncture.	Bicaval and short-axis views of the interatrial septum	Transseptal puncture should be low and posterior to allow for the best angle into the LAA.	Transseptal puncture should be low and posterior to allow for the best angle into the LAA.
Assess device after implantation.	Device shape and size can be assessed.	Ensure that the threaded insert (release anchor point) is visible, and measure the widest diameter of the device. The implanted device diameter should be 80%–92% of the original size. If it is > 92%, the device should be repositioned or a larger device chosen because there is a risk that it will dislodge.	The lobe of the device should be tire shaped, adjacent to the circumflex artery, and with some separation between the lobe and disc. The shape of the disc should be concave in the ostium.
Assess device depth.	The device should be located at or just distal to the ostium. Further extension into the LAA increases the risk of device embolization. It should not be too deep into the LAA because it may not cover a side lobe.	Depending on device size, the tip may protrude out of the LAA by 4.2 to 6.6 mm. The Watchman needs a landing zone depth at least equal to the diameter of the device as measured to the LAA apex.	Depth is measured toward the back wall of the LAA. There needs to be 10 mm for 16–22 mm devices and 12 mm for 25–34 mm devices.
Ensure device is anchored.	Usually, 135 degrees provides the best view, but any view can be used. Operator performs a slight tug on the device before deployment.	The device and LAA pull back in tandem. If the device alone pulls back, it is not anchored and needs to be redeployed. Too firm a tug may cause dislodgement or perforation.	The device and LAA pull back in tandem. If the device alone pulls back, it is not anchored and needs to be redeployed. Too firm a tug may cause dislodgement or perforation.
Assess for LAA seal.	Use color Doppler to assess flow between the device and the LAA wall.	Lowering the Nyquist limit to 20–30 cm/s is recommended to assess peridevice leaks using color-flow Doppler. Although there is no acceptable definition, the goal is a leak of ≤ 3 mm, and a small residual leak of ≤ 5 mm is acceptable. If it is greater, the device should be retrieved, repositioned, and redeployed. A larger size may be needed.	Lowering the Nyquist limit to 35–45 cm/s is recommended to assess for peridevice leaks using color-flow Doppler. Although there is no acceptable definition, the goal is a leak of ≤3 mm, a small residual leak of ≤ 5 mm is acceptable. If it is greater, the device should be retrieved, repositioned, and redeployed. A larger size may be needed.
Release device.	Reassess device position, size, and seal after the device has been released.	If the device is unstable or protruding out into the LA too far, it may need to be snared and a new one implanted.	If the device is unstable or protruding out into the LA too far, it may need to be snared and a new one implanted.
Evaluate for other complications.	During and after device implantation, imaging of the intraprocedural thrombus or pericardial effusion should be completed, especially if there are hemodynamic changes.	Management of a thrombus may include removing it by suction through the sheath, increasing the heparin dose, or pulling the sheath back into the RA. A pericardial effusion may need to be managed by pericardiocentesis or cardiac surgery.	Management of a thrombus may include removing it by suction through the sheath, increasing the heparin dose, or pulling the sheath back into the RA. A pericardial effusion many need to be managed by pericardiocentesis or cardiac surgery.

[a]For all steps, unless otherwise stated, imaging of the LAA should be completed at 0, 45, 90, and 135 degrees.
LAA, Left atrial appendage; *LSPV*, left superior pulmonary vein.

With more experience, there has been improvement in outcomes, with data suggesting significant reductions in thromboembolic rates.[92] It is thought that LAA exclusion may reduce AF burden in those undergoing pulmonary vein isolation, and the randomized aMAZE trial (NCT02513797) is testing the Lariat device versus no additional treatment for reduction in AF burden at 12 months.

TEE is used,[93] and one study suggested that 3D TEE may improve visualization of the catheter and wires.[94] It can assess the maximum LAA width, which should be 45 mm or less (best seen at 135 degrees) and can determine whether the LAA apex is behind the pulmonary trunk, which makes the procedure very difficult.[79] TEE can be used during the epicardial access portion of the procedure to ensure that the needle and wire are in the epicardial space, rather than the RV (seen best in the mid-esophageal short-axis view).[79] After transseptal puncture, TEE can show that the catheter, magnet-tipped wire, and endocardially inflated balloon are placed in the LAA. TEE can be used to assess residual leaks of the LAA after it has been excluded (Fig. 39.15).[94] It is also used to evaluate pericardial effusion, which may occur in up to 10% of cases.[95]

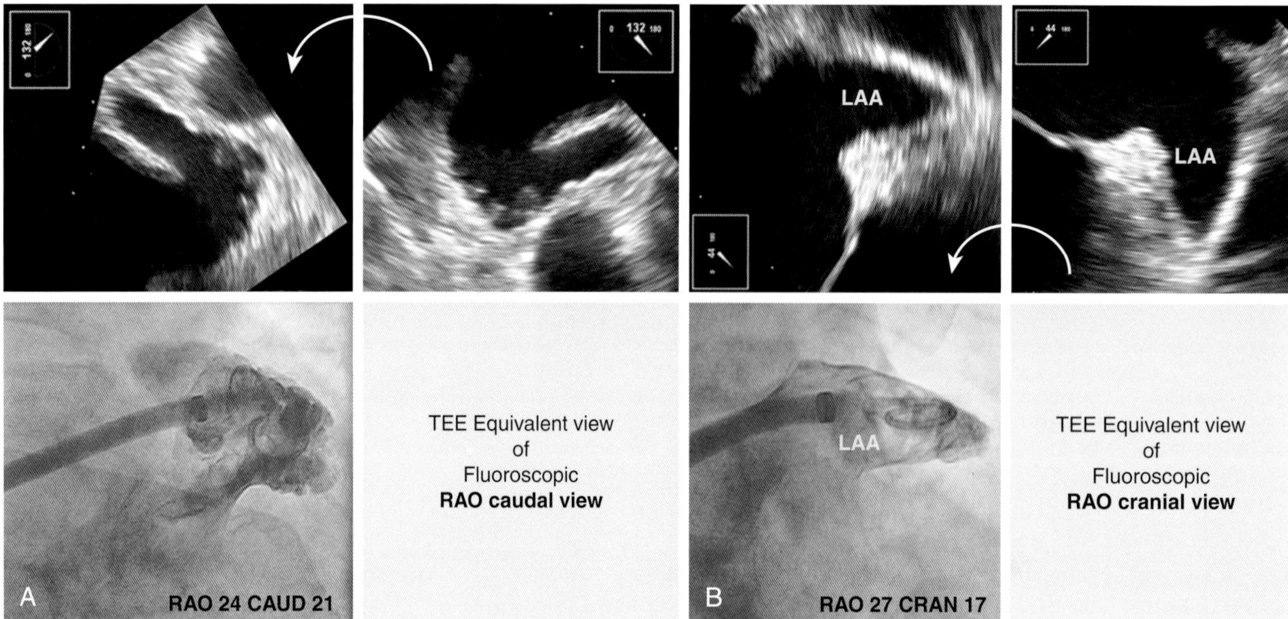

Fig 39.14 Fluoroscopic versus TEE views. (A) The right anterior oblique (RAO) caudal view is similar to a view at about 135 degrees rotated counterclockwise. (B) The RAO cranial view is similar to about 45 degrees rotated counterclockwise. (From Vainrib AF, Harb SC, Jaber W, et al. Left atrial appendage occlusion/exclusion: procedural image guidance with transesophageal echocardiography. *J Am Soc Echocardiogr*. 2018;31[4]:454–474.)

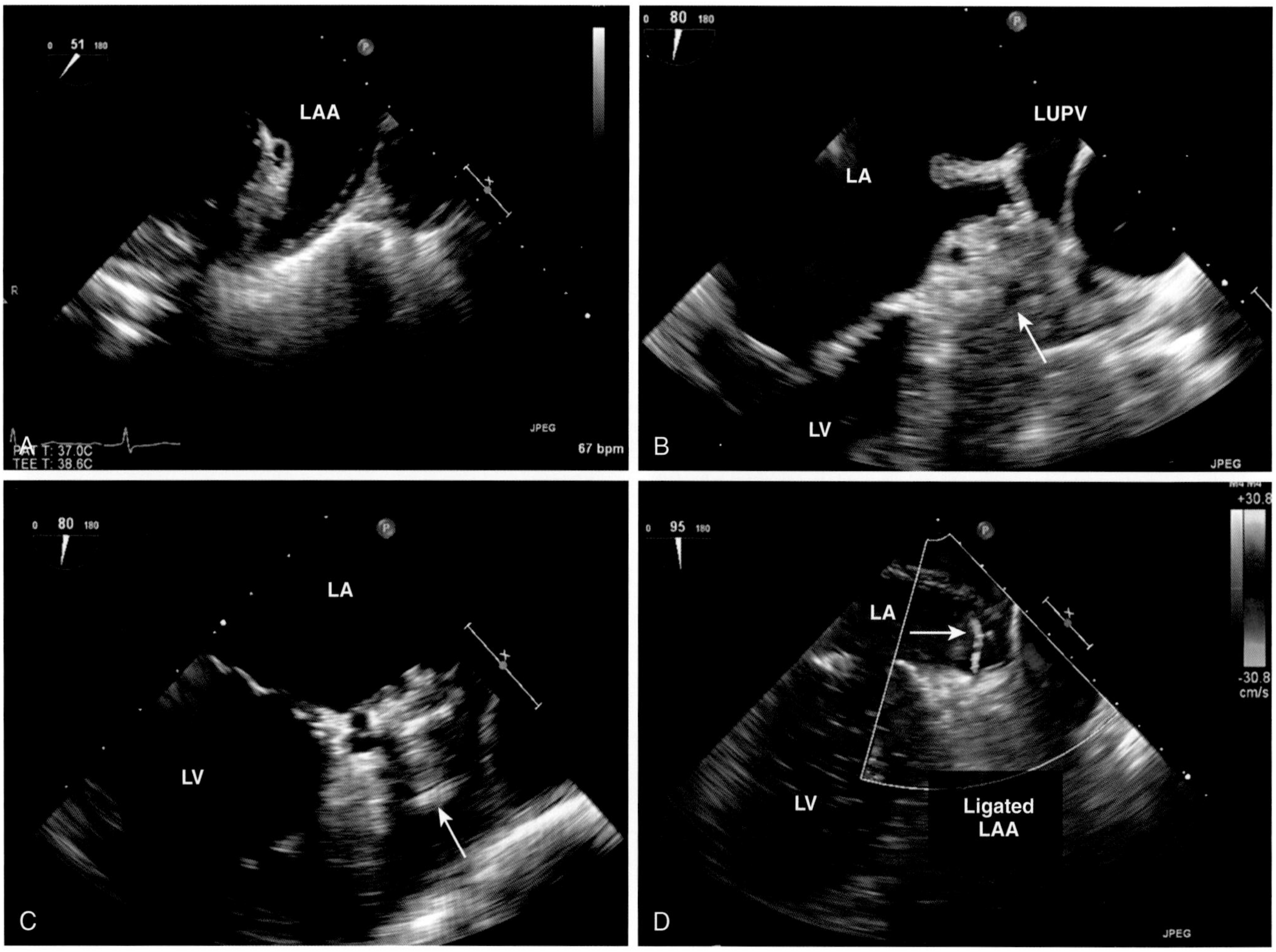

Fig. 39.15 TEE of Lariat procedure. (A) Left atrial appendage (LAA) seen before occlusion. (B) The LAA after the Lariat has been deployed and ligated. The relationships to the left upper pulmonary vein (LUPV), LA, and LV are seen. Pericardial effusion is indicated by the *arrow*. (C) A small pericardial effusion is present and outlines the LAA *(white arrow)*. (D) A small leak is seen on color Doppler *(white arrow)* after the LAA has been ligated but before the endocardial catheter has been removed (see Video 39.15). (From Laura DM, Chinitz LA, Aizer A, et al. The role of multimodality imaging in percutaneous left atrial appendage suture ligation with the Lariat device. *J Am Soc Echocardiogr*. 2014;27: 699–708.)

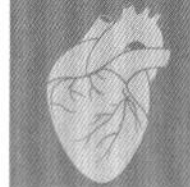

SUMMARY Imaging the Left Atrial Appendage

Imaging Modality	Probe Location	Imaging Angle or Direction	Purpose or Measurement	Limitations
TEE	High esophageal location in a 4-chamber, 2-chamber, and long-axis view. Biplane imaging may be helpful.	The LAA should be imaged at 0, 45, 90, and 135 degrees. It is better to use a high frequency transducer (typically 7 MHz), in zoom mode, with a narrow field of view.	Exclusion of LAA thrombus.	It is important to image the entire LA and not just the LAA, because 10% of thrombi occur outside of the appendage. Reverberation artifact from the ridge between the left superior pulmonary vein and LAA may falsely give the appearance of thrombus and should be excluded.
	Pulsed wave Doppler		LAA velocities should be measured with a sample volume about 1 cm into the ostium of the appendage. A normal LAA velocity is >0.4 m/s.	
ICE	RV outflow tract	Rotate clockwise for a long-axis view of the LAA and side lobes.	Exclusion of LAA thrombus.	Stiff catheter must be maneuvered carefully to prevent perforation.
	Pulmonary artery	Maneuver inferior medially for a short-axis view of the LAA. Clockwise rotation and further inferior imaging may also be helpful.	Exclusion of LAA thrombus.	Stiff catheter must be maneuvered carefully to prevent perforation.
	Coronary sinus	Advancing and retracting the catheter with rotation can demonstrate a long- and short-axis view of the LAA.	Exclusion of LAA thrombus.	Difficult catheter manipulation due to coronary sinus size and anatomy.
	LA	Directly access the LA after transseptal puncture.	Exclusion of LAA thrombus.	This runs the risk of dislodging a thrombus if one is present.

REFERENCES

1. Roger VL, Go AS, Lloyd-Jones DM, et al. Heart disease and stroke statistics—2012 update: a report from the American Heart Association. *Circulation*. 2012;125:e2–e220.
2. Go AS, Hylek EM, Phillips KA, et al. Prevalence of diagnosed atrial fibrillation in adults: national implications for rhythm management and stroke prevention: the AnTicoagulation and Risk Factors in Atrial Fibrillation (ATRIA) Study. *J Am Med Assoc*. 2001;285:2370–2375.
3. Owan TE, Hodge DO, Herges RM, Jacobsen SJ, Roger VL, Redfield MM. Trends in prevalence and outcome of heart failure with preserved ejection fraction. *N Engl J Med*. 2006;355:251–259.
4. Dulli DA, Stanko H, Levine RL. Atrial fibrillation is associated with severe acute ischemic stroke. *Neuroepidemiology*. 2003;22:118–123.
5. Mary-Rabine L, Albert A, Pham TD, et al. The relationship of human atrial cellular electrophysiology to clinical function and ultrastructure. *Circ Res*. 1983;52:188–199.
6. Kottkamp H. Human atrial fibrillation substrate: towards a specific fibrotic atrial cardiomyopathy. *Eur Heart J*. 2013;34:2731–2738.
7. Damy T, Kallvikbacka-Bennett A, Goode K, et al. Prevalence of, associations with, and prognostic value of tricuspid annular plane systolic excursion (TAPSE) among out-patients referred for the evaluation of heart failure. *J Card Fail*. 2012;18:216–225.
8. Ausma J, Wijffels M, Thone F, Wouters L, Allessie M, Borgers M. Structural changes of atrial myocardium due to sustained atrial fibrillation in the goat. *Circulation*. 1997;96:3157–3163.
9. Lang RM, Bierig M, Devereux RB, et al. Recommendations for chamber quantification: a report from the American Society of Echocardiography's Guidelines and Standards Committee and the Chamber Quantification Writing Group, developed in conjunction with the European Association of Echocardiography, a branch of the European Society of Cardiology. *J Am Soc Echocardiogr*. 2005;18:1440–1463.
10. Fuster V, Ryden LE, Asinger RW, et al. ACC/AHA/ESC guidelines for the management of patients with atrial fibrillation: executive

summary. A report of the American College of Cardiology/American Heart Association Task Force on Practice Guidelines and the European Society of Cardiology Committee for Practice Guidelines and Policy Conferences (Committee to Develop Guidelines for the Management of Patients with Atrial Fibrillation): developed in collaboration with the North American Society of Pacing and Electrophysiology. *J Am Coll Cardiol.* 2001;38:1231–1266.

11. Vandenberg BF, Weiss RM, Kinzey J, et al. Comparison of left atrial volume by two-dimensional echocardiography and cine-computed tomography. *Am J Cardiol.* 1995;75:754–757.
12. Gabor GE, Winsberg F. Motion of mitral valves in cardiac arrythmias: ultrasonic cardiographic study. *Invest Radiol.* 1970;5:355–360.
13. Manning WJ, Silverman DI, Katz SE, Douglas PS. Atrial ejection force: a noninvasive assessment of atrial systolic function. *J Am Coll Cardiol.* 1993;22:221–225.
14. Cameli M, Caputo M, Mondillo S, et al. Feasibility and reference values of left atrial longitudinal strain imaging by two-dimensional speckle tracking. *Cardiovasc Ultrasound.* 2009; 7:6.
15. Di Salvo G, Caso P, Lo Piccolo R, et al. Atrial myocardial deformation properties predict maintenance of sinus rhythm after external cardioversion of recent-onset lone atrial fibrillation: a color Doppler myocardial imaging and transthoracic and transesophageal echocardiographic study. *Circulation.* 2005;112:387–395.
16. Kuppahally SS, Akoum N, Burgon NS, et al. Left atrial strain and strain rate in patients with paroxysmal and persistent atrial fibrillation: relationship to left atrial structural remodeling detected by delayed-enhancement MRI. *Circ Cardiovasc Imaging.* 2010;3: 231–239.
17. Habibi M, Lima JA, Khurram IM, et al. Association of left atrial function and left atrial enhancement in patients with atrial fibrillation: cardiac magnetic resonance study. *Circ Cardiovasc Imaging.* 2015;8. e002769.
18. Vasan RS, Larson MG, Levy D, Galderisi M, Wolf PA, Benjamin EJ. Doppler transmitral flow indexes and risk of atrial fibrillation (the Framingham Heart Study). *Am J Cardiol.* 2003;91:1079–1083.
19. Vaziri SM, Larson MG, Benjamin EJ, Levy D. Echocardiographic predictors of nonrheumatic atrial fibrillation. The Framingham Heart Study. *Circulation.* 1994;89:724–730.
20. Tsang TS, Gersh BJ, Appleton CP, et al. Left ventricular diastolic dysfunction as a predictor of the first diagnosed nonvalvular atrial fibrillation in 840 elderly men and women. *J Am Coll Cardiol.* 2002;40:1636–1644.
21. Tsang TS, Barnes ME, Gersh BJ, Bailey KR, Seward JB. Risks for atrial fibrillation and congestive heart failure in patients >/=65 years of age with abnormal left ventricular diastolic relaxation. *Am J Cardiol.* 2004;93:54–58.
22. Wolf PA, Abbott RD, Kannel WB. Atrial fibrillation as an independent risk factor for stroke: the Framingham Study. *Stroke.* 1991;22: 983–988.
23. Mozaffarian D, Benjamin EJ, Go AS, et al. Heart disease and stroke statistics—2015 update: a report from the American Heart Association. *Circulation.* 2015;131:e29–322.
24. Al-Saady N, Obel O, Camm A. Left atrial appendage: structure, function, and role in thromboembolism. *Heart (British Cardiac Society).* 1999;82:8.
25. Veinot JP, Harrity PJ, Gentile F, et al. Anatomy of the normal left atrial appendage: a quantitative study of age-related changes in 500 autopsy hearts: implications for echocardiographic examination. *Circulation.* 1997;96: 3112–3115.
26. Willens HJ, Qin JX, Keith K, Torres S. Diagnosis of a bilobed left atrial appendage and pectinate muscles mimicking thrombi on real-time 3-dimensional transesophageal echocardiography. *J Ultrasound Med.* 2010;29:975–980.
27. Di Biase L, Santangeli P, Anselmino M, et al. Does the left atrial appendage morphology correlate with the risk of stroke in patients with atrial fibrillation?: results from a multicenter study. *J Am Coll Cardiol.* 2012;60:531–538.
28. Kimura T, Takatsuki S, Inagawa K, et al. Anatomical characteristics of the left atrial appendage in cardiogenic stroke with low CHADS2 scores. *Heart Rhythm.* 2013;10:921–925.
29. Shirani J, Alaeddini J. Structural remodeling of the left atrial appendage in patients with chronic non-valvular atrial fibrillation: implications for thrombus formation, systemic embolism, and assessment by transesophageal echocardiography. *Cardiovasc Pathol.* 2000;9:95–101.
30. Tabata T, Oki T, Fukuda N, et al. Influence of aging on left atrial appendage flow velocity patterns in normal subjects. *J Am Soc Echocardiogr.* 1996;9:274–280.
31. Goldsmith I, Kumar P, Carter P, Blann AD, Patel RL, Lip GYH. Atrial endocardial changes in mitral valve disease: a scanning electron microscopy study. *Am Heart J.* 2000;140:777–784.
32. Lim HS, Willoughby SR, Schultz C, et al. Effect of atrial fibrillation on atrial thrombogenesis in humans: impact of rate and rhythm. *J Am Coll Cardiol.* 2013;61:852–860.
33. Calkins H, Kuck KH, Cappato R, et al. 2012 HRS/EHRA/ECAS expert consensus statement on catheter and surgical ablation of atrial fibrillation: recommendations for patient selection, procedural techniques, patient management and follow-up, definitions, endpoints, and research trial design. *Europace.* 2012.
34. Aschenberg W, Schluter M, Kremer P, Schroder E, Siglow V, Bleifield W. Transesophageal two-dimentional echocardiography for the detection of left atrial appendage thrombus. *J Am Coll Cardiol.* 1986;7:4.
35. January CT, Wann LS, Alpert JS, et al. 2014 AHA/ACC/HRS guideline for the management of patients with atrial fibrillation: a report of the American College of Cardiology/ American Heart Association Task Force on Practice Guidelines and the Heart Rhythm Society. *J Am Coll Cardiol.* 2014;64:e1–76.
36. Nishimura RA, Otto CM, Bonow RO, et al. 2014. AHA/ACC guideline for the management of patients with valvular heart disease: a report of the American College of Cardiology/American Heart Association Task Force on Practice Guidelines. *J Am Coll Cardiol.* 2014;63:e57–185.
37. Vahanian A, Alfieri O, Andreotti F, et al. Guidelines on the management of valvular heart disease (version 2012): the Joint Task Force on the Management of Valvular Heart Disease of the European Society of Cardiology (ESC) and the European Association for Cardio-Thoracic Surgery (EACTS). *Eur J Cardio Thorac Surg.* 2012;42:S1–S44.
38. Whitlock RP, Sun JC, Fremes SE, Rubens FD, Teoh KH, Physicians ACC. Antithrombotic and Thrombolytic Therapy for Valvular Disease: Antithrombotic Therapy and Prevention of Thrombosis, 9th ed: American College of chest Physicians evidence-based clinical practice guidelines. *Chest.* 2012;141:e576S–600S.
39. Connolly SJ, Ezekowitz MD, Yusuf S, et al. Dabigatran versus warfarin in patients with atrial fibrillation. *N Engl J Med.* 2009;361:1139–1151.
40. Giugliano RP, Ruff CT, Braunwald E, et al. Edoxaban versus warfarin in patients with atrial fibrillation. *N Engl J Med.* 2013;369:2093–2104.
41. Granger CB, Alexander JH, McMurray JJV, et al. Apixaban versus warfarin in patients with atrial fibrillation. *N Engl J Med.* 2011;365:981–992.
42. Patel MR, Mahaffey KW, Garg J, et al. Rivaroxaban versus warfarin in nonvalvular atrial fibrillation. *N Engl J Med.* 2011;365:883–891.
43. Eikelboom JW, Connolly SJ, Brueckmann M, et al. Dabigatran versus warfarin in patients with mechanical heart valves. *N Engl J Med.* 2013;369:1206–1214.
44. Haissaguerre M, Jais P, Shah DC, et al. Spontaneous initiation of atrial fibrillation by ectopic beats originating in the pulmonary veins. *N Engl J Med.* 1998;339:659–666.
45. Calkins H, Hindricks G, Cappato R, et al. 2017. HRS/EHRA/ECAS/APHRS/SOLAECE expert consensus statement on catheter and surgical ablation of atrial fibrillation. *Heart Rhythm.* 2017;14:e275–e444.
46. Lerman BB, Markowitz SM, Liu CF, Thomas G, Ip JE, Cheung JW. Fluoroless catheter ablation of atrial fibrillation. *Heart Rhythm.* 2017;14:928–934.
47. Lyan E, Tsyganov A, Abdrahmanov A, et al. Nonfluoroscopic catheter ablation of paroxysmal atrial fibrillation. *Pacing Clin Electrophysiol.* 2018;41:611–619.
48. Santangeli P, Di Biase L, Burkhardt JD, et al. Transseptal access and atrial fibrillation ablation guided by intracardiac echocardiography in patients with atrial septal closure devices. *Heart Rhythm: The Official Journal of the Heart Rhythm Society.* 2011;8:1669–1675.
49. Lakkireddy D, Rangisetty U, Prasad S, et al. Intracardiac echo-guided radiofrequency catheter ablation of atrial fibrillation in patients with atrial septal defect or patent foramen ovale repair: a feasibility, safety, and efficacy study. *J Cardiovasc Electrophysiol.* 2008;19:1137–1142.
50. Baran J, Stec S, Pilichowska-Paszkiet E, et al. Intracardiac echocardiography for detection of thrombus in the left atrial appendage: comparison with transesophageal echocardiography in patients undergoing ablation for atrial fibrillation: the Action-Ice I Study. *Circ Arrhythm Electrophysiol.* 2013;6:1074–1081.
51. Ren JF, Marchlinski FE, Supple GE, et al. Intracardiac echocardiographic diagnosis of thrombus formation in the left atrial appendage: a complementary role to transesophageal echocardiography. *Echocardiography.* 2013;30:72–80.
52. Reddy VY, Neuzil P, Ruskin JN. Intracardiac echocardiographic imaging of the left atrial appendage. *Heart Rhythm: The Official Journal of the Heart Rhythm Society.* 2005;2:1272–1273.
53. Ren JF, Callans DJ. Intracardiac echocardiography with different approaches for imaging of left atrial appendage. *Heart Rhythm: The Official Journal of the Heart Rhythm Society.* 2006;3:623. author reply -4.
54. Saksena S, Sra J, Jordaens L, et al. A prospective comparison of cardiac imaging using intracardiac echocardiography with transesophageal echocardiography in patients with atrial fibrillation: the intracardiac echocardiography

guided cardioversion helps interventional procedures study. *Circulation Arrhythmia and electrophysiology*. 2010;3:571–577.
55. Anter E, Silverstein J, Tschabrunn CM, et al. Comparison of intracardiac echocardiography and transesophageal echocardiography for imaging of the right and left atrial appendages. *Heart Rhythm*. 2014;11:1890–1897.
56. Ren JF, Marchlinski FE, Callans DJ. Left atrial thrombus associated with ablation for atrial fibrillation: identification with intracardiac echocardiography. *J Am Coll Cardiol*. 2004;43:1861–1867.
57. Lakhani M, Saiful F, Bekheit S, Kowalski M. Use of intracardiac echocardiography for early detection of phrenic nerve injury during cryoballoon pulmonary vein isolation. *J Cardiovasc Electrophysiol*. 2012;23:874–876.
58. Wilson L, Brooks AG, Lau DH, et al. Real-time CartoSound imaging of the esophagus: a comparison to computed tomography. *Int J Cardiol*. 2012;157:260–262.
59. Schmidt M, Daccarett M, Marschang H, et al. Intracardiac echocardiography improves procedural efficiency during cryoballoon ablation for atrial fibrillation: a pilot study. *J Cardiovasc Electrophysiol*. 2010;21:1202–1207.
60. Catanzariti D, Maines M, Angheben C, Centonze M, Cemin C, Vergara G. Usefulness of contrast intracardiac echocardiography in performing pulmonary vein balloon occlusion during cryo-ablation for atrial fibrillation. *Indian Pacing Electrophysiol J*. 2012;12:237–249.
61. Schwartzman D, Zhong H. On the use of CartoSound for left atrial navigation. *J Cardiovasc Electrophysiol*. 2010;21:656–664.
62. Steinberg BA, Hammill BG, Daubert JP, et al. Periprocedural imaging and outcomes after catheter ablation of atrial fibrillation. *Heart (British Cardiac Society)*. 2014;100:1871–1877.
63. Lee G, Sparks PB, Morton JB, et al. Low risk of major complications associated with pulmonary vein antral isolation for atrial fibrillation: results of 500 consecutive ablation procedures in patients with low prevalence of structural heart disease from a single center. *J Cardiovasc Electrophysiol*. 2011;22:163–168.
64. Ottaviano L, Chierchia G-B, Bregasi A, et al. Cryoballoon ablation for atrial fibrillation guided by real-time three-dimensional transoesophageal echocardiography: a feasibility study. *Europace*. 2013;15:944–950.
65. Acena M, Regoli F, Faletra FF, et al. 3D real-time TEE during pulmonary vein isolation in atrial fibrillation. *JACC Cardiovasc Imaging*. 2014;7:737–738.
66. Kumar S, Brown G, Sutherland F, et al. The transesophageal echo probe may contribute to esophageal injury after catheter ablation for paroxysmal atrial fibrillation under general anesthesia: a preliminary observation. *J Cardiovasc Electrophysiol*. 2015;26:119–126.
67. O'Shea JP, Southern JF, D'Ambra MN, et al. Effects of prolonged transesophageal echocardiographic imaging and probe manipulation on the esophagus—an echocardiographic-pathologic study. *J Am Coll Cardiol*. 1991;17:1426–1429.
68. Chavez P, Messerli FH, Casso Dominguez A, et al. Atrioesophageal fistula following ablation procedures for atrial fibrillation: systematic review of case reports. *Open Heart*. 2015;2. e000257.
69. Bhargava M, Di Biase L, Mohanty P, et al. Impact of type of atrial fibrillation and repeat catheter ablation on long-term freedom from atrial fibrillation: results from a multicenter study. *Heart Rhythm*. 2009;6:1403–1412.
70. Di Biase L, Fahmy TS, Wazni OM, et al. Pulmonary vein total occlusion following catheter ablation for atrial fibrillation: clinical implications after long-term follow-up. *J Am Coll Cardiol*. 2006;48:2493–2499.
71. Schneider C, Ernst S, Malisius R, et al. Transesophageal echocardiography: a follow-up tool after catheter ablation of atrial fibrillation and interventional therapy of pulmonary vein stenosis and occlusion. *J Interv Card Electrophysiol*. 2007;18:195–205.
72. Scaglione M, Caponi D, Di Donna P, et al. Typical atrial flutter ablation outcome: correlation with isthmus anatomy using intracardiac echo 3D reconstruction. *Europace*. 2004;6:407–417.
73. Bencsik G. Novel strategies in the ablation of typical atrial flutter: role of intracardiac echocardiography. *Curr Cardiol Rev*. 2015;11:127–133.
74. Okumura Y, Watanabe I, Ashino S, et al. Anatomical characteristics of the cavotricuspid isthmus in patients with and without typical atrial flutter: analysis with two- and three-dimensional intracardiac echocardiography. *J Interv Card Electrophysiol*. 2006;17:11–19.
75. Kanderian AS, Gillinov AM, Pettersson GB, Blackstone E, Klein AL. Success of surgical left atrial appendage closure: assessment by transesophageal echocardiography. *J Am Coll Cardiol*. 2008;52:924–929.
76. Holmes DR, Doshi SK, Kar S, et al. Left atrial appendage closure as an alternative to warfarin for stroke prevention in atrial fibrillation: a patient-level meta-analysis. *J Am Coll Cardiol*. 2015;65:2614–2623.
77. Subramaniam K, Ibarra A, Boisen ML. Echocardiographic guidance of Amplatzer Amulet left atrial appendage occlusion device placement. *Semin CardioThorac Vasc Anesth*. 2019;23:248–255.
78. Wunderlich NC, Beigel R, Swaans MJ, Ho SY, Siegel RJ. Percutaneous interventions for left atrial appendage exclusion: options, assessment, and imaging using 2D and 3D echocardiography. *JACC Cardiovasc Imaging*. 2015;8:472–488.
79. Vainrib AF, Harb SC, Jaber W, et al. Left atrial appendage occlusion/exclusion: procedural image guidance with transesophageal echocardiography. *J Am Soc Echocardiogr*. 2018;31:454–474.
80. Mráz T, Neuzil P, Mandysová E, Niederle P, Reddy VY. Role of echocardiography in percutaneous occlusion of the left atrial appendage. *Echocardiography*. 2007;24:401–404.
81. Palios J, Paraskevaidis I. Thromboembolism prevention via transcatheter left atrial appendage closure with transeosophageal echocardiography guidance. *Thrombosis*. 2014;2014:832752.
82. Chue CD, de Giovanni J, Steeds RP. The role of echocardiography in percutaneous left atrial appendage occlusion. *Eur J Echocardiogr*. 2011;12:i3–10.
83. Velagapudi P, Turagam MK, Kolte D, et al. Intracardiac vs transesophageal echocardiography for percutaneous left atrial appendage occlusion: a meta-analysis. *J Cardiovasc Electrophysiol*. 2019;30:461–467.
84. Goebel B, Wieg S, Hamadanchi A, et al. Interventional left atrial appendage occlusion: added value of 3D transesophageal echocardiography for device sizing. *Int J Cardiovasc Imaging*. 2016;32:1363–1370.
85. Schmidt-Salzmann M, Meincke F, Kreidel F, et al. Improved algorithm for ostium size assessment in Watchman left atrial appendage occlusion using three-dimensional echocardiography. *J Invasive Cardiol*. 2017;29: 232–238.
86. Sedaghat A, Al-Kassou B, Vij V, et al. Contrast-free, echocardiography-guided left atrial appendage occlusion (LAAo): a propensity-matched comparison with conventional LAAo using the Amplatzer Amulet device. *Clin Res Cardiol*. 2019;108:333–340.
87. Tzikas A, Holmes Jr DR, Gafoor S, et al. Percutaneous left atrial appendage occlusion: the Munich consensus document on definitions, endpoints, and data collection requirements for clinical studies. *Europace*. 2017;19:4–15.
88. Landmesser U, Tondo C, Camm J, et al. Left atrial appendage occlusion with the Amplatzer Amulet device: one-year follow-up from the prospective global Amulet observational registry. *EuroIntervention*. 2018;14:e590–e597.
89. Jazayeri MA, Vuddanda V, Parikh V, Lakkireddy DR. Percutaneous left atrial appendage closure: current state of the art. *Curr Opin Cardiol*. 2017;32:27–38.
90. Lakkireddy D, Afzal MR, Lee RJ, et al. Short and long-term outcomes of percutaneous left atrial appendage suture ligation: results from a US multicenter evaluation. *Heart Rhythm*. 2016;13:1030–1036.
91. Turagam M, Atkins D, Earnest M, et al. Anatomical and electrical remodeling with incomplete left atrial appendage ligation: results from the LAALA-AF registry. *J Cardiovasc Electrophysiol*. 2017;28:1433–1442.
92. Litwinowicz R, Bartus M, Burysz M, et al. Long term outcomes after left atrial appendage closure with the Lariat device-stroke risk reduction over five years follow-up. *PLoS One*. 2018;13. e0208710.
93. Lasala JD, Tolpin DA, Collard CD, Pan W. Real-time transesophageal echocardiography for left atrial appendage ligation using the Lariat snare device. *Anesth Analg*. 2015;120: 1204–1207.
94. Laura DM, Chinitz LA, Aizer A, et al. The role of multimodality imaging in percutaneous left atrial appendage suture ligation with the Lariat device. *J Am Soc Echocardiogr*. 2014;27: 699–708.
95. Price MJ, Gibson DN, Yakubov SJ, et al. Early safety and efficacy of percutaneous left atrial appendage suture ligation: results from the U.S. transcatheter LAA ligation consortium. *J Am Coll Cardiol*. 2014;64:565–572.

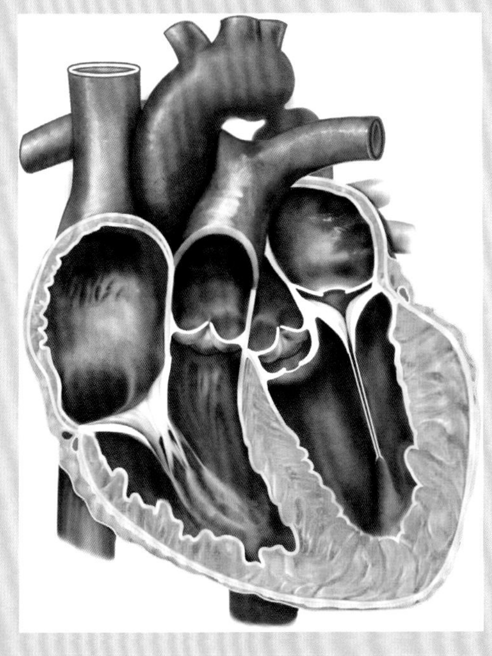

PART Ⅶ
第七部分

Adult Congenital Heart Disease and the Pregnant Patient
成人先天性心脏病和妊娠患者

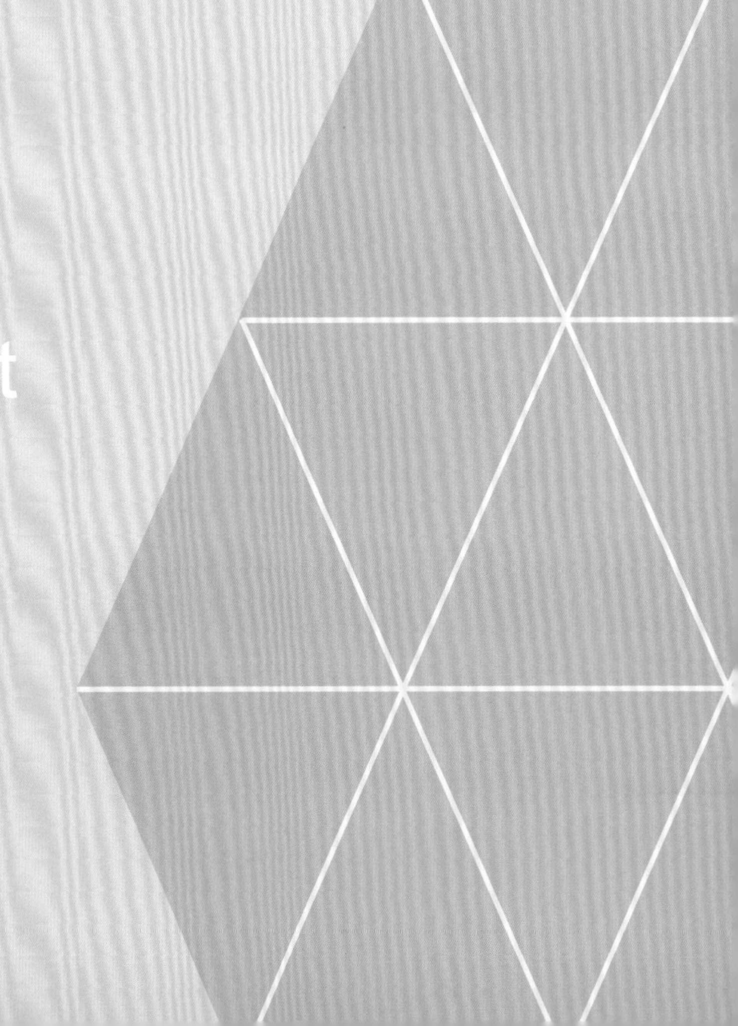

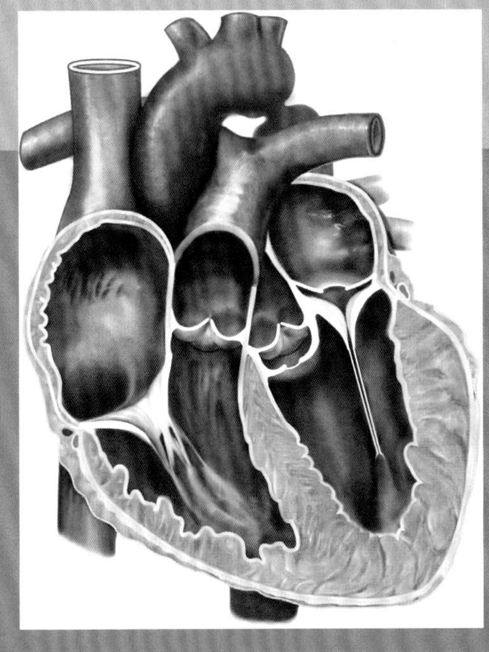

中文导读

第40章 妊娠期心脏病

患有心脏病的孕妇随着妊娠周数的增加，心脏负担加重容易诱发心力衰竭，影响孕妇和胎儿的安全。因此对已有心脏病理改变的妇女在围孕期对心脏结构和功能进行整体风险评估非常重要。超声心动图具有无创性、便捷性等优点，是评估妊娠妇女心脏结构和功能的首选重要检查技术，能在妊娠前、妊娠期和妊娠后不同时期，对心脏结构、功能和血流动力学进行全方位检测评价。超声心动图为妊娠期间的风险分级评估、妊娠期间的随访及是否需要临床干预等决策，提供重要参考依据，对于提高妊娠妇女和胎儿生存率有重要临床意义。本章简要介绍了正常妊娠期、分娩期和妊娠后母体生理变化，详细阐述了各种先天性和后天获得性心脏病孕妇妊娠期的病理生理变化、妊娠风险分级、超声心动图评估要点和孕妇的常规管理原则。

陈慧婷

40 Heart Disease in Pregnancy

CANDICE K. SILVERSIDES, MD | SAMUEL C. SIU, MD

Echocardiography is safe for use during pregnancy and is an important tool in evaluation of pregnant women with heart disease. It is used for risk stratification, follow-up during pregnancy, and diagnosis of women who develop complications during pregnancy. The signs and symptoms of pregnancy can mimic those of heart disease, and transthoracic echocardiography (TTE) is an important tool for differentiating normal pregnancy changes from pathologic cardiac disease. Understanding the effects of pregnancy on the heart, pregnancy risks, and role of echocardiography in the management of pregnant women with heart disease is fundamental for patient management. This chapter reviews the physiologic and echocardiographic changes of pregnancy, the risks of pregnancy, the role of echocardiography, and the general management principles for pregnant women with heart disease.

PHYSIOLOGIC CHANGES DURING PREGNANCY

Pregnancy is accompanied by adaptive changes in maternal circulating blood volume, red cell mass, peripheral vascular compliance and resistance, heart rate, and cardiac output (Fig. 40.1).[1] Although these hemodynamic changes are usually well tolerated by women without heart disease, they can result in maternal or fetal decompensation in women with preexisting heart disease. Some cardiac conditions, such as peripartum cardiomyopathy (PPCM), preeclampsia, and coronary dissection, develop de novo during pregnancy.

BLOOD VOLUME

The increase in blood volume begins as early as the 6th week of gestation and peaks at an average of 50% more than in the pre-pregnant state by the end of the 2nd trimester. Blood volume plateaus in the 3rd trimester. Red cell mass increases during pregnancy to as much as 40% above pre-pregnancy levels. *Physiologic anemia of pregnancy* results because the increase in plasma volume is proportionately greater than the increase in red blood cell mass. Increased levels of clotting factors and decreased fibrinolytic activity contribute to the increased risk for thromboembolism during pregnancy.

SYSTEMIC VASCULAR RESISTANCE

Concomitant with the physiologic hypervolemic state, a decrease in systemic arterial pressure occurs during the 1st trimester as a result of a decrease in systemic vascular resistance (SVR). This decrease in systemic arterial pressure reaches its nadir in mid-pregnancy, after which blood pressure stabilizes.[2,3] After the 32nd week of gestation, the SVR slowly increases until term and is accompanied by recovery of systemic arterial pressure, which ultimately reaches or exceeds pre-pregnancy levels.

CARDIAC OUTPUT

Increase in cardiac output begins as early as the 5th week of gestation and reaches its zenith near the end of the 2nd trimester, typically after the 24th week of gestation, It then plateaus until term at 30% to 50% above pre-pregnancy levels.[2,4–6] Most of the early increase in cardiac output is caused by a progressive increase in stroke volume, whereas later in pregnancy the heart rate continues to rise while the stroke volume reaches a plateau.[2,7] The mean heart rate at term is approximately 10 to 20 beats/min above pre-pregnancy levels. Cardiac output can fall acutely if the inferior vena cava is compressed by the gravid uterus in the supine position; this phenomenon can be reversed by assuming the left lateral decubitus position.

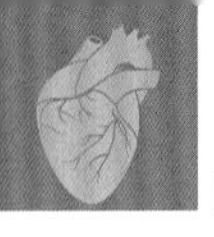

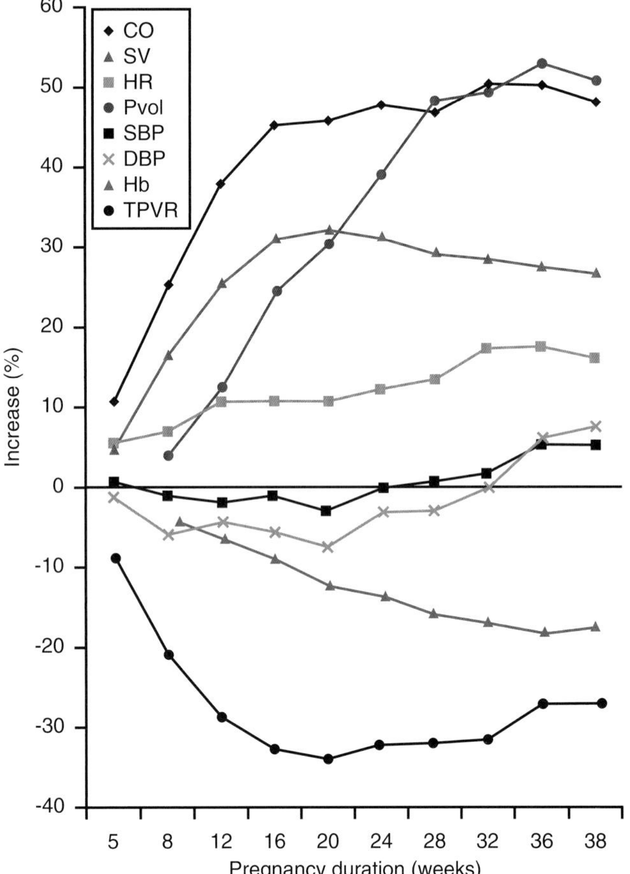

Fig. 40.1 The hemodynamic changes of pregnancy. Pregnancy is accompanied by adaptive changes in maternal circulating blood volume, red cell mass, peripheral vascular compliance and resistance, heart rate, and cardiac output. *CO*, Cardiac output; *DBP*, diastolic blood pressure; *Hb*, hemoglobin concentration; *HR*, heart rate; *Pvol*, plasma volume; *SV*, stroke volume; *SBP*, systolic blood pressure; *TPVR*, total peripheral vascular resistance. (From Karamermer Y, Roos-Hesselink JW. Pregnancy and adult congenital heart disease. *Expert Rev Cardiovasc Ther.* 2007;5[5]:859–869.)

During labor, there is an additional increase in cardiac output that is mediated by increases in heart rate and stroke volume and augmented by a further increase in response to each uterine contraction, with maximal augmentation occurring during the second stage of labor. Immediately after delivery, cardiac output may transiently increase to as much as 80% above pre-labor values due to relief of inferior vena cava compression and autotransfusion from the placenta. Thereafter, the hemodynamic changes that developed during pregnancy return toward baseline values. Most of the changes resolve early after delivery, although complete resolution of all measurable pregnancy-associated effects may take as long as 6 months.[8] Early published data on serial changes in cardiac structure and function during pregnancy were mostly derived from small samples of women without heart disease, and postpartum measurements were assumed to be a surrogate for prepregnancy values.

In a small study, pregnant women with valvular disease had lower cardiac output than pregnant women with normal cardiac function.[9] In a study that prospectively measured cardiac outputs serially in 127 pregnant women with a spectrum of preexistent heart disease and 45 healthy pregnant women, there were no significant differences in baseline and 3rd trimester cardiac output values between the two groups. However, within the heart disease group, those who experienced a reduction in cardiac output during later pregnancy were at increased risk for neonatal complications.[10] The absence of difference in cardiac output between the two groups in this study, in contrast to the earlier study, may reflect differences in lesion severity between contemporary and historical populations.

ECHOCARDIOGRAPHIC FINDINGS IN NORMAL PREGNANCY

CARDIAC CHAMBER SIZE

Echocardiographic studies during normal pregnancy reveal that dimensions of all four cardiac chambers increase and there is an increase in left ventricular (LV) wall thickness and mass.[5,8,11] Table 40.1 displays the common structural parameters during advanced pregnancy compared with nonpregnant controls or postpartum measurements. If the upper limits of the 95% confidence interval (mean + 2 standard deviations) are calculated for the normal ranges during pregnancy, the upper values overlap with the mildly abnormal range in the nonpregnant patient. Knowledge of these pregnancy-associated changes minimizes the risk of giving a false-positive diagnosis of cardiac dysfunction.

DOPPLER FLOWS

Increases in transvalvular flow velocities are seen during pregnancy. The decrease in SVR may decrease the severity of regurgitant valve lesions. However, there is also an increase in plasma volume, and one study showed that mitral, tricuspid, and pulmonic annular diameters increase during pregnancy, which may result in increasing degrees of mitral, tricuspid, and pulmonic regurgitation, respectively.[12] This finding was not replicated in all studies. Table 40.2 lists the common Doppler velocity measures during advanced pregnancy compared with nonpregnant controls and with baseline measurements.

SYSTOLIC AND DIASTOLIC FUNCTION

Although increases in LV ejection fraction during pregnancy have been reported by some,[2,5] other studies have not demonstrated this finding.[6,13,14] Whether measured by mitral inflow or by tissue Doppler, there is an increase in the contribution from atrial filling during late pregnancy; this is attributed to a change in LV compliance due to increased LV dimensions and mass.[7,15] These changes should be interpreted as a physiologic adaptation to the hemodynamic state of advanced pregnancy rather than an example of diastolic dysfunction.

Using 2D and 3D speckle-tracking echocardiography, studies of pregnant women without heart disease and nonpregnant controls have reported changes in LV strain, LV twist, LV untwisting, and left atrial (LA) strain with progression of pregnancy. Progressive eccentric hypertrophy accompanied by reduced global longitudinal, global circumferential, global area, and global radial strain in the 3rd trimester was reported in a 3D speckle tracking study.[16] In contrast, a 2D speckle tracking study reported reduced global longitudinal and global circumferential strain but elevated global radial strain relative to nonpregnant controls. Changes in the latter report were adjusted to account for hemodynamic conditions at the time of the study.[17]

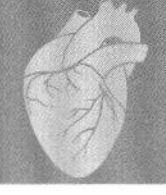

TABLE 40.1 Echocardiographic Changes in Cardiac Dimensions in Normal Pregnancy.

Parameter	Modality	Mean ± SD	Timing in Pregnancy	Comparison	Timing of Comparison	No. of Pregnant Patients	Study
LVOT area (cm^2)	2D	3.5 ± 0.3	36–40 weeks	3.2 ± 0.3	Postpartum	$n = 15$	Vered et al.[108]
LA dimension (cm)	M-mode	3.8 ± 0.4	36–40 weeks	3.4 ± 0.5	Postpartum	$n = 15$	Vered et al.[108]
LA area (cm^2)	2D	18 ± 2	32–33 weeks	15 ± 2	Nonpregnant controls ($n = 10$)	$n = 51$	Savu et al.[109]
RA area (cm^2)	2D	14.1 ± 3.8	3rd trimester	13.1 ± 1.8	Postpartum	$n = 28$	Sadaniantz et al.[110]
LVEDD (mm)	2D	47 ± 3	32–33 weeks	44 ± 3	Nonpregnant controls ($n = 10$)	$n = 51$	Savu et al.[109]
LVESD (mm)	2D	30 ± 3	32–33 weeks	26 ± 2	Nonpregnant controls ($n = 10$)	$n = 51$	Savu et al.[109]
LVEDV (mL)	Biplane, Simpson	92 ± 14	32–33 weeks	69 ± 10	Nonpregnant controls ($n = 10$)	$n = 51$	Savu et al.[109]
LVESV (mL)	Biplane, Simpson	34 ± 6	32–33 weeks	26 ± 5	Nonpregnant controls ($n = 10$)	$n = 51$	Savu et al.[109]
LV septal thickness (cm)	M-mode	0.85 ± 0.2	36–39 weeks	0.71 ± 0.1	12 weeks postpartum	$n = 18$	Mabie et al.[7]
LV posterior wall thickness (cm)	M-mode	1.0 ± 0.1	36–39 weeks	0.84 ± 0.1	12 weeks postpartum	$n = 18$	Mabie et al.[7]
LV mass (g)	2D	151 ± 27	32–33 weeks	115 ± 30	Nonpregnant controls ($n = 10$)	$n = 51$	Savu et al.[109]
LV mass index (g/m^2)	M-mode	97 ± 17	36–39 weeks	79 ± 9	12 weeks postpartum	$n = 18$	Mabie et al.[7]
Sphericity index	2D	1.7 ± 0.2	32–33 weeks	2.0 ± 0.1	Nonpregnant controls ($n = 10$)	$n = 51$	Savu et al.[109]
Mitral annulus diameter	2D	2.4 ± 0.5	3rd trimester	2.1 ± 0.4	Postpartum	$n = 28$	Sadaniantz et al.[110]
Tricuspid annulus diameter	2D	2.7 ± 3.2	3rd trimester	1.8 ± 0.3	Postpartum	$n = 28$	Sadaniantz et al.[110]

LVEDD, Left ventricular end-diastolic dimension; *LVEDV*, left ventricular end-diastolic volume; *LVESD*, left ventricular end-systolic dimension; *LVESV*, left ventricular end-systolic volume; *LVOT*, left ventricular outflow tract; *SD*, standard deviation.

TABLE 40.2 Echocardiographic Changes in Functional Parameters During Normal Pregnancy.

Parameters	Modality	Mean ± SD	Timing in Pregnancy	Comparison	Timing of Comparison	No. of Pregnant Patients	Study
Myocardial diastolic E-wave velocity (cm/s)	Color-coded TDI free wall of LV	12.1 ± 2.4	3rd trimester	14.0 ± 2.4	1st trimester	$n = 47$	Vogt et al.[15]
Myocardial diastolic A-wave velocity (cm/s)	Color-coded TDI free wall of LV	6.2 ± 2.0	3rd trimester	5.2 ± 1.6	1st trimester	$n = 47$	Vogt et al.[15]
Average systolic longitudinal strain	Color-coded TDI of LV at basal, middle, and apical levels	−17.6 ± 1.5	32–33 weeks	−19.1 ± 1.5	Nonpregnant controls ($n = 10$)	$n = 51$	Savu et al.[109]
E/A ratio	Mitral inflow	1.3 ± 0.3	3rd trimester	1.6 ± 0.4	Postpartum	$n = 28$	Sadaniantz et al.[110]
AoV velocity (m/s)	Continuous wave	1.4 ± 0.2	36–39 weeks	1.1 ± 0.1	12 weeks postpartum	$n = 18$	Mabie et al.[7]
Mitral A velocity	Pulsed-wave Doppler	0.54 ± 0.11	36–39 weeks	0.46 ± 0.07	12 weeks postpartum	$n = 18$	Mabie et al.[7]
LV ejection fraction	3D	57.1% ± 4.6%	3rd trimester	59.5% ± 5.8%	1st trimester	$n = 68$	Cong et al.[16]
LV global longitudinal strain	2D speckle tracking	−17.2% ± 2.8%	3rd trimester	−18.7% ± 2.5%	1st trimester	$n = 35$	Sengupta et al.[17]
LV twist	2D speckle tracking	16.8 ± 3.7 degrees	3rd trimester	13.0 ± 5.3 degrees	Nonpregnant controls ($n = 11$)	$n = 27$	Papadopoulou et al.[18]
LV untwisting rate	2D speckle tracking	−144.3 ± 45.1 °/s	3rd trimester	−96.7 ± 55.0 °/s	Nonpregnant controls ($n = 11$)	$n = 27$	Papadopoulou et al.[18]
LA reservoir phase strain	2D speckle tracking	33.5% ± 9.0%	3rd trimester	40.3% ± 11.7%	1st trimester	$n = 47$	Tasar et al.[19]

AoV, Aortic valve; *SD*, standard deviation; *TDI*, tissue Doppler imaging.

Other studies have reported increased LV twist and increased LV untwisting rate during pregnancy that were attributed to changes in LV end-systolic and end-diastolic volume.[18] LA reservoir phase strain and LA pump function strain gradually decreased from the 1st to the 3rd trimester and then rose to the initial level after delivery.[19] Changes in cardiac mechanics should be seen as adaptive responses to pregnancy-associated changes in LV volumes, LV mass, and loading conditions.[20]

INTERPRETATION OF ECHOCARDIOGRAPHIC FINDINGS DURING PREGNANCY

Timing of the pregnancy (i.e., gestational age) should be reported to help the referring physician place the echocardiographic findings in context. For example, the magnitude of valvular regurgitation may be reduced along with the reduced SVR during mid-pregnancy; it then increases during late pregnancy as SVR approaches pre-pregnancy levels. Similarly, mild mitral valve prolapse may be masked by the chamber dilation of pregnancy. For women with lesions known to be masked by the physiologic changes of pregnancy, the echocardiogram should be repeated after the 6th postpartum month, when the hemodynamic changes have returned to baseline.

PREGNANCY RISKS

Preconception counseling should be offered to all women with cardiac disease who are contemplating pregnancy. The risk assessment should be performed by a cardiologist with expertise in pregnancy and heart disease. Counseling should include assessment of the maternal risks of pregnancy and the effects of the maternal cardiac condition on fetal health. Some women may require cardiac procedures before pregnancy to minimize pregnancy risks. The long-term effects of pregnancy on the heart, if known, should be discussed. The role of the echocardiographic laboratory is crucial in preconceptual counseling because risk stratification depends on characterization of the severity and nature of the underlying cardiac lesion, the feasibility of intervention before pregnancy, and the potential long-term prognosis.

Factors other than maternal cardiac risk must be addressed. The benefits of medical therapy for the mother and the potential adverse effects of the medications on the fetus should be considered. Exposure to teratogens such as alcohol, warfarin, hydantoin, lithium, and valproic acid is associated with cardiovascular defects in offspring, and use of such agents should be stopped if possible. Drug dosing and frequency of administration of continued medications may need adjustment during pregnancy because of changes in volume of distribution, glomerular filtration rate, and hepatic metabolism. Risk assessment should include a genetics evaluation for women with inherited conditions.

To estimate the risk of developing cardiac complications during pregnancy, several factors need to be integrated into the assessment, including the general predictors of cardiac complications, lesion-specific data, and individual patient factors. General risk predictors, such as having a cardiac event (i.e., heart failure or arrhythmia) during pregnancy, poor functional capacity, and significant ventricular and valve dysfunction, apply to all women with heart disease.

Several derived risk scores use general risk predictors to estimate maternal cardiac risks during pregnancy. They include the CARPREG (Cardiac Disease in Pregnancy) I and II risk scores[21,22] (Fig. 40.2), the ZAHARA (Dutch: Zwangerschap bij vrouwen met een Aangeboren HARtAfwijking) risk score,[23] and the BACH (Boston Adult Congenital Heart) risk score.[24]

Table 40.3 shows the general risk predictors identified from large cohort studies.[21–26] These general risk scores should act as a starting point for estimating cardiac risk during pregnancy. Lesion-specific risks, when available, should be incorporated into the risk estimate. Lesion-specific risks are known for many congenital[27] and acquired[28–32] cardiac conditions and are discussed in detail elsewhere. The modified World Health Organization (WHO) classification, which stratifies cardiac risk by lesion, is shown in Table 40.4.[33–35] The WHO classification can be further stratified by incorporating general risk predictors from the CARPREG risk score[22] (Fig. 40.3). When the risk index and individual lesion-specific risk estimates are discordant, it is reasonable to assume the higher risk estimate.

Some important clinical variables may not be included in risk scores and may need to be incorporated into the risk assessment. They include variables such as maternal comorbidities, other cardiac test results (e.g., cardiopulmonary tests, magnetic resonance imaging [MRI]), genetic information, and patient compliance and access to care.

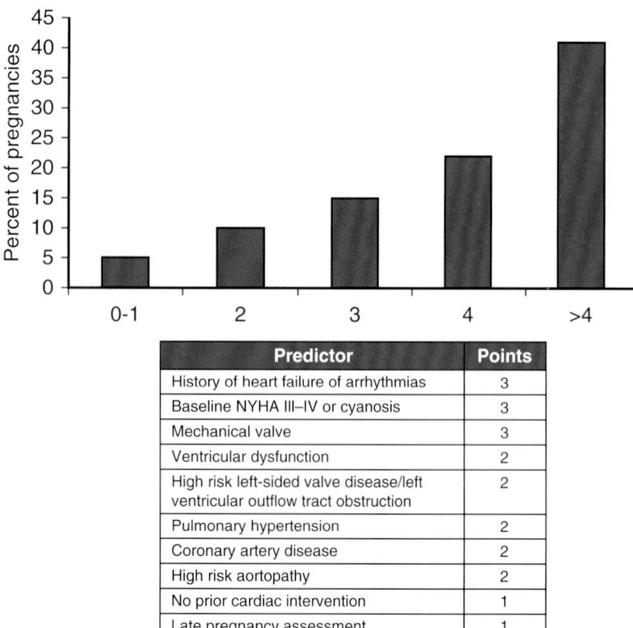

Predictor	Points
History of heart failure of arrhythmias	3
Baseline NYHA III–IV or cyanosis	3
Mechanical valve	3
Ventricular dysfunction	2
High risk left-sided valve disease/left ventricular outflow tract obstruction	2
Pulmonary hypertension	2
Coronary artery disease	2
High risk aortopathy	2
No prior cardiac intervention	1
Late pregnancy assessment	1

Fig. 40.2 Frequency of primary maternal cardiac events as predicted by the CARPREG II risk score. The percentage of pregnancies likely to experience adverse maternal cardiac events as predicted by the Canadian Cardiac Disease in Pregnancy (CARPREG) II risk score. The risk predictors are weighted as shown in the box. The total point score correlates with the risk of a cardiac event as follows: 0–1 point, 5%; 2 points, 10%; 3 points, 15%; 4 points, 22%; and more than 4 points, 41%. (Adapted from Silversides CK, Grewal J, Mason J, et al. Pregnancy outcomes in women with heart disease: the CARPREG II study. *J Am Coll Cardiol*. 2018;71[21]:2419–2430.)

CARDIAC SHUNTS

Women with uncorrected, small to moderate, left-to-right shunts from secundum atrial septal defects (ASDs), restrictive ventricular septal defects (VSDs), or patent ductus arteriosus (PDA) may be identified for the first time during pregnancy when a murmur is detected. Women with large shunts are more likely to be aware of the diagnosis or to have undergone cardiac repair as a child. Eisenmenger syndrome, which occurs in the setting of large shunts with irreversible pulmonary artery hypertension (PAH) and shunt flow reversal, results in chronic cyanotic heart disease (discussed later).

Women with uncorrected left-to-right shunts are at low risk for adverse maternal cardiac events during pregnancy if they have preserved ventricular function and no evidence of PAH (Fig. 40.4). Rarely, atrial arrhythmias develop.[21,25,27,36,37] For women with ASD or patent foramen ovale, there is the potential for paradoxical embolization if there is a thrombus and systemic vasodilation and/or elevation of pulmonary resistance results in transient right-to-left shunting.

Atrioventricular septal defects (AVSDs) are complex lesions. The echocardiographer should be aware of the associations among AVSD, cleft mitral valve lesions, and left ventricular outflow tract (LVOT) obstruction. In a study of 62 pregnancies in women with AVSD, persistent New York Heart Association (NYHA) functional class deterioration, arrhythmias, and heart

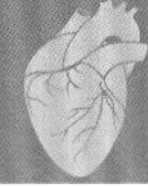

TABLE 40.3 Risk Factors for Maternal and Perinatal Complications During Pregnancy.

Predictor	*CARPREG*[21,25]	*CARPREG II*[22]	*BACH*[24]	*ZAHARA 1*[23]	*ROPAC*[35]	*Shanghai*[26]
Maternal Cardiac Complications						
Cardiac events before pregnancy	Yes	Yes	Yes	Yes	—	Yes
No prior cardiac interventions	—	Yes	—	—	—	—
Cardiac medications before pregnancy	—	—	—	Yes	—	—
Systemic ventricular systolic dysfunction	Yes	Yes	Yes	—	—	—
NYHA functional class III or IV	Yes	Yes	Yes	Yes	—	Yes
Cyanosis or oxygen saturation <90%	Yes	Yes	Yes	Yes	—	Yes
Left heart obstruction	Yes	Yes	Yes	Yes	—	Yes
Pulmonary atrioventricular valve regurgitation (moderate/severe)	—	—	—	Yes	—	—
Systemic atrioventricular valve regurgitation (moderate/severe)	—	—	—	Yes	—	—
Pulmonary regurgitation or depressed subpulmonary ventricular function	—	—	Yes	—	—	—
High-risk aortopathy	—	Yes	—	—	—	—
Coronary artery disease	—	Yes	—	—	—	—
Pulmonary hypertension	—	Yes	—	—	—	—
Mechanical prosthesis	—	Yes	—	Yes	—	—
Modified WHO classification	—	—	—	—	Yes	—
Smoking during pregnancy	—	—	Yes	—	—	—
Late presentation for care	—	Yes	—	—	—	—
Fetal and Neonatal Complications						
Cardiac medications before pregnancy	—	—	—	Yes	—	—
Left heart obstruction	Yes	—	Yes	—	—	—
NYHA functional class III or IV	Yes	—	—	—	—	Yes
Cyanosis or oxygen saturation <0%	Yes	—	—	—	—	—
Smoking during pregnancy	Yes	—	—	Yes	—	—
Multiple gestation	Yes	—	—	Yes	—	—
Anticoagulation	Yes	—	—	—	—	—
Mechanical prosthesis	—	—	—	Yes	—	—
Cyanotic heart disease	—	—	—	Yes	—	—
Pulmonary artery hypertension (systolic PAP ≥ 50 mmHg)	—	—	—	—	—	Yes

BACH, Boston Adult Congenital Heart; *CARPREG*, Cardiac Disease in Pregnancy; *NYHA*, New York Heart Association; *PAP*, pulmonary artery pressure; *ROPAC*, Registry Of Pregnancy and Cardiac Disease; *WHO*, World Health Organization; *ZAHARA*, Zwangerschap bij vrouwen met een Aangeboren HARtAfwijking.

failure were observed in 23%, 19%, and 2% of subjects, respectively.[38] If cardiac shunts are associated with pulmonary hypertension, the risk is dominated by the impact of the elevated pulmonary vascular resistance (discussed later).

Large left-to-right shunts can usually be detected with color Doppler imaging. A large shunt is associated with volume overload of the ventricle (i.e., right ventricular [RV] dilation in women with ASD, and LV dilation in women with VSD or PDA) or with elevations in the pulmonary artery systolic pressure (PASP). The echocardiographic examination of ASD or VSD through a subcostal window can be challenging in later pregnancy because of the gravid uterus. The increase in cardiac output also results in prominent caval flow entering the right atrium (RA), which can lead to a false-positive diagnosis of interatrial shunting. Off-axis views such as the right parasternal and low parasternal long-axis views are often helpful alternatives when the subcostal view is not feasible or optimal.

TETRALOGY OF FALLOT

Women of childbearing age with tetralogy of Fallot usually have undergone surgical repair in childhood. Residual pulmonary regurgitation is common in those who had transannular patch repairs, and it can be associated with RV dilation and dysfunction. Some women have had a pulmonary valve implant for treatment of pulmonary regurgitation. Women who have undergone annular sparing operations may have residual right ventricular outflow tract (RVOT) obstruction. Atrial and, less commonly, ventricular arrhythmias can occur late after repair. Rarely, women with unrepaired tetralogy of Fallot become pregnant. These women have cyanotic heart disease and are at high risk for pregnancy complications.

The volume overload of pregnancy may be poorly tolerated by women with significant RVOT lesions and RV dilation or dysfunction. Two risk indices (i.e., BACH and ZAHARA) identified pulmonary regurgitation as an independent predictor of adverse outcomes during pregnancy.[24,23] Although the rate of complications during pregnancy has varied, women with preserved ventricular function and without major residual lesions usually do well.[39,40] Overall, the risk of developing an arrhythmia during pregnancy is 6%, and the risk of developing heart failure during pregnancy is 2%.[41]

Women with repaired tetralogy of Fallot who have severe pulmonic regurgitation with RV dysfunction or branch pulmonary artery stenosis are at higher risk for heart failure during pregnancy.[39,40] Although it is less common in young women with tetralogy of Fallot, women with LV dysfunction are at risk for pregnancy-related complications.

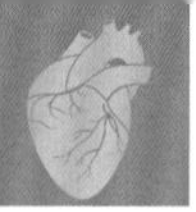

TABLE 40.4 Pregnancy Risk According to the Modified World Health Organization (mWHO) Classification.

mWHO classification I[a]
- Small or mild pulmonary stenosis
- Patent ductus arteriosus
- Mitral valve prolapse
- Successfully repaired simple lesions (e.g., atrial or ventricular septal defect, patent ductus arteriosus, anomalous pulmonary venous connection)
- Atrial or ventricular ectopic beats, isolated

mWHO classification II (if otherwise well and uncomplicated)[b]
- Unoperated atrial or ventricular septal defect
- Repaired tetralogy of Fallot
- Most arrhythmias (supraventricular arrhythmias)
- Turner syndrome without aortic dilation

mWHO classification II–III (depending on individual)[c]
- Mild LV impairment (LVEF > 45%)
- Hypertrophic cardiomyopathy
- Native or tissue valvular heart disease not considered WHO I or IV (mild mitral stenosis, moderate aortic stenosis)
- Marfan syndrome or other heritable thoracic aortic disease without aortic dilation
- Aorta < 45 mm in association with bicuspid aortic valve pathology
- Repaired coarctation
- Atrioventricular septal defects

mWHO classification III[d]
- Moderate LV impairment (LVEF 30%–45%)
- Previous peripartum cardiomyopathy without any residual LV impairment
- Mechanical valve
- Systemic RV with good or mildly decreased ventricular function
- Fontan circulation if the patient is otherwise well and the cardiac condition is uncomplicated
- Unrepaired cyanotic heart disease
- Other complex heart disease
- Moderate mitral stenosis
- Severe asymptomatic aortic stenosis
- Moderate aortic dilation (40–45 mm in Marfan syndrome or other heritable thoracic aortic disease; 45–50 mm in bicuspid aortic valve; Turner syndrome aortic size index of 20–25 mm/m^2; tetralogy of Fallot < 50 mm)
- Ventricular tachycardia

mWHO classification IV (pregnancy contraindicated)[e]
- Pulmonary artery hypertension
- Severe systemic ventricular dysfunction (EF < 30% or NYHA class III–IV)
- Previous peripartum cardiomyopathy with any residual LV impairment
- Severe mitral stenosis
- Severe symptomatic aortic stenosis
- Systemic RV with moderate or severely decreased ventricular function
- Severe aortic dilation (>45 mm in Marfan syndrome or other heritable thoracic aortic disease, > 50 mm in bicuspid aortic valve, Turner syndrome aortic size index > 25 mm/m^2, tetralogy of Fallot > 50 mm)
- Vascular Ehlers-Danlos syndrome
- Severe (re)coarctation
- Fontan with any complication

[a]mWHO classification I: no detectable increased risk of maternal death and no or mild increase in morbidity.
[b]mWHO classification II: small increase in risk of maternal death or moderate increase in morbidity.
[c]mWHO classification II–III: intermediate increased risk of maternal death or moderate to severe increase in morbidity.
[d]mWHO classification III: significantly increased risk of maternal death or severe morbidity. Expert counseling is required, and care should occur at an expert center for pregnancy and cardiac disease.
[e]mWHO classification IV: extremely high risk of maternal death or severe morbidity, and pregnancy is contraindicated. If pregnancy occurs, termination should be discussed. If pregnancy continues, care should occur at an expert center for pregnancy and cardiac disease.
LVEF, Left ventricular ejection fraction; *NYHA*, New York Heart Association.
From Regitz-Zagrosek V, Roos-Hesselink JW, Bauersachs J, et al. 2018 ESC Guidelines for the management of cardiovascular diseases during pregnancy. *Eur Heart J*. 2018;39[34]:3165–3241.)

TTE is helpful for risk stratification during preconception counseling or at the time of the first antenatal visit. Assessment of RV size and systolic function during pregnancy is important for women with significant pulmonary regurgitation. For those with RVOT obstruction, RVOT gradients and RV systolic pressure should be monitored during pregnancy. The prolonged hemodynamic stress of pregnancy can have an adverse effect on the RV. RV dilation and adverse outcomes are more common among women with tetralogy of Fallot who have been pregnant compared with those who have never been pregnant.[42–44] In view of these findings, echocardiographic assessment should be repeated after delivery.

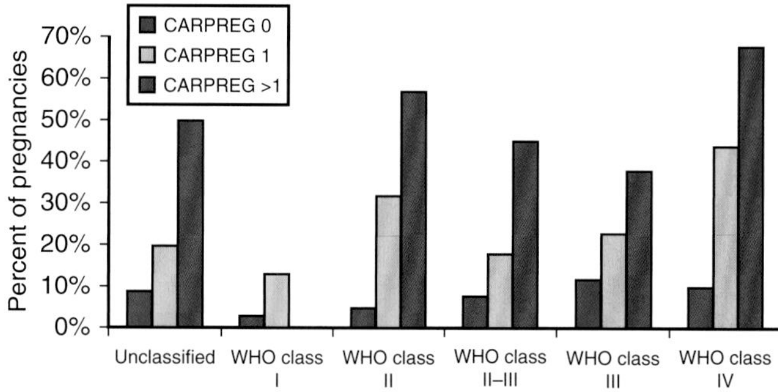

Fig. 40.3 Frequency of maternal cardiac events by the mWHO classification based on the CARPREG risk score. Bar graph shows the percentage of pregnancies likely to be affected by adverse maternal cardiac events as predicted by the Cardiac Disease in Pregnancy (CARPEG) risk score (0, 1, or > 1) for each modified World Health Organization (mWHO) classification. (Adapted from Silversides CK, Grewal J, Mason J, et al. Pregnancy outcomes in women with heart disease: the CARPREG II study. *J Am Coll Cardiol*. 2018;71[21]:2419–2430.)

COARCTATION OF THE AORTA

Unrepaired coarctation of the aorta is rare in young women. Significant coarctation of the aorta impedes delivery of blood to the arterial tree distal to the coarctation site. During pregnancy, this reduction in distal perfusion may affect the placental circulation; intrauterine growth restriction and premature labor are more common among women with unrepaired coarctation. Most women with coarctation of the aorta have undergone surgical repair or stenting. Even when the coarctation has been successfully repaired, persistent or recurrent systemic hypertension is common. Hypertension, concomitant bicuspid aortic valve disease, or aneurysms at the site of the repair pose additional risks.

Maternal death is rare in contemporary series, in which most women with coarctation have undergone surgical repair or stenting.[45,46] The most common complication in women with repaired coarctation is pregnancy-induced hypertension and preeclampsia.[21,25,47] The risk of hypertension is highest among women with unrepaired coarctation in proportion to the degree of residual gradient.[45,46]

As in the case of aortic stenosis, the gradient across the stent or coarctation site increases during pregnancy (Fig. 40.5). It is important not to overdiagnose coarctation based on an elevated velocity or gradient because hypoplastic aorta and flow acceleration are alternative causes of an elevated velocity.

Although they are not well established for pregnancy, factors that favor a gradient's being true coarctation include spillover of the color-flow turbulence into diastole or persistent elevated gradient into diastole in the descending thoracic aorta or in the subcostal long-axis view of the abdominal aorta.[48] In some cases, additional aortic imaging such as MRI or invasive catheterization is necessary to differentiate a true coarctation from a pseudocoarctation, recognizing that the use of these alternative modalities may be limited during pregnancy. Aneurysms at the site of coarctation repair are often not well seen by echocardiography; if they are suspected, an MRI may need to be performed during pregnancy.

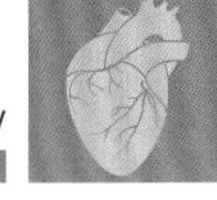

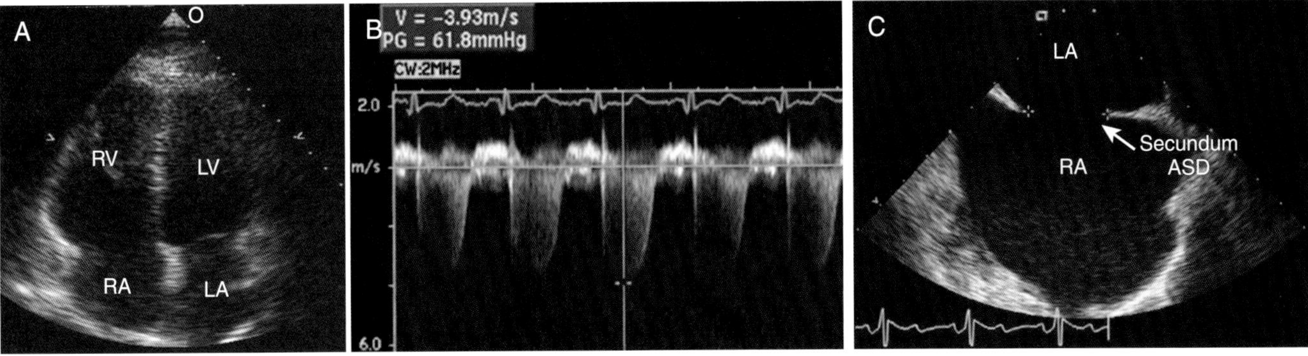

Fig. 40.4 Secundum atrial septal defect. (A) TTE of a 36-year-old woman diagnosed with a secundum atrial septal defect *(ASD)*, a dilated RV, and an elevated RV systolic pressure of 70 mmHg during pregnancy. (B) In the 3rd trimester, her RV systolic pressure increased to 90 mmHg. She had no cardiac complications during the pregnancy. (C) Her postpartum TEE showed a 2.4-cm ASD. She had a pericardial patch closure of the ASD after an attempt at percutaneous device closure was unsuccessful. In the late follow-up period, she had no residual pulmonary artery hypertension.

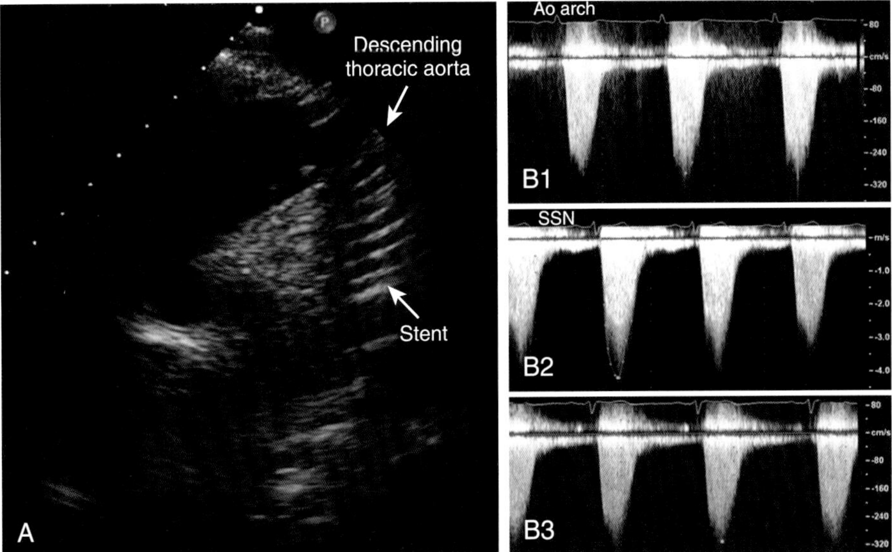

Fig. 40.5 Coarctation of the aorta. Serial TTE studies of a 27-year-old woman with coarctation of the aorta who had a covered stent inserted as an adult. (A) Her stent is seen on the TTE. (B) The serial Doppler studies show her increase in baseline gradients across the stent (B1) and during pregnancy (B2) and return of the gradients to baseline in the postpartum period (B3).

EBSTEIN ANOMALY

There is substantial variation in the severity of Ebstein anomaly. Some women have very mild forms of the disease with minimal involvement of the tricuspid valve, mild tricuspid regurgitation, and excellent RV systolic function. More severe forms of Ebstein anomaly are associated with significant tricuspid valve dysmorphogenesis, severe tricuspid regurgitation, and RV systolic dysfunction. In this setting, Ebstein anomaly is associated with high cardiac morbidity and mortality rates.

The ability of the heart to tolerate the hemodynamic changes of pregnancy varies according to the severity of the disease. Women with mild variants can expect to have an uncomplicated pregnancy, whereas women with severe Ebstein anomaly may be unable to tolerate the increased preload of pregnancy. These women are at risk for functional deterioration, right heart failure, and arrhythmias.[49,50] In one large series of 111 pregnancies, no serious maternal cardiac complications were reported, but there were increases in fetal loss, prematurity, and congenital heart disease in the offspring.[49] Women with interatrial shunts may demonstrate reversal of or an increase in right-to-left shunting, which increases cyanosis during pregnancy, and they are at high risk for complications as a consequence.

For the echocardiographic laboratory, the main role is the diagnosis of Ebstein anomaly and delineation of interatrial communication. Diagnosis of Ebstein anomaly in pregnant women is no different from that in nonpregnant women. During pregnancy, surveillance TTE should be performed. The frequency of TTE during pregnancy is based on the severity of the Ebstein anomaly. The echocardiographer should be aware of the institution's criteria for deciding whether the tricuspid valve is reparable so that these parameters can be included in the study report.

TRANSPOSITION OF THE GREAT ARTERIES

Women with complete transposition of the great arteries have had an atrial switch operation (i.e., Mustard or Senning procedure), a Rastelli operation, or an arterial switch operation (i.e., Jatene operation). Women with atrial switch operations have blood flow redirected at the atrial level using baffles. This leaves the morphologic RV in the subaortic position. These operations

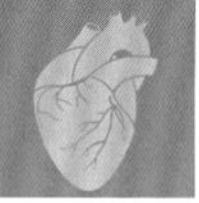

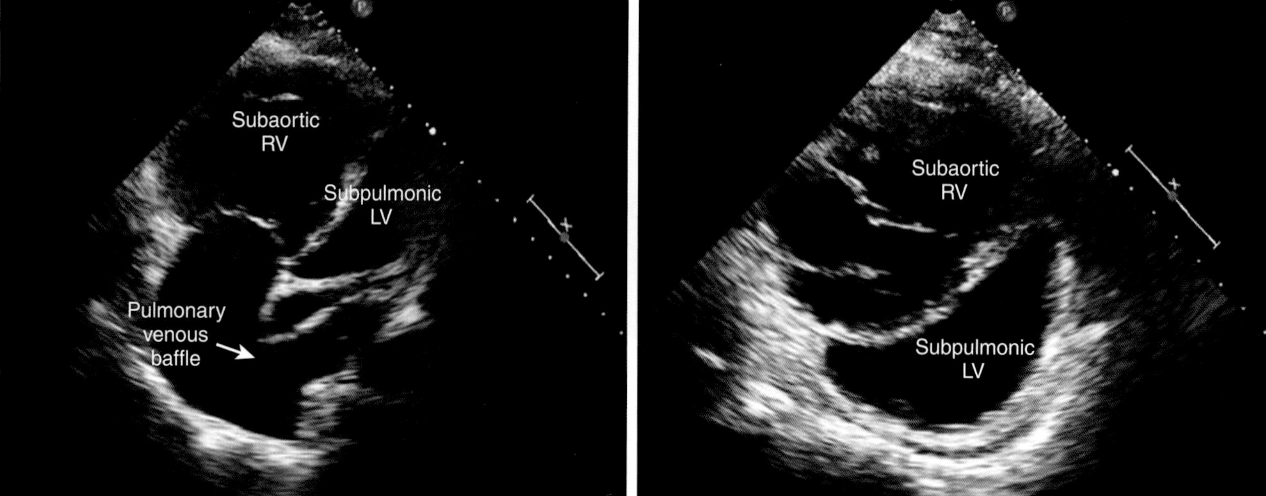

Fig. 40.6 Mustard operation. TTE of a 30-year-old woman with complete transposition of the great arteries; apical 4-chamber *(left)* and parasternal short-axis *(right)* views after Mustard operation. The patient had a Blalock-Hanlon atrial septectomy followed by an atrial switch operation (i.e., Mustard operation). She had moderate to severe subaortic RV dilation and systolic dysfunction (see Video 40.6) and moderate systemic atrioventricular valve regurgitation. She had no cardiac complications during pregnancy. She had a spontaneous vaginal delivery at 35 weeks' gestation. There was no change in her subaortic ventricular size, systolic function, or atrioventricular valve regurgitation during pregnancy.

are associated with several late sequelae, including subaortic ventricular dysfunction, atrioventricular valve regurgitation, baffle leaks or stenosis, sinus node dysfunction, and atrial and ventricular arrhythmias (Fig. 40.6). Rarely, PASPs may be elevated.

The residual lesions are important determinants of pregnancy risk. The most common complications during pregnancy are atrial arrhythmias, which occur in as many as 22% of pregnancies.[51] Less commonly, women develop heart failure or deterioration of ventricular function.[52–54] In one study, progressive RV dilation (31%) and subaortic ventricular deterioration (25%) were common during pregnancy and often irreversible.[54] Maternal death of women with atrial switch operations is rare, but it has been described.

Women with transposition of the great arteries and a VSD may have a Rastelli operation. The Rastelli operation involves the creation of an LV-to-aorta tunnel and insertion of an RV-to–pulmonary artery conduit. There are few data on pregnancy outcomes for women with a Rastelli operation. Progressive LVOT obstruction during pregnancy has been reported.[55] Atrial switch operations became the surgical repair strategy of choice in the 1980s, and many of these patients have since reached childbearing age. Although most women with arterial switches do well during pregnancy, adverse outcomes have been reported for women with residual cardiac disease after surgery.[56,57]

Congenitally corrected transposition of the great arteries may be isolated (i.e., simple) or associated with other congenital defects (i.e., complex), most commonly VSDs and pulmonary stenosis. Women with congenitally corrected transposition of the great arteries have a subaortic morphologic RV with various degrees of subaortic ventricular dilation and dysfunction. Pregnancy risk is related to the degree of subaortic systolic ventricular function, severity of systemic atrioventricular valve regurgitation, and associated defects. Most women with good subaortic ventricular function and normal functional capacity do well, but heart failure, arrhythmias, stroke, endocarditis, and myocardial infarction have been reported during pregnancy.[58]

For women with Mustard or Senning operations and those with congenitally corrected transposition of the great arteries, frequent serial TTE assessment during pregnancy is essential to detect changes in subaortic ventricular size, altered systolic function, and atrioventricular valve regurgitation.[34] RV systolic pressure may be elevated in women who had Rastelli operations and RV-to–pulmonary artery conduit stenosis and should be monitored during pregnancy.

FONTAN CIRCULATION

The Fontan operation for the functionally single ventricle directs RA or caval blood into the pulmonary artery. It most often leaves no subpulmonary ventricle in the circuit. Although the operation improves oxygenation and volume overload for the subaortic ventricle, the ability of the heart to increase cardiac output is limited, systemic venous pressure is chronically elevated, and the risk of thromboembolic complications is increased. Scarring and remodeling of the atria contribute to atrial arrhythmias. The hemodynamic changes of pregnancy may be poorly tolerated, especially in women with poor functional capacity, systolic ventricular dysfunction, severe atrioventricular valve regurgitation, or recurrent arrhythmias.

Preconception risk stratification of women who have undergone the Fontan operation is important because some (i.e., those with single ventricle physiology and ventricular dysfunction or recurrent arrhythmias) have a very high pregnancy risk and should be advised accordingly. The incidence of 1st trimester miscarriage is high. In one series, only 45% of pregnancies resulted in live births.[59] The most common complications are postpartum hemorrhage (14% of pregnancies), prematurity (59% of pregnancies), and infants who were small for gestational age (20%).[60] Supraventricular arrhythmias and heart failure occur in 8.4% and 3.9% of pregnancies, respectively. Other cardiac complications are deterioration in NYHA functional class, thromboembolic complications, and gestational hypertension.[59–62]

The role of echocardiographic services for pregnant women who have had a Fontan operation is usually limited to confirmation of cardiac anatomy in the newly presenting patient, assessment of ventricular function and valve regurgitation for

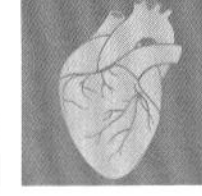

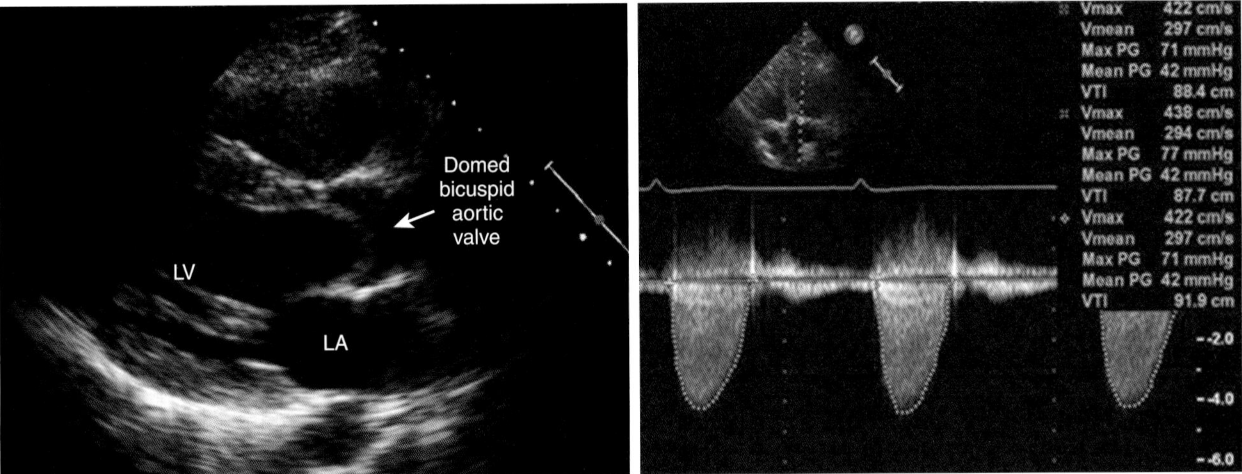

Fig. 40.7 Bicuspid valve with severe aortic stenosis. *Left,* Parasternal long-axis view, *Right,* Apical 5-chamber view. A 31-year-old woman with a bicuspid aortic valve underwent balloon valvuloplasty for severe aortic stenosis as a teenager. At the time of her first antenatal visit, she had severe aortic stenosis, normal LV systolic function, LV hypertrophy, and a mildly dilated aortic root (see Video 40.7 ▶). Her baseline peak and mean aortic valve gradients were 71/42 mmHg, and her calculated aortic valve area was 0.8 cm^2. The aortic valve gradients increased to 120/75 mmHg during pregnancy. At 35 weeks' gestation she developed preeclampsia and had an urgent cesarean delivery. Her infant daughter had a small ventricular septal defect.

preconception counseling, and surveillance during pregnancy. Complex anatomy resulting from Fontan circulation and repair and the limited acoustical access in a patient with multiple cardiac operations frequently necessitates a multimodality imaging approach that includes echocardiography and cardiac MRI. TEE is often indicated before cardioversion because patients with Fontan physiology do not tolerate atrial fibrillation well and are at high risk for formation of thrombi.

CYANOTIC HEART DISEASE

Pregnancies in women with cyanotic congenital heart disease or Eisenmenger syndrome are rare. Miscarriages are common in both groups because of chronic hypoxemia. Both conditions are associated with significant maternal and fetal risks.

Cyanotic heart disease is seen in women with unrepaired tetralogy of Fallot, pulmonary atresia with aortopulmonary collaterals, Ebstein anomaly with ASDs, and single ventricles (i.e., tricuspid atresia). These cardiac lesions are different from those seen in Eisenmenger syndrome, in which there is typically no associated elevation in the PASP. Overall pregnancy risk, although high, is less than that in Eisenmenger syndrome. In one study of 96 pregnancies in women with cyanotic heart disease, cardiac complications occurred in 32% of pregnancies and included heart failure, arrhythmias, and cerebral infarction.[63] Maternal deaths, although rare, have been reported.[63] Women with cyanotic heart disease have low live birth rates (43%), and when the maternal oxygen saturation is 85% or less, the live birth rate is only 12%.[63]

Eisenmenger syndrome is a multisystem disorder with hematologic, renal, neurologic, and musculoskeletal involvement. It occurs when severe PAH leads to shunt reversal and chronic cyanosis. Pregnancy is very poorly tolerated by women with Eisenmenger syndrome due to fixed pulmonary resistance, volume loading on the right heart, and decreases in afterload that can lead to increases in right-to-left intracardiac shunting. Pregnancy is contraindicated for women with Eisenmenger syndrome because of the high risk of maternal death, which occurs in 28% to 36% of pregnancies.[64–66] Causes of death are related to right heart failure, pulmonary hypertensive crisis, sudden death, pulmonary emboli, and pulmonary artery dissection. Pulmonary vasodilators are being increasingly used during pregnancy for women with PAH of any cause.

Women are likely to be diagnosed with cyanotic heart disease or Eisenmenger syndrome before pregnancy because they are chronic conditions. For women who decide on pregnancy, a preconception or early pregnancy TTE study is important to define cardiac anatomy, estimate pulmonary artery pressures, and assess systolic ventricular function for future comparisons. Complications are common during pregnancy, and frequent TTE surveillance, as often as every 4 to 6 weeks, should be performed to monitor RV function and pulmonary artery pressures during pregnancy and the postpartum period. For women with Eisenmenger syndrome, ongoing clinical and echocardiographic surveillance is required because most maternal deaths occur within the first month after delivery.

AORTIC VALVE DISEASE

Significant aortic stenosis limits the ability of the heart to increase cardiac output. The hypertrophied, noncompliant ventricle is also more sensitive to a fall in preload. During pregnancy, these factors contribute to an increased propensity for heart failure, hypotension, angina, and arrhythmias. Aortic stenosis in women of childbearing age most commonly results from bicuspid aortic valve disease. Bicuspid aortic valve disease is sometimes associated with ascending aortopathy or coarctation of the aorta, which confer additional risks during pregnancy.

Women with symptomatic aortic stenosis should undergo surgical correction before pregnancy.[67] Management of asymptomatic women with severe aortic stenosis is more controversial, and careful risk stratification is required before pregnancy. In selected patients, aortic balloon valvuloplasty may provide short-term palliation before a planned pregnancy.

Although the maternal mortality rate is generally low, women with significant aortic stenosis are at risk for heart failure, arrhythmias, and angina during pregnancy[27,68–72] (Fig. 40.7). Asymptomatic women with mild or moderate aortic stenosis

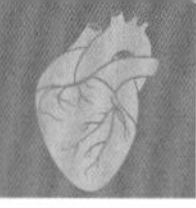

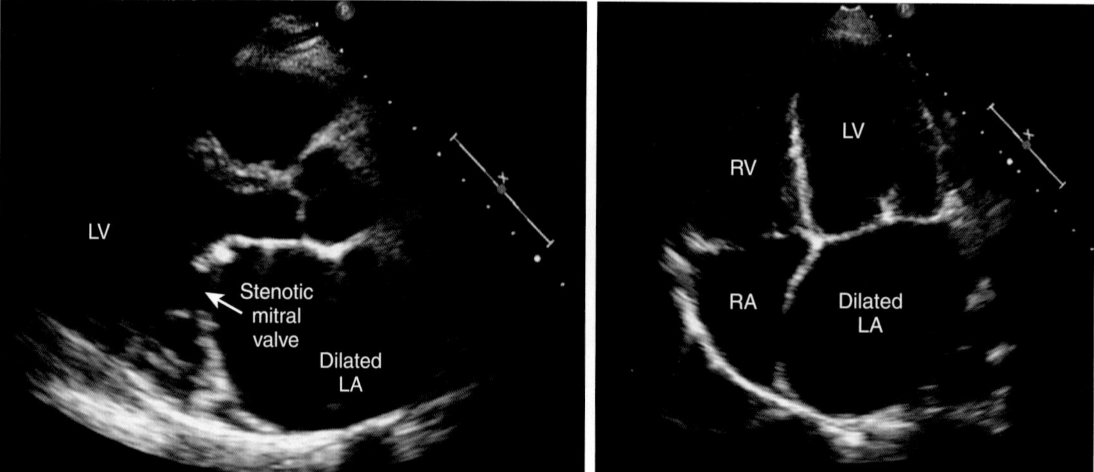

Fig. 40.8 Rheumatic mitral stenosis. *Left*, Parasternal long-axis view. *Right*, Apical 4-chamber view. A 43-year-old woman had moderate rheumatic mitral valve stenosis, mild mitral regurgitation, severely dilated LA, and mild pulmonary artery hypertension. In the 3rd trimester, she developed congestive heart failure. She was successfully treated with a β-blocker and diuretics.

typically do well. One study reported cardiac complication rates of 10% for women with severe aortic stenosis, although higher rates have been reported.[70] A review of the literature revealed a 9% risk of heart failure and a 4% risk of new or recurrent arrhythmias in women with severe aortic stenosis.[32] For pregnant women with severe aortic stenosis and persistent symptoms despite bed rest and medical therapy, palliation by balloon valvuloplasty may be considered if the valve anatomy is suitable.

Pregnancy may increase long-term risks for women with aortic stenosis. Women with moderate or severe aortic stenosis who had been pregnant were more likely to require aortic valve replacement than a matched control group of women who had not been pregnant.[70,73]

Aortic regurgitation in young women is most commonly caused by bicuspid aortic valve disease. Most women with mild or moderate aortic regurgitation and normal LV systolic function do well during pregnancy. The increased plasma volume and cardiac output may not be tolerated in women with severe aortic regurgitation and LV systolic dysfunction.

Frequent TTE monitoring during pregnancy is recommended for women with severe aortic stenosis. Increased cardiac output in pregnancy leads to an increase in the transaortic velocity and pressure gradient with advancing gestation.[70] The calculated aortic valve area should be unchanged and can be used to assess stenosis if women present for the first time later in pregnancy. In a preliminary study, an increase in LV twist was seen during pregnancy, and the absence of increased LV twist was associated with cardiac deterioration necessitating balloon valvuloplasty.[74]

MITRAL VALVE DISEASE

Rheumatic heart disease is the most common cause of mitral stenosis in young women. Rarely, mitral stenosis may result from congenital mitral valve malformations such as parachute mitral valve. During pregnancy, increased blood volume, cardiac output, and heart rate (i.e., shortened diastolic filling time) can lead to elevated LA pressure and the development of symptoms. Mitral stenosis sometimes first manifests during pregnancy. Other factors that increase heart rate (e.g., atrial fibrillation) can contribute to decompensation and development of pulmonary edema. Pulmonary edema and atrial arrhythmias are common in pregnant women with moderate or severe mitral stenosis[35,69,75,76] (Fig. 40.8).

A systematic review of the literature of pregnancy outcomes in developed countries revealed that overall rates of maternal mortality, heart failure, and new or recurrent arrhythmias in women with severe mitral stenosis were 3%, 37%, and 16%, respectively.[32] Transient ischemic attacks and strokes can occur but are less common. In two large North American series, women with mild, moderate, and severe mitral stenosis developed pulmonary edema in 20%, 45%, and 67% of pregnancies and atrial arrhythmias in 8%, 15%, and 33% of pregnancies, respectively. There were no maternal deaths in the North American series.[69,75] Although maternal deaths during pregnancy are rare in developed countries, in some regions such as sub-Saharan Africa, the maternal mortality rate is very high.[77]

Treatment of mitral stenosis involves slowing the heart rate with β-blockers and treating pulmonary edema.[78] For women with suitable valve anatomy who remain symptomatic despite medial therapy, percutaneous balloon valvuloplasty has been used during pregnancy.[78,79] TEE guidance can be used during pregnancy to minimize fluoroscopy time.

In women of childbearing age, mitral regurgitation can be the result of rheumatic heart disease, congenital heart disease, or mitral valve prolapse. Women with mild or moderate mitral regurgitation and normal LV systolic function tend to do well during pregnancy. As with aortic regurgitation, the increased plasma volume and cardiac output may be poorly tolerated when the mitral regurgitation is severe and there is associated ventricular dysfunction.

For women presenting for the first time during pregnancy, TTE is necessary for risk stratification. Risk is based on the severity of the valve lesion, the PASP, the LA size, and the presence of concomitant valve lesions. The increased cardiac output and heart rate during pregnancy contribute to increased transmitral flow velocities and pressure gradients in women with mitral stenosis. The mitral valve pressure half-time area remains unchanged during pregnancy and can be used to assess valve lesion severity.[75] Serial TTE studies should be performed to monitor transmitral Doppler gradients, PASP, and systolic ventricular function during pregnancy and the early postpartum period.

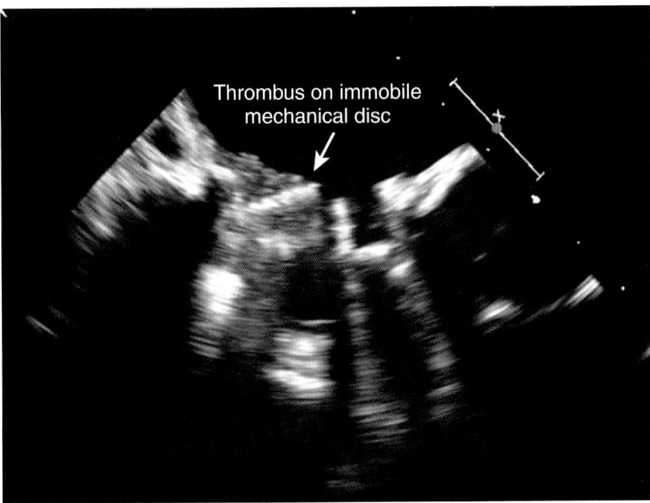

Fig. 40.9 Mechanical mitral valve with valve thrombosis. TEE of a 23-year-old woman with a bileaflet mechanical mitral valve. She had been noncompliant with her warfarin during the pregnancy. After an uncomplicated delivery at term, she had a transient ischemic attack. Her echocardiogram showed an increase in mitral valve gradients, an increase in the pulmonary artery systolic pressure, and a thrombus on the atrial side of an immobile disc (see Video 40.9B). She underwent urgent mitral valve replacement.

PROSTHETIC HEART VALVES

There are two types of prosthetic heart valves; mechanical and tissue. Pregnancy in women with mechanical heart valves is high risk due to the potential for thromboembolic complications, specifically valve thrombosis, which can be fatal. The prothrombotic state of pregnancy increases the risk of thromboembolic complications during pregnancy (Fig. 40.9). Maintenance of therapeutic anticoagulation can be difficult with increases in body weight, changes in anticoagulants, and difficulty monitoring heparin levels. Women with mechanical valves are also at risk for heart failure and arrhythmias. Maternal complications depend on many factors, including the underlying cardiac condition, the type of valve (i.e., new bileaflet valves are less thrombogenic), the position of the valve (i.e., mitral valves are associated with more thromboembolic complications than aortic valves), the function of the prosthesis, the type of anticoagulant used (i.e., lowest thromboembolic complications with warfarin and highest with unfractionated heparin), and the LV systolic function.

The type of anticoagulation is a major determinant of thromboembolic complications. Warfarin is associated with the lowest rates of maternal complications, but it is associated with warfarin embryopathy. Heparin does not cross the placenta and therefore is not associated with embryopathy, but it is associated with significantly higher rates of maternal complications. Low-molecular-weight heparin is used during pregnancy as an alternative to unfractionated heparin[80–82] because of the high rates of valve thrombosis with unfractionated heparin.

Maternal deaths and thromboembolic complications occur in 0.9% and 2.7% of pregnancies of women with mechanical valves using warfarin and in 2.9% and 8.7% of pregnancies of women using low-molecular-weight heparin, respectively.[82] Management of anticoagulation at the time of labor and delivery is complex because warfarin must be switched to heparin before delivery. Guidelines on the management of anticoagulation of pregnant women with mechanical valves are available from the European Society of Cardiology,[34] the American College of Cardiology/American Heart Association,[67] and the American College of Chest Physicians.[83]

Women with normally functioning bioprosthetic valves generally do well during pregnancy. Although there had been discrepant reports on the effect of pregnancy on valve degeneration, larger studies suggested that pregnancy did not accelerate valve degeneration.[84]

TTE is used to determine pregnancy risk and provide information on valve function, ventricular function, and PASPs. Baseline valve gradients are helpful references because flow velocities and pressure gradients increase as pregnancy progresses. Serial follow-up examinations during pregnancy are important. In women with mechanical valves, dyspnea, heart failure, muffled mechanical heart sounds, and increasing valve gradients may represent valve thrombosis. These findings should prompt an immediate echocardiographic assessment of valve function. Women with mechanical valves in whom symptoms suggest valve thrombosis should have a TEE study. Fluoroscopy with abdominal shielding should be used to assess leaflet mobility if the TEE does not establish a diagnosis.

AORTOPATHIES

Although some women come to attention during pregnancy when they present with aortic dissection, many women with aortopathies are aware of their diagnosis before pregnancy. The most common causes of dilated thoracic aortas in young women are related to bicuspid valves, Marfan syndrome, and coarctation of the aorta. Other aortic syndromes such as Ehlers-Danlos syndrome, Turner syndrome, Loeys-Dietz syndrome, and familial thoracic aneurysm syndrome and dissection are rare. The increased blood volume, cardiac output, and changing hormones of pregnancy increase the risk of progressive aortic dilation and dissection.[85]

The risk of dissection or dilation during pregnancy varies considerably by lesion.[31] Aortic dissection has been reported in women with bicuspid aortic valves, although much less commonly than in women with Marfan syndrome.[85] The risk of dissection and other serious obstetric complications is higher for women with Marfan syndrome who have dilated aortas and those with vascular Ehlers-Danlos or Loeys-Dietz syndrome.[31] Overall, the risk of aortic dissection during pregnancy is approximately 3% for women with Marfan syndrome,[86] although some groups have reported lower dissection rates.[87]

The risk of aortic dissection is related to the aortic diameter, and women with aortic diameters less than 4.0 cm have the lowest risk of dissection (1%). Women with aortic diameters greater than 4.5 cm are at high risk for rapid dilation or dissection, and pregnancy is not advised (Fig. 40.10). There is debate about the pregnancy risk when the aortic dimensions are 4.0 to 4.5 cm; some groups have reported no dissection for this group of women.[88] Prophylactic root replacement before pregnancy is advised if the aortic diameter is 4.4 cm or larger.[34] Aortic dissection has been reported after prophylatic root replacement. Women with Marfan syndrome and other connective tissue disorders may also have aortic regurgitation, mitral valve prolapse, and mitral valve regurgitation.

TTE is used for serial pregnancy assessment of aortic dimensions in women who are at risk for or have proven aortic dilation. It is important to perform standardized measurements of the aorta at multiple levels (i.e., aortic root, ascending aorta, arch, and proximal descending aorta) serially during pregnancy.

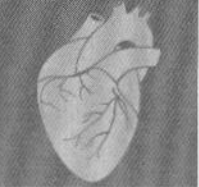

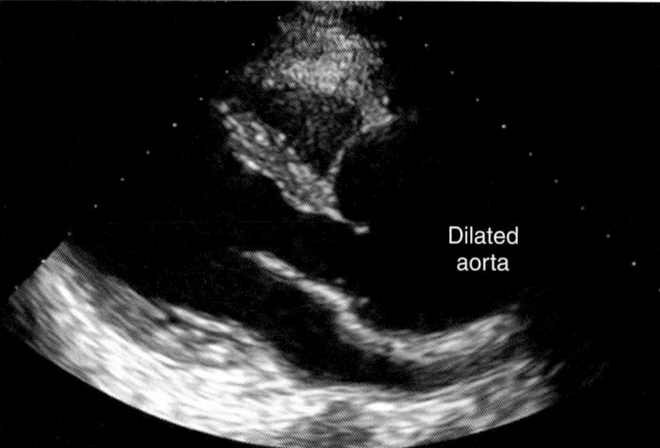

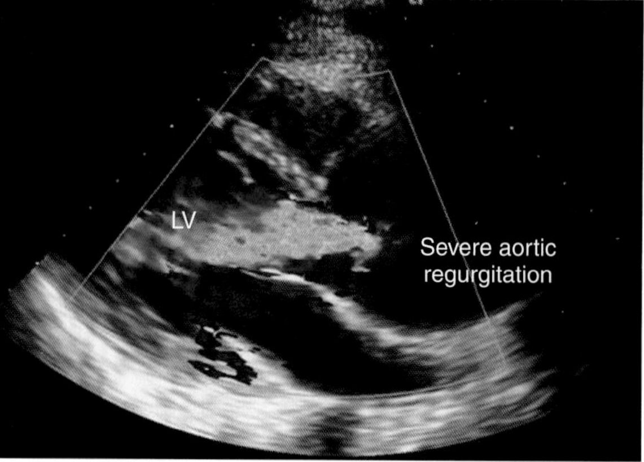

Fig. 40.10 Marfan syndrome. TTE of a 29-year-old woman with Marfan syndrome, severe dilation of the aortic root, and severe aortic regurgitation (2D *[left]* and color *[right]* parasternal long-axis views) (see Video 40.10). The patient presented for the first time late in the 1st trimester. She had a successful valve-sparing root replacement at 12 weeks' gestation.

Guidelines recommend evaluations every 6 to 8 weeks during pregnancy for women with Marfan syndrome or bicuspid aortic valve.[34]

Although computed tomography (CT) and MRI may provide a more comprehensive assessment of the aorta, their role is mainly in preconception counseling and in evaluating those with suspected aortic complications during pregnancy. Postpartum aortic complications can develop, and clinical and TTE monitoring should be continued for up to 6 months after delivery.

CARDIOMYOPATHIES

For women with *idiopathic dilated cardiomyopathy*, the increased plasma volume and cardiac output can lead to deterioration in LV systolic function, heart failure, or arrhythmias[89–91] (Fig. 40. 11). During labor and delivery, relief of inferior vena cava compression and autotransfusions from the contracting uterus can further contribute to complications. Heart failure most commonly occurs later in pregnancy or within the first month after delivery.[22] In one study of 36 pregnancies in women with dilated cardiomyopathy, maternal cardiac complications occurred in 14 pregnancies (39%).[91]

Women with a history of clinical heart failure, moderate or severe LV systolic dysfunction, or NYHA functional class III or IV indications were at high risk for complications during pregnancy. During postpartum follow-up, the complication rates for women with dilated cardiomyopathy and moderate or severe LV systolic dysfunction were significantly higher compared with a control group of nonpregnant women with dilated cardiomyopathy and similar ventricular function.[91]

Acute heart failure is treated with diuretics and afterload reduction. Hydralazine and nitrates can be used in pregnancy for afterload reduction. Angiotensin-converting enzyme inhibitors and angiotensin receptor blockers should not be used in pregnancy because of the effect on fetal renal function. Women with preexisting LV systolic dysfunction treated with β-blockers should continue their β-blocker therapy during pregnancy.

Peripartum cardiomyopathy (PPCM) is an idiopathic cardiomyopathy that occurs near the end of pregnancy or during the months after delivery, abortion, or miscarriage, without other causes, and with an LV ejection fraction of less than 45%.[92] PPCM is rare condition. Risk factors associated with

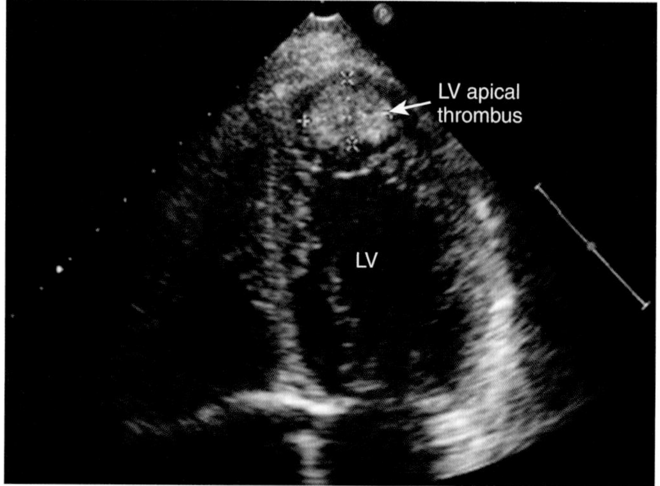

Fig. 40.11 Cardiomyopathy and an LV thrombus on apical 4-chamber view. TTE of a 35-year-old woman with anthracycline cardiomyopathy. Early in pregnancy, her LV systolic function was mildly hypokinetic. Her LV systolic function remained unchanged during pregnancy. She delivered twins near term. At 8 weeks' postpartum, she presented with congestive heart failure, and her TTE showed severe LV systolic function and new LV apical thrombus (see Video 40.11).

the condition include multiparity, twin gestation, extremes of reproductive age, preeclampsia, and prolonged tocolysis.[93] There is likely also a genetic predisposition to the condition.

Timing and onset of symptoms and TTE findings confirm the diagnosis of PPCM. The presentation varies. Some women present with mild heart failure symptoms, and others present with cardiogenic shock. Reported maternal mortality rates are 1% to 30%.[94] LV thrombus is seen in as many as 20% of cases at presentation.

For women who present during pregnancy, modifications in heart failure treatment are required, as previously described for women with idiopathic dilated cardiomyopathy.[34,92] For those who present in the postpartum period, heart failure is treated in the standard fashion. A small study demonstrated a benefit for bromocriptine treatment when added to standard heart failure therapies.[95] Anticoagulation should be started in women with LV thrombus. Women with PPCM should be treated at a high-risk cardiac center with LV assist device and transplantation capabilities.

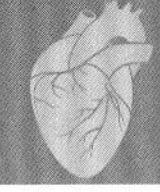

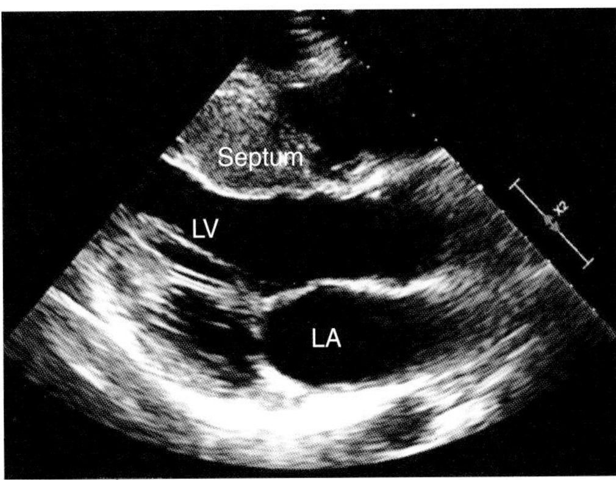

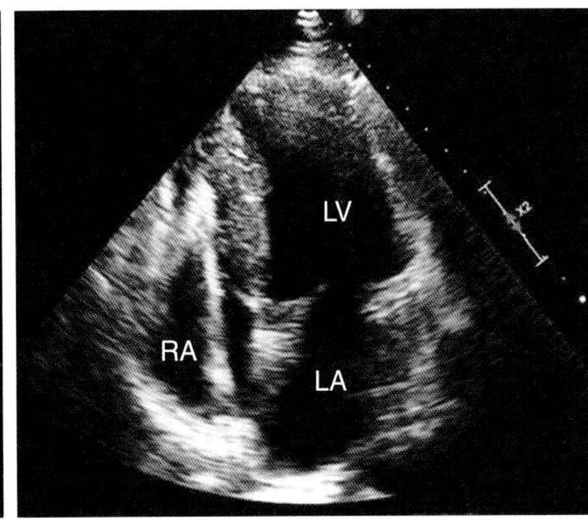

Fig. 40.12 Hypertrophic cardiomyopathy. *Left*, Parasternal long-axis view showing a thickened ventricular septum. *Right*, Apical 4-chamber view. TTE of a 30-year-old woman with nonobstructive hypertrophic cardiomyopathy and an *MYH7* gene mutation. She had a surgical myectomy as a teenager. After the myectomy, she required a permanent pacemaker to remedy complete heart block. She received a prophylactic implantable cardioverter-defibrillator before pregnancy and was given β-blocker therapy before and during pregnancy. She had an uncomplicated spontaneous vaginal delivery. The infant was found to have hypoglycemia at the time of delivery. Exposure to β-blockers in utero is associated with an increased risk of hypoglycemia in neonates.

In a contemporary North American population, spontaneous recovery of LV systolic function occurred in most women with PPCM.[93] Those women who have had full recovery of LV systolic function and are considering further pregnancies must be advised of the risks of recurrence. Pregnancy is contraindicated for women with residual LV systolic dysfunction because of the associated 19% maternal mortality rate.[96]

Hypertrophic cardiomyopathy is the most common inherited cardiomyopathy among women of childbearing age. Hypertrophic cardiomyopathy is associated with various degrees of LV hypertrophy with or without a dynamic LVOT obstruction. The clinical status of women with hypertrophic cardiomyopathies varies; some women are asymptomatic, but others have heart failure, ventricular arrhythmias, or sudden death (Fig. 40.12).

At the time of labor and delivery, anesthetics, expulsive efforts (e.g., Valsalva maneuver), and blood loss can contribute to worsening LVOT gradients in women with obstructive hypertrophic cardiomyopathy. Those with good functional capacity, preserved LV systolic function, and no significant LVOT obstruction or arrhythmias often do well in pregnancy. The hemodynamic changes of pregnancy may be poorly tolerated in women with more severe disease. Ventricular tachycardia, atrial fibrillation, heart failure, angina, and syncope have been described during pregnancy.[89,97–99] Maternal deaths are rare but have been reported for women with high-risk features.[97] Precautions at the time of labor and delivery are necessary to prevent the complications that can occur with anesthesia and blood loss.

TTE is used for diagnosis when women present during pregnancy with symptoms suggesting cardiomyopathy. For women with preexisting cardiomyopathy, TTE is used for risk stratification and follow-up during pregnancy. TTE should be performed frequently during pregnancy to assess LV systolic function and PASPs.[34] The degree of LVOT obstruction should be documented in women with obstructive hypertrophic cardiomyopathy. TTE should include assessment for LV thrombus, particularly in women with PPCM.

FETAL AND NEONATAL RISK

Along with focusing on the mother, it is equally important to assess the significant fetal and neonatal risks in pregnancies of women with heart disease. Compared with pregnant women without heart disease, pregnant women with heart disease have higher risks of miscarriage, fetal or neonatal death, small for gestational age infant, premature birth, and the associated complications of respiratory distress syndrome and interventricular hemorrhage.[100] For example, a palliated or uncorrected cyanotic cardiac lesion portends a high risk of fetal death, regardless of the presence or absence of Eisenmenger syndrome. Table 40.3 lists the risk factors for fetal and neonatal complications in pregnant women with heart disease, many of which are the same factors that predict maternal complications in pregnancy.

Uteroplacental insufficiency due to reduction in maternal cardiac output has been the purported link between maternal heart disease and fetal or neonatal complications. Although there are preliminary studies linking abnormalities in maternal cardiac structure and function to fetal and neonatal complications and abnormal obstetric Doppler imaging, the mechanistic role of cardiac output has been assumed.[101] Cardiac output and abnormal umbilical artery Doppler findings (representing the downstream effect of uteroplacental insufficiency) have been identified as independent predictors of neonatal complications.[10]

For patients with congenital heart disease who do not have specific genetic syndromes, the recurrence risk of congenital heart disease in offspring is approximately 3% to 5%. Parental left heart obstructive lesions are associated with higher rates of transmission (13%–18%). Autosomal dominant conditions such as Noonan syndrome, Williams syndrome, Holt-Oram syndrome, Marfan syndrome, or 22q11.2 deletion syndrome confer a 50% risk of recurrence in offspring. The role of adult echocardiography is the diagnosis of lesions with a congenital basis, particularly those with an autosomal dominant or familial basis. Fetal echocardiograms at 18 to 22 weeks' gestation are offered to women with congenital heart disease and other inherited cardiac conditions.[34]

MANAGEMENT PRINCIPLES

Various guidelines address risk stratification and the management of pregnant women with heart disease. The most comprehensive guideline is from the European Society of Cardiology Task Force on the Management of Cardiovascular Diseases During Pregnancy.[34] Other guidelines by the American College of Cardiology/American Heart Association, American College

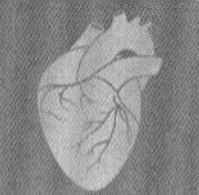

TABLE 40.5 Clinical Guidelines Addressing Risk Stratification and Management of Pregnant Women With Heart Disease: Recommendations Pertaining to Cardiac Imaging.

Guidelines	*Year*	*Key Recommendations for Cardiac Imaging*
European Society of Cardiology guidelines for the management of cardiovascular disease during pregnancy[34]	2018	• TTE is the preferred imaging method in pregnancy. • Echocardiography is recommended in any pregnant patient with unexplained or new cardiovascular signs or symptoms. • MRI (without gadolinium) should be considered if echocardiography is insufficient for a definite diagnosis.
2018 AHA/ACC guideline for the management of adults with congenital heart disease: a report of the American College of Cardiology/American Heart Association Task Force on Clinical Practice Guidelines[113]	2019	• No specific recommendations pertaining to cardiac imaging.
American College of Cardiology/American Heart Association guidelines for the management of patients with valvular heart disease[67]	2014	• Criteria for intervention on stenotic lesions before pregnancy include TTE thresholds (AS peak velocity > 4 m/s or mean gradient ≥40 mmHg, MS mitral valve area ≤1.5 cm^2. • TTE should be performed in women with native valve disease or prosthetic valves before pregnancy; if not before, then during pregnancy. • TEE should be performed in pregnant women with mechanical valves who have suspected valve obstruction or an embolic event.
Canadian Cardiovascular Society position statement on the management of thoracic aortic disease[111]	2014	• Cardiac CT is the preferred initial imaging study for acute aortic syndromes. • TEE is an appropriate alternative for acute aortic syndromes (1) when CT results are indeterminate, (2) if transport to CT is not feasible because of hemodynamic instability, or (3) if intraoperative TEE is needed when a dissection flap is seen on the initial TEE. • Recommendations for management of specific aortic disease during pregnancy are provided in supplemental S3 of guideline document.
American College of Chest Physicians evidence-based clinical practice guidelines on antithrombotic therapy and prevention of thrombosis[83]	2012	• Provides updated recommendations on the anticoagulation options for pregnant women with mechanical heart valves. • No specific recommendations pertaining to cardiac imaging.
American College of Cardiology/American Heart Association guidelines for the diagnosis and management of patients with thoracic aortic disease[112]	2010	• For measurements of the aorta by echocardiography, the internal diameter should be measured perpendicular to the axis of blood flow. • Widest diameter, typically at mid-sinus level, should be used for aortic root measurements. • Thresholds for treatment of asymptomatic ascending aortic aneurysm include absolute size, growth rate over time, and/or ratio of aorta area indexed by patient's height.

AS, Aortic stenosis; *CT*, cardiac tomography; *MRI*, magnetic resonance imaging; *MS*, mitral stenosis.

of Chest Physicians, European Society of Cardiology, and Canadian Cardiovascular Society are available (Table 40.5).

ANTEPARTUM PERIOD

Women who are at intermediate or high risk for complications during pregnancy should receive care from a multidisciplinary team at a center with expertise in pregnancy and heart disease. The team should include a cardiologist, maternal fetal medicine specialists, and anesthetists with expertise in pregnancy and heart disease. In specific cases, a hematologist, geneticist, and neonatologist should be involved. Fetal monitoring during pregnancy is an important aspect of care.

Differentiating cardiac signs and symptoms from the normal physiologic changes of pregnancy can be challenging. Pregnant women often have symptoms of fatigue, dyspnea, palpitations, dizziness, and pedal edema. On physical examination, women may have sinus tachycardia, a displaced apical impulse, prominence of the jugular venous pulsation, wide splitting of the first or second heart sound, systolic flow murmurs or continuous murmurs, and pedal edema. TTE is often used to differentiate cardiac conditions from normal pregnancy changes.

All women with heart disease should have an early pregnancy assessment, and a pregnancy plan should be established. The frequency of follow-up during pregnancy is individualized and is based on the pregnancy risk. Pregnancy surveillance includes TTE. For most cardiac lesions, TTE is performed at the first antenatal visit to assist in risk stratification, in the 3rd trimester at the time of the peak hemodynamic stress, and after delivery to reestablish a baseline. Women with high-risk cardiac lesions and those who develop symptoms during pregnancy need more frequent TTE monitoring.

LABOR AND DELIVERY

Vaginal delivery is the preferred mode of delivery because it is associated with less blood loss, thrombosis, and infection. Cesarean delivery is performed for women with Marfan syndrome who have a dilated aortic root (>4.5 cm) and for women who present in preterm labor while taking anticoagulants. Some groups suggest cesarean delivery for women with severe aortic stenosis and Eisenmenger syndrome.[34]

For women with high-risk cardiac conditions who require an experienced team at the time of delivery, induction of labor should be considered to better predict the timing of delivery. Preterm induction of labor is not usually indicated for women with cardiac conditions. For women undergoing a vaginal delivery, early epidural anesthesia is used to minimize pain, catecholamine surges, and hemodynamic fluctuations. Labor is often conducted in the left lateral decubitus position to avoid aortocaval compression. An assisted second stage of labor, with vacuum extraction or forceps, is used to minimize maternal explusive efforts by women with high-risk cardiac conditions.[102] Oxytocin can lead to vasodilation and hypotension and should be used with caution in women with significant cardiac disease.

Hemodynamic monitoring during labor and delivery should be individualized. Continuous electrocardiographic monitoring and pulse oximetry can be used as necessary. Arterial monitoring may be useful for women with severe ventricular systolic dysfunction, severe aortic stenosis, or PAH. Air and particulate filters are used on intravenous lines for women with intracardiac shunts to prevent paradoxical emboli. Endocarditis prophylaxis for uncomplicated vaginal deliveries is not recommended.[103]

The hemodynamic changes of labor and delivery do not return to baseline levels immediately after delivery. Women with high-risk cardiac lesions require additional monitoring before hospital discharge. Most women do not need a TTE evaluation immediately after delivery, but for women with PAH or severe LV systolic dysfunction, an early TTE before discharge may be helpful to examine ventricular function and exclude other complications. The safety of medications with breast feeding should be addressed before hospital discharge.[34]

POSTPARTUM PERIOD

The risk of cardiac complications extends into the postpartum period. Women are typically seen 1 to 2 months after delivery. Postpartum complications are particularly common in women with Eisenmenger syndrome and PAH from other causes, Marfan syndrome, and cardiomyopathies. These women should be seen earlier and more frequently in the postpartum period. TTE studies are an important aspect of postpartum assessment to reestablish a baseline and exclude important cardiac changes.

MANAGEMENT OF COMPLICATIONS

Any woman with heart disease who has signs of clinical deterioration should have a TTE. Table 40.6 shows common clinical presentations during pregnancy and associated cardiac lesions. When necessary, there are cardiac medications that are relatively safe to use during pregnancy. They include β-blockers, sotolol, digoxin, hydralazine, and furosemide (Lasix).

In women who develop arrhythmias, cardioversions are safe during pregnancy. Ablation without fluoroscopic exposure can be considered.[104] Catheter interventions during pregnancy include valvuloplasty, cardiac catheterization, and percutaneous coronary intervention. These interventions can be successfully performed during pregnancy, but radiation exposure to the fetus should be minimized by using appropriate shielding, shorter imaging durations, and the radial approach when possible. Radiation exposure dosages incurred with common cardiac interventions are available in published guidelines.[34]

Cardiovascular surgery during pregnancy is associated with maternal and fetal mortality rates of approximately 6% and 14% to 30%, respectively, and it should be avoided when possible.[105,106] Maternal hypotension and uterine contractions during extracorporeal circulation and consequent placental hypoperfusion contribute, with these factors conspiring to promote fetal hypoperfusion, hypoxia, and bradycardia. Fetal death during maternal cardiac surgery is predicted by maternal age, maternal functional class, reoperation, emergency surgery, type of myocardial protection, and anoxic time.[107] To minimize fetal risks, tailored anesthetic and bypass techniques can be used during cardiac surgery. In exceptional circumstances, cardiac surgery can be combined with elective cesarean delivery immediately before bypass.

TABLE 40.6 Clinical Presentations During Pregnancy and Associated Cardiac Lesions.

Clinical Presentation	*Cardiac Lesion*
Cardiac arrest	Cardiomyopathies Complex congenital heart disease Aortopathies Stenotic valve lesions
Heart failure	Cardiomyopathies Congenital heart disease Stenotic valve lesions Preeclampsia
Hypertension	Gestational hypertension Preeclampsia Coarctation of the aorta
Arrhythmias	Cardiomyopathies Valvular heart disease, stenotic lesions Congenital heart disease Long QT and other primary arrhythmias
Syncope	Stenotic valve lesions Congenital heart disease Hypertrophic cardiomyopathy Long QT and other primary arrhythmias
Stroke or transient ischemic attack	Eisenmenger syndrome Ebstein anomaly with larger PFOs or ASDs Intracardiac shunts (ASD or PFO)
Myocardial infarction	Coronary dissection Preexisting coronary disease Thromboembolism
Aortic dissection	Marfan syndrome and other inherited aortopathies Bicuspid valve disease
New or worsening cyanosis	Eisenmenger syndrome Cyanotic heart disease Ebstein anomaly with larger PFOs or ASDs Large intracardiac shunts (ASD or VSD)

ASD, Atrial septal defect; *PFO*, patent foramen ovale; *VSD*, ventricular septal defect.

LIMITATIONS OF ECHOCARDIOGRAPHY AND ALTERNATIVE APPOACHES

The gravid uterus can limit the ability to acquire standard views. Subcostal views are difficult to obtain when the gravid uterus is large. Off-axis views may be needed. LV wall thickness, LV mass, ventricular dimensions, transvalvular gradients, and the severity of regurgitant lesions can be affected by pregnancy. If values are abnormal, measurement of these parameters should be repeated after delivery.

Contrast agents are not used during pregnancy because no safety data are available. TEE is possible during pregnancy, although rarely necessary. It is sometimes used before cardioversion to exclude LA thrombus, to assess mechanical valve function in women with suspected valve thrombosis, or during cardiac interventions. Late in pregnancy, gastric emptying is delayed, and techniques to avoid aspiration are necessary. Fetal monitoring should be considered in women who receive sedation during TEE.[34]

When echocardiography cannot adequately answer an important clinical question, cardiac MRI or CT should be considered. For instance, women with inherited aortopathies such as Marfan syndrome and chest pain may require cardiac MRI or CT. Ideally, MRI scans should be performed after the 1st trimester, when the magnetic field is less likely to affect the developing fetus. Gadolinium is contraindicated during pregnancy.

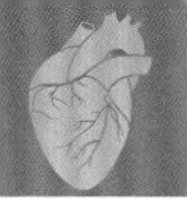

SUMMARY Heart Disease in Pregnancy.

Cardiac Lesion	Potential Cardiac Complications During Pregnancy	Echocardiographic Assessment
ASD (repaired and unrepaired)	Arrhythmias Paradoxical emboli	Type of ASD Size of ASD RV size and function RVSP
VSD (repaired and unrepaired)	Arrhythmias Congestive heart failure	Type of VSD Gradient across VSD LV size and function RVSP
PDA (repaired and unrepaired)	Arrhythmias Congestive heart failure	Gradient across PDA LV size and function RVSP
Repaired tetralogy of Fallot	Arrhythmias Right heart failure	RV size and function LV systolic function Severity of pulmonary regurgitation RV outflow tract gradient Severity of tricuspid regurgitation RVSP
Coarctation of the aorta (repaired and unrepaired)	Hypertensive disorders of pregnancy, including preeclampsia Aortic dissection Congestive heart failure	Coarctation gradient Aneurysms at the site of coarctation repair LV hypertrophy LV systolic function Assessment for bicuspid valve disease
Ebstein anomaly (repaired and unrepaired)	Arrhythmias Right heart failure Paradoxical emboli Cyanosis	Assessment of the tricuspid valve Severity of tricuspid regurgitation RV size and function Presence of ASD or PFO
Transposition of the great arteries with atrial switch operation and a Mustard or Senning operation	Congestive heart failure Deterioration in subaortic RV systolic function Arrhythmias Endocarditis	Subaortic RV size and function Severity of subaortic atrioventricular valve regurgitation Baffle leaks and stenosis LV systolic pressure (subpulmonic)
Transposition of the great arteries with arterial switch operation and a Jatene operation	Arrhythmias Progressive aortic dilation	LV size and systolic function Regional wall motion abnormalities Severity of aortic regurgitation Aortic root dimensions Severity of pulmonary stenosis
Fontan circulation	Arrhythmias Heart failure Thromboembolic complications Bleeding complications	Subaortic ventricle size and function Severity of atrioventricular valve regurgitation Atrial size Atrial thrombus Patency of Fontan connections
Eisenmenger syndrome	Maternal deaths Heart failure Arrhythmias Worsening cyanosis Pulmonary embolism Pulmonary artery rupture Bleeding complications	Intracardiac shunts RV size and function LV size and systolic function Severity of tricuspid regurgitation RVSP
Aortic stenosis	Congestive heart failure Syncope Arrhythmias, including sudden death Angina	Severity of aortic stenosis LV size and systolic function LV hypertrophy

Continued

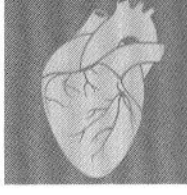

SUMMARY Heart Disease in Pregnancy.—cont'd

Cardiac Lesion	Potential Cardiac Complications During Pregnancy	Echocardiographic Assessment
Mitral stenosis	Arrhythmias, most commonly atrial fibrillation Congestive heart failure Thromboembolic complications	Severity of mitral stenosis LV size and systolic function RV size and systolic function LA size RVSP
Bioprosthetic heart valves	Arrhythmias Congestive heart failure	Bioprosthetic valve function LV and RV size and systolic function RVSP
Mechanical heart valves	Thromboembolic complications, including valve thrombosis Arrhythmias Heart failure Bleeding complications	Mechanical valve function LV and RV size and systolic function RVSP
Aortopathies	Aortic dissection or progressive aortic dilation Congestive heart failure in women with aortic or mitral regurgitation Other medium-sized vessel rupture Uterine rupture	Aortic dimensions Severity of aortic regurgitation Mitral valve prolapse Severity of mitral regurgitation
Idiopathic dilated cardiomyopathy	Heart failure Arrhythmias, including sudden death	LV size and systolic function Severity of mitral regurgitation Severity of tricuspid regurgitation RVSP
Peripartum cardiomyopathy	Maternal death Heart failure Arrhythmias, including sudden death Thromboembolic complications (e.g., LV thrombus)	LV size and systolic function LV thrombus Severity of mitral regurgitation Severity of tricuspid regurgitation RVSP
Hypertrophic cardiomyopathy	Heart failure Arrhythmias, including sudden death Syncope	LV hypertrophy LV outflow tract obstruction Systolic anterior motion of the anterior mitral valve leaflet Mitral regurgitation LV size and systolic function LA size

ASD, Atrial septal defect; *PDA*, patent ductus arteriosus; *PFO*, patent foramen ovale; *RVSP*, right ventricular systolic pressure; *VSD*, ventricular septal defect.

REFERENCES

1. Karamermer Y, Roos-Hesselink JW. Pregnancy and adult congenital heart disease. *Expert Rev Cardiovasc Ther*. 2007;5:859–869.
2. Robson SC, Hunter S, Boys RJ, Dunlop W. Serial study of factors influencing changes in cardiac output during human pregnancy. *Am J Physiol*. 1989;256:H1060–H1065.
3. Duvekot JJ, Cheriex EC, Pieters FA, Menheere PP, Peeters LH. Early pregnancy changes in hemodynamics and volume homeostasis are consecutive adjustments triggered by a primary fall in systemic vascular tone. *Am J Obstet Gynecol*. 1993;169:1382–1392.
4. Clark SL, Cotton DB, Lee W, et al. Central hemodynamic assessment of normal term pregnancy. *Am J Obstet Gynecol*. 1989;161:1439–1442.
5. Rubler S, Damani PM, Pinto ER. Cardiac size and performance during pregnancy estimated with echocardiography. *Am J Cardiol*. 1977;40:534–540.
6. Katz R, Karliner JS, Resnik R. Effects of a natural volume overload state (pregnancy) on left ventricular performance in normal human subjects. *Circulation*. 1978;58:434–441.
7. Mabie WC, DiSessa TG, Crocker LG, Sibai BM, Arheart KL. A longitudinal study of cardiac output in normal human pregnancy. *Am J Obstet Gynecol*. 1994;170:849–856.
8. Robson SC, Hunter S, Moore M, Dunlop W. Haemodynamic changes during the puerperium: a Doppler and M-mode echocardiographic study. *Br J Obstet Gynaecol*. 1987;94:1028–1039.
9. Ueland K, Novy MJ, Metcalfe J. Hemodynamic responses of patients with heart disease to pregnancy and exercise. *Am J Obstet Gynecol*. 1972;113:47–59.
10. Wald RM, Silversides CK, Kingdom J, et al. Maternal cardiac output and fetal Doppler predict adverse neonatal outcomes in pregnant women with heart disease. *J Am Heart Assoc*. 2015;4.
11. Campos O. Doppler echocardiography during pregnancy: physiological and abnormal findings. *Echocardiography*. 1996;13:135–146.
12. Campos O, Andrade JL, Bocanegra J, et al. Physiologic multivalvular regurgitation during pregnancy: a longitudinal Doppler echocardiographic study. *Int J Cardiol*. 1993;40:265–272.

13. Mashini IS, Albazzaz SJ, Fadel HE, et al. Serial noninvasive evaluation of cardiovascular hemodynamics during pregnancy. *Am J Obstet Gynecol.* 1987;156:1208–1213.
14. Geva T, Mauer MB, Striker L, Kirshon B, Pivarnik JM. Effects of physiologic load of pregnancy on left ventricular contractility and remodeling. *Am Heart J.* 1997;133:53–59.
15. Vogt M, Muller J, Kuhn A, Elmenhorst J, Muhlbauer F, Oberhoffer R. Cardiac adaptation of the maternal heart during pregnancy: a color-coded tissue Doppler imaging study - feasibility, reproducibility and course during pregnancy. *Ultraschall der Med.* 2015;36:270–275.
16. Cong J, Fan T, Yang X, et al. Structural and functional changes in maternal left ventricle during pregnancy: a three-dimensional speckle-tracking echocardiography study. *Cardiovasc Ultrasound.* 2015;13:6.
17. Sengupta SP, Bansal M, Hofstra L, Sengupta PP, Narula J. Gestational changes in left ventricular myocardial contractile function: new insights from two-dimensional speckle tracking echocardiography. *Int J Cardiovasc Imaging.* 2017;33:69–82.
18. Papadopoulou E, Kaladaridou A, Agrios J, Matthaiou J, Pamboukas C, Toumanidis S. Factors Influencing the twisting and untwisting properties of the left ventricle during normal pregnancy. *Echocardiography.* 2014;31:155–163.
19. Tasar O, Kocabay G, Karagoz A, et al. Evaluation of left atrial functions by 2-dimensional speckle-tracking echocardiography during healthy pregnancy. *J Ultrasound Med.* 2019. https://doi:10.1002/jum.15004.
20. Mor-Avi V, Lang RM, Badano LP, et al. Current and evolving echocardiographic techniques for the quantitative evaluation of cardiac mechanics: ASE/EAE consensus statement on methodology and indications endorsed by the Japanese Society of Echocardiography. *J Am Soc Echocardiogr.* 2011;24:277–313.
21. Siu SC, Sermer M, Colman JM, et al. Prospective multicenter study of pregnancy outcomes in women with heart disease. *Circulation.* 2001;104:515–521.
22. Silversides CK, Grewal J, Mason J, et al. Pregnancy outcomes in women with heart disease: the CARPREG II study. *J Am Coll Cardiol.* 2018;71:2419–2430.
23. Drenthen W, Boersma E, Balci A, et al. Predictors of pregnancy complications in women with congenital heart disease. *Eur Heart J.* 2010;31:2124–2132.
24. Khairy P, Ouyang DW, Fernandes SM, Lee-Parritz A, Economy KE, Landzberg MJ. Pregnancy outcomes in women with congenital heart disease. *Circulation.* 2006;113:517–524.
25. Siu SC, Sermer M, Harrison DA, et al. Risk and predictors for pregnancy-related complications in women with heart disease. *Circulation.* 1997;96:2789–2794.
26. Liu H, Huang T, Zhao W, Shen Y, Lin J. Pregnancy outcomes and relative risk factors among Chinese women with congenital heart disease. *Int J Gynaecol Obstet.* 2013;120:245–248.
27. Drenthen W, Pieper PG, Roos-Hesselink JW, et al. Outcome of pregnancy in women with congenital heart disease: a literature review. *J Am Coll Cardiol.* 2007;49:2303–2311.
28. Krul SP, van der Smagt JJ, van den Berg MP, Sollie KM, Pieper PG, van Spaendonck-Zwarts KY. Systematic review of pregnancy in women with inherited cardiomyopathies. *Eur J Heart Fail.* 2011;13:584–594.
29. Stergiopoulos K, Shiang E, Bench T. Pregnancy in patients with pre-existing cardiomyopathies. *J Am Coll Cardiol.* 2011;58:337–350.
30. Lameijer H, Burchill LJ, Baris L, et al. Pregnancy in women with pre-existent ischaemic heart disease: a systematic review with individualised patient data. *Heart.* 2019;105:873–880.
31. Wanga S, Silversides C, Dore A, de Waard V, Mulder B. Pregnancy and thoracic aortic disease: managing the risks. *Can J Cardiol.* 2016;32:78–85.
32. Ducas R, Javier D, D'Souza R, Silversides CK, Tsang W. Pregnancy outcomes in women with significant valve disease: a systematic review and meta-analysis. *Heart.* 2020;106(7):512–519. 2019.
33. Thorne S, MacGregor A, Nelson-Piercy C. Risks of contraception and pregnancy in heart disease. *Heart.* 2006;92:1520–1525.
34. Regitz-Zagrosek V, Roos-Hesselink JW, Bauersachs J, ESC Scientific Document Group, et al. 2018 ESC Guidelines for the management of cardiovascular diseases during pregnancy. *Eur Heart J.* 2018;39(34):3165–3241.
35. Roos-Hesselink JW, Ruys TP, Stein JI, et al. Outcome of pregnancy in patients with structural or ischaemic heart disease: results of a registry of the European Society of Cardiology. *Eur Heart J.* 2013;34:657–665.
36. Yap SC, Drenthen W, Pieper PG, et al. Pregnancy outcome in women with repaired versus unrepaired isolated ventricular septal defect. *BJOG.* 2010;117:683–689.
37. Yap SC, Drenthen W, Meijboom FJ, et al. Comparison of pregnancy outcomes in women with repaired versus unrepaired atrial septal defect. *BJOG.* 2009;116:1593–1601.
38. Drenthen W, Pieper PG, van der Tuuk K, et al. Cardiac complications relating to pregnancy and recurrence of disease in the offspring of women with atrioventricular septal defects. *Eur Heart J.* 2005;26:2581–2587.
39. Veldtman GR, Connolly HM, Grogan M, Ammash NM, Warnes CA. Outcomes of pregnancy in women with tetralogy of Fallot. *J Am Coll Cardiol.* 2004;44:174–180.
40. Greutmann M, Von Klemperer K, Brooks R, Peebles D, O'Brien P, Walker F. Pregnancy outcome in women with congenital heart disease and residual haemodynamic lesions of the right ventricular outflow tract. *Eur Heart J.* 31:1764–1770.
41. Balci A, Drenthen W, Mulder BJ, et al. Pregnancy in women with corrected tetralogy of Fallot: occurrence and predictors of adverse events. *Am Heart J.* 2011;161:307–313.
42. Uebing A, Arvanitis P, Li W, et al. Effect of pregnancy on clinical status and ventricular function in women with heart disease. *Int J Cardiol.* 2010;139:50–59.
43. Egidy Assenza G, Cassater D, Landzberg M, et al. The effects of pregnancy on right ventricular remodeling in women with repaired tetralogy of Fallot. *Int J Cardiol.* 2013;168:1847–1852.
44. Metz TD, Hayes SA, Garcia CY, Yetman AT. Impact of pregnancy on the cardiac health of women with prior surgeries for pulmonary valve anomalies. *Am J Obstet Gynecol.* 209:370 e1–6.
45. Beauchesne LM, Connolly HM, Ammash NM, Warnes CA. Coarctation of the aorta: outcome of pregnancy. *J Am Coll Cardiol.* 2001;38: 1728–1733.
46. Vriend JW, Drenthen W, Pieper PG, et al. Outcome of pregnancy in patients after repair of aortic coarctation. *Eur Heart J.* 2005;26:2173–2178.
47. Krieger EV, Landzberg MJ, Economy KE, Webb GD, Opotowsky AR. Comparison of risk of hypertensive complications of pregnancy among women with versus without coarctation of the aorta. *Am J Cardiol.* 2011;107:1529–1534.
48. Tan JL, Babu-Narayan SV, Henein MY, Mullen M, Li W. Doppler echocardiographic profile and indexes in the evaluation of aortic coarctation in patients before and after stenting. *J Am Coll Cardiol.* 2005;46:1045–1053.
49. Connolly HM, Warnes CA. Ebstein's anomaly: outcome of pregnancy. *J Am Coll Cardiol.* 1994;23:1194–1198.
50. Donnelly JE, Brown JM, Radford DJ. Pregnancy outcome and Ebstein's anomaly. *Br Heart J.* 1991;66:368–371.
51. Drenthen W, Pieper PG, Ploeg M, et al. Risk of complications during pregnancy after Senning or Mustard (atrial) repair of complete transposition of the great arteries. *Eur Heart J.* 2005;26:2588–2595.
52. Clarkson PM, Wilson NJ, Neutze JM, North RA, Calder AL, Barratt-Boyes BG. Outcome of pregnancy after the Mustard operation for transposition of the great arteries with intact ventricular septum. *J Am Coll Cardiol.* 1994;24:190–193.
53. Genoni M, Jenni R, Hoerstrup SP, Vogt P, Turina M. Pregnancy after atrial repair for transposition of the great arteries. *Heart.* 1999;81:276–277.
54. Guedes A, Mercier LA, Leduc L, Berube L, Marcotte F, Dore A. Impact of pregnancy on the systemic right ventricle after a Mustard operation for transposition of the great arteries. *J Am Coll Cardiol.* 2004;44:433–437.
55. Radford DJ, Stafford G. Pregnancy and the Rastelli operation. *Aust N Z J Obstet Gynaecol.* 2005;45:243–247.
56. Tobler D, Fernandes SM, Wald RM, et al. Pregnancy outcomes in women with transposition of the great arteries and arterial switch operation. *Am J Cardiol.* 106:417–420.
57. Horiuchi C, Kamiya CA, Ohuchi H, et al. Pregnancy outcomes and mid-term prognosis in women after arterial switch operation for dextro-transposition of the great arteries - Tertiary hospital experiences and review of literature. *J Cardiol.* 2019;73(3):247–254.
58. Connolly HM, Grogan M, Warnes CA. Pregnancy among women with congenitally corrected transposition of great arteries. *J Am Coll Cardiol.* 1999;33:1692–1695.
59. Canobbio MM, Mair DD, van der Velde M, Koos BJ. Pregnancy outcomes after the Fontan repair. *J Am Coll Cardiol.* 1996;28:763–767.
60. Garcia Ropero A, Baskar S, Roos Hesselink JW, et al. Pregnancy in women with a Fontan circulation: a systematic review of the literature. *Circ Cardiovasc Qual Outcomes.* 2018;11. e004575.
61. Gouton M, Nizard J, Patel M, et al. Maternal and fetal outcomes of pregnancy with Fontan circulation: a multicentric observational study. *Int J Cardiol.* 2015;187:84–89.
62. Drenthen W, Pieper PG, Roos-Hesselink JW, et al. Pregnancy and delivery in women after Fontan palliation. *Heart.* 2006;92:1290–1294.
63. Presbitero P, Somerville J, Stone S, Aruta E, Spiegelhalter D, Rabajoli F. Pregnancy in cyanotic congenital heart disease. Outcome of mother and fetus. *Circulation.* 1994;89:2673–2676.

64. Gleicher N, Midwall J, Hochberger D, Jaffin H. Eisenmenger's syndrome and pregnancy. *Obstet Gynecol Surv*. 1979;34:721–741.
65. Weiss BM, Zemp L, Seifert B, Hess OM. Outcome of pulmonary vascular disease in pregnancy: a systematic overview from 1978 through 1996. *J Am Coll Cardiol*. 1998;31:1650–1657.
66. Bedard E, Dimopoulos K, Gatzoulis MA. Has there been any progress made on pregnancy outcomes among women with pulmonary arterial hypertension? *Eur Heart J*. 2009;30:256–265.
67. Nishimura RA, Otto CM, Bonow RO, et al. 2014 AHA/ACC guideline for the management of patients with valvular heart disease: executive summary: a report of the American College of Cardiology/American Heart Association Task Force on Practice Guidelines. *J Am Coll Cardiol*. 2014;63:2438–2488.
68. Lao TT, Sermer M, MaGee L, Farine D, Colman JM. Congenital aortic stenosis and pregnancy—a reappraisal. *Am J Obstet Gynecol*. 1993;169:540–545.
69. Hameed A, Karaalp IS, Tummala PP, et al. The effect of valvular heart disease on maternal and fetal outcome of pregnancy. *J Am Coll Cardiol*. 2001;37:893–899.
70. Silversides CK, Colman JM, Sermer M, Farine D, Siu SC. Early and intermediate-term outcomes of pregnancy with congenital aortic stenosis. *Am J Cardiol*. 2003;91:1386–1389.
71. Yap SC, Drenthen W, Pieper PG, et al. Risk of complications during pregnancy in women with congenital aortic stenosis. *Int J Cardiol*. 2008;126:240–246.
72. Tzemos N, Silversides CK, Colman JM, et al. Late cardiac outcomes after pregnancy in women with congenital aortic stenosis. *Am Heart J*. 2009;157:474–480.
73. Tzemos N, Harris L, Carasso S, et al. Adverse left ventricular mechanics in adults with repaired tetralogy of Fallot. *Am J Cardiol*. 2009;103:420–425.
74. Tzemos N, Silversides CK, Carasso S, Rakowski H, Siu SC. Effect of pregnancy on left ventricular motion (twist) in women with aortic stenosis. *Am J Cardiol*. 2008;101:870–873.
75. Silversides CK, Colman JM, Sermer M, Siu SC. Cardiac risk in pregnant women with rheumatic mitral stenosis. *Am J Cardiol*. 2003;91:1382–1385.
76. Sawhney H, Aggarwal N, Suri V, Vasishta K, Sharma Y, Grover A. Maternal and perinatal outcome in rheumatic heart disease. *Int J Gynaecol Obstet*. 2003;80:9–14.
77. Diao M, Kane A, Ndiaye MB, et al. Pregnancy in women with heart disease in sub-Saharan Africa. *Arch Cardiovasc Dis*. 2011;104:370–374.
78. al Kasab SM, Sabag T, al Zaibag M, et al. Beta-adrenergic receptor blockade in the management of pregnant women with mitral stenosis. *Am J Obstet Gynecol*. 1990;163:37–40.
79. Iung B, Cormier B, Elias J, et al. Usefulness of percutaneous balloon commissurotomy for mitral stenosis during pregnancy. *Am J Cardiol*. 1994;73:398–400.
80. McLintock C, McCowan LM, North RA. Maternal complications and pregnancy outcome in women with mechanical prosthetic heart valves treated with enoxaparin. *BJOG*. 2009;116:1585–1592.
81. Yinon Y, Siu SC, Warshafsky C, et al. Use of low molecular weight heparin in pregnant women with mechanical heart valves. *Am J Cardiol*. 2009;104:1259–1263.
82. D'Souza R, Ostro J, Shah PS, et al. Anticoagulation for pregnant women with mechanical heart valves: a systematic review and meta-analysis. *Eur Heart J*. 2017;38:1509–1516.
83. Bates SM, Greer IA, Middeldorp S, Veenstra DL, Prabulos AM, Vandvik PO. VTE, thrombophilia, antithrombotic therapy, and pregnancy: antithrombotic therapy and prevention of thrombosis, 9th ed: American College of Chest Physicians Evidence-Based Clinical Practice Guidelines. *Chest*. 2012;141:e691S–736S.
84. North RA, Sadler L, Stewart AW, McCowan LM, Kerr AR, White HD. Long-term survival and valve-related complications in young women with cardiac valve replacements. *Circulation*. 1999;99:2669–2676.
85. Immer FF, Bansi AG, Immer-Bansi AS, et al. Aortic dissection in pregnancy: analysis of risk factors and outcome. *Ann Thorac Surg*. 2003;76:309–314.
86. Goland S, Elkayam U. Cardiovascular problems in pregnant women with marfan syndrome. *Circulation*. 2009;119:619–623.
87. Donnelly RT, Pinto NM, Kocolas I, Yetman AT. The immediate and long-term impact of pregnancy on aortic growth rate and mortality in women with Marfan syndrome. *J Am Coll Cardiol*. 2012;60:224–229.
88. Meijboom LJ, Vos FE, Timmermans J, Boers GH, Zwinderman AH, Mulder BJ. Pregnancy and aortic root growth in the Marfan syndrome: a prospective study. *Eur Heart J*. 2005;26:914–920.
89. Avila WS, Rossi EG, Ramires JA, et al. Pregnancy in patients with heart disease: experience with 1,000 cases. *Clin Cardiol*. 2003;26:135–142.
90. Ruys TP, Roos-Hesselink JW, Hall R, et al. Heart failure in pregnant women with cardiac disease: data from the ROPAC. *Heart*. 2014;100:231–238.
91. Grewal J, Siu SC, Ross HJ, et al. Pregnancy outcomes in women with dilated cardiomyopathy. *J Am Coll Cardiol*. 2009;55:45–52.
92. Bauersachs J, Konig T, van der Meer P, et al. Pathophysiology, diagnosis and management of peripartum cardiomyopathy: a position statement from the Heart Failure Association of the European Society of Cardiology Study Group on peripartum cardiomyopathy. *Eur J Heart Fail*. 2019;21:827–843.
93. McNamara DM, Elkayam U, Alharethi R, et al. Clinical outcomes for peripartum cardiomyopathy in North America: results of the IPAC study (Investigations of pregnancy-associated cardiomyopathy). *J Am Coll Cardiol*. 2015;66:905–914.
94. Elkayam U. Clinical characteristics of peripartum cardiomyopathy in the United States: diagnosis, prognosis, and management. *J Am Coll Cardiol*. 2011;58:659–670.
95. Sliwa K, Blauwet L, Tibazarwa K, et al. Evaluation of bromocriptine in the treatment of acute severe peripartum cardiomyopathy: a proof-of-concept pilot study. *Circulation*. 2011;121:1465–1473.
96. Elkayam U, Tummala PP, Rao K, et al. Maternal and fetal outcomes of subsequent pregnancies in women with peripartum cardiomyopathy. *N Engl J Med*. 2001;344:1567–1571.
97. Autore C, Conte MR, Piccininno M, et al. Risk associated with pregnancy in hypertrophic cardiomyopathy. *J Am Coll Cardiol*. 2002;40:1864–1869.
98. Avila WS, Amaral FM, Ramires JA, et al. Influence of pregnancy on clinical course and fetal outcome of women with hypertrophic cardiomyopathy. *Arq Bras Cardiol*. 2007;88:480–485.
99. Thaman R, Varnava A, Hamid MS, et al. Pregnancy related complications in women with hypertrophic cardiomyopathy. *Heart*. 2003;89:752–756.
100. Siu SC, Colman JM, Sorensen S, et al. Adverse neonatal and cardiac outcomes are more common in pregnant women with cardiac disease. *Circulation*. 2002;105:2179–2184.
101. Pieper PG, Balci A, Aarnoudse JG, et al. Uteroplacental blood flow, cardiac function, and pregnancy outcome in women with congenital heart disease. *Circulation*. 2013;128:2478–2487.
102. Robertson JE, Silversides CK, Mah ML, et al. A contemporary approach to the obstetric management of women with heart disease. *J Obstet Gynaecol Can*. 2012;34:812–819.
103. Wilson W, Taubert KA, Gewitz M, et al. Prevention of infective endocarditis: guidelines from the American Heart Association: a Guideline From the American Heart Association Rheumatic Fever, Endocarditis and Kawasaki Disease Committee, Council on Cardiovascular Disease in the Young, and the Council on Clinical Cardiology, Council on Cardiovascular Surgery and Anesthesia, and the Quality of Care and Outcomes Research Interdisciplinary Working Group. *J Am Dent Assoc*. 2008;139(Suppl):3S–24S.
104. Li MM, Sang CH, Jiang CX, et al. Maternal arrhythmia in structurally normal heart: Prevalence and feasibility of catheter ablation without fluoroscopy. *Pacing Clin Electrophysiol*. 2019 Oct 17. https://doi.org/10.1111/pace.13819. (Epub ahead of print).
105. Weiss BM, von Segesser LK, Alon E, Seifert B, Turina MI. Outcome of cardiovascular surgery and pregnancy: a systematic review of the period 1984-1996. *Am J Obstet Gynecol*. 1998;179:1643–1653.
106. John AS, Gurley F, Schaff HV, et al. Cardiopulmonary bypass during pregnancy. *Ann Thorac Surg*. 2011;91:1191–1196.
107. Arnoni RT, Arnoni AS, Bonini RC, et al. Risk factors associated with cardiac surgery during pregnancy. *Ann Thorac Surg*. 2003;76:1605–1608.
108. Vered Z, Poler SM, Gibson P, Wlody D, Perez JE. Noninvasive detection of the morphologic and hemodynamic changes during normal pregnancy. *Clin Cardiol*. 1991;14:327–334.
109. Savu O, Jurcut R, Giusca S, et al. Morphological and functional adaptation of the maternal heart during pregnancy. *Circ Cardiovasc Imaging*. 2012;5:289–297.
110. Sadaniantz A, Kocheril AG, Emaus SP, Garber CE, Parisi AF. Cardiovascular changes in pregnancy evaluated by two-dimensional and Doppler echocardiography. *J Am Soc Echocardiogr*. 1992;5:253–258.
111. Boodhwani M, Andelfinger G, Leipsic J, et al. Canadian Cardiovascular Society position statement on the management of thoracic aortic disease. *Can J Cardiol*. 2014;30:577–589.
112. Hiratzka LF, Bakris GL, Beckman JA, et al. 2010 ACCF/AHA/AATS/ACR/ASA/SCA/SCAI/SIR/STS/SVM guidelines for the diagnosis and management of patients with thoracic aortic disease. A report of the American

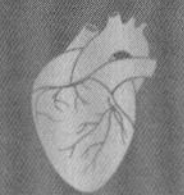

College of Cardiology Foundation/American Heart Association Task Force on Practice Guidelines, American Association for Thoracic Surgery, American College of Radiology, American Stroke Association, Society of Cardiovascular Anesthesiologists, Society for Cardiovascular Angiography and Interventions, Society of Interventional Radiology, Society of Thoracic Surgeons, and Society for Vascular Medicine. *J Am Coll Cardiol.* 2010;55:e27–e129.

113. Stout KK, Daniels CJ, Aboulhosn JA, et al. 2018 AHA/ACC guideline for the management of adults with congenital heart disease: a report of the American College of Cardiology/American Heart Association Task Force on Clinical Practice Guidelines. *J Am Coll Cardiol.* 2019;73(12):e81–e192.

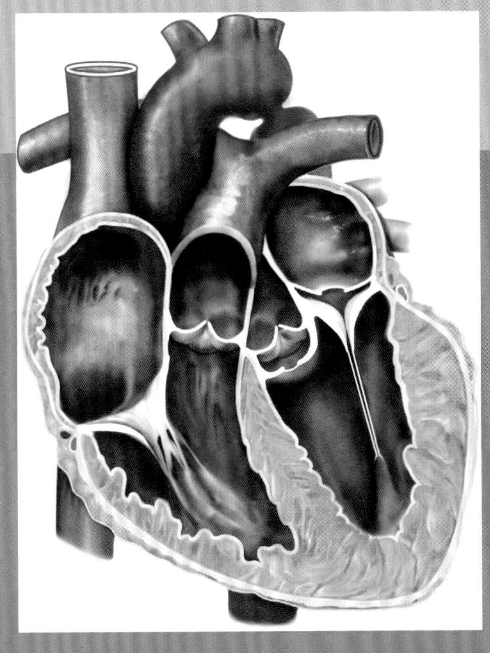

中文导读

第41章 先天性分流疾病

超声心动图在先天性分流疾病的筛查和诊断中起着核心作用，本章介绍了先天性分流型心脏病的定义、病理解剖、病理生理、超声心动图表现特点、外科及介入干预治疗指征。具体介绍了房水平分流中的继发孔型房间隔缺损、原发孔型房间隔、静脉窦缺损、无顶冠状静脉窦综合征、肺静脉异位引流，还有膜周部、肌部室间隔缺损等不同种类的室间隔缺损、动脉导管未闭、主动脉窦瘤破裂（瓦氏瘤窦破裂）、冠状动脉瘘等常见先天性分流心脏病的常用切面和超声特点。经胸、经食管二维、三维超声心动图及心腔内超声心动图等多普勒超声心动图技术的综合应用有助于无创评估先天性分流疾病的确切分流部分、缺损大小及数目、测量流速，以及计算跨分流的梯度、心室和瓣膜功能、心房室大小、肺静脉和腔静脉的连接，外科及介入治疗术前超声心动图特点及表现、评估要点及图像展示，检测干预术后残余分流和并发症的存在和程度。

王　燕

41 Congenital Shunts

JEANNETTE LIN, MD | JAMIL A. ABOULHOSN, MD

Approximately 1 in 100 adults have congenital heart disease. Congenital heart defects (CHDs) can be characterized as simple, moderate, or severe in complexity, based on the morbidity and mortality associated with each of these lesions.[1]

Echocardiography plays a central role in the screening and diagnosis of congenital shunts, and all pediatric and adult echocardiography laboratories should be accustomed to evaluating CHDs. Evaluation and management of adult CHDs requires detailed knowledge of (1) the original anatomy and physiology; (2) dynamic changes in anatomy and physiology that occur with time; (3) effects of adult diseases (e.g., systemic arterial hypertension, coronary artery disease) or conditions (e.g., pregnancy) on that physiology; (4) types of operative or transcatheter repair for each lesion, both current and historic; (5) presence and extent of possible postoperative residua, sequelae, and complications; (6) the echocardiographic appearance of different types of devices, expected sequelae, and potential complications; and (7) proper selection, performance, and interpretation of modalities required for anatomic imaging and hemodynamic assessment.

The goal of the echocardiographer is to define the defect, comment on the presence or absence of associated CHDs, and evaluate the residua or sequelae of unrepaired and repaired defects. Comprehensive use of echocardiography with Doppler facilitates the noninvasive assessment of ventricular and valvular function, atrial size, interatrial and intraatrial anatomy, connections of the pulmonary and systemic veins, and estimated intracardiac systolic and diastolic pressures. Used in combination with two-dimensional (2D) imaging, spectral and color Doppler echocardiography enable localization of native shunts, detection of residual shunts after intervention, measurement of flow velocity, and calculation of gradients across the shunts.

Transthoracic echocardiography (TTE) is the recommended modality for the initial evaluation of asymptomatic patients with an abnormal electrocardiogram or chest radiograph that is concerning for structural heart disease or an abnormal murmur auscultated during a physical examination.[2] To avoid late sequelae of chronic volume or pressure loading, even asymptomatic patients with unrepaired defects should be referred for consideration of repair if there is significant chamber dilation or the next left-to-right shunt is sufficiently large enough to cause physiologic sequelae.[1]

Repaired and unrepaired patients should have regular cardiology follow-up and lifelong surveillance echocardiograms because shunts may lead to late sequelae such as arrhythmias, heart failure, or residual or recurrent shunts from patch leaks.[1] Echocardiography is the recommended imaging modality for initial and serial evaluation of symptomatic patients with symptoms of right- or left-sided heart failure, evidence of pulmonary hypertension, atrial arrhythmias, or endocarditis.[1]

Transesophageal echocardiography (TEE) and intracardiac echocardiography (ICE) enable improved visualization of left-sided valves and the more posterior aspects of the heart. They can provide valuable information for diagnostic assessment and interventional guidance in CHDs. When questions remain, particularly regarding visualization of extracardiac structures, magnetic resonance imaging (MRI) or computed tomography (CT) provides useful additional information. Diagnostic cardiac catheterization remains important for confirmation of intracardiac and pulmonary artery pressures, confirmation of the degree of shunting, and preoperative evaluation of coronary arteries in the older adult.

When approaching cardiac shunts, it is helpful to differentiate between *pre-tricuspid* and *post-tricuspid* shunts based on whether the chamber receiving the flow is proximal or distal to the tricuspid valve (TV) (Table 41.1). Pre-tricuspid shunts result in volume loading of the right heart and therefore in symptoms and echocardiographic findings of right heart dilation. Pre-tricuspid shunts do not frequently lead to significant pulmonary vascular disease.

The degree of shunting across pre-tricuspid shunts depends on the size of the defect and relative right ventricle (RV) and left ventricle (LV) compliance. Post-tricuspid shunts result in pressure loading of the RV and volume loading of the left atrium (LA) and LV. Patients with moderate or large post-tricuspid shunts may have symptoms of left heart failure, RV hypertrophy with eventual dysfunction and dilation due to chronically increased pressure afterload, and LA or LV dilation due to volume loading.

The degree of shunting across a post-tricuspid shunt depends on the size of the defect and relative pulmonary and systemic vascular resistance. Nonrestrictive post-tricuspid shunts result in progressive elevation of pulmonary vascular resistance and

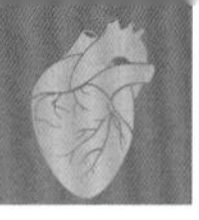

TABLE 41.1 Characteristics of Pre-tricuspid Versus Post-tricuspid Shunts.

Parameters	*Pre-Tricuspid Shunts*	*Post-Tricuspid Shunts*
Chamber receiving shunt flow	Systemic veins (IVC, SVC) RA Coronary sinus	RV Pulmonary artery
Examples	Atrial-level shunts Secundum ASD Primum ASD Sinus venous defects Unroofed coronary sinus LV-RA septal defect Anomalous pulmonary venous return Partial anomalous pulmonary veins Total anomalous pulmonary veins	VSD PDA Ruptured sinus of Valsalva aneurysm (aorta-to-RV shunt)
Hemodynamics	Right heart volume loading	RV pressure loading Left heart volume loading
Echocardiographic findings	RA dilation RV dilation Tricuspid regurgitation Mildly to moderately elevated pulmonary pressures Diastolic flattening of the ventricular septum	RV hypertrophy LA dilation LV dilation Severely elevated pulmonary pressures if large shunt, and shunt reversal (Eisenmenger syndrome) Systolic and diastolic flattening, ventricular septum

ASD, Atrial septal defect; *IVC*, inferior vena cava; *PDA*, patent ductus arteriosus; *SVC*, superior vena cava; *VSD*, ventricular septal defect.

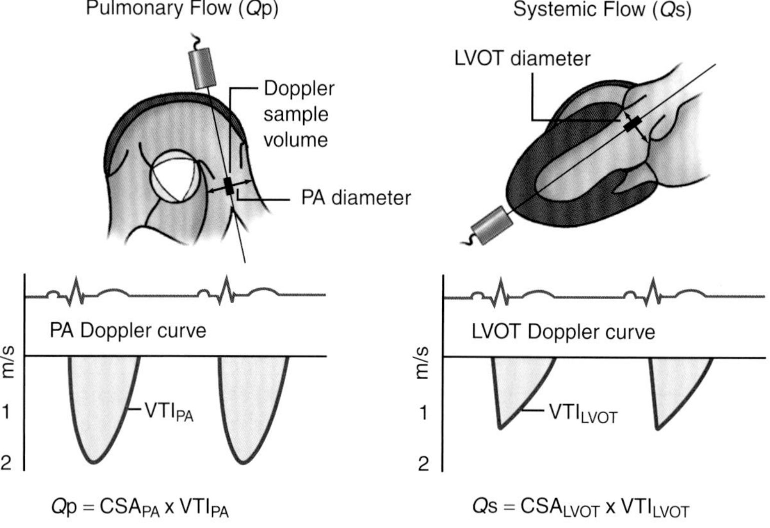

Fig. 41.1 Calculation of pulmonary blood flow *(Qp)* and systemic blood flow *(Qs)*. Pulmonary blood flow is equal to the cross-sectional area *(CSA)* of the pulmonary artery *(PA)* multiplied by the velocity–time integral *(VTI)* of pulmonary artery blood flow measured at the same site. Systemic blood flow is similarly measured using the LV outflow tract *(LVOT)* diameter and LVOT VTI.

eventual shunt reversal (Eisenmenger syndrome) if not corrected during the first few years of life. Both types of pre-tricuspid and post-tricuspid shunts may lead to right heart failure. Coronary artery fistulas are typically small and do not result in significant volume load but may cause symptoms of coronary insufficiency.

The ratio of pulmonary blood flow (Qp) to systemic blood flow (Qs) can be determined noninvasively with Doppler echocardiographic measurements of stroke volume at two intracardiac sites (Fig. 41.1). Most commonly, the Qp is calculated from the cross-sectional area (CSA) of the pulmonary artery and the velocity–time integral (VTI) gathered by a pulsed-wave Doppler sample at the site of area calculation; in patients with pulmonic valve stenosis, measurements may be made at the RVOT. In patients with pulmonary regurgitation, echocardiography should not be used to calculate Qp:Qs ratio. The Qs is calculated from the CSA of the left ventricular outflow tract (LVOT) and the LVOT VTI measured by PW Doppler. This method is reliable when 2D images are of sufficient quality for accurate measurements of the LVOT and right ventricular outflow tract (RVOT) or pulmonary artery diameters and when Doppler tracings are obtained parallel to flow. Small errors in 2D measurements can result in unreliable calculated values. If there are inconsistencies between the Qp:Qs ratio calculated from echocardiographic measurements and other echocardiographic or clinical findings, a cardiac catheterization should be performed, and pulmonary and systemic blood flow should be calculated using the Fick equation.

ATRIAL-LEVEL SHUNTS

OVERVIEW

Atrial septal defects (ASDs) account for approximately 10% of all congenital cardiac defects[3] and occur in approximately 4 of every 100,000 newborns. ASDs account for 25% to 30% of CHDs diagnosed in adults.[4] Three common types of defects result in interatrial shunts: secundum ASD, primum ASD, and sinus venosus defects (Fig. 41.2). A fourth type, the unroofed coronary sinus, is rare.

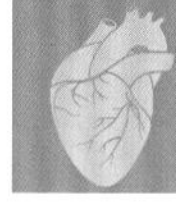

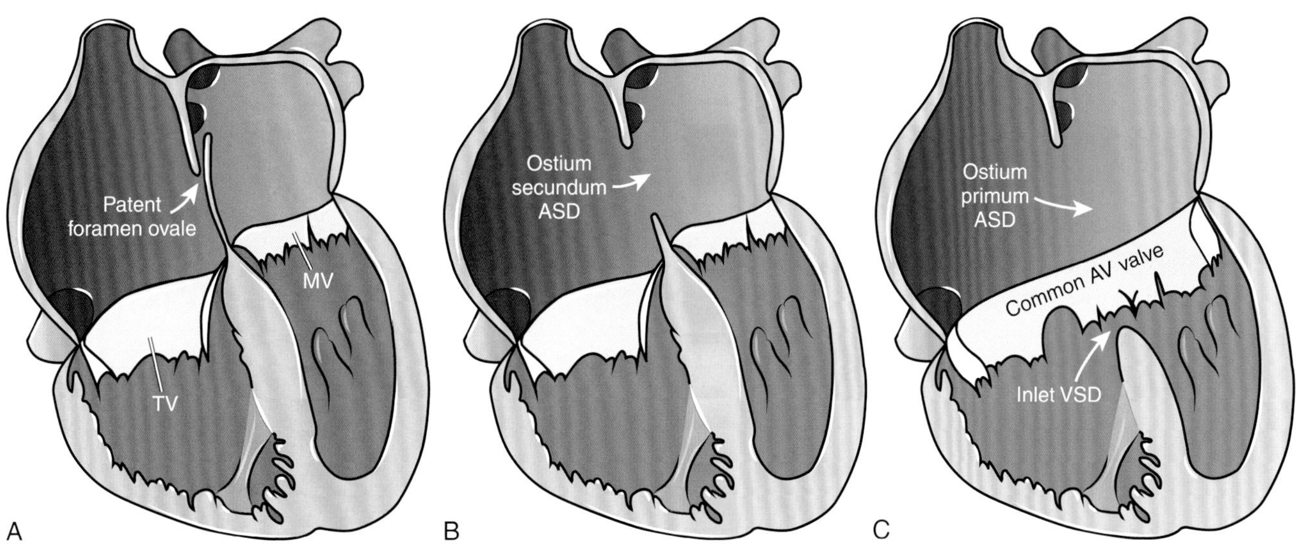

Fig. 41.2 Atrial-level shunts. (A) Patent foramen ovale. (B) An ostium secundum atrial septal defect *(ASD)*. (C) Ostium primum ASD with a common atrioventricular *(AV)* valve and associated inlet ventricular septal defect (*VSD*). *MV*, Mitral valve; *TV*, tricuspid valve.

The degree of shunting depends on relative ventricular compliance, which is determined by ventricular afterload. In a newborn with an isolated ASD, the RV is relatively thick and noncompliant due to elevated pulmonary vascular resistance in the fetal circulation. As the pulmonary vascular resistance decreases in the first months of life, RV hypertrophy regresses and the RV becomes more compliant than the LV, resulting in increased left-to-right shunting.

Individuals with small- to moderate-sized defects may remain asymptomatic until adulthood. As individuals age, the compliance of the LV decreases and LA pressures increase, resulting in even greater left-to-right shunting. After several decades of chronic right heart volume overload, patients may present with atrial arrhythmias or right heart failure.

Unexplained dilation of the RA and RV on TTE should trigger further evaluation for pre-tricuspid shunting. If no shunt is readily apparent on TTE, a TEE and/or cardiac CT or MRI should be considered. Atrial arrhythmias are uncommon in patients younger than 40 years of age.[5] Mild to moderate pulmonary hypertension is common; severe pulmonary hypertension occurs in 5% to 10% of patients with unrepaired ASDs, predominantly in women.[6] The cause of severe pulmonary hypertension in this minority of patients with ASDs is unclear. It appears to be unrelated to the degree of shunting and may represent the coexistence of idiopathic pulmonary arterial hypertension and an atrial-level communication.

MANAGEMENT

For all types of ASDs, repair is indicated if symptoms are present. For asymptomatic patients, repair should be considered to avoid late sequelae if right heart enlargement is identified or the Qp:Qs ratio is greater than 1.5:1.[1] Severe pulmonary hypertension (i.e., pulmonary artery systolic pressure or pulmonary vascular resistance greater than two thirds of the systemic resistance) and net right-to-left shunting are contraindications to ASD closure.[1] In selected cases, pulmonary vasodilators may decrease the pulmonary vascular resistance sufficiently to allow closure, and closure may improve functional capacity.[7]

There are unusual cases of right-to-left shunting through an atrial communication in the absence of pulmonary hypertension; a variety of mechanisms may cause this, including medially directed tricuspid regurgitation, inferior vena cava (IVC) flow directed toward the atrial communication by the eustachian valve, and decreased right heart compliance, as in repaired pulmonary atresia with an intact ventricular septum. In such cases, patients may benefit from ASD closure, but provocative testing with transient defect balloon occlusion and volume loading may be necessary to avoid subsequent elevations in RA pressure.

Post-repair TTE should include evaluation of chamber sizes and tricuspid regurgitation, evaluation for new or worsening mitral regurgitation, and evaluation for residual shunting. RA and RV dilation typically improves in the first 3 to 6 months after ASD closure, although persistent dilation and tricuspid regurgitation are common in patients with large shunts repaired later in life. Mitral regurgitation may increase after ASD closure in 10% to 30% of patients; this occurs more often in older patients and in those with atrial fibrillation, LA dilation, or tricuspid regurgitation.[8,9] Late postoperative recurrence of RA and RV dilation warrants close echocardiographic evaluation for residual shunting from the device or surgical patch leaks or the worsening of pulmonary arterial hypertension. Comprehensive echocardiographic assessment of chamber sizes, ventricular function, and pressure estimation is imperative before and after ASD closure.

SECUNDUM ATRIAL SEPTAL DEFECT

Overview

Secundum ASDs are the most common type of ASDs, accounting for approximately 75% of cases. The ostium secundum is a normal gap in septum that allows blood to bypass the lungs in the fetal circulation. During embryologic atrial septation, the ostium secundum is normally occluded by the septum secundum as it grows from the roof of the common atrium toward the crux of the heart. Secundum ASDs may result from inadequate growth of the septum secundum, which leads to persistence of the ostium secundum.

The size of secundum ASDs varies widely, from small fenestrations in the fossa ovalis to very large defects with minimal rims. They can be round or oval and may be single or multiple. Small defects typically do not result in any measurable degree of right heart enlargement or pulmonary hypertension and may not be readily apparent on TTE. Moderate to large defects can usually be identified on TTE. Dropout in the area of the fossa ovalis is common, and the presence of a shunt should be

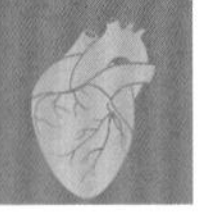

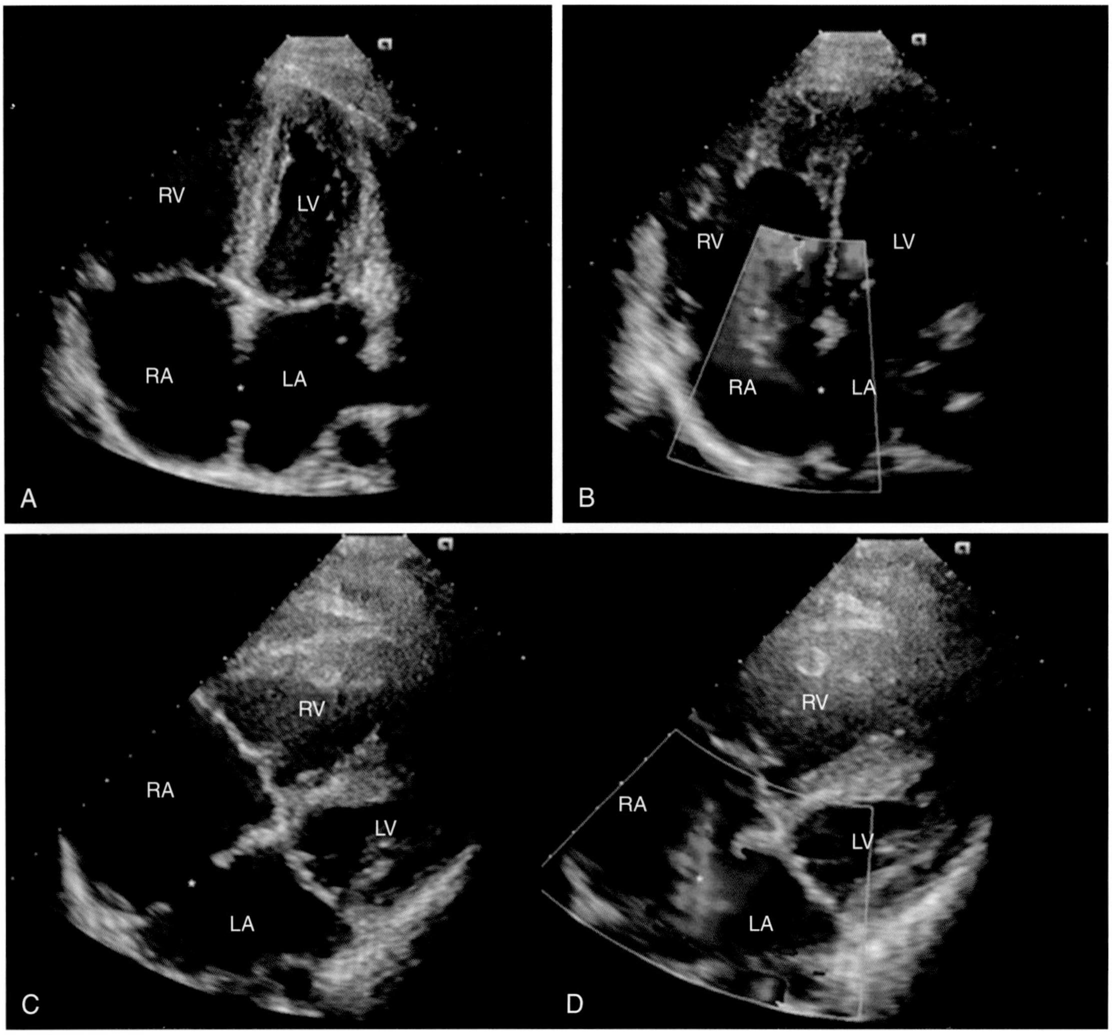

Fig. 41.3 Secundum atrial septal defect. TTE images demonstrate secundum atrial septal defect, denoted by an asterisk *(*)*. Apical 4-chamber view (A) and apical 4-chamber view with color (B). Notice that the interatrial shunting is not well visualized with color Doppler from the apical view because the flow is perpendicular to the angle of interrogation (see Videos 41.3A ▶ and 41.3B ▶). Subcostal view (C) and subcostal view with color flow (D). The interatrial shunting is well visualized from the subcostal view, with left-to-right shunting across the septum (see Videos 41.3C ▶ and 41.3D ▶).

confirmed with color Doppler. Spectral Doppler should then be used to confirm the direction of flow across the shunt, which can be predominantly left-to-right, right-to-left, or bidirectional (Fig. 41.3). The subcostal view is optimal for color imaging of flow across the ASD because the direction of flow is parallel to the ultrasound beam.

Agitated saline contrast studies can be used to confirm right-to-left interatrial shunting when there is uncertainty about the presence of an interatrial shunt on 2D imaging and color Doppler, but differentiating a patent foramen ovalis from a small ASD requires TEE for most adult patients. During an agitated saline contrast study, absence of agitated saline contrast adjacent to the interatrial septum due to inflow of blood without agitated saline contrast is called *negative contrast*. However, because superior vena cava (SVC) flow also streams along the interatrial septum, the presence or absence of negative contrast should be considered together with other echocardiographic findings to confirm an ASD.

Management

Transcatheter closure of secundum ASDs has replaced traditional surgical ASD closure in most cases. The feasibility of device closure depends on the size of the defect, adequacy of the tissue rims, proximity to valves and pulmonary veins, and whether any other CHD (e.g., anomalous pulmonary veins) is present (Table 41.2). These data are readily obtained with TEE imaging. The echocardiographer should interrogate the ASD at multiple angles to assess all rims (Fig. 41.4). ASDs are dynamic, and their dimensions vary throughout the cardiac cycle. The echocardiographer should report the maximal diameter of the defect in two orthogonal planes to assist with device selection.

TABLE 41.2 Echocardiographic Evaluation of Secundum Atrial Septal Defects.
Presence and depth of rims
Relationship to atrioventricular valves, SVC, IVC, pulmonary veins
Dimensions (often oval and dynamic)
RA and RV size and function
Tricuspid and pulmonic regurgitation
Pulmonary artery dilation
RV and pulmonary artery pressure estimation

IVC, Inferior vena cava; *PDA*, patent ductus arteriosus; *SVC*, superior vena cava; *VSD*, ventricular septal defect.

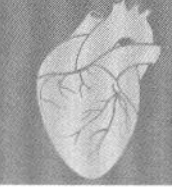

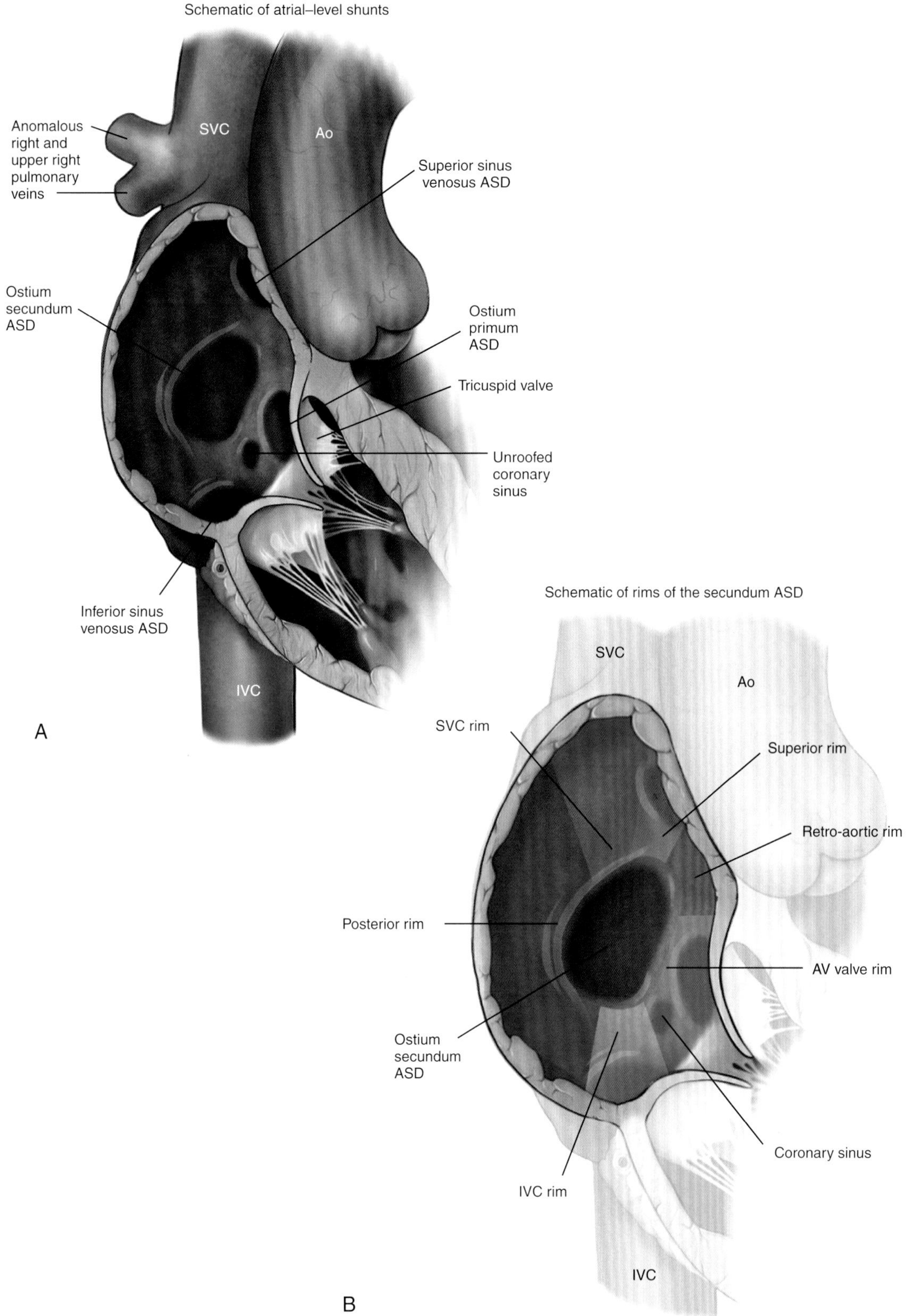

Fig. 41.4 Atrial-level shunts, en face view. (A) RA view of the interatrial septum demonstrates the locations of different types of atrial septal defects *(ASDs)*. (B) Schematic of the rims of the secundum ASD. *Ao,* Aorta; *AV,* atrioventricular; *IVC,* inferior vena cava; *SVC,* superior vena cava.

Three-dimensional (3D) TEE imaging is an important adjunct to 2D imaging. Multiplanar reconstruction ensures that the defect is measured accurately.[10] TEE images can be rotated to demonstrate the defect from the RA or LA side. If 3D images are being used to guide intervention, it is recommended that images be displayed in a standard format with the SVC at 12 o'clock from the RA view and the right upper pulmonary vein at 1 o'clock from the LA view to orient the image for the operator performing the transcatheter interventions[11] (Fig. 41.5).

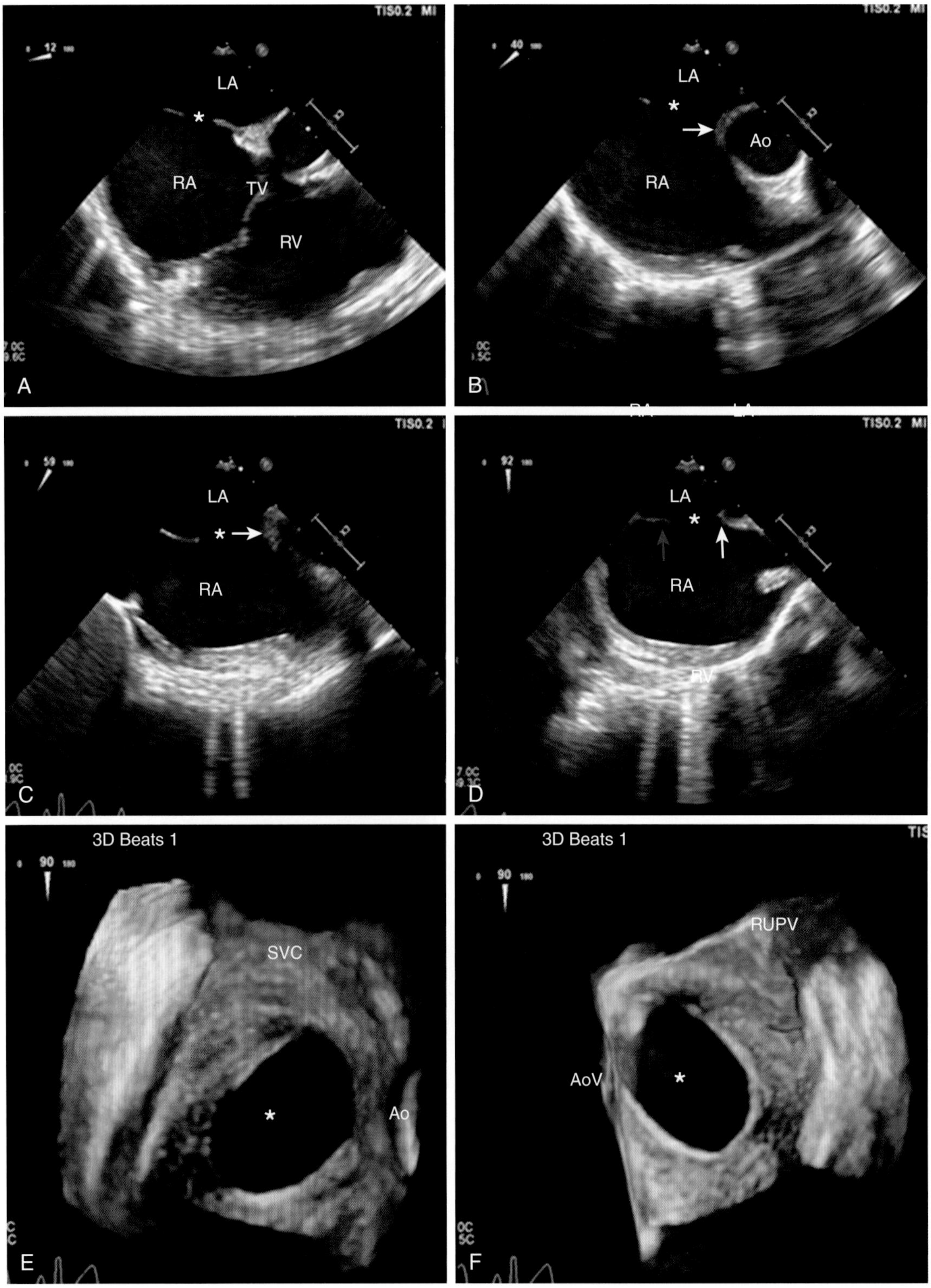

Fig. 41.5 **Evaluation of atrial septal defect by TEE.** TEE images from the mid-esophageal view demonstrate a complete evaluation of the rims of the atrial septal defect, which is denoted by an *asterisk (*)*. (A) Multiplane image at 0 to 15 degrees shows the atrioventricular valve rim and posterior rim (see Video 41.5A). (B) Multiplane image at 30 to 50 degrees shows the aortic rim *(arrow)* and posterior rim (see Video 41.5B). (C) Multiplane image at 60 to 80 degrees shows the superior rim *(arrow)* (see Video 41.5C). (D) Multiplane image at 90 to 120 degrees shows the SVC rim *(white arrow)* and IVC rim *(red arrow)* (see Video 41.5D). (E) 3D TEE view of the interatrial septum from the RA, with the SVC at 12 o'clock (see Video 41.5E). (F) 3D TEE view of the interatrial septum from the LA, with the RUPV at 1 o'clock (see Video 41.5F). *Ao*, Aorta; *AoV*, aortic valve; *RUPV*, right upper pulmonary vein; *SVC*, superior vena cava; *TV*, tricuspid valve.

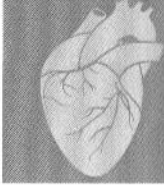

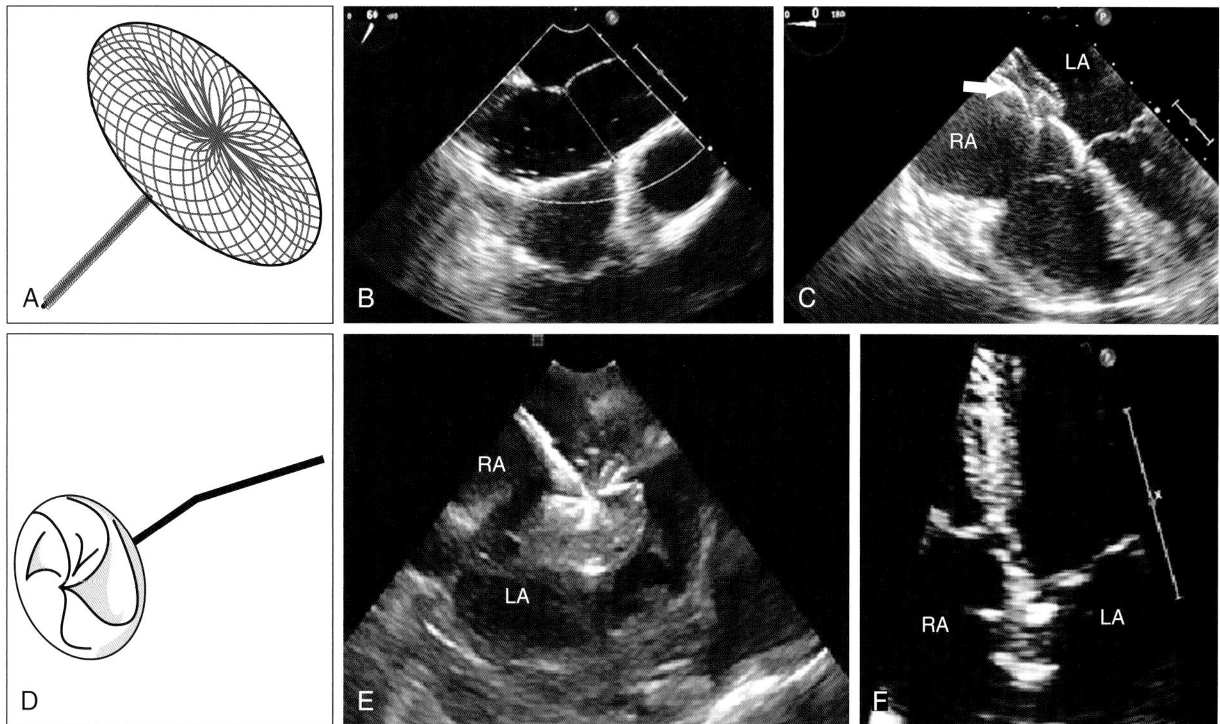

Fig. 41.6 Atrial septal occluder devices. (A) Amplatzer (Abbott, St. Paul, MN) atrial septal occluder. (B) Intraoperative balloon sizing of an atrial septal defect (see Video 41.6B). (C) TEE mid-esophageal 4-chamber view demonstrates the deployed Amplatzer occluder *(arrow)*. (D) Gore Cardioform septal occluder (W.L. Gore & Associates, Medical Products Division, Flagstaff, AZ). (E) Intracardiac echocardiogram obtained during device deployment (see Video 41.6E). (F) TTE apical 4-chamber view with the Gore device well seated in the interatrial septum (see Video 41.6F).

Amplatzer septal occluders and Gore ASD occluders are approved by the US Food and Drug Administration (FDA) for percutaneous ASD closure (Fig. 41.6). Previously, percutaneous ASD closure was limited to ASDs that are smaller than 30 mm in diameter and have at least 5 mm of circumferential rims. However, larger defects and defects with deficient rims have been closed successfully and with minimal complications.[12] Potential complications of ASDs include arrhythmias, device erosion, perforation, pericardial effusion, thromboembolic events, device embolization, and allergic reactions to the nickel alloy contained in the device.

ASD closures can be performed under ultrasound guidance with TEE or ICE. The advantage of ICE is that a single operator can maneuver the ICE catheter and deploy the device with the patient under moderate sedation. Disadvantages are the learning curve associated with operating the ICE catheter, difficulty visualizing and assessing all rims and pulmonary venous connections, and limited sector width for guiding closure of larger defects. TEE guidance requires a second operator, and patients require deep sedation or general anesthesia for the duration of the procedure because of the discomfort of prolonged intubation with the TEE probe. However, TEE allows a more comprehensive evaluation of the rims in larger defects.

During transcatheter ASD closure, a right heart catheterization is performed, and measurements of hemodynamics and saturations are obtained. A wire is advanced from a femoral vein, across the ASD, and into the left upper pulmonary vein under TEE/ICE and fluoroscopic guidance. A sizing balloon is advanced over the wire across the defect and inflated with a mixture of saline and iodinated contrast until flow across the ASD is completely obstructed by the inflated balloon and a discrete narrowing (i.e., waist) is seen in the balloon. The diameter of the waist is referred to as the *stretched diameter* of the defect; it is measured on both TEE and fluoroscopic images to guide device selection. The stretched diameter is typically 10% to 20% larger than the corresponding diameter on baseline images.

The echocardiographer must ensure that there is no residual shunting at this point. If flow continues to occur across the septum, a second defect could be present, or the balloon may need to be inflated further to seal the defect completely and give the most accurate measurement. The balloon is then slowly deflated until a small amount of flow is observed and then reinflated another few milliliters until cessation of flow is again seen; the balloon waist at this point is called the *stop flow diameter*. The stop flow diameter is typically used to guide selection of the device size.

The delivery sheath is advanced over a wire, across the defect, and into the LA, and the closure device is then advanced through the sheath into the LA. The LA portion of the device is deployed with the catheter in the LA, and the catheter and device are then retracted together until the LA disk is flush with the LA aspect of the interatrial septum. The RA disk is then deployed. Before the device is released from the catheter, appropriate positioning is confirmed by interrogating all rims with 2D and color Doppler, and push/pull maneuvers are performed to confirm device stability. After the device is released, trace residual flow is expected and normal.

Repeat TTE is recommended within the first week after the procedure to ensure that a pericardial effusion has not developed and that the device is well seated. Agitated saline studies may remain positive at this first follow-up study, but residual shunting across the device typically resolves after the device is endothelialized, several months after the procedure.

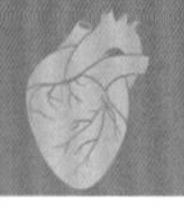

PRIMUM ATRIAL SEPTAL DEFECTS

Overview

Primum ASDs are part of the spectrum of atrioventricular septal defects (AVSDs), which are commonly called *atrioventricular canal defects* or *endocardial cushion defects*. AVSDs are caused by deficient formation of the atrioventricular (AV) septum from embryonic endocardial cushions, which results in a distinct malformation of the central fibrous cardiac crux.

AVSDs are characterized as partial, transitional, or complete. Isolated primum ASDs and isolated inlet VSDs are considered to be partial AVSDs. A transitional AVSD has a primum ASD and two AV valve annuli but abnormal left AV valve morphology. There is often a small inlet VSD that may be partly or completed closed by the chordal tissue of the AV valves. In the complete form of AVSD, a primum ASD and an inlet VSD exist, and there is one common AV valve. AVSDs are associated with trisomy 21 (i.e., Down syndrome), DiGeorge syndrome, Holt-Oram syndrome, and Ellis-van Creveld syndrome. Secundum-type ASDs and persistent left SVC are the most common anomalies associated with AVSD.

Unlike secundum ASDs, which are commonly diagnosed in adulthood, primum ASDs are more commonly diagnosed early in life because the atrial defect is usually large and the associated malformation of the AV valves often results in significant left AV valve regurgitation and heart failure symptoms. However, patients may be asymptomatic until adulthood if the degree of AV valve regurgitation is mild.

The cardiac crux and primum ASDs are well visualized in the apical 4-chamber view with TTE imaging. TEE is rarely necessary to establish the diagnosis, although it may be useful for further characterization of the AV valve. In AVSD, there is a common AV valve with five leaflets, rather than distinct mitral and tricuspid valves (Fig. 41.7). The common AV valve is divided into left and right AV valves by the atrial or ventricular septum (Table 41.3). The common AV valve may override both ventricles, or it may be unbalanced, predominantly draining into one fully formed ventricle and draining only partially into a hypoplastic second ventricle. Abnormal septal attachments are common.

The common AV valve results in anterior displacement of the aortic valve and elongation of the LVOT, and distortion of the LVOT may result in tunnel-like subaortic stenosis (Fig. 41.8). Pulsed-wave Doppler imaging of the LVOT demonstrates flow acceleration in these cases. The term *gooseneck deformity* has been used to describe the angiographic appearance of the LVOT in patients with AVSD.

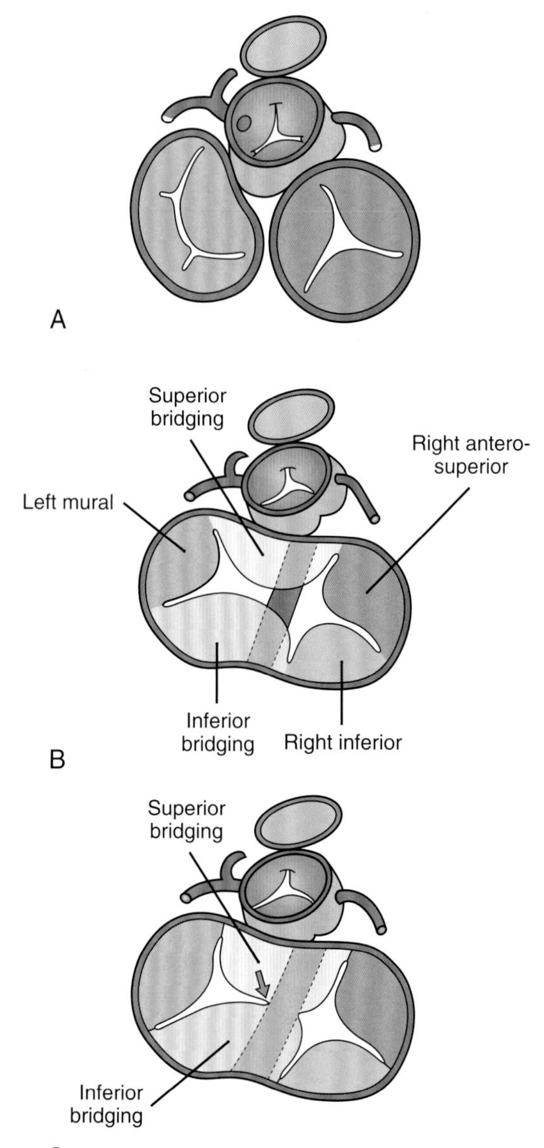

Fig. 41.7 Atrioventricular septal defect. The atrioventricular (AV) junction viewed from the atrial aspect. (A) Normal configuration. Notice the wedged position of the aortic valve between the mitral and tricuspid valves. (B) Complete atrioventricular septal defect (AVSD) with inlet ventricular septal defect (VSD) and primum atrial septal defect (ASD). (C) Partial AVSD (i.e., inlet VSD or primum ASD) with a divided orifice. Fusion between the anterior leaflets and bridging leaflets results in two separate valve orifices with the so-called cleft in the left AV valve. (From Shinebourne E, Ho SY. Atrioventricular septal defect. In: Gatzoulis M, Webb G, Daubeney P, eds. *Diagnosis and Management of Adult Congenital Heart Disease*, Philadelphia, PA: Elsevier; 2011.)

Management

Primum ASDs are not amenable to percutaneous closure because there is no AV valve rim. They require surgical patch closure, usually with concurrent repair of the regurgitant left AV valve. Additional surgical intervention with a Konno-type procedure may be required to relieve LVOT obstruction.

SINUS VENOSUS DEFECTS

Overview

Sinus venosus defects result from incomplete embryologic resorption of the sinus venosus, which causes a deficiency in the wall separating the right pulmonary veins from the SVC, IVC, and RA. The interatrial communication is the orifice of the unroofed right pulmonary veins as they pass posterior to the RA.[13] In this sense, sinus venosus defects are not true ASDs because they do not result from defects in the septum primum or septum secundum, but they are often referred to as *sinus venosus atrial septal defects* because they result in interatrial shunting with hemodynamic and clinical consequences similar to those of primum and secundum ASDs. In this classification, they constitute approximately 5% of ASDs.[14] The superior sinus venosus defect is much more common than the inferior sinus venosus defect. Partial anomalous pulmonary venous return (PAPVR) of right upper pulmonary vein or both right pulmonary veins occurs in approximately 95% of sinus venosus defects.

Both superior and inferior types are difficult to identify on TTE. Superior sinus venosus defects are superior and posterior and may be seen in the subcostal view. Sinus venosus defects are readily identified by TEE in the bicaval view (Fig. 41.9). Superior sinus venosus defects are visualized immediately inferior to the entry of the SVC into the atrium; the SVC typically appears to straddle the atrial septum. Inferior sinus venosus defects are located immediately superior to the entry of the IVC into the RA. CT or MRI is a useful adjunct, particularly if the pulmonary veins are not well seen on TEE.

Management

As with primum ASDs, correction of sinus venosus defects requires surgery. If the anomalous pulmonary veins lie close to the RA, a baffle is used to "reroof" the pulmonary veins to the LA, taking care to avoid obstructing SVC flow into the RA. However, if the pulmonary veins enter the SVC more than 2 cm above the atriocaval junction, the Warden procedure may be performed. In this procedure, the SVC is transected above the entry of the right upper/middle pulmonary veins and then anastomosed to the right atrial appendage. The right pulmonary vein flow is redirected to the LA using a baffle. Long-term follow-up after a Warden procedure should include evaluation for signs of stenosis of the pulmonary venous baffle and SVC-RA anastomosis. If stenosis is suspected, further imaging with TEE, CT, or MRI should be obtained.

TABLE 41.3 Differences Between Normal Mitral/Tricuspid Valves and Atrioventricular Valves in Patients With Atrioventricular Septal Defects.

Normal Valve Anatomy	*Atrioventricular Septal Defect*
Septal attachment of the tricuspid valve is more apical than septal attachment of the mitral valve.	Septal attachment points are at the same level.
Each mitral valve or tricuspid valve has its own annulus. The mitral valve annulus is saddle shaped.	A common annulus encompasses the left and right valves.
Mitral valve morphology comprises anterior and posterior leaflets.	Left AV valve has a cleft between the left-sided portion of the superior bridging leaflet and the left mural leaflet, leading to regurgitation. The inferior bridging leaflet serves as the posterior leaflet.
The tricuspid valve comprises septal, anterior, and posterior leaflets.	Right AV valve comprises portions of the superior and inferior bridging leaflets, the right anterosuperior leaflet, and the right inferior leaflet.

AV, Atrioventricular.

UNROOFED CORONARY SINUS

Overview

The coronary sinus defect, or unroofed coronary sinus, is a rare type of defect that allows interatrial shunting through the coronary sinus and is strongly associated with a persistent left SVC, with or without a bridging vein connecting the right and left SVCs (Fig. 41.10). Like the sinus venosus defect, the unroofed coronary sinus does not represent a true defect in the septum primum or septum secundum but is often classified as an ASD because it permits shunting at the atrial level.

It is a rare finding, accounting for less than 1% of atrial-level shunts, and it is usually associated with heterotaxy syndromes. Kirklin and Barratt-Boyes described four morphologies of the coronary sinus ASD: type I, completely unroofed with a left SVC; type II, completely unroofed without left SVC; type III, partially unroofed midportion; and type IV, partially unroofed terminal portion.[14]

Management

Surgery for an isolated unroofed coronary sinus is rarely required because of the restrictive nature of these shunts. However, it may be undertaken in patients who are undergoing surgical intervention for associated CHDs.

ANOMALOUS PULMONARY VENOUS RETURN

Overview

Anomalous pulmonary veins encompass a broad range of CHDs in which some or all of the pulmonary veins fail to drain normally to the LA. Every possible combination of anomalous

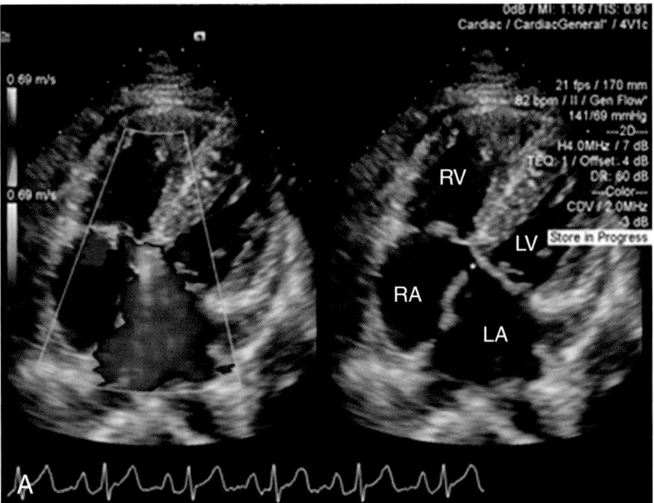

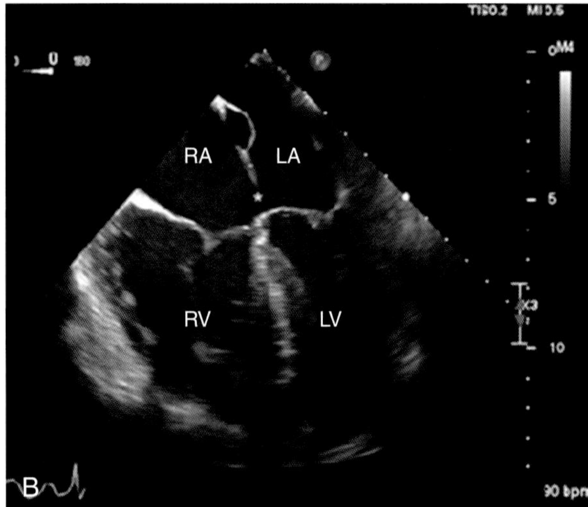

Fig. 41.8 Transitional atrioventricular septal defect. (A) Apical 4-chamber view. Notice the primum-type atrial septal defect *(asterisk)* and the common atrioventricular (AV) valve with insertion of the left and right AV valves at the same level (see Video 41.8A). (B) Mid-esophageal 4-chamber view demonstrates the primum-type atrial septal defect and common AV valve. The very small inlet ventricular septal defect is closed by septal insertion of the AV valves (see Video 41.8B).

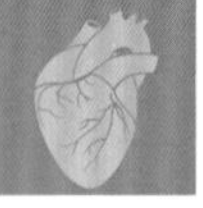

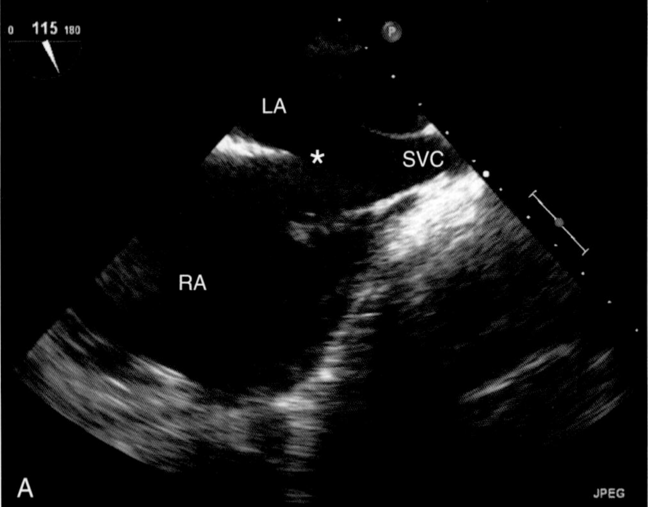

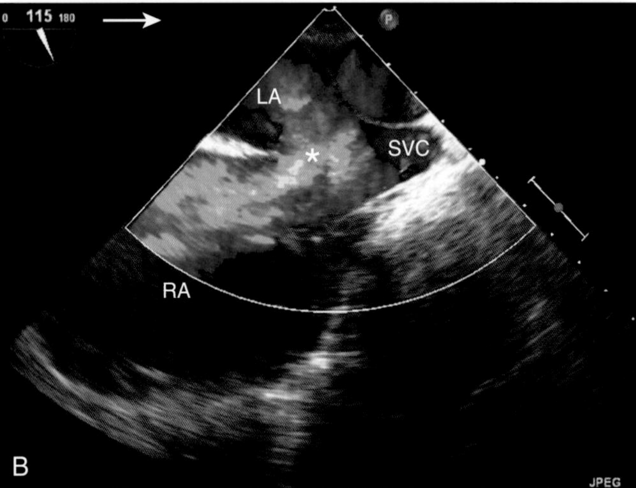

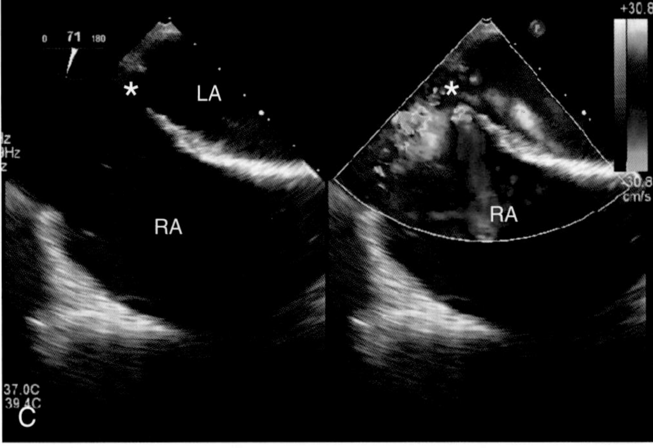

Fig. 41.9 TEE imaging of sinus venosus defects. (A) Superior sinus venosus defect *(asterisk)* is seen in the mid-esophageal bicaval view. (B) Color Doppler imaging demonstrates flow from the LA to the RA across the defect in the mid-esophageal bicaval view. (C) Inferior sinus venosus defect *(asterisk)* in the mid-esophageal bicaval view; color Doppler demonstrates flow from the LA to the RA across the defect. *SVC,* Superior vena cava.

veins, draining to a broad spectrum of receiving chambers, with or without stenosis, has been reported in the literature.

In total anomalous pulmonary venous return (TAPVR), all of the pulmonary veins drain abnormally. This defect is further classified as supracardiac, cardiac, or infracardiac, based on the position of the drainage in relation to the heart (Table 41.4). Patients with this condition almost always undergo surgical repair in infancy. If extensive baffle material was used in the repair, the patient may be at increased risk for stenosis or baffle leaks related to the initial repair. Because there are inadequate TTE windows in the adult for complete visualization of pulmonary venous connections, CT or MRI imaging is recommended for evaluation.[1]

PAPVR can manifest in adulthood. One or more pulmonary veins may connect abnormally to systemic veins, the coronary sinus, or the RA. There are three common patterns of PAPVR (Table 41.5). RA and RV dilation is seen on TTE imaging. PAPVR defects with cardiac connections are usually appreciable on TTE (Fig. 41.11). Extracardiac connections may be difficult to identify on TTE and typically require CT or MRI imaging.

Management

Surgery is indicated for PAPVR if patients are symptomatic, there is right heart volume enlargement, there is a physiologically significant left-to-right shunt, and the patient has a pulmonary artery systolic pressure less than 50% of the systemic pressure.[7] Patients with a single anomalous pulmonary vein rarely require intervention because the degree of shunting is modest.

After repair, patients should be monitored for signs and symptoms of pulmonary venous obstruction. TEE, CT, and MRI are useful to assess for patency of the surgical anastomosis and to evaluate pulmonary venous obstruction or residual atrial shunting after TAPVR or PAPVR repair.

VENTRICULAR SEPTAL DEFECTS

OVERVIEW

Ventricular septal defects (VSDs) are among the most common forms of CHD in childhood. The reported incidence of VSDs varies widely in the literature; many patients are asymptomatic, and many small defects close spontaneously. An estimated 10,000 to 11,000 isolated VSDs are diagnosed in infants in the United States annually.[15,16]

TTE is essential in identifying the location of the defects, number of defects, size of defects, direction and velocity of shunting, and associated defects. Small defects can be difficult to visualize with 2D imaging. Because the VSD jet can be eccentric, it should be interrogated from multiple angles to obtain a parallel intercept, and the highest velocity obtained should be used to calculate the LV-RV systolic VSD gradient. Assuming absence of RVOT or LVOT obstruction, the RV pressure and therefore the pulmonary artery pressure can be estimated by subtracting the VSD gradient from the systolic blood pressure. TEE can be a useful adjunct when transthoracic acoustic windows are suboptimal. TEE is also useful in the guidance of percutaneous VSD closure.

The interventricular septum is a complex, nonplanar structure. Multiple classification systems for VSDs have been proposed; the scheme described in this chapter is based on the Congenital Heart Surgery Nomenclature and Database Project.[17–20] Although autopsy examination allows precise description of VSD in relation to anatomic landmarks and dozens of subclassifications exist from an echocardiographic perspective, VSD may be classified in four broad groups: perimembranous, muscular, inlet, and supracristal. The location can be confirmed with TTE interrogation in multiple views (Fig. 41.12).

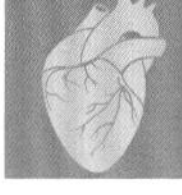

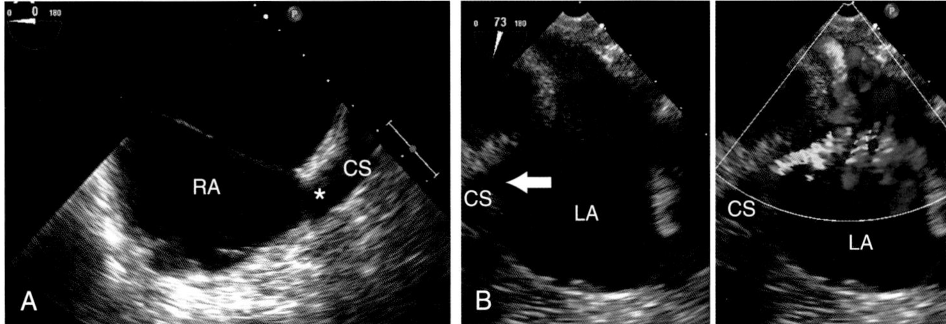

Fig. 41.10 **Unroofed coronary sinus.** Patient with tricuspid atresia, classic RA–pulmonary artery Fontan anatomy, and unroofed coronary sinus *(CS)*. In this example, the RA pressure is higher than the LA pressure because of the Fontan physiology, resulting in shunting from the RA to the LA. (A) Normal coronary sinus ostium *(asterisk)* in the RA (see Video 41.10A). (B) 2D *(left)* and color Doppler *(right)* images of the LA demonstrate an abnormal communication of the coronary sinus *(arrow)* into the LA (see Video 41.10B).

TABLE 41.4 Total Anomalous Pulmonary Venous Connection Subtypes and Site of Drainage of the Common Pulmonary Venous Connection.

Classification	*Site of Common Pulmonary Venous Connection*
Supracardiac	Innominate Azygos Superior vena cava
Cardiac	Cardiac chamber Coronary sinus
Infracardiac	Hepatic circulation through the descending draining vein

TABLE 41.5 Most Common Patterns of Partial Anomalous Pulmonary Venous Drainage.

Pulmonary Venous Drainage	*Association*
Right upper and middle veins to the SVC or RA	Sinus venosus defect
Right pulmonary veins or right lower pulmonary vein to a vertical draining vein to the IVC	Scimitar syndrome Hypoplasia of the right lung Intact atrial septum
Left pulmonary veins to vertical vein to the brachiocephalic vein or coronary sinus	

IVC, Inferior vena cava; *SVC*, superior vena cava.

Perimembranous VSDs account for approximately 80% of VSDs.[21] The membranous septum is a small, fibrous membrane located at the base of the heart; it is contiguous with the tricuspid-mitral-aortic fibrous continuity. It can be further divided into two components (interventricular and AV), which are separated by the septal leaflet of the TV. The AV aspect of the membranous septum lies between the septal insertion points of the mitral valve and TV. Because the TV septal insertion point is more apically placed than the mitral annulus, the AV component of the membranous septum is defined by the RA and the LV.[22]

An LV-RA shunt is also known as a *Gerbode defect*.[23] The interventricular component is bordered superiorly by the AV component of the membranous septum, anteriorly by the outlet septum, inferiorly by the trabecular septum, and posteriorly by the inlet septum. Perimembranous VSDs are located in this region, inferomedial to the aortic valve and lateral to the septal leaflet of the TV.

Perimembranous VSDs are best visualized in a parasternal long-axis view that is angulated slightly medially. In the short-axis view just below the aortic valve level, the perimembranous VSD is seen in the 9- to 10-o'clock position, inferior to the right coronary cusp of the aortic valve and adjacent to the septal leaflet of the TV (Fig. 41.13A–C). Careful attention should be paid to the septal leaflet of the TV, which may partially obstruct the flow across a perimembranous VSD, reducing the degree of left-to-right shunting. The septal leaflet may completely close the VSD, in which case the VSD may be undetectable or visualized as a ventricular septal aneurysm.

Muscular VSDs constitute approximately 5% to 10% of VSDs.[24] They may occur in any location in the muscular portion of the ventricular septum, which is divided into inlet, trabecular, and infundibular portions. Muscular VSDs can be multiple. Very small VSDs may not be visualized on 2D imaging, and they may be detectable only by the presence of color flow across the septum. In these cases, the VSD flow may terminate in mid-systole as the thickening of the myocardium transiently obliterates the VSD.

Inlet VSDs account for approximately 5% of VSDs. They result from failure of complete formation of the central fibrous body and are associated with a common AV valve (see earlier discussion of primum ASDs). The inlet septum is inferior and posterior to the membranous septum. The basal and apical borders of the inlet septum are the AV valves and the chordal attachments of the AV valves, respectively. Inlet VSDs are best evaluated in the apical 4-chamber and subcostal views.

Supracristal VSDs comprise approximately 5% to 7% of VSDs.[25] The infundibular septum resides below both semilunar valves and divides the RVOT and LVOT. On the right side, the membranous septum, the papillary muscle of the conus, and the semilunar valves form the border of the infundibular septum. This defect is seen in the long-axis view with slight medial angulation and in the short-axis view at the 2-o'clock position, inferior to the aortic valve and adjacent to the pulmonic valve. Flow courses from the LVOT into the RV outflow region of the RV.

MANAGEMENT

Small, restrictive VSDs do not result in hemodynamically significant shunting. Pulmonary artery pressure and left heart volumes remain normal. They may close spontaneously in childhood. Although most patients with restrictive perimembranous VSDs do not require intervention, regular surveillance is required because patients are at risk for TV

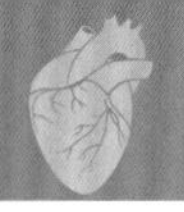

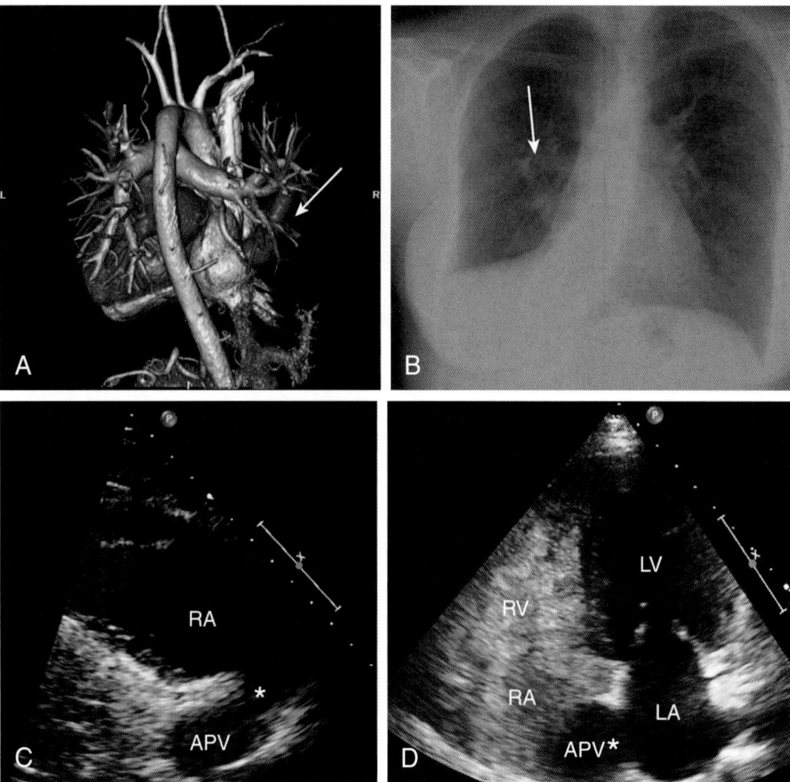

Fig. 41.11 Partial anomalous pulmonary venous return. In this 50-year-old woman with exertional dyspnea, all right pulmonary veins drain to the RA. (A) 3D reconstruction of a cardiac CT image, rotated to view the posterior aspect of the heart; pulmonary veins are *red*. All of the right-sided pulmonary veins *(arrow)* are seen draining by a common vertical vein to the RA. (B) Chest radiograph shows the characteristic scimitar appearance of the vertical vein in the right chest *(arrow)*. (C) RV inflow view shows the large anomalous pulmonary vein *(APV)* draining into the RA *(asterisk)* (see Video 41.11C). (D) Agitated saline contrast study, apical 4-chamber view. Notice the negative contrast of unopacified blood where the pulmonary vein drains to the RA *(asterisk)* (see Video 41.11D).

endocarditis, double-chambered RV (see Fig. 41.13D–F), and aortic regurgitation.

Because of the relationship of the septal leaflet and the membranous septum, the high-velocity flow across the VSD often impinges on this leaflet, predisposing the patient to endocarditis. TEE is useful for evaluation of the TV in cases of suspected endocarditis. Surgical VSD closure may be considered in patients with infective endocarditis.[1] If a patient develops significant tricuspid regurgitation after infective endocarditis, TV repair or replacement should be considered after completion of antibiotic therapy or sooner if septic pulmonary emboli or symptomatic severe tricuspid regurgitation is diagnosed.

In some patients, the high-velocity VSD jet impinges on a mid-RV muscle bundle, causing progressive thickening and fibrosis. The thickened muscle bundle causes a mid-cavitary obstruction, which promotes further hypertrophy of the muscle bundle. The RV is therefore effectively divided into two compartments: a hypertrophied, high-pressure inlet chamber and a thin-walled, low-pressure outlet chamber.[26]

Perimembranous and supracristal VSDs are associated with aortic regurgitation because the proximity of the defect to the aortic valve leaves the aortic valve leaflets somewhat unsupported and prone to prolapse into the LVOT (i.e., perimembranous VSDs) or directly into the VSD (i.e., supracristal VSDs). To preserve the integrity of the aortic valve and avoid eventual aortic valve replacement, early repair of a perimembranous or supracristal VSD should be considered if aortic regurgitation is worsening.[1]

Patients with moderate-sized VSDs may have moderate pulmonary hypertension and mild dilation of the LA and LV. Cardiac catheterization can be useful for quantification of shunting, measurement of pulmonary pressure and resistance, and testing for reversibility of pulmonary arterial hypertension. VSD closure is indicated if the Qp:Qs ratio is 1.5 or greater.[1]

Patients with large, nonrestrictive VSDs may develop heart failure early in life due to left heart volume overload and should undergo repair in the first 6 to 12 months of life. Thereafter, pulmonary vascular disease is progressive. Closure during the first several years of life is typically still feasible as long as the pulmonary artery pressure is less than two thirds of the systemic pressure and pulmonary vascular resistance is less than two thirds of systemic vascular resistance. Severe pulmonary hypertension develops in most individuals with nonrestrictive VSDs by 8 to 10 years of age.

VSD closure is contraindicated for patients with Eisenmenger syndrome. Doppler interrogation demonstrates low-velocity right-to-left or bidirectional shunting, RV hypertrophy, and RV dilation. Pulmonary vasodilators have markedly improved morbidity and mortality rates for this group of patients and may result in decreased pulmonary arterial resistance with improved RV systolic and diastolic function.

When VSD closure is indicated, surgical repair is required for inlet and supracristal types because of their proximity to the cardiac valves. Transcatheter VSD closure has become an accepted alternative to surgery for closure of muscular VSDs. In the United States, the Amplatzer muscular VSD occluder is the

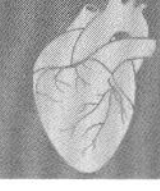

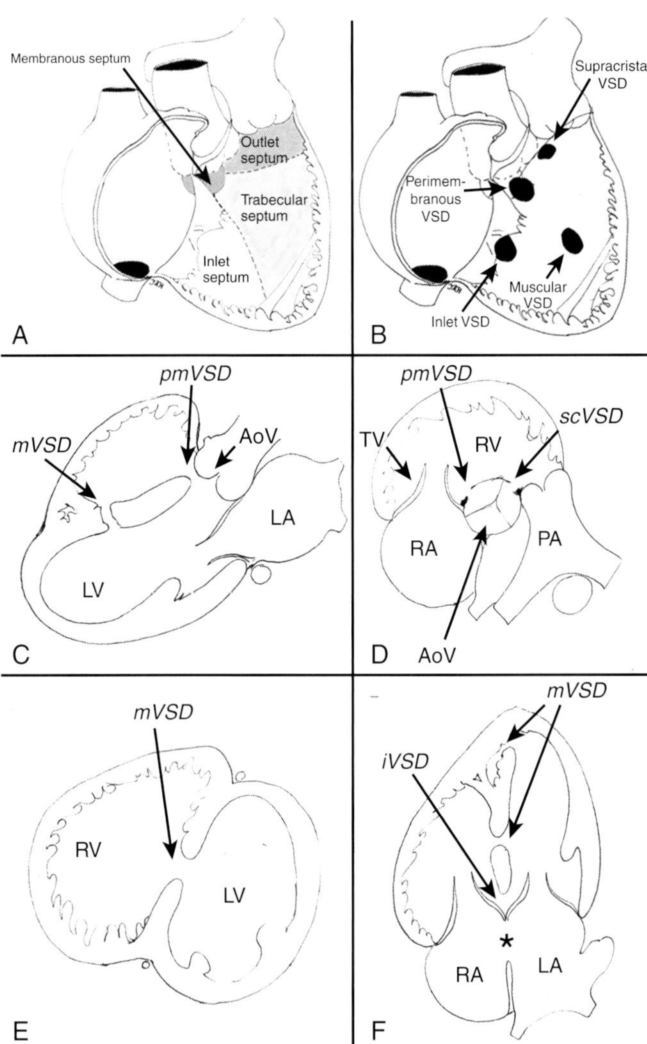

Fig. 41.12 Ventricular septum and ventricular septal defects. (A) Schematic of the ventricular septum. The smooth-walled inlet septum is bordered superiorly and posteriorly by the septal attachment of the tricuspid valve *(TV)* and extends inferiorly and posteriorly to the septal attachment of the TV papillary muscle. The trabecular septum lies inferior and anterior to the inlet septum and is characterized by coarse trabeculations on the RV side. The outlet septum is separated from the trabecular septum by the septal band. It extends from the septal band anterosuperiorly to the pulmonic valve. The membranous septum is a small, translucent area bordered anteriorly by the subaortic outlet septum, inferiorly by the trabecular septum, and posteriorly by the inlet septum. (B) Ventricular septal defects *(VSDs)* are defined by their location in the interventricular septum but may span more than one component of the interventricular septum. (C) Parasternal long-axis view demonstrates a perimembranous VSD *(pmVSD)* below the aortic valve *(AoV)* and a mid-muscular VSD *(mVSD)*. (D) Parasternal short-axis view at the level of the AoV demonstrates a pmVSD at 10 o'clock. Notice the proximity of the septal leaflet of the TV to this defect and a supracristal VSD *(scVSD)* at 1 o'clock just below the pulmonic valve. (E) Parasternal short-axis view at the level of the LV and RV demonstrates a muscular VSD (mVSD). (F) Apical 4-chamber view demonstrates an apical and a mid-muscular mVSD and an inlet-type VSD *(iVSD)*. In patients with an iVSD caused by an endocardial cushion defect, the TV and mitral valve are at the same level, and these patients often have a concomitant primum-type atrial septal defect *(asterisk)*.

only device approved for VSD closure. Perimembranous VSDs have also been closed with the use of transcatheter devices, although devices are not FDA approved for this indication in the United States. In a meta-analysis, the risk of major complications (i.e., early death, reoperation, or permanent pacemaker) was similar for patients who had transcatheter closure and those who underwent surgery.[27]

Similar to device closure of secundum ASDs, percutaneous VSD closure may be performed under TEE or ICE guidance to ensure that the device is well seated, evaluate for residual shunting, and ensure normal function of adjacent valves. After device or surgical VSD closure, the repair should be evaluated carefully to assess for residual shunting across the device or VSD patch leaks.

RUPTURED SINUS OF VALSALVA ANEURYSM

Aneurysms of the sinus of Valsalva (SOV) may be congenital, or they may result from infection, connective tissue disease, or prior surgery. Congenital SOV aneurysm appears as a thin, focal dilation of the aorta that prolapses into adjacent structures, often described as a windsock shape.

An SOV aneurysm may rupture, forming a fistulous communication. An aneurysm of the noncoronary cusp projects into the RA, the left coronary cusp into the LA, and the right coronary cusp into the RA. In patients without pulmonary hypertension or RVOT obstruction, SOV aneurysms result in continuous left-to-right shunting from the aortic root to the RVOT as aortic pressures exceed RV pressures throughout the cardiac cycle.

The diagnosis may be made on TTE imaging. TEE is essential for assessing the proximity of the defect to the aortic valve and coronary arteries. SOV aneurysms can be closed surgically or with transcatheter techniques under TEE guidance (Fig. 41.14).

PATENT DUCTUS ARTERIOSUS

A patent ductus arteriosus (PDA) is an arterial communication between the upper descending aorta and the distal main pulmonary artery. It is an important part of normal fetal cardiac anatomy and usually closes spontaneously within a few days after birth, but in some cases it remains patent (open). The estimated incidence of PDA is 56.7 cases per 100,000 live births.[16]

Most PDAs are small and difficult to appreciate by 2D imaging but easily detected by the abnormal color Doppler signal in the parasternal short-axis and RVOT views. From the parasternal short-axis view, moving the transducer superiorly into a high-parasternal window and rotating it clockwise demonstrates the pulmonary artery bifurcation. From this view, counterclockwise rotation of the transducer then yields the so-called *ductal view* of the ductus in the long axis. From the suprasternal window, the aortic arch can be visualized. Leftward tilt and clockwise rotation of the transducer brings the left pulmonary artery and descending aorta into the same plane. A PDA can be visualized in this plane.

In patients with normal pulmonary pressures, the spectral Doppler tracing demonstrates continuous flow from the aorta into the pulmonary artery. Flow velocity may be used to estimate pulmonary artery pressures.

CORONARY ARTERY FISTULA

A coronary artery fistula is an abnormal termination of a coronary artery; it can occur between a coronary artery and the cardiac chambers or a great vessel. Coronary artery fistulas may originate at any part of the coronary arterial tree and may have multiple origins. They may form a complex network before draining into a lower-pressure receiving chamber or vessel.

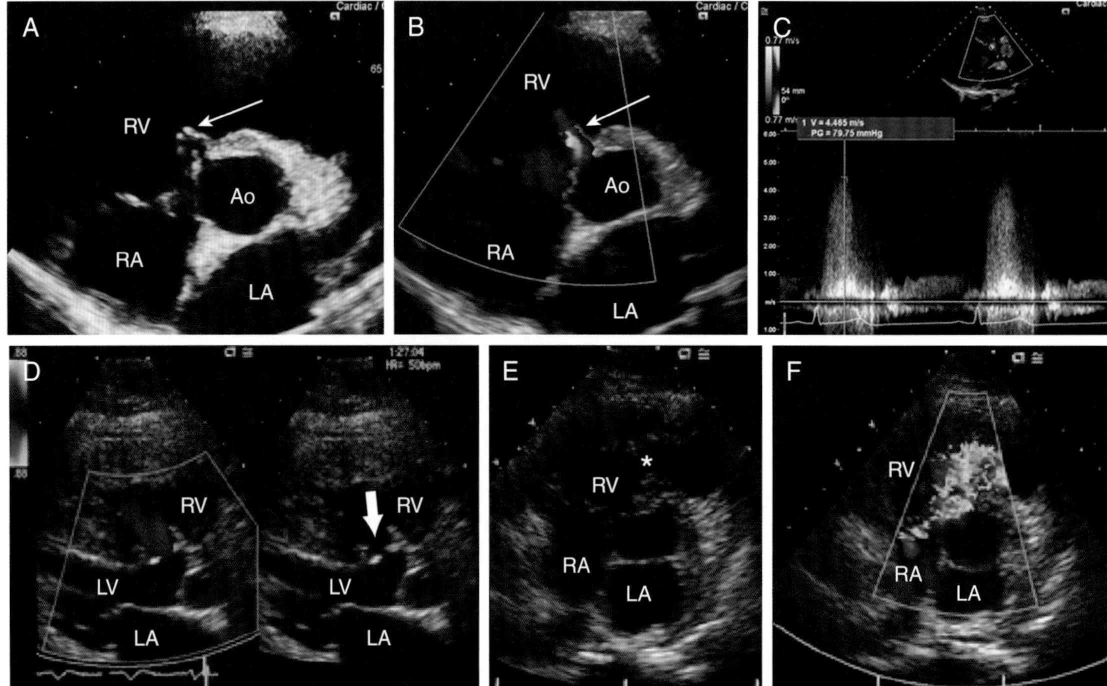

Fig. 41.13 Perimembranous ventricular septal defect. (A–C) An asymptomatic, 20-year-old woman with a restrictive perimembranous ventricular septal defect (VSD) *(arrow)*. (A) Parasternal short-axis view demonstrates an aneurysmal septal leaflet of the tricuspid valve causing partial closure of the VSD (see Video 41.13A). (B) Parasternal short-axis view with color Doppler demonstrates flow across the VSD into the aneurysmal septal leaflet of the tricuspid valve (see Video 41.13B). (C) Spectral Doppler tracing obtained parallel to the shunt flow in the parasternal long-axis view shows left-to-right shunting by a high-velocity jet and an LV-RV gradient of 80 mmHg. (D–F) A 50-year-old woman with Down syndrome, restrictive perimembranous inlet VSD, and double-chambered RV. (D) Parasternal low-axis view with *(left)* and without *(right)* color Doppler. Notice the VSD *(arrow)* with left-to-right shunting and severe hypertrophy of the inlet portion of the RV (see Video 41.13D). (E) Parasternal short-axis view shows hypertrophy of the proximal inlet portion of the RV with a hypertrophied muscle bundle causing narrowing at the mid-ventricle *(asterisk)*. The low-pressure outlet portion of the RV is thin walled (see Video 41.13E). (F) Parasternal short-axis view with color Doppler shows the VSD and aliasing of the intracavitary flow due to mid-ventricular flow obstruction from the muscle bundle (see Video 41.13F). *Ao,* Aorta.

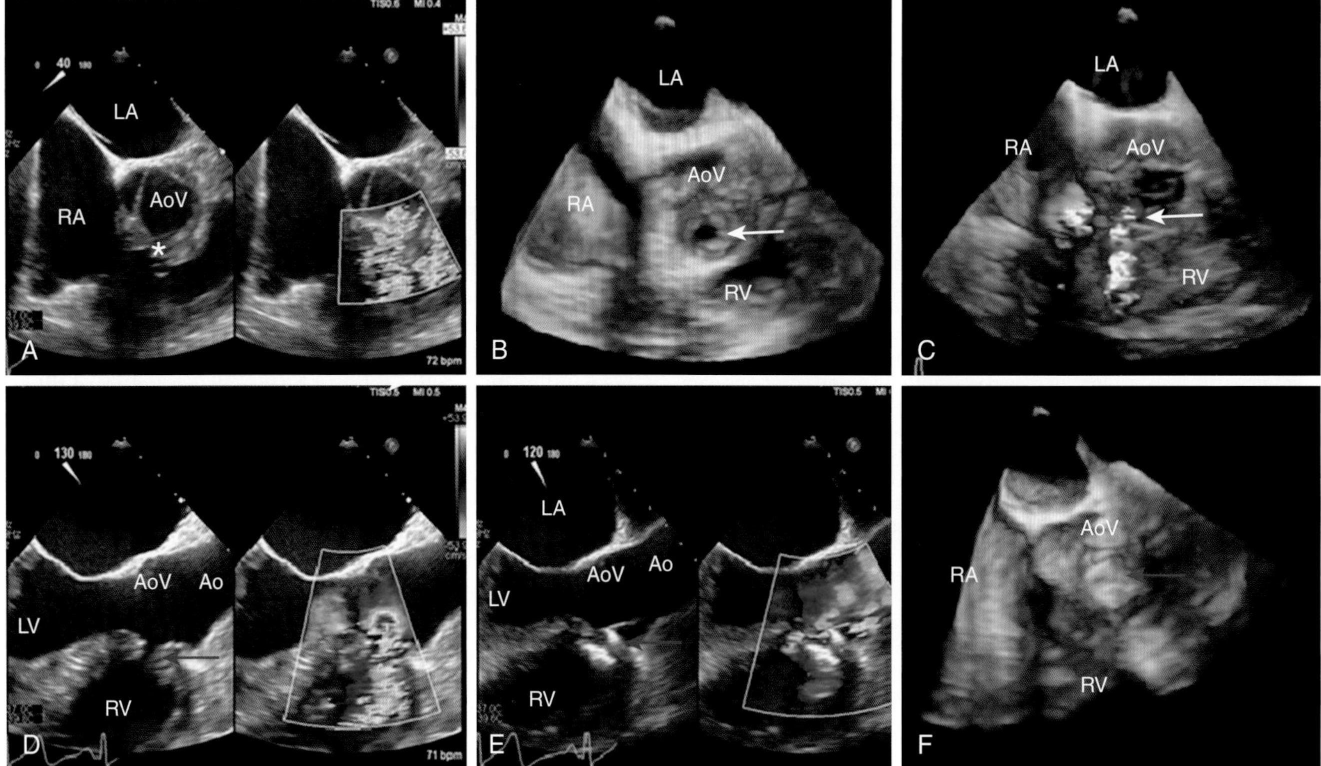

Fig. 41.14 Ruptured sinus of Valsalva aneurysm. (A) TEE mid-esophageal short-axis view of the ruptured sinus of Valsalva (SOV) aneurysm with left-to-right flow from the aortic root into the RV outflow tract. 3D TEE views with (B) and without (C) color flow demonstrate the defect within the right coronary sinus *(arrow)* (see Videos 41.14A, 41.14B, and 41.14C). (D) Mid-esophageal long-axis view of the ruptured SOV *(red arrow)* (see Video 41.14D). (E) A 6-mm Amplatzer VSD occluder is deployed across the ruptured SOV aneurysm *(red arrow)*. A residual VSD is identified (see Video 41.14E). (F) 3D TEE view demonstrates the VSD occluder in the ruptured SOV aneurysm *(red arrow)* (see Video 41.14F). *Ao,* Aorta; *AoV,* aortic valve.

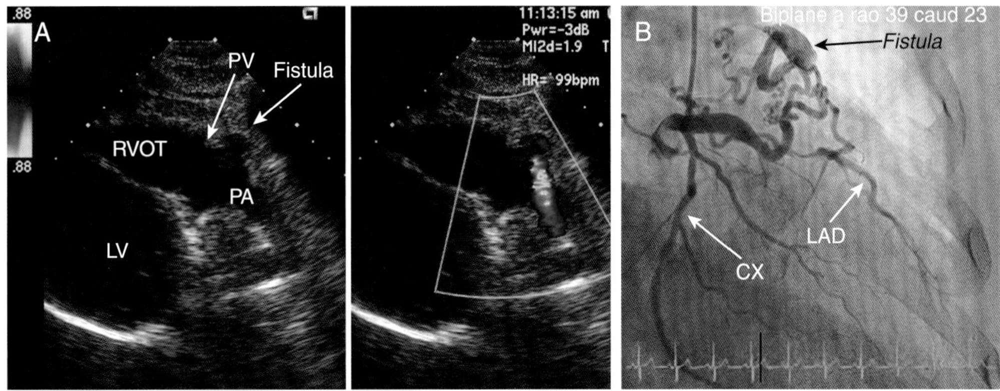

Fig. 41.15 Coronary artery fistula. A 50-year-old man with chest pain. (A) Parasternal RV outflow view demonstrates the pulmonic valve *(PV)* and main pulmonary artery *(PA)*. A small echolucency is seen above the PV, representing the aneurysmal coronary artery fistula draining to the PA. Color Doppler demonstrates continuous flow into the PA at this site (see Video 41.15A). (B) Coronary angiography demonstrates severe left anterior descending artery *(LAD)* stenosis, with a coronary artery fistula arising proximal and distal to the stenosis and draining to the PA. The saccular aneurysm on coronary angiography corresponds with the aneurysm seen on the echocardiogram (see Video 41.15B). *CX*, Circumflex artery; *RVOT*, RV outflow tract.

Although they are usually discovered incidentally, a coronary fistula can sometimes be detected by echocardiography, particularly if the fistula is large and/or portions of the coronary artery are aneurysmal. Color Doppler imaging demonstrates continuous flow (Fig. 41.15).

Surgical ligation or percutaneous coiling or device occlusion of the coronary fistula can be considered if the patient is symptomatic due to coronary steal (or, rarely, volume overload) and the anatomy is amenable to intervention.

SUMMARY Congenital Cardiac Shunts.

Congenital Defect	Definition	Echocardiographic/Doppler Findings	Indications for Intervention
Patent foramen ovale	Incomplete fusion of the septum secundum and septum primum	Continuous or intermittent color flow across the PFO, usually predominantly from left to right Shunt may be right to left with Valsalva release or cough or if right heart pressures are elevated.	Hypoxemia Recurrent embolic events
Atrial-level shunts	Pre-tricuspid shunts, resulting in volume loading of the right heart	RA/RV dilation, diastolic flattening of the ventricular septum Color Doppler shows shunting across the defect, usually left to right. Qp:Qs is calculated using RVOT CSA/VTI and LVOT CSA/VTI.	Heart failure Qp:Qs > 1.5 Evidence for RA/RV dilation Closure contraindicated if severe PAH or PVR > 7–8 WU
Secundum ASD	Defect in the region of the fossa ovalis	TTE: subcostal 4C view for visualization of defect and color flow; parasternal short-axis, apical 4C views to assess rims TEE: ME view, multiplane to assess all rims when considering transcatheter closure	Transcatheter closure: preferred if >3 mm circumferential rims, may be considered if <3 mm rims Surgical closure if very large defect (>30–32 mm diameter), deficient rims

Continued

SUMMARY Congenital Cardiac Shunts.—cont'd

Congenital Defect	Definition	Echocardiographic/Doppler Findings	Indications for Intervention
Primum ASD	Defect involving the crux of the heart, bordered inferiorly by the AV valves; part of the spectrum of AVSD	Best visualized in apical 4C view; may have concomitant AV valve regurgitation from cleft and LVOT obstruction	Requires surgical repair
Sinus venosus defect	Defect at the junction of the vena cava and RA Often associated with anomalous pulmonary veins	Poorly visualized by TTE TEE imaging recommended to visualize defect and assess pulmonary venous return	Requires surgical repair
Unroofed coronary sinus	Defect in the roof of the CS, allowing left-to-right shunting through the CS	TTE: CS may be dilated; persistent left SVC may exist TEE: ME view, posterior angulation, 100–110 degrees to demonstrate roof of the CS	Requires surgical repair
Anomalous pulmonary venous return	Varies widely depending on number of anomalous veins and chamber receiving drainage TAPVR usually diagnosed and repaired in neonatal period PAPVR may be diagnosed in adulthood; associated with sinus venosus defects	RA/RV dilation, flattening of the interventricular septum TTE may demonstrate cardiac connection to RA or IVC. TEE useful for demonstrating connection to SVC, RA, CS	Consider surgical repair for heart failure symptoms or for RA/RV enlargement. PAPVR of a single pulmonary vein usually does not require repair
VSDs	Post-tricuspid shunts, result in pressure loading of the RV and volume loading of the left heart.	RV hypertrophy, dilation, dysfunction; elevated RV/PA systolic pressures; LA/LV dilation Left-to-right shunting if defect is small or moderate; for bidirectional or right-to-left shunting, suspect severe pulmonary hypertension	Closure indicated if Qp:Qs > 2.0 and LA/LV dilated Closure reasonable if Qp:Qs > 1.5, PAP < 2/3 systemic pressure and PVR < 2/3 SVR, or in setting of LV systolic/diastolic failure Closure indicated if associated DCRV, endocarditis, or AR
Perimembranous VSD	Defect adjacent to the membranous septum at the base of the heart	PLAX view, located inferior to the aortic valve; PSAX view, located at the 9- to 10-o'clock position May be partially closed by septal leaflet of the TV	Surgery recommended using a transcatheter approach due to higher risk of heart block
Muscular VSD	Defect in the muscular septum; may be multiple	PLAX and apical 4C views Small defects difficult to identify on 2D but may be diagnosed by color Doppler	Percutaneous device closure is reasonable if small to moderate defect is remote from TV and aorta
Inlet VSD	Defect involving the crux of the heart, bordered superiorly by the AV valves Part of spectrum of AVSD	Apical 4C view, immediately inferior to AV valves May have concomitant AV valve regurgitation from cleft and LVOT obstruction	Requires surgical repair
Supracristal VSD	Defect in the infundibular septum, inferior to the aortic valve and adjacent to the pulmonic valve	PLAX view with medial angulation; PSAX view, located at 2-o'clock position	Requires surgical repair

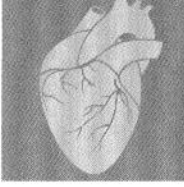

SUMMARY Congenital Cardiac Shunts.—cont'd

Congenital Defect	Definition	Echocardiographic/Doppler Findings	Indications for Intervention
Ruptured sinus of Valsalva aneurysm	Usually restrictive shunt with varied location: right CS to RV, left CS to LA, noncoronary sinus to RA	High PSAX view, immediately above the aortic valve level Continuous, usually high-velocity left-to-right shunting throughout the cardiac cycle	Closure recommended at any size given risk for increase in size of defect Surgical or transcatheter closure acceptable, depending on available expertise Sufficient distance between defect and the coronary arteries and aortic valve required for transcatheter approach
Patent ductus arteriosus	Shunt between the upper descending aorta and the distal main PA	High PSAX view, transducer rotated counterclockwise for PA bifurcation SSN view of aortic arch, modified to view LPA and descending aorta Continuous left-to-right flow if small or moderate PDA Low-velocity bidirectional or right-to-left flow for severe PAH (Eisenmenger)	Closure indicated for left-to-right shunt and symptoms of LA/LV dilation, PAH, or heart failure symptoms Closure contraindicated for patients with PAH and right-to-left shunting
Coronary artery fistula	Abnormal termination of a coronary artery Originates at any part of coronary arterial tree May have multiple origins and/or meshlike network before terminating in any cardiac chamber, SVC, PA, or CS	Dilated coronary artery may be visible; color and spectral Doppler confirm abnormal flow signals, which vary depending on size of fistula and receiving chamber	Closure indicated if patient has symptoms of coronary steal and anatomy is suitable for surgical ligation or catheter coil embolization

4C, 4-Chamber; *AR,* atrial regurgitation; *ASD,* atrial septal defect; *AV,* atrioventricular; *AVSD,* atrioventricular septal defects; *CS,* coronary sinus; *CSA,* cross-sectional area; *DCRV,* double-chambered RV; *IVC,* inferior vena cava; *LPA,* left pulmonary artery; *LVOT,* LV outflow tract; *ME,* mid-esophageal; *PA,* pulmonary artery; *PAH,* pulmonary arterial hypertension; *PAPVR,* partial anomalous pulmonary venous return; *PDA,* patent ductus arteriosus; *PFO,* patent foramen ovale; *PLAX,* parasternal long axis; *PSAX,* parasternal short axis; *PVR,* pulmonary vascular resistance; *Qp,* pulmonary blood flow; *Qs,* systemic blood flow; *RVOT,* RV outflow tract; *SSN,* suprasternal notch; *SVC,* superior vena cava; *TAPVR,* total anomalous pulmonary venous return; *TV,* tricuspid valve; *VSD,* ventricular septal defect; *VTI,* velocity–time integral; *WU,* Wood units.

REFERENCES

1. Stout KK, Daniels CJ, Aboulhosn JA, et al. 2018. AHA/ACC guideline for the management of adults with congenital heart disease: executive summary: a report of the American College of Cardiology/American Heart Association Task Force on Clinical Practice Guidelines. *J Am Coll Cardiol.* 2019;73(12):1494–1563.
2. American College of Cardiology Foundation Appropriate Use Criteria Task Force, American Society of Echocardiography, American Heart Association, et al. ACCF/ASE/AHA/ASNC/HFSA/HRS/SCAI/SCCM/SCCT/SCMR 2011 Appropriate Use Criteria for Echocardiography. A Report of the American College of Cardiology Foundation Appropriate Use Criteria Task Force, American Society of Echocardiography, American Heart Association, American Society of Nuclear Cardiology, Heart Failure Society of America, Heart Rhythm Society, Society for Cardiovascular Angiography and Interventions, Society of Critical Care Medicine, Society of Cardiovascular Computed Tomography, and Society for Cardiovascular Magnetic Resonance Endorsed by the American College of Chest Physicians. *J Am Coll Cardiol.* 2011;57(9):1126–1166.
3. Campbell M. Natural history of atrial septal defect. *Br Heart J.* 1970;32(6):820–826.
4. Lindsey JB, Hillis LD. Clinical update: atrial septal defect in adults. *Lancet.* 2007;369(9569): 1244–1246.
5. Gatzoulis MA, Freeman MA, Siu SC, Webb GD, Harris L. Atrial arrhythmia after surgical closure of atrial septal defects in adults. *N Engl J Med.* 1999;340(11):839–846.
6. Steele PM, Fuster V, Cohen M, Ritter DG, McGoon DC. Isolated atrial septal defect with pulmonary vascular obstructive diseaselong-term follow-up and prediction of outcome after surgical correction. *Circulation.* 1987;76(5):1037–1042.
7. Bradley EA, Ammash N, Martinez SC, et al. "Treat-to-close": Non-repairable ASD-PAH in the adult: results from the North American ASD-PAH (NAAP) Multicenter Registry. *Int J Cardiol.* 2019;291:127–133.
8. Park JJ, Lee SC, Kim JB, et al. Deterioration of mitral valve competence after the repair of atrial septal defect in adults. *Ann Thorac Surg.* 2011;92(5):1629–1633.
9. Takaya Y, Kijima Y, Akagi T, et al. Fate of mitral regurgitation after transcatheter closure of atrial septal defect in adults. *Am J Cardiol.* 2015;116(3):458–462.
10. Silvestry FE, Cohen MS, Armsby LB, et al. Guidelines for the echocardiographic assessment of atrial septal defect and patent foramen ovale: from the American Society of Echocardiography and Society for Cardiac Angiography and Interventions. *J Am Soc Echocardiogr.* 2015;28(8):910–958.
11. Saric M, Perk G, Purgess JR, Kronzon I. Imaging atrial septal defects by real-time three-dimensional transesophageal echocardiography: step-by-step approach. *J Am Soc Echocardiogr.* 2010;23(11): 1128–1135.

12. Kijima Y, Akagi T, Takaya Y, et al. Deficient surrounding rims in patients undergoing transcatheter atrial septal defect closure. *J Am Soc Echocardiogr*. 2016;29(8):768–776.
13. Van Praagh S, Carrera ME, Sanders SP, Mayer JE, Van Praagh R. Sinus venosus defects: unroofing of the right pulmonary veinsanatomic and echocardiographic findings and surgical treatment. *Am Heart J*. 1994;128(2):365–379.
14. Kirklin JW, Barratt-Boyes BG. *Cardiac Surgery: Morphology, Diagnostic Criteria, Natural History, Techniques, Results, and Indications*. New York: Wiley; 1986.
15. Mitchell SC, Korones SB, Berendes HW. Congenital heart disease in 56,109 births. Incidence and natural history. *Circulation*. 1971;43(3):323–332.
16. Hoffman JI, Christianson R. Congenital heart disease in a cohort of 19,502 births with long-term follow-up. *Am J Cardiol*. 1978;42(4):641–647.
17. Anderson RH, Wilcox BR. The surgical anatomy of ventricular septal defect. *J Card Surg*. 1992;7(1):17–35.
18. Soto B, Becker AE, Moulaert AJ, Lie JT, Anderson RH. Classification of ventricular septal defects. *Br Heart J*. 1980;43(3):332–343.
19. Van Praagh R, Geva T, Kreutzer J. Ventricular septal defects: how shall we describe, name and classify them? *J Am Coll Cardiol*. 1989;14(5):1298–1299.
20. Jacobs JP, Burke RP, Quintessenza JA, Mavroudis C. Congenital Heart Surgery Nomenclature and Database Project: ventricular septal defect. *Ann Thorac Surg*. 2000;69(4 Suppl):S25–S35.
21. Soto B, Ceballos R, Kirklin JW. Ventricular septal defects: a surgical viewpoint. *J Am Coll Cardiol*. 1989;14(5):1291–1297.
22. Ho SY, McCarthy KP, Rigby ML. Morphology of perimembranous ventricular septal defects: implications for transcatheter device closure. *J Intervent Cardiol*. 2004;17(2):99–108.
23. Gerbode F, Hultgren H, Melrose D, Osborn J. Syndrome of left ventricular-right atrial shunt; successful surgical repair of defect in five cases, with observation of bradycardia on closure. *Annals of surgery*. 1958;148(3):433–446.
24. Ramaciotti C, Vetter JM, Bornemeier RA, Chin AJ. Prevalence, relation to spontaneous closure, and association of muscular ventricular septal defects with other cardiac defects. *Am J Cardiol*. 1995;75(1):61–65.
25. Lincoln C, Jamieson S, Joseph M, Shinebourne E, Anderson RH. Transatrial repair of ventricular septal defects with reference to their anatomic classification. *J Thorac Cardiovasc Surg*. 1977;74(2):183–190.
26. Wong PC, Sanders SP, Jonas RA, et al. Pulmonary valve-moderator band distance and association with development of double-chambered right ventricle. *Am J Cardiol*. 1991;68(17):1681–1686.
27. Saurav A, Kaushik M, Mahesh Alla V, et al. Comparison of percutaneous device closure versus surgical closure of peri-membranous ventricular septal defects: a systematic review and meta-analysis. *Cathet Cardiovasc Interv*. 2015;86(6):1048–1056.

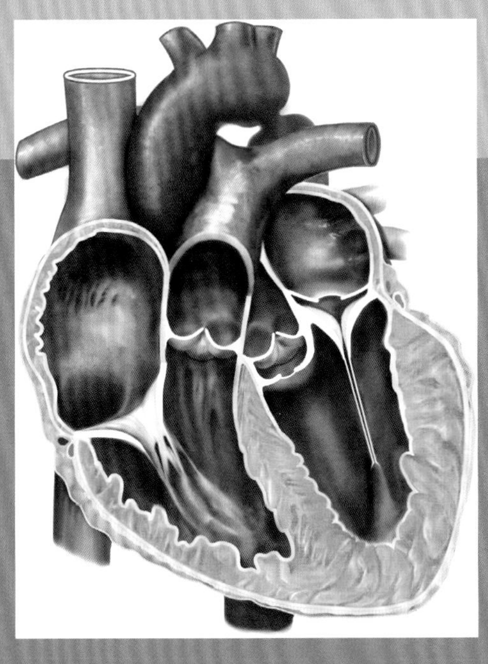

中文导读

第42章
左心异常

左心异常在成人先天性心脏病中普遍存在，其可单独发生或存在相关缺陷。患者通常需要终生监测，因为自体病变可能进展而干预后可能出现并发症。超声心动图对于诊断、治疗和长期随访至关重要，其越来越多地在了解左心系统异常的生理变化和干预时机方面发挥作用。本章回顾介绍了先天性左心异常，包括左心房、二尖瓣、左心室、左心室流出道、主动脉和冠状动脉异常，包括三房心、先天性二尖瓣瓣上隔膜、二尖瓣前叶裂、双孔二尖瓣、降落伞式二尖瓣、主动脉瓣畸形、主动脉瓣下狭窄、主动脉瓣上狭窄、主动脉弓缩窄、主动脉弓离断、双主动脉弓、冠状动脉起源异常等先天性左心疾病的定义、病理解剖、病理生理、超声心动图常用切面、二维超声、彩色多普勒超声表现特点及典型图像、常见相关并发症及手术干预治疗指征等。

王　燕

42

Left Heart Anomalies

JENNIFER COHEN, MD | KENAN W.D. STERN, MD | ALI N. ZAIDI, MD

Left-sided anomalies are prevalent among adults with congenital heart disease. They can occur in isolation or with associated defects (Fig. 42.1). Patients usually require lifelong monitoring because native lesions may progress and postintervention complications may develop. Echocardiography is essential for diagnosis, management, and long-term follow-up, and it increasingly plays a role in understanding the physiologic changes of left-sided anomalies and the timing for intervention. We review left heart congenital anomalies, including those of the left atrium (LA), mitral valve, left ventricle (LV), left ventricular outflow tract (LVOT), aorta, and coronary arteries.

COR TRIATRIATUM

Cor triatriatum sinister is a rare diagnosis, accounting for only 0.1% to 0.4% of all congenital heart disease.[1,2] The incidence is similar for men and women, and no related genetic disorders have been described.[2]

Cor triatriatum (i.e., triatrial heart) results when the atrium is divided by a membrane into a posterior pulmonary venous chamber and an anterior anatomic LA chamber that contains the left atrial appendage (LAA) and the true atrial septum that bears the fossa ovalis. The membrane can vary significantly in size and shape. It may appear similar to a diaphragm or be funnel shaped, bandlike, or imperforate and can contain one or more fenestrations of various sizes. Classically, the posterior portion of this condition should be distinguished from a supramitral ring, in which the LAA is located proximal to the membrane.[3]

Atrial septal defects (ASDs) are common, with about 70% of patients having a patent foramen ovale or ASD. The ASD allows communication between the right atrium and the pulmonary venous chamber or the distal LA chamber. Associated anomalous pulmonary venous connections can occur, and cor triatriatum sometimes involves veins from only one lung. Other associations include a persistent left superior vena cava to the coronary sinus and coarctation of the aorta (CoA).[4]

Cor triatriatum in adults has been diagnosed incidentally or in the setting of atrial arrhythmias. There may also be chronic pulmonary venous hypertension leading to heart failure and the development of secondary pulmonary arterial hypertension.[5]

Echocardiographic imaging of cor triatriatum with two-dimensional (2D) transthoracic echocardiography (TTE) is often best demonstrated in apical views. It is seen as a curvilinear membrane in the midportion of the LA. The membrane is often thin and may move in response to changes in atrial pressures. The membrane also can be seen in the parasternal long-axis view as a vertical linear structure within the LA that is perpendicular to the ascending aorta. Color Doppler imaging is used to assess turbulent diastolic flow, and spectral Doppler can document any gradient across the membrane (Fig. 42.2).

The relationship between the LAA and the membrane is most easily seen in parasternal short-axis views. The position of the septum primum should also be assessed because malattachment of the septum primum can be confused with cor triatriatum in some views. All four pulmonary venous connections are assessed from high parasternal short-axis views, and the atrial septum is carefully evaluated from subxiphoid, parasternal short-axis, and high right parasternal views. Evaluation also includes measurement of the coronary sinus size, assessment for left-sided superior vena cava, and acquisition of suprasternal notch views of the aortic arch with Doppler for CoA. RV pressures should be carefully assessed. Three-dimensional (3D) reconstruction of echocardiographic images can improve definition of the accessory membrane, detection of fenestrations, and characterization of the membrane's relationship with surrounding structures.[6]

CONGENITAL MITRAL VALVE DISEASE

Congenital mitral valve disease (excluding mitral valve prolapse) is rare, but it is associated with increased morbidity and mortality rates due to mitral stenosis, regurgitation, or both. Mitral valve anomalies can involve one or more of its

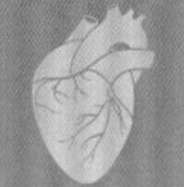

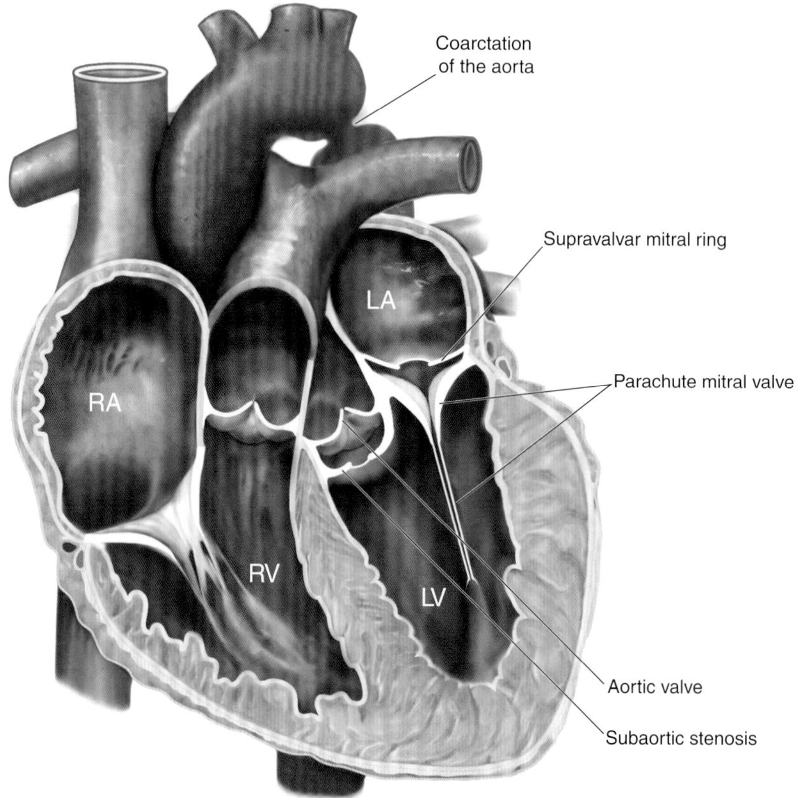

Fig. 42.1 Congenital left-sided obstructions. Several left-sided obstructions are shown. The Shone complex comprises a supramitral ring, parachute mitral valve, subaortic membrane, and coarctation of the aorta.

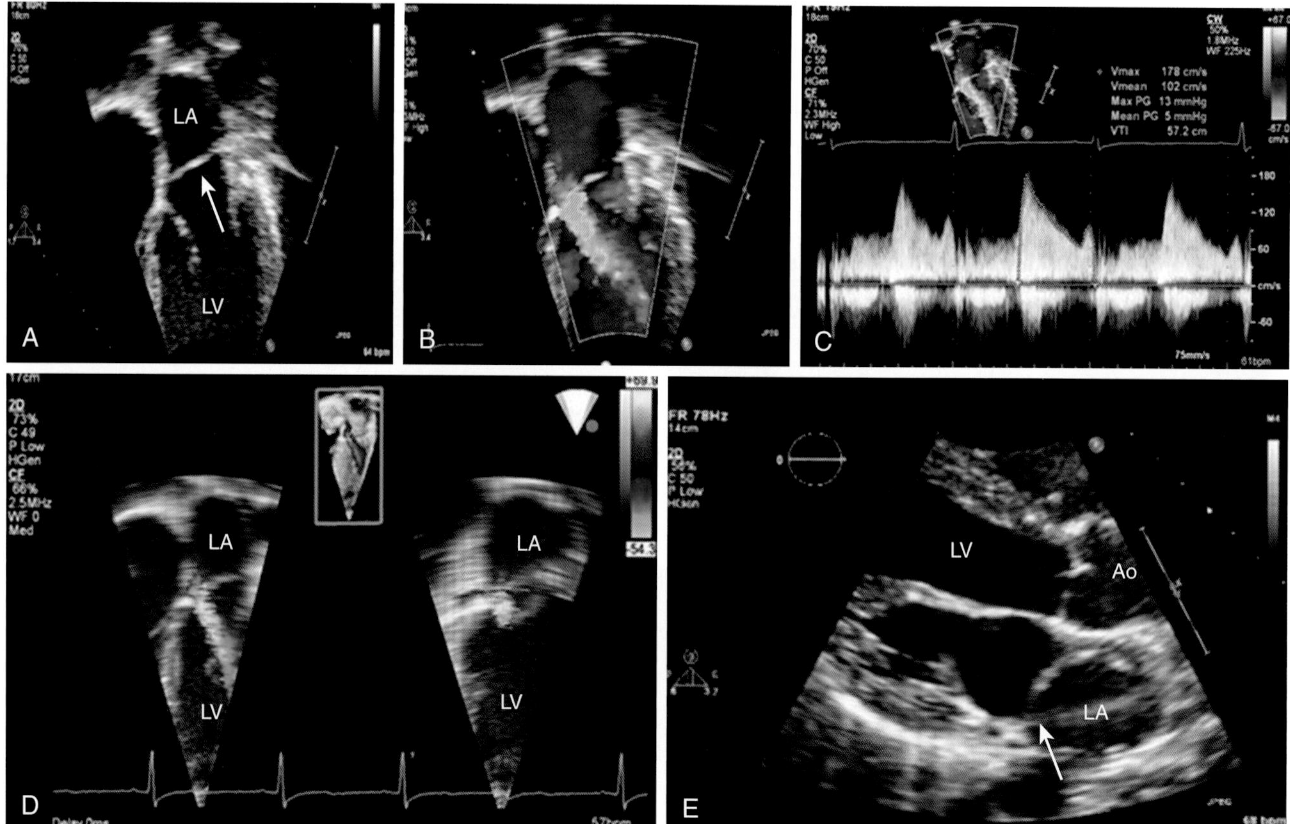

Fig. 42.2 Cor triatriatum. (A) The apical 4-chamber view demonstrates a membrane *(arrow)* bisecting the LA, separating the pulmonary venous atrium from the mitral inflow portion of the atrium (see Video 42.2A). (B) Color Doppler image demonstrates color flow acceleration across the membrane (see Video 42.2B). (C) Continuous-wave Doppler through the accelerated flow jet demonstrates a mean gradient of 5 mmHg. (D) 3D imaging shows accelerated flow jet across the membrane. (E) The membrane is also well seen in the parasternal long-axis view *(arrow)* (see Video 42.2E). *Ao*, Aorta.

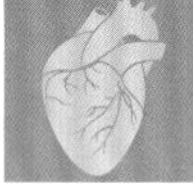

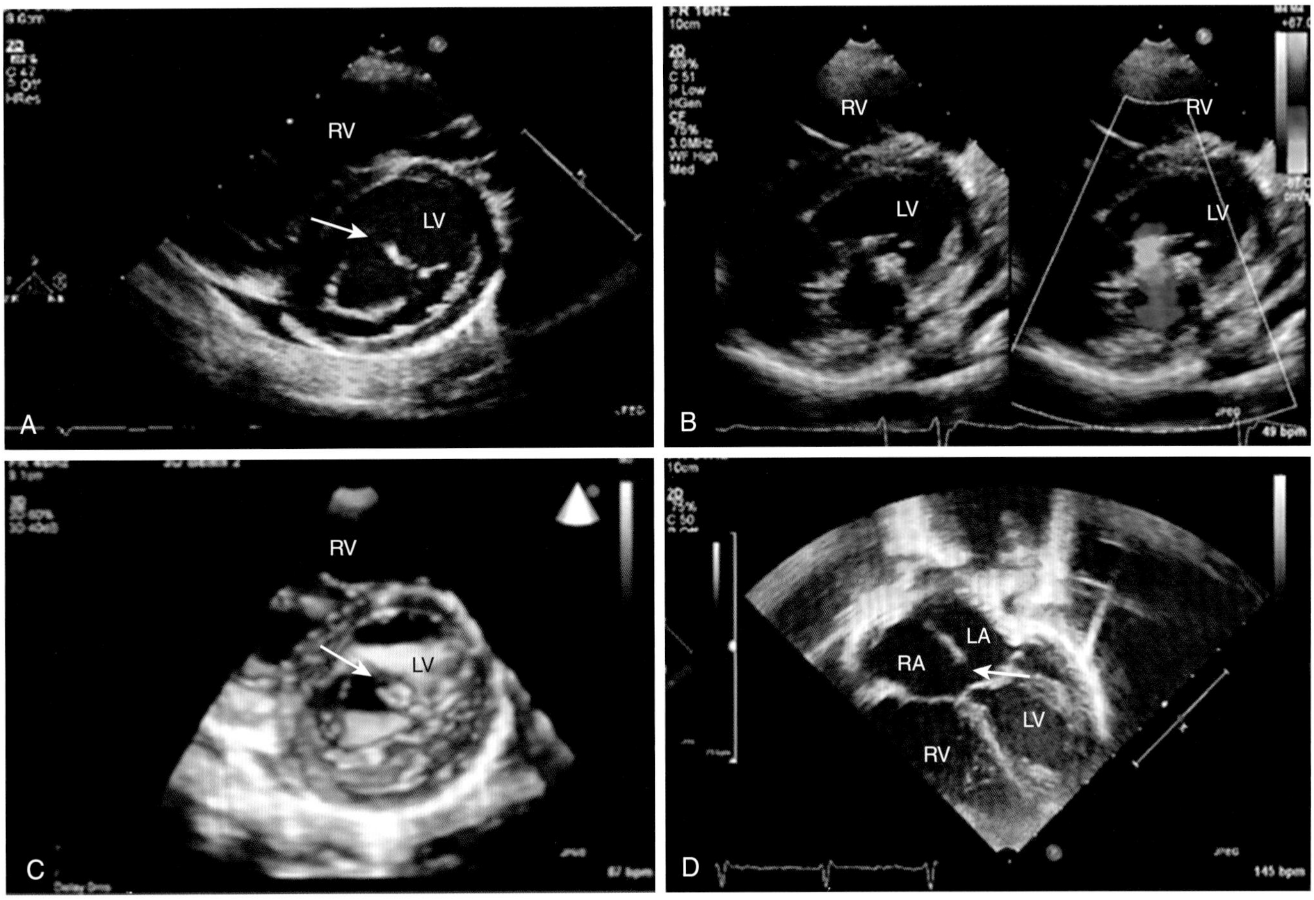

Fig. 42.3 Cleft mitral valve. (A) In the parasternal short-axis view, the cleft mitral valve is seen with a discontinuity in the anterior mitral valve leaflet *(arrow)* (see Video 42.3A ▶). (B). Color imaging demonstrates posteriorly directed mitral regurgitation originating from the mitral valve cleft (see Video 42.3B ▶). (C) 3D imaging demonstrates the mitral valve cleft *(arrow)* (see Video 42.3C ▶). (D) An apex-down apical 4-chamber view shows a primum atrial septal defect *(arrow)*, which is associated with a mitral valve cleft in the setting of a partial atrioventricular canal defect (see Video 42.3D ▶).

components, including the mitral annulus, valve leaflets, chordae tendineae, and papillary muscles. Congenital mitral valve disease commonly occurs in conjunction with other left heart obstructive lesions, including the Shone complex (i.e., supravalvular mitral ring, parachute mitral valve, subvalvular aortic stenosis, and CoA).[7] 3D evaluation often can provide added insight to assess complex mitral morphology for surgical or percutaneous intervention.

CLEFT MITRAL VALVE

A cleft mitral valve is a cleft (split) of the anterior leaflet into two separate leaflet components, with each attached to a separate papillary muscle group (Fig. 42.3). Cleft mitral valves are most commonly encountered in atrioventricular septal defects (AVSDs), in which the cleft represents the deficiency of atrioventricular valve tissue where the superior and inferior bridging leaflets meet at the ventricular septum. In this setting, the cleft is oriented toward the mid-interventricular septum.

An isolated cleft mitral valve is not associated with an AVSD. Isolated clefts are typically oriented toward the LVOT. This is an uncommon congenital anomaly that can occasionally be associated with ventricular septal defects (VSDs) or conotruncal anomalies.[7]

Cleft mitral valves tend to be regurgitant. The mitral regurgitation jet typically originates from the anterior cleft and is directed posteriorly. The cleft is best visualized from a subxiphoid short-axis or parasternal short-axis view. It is important to determine whether the cleft attachments are contributing to LVOT obstruction. An isolated cleft can be diagnosed adequately by means of 2D echocardiography and Doppler interrogation or by 3D echocardiography.[8]

Closure of the cleft improves coaptation, but there is a tradeoff between coaptation and adequacy of the flow orifice, and mitral stenosis can sometimes occur.[9] When the cleft mitral valve is the only defect, repair must be initiated on the basis of the usual clinical and echocardiographic criteria. If the degree of regurgitation is only mild to moderate, surgical repair is not urgent because the regurgitation does not progress over the intermediate term.[10]

SUPRAMITRAL RING

A *supramitral ring* is an abnormal membranous tissue growth on the LA side of the mitral valve that appears as a shelf-like membrane located just above the mitral annulus but distal to the LAA, resulting in mitral inflow obstruction. The supramitral ring may be associated with other left-sided obstructive lesions.[7] The ring, which is often circumferential, may encroach on the orifice of the mitral valve and adhere to the leaflets of the valve, restricting their movements.

An *intramitral ring* is located within the mitral tunnel, is closely adherent to the mitral leaflets, and occurs with a high incidence of structural mitral abnormalities, including restricted

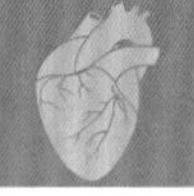

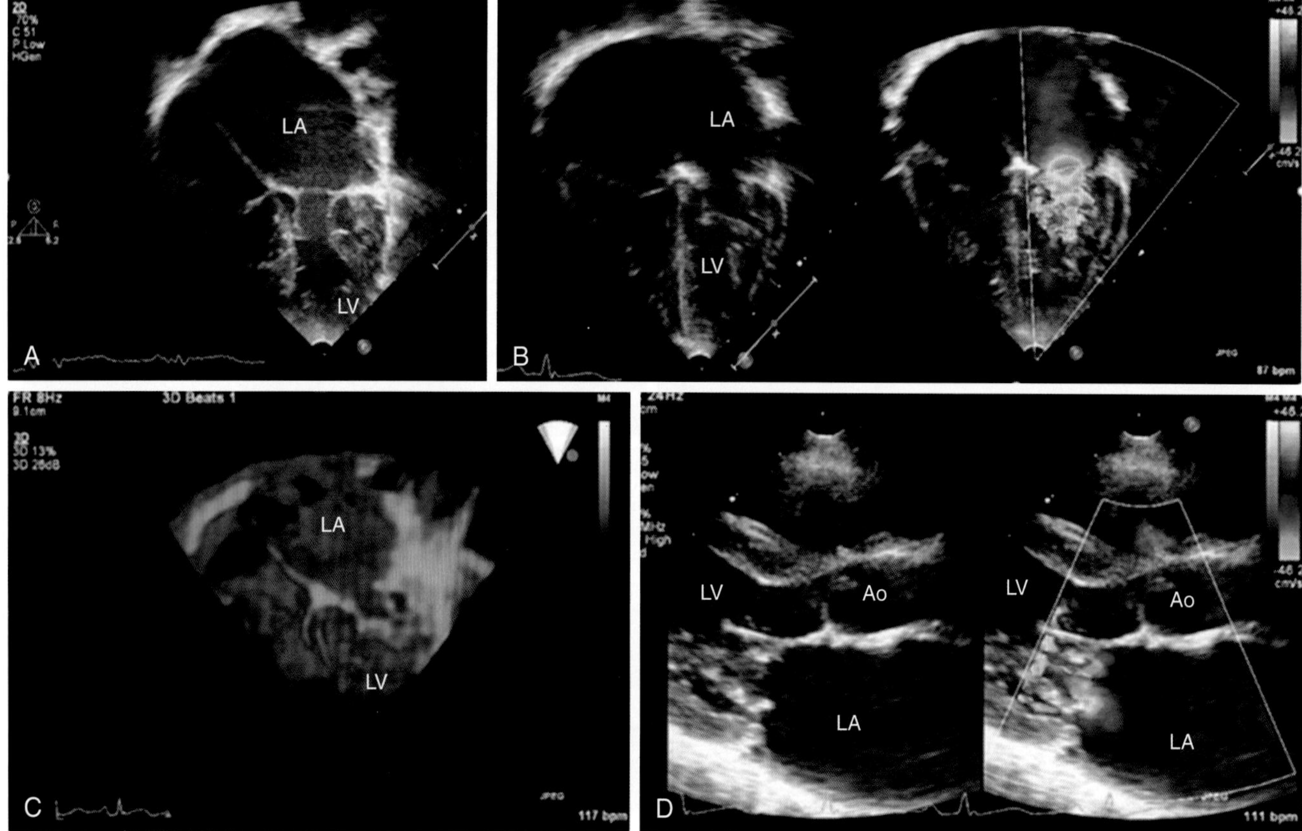

Fig. 42.4 Supramitral ring. (A) In the apical 4-chamber view, 2D imaging shows a supramitral membrane with significant LA dilation (see Video 42.4A). (B) Color imaging in a different patient with a supramitral ring shows color flow acceleration beginning just above the level of the mitral annulus (see Videos 42.4B1 and B2). (C) 3D image of a supramitral ring in an apical view (see Video 42.4C). (D) Parasternal long-axis color view shows color flow acceleration beginning above the level of the mitral valve annulus. The mitral valve is abnormal in this patient. It has shortened chordae, and the LA is significantly dilated (see Video 42.4D). *Ao*, Aorta.

mobility of the mitral leaflets, reduced chordal length, reduced interpapillary muscle distance, single papillary muscle, and hypoplastic mitral annulus. The intramitral type is frequently part of the Shone complex.

Unlike rheumatic mitral disease, restriction occurs at the base of the leaflet, and the leaflet tips open freely in parallel and are unrestricted (Fig. 42.4). The 4-chamber apical view provides an angle of interrogation perpendicular to the membrane. Color Doppler demonstrates flow acceleration beginning at the annular level, not at the leaflet tips. Parasternal long-axis views can also be helpful. If there is uncertainty after a thorough TTE, transesophageal echocardiography (TEE) should be performed.

Stenosis in the setting of a supramitral ring tends to increase over time. Surgical intervention should be considered for all patients with symptoms of obstruction, and it has an overall good outcome.[11,12] In all cases of supramitral obstruction and in one half of cases of intramitral obstruction, ring resection led to excellent long-term results.[13]

DOUBLE-ORIFICE MITRAL VALVE

A double-orifice mitral valve (DOMV) occurs when there are two separate mitral valve orifices, and each is supported by its own chordae and papillary muscles. Orifices may be equal in size, or one may be significantly smaller than the other. DOMV is more common among patients with AVSD, but it can rarely be seen in isolation (7% of all DOMV cases).

When DOMV occurs in isolation, the valve typically functions well, and the defect is clinically insignificant. In the setting of DOMV associated with AVSD, regurgitation typically occurs through the posteromedial orifice. DOMV can be best seen from a short-axis view, which allows en face imaging of the double orifice and comparison of the size of each orifice.[14] 3D echocardiography can provide additional detail to confirm orifice size and shape (Fig. 42.5).

PARACHUTE MITRAL VALVE

A true parachute mitral valve occurs when all chordae insert into a single papillary muscle, With a parachute-like mitral valve, the chordae are distributed unequally between two identifiable papillary muscles, but most converge on a dominant papillary muscle.[15] This typically results in mitral stenosis due to restricted leaflet motion and restriction at the chordal apparatus.[15] The other papillary muscle may be present without any chordal attachment, or it may be aberrant, small, or absent.

There is a strong correlation with other left-sided obstructive lesions. Parachute mitral valves associated with the Shone complex tend to connect to the posteromedial papillary muscles, whereas those associated with AVSDs tend to connect to the anterolateral papillary muscle. Abnormalities in papillary muscle formation can lead to a parachute mitral valve, likely because of underdeveloped space between the papillary muscles.

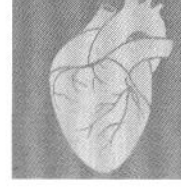

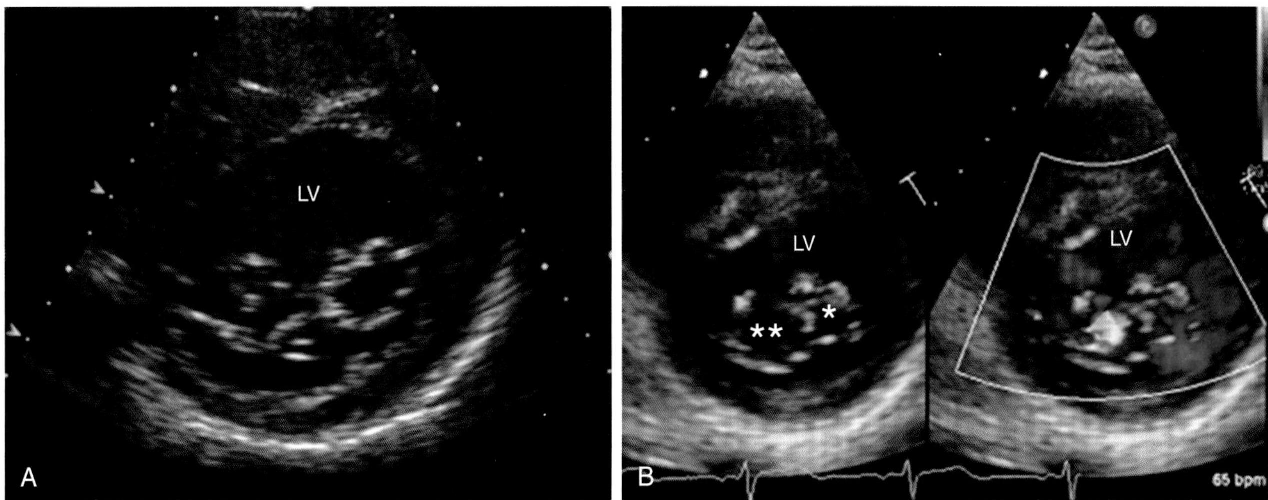

Fig. 42.5 **Double-orifice mitral valve.** (A) 2D parasternal short-axis imaging demonstrates a double-orifice mitral valve with relatively equal orifices (see Video 42.5A). (B) Color parasternal short-axis imaging demonstrates a double-orifice mitral valve with a smaller anterior orifice *(single asterisk)* and larger posterior orifice *(double asterisks)* (see Video 42.5B).

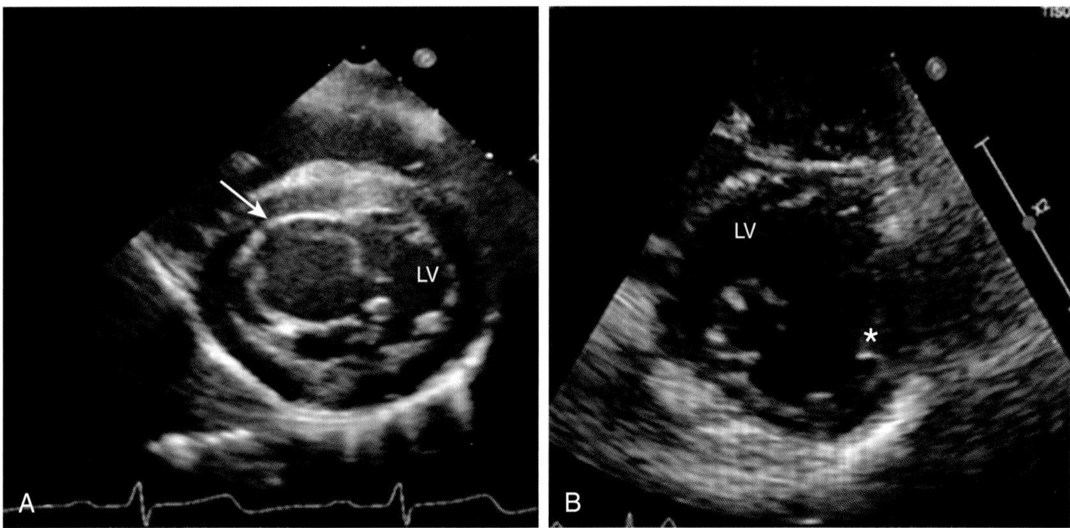

Fig. 42.6 **Parachute mitral valve.** (A) 2D parasternal short-axis view demonstrates a parachute mitral valve in the setting of a repaired atrioventricular canal defect and mitral valve attachments to the anterolateral papillary muscle. There is also a mitral valve cleft *(arrow)* (see Video 42.6A). (B) 2D short-axis view demonstrates a parachute mitral valve in a patient with multiple left-sided obstructed lesions. The mitral valve has attachments to the posteromedial papillary muscle. There is an anterolateral papillary muscle *(asterisk)* that is not receiving any mitral valve attachments (see Video 42.6B).

The diagnosis is made with parasternal short-axis imaging, which is used to assess the size and location of papillary muscles, mitral valve leaflets, and chordal attachments. Imaging must also carefully assess for other left-sided obstructive lesions, including LVOT obstruction and aortic arch imaging to rule out CoA[16] (Fig. 42.6).

MITRAL ARCADE

Mitral arcade is a rare entity that involves muscularization of the chordal apparatus, with the leaflets appearing to insert directly into the papillary muscles. Chordae are shortened or absent, and leaflets are often thickened. This is also known as a *hammock valve,* and it can result in mitral stenosis or regurgitation.[17] This lesion often manifests early in life and has an overall poor outcome.[18]

CONGENITAL LV OUTFLOW TRACT OBSTRUCTION

LVOT obstruction (LVOTO) occurs when blood flow from the LV is obstructed. It can occur below the aortic valve (i.e., subaortic stenosis), at the level of the aortic valve (i.e., valvular aortic stenosis), or above the aortic valve (i.e., supravalvular aortic stenosis). Other types of congenital heart disease can have some degree of obstruction to systemic blood flow resulting from malposed great arteries associated with a hypoplastic ventricle.

SUBAORTIC OBSTRUCTION

Subvalvular aortic stenosis (SAS) is the second most common type of aortic stenosis, accounting for 14% of LVOTO. Valvular aortic stenosis is the most common cause (70%).[20,21] SAS

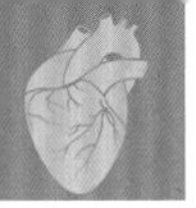

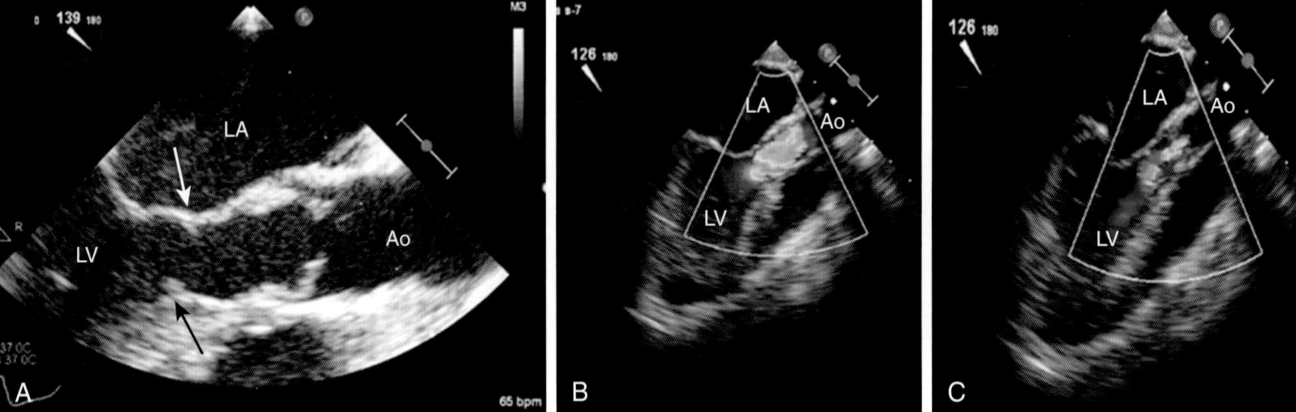

Fig. 42.7 **Subaortic membrane.** (A) TEE demonstrates a discrete circumferential subaortic membrane *(arrows)*. The membrane extends from the base of the anteroseptum to the anterior mitral valve leaflet. This patient also has a bicuspid aortic valve, and the aortic valve leaflets appear thickened and doming (see Video 42.7A). (B) TEE with color shows color flow aliasing starting below the level of the aortic valve that is consistent with subaortic stenosis (see Video 42.7B). (C) TEE with color shows mild aortic regurgitation in diastole, which is typically an indication for surgical membrane resection. *Ao*, Aorta.

accounts for 10% to 20% of cases of LVOTO in the pediatric population, with a male predominance.[21] Associated defects occur in slightly more than one half of cases and can include VSDs, valvular aortic stenosis, CoA, and AVSDs. Mitral valve anomalies sometimes contribute to the pathophysiology of the obstruction. With the exception of posterior malaligned VSDs, fixed subaortic stenosis is rarely seen in the neonatal heart and is thought by some to be an acquired rather than a congenital lesion.[22]

SAS may develop after patch closure of a perimembranous or malaligned VSD or AVSD. Hypertrophic cardiomyopathy can result in septal hypertrophy, which causes a muscular obstruction of the LVOT. This can be accompanied by abnormal systolic anterior motion of the mitral valve. Rarely, abnormal mitral valve chords can cause outflow tract obstruction that mimics SAS. A thick fibromuscular ridge or tunnel-like obstruction with a long, narrow fibromuscular channel along the LVOT also can result in SAS.

Another type of SAS is the discrete or membranous form (Fig. 42.7), which usually manifests during childhood. It is often associated with a membranous VSD, and the growth of fibrous tissue may result from the abnormal shear stresses of VSD flow. Discrete ASA also can be associated with bicuspid aortic valve (BAV) and CoA. The tissue is typically attached to the superior aspect of the ventricular septum, but it may also extend onto the anterior mitral valve leaflet.

SAS less frequently occurs as a longer, tunnel-like obstruction. Muscular narrowing can involve septal hypertrophy, an accessory anterolateral papillary muscle, or both. This is often associated with other forms of left heart obstruction and involves a hypoplastic LVOT and aortic valve annulus.[23,24] Subaortic obstruction can also occur after repair of more complex forms of congenital heart disease, including subaortic obstruction after a Rastelli repair, in which a VSD is closed and the LV is baffled to a malpositioned aorta.

The American Heart Association and American College of Cardiology (AHA/ACC) guidelines combine the indications for surgical repair of subaortic membrane and subaortic tunnel. The class I indications for surgical membrane resection are a peak instantaneous gradient of 50 mmHg or a mean gradient of 30 mmHg or greater, determined by echocardiography. Lesser gradients with progressive aortic regurgitation, decreased LV function, or symptoms attributable to SAS are also indications for surgery.

TABLE 42.1 **Left-Sided Heart Anomalies and Associated Findings.**

Diagnosis	*Associated Findings*	*Associated Congenital Lesions*
Subaortic membrane	Subaortic obstruction, aortic regurgitation	BAV, supramitral ring, CoA, ventricular septal defect, double-chambered RV
Bicuspid aortic valve	Aortic stenosis, regurgitation aortic dilation	CoA
CoA	Recurrent coarctation, poststenotic dilation, diminutive transverse arch, collaterals	BAV, abdominal coarctation, mitral valve anomalies

BAV, Bicuspid aortic valve; *CoA*, coarctation of the aorta.

Oliver et al.[25] compared SAS in adult and pediatric populations. There was a slower rate of progression of LVOTO in adults, and aortic regurgitation was common but usually mild and nonprogressive. These differences suggest that there should be different indications for surgery for adults and children.[25]

The criteria and exact timing of intervention for SAS are controversial. Regrowth of tissue may lead to recurrent subaortic obstruction, which makes regular clinical and echocardiographic monitoring mandatory. Repair of a subaortic tunnel is complex and may involve a more complicated surgical repair. In selected patients with a hypoplastic LVOT, extensive subaortic resection may need to be combined with insertion of the patient's pulmonary valve into the aortic position (i.e., Ross-Konno operation).[26] Degeneration of the aortic valve in response to subvalvular turbulence or involvement of the base of the mitral valve by the membrane may require aortic or mitral valve reconstruction or replacement.

Physical examination of adults reveals a systolic outflow murmur, absence of systolic ejection clicks, and the murmur of aortic regurgitation (Table 42.1). Echocardiography is the best method for diagnosing SAS. It can be used to characterize the anatomy of the subaortic lesion, assess LVOT involvement, determine the dimensions and function of the LV, and evaluate the integrity of the aortic and mitral valves.

The LVOT is best assessed with 2D echocardiographic imaging using parasternal long- and short-axis views. A subaortic membrane is most commonly visible adherent to the basal anteroseptal LV surface at various distances below the aortic annulus. Although membranes may also be located immediately below the leaflets or adherent to the ventricular surface of the aortic leaflets, they are most commonly identified approximately 1.0 to 1.5 cm below the aortic annulus. They may extend from the base of the anteroseptum around the LVOT and insert onto the basal portion of the anterior mitral leaflet, or they may be completely circumferential within the LVOT. 3D imaging allows for en face views of the subaortic obstruction.

Color-flow Doppler imaging demonstrates flow acceleration in the LVOT at the membrane below the level of the aortic valve, with 2D imaging often demonstrating normal aortic valve leaflet excursion. Although secondary hypertrophy of the septum may develop below the subaortic membrane, echocardiographically mimicking hypertrophic cardiomyopathy, pulsed-wave (PW) and continuous-wave (CW) Doppler across the LVOT in patients with subaortic membranes typically does not demonstrate a late peaking gradient as is the case for dynamic LVOTO. The high-velocity systolic jet across the LVOT collides with the aortic valve leaflets, resulting in aortic leaflet scarring that can promote aortic regurgitation. There may be flutter of aortic valve leaflets during systole as they are hit by the turbulent jet from the subaortic region. The aortic valve damage can lead to clot and vegetation formation. Detailed mitral valve assessment also is essential.

To accurately assess the gradient across the LVOT, CW Doppler should be used with an optimal angle of interrogation as parallel to the flow jet as possible. Assessment should use the apical views and a suprasternal view, which often produces the highest gradient. PW Doppler should be performed at various levels of the LVOT to ascertain their relative contributions to obstruction. In the postoperative setting, TEE is useful in assessing the adequacy of subaortic muscle resection, evaluating mitral and aortic valves for dysfunction due to surgical procedures, and evaluating the ventricular septum for iatrogenic VSDs.[22,27]

VALVULAR CONGENITAL AORTIC DISEASE

Aortic valve disease in children or young adults is typically caused by commisssural underdevelopment, hypoplasia of the annulus, myxomatous thickening of the valve, or some combination. If it is a result of commissural underdevelopment, the aortic valve may be unicommissural or bicommissural. Unicommisural valves occur only when the commissure is well formed. Typically, it is the left noncoronary commissure. Unicommisural valves are rare and usually manifest in the third to fifth decade of life with severe aortic stenosis or regurgitation.

In bicommissural aortic valves, one commissure is underdeveloped, and the other two are well formed. BAV is the most common congenital cardiac abnormality, with an estimated occurrence of 1% to 2%. It can manifest as many morphologic variants. The most common anatomic form of BAV consists of two cusps with a false raphe (between the right and left coronary cusps) and two commissures.

Quadricuspid aortic valves are rarely seen and typically manifest with regurgitation. The prevalence of quadricuspid aortic valve at autopsy is about 0.01%.

Congenitally abnormal aortic valves may manifest with stenosis or regurgitation. They have abnormal aortic wall architecture that predisposes patients to aortopathy and risk of aortic dilation, aneurysm formation, and sometimes aortic dissection, particularly in those older than 50 years of age and those with significantly dysfunctional valves.[30] This lesion mandates adequate echocardiographic assessment of the aortic root and ascending aorta in individuals with congenital aortic valve disease.[31]

Aortic pathology does not depend on the degree of valvular disease, and aortic assessment is essential even for congenitally abnormal valves with minimal valvular dysfunction.[32–35] Physical examination of young patients may demonstrate a prominent mid-systolic ejection click and the murmur of aortic stenosis or regurgitation.

Percutaneous aortic valvuloplasty is the therapy of choice for children and young adults with congenital aortic stenosis without significant regurgitation. For adult patients with congenital aortic stenosis, practice guidelines suggest that percutaneous balloon valvuloplasty is indicated if the symptoms of angina, syncope, or dyspnea are identified and the peak-to-peak gradient determined by catheterization is 50 mmHg or higher, or for asymptomatic patients with electrocardiographic changes or a peak-to-peak gradient of 60 mmHg.[36]

Complications of percutaneous aortic valvuloplasty include significant increase in aortic regurgitation (10%–30%) and stroke or other embolic complication if there is aortic calcification. After the fourth or fifth decade, the aortic valve may become thickened and calcified (commensurate with loss of the systolic ejection click), and it may be less amenable to valvuloplasty.[35]

Parasternal views provide the best images of aortic valve morphology. Parasternal long-axis views demonstrate BAV leaflets that dome at the tips and asymmetric closure in diastole. Valve morphology, including the number of commissures, can be determined on parasternal short-axis imaging in systole, and the raphe can be seen in diastole (Table 42.2). The most common morphology is fusion of the intercoronary commissure, followed by fusion of the non/right commissure. The least common case is underdevelopment of the non/left commissure. Fusion of the intercoronary commissure is more often associated with CoA and other congenital heart disease, whereas fusion of the right/non commissure is more often associated with aortic valve dysfunction and aortic dilation. In another variant, the valve is truly bicuspid, with two relatively equal leaflets and one commissure.[33–35]

Doppler echocardiography should be used for all congenitally abnormal aortic valves to determine the peak and mean transvalvular gradients. As with evaluation of SAS, gradients should be obtained in apical and suprasternal views; suprasternal views often give the highest gradients.

Mild stenosis is defined as a peak Doppler velocity of less than 3 m/s (mean gradient <20 mmHg), moderate stenosis as a peak velocity of 3 to 4 m/s (mean, 20–40 mmHg), and severe stenosis as a peak velocity more than 4 m/s (mean >40 mmHg). For older children and adults, the valve area can be assessed using the continuity equation. It is important to assess LV function when considering Doppler gradients because the Doppler gradient underestimates the degree of stenosis in those with reduced function.[37,38] Imaging of the aortic root and ascending aorta must be obtained in a parasternal long-axis view to assess for aortopathy.

For all patients with a BAV, the aortic arch must be assessed along with Doppler imaging of the abdominal aorta at the level of the diaphragm to exclude CoA.[39] A BAV may also be

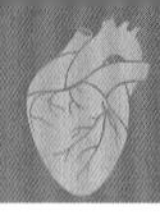

TABLE 42.2 Physical Examination Findings and Echocardiographic Correlates for Left Heart Obstruction.

Diagnosis	*Physical Examination Findings*	*Echocardiographic Correlates*	*Additional Modalities*
Subaortic stenosis	Holosystolic to mid-systolic murmur at the LUSB/RUSB, radiation to carotids, sustained LV apical impulse May be associated with aortic diastolic murmur at LSB	Flow acceleration beginning below the aortic valve Normal excursion of aortic valve leaflets Echo-bright ridge at the base of the anteroseptum that is best seen in parasternal long-axis, apical 3-chamber, and apical 5-chamber views and may extend to the base of the anterior mitral leaflet Aortic regurgitation Aortic leaflet fluttering	TEE
BAV	Systolic ejection murmur with progressively late peaking and progressive carotid pulse delay and volume reduction with severity Systolic click may diminish with increased gradient. AR may be detected	Leaflet doming in parasternal long-axis view Two patent commissures in PSAX view at the level of the aortic valve Raphae may or may not be present Cusp asymmetry, dilation of the sinuses of Valsalva, effacement of the STJ, and ascending aortic dilation CoA must be excluded	—
Supravalvulvar aortic stenosis	Mid-systolic murmur at RUSB that often radiates to carotids	Proximal ascending aortic narrowing at and just above the STJ; flow acceleration at this level Screen for branch pulmonic stenosis	Cardiac CT or MRI
CoA	Radial femoral pulse delay Diminished lower extremity pulses Continuous murmur at left sternal border or mid-scapular region	Suprasternal notch imaging of arch, branch, and proximal descending aorta with PW and CW Doppler imaging Abdominal aortic imaging with color to assess for persistent diastolic flow PW Doppler in the abdominal aorta demonstrates delayed upstroke and anterograde diastolic runoff Screen for bicuspid aortic valve, VSD, and mitral anomalies	Cardiac MRI or CT

AR, Aortic regurgitation; *BAV*, bicuspid aortic valve; *CoA*, coarctation of the aorta; *CT*, computed tomography; *LSB*, lower sternal border; *LUSB*, left upper sternal boarder; *MRI*, magnetic resonance imaging; *PSAX*, parasternal short axis; *PW*, pulsed-wave; *RUSB*, right upper sternal border; *STJ*, sinotubular junction; *TEE*, transesophageal echocardiography; *VSD*, ventricular septal defect.

associated with an ASD, a VSD, or mitral prolapse. 3D echocardiography can provide accurate measurements of aortic valve annulus dimensions, determine the number of valve leaflets, identify sites of fusion of the leaflets, and reveal nodules and excrescences that characterize dysplastic valves. Because familial clusters of BAV have been described, screening of first-degree relatives is recommended. Aortic valve morphology and aortic dimensions should be assessed when screening first-degree relatives because aortopathy can exist without a bicuspid valve.[39,40]

Unicuspid unicommissural aortic valve leaflets appear abnormal, deformed, or dysplastic, and parasternal long-axis imaging can show that they dome at the tips (Fig. 42.8). In high parasternal short-axis imaging, a single open commissure is visualized between the left and noncoronary leaflets, and in systole, there is a rounded opening with the typical keyhole or teardrop appearance. As leaflets dome, the minimal cross-sectional area is at the tips, and the plane in traditional 2D parasternal short-axis imaging from which to optimally view leaflet morphology commonly falls below this level. The cross-sectional valve area as measured in standard parasternal short-axis imaging may therefore overestimate the minimal cross-sectional area at the leaflet tips. 3D echocardiography also provides the opportunity to identify the minimal cross-sectional opening, and planimetry from 3D-generated images may provide a more accurate assessment of the valve area.[41]

Aortic valve disease is usually treated with valvotomy in infancy or childhood or with valve repair or replacement later in life, sometimes with the Ross procedure, in which the pulmonic valve is transplanted to the aortic position and the patient receives a homograft to the pulmonic annulus with coronary reimplantation. For patients with congenital aortic valve disease deemed appropriate for aortic valve replacement using the Ross procedure, echocardiography is essential for detailed measurements of the aortic and pulmonary annulus and for functional evaluation of the pulmonic valve to exclude pulmonic regurgitation or cusp abnormalities that can lead to suboptimal function in the aortic position. It is also critical to assess coronary artery origins preoperatively. Preoperative and postoperative assessment and long-term follow-up of LV function are also essential for coronary artery reimplantation.[40]

SUPRAVALVULAR AORTIC STENOSIS

There are at least two anatomic forms of supravalvular aortic stenosis. Between 60% and 75% of patients have an hourglass deformity, consisting of a discrete constriction of a thickened ascending aorta at the superior aspect of the sinuses of Valsalva. More diffuse narrowing for some distance along the ascending aorta is seen in 25% to 40% of patients. There are rare reports of a discrete membranous stenosis, which may be a variant of the hourglass deformity.[42] Discrete narrowing at the sinotubular junction is most commonly seen in the setting of Williams syndrome, which is a deletion on chromosome 7 that involves the elastin gene [43] (Table 42.3). SAS may also occur as an isolated finding.

Other cardiac manifestations of Williams syndrome include various degrees of hypoplasia of the ascending aorta, aortic arch, a more distal aorta, and stenosis of the head and neck vessels. Patients may have coronary ostial stenosis, which can be worsened by tethering of the aortic valve leaflets. Extracardiac manifestations of Williams syndrome include significant developmental delays and hypercalcemia. Hypertension is prevalent, likely due to the decreased aortic compliance resulting from the elastin gene *(ELN)* mutation.[44,45]

SAS is associated with several other cardiovascular anomalies, including thickened and redundant aortic valve leaflets with reduced mobility.[46] Rarely, coronary artery stenosis can result from focal or diffuse coronary narrowing or from obstruction by redundant, dysplastic aortic valve leaflets.[47] CoA and ostial stenosis of the carotid, renal, iliac, and other

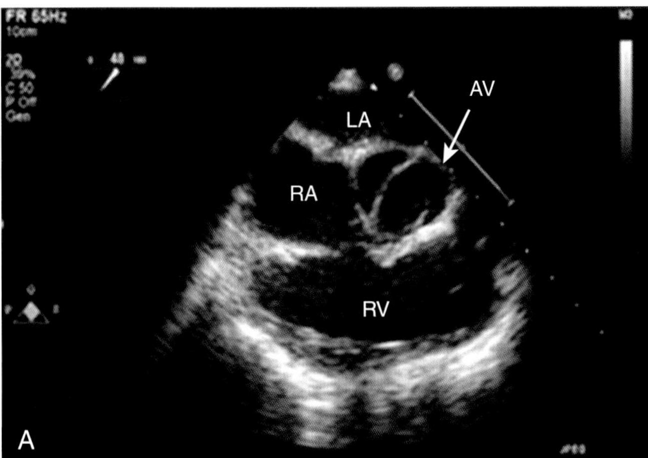

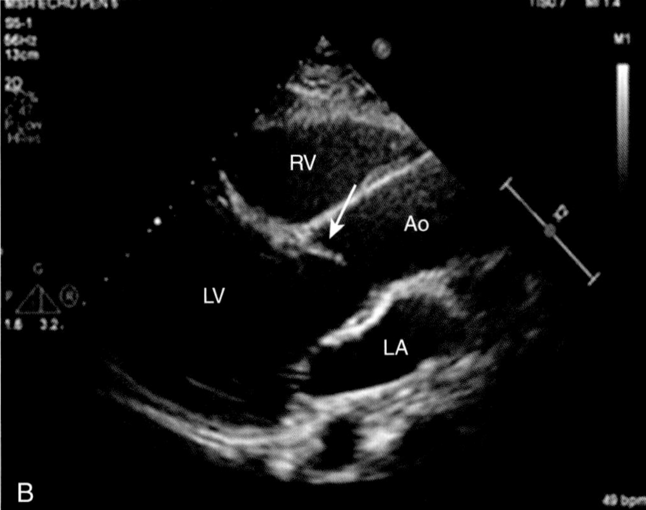

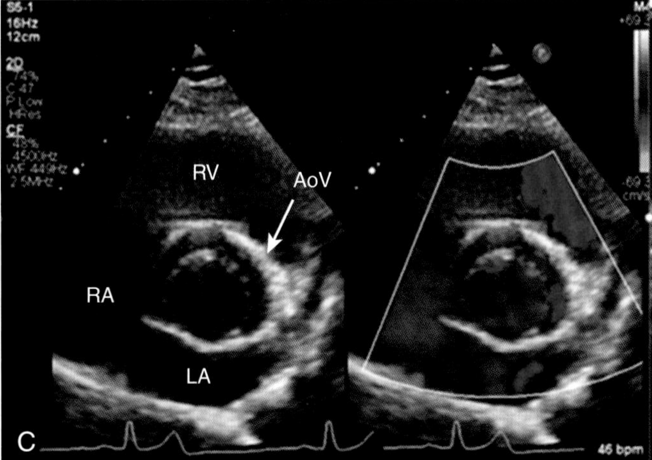

Fig. 42.8 Bicuspid and unicuspid aortic valves. (A) TEE shows an example of a true bicuspid aortic valve *(arrow)* with relatively equal cusps (see Video 42.8A). (B) Parasternal long-axis view in a patient with a unicuspid aortic valve shows doming of the anterior aortic valve leaflet *(arrow)*. The posterior leaflet is flush against the wall, while the anterior leaflet is still in the aortic lumen (see Video 42.8B). (C) Color parasternal short-axis view shows a unicommissural aortic valve *(arrow)* with fusion of the intercoronary and non/right commissures (see Video 42.8C). *AoV*, Aortic valve.

peripheral arteries have been reported for some patients.[48] Stenosis of the main pulmonary artery or branch pulmonary arteries is common, occurring in approximately one half of patients. In contrast to the systemic arterial stenosis described previously, pulmonary artery stenosis typically decreases in severity over time.

Percutaneous approaches are usually unsuccessful, and open surgical repair is preferred when repair is necessary.[49] TTE typically demonstrates the normal size of the sinuses of Valsalva with narrowing of the sinotubular junction and proximal ascending aorta; this is best seen in the parasternal long-axis view (Fig. 42.9).[46] Doppler echocardiography is useful for deriving peak instantaneous and mean pressure gradients across this region; the most accurate gradient is typically obtained with the suprasternal view (see Table 42.2). The full extent of the ascending aorta is difficult to visualize in adults with TTE, and TEE or magnetic resonance imaging (MRI) may be superior.

Aortic valve abnormalities can occur and should be evaluated. Stress and shear forces are increased on the aortic valve leaflets in the setting of a poorly distensible sinotubular junction, resulting in leaflet thickening and damage. Careful evaluation for branch pulmonic stenosis should be performed. The full aortic arch should be imaged from suprasternal views, and the coronary ostia should be assessed by 2D and color Doppler imaging.[44,45]

COARCTATION OF THE AORTA

CoA is a relatively common defect, comprising 6% to 8% of all congenital heart disease. It affects 4 of 10,000 live births and has a male predominance (1.7:1).[50,51] CoA may be defined as a constricted aortic segment with localized medial thickening and some infoldings of the medial and superimposed neointimal tissue. The localized constriction may form a shelf-like structure with an eccentric opening or may be a membranous structure with a central or eccentric opening. The coarctation is usually discrete, although sometimes a long segment of the aorta is narrowed.

Classic coarctation is located in the thoracic aorta distal to the origin of the left subclavian artery, at about the level of insertion of the ductus arteriosus. Other types of coarctation involve narrowing of the aorta above or below the ductus arteriosus. About 64% of patients present shortly after birth. In older children and adults, aortic arch hypoplasia is less common, and the coarctation is usually discrete. Typically, there are collateral arteries bypassing the region of coarctation; these collateral vessels develop in response to increased flow through the internal mammary and intercostal arteries.

Associated cardiac abnormalities are common, including BAV (50%–60%), mitral valve abnormalities, subaortic membrane, and VSD. Up to 10% of individuals have cerebral aneurysms in the circle of Willis (i.e., berry aneurysm), and one-time arterial screening of the brain is recommended for all patients.[52–55]

Complications include persistent hypertension, early-age hypertension, and in some cases, isolated exercise-induced hypertension, even among patients who have undergone repair. For patients with native unrepaired coarctation or restenosis at a prior repair site, physical examination results may be notable for upper extremity hypertension, reduced blood pressure in the legs, radial-femoral delay, and the systolic ejection click of a BAV.

The initial imaging and hemodynamic evaluation of patients with suspected CoA depends on TTE (Table 42.4). Evaluation for CoA is best done with the suprasternal notch view (Fig. 42.10) and should include color and CW Doppler assessment of the distal aortic arch and isthmus. A hemodynamically significant coarctation has a typical CW Doppler profile demonstrating continuing anterograde flow tapering off during diastole.[57] If elevated, the proximal velocity should be accounted for using the Bernoulli equation for pressure

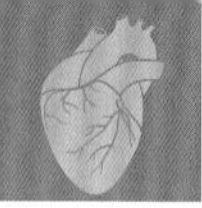

TABLE 42.3 **Syndromes Associated With Left Heart Anomalies.**

Syndrome	*Left Heart Anomaly*	*Associated Cardiovascular Anomalies*	*Systemic Processes Affecting Cardiac Function*
Williams-Beuren	Supravalvular ASD	Coronary origin stenosis; carotid, renal, subclavian, celiac artery stenoses; pulmonary arterial stenoses, hypoplastic aorta	Hypertension (important to evaluate for LV hypertrophy and diastolic function), hypercalcemia, QT prolongation, abnormal glucose metabolism
Turner	CoA, BAV, mitral valve anomalies, rarely HLHS	Aortic dilation, PAPVR, ASD, VSD	Hypertension, risk of aortic event in pregnancy, QT prolongation
22q11.2 deletion	IAA type B, truncus arteriosus, isolated arch anomaly (cervical arch, RAA, aberrant origin of the SCA)	Tetralogy of Fallot, conoventricular VSD	—
Down syndrome	LV outflow obstruction after repair of AVSD, residual MR, MS from cleft repair	ASD, VSD, AVSD, PDA, TOF, DORV, mitral valve prolapse	Diabetes, overweight, pulmonary hypertension

ASD, Atrial septal defect; *AVSD,* atrioventricular septal defect; *BAV,* bicuspid aortic valve; *CoA,* coarctation of the aorta; *DORV,* double-outlet right ventricle; *HLHS,* hypoplastic left heart syndrome; *IAA,* interrupted aortic arch; *MR,* mitral regurgitation; *MS,* mitral stenosis; *PAPVR,* partial anomalous pulmonary venous drainage; *PDA,* patent ductus arteriosus; *RAA,* right aortic arch; *SCA,* subclavian artery; *TOF,* tetralogy of Fallot; *VSD,* ventricular septal defect.
From Lin AE, Basson CT, Goldmuntz E, et al. Adults with genetic syndromes and cardiovascular abnormalities: clinical history and management. *Genet Med.* 2008;10:469–494.

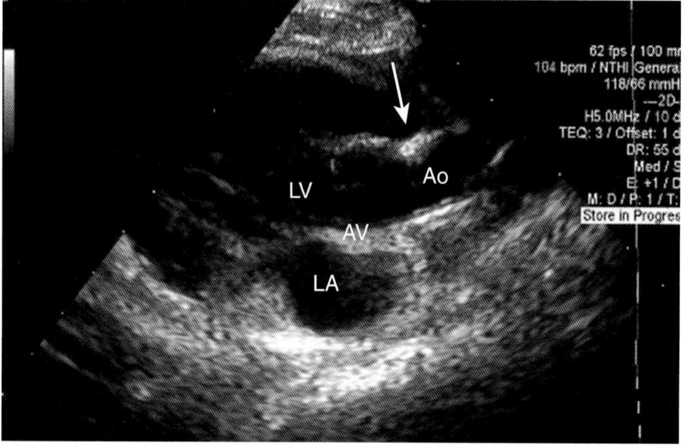

Fig. 42.9 Supravalvular aortic stenosis. Mild narrowing *(arrow)* at the sinotubular junction in a patient with Williams syndrome (see Video 42.9). *Ao,* Aorta.

gradient assessment. Among patients with native coarctation, the jet direction may be highly eccentric, and it can be challenging to align the ultrasound beam and jet direction. The mean gradient through the region of narrowing seems to correlate better with peak-to-peak gradients derived from catheterization compared with peak echocardiographic gradients.

Interrogation of the abdominal aorta is done to assess flow pattern. Delay in systolic upstroke and persistent antegrade flow in diastole constitute the hallmark of significant aortic obstruction. In addition to evaluation of the coarctation gradient and anatomy, echocardiography should be used to assess for commonly associated lesions and dilation of the ascending aorta.[58] Advanced imaging such as cardiac MRI or computed tomography (CT) is typically needed to evaluate the entire aortic arch, site of CoA, and location of collaterals.[59]

Congenital heart defects that cause LVOTO (see Table 42.1) result in chronic pressure overload, LV hypertrophy, myocardial fibrosis, and diastolic dysfunction, predisposing patients to clinical heart failure. Studies have validated 3D echocardiography as an accurate method for measuring an LV mass in adults.[60] Although studies of LV mass in children have been limited in number and scope, Riehle et al. demonstrated excellent correlations between LV mass measured by 3D echocardiography and by MRI.[61] Assessment of LV diastolic parameters has become increasingly important for the adult population with congenital heart disease. Patients who have sustained left heart obstructive processes over years often demonstrate delayed relaxation or more advanced restrictive diastolic filling patterns. Arterial stiffness is prevalent in this population, and ventriculoarterial interaction likely contributes to abnormalities of myocardial relaxation. Echocardiography can be used to assess arterial compliance, but it is not done routinely in clinical practice.[62]

AORTIC ARCH ANOMALIES

Congenital aortic arch anomalies are rare but are more prevalent among patients with congenital heart disease. The anomalies can be incidentally identified radiographically in asymptomatic adult patients. Occasionally an adult patient presents with subacute symptoms of dysphagia or respiratory distress.

The aortic arch begins to develop in the fourth week of embryogenesis from six symmetric, paired aortic arch vessels and the paired dorsal aortae. Remodeling and rearrangement of these structures occur to form a normal left aortic arch.[65,66] In Edwards' hypothetical double aortic arch system, in which there is an aortic arch and a ductus arteriosus on each side, the right carotid and subclavian arteries arise from the right arch, and the left carotid and subclavian arteries originate from the left arch.[67] Normal arch development results from interruption of the dorsal segment of the right arch between the right subclavian and the descending aorta, with regression of the right ductus arteriosus (Fig. 42.11). Interruption of this arch system at different locations can explain the various aortic arch anomalies.[68] Abnormal development results in arch malformations and a wide range of anatomic variations in vascular rings. Abnormalities in aortic arch development are associated with genetic abnormalities, particularly a 22q11 deletion.[68]

A *complete vascular ring* is an aortic arch anomaly in which the trachea and esophagus are completely surrounded by vascular structures. These vascular structures do not need to be patent (e.g., ligamentum arteriosus, atretic aortic arch segment). These patients may present with symptoms of tracheal compression such as stridor or frequent respiratory infections or with compression of the esophagus along with feeding difficulties or

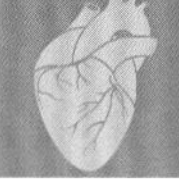

TABLE 42.4 Echocardiography for Coarctation of the Aorta.

Type of Imaging	*Anatomic Imaging*	*Physiologic Imaging*
Suprasternal notch	2D and color imaging of the entire aortic arch for anatomy and turbulent flow	Doppler-derived pressure gradient Mean gradient often correlates better with catheterization-derived peak-to-peak gradient
High parasternal view	Displays aorta in sagittal plane	May demonstrate poststenotic dilation, although not an ideal imaging mechanism for aneurysm assessment
Abdominal aorta	2D and color imaging of distal aorta	Persistent diastolic flow or delayed upstroke in abdominal aorta from severe coarctation
Parasternal short- and long-axis views	Assessment of aortic valve morphology, severity of stenosis or regurgitation, aortic root size, and ascending aorta size	Quantifies LV hypertrophy and LV dimensions
Apical views	Assessment of aortic valve and LV outflow (5-chamber views)	LV systolic and diastolic function (4- and 2-chamber views)
TEE	Excellent 2D and 3D imaging of anatomy	Poor Doppler-derived gradient due to inadequate alignment

LVOT, left ventricular outflow tract.

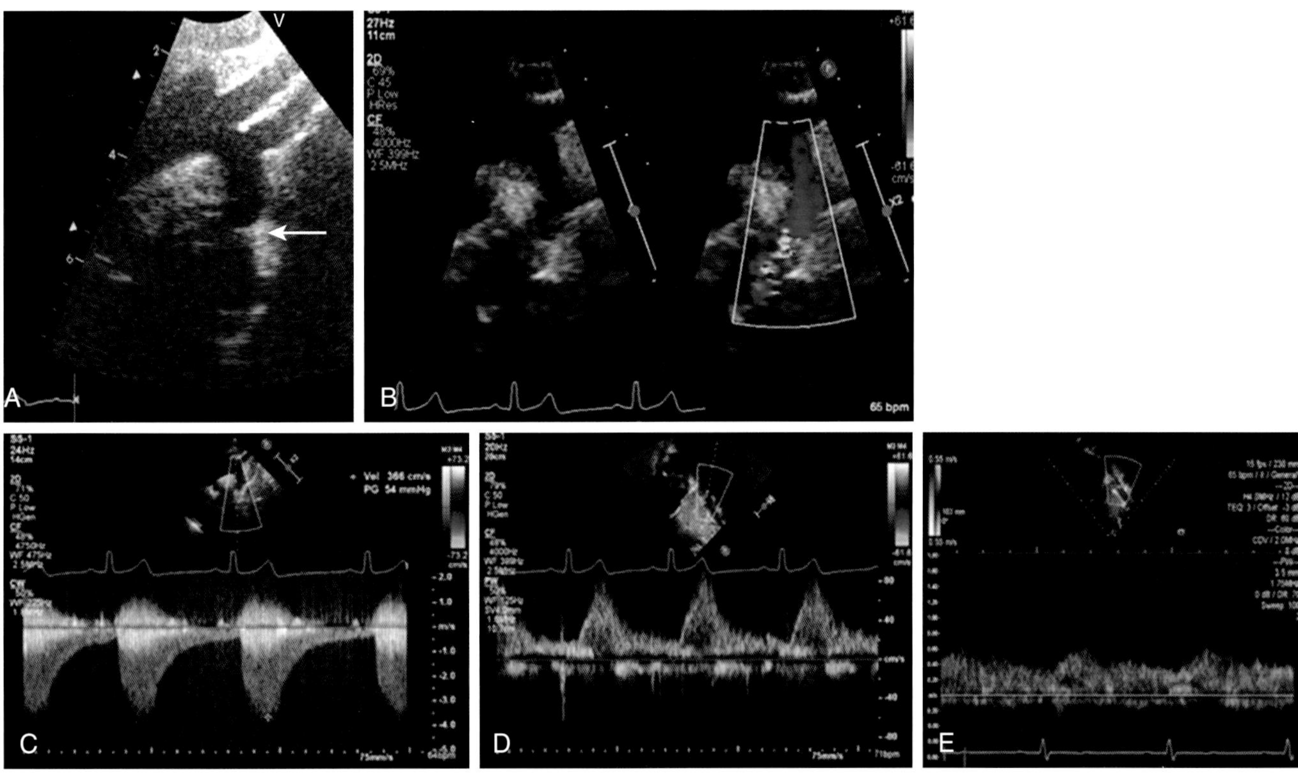

Fig. 42.10 Coarctation of the aorta. (A) 2D suprasternal notch imaging demonstrates a posterior shelf at the aortic isthmus *(arrow)*, consistent with coarctation of the aorta. (B) Color view demonstrates flow aliasing at the level of narrowing of the aortic isthmus. (C) CW Doppler imaging at the area of narrowing demonstrates a significant gradient across the aortic isthmus. (D) Abdominal aortic Doppler imaging in a patient with mild coarctation shows slightly increased flow during diastole. (E) Abdominal aortic Doppler imaging in a patient with severe coarctation shows limited pulsatility and significant flow during diastole.

dysphagia. Complete rings include a double aortic arch and a right arch with an aberrant left subclavian artery with a left ductus arteriosus or ligamentum.

An *incomplete vascular ring* is an arch anomaly that does not completely encircle the trachea and esophagus and includes a pulmonary artery sling, innominate artery compression, and an aberrant right subclavian artery. Clear definition of arch anomalies can be challenging echocardiographically; CT angiography and cardiac MRI are ideal for defining the anatomy of the arch and its relation to other intrathoracic structures.[69]

Echocardiographic imaging of the aortic arch focuses on suprasternal views. Imaging is optimized by elevating the patient's shoulders and extending the neck. A transverse sweep of the transducer (with the marker toward the patient's left) should begin at the level of the cross section of the ascending aorta and superior vena cava, and then continue superiorly to image the aortic arch branching. A long-axis suprasternal view of the arch should also be obtained. From these images, the arch sidedness and branching pattern can be determined.[70]

INTERRUPTED AORTIC ARCH

An interrupted aortic arch (IAA) is a rare anomaly, comprising 1% of all critically ill infants with congenital heart disease and

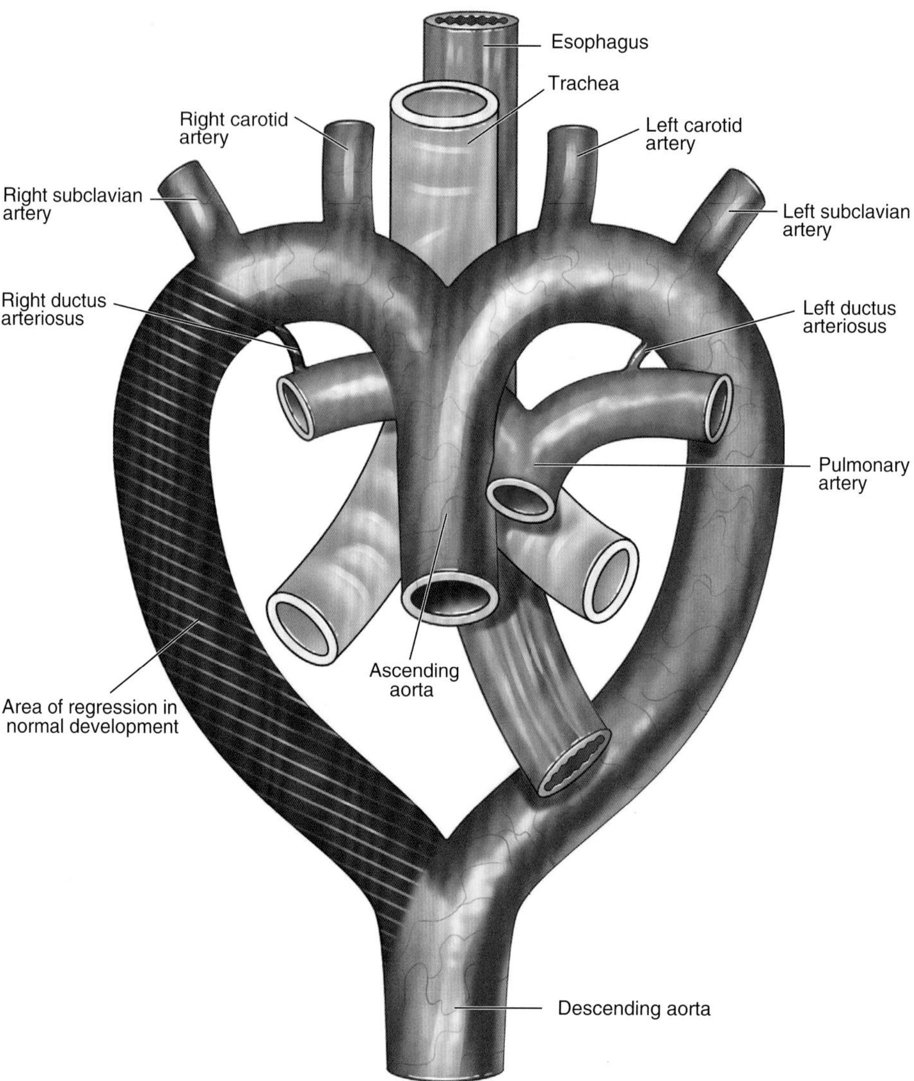

Fig. 42.11 Aortic arch embryology. The Edward system for understanding aortic arch embryology (see Videos 42.11A and 42.11B).

characterized by discontinuity between two adjacent segments of the aortic arch. Three types of IAA are classified according to the site of interruption in relation to the head and neck vessels. Type A is an interruption distal to the origin of the left subclavian artery. This is the second most common type. It is very similar to severe coarctation and is differentiated only by the absence of luminal continuity of the aortic isthmus.

Type B IAA, the most common type, is defined as interruption between the left common carotid and the left subclavian artery. It is highly associated with an aberrant right subclavian artery distal to the interruption. Most patients have an associated VSD (often with posterior deviation of the conal septum underneath the aortic valve). There is also a strong association with the 22q11 deletion (see Table 42.3).

Type C IAA is an interruption between the right innominate and left common carotids and is rare.[42] IAA is almost universally diagnosed in the newborn period because of the requirement of a patent ductus arteriosus for survival. There are rare cases of interrupted aortic arch associated with hypertension in adults with aortopulmonary collateral flow bypassing the obstruction. More often, adults present after surgical repair in infancy.

Echocardiographic evaluation is similar to that for CoA. It involves abdominal aortic Doppler assessment, detailed arch imaging from the suprasternal notch view, assessment of LV mass and systolic/diastolic function, and evaluation of any associated lesions.[63,64]

DOUBLE AORTIC ARCH

A double aortic arch is a variant of a complete vascular ring in which the ascending aorta divides into two separate arches (Fig. 42.12). The right arch gives rise to the right common carotid and right subclavian artery, and the left arch gives rise to the left common carotid and left subclavian artery. The two arches join and form the descending aorta (although one arch may be atretic, with only a remnant ligament). Typically, the right arch is larger than the left, and it is often positioned slightly more superiorly than the left. There is also typically a left-sided ductal ligament that contributes to the ring. This anomaly is the most common cause of a complete vascular ring and is rarely associated with intracardiac congenital heart disease.

The onset and severity of symptoms vary and depend on the diameter of the ring. Patients may present with dysphagia, stridor, or recurrent respiratory infections early in infancy. The complete ring is often incidentally identified in adulthood.[71]

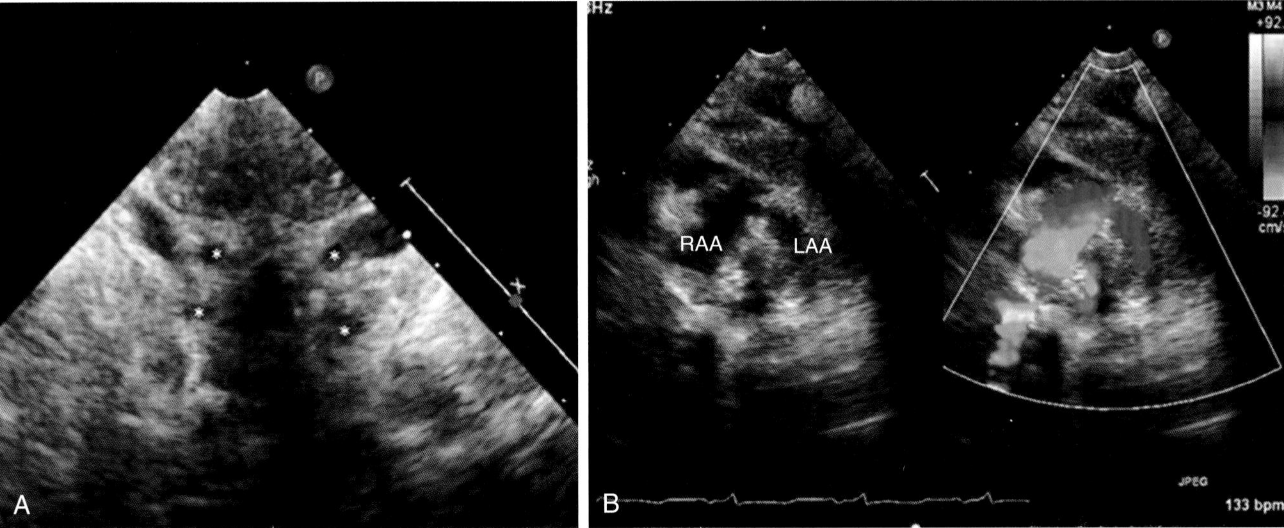

Fig. 42.12 **Double aortic arch.** (A) Suprasternal notch image shows the symmetric head and neck vessel arrangement in a patient with a double aortic arch. Each head and neck vessel is marked by an *asterisk* (see Video 42.12A). (B) Suprasternal image (more inferior than in A) shows a dominant right aortic arch. This patient had an atretic segment between the origin of the left subclavian artery and the descending aorta (see Video 42.12B). *LAA*, Left aortic arch; *RAA*, right aortic arch.

RIGHT AORTIC ARCH

A right aortic arch is a relatively common anomaly that occurs in approximately 0.1% of the population.[72] The two most common types are a right aortic arch with mirror-image branching and a right aortic arch with an aberrant left subclavian artery. Less common variants include isolation of the left subclavian artery and a right arch with a left descending aorta (i.e., circumflex arch).

In a right aortic arch with mirror-image branching, the branching pattern mirrors that of a normal left arch. The first branch is a left innominate artery that bifurcates into a left common carotid and left subclavian artery, followed by the right common carotid and right subclavian artery. This type of aortic arch tends to be associated with conotruncal defects such as tetralogy of Fallot and truncus arteriosus. A right aortic arch with these conotruncal defects increases the risk of identifying a genetic disorder such as DiGeorge syndrome. The ductus in this type of aortic arch is typically a left anterior ductus (arising from the base of the left innominate artery), rather than a ductus that arises posteriorly from the descending aorta. Most right aortic arches with mirror-image branching do not form a vascular ring. Rarely, the ductus (or ligament) can arise from the right-sided descending aorta and course leftward to connect to the proximal left pulmonary artery and form a vascular ring.[73]

A right aortic arch with aberrant left subclavian artery results from interruption of the dorsal segment of the left arch between the left common carotid and left subclavian arteries, with regression of the right ductus arteriosus. The first branch arising from the aortic arch is the left carotid artery, followed by the right carotid artery, the right subclavian artery, and the anomalous left subclavian artery. The descending aorta is usually to the right of midline. The left ductus (or ductal ligament) usually originates from a dilation at the base of the left subclavian artery and attaches to the proximal left pulmonary artery, completing the vascular ring. The bulbous dilation at the base of the left subclavian artery is called a *diverticulum of Kommerell*. It indicates the site of the ductal ligament when the ductus arteriosus is closed. These diverticula can be associated with an increased risk of dissection, and surgical repair is often considered.[53]

Rarely, the ductus can be right sided, in which case there is no vascular ring. In these cases, there is no diverticulum of Kommerell, and the left subclavian artery caliber is uniform throughout. A right aortic arch with aberrant left subclavian artery is more likely to be associated with normal intracardiac anatomy compared with a right aortic arch with mirror-image branching.[51]

CERVICAL AORTIC ARCH

A cervical aortic arch is a rare anomaly in which the aortic arch is situated cervically above the clavicle. This lesion is often isolated, but it may occur with CoA and may be prone to aneurysmal change.[74] Cervical arches are easily identified with suprasternal notch imaging. Typically, there are several centimeters between the inferior border of the arch and the right pulmonary artery in cross section. There may be kinking at the isthmus and acceleration of flow because the flow makes an almost 180-degree turn from the ascending aorta to the proximal descending aorta.[75]

CORONARY ARTERY ANOMALIES

ANOMALIES OF CORONARY ARTERY ORIGINS

Assessment of coronary artery origins is recommended for all pediatric and young adult patients and for any adult patient with known or suspected congenital heart disease. Not all coronary anomalies carry clinical consequences, and most are benign and incidentally identified. Coronary artery origins may be difficult to assess by echocardiography, particularly in adults, and cardiac CT or MRI may be necessary for more definitive diagnosis.[76–78]

Anomalous Coronary Artery Origin From the Opposite Sinus

An anomalous coronary artery origin from the opposite sinus is a rare but an important cause of sudden cardiac

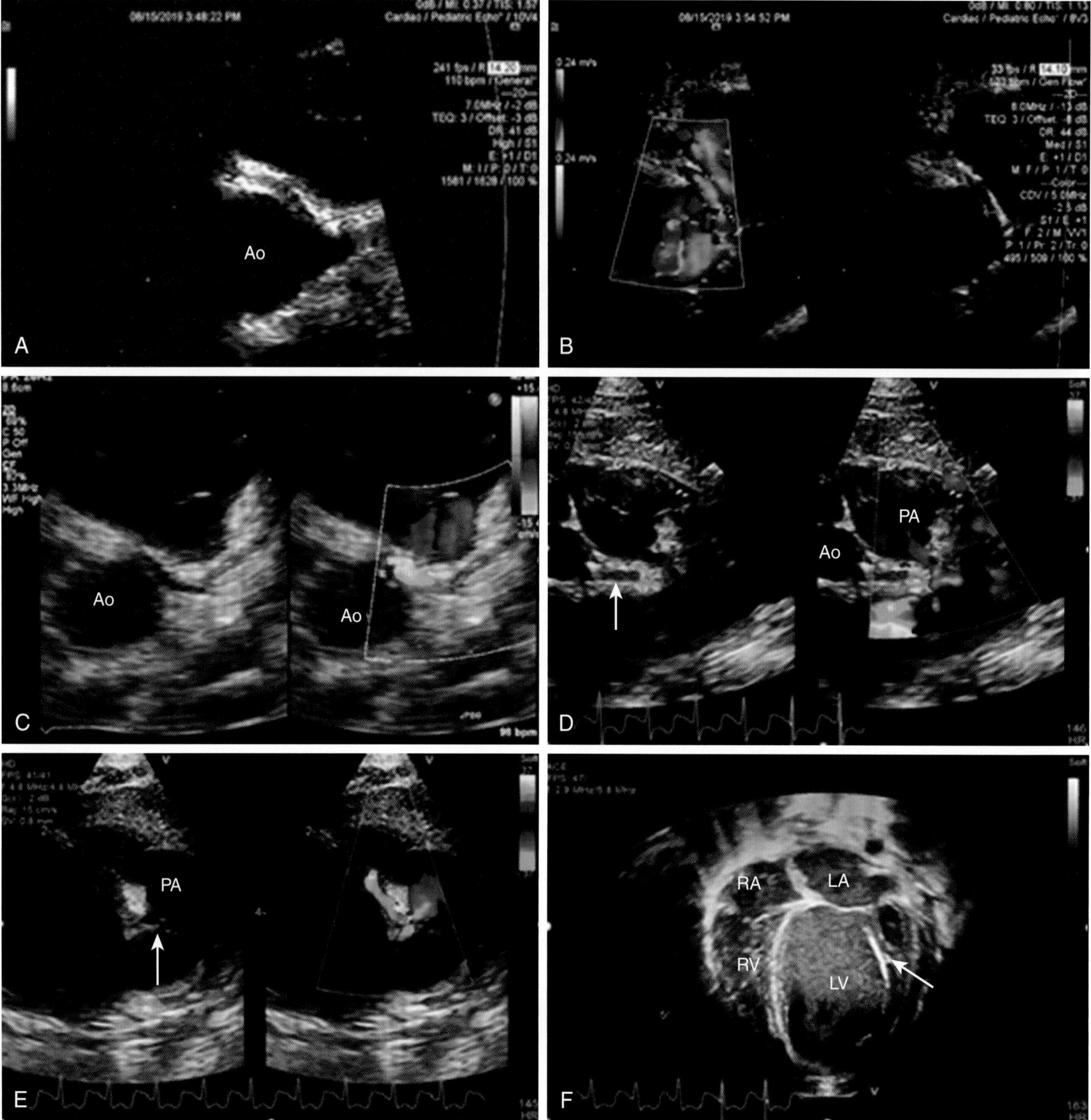

Fig. 42.13 Anomalous coronary artery origins. Anomalous coronary origins. (A and B) Parasternal short-axis imaging demonstrates the anomalous origin of the right coronary artery from the left sinus of Valsalva (see Videos 42.13A and 42.13B). (C) Parasternal short-axis view demonstrates an anomalous left coronary artery arising from the right sinus of Valsalva (see Video 42.13C). (D) Parasternal short-axis view demonstrates the anomalous origin of the left coronary artery from the pulmonary artery (ALCAPA) *(arrow)* (see Video 42.13D). (E) Parasternal long-axis view demonstrates ALCAPA *(arrow)* (see Video 42.13E). (F) Apical view demonstrates a severely dilated LV and bright mitral valve apparatus *(arrow)*, consistent with LV ischemia associated with ALCAPA (see Video 42.13F). *Ao*, Aorta; *PA*, pulmonary artery.

death in otherwise healthy young people. Anomalous left main coronary arteries arising from the right sinus of Valsalva typically course between the aorta and pulmonary artery (i.e., interarterial course). In an intramural course, the anomalous coronary artery courses within the aortic wall. This carries a risk of sudden death and ventricular tachycardia. When identified, these cases are typically treated surgically.[61] Anomalous right coronary arteries arising from the left sinus of Valsalva also carry a risk of sudden death for young patients, but significantly less so than an anomalous left coronary artery (Fig. 42.13). These anomalous coronary arteries may be incidentally identified in older adults, and in the absence of concerning clinical symptoms, they may often be followed without surgical intervention, although the optimal approach to diagnostic imaging assessment and management remains controversial.[79]

On echocardiography, the coronary artery origins are best visualized in the parasternal short-axis view at the level of the aortic sinuses. The location of the coronary artery origin and the relation to the aortic commissures can be appreciated in this view.

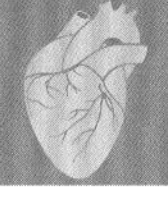

Imaging of coronary artery origins must be confirmed on 2D and color imaging. The parasternal long-axis view between the aorta and the pulmonary artery may demonstrate an anomalous, interarterial coronary artery with an anterior, steep-angled course. Incorporation of these modified views may increase sensitivity for detection of an anomalous coronary artery origin from the opposite sinus.[80]

A retroaortic left circumflex artery course is a common coronary anomaly in which the circumflex artery arises from the right sinus of Valsalva and courses posterior to the aortic root. This lesion does not carry an increased risk of sudden death and is most often incidentally identified. It may be visualized in the 4-chamber view with the probe tipped anteriorly to identify a narrow tubular structure parallel to the left atrioventricular groove.

Anomalous Coronary Artery Origin From the Pulmonary Artery

An anomalous left or right coronary artery arising from the pulmonary artery (ALCAPA or ARCAPA, respectively) is rare, especially in the adult population. The more common echocardiographic findings for patients who have not undergone repair include LV dilation and regional dysfunction, functional mitral regurgitation, echogenicity of mitral valve papillary muscles, and retrograde flow through collateral vessels supplied by the coronary artery with an aortic origin (see Fig. 42.13).[81,82]

CORONARY-CAMERAL FISTULAS

Coronary-cameral fistulas are rare congenital vascular anomalies resulting in communication between the coronary arteries and the cardiac chambers. They are most commonly incidental findings on imaging studies, although they may cause chamber enlargement.[83] Echocardiographic evidence of holodiastolic flow from the epicardial surface into the cardiac chambers on color Doppler imaging should raise suspicion for these fistulas.[84] Significant chamber enlargement and coronary steal are indications for intervention.

SUMMARY Left Heart Anomalies.

Anomaly	Imaging	Doppler	Associated Findings	Other Imaging
Cor triatriatum	Thin membrane divides LA, may be complete or perforated in adulthood	Color Doppler and velocity show degree of obstruction. Pulmonary venous HTN may be reflected in RVSP.	PFO, ASD, anomalous pulmonary veins, persistent left SVC, aortic coarctation	3D echocardiography if fenestrations present
Congenital mitral valve disease	Various forms, including cleft anterior leaflet, supramitral ring, double-orifice valve, parachute valve, abnormal papillary muscle arrangement Assessment of LA and LV size	Doppler evaluation of stenosis and/or regurgitation RVSP assessment for pulmonary arterial HTN	Shone complex, AVSD, CoA	—
Congenital aortic stenosis	Obstruction may be subaortic, valvular, or supravalvular.	PW and CW Doppler to assess severity of obstruction, levels of obstruction, and associated aortic regurgitation	VSDs, aortic coarctation, double-chambered RV, aortopathy	—
Aortic arch abnormalities	Anatomic variations, including complete vascular ring, double aortic arch, right aortic arch, cervical aortic arch, and interrupted aortic arch	Color, PW, and CW Doppler imaging allows assessment of flow patterns.	—	Cardiac MRI or CT imaging allows better definition of arch and vascular anatomy.

SUMMARY Left Heart Anomalies.—cont'd

Anomaly	Imaging	Doppler	Associated Findings	Other Imaging
CoA	Anatomy ranges from localized stricture to long, tubular narrowing.	CW Doppler shows increased flow velocity in systole with persistent antegrade flow in diastole. PW Doppler of abdominal aorta shows delayed upstroke or persistent diastolic flow.	BAV in > 50% of patients with aortic coarctation Berry aneurysm screening recommended HTN is prevalent.	Cardiac MRI or CT imaging allows better definition of coarctation anatomy, location, and severity and aortic dilation.
Coronary artery anomalies	Anatomy includes anomalous coronary artery from opposite sinus, anomalous coronary artery from PA, and coronary-cameral fistulas.	Color Doppler helps identify coronary ostia. Retrograde flow in coronary artery if it arises from PA Continuous flow seen with coronary-cameral fistula.	—	Cardiac CT with contrast is the reference standard for diagnosis of coronary anomalies. Coronary angiography also may be appropriate.

ASD, Atrial septal defect; *AVSD,* atrioventricular septal defect; *BAV,* bicuspid aortic valve; *CT,* computed tomography; *CW,* continuous wave; *CoA,* coarctation of the aorta; *HTN,* hypertension; *MRI,* magnetic resonance imaging; *PA,* pulmonary artery; *PFO,* patent foramen ovale; *PW,* pulsed wave; *RVSP,* right ventricular systolic pressure; *SVC,* superior vena cava; *VSD,* ventricular septal defect.

REFERENCES

1. Rozema TK, Arruda J, Snyder CS. Cor triatriatum: a tale of two membranes. *CASE (Phila).* 2019;3(1):25–27.
2. Nassar PN, Hamdan RH. Cor triatriatum Sinistrum: classification and imaging modalities. *Eur J Cardiovasc Med.* 2011;1(3):84–87.
3. Niwayama G. Cor triatriatum. *Am Heart J.* 1960;59:291–317.
4. Marin-Garcia J, et al. Cor triatriatum: study of 20 cases. *Am J Cardiol.* 1975;35(1):59–66.
5. Ather B, Siddiqui WJ. *Cor Triatriatum.* Treasure Island, FL: StatPearls; 2020.
6. Wolf WJ. Diagnostic features and pitfalls in the two-dimensional echocardiographic evaluation of a child with cor triatriatum. *Pediatr Cardiol.* 1986;6(4):211–213.
7. Shone JD, et al. The developmental complex of "parachute mitral valve," supravalvular ring of left atrium, subaortic stenosis, and coarctation of aorta. *Am J Cardiol.* 1963;11:714–725.
8. Kuperstein R, et al. The added value of real-time 3-dimensional echocardiography in the diagnosis of isolated cleft mitral valve in adults. *J Am Soc Echocardiogr.* 2006;19(6):811–814.
9. Tamura M, Menahem S, Brizard C. Clinical features and management of isolated cleft mitral valve in childhood. *J Am Coll Cardiol.* 2000;35(3):764–770.
10. Zhu D, et al. Isolated cleft of the mitral valve: clinical spectrum and course. *Tex Heart Inst J.* 2009;36(6):553–556.
11. LaCorte M, Harada K, Williams RG. Echocardiographic features of congenital left ventricular inflow obstruction. *Circulation.* 1976;54(4):562–566.
12. Perier P, Clausnizer B. Isolated cleft mitral valve: valve reconstruction techniques. *Ann Thorac Surg.* 1995;59(1):56–59.
13. Toscano A, et al. Congenital supravalvar mitral ring: an underestimated anomaly. *J Thorac Cardiovasc Surg.* 2009;137(3):538–542.
14. Trowitzsch E, et al. Two-dimensional echocardiographic findings in double orifice mitral valve. *J Am Coll Cardiol.* 1985;6(2):383–387.
15. Oosthoek PW, et al. The parachute-like asymmetric mitral valve and its two papillary muscles. *J Thorac Cardiovasc Surg.* 1997;114(1):9–15.
16. Marino BS, et al. Parachute mitral valve: morphologic descriptors, associated lesions, and outcomes after biventricular repair. *J Thorac Cardiovasc Surg.* 2009;137(2):385–393 e4.
17. Myers ML, et al. Anomalous mitral arcade: a rare cause of mitral valve disease in an adult. *Can J Cardiol.* 1987;3(2):60–62.
18. Layman TE, Edwards JE. Anomalous mitral arcade. A type of congenital mitral insufficiency. *Circulation.* 1967;35(2):389–395.
19. Gaynor JW, Elliott MJ. Congenital left ventricular outflow tract obstruction. *J Heart Valve Dis.* 1993;2(1):80–93.
20. Barekatain A, et al. Subvalvular aortic stenosis. *Del Med J.* 2015;87(11):346–348.
21. Etnel JR, et al. Paediatric subvalvular aortic stenosis: a systematic review and meta-analysis of natural history and surgical outcome. *Eur J Cardio Thorac Surg.* 2015;48(2):212–220.
22. Kleinert S, Geva T. Echocardiographic morphometry and geometry of the left ventricular outflow tract in fixed subaortic stenosis. *J Am Coll Cardiol.* 1993;22(5):1501–1508.
23. Gersony WM. Natural history of discrete subvalvar aortic stenosis: management implications. *J Am Coll Cardiol.* 2001;38(3):843–845.
24. Serraf A, et al. Surgical treatment of subaortic stenosis: a seventeen-year experience. *J Thorac Cardiovasc Surg.* 1999;117(4):669–678.
25. Oliver JM, et al. Discrete subaortic stenosis in adults: increased prevalence and slow rate of progression of the obstruction and aortic regurgitation. *J Am Coll Cardiol.* 2001;38(3):835–842.
26. Matsuzaki Y, et al. Long-term outcomes of Ross and Ross-Konno operations in patients under 15 years of age. *Gen Thorac Cardiovasc Surg.* 2019;67(5):420–426.
27. Barkhordarian R, et al. Geometry of the left ventricular outflow tract in fixed subaortic stenosis and intact ventricular septum: an echocardiographic study in children and adults. *J Thorac Cardiovasc Surg.* 2007;133(1):196–203.
28. Hurwitz LE, Roberts WC. Quadricuspid semilunar valve. *Am J Cardiol.* 1973;31(5):623–626.
29. Kovar J, Runt V, Cerny B. The quadricuspid semilunar valve of the aorta. *Folia Morphol (Praha).* 1982;30(3):255–259.
30. Wedin J, et al. Bicuspid aortic valve - a common congenital cardiac malformation associated with serious. *Lakartidningen.* 2019:116.
31. Liu T, et al. Bicuspid aortic valve: an update in morphology, genetics, biomarker, complications, imaging diagnosis and treatment. *Front Physiol.* 2018;9:1921.
32. Fedak PW, et al. Clinical and pathophysiological implications of a bicuspid aortic valve. *Circulation.* 2002;106(8):900–904.
33. Nishimura RA, et al. 2014 AHA/ACC guideline for the management of patients with valvular heart disease: a report of the American College of Cardiology/American Heart Association Task Force on Practice Guidelines. *J Am Coll Cardiol.* 2014;63(22):e57–185.
34. Nishimura RA, et al. 2017 AHA/ACC focused update of the 2014 AHA/ACC guideline for the management of patients with valvular

heart disease: a report of the American College of Cardiology/American Heart Association Task Force on Clinical Practice Guidelines. *J Am Coll Cardiol.* 2017;70(2):252–289.
35. Grayburn PA, et al. Pivotal role of aortic valve area calculation by the continuity equation for Doppler assessment of aortic stenosis in patients with combined aortic stenosis and regurgitation. *Am J Cardiol.* 1988;61(4):376–381.
36. Ananthakrishna Pillai A, Rangaswamy Balasubramanian V, Kanshilal Sharma D. Immediate and long-term follow up results of balloon aortic valvuloplasty in congenital bicuspid aortic valve stenosis among young patients. *J Heart Valve Dis.* 2018;27(1):17–23.
37. Zoghbi WA, et al. Accurate noninvasive quantification of stenotic aortic valve area by Doppler echocardiography. *Circulation.* 1986;73(3):452–459.
38. Biner S, et al. Aortopathy is prevalent in relatives of bicuspid aortic valve patients. *J Am Coll Cardiol.* 2009;53(24):2288–2295.
39. Hardikar AA, Marwick TH. The natural history of guidelines: the case of aortopathy related to bicuspid aortic valves. *Int J Cardiol.* 2015;199:150–153.
40. Ross D, Jackson M, Davies J. Pulmonary autograft aortic valve replacement: long-term results. *J Card Surg.* 1991;6(4 Suppl):529–533.
41. Michelena HI, et al. Incidence of aortic complications in patients with bicuspid aortic valves. *J Am Med Assoc.* 2011;306(10):1104–1112.
42. Flaker G, et al. Supravalvular aortic stenosis. A 20-year clinical perspective and experience with patch aortoplasty. *Am J Cardiol.* 1983;51(2):256–260.
43. Lee JU, et al. Early manifestation of supravalvular aortic and pulmonary artery stenosis in a patient with Williams syndrome. *Korean J Thorac Cardiovasc Surg.* 2016;49(2):115–118.
44. Bruno E, et al. Cardiovascular findings, and clinical course, in patients with Williams syndrome. *Cardiol Young.* 2003;13(6):532–536.
45. Ewart AK, et al. Supravalvular aortic stenosis associated with a deletion disrupting the elastin gene. *J Clin Invest.* 1994;93(3):1071–1077.
46. McElhinney DB, et al. Issues and outcomes in the management of supravalvar aortic stenosis. *Ann Thorac Surg.* 2000;69(2):562–567.
47. Thistlethwaite PA, et al. Surgical management of congenital obstruction of the left main coronary artery with supravalvular aortic stenosis. *J Thorac Cardiovasc Surg.* 2000;120(6):1040–1046.
48. Stamm C, et al. Congenital supravalvar aortic stenosis: a simple lesion? *Eur J Cardio Thorac Surg.* 2001;19(2):195–202.
49. Wu FY, et al. Long-term surgical prognosis of primary supravalvular aortic stenosis repair. *Ann Thorac Surg.* 2019;108(4):1202–1209.
50. Hoffman JI, Kaplan S. The incidence of congenital heart disease. *J Am Coll Cardiol.* 2002;39(12):1890–1900.
51. Gurvitz M, et al. Prevalence and predictors of gaps in care among adult congenital heart disease patients: HEART-ACHD (The Health, Education, and Access Research Trial). *J Am Coll Cardiol.* 2013;61(21):2180–2184.
52. Campbell M, Polani PE. The aetiology of coarctation of the aorta. *Lancet.* 1961;1(7175):463–468.
53. Edwards JE, Christensen NA, et al. Pathologic considerations of coarctation of the aorta. *Proc Staff Meet Mayo Clin.* 1948;23(15):324–332.
54. Nguyen L, Cook SC. Coarctation of the aorta: Strategies for improving outcomes. *Cardiol Clin.* 2015;33(4):521–530 (vii).
55. Cook SC, et al. Assessment of the cerebral circulation in adults with coarctation of the aorta. *Congenit Heart Dis.* 2013;8(4):289–295.
56. Rudolph AM, Heymann MA, Spitznas U. Hemodynamic considerations in the development of narrowing of the aorta. *Am J Cardiol.* 1972;30(5):514–525.
57. Child JS. Echo-Doppler and color-flow imaging in congenital heart disease. *Cardiol Clin.* 1990;8(2):289–313.
58. Nielsen JC, et al. Magnetic resonance imaging predictors of coarctation severity. *Circulation.* 2005;111(5):622–628.
59. Muzzarelli S, et al. Prediction of hemodynamic severity of coarctation by magnetic resonance imaging. *Am J Cardiol.* 2011;108(9):1335–1340.
60. Armstrong AC, et al. LV mass assessed by echocardiography and CMR, cardiovascular outcomes, and medical practice. *JACC Cardiovasc Imaging.* 2012;5(8):837–848.
61. Riehle TJ, et al. Real-time three-dimensional echocardiographic acquisition and quantification of left ventricular indices in children and young adults with congenital heart disease: comparison with magnetic resonance imaging. *J Am Soc Echocardiogr.* 2008;21(1):78–83.
62. Lombardi KC, et al. Aortic stiffness and left ventricular diastolic function in children following early repair of aortic coarctation. *Am J Cardiol.* 2013;112(11):1828–1833.
63. Kaulitz R, Jonas RA, van der Velde ME. Echocardiographic assessment of interrupted aortic arch. *Cardiol Young.* 1999;9(6):562–571.
64. Rein AJ, Gotsman MS, Simcha A. Echocardiographic diagnosis of interrupted aortic arch with an aortopulmonary communication. *Int J Cardiol.* 1989;24(2):238–241.
65. Davies M, Guest PJ. Developmental abnormalities of the great vessels of the thorax and their embryological basis. *Br J Radiol.* 2003;76(907):491–502.
66. Licari A, et al. Congenital vascular rings: a clinical challenge for the pediatrician. *Pediatr Pulmonol.* 2015;50(5):511–524.
67. Edwards JE. Anomalies of the derivatives of the aortic arch system. *Med Clin North Am.* 1948;32:925–949.
68. McElhinney DB, et al. Association of chromosome 22q11 deletion with isolated anomalies of aortic arch laterality and branching. *J Am Coll Cardiol.* 2001;37(8):2114–2119.
69. Beekman RP, et al. A new diagnostic approach to vascular rings and pulmonary slings: the role of MRI. *Magn Reson Imaging.* 1998;16(2):137–145.
70. Murdison KA, Andrews BA, Chin AJ. Ultrasonographic display of complex vascular rings. *J Am Coll Cardiol.* 1990;15(7):1645–1653.
71. Ruiz Pizarro V, Deiros L, Uceda A. [Evaluation of double aortic arch by ultrasound and computed tomography]. *An Pediatr.* 2019;91(6):419–421.
72. D'Antonio F, et al. Fetuses with right aortic arch: a multicenter cohort study and meta-analysis. *Ultrasound Obstet Gynecol.* 2016;47(4):423–432.
73. McElhinney DB, et al. Patterns of right aortic arch and mirror-image branching of the brachiocephalic vessels without associated anomalies. *Pediatr Cardiol.* 2001;22(4):285–291.
74. Pearson GD, et al. Cervical aortic arch with aneurysm formation. *Am J Cardiol.* 1997;79(1):112–114.
75. Noguchi M, Shibata R, Iwamatsu M. Surgical treatment for cervical aortic arch with aneurysm formation. *Jpn J Thorac Cardiovasc Surg.* 2003;51(7):314–318.
76. Goo HW, et al. CT of congenital heart disease: normal anatomy and typical pathologic conditions. *Radiographics.* 2003;23:S147–S165. Spec No.
77. Gilkeson RC, Ciancibello L, Zahka K. Pictorial essay. Multidetector CT evaluation of congenital heart disease in pediatric and adult patients. *AJR Am J Roentgenol.* 2003;180(4):973–980.
78. Pandey NN, et al. Anomalies of coronary artery origin: evaluation on multidetector CT angiography. *Clin Imaging.* 2019;57:87–98.
79. Brothers JA, et al. Expert consensus guidelines: anomalous aortic origin of a coronary artery. *J Thorac Cardiovasc Surg.* 2017;153(6):1440–1457.
80. Thankavel PP, Lemler MS, Ramaciotti C. Utility and importance of new echocardiographic screening methods in diagnosis of anomalous coronary origins in the pediatric population: assessment of quality improvement. *Pediatr Cardiol.* 2015;36(1):120–125.
81. Saedi S, et al. The role of echocardiography in anomalous origin of coronary artery from pulmonary artery (ALCAPA): simple tool for a complex diagnosis. *Echocardiography.* 2019;36(1):177–181.
82. Kamperidis V, et al. ALCAPA syndrome and risk of sudden death in young people. *QJM.* 2019;112(4):291–292.
83. Nagpal P, et al. Symptomatic coronary cameral fistula. *Heart Views.* 2015;16(2):65–67.
84. Alur I, Gunes T, Goksin I. Evaluating coronary-cameral fistulas. *Tex Heart Inst J.* 2016;43(6):562–563.

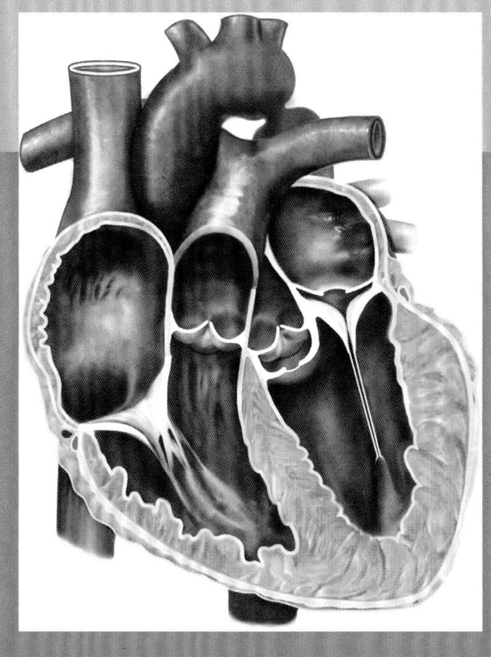

中文导读

第43章 右心疾病

本章所介绍的右心疾病包括：肺动脉瓣狭窄、肺动脉瓣下狭窄、肺动脉瓣上狭窄和三尖瓣下移畸形等。肺动脉瓣狭窄是最常见的右心梗阻形式，本章介绍了其自然病史与临床表现，超声心动图作为评估肺动脉瓣狭窄的主要影像学手段，如何对其观察和评估狭窄程度。比较了经皮腔内球囊瓣膜成形术和瓣膜切开术两种干预方法，介绍了其适应证和术后反流的评估。肺动脉瓣下狭窄和右室双腔心的临床表现与肺动脉瓣狭窄相似，取决于梗阻的程度及相关的房间隔缺损或其他合并畸形。本章对其超声评估和手术指征也做了介绍，并简单介绍了肺动脉瓣上狭窄。

三尖瓣下移畸形作为一种少见畸形，本章从胚胎发育、病理解剖、临床体征、超声观察方法和注意事项等方面做了详细介绍。三尖瓣下移畸形的手术方式有多种，本章做了详细介绍并从手术治疗角度介绍了相应超声观察要点。

王剑鹏

43 Right Heart Anomalies

YULI Y. KIM, MD

PULMONIC VALVE, SUBPULMONIC, AND SUPRAVALVULAR PULMONARY STENOSIS

PULMONIC VALVE STENOSIS

Pulmonic valve stenosis is usually an isolated lesion. It occurs in 8% to 10% of individuals with congenital heart disease (CHD) and is the most common form of right-sided obstruction.[1]

The pulmonic valve is often dome shaped, with a narrow central opening and leaflet fusion. It can be calcified in older adults. Pulmonic valve dysplasia is less common and is characterized by thickened, poorly mobile leaflets and no commissural fusion. Dysplastic pulmonic valves are more often found with other cardiac and noncardiac abnormalities. Unicuspid or bicuspid pulmonic valves are rarely isolated and are usually associated with complex CHD such as tetralogy of Fallot (TOF). Pulmonic stenosis may be associated with genetic syndromes, including Noonan, Alagille, and Williams syndromes, and with congenital rubella.[1]

The physiologic consequence of valvular pulmonic stenosis (and subpulmonic stenosis) is right ventricular outflow tract (RVOT) obstruction with increased right ventricular (RV) pressure. Maintenance of RV output is accomplished by development of RV hypertrophy. Severe RV hypertrophy leads to diminished compliance of the RV and can result in increased RV end-diastolic and right atrial (RA) pressures. Right-to-left shunting may occur if there is an interatrial communication. The main pulmonary artery is often dilated, with the poststenotic jet favoring the left pulmonary artery. However, the degree of pulmonary artery dilation is not necessarily related to the severity of pulmonic valve stenosis.

Natural History and Clinical Presentation

Progression of mild pulmonic stenosis is unusual after early childhood. The Second Natural History Study of Congenital Heart Defects[2] demonstrated that survival was comparable to that for the general population, regardless of medical versus surgical management strategy, and most patients were asymptomatic. Those with a gradient between 25 and 49 mmHg had a 20% chance of needing an intervention, and most of those with gradients of 50 mmHg or more had progressive stenosis that required intervention.[2]

Severe valvular pulmonic stenosis can manifest with dyspnea on exertion, fatigue, chest pain, palpitations, and syncope. Exertional chest discomfort can be attributed to relative RV ischemia or coexistent coronary atherosclerosis. Compression of the left coronary artery by an aneurysmal pulmonary artery in pulmonic valve stenosis has been reported.[3] Patients may be cyanotic and may have clubbed fingers due to right-to-left shunting at the atrial level.

Results of the physical examination of an adult with pulmonic valve stenosis depend on the severity of the stenosis and any associated lesions. In mild pulmonic stenosis, the jugular venous waveforms are normal, and the precordium is quiet. There is a systolic ejection murmur heard in the pulmonary position that increases with inspiration and usually ends in midsystole. There may be a pulmonic ejection click that decreases with inspiration.

In severe pulmonic stenosis, the jugular venous pressure may be elevated with a prominent a wave. There may be an RV lift and a loud, harsh ejection murmur with associated thrill that radiates to the back. The degree of second heart sound (S2) splitting is proportional to the degree of stenosis; it may be widely split and fixed. The P2 (pulmonic) component may be reduced or absent with severe stenosis, which can make S2 splitting difficult to appreciate. A right-sided S4 gallop may be auscultated.

Echocardiography for Pulmonic Valve Stenosis

Echocardiography is considered the mainstay of imaging for the assessment of pulmonic valve stenosis. The goals of the echocardiographic evaluation of pulmonic valve stenosis are summarized in Table 43.1.

The key views for assessing the pulmonic valve are the parasternal short-axis view at the base and the parasternal long-axis RVOT view. The valve leaflets are thickened, with restricted systolic motion of the leaflet tips producing a domed appearance (Fig. 43.1). A dysplastic pulmonic valve is thickened with rudimentary, immobile leaflet tissue associated with a hypoplastic annulus and often with supravalvular pulmonary artery narrowing. The high right parasternal view can image the pulmonic valve en face and provide greater detail on morphology, but it is challenging to acquire in adults.

TABLE 43.1 Echocardiographic Goals in the Evaluation of Pulmonic Valve Stenosis.

Structure	*Assessment*	*Imaging Plane and Technique*
Pulmonic valve morphology	Doming, leaflet hypoplasia or dysplasia, mobility	Parasternal long-axis RVOT and parasternal short-axis; high right parasternal axis to view en face
Other levels of obstruction	Infundibular (subvalvular), supravalvular, branch pulmonary artery	Parasternal long-axis RVOT and parasternal short-axis at the base using PW and CW Doppler to localize and estimate severity of obstruction Subcostal RAO with counterclockwise 45-degree rotation from long axis to get RV inflow-outflow view
Pulmonic valve function	Pulmonic stenosis severity, degree of pulmonic regurgitation	Parasternal short-axis at the base and modified apical with anterior angulation using PW and CW Doppler
Pulmonic valve annulus	Pulmonic annulus dimension	Parasternal short-axis at the base focused over the pulmonic valve and bifurcation
RV	RV hypertrophy, size, and function	Subcostal long-axis or parasternal long-axis by M-mode or 2D echocardiography with RV diastolic wall thickness >5 mm consistent with hypertrophy (Refer to Table 44.3 on RV size and function assessment in tetralogy of Fallot.)
Interventricular septum	Systolic septal flattening consistent with RV pressure overload	Parasternal short-axis at the mid-ventricular level
Tricuspid valve	Degree of regurgitation and RV systolic pressure estimate	Apical 4-chamber, parasternal long-axis RV inflow, and parasternal short-axis at the base focused over the tricuspid valve
RA	RA size	Apical 4-chamber with upper limit of normal of 18 cm^2
Inferior vena cava	Size and inspiratory collapse to assess RA pressure	Subcostal long-axis with measurement of inferior vena cava diameter at end-expiration
Interatrial septum	Atrial septal defect or patent foramen ovale, bowing of interatrial septum	Subcostal long-axis, short-axis, and in-between views; parasternal short-axis; high right parasternal axis

PW, Pulsed-wave; *RAO*, right anterior oblique; *RVOT*, right ventricular outflow tract.

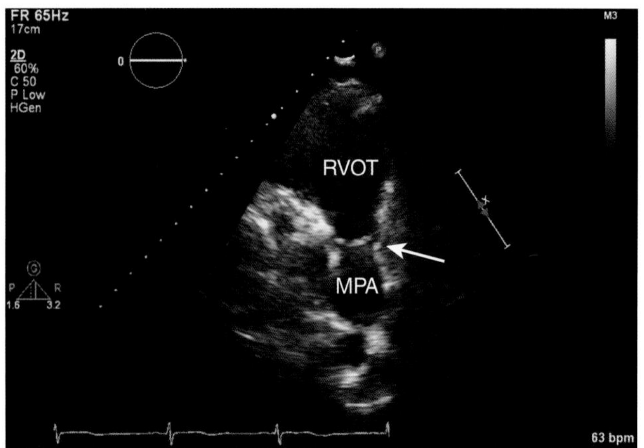

Fig. 43.1 Valvular pulmonic stenosis. Parasternal short-axis view focused over the main pulmonary artery *(MPA)* shows a thickened pulmonic valve that domes in systole *(arrow)*. *RVOT*, Right ventricular outflow tract (see Video 43.1).

TABLE 43.2 Severity of Pulmonic Valve Stenosis.

Parameter	*Mild*	*Moderate*	*Severe*
Peak Doppler velocity (m/s)	<3	3–4	>4
Peak Doppler gradient (mmHg)	<36	36–64	>64
Mean Doppler gradient (mmHg)	—	—	>35
RV systolic pressure/LV systolic pressure (%)	<50	50–74	≥75

Adapted from Stout KK, Daniels CJ, Aboulhosn JA, et al. 2018 AHA/ACC guideline for the management of adults with congenital heart disease: a report of the American College of Cardiology/American Heart Association Task Force on Clinical Practice Guidelines. *J Am Coll Cardiol.* 2019;73(12):e81–e192; Cuypers JA, Wisenbrug M, vander Linde D, Roos-Hesselink JW. Pulmonary stenosis: update on diagnosis and therapeutic options. *Heart.* 2013;99:339–347.

Pulsed-wave and continuous-wave Doppler imaging are used to evaluate the degree of pulmonic stenosis and define the level of obstruction. In addition to the parasternal short-axis view at the base focused on the pulmonic valve and branch pulmonary arteries, a modified apical view with the transducer placed more medially or a subcostal view with anterior angulation can provide an another approach for assessment of gradients.

Physiologic conditions that alter flow across the pulmonic valve affect the accuracy of gradient estimation by the modified Bernoulli equation, which is most accurate when there is isolated, discrete valve stenosis. For example, if there is severe RV systolic dysfunction with RV failure, the RV cannot generate sufficient pressure to overcome significant stenosis, yielding a peak instantaneous gradient that underestimates the true severity of the stenosis. Similarly, left-to-right flow across an atrial septal defect (ASD) or concomitant pulmonic regurgitation increases flow across the pulmonic valve, thereby increasing the transpulmonic gradient and overestimating the severity of pulmonic valve stenosis. Long-segment stenosis and serial obstructions (i.e., associated subvalvular and/or supravalvular pulmonic stenosis) are other conditions in which Doppler-derived gradients are less reliable.

According to the 2014 American Heart Association and American College of Cardiology (AHA/ACC) guidelines for the management of patients with valvular heart disease[4] and the AHA/ACC 2018 guidelines for the management of adults with CHD,[5] the definition of severe pulmonic valve stenosis is a maximum velocity greater than 4 m/s or a peak instantaneous gradient greater than 64 mmHg (Table 43.2). Echocardiography provides excellent anatomic characterization for diagnosis and for estimates of RV pressure and assessment of RV size and function.

There are mixed data on the accuracy of peak instantaneous gradients derived by echocardiography compared with invasive gradients measured by cardiac catheterization for

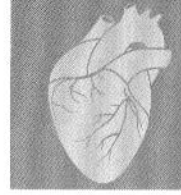

assessment of pulmonic stenosis. Some studies have demonstrated excellent correlation with peak-to-peak gradients,[6,7] whereas others have determined that peak instantaneous gradients overestimate peak-to-peak gradients but are comparable with catheter-derived maximal instantaneous gradients.[8,9] Mean Doppler gradients have the best correlation with peak-to-peak gradients in isolated[10] and complex[11] pulmonic valve stenosis.

In our experience, peak instantaneous gradients obtained by echocardiography overestimate peak-to-peak gradients in the catheterization laboratory and may be exaggerated by effects of sedation. Other echocardiographic methods can indirectly assess the degree of pulmonic stenosis. Tricuspid regurgitation peak velocity, or v, can be used to measure RV systolic pressure (as opposed to pulmonary artery systolic pressure) by using the modified Bernoulli equation $4v^2$ and adding RA pressure estimates. The latter is estimated by assessing IVC size and inspiratory collapse. Although the exact gradient across the pulmonic valve is not calculated, the pressure load to the RV relative to the left ventricular (LV) systolic pressure assessed by blood pressure cuff measurement can be compared. Qualitative assessment of septal position and degree of RV hypertrophy can provide additional information on relative pulmonic stenosis severity. Correlation between the Doppler gradient derived by echocardiography and clinical findings is recommended.

Indications for Intervention and Assessment After Intervention

Indications for intervention in pulmonic valve stenosis are summarized in Table 43.3.[5] Successful percutaneous balloon valvuloplasty was initially reported in 1982, and it is the treatment of choice for classic domed pulmonic valve stenosis[12] (Fig. 43.2). The mechanism for relief of stenosis is commissural splitting, and outcomes are typically excellent.[13,14] Although outcomes are not optimal compared with those for classic domed pulmonic valve stenosis, balloon valvuloplasty may provide some degree of relief for dysplastic pulmonic valves and is a reasonable first-line option.

A large, multicenter registry of 533 patients followed for a median of 33 months (range, 1 month to 8.7 years) after balloon valvuloplasty showed that 23% had suboptimal results, defined as a residual gradient of 36 mmHg or more or repeat balloon valvuloplasty or surgical valvotomy. Predictors of suboptimal outcome included earlier study year of intervention, higher residual postprocedural gradient, and valvular anatomy.[15] In 2012, long-term outcomes were reported for 139 patients with a median follow-up of 6 years (range, 0–21 years) and showed that reintervention was required in only 9.4% of patients, mostly for restenosis. In the same study, 79 patients who had undergone surgical valvotomy were identified; after a median follow-up of 22.5 years (range, 0–45 years), 20.3% required reintervention,

TABLE 43.3 AHA/ACC Recommendations for Intervention in Pulmonary Valve Stenosis.

Class I

1. In adults with moderate or severe valvular pulmonic stenosis and otherwise unexplained symptoms of HF, cyanosis from interatrial right-to-left communication, and/or exercise intolerance, balloon valvuloplasty is recommended (level of evidence: B).
2. In adults with moderate or severe valvular pulmonic stenosis and otherwise unexplained symptoms of HF, cyanosis, and/or exercise intolerance who are ineligible for or who have failed balloon valvuloplasty, surgical repair is recommended (level of evidence: B).

Class IIa

1. In asymptomatic adults with severe valvular pulmonic stenosis, intervention is reasonable (level of evidence: C).

AHA/ACC, American Heart Association and American College of Cardiology; *HF*, heart failure.

From Stout KK, Daniels CJ, Aboulhosn JA, et al. 2018 AHA/ACC guideline for the management of adults with congenital heart disease: a report of the American College of Cardiology/American Heart Association Task Force on Clinical Practice Guidelines. *J Am Coll Cardiol*. 2019;73(12):e81–e192.

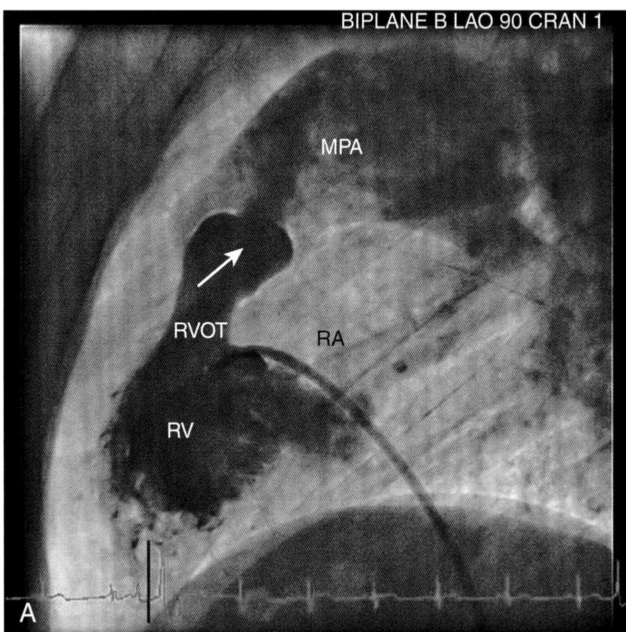

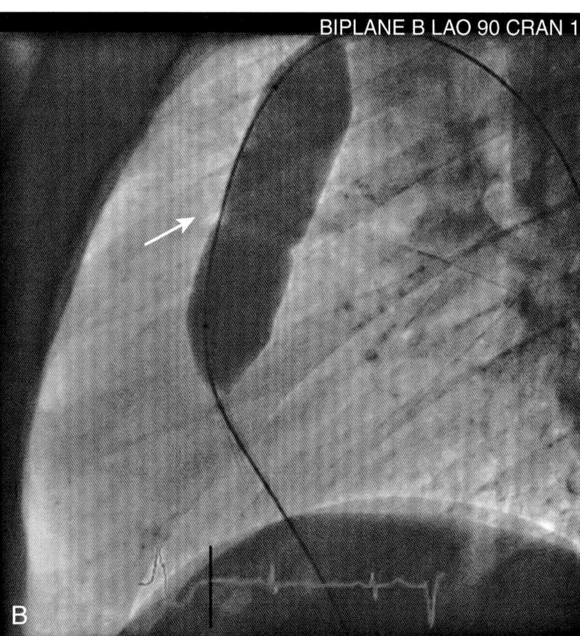

Fig. 43.2 Balloon valvuloplasty of pulmonic stenosis. (A) Lateral projection of a right ventriculogram demonstrates doming pulmonic valve leaflets *(arrow)*. Notice the dilated main pulmonary artery *(MPA)*. (B) Lateral projection of balloon inflation across the pulmonic valve. There is a mild waist at the level of pulmonic valve obstruction *(arrow)*. *RVOT*, Right ventricular outflow tract.

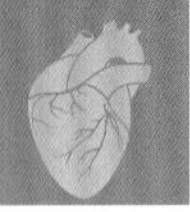

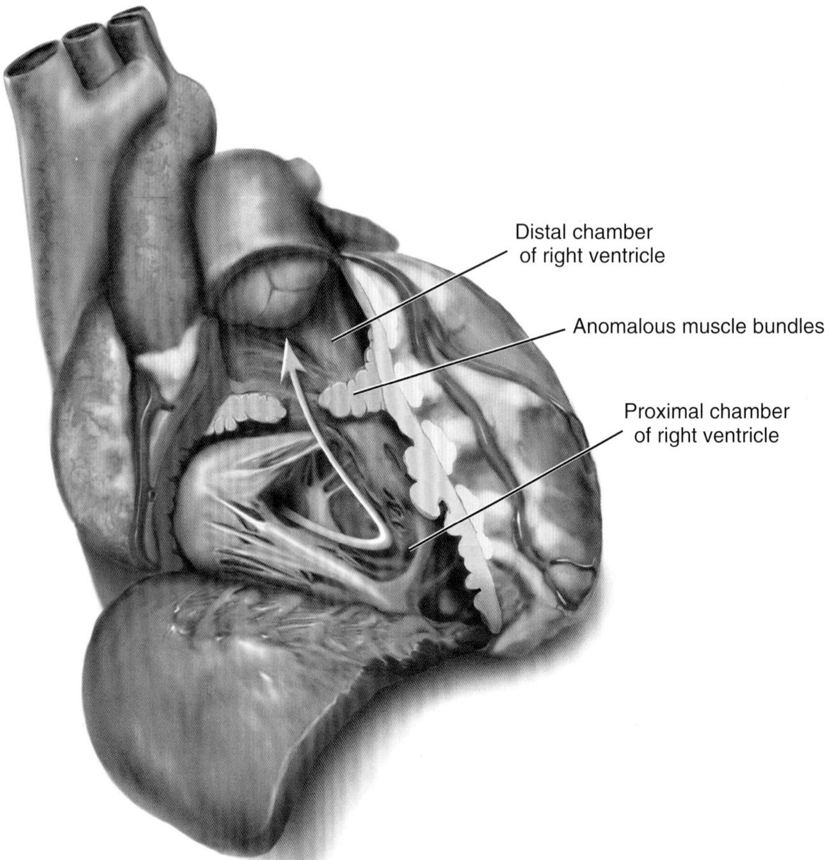

Fig. 43.3 Double-chambered RV caused by hypertrophied muscle bundles. Double-chambered RV results from anomalous muscle bundles that divide the RV into proximal and distal chambers. (From Loukas M, Housman B, Blaak C, et al. Double-chambered right ventricle: a review. *Cardiovasc Pathol.* 2013;22:417–423.)

mostly for pulmonic regurgitation.[16] Other studies showed a significant incidence of pulmonic regurgitation after surgical valvotomy, necessitating repeat surgical intervention (e.g., pulmonic valve replacement) later in life. Balloon valvuloplasty was supported as the treatment of choice in patients with anatomically suitable substrates.[17–20]

The severity of residual obstruction and location and severity of pulmonic regurgitation should be documented during echocardiographic evaluation of patients after percutaneous balloon valvuloplasty or surgical valvotomy. Worsening of infundibular obstruction after relief of pulmonic valve stenosis is a well-documented phenomenon of surgical valvotomy and balloon valvuloplasty, but it improves over time with regression of RV hypertrophy.[21,22]

Pulmonic regurgitation is not uncommon, especially after surgical intervention in cases of pulmonic valve stenosis. Indications for valve replacement for severe regurgitation after pulmonic valvotomy are not well established. Data suggest that despite the comparable extent of RV remodeling in response to chronic pulmonic regurgitation, reverse remodeling may be different, and guidelines used to determine the timing for pulmonic valve replacement in TOF should not be extrapolated to patients with pulmonic valve stenosis.[23,24] Pulmonary valve replacement may be reasonable in the asymptomatic patient with moderate or greater pulmonic regurgitation if there is evidence of progressive RV dilation and/or dysfunction.[5]

SUBPULMONIC STENOSIS

Background

The anatomic RV is tripartite and comprises the inflow, the trabecular apex or sinus portion, and the outflow, also known as the infundibulum. Subpulmonic stenosis is an uncommon form of right-sided CHD. It is caused by (1) RVOT (infundibular) stenosis due to a discrete fibromuscular ridge or ring or by (2) hypertrophied muscle bundles resulting in a double-chambered RV. Infundibular stenosis can be located anywhere within the RVOT, from the ostium of the infundibulum to just below the pulmonic valve, whereas obstruction in a double-chambered RV occurs at the os infundibulum, effectively dividing the RV into a proximal high-pressure RV sinus chamber and a distal low-pressure infundibular chamber (Fig. 43.3).

A double-chambered RV is associated with a ventricular septal defect (VSD), most commonly the membranous type, in 60% to 90% of patients. There usually is a communication between the LV and the proximal high-pressure chamber. Pulmonic valve stenosis is seen in approximately 40% of cases, and ASD exists in approximately 17%; double-chambered RV can be associated with complex CHD such as double-outlet RV or TOF,[25,26] with LV outflow tract obstruction or subaortic stenosis an uncommon association.

Pathophysiology and Clinical Presentation

The pathophysiology of both forms of subpulmonic stenosis involves increased pressure in the proximal portion of the

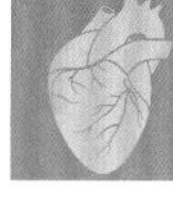

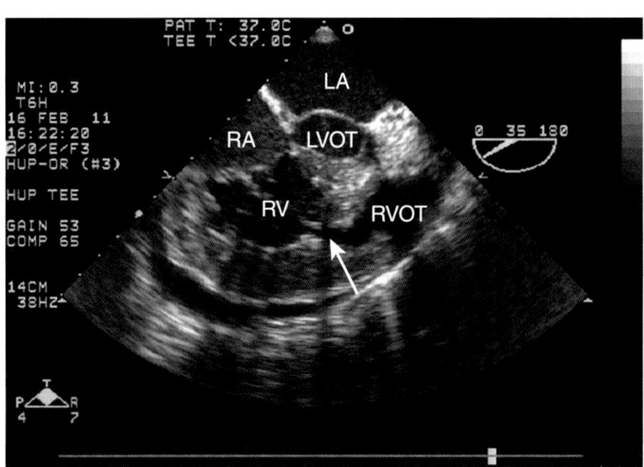

Fig. 43.4 Double-chambered RV caused by obstruction at the os infundibulum. Mid-esophageal short-axis view demonstrates obstruction in the RV at the os infundibulum *(arrow)*. *LVOT,* Left ventricular outflow tract; *RVOT,* right ventricular outflow tract (see Video 43.4).

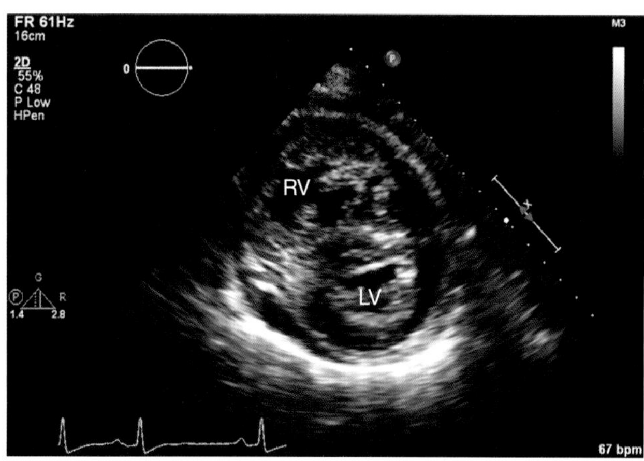

Fig. 43.5 RV dilation and hypertrophy in double-chambered RV. Parasternal short-axis view at the mid-ventricle in a double-chambered RV shows RV dilation and severe RV hypertrophy with a flattened, D-shaped septum in systole (see Video 43.5).

RV, with ensuing RV hypertrophy and elevated end-diastolic and RA pressures. RV obstruction in double-chambered RV is progressive and is caused by muscle bundle hypertrophy over time, but the rate of obstruction varies.[27,28] It is hypothesized that adults who present with double-chambered RV in isolation later in life may have had an associated VSD that spontaneously closed. In the setting of a VSD located proximal to the obstruction, elevated RV pressures can diminish the degree of left-to-right shunting and can cause right-to-left shunting and cyanosis in severe cases.

The clinical presentation of subpulmonic stenosis is similar to that of pulmonic valve stenosis and depends on the degree of obstruction and the associated VSD or other anomalies. The physical examination is distinct from that of pulmonic valve stenosis in that there is no ejection click and the P2 component of the S2 is normal. The ejection murmur across the obstruction is associated with a thrill in approximately 25% of patients who have double-chambered RV.[26]

Echocardiography of Subpulmonic Stenosis

Echocardiography is usually diagnostic, especially in young patients, but it can be challenging in older adults, and transesophageal echocardiography (TEE) may be required[25] (Fig. 43.4). Cardiac magnetic resonance imaging (MRI) is increasingly used and provides excellent visualization of anatomy.[29,30] The goals of the echocardiographic evaluation of subpulmonic stenosis are similar to those for pulmonic valve stenosis, except that a VSD should be sought and evaluated for type, location, and transseptal gradient. The LV outflow tract should be evaluated for evidence of obstruction.

Similar to the assessment of pulmonic valve stenosis, key views for evaluating subpulmonic stenosis are the parasternal short-axis view at the base and the parasternal long-axis RVOT view. Doppler gradients across the RVOT may not be perpendicular to the angle of insonation in the parasternal short-axis view, and a modified apical view obtained by sliding the transducer medially with anterior angulation may offer better alignment. The location and relationship of the subpulmonic stenosis to the tricuspid and pulmonic valves are best assessed in the subcostal views, which offer excellent assessment of gradients across the RVOT in the short-axis view but are often difficult to obtain in adults. Elevated RV systolic pressures based on tricuspid regurgitation jet velocity and severe RV hypertrophy in the setting of a normal pulmonic valve may be mistakenly diagnosed as pulmonary hypertension if this form of RVOT obstruction is not recognized (Fig. 43.5).

Defining the location of a VSD in relation to the obstructive muscle bundles is important. If the VSD communicates with the high-pressure RV sinus chamber, the transseptal velocity across the VSD will be relatively low when there is significant RVOT obstruction, even if the VSD is small and restrictive to flow.

Indication for Surgical Repair

Treatment of discrete infundibular obstruction, whether caused by a membranous ridge or by obstructive muscle bundles, is surgical. Delaying surgical repair for a double-chambered RV is not recommended, unless the degree of obstruction is mild, because of the progressive nature of the obstruction. Outcomes of surgical repair are excellent with minimal residua.[31,32] Surgical repair of double-chambered RV is recommended in patients with symptoms and may be considered in asymptomatic patients with a severe gradient.[5]

SUPRAVALVULAR PULMONARY STENOSIS

Background

Supravalvular pulmonary stenosis of the pulmonary artery trunk occurs in 1% to 2% of CHD and peripheral branch pulmonary artery stenosis in 2% to 5%.[33,34] Although isolated peripheral pulmonary stenosis can occur, in 60% of cases it is seen with other congenital cardiac malformations such as valvar pulmonic stenosis, ASD, VSD, and patent ductus arteriosus.[33]

Developmental and genetic factors play a role, and supravalvular pulmonary stenosis can be associated with Noonan, Williams, Alagille, or Keutel syndromes; with complex CHD such as TOF; or with congenital rubella syndrome. It also may be seen postoperatively at the site of a prior pulmonary artery band or after arterial switch operation for dextro-transposition of the great arteries (D-TGA). Focal left pulmonary artery stenosis is associated with TOF after repair (see Chapter 44). Morphology and severity can range from focal single stenosis to multiple stenoses of the main pulmonary artery out to the peripheral branches. Diffuse hypoplasia or near-atresia also can occur.

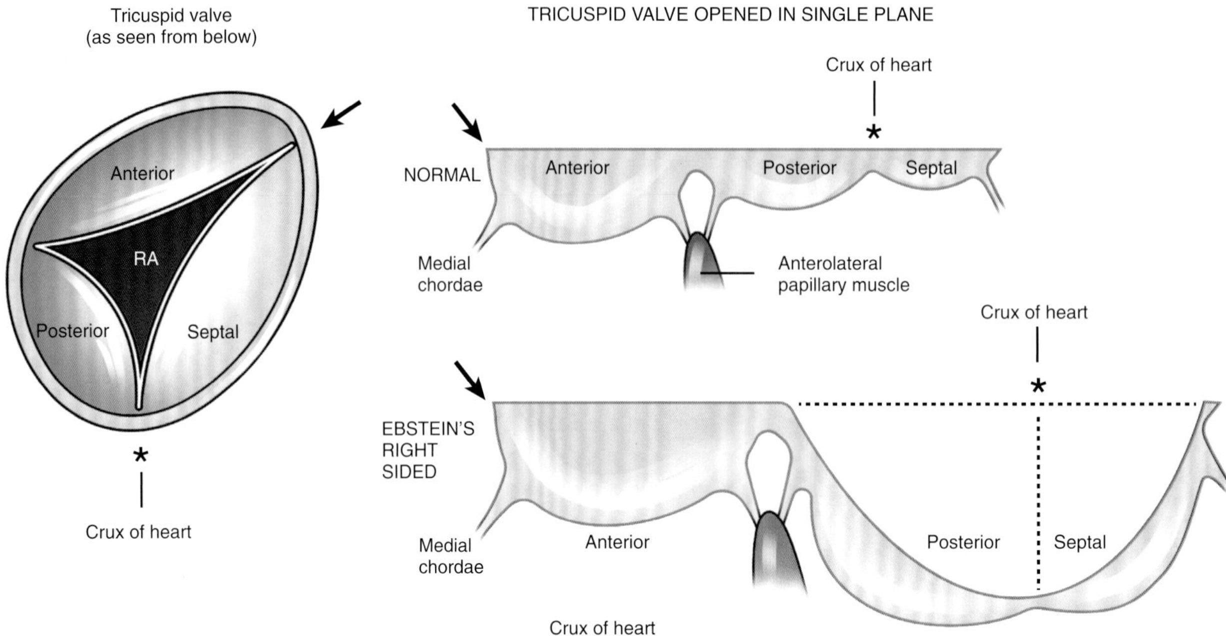

Fig. 43.6 Ebstein anomaly. The tricuspid valve is opened to show the leaflets in a single plane. The normal tricuspid valve has all three leaflets along one plane. In the right-sided Ebstein anomaly, the septal and posterior leaflets are displaced from the crux of the heart. The Ebstein anomaly of the left-sided atrioventricular valve in a physiologically corrected transposition of the great vessels has similar displacement of the septal and posterior leaflets. (From Anderson KR, Zuberbuhler JR, Anderson RH, et al. Morphologic spectrum of Ebstein's anomaly of the heart: a review. *Mayo Clin Proc.* 1979;54:174–180.)

Clinical Presentation and Physical Examination

Patients with mild to moderate bilateral or unilateral branch pulmonary artery stenosis are usually asymptomatic. In cases of severe obstruction, patients can present with exertional intolerance or even right heart failure akin to pulmonic or subpulmonic valve stenosis as a result of increased RV afterload.

The auscultatory findings are notable for lack of an ejection click. S2 is normally split and can have a prominent P2 component. In cases of severe stenosis, RV ejection is prolonged and pulmonic valve closure is delayed. The systolic ejection murmur is appreciated at the left upper sternal border and transmits to the back and peripheral lung fields. A continuous murmur may be heard, representing a significant diastolic gradient of severe obstruction.

Imaging and Management

The echocardiographic evaluation of supravalvular and peripheral pulmonary stenosis can be challenging in the adult with suboptimal windows. The right pulmonary artery can be seen along its length in the high left parasternal short-axis or suprasternal short-axis view, but the left pulmonary artery is often difficult to visualize, and alternative modes of imaging such as cardiac MRI or computed tomography are recommended. Echocardiography is useful for estimating RV pressure and RV function.

Balloon dilation with or without stenting can be useful in cases of clinically significant peripheral pulmonary stenosis.[5] However, it often requires further intervention in the future, necessitating regular surveillance and monitoring.

EBSTEIN ANOMALY

BACKGROUND AND MORPHOLOGY

Ebstein anomaly of the tricuspid valve is a rare congenital lesion with a prevalence of 5.2 cases per 100,000 live births, accounting for less than 1% of congenital heart defects.[35] Most cases of Ebstein anomaly are sporadic, but genetic, reproductive, and environmental risk factors have been implicated, including maternal lithium use.[35,36]

It is characterized by adherence of the septal and posterior leaflets to the RV myocardium due to failure of leaflet delamination during embryologic development, which leads to displacement of the leaflet hinge-points.[37] The anterior leaflet is redundant and may be fenestrated with abnormal chordae tendineae, but it is not usually displaced[38] (Fig. 43.6). The previously described apical or downward displacement of the annulus is therefore more accurately described as a rotational, rightward, and anterior annular displacement toward the RVOT[39] (Fig. 43.7).

The anatomic tripartite RV becomes divided into the atrialized portion of the RV and the functional RV chamber. In severe cases, the functional RV may comprise an infundibular chamber only. The anatomic tricuspid annulus may be severely dilated. The degree of tricuspid regurgitation varies, but the valve may be stenotic or, rarely, imperforate.[40]

Other cardiovascular anomalies are commonly associated with Ebstein anomaly and are summarized in Table 43.4.[41] Ebstein anomaly has occasionally been seen in TOF and pulmonary atresia with an intact ventricular septum. The left atrioventricular valve in physiologically (or congenitally) corrected TGA meets criteria for Ebstein anomaly in up to 50% of cases.[42] From a conduction standpoint, right bundle branch block is common, and preexcitation is found in 18% to 44% of patients.[43–45]

CLINICAL PRESENTATION AND PHYSICAL EXAMINATION

Ebstein anomaly has a wide spectrum; more severe forms of the disease are detected in the fetus, and relatively milder forms are

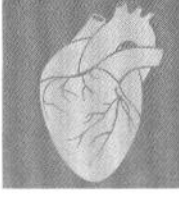

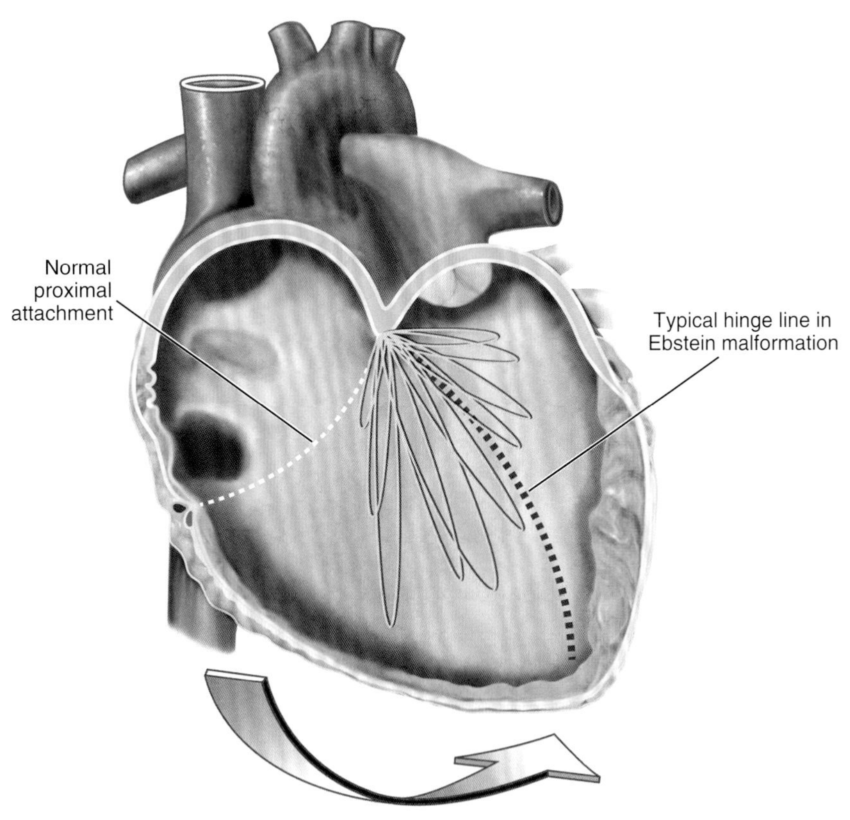

Fig. 43.7 Spectrum of annular anatomy in Ebstein anomaly. Annular orifice rotation in Ebstein anomaly was observed in a series of 23 heart specimens by Schreiber and colleagues.[38] *Green ellipses* indicate the angle of tilt of the effective valvular orifice for each specimen, and their magnitudes represent the maximal width of the orifice as a percentage of the distance between the atrioventricular junction and the apex of the RV measured along the acute margin. (From Martinez RM, O'Leary PW, Anderson RH. Anatomy and echocardiography of the normal and abnormal tricuspid valve. *Cardiol Young.* 2006;16 Suppl 3:4–11.)

TABLE 43.4 Congenital Anomalies Associated With Ebstein Anomaly.

Associated Anomaly	*Percentage of Cases (%)*	*Study*
Atrial communication (patent foramen ovale or atrial septal defect)	50–89	Attie et al.[43] Barbara et al.[44] Silva et al.[45]
Ventricular septal defect	3	Barbara et al.[44]
Tricuspid stenosis		
RV outflow tract obstruction (functional or anatomic pulmonary atresia)	6	Silva et al.[45]
Mitral valve prolapse (cleft mitral valve, parachute mitral valve, double-outlet mitral valve)	13	Barbara et al.[44]
Bicuspid aortic valve	5	Barbara et al.[44]
LV abnormalities (noncompaction, systolic and diastolic dysfunction)	2 (noncompaction)	Barbara et al.[44]
Partial anomalous pulmonary venous drainage	2	Silva et al.[45]

Adapted from Arya P, Beroukhim R. Ebstein anomaly: assessment, management, and timing of intervention. *Curr Treat Options Cardiovasc Med.* 2014;16:338.

detected in adolescence or adulthood.[46] Patients may be asymptomatic or may present with right-sided heart failure, arrhythmias, paradoxical embolism, or even sudden cardiac death.[41]

On physical examination, patients may be cyanotic due to right-to-left shunting at the atrial level. There is an RV lift and a holosystolic murmur of tricuspid regurgitation. The first heart sound (S1) is widely split with a loud, delayed tricuspid (T1) component, and S2 also may be widely split. Systolic clicks can be appreciated and are caused by redundant anterior leaflet motion. The jugular venous waveform is notable for the absence of prominent venous filling (v) waves, despite severe tricuspid regurgitation, due to the damping effect of a severely dilated and compliant RA.

ECHOCARDIOGRAPHY OF EBSTEIN ANOMALY

Echocardiography is the mainstay of diagnosis and evaluation of Ebstein anomaly. It is also essential for preoperative planning and should be used routinely in the intraoperative setting. Echocardiographic assessment of valve morphology and

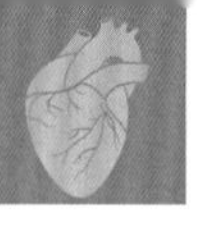

TABLE 43.5 Echocardiographic Goals in the Evaluation of Ebstein Anomaly.

Structure	*Assessment*	*Imaging Plane and Technique*
Septal and posterior leaflet	Displacement, thickening, dysplasia, chordae and tethering of septal leaflet, absence of septal leaflet in severe Ebstein anomaly[58]	Septal leaflet displacement > 8 mm/m^2 in apical 4-chamber view, also seen in parasternal short-axis view Posterior leaflet seen in parasternal RV inflow
Anterior leaflet	Elongation or redundancy, mobility, chordae and tethering to free wall, substrate for RVOT obstruction, fenestrations, displacement (rare)[47]	Anterior leaflet seen in apical 4-chamber, parasternal short-axis, and parasternal RV inflow views Attachments to RVOT seen in the parasternal RVOT view
Tricuspid valve orifice	Leaflet coaptation, effective regurgitant orifice, orifice orientation that may be toward apex or RVOT	Subcostal LAO or en face view obtained by rotating transducer 30–45 degrees from the subcostal long-axis view
Anatomic tricuspid annulus	Annulus dimension for preoperative planning	Apical 4-chamber and parasternal long-axis views
Tricuspid regurgitation	Number of jets, location, leaflet/chordal pathology, vena contracta, RV systolic pressure (may be underestimated in severe regurgitation)	Apical 4-chamber view, parasternal long-axis RV inflow view, and parasternal short-axis view at the base focused over the tricuspid valve
RA	Anatomic and atrialized portion	Apical 4-chamber and parasternal short-axis views
RV	Anatomic and physiologic RV size and function	Apical 4-chamber optimized over the RV, parasternal short-axis, parasternal long-axis, parasternal long-axis RV inflow, and parasternal long-axis RVOT views
Right ventricular outflow tract, pulmonic valve	RVOT obstruction or pulmonic stenosis	Parasternal long-axis RVOT view and parasternal short-axis view at the base focused over the pulmonic valve and bifurcation
Inferior vena cava	Size and inspiratory collapse to assess RA pressure	Subcostal long-axis with measurement of inferior vena cava diameter at end-expiration
Interatrial septum	Atrial septal defect or patent foramen ovale, location and direction of shunt, bowing of interatrial septum	Subcostal long-axis, short-axis, and in-between views, parasternal short-axis view, high right parasternal view
Ventricular septum	Ventricular septal defect, paradoxical septal motion, septal position for RV systolic pressure estimate	Parasternal short-axis view from base to apex, parasternal long-axis view, apical 4-chamber and sweep to apical 5-chamber view with color Doppler to assess direction of flow Paradoxical septal motion in parasternal short-axis view at basal ventricular septum
LV	LV noncompaction, LV systolic and diastolic function	Apical 4-chamber, apical 2-chamber, apical 3-chamber, parasternal long-axis, and parasternal short-axis views

LAO, Left anterior oblique; *RVOT*, right ventricular outflow tract.

disease severity is also prognostic. Morphology is associated with outcomes such as functional capacity and death.[46–48] The echocardiographic goals in the evaluation of Ebstein anomaly are summarized in Table 43.5.[41,49]

In the apical 4-chamber view, apical displacement of the septal leaflet from the insertion of the anterior mitral valve leaflet by more than 8 mm/m2 is diagnostic of Ebstein anomaly[47] (Fig. 43.8). The septal leaflet may be hypoplastic with restricted motion due to shortened chordae tendineae. The RV inflow view demonstrates the anterior and posterior leaflets and the hinge points and attachments. The sail-like movement of the anterior leaflet can be appreciated in the parasternal short-axis view and the parasternal RV inflow view. If the patient has adequate acoustic windows, the subcostal short-axis view may depict distal attachments of the anterior leaflet and fenestrations and RVOT obstruction.

The subcostal en face view, achieved by rotating the transducer 30 to 45 degrees from the subcostal long axis, is the only view in which all three leaflets may be seen by transthoracic echocardiography (TTE) (Fig. 43.9). TEE can offer en face imaging in the transgastric short-axis view and can provide excellent assessment of the subvalvular apparatus, including the chordae tendineae and papillary muscles, in the transgastric RV inflow view.[39]

The size and function of the RV correlate with disease severity and are prognostic. With increasing displacement of the tricuspid annulus, the atrialized portion of the RV increases, and the size of the functional RV decreases. The severity of Ebstein anomaly may be described as a ratio between the area of the functional RV and the area of the RA plus the atrialized RV. The larger the atrialized RV portion or the smaller the ratio (<35%), the poorer the prognosis.[46,47]

The echocardiographic evaluation of LV function is challenging in Ebstein anomaly because of alterations in LV geometry

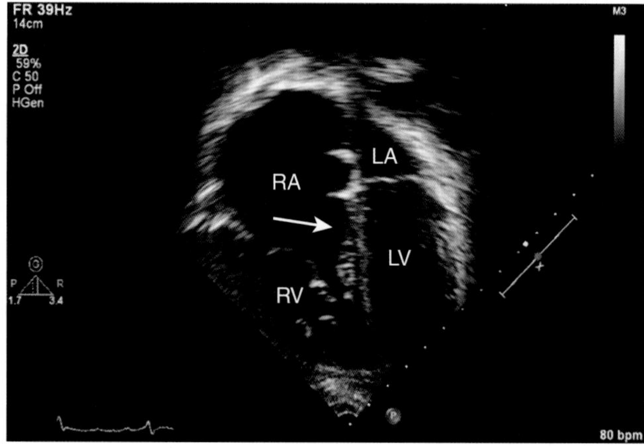

Fig. 43.8 Ebstein anomaly in apical 4-chamber view. Apical 4-chamber view demonstrates apical displacement of the septal leaflet of the tricuspid valve *(arrow)*. There is tethering of the septal leaflet, and the anterior leaflet is redundant (see Video 43.8).

related to ventricular interdependence.[49] The interventricular septum can exhibit paradoxical motion, which impairs LV diastolic filling. A septal bulge into the LV cavity creates a crescent-shaped chamber that is compressed. For this reason, it may be necessary to assess LV systolic function qualitatively or semi-quantitatively using fractional shortening.[49]

The assessment of Ebstein anomaly by two-dimensional (2D) TTE can be limited because it visualizes only two of three leaflets at once in the standard views, and definition of the tricuspid valve commissural anatomy and leaflet commissures may be difficult. Three-dimensional (3D) echocardiography is helpful

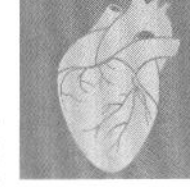

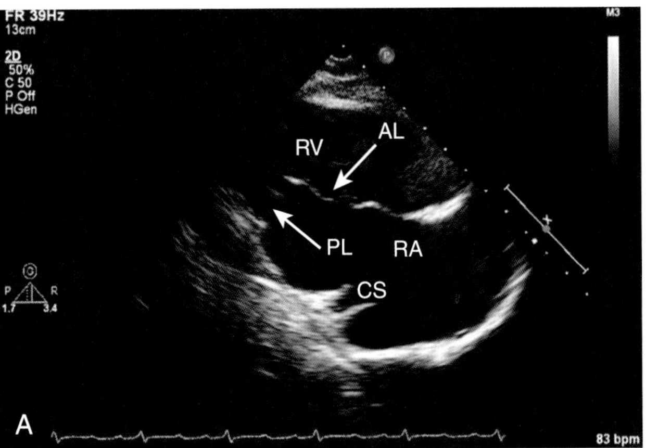

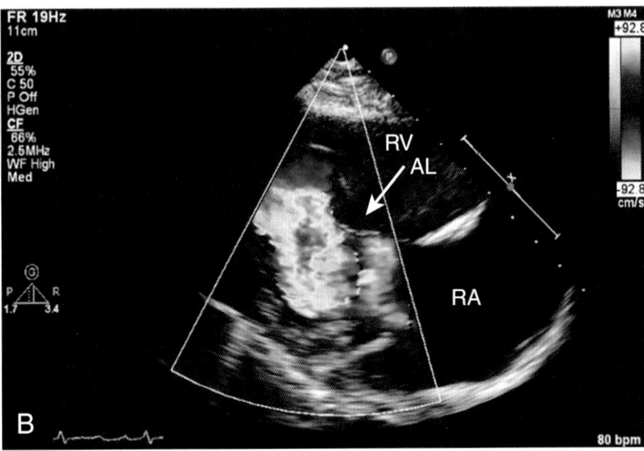

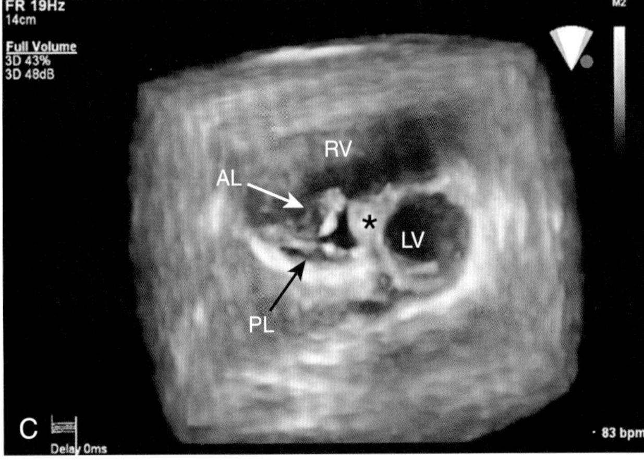

Fig. 43.9 Ebstein anomaly of the tricuspid valve. (A) Parasternal long-axis RV inflow view of the anterior leaflet *(AL)* and posterior leaflet *(PL)* of the tricuspid valve (see Video 43.9A). (B) Parasternal long-axis RV inflow view with color Doppler shows severe tricuspid regurgitation (see Video 43.9B). (C) Subcostal en face view of Ebstein anomaly. There is a thickened septal leaflet *(asterisk)* and a small PL. Notice the large central coaptation defect (see Video 43.9C). *CS*, Coronary sinus.

in defining valve morphology and in displaying the degree of rotation of the effective annulus toward the RVOT.[50,51]

Cardiac MRI is a complementary imaging modality for Ebstein anomaly, especially in cases with difficult acoustic windows.[52] It can offer improved visualization of valve anatomy and superior visualization of the posterior leaflet.[52] Volumetric data on anatomic and physiologic RV size and function can be obtained, as can tricuspid valve regurgitant fraction and shunt fraction if there is an interatrial communication. Cardiac MRI is uniquely suited for tissue characterization, including myocardial delayed-enhancement imaging and assessment of LV noncompaction.

TABLE 43.6 ACC/AHA Recommendations for Surgery in Ebstein Anomaly.

Class I

1. Surgical repair or reoperation for adults with Ebstein anomaly and significant TR is recommended when one or more of the following are present: heart failure symptoms, objective evidence of worsening exercise capacity, progressive RV systolic dysfunction by echocardiography or cardiac magnetic resonance imaging (level of evidence: B).

Class IIa

1. Surgical repair or reoperation for adults with Ebstein anomaly and significant TR can be beneficial in the presence of progressive RV enlargement, systemic desaturation from right-to-left atrial shunt, paradoxical embolism, and/or atrial tachyarrhythmias (level of evidence: B).

Class IIb

1. Bidirectional superior cavopulmonary (Glenn) anastomosis at the time of Ebstein anomaly repair may be considered for adults when severe RV dilation or severe RV systolic dysfunction is present, LV function is preserved, and LA pressure and LV end-diastolic pressure are not elevated (level of evidence: B).

AHA/ACC, American Heart Association and American College of Cardiology; *TR*, tricuspid regurgitation.

From Stout KK, Daniels CJ, Aboulhosn JA, et al. 2018 AHA/ACC guideline for the management of adults with congenital heart disease: a report of the American College of Cardiology/American Heart Association Task Force on Clinical Practice Guidelines. *J Am Coll Cardiol*. 2019;73(12):e81–e192.

SURGICAL REPAIR AND OUTCOMES

Indications for surgical repair are summarized in Table 43.6. The optimal timing for surgery is debated, however, and decisions must be made on an individualized basis.

Surgery involves tricuspid valve repair or replacement to improve the degree of tricuspid regurgitation, closure of any interatrial communication, surgical ablation procedures for arrhythmias, and possible RV plication.[53] Tricuspid valve repair is preferred if anatomically suitable and should be performed by surgeons with training and expertise in CHD.[5] Tricuspid valve repair has evolved over the past 30 years and involves reducing annulus size with or without an annuloplasty ring, repositioning tricuspid valve leaflet tissue to improve coaptation, and reducing RA and atrialized RV size.

The cone procedure, pioneered by da Silva, is a technically challenging operation that results in a cone-shaped leaflet that coapts as a bileaflet valve and has excellent short and midterm outcomes[45,54] (Fig. 43.10). Other operations include monocusp repair and bioprosthetic tricuspid valve replacement. In cases of severe RV dilation and/or low cardiac output, a bidirectional cavopulmonary anastomosis (i.e., bidirectional Glenn repair in which the superior vena cava is anastomosed to the ipsilateral branch pulmonary artery to unload the RV) may be required and is known as a "one-and-a-half repair" if there is simultaneous antegrade pulmonary blood flow.

The echocardiographic assessment of Ebstein anomaly is critical for surgical planning, and TEE may be required. From an anatomic standpoint, mobility of the anterior leaflet with identification of a free leading edge is key to successful surgical repair.[53] Patients with highly muscularized anterior leaflets or severely hypoplastic or absent septal leaflets are not candidates for cone repair. Multiple separate jets of tricuspid regurgitation, direct muscular insertions into the leading edge of the anterior leaflet, and inflow orientation positioned toward the RVOT also make successful repair less likely.[39]

Tricuspid valve surgery leads to decreased tricuspid regurgitation and RV size with concomitant improvement in exercise capacity.[54,55] LV systolic function can improve postoperatively.[55,56] Long-term outcomes for Ebstein surgery have been

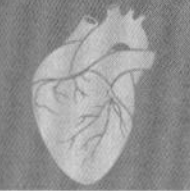

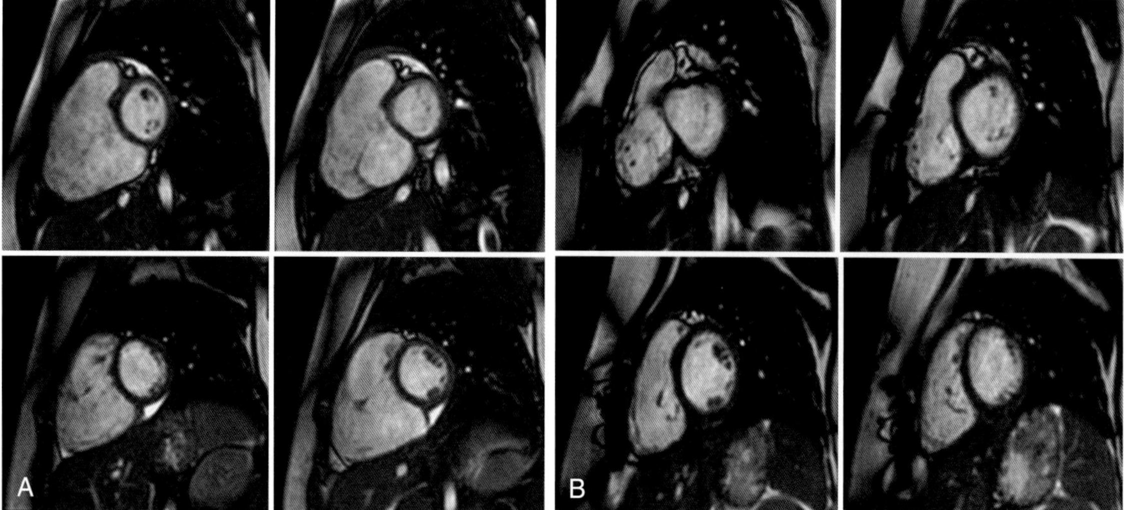

Fig. 43.10 Cardiac magnetic resonance imaging of Ebstein anomaly. (A) Short-axis preoperative views (see Video 43.10A). (B) Short-axis views after cone repair (see Video 43.10B),

reported with good survival and functional status. However, fatigue and dyspnea are common, as are atrial arrhythmias.[57]

REVIEW

- The RV is a tripartite structure consisting of inlet, sinus, and outlet portions. The RVOT is also known as the infundibulum.
- The most common right-sided congenital anomaly is valvular pulmonic stenosis. Classic domed-shape pulmonic stenosis is rarely progressive when mild; if severe, it can be treated by transcatheter balloon valvuloplasty with good results.
- Peak instantaneous gradients by spectral Doppler across the RVOT and/or pulmonic valve often overestimate invasive gradients obtained by catheterization. Other ways to estimate the severity of obstruction include calculation of RV systolic pressure from the tricuspid regurgitant velocity, septal position, and degree of RV hypertrophy. Regurgitant right-sided lesions and left-to-right shunting can lead to increased flow across the pulmonary valve and overestimation of the degree of stenosis.
- Tricuspid regurgitation jet velocity is predictive of RV systolic pressures and should not be confused with pulmonary artery systolic pressure in the setting of RV outflow obstruction.
- Multiple levels of obstruction across the RVOT, pulmonary valve, and main and branch pulmonary arteries in right-sided congenital anomalies can occur and should be sought in the echocardiographic examination.
- The forms of Ebstein anomaly of the tricuspid valve vary, and prognosis depends on morphologic severity. Apical and downward displacement of the annulus may be more accurately thought of as rotational displacement of the annulus into the infundibulum.
- TEE and cardiac MRI are useful imaging techniques in the preoperative assessment of Ebstein anomaly for surgical planning. Certain patients may be candidates for the da Silva cone procedure, which results in a bileaflet valve but should be performed by surgeons with training in CHD.

SUMMARY Congenital Right Heart Anomalies.

Structural and Functional Assessment	Imaging Plane and Techniques	Measurement and Interpretation
Right atrium	Apical 4-chamber	Upper limit of normal is 18 cm^2 or 25 ± 7 mL/m^2 in men and 21 ± 6 mL/m^2 in women Anatomic and atrialized portion in Ebstein anomaly
Tricuspid valve morphology	Apical 4-chamber (septal and anterior leaflets), parasternal long-axis RV inflow (anterior and posterior leaflets), parasternal short-axis at the base (anterior and septal leaflets) Subcostal LAO or en face view obtained by rotating transducer 30–45 degrees from the subcostal long-axis (all three leaflets)	Septal leaflet displacement >8 mm/m^2 in apical 4-chamber view is consistent with Ebstein anomaly Leaflet and chordal pathology, abnormal attachments Septal leaflet compromise from a ventricular septal defect patch

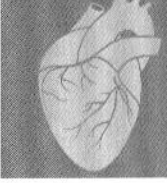

SUMMARY Congenital Right Heart Anomalies.—cont'd

Structural and Functional Assessment	Imaging Plane and Techniques	Measurement and Interpretation
Tricuspid regurgitation	Apical 4-chamber, parasternal long-axis RV inflow, and parasternal short-axis at the base focused over the tricuspid valve Subcostal LAO or en face view obtained by rotating transducer 30–45 degrees from the subcostal long-axis view	Jet area >10 cm^2 and vena contracta width >0.7 cm consistent with severe TR Annular dilation, RA size, diastolic interventricular septal flattening, effective orifice area in en face view RVSP estimate
RV size and hypertrophy	Subcostal long-axis or parasternal long-axis by M-mode or 2D echocardiography for hypertrophy Apical 4-chamber optimized over the RV, parasternal short-axis, parasternal long-axis, parasternal long-axis RV inflow, parasternal long-axis RV outflow for size	RV diastolic wall thickness >5 mm consistent with RV hypertrophy RV basal diameter >4.1 cm and parasternal long-axis RVOT proximal diameter >3.0 cm are abnormal in noncongenital RV
RV function	Apical 4-chamber optimized over the RV, parasternal short-axis, parasternal long-axis, parasternal long-axis RV inflow, parasternal long-axis RV outflow	Fractional area of change, TAPSE, color tissue Doppler, myocardial performance index, and 3D echocardiography with limited applicability to RV function in CHD
RV outflow tract	Parasternal long-axis RVOT view and parasternal short-axis at the base Subcostal RAO view with counterclockwise 45-degree rotation from long axis to get RV inflow-outflow view	Assessment of anatomy and severity of obstruction from membrane, muscle bundles, or chordal attachments Anterior infundibular akinesis from RVOT or transannular patch RVOT aneurysm with echo-free space
Pulmonic valve morphology	Parasternal long-axis RVOT and parasternal short-axis views High right parasternal axis to view en face	Assessment of morphology, including doming, leaflet hypoplasia or dysplasia, and leaflet mobility Pulmonary annulus dimension with normal range of 17–26 mm
Pulmonic valve function	Parasternal short-axis at the base and modified apical with anterior angulation	Peak Doppler gradient >4 m/s, mean Doppler gradient >40 mmHg, or RVSP ≥75% of LV systolic pressure consistent with severe PS Regurgitant jet width >70% of the annulus, color flow reversal in branch pulmonary arteries, and pressure half-time <100 ms correlate with significant PR
Main and branch pulmonary arteries	Parasternal short-axis at the base focused over the pulmonic valve and bifurcation Suprasternal short-axis and high left parasternal axis for central pulmonary artery and RPA Suprasternal long-axis and high left parasternal axis for LPA	Assessment of size, hypoplasia, continuity, stenosis Main pulmonary artery is measured at its midpoint during systole. Assessment of residual shunt flow
Ventricular septal defect	Parasternal short-axis from base to apex, parasternal long-axis, apical 4-chamber, and sweep to apical 5-chamber	Residual or unrepaired ventricular septal defect Location, including relationship to tricuspid, aortic, and pulmonic valves and infundibulum Color Doppler to assess direction of flow and CW Doppler for transseptal gradient If left-to-right flow, RV systolic pressure = LV systolic pressure (cuff systolic pressure in the absence of LV outflow tract obstruction) − peak transseptal gradient
Inferior vena cava	Subcostal long-axis	Inferior vena cava diameter at end-expiration and inspiratory collapse to assess RA pressure
Interatrial septum	Subcostal long-axis, short-axis, and in-between views Parasternal short-axis and high right parasternal-axis	Atrial septal defect or patent foramen ovale, bowing of interatrial septum

CHD, Congenital heart disease; *LAO*, left anterior oblique; *LPA*, left pulmonary artery; *PR*, pulmonic regurgitation; *PS*, pulmonic stenosis; *RAO*, right anterior oblique; *RPA*, right pulmonary artery; *RVOT*, right ventricular outflow tract; *RVSP*, right ventricular systolic pressure; *TAPSE*, tricuspid annular plane systolic excursion; *TR*, tricuspid regurgitation.

REFERENCES

1. Prieto LR, Latson LA. Pulmonary stenosis. In: Allen HD, Driscoll DJ, Shaddy RE, Feltes TF, eds. *Moss and Adams' Heart Disease in Infants, Children, and Adolescents: Including the Fetus and Young Adult*. Vol 2, 9th ed. Philadelphia: Lippincott Williams & Wilkins; 2016.
2. Hayes CJ, Gersony WM, Driscoll DJ, et al. Second natural history study of congenital heart defects. Results of treatment of patients with pulmonary valvar stenosis. *Circulation*. 1993;87(2 suppl):I28–37.
3. Jurado-Roman A, Hernandez-Hernandez F, Ruiz-Cano MJ, et al. Compression of the left main coronary artery by a giant pulmonary artery aneurysm. *Circulation*. 2013;127(12): 1340–1341.
4. Nishimura RA, Otto CM, Bonow RO, et al. 2014. AHA/ACC Guideline for the Management of Patients With Valvular Heart Disease: a report of the American College of Cardiology/American Heart Association Task Force on Practice Guidelines. *Circulation*. 2014;129(23): e521–e643.
5. Stout KK, Daniels CJ, Aboulhosn JA, et al. 2019. AHA/ACC Guideline for the Management of Adults With Congenital Heart Disease: A Report of the American College of Cardiology/American Heart Association Task Force on Clinical Practice Guidelines. *J Am Coll Cardiol*. 2018;73(12):e81–e192.
6. Frantz EG, Silverman NH. Doppler ultrasound evaluation of valvar pulmonary stenosis from multiple transducer positions in children requiring pulmonary valvuloplasty. *Am J Cardiol*. 1988;61(10):844–849.
7. Lima CO, Sahn DJ, Valdes-Cruz LM, et al. Noninvasive prediction of transvalvular pressure gradient in patients with pulmonary stenosis by quantitative two-dimensional echocardiographic Doppler studies. *Circulation*. 1983; 67(4):866–871.
8. Aldousany AW, DiSessa TG, Dubois R, Alpert BS, Willey ES, Birnbaum SE. Doppler estimation of pressure gradient in pulmonary stenosis: maximal instantaneous vs peak-to-peak, vs mean catheter gradient. *Pediatr Cardiol*. 1989;10(3):145–149.
9. Currie PJ, Hagler DJ, Seward JB, et al. Instantaneous pressure gradient: a simultaneous Doppler and dual catheter correlative study. *J Am Coll Cardiol*. 1986;7(4):800–806.
10. Silvilairat S, Cabalka AK, Cetta F, Hagler DJ, O'Leary PW. Echocardiographic assessment of isolated pulmonary valve stenosis: which outpatient Doppler gradient has the most clinical validity? *J Am Soc Echocardiogr*. 2005;18(11):1137–1142.
11. Silvilairat S, Cabalka AK, Cetta F, Hagler DJ, O'Leary PW. Outpatient echocardiographic assessment of complex pulmonary outflow stenosis: Doppler mean gradient is superior to the maximum instantaneous gradient. *J Am Soc Echocardiogr*. 2005;18(11):1143–1148.
12. Kan JS, White Jr RI, Mitchell SE, Gardner TJ. Percutaneous balloon valvuloplasty: a new method for treating congenital pulmonary-valve stenosis. *N Engl J Med*. 1982;307(9):540–542.
13. Ananthakrishna A, Balasubramonium VR, Thazhath HK, et al. Balloon pulmonary valvuloplasty in adults: immediate and long-term outcomes. *J Heart Valve Dis*. 2014;23(4):511–515.
14. Chen CR, Cheng TO, Huang T, et al. Percutaneous balloon valvuloplasty for pulmonic stenosis in adolescents and adults. *N Engl J Med*. 1996;335(1):21–25.
15. McCrindle BW. Independent predictors of long-term results after balloon pulmonary valvuloplasty. Valvuloplasty and Angioplasty of Congenital Anomalies (VACA) Registry Investigators. *Circulation*. 1994;89(4):1751–1759.
16. Voet A, Rega F, de Bruaene AV, et al. Long-term outcome after treatment of isolated pulmonary valve stenosis. *Int J Cardiol*. 2012;156(1): 11–15.
17. Earing MG, Connolly HM, Dearani JA, Ammash NM, Grogan M, Warnes CA. Long-term follow-up of patients after surgical treatment for isolated pulmonary valve stenosis. *Mayo Clin Proc*. 2005;80(7):871–876.
18. O'Connor BK, Beekman RH, Lindauer A, Rocchini A. Intermediate-term outcome after pulmonary balloon valvuloplasty: comparison with a matched surgical control group. *J Am Coll Cardiol*. 1992;20(1):169–173.
19. Peterson C, Schilthuis JJ, Dodge-Khatami A, Hitchcock JF, Meijboom EJ, Bennink GB. Comparative long-term results of surgery versus balloon valvuloplasty for pulmonary valve stenosis in infants and children. *Ann Thorac Surg*. 2003;76(4):1078–1082; discussion 1082–1073.
20. Roos-Hesselink JW, Meijboom FJ, Spitaels SE, et al. Long-term outcome after surgery for pulmonary stenosis (a longitudinal study of 22–33 years). *Eur Heart J*. 2006;27(4):482–488.
21. Ben-Shachar G, Cohen MH, Sivakoff MC, Portman MA, Riemenschneider TA, Van Heeckeren DW. Development of infundibular obstruction after percutaneous pulmonary balloon valvuloplasty. *J Am Coll Cardiol*. 1985;5(3):754–756.
22. Engle MA, Holswade GR, Goldberg HP, Lukas DS, Glenn F. Regression after open valvotomy of infundibular stenosis accompanying severe valvular pulmonic stenosis. *Circulation*. 1958;17(5):862–873.
23. Bokma JP, Winter MM, Oosterhof T, et al. Pulmonary valve replacement after repair of pulmonary stenosis compared with tetralogy of Fallot. *J Am Coll Cardiol*. 2016;67(9):1123–1124.
24. Zdradzinski MJ, Qureshi AM, Stewart R, Pettersson G, Krasuski RA. Comparison of long-term postoperative sequelae in patients with tetralogy of Fallot versus isolated pulmonic stenosis. *Am J Cardiol*. 2014;114(2):300–304.
25. Hoffman P, Wojcik AW, Rozanski J, et al. The role of echocardiography in diagnosing double chambered right ventricle in adults. *Heart*. 2004;90(7):789–793.
26. Singh MN, McElhinney DB. Double-chambered right ventricle. In: Gatzoulis MA, Webb G, Daubeney PEF, eds. *Diagnosis and Management of Adult Congenital Heart Disease*. 2nd ed. Philadelphia, PA: Elsevier Saunders; 2011.
27. Oliver JM, Garrido A, Gonzalez A, et al. Rapid progression of midventricular obstruction in adults with double-chambered right ventricle. *J Thorac Cardiovasc Surg*. 2003;126(3):711–717.
28. Pongiglione G, Freedom RM, Cook D, Rowe RD. Mechanism of acquired right ventricular outflow tract obstruction in patients with ventricular septal defect: an angiocardiographic study. *Am J Cardiol*. 1982;50(4):776–780.
29. Bashore TM. Adult congenital heart disease: right ventricular outflow tract lesions. *Circulation*. 2007;115(14):1933–1947.
30. Kilner PJ, Geva T, Kaemmerer H, Trindade PT, Schwitter J, Webb GD. Recommendations for cardiovascular magnetic resonance in adults with congenital heart disease from the respective working groups of the European Society of Cardiology. *Eur Heart J*. 2010;31(7): 794–805.
31. Kahr PC, Alonso-Gonzalez R, Kempny A, et al. Long-term natural history and postoperative outcome of double-chambered right ventricle–experience from two tertiary adult congenital heart centres and review of the literature. *Int J Cardiol*. 2014;174(3):662–668.
32. Said SM, Burkhart HM, Dearani JA, O'Leary PW, Ammash NM, Schaff HV. Outcomes of surgical repair of double-chambered right ventricle. *Ann Thorac Surg*. 2012;93(1):197–200.
33. Bacha EA, Kreutzer J. Comprehensive management of branch pulmonary artery stenosis. *J Interv Cardiol*. 2001;14(3):367–375.
34. Cuypers JA, Witsenburg M, van der Linde D, Roos-Hesselink JW. Pulmonary stenosis: update on diagnosis and therapeutic options. *Heart*. 2013;99(5):339–347.
35. Correa-Villasenor A, Ferencz C, Neill CA, Wilson PD, Boughman JA. Ebstein's malformation of the tricuspid valve: genetic and environmental factors. The Baltimore-Washington Infant Study Group. *Teratology*. 1994;50(2):137–147.
36. Cohen LS, Friedman JM, Jefferson JW, Johnson EM, Weiner ML. A reevaluation of risk of in utero exposure to lithium. *JAMA*. 1994;271(2):146–150.
37. Van Mierop LH, Gessner IH. Pathogenetic mechanisms in congenital cardiovascular malformations. *Prog Cardiovasc Dis*. 1972;15(1):67–85.
38. Schreiber C, Cook A, Ho SY, Augustin N, Anderson RH. Morphologic spectrum of Ebstein's malformation: revisitation relative to surgical repair. *J Thorac Cardiovasc Surg*. 1999;117(1):148–155.
39. Martinez RM, O'Leary PW, Anderson RH. Anatomy and echocardiography of the normal and abnormal tricuspid valve. *Cardiol Young*. 2006;16(suppl 3):4–11.
40. Anderson KR, Zuberbuhler JR, Anderson RH, Becker AE, Lie JT. Morphologic spectrum of Ebstein's anomaly of the heart: a review. *Mayo Clin Proc*. 1979;54(3):174–180.
41. Arya P, Beroukhim R. Ebstein anomaly: assessment, management, and timing of intervention. *Curr Treat Options Cardiovasc Med*. 2014;16(10):338.
42. Attenhofer Jost CH, Connolly HM, Dearani JA, Edwards WD, Danielson GK. Ebstein's anomaly. *Circulation*. 2007;115(2):277–285.
43. Attie F, Rosas M, Rijlaarsdam M, et al. The adult patient with Ebstein anomaly. Outcome in 72 unoperated patients. *Medicine (Baltimore)*. 2000;79(1):27–36.
44. Barbara DW, Edwards WD, Connolly HM, Dearani JA. Surgical pathology of 104 tricuspid valves (2000–2005) with classic right-sided Ebstein's malformation. *Cardiovasc Pathol*. 2008;17(3):166–171.
45. Silva JP, Silva Lda F, Moreira LF, et al. Cone reconstruction in Ebstein's anomaly repair: early and long-term results. *Arq Bras Cardiol*. 2011;97(3):199–208.

46. Celermajer DS, Bull C, Till JA, et al. Ebstein's anomaly: presentation and outcome from fetus to adult. *J Am Coll Cardiol.* 1994;23(1):170–176.
47. Shiina A, Seward JB, Edwards WD, Hagler DJ, Tajik AJ. Two-dimensional echocardiographic spectrum of Ebstein's anomaly: detailed anatomic assessment. *J Am Coll Cardiol.* 1984;3(2 Pt 1):356–370.
48. Trojnarska O, Szyszka A, Gwizdala A, et al. Adults with Ebstein's anomaly—cardiopulmonary exercise testing and BNP levels exercise capacity and BNP in adults with Ebstein's anomaly. *Int J Cardiol.* 2006;111(1):92–97.
49. Oechslin E, Buchholz S, Jenni R. Ebstein's anomaly in adults: Doppler-echocardiographic evaluation. *Thorac Cardiovasc Surg.* 2000;48(4):209–213.
50. Bharucha T, Anderson RH, Lim ZS, Vettukattil JJ. Multiplanar review of three-dimensional echocardiography gives new insights into the morphology of Ebstein's malformation. *Cardiol Young.* 2010;20(1):49–53.
51. Muraru D, Badano LP, Sarais C, Solda E, Iliceto S. Evaluation of tricuspid valve morphology and function by transthoracic three-dimensional echocardiography. *Curr Cardiol Rep.* 2011;13(3):242–249.
52. Attenhofer Jost CH, Edmister WD, Julsrud PR, et al. Prospective comparison of echocardiography versus cardiac magnetic resonance imaging in patients with Ebstein's anomaly. *Int J Cardiovasc Imaging.* 2012;28(5):1147–1159.
53. Dearani JA, Danielson GK. Surgical management of Ebstein's anomaly in the adult. *Semin Thorac Cardiovasc Surg.* 2005;17(2):148–154.
54. Holst KA, Dearani JA, Said S, et al. Improving results of surgery for Ebstein anomaly: Where are we after 235 cone repairs? *Ann Thorac Surg.* 2018;105(1):160–168.
55. Kuhn A, De Pasquale Meyer G, Muller J, et al. Tricuspid valve surgery improves cardiac output and exercise performance in patients with Ebstein's anomaly. *Int J Cardiol.* 2013;166(2):494–498.
56. Brown ML, Dearani JA, Danielson GK, et al. Effect of operation for Ebstein anomaly on left ventricular function. *Am J Cardiol.* 2008;102(12):1724–1727.
57. Brown ML, Dearani JA, Danielson GK, et al. Functional status after operation for Ebstein anomaly: the Mayo Clinic experience. *J Am Coll Cardiol.* 2008;52(6):460–466.
58. Rusconi PG, Zuberbuhler JR, Anderson RH, Rigby ML. Morphologic-echocardiographic correlates of Ebstein's malformation. *Eur Heart J.* 1991;12(7):784–790.

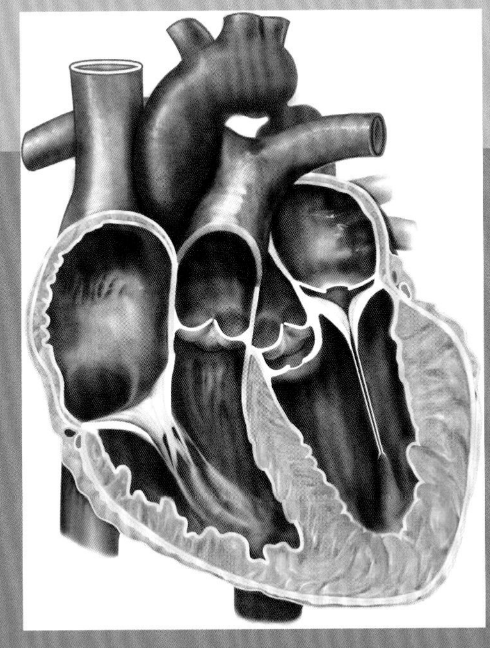

中文导读

第44章 复杂圆锥动脉干异常

圆锥动脉干发育异常导致累及心室流出道和大动脉的缺陷。圆锥动脉干发育异常可能导致：①心室-动脉排列和连接异常；②流出道间隔缺损；③流出道发育不良、狭窄或闭锁。复杂圆锥动脉干异常的精确诊断通常具有挑战性，因为每个疾病有不同特点，其细节对于构建可行的手术计划至关重要。本章重点从复杂圆锥动脉干异常的胚胎时期发育、相关的染色体异常、如何用全面的节段性分析法分析房室水平连接及心室大动脉水平连接、超声诊断要点及注意事项和典型图像显示等方面详细介绍了其他复杂的圆锥动脉干异常，包括法洛四联症、永存动脉干、右心室双出口、左心室双出口、解剖学矫正的大动脉畸形和主肺动脉窗。详细介绍了复杂圆锥动脉干异常的病理解剖及分类、术前超声评价不同节段的连接关系、合并畸形如室间隔缺损及流出道狭窄的部位、左右心室及瓣膜功能、术后流出道狭窄、残余分流等畸形矫正情况评估。

王　燕

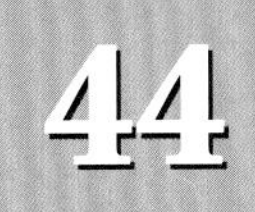

Complex Conotruncal Anomalies

ANNE MARIE VALENTE, MD | YULI Y. KIM, MD | STEPHEN P. SANDERS, MD

Abnormal conotruncal development results in defects involving the ventricular outflow tracts and great arteries. Developmental abnormalities in the conotruncus may result in (1) abnormal ventriculoarterial alignments and connections; (2) outlet septation defects; or (3) outlet hypoplasia, stenosis, or atresia.[1] The category of *conotruncal anomalies* includes many defects, some of which, including transposition of the great arteries (TGA) (see Chapter 45), interrupted aortic arch (see Chapter 45), and semilunar valve abnormalities (see Chapter 42), are covered elsewhere in this textbook. This chapter focuses on other complex conotruncal anomalies, including tetralogy of Fallot (TOF), truncus arteriosus (TA), double-outlet ventricle, anatomically corrected malposition of the great arteries, and aortopulmonary window.

Precise diagnosis of a conotruncal defect is often challenging because there are many variations of each defect, the details of which are essential for construction of a coherent and workable surgical plan. The diagnosis of conotruncal defects is usually made in early childhood when a complete echocardiographic examination, including subxiphoid views, is feasible.[2] Although these defects are complex, multiple-plane imaging with two-dimensional (2D) echocardiography is reliable in ascertaining the anatomy when a comprehensive, segmental analysis is applied. As patients age, echocardiographic windows may become limited, and alternative imaging modalities, such as cardiac magnetic resonance imaging (MRI), are increasingly used.[3]

CONOTRUNCAL DEVELOPMENT

Imaging of patients with conotruncal defects is aided by an understanding of cardiac development. The heart starts to form in the third week of gestation and is more or less fully formed by 8 weeks. Mesodermal precardiac cells migrate to form the cardiac crescents (i.e., primary heart fields) in anterior lateral plate mesoderm, and they are then brought together to form a primary linear heart tube by ventral closure of the embryo. Cells of the second heart field continue to proliferate outside the heart and are added to the heart tube over the course of embryogenesis, contributing to the atria, the right ventricle (RV), and the outflow tract.

Cardiac neural crest cells migrate into the developing heart in the fifth to sixth weeks and are essential for septation of the outflow, formation of the semilunar valves, and patterning of the aortic arches. Once formed, the heart tube grows and elongates by the addition of cells from the second heart field. The ends of the heart tube are relatively fixed by the pericardial sac so that as it elongates, it must bend or loop. In most hearts, the loop falls to the right (D-loop). Further elongation pushes the midportion of the tube (i.e., future ventricles) inferior or caudal to the inflow, resulting in the normal relationship between the atria and ventricles. Further growth pushes the outflow medially and is associated with outflow rotation; both processes are essential for normal alignment of the outflow. The proximal part of the outflow is incorporated into the RV, shortening the outflow in association with further rotation.

While this remodeling is occurring, the outflow is undergoing septation under the influence of cardiac neural crest cells. Septation proceeds from distal to proximal, culminating in formation and muscularization of the infundibular or muscular outflow septum, which inserts onto the superior endocardial cushion at the rightward rim of the outflow foramen, walling the aorta into the left ventricle (LV) by means of the outflow foramen and the pulmonary artery (PA) directly into the RV. Failure of any of these processes, including outflow elongation, rotation, shortening, and septation, results in a conotruncal anomaly.[4,5]

NOMENCLATURE FOR CONGENITAL HEART DEFECTS

Congenital heart defects are complex anomalies, and a segmental approach is used for their analysis and description. The heart is composed of several parts, or *segments*. In the segmental approach, the cardiac anatomy is assessed first by dividing the heart into three distinct segments, based on 10 embryologic regions, which are analyzed separately before formulating a comprehensive diagnosis. The principal segments are the atria, the ventricles, and the great arteries, which are joined together by the atrioventricular (AV) canal and the conus or infundibulum.

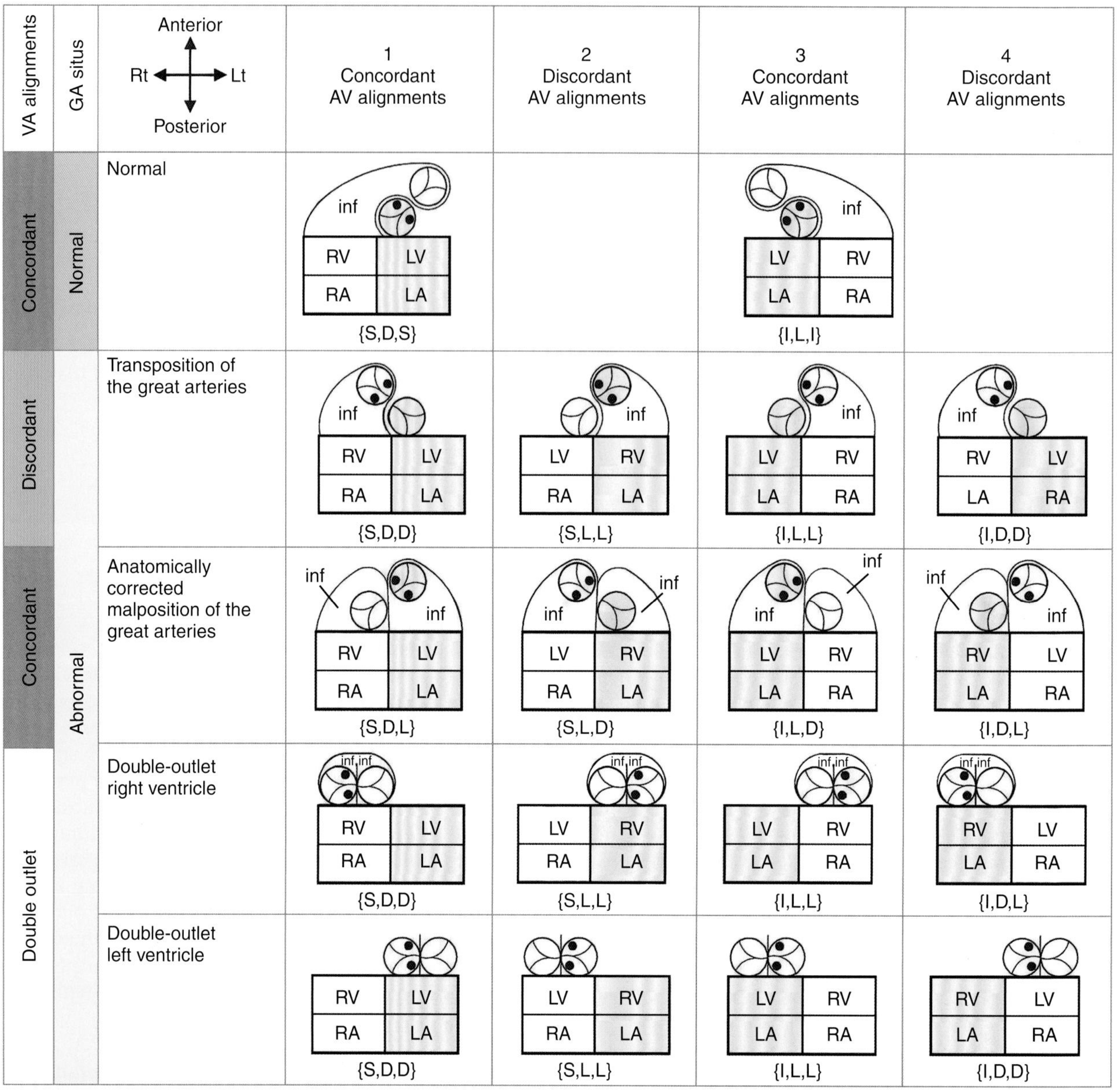

VA alignments	GA situs	Anterior Rt ↔ Lt Posterior	1 Concordant AV alignments	2 Discordant AV alignments	3 Concordant AV alignments	4 Discordant AV alignments
Concordant	Normal	Normal	inf RV LV RA LA {S,D,S}		inf LV RV LA RA {I,L,I}	
Discordant	Abnormal	Transposition of the great arteries	inf RV LV RA LA {S,D,D}	inf LV RV RA LA {S,L,L}	inf LV RV LA RA {I,L,L}	inf RV LV LA RA {I,D,D}
Concordant	Abnormal	Anatomically corrected malposition of the great arteries	inf inf RV LV RA LA {S,D,L}	inf inf LV RV RA LA {S,L,D}	inf inf LV RV LA RA {I,L,D}	inf inf RV LV LA RA {I,D,L}
Double outlet	Abnormal	Double-outlet right ventricle	inf,inf RV LV RA LA {S,D,D}	inf,inf LV RV RA LA {S,L,L}	inf,inf LV RV LA RA {I,L,L}	inf,inf RV LV LA RA {I,D,L}
Double outlet	Abnormal	Double-outlet left ventricle	RV LV RA LA {S,D,D}	LV RV RA LA {S,L,L}	LV RV LA RA {I,L,L}	RV LV LA RA {I,D,D}

Fig. 44.1 Representation of the situs, alignments, and connections of various conotruncal anomalies. The pulmonary artery is normally connected to the RV by the muscular infundibulum or conus *(inf)*, whereas the aorta is connected to the LV by aortic-mitral fibrous continuity. Anatomically corrected malposition exemplifies normal (i.e., concordant) ventriculoarterial alignment but abnormal connection—a large infundibulum connecting the aorta to the LV but a deficient or even absent subpulmonary infundibulum. The connections in double-outlet ventricle vary; double-outlet RV typically but not uniformly has a bilateral subarterial conus, whereas double-outlet LV usually has a deficient or absent subarterial conus. (Modified with permission from Ezon DS, Goldberg JF, Kyle WB. *The Atlas of Congenital Heart Disease Nomenclature: an Illustrated Guide to the Van Praagh and Anderson Approaches to Describing Congenital Cardiac Pathology*. Seattle, WA: CreateSpace Independent Publishing Platform; 2015.)

Segmental classification of congenital heart disease (CHD) uses specific set notation to describe cardiac anatomy. The notation system, which is a series of three letters separated by commas and enclosed within curly brackets (e.g., {S,D,L}), is used to describe the visceroatrial situs, the orientation of the ventricular loop, and the positions and relationships of the great vessels. For example, {S,D,S} describes the normal anatomic configuration, in which the right atrium (RA) and largest hepatic lobe are on the patient's right side and the left atrium, stomach, and spleen are on the left side (situs *s*olitus [S]); the ventricular loop is curved rightward (dextro- or D-loop [D]); and the aortic valve is posterior to and to the right of the pulmonary valve (situs *s*olitus [S]).

In practice, the situs, or organization, of the three main segments is determined first. For example, in the normal heart, the RV is right sided with right-hand chirality and is organized inflow-to-outflow from right to left; the LV is left sided with left-hand chirality and is organized inflow-to-outflow from left to right. Second, the segmental alignments are determined (i.e., what drains into what). For example, in the normal heart, the RA is aligned with (drains into) the RV and the LV with the aorta. Third, the segmental connections (i.e., the ways in which adjacent segments are physically connected to each other) are described. For example, in the normal heart, the PA is connected to the RV by a complete muscular conus or infundibulum, whereas the aorta is connected to the LV by aortic-mitral fibrous continuity (i.e., without a complete conus).

Alignment and connection are different concepts, and both are important, especially in complex defects. Fig. 44.1 is a diagrammatic summary of the types of situs, alignment, and connection seen in a variety of congenital heart defects.

GENETICS CONSIDERATIONS

Conotruncal defects are associated with several chromosomal abnormalities, most notably a deletion at chromosome 22q11 (i.e., DiGeorge syndrome). Echocardiographic clues to this association in patients with a conotruncal defect include an associated right aortic arch or aberrant subclavian artery and the absence of thymic tissue in infants.

Many adults living with conotruncal defects may not have undergone testing for DiGeorge syndrome. This condition is important to recognize because a variety of psychiatric disorders and disabilities in cognitive function may be present and untreated.[6] Comparative genomic hybridization was used to match DNA copy variations in 60 patients with conotruncal defects with the data from genomic databases. The study revealed that 38% of subjects had some genetic imbalance. These results emphasize the growing importance of genome-wide assays for patients with CHD.[7]

AORTOPATHY IN CONOTRUNCAL ANOMALIES

It should not be surprising that aortopathy is a common finding in patients with conotruncal anomalies because the arterial walls are derived from cardiac neural crest and second heart field cells, either or both of which can be abnormal in these defects.[8] For example, marked histologic abnormalities have been documented in the aortic root and ascending aorta that are present from infancy in patients with TOF.[9] Aortic dilation is common in adults with repaired TOF, and risk factors include older age, male gender, right aortic arch, pulmonary atresia, prior aortopulmonary shunt, and 22q11 deletion.[10,11] Up to 25% of adults with repaired TOF have an aortic root diameter larger than 4 cm but only 6.6% have *indexed* aortic values above the expected limits.[11]

An aortic root dimension of 5.5 cm has been suggested as the threshold for consideration of aortic repair,[12,13] but there is no universally accepted size that triggers the decision for surgery. Only four cases of aortic dissection have been reported in the literature on TOF, suggesting that the risk of dissection is low.[14–17]

Similarly, 50% of children with D-loop TGA have aortic root dilation 10 years after an arterial switch operation; however, this dilation does not appear to be progressive.[18] In a single-center retrospective review of 76 patients with TA, the truncal root was dilated in all but three patients, with a mean truncal root Z score of 5.1 ± 2.3.[19] Despite the high prevalence of dilated ascending aorta in patients with conotruncal anomalies, aortic dissection is rare.[20]

Echocardiography laboratories have various imaging protocols for aortic measurements that must be taken into account when comparing serial studies. The current multimodality imaging guidelines for the thoracic aorta in adults advocate obtaining aortic root measurements at end-diastole with a leading edge–to–leading edge technique,[21] whereas imaging guidelines for pediatric echocardiograms, which are often used in echocardiography laboratories specializing in CHD, suggest obtaining aortic root measurements in mid-systole with an inner edge–to–inner edge technique.[22]

SPECIFIC COMPLEX CONOTRUNCAL ANOMALIES

TETRALOGY OF FALLOT

TOF is the most common cyanotic heart defect, with an incidence of 0.33 cases per 1000 live births; it accounts for 6.7% of all forms of CHD.[23] It comprises (1) a ventricular septal defect (VSD), (2) an aorta overriding the VSD, (3) an RV outflow tract (RVOT) obstruction, and (4) RV hypertrophy (Fig. 44.2).

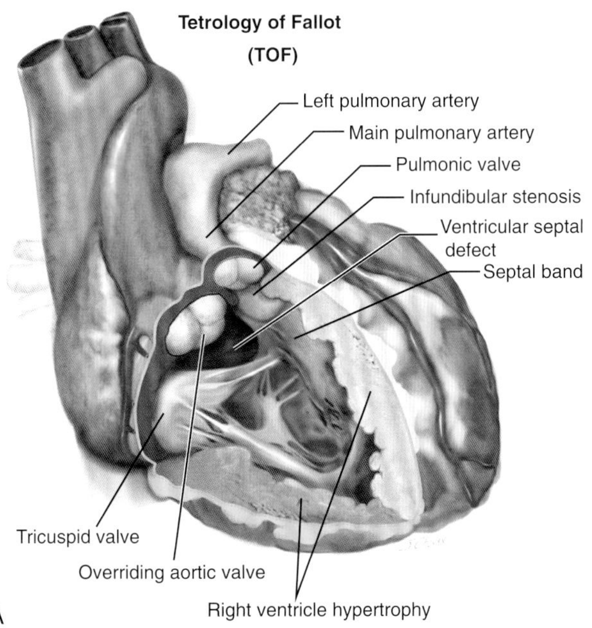

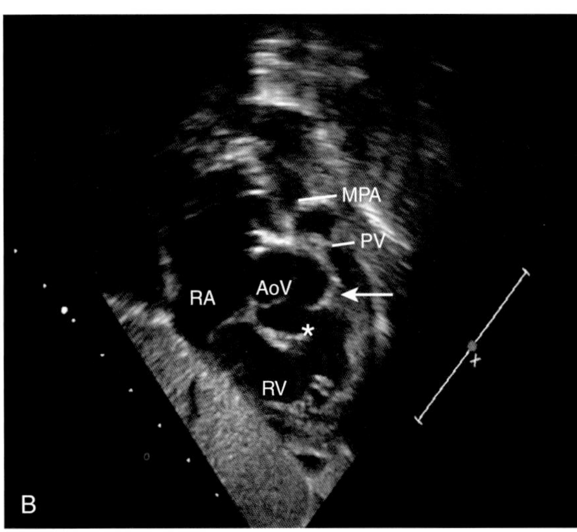

Fig. 44.2 Tetralogy of Fallot (TOF). (A) TOF with anterior deviation of the infundibular septum *(Inf)*, infundibular stenosis *(IS)*, malalignment ventricular septal defect *(VSD)*, overriding aortic valve *(AoV)*, and RV hypertrophy. (B) Unrepaired TOF. The subcostal right anterior oblique view demonstrates the anteriorly malaligned infundibular septum *(arrow)* with resulting VSD *(asterisk)*, overriding AoV, and hypoplastic pulmonic valve *(PV)*. The transducer is rotated approximately 45 degrees clockwise from the subcostal long-axis view, with the notch positioned at approximately 1 to 2 o'clock. *MPA*, Main pulmonary artery. (A, From Srivastava S, Parness IA. Tetralogy of Fallot. In: Lai WW, Mertens L, Cohen MS, Geva T, eds. *Echocardiography in Pediatric and Congenital Heart Disease: From Fetus to Adult.* Hoboken, NJ: Wiley-Blackwell; 2009:362–384.)

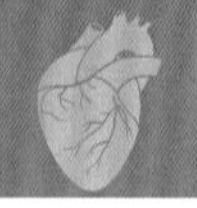

TABLE 44.1 **Preoperative Echocardiographic Evaluation of Tetralogy of Fallot.**

Structure	*Assessment*	*Imaging Plane and Technique*
RVOT	Aneurysm or obstruction	Parasternal long-axis RVOT and parasternal short-axis at the base using pulsed-wave and CW Doppler to localize and estimate severity of obstruction Subcostal RAO with counterclockwise 45-degree rotation from the long axis to get RV inflow-outflow view
Pulmonic valve	Annulus size, residual leaflet tissue, pulmonic stenosis, pulmonic regurgitation, or evaluation of RV-to-PA conduit	Parasternal long-axis RVOT, parasternal short-axis at the base, and modified apical with anterior angulation Diastolic color flow reversal in branch PAs to assess pulmonic regurgitation Pulsed-wave and CW Doppler for peak and mean gradients, pressure half-time, and antegrade diastolic flow to assess restrictive RV physiology
Main and branch PAs	Size, hypoplasia, continuity, stenosis, residual shunt	Parasternal short-axis at the base focused over the pulmonic valve and bifurcation Main PA measured at its midpoint during systole Suprasternal short-axis and high left parasternal axis for central PA and RPA Suprasternal long-axis and high left parasternal axis for LPA
RV	Size, hypertrophy, and function	Subcostal long-axis or parasternal long-axis by M-mode or 2D echocardiography with RV diastolic wall thickness > 5 mm, consistent with hypertrophy Apical 4-chamber optimized over the RV, parasternal short-axis, parasternal long-axis, parasternal long-axis RV inflow, parasternal long-axis RV outflow for size and function
Interventricular septal position	RV volume overload (diastolic flattening), pressure overload (systolic flattening)	Parasternal short-axis at the mid-ventricular level
Ventricular septal defect	Residual ventricular septal defect, relation to tricuspid and aortic valves	Parasternal short-axis from base to apex, parasternal long-axis, apical 4-chamber, and sweep to apical 5-chamber with color Doppler to assess direction of flow and CW Doppler for transseptal gradient For left-to-right flow, RV systolic pressure = LV systolic pressure (cuff systolic pressure in the absence of LV outflow tract obstruction) − transseptal gradient
Tricuspid valve	Degree of regurgitation and RV systolic pressure estimate	Apical 4-chamber, parasternal long-axis RV inflow, and parasternal short-axis at the base focused over the tricuspid valve
RA	RA size	Apical 4-chamber with upper limit of normal of 18 cm^2
Inferior vena cava	Size and inspiratory collapse to assess RA pressure	Subcostal long-axis with measurement of inferior vena cava diameter at end-expiration
Interatrial septum	Atrial septal defect or patent foramen ovale, direction of flow, bowing of interatrial septum	Subcostal long-axis, short-axis, and in-between views; parasternal short-axis, high right parasternal-axis
LV	Size and function	Apical 4-chamber with DTI over lateral and medial mitral valve annulus, apical 2-chamber, apical 3-chamber, parasternal long-axis, parasternal short-axis
Aortic valve	Aortic regurgitation	Parasternal long-axis, apical 5-chamber, apical 3-chamber, parasternal short-axis at base, subcostal short-axis or suprasternal long-axis focused on descending aorta with pulsed-wave Doppler for diastolic runoff pattern
Aorta	Aortic root and ascending dilation, arch sidedness, aortopulmonary collaterals	Parasternal long-axis for aortic root and ascending aortic dimensions, suprasternal long-axis for aortic arch, suprasternal short-axis sweep for arch sidedness, subcostal short-axis or suprasternal long-axis focused on descending aorta with pulsed-wave Doppler for diastolic runoff pattern

DTI, Doppler tissue imaging; *LPA*, left pulmonary artery; *PA*, pulmonary artery; *RAO*, right anterior oblique; *RPA*, right pulmonary artery; *RVOT*, RV outflow tract.

The VSD in TOF is a malalignment VSD, in which the infundibular septum is deviated anteriorly and superiorly out of the plane with the rest of the ventricular septum. This results in infundibular obstruction that can be exacerbated by anomalous muscle bundles crossing the RVOT. The pulmonic valve is often hypoplastic and can be bicuspid or unicuspid with various degrees of stenosis. The most extreme form is TOF with pulmonary atresia, which can be associated with discontinuous branch PAs and major aortopulmonary collateral arteries that supply portions of the lung. Other variants include TOF with a common AV canal defect (often seen in Down syndrome) and TOF with an absent pulmonic valve. Table 44.1 lists the main anatomic and physiologic features to be delineated in patients with TOF before surgical repair.

Most adults with TOF have undergone surgical repair, and the echocardiographic assessment depends on knowledge of palliative surgical strategies. In the era when neonatal cardiopulmonary bypass was not readily available, a staged approach was used in which patients underwent an aortopulmonary shunt procedure to augment pulmonary blood flow before complete repair. Primary complete repair became the standard of care in the 1980s, but palliative shunts may still be performed for infants with pulmonary atresia, for symptomatic neonates, or in centers where neonatal primary repair is not performed.

Complete repair involves VSD closure, relief of RVOT obstruction, and takedown of the shunt if previously palliated. RVOT obstruction is addressed in a variety of ways, including muscle bundle resection, patch augmentation of the RVOT, transannular patch, pulmonic valvotomy or valvectomy, and a conduit between the RV and PA in cases of pulmonary atresia or anomalous coronary artery crossing the RVOT. Historically, patients underwent repair by right ventriculotomy with a generous transannular patch, which effectively relieved the RVOT obstruction but resulted in severe pulmonic regurgitation, RV dysfunction, and scar.

Postoperative residual structural and functional abnormalities are the norm, with pulmonic regurgitation being one of the most common and clinically significant postoperative residua. The goals of the echocardiographic evaluation of TOF are summarized in Table 44.2 in relation to the previously described postoperative anatomic and functional sequelae. Published guidelines for echocardiographic imaging in TOF recommend comprehensive evaluation for longitudinal follow-up of patients with repaired TOF.[24]

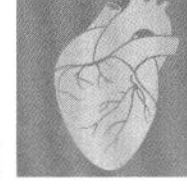

TABLE 44.2 Postoperative Imaging Evaluation of Tetralogy of Fallot.

Structural Abnormalities	*Functional Abnormalities*
Inherent to TOF repair • Partial or complete removal of pulmonic valve tissue • Infundibulotomy scar • Resection of RV/infundibular muscle bundles • Right atriotomy scar • Ventricular septal defect patch	RV volume overload • Pulmonic regurgitation • Tricuspid regurgitation • Left-to-right shunt from ventricular septal defect, atrial septal defect, or aortopulmonary collaterals
Residual or recurrent lesions • RV outflow tract obstruction • Main or branch PA stenosis • Ventricular septal defect • Atrial septal defect	RV pressure overload • RV outflow tract or PA stenosis • Pulmonary vascular disease • Pulmonary venous hypertension from LV dysfunction
Acquired lesions • Tricuspid valve abnormalities • RV outflow tract aneurysm • RV fibrosis	RV systolic and diastolic dysfunction
Other • Dilated aorta	LV dysfunction

PA, Pulmonary artery; *TOF*, tetralogy of Fallot.
Adapted from Geva T. Repaired tetralogy of Fallot: the roles of cardiovascular magnetic resonance in evaluating pathophysiology and for pulmonary valve replacement decision support. *J Cardiovasc Magn Reson*. 2011;13:9.

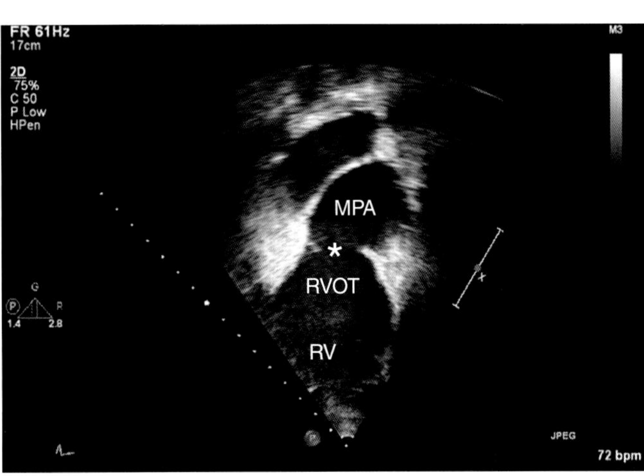

Fig. 44.3 Tetralogy of Fallot RV outflow tract. Modified apical view with anterior angulation across the RV outflow tract *(RVOT)* and pulmonary annulus *(asterisk)* provides an excellent angle of insonation for spectral Doppler imaging. *MPA*, Main pulmonary artery.

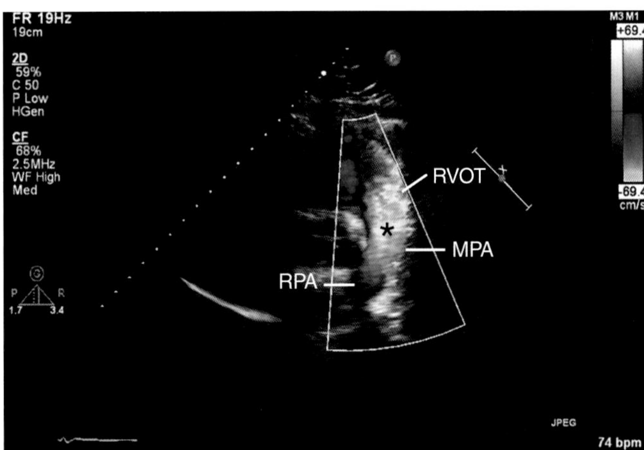

Fig. 44.4 Severe pulmonic regurgitation in tetralogy of Fallot. Parasternal short-axis view at the base with color Doppler imaging demonstrates severe pulmonic regurgitation with color flow reversal in the right pulmonary artery *(RPA)*. The width of the regurgitant jet occupies the entire pulmonary annulus *(asterisk)*. *MPA*, Main pulmonary artery; *RVOT*, RV outflow tract.

Assessment of the RVOT and pulmonic valve is similar to that for the pulmonic and subpulmonic valve stenosis described previously. Residual obstruction should be sought, with a goal of defining the levels and extent of obstruction across the infundibulum, annulus, and main PA. Aneurysm of the RVOT is characterized by a large echo-free space anterior or lateral to the outflow tract and main PA with associated thinning and dyskinesia.

The pulmonary annulus or conduit diameter should be measured for surgical or interventional planning. In adults, the normal pulmonary annulus size ranges from 17 to 26 mm.[25] Conduits are notoriously difficult to profile in adults due to the varied and often retrosternal location. Multiple views are required to adequately profile the conduit. Doppler echocardiography is often helpful for conduit localization and necessary for gradient measurements.

Pulmonic regurgitation severity is determined by regurgitant orifice size, RV compliance, and RV afterload. It is best evaluated in the parasternal long-axis RVOT view and parasternal short-axis view at the base. In adults with good acoustic windows, a modified apical view with the transducer positioned medially with anterior angulation can provide excellent visualization of the RVOT and pulmonic valve (Fig. 44.3). Echocardiographic assessment of pulmonic regurgitation severity is qualitative and is best at distinguishing between mild and severe pulmonic regurgitation; many studies use cardiac MRI as the ideal standard.

Diastolic flow reversal in the branch PAs[26,27] and width of the regurgitant jet greater than 70% of the annulus diameter[26] are associated with severe pulmonic regurgitation (Fig. 44.4). One scheme for grading pulmonic regurgitation uses a ratio of regurgitant jet width to annulus diameter as an index of severity.[28] A pressure half-time shorter than 100 ms correlates with hemodynamically significant pulmonic regurgitation, but a noncompliant RV chamber with diastolic dysfunction can overestimate the degree of regurgitation by this measure due to rapid equilibration of end-diastolic pressures. Other echocardiographic indices have been explored with various degrees of sensitivity and specificity or have not been validated.[29–31]

The combination of several echocardiographic parameters may provide the best assessment of pulmonic regurgitation severity. Studies have demonstrated high positive predictive value using pressure half-time and diastolic color flow reversal in the branch PAs or pressure half-time with pulmonic regurgitation jet width–to–annulus ratio for identifying severe pulmonic regurgitation.[32,33]

Careful assessment of the main and branch PAs is a key component of the echocardiographic evaluation of TOF, but it can be challenging in adults with suboptimal windows. The main and branch PAs can be imaged in the parasternal short-axis view at the base, but aligning the transducer in the high parasternal and infraclavicular positions is often necessary for adequate imaging of the branch PAs and for a Blalock-Taussig shunt. The right PA can be seen along its length in the high left parasternal short-axis or suprasternal short-axis view. The left PA is often difficult to visualize but can sometimes be seen by rotating the transducer counterclockwise from a high parasternal short-axis view.

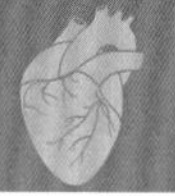

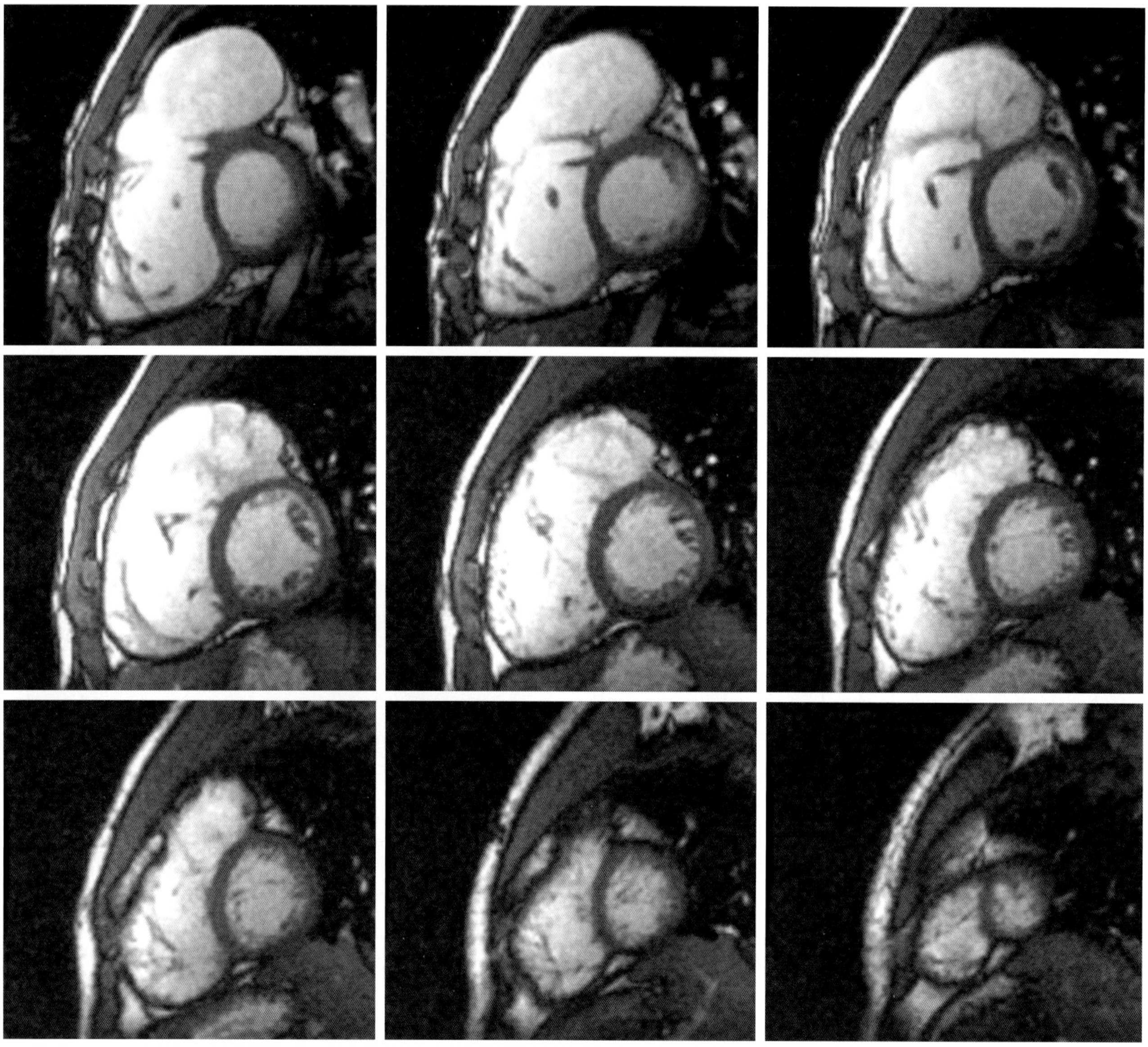

Fig. 44.5 Cardiac magnetic resonance imaging of tetralogy of Fallot. Short-axis stack of cine steady-state free precession cardiac magnetic resonance imaging (MRI) in repaired tetralogy of Fallot from base *(top row)*, mid-ventricle *(middle row)*, and apex *(bottom row)*. The RV volume and ejection fraction are calculated by tracing the endocardial border at end-diastole and end-systole for each slice. Notice the severely dilated RV and thin-walled anterior infundibulum *(top row)*, consistent with prior patch.

RV assessment by echocardiography is challenging because of its complex and highly varied geometry and its retrosternal location. Surgical repair of the RVOT results in regional variation in function of the RV sinus compared with the infundibulum. For these reasons, cardiac MRI is considered the standard for imaging of the RV in TOF[24,25] (Fig. 44.5). Even so, echocardiography remains an important first-line modality for qualitative assessment of the RV.[34] Accepted criteria for RV size and function that specifically exclude CHD have been reported and can serve as a reference point.[25,35] Table 44.3 summarizes published reference values and specific data for TOF.

Three-dimensional (3D) echocardiography promises an accurate determination of RV volume and function. Studies have shown good correlation between 3D echocardiography and cardiac MRI in cases of repaired TOF, but 3D echocardiography typically underestimates RV size and function in larger, more dilated RVs.[36–41] A newer method, knowledge-based 3D reconstruction, involves 2D-based 3D reconstruction using a magnetic tracking device and results in less discrepancy in RV volumes, but it is time-consuming and requires specialized hardware and software.[42] Contrast-enhanced imaging for better definition of endocardial borders and newer software using RV-focused volumetric analytics may produce more accurate measurements.[43,44]

Strain and strain rate can be used to assess RV function but are not considered a standard part of the echocardiographic evaluation in CHD and particularly in the evaluation of the RV, partly due to the lack of widely available RV-specific software and consensus on normative values of RV strain. Limited studies demonstrate a wide variation in longitudinal strain and strain rate, depending on age and degree of pulmonic regurgitation.[45] Nevertheless, peak global and RV free wall longitudinal strain may be a marker of RV dysfunction despite preserved ejection fraction,[46] and longitudinal RV strain correlates with exercise performance of patients with repaired TOF.[47]

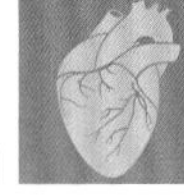

TABLE 44.3 RV Size and Function in the Normal Heart and Applicability to Tetralogy of Fallot.

Measurement of Right Heart Size and Function	*Threshold for Abnormal (Non-TOF)*	*Applications for TOF*
RV basal diameter	>4.1 cm	RV end-diastolic area indexed to body surface area correlates well with MRI-derived end-diastolic volumes in repaired TOF.
RVOT PLAX proximal diameter	>3.0 cm	—
Fractional area of change	<35%	Fractional area of change <30% with RVOT shortening fraction <25% correlates well with RV ejection fraction <35% by cardiac MRI for adults with TOF.
TAPSE	<1.7 cm	Weak to no correlation between TAPSE and RVEF in TOF
Pulsed Doppler S-wave peak velocity	<9.5 cm/s	May not be accurate, with better correlation between pulsed Doppler S-wave velocity and global RVEF in those with infundibular ejection fraction ≥30%
Color Doppler S-wave peak velocity	<6.0 cm/s	Scant data on color tissue Doppler imaging for assessing RVEF in TOF
Pulsed-wave Doppler MPI	>0.43	Mixed data on the accuracy and clinical utility of MPI for assessing RV function in TOF with limited applicability
Tissue Doppler MPI	>0.54	As for pulsed-wave Doppler MPI
Global longitudinal RV free wall strain	>−20%	Few data on repaired TOF
3D-derived RVEF	<45%	3D echocardiography underestimates RV volumes and function compared with cardiac MRI and is most pronounced in those with larger a RV.[36,38,40]

MPI, Myocardial performance index; *MRI*, magnetic resonance imaging; *PLAX*, parasternal long-axis; *RVEF*, right ventricular ejection fraction; *RVOT*, right ventricular outflow tract; *TAPSE*, tricuspid annular plane systolic excursion; *TOF*, tetralogy of Fallot.

Adapted from Portnoy SG, Rudski LG. Echocardiographic evaluation of the right ventricle: a 2014 perspective. *Curr Cardiol Rep*. 2015;17:21; Lang RM, Badano LP, Mor-Avi V, et al. Recommendations for cardiac chamber quantification by echocardiography in adults: an update from the American Society of Echocardiography and the European Association of Cardiovascular Imaging. *J Am Soc Echocardiogr*. 2015;28(1):1.e14–39.e14.

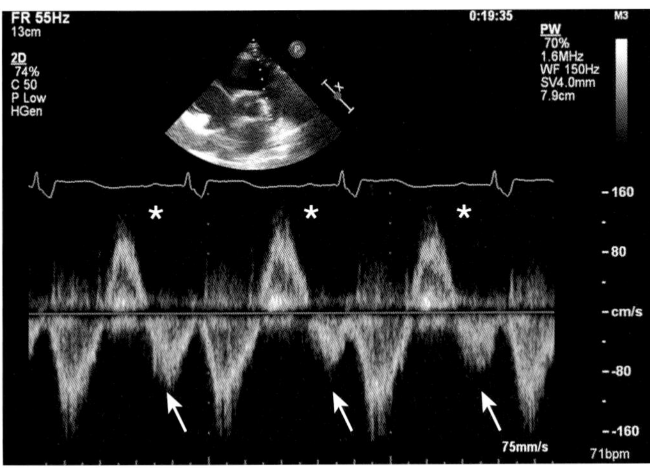

Fig. 44.6 Restrictive RV. Pulsed-wave Doppler imaging of the main pulmonary artery demonstrates antegrade diastolic flow with atrial contraction *(arrows)*. Notice the relationship to the p wave on the electrocardiogram *(asterisks)*.

Restrictive RV physiology is characterized by poor diastolic function due to severe hypertrophy and fibrosis from chronic pressure overload. Late surgical repair has been identified as a risk factor. Restrictive physiology can limit the degree of pulmonic regurgitation because of increased middle to late diastolic pressure that equilibrates with PA pressure, and end-diastolic forward flow may be observed after atrial contraction. The restrictive RV acts as a passive conduit between the RA and PA during atrial systole. End-diastolic forward flow can be seen normally during inspiration and therefore should be detected during the entire respiratory cycle to be considered pathologic (Fig. 44.6). There are mixed data on the relationship between restrictive RV physiology and RV size and outcomes such as exercise tolerance, likely due to differences in patient age and era of repair.[48,49]

Tricuspid regurgitation is commonly seen in TOF and can develop as a result of RV and tricuspid annular dilation (i.e., functional tricuspid regurgitation). It may also arise from disruption of tricuspid valve integrity by the VSD patch or from leaflet pinning by a transvenous device wire. The additional volume load of tricuspid regurgitation can exacerbate RV volume overload from pulmonic regurgitation and further compromise RV function.

Assessment of tricuspid regurgitation severity by echocardiography is semiquantitative at best. A vena contracta jet width greater than 0.7 cm is consistent with severe tricuspid regurgitation. Whether the tricuspid valve should be repaired at the time of pulmonic valve replacement is debatable, but severe preoperative tricuspid regurgitation has been shown to correlate with adverse outcomes after pulmonic valve replacement, regardless of the degree of postoperative tricuspid regurgitation.[50]

The left-sided structures in TOF should be part of the standard echocardiographic evaluation of an adult with TOF. In a cross-sectional study, LV systolic dysfunction was found in approximately 20% of adults with TOF.[51] The cause is multifactorial and attributable to ventricular interdependence, late repair, tissue hypoxia, volume overload, patch repair of the VSD, and myocardial fibrosis.[51,52]

Ventricular interdependence refers to forces transmitted from one ventricle to the other through shared structures such as myofibers, interventricular septum, and pericardium. For example, RV ejection fraction correlates with LV ejection fraction in TOF.[53] Diastolic filling of the LV can be impaired by RV dilation from volume overload due to severe pulmonic regurgitation with little effect on contractility but a decrease in LV ejection fraction due to reduced preload. Abnormal LV rotational mechanics such as twist and torsion are associated with RV dilation and biventricular dysfunction and may mechanistically explain this effect of RV size on LV filling.[54,55] Decreased LV function is a strong risk factor for sudden cardiac death.[56,57] Other echocardiographic measures of LV performance, such as LV longitudinal strain and mitral annular plane systolic excursion distance, have been associated with adverse arrhythmic outcomes in adults with TOF.[58]

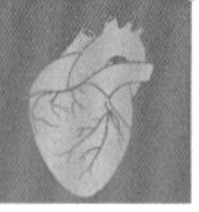

Late survival rates after repair are excellent, reaching 86% up to 40 years after surgery.[59] However, morbidity is substantial, with almost one half of patients requiring reintervention; most commonly pulmonic valve replacement.[59] RV size and function in the setting of significant pulmonic regurgitation is prognostic in repaired TOF, and accurate assessment is critical in determining appropriate timing for pulmonic valve replacement. RV size thresholds for pulmonic valve replacement are determined by cardiac MRI and based on reverse RV remodeling after surgery, with a goal of normalization of RV size. Optimal timing is still under debate, but the accepted RV size and function thresholds measured by cardiac MRI in asymptomatic patients are as follows[34,60]:

- RV end-diastolic volume index greater than 160 mL/m^2
- RV/LV end-diastolic volume ratio greater than 2
- RV end-systolic volume index greater than 80 mL/m^2
- RV ejection fraction less than 47%
- LV ejection fraction less than 55%

Transcatheter pulmonic valve replacement can be performed in patients with an RV-to-PA conduit or prestented RVOT with good outcomes and is considered a viable alternative to surgical pulmonic valve replacement. The Medtronic Melody transcatheter pulmonic valve (Medtronic, Minneapolis, MN) has been commercially available since 2010 and received premarket approval in 2015 by the U.S. Food and Drug Administration (FDA) for this indication. Reductions in pulmonic regurgitation and RV volumes appear similar to those of surgical cohorts, although no randomized controlled trials have compared the two approaches.[61–63] A 5-year rate of freedom from reintervention of 76% has been reported, which was largely mitigated by conduit prestenting.[64] Increased rates of infective endocarditis have been reported with the Melody valve,[65] which may be related to the bovine jugular venous component of the prosthesis.[66]

The Edwards Sapien valve (Edwards Lifesciences, Irvine, CA) can be used up to a maximum diameter of 26 mm in the pulmonic position,[67] and the Sapien XT has been approved for use in conduits or in the valve-in-valve position. Several newer and larger transcatheter valves using self-expanding technology (i.e., Medtronic Harmony Valve, Venus P-Valve, and Alterra Adaptive Prestent) are being tested in the native RVOT. Whether these valves are at similarly increased risk for prosthetic valve endocarditis as the Melody valve remains to be seen.

Recommendations regarding surgical indications for residual lesions in repaired TOF are summarized in Table 44.4.[34]

TABLE 44.4 AHA/ACC Guidelines on Recommendations for Surgery in Repaired Tetralogy of Fallot.

Class I

1. Pulmonic valve replacement (surgical or percutaneous) for relief of symptoms is recommended for patients with repaired TOF and moderate or greater PR with cardiovascular symptoms not otherwise explained (level of evidence: B).

Class IIa

2. Pulmonic valve replacement (surgical or percutaneous) is reasonable for preservation of ventricular size and function in asymptomatic patients with repaired TOF and ventricular enlargement or dysfunction and moderate or greater PR (level of evidence: B).

Class IIb

1. Surgical pulmonary valve replacement may be reasonable for adults with repaired TOF and moderate or greater PR with other lesions requiring surgical interventions (level of evidence: C).
2. Pulmonary valve replacement, in addition to arrhythmia management, may be considered for adults with repaired TOF and moderate or greater PR and ventricular tachyarrhythmia (level of evidence: C).

PR, Pulmonic regurgitation; *RVOT*, RV outflow tract; *TOF*, tetralogy of Fallot.
From Stout KK, Daniels CJ, Aboulhosn JA, et al. 2018 AHA/ACC guideline for the management of adults with congenital heart disease: a report of the American College of Cardiology/American Heart Association Task Force on Clinical Practice Guidelines. *J Am Coll Cardiol.* 2019;73(12):e81–e192.

TRUNCUS ARTERIOSUS

TA is an uncommon type of congenital heart defect in which a single arterial trunk arises from the heart, giving origin to the coronary arteries, PAs, and systemic arteries, in that order. In most cases, a VSD and single semilunar valve are present. This semilunar valve may consist of two, three, four, or more leaflets and usually overrides the ventricular septum through an outlet VSD.

Two principal classification systems have been proposed (Fig. 44.7). The older Collett and Edwards classification is used less often now because it does not include TA with interrupted aortic arch and does include TOF with pulmonary atresia, which has been recognized not to be a form of TA. The Van Praagh classification is more inclusive and recognizes rare cases of TA without a VSD.[68]

Without treatment, the mean age at death is 2.5 months, and 80% of children with unrepaired TA die within the first year of life. However, survival into adulthood with unrepaired TA has been described.[69–71]

Table 44.5 lists the main anatomic and physiologic features to be delineated in patients with TA before undergoing surgical repair. As in most infants and children, the examination is begun with subxiphoid long-axis (Fig. 44.8A) and short-axis views, which provide an excellent overview of the cardiac anatomy. The long-axis view shows the truncal root dividing into aortic and PA components, and the short-axis view shows the VSD with overriding truncal root. Parasternal views (see Fig. 44.8B) are most useful for studying the morphology and function of the truncal valve and for imaging the branch PAs. Suprasternal views show the aortic arch anatomy (Fig. 44.9) and the ductus arteriosus in the rare cases in which it is present.

The surgical repair involves removal of the PAs from the truncal root, patch closure of the VSD, and placement of a conduit between the RV and PAs. In cases in which the truncal valve is dysfunctional, repair or replacement with a homograft is performed. In a small series of patients undergoing truncal valve intervention, Kaza et al. reported that truncal valve repair is a durable option with an acceptable reoperation rate, good function, and a low likelihood of needing truncal valve replacement.[72] Postoperatively, patients are followed with serial imaging to monitor for conduit dysfunction, branch PA obstruction, truncal valve dysfunction, and root dilation (Fig. 44.10). Table 44.6 lists the major imaging findings that should be assessed in patients who have undergone TA repair.

DOUBLE-OUTLET VENTRICLE

Double-outlet ventricle describes a type of ventriculoarterial alignment, not a specific heart defect. Double-outlet ventricle occurs when both great arteries are completely or almost completely aligned with one ventricle or outflow chamber.[73] The other ventricle may be normally formed, hypoplastic, or absent. Both great arteries may be patent, or there can be valvar atresia of one great artery. The anatomy and physiology of double-outlet ventricle vary widely, as does the clinical presentation. The VSD size, relationship of the VSD to the great arteries, conal morphology, existence

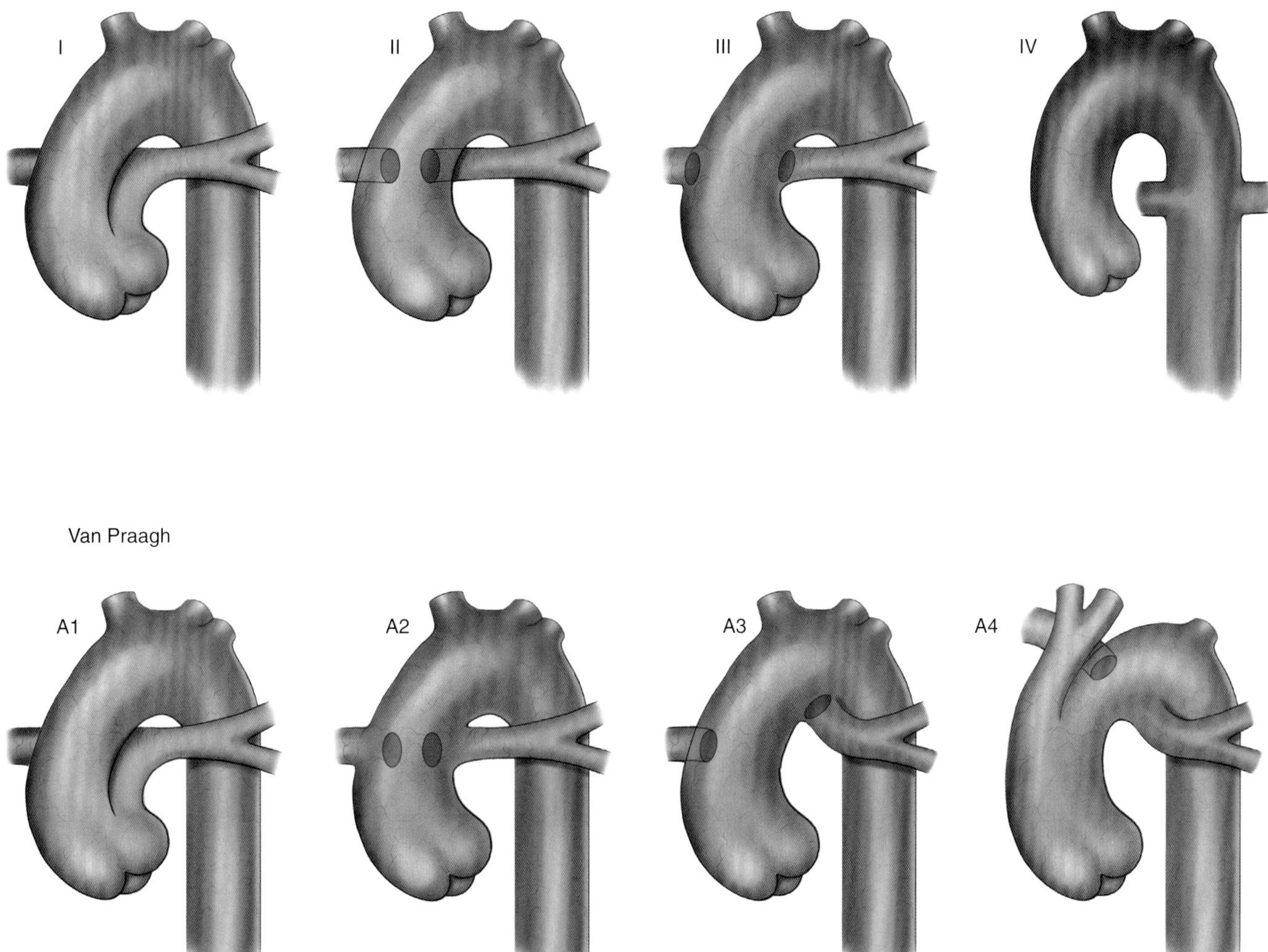

Fig. 44.7 Two classification schemes of truncus arteriosus. Note that in the Van Praagh type A3 truncus arteriosus, either branch pulmonary artery can be fed by the ductus arteriosus. (Reproduced with permission from Lai WW, Mertens LL, Cohen MS, Geva T, eds, *Echocardiography in Pediatric and Congenital Heart Disease: From Fetus to Adult*. Hoboken, NJ: Wiley-Blackwell; 2009.)

TABLE 44.5 Preoperative Echocardiographic Evaluation of Truncus Arteriosus.

Type of truncus arteriosus (see Fig. 44.7)
Pulmonary artery location and size
Coronary artery origins and proximal courses
Truncal valve morphology
Quantification of truncal valve stenosis
Quantification of truncal valve regurgitation
Associated anomalies
Right aortic arch
Interrupted aortic arch
VSD
ASD
LSVC
Absence of PDA

ASD, Atrial septal defect; *LSVC*, left superior vena cava; *PDA*, patent ductus arteriosus; *VSD*, ventricular septal defect.

of outflow tract obstruction, and associated cardiovascular defects primarily determine the physiology and treatment strategy.

Double-Outlet Right Ventricle

Double-outlet RV (DORV) is a conotruncal anomaly in which both great arteries are completely or almost completely aligned with the RV. DORV varies in complexity from a simple form that is physiologically like a VSD to extremely complex defects with heterotaxy syndrome.

The key anatomic features of DORV are the VSD, the infundibular septum, and the position of the arterial roots.[74] The location of the VSD is almost always between the limbs of the septal band. The commitment of the VSD to an arterial root depends on the orientation and size of the infundibular septum and the position of the arterial roots (Fig. 44.11).

Fig. 44.12 shows the relationship between the VSD and arterial roots in some common forms of DORV. Most often the VSD is aligned with the rightward aorta because the infundibular

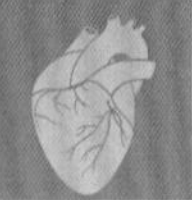

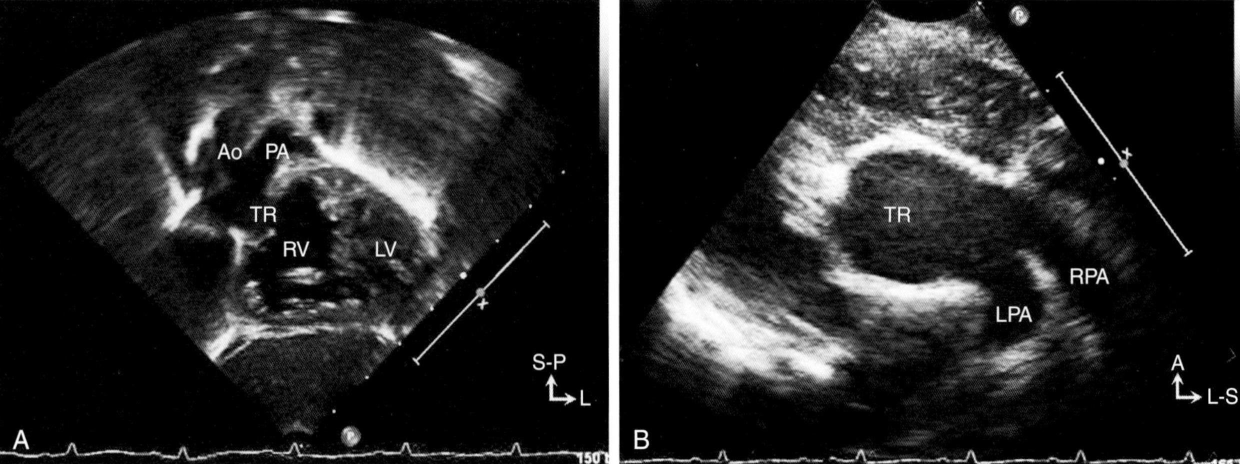

Fig. 44.8 Truncus arteriosus. (A) Subxiphoid long-axis view of a neonate with truncus arteriosus (TA) demonstrates the aorta and pulmonary trunk arising from the truncal root. (B) Oblique parasternal short-axis view of a neonate with TA type I. *A*, Anterior; *Ao*, aorta; *L*, left; *L-S*, left-superior; *LPA*, left pulmonary artery; *PA*, pulmonary artery; *RPA*, right pulmonary artery; *S-P*, superior-posterior; *TR*, truncal root.

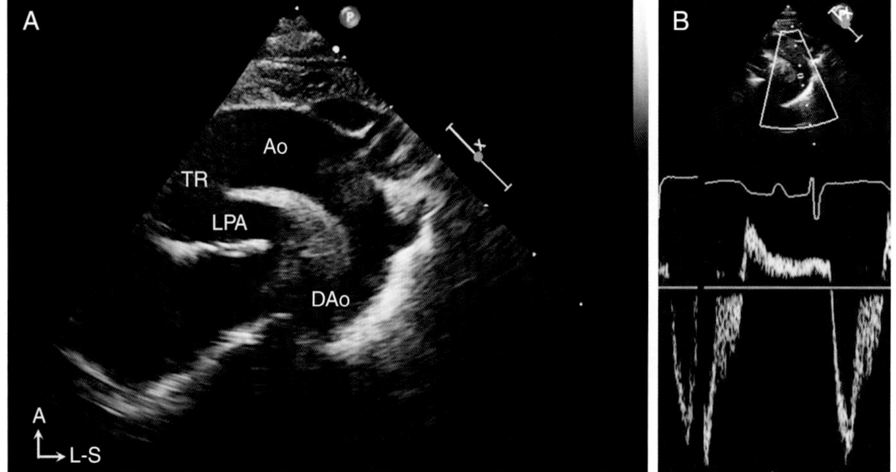

Fig. 44.9 Aortic arch in truncus ateriosus. (A) High parasternal parasagittal view of a child with truncus arteriosus (TA) demonstrates the aortic arch. (B) Pulsed-wave Doppler imaging of the distal aortic arch demonstrates pandiastolic retrograde flow due to runoff into the branch pulmonary arteries from the truncal root, which is typical of TA. *A*, Anterior; *Ao*, aorta; *DAo*, descending aorta; *L-S*, left-superior; *LPA*, left pulmonary artery; *TR*, truncal root.

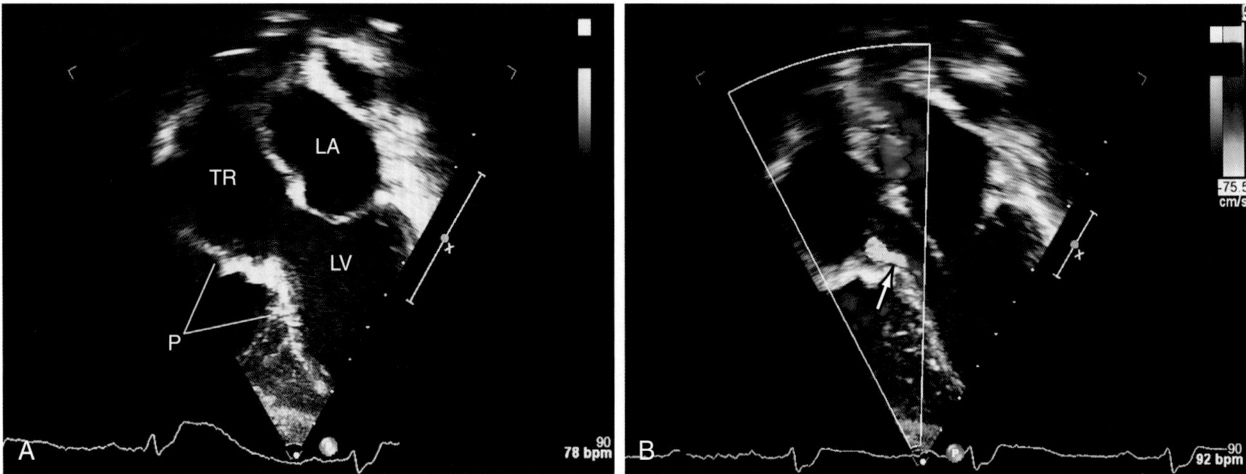

Fig. 44.10 Prior truncus arteriosus repair. (A) Apical long-axis view demonstrates aortic root dilation in an adolescent with prior truncus arteriosus repair. (B) Color Doppler imaging demonstrates moderate aortic regurgitation *(arrow)* in this patient. *P*, Ventricular septal defect patch.

septum attaches to the muscular septum leftward and superior to the VSD, shielding the PA from the VSD. In 30% of cases, the VSD is aligned with the PA because the infundibular septum extends anterior and rightward, away from the muscular septum and under the aorta, shielding it from the VSD. If the infundibular septum is hypoplastic or absent, there is nothing to shield either arterial root from the VSD, and it is doubly committed. In rare cases, the VSD is distant from the arterial roots and uncommitted to either. These are usually muscular or inlet defects.

The position of the great arteries is also important in determining the relationship between the VSD and the arterial roots. The aorta is usually posterior to or side-by-side with the PA if there is a subaortic VSD. However, in cases with a subpulmonic VSD, the aorta is usually side-by-side or anterior to the PA. In rare cases, the aorta is to the left of the PA (i.e., DORV {S,D,L}), and what would usually be a subpulmonary VSD becomes subaortic and vice versa.

Four common physiologic variations of DORV dictate the clinical presentation and approach to surgical repair:

1. VSD physiology: DORV with large subaortic VSD and no pulmonic stenosis
2. TOF physiology: DORV with subaortic VSD and pulmonic stenosis
3. TGA physiology: DORV with subpulmonary VSD with or without aortic obstruction
4. Single-ventricle physiology: DORV with mitral atresia, severely unbalanced AV canal defect, or other cause of significant ventricular hypoplasia

DORV with a subpulmonary VSD, bilateral conus, and side-by-side semilunar valves is known as the *Taussig-Bing anomaly.*[75] These patients often require repeated interventions in adult life to address residual obstruction in both outflow tracts.[76]

Outflow tract obstruction occurs in up to 70% of DORV patients; it most often involves the pulmonary outflow tract.[77] Subaortic stenosis or aortic arch obstruction occurs in up to 50% of patients with a subpulmonary VSD. DORV patients may also have abnormalities of the AV valves, including a common AV valve (i.e., AV canal defect), straddling AV valve, or AV valve atresia. Abnormalities of the mitral valve are associated with worse outcomes because a straddling mitral valve may complicate surgical repair. Patients with DORV and mitral valve atresia undergo staged palliation, leading to a Fontan operation. DORV may also be associated with atrial septal defect (ASD), persistent left superior vena cava, and left juxtaposition of the atrial appendages. DORV is common in patients with the asplenia type of heterotaxy syndrome.[78]

An organized, comprehensive, and segmental examination of the heart is essential for a complete and accurate diagnosis. We usually begin with the subxiphoid long- and short-axis views because they provide an overview of the cardiac anatomy and direct visualization of the ventriculoarterial alignment (Fig. 44.13).[79] Additional details of the anatomy are obtained in the apical views (e.g., AV valve size and function, muscular VSD), parasternal views (e.g., semilunar valve and root anatomy and function, branch PAs), and suprasternal notch views (e.g., aortic arch, ductus arteriosus, other sources of pulmonary blood flow).[80]

Table 44.7 lists the main anatomic details that should be delineated in patients with DORV before surgical repair. The distance between the tricuspid valve and the pulmonic valve and/or infundibular septum is an important measurement in patients with a subaortic VSD because it defines the minimum dimension of the LV outflow after VSD closure. This distance is

TABLE 44.6 Postoperative Imaging Evaluation of Truncus Arteriosus.

RV-PA conduit
Quantification of stenosis
Quantification of regurgitation
Estimation of RV systolic pressure
Residual VSD
Proximal branch PA caliber
Truncal valve morphology
Quantification of truncal valve stenosis
Quantification of truncal valve regurgitation
LV outflow tract obstruction
Aortic arch morphology
Ventricular size and function

PA, Pulmonary artery; *VSD*, ventricular septal defect.

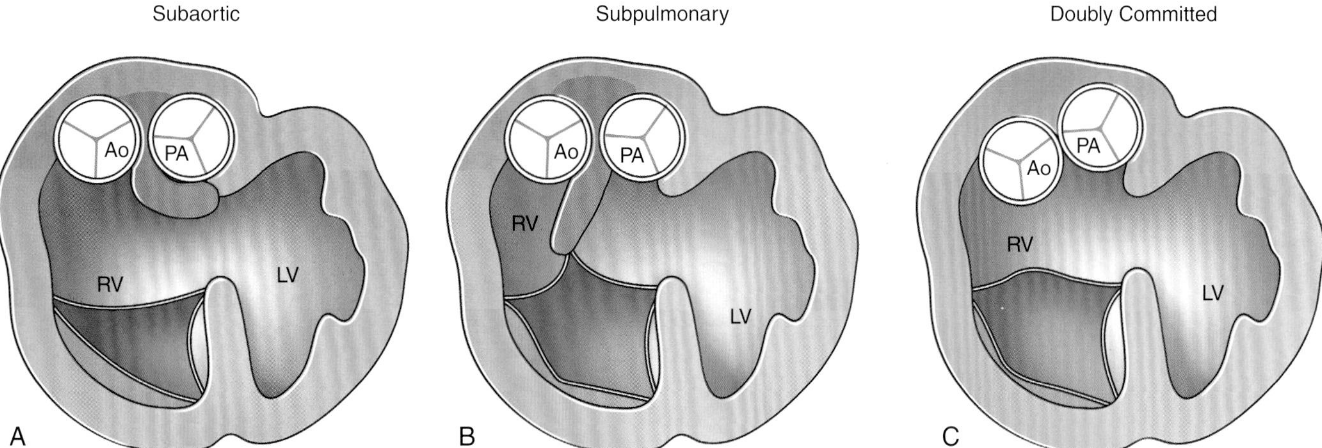

Fig. 44.11 Double-outlet RV anatomy. Position of the conal septum *(brown)* in the short-axis view in various types of double-outlet RVs: subaortic (A), subpulmonary (B), and doubly committed (C). *Ao*, Aorta; *PA*, pulmonary artery.

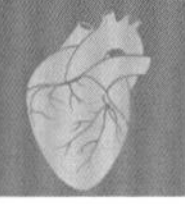

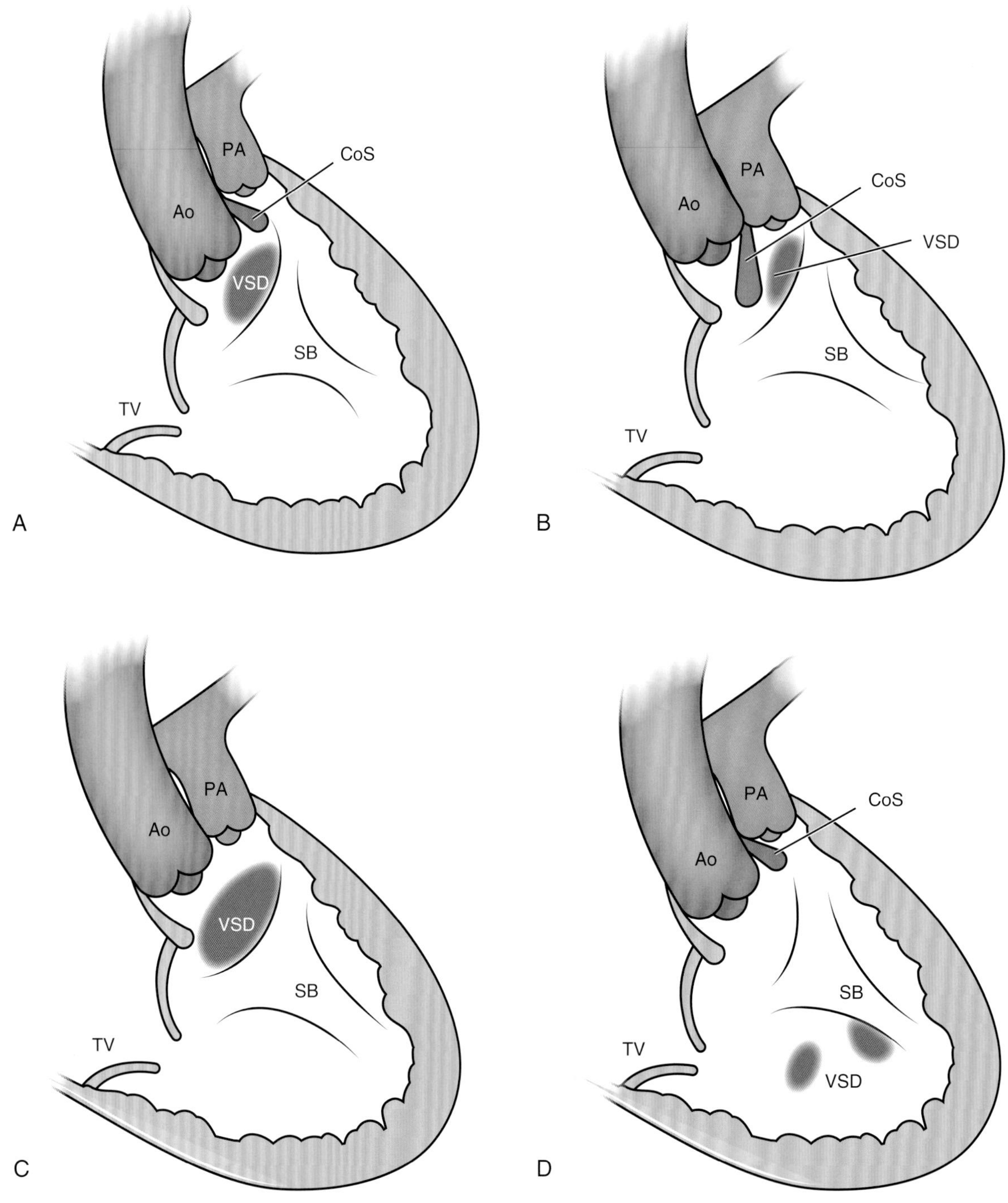

Fig. 44.12 Relationship between the ventricular septal defect *(VSD)* and arterial roots in common forms of double-outlet RV. (A) Subaortic VSD. (B) Subpulmonary VSD. (C) Doubly committed VSD. (D) Remote VSD. *Ao,* Aorta *(red)*; *CoS,* conal septum *(brown)*; *PA,* pulmonary artery *(purple)*; *SB,* septal band; *TV,* tricuspid valve; *VSD,* ventricular septal defect *(gray)*. (Modified with permission from Lopez L. Double-outlet ventricles. In: Lai WW, Mertens LL, Cohen MS, Geva T, eds. *Echocardiography in pediatric and Congenital Heart Disease: from Fetus to Adult.* Hoboken, NJ: Wiley-Blackwell; 2009.)

the primary determinant of whether an intraventricular baffle can be constructed between the VSD and the aorta.

In the most common form of DORV (i.e., subaortic VSD), the surgical goal is to establish LV-to-aortic continuity by patching the VSD to the aorta. In some cases, the VSD must be enlarged to allow creation of an adequate systemic outflow tract.[77] Subaortic stenosis is more likely to result if the distance between the tricuspid valve and the pulmonary annulus is less than the aortic annulus diameter and the pulmonary outflow is left in its native position.

When pulmonic stenosis exists, relief of obstruction can be accomplished by patch enlargement of the pulmonary outflow, valvotomy, or insertion of a conduit to establish RV-to-PA continuity. For patients with DORV and a subpulmonary VSD, the VSD is patched to the pulmonic valve, and an arterial switch operation is performed. Patients with unfavorable anatomy for a biventricular repair are staged to a Fontan palliation.[81]

Residual hemodynamic lesions are common after DORV repair, and postoperative imaging surveillance plays an

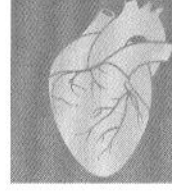

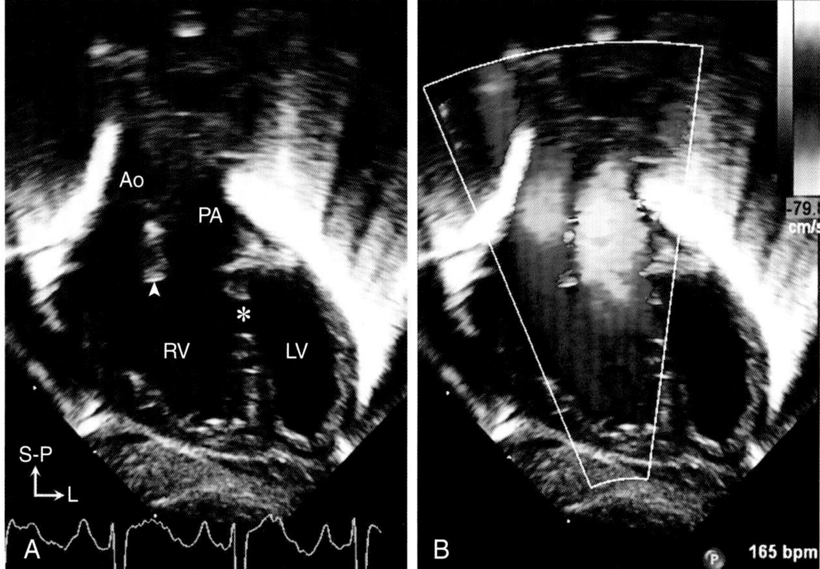

Fig. 44.13 Double-outlet RV on echocardiography. (A) Subxiphoid long-axis view in a neonate with double-outlet RV and subpulmonary ventricular septal defect *(asterisk)*. The ventricular septal defect sees the pulmonary artery *(PA)* because of rightward and anterior deviation of the infundibular septum *(arrowhead)*. (B) Color Doppler image in the same patient (see Video 44.13). *Ao*, Aorta; *L*, left; *S-P*, superior-posterior.

TABLE 44.7 Preoperative Echocardiographic Evaluation of Double-Outlet RV.

VSD location, size, and relationship to the semilunar valves
Conal morphology
Spatial relationship of the great arteries to each other
Associated cardiac lesions
Outflow tract obstruction
Atrioventricular valve abnormalities
Ventricular hypoplasia
Coronary artery origins and proximal courses

VSD, Ventricular septal defect.

important role in the long-term management of these patients. Table 44.8 lists the major imaging questions that should be addressed for patients who have undergone DORV repair. LV outflow tract obstruction can result from inadequate VSD, distortion of the outflow baffle, buildup of fibrous tissue in the VSD or outflow tunnel, or hypoplasia of the aortic annulus.[82,83]

Intramural residual interventricular defects may be present (Figs. 44.14 and 44.15) in patients with a subaortic VSD. They are located within trabeculae at the margin between the VSD patch and the RV free wall, often just below the aortic valve. These defects are often not obvious immediately after surgical repair but increase in size as RV hypertrophy regresses. The defects are particularly difficult to diagnose by all imaging modalities, and a high index of suspicion is needed. Transcatheter device closure is often effective to obliterate or reduce the left-to-right shunt. Successful surgical closure may require removal and reattachment of the anterior portion of the patch.[84,85]

Double-Outlet LV

Double-outlet LV (DOLV) is a rare conotruncal anomaly in which both great arteries are completely or almost completely aligned with the LV. It has many features in common with DORV. Until the first description in 1967, DOLV was considered to be impossible.[86] Since that time, at least 15 distinct anatomic types have been described.[87] About 75% of cases of DOLV have two well-formed ventricles, and the remainder have tricuspid atresia, mitral atresia, double-inlet LV, common-inlet LV, or severe Ebstein malformation of the tricuspid valve. Most patients with DOLV are diagnosed in childhood; however, noninvasive imaging of unrepaired defects in adults has been reported in the literature.[88]

The most common type is DOLV {S,D,D}, with a subaortic VSD and pulmonic stenosis (i.e., TOF type) (Fig. 44.16). The VSD is subpulmonary in 10% and doubly committed in 6%. Outflow tract obstruction may exist. It is subpulmonary in more than 25% of cases (i.e., physiology resembling TOF), and it is subaortic in 4%. Other segmental combinations are less common. In patients with two adequate ventricles, the pathophysiology is dictated by the relation of the VSD to the great arteries and the presence or absence of outflow obstruction. For example, a patient with DOLV{S,D,D} and a subaortic VSD

TABLE 44.8 Postoperative Imaging Evaluation of Double-Outlet RV.

Residual VSD, including intramural VSDs (see Fig. 44.15)
Subaortic stenosis
Subvalvular pulmonic stenosis
Pulmonic regurgitation
Ventricular size and function
AV valve function (particularly in patients who have undergone an AV canal repair)
For those who have undergone aortic arch reconstruction:
• Aortic arch morphology and quantification of obstruction
For those who have undergone an arterial switch operation:
• Neo-aortic valve regurgitation
• Supravalvar aortic stenosis
• Neo-aortic root dilation
• Supravalvular pulmonic stenosis or branch proximal PA stenosis

AV, Atrioventricular; *PA*, pulmonary artery; *VSD*, ventricular septal defect.

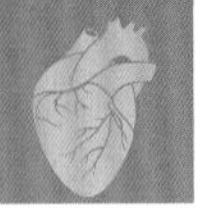

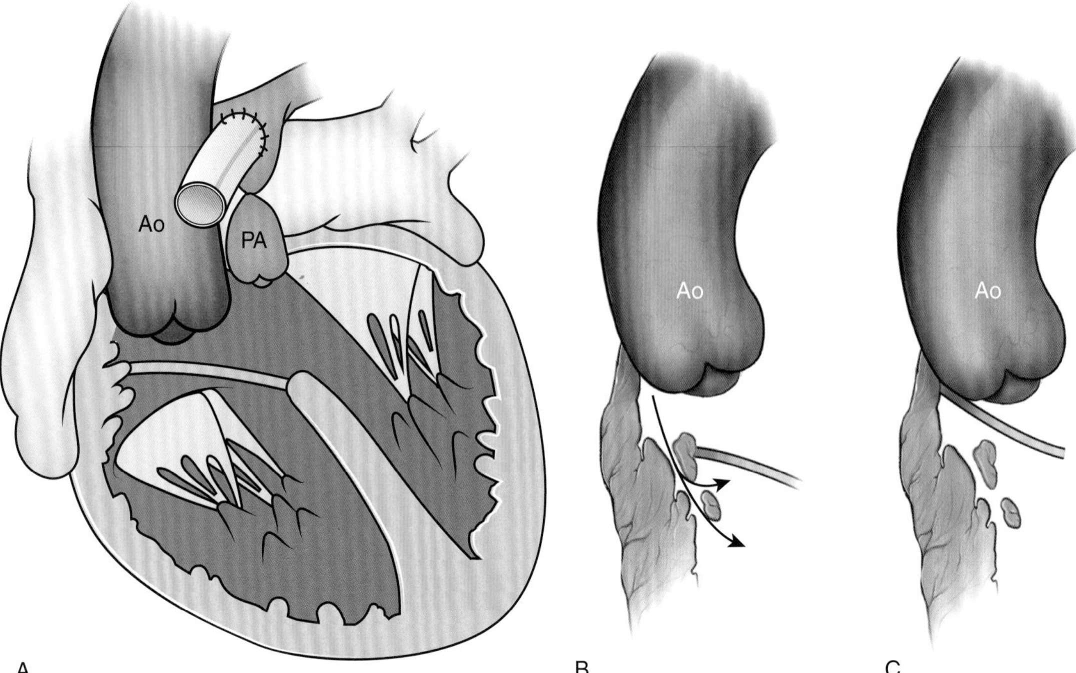

Fig. 44.14 Intramural defects. (A) The ventricular septal defect patch that directs the LV to the aorta *(Ao)* is anchored to RV trabeculations rather than the free wall. (B) Blood can pass between the trabeculae from the neo-LV outflow tract to the RV cavity. The channels may be small early after surgical repair of the conotruncal anomaly because of RV hypertrophy, but they enlarge to become hemodynamically significant, and hypertrophy regresses after RV decompression. (C) Treatment involves repositioning the patch and attaching it firmly to the solid RV free wall. *PA,* Pulmonary artery. (With permission from Preminger TJ, Sanders SP, van der Velde ME, et al. "Intramural" residual interventricular defects after repair of conotruncal malformations. *Circulation.* 1994;89:236–242.)

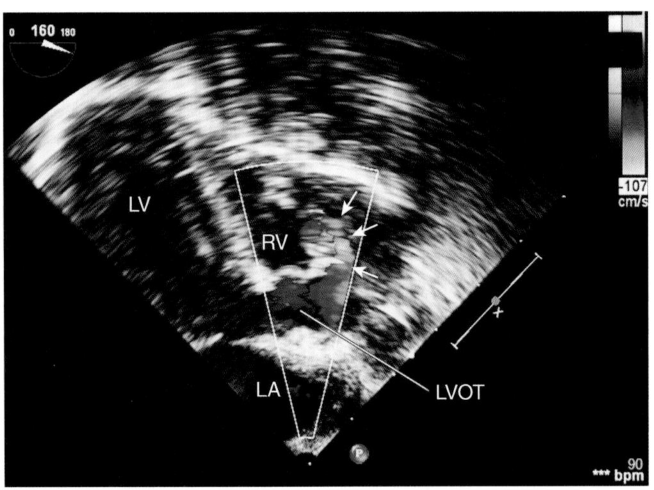

Fig. 44.15 Intramural ventricular septal defect. TEE demonstrates an intramural ventricular septal defect *(arrows)* in a patient with a repaired double-outlet RV (see Video 44.15). *LVOT,* LV outflow tract.

with no outflow tract obstruction has mild to moderate cyanosis and pulmonary overcirculation, similar to TGA with VSD and no pulmonic stenosis. Conversely, patients with a subpulmonary VSD are usually pink and present with heart failure from a large left-to-right shunt. Patients with pulmonary outflow tract obstruction are cyanotic like those with TOF, whereas patients with LV outflow tract obstruction or arch obstruction may present in neonatal shock from inadequate systemic cardiac output.

The imaging approach to DOLV is similar to that for DORV and is best done by following an organized, comprehensive approach. The subxiphoid long- and short-axis views provide an overview of the cardiac anatomy and direct visualization of the ventriculoarterial alignment. Additional details of the anatomy are obtained in the apical, parasternal, and suprasternal notch views, as previously described for DORV.

The surgical approach to DOLV is similar to that of DORV. It depends on the intracardiac anatomy.[89] Surgical options include the following:

1. VSD closure with RV-to-PA conduit placement
2. VSD closure with translocation of the pulmonary root to the RV
3. Baffling of the RV to the PA through the VSD with potential enlargement of the VSD
4. Single-ventricle palliation (Fontan surgery)

Postoperative imaging surveillance plays a large role in the long-term management of patients with DOLV.

ANATOMICALLY CORRECTED MALPOSITION OF THE GREAT ARTERIES

Anatomically corrected malposition of the great arteries is a rare congenital heart defect in which the great arteries are normally aligned with the ventricles (i.e., ventriculoarterial concordance) but abnormally connected to the ventricles (Figs. 44.17 and 44.18). In the most common type, anatomically corrected malposition {S,D,L}, the PA is aligned with the RV but connected by a deficient subpulmonary conus, and the aorta is aligned with the LV but connected by a large subaortic conus. This

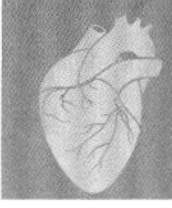

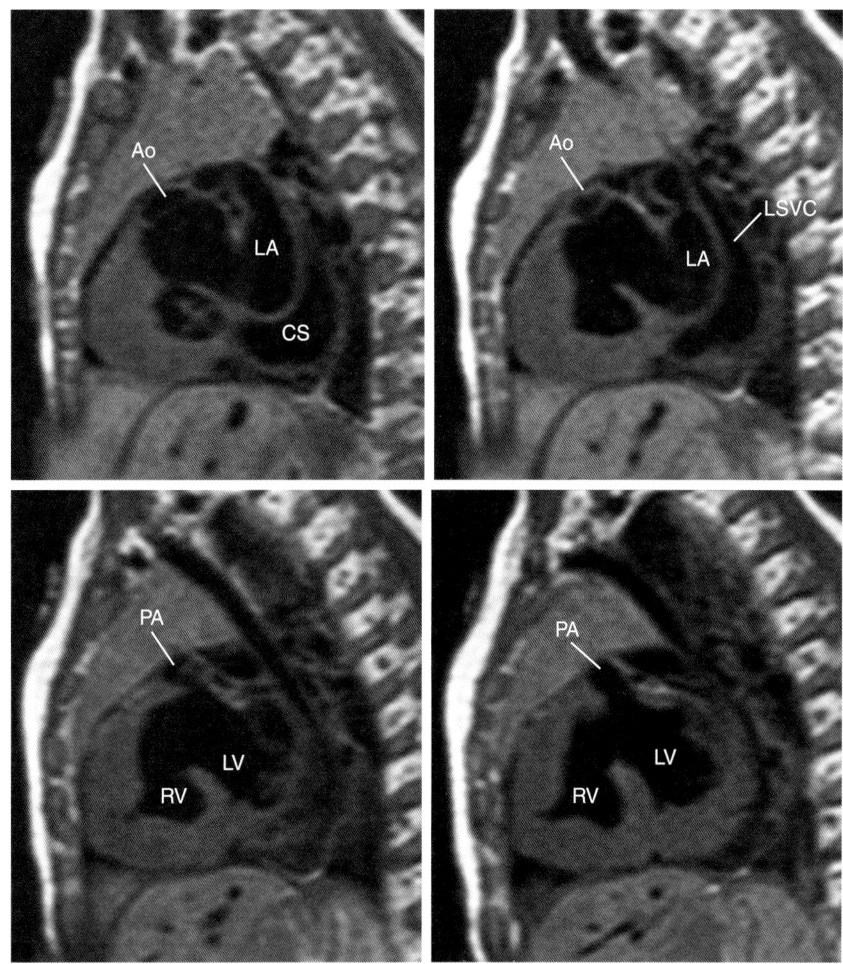

Fig. 44.16 **Double-outlet LV.** Cardiac magnetic resonance turbo-spin short-axis images of a child with a double-outlet LV and a persistent left superior vena cava *(LSVC)*–to–coronary sinus *(CS)* drainage, causing dilation of the CS. *Ao,* Aorta; *PA,* pulmonary artery.

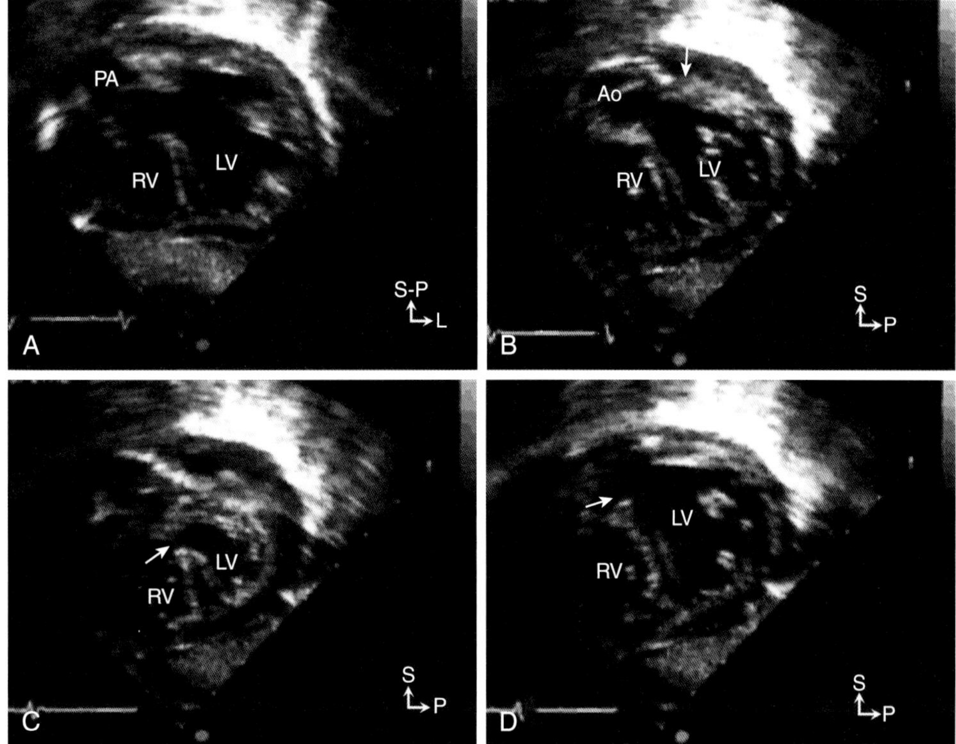

Fig. 44.17 **Anatomically corrected malposition of the great arteries.** Subxiphoid long-axis (A) and short-axis (B–D) views show anatomically corrected malposition of the great arteries ({S,D,L}) in a child. In B, a long subaortic conus *(arrow)* separates the aortic and mitral valves. The two VSDs *(arrows)* usually present in this defect are a typical conoventricular defect (C, *arrow*) and an anterior defect between the subaortic infundibulum and the RV (D, *arrow*) (see Video 44.17). *Ao,* Aorta; *L,* left; *P,* posterior; *PA,* pulmonary artery; *S,* superior; *S-P,* superior-posterior.

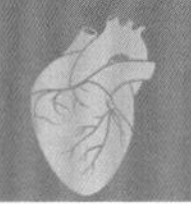

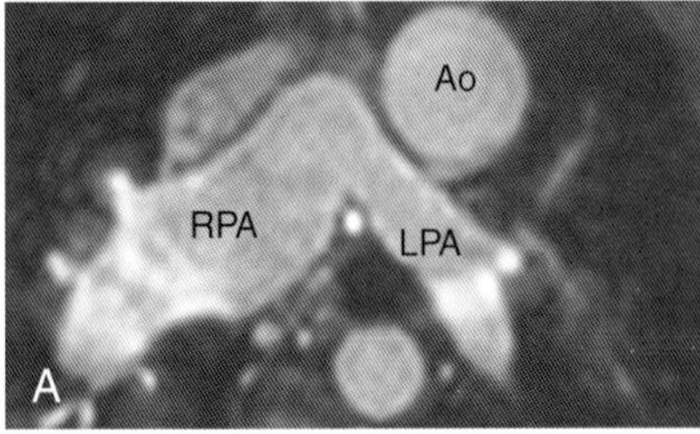

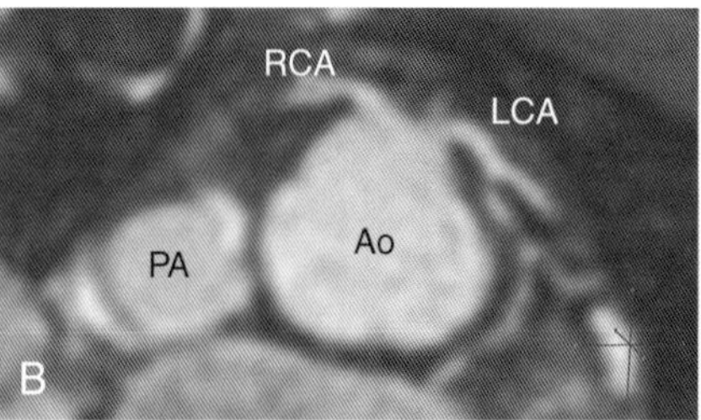

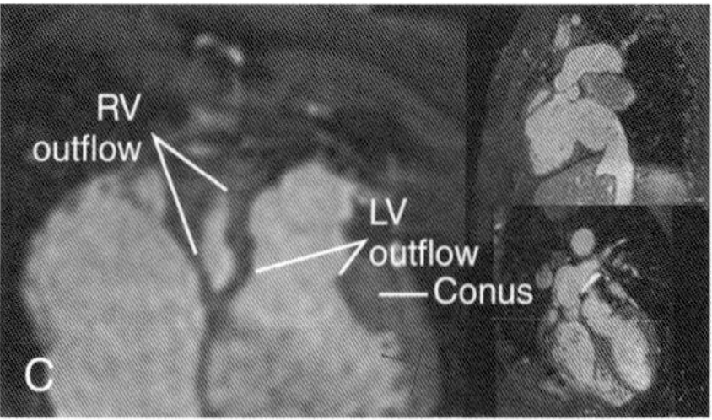

Fig. 44.18 Cardiac magnetic resonance bright blood images from a patient with repaired, anatomically corrected malposition {S,D,L}. (A) Axial view demonstrates the ascending aorta *(Ao)* leftward of and anterior to the pulmonary bifurcation. (B) Short-axis view demonstrates the coronary origins from the aorta, which is leftward of and anterior to the pulmonary artery *(PA)*. Both coronary arteries arise from the anterior-facing sinus, and the right coronary artery *(RCA)* typically passes anterior to the RV outflow tract, limiting options for surgical enlargement. (C) 3D steady-state free precession (SSFP) acquisition was reformatted to show the narrowed RV outflow tract *(RV outflow)*, LV outflow tract *(LV outflow)*, and subaortic conus. *LCA*, Left coronary artery; *LPA*, left pulmonary artery; *RPA*, right pulmonary artery.

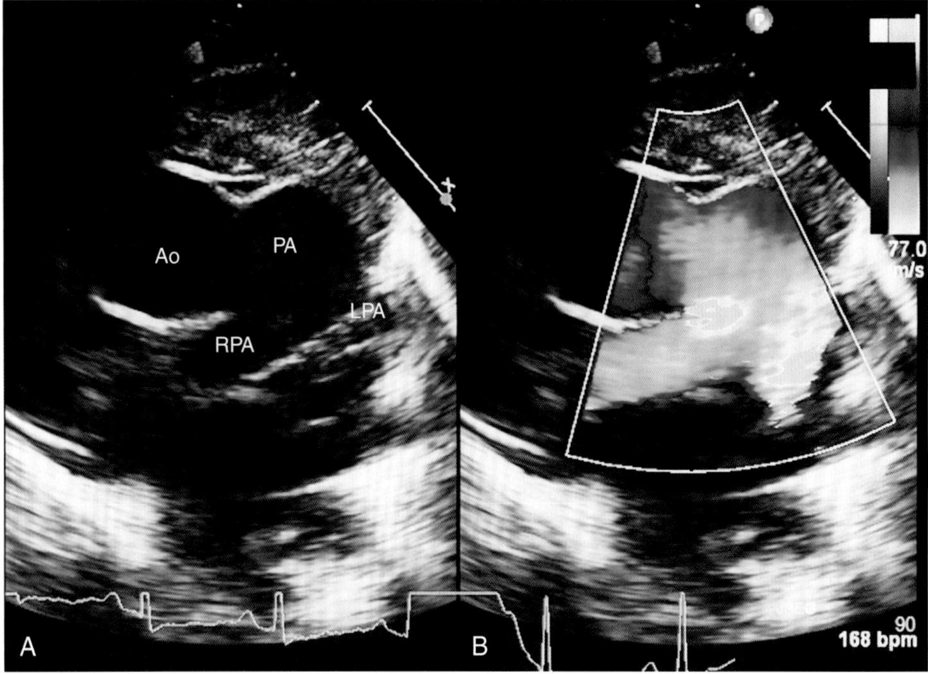

Fig. 44.19 Aortopulmonary window. (A) Parasternal short-axis view demonstrates a distal aortopulmonary window at the pulmonary bifurcation. (B) Color Doppler imaging demonstrates antegrade flow in the distal main and proximal branch pulmonary arteries through this defect (see Video 44.19). *Ao*, Aorta; *LPA*, left pulmonary artery; *PA*, pulmonary artery; *RPA*, right pulmonary artery.

condition was first reported in 1895 by Theremin and was further characterized by Van Praagh et al. in 1971. In rare cases of anatomically corrected malposition {S,D,L} without associated malformations, the physiology is normal and incidental detection has been reported.[90] Usually, this type is associated with VSD and often with pulmonic stenosis. Patients can undergo VSD closure with or without relief of pulmonic stenosis with good results.

In another type, anatomically corrected malposition {S,L,D}, there is AV discordance with ventriculoarterial concordance, which results in cyanosis because systemic venous blood drains from the RA to the right-sided LV and aorta, and pulmonary venous blood passes from the LA into the left-sided RV and PA. In these cases, an atrial switch operation is necessary to correct the AV discordance along with VSD closure and possibly relief of outflow obstruction. An important imaging consideration for patients with anatomically corrected malposition is that there are almost always two VSDs present: the usual outflow defect between the limbs of the septal band and a higher defect in the anterior muscular septum between the subaortic infundibulum and the RV.

AORTOPULMONARY WINDOW

An aortopulmonary window is a rare congenital heart defect consisting of a communication between the PA and the intrapericardial portion of the ascending aorta in the setting of two separate semilunar valves. Approximately 50% of patients with aortopulmonary window have associated anomalies such as a right aortic arch, type A interruption of the aortic arch, anomalous origin of a coronary artery from the PA, TOF, TGA, VSD, or origin of the right PA from the aorta. Children usually present with symptoms of heart failure and pulmonary hypertension.

An aortopulmonary window can be imaged in the parasternal short-axis (Fig. 44.19), subxiphoid, or suprasternal view. Careful imaging is key to differentiating an aortopulmonary window from other abnormal aortopulmonary connections such as a persistent ductus arteriosus or origin of a branch PA from the aorta (i.e., hemitruncus). Color Doppler echocardiography is useful for demonstrating left-to-right shunt flow across the window.

Irreversible pulmonary vascular disease can develop as early as the first year of life, making a timely diagnosis important. Patients with an isolated, small aortopulmonary window may be candidates for percutaneous closure. Larger defects are typically closed surgically. The surgical repair techniques of this defect have varied by center and era. Backer and Mavroudis described the single-center experience of 22 cases of aortopulmonary window over a 40-year period.[91] There were five early deaths and one late death (i.e., pulmonary hypertension) among the first 16 patients, for whom the primary strategy was aortopulmonary window division (37% mortality rate). However, no deaths were reported among the most recent six patients, who had undergone transaortic patch closure.

Rarely, aortopulmonary window manifests in adulthood. There have been reports of successful closure in adulthood; however, reversibility of elevated pulmonary vascular resistance must be demonstrated with pharmacologic testing before surgical closure.[92] Adults who have undergone aortopulmonary window closure in childhood should undergo periodic imaging for surveillance of a recurrent defect, stenosis of the ascending aorta or a PA, and pulmonary hypertension.

CONCLUSIONS

Complex conotruncal defects are rare and often challenging to diagnose because there are many variations for each diagnosis that must be clearly delineated. A complete echocardiographic examination is essential, and the surgical plan is often dictated by details specific to the individual patient. All patients with conotruncal anomalies should be followed throughout life with serial imaging. Specific attention to aortic size and function is important because aortopathy is common among these patients.

SUMMARY Complex Conotruncal Abnormalities.

Condition	Echocardiographic Findings	Postoperative Imaging Findings
Tetralogy of Fallot	Outlet VSD Deviation of the conal septum anteriorly, superiorly, and leftward Overriding aorta	Pulmonary regurgitation Residual stenosis of the RVOT, main and branch PAs Tricuspid regurgitation RA size Residual VSD Ventricular size and function Aortic root dilation
Truncus arteriosus	A single common arterial trunk arises from the heart, giving origin to the coronary arteries, PAs, and systemic arteries.	RV-PA conduit Quantification of stenosis Quantification of regurgitation Estimation of RV systolic pressure Residual VSD Proximal branch PA caliber Truncal valve morphology Quantification of truncal valve stenosis Quantification of truncal valve regurgitation LV outflow tract obstruction Aortic arch morphology Ventricular size and function
Double-outlet RV	Both great arteries are completely or almost completely aligned with the RV. Associated anomalies: • VSD • Outflow tract obstruction • Anomalies of the AV valves • Heterotaxy syndrome	Residual VSD, including intramural VSDs (see Fig. 44.15) Subaortic stenosis Subvalvular PS Pulmonic regurgitation Ventricular size and function AV valve function (particularly in patients who have undergone AV canal repair) For those who have undergone aortic arch reconstruction: • Aortic arch morphology and quantification of obstruction For those who have undergone an arterial switch operation: • Neo-aortic valve regurgitation • Supravalvular aortic stenosis • Neo-aortic root dilation • Supravalvular PS or branch PA stenosis

Continued

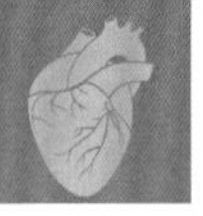

SUMMARY Complex Conotruncal Abnormalities.—cont'd

Condition	Echocardiographic Findings	Postoperative Imaging Findings
Double-outlet LV	Both great arteries are completely or almost completely aligned with the LV. Associated anomalies: • VSD • Outflow tract obstruction • Anomalies of the AV valves	Similar to DORV

Anatomically corrected malposition	The great arteries are aligned with the correct ventricle (RV → PA, LV → Ao) but are abnormally connected to the ventricles (subaortic conus, deficient or absent subpulmonary conus).
	Associated anomalies:
	• VSD
	• Outflow tract obstruction
	• Some types have AV discordance
		Depends on the surgical repair:
		• Residual VSD
		• Ventricular size and function
		• If atrial switch procedure
		  • Atrial baffle obstruction
		  • Atrial baffle leaks

AP window	Communication between the PA and the intrapericardial ascending aorta in the setting of two separate semilunar valves	Residual defects: • Stenosis of the ascending aorta • Stenosis of a PA • Pulmonary hypertension

Ao, Aorta; *AP*, aortopulmonary; *AV*, atrioventricular; *DORV*, double-outlet RV; *PA*, pulmonary artery; *PS*, pulmonary stenosis; *RVOT*, right ventricular outflow tract; *VSD*, ventricular septal defect.

REFERENCES

1. Hutson MR, Kirby ML. Model systems for the study of heart development and disease. Cardiac neural crest and conotruncal malformations. *Semin Cell Dev Biol*. 2007;18(1):101–110.
2. Johnson TR. Conotruncal cardiac defects: a clinical imaging perspective. *Pediatr Cardiol*. 2010;31(3):430–437.
3. Frank L, Dillman JR, Parish V, et al. Cardiovascular MR imaging of conotruncal anomalies. *Radiographics*. 2010;30(4):1069–1094.
4. Schleich JM, Abdulla T, Summers R, Houyel L. An overview of cardiac morphogenesis. *Arch Cardiovasc Dis*. 2013;106(11):612–623.
5. Bajolle F, Zaffran S, Kelly RG, et al. Rotation of the myocardial wall of the outflow tract is implicated in the normal positioning of the great arteries. *Circ Res*. 2006;98(3):421–428.
6. Vogels A, Schevenels S, Cayenberghs R, et al. Presenting symptoms in adults with the 22q11 deletion syndrome. *Eur J Med Genet*. 2014;57(4):157–162.
7. de Souza KR, Mergener R, Huber J, Campos Pellanda L, Riegel M. Cytogenomic evaluation of subjects with syndromic and nonsyndromic conotruncal heart defects. *BioMed Res Int*. 2015;2015:401941.
8. Trippel A, Pallivathukal S, Pfammatter JP, Hutter D, Kadner A, Pavlovic M. Dimensions of the ascending aorta in conotruncal heart defects. *Pediatr Cardiol*. 2014;35(5):831–837.
9. Tan JL, Davlouros PA, McCarthy KP, Gatzoulis MA, Ho SY. Intrinsic histological abnormalities of aortic root and ascending aorta in tetralogy of Fallot: evidence of causative mechanism for aortic dilatation and aortopathy. *Circulation*. 2005;112(7):961–968.
10. John AS, Rychik J, Khan M, Yang W, Goldmuntz E. 22q11.2 deletion syndrome as a risk factor for aortic root dilation in tetralogy of Fallot. *Cardiol Young*. 2014;24(2):303–310.
11. Mongeon FP, Gurvitz MZ, Broberg CS, et al. Aortic root dilatation in adults with surgically repaired tetralogy of Fallot: a multicenter cross-sectional study. *Circulation*. 2013;127(2):172–179.
12. Silversides CK, Kiess M, Beauchesne L, et al. Canadian Cardiovascular Society 2009 Consensus Conference on the management of adults with congenital heart disease: outflow tract obstruction, coarctation of the aorta, tetralogy of Fallot, Ebstein anomaly and Marfan's syndrome. *Can J Cardiol*. 2010;26(3):e80–97.
13. Stulak JM, Dearani JA, Burkhart HM, Sundt TM, Connolly HM, Schaff HV. Does the dilated ascending aorta in an adult with congenital heart disease require intervention? *J Thorac Cardiovasc Surg*. 2010;140(6 suppl):S52–S57, discussion S86–S91.
14. Kim WH, Seo JW, Kim SJ, Song J, Lee J, Na CY. Aortic dissection late after repair of tetralogy of Fallot. *Int J Cardiol*. 2005;101(3):515–516.
15. Konstantinov IE, Fricke TA, d'Udekem Y, Robertson T. Aortic dissection and rupture in adolescents after tetralogy of Fallot repair. *J Thorac Cardiovasc Surg*. 2010;140(5):e71–73.
16. Rathi VK, Doyle M, Williams RB, Yamrozik J, Shannon RP, Biederman RW. Massive aortic aneurysm and dissection in repaired tetralogy of Fallot; diagnosis by cardiovascular magnetic resonance imaging. *Int J Cardiol*. 2005;101(1):169–170.
17. Wijesekera VA, Kiess MC, Grewal J, et al. Aortic dissection in a patient with a dilated aortic root following tetralogy of Fallot repair. *Int J Cardiol*. 2014;174(3):833–834.
18. Schwartz ML, Gauvreau K, del Nido P, Mayer JE, Colan SD. Long-term predictors of aortic root dilation and aortic regurgitation after arterial switch operation. *Circulation*. 2004;110(11 suppl 1):II128–132.
19. Carlo WF, McKenzie ED, Slesnick TC. Root dilation in patients with truncus arteriosus. *Congenit Heart Dis*. 2011;6(3):228–233.
20. Frischhertz BP, Shamszad P, Pedroza C, Milewicz DM, Morris SA. Thoracic aortic dissection and rupture in conotruncal cardiac defects: a population-based study. *Int J Cardiol*. 2015;184:521–527.
21. Goldstein SA, Evangelista A, Abbara S, et al. Multimodality imaging of diseases of the thoracic aorta in adults: from the American Society of Echocardiography and the European Association of Cardiovascular Imaging: Endorsed by the Society of Cardiovascular Computed Tomography and Society for Cardiovascular Magnetic Resonance. *J Am Soc Echocardiogr*. 2015;28(2):119–182.
22. Lopez L, Colan SD, Frommelt PC, et al. Recommendations for quantification methods during the performance of a pediatric echocardiogram: a report from the Pediatric Measurements Writing Group of the American Society of Echocardiography Pediatric and Congenital Heart Disease Council. *J Am Soc Echocardiogr*. 2010;23(5):465–495. quiz 576–577.
23. Nies M, Brenner JI. Tetralogy of Fallot: epidemiology meets real-world management: lessons from the Baltimore-Washington Infant Study. *Cardiol Young*. 2013;23(6):867–870.
24. Valente AM, Cook S, Festa P, et al. Multimodality imaging guidelines for patients with repaired tetralogy of Fallot: a report from the American Society of Echocardiography: developed in collaboration with the Society for Cardiovascular Magnetic Resonance and the Society for Pediatric Radiology. *J Am Soc Echocardiogr*. 2014;27(2):111–141.
25. Rudski LG, Lai WW, Afilalo J, et al. Guidelines for the echocardiographic assessment of the right heart in adults: a report from the Ameri-

can Society of Echocardiography endorsed by the European Association of Echocardiography, a registered branch of the European Society of Cardiology, and the Canadian Society of Echocardiography. *J Am Soc Echocardiogr.* 2010;23(7):685–713, quiz 786–788.
26. Puchalski MD, Askovich B, Sower CT, Williams RV, Minich LL, Tani LY. Pulmonary regurgitation: determining severity by echocardiography and magnetic resonance imaging. *Congenit Heart Dis.* 2008;3(3):168–175.
27. Renella P, Aboulhosn J, Lohan DG, et al. Two-dimensional and Doppler echocardiography reliably predict severe pulmonary regurgitation as quantified by cardiac magnetic resonance. *J Am Soc Echocardiogr.* 2010;23(8):880–886.
28. Srivastava S, Parness IA. Tetralogy of Fallot. In: Lai WW, Mertens L, Cohen MS, Geva T, eds. *Echocardiography in Pediatric and Congenital Heart Disease: From Fetus to Adult.* Hoboken, NJ: Wiley-Blackwell; 2009.
29. Festa P, Ait-Ali L, Minichilli F, Kristo I, Deiana M, Picano E. A new simple method to estimate pulmonary regurgitation by echocardiography in operated Fallot: comparison with magnetic resonance imaging and performance test evaluation. *J Am Soc Echocardiogr.* 2010;23(5):496–503.
30. Mercer-Rosa L, Yang W, Kutty S, Rychik J, Fogel M, Goldmuntz E. Quantifying pulmonary regurgitation and right ventricular function in surgically repaired tetralogy of Fallot: a comparative analysis of echocardiography and magnetic resonance imaging. *Circ Cardiovasc Imaging.* 2012;5(5):637–643.
31. Pothineni KR, Wells BJ, Hsiung MC, et al. Live/real time three-dimensional transthoracic echocardiographic assessment of pulmonary regurgitation. *Echocardiography.* 2008;25(8):911–917.
32. Beurskens NEG, Gorter TM, Pieper PG, et al. Diagnostic value of Doppler echocardiography for identifying hemodynamic significant pulmonary valve regurgitation in tetralogy of Fallot: comparison with cardiac MRI. *Int J Cardiovasc Imaging.* 2017;33(11):1723–1730.
33. Van Berendoncks A, Van Grootel R, McGhie J, et al. Echocardiographic parameters of severe pulmonary regurgitation after surgical repair of tetralogy of Fallot. *Congenit Heart Dis.* 2019 14(4):628–637.
34. Stout KK, Daniels CJ, Aboulhosn JA, et al. 2018 AHA/ACC guideline for the management of adults with congenital heart disease: a report of the American College of Cardiology/American Heart Association task force on Clinical Practice Guidelines. *J Am Coll Cardiol.* 2019;73(12):e81–e192.
35. Lang RM, Badano LP, Mor-Avi V, et al. Recommendations for cardiac chamber quantification by echocardiography in adults: an update from the American Society of Echocardiography and the European Association of Cardiovascular Imaging. *J Am Soc Echocardiogr.* 2015;28(1):1–39. e14.
36. Crean AM, Maredia N, Ballard G, et al. 3D Echo systematically underestimates right ventricular volumes compared to cardiovascular magnetic resonance in adult congenital heart disease patients with moderate or severe RV dilatation. *J Cardiovasc Magn Reson.* 2011;13:78.
37. Grewal J, Majdalany D, Syed I, Pellikka P, Warnes CA. Three-dimensional echocardiographic assessment of right ventricular volume and function in adult patients with congenital heart disease: comparison with magnetic resonance imaging. *J Am Soc Echocardiogr.* 2010;23(2):127–133.
38. Iriart X, Montaudon M, Lafitte S, et al. Right ventricle three-dimensional echography in corrected tetralogy of Fallot: accuracy and variability. *Eur J Echocardiogr.* 2009;10(6):784–792.
39. Khoo NS, Young A, Occleshaw C, Cowan B, Zeng IS, Gentles TL. Assessments of right ventricular volume and function using three-dimensional echocardiography in older children and adults with congenital heart disease: comparison with cardiac magnetic resonance imaging. *J Am Soc Echocardiogr.* 2009;22(11):1279–1288.
40. Shimada YJ, Shiota M, Siegel RJ, Shiota T. Accuracy of right ventricular volumes and function determined by three-dimensional echocardiography in comparison with magnetic resonance imaging: a meta-analysis study. *J Am Soc Echocardiogr.* 2010;23(9):943–953.
41. van der Zwaan HB, Helbing WA, McGhie JS, et al. Clinical value of real-time three-dimensional echocardiography for right ventricular quantification in congenital heart disease: validation with cardiac magnetic resonance imaging. *J Am Soc Echocardiogr.* 2010;23(2):134–140.
42. Dragulescu A, Grosse-Wortmann L, Fackoury C, et al. Echocardiographic assessment of right ventricular volumes after surgical repair of tetralogy of Fallot: clinical validation of a new echocardiographic method. *J Am Soc Echocardiogr.* 2011;24(11):1191–1198.
43. Medvedofsky D, Addetia K, Patel AR, et al. Novel approach to three-dimensional echocardiographic quantification of right ventricular volumes and function from focused views. *J Am Soc Echocardiogr.* 2015;28(10):1222–1231.
44. Medvedofsky D, Mor-Avi V, Kruse E, et al. Quantification of right ventricular size and function from contrast-enhanced three-dimensional echocardiographic images. *J Am Soc Echocardiogr.* 2017;30(12):1193–1202.
45. Xie M, Li Y, Cheng TO, et al. The effect of right ventricular myocardial remodeling on ventricular function as assessed by two-dimensional speckle tracking echocardiography in patients with tetralogy of Fallot: a single center experience from China. *Int J Cardiol.* 2015;178:300–307.
46. Scherptong RW, Mollema SA, Blom NA, et al. Right ventricular peak systolic longitudinal strain is a sensitive marker for right ventricular deterioration in adult patients with tetralogy of Fallot. *Int J Cardiovasc Imaging.* 2009;25(7):669–676.
47. Alghamdi MH, Mertens L, Lee W, Yoo SJ, Grosse-Wortmann L. Longitudinal right ventricular function is a better predictor of right ventricular contribution to exercise performance than global or outflow tract ejection fraction in tetralogy of Fallot: a combined echocardiography and magnetic resonance study. *Eur Heart J Cardiovasc Imaging.* 2013;14(3):235–239.
48. Gatzoulis MA, Clark AL, Cullen S, Newman CG, Redington AN. Right ventricular diastolic function 15 to 35 years after repair of tetralogy of Fallot. Restrictive physiology predicts superior exercise performance. *Circulation.* 1995;91(6):1775–1781.
49. Samyn MM, Kwon EN, Gorentz JS, et al. Restrictive versus nonrestrictive physiology following repair of tetralogy of Fallot: is there a difference? *J Am Soc Echocardiogr.* 2013;26(7):746–755.
50. Bokma JP, Winter MM, Oosterhof T, et al. Severe tricuspid regurgitation is predictive for adverse events in tetralogy of Fallot. *Heart.* 2015;101(10):794–799.
51. Broberg CS, Aboulhosn J, Mongeon FP, et al. Prevalence of left ventricular systolic dysfunction in adults with repaired tetralogy of Fallot. *Am J Cardiol.* 2011;107(8):1215–1220.
52. Hausdorf G, Hinrichs C, Nienaber CA, Schark C, Keck EW. Left ventricular contractile state after surgical correction of tetralogy of Fallot: risk factors for late left ventricular dysfunction. *Pediatr Cardiol.* 1990;11(2):61–68.
53. Geva T, Sandweiss BM, Gauvreau K, Lock JE, Powell AJ. Factors associated with impaired clinical status in long-term survivors of tetralogy of Fallot repair evaluated by magnetic resonance imaging. *J Am Coll Cardiol.* 2004;43(6):1068–1074.
54. Dragulescu A, Friedberg MK, Grosse-Wortmann L, Redington A, Mertens L. Effect of chronic right ventricular volume overload on ventricular interaction in patients after tetralogy of Fallot repair. *J Am Soc Echocardiogr.* 2014;27(8):896–902.
55. Menting ME, Eindhoven JA, van den Bosch AE, et al. Abnormal left ventricular rotation and twist in adult patients with corrected tetralogy of Fallot. *Eur Heart J Cardiovasc Imaging.* 2014;15(5):566–574.
56. Ghai A, Silversides C, Harris L, Webb GD, Siu SC, Therrien J. Left ventricular dysfunction is a risk factor for sudden cardiac death in adults late after repair of tetralogy of Fallot. *J Am Coll Cardiol.* 2002;40(9):1675–1680.
57. Valente AM, Gauvreau K, Assenza GE, et al. Contemporary predictors of death and sustained ventricular tachycardia in patients with repaired tetralogy of Fallot enrolled in the INDICATOR cohort. *Heart.* 2014;100(3):247–253.
58. Diller GP, Kempny A, Liodakis E, et al. Left ventricular longitudinal function predicts life-threatening ventricular arrhythmia and death in adults with repaired tetralogy of fallot. *Circulation.* 2012;125(20):2440–2446.
59. Cuypers JA, Menting ME, Konings EE, et al. Unnatural history of tetralogy of Fallot: prospective follow-up of 40 years after surgical correction. *Circulation.* 2014;130(22):1944–1953.
60. Geva T. Repaired tetralogy of Fallot: the roles of cardiovascular magnetic resonance in evaluating pathophysiology and for pulmonary valve replacement decision support. *J Cardiovasc Magn Reson.* 2011;13:9.
61. McElhinney DB, Hellenbrand WE, Zahn EM, et al. Short- and medium-term outcomes after transcatheter pulmonary valve placement in the expanded multicenter US Melody valve trial. *Circulation.* 2010;122(5):507–516.
62. Zahn EM, Hellenbrand WE, Lock JE, McElhinney DB. Implantation of the Melody transcatheter pulmonary valve in patients with a dysfunctional right ventricular outflow tract conduit early results from the U.S. clinical trial. *J Am Coll Cardiol.* 2009;54(18):1722–1729.
63. Steinberg ZL, Jones TK, Verrier E, Stout KK, Krieger EV, Karamlou T. Early outcomes in patients undergoing transcatheter versus surgical pulmonary valve replacement. *Heart.* 2017;103(18):1455–1460.
64. Cheatham JP, Hellenbrand WE, Zahn EM, et al. Clinical and hemodynamic outcomes up to 7 years after transcatheter pulmonary valve replacement in the US Melody valve investigational device exemption trial. *Circulation.* 2015;131(22):1960–1970.

65. Abdelghani M, Nassif M, Blom NA, et al. Infective endocarditis after Melody valve implantation in the pulmonary position: a systematic review. *J Am Heart Assoc*. 2018; https://doi.org/10.1161/JAHA.117.008163.
66. Sharma A, Cote AT, Hosking MCK, Harris KC. A systematic review of infective endocarditis in patients with bovine jugular vein valves compared with other valve types. *JACC Cardiovasc Interv*. 2017;10(14):1449–1458.
67. Kenny D, Rhodes JF, Fleming GA, et al. 3-Year outcomes of the Edwards SAPIEN transcatheter heart valve for conduit failure in the pulmonary position from the COMPASSION multicenter clinical trial. *JACC Cardiovasc Interv*. 2018;11(19):1920–1929.
68. Jacobs ML. Congenital Heart Surgery Nomenclature and Database Project: truncus arteriosus. *Ann Thorac Surg*. 2000;69(4 suppl):S50–S55.
69. Lopes LM, Silva JP, Fonseca L, Meiken S, Salvador AB, Fernandes GS. Atypical truncus arteriosus operated at 28 years of age: importance of differential diagnosis. *Arq Bras Cardiol*. 2011;97(2):e29–32.
70. Guenther F, Frydrychowicz A, Bode C, Geibel A. Cardiovascular flashlight. Persistent truncus arteriosus: a rare finding in adults. *Eur Heart J*. 2009;30(9):1154.
71. Abid D, Daoud E, Ben Kahla S, et al. Unrepaired persistent truncus arteriosus in a 38-year-old woman with an uneventful pregnancy. *Cardiovasc J Afr*. 2015;26(4):e6–8.
72. Kaza AK, Burch PT, Pinto N, Minich LL, Tani LY, Hawkins JA. Durability of truncal valve repair. *Ann Thorac Surg*. 2010;90(4):1307–1312, discussion 1312.
73. Lev M, Bharati S, Meng CC, Liberthson RR, Paul MH, Idriss F. A concept of double-outlet right ventricle. *J Thorac Cardiovasc Surg*. 1972;64(2):271–281.
74. Anderson RH, Becker AE, Wilcox BR, Macartney FJ, Wilkinson JL. Surgical anatomy of double-outlet right ventriclea reappraisal. *Am J Cardiol*. 1983;52(5):555–559.
75. Van Praagh R. What is the Taussig-Bing malformation? *Circulation*. 1968;38(3):445–449.
76. Schwarz F, Blaschczok HC, Sinzobahamvya N, et al. The Taussig-Bing anomaly: long-term results. *Eur J Cardio Thorac Surg*. 2013;44(5):821–827.
77. Belli E, Serraf A, Lacour-Gayet F, et al. Biventricular repair for double-outlet right ventricle. Results and long-term follow-up. *Circulation*. 1998;98(19 suppl):II360–II365, discussion II365–II367.
78. Artrip JH, Sauer H, Campbell DN, et al. Biventricular repair in double outlet right ventricle: surgical results based on the STS-EACTS International Nomenclature classification. *Eur J Cardio Thorac Surg*. 2006;29(4):545–550.
79. Sanders SP, Bierman FZ, Williams RG. Conotruncal malformations: diagnosis in infancy using subxiphoid 2-dimensional echocardiography. *Am J Cardiol*. 1982;50(6):1361–1367.
80. Hagler DJ, Tajik AJ, Seward JB, Mair DD, Ritter DG. Double-outlet right ventricle: wide-angle two-dimensional echocardiographic observations. *Circulation*. 1981;63(2):419–428.
81. Ruzmetov M, Rodefeld MD, Turrentine MW, Brown JW. Rational approach to surgical management of complex forms of double outlet right ventricle with modified Fontan operation. *Congenit Heart Dis*. 2008;3(6):397–403.
82. Aoki M, Forbess JM, Jonas RA, Mayer Jr JE, Castaneda AR. Result of biventricular repair for double-outlet right ventricle. *J Thorac Cardiovasc Surg*. 1994;107(2):338–349, discussion 349–350.
83. Chaitman BR, Grondin CM, Theroux P, Bourassa MG. Late development of left ventricular outflow tract obstruction after repair of double-outlet right ventricle. *J Thorac Cardiovasc Surg*. 1976;72(2):265–268.
84. Preminger TJ, Sanders SP, van der Velde ME, Castaneda AR, Lock JE. "Intramural" residual interventricular defects after repair of conotruncal malformations. *Circulation*. 1994;89(1):236–242.
85. Patel JK, Glatz AC, Ghosh RM, et al. Intramural ventricular septal defect is a distinct clinical entity associated with postoperative morbidity in children after repair of conotruncal anomalies. *Circulation*. 2015;132(15):1387–1394.
86. Sakakibara STA, Arai T, Hashimoto A, Nogi M. Both great vessels arising from the left ventricle (double outlet left ventricle) (origin of both great vessels from the left ventricle). *Bull Heart Inst Jap*. 1967:66–86.
87. Van Praagh R, Weinberg PM, Srebro JP. Double-outlet left ventricle. In: Moss AJ, Adams FH, Emmanouilides GC, eds. *Heart Disease in Infants, Children, and Adolescents*. 3 rd ed. Baltimore, MD: Williams & Wilkins; 1988.
88. Karavelioglu Y, Turan B, Karapinar H. Noninvasive diagnosis of an adult patient with double-outlet left ventricle. *Eur J Cardio Thorac Surg*. 2011;40(4):e154–155.
89. Bharati S, Lev M, Stewart R, McAllister Jr HA, Kirklin JW. The morphologic spectrum of double outlet left ventricle and its surgical significance. *Circulation*. 1978;58(3 Pt 1):558–565.
90. Blume ED, Chung T, Hoffer FA, Geva T. Images in cardiovascular medicine. Anatomically corrected malposition of the great arteries [S,D,L]. *Circulation*. 1998;97(12):1207.
91. Backer CL, Mavroudis C. Surgical management of aortopulmonary window: a 40-year experience. *Eur J Cardio Thorac Surg*. 2002;21(5):773–779.
92. Aggarwal SK, Mishra J, Sai V, Iyer VR, Panicker BK. Aortopulmonary window in adults: diagnosis and treatment of late-presenting patients. *Congenit Heart Dis*. 2008;3(5):341–346.

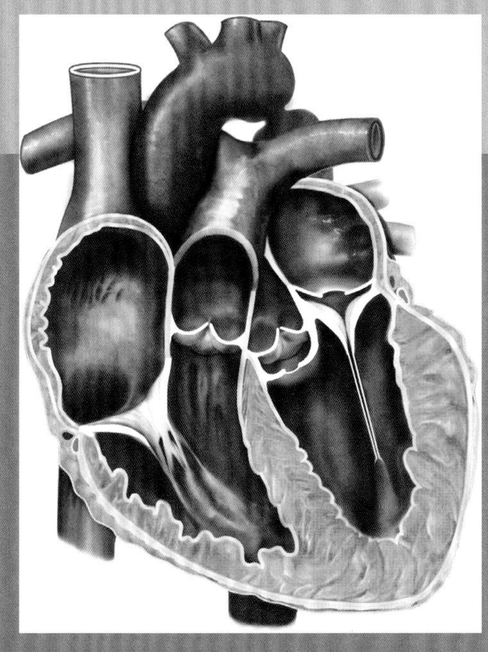

中文导读

第45章 大动脉转位

完全型大动脉转位是一种比较常见的紫绀型先天性心脏畸形，有两个平行的循环，含氧血液通过肺部运输，缺氧血液通过体循环运输，需要及时修复，否则通常会在1岁内死亡。大约50%的完全型大动脉转位患者出生时同时存在先天性异常，包括室间隔缺损、左心室流出道梗阻、肺动脉瓣狭窄，以及冠状动脉异常，相关畸形可增加手术风险并影响修复后的晚期预后。手术修复的目标是将平行的肺循环和体循环重新串联起来，使含氧血液流向主动脉，缺氧血液流向肺动脉。本章系统介绍了大动脉转位的各种手术方式，包括心房调转手术（Mustard或Senning手术）、ASO手术、Rastelli手术、Nikaidoh手术等手术方式和术后情况观察，以及术后并发症情况的超声观察。

本章还从病理解剖、病理生理、临床表现、流行病学等方面介绍了矫正型大动脉转位，并介绍了双调转手术和生理修复两种手术策略，以及术后可能出现的各类异常情况的超声评估方法。

王剑鹏

45

Transposition of the Great Arteries

ERIC V. KRIEGER, MD | JASON F. DEEN, MD

COMPLETE TRANSPOSITION OF THE GREAT ARTERIES

BACKGROUND

Complete transposition of the great arteries (TGA, also called D-loop TGA [D-TGA]) is a relatively common cyanotic congenital heart defect that accounts for 5% to 7% of congenital heart disease and affects 3 in 10,000 live births. It affects males more commonly than females. In TGA, there are two parallel circulations that transport oxygenated blood through the lungs and deoxygenated blood through the systemic circulation. Unless it is repaired promptly, death in the first year is almost universal.[1]

Most commonly, patients with TGA have normal systemic venous return, normal atrial situs, and normal atrioventricular (AV) connections. The aortic valve typically arises from the morphologic right ventricle (RV) anteriorly and rightward from the pulmonic valve, which arises from the morphologic left ventricle (LV). Approximately 50% of patients born with TGA have coexisting congenital anomalies, including ventricular septal defect (VSD), left ventricular outflow tract obstruction (LVOTO) (i.e., subpulmonic stenosis), and coronary anomalies (Table 45.1). The associated defects can increase the surgical risk and affect late outcomes after repair.[2–4]

This chapter focuses on the adult with repaired TGA. Discussions of fetal echocardiography, neonatal diagnosis, and perioperative echocardiography can be found elsewhere.[5]

OVERVIEW OF SURGICAL APPROACHES

A baby born with TGA cannot survive unless mixing allows oxygenated blood to reach the systemic circulation. Mixing is most reliably achieved at the atrial level. For babies born with a restrictive atrial communication, balloon atrial septostomy can augment the atrial shunt until definitive surgical treatment can be performed.

The goal of surgical repair is to bring the parallel pulmonary and systemic circulations back into series such that oxygenated blood flows to the aorta and deoxygenated blood flows to the pulmonary arteries. The corrective surgical techniques have depended on the year of repair, associated cardiac defects, era of repair, and local institutional preferences (Table 45.2).

The atrial switch procedure (i.e., Mustard or Senning operation) was widely used from the 1960s until the late 1980s, when it was replaced by the arterial switch operation (ASO).[6,7] Although the atrial switch operation is no longer performed for TGA, there is a large population of adults who have undergone an atrial switch procedure. In this operation, intraatrial baffles reroute deoxygenated systemic venous return leftward to the mitral valve and LV, and the oxygenated pulmonary venous blood is routed to the tricuspid valve and systemic right ventricle (sRV) (Figs. 45.1 and 45.2).

The atrial switch procedure relieved cyanosis but left the patient with an sRV, systemic tricuspid valve, and intraatrial baffles, which could develop leaks or stenosis and limit preload capacity. Pulmonary hypertension has been described as a late complication.[8] The late sequelae led to increased morbidity and premature mortality for patients who underwent an atrial switch operation.

The ASO was introduced in the 1970s but was not widely adopted until the early 1990s.[9,10] This operation is conceptually simple but technically challenging, requiring reimplantation of coronary arteries, mobilization of the pulmonary arteries, and neonatal surgery. Late outcomes have been excellent, and it is superior to the atrial switch procedure.[11,12] Nonetheless, patients are at risk for coronary ischemia, supravalvular pulmonic stenosis, dilation of the aortic root, and aortic regurgitation.

The Rastelli operation is typically used for the large subset of patients with TGA, VSD, and pulmonary valve stenosis. In this procedure, a VSD patch is baffled to direct oxygenated blood from the LV, across the VSD, and out the anterior aortic valve. The native stenotic pulmonic valve is oversewn, and a conduit is placed between the RV and pulmonary artery (PA).

The Rastelli operation is appealing because it relieves cyanosis, creates a systemic LV, and does not require coronary reimplantation. However, babies and children rapidly outgrow the pulmonary conduit, necessitating frequent reoperations in childhood and the risk of multiple median sternotomies. Conduit dysfunction, VSD baffle stenoses, and ventricular dysfunction can occur in adults after the Rastelli operation. The postoperative anatomy and associated complications of each surgical approach are shown in Table 45.2.

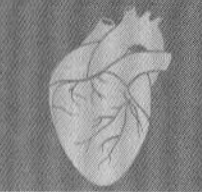

TABLE 45.1 Incidence of Associated Anomalies in Patients With Complete Transposition of the Great Arteries.

Defect Type	*Incidence (%)*	*Comments*
VSD	40–45	Perimembranous type is most common. Muscular defects are often hemodynamically insignificant. Inlet VSDs may be associated with straddling atrioventricular valves. Anterior malalignment VSDs are associated with RVOT and aortic hypoplasia. Posterior malalignment VSDs are associated with LVOTO and pulmonic hypoplasia.
Coronary anomalies	35	Most common pattern is left coronary from left posterior sinus and right coronary from right posterior sinus. In 14% of patients, the circumflex arises from the right posterior sinus; 8% of patients have a single right coronary artery. Anomalous coronary artery patterns can pose technical challenges to coronary reimplantation in the ASO.
LVOTO	20–30	Many possible mechanisms of LVOTO include discrete subpulmonic ridge, posterior malalignment VSD, anomalous insertion of mitral chords to the interventricular septum, and focal septal hypertrophy.
Coarctation or aortic arch abnormalities	5	More commonly seen in patients with double-outlet RV with transposition physiology (i.e., Taussig-Bing anomaly)

ASO, Arterial switch operation; *LVOTO*, LV outflow tract obstruction; *RVOT*, RV outflow tract obstruction; *VSD*, ventricular septal defect.

TABLE 45.2 Repairs for Complete Transposition of the Great Arteries.

Name (Eponyms)	*Description*	*Figure*	*Late Sequelae*
Atrial switch operation (Mustard procedure, Senning procedure)	Intraatrial baffles redirect systemic venous return to the mitral valve and LV and the pulmonary venous return to the tricuspid valve and RV.	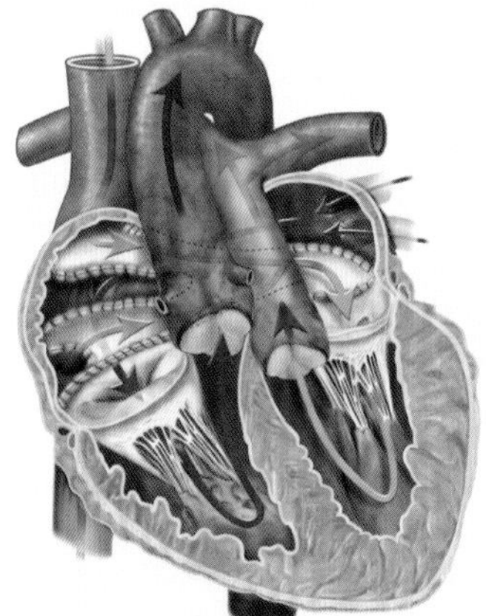	• Systemic RV systolic dysfunction • Tricuspid regurgitation • Baffle leak • SVC baffle stenosis • Atrial arrhythmia • Sudden death
Arterial switch operation (Jatene procedure, Lecompte maneuver)	Aorta and PA are transected above the sinuses. The aorta is brought posterior to the native pulmonic valve, and PAs are anastomosed to the native aortic valve. Coronary arteries are reimplanted in the neoaortic root.	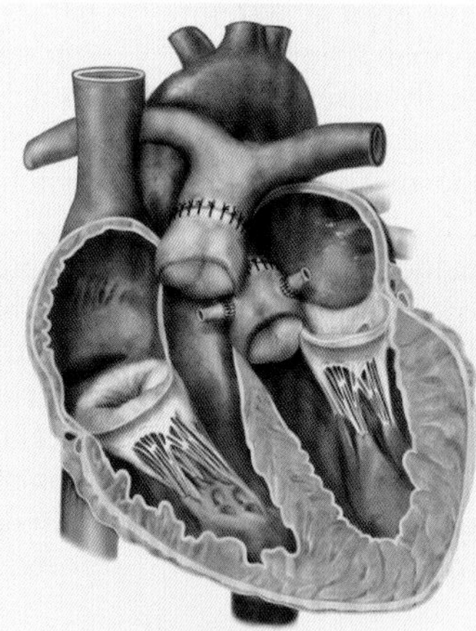	• Coronary artery ischemia or occlusion • Neoaortic root dilation • Neoaortic valve regurgitation • Supravalvular pulmonic stenosis • Supravalvular aortic stenosis • Branch PA stenosis
Rastelli operation	Performed in patients with TGA, VSD, and pulmonic stenosis. VSD patch is angled to direct blood across the VSD to the anterior aorta. The native pulmonic valve is oversewn, and an RV-to-PA conduit is placed.	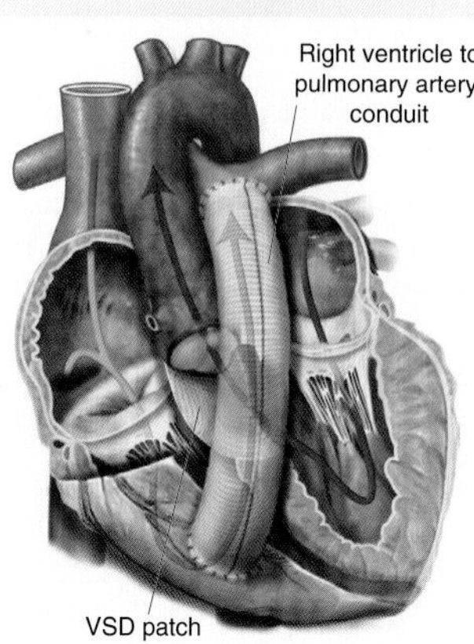	• RV-to-PA conduit stenosis and regurgitation • RV hypertension and dysfunction due to conduit obstruction • Multiple conduit replacements • VSD patch leak

PA, Pulmonary artery; *SVC*, superior vena cava; *TGA*, transposition of the great arteries; *VSD*, ventricular septal defect.

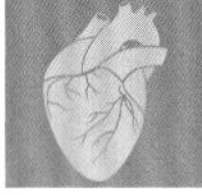

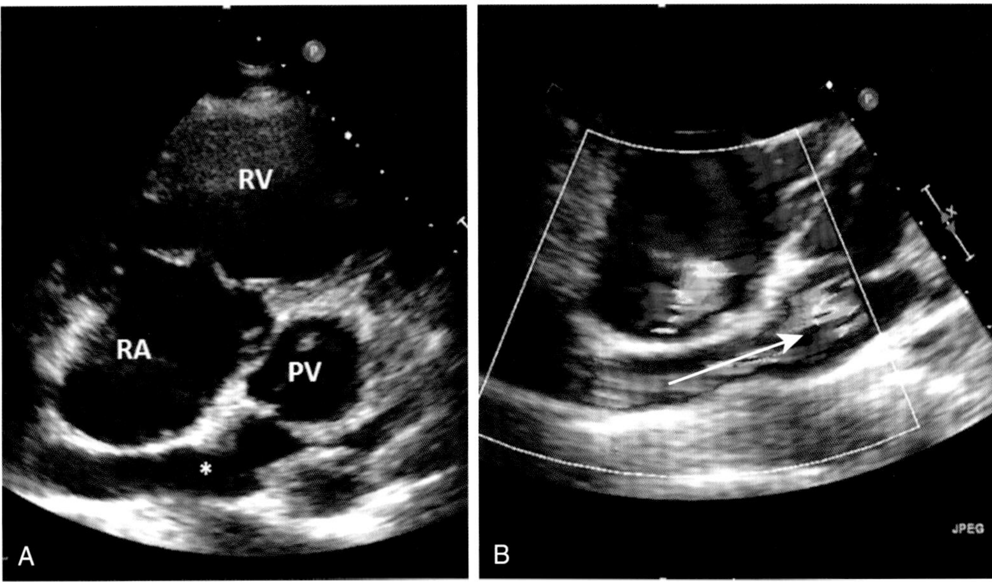

Fig. 45.1 **Systemic venous pathway after Mustard procedure.** 2D (A) and color Doppler (B) images of the superior limb of the systemic venous pathway in a patient with complete transposition of the great arteries who underwent a Mustard procedure (see Videos 45.1A and 45.1B). *PV*, Pulmonic valve.

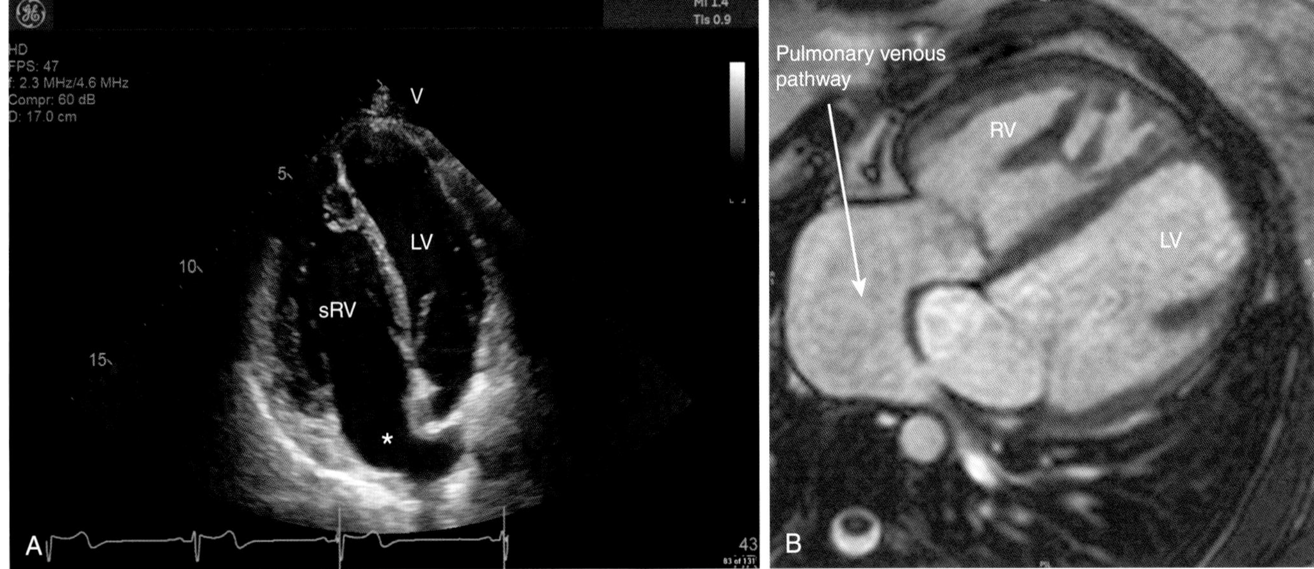

Fig. 45.2 **Pulmonary venous pathway after atrial switch procedure.** (A) Pulmonary venous pathway *(asterisk)* seen from an apical 4-chamber view in a patient with complete transposition of the great arteries and atrial switch procedure (see Video 45.2A). (B) Bright blood cardiac magnetic resonance image shows the pulmonary venous pathway (see Video 45.2B). *sRV*, Systemic RV, *LV*, subpulmonic LV.

EVALUATION OF THE POSTOPERATIVE PATIENT

Evaluation of the Patient After a Mustard or Senning Atrial Switch Procedure

The Mustard and Senning procedures were widely used from the 1960s to the late 1980s. Despite the inherent disadvantages of an sRV, a systemic tricuspid valve, and intraatrial baffles, the early and intermediate prognoses for children were very good. In one series of 132 patients who underwent a Senning operation, the surgical mortality rate was 5%. At 10 years of follow-up, more than 95% of the children had normal sRV systolic function, and very few had regurgitation of the systemic tricuspid valve. However, after 30 years, there is a frequent need for reintervention, onset of atrial arrhythmias, and a precipitous decline in ventricular function.[13,14] Patients with symptoms, RV dysfunction, or a pacemaker are at increased risk for death and ventricular arrhythmia (Fig. 45.3).

After an atrial switch procedure (i.e., Mustard or Senning operation), sinus node dysfunction occurs in more than one half of patients late after repair, likely due to scar and suture lines from the intraatrial baffles.[2,15,16] Approximately 5% to 10% of patients require a pacemaker, which can be technically challenging and can predispose to superior vena cava (SVC) limb obstruction. Reentrant atrial tachyarrhythmias are also common after the atrial switch procedure, occurring in 9% to 14% of patients, and they usually result from atrial scar and suture lines.[2,16]

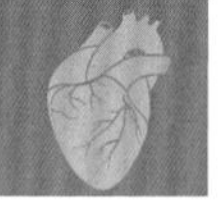

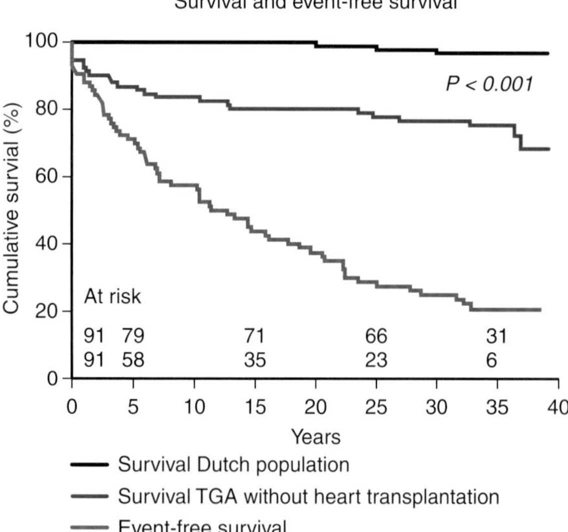

Fig. 45.3 Event-free survival after the Mustard procedure. Kaplan-Meier curves for survival without heart transplantation and event-free survival (i.e., free of heart transplantation, cardiac reinterventions, symptomatic arrhythmias, heart failure, or death). Results were compared with the survival curve for the Dutch population. (From Cuypers JA, Eindhoven JA, Slager MA, et al. The natural and unnatural history of the Mustard procedure: long-term outcome up to 40 years. *Eur Heart J.* 2014;35:1666–1674.)

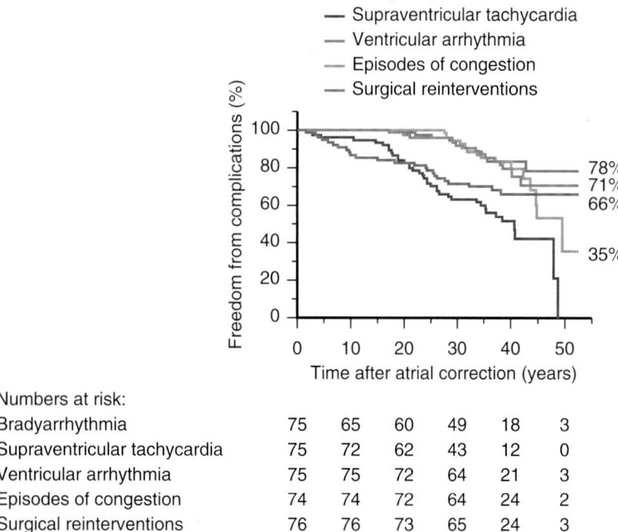

Numbers at risk:						
Bradyarrhythmia	75	65	60	49	18	3
Supraventricular tachycardia	75	72	62	43	12	0
Ventricular arrhythmia	75	75	72	64	21	3
Episodes of congestion	74	74	72	64	24	2
Surgical reinterventions	76	76	73	65	24	3

Fig. 45.4 Freedom from adverse events after an atrial switch procedure. Survival curves for freedom from adverse events for adults after atrial correction for transposition of the great arteries. (From Couperus LE, Vliegen HW, Zandstra TE, et al. Long-term outcome after atrial correction for transposition of the great arteries. *Heart.* 2019;105:790–796.)

Atrial arrhythmias are not well tolerated after the atrial switch procedure because rigid intraatrial baffles are limited in their ability to provide preload to the sRV and stroke volume decreases during tachycardia, regardless of contractility.[17] Likely for this reason, reentrant atrial tachycardia has been strongly linked to sudden death in this population.[18–20] Atrial arrhythmias typically manifest earlier, and ventricular arrhythmia and heart failure tend to manifest later[14] (Fig. 45.4).

Evaluation of exercise intolerance is important for patients with repaired TGA. Not surprisingly, symptomatic patients have a worse prognosis.[18] Exercise testing can often uncover impairment, even in patients who consider themselves to be well.[21] After an atrial switch procedure, impaired exercise performance has been associated with worse survival. Patients with ventilatory inefficiency (i.e., slope of minute ventilation vs. carbon dioxide production [V_E/V_{CO_2}] ≥ 35.4) or poor aerobic capacity (maximum oxygen uptake < 52% of predicted) have an increased 4-year risk of death or cardiac hospitalization.[22]

There are several goals of echocardiographic evaluation after an atrial switch procedure:

1. Determination of baffle stenosis and baffle leak
2. Qualitative and semiquantitative evaluation of sRV systolic function
3. Evaluation of severity and mechanisms of tricuspid valve regurgitation
4. Presence and severity of LVOTO (i.e., subpulmonic obstruction)
5. Estimation of subpulmonic LV systolic pressure and PA pressures
6. Evaluation of residual shunts

Baffle Complications

Stenosis in Venous Pathways. Baffle complications are common after an atrial switch procedure and are the most common indication for a repeat intervention. The prevalence of baffle complications depends on the definitions used. Partial obstruction of the systemic venous pathway (i.e., gradient of > 3 mmHg) occurred in more than 35% of patients, and was more common after a Mustard procedure than a Senning procedure.[2,23,24] Transvenous pacemaker or defibrillator leads also pose a risk for the development of pathway stenosis.[25]

Systemic venous pathway obstruction usually occurs in the SVC limb. Patients may present with symptoms of SVC syndrome, but many are asymptomatic because the SVC flow can decompress down the azygous vein. Pulmonary venous pathway obstruction is less common, occurring in approximately 5% of patients. Despite the high incidence of SVC limb pathway stenosis, most patients can be treated conservatively, and many do not require intervention, even in the setting of complete obstruction of the SVC limb. However, some patients develop symptoms, and many need a pacemaker after an atrial switch procedure, which sometimes necessitates treatment of SVC pathway stenosis.

Because venous pathways impose an important preload restriction on the heart, particularly during exercise, obstruction may manifest as exercise intolerance, exertional hypotension, or syncope.[17] In one series of 478 patients, 5% required reoperation for obstruction over a follow-up period of 12 years.[26] In the modern era, most baffle obstructions can be treated percutaneously with angioplasty and stents. In patients with transvenous pacemaker leads, leads typically are extracted before stenting to avoid jailing leads in the SVC limb.[27,28]

Obstruction within the venous pathways or stenosis is difficult to evaluate by transthoracic echocardiography (TTE), particularly in adults. Alternative imaging is usually necessary. The SVC is difficult to visualize by TTE after atrial switch procedures. The SVC limb should measure more than 0.8 × 1 cm by two-dimensional (2D) echocardiography, and the inferior vena cava (IVC) limb typically is slightly larger.[24,29] If the diameter is less than 0.5 cm, stenosis should be suspected.[24]

The SVC is seen from the suprasternal notch view, and color Doppler can show flow acceleration, which is specific but insensitive for baffle obstruction. By spectral Doppler, gradients of as low as 3 to 5 mmHg can be important in the venous system. Flow reversal in the azygous vein is seen in SVC obstruction. If the SVC flow is draining through the azygous system due to SVC limb obstruction, a gradient will not be seen. If SVC obstruction is suspected, injecting agitated saline in the arm while observing the IVC can be useful to see if the microbubbles return through the IVC, which confirms SVC limb obstruction.[30]

Despite these various techniques, the sensitivity of TTE is poor for the detection of obstruction. In one study of 49 patients with SVC limb stenosis, TTE had only a 16% sensitivity for detecting baffle stenosis.[31,32] Computed tomography (CT) or magnetic resonance imaging (MRI) can show pathway dimensions, and three-dimensional (3D) reconstructions can be made. Cardiac MRI using through-plane flow measurements through the azygous vein can demonstrate flow reversal; the flow should be traveling in the opposite direction to flow in the descending aorta, which can be used as a reference. If flow in the azygous is caudal, SVC limb obstruction is present.

Pulmonary venous pathway obstruction is less common than SVC limb obstruction. It usually occurs at the level where the systemic venous pathway impinges on the anastomosis between the right pulmonary veins and the right atrial (RA) free wall.[29] Pulmonary venous obstruction manifests as pulmonary hypertension, pulmonary edema, or exertional intolerance. Surgery is often used to relieve pulmonary venous pathway obstruction, but there are several reports of successful angioplasty and stent deployment.[27,33]

Baffle Leaks. Baffle leaks represent a defect between the pulmonary venous pathway and the systemic venous pathway. Shunt direction depends on the relative ventricular compliance of the sRV and subpulmonic LV. In most adults who have undergone an atrial switch procedure, the sRV is dilated and dysfunctional, and it has a higher diastolic pressure. Shunt direction is typically from the pulmonary venous pathway into the systemic venous pathway and does not lead to cyanosis. Shunts can be detected by color Doppler imaging from a posteriorly angulated 4-chamber apical view.

If a baffle leak is suspected, an agitated saline injection should be performed. Shunts often occur at the junction between the pulmonary venous and systemic venous pathways. Agitated saline injection can aid in the detection of shunts; bubbles should not appear in the sRV. A baffle leak typically leads to volume loading of the subpulmonic LV and reduced systemic cardiac output.

Baffle leaks can be bidirectional, and the shunt direction can depend on activity. Due to loading conditions, the shunt may go from right to left during exercise, causing desaturation even with minimal exertion. Erythrocytosis can be a clue to a baffle leak with a right-to-left component, and desaturation with exercise should be elicited.[34] Baffle leaks also pose a risk of paradoxical embolization, particularly in patients with thrombogenic transvenous pacing leads.[35] Like baffle stenosis, baffle leaks are more common in the SVC limb than in the IVC limb.[27]

Clinically important baffle leaks can usually be closed with covered stents or with an atrial septal occluder device.[34] Periprocedurally, transesophageal echocardiography (TEE) or intracardiac echocardiography can be used to guide closure (Fig. 45.5).

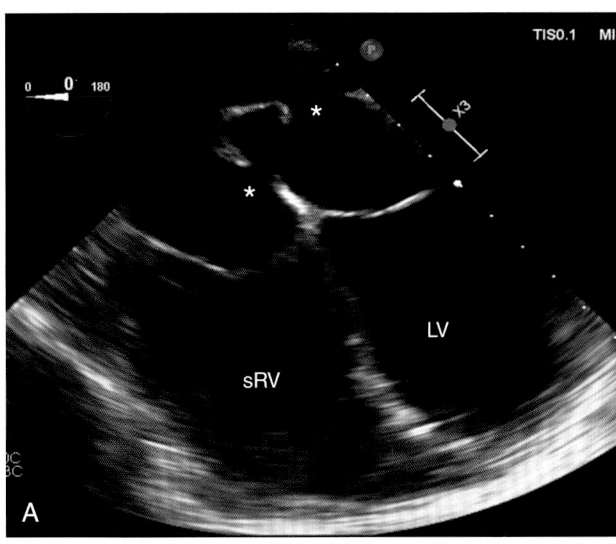

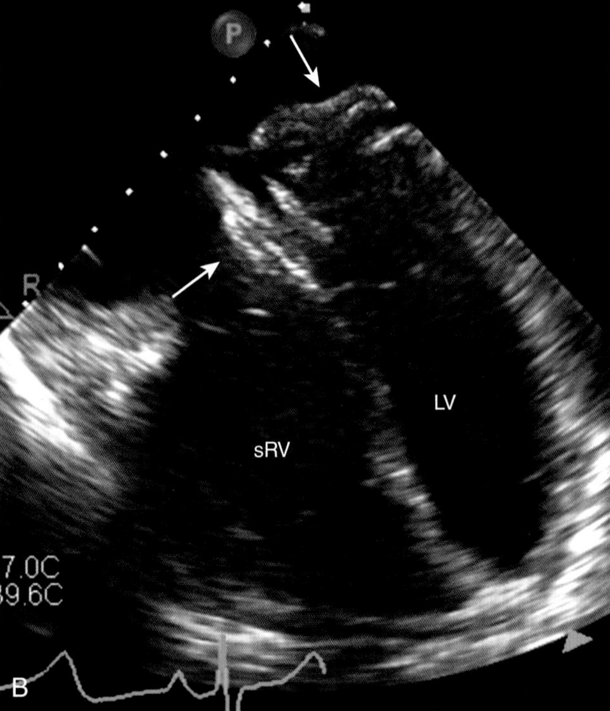

Fig. 45.5 **Baffle leak after an atrial switch procedure.** TEE of a patient with two baffle leaks between the pulmonary venous pathway and the systemic venous pathway. (A) Baffle leaks are denoted by *asterisks*. (see Video 45.5A). (B) Both leaks were closed with atrial septal defect closure devices *(arrows)* (see Video 45.5B). *sRV*, Systemic RV.

Evaluation of the Systemic RV and Tricuspid Valve

Patients who have undergone an atrial switch procedure for complete TGA have an sRV pumping to the aorta. sRV function remains normal in most children after an atrial switch procedure, which contributed to early enthusiasm for the procedure.[36] However, sRV systolic function deteriorates over time. By the fourth decade, approximately 25% of patients who had a Mustard procedure developed systolic dysfunction and heart failure.[2,19]

In a longitudinal study of 91 atrial switch patients followed for more than 40 years, most developed sRV systolic dysfunction. At 36 years of age, only 2% of patients had normal sRV function. sRV systolic dysfunction was mild in 23%, moderate in 60%, and severe in 15% of patients at late follow-up.[2]

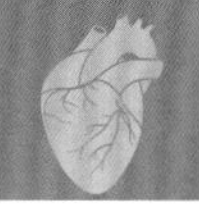

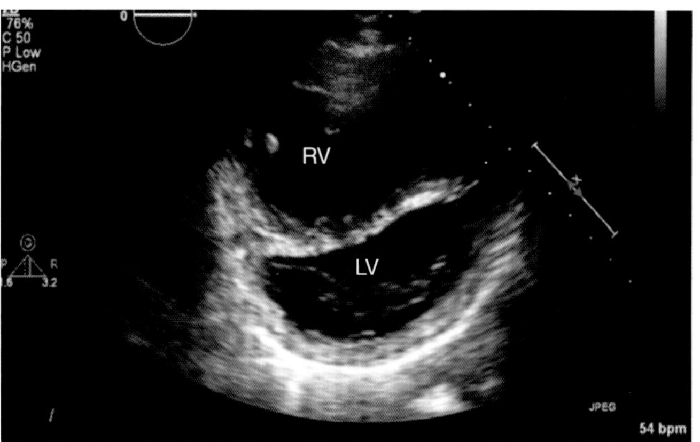

Fig. 45.6 Parasternal short-axis view after atrial switch procedure. Parasternal short-axis view of a patient with complete transposition of the great arteries shows that the RV is large and hypertrophied and the LV is compressed. The flattened interventricular septum is consistent with RV pressure overload (see Video 45.6). *LV*, Subpulmonic LV; *RV*, systemic RV.

Other than older age, there have been discrepant reports about risk factors for the development of RV dysfunction; some studies found that older age of the patient at the time of repair, tricuspid regurgitation (TR), and VSD were associated with sRV deterioration.[2,19,37] Some reports suggest that sRV function may be superior after the Senning operation, but these results are speculative.[19]

Quantitative evaluation of sRV function by echocardiography is difficult. Because interobserver variability is high for measurements such as RV ejection fraction and fractional shortening, they are of limited use for developing normative data or monitoring a patient over time.[38] Quantitative measures such as fractional area change correlate poorly with the MRI-derived ejection fraction ($r^2 = 0.2$), and other measures perform even worse.[39] 3D echocardiography from multiple planes can add to accuracy, but it is rarely performed because it requires specialized software and is time-consuming.[40]

In clinical practice, description of sRV function by echocardiography is usually qualitative. In short-axis views, the RV is large and hypertrophied. The septum bows from right to left, and the LV is often compressed (Fig. 45.6). Reference values for normal sRV function are lacking. In a large cross-sectional study of adults late after the Mustard procedure, the mean fractional area change of the RV was 25%, the mean tricuspid annular plane systolic excursion (TAPSE) was 1.3 cm, and the mean systolic tissue velocity at the tricuspid annulus (S′) was 7.5 cm/s; similar values have been found by others.[41,42] Compared with other quantitative markers, TAPSE has the strongest association with clinical status and exercise performance.[42] Compared with cardiac MRI, echocardiography typically underestimates the sRV ejection fraction.[43]

Evaluation of Tricuspid Regurgitation

After an atrial switch procedure, the tricuspid valve functions as the systemic AV valve. Like sRV dysfunction, TR progresses over time. Only 2% of adolescents have severe TR, but by the fourth decade 38% have severe TR.[2] TR typically results from sRV dysfunction (i.e., functional TR). In almost all cases, sRV dysfunction precedes severe TR, suggesting that TR results from ventricular dilation. In contrast, patients with congenitally corrected TGA are more likely to have a morphologically abnormal tricuspid valve and primary TR that precipitates sRV dysfunction.

A mechanism of TR in this population is a leftward septal shift due to sRV pressure overload. This pulls the leaflets of the tricuspid valve apart and can lead to TR, which contributes to sRV failure. Occasionally, PA banding can be used to pressure-load the subpulmonic LV, shift the septum rightward, and reduce the degree of TR. Because this procedure carries a high surgical risk, is palliative, and can precipitate LV failure, it is rarely performed.[44,45]

TR should be evaluated using an integrated approach, including color Doppler, pulmonary vein flow pattern, and density of the spectral Doppler jet. Because the tricuspid valve is the systemic AV valve, the velocity of the tricuspid jet cannot be used to estimate PA pressures.

Evaluation of LV Outflow Tract Obstruction

LVOTO occurs in 20% to 30% of patients with TGA. After an atrial switch procedure, LVOTO is functionally subpulmonic stenosis. The various mechanisms of LVOTO include a discrete subpulmonic ridge, posterior malalignment VSD, anomalous insertion of mitral chords in the interventricular septum, focal septal hypertrophy, and systolic anterior motion of the mitral valve.

Conceptually, LVOTO can be beneficial in some patients after an atrial switch procedure because a pressure-loaded LV can maintain an interventricular septum position more in the midline and therefore can prevent TR due to unfavorable septal position. Nonetheless, LVOTO is a common reason for reoperation after an atrial switch operation.[19]

LVOTO can be evaluated using 2D and Doppler echocardiography. From parasternal long-axis views, the LVOT can be evaluated to determine the mechanism of obstruction. Pulsed-wave (PW) spectral Doppler with apical views can be used to "march through" the LVOT to determine the level of obstruction. Continuous-wave (CW) Doppler should be used to determine the maximum instantaneous gradient through the LVOT. In the context of LVOTO, the LVOT gradient should be subtracted from the mitral regurgitation jet velocity to estimate the PA systolic pressure.

Evaluation of the Patient After an Arterial Switch Operation

In the ASO, the aorta and main PA are transected above the sinotubular junction. The aorta is brought posterior and anastomosed to the native pulmonic root (which becomes the *neoaortic root*). The pulmonary arteries are brought anterior, the PA bifurcation is typically draped across the ascending aorta (i.e., Lecompte maneuver), and the PA is anastomosed to the native aortic valve, which becomes the *neopulmonic valve* (Fig. 45.7). In the most technically demanding part of the operation, the coronary arteries are transposed from the native aortic root to the neoaortic root, which can lead to coronary artery injury or kinking.

The ASO became the operation of choice for complete TGA in most centers by the early 1990s. The appeal of the ASO over the atrial switch procedure is that patients have a systemic LV and the mitral valve serves as the systemic AV valve. However, the operation is technically challenging, requiring coronary artery transfer, anterior translocation of the PA bifurcation, and intracardiac surgery for those with associated defects. In the first 5 years of the ASO, the operative mortality rate was high, particularly at centers with low surgical volumes.[10,46] With experience, surgical results improved by the late 1990s. In contemporary series, the operative mortality rate is less than 3%

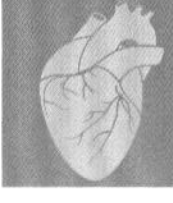

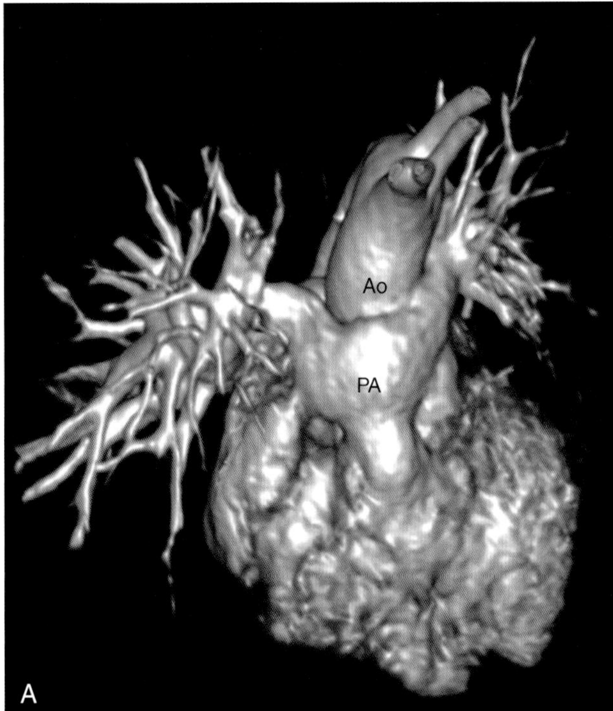

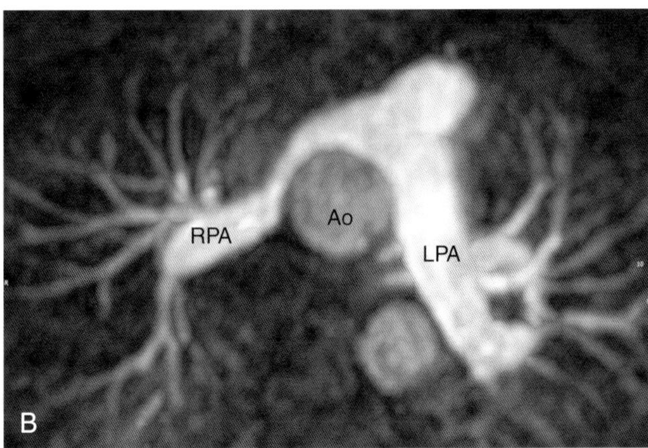

Fig. 45.7 Lecompte maneuver. (A) 3D volume-rendered magnetic resonance angiogram in a patient with complete transposition of the great arteries who underwent an arterial switch operation *(ASO)* shows the pulmonary arteries *(PAs)* draped over the aorta after the Lecompte maneuver (see Video 47.7A). (B) Contrast-enhanced magnetic resonance angiogram in the axial plane shows the pulmonary arteries draped over the aorta after the Lecompte maneuver as part of the arterial switch operation. The right pulmonary artery *(RPA)* is narrowed. *Ao*, Ascending aorta; *LPA*, left pulmonary artery; *TGA*, transposition of the great arteries.

for patients without complex associated defects. Surgical risk is higher for those who have associated defects, patients who require aortic arch reconstruction, or those who have coronary anomalies.[12,47]

Long-term results after the ASO are better than late outcomes after a Mustard or Senning procedure. The late mortality rate is less than 1%.[12] At age 20, almost all patients with an ASO are asymptomatic, whereas 58% of patients with a Mustard procedure have New York Heart Association (NYHA) class II or III symptoms. Atrial switch patients have a higher N-terminal pro B-type natriuretic peptide (NT-proBNP) level than patients who underwent an ASO. Pacemakers are rare after an ASO, but about 40% of patients undergoing an atrial switch procedure require a pacemaker.[11,48]

TABLE 45.3 Postoperative Sequelae After the Arterial Switch Operation.

Long-Term Postoperative Sequelae	*Incidence (%)*
Supravalvular pulmonary stenosis	10
Supravalvular aortic stenosis	5
Neoaortic dilation	>75
Neoaortic regurgitation	~50
Coronary artery obstruction	2–7

Modified from Villafane J, Lantin-Hermoso MR, Bhatt AB, et al. d-Transposition of the great arteries: the current era of the arterial switch operation. *J Am Coll Cardiol.* 2014;64(5):498–511.

It is a truism of adult congenital heart disease that no patient with complex disease is ever cured, no matter how good the surgical technique, and the ASO is no exception. Several late complications undergoing ASO require surveillance and, occasionally, intervention (Table 45.3).

Goals of the echocardiogram after an ASO include the following:

1. Assess for neoaortic dilation
2. Assess for neoaortic regurgitation
3. Assess for supravalvular and branch pulmonic stenosis
4. Evaluate LV function and regional wall motion abnormalities suggesting coronary artery disease

Neoaortic Root After an Arterial Switch Operation

After an ASO, the neoaortic root (which is native PA tissue) is prone to dilation when subjected to systemic arterial pressure. Late dilation of the neoaortic root occurs, but is not severe, in most adults after an ASO.[49] At 15 years of follow-up, only 32% to 56% of patients have normal aortic dimensions, but only 5% of patients have a maximum dimension greater than 4 cm.[50,51] The rate of growth of the neoaortic root is slow for most, and growth further stabilizes in adulthood.[51] Significant neoaortic dilation of more than 4.5 cm occurs in 13% of patients, and neoaortic dilation of more than 5 cm occurs in 5%. Fortunately, dissection and rupture are rare, and there have been only isolated case reports.

The neoaortic root can be evaluated by echocardiography using conventional techniques such as 2D TTE with the parasternal long-axis view and M-mode echocardiography.[52] Conventionally, most pediatric echocardiographic laboratories report aortic dimensions in systole, when dimensions are largest, but adult laboratories report dimensions in diastole, and these measurements are most reproducible. For patients transitioning from a pediatric to an adult program, the providers should compare side-by-side images.

Neoaortic Regurgitation

After an ASO, the native pulmonic valve functions as the neoaortic valve. Like neoaortic dilation, neoaortic valve regurgitation occurs after the ASO. Risk factors for neoaortic regurgitation include aortic regurgitation at the time of hospital discharge, a VSD, a bicuspid neoaortic valve, previous PA banding, perioperative neoaortic regurgitation, and a discrepancy between the size of the native PA and that of the aorta before surgery.[10,51–53]

The prevalence of at least moderate neoaortic regurgitation varies between 3% and 25% at 15 years of follow-up.[51,53,54] However, severe aortic regurgitation is rare, and less than 5% of patients need reoperation for aortic valve dysfunction at 20 years of follow-up.[53]

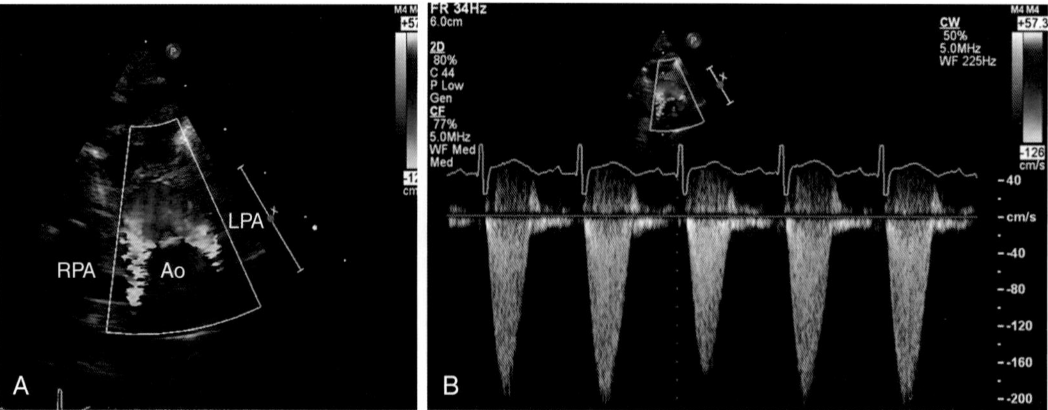

Fig. 45.8 Color and spectral Doppler of the arterial switch procedure. (A) Color Doppler imaging shows the branch pulmonary arteries draped over the aorta after the Lecompte maneuver in a patient with complete transposition of the great arteries. (B) Spectral Doppler shows mild flow acceleration across the right pulmonary artery. *Ao*, Aorta; *LPA*, left pulmonary artery; *RPA*, right pulmonary artery.

Aortic regurgitation should be evaluated from multiple windows, including the parasternal short-axis, long-axis, and apical windows. The color Doppler signal gives clues to the severity of aortic regurgitation, which is usually central and probably related to annular dilation. The deceleration slope and density of the spectral Doppler signal should be evaluated, and flow reversal in the descending aorta should be sought.

Supravalvular and Branch Pulmonary Artery Stenosis

PA stenosis occurs in more than one half of patients by 20 years after an ASO, and it is the most common reason for late reintervention.[54] Two areas can be affected by supravalvular pulmonic stenosis. PA trunk stenosis occurs at the anastomosis of the native aorta and PA, and branch PA stenosis occurs beyond the PA bifurcation, where the branches drape across the ascending aorta.

PA trunk stenosis can occur after the coronary arteries are excised from the native aortic root and transferred to the neoaortic root. This can cause narrowing in the neopulmonic root, particularly if the entire sinus is removed with the coronary arteries and patch reconstruction of the neopulmonic valve is required. When smaller coronary artery buttons are used, the risk of supravalvular pulmonic stenosis is lower.[55,56] Color Doppler imaging can show flow disturbance just above the level of the neopulmonic valve. Marching PW Doppler through the right ventricular outflow tract (RVOT) and the valve can delineate the level of obstruction. Balloon dilation is sometimes successful in managing supravalvular PA stenosis, although rebound is common.

Branch PA narrowing can occur in the PA because of the Lecompte maneuver. The PA bifurcation is very anterior after an ASO, and evaluation by echocardiography is difficult. The branch PAs can be seen from the high parasternal window or the suprasternal notch. PW and CW Doppler imaging should be performed in the branch PAs to assess for stenosis (Fig. 45.8). Gradients may not be very high in unilateral PA stenosis because flow can be diverted to the contralateral PA and low flow generates a low gradient.

Peripheral PA stenosis can be evaluated using alternative imaging techniques. Through-plane MRI in the right and left PAs or nuclear perfusion scans can demonstrate asymmetric pulmonary blood flow. Hemodynamically significant unilateral PA stenosis typically causes at least 70% of the blood flow to go to the contralateral lung.

Peripheral PA stenosis can usually be successfully treated with stent implantation. In the setting of PA stenosis, it is difficult to estimate distal PA pressure from the TR jet.

Coronary Artery Disease After the Arterial Switch Operation

Coronary artery transfer is the most technically difficult component of the ASO, particularly in the 35% of TGA patients with coronary anomalies. In the early era of the ASO, coronary artery complications were a common cause of early death after the operation. Coronary complications typically manifest within the first year of life but can manifest later.

The risk of clinically significant late coronary complications is less well defined. Coronary artery obstruction appears in 5% to 7% of ASO survivors, although this complication is likely declining as surgical technique improves.[10,54,57] Spontaneous coronary events in adults are rare after an ASO. In one study with 20 years of follow-up, coronary artery disease was identified in 5% of patients, but there were no acute coronary events beyond infancy.[54] Previously, centers performed routine angiography for all survivors of the ASO, leading to high rates of detection of asymptomatic coronary artery stenosis.[58]

The optimal protocol for surveillance of coronary complications is unknown. Resting wall motion abnormalities or LV systolic dysfunction should raise suspicion for coronary artery disease. The 2018 consensus guidelines on the management of adults with congenital heart disease suggest that it is reasonable to perform an evaluation of the coronary arteries with angiography, coronary CT, or MRI after an ASO. Symptomatic patients can be evaluated with functional testing or angiography.[59]

Evaluation of the Patient After a Rastelli Operation

The Rastelli operation is performed for patients with a complete TGA, VSD, and LVOTO (subpulmonic stenosis). A VSD patch is aligned to direct oxygenated blood across the VSD to the anterior aorta. The native pulmonic valve is oversewn, and an RV-to-PA conduit is placed to establish a pulmonary circulation (see Table 45.2). After the Rastelli operation, the patient has relief of cyanosis, a systemic LV, and a subpulmonic RV.

Late complications include dysfunction of the RV-to-PA conduit, VSD baffle stenosis, or complete heart block, particularly if the VSD needs to be enlarged at the time of surgical repair. Some centers have moved away from the Rastelli procedure in favor of an aortic translocation (Nikaidoh) procedure with reconstruction of the RVOT to avoid late outflow tract obstruction.

Conduit dysfunction is common. Most patients require reoperation for conduit stenosis before adulthood, with up to 40% needing reoperation in early childhood.[60] Multiple reoperations are common, and this increases the risk of a surgical mishap in patients undergoing repeated sternotomy incisions, particularly because the conduit can become adherent to the underside of the sternum.

Evaluation of the conduit by echocardiography should assess for stenosis and regurgitation. Because the conduit is located very anteriorly, extreme angulation of the transducer may be required to align the image with the direction of the conduit. A peak conduit velocity of 2 to 3 m/s is typical for a normally functioning conduit. A velocity of more than 4 m/s suggests significant conduit stenosis. Mean Doppler gradients correlate better with catheter-measured gradients. The RV systolic pressure is evaluated by tricuspid regurgitant jet assessment. An elevated RV pressure is seen with conduit stenosis. Most adults with dysfunctional PA conduits can be treated with percutaneous valve implantation.

LVOTO can occur after the Rastelli procedure. If the VSD was not large enough, subaortic obstruction can occur. To image the LVOT, the echocardiographer needs to know that the aorta is located anteriorly, and the image planes should be adjusted to show the flow across the VSD to the anterior aorta.

CONGENITALLY CORRECTED TRANSPOSITION OF THE GREAT ARTERIES

ANATOMY AND DEFINITIONS

Congenitally corrected transposition of the great arteries (CCTGA) is also called L-loop transposition of the great arteries or physiologically corrected transposition of the great arteries. CCTGA is a rare congenital heart lesion defined as AV discordance with ventriculoarterial discordance (Fig. 45.9). Blood returns to the heart through the systemic veins to the RA and flows through the mitral valve to the right-sided morphologic LV before being ejected into the PA. In a similar fashion, pulmonary veins return to the left atrium, and blood flows through the tricuspid valve into the left-sided systemic morphologic RV and is ejected into the aorta.

The circulation is physiologically correct because deoxygenated blood is delivered to the lungs and oxygenated blood is delivered to the systemic circulation. However, because of abnormal ventricular looping leading to ventricular inversion, the RV acts as the systemic ventricle. Because the AV valves are derived embryologically from their respective ventricles, the subpulmonic AV valve in CCTGA is the mitral valve, and the systemic AV valve is the tricuspid valve. Although CCTGA can occur in isolation, it is more commonly associated with other congenital cardiac defects (Table 45.4).

Approximately 10% of patients with CCTGA have dextrocardia. The coronary arteries are almost always inverted and follow their anatomic ventricles: the left coronary artery arises from the right anterior aortic sinus, and the right coronary artery arises from the left posterior aortic sinus. The conduction system is characterized by dual AV node physiology with inverted His bundle branches. As a consequence, patients with CCTGA experience a high incidence of AV block.

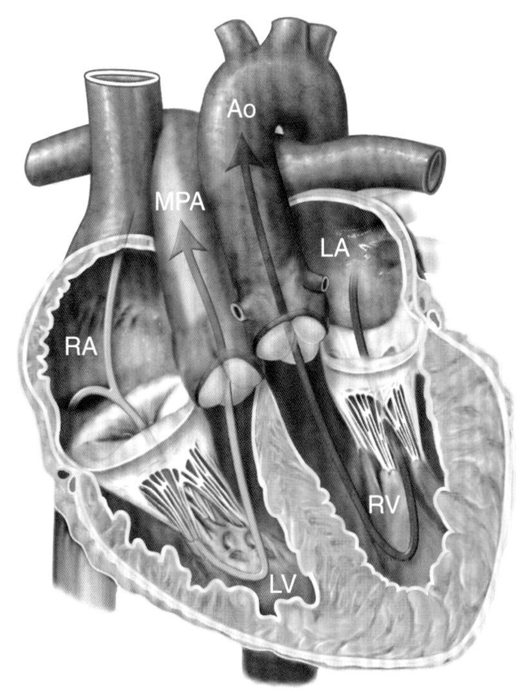

Fig. 45.9 Anatomy of congenitally corrected transposition of the great arteries. In congenitally corrected transposition of the great arteries, there is ventricular inversion along with transposed great arteries. Blood flow is physiologically correct, but the RV is the systemic ventricle, and the tricuspid valve is the systemic atrioventricular valve. *Ao*, Aorta; *MPA*, main pulmonary artery.

TABLE 45.4 Anomalies Associated With Congenitally Corrected Transposition of the Great Arteries.

Defect Type	*Incidence (%)*	*Comments*
Ventricular septal defect	60–80	Perimembranous type most common
Pulmonary outflow obstruction	30–50	Often found with ventricular septal defect May be valvular or subvalvular
Tricuspid valve abnormalities	14–56	Ebstein-like malformation of the tricuspid valve Predisposes to RV dysfunction

The clinical presentation of patients with CCTGA is dictated by the associated cardiac anomalies. A patient without associated anomalies may escape detection until an older age, but patients with a VSD or LVOTO are most commonly diagnosed prenatally or shortly after birth. RV systolic dysfunction and congestive heart failure are common among patients with CCTGA, particularly for those with TR. sRV failure may be the initial presenting symptom[61] (Fig. 45.10).

EPIDEMIOLOGY

CCTGA is rare, accounting for less than 0.5% of congenital heart disease, and there is a slight male predominance. It is 10 times less common than complete TGA. Although an underlying genetic cause for CCTGA is unknown, recurrence rates for congenital heart disease are elevated among siblings of patients with CCTGA from unaffected parents.[62]

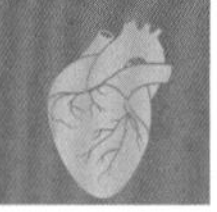

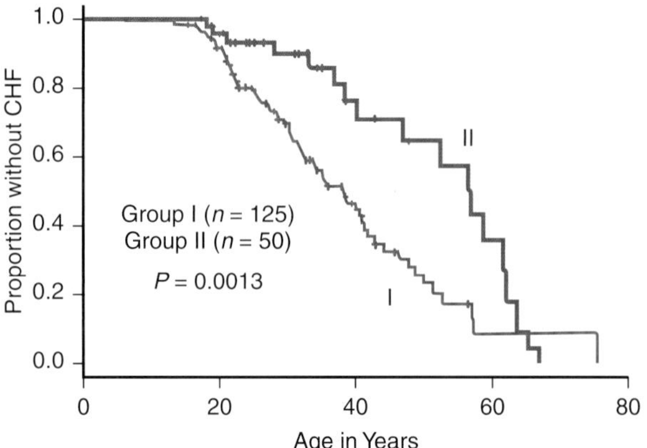

Fig. 45.10 Freedom from congestive heart failure in patients with congenitally corrected transposition of the great arteries with or without associated lesions. Probability of freedom from congestive heart failure *(CHF)* is plotted for group I (patients with associated lesions) and group II (patients with no significant associated lesions) as a function of increasing age. *N* = 175 instead of 182 because it was unclear whether 7 patients had clinical CHF. (From Graham TP Jr, Bernard YD, Mellen BG, et al. Long-term outcome in congenitally corrected transposition of the great arteries: a multiinstitutional study. *J Am Coll Cardiol.* 2000;36:255–261.)

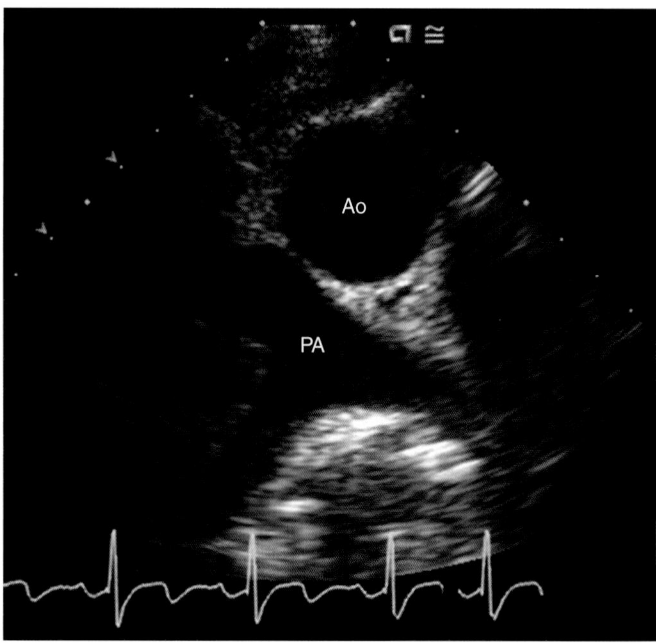

Fig. 45.11 Relationship of the aorta and pulmonary artery in congenitally corrected transposition of the great arteries. High parasternal short-axis view shows that the aorta is anterior and leftward (L-transposed great arteries) in a patient with congenitally corrected transposition of the great arteries (see Video 45.11). *Ao,* Aorta; *PA,* pulmonary artery.

TABLE 45.5 Surgical Strategies for Congenitally Corrected Transposition of the Great Arteries.

Associated Defect	*Physiologic Repair*	*Anatomic Repair (Double-Switch)*
None	No repair needed	Arterial switch and atrial switch procedures
VSD	VSD closure	VSD closure, arterial switch and atrial switch
VSD with pulmonary stenosis or atresia	VSD closure with LV-to-PA conduit	Atrial switch plus Rastelli with RV-to-PA conduit *or* hemi-Mustard with cavopulmonary anastomosis plus Rastelli procedure

PA, Pulmonary artery; *VSD,* ventricular septal defect.

SURGICAL REPAIR

Babies born with CCTGA and no associated defects do not require operations. There are two strategies for surgical management for babies born with CCTGA (Table 45.5):

1. A physiologic approach repairs associated lesions (e.g., VSDs, LVOTO) but maintains the RV as the systemic ventricle and the LV as the subpulmonic ventricle.
2. An anatomic approach (i.e., double-switch operation) reorients the LV to the systemic circulation and the RV to the subpulmonic position. This is done through a combination of atrial venous baffles with ventricular rerouting by a surgically created baffle (i.e., Rastelli operation) or an ASO.

The surgical strategy is influenced by the age of the patient, the feasibility of anatomic repair, and the preferences of the center and patient. Occasionally, distinct features of associated cardiac abnormalities preclude a particular strategy (e.g., a coronary abnormality may be a contraindication to an ASO), making a physiologic repair more appealing.

Patients with isolated CCTGA may not be diagnosed in childhood, coming to medical attention only at an older age with symptoms of a failing sRV or heart block. A late double-switch operation is rarely performed because the subpulmonic LV becomes detrained after prolonged exposure to low pulmonary arterial pressures.[63,64] Intermediate and long-term morbidity and mortality rates were comparable for anatomic and physiologic repairs.[65,66]

The two surgical strategies are different in terms of needing reoperation. Patients after physiologic repair may require repeat operations—most commonly conduit replacement, tricuspid valve replacement, and pacemaker implantation—at approximately 10 years after the initial procedure. Patients who have had a physiologic repair also have more systemic AV valve regurgitation and more systemic ventricular systolic dysfunction.[65]

Late Outcomes and Echocardiographic Evaluation

Physiologic Repair

Evaluation of Anatomy. The basic anatomy of CCTGA with levocardia after physiologic repair is identified by TTE; L-looping of the ventricles and L-transposition of the great arteries (i.e., the aorta is anterior and leftward of the PA) should be demonstrated. The morphologic LV with its corresponding mitral valve is on the right, and the morphologic RV and tricuspid valve are on the left. A morphologic LV has fine apical trabeculations and a smooth septal surface; the AV valve should have the typical morphology of a mitral valve without septal chordal attachments. A morphologic RV is coarsely trabeculated with a moderator band. The AV valve of the RV is the tricuspid valve with chordal attachments to the septum. The aorta arises from the sRV, anterior to and leftward of the PA, which arises from the subpulmonic LV (Fig. 45.11).

Attention should also focus on the residual VSD, the LVOTO, and the structure and function of the AV valves, particularly the systemic tricuspid valve. RV systolic function should be evaluated (see later discussion). Acoustic windows can be difficult, particularly in patients with mesocardia or dextrocardia. TEE or cardiac MRI should be considered if the quality of TTE is poor.[67]

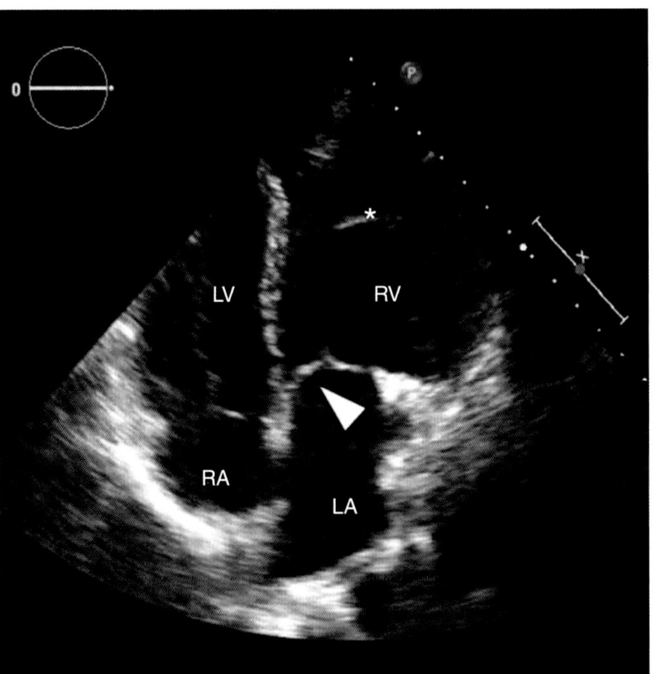

Fig. 45. 12 **Apical 4-chamber view of congenitally corrected transposition of the great arteries.** Apical 4-chamber view shows the atrial and ventricular orientations in congenitally corrected transposition of the great arteries (see Video 45.12). The apically offset tricuspid valve *(ar)* and moderator band *(asterisk)* are shown.

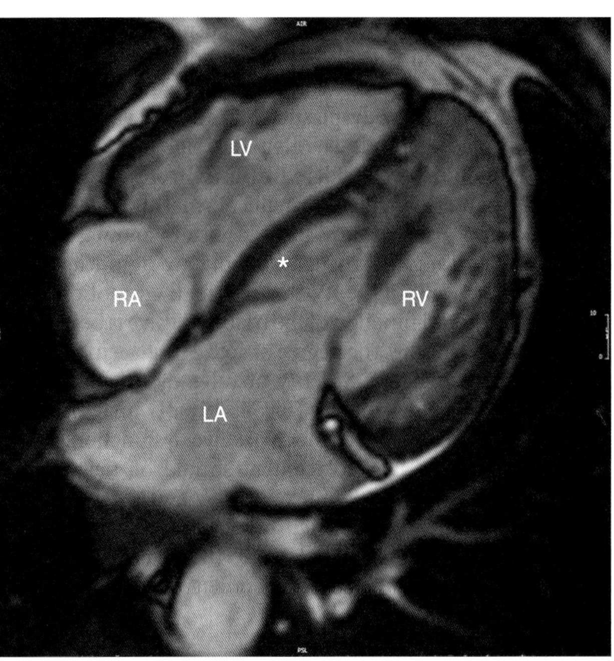

Fig. 45.13 **A 4-chamber cardiac MRI of congenitally corrected transposition of the great arteries.** Bright blood cine MRI 4-chamber view shows the atrial and ventricular orientation in congenitally corrected transposition of the great arteries. *Asterisk* indicates the apically offset septal leaflet of the tricuspid valve. *LV,* Subpulmonic left ventricle; *RV,* systemic right ventricle.

In patients with good subcostal windows, the long-axis plane can demonstrate ventricular looping and the distinct morphologic features of the ventricles. A long-axis sweep can demonstrate the position of the great arteries. The posterior vessel arises from the right-sided LV and bifurcates, identifying it as the PA. The aorta arises anteriorly from the morphologic RV, which can also be identified as the great vessel that gives rise to the head and neck vessels. The outflow tracts have a side-by-side configuration and do not cross each other as in normally related great arteries.

The LVOTO (i.e., subpulmonic stenosis) is identified by the application of color and spectral Doppler. A subcostal short-axis sweep should also be performed and should confirm the ventricular morphology by identification of the presence or absence of chordal attachments to the septum. The position of the great artery can be confirmed in the short-axis view, and an anterior and leftward aorta is seen. The parallel configuration of the great arteries can be seen. Residual VSDs can be assessed by color Doppler focused on the ventricular septum. Color and spectral Doppler imaging can demonstrate outflow tract obstruction or valve insufficiency.

Apical imaging should demonstrate ventricular morphology and systolic function (Fig. 45.12), and it is useful for AV valve assessment. Any apical displacement of the right-sided tricuspid valve should be noted, and a functional assessment should be carried out with Doppler imaging. A residual VSD or outflow tract obstruction also can be demonstrated. Anterior angulation brings the outflow tracts into view and can demonstrate outflow tract obstruction or valve regurgitation.

Parasternal imaging in the long axis is usually challenging in CCTGA because of the loss of the normal anterior-posterior relationship of the ventricles. It is difficult to align the outflow tract with its respective AV valve because of a side-by-side orientation of the ventricles. It is common for an echocardiographer unfamiliar with CCTGA to align the right-sided pulmonary valve with the left-sided tricuspid valve, giving a false impression of ventricular-arterial concordance. To prevent this, the transducer should be more aligned to the plane of the body.

RV Dysfunction. Congestive heart failure resulting from sRV dysfunction is common, particularly in patients with TR.[61] Given the natural history of progressive sRV dysfunction, functional assessment of the sRV is paramount in the evaluation CCTGA after physiologic repair. There are several mechanisms of sRV systolic dysfunction. They include inherent morphologic characteristics of the RV, which make it inefficient at pumping against systemic pressures, and the tricuspid valve, which predisposes it to regurgitation when exposed to systemic arterial pressures. The sRV in CCTGA may have impaired myocardial blood flow as a contributor to systolic dysfunction.[68]

Echocardiographic assessment of sRV function is difficult. Because of the geometric changes of the sRV and its contractility pattern, conventional echocardiography parameters used to evaluate RV systolic function may not be applicable in patients with an sRV. Cardiac MRI has become the gold standard because of its reproducibility for quantitative RV assessment[38,69] (Figs. 45.13 and 45.14). However, some echocardiographic techniques may identify patients with an abnormal sRV ejection fraction (Table 45.6). They include an sRV fractional area change of less than 33%, *dP/dt* assessment of less than 1000 mmHg/s, and a myocardial performance index of less than 0.4 to 0.53.[39,70,71]

Some studies have found that a TAPSE value of less than 14 mm is associated with an abnormal sRV ejection fraction.[38,39,70] A global longitudinal strain of less than −14.2% is associated with a normal sRV ejection fraction.[70,72] Impaired global longitudinal strain correlates with an elevated NT-proBNP level and worsening NYHA class.[73]

Tricuspid Valve Regurgitation. Tricuspid valve dysfunction is strongly associated with the development of heart failure and sRV dysfunction in patients with CCTGA.[61] The tricuspid valve in CCTGA is frequently dysplastic and can have various degrees of apical displacement. It is often described as Ebstein-like, although it should be considered distinct from classic Ebstein anomaly. The anterior leaflet is usually normal and does not have the sail-like appearance found in true Ebstein anomaly, and the septal and posterior leaflets usually do not have significant attachments along the walls of the RV that restrict their motion.

The structure and function of the tricuspid valve is best assessed from the apical window. The degree of apical displacement is demonstrated by 2D imaging. Severity of valve dysfunction may be demonstrated by color Doppler (Fig. 45.15). 3D imaging may be helpful in qualifying the mechanism of valve dysfunction.[74]

Early tricuspid valve replacement should be performed in patients with significant TR to prevent sRV systolic dysfunction. Although sRV function and tricuspid valve function are linked, the degree of TR may not be related to the severity of sRV dysfunction.[75] Tricuspid replacement is preferred to tricuspid valve repair, which is rarely durable.[65,76,77]

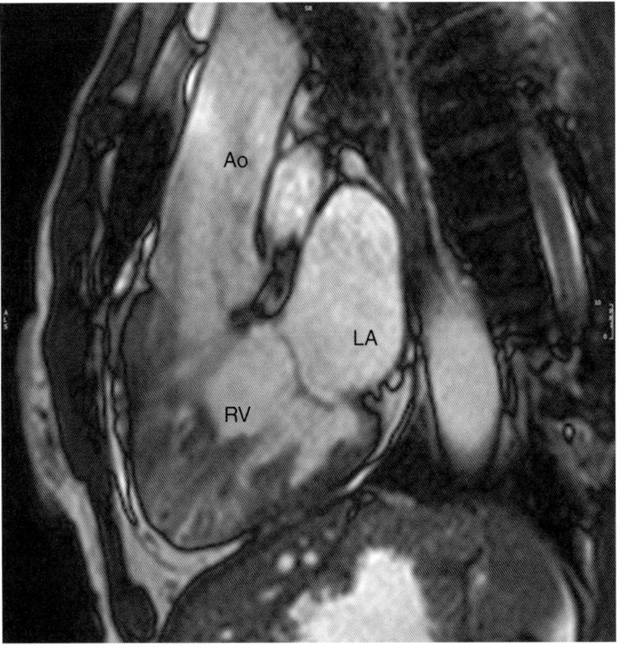

Fig. 45.14 Systemic RV inflow and outflow in a patient with congenitally corrected transposition of the great arteries. Bright blood cine MRI shows RV inflow and outflow in a patient with congenitally corrected transposition of the great arteries, including ejection from the RV into the anterior aorta. *Ao*, aorta.

The preoperative sRV ejection fraction should ideally be normal because the ejection fraction typically declines postoperatively.[78] The most favorable results support early tricuspid valve replacement, with an sRV ejection fraction of 40% or greater and LV systolic pressure less than 50 mmHg. In patients with complete heart block and transvenous pacing systems, univentricular LV pacing may exacerbate sRV systolic dysfunction and is associated with increased sRV size and worsening of sRV function.[79] Cardiac resynchronization should be considered in these patients to see if TR severity improves.

LV Outflow Tract Obstruction. In patients who have undergone a pulmonary valve intervention, pulmonary stenosis or insufficiency (or both) may be seen. Color Doppler imaging is used to confirm increased flow velocity or valve incompetence. Spectral Doppler is then used to quantify the dysfunction.

Many patients with CCTGA with pulmonary atresia or critical pulmonary stenosis are treated with placement of an LV-to-PA conduit. The conduit is prone to dysfunction (i.e., stenosis and insufficiency) and can lead to a pressure-loaded subpulmonary LV. Alleviation of conduit dysfunction causes the interventricular septum to shift toward the subpulmonic LV and away from the sRV. This septal displacement applies tension to the tricuspid valve leaflets because of their septal chordal attachments, and this affects tricuspid valve function. Adverse tricuspid valve function may worsen sRV function over time.[80]

Residual Ventricular Septal Defect. VSDs may be demonstrated in any of the listed acoustic windows, although they should be confirmed in bisecting orthogonal planes. Color Doppler imaging shows the direction of the shunt. The peak velocity should be obtained by spectral Doppler using the view that aligns the shunt flow with the transducer.

Anatomic Repair

Goals and Outcomes. Anatomic repair for CCTGA is performed to leave the patient with a systemic LV. It requires venous and arterial redirection and has therefore been called a *double-switch* operation. Surgical technique is influenced by the underlying cardiac anatomy and the location of associated cardiac defects. An intraatrial baffle (i.e., Mustard or Senning procedure) brings pulmonary venous blood to the LV and systemic venous blood to the RV.

There are two options for routing ventricular output to the correct great artery. An ASO can be performed if the coronary artery anatomy is favorable, or a Rastelli operation (i.e., interventricular baffle from the LV to the aorta and an RV-to-PA conduit) is performed if the VSD is favorable for rerouting. A bidirectional superior cavopulmonary anastomosis (i.e., Glenn anastomosis) is sometimes used to simplify surgery and prevent

TABLE 45.6 Echocardiographic Parameters for RV Functional Assessment.

Modality	*Method*	*Comments*
RV FAC	Change in RV area between end-diastole and end-systole	FAC < 33% predicts RV EF with 77% sensitivity and 58% specificity Correlates strongly with RV EF measured by cardiac MRI
RV *dP/dT*	Rate of pressure rise in the ventricle	*dP/dt* < 1000 mmHg/s predicts RV EF < 50% with 69% sensitivity and 87% specificity
MPI	Ratio of total isovolumic time divided by ejection time	Predicts RV EF = 65% (45 2 × MPI)
TAPSE	Distance of systolic movement of tricuspid valve annulus	TAPSE < 14 mm predicts RV EF < 50% with 67% sensitivity and 61% specificity ± correlation with RV EF
GLS	Myocardial deformation measurement	Predicts RV EF < 45% with 96% sensitivity and 93% specificity May have prognostic value; correlates with New York Heart Association class

EF, Ejection fraction; *FAC*, fractional area change; *GLS*, global longitudinal strain; *MPI*, myocardial performance index; *TAPSE*, tricuspid annular plane systolic excursion.

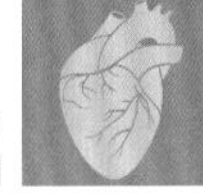

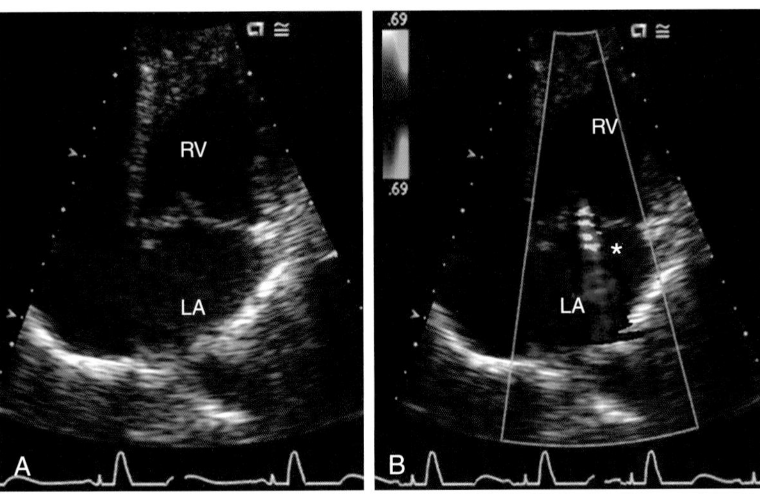

Fig. 45.15 **Tricuspid valve regurgitation in a patient with congenitally corrected transposition of the great arteries.** Apical 4-chamber (A) and color Doppler (B) views show tricuspid valve (i.e., systemic atrioventricular valve *[asterisk]*) regurgitation (see Videos 45.15A and 45.15B).

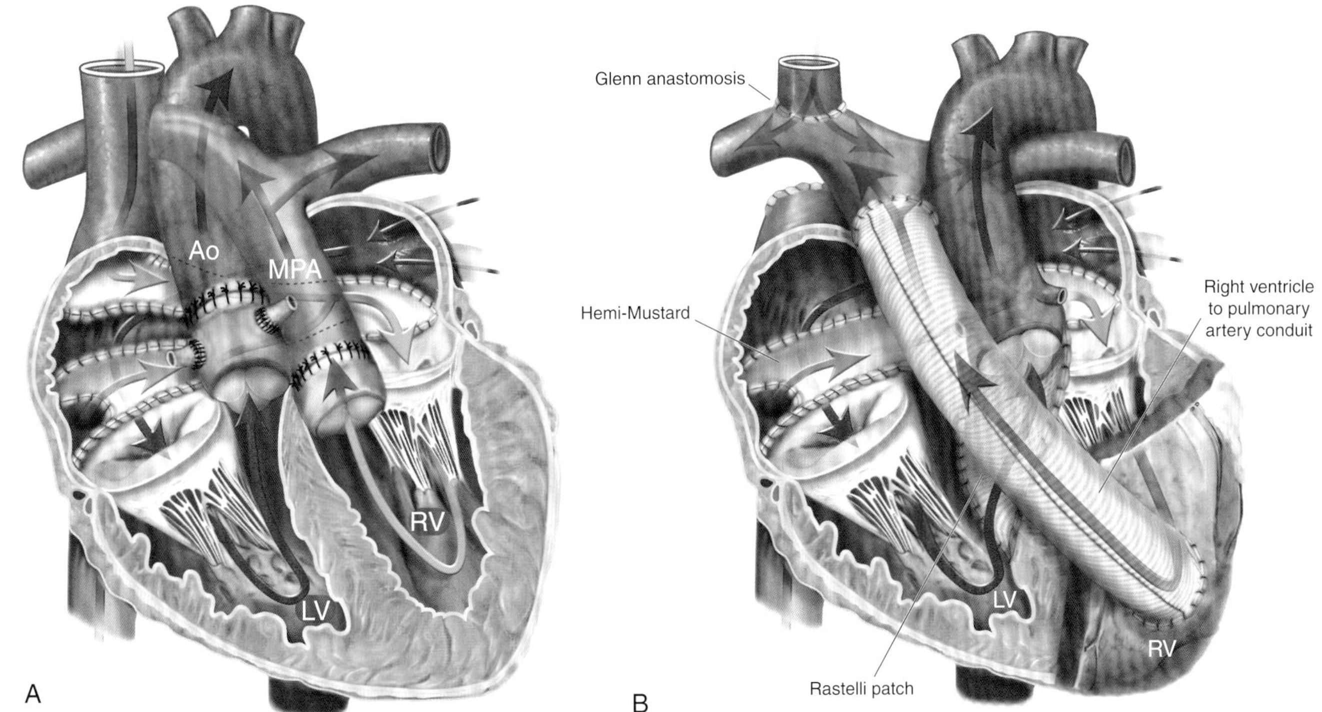

Fig. 45.16 **Anatomic repair of congenitally corrected transposition of the great arteries.** (A) Double-switch (anatomic repair) with a Mustard procedure and an arterial switch operation. Intraatrial baffles reroute deoxygenated blood to the RV and oxygenated blood to the LV. After an arterial switch operation, the aorta arises from the LV, and the pulmonary artery (PA) arises from the RV. (B) Double-switch using hemi-Mustard and Rastelli procedures. The inferior vena cava flow is baffled to the RV, which ejects blood across an RV-to-PA conduit. The superior vena cava is anastamosed to the right PA (i.e., Glenn operation). The LV is baffled across a ventricular septal defect to the anterior aorta. *Arrows* indicate blood flow.

late SVC stenosis and sinus node dysfunction and to prolong the lifespan of the RV-to-PA conduit[81] (Fig. 45.16).

The operative mortality rate is high for the double-switch procedure, but long-term survival after anatomic repair is good, with 20-year survival rates of 83% after atrial switch with ASO and 76% after atrial switch with an interventricular baffle.[82] Midterm results for the atrial switch modification with Glenn anastomosis are promising, with improved tricuspid valve function and prolonged RV-to-PA conduit longevity because one half of the cardiac output does not go through the conduit. This technique should be considered if an RV-to-PA conduit is planned as part of the anatomic repair.[81] Late LV dysfunction after appropriately timed anatomic repair (without the need for LV training) is a known complication and is associated with pacemaker implantation, a widened QRS duration, and older age at primary repair.[83,84]

Echocardiographic Evaluation of Postoperative Complications. Long-term complications of anatomic repair are undefined, although they undoubtedly encompass a combination of atrial baffle, ventricular baffle, and ASO issues, as discussed in previous sections on complete TGA. For patients who underwent the modified atrial switch repair with a Glenn anastomosis, assessment of the superior cavopulmonary anastomosis for obstruction should be done with a high right parasternal view. Color Doppler interrogation should show laminar flow. Spectral Doppler application reveals low-velocity venous flow with respiratory phasic variation in an unobstructed Glenn anastomosis.

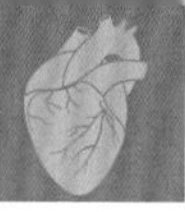

SUMMARY Echocardiographic Evaluation of Postoperative Problems in Patients With Complete or Congenitally Corrected Transposition of the Great Arteries.

Surgical Procedure	Problems	Echocardiographic Views	Interpretation and Measurements
Atrial switch	Baffle stenosis	SVC is visualized from the suprasternal notch. Color Doppler can show flow acceleration. Obstruction of the IVC baffle is less common.	Baffle diameter <0.5 cm suggests stenosis. Spectral Doppler gradients >3 mmHg may be significant. Retrograde flow into the azygous vein is seen in cases with significant obstruction.
	Baffle leak	Best visualized from the apical 4-chamber view with posterior angulation. Agitated saline injection aids in detection of shunts.	Shunting is usually from the pulmonary venous to the systemic venous baffle. During agitated saline injection, saline should not appear in the sRV. Significant baffle leaks can lead to a volume load on the subpulmonary LV.
	LV outflow tract obstruction (i.e., subpulmonic obstruction)	Parasternal long-axis view shows mechanism of obstruction. Spectral Doppler from apical views can measure pressure gradient.	Severe obstruction is defined by a velocity ≥4.0 m/s. Moderate obstruction is 3.0–3.9 m/s. Mild obstruction is <3 m/s.
	Tricuspid regurgitation	Apical 4-chamber view with color and spectral Doppler.	In many with TGA, the tricuspid valve is the systemic AV valve, so it cannot be used to estimate PA pressures.
	sRV systolic function	Qualitative assessment from parasternal short-axis view and apical 4-chamber view.	sRV is typically large and hypertrophied, with bowing on the ventricular septum into the LV.
Arterial switch (ASO)	Neoaortic dilation	The neoaortic root is measured from the parasternal long-axis view using conventional techniques (2D vs. M-mode measurement).	Most pediatric echocardiography laboratories measure during systole, whereas adult laboratories report measurements obtained in diastole.
	Neoaortic regurgitation	Parasternal long- and short-axis views with color and spectral Doppler.	Neoaortic regurgitation is often progressive.
	Pulmonary stenosis (supravalvular and branch)	Pulmonary anastomosis is best seen in the parasternal short-axis view. The PA bifurcation is anterior after an ASO; the branch PAs are best evaluated from a high parasternal or suprasternal view. Imaging of branch PAs is often difficult.	Lecompte maneuver drapes the branch PAs around the ascending aorta. Unilateral stenosis may not produce a high pressure gradient because flow may be diverted to the contralateral PA.
	LV systolic function	Standard assessment of LV systolic function, including assessment of wall motion abnormalities, is important after ASO.	ASO requires a coronary artery transfer, and obstruction is common. Resting wall motion abnormalities or LV systolic dysfunction should raise suspicion for coronary obstruction.

Continued

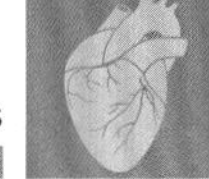

SUMMARY Echocardiographic Evaluation of Postoperative Problems in Patients With Complete or Congenitally Corrected Transposition of the Great Arteries.—cont'd

Surgical Procedure	Problems	Echocardiographic Views	Interpretation and Measurements
Rastelli operation	Conduit dysfunction	The anterior RV-to-PA conduit may be difficult to visualize in 2D. Anterior angulation of a high parasternal short-axis or apical view may work. Spectral Doppler should be used to assess the pressure gradient. CW Doppler should be obtained from the suprasternal notch using a nonimaging transducer.	A peak conduit velocity of 2.0–3.0 m/s is typical for a normally functioning conduit. A velocity of > 4.0 m/s indicates severe conduit stenosis.
	LV outflow tract obstruction	The apical 3-chamber view shows the relationship between the ventricular septal defect and the anterior aorta. Pulsed-wave and CW Doppler should be used to assess the level and severity of obstruction.	Severe obstruction is indicated by a velocity ≥ 4.0 m/s. Moderate obstruction is 3.0–3.9 m/s. Mild obstruction is 2.0–2.9 m/s.
Glenn anastomosis	Superior cavopulmonary anastomosis obstruction	The Glenn anastomosis can be visualized in a high right parasternal view. The anastomosis should be interrogated by color and spectral Doppler.	The color Doppler signal should be laminar. A normal spectral Doppler pattern is a low-velocity venous signal with respiratory variation.

ASO, Arterial switch operation; *AV*, atrioventricular; *IVC,* inferior vena cava; *PA*, pulmonary artery; *sRV*, systemic right ventricle; *SVC,* superior vena cava; *TGA,* transposition of the great arteries.

REFERENCES

1. Liebman J, Cullum L, Belloc NB. Natural history of transpositon of the great arteries. Anatomy and birth and death characteristics. *Circulation.* 1969;40(2):237–262.
2. Cuypers JA, Eindhoven JA, Slager MA, et al. The natural and unnatural history of the Mustard procedure: long-term outcome up to 40 years. *Eur Heart J.* 2014;35(25):1666–1674.
3. Lange R, Horer J, Kostolny M, et al. Presence of a ventricular septal defect and the Mustard operation are risk factors for late mortality after the atrial switch operation: thirty years of follow-up in 417 patients at a single center. *Circulation.* 2006;114(18):1905–1913.
4. Pasquali SK, Hasselblad V, Li JS, Kong DF, Sanders SP. Coronary artery pattern and outcome of arterial switch operation for transposition of the great arteries: a meta-analysis. *Circulation.* 2002;106(20):2575–2580.
5. Lai WW. *Echocardiography in Pediatric and Congenital Heart Disease: From Fetus to Adult.* Oxford: Wiley-Blackwell; 2009.
6. Senning A. Surgical correction of transposition of the great vessels. *Surgery.* 1959;45(6):966–980.
7. Mustard WT. Successful two-stage correction of transposition of the great vessels. *Surgery.* 1964;55:469–472.
8. Chaix MA, Dore A, Mercier LA, et al. Late onset postcapillary pulmonary hypertension in patients with transposition of the great arteries and mustard or senning baffles. *J Am Heart Assoc.* 2017;6(10):e006481.
9. Jatene AD, Fontes VF, Paulista PP, et al. Anatomic correction of transposition of the great vessels. *J Thorac Cardiovasc Surg.* 1976;72(3):364–370.
10. Villafane J, Lantin-Hermoso MR, Bhatt AB, et al. D-transposition of the great arteries: the current era of the arterial switch operation. *J Am Coll Cardiol.* 2014;64(5):498–511.
11. Junge C, Westhoff-Bleck M, Schoof S, et al. Comparison of late results of arterial switch versus atrial switch (mustard procedure) operation for transposition of the great arteries. *Am J Cardiol.* 2013;111(10):1505–1509.
12. Fricke TA, d'Udekem Y, Richardson M, et al. Outcomes of the arterial switch operation for transposition of the great arteries: 25 years of experience. *Ann Thorac Surg.* 2012;94(1):139–145.
13. Dennis M, Kotchetkova I, Cordina R, Celermajer DS. Long-term follow-up of adults following the atrial switch operation for transposition of the great arteries - a contemporary cohort. *Heart Lung Circ.* 2018;27(8):1011–1017.
14. Couperus LE, Vliegen HW, Zandstra TE, et al. Long-term outcome after atrial correction for transposition of the great arteries. *Heart.* 2019;105(10):790–796.
15. Warnes CA. Transposition of the great arteries. *Circulation.* 2006;114(24):2699–2709.
16. Dos L, Teruel L, Ferreira IJ, et al. Late outcome of Senning and Mustard procedures for correction of transposition of the great arteries. *Heart.* 2005;91(5):652–656.
17. Derrick GP, Narang I, White PA, et al. Failure of stroke volume augmentation during exercise and dobutamine stress is unrelated to load-independent indexes of right ventricular performance after the Mustard operation. *Circulation.* 2000;102(19 suppl 3):III154–159.
18. Kammeraad JA, van Deurzen CH, Sreeram N, et al. Predictors of sudden cardiac death after Mustard or Senning repair for transposition of the great arteries. *J Am Coll Cardiol.* 2004;44(5):1095–1102.
19. Roubertie F, Thambo JB, Bretonneau A, et al. Late outcome of 132 Senning procedures after 20 years of follow-up. *Ann Thorac Surg.* 2011;92(6):2206–2213, Discussion 2213–2214.
20. Khairy P, Harris L, Landzberg MJ, et al. Sudden death and defibrillators in transposition of the great arteries with intra-atrial baffles: a multicenter study. *Circ Arrhythm Electrophysiol.* 2008;1(4):250–257.
21. Diller GP, Dimopoulos K, Okonko D, et al. Exercise intolerance in adult congenital heart disease: comparative severity, correlates, and prognostic implication. *Circulation.* 2005;112(6):828–835.
22. Giardini A, Hager A, Lammers AE, et al. Ventilatory efficiency and aerobic capacity predict event-free survival in adults with atrial repair for complete transposition of the great arteries. *J Am Coll Cardiol.* 2009;53(17):1548–1555.
23. Khairy P, Landzberg MJ, Lambert J, O'Donnell CP. Long-term outcomes after the atrial switch for surgical correction of transposition:

a meta-analysis comparing the Mustard and Senning procedures. *Cardiol Young*. 2004; 14(3):284–292.

24. Bottega NA, Silversides CK, Oechslin EN, et al. Stenosis of the superior limb of the systemic venous baffle following a Mustard procedure: an under-recognized problem. *Int J Cardiol*. 2012;154(1):32–37.
25. Chintala K, Forbes TJ, Karpawich PP. Effectiveness of transvenous pacemaker leads placed through intravascular stents in patients with congenital heart disease. *Am J Cardiol*. 2005;95(3):424–427.
26. Horer J, Karl E, Theodoratou G, et al. Incidence and results of reoperations following the Senning operation: 27 years of follow-up in 314 patients at a single center. *Eur J Cardio Thorac Surg*. 2008;33(6):1061–1067, Discussion 1067–1068.
27. Hill KD, Fleming G, Curt Fudge J, Albers EL, Doyle TP, Rhodes JF. Percutaneous interventions in high-risk patients following Mustard repair of transposition of the great arteries. *Catheter Cardiovasc Interv*. 2012;80(6):905–914.
28. Brown SC, Eyskens B, Mertens L, Stockx L, Dumoulin M, Gewillig M. Self expandable stents for relief of venous baffle obstruction after the Mustard operation. *Heart*. 1998;79(3):230–233.
29. Chin AJ, Sanders SP, Williams RG, Lang P, Norwood WI, Castaneda AR. Two-dimensional echocardiographic assessment of caval and pulmonary venous pathways after the Senning operation. *Am J Cardiol*. 1983;52(1):118–126.
30. Lewin MB, Stout KK. *Echocardiography in Congenital Heart Disease: Expert Consult*. Elsevier Saunders; 2012.
31. Cook SC, McCarthy M, Daniels CJ, Cheatham JP, Raman SV. Usefulness of multislice computed tomography angiography to evaluate intravascular stents and transcatheter occlusion devices in patients with D-transposition of the great arteries after mustard repair. *Am J Cardiol*. 2004;94(7):967–969.
32. Fogel MA, Hubbard A, Weinberg PM. A simplified approach for assessment of intracardiac baffles and extracardiac conduits in congenital heart surgery with two- and three-dimensional magnetic resonance imaging. *Am Heart J*. 2001;142(6):1028–1036.
33. Parekh DR, Cabrera MS, Ing FF. Simultaneous transcatheter implantation of systemic and pulmonary venous baffle stents after mustard operation for d-transposition of the great arteries. *Catheter Cardiovasc Interv*, 2015;86(4):708–713: https://doi.org/10.1002/ccd.25951.
34. Bentham J, English K, Hares D, Gibbs J, Thomson J. Effect of transcatheter closure of baffle leaks following senning or mustard atrial redirection surgery on oxygen saturations and polycythaemia. *Am J Cardiol*. 2012;110(7):1046–1050.
35. Khairy P, Landzberg MJ, Gatzoulis MA, et al. Transvenous pacing leads and systemic thromboemboli in patients with intracardiac shunts: a multicenter study. *Circulation*. 2006;113(20):2391–2397.
36. Hurwitz RA, Caldwell RL, Girod DA, Brown J. Right ventricular systolic function in adolescents and young adults after Mustard operation for transposition of the great arteries. *Am J Cardiol*. 1996;77(4):294–297.
37. Kirjavainen M, Happonen JM, Louhimo I. Late results of Senning operation. *J Thorac Cardiovasc Surg*. 1999;117(3):488–495.
38. Iriart X, Horovitz A, van Geldorp IE, et al. The role of echocardiography in the assessment of right ventricular systolic function in patients with transposition of the great arteries and atrial redirection. *Arch Cardiovasc Dis*. 2012;105(8–9):432–441.
39. Khattab K, Schmidheiny P, Wustmann K, Wahl A, Seiler C, Schwerzmann M. Echocardiogram versus cardiac magnetic resonance imaging for assessing systolic function of subaortic right ventricle in adults with complete transposition of great arteries and previous atrial switch operation. *Am J Cardiol*. 2013;111(6):908–913.
40. Moroseos T, Mitsumori L, Kerwin WS, et al. Comparison of Simpson's method and three-dimensional reconstruction for measurement of right ventricular volume in patients with complete or corrected transposition of the great arteries. *Am J Cardiol*. 2010;105(11):1603–1609.
41. Wheeler M, Grigg L, Zentner D. Can we predict sudden cardiac death in long-term survivors of atrial switch surgery for transposition of the great arteries? *Congenit Heart Dis*. 2014;9(4):326–332.
42. Li W, Hornung TS, Francis DP, et al. Relation of biventricular function quantified by stress echocardiography to cardiopulmonary exercise capacity in adults with Mustard (atrial switch) procedure for transposition of the great arteries. *Circulation*. 2004;110(11):1380–1386.
43. Ho JG, Cohen MD, Ebenroth ES, et al. Comparison between transthoracic echocardiography and cardiac magnetic resonance imaging in patients status post atrial switch procedure. *Congenit Heart Dis*. 2012;7(2):122–130.
44. van Son JA, Reddy VM, Silverman NH, Hanley FL. Regression of tricuspid regurgitation after two-stage arterial switch operation for failing systemic ventricle after atrial inversion operation. *J Thorac Cardiovasc Surg*. 1996;111(2):342–347.
45. Winlaw DS, McGuirk SP, Balmer C, et al. Intention-to-treat analysis of pulmonary artery banding in conditions with a morphological right ventricle in the systemic circulation with a view to anatomic biventricular repair. *Circulation*. 2005;111(4):405–411.
46. Karamlou T, Jacobs ML, Pasquali S, et al. Surgeon and center volume influence on outcomes after arterial switch operation: analysis of the STS Congenital Heart Surgery Database. *Ann Thorac Surg*. 2014;98(3):904–911.
47. Stoica S, Carpenter E, Campbell D, et al. Morbidity of the arterial switch operation. *Ann Thorac Surg*. 2012;93(6):1977–1983.
48. Vandekerckhove KD, Blom NA, Lalezari S, Koolbergen DR, Rijlaarsdam ME, Hazekamp MG. Long-term follow-up of arterial switch operation with an emphasis on function and dimensions of left ventricle and aorta. *Eur J Cardio Thorac Surg*. 2009;35(4):582–587, Discussion 587–588.
49. McMahon CJ, Ravekes WJ, Smith EO, et al. Risk factors for neo-aortic root enlargement and aortic regurgitation following arterial switch operation. *Pediatr Cardiol*. 2004;25(4):329–335.
50. van der Bom T, van der Palen RL, Bouma BJ, et al. Persistent neo-aortic growth during adulthood in patients after an arterial switch operation. *Heart*. 2014;100(17):1360–1365.
51. Co-Vu JG, Ginde S, Bartz PJ, Frommelt PC, Tweddell JS, Earing MG. Long-term outcomes of the neoaorta after arterial switch operation for transposition of the great arteries. *Ann Thorac Surg*. 2013;95(5):1654–1659.
52. Lang RM, Badano LP, Mor-Avi V, et al. Recommendations for cardiac chamber quantification by echocardiography in adults: an update from the American Society of Echocardiography and the European Association of Cardiovascular Imaging. *J Am Soc Echocardiogr*. 2015;28(1):1–39 e14.
53. Lo Rito M, Fittipaldi M, Haththotuwa R, et al. Long-term fate of the aortic valve after an arterial switch operation. *J Thorac Cardiovasc Surg*. 2015;149(4):1089–1094.
54. Khairy P, Clair M, Fernandes SM, et al. Cardiovascular outcomes after the arterial switch operation for D-transposition of the great arteries. *Circulation*. 2013;127(3):331–339.
55. Swartz MF, Sena A, Atallah-Yunes N, et al. Decreased incidence of supravalvar pulmonary stenosis after arterial switch operation. *Circulation*. 2012;126(11 suppl 1):S118–S122.
56. Moll JJ, Michalak KW, Mludzik K, et al. Long-term outcome of direct neopulmonary artery reconstruction during the arterial switch procedure. *Ann Thorac Surg*. 2012;93(1):177–184.
57. Legendre A, Losay J, Touchot-Kone A, et al. Coronary events after arterial switch operation for transposition of the great arteries. *Circulation*. 2003;108(suppl 1):II186–190.
58. El-Segaier M, Lundin A, Hochbergs P, Jogi P, Pesonen E. Late coronary complications after arterial switch operation and their treatment. *Catheter Cardiovasc Interv*. 2010;76(7):1027–1032.
59. Stout KK, Daniels CJ, Aboulhosn JA, et al. AHA/ACC guideline for the management of adults with congenital heart disease: Executive summary: a report of the American College of Cardiology/American Heart Association Task Force on Clinical Practice Guidelines. *Circulation*. 2018;139(14):e637–e697. 2019.
60. Brown JW, Ruzmetov M, Huynh D, Rodefeld MD, Turrentine MW, Fiore AC. Rastelli operation for transposition of the great arteries with ventricular septal defect and pulmonary stenosis. *Ann Thorac Surg*. 2011;91(1):188–193, Discussion 193–194.
61. Graham Jr TP, Bernard YD, Mellen BG, et al. Long-term outcome in congenitally corrected transposition of the great arteries: a multi-institutional study. *J Am Coll Cardiol*. 2000;36(1):255–261.
62. Piacentini G, Digilio MC, Capolino R, et al. Familial recurrence of heart defects in subjects with congenitally corrected transposition of the great arteries. *Am J Med Genet*. 2005;137(2):176–180.
63. Myers PO, del Nido PJ, Geva T, et al. Impact of age and duration of banding on left ventricular preparation before anatomic repair for congenitally corrected transposition of the great arteries. *Ann Thorac Surg*. 2013;96(2):603–610.
64. Quinn DW, McGuirk SP, Metha C, et al. The morphologic left ventricle that requires training by means of pulmonary artery banding before the double-switch procedure for congenitally corrected transposition of the great arteries is at risk of late dysfunction. *J Thorac Cardiovasc Surg*. 2008;135(5):1137–1144, e1131–e1132.
65. Lim HG, Lee JR, Kim YJ, et al. Outcomes of biventricular repair for congenitally corrected transposition of the great arteries. *Ann Thorac Surg*. 2010;89(1):159–167.
66. Murtuza B, Barron DJ, Stumper O, et al. Anatomic repair for congenitally corrected

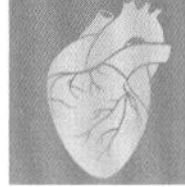

transposition of the great arteries: a single-institution 19-year experience. *J Thorac Cardiovasc Surg*. 2011;142(6):1348–1357. e1341.

67. Caso P, Ascione L, Lange A, Palka P, Mininni N, Sutherland GR. Diagnostic value of transesophageal echocardiography in the assessment of congenitally corrected transposition of the great arteries in adult patients. *Am Heart J*. 1998;135(1):43–50.
68. Hauser M, Bengel FM, Hager A, et al. Impaired myocardial blood flow and coronary flow reserve of the anatomical right systemic ventricle in patients with congenitally corrected transposition of the great arteries. *Heart*. 2003;89(10):1231–1235.
69. Geva T. Is MRI the preferred method for evaluating right ventricular size and function in patients with congenital heart disease?: MRI is the preferred method for evaluating right ventricular size and function in patients with congenital heart disease. *Circ Cardiovasc Imaging*. 2014;7(1):190–197.
70. Focardi M, Cameli M, Carbone SF, et al. Traditional and innovative echocardiographic parameters for the analysis of right ventricular performance in comparison with cardiac magnetic resonance. *Eur Heart J Cardiovasc Imaging*. 2015;16(1):47–52.
71. Salehian O, Schwerzmann M, Merchant N, Webb GD, Siu SC, Therrien J. Assessment of systemic right ventricular function in patients with transposition of the great arteries using the myocardial performance index: comparison with cardiac magnetic resonance imaging. *Circulation*. 2004;110(20):3229–3233.
72. Lipczynska M, Szymanski P, Kumor M, Klisiewicz A, Mazurkiewicz L, Hoffman P. Global longitudinal strain may identify preserved systolic function of the systemic right ventricle. *Can J Cardiol*. 2015;31(6):760–766.
73. Eindhoven JA, Menting ME, van den Bosch AE, et al. Quantitative assessment of systolic right ventricular function using myocardial deformation in patients with a systemic right ventricle. *Eur Heart J Cardiovasc Imaging*. 2015;16(4):380–388.
74. Abadir S, Leobon B, Acar P. Assessment of tricuspid regurgitation mechanism by three-dimensional echocardiography in an adult patient with congenitally corrected transposition of the great arteries. *Arch Cardiovasc Dis*. 2009;102(5):459–460.
75. Lewis M, Ginns J, Rosenbaum M. Is systemic right ventricular function by cardiac MRI related to the degree of tricuspid regurgitation in congenitally corrected transposition of the great arteries? *Int J Cardiol*. 2014;174(3):586–589.
76. Hirose K, Nishina T, Kanemitsu N, et al. The long-term outcomes of physiologic repair for ccTGA (congenitally corrected transposition of the great arteries). *Gen Thorac Cardiovasc Surg*. 2015;63(9):496–501.
77. Scherptong RW, Vliegen HW, Winter MM, et al. Tricuspid valve surgery in adults with a dysfunctional systemic right ventricle: repair or replace? *Circulation*. 2009;119(11):1467–1472.
78. Mongeon FP, Connolly HM, Dearani JA, Li Z, Warnes CA. Congenitally corrected transposition of the great arteries ventricular function at the time of systemic atrioventricular valve replacement predicts long-term ventricular function. *J Am Coll Cardiol*. 2011;57(20):2008–2017.
79. Yeo WT, Jarman JW, Li W, Gatzoulis MA, Wong T. Adverse impact of chronic subpulmonary left ventricular pacing on systemic right ventricular function in patients with congenitally corrected transposition of the great arteries. *Int J Cardiol*. 2014;171(2):184–191.
80. Buber J, McElhinney DB, Valente AM, Marshall AC, Landzberg MJ. Tricuspid valve regurgitation in congenitally corrected transposition of the great arteries and a left ventricle to pulmonary artery conduit. *Ann Thorac Surg*. 2015;99(4):1348–1356.
81. Malhotra SP, Reddy VM, Qiu M, et al. The hemi-Mustard/bidirectional Glenn atrial switch procedure in the double-switch operation for congenitally corrected transposition of the great arteries: rationale and midterm results. *J Thorac Cardiovasc Surg*. 2011;141(1):162–170.
82. Hiramatsu T, Matsumura G, Konuma T, Yamazaki K, Kurosawa H, Imai Y. Long-term prognosis of double-switch operation for congenitally corrected transposition of the great arteries. *Eur J Cardio Thorac Surg*. 2012;42(6):1004–1008.
83. Bautista-Hernandez V, Marx GR, Gauvreau K, Mayer Jr JE, Cecchin F, del Nido PJ. Determinants of left ventricular dysfunction after anatomic repair of congenitally corrected transposition of the great arteries. *Ann Thorac Surg*. 2006;82(6):2059–2065, Discussion 2065–2066.
84. Bautista-Hernandez V, Myers PO, Cecchin F, Marx GR, Del Nido PJ. Late left ventricular dysfunction after anatomic repair of congenitally corrected transposition of the great arteries. *J Thorac Cardiovasc Surg*. 2014;148(1):254–258.

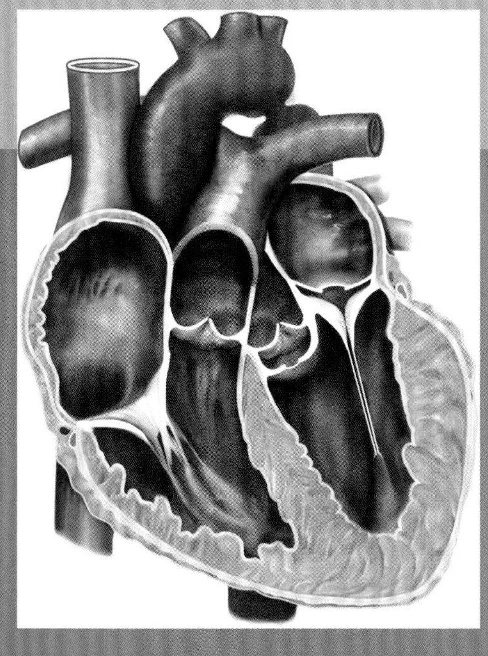

中文导读

第46章
单心室

单心室是一组包含多种畸形的复杂先天性心脏畸形，其具有一个共同的特征：单个主导心室支持体循环和肺循环，与单心室生理类似的畸形有三尖瓣闭锁、左心发育不良综合征、双入口心室和双出口右心室。大多数出生时就患有单心室畸形的患者都会接受Fontan手术。Fontan手术有几种变体，但常见的结果是依赖静脉压力让全身静脉血回流到肺循环，而不是依赖于心室的收缩。

本章回顾了单心室畸形、Fontan手术的手术演变，包括右心房–右心室连接术、格林手术、全腔手术和外管道开窗等相关手术，以及Fontan手术前后心室功能的变化。另外介绍了超声心动图如何评估所需要了解的心脏解剖，心室功能和房室瓣反流情况，Fontan手术静脉连接情况，以及该类患者检查所需注意的其他情况和检查步骤，确保了对单心室循环患者进行系统和全面的超声心动图评估。

王剑鹏

46 Single Ventricles

LUKE J. BURCHILL, MBBS, PhD | RACHEL M. WALD, MD

Single-ventricle anomalies are a diverse group of congenital heart defects with one common feature: a single dominant ventricle supports the systemic and pulmonary circulations. Most patients born with single-ventricle anomalies undergo the Fontan operation. The Fontan operation has several variations, but the common result is passive systemic venous return to the pulmonary circulation without reliance on an interposing subpulmonary ventricle.

This chapter reviews single-ventricle anomalies, the surgical evolution of the Fontan operation, and changes in ventricular function before and after the Fontan operation. A stepwise approach to echocardiographic assessment requires an understanding of cardiac anatomy and an evaluation of the Fontan connections. This ensures an organized and comprehensive echocardiographic assessment of patients with a single-ventricle circulation.

BASIC PRINCIPLES

CONGENITAL HEART DEFECTS ASSOCIATED WITH SINGLE-VENTRICLE PHYSIOLOGY

Most patients with single-ventricle physiology have two ventricles, one large (i.e., dominant) and the other small (i.e., codominant).[1] The term *single-ventricle circulation* is best used to describe the physiologic state rather than the anatomic condition because a true single ventricle is rare. Congenital heart defects associated with single-ventricle physiology are listed in Table 46.1. Tricuspid atresia, hypoplastic left heart syndrome (HLHS), double-inlet left ventricle, and double-outlet right ventricle (DORV) account for most of the anatomic defects leading to single-ventricle physiology.

In tricuspid atresia (Fig. 46.1), there is no connection between the right atrium (RA) and the right ventricle (RV) because the atrioventricular (AV) valve is imperforate or absent. This appears on the echocardiogram as a fibrous band or plate with no connection between the RA and RV. Tricuspid atresia is typically associated with an atrial septal defect (ASD) with right-to-left shunting, a hypoplastic RV, and a ventricular septal defect (VSD). The great vessels are usually normally related (70% of patients) or transposed (30%), often with obstruction to pulmonary and/or systemic blood flow. If the great vessels are normally related, the pulmonary artery (PA) arises from the RV and is usually associated with pulmonary or subpulmonary stenosis. In transposition of the great arteries, the PA arises from the left ventricle (LV), and the aorta arises from the RV. There may be obstruction to aortic outflow due to a muscular infundibulum or a restrictive VSD.

Patients with tricuspid atresia typically require a modified Blalock-Taussig shunt (subclavian-to-PA anastomosis using a synthetic tube), which is followed by a bidirectional Glenn shunt and a Fontan operation.

HLHS encompasses a spectrum of defects associated with a severely underdeveloped left heart and aortic arch. The mitral and aortic valves have severe stenosis and/or atresia. Typically, the ascending aorta is hypoplastic, and coarctation exists (Fig. 46.2). The goal of surgical palliation in HLHS is to establish an RV-based systemic circulation, in which the RV becomes the dominant ventricle supporting the systemic circulation. Children born with HLHS typically undergo a series of three operations, beginning with a Norwood operation in the neonatal period (stage 1) and followed by a bidirectional cavopulmonary anastomosis (stage 2, around 6 months) and a Fontan operation completion between 2 and 3 years of age (stage 3) (Fig. 46.3).

In the Norwood operation, the pulmonary valve becomes the new or neoaortic valve, and the aorta is reconstructed using the trunk of the PA, the original hypoplastic aorta, and graft tissue. The RV becomes the systemic chamber responsible for pumping blood to the brain and body. The PAs are disconnected from the RV, and pulmonary blood flow is provided by a Blalock-Taussig shunt or an RV-to-PA conduit (i.e., Sano modification). HLHS and its management are reviewed in several excellent articles.[2–4]

Double-inlet LV refers to hearts in which both atria connect to one dominant LV. Double-inlet LV is often associated with transposition of the great arteries. When double-inlet LV occurs with normally related great arteries, it is called the *Holmes heart.* VSDs are usually detected, and they connect the dominant LV to

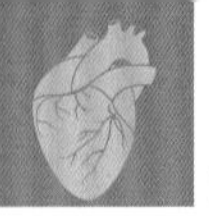

a small hypoplastic RV. Depending on whether the great arteries are normally related or transposed, a restrictive VSD may cause obstruction to systemic or pulmonary blood flow. Other associations include pulmonary stenosis (i.e., valvular and subvalvular), coarctation of the aorta, and interrupted aortic arch (Fig. 46.4).

TABLE 46.1 Congenital Heart Defects Associated With Single-Ventricle Physiology.

Cardiac Anatomic Diagnosis	*Prevalence*[a]
Tricuspid atresia	22%
Hypoplastic left heart	21%
Double-inlet LV	15%
Heterotaxy	8%
Double-outlet RV	8%
Pulmonary atresia intact ventricular septum	6%
Mitral atresia	6%
Abnormal tricuspid valve	4%
Atrioventricular septal defect, unbalanced	4%
Other	7%

[a]Prevalence of cardiac anatomic diagnoses among 546 Fontan cross-sectional study subjects.

Adapted from Anderson PA, Sleeper LA, Mahony L, et al. Contemporary outcomes after the Fontan procedure: a Pediatric Heart Network multicenter study. *J Am Coll Cardiol.* 2008;52:85–98.

Patients with double-inlet LV and transposition of the great arteries usually require a Norwood-type operation in the neonatal period. This is followed by a bidirectional cavopulmonary anastomosis and a Fontan operation.

DORV describes hearts in which the aorta and PA originate from the RV. The three types of DORV are a less complex DORV with a single VSD, normal-sized ventricles, and no major PA anomalies (group 1); a DORV with transposition of the great arteries and a subpulmonary VSD (i.e. Taussig-Bing anomaly; group 2); and a complex DORV that includes AV septal defects (which may or may not straddle the VSD) and/or a hypoplastic valve or ventricle (group 3).

Complete surgical repair (i.e., biventricular repair) is achievable in most DORV patients in groups 1 and 2. The Rastelli operation is performed for group 1 DORV patients. It comprises an intraventricular tunnel or baffle from the VSD to the aorta with or without placement of a conduit from the RV to the main PA. Group 2 DORV patients undergo the arterial switch operation, with tunneling of the VSD to the neoaorta. Because of the complexity, group 3 patients are not suitable for complete repair and usually require a Fontan operation (Fig. 46.5).

SURGICAL EVOLUTION AFTER THE FONTAN OPERATION

First reported in 1971,[5] the Fontan operation has given rise to a new generation of children born with very complex forms of

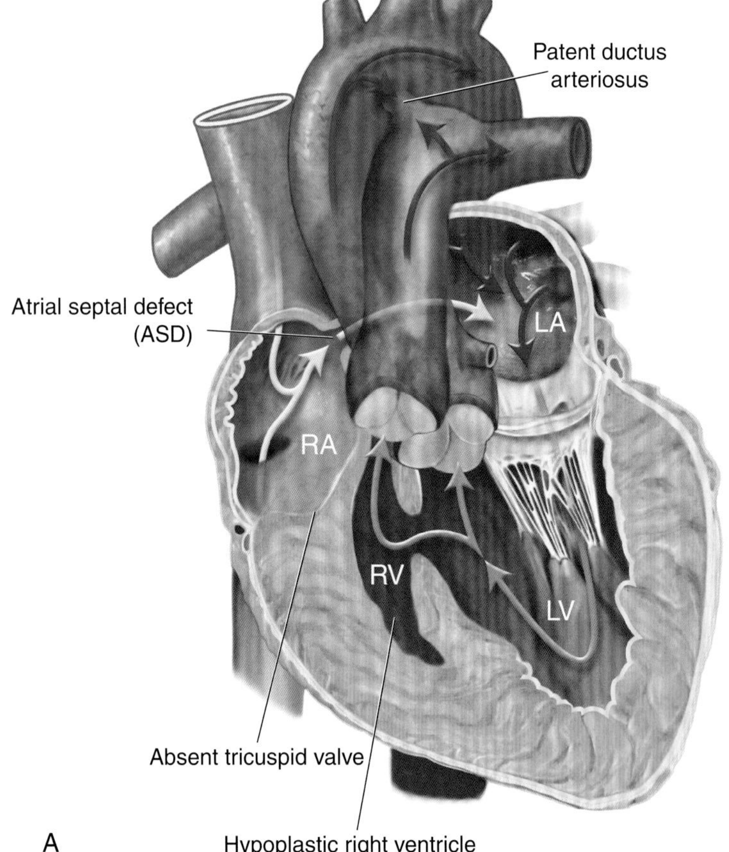

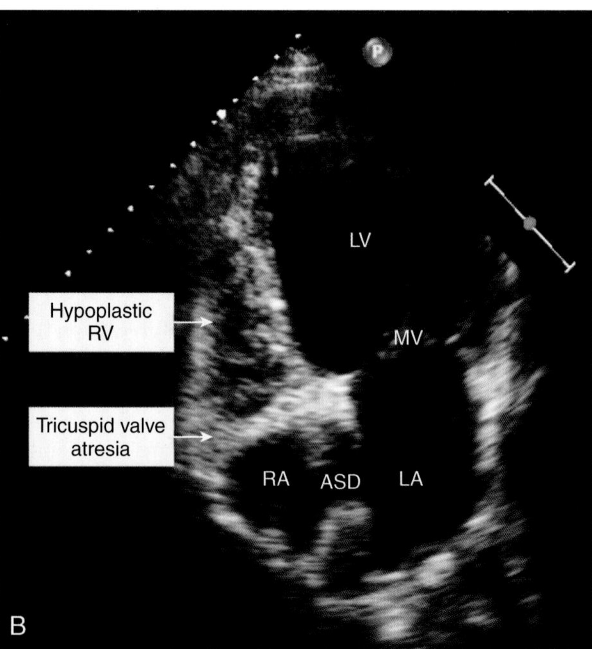

Fig. 46.1 Tricuspid atresia. (A) In patients with tricuspid atresia, the connection between the RA and RV is absent due to an atretic (absent) tricuspid valve. Blood that returns from the body to the RA must pass through an atrial septal defect *(ASD)* into the LA. Blood then enters the LV through the mitral (left atrioventricular) valve. There is usually a ventricular septal defect, leading to a small or hypoplastic RV. Ventriculoarterial connections may be concordant (70% of cases, as shown in the diagram) or discordant with transposition of the great arteries (30% of cases). (B) 2D apical 4-chamber echocardiogram demonstrates an atretic tricuspid valve that appears as a thick echogenic muscular band separating the RA and RV. The RV is hypoplastic, and an ASD is seen. *MV*, Mitral valve.

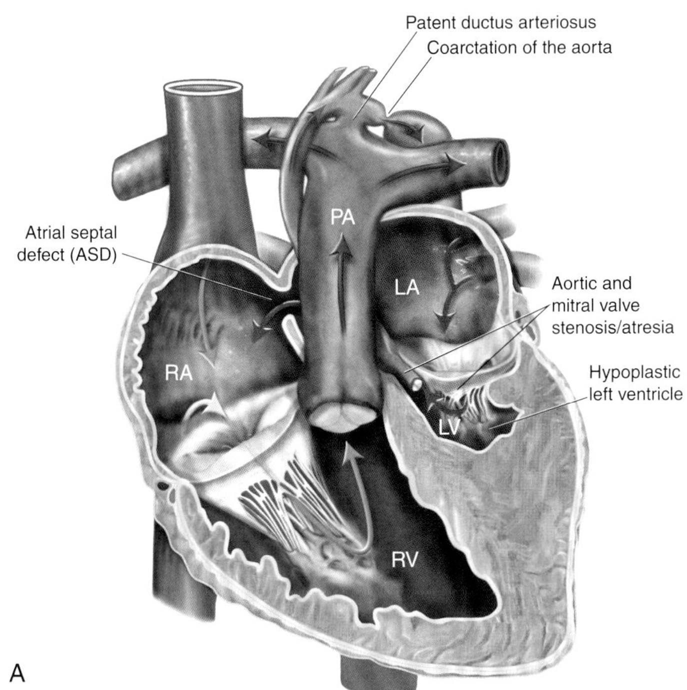

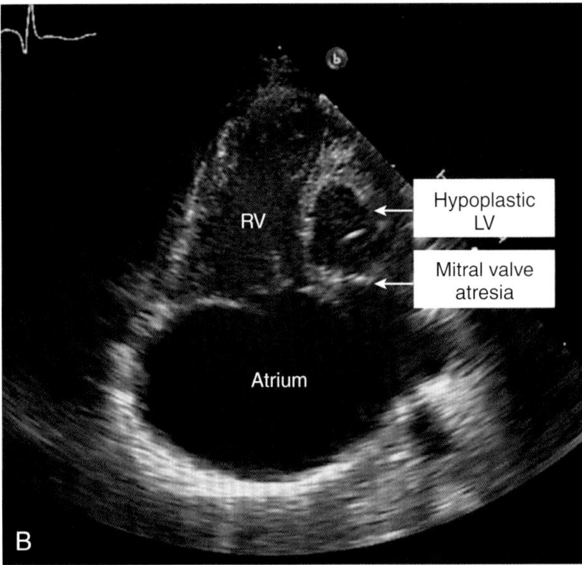

Fig. 46.2 Hypoplastic left heart syndrome. (A) In hypoplastic left heart syndrome (HLHS), all of the structures on the left side of the heart, including the aorta and aortic arch, are severely underdeveloped. The left side of the heart cannot support the circulation. In addition to mitral and aortic valve stenosis or atresia, the LV is very small, and the first part of the aorta is often only millimeters in diameter. Blood that returns from the lungs to the LA must pass through an atrial septal defect to the right side of the heart. The RV pumps blood to the lungs through the pulmonary artery *(PA)*. The RV is also the sole source of blood supply to the body via a patent ductus arteriosus. (B) 2D echocardiogram apical 4-chamber view in a patient with HLHS demonstrates an atretic mitral valve that appears as a thick echogenic muscular band separating the atrium and LV. The LV is hypoplastic. The RV is the dominant chamber. The atria appear as one common atrium after atrial septectomy.

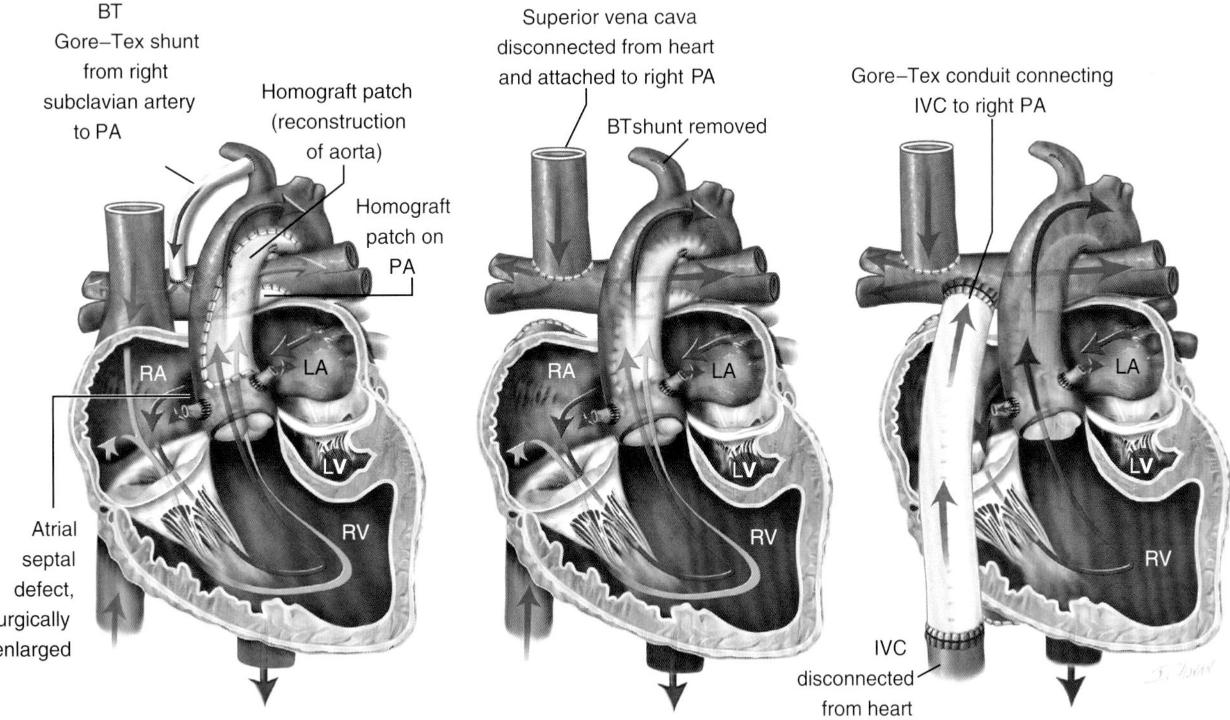

Fig. 46.3 Stages of Fontan palliation for hypoplastic left heart syndrome. (A) Stage 1: Norwood procedure. This operation is performed during the first week after birth. The purpose of the Norwood procedure is to provide a stable source of blood flow to the body and lungs. The native pulmonary artery *(PA)* becomes the neoaortic valve, and the aorta is reconstructed using a homograft patch. The morphologic RV becomes the systemic ventricle. Pulmonary blood flow is provided by a Blalock-Taussig Gore-Tex shunt between the subclavian and PA or a Sano shunt, providing a direct shunt from the RV to the PA. (B) Stage 2: Bidirectional Glenn procedure. This operation is usually performed within the first 6 months after birth. The superior vena cava is ligated and disconnected from the heart and then anastomosed to the PA. Deoxygenated blood from the upper body goes to the lungs. (C) Stage 3: Fontan operation. The Fontan operation occurs at approximately 1.5 to 3 years of age. The inferior vena cava *(IVC)* is disconnected from the heart and attached to the PA. After the Fontan operation, all deoxygenated blood from the upper and lower body goes to the lungs without passing through the heart. *BT*, Blalock-Taussig; *PDA*, patent ductus arteriosus.

congenital heart disease who survived to adulthood. The Fontan operation is the most common surgery for children with complex congenital heart defects not suitable for biventricular repair.[6]

The Fontan operation directs the systemic venous return into the pulmonary circulation, usually without an interposing RV. The objectives of surgical palliation are to provide adequate pulmonary and systemic blood flow while alleviating cyanosis and ventricular volume overload. In the absence of a subpulmonary chamber or pump, systemic venous flow to the pulmonary circulation is passive. Postcapillary energy and systemic venous pressure are the driving forces for pulmonary blood flow,[7] augmented by respirophasic changes in intrathoracic pressure.[8] In 2019, the American Heart Association's *Scientific Statement for Evaluation and Management of the Child and Adult With Fontan Circulation* reported that there may be up to 70,000 patients alive today with a Fontan circulation, and that this population is expected to double in the next 20 years.[9]

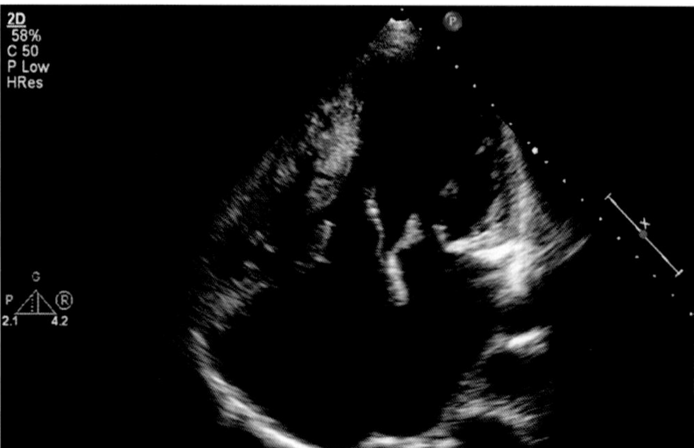

Fig. 46.4 Double-inlet LV. (A) Both atria connect to the dominant LV. The RV is small and hypoplastic. A ventricular septal defect usually exists, and ventriculoarterial connections are often discordant (i.e., transposition of the great arteries). Other defects such as coarctation of the aorta, pulmonary or subpulmonary stenosis, and pulmonary atresia are common. (B) Double-inlet LV 2D echocardiogram in an apical 4-chamber view demonstrates the left and right atrioventricular valves connecting to the LV. The atrioventricular valves are seen in the open position. The hypoplastic RV is not seen in this image. A small atrial septal defect is seen.

Over time, the Fontan operation has evolved to facilitate more efficient venous flow from the systemic circulation to the pulmonary circulation. The first Fontan connections were RA-to-PA connections, called the *atriopulmonary Fontan procedure* (Fig. 46.6). Valves and conduits were used in some patients but were found to impede flow through Fontan connections. The Bjork modification comprised a conduit (often valved) between the RA and RV in cases of tricuspid atresia.[10]

The elevated RA pressures associated with atriopulmonary Fontan connections resulted in progressive RA enlargement along with arrhythmia, thrombus formation, and pulmonary venous obstruction. Consequently, the atriopulmonary Fontan connection was abandoned in favor of a circuit that largely excluded the RA from the Fontan connection. Introduced in 1988 and still used today, the lateral tunnel Fontan connection comprises a synthetic tunnel sutured within the RA, extending from the inferior vena cava (IVC) to the PA (Fig. 46.7).[11,12]

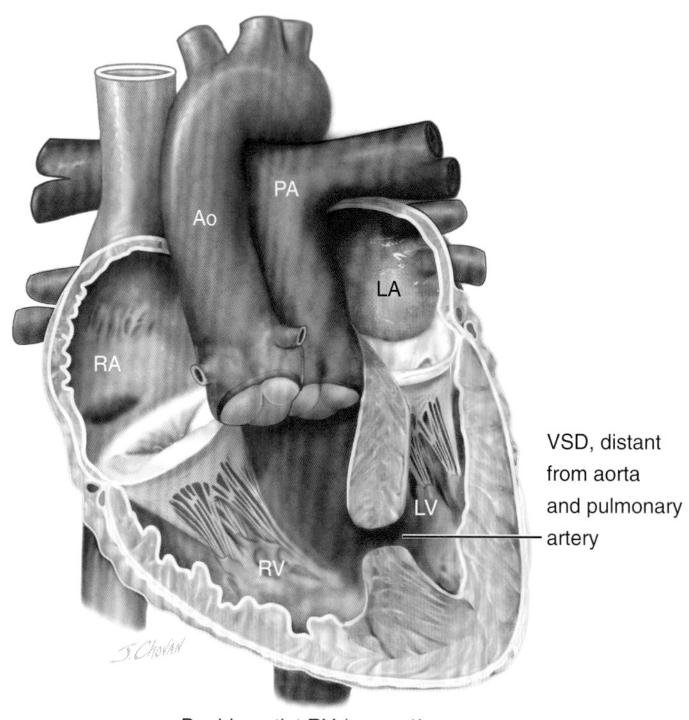

Fig. 46.5 Double-outlet RV. Both great vessels arise from the RV. Blood from the LV passes across a ventricular septal defect *(VSD)* into the RV to reach the great arteries. The clinical manifestations of double-outlet RV vary according to the site of the VSD. *Ao,* Aorta.

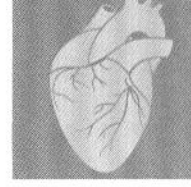

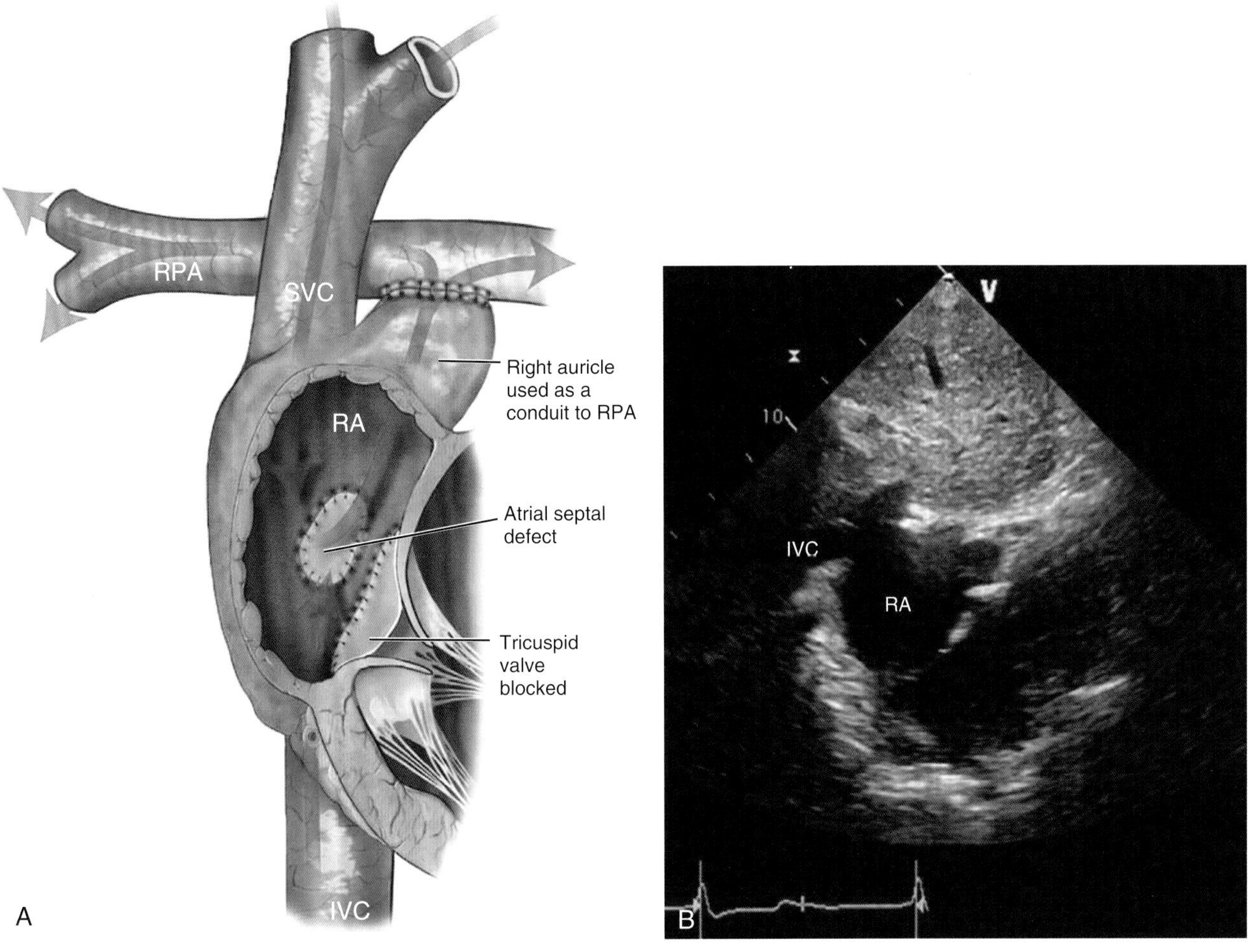

Fig. 46.6 Atriopulmonary Fontan procedure. (A) The RA is isolated by closure of the atrial septal defect and the hypoplastic tricuspid valve. The RA appendage is anastomosed to the right pulmonary artery *(RPA)*. (B) 2D subcostal-view echocardiogram shows the inferior vena cava *(IVC)* connecting to the RA in a patient with tricuspid atresia after an atriopulmonary Fontan operation. The RA is dilated, and the RV is hypoplastic. *SVC*, Superior vena cava.

Because the intraatrial conduit was still associated with RA dilation, scarring, and atrial arrhythmia, it was superseded by the extracardiac Fontan operation, which bypasses the RA altogether.[13] IVC blood flows through a synthetic conduit located external to the RA (Fig. 46.8). The simplicity of the extracardiac Fontan operation, reduced suture burden, and avoidance of aortic cross-clamping led to its becoming the procedure of choice in many congenital heart centers.

A 2019 meta-analysis included 3300 patients, 1729 with an extracardiac Fontan operation and 1601 with a lateral tunnel Fontan procedure. Those with an extracardiac Fontan operation had improved survival (93% vs. 89% at 20 years, respectively; $P = 0.007$) and greater freedom from tachyarrhythmia (92% vs. 83% at 15 years; $P < 0.0001$).[14] The extracardiac Fontan operation was also associated with a lower thromboembolic risk than the lateral tunnel and atriopulmonary Fontan types.[15]

A staged approach to the Fontan operation completion is preferred. Typically, patients with a single ventricle undergo a shunt or PA banding first, followed by a cavopulmonary anastomosis or Glenn shunt. The Glenn shunt is a surgical anastomosis between the superior vena cava (SVC) and the pulmonary circulation. Older patients undergoing echocardiographic assessment may have a classic Glenn shunt (Fig. 46.9), whereas younger patients are more likely to have a bidirectional Glenn shunt (Fig. 46.10). The *classic Glenn shunt* refers to a unilateral anastomosis of the SVC to the right PA; the left and right PAs are disconnected.[15] Pulmonary arteriovenous malformations (AVMs) are common in patients with a classic Glenn procedure; they are thought to arise from the absence of hepatic venous flow to the right lung because regression of AVMs can occur after hepatic flow is restored.[16] The bidirectional Glenn shunt comprises end-to-side anastomosis of the SVC to the undivided PA.[17] These connections ensure that systemic venous return from the upper half of the body flows passively into the lungs.

The bidirectional Glenn shunt typically is performed in patients between 4 and 6 months of age. Fontan completion connecting the IVC to the PAs is performed in patients between 2 and 4 years of age.

The Kawashima operation is a type of bidirectional Glenn connection that is performed in patients with left atrial (LA) isomerism and an interrupted IVC with azygous continuation to the right SVC or hemiazygos continuation to a persistent left SVC.[18] Those with a persistent left SVC have bilateral Glenn shunts. This routes all of the systemic venous return, except hepatic and mesenteric flow, to the PAs (Fig. 46.11). As in patients with a classic Glenn shunt who do not receive hepatic venous flow, a significant percentage of patients who have undergone the Kawashima operation develop pulmonary AVMs as a cause of progressive cyanosis.

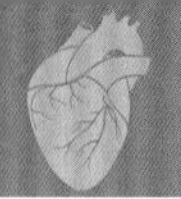

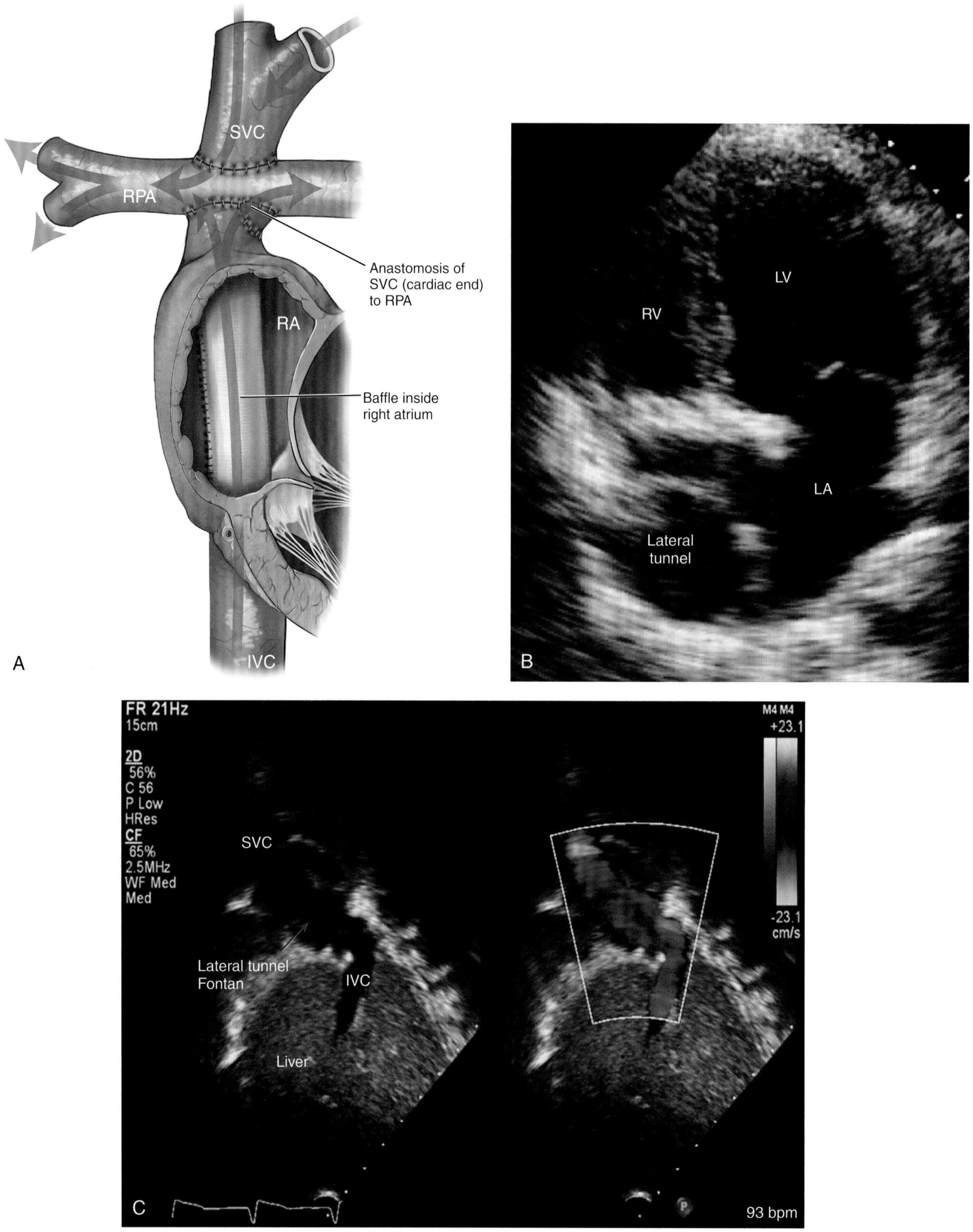

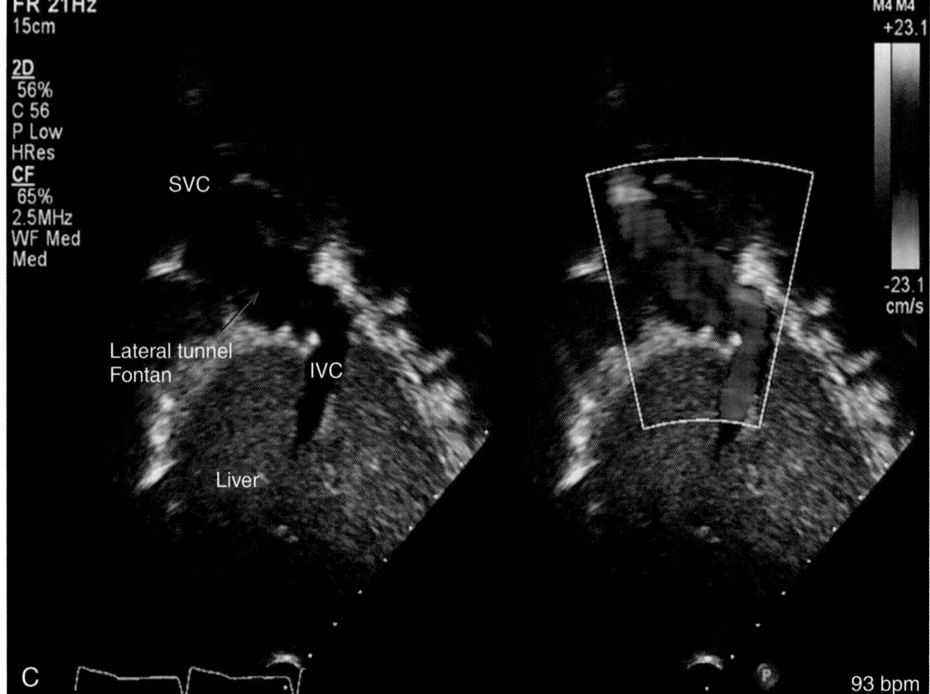

Fig. 46.7 Lateral tunnel Fontan operation. (A) Inferior vena cava *(IVC)* flow is directed by a synthetic tunnel or baffle placed within the RA. The lower portion of the superior vena cava *(SVC)* is sutured directly to the right pulmonary artery *(RPA)*. The upper part of the SVC is connected to the superior aspect of the RPA as a bidirectional Glenn shunt. Most of the RA is excluded from the Fontan circuit. (B) 2D apical 4-chamber echocardiogram shows the lateral tunnel Fontan connection within the RA. There is also a tricuspid atresia and a hypoplastic RV. (C) Side-by-side 2D echocardiogram and color subcostal view of a lateral tunnel Fontan *(arrow)* directing low-velocity IVC flow to the lower portion of the divided SVC.

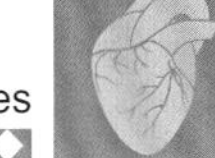

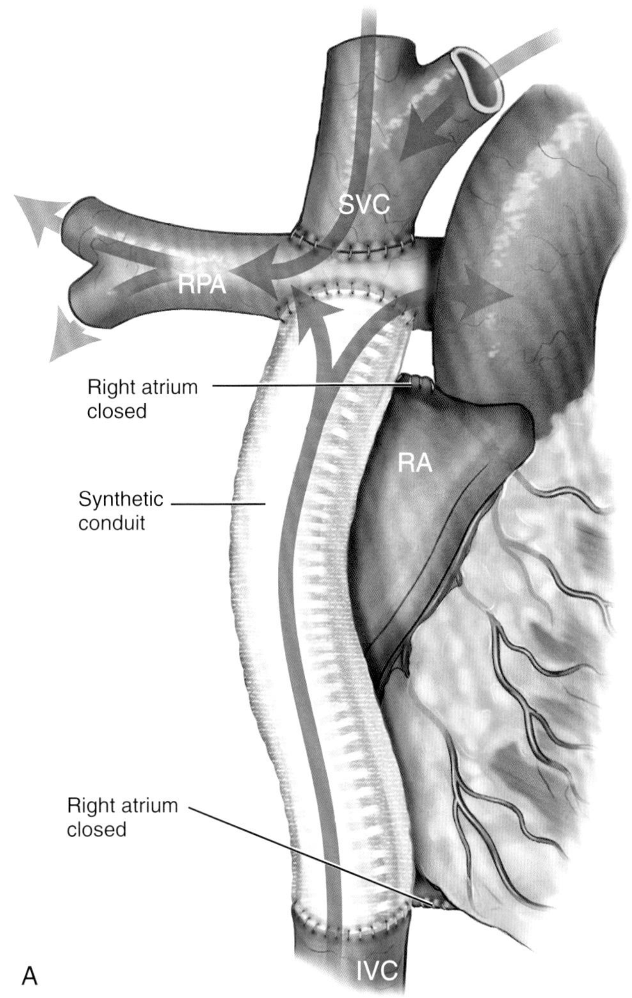

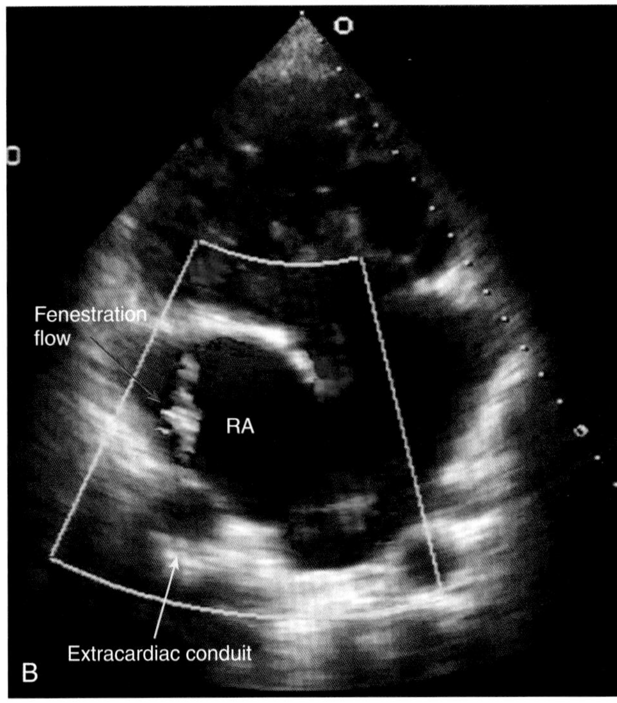

Fig. 46.8 Extracardiac Fontan operation. (A) Inferior vena cava *(IVC)* flow is directed to the pulmonary artery by an extracardiac synthetic conduit that sits entirely outside of the RA. The extracardiac conduit is anastomosed to the inferior portion of the right pulmonary artery *(RPA)*. The superior vena cava *(SVC)* is anastomosed to the superior aspect of the pulmonary artery as a bidirectional Glenn shunt. (B) 2D apical 4-chamber echocardiogram of the extracardiac Fontan conduit. Notice that the conduit sits outside of the RA. A fenestration is demonstrated with color Doppler as flow from the extracardiac conduit into the RA.

The Fontan operation separates systemic venous and pulmonary venous blood flow, resulting in normal arterial saturations. The flow through the pulmonary circulation is passive and therefore limits any increase in cardiac output, especially during exercise. The Fontan circulation results in chronic volume unloading of the single ventricle at the expense of increased systemic venous pressures. Short- and medium-term outcomes after the Fontan procedure are excellent, with operative mortality rates approaching 1% and reported transplantation-free survival rates of 95% and 90% at 5 and 10 years, respectively.[19,20]

Late complications in adulthood are common, including systemic venous hypertension, reduced cardiac output, and limited cardiac reserve during exercise. Other complications include atrial arrhythmias, atrial thrombus, hepatic congestion, liver cirrhosis, and ascites. Protein-losing enteropathy, which affects 4% of Fontan operation survivors, is characterized by chronic diarrhea and gastrointestinal protein loss, which leads to peripheral edema, pleural effusions, ascites, impaired immunity, and increased mortality rates.[21] Another rare complication is plastic bronchitis, in which bronchial casts of a gelatinous consistency obstruct the tracheobronchial tree.

By creating a right-to-left shunt between the Fontan circulation and the RA, a fenestration can relieve elevated Fontan pressures, improve ventricular preload, and increase cardiac output (Fig. 46.12). This is most relevant in the postoperative period, when the risk of early Fontan failure and chronic pleural effusions is high. In later years, fenestrations may be closed to reduce the cyanosis associated with the right-to-left shunting.

VENTRICULAR FUNCTION BEFORE AND AFTER A FONTAN OPERATION

During fetal life, the dominant ventricle is responsible for the combined output of the systemic and pulmonary circulations. The parallel circulations cause a persistent, chronic volume load, leading to prenatal eccentric remodeling and ventricular dilation in the single ventricle at birth.[22] The bidirectional Glenn shunt procedure performed at 4 to 8 months of age reduces the chronic volume load, leading to reverse remodeling and improved ejection fraction.[23] After the Fontan operation, further volume unloading occurs,

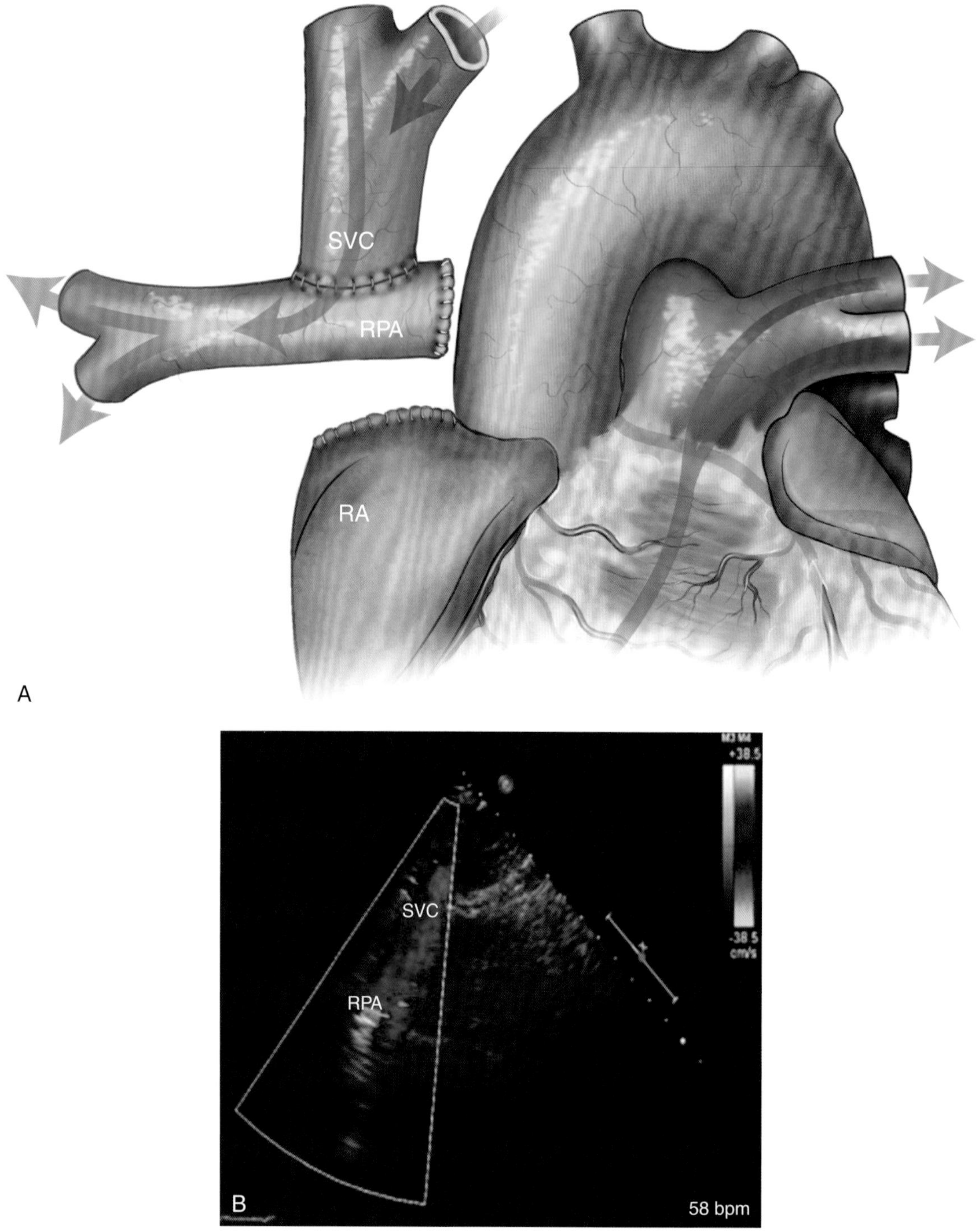

Fig. 46.9 Classic Glenn procedure. (A) The superior vena cava *(SVC)* is anastomosed to the distal end of the divided right pulmonary artery *(RPA)*. The right and left pulmonary arteries are disconnected. The inferior portion of the SVC is ligated below the anastomosis. (B) 2D echocardiogram with color flow shows a classic Glenn connection with venous flow from the SVC to the divided RPA.

which in the face of unchanging ventricular mass leads to an acquired hypertrophy that impairs ventricular diastolic performance.[24–26]

The incidence of heart failure increases with age. Up to 40% of adult Fontan patients meet the Framingham criteria for a diagnosis of heart failure.[27] Male sex, a common AV valve, older age at the time of a Fontan operation, elevated preoperative and early postoperative PA pressures, concomitant surgery at the time of the Fontan operation, and prolonged pleural effusions after Fontan completion have been associated with worse late survival rates.[28,29]

Early recognition of heart failure in Fontan patients remains a major clinical challenge, as does accurate assessment of ventricular function. The accuracy of echocardiographically derived measurements has been questioned because assumptions of uniform geometry do not apply in those with single-ventricle physiology. Reduced ventricular preload after the Fontan operation also raises questions about the relevance of ejection fraction as a load-dependent measure of ventricular function. Echocardiographers face the additional challenges of limited views, chest wall deformities, unpredictable orientation of the heart in the thorax, and abnormal chamber geometry.

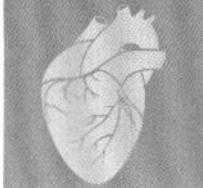

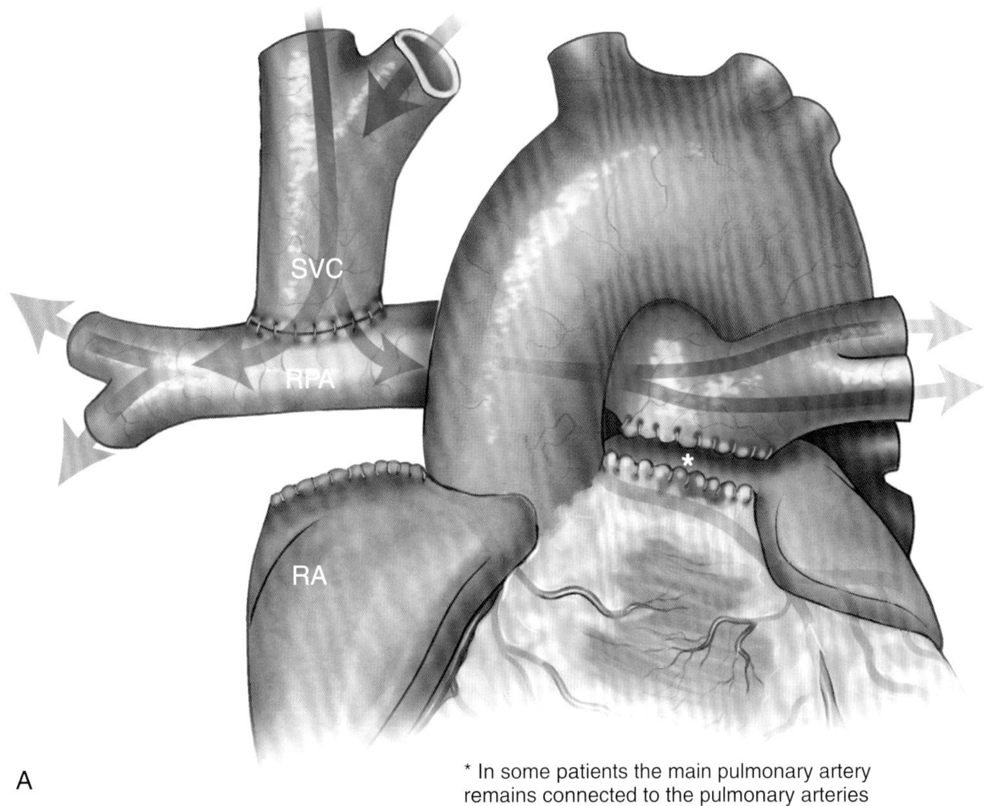

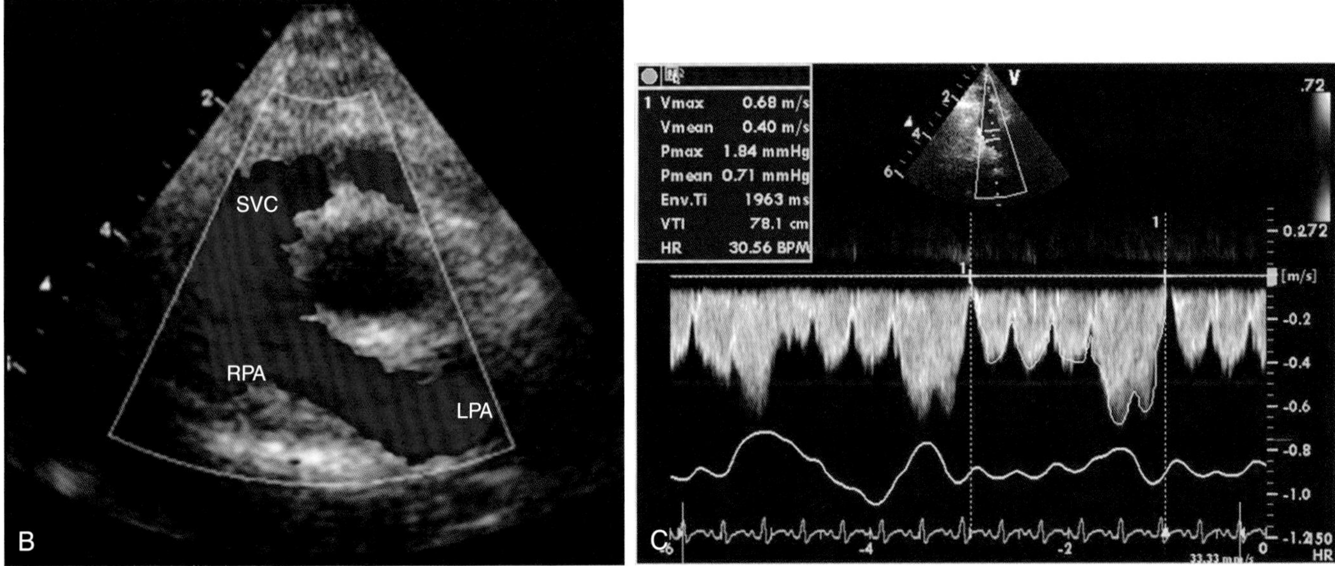

Fig. 46.10 Bidirectional Glenn procedure. (A) End-to-side anastomosis of the divided superior vena cava *(SVC)* to the undivided pulmonary artery. The right *(RPA)* and left *(LPA)* pulmonary arteries are connected. (B) 2D echocardiogram with color flow shows a bidirectional Glenn connection with venous flow from the SVC to the RPA and LPA. (C) Pulsed-wave Doppler imaging of the SVC in a classic Glenn procedure shows normal low-velocity venous flow with respirophasic variation. Peak and mean velocities and pressures can be estimated by averaging flow velocities over five beats.

Given these challenges, a range of techniques, including cardiac magnetic resonance imaging (MRI), are being used to better understand ventricular function in patients with single-ventricle physiology.

PREPARATION FOR THE SCAN

Echocardiographic assessment of adults with congenital heart disease requires preparation and planning. Understanding the patient's cardiac history, including review of surgical operative reports, is invaluable for planning the echocardiographic examination. Special attention is given to the type of Fontan connection and other cardiac operations, including prior shunts, valve repair or replacement, arch reconstruction, and interventions involving the PAs and veins (Table 46.2). Review of prior echocardiograms may identify technical challenges associated with scanning, including the need for nonstandard imaging planes to account for variations in cardiac position and anatomy.

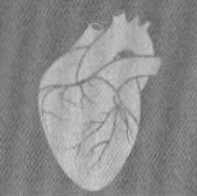

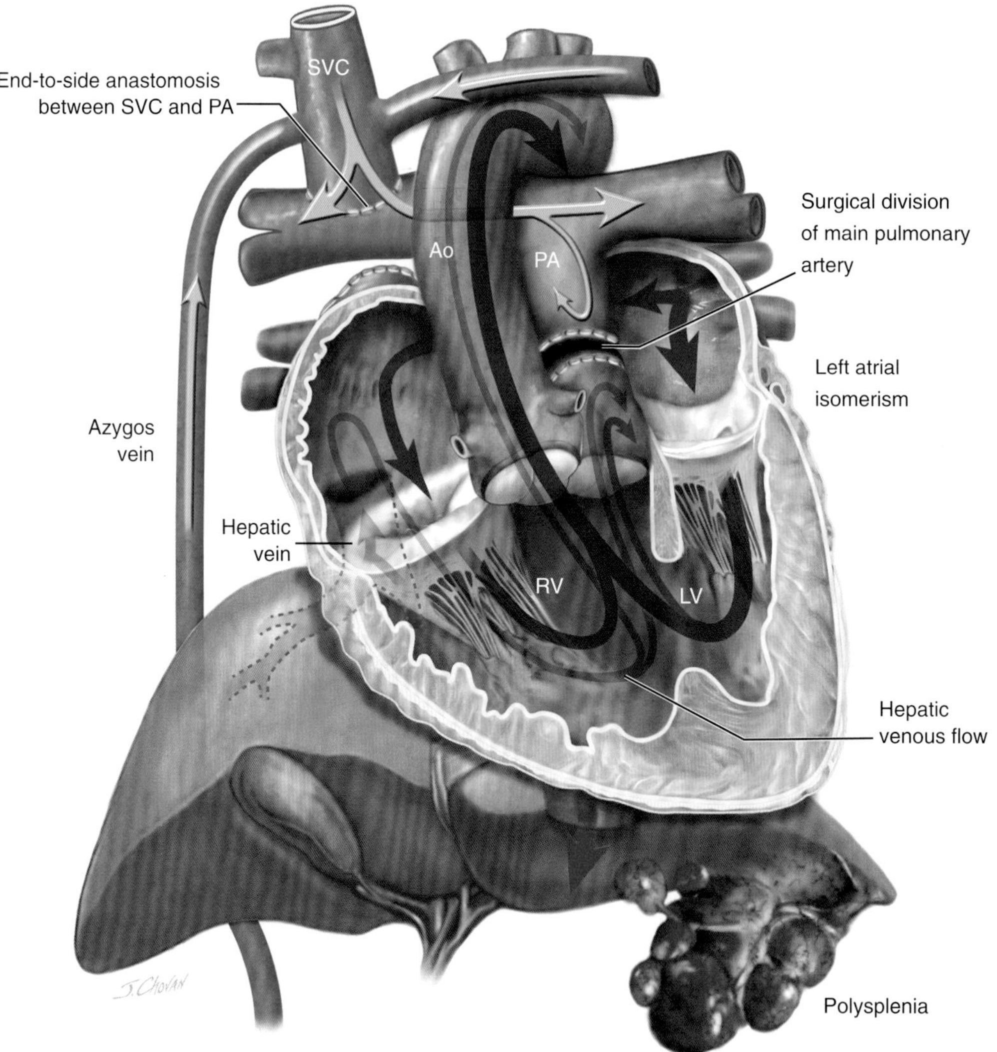

Fig. 46.11 Kawashima operation. The Kawashima operation is performed in patients with LA isomerism and an interrupted inferior vena cava. The operation involves end-to-side anastomosis between the superior vena cava *(SVC)* with azygos or hemiazygos continuation and the pulmonary arteries *(PA)*. The main PA is surgically divided. Total venous return, except for hepatic venous and coronary sinus flow, drains directly into the PA. Pulmonary arteriovenous malformations are common in patients after the Kawashima operation and are thought to result from an absence of hepatic venous flow to the lungs. *Ao*, Aorta.

SEQUENTIAL AND SEGMENTAL APPROACH

TERMINOLOGY

Segmental analysis refers to the stepwise assessment of the connections between the three segments of the heart: atria, ventricles, and great arteries. Variations in these segmental arrangements are common in congenital heart disease.

Concordance describes situations in which one anatomic segment connects appropriately with the next. A concordant AV connection describes an appropriate connection of the morphologic RA to the morphologic RV and the morphologic LA to the morphologic LV. Concordant ventriculoarterial connections describe an appropriate origin of the pulmonary trunk from the morphologic RV and of the aorta from the morphologic LV.

A *discordant* AV connection involves connection of the morphologic RA with the morphologic LV. Discordant ventriculoarterial connections describe mismatched great arteries and ventricles such that the PA arises from the LV and the aorta arises from the RV.

Depending on its relation to the thoracic (spine) midline, the *cardiac position* may be in the left chest (normal or levoposition), in the right chest (dextroposition), or in the midline (mesoposition). Levoposition is confirmed when the heart is identified 30 to 45 degrees to the left of the midline (i.e., midline marked posteriorly by the vertebral body). Mesoposition indicates that the heart occupies a midline position. Dextroposition is seen when the heart is 30 to 45 degrees to the right of the central plane.

Cardia denotes the location of the apex. Levocardia indicates a normal leftward apex, whereas dextrocardia means the apex points to the right.

Situs refers to the right-left position of the body's organs. Situs solitus denotes normal position (i.e., the right lung and liver are to the right, and the left lung, heart, spleen, and stomach are to the left). In situs inversus (1 case in every 5000 to 10,000 individuals),[30] the right-left orientation of the unpaired viscera (including the heart) is inverted.

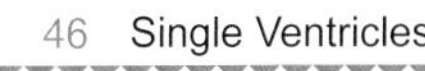

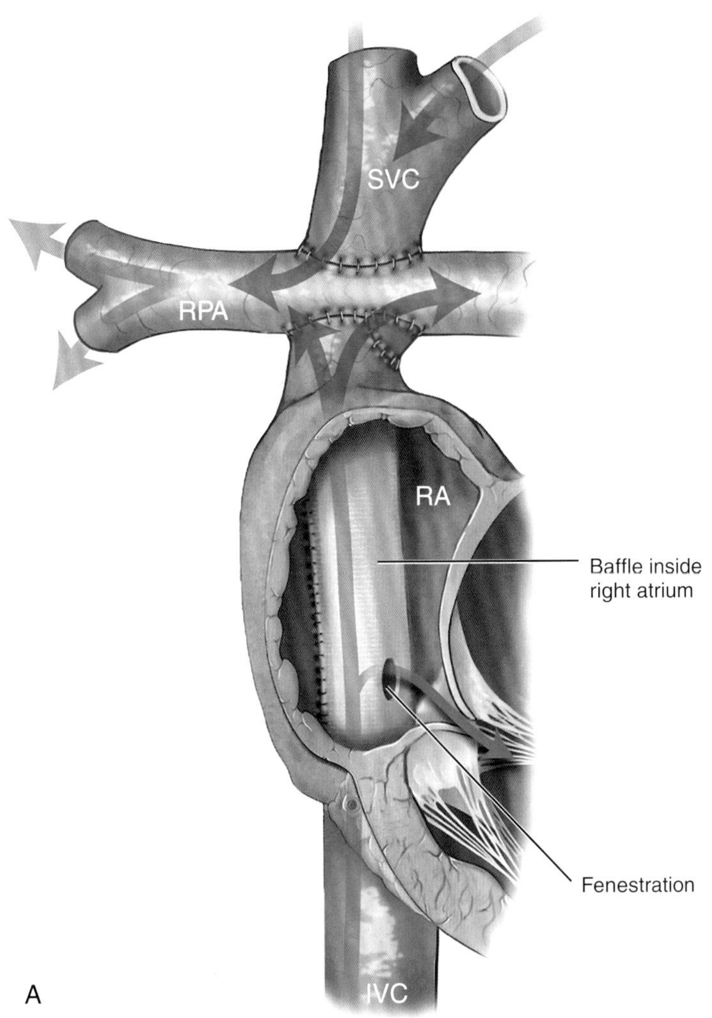

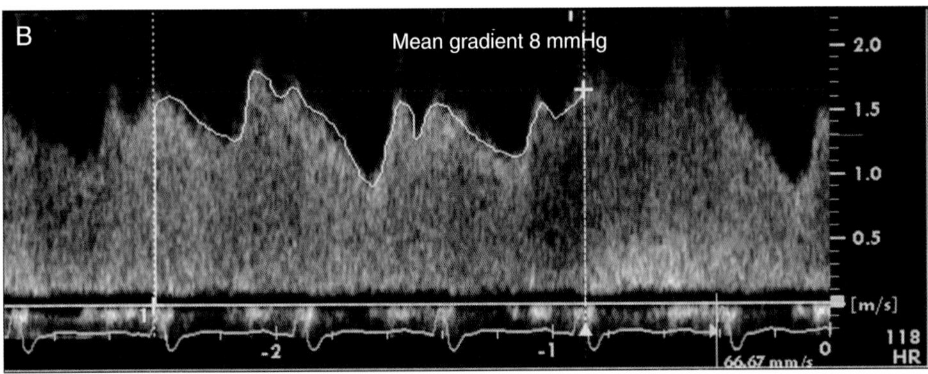

Fig. 46.12 Lateral tunnel fenestration. (A) Fenestrations in the lateral tunnel and extracardiac Fontan conduits enable right-to-left shunting between the Fontan connection and the RA. Fenestrations can relieve elevated Fontan pressures, which may be protective against early Fontan failure (see Fig. 49.6B). (B) CW Doppler assessment of fenestration flow enables estimation of the mean Fontan gradient. The mean fenestration gradient equals the transpulmonary gradient because it reflects the pressure difference between the Fontan and pulmonary venous chamber. *IVC*, Inferior vena cava; *RPA*, right pulmonary artery; *SVC*, superior vena cava.

Using this terminology, the finding of a normal cardiac position with normal visceral arrangements is classified as levocardia with situs solitus. Alternatively, if the heart occupies the right chest with reversal of the body's organs (i.e., liver present on the left and stomach on the right), the classification is dextrocardia with situs inversus.

Dextrocardia has three causes: (1) situs inversus; (2) loss of normal lung volume in the right chest leading to mediastinal shift; and (3) dextroversion, in which the apex fails to rotate normally during fetal development. Situs inversus is distinguished by the reversed position of the right and left heart structures. When dextrocardia occurs due to mediastinal shift or dextroversion, the RA and RV are still on the right, and the LA and LV are on the left. Most people with dextrocardia and situs inversus have otherwise normal hearts.

In patients with single-ventricle physiology, the congenital heart defect most commonly associated with dextrocardia and situs inversus is congenitally corrected transposition of the great arteries.[31] *Situs ambiguous* refers to situations in which situs cannot be clearly defined and commonly coincides with atrial isomerism (i.e., mirror-image atria). LA isomerism is associated with paired morphologically left structures: bilateral left bronchi, bilateral bilobed lungs, and bilateral spleens. RA isomerism is associated with paired morphologically right structures;

TABLE 46.2 **Common Surgical Interventions in Patients With Single-Ventricle Physiology.**

Operation	*Objective, Description, and Approach*
Atrial septectomy	Objective: To improve arterial oxygen saturation in patients with D-transposition of the great arteries and HLHS Description: Excision of the atrial septum enables blood from the systemic and pulmonary venous blood to mix at the atrial level Approach: Lateral thoracotomy
Blalock-Taussig shunt (i.e., Blalock-Taussig-Thomas shunt)	Objective: To improve arterial oxygen saturation by increasing pulmonary blood flow. In the classic BT shunt, the subclavian artery is anastomosed to the ipsilateral PA. In the modified BT shunt, a synthetic interposition graft is placed between the subclavian artery and the ipsilateral PA. Description: Anastomosis between the subclavian artery and the PA directly or by using a synthetic tube graft Approach: Lateral thoracotomy
Damus-Kaye-Stansel operation	Objective: To relieve systemic ventricular outflow obstruction in patients with transposition of the great arteries, subaortic stenosis, and HLHS with aortic atresia Description: Anastomosis of the proximal PA to the side of the ascending aorta ensures unobstructed flow to the systemic circulation through the pulmonary valve functioning as the neoaortic valve. Pulmonary blood flow is established by a Fontan procedure or, in patients undergoing biventricular repair, a conduit between the RV and distal PA. Approach: Midline sternotomy
Glenn anastomosis	Objective: To direct SVC flow to the pulmonary circulation and improve arterial oxygenation Description: Anastomosis between the SVC and the PAs (also called a cavopulmonary anastomosis). See text for description of classic versus bidirectional Glenn. Approach: Midline sternotomy
Kawashima repair	Objective: To direct SVC flow to the pulmonary circulation and improve arterial oxygenation Description: Glenn anastomosis in the setting of an interrupted IVC with azygous continuation, ensuring SVC and IVC (excluding hepatic veins) flow to the PA Approach: Midline sternotomy
Norwood procedure	Objective: To provide the first step toward Fontan palliation in patients with HLHS. Components of the Norwood procedure are atrial septectomy, Blalock-Taussig shunt, a Damus-Kaye-Stansel connection, and ligation of the patent ductus arteriosus. Description: A systemic-to-PA shunt is created to maintain pulmonary blood flow, and the main PA and aortic arch repair is anastomosed to a reconstructed aorta to provide systemic blood flow. Approach: Midline sternotomy
PA banding	Objective: To balance systemic and pulmonary blood flow and reduce the risk of pulmonary hypertension Description: Surgical insertion of a synthetic band around the branch PAs that can be tightened to reduce pulmonary blood flow and pressure Approach: Midline sternotomy, thoracotomy
Potts shunt	Objective: To improve arterial oxygen saturation by increasing pulmonary blood flow Description: Creation of a communication between the left PA and descending thoracic aorta. This type of shunt is now rarely performed due to the risk of pulmonary hypertension arising from exposure of the pulmonary vessels to systemic pressures. Approach: Midline sternotomy, thoracotomy
Sano shunt	Objective: Used in HLHS to improve arterial oxygen saturation by increasing pulmonary blood flow. Description: Synthetic homograft from the free wall of the single ventricle to the PA. Approach: Midline sternotomy
Waterston shunt	Objective: To improve arterial oxygen saturation by increasing pulmonary blood flow Description: Creation of a communication between the right PA and ascending aorta. This type of shunt is now rarely performed due to the risk of pulmonary hypertension arising from exposure of the pulmonary vessels to systemic pressures. Approach: Midline sternotomy

BT, Blalock-Taussig; *HLHS*, hypoplastic left heart syndrome; *IVC*, inferior vena cava; *PA*, pulmonary artery; *SVC*, superior vena cava.

bilateral right bronchi, bilateral trilobed lungs, and congenital absence of the spleen.

TECHNICAL ASPECTS

Although the standard examination begins with the parasternal long-axis view for most adults, echocardiographic evaluation for adults with single-ventricle physiology is most informative when commenced in the subcostal imaging plane. With the transducer placed midline beneath the xiphoid process, it is possible to determine atrial and visceral situs and the cardiac position.

Atrial situs is most reliably assessed by the position of the liver and the relationship of the IVC and abdominal aorta. Atrial situs is concordant with visceral situs in 99% of patients. Identification of a right-sided liver usually establishes situs solitus, which can be confirmed by evaluating the arrangement of the great vessels. From the subcostal view, the imaging plane is adjusted to identify three structures: aorta, IVC, and vertebral body. The vertebral body signifies the midline. Situs solitus is diagnosed when the aorta lies in its normal position left of the midline with the IVC to the right. Scanning toward the liver, the IVC is seen inserting into the RA. Identification of the liver on the left side and an IVC left of the midline confirms the diagnosis of atrial situs inversus (i.e., the RA is left-sided and the LA is right-sided).

In situs ambiguous, which is seen in patients with heterotaxy syndrome with atrial isomerism, the IVC and aorta lie on the same side of the vertebral body, one in front of the other (Fig. 46.13). In heterotaxy, the IVC is commonly interrupted with a hemiazygos vein connecting the subhepatic IVC to the SVC. In cases of heterotaxy, the hepatic vein commonly drains directly to the RA.

After the cardiac position and atrial situs are established, the morphology of the dominant ventricle and its codominant or accessory chamber is assessed. From a subcostal or parasternal location, the short-axis view of the ventricles is used to understand the ventricular arrangements (Fig. 46.14). A small accessory chamber, typically the outlet part of the ventricle, is seen arising from the larger dominant ventricle. When the accessory chamber is anterior, it represents the rudimentary RV. The dominant (posteriorly located) ventricle is the LV. A posteriorly positioned accessory chamber signifies the rudimentary LV, and the dominant anterior chamber is the RV. Additional features that define the dominant ventricle as an RV are a moderator band and chordal attachments of the AV valve to the septal surface. Uncommonly, there is no accessory chamber and no other distinguishing anatomic features, and the ventricle is said to be of indeterminate morphology.

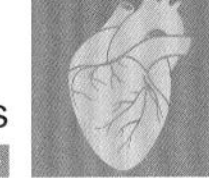

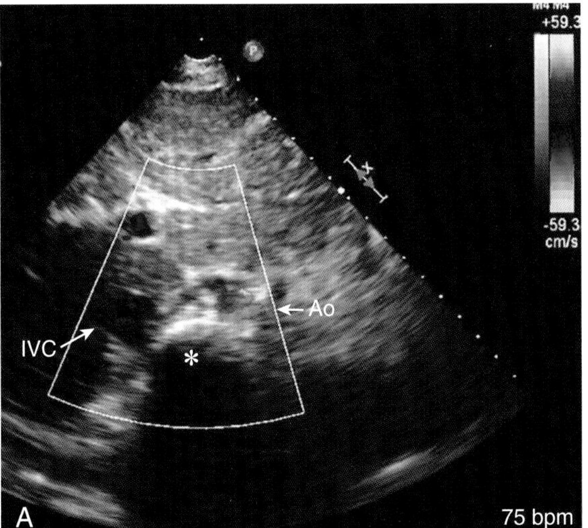

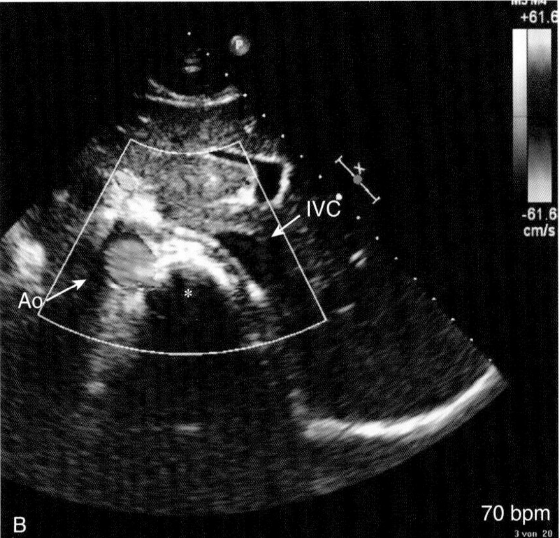

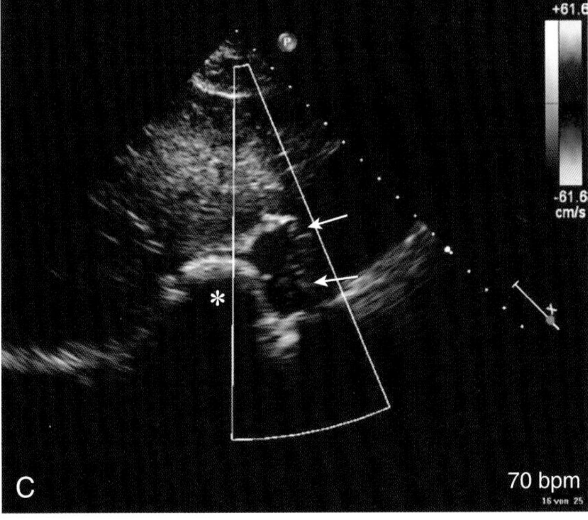

Fig. 46.13 Establishing situs using the inferior vena cava and aorta. (A) Situs solitus (normal arrangement). Subcostal 2D echocardiogram and color Doppler in a short-axis orientation with the vertebral body located posteriorly in the center of the image *(asterisk)* demonstrates situs solitus with the inferior vena cava *(IVC)* on the right of the vertebral body and the aorta *(Ao)* on the left (see Video 46.13A). (B) Situs inversus. Subcostal 2D echocardiogram and color Doppler demonstrate situs inversus, in which the normal positions of the IVC and Ao are reversed (see Video 46.13B). (C) Heterotaxy. Subcostal 2D echocardiogram and color Doppler demonstrate the IVC and Ao *(arrows)* positioned on the same (left) side of the vertebral body (see Video 46.13C).

After the atrial situs and morphology of the ventricles are established, the AV connections can be described. AV connections can be categorized as univentricular or biventricular. Univentricular AV connections occur when the AV junction or junctions lead to a dominant ventricle with or without a small accessory chamber. Univentricular connections can be further subdivided into three groups: double inlet (most common), single inlet, or common AV valve.

In double-inlet anatomy, the left and right AV valves are usually connected to a morphologic LV (see Fig. 46.4). In single-inlet anatomy, one AV valve is functional, and the other is atretic. When the right-sided valve is atretic, it is called *tricuspid atresia* (see Fig. 46.1); when the left is atretic, it is called *mitral atresia* (see Fig. 46.2).

A common AV valve is less frequently encountered than double- or single-inlet anatomy and is usually associated with a primum ASD or common atrium. When two ventricles are present, the AV connection can be described as *biventricular*. Biventricular AV connections encompass a diverse range of congenital heart defects in which septation (i.e., surgical division) of the left and right heart chambers is not possible. Anatomic factors precluding biventricular repair include AV valves and attachments that straddle the ventricular septum, very large VSDs, and hypoplastic left or right heart syndromes.

Ventricular outflow is examined to determine the orientation and identity of each great artery. The best imaging planes for evaluating the great vessels are the subcostal long- and short-axis views, which are aligned, respectively, with the coronal and sagittal planes of the heart. Normally, the great vessels cross one another obliquely as they exit the heart. In echocardiographic terms, when one vessel is seen in the long axis, the other is seen in the short axis (Fig. 46.15). The parasternal short-axis view demonstrates this arrangement, with the aortic valve seen in the short-axis view, and the RV outflow tract and PA seen in the long-axis view.

In transposition of the great arteries, the great vessels are arranged in parallel and simultaneously appear in long- or short-axis views on echocardiography. In the short-axis view, the aorta is usually located anterior and to either the left or the right of the PA. The great vessels are also recognized according to their direction, shape, and branching pattern. The ascending aorta courses superiorly toward the head and neck, giving rise to the brachiocephalic vessels before arching as it becomes the descending thoracic aorta. The PA is straight and courses posteriorly before bifurcating into the left and right PAs. In patients seen after a Fontan procedure, the PA terminates in a blind-ending stump, having been surgically divided from the distal main PA (now part of the Fontan circuit).

The possible alignments between the great arteries and underlying ventricles exist across a spectrum, although four major patterns can be described: (1) concordant ventriculoarterial connections, (2) discordant ventriculoarterial connections (i.e., transposition of the great arteries and congenitally corrected transposition), (3) double outlet, and (4) single outlet. Double-outlet anatomy occurs when both chambers arise from the dominant chamber. A single outlet may occur when one great vessel arises from the ventricle and gives rise to the aorta and PA (i.e., truncus arteriosus) or in the setting of pulmonary or aortic atresia. The ascending aorta varies in size and is related to the degree of antegrade flow. In aortic atresia, the ascending aorta may be markedly hypoplastic. Coarctation of the aorta is also common in patients with HLHS.

The final step in the segmental assessment is identification of intracardiac shunts. If an ASD or VSD exists, any restriction to flow must be excluded. A severely restrictive VSD is equivalent

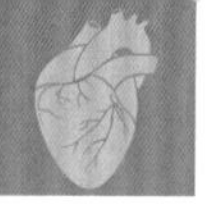

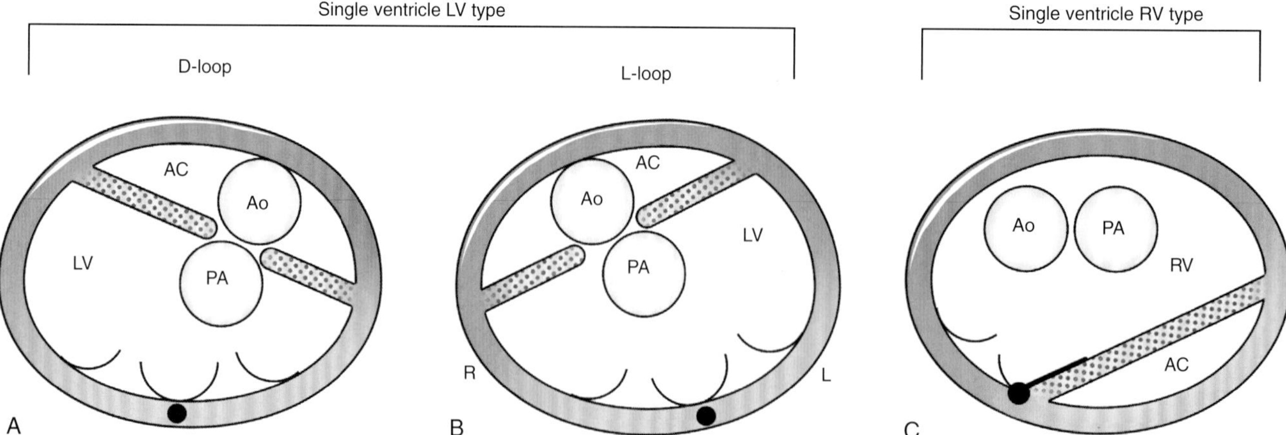

Fig. 46.14 Arrangement of the dominant ventricle and accessory chambers. (A) Single ventricle, LV type, D-loop. An anteriorly positioned hypoplastic ventricle represents the rudimentary RV; the dominant ventricle has LV morphology. In a D-looped ventricle, the hypoplastic RV and aorta *(Ao)* are positioned anterior and to the right. (B) Single ventricle, LV type, L-loop. An anteriorly positioned hypoplastic ventricle represents the rudimentary RV; the dominant ventricle has LV morphology. In an L-looped ventricle, the hypoplastic RV and Ao are positioned anterior and to the left. (C) Single ventricle, RV type. A posteriorly positioned accessory chamber *(AC)* signifies the rudimentary LV; the dominant chamber has RV morphology. *PA*, Pulmonary artery.

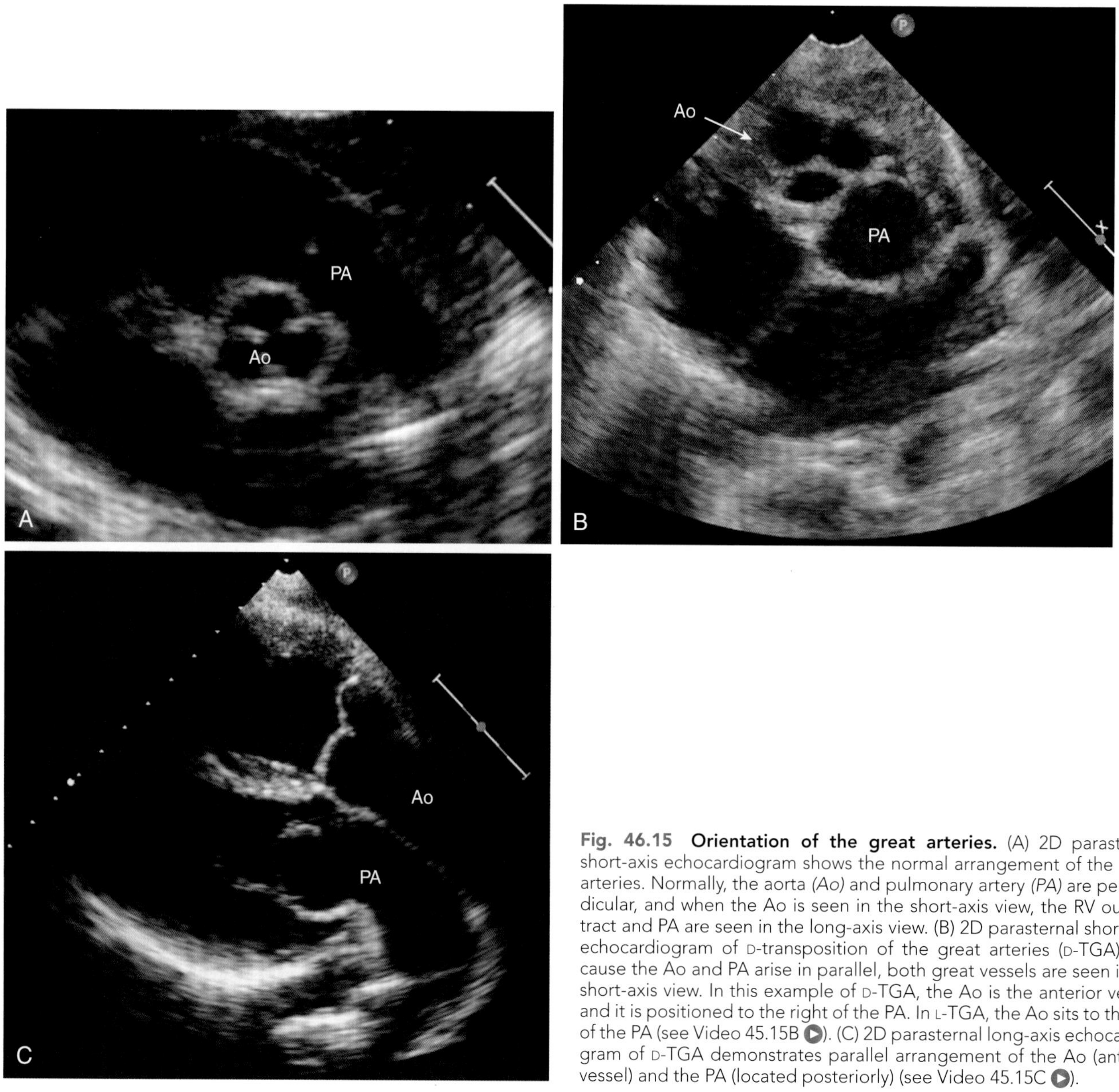

Fig. 46.15 Orientation of the great arteries. (A) 2D parasternal short-axis echocardiogram shows the normal arrangement of the great arteries. Normally, the aorta *(Ao)* and pulmonary artery *(PA)* are perpendicular, and when the Ao is seen in the short-axis view, the RV outflow tract and PA are seen in the long-axis view. (B) 2D parasternal short-axis echocardiogram of D-transposition of the great arteries (D-TGA). Because the Ao and PA arise in parallel, both great vessels are seen in the short-axis view. In this example of D-TGA, the Ao is the anterior vessel, and it is positioned to the right of the PA. In L-TGA, the Ao sits to the left of the PA (see Video 45.15B). (C) 2D parasternal long-axis echocardiogram of D-TGA demonstrates parallel arrangement of the Ao (anterior vessel) and the PA (located posteriorly) (see Video 45.15C).

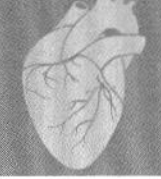

TABLE 46.3 Segmental Analysis for Complex Congenital Heart Disease.

Anatomic Structure	*Questions to Be Answered in a Sequential and Segmental Analysis*
Heart position in the chest	What is the position of the heart in the chest? • Levoposition = left chest • Dextroposition[a] = right chest • Mesoposition = midline
Cardiac apex direction	In which direction does the apex of the heart point? • Levocardia = left chest • Dextrocardia[a] = right chest • Mesocardia = midline
Atrial location or situs	Is the RA located normally on the right side? • Situs solitus = morphologic RA is on the right side • Situs inversus = morphologic RA is on the left side • Situs ambiguous = indeterminate (usually in the setting of atrial isomerism)
Ventricles	What is the morphology of the dominant ventricle? Is there an accessory chamber, and if so, what is its location? • LV type • RV type • Indeterminate
AV connection	What are the AV connections (where applicable)? • Univentricular vs. biventricular • Univentricular = AV junction or junctions lead to a dominant single ventricle • Biventricular = AV connection or junctions lead to two ventricular chambers
Great vessels	What is the alignment of the aorta vs. pulmonary artery? • Oblique alignment = normal • Parallel alignment = transposition of the great arteries
VA connection	Are VA connections concordant or discordant? Is there a double or single outlet? What is the aortic arch anatomy, including coarctation?
Intracardiac shunts	Is there an ASD or VSD? If so, is there evidence of a restrictive ASD or VSD?

[a]Dextrocardia has three subtypes: (1) dextrocardia with situs inversus, (2) dextrocardia due to mediastinal shift (i.e., right lung hypoplasia), and (3) dextroversion. Only situs inversus is associated with mirror-image switching of the left and right heart chambers.
ASD, Atrial septal defect; *AV*, atrioventricular; *VA*, ventriculoarterial; *VSD*, ventricular septal defect.

to severe aortic or pulmonary stenosis and may require intervention to relieve outflow obstruction. The key questions to be answered and terminology relevant to undertaking a segmental analysis are summarized in Table 46.3.

TABLE 46.4 Goals of Echocardiographic Assessment of Single-Ventricle Patients After the Fontan Operation.

Echocardiographic Assessment Goals	*Clinical Correlate*
Assessment of the Fontan Pathway	
Presence and size of fenestration	Right-to-left shunt suggests elevated Fontan pressures and contributes to cyanosis.
Presence and size of thrombus	Thrombus impedes Fontan flow and increases risk of pulmonary emboli, pulmonary HT, and Fontan failure.
Fontan-to-PA anastomosis	Any impediment to flow (i.e., stenosis or obstruction) increases Fontan pressures, systemic venous congestion, ascites, and atrial arrhythmias.
Branch pulmonary arteries	Branch PA stenosis reduces pulmonary flow and increases Fontan and systemic venous pressures.
Assessment of the Pulmonary Venous Chamber	
Atrial communication (mixing) Pulmonary venous obstruction	Restriction to pulmonary venous return and reduced ventricular filling decreases ventricular preload, leading to low cardiac output, exercise intolerance, circulatory dysfunction, and Fontan failure.
Assessment of AV Valve Function	
AV valve regurgitation severity AV valve regurgitation mechanism	AV valve regurgitation is associated with ventricular volume overload and Fontan failure.
AV valve stenosis (i.e., after repair, prosthetic valve replacement)	Ventricular function may decline after AV valve repair and is associated with worse clinical outcomes.
Assessment of Dominant Ventricular Function	
Systolic function Diastolic function	Higher grades of systolic dysfunction, although uncommon, are associated with worse outcomes.
Assessment of Outflow Tract	
Semilunar valve regurgitation or stenosis	Semilunar valve regurgitation contributes to volume overload and ventricular dysfunction.
Residual or recurrent arch obstruction	Semilunar valve stenosis and outflow tract obstruction cause chronic pressure loading, hypertrophy, and ventricular diastolic and systolic dysfunction. Residual arch obstruction and coarctation of the aorta causes arterial hypertension.

AV, Atrioventricular; *HT*, hypertension; *PA*, pulmonary artery.

ECHOCARDIOGRAPHIC EVALUATION

FONTAN CONNECTIONS

Echocardiographic evaluation of Fontan connections begins in the subcostal window with the transducer midline immediately beneath the xiphoid process. The goals of echocardiographic assessment of patients with a single ventricle after the Fontan procedure are listed in Table 46.4. Technical details of echocardiographic acquisition and measurement are summarized in Table 46.5.

Taking an anatomic approach, the goal of the examination is to assess (1) the Fontan connection, (2) the pulmonary venous chamber, (3) AV and semilunar valve function, (4) dominant ventricular function, (5) the outflow tract (including the aortic arch), and (6) intracardiac shunts (typically at the atrial and/or ventricular levels). Guidelines for imaging and timing of intervention in Fontan patients are summarized in Table 46.6.

Connection Between the Inferior Vena Cava and Fontan Circulation

Using two-dimensional (2D) Doppler in the subcostal view, the IVC and its connection to the Fontan circulation is identified (see Fig. 46.6B and C). Normally, blood flow in the Fontan connections is laminar and has a low velocity (<20–30 cm/s) with respirophasic variation. The flow increases with inspiration as intrathoracic pressure falls and decreases during expiration as intrathoracic pressure rises. Color-flow imaging and pulsed-wave Doppler are used to confirm normal Fontan flow. To enable color-flow imaging, the Nyquist setting should be lowered (typically to <30 cm/s). For pulsed-wave Doppler, the sweep speed is decreased to record flow throughout the respiratory cycle (see Fig. 46.10C).

Flow reversal or lack of respiratory variation indicates abnormal flow and should raise concerns for obstruction. If evidence of obstruction is demonstrated without a clear cause on transthoracic echocardiography (TTE), additional cardiac imaging with MRI, computed tomography (CT), or transesophageal echocardiography (TEE) should be performed. Thrombus is usually well visualized on TEE.[29] A fenestration is seen by color-flow imaging as turbulent flow between the Fontan repair and pulmonary venous atrium (see Fig. 46.8B).

TABLE 46.5 Echocardiographic Validation Studies of Ventricular Function in Fontan Patients.

Study Design	*Study*	*Reproducibility*	*Correlation With MRI*
Geometric			
Qualitative assessment of ventricular function	Bellsham-Revell et al.[23]	Not assessed	Qualitative assessment with 2D echocardiography correlates poorly with quantitative assessment by MRI Qualitative assessment to detect reduced function (MRI-derived EF < 50%) is associated with high sensitivity but low specificity
	Margossian et al.[38]	Modest for LV morphology Weak for RV morphology	Agreement between qualitative assessment and MRI was weak
Modified biplane Simpson method	Margossian et al.[38]	Modest	Agreement between Simpson biplane and quantitative assessment by MRI was weak Ventricular volumes underestimated by echocardiography
3D Simpson biplane	Soriano et al.[40]	Good	Not yet validated
Nongeometric			
dP/dt	Rhodes et al.[41]	High	Weak correlation with MRI-based measurement of EF
Tissue Doppler velocities	Rhodes et al.[41]	S′ has excellent intraobserver and moderate interobserver agreement.	No correlation between S′ and EF
MPI or Tei index	Williams et al.[49]	Not assessed	Correlation with MRI not assessed However, a weak positive correlation was observed between MPI and end-diastolic pressure
	Bellsham-Revell et al.[43]	Good	MPI did not correlate with EF in patients with HLHS
Echocardiography-derived 2D strain imaging	Singh et al.[50]	Not reliable for tachycardia; reproducibility is best with frame rates between 60 and 90 frames/s Reproducibility is highest in basal compared with apical segments	Good correlation with MRI-based myocardial tagging Agreement is better for longitudinal than circumferential strain

EF, Ejection fraction; *HLHS,* hypoplastic left heart syndrome; *MPI,* myocardial performance index; *MRI,* magnetic resonance imaging; *S′*, peak annular systolic velocity.

TABLE 46.6 Guidelines for Cardiovascular Imaging Surveillance of Fontan Patients.

Test	*Child*	*Adolescent*	*Adult*
Echocardiogram	Yearly	Yearly	Yearly
Cardiac MRI	Once every 3 y	Once every 2–3 y	Once every 2–3 y
CT angiography	As clinically indicated	As clinically indicated	As clinically indicated
Cardiac catheterization	As clinically indicated	Once every 10 y	Once every 10 y

Data from Rychik J, Atz A, Deal B, et al. Evaluation and management of the child and adult with Fontan circulation. A scientific statement from the American Heart Association. *Circulation.* 2019;140:e234–e284.

Pulsed-wave Doppler is used to estimate the fenestration gradient. The velocity is usually low (<4 m/s).[32] The mean fenestration gradient equals the transpulmonary gradient because it reflects the pressure difference between the Fontan circulation and the pulmonary venous chamber (see Fig. 46.12B).

Connection Between the Superior Vena Cava and Fontan Circulation

The superior Fontan connections are those between the SVC and one or both PAs. Whether the PAs are connected or disconnected depends on the type of Glenn anastomosis (see Table 46.2). These connections are best seen from the suprasternal notch, supraclavicular, or high parasternal view (see Figs. 46.9A and B and 46.10A and B).

For the IVC-to-Fontan connections, flow is low velocity, and respirophasic variation should be seen (see Fig. 46.10C).[8] If flow acceleration is seen, a pulsed-Doppler tracing can be used to determine the mean gradient. In patients with bilateral SVCs, both anastamotic connections should be visualized.

Connection Between the Fontan Circulation and Branch Pulmonary Arteries

The Fontan connection is followed throughout its course. The branch PAs are best seen from the suprasternal notch or high parasternal positions. Doppler flow is low velocity and nonpulsatile due to the absence of a subpulmonic ventricle. Stenosis is indicated by a continuous-flow pattern with an elevated mean gradient. Flow reversal may be seen with increased pulmonary vascular resistance or significant aortopulmonary collaterals.

PULMONARY VENOUS RETURN

The chambers receiving the pulmonary venous return may take many forms, but they most commonly involve a large common atrium or right RA and LA with a large ASD. A lateral tunnel can be seen within the atria, and an extracardiac Fontan conduit is positioned outside the atrial wall. Pulmonary vein compression may result from an extracardiac conduit or significant atrial dilation.

Assessment of the chamber receiving the pulmonary venous return uses 2D color-flow imaging and pulsed-wave Doppler imaging to rule out thrombus in either chamber receiving systemic or pulmonary venous return (Fig. 46.16). Imaging also is used to detect pulmonary vein compression (Fig. 46.17).

ATRIOVENTRICULAR VALVE FUNCTION

Progressive AV regurgitation is seen in a subset of patients with a Fontan circulation and is associated with increased morbidity and mortality rates.[33] AV connections can be categorized as univentricular or biventricular.

The anatomy and function of the AV valves are assessed from multiple views, including the subcostal, parasternal long-axis, apical 4-chamber, and apical 2-chamber views. 2D and color-flow imaging are used to evaluate the severity and mechanism of AV valve regurgitation.

AV valve dysplasia is a common mechanism for regurgitation, particularly in patients with HLHS, and tricuspid regurgitation is a predictor of adverse outcomes.[34] Other mechanisms of AV valve regurgitation include volume overload, annular dilation, and abnormal chordae and papillary muscles. The area, width, and length of the regurgitant jet enable qualitative assessment of regurgitation severity. More-than-mild regurgitation is significant and warrants further assessment with three-dimensional (3D) echocardiography,[35] TEE, and/or cardiac MRI, along with consideration of invasive hemodynamic assessment if deemed significant on noninvasive imaging.

AV valve stenosis may be found after AV valve repair or after prosthetic valve replacement. After achieving optimal alignment between the ultrasound beam and the AV valve (i.e., apical 4-chamber view), continuous-wave (CW) Doppler should be used to obtain a transvalvular mean gradient. Pressure half-time may also be useful.

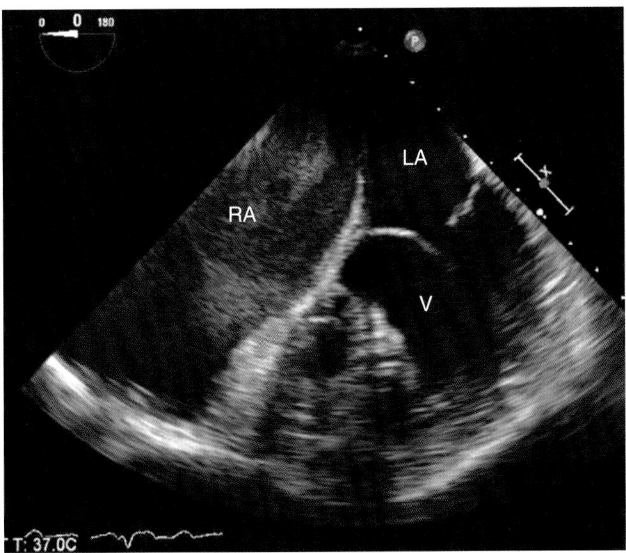

Fig. 46.16 Atriopulmonary Fontan operation with spontaneous echocardiographic contrast. TEE in a patient with tricuspid atresia after an atriopulmonary Fontan operation shows that the RA is severely dilated, and spontaneous echocardiographic contrast indicates low-velocity flow with a high thrombus potential. The interatrial septum is displaced rightward, indicating elevated RA pressure (see Video 46.16). *V*, Ventricle.

VENTRICULAR SYSTOLIC FUNCTION

Ventricular function is assessed from multiple views, including the subcostal, parasternal long-axis, apical 5-chamber, and apical 2-chamber views. Cardiac anatomy and segments are evaluated using 2D echocardiography followed by assessment of ventricular function.

Studies evaluating the role of echocardiography for assessment of ventricular function after the Fontan operation can be broadly grouped as those of (1) ventricular systolic function, (2) ventricular diastolic function, or (3) ventricular dyssynchrony. Studies evaluating the reproducibility or reliability of echocardiographic assessment of ventricular function in Fontan patients are summarized in Table 46.4.

Qualitative Assessment

Qualitative assessment is the most commonly used technique to grade ventricular systolic function in patients with single-ventricle physiology. Ventricular function is rated as normal (>55%), mild (41%–55%), moderate (31%–40%), or severely reduced (≤30%) based on the echocardiographic reader's subjective evaluation. This grading system has been adopted from guidelines for echocardiographic assessment of adults with acquired heart disease.[36] As such, its reliability for grading ventricular function in patients with a single ventricle is questionable.

Qualitatively graded ventricular function correlates poorly with cardiac MRI, which is the current standard technique for assessing single-ventricle function.[37,38] Using an MRI-derived ejection fraction of less than 50% as a cutoff, subjective assessment to detect reduced function is associated with high sensitivity but low specificity. This likely reflects a tendency for echocardiographic readers to overcall ventricular dysfunction to avoid missing patients with clinically significant ventricular dysfunction.[37] As ventricular dysfunction progresses to the mild or moderately impaired range, the levels of disagreement between readers increases, suggesting that qualitative

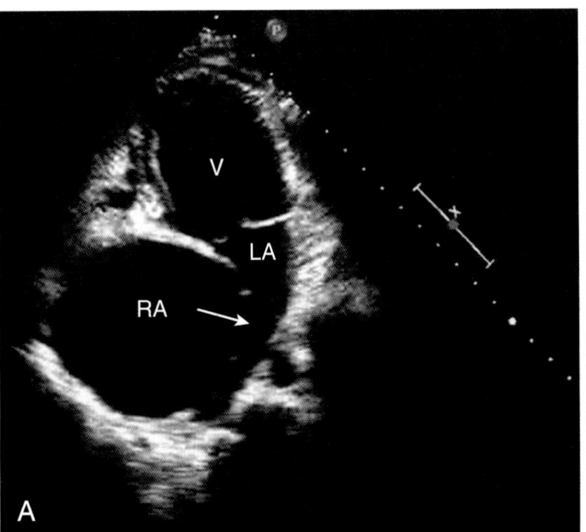

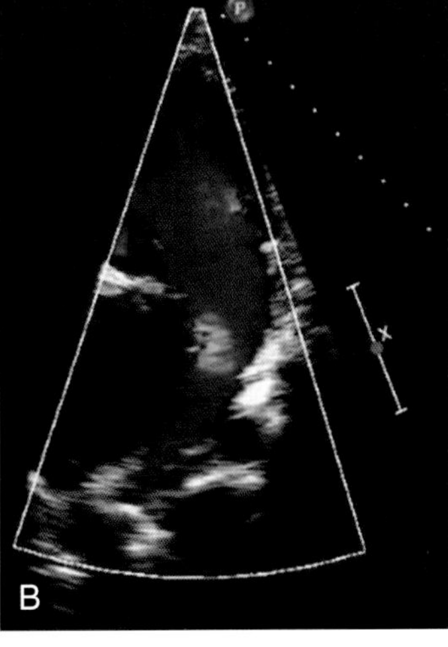

Fig. 46.17 Pulmonary vein compression after an atriopulmonary Fontan operation. (A) 2D apical 4-chamber TTE shows a severely dilated RA in a patient with tricuspid atresia and RV hypoplasia after an atriopulmonary Fontan operation. There is concern about compression of the LA and right upper pulmonary vein (see Video 46.17A). (B) A color Doppler image is focused on the LA and right upper pulmonary vein. High-velocity flow indicates pulmonary vein compression (see Video 46.17B). *V*, Ventricle.

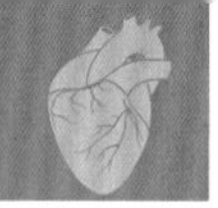

assessment is insensitive to more subtle progression in single-ventricle dysfunction. Dyssynchrony and variation in cardiac morphology further affect qualitative assessment of ventricular systolic function; RV morphology is less reproducible than LV morphology.[38]

Quantitative Assessment

Quantitative measures overcome the limitations seen with qualitative assessment. Using the modified biplane Simpson method, the mean ejection fraction in children and adolescents after the Fontan procedure is 59% ± 10%. Compared with qualitative assessment, the Simpson method is more reproducible, although agreement with the MRI-derived ejection fraction remains weak.[38] Ventricular dilation is almost universal; mean diastolic volumes in patients with a single ventricle are 79 ± 29 mL/m^2 for LV-dominant circulation and 93 ± 29 mL/m^2 for RV-dominant circulation.[24]

Difficulties in acquiring true long- and short-axis imaging planes is a key weakness of the Simpson method that leads to systematic underestimation of the single-ventricle volume. The Simpson method assumes that the heart has an ellipsoid shape, which is not the case in a geometrically complex single ventricle. 3D echocardiography requires no geometric assumptions and has significantly closer agreement with MRI than with 2D echocardiography,[39,40] although volumes continue to be underestimated and data sets are limited by low frame rates. Despite promising data from pediatric populations, 3D imaging is often more challenging in adults, among whom obesity and ventricular dilation are more prevalent.

Nongeometric Indices

Because they are not reliant on volumetric measures, nongeometric methods overcome the limitations associated with 2D and 3D imaging. Methods evaluated for Fontan patients include *dP/dt*,[41] myocardial performance (Tei) index,[42] tissue Doppler velocities,[43] and the ratio of systolic to diastolic duration.[44] Although reproducibility is high for many of these methods, they often correlate poorly with the MRI-derived ejection fraction. The clinical relevance of these methods for patients with a single ventricle is therefore unclear.

VENTRICULAR DIASTOLIC FUNCTION

Abnormal diastolic dysfunction is common among Fontan patients.[24] However, it is unclear whether conventional echocardiographic parameters apply to the Fontan circulation.[45] When standard adult criteria for diastolic dysfunction are applied, more than 70% of Fontan patients have some evidence of diastolic dysfunction.[24] However, conventional echocardiographic measures of diastolic function remain poorly validated, and caution is needed when applying standard grading systems because they do not take into account important differences in single-ventricle physiology.

In the normal adult heart, a ratio of mitral inflow to mitral annulus velocity (E/e′) greater than 15 is useful for identifying an elevated ventricular end-diastolic pressure of more than 12 mmHg.[46] Studies of patients with a single ventricle have given mixed results, with some groups reporting weak[47] and others moderate correlations between E/e′ and ventricular end-diastolic pressure.[45] In a study of 32 patients with single-ventricle physiology undergoing echocardiography and cardiac catheterization, an E/e′ value of 12 or more had a sensitivity of 90% and a specificity of 75% for recognizing ventricular end-diastolic pressure greater than 10 mmHg.

Pulmonary venous flow reversal may also be helpful, with atrial systolic pulmonary vein reversal being more highly correlated with end-diastolic pressure than E/e′ (r = 0.77 vs. 0.44, respectively).[45] Among 15 patients who underwent transthoracic assessment within 12 months of direct measurement of ventricular end-diastolic pressure, the AV valve systolic-to-diastolic ratio (AVV S/D ratio) had the strongest correlation with ventricular end-diastolic pressure (r = 0.8, P = 0.001). An AVV S/D ratio greater than 1.1 had 100% positive predictive value and 92% negative predictive value for predicting a ventricular end-diastolic pressure greater than 10 mmHg.[48] Larger multicenter studies are needed to confirm these findings before they can be recommended for daily clinical practice.

OUTFLOW TRACTS

After the Fontan operation, the outflow tract connects the ventricular chamber to the aorta. The most common mechanism for outflow tract obstruction is subvalvular obstruction due to a restrictive VSD. Less commonly, patients may have a subaortic membrane, chord, valvular stenosis, arch hypoplasia, or recurrent coarctation. Chronic pressure overload contributes to ventricular systolic and diastolic dysfunction and impaired Fontan flow.

The outflow tracts should be imaged from multiple acoustic windows, including the subcostal, apical, and parasternal long-axis views. Color-flow imaging and pulsed-wave and CW Doppler are used to identify flow acceleration, turbulence, and increased peak and mean gradients. Alignment of the ultrasound beam with the outflow tract is vital for accurate measurement of outflow tract gradients.

A Damus-Kaye-Stansel connection is used to relieve systemic outflow obstruction in patients with transposition of the great arteries and as part of the Norwood operation for HLHS. The proximal PA is anastomosed to the side of the ascending aorta, ensuring unobstructed flow to the systemic circulation through the pulmonary valve functioning as the neoaortic valve.

The Damus-Kaye-Stansel connection between the ascending aorta and previous pulmonary trunk should be imaged to exclude obstruction, which could compromise coronary blood flow, producing ischemia and ventricular dysfunction. Semilunar valve function should be evaluated. When the pulmonary valve is assigned to the aortic position (i.e., neoaorta), regurgitation is prevalent. A Damus-Kaye-Stansel connection can distort one or both semilunar valves and cause regurgitation, although it is usually mild.

Evaluation of the aortic arch is essential in all single-ventricle patients but especially in those with HLHS. The aortic arch is best seen from the suprasternal view, using color and CW Doppler to determine the peak gradient across the arch and descending aorta. For adults in whom the arch is not well seen, it can be useful to rule out significant arch obstruction by applying pulsed-wave Doppler to the abdominal aorta. The absence of diastolic antegrade flow in the abdominal aorta excludes significant obstruction.

CONCLUSIONS

Echocardiographic assessment of adult patients with a single ventricle requires knowledge of the congenital heart defects and familiarity with sequential and segmental analysis of the heart and its connections, including the Fontan connection, pulmonary venous chamber, AV valve, ventricles, and outflow tract. TEE, cardiac MRI, and CT remain important complementary modalities, particularly for patients with significant valvular or ventricular dysfunction or suspicion of thrombus.

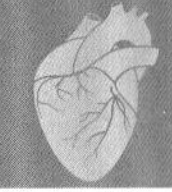

SUMMARY Practical Guide for Imaging Single-Ventricle Anatomy.

Imaging Target	Anatomic Structures	Imaging Planes	Echocardiographic Goals and Techniques
Assessment of Fontan pathway	IVC connection to Fontan circulation	Subcostal	2D for dilation, spontaneous contrast, thrombus Color flow: lower Nyquist settings to detect low-velocity flow PW Doppler: use low sweep speed to compare flow throughout the respiratory cycle
	Fontan baffle	Subcostal, apical, parasternal	As above and identify fenestrations PW Doppler for estimate of fenestration gradient (mean fenestration gradient = transpulmonary gradient)
	SVC-to-PA connection (Glenn anastomosis)	Suprasternal notch High parasternal	2D for thrombus in the SVC Color flow as for IVC connection PW Doppler as for IVC connection
	Branch PAs	Suprasternal notch	2D for PA branch stenosis Color flow: flow reversal suggests increased pulmonary vascular resistance or competitive aortopulmonary collateral flow PW Doppler: stenosis suggested by continuous flow pattern and elevated mean gradient
Assessment of pulmonary venous chamber	Pulmonary venous connections	Apical 4-chamber	2D: pulmonary vein compression, restrictive ASD Color: flow acceleration at site of pulmonary vein compression, rule out restrictive ASD PW Doppler: increased velocity
Assessment of AV valve function	Common AV valve Dominant tricuspid valve	Apical 4-chamber Apical 2-chamber Parasternal long axis Short axis[a]	2D: Valve appearance and function, planimetry for valve stenosis Color flow: jet length, width, and area CW Doppler: peak/mean gradients in valve stenosis, pressure half-time
Assessment of ventricular function	Dominant ventricle[b]	Apical 4-chamber Apical 2-chamber Parasternal long axis Short axis Subcostal	*Systolic function* 2D: Simpson biplane unreliable for nonuniform ventricular geometry Nongeometric techniques: tissue Doppler velocities, *dP/dt*, isovolumic contraction time, myocardial performance index, strain imaging *Diastolic function* PW Doppler: ventricular inflow velocities, E/E′
Assessment of outflow tract	Ventricular outflow tract Aortic valve Aortic arch and descending aorta	Parasternal long axis Apical long axis Subcostal off-axis Suprasternal for coarctation	2D: mechanism of obstruction or regurgitation Color flow: site of obstruction, vena contracta for aortic regurgitation PW Doppler: localize peak gradient CW Doppler: peak/mean gradients

[a]Different imaging planes are important for assessing the regurgitant jet in three dimensions.
[b]Most forms of single-ventricle physiology have two morphologically distinct ventricles, although there is functionally only one chamber. The second, smaller chamber has been described as the codominant ventricle, the bulboventricular chamber, and the outlet chamber.
ASD, Atrial septal defect; *AV*, atrioventricular; *CW*, continuous wave; *IVC*, inferior vena cava; *PA*, pulmonary artery; *PW*, pulsed wave; *SVC*, superior vena cava.

REFERENCES

1. Cook AC, Anderson RH. The functionally univentricular circulation: anatomic substrates as related to function. *Cardiol Young*. 2005;15(suppl 3):7–16.
2. Barron DJ, Kilby MD, Davies B, Wright JG, Jones TJ, Brawn WJ. Hypoplastic left heart syndrome. *Lancet*. 2009;374(9689):551–564.
3. Bondy CA. Hypoplastic left heart syndrome. *N Engl J Med*. 2010;362(21):2026–2028.
4. Ohye RG, Schranz D, D'Udekem Y. Current therapy for hypoplastic left heart syndrome and related single ventricle lesions. *Circulation*. 2016;134(17):1265–1279.
5. Fontan F, Baudet E. Surgical repair of tricuspid atresia. *Thorax*. 1971;26(3):240–248.
6. Gersony WM. Fontan operation after 3 decades: what we have learned. *Circulation*. 2008;117(1):13–15.
7. Gewillig M. The Fontan circulation. *Heart*. 2005;91(6):839–846.
8. Penny DJ, Redington AN. Doppler echocardiographic evaluation of pulmonary blood flow after the Fontan operation: the role of the lungs. *Br Heart J*. 1991;66(5):372–374.
9. Rychik J, Atz AM, Celermajer DS, et al. Evaluation and management of the child and adult with Fontan circulation: a scientific statement

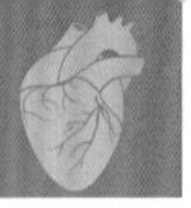

from the American heart association. *Circulation*. 2019. CIR0000000000000696.

10. Bjork VO, Olin CL, Bjarke BB, Thoren CA. Right atrial-right ventricular anastomosis for correction of tricuspid atresia. *J Thorac Cardiovasc Surg*. 1979;77(3):452–458.
11. Laks H, Ardehali A, Grant PW, et al. Modification of the Fontan procedure. Superior vena cava to left pulmonary artery connection and inferior vena cava to right pulmonary artery connection with adjustable atrial septal defect. *Circulation*. 1995;91(12):2943–2947.
12. Puga FJ, Chiavarelli M, Hagler DJ. Modifications of the Fontan operation applicable to patients with left atrioventricular valve atresia or single atrioventricular valve. *Circulation*. 1987;76(3 Pt 2):III53–60.
13. Marcelletti CF, Hanley FL, Mavroudis C, et al. Revision of previous Fontan connections to total extracardiac cavopulmonary anastomosis: a multicenter experience. *J Thorac Cardiovasc Surg*. 2000;119(2):340–346.
14. Ben Ali W, Bouhout I, Khairy P, Bouchard D, Poirier N. Extracardiac versus lateral tunnel Fontan: a meta-analysis of long-term results. *Ann Thorac Surg*. 2019;107(3):837–843.
15. Deshaies C, Hamilton RM, Shohoudi A, et al. Thromboembolic risk after atriopulmonary, lateral tunnel, and extracardiac conduit Fontan surgery. *J Am Coll Cardiol*. 2019;74(8):1071–1081.
16. Lee J, Menkis AH, Rosenberg HC. Reversal of pulmonary arteriovenous malformation after diversion of anomalous hepatic drainage. *Ann Thorac Surg*. 1998;65(3):848–849.
17. Haller Jr JA, Adkins JC, Worthington M, Rauenhorst J. Experimental studies on permanent bypass of the right heart. *Surgery*. 1966;59(6):1128–1132.
18. Kawashima Y, Kitamura S, Matsuda H, Shimazaki Y, Nakano S, Hirose H. Total cavopulmonary shunt operation in complex cardiac anomalies. A new operation. *J Thorac Cardiovasc Surg*. 1984;87(1):74–81.
19. Downing TE, Allen KY, Glatz AC, et al. Long-term survival after the Fontan operation: twenty years of experience at a single center. *J Thorac Cardiovasc Surg*. 2017;154(1):243–253 e2.
20. Iyengar AJ, Winlaw DS, Galati JC, et al. Trends in Fontan surgery and risk factors for early adverse outcomes after Fontan surgery: the Australia and New Zealand Fontan Registry experience. *J Thorac Cardiovasc Surg*. 2014;148(2):566–575.
21. Mertens L, Hagler DJ, Sauer U, Somerville J, Gewillig M. Protein-losing enteropathy after the Fontan operation: an international multicenter study. PLE study group. *J Thorac Cardiovasc Surg*. 1998;115(5):1063–1073.
22. Brooks PA, Khoo NS, Mackie AS, Hornberger LK. Right ventricular function in fetal hypoplastic left heart syndrome. *J Am Soc Echocardiogr*. 2012;25(10):1068–1074.
23. Bellsham-Revell HR, Tibby SM, Bell AJ, et al. Serial magnetic resonance imaging in hypoplastic left heart syndrome gives valuable insight into ventricular and vascular adaptation. *J Am Coll Cardiol*. 2013;61(5):561–570.
24. Anderson PA, Sleeper LA, Mahony L, et al. Contemporary outcomes after the Fontan procedure: a Pediatric Heart Network Multicenter Study. *J Am Coll Cardiol*. 2008;52(2):85–98.
25. Fogel MA, Weinberg PM, Chin AJ, Fellows KE, Hoffman EA. Late ventricular geometry and performance changes of functional single ventricle throughout staged Fontan reconstruction assessed by magnetic resonance imaging. *J Am Coll Cardiol*. 1996;28(1):212–221.
26. Penny DJ, Redington AN. Diastolic ventricular function after the Fontan operation. *Am J Cardiol*. 1992;69(9):974–975.
27. Piran S, Veldtman G, Siu S, Webb GD, Liu PP. Heart failure and ventricular dysfunction in patients with single or systemic right ventricles. *Circulation*. 2002;105(10):1189–1194.
28. d'Udekem Y, Iyengar AJ, Galati JC, et al. Redefining expectations of long-term survival after the Fontan procedure: twenty-five years of follow-up from the entire population of Australia and New Zealand. *Circulation*. 2014;130(11 suppl 1):S32–S38.
29. Pundi KN, Johnson JN, Dearani JA, et al. 40-Year follow-up after the Fontan operation: long-term outcomes of 1,052 patients. *J Am Coll Cardiol*. 2015;66(15):1700–1710.
30. Moller THNW. *Heart Disease in Infancy*. New York: Appleton-Century-Crofts; 1978.
31. Campbell M, Deuchar DC. Dextrocardia and isolated laevocardia. II. Situs inversus and isolated dextrocardia. *Br Heart J*. 1966;28(4):472–487.
32. Stumper O, Sutherland GR, Geuskens R, Roelandt JR, Bos E, Hess J. Transesophageal echocardiography in evaluation and management after a Fontan procedure. *J Am Coll Cardiol*. 1991;17(5):1152–1160.
33. King G, Gentles TL, Winlaw DS, et al. Common atrioventricular valve failure during single ventricle palliationdagger. *Eur J Cardio Thorac Surg*. 2017;51(6):1037–1043.
34. Bharucha T, Honjo O, Seller N, et al. Mechanisms of tricuspid valve regurgitation in hypoplastic left heart syndrome: a case-matched echocardiographic-surgical comparison study. *Eur Heart J Cardiovasc Imaging*. 2013;14(2):135–141.
35. Takahashi K, Inage A, Rebeyka IM, et al. Real-time 3-dimensional echocardiography provides new insight into mechanisms of tricuspid valve regurgitation in patients with hypoplastic left heart syndrome. *Circulation*. 2009;120(12):1091–1098.
36. Lang RM, Bierig M, Devereux RB, et al. Recommendations for chamber quantification: a report from the American Society of Echocardiography's Guidelines and Standards Committee and the Chamber Quantification Writing Group, Developed in Conjunction with the European Association of Echocardiography, a Branch of the European Society of Cardiology. *J Am Soc Echocardiogr*. 2005;18(12):1440–1463.
37. Bellsham-Revell HR, Simpson JM, Miller OI, Bell AJ. Subjective evaluation of right ventricular systolic function in hypoplastic left heart syndrome: how accurate is it? *J Am Soc Echocardiogr*. 2013;26(1):52–56.
38. Margossian R, Schwartz ML, Prakash A, et al. Comparison of echocardiographic and cardiac magnetic resonance imaging measurements of functional single ventricular volumes, mass, and ejection fraction (from the Pediatric Heart Network Fontan Cross-Sectional Study). *Am J Cardiol*. 2009;104(3):419–428.
39. Altmann K, Shen Z, Boxt LM, et al. Comparison of three-dimensional echocardiographic assessment of volume, mass, and function in children with functionally single left ventricles with two-dimensional echocardiography and magnetic resonance imaging. *Am J Cardiol*. 1997;80(8):1060–1065.
40. Soriano BD, Hoch M, Ithuralde A, et al. Matrix-array 3-dimensional echocardiographic assessment of volumes, mass, and ejection fraction in young pediatric patients with a functional single ventricle: a comparison study with cardiac magnetic resonance. *Circulation*. 2008;117(14):1842–1848.
41. Rhodes J, Margossian R, Sleeper LA, et al. Non-geometric echocardiographic indices of ventricular function in patients with a Fontan circulation. *J Am Soc Echocardiogr*. 2011;24(11):1213–1219.
42. Cheung MM, Smallhorn JF, Redington AN, Vogel M. The effects of changes in loading conditions and modulation of inotropic state on the myocardial performance index: comparison with conductance catheter measurements. *Eur Heart J*. 2004;25(24):2238–2242.
43. Bellsham-Revell HR, Tibby SM, Bell AJ, et al. Tissue Doppler time intervals and derived indices in hypoplastic left heart syndrome. *Eur Heart J Cardiovasc Imaging*. 2012;13(5):400–407.
44. Friedberg MK, Silverman NH. The systolic to diastolic duration ratio in children with hypoplastic left heart syndrome: a novel Doppler index of right ventricular function. *J Am Soc Echocardiogr*. 2007;20(6):749–755.
45. Menon SC, Gray R, Tani LY. Evaluation of ventricular filling pressures and ventricular function by Doppler echocardiography in patients with functional single ventricle: correlation with simultaneous cardiac catheterization. *J Am Soc Echocardiogr*. 2011;24(11):1220–1225.
46. Ommen SR, Nishimura RA, Appleton CP, et al. Clinical utility of Doppler echocardiography and tissue Doppler imaging in the estimation of left ventricular filling pressures: a comparative simultaneous Doppler-catheterization study. *Circulation*. 2000;102(15):1788–1794.
47. Husain N, Gokhale J, Nicholson L, Cheatham JP, Holzer RJ, Cua CL. Noninvasive estimation of ventricular filling pressures in patients with single right ventricles. *J Am Soc Echocardiogr*. 2013;26(11):1330–1336.
48. Cordina R, Nasir Ahmad S, Kotchetkova I, et al. Management errors in adults with congenital heart disease: prevalence, sources, and consequences. *Eur Heart J*. 2018;39(12):982–989.
49. Williams RV, Ritter S, Tani LY, et al. Quantitative assessment of ventricular function in children with single ventricles using the Doppler myocardial performance index. *Am J Cardiol*. 2000;86(10):1106–1110.
50. Singh GK, Cupps B, Pasque M, et al. Accuracy and reproducibility of strain by speckle tracking in pediatric subjects with normal heart and single ventricular physiology: a two-dimensional speckle-tracking echocardiography and magnetic resonance imaging correlative study. *J Am Soc Echocardiogr*. 2010;23(11):1143–1152.